General Dilution Chart (mg to mcg)							
Amount of Drug Required in Grams	Amount of Diluent						
	1,000 mL	500 mL	250 mL	125 mL	100 mL	50 mL	25 mL
	mcg/mL	mcg/mL	mcg/mL	mcg/mL	mcg/mL	mcg/mL	mcg/mL
20 mg	20	40	80	160	200	400	800
19 mg	19	38	76	152	190	380	760
18 mg	18	36	72	144	180	360	720
17 mg	17	34	68	136	170	340	680
16 mg	16	32	64	128	160	320	640
15 mg	15	30	60	120	150	300	600
14 mg	14	28	56	112	140	280	560
13 mg	13	26	52	104	130	260	520
12 mg	12	24	48	96	120	240	480
11 mg	11	22	44	88	110	220	440
10 mg	10	20	40	80	100	200	400
9 mg	9	18	36	72	90	180	360
8 mg	8	16	32	64	80	160	320
7 mg	7	14	28	56	70	140	280
6 mg	6	12	24	48	60	120	240
5 mg	5	10	20	40	50	100	200
4.5 mg	4.5	9	18	36	45	90	180
4 mg	4	8	16	32	40	80	160
3.5 mg	3.5	7	14	28	35	70	140
3 mg	3	6	12	24	30	60	120
2.5 mg	2.5	5	10	20	25	50	100
2 mg	2	4	8	16	20	40	80
1.5 mg	1.5	3	6	12	15	30	60
1 mg	1	2	4	8	10	20	40
0.5 mg	0.5	1	2	4	5	10	20
0.25 mg	0.25	0.5	1	2	2.5	5	10

To use chart:
1. Find mcg/mL desired, track to amount of diluent desired and amount of drug in mg required.
2. Find amount of drug in mg required, track to diluent desired and/or mcg/mL desired.
3. Find amount of diluent required, track to amount of drug in mg and/or mcg/mL desired.

Formula: Substitute any number for X

X mg diluted in 1,000 mL = X mcg/mL (1 mg in 1,000 mL = 1 mcg/mL)
X mg diluted in 500 mL = 2 X mcg/mL (1 mg in 500 mL = 2 mcg/mL)
X mg diluted in 250 mL = 4 X mcg/mL (1 mg in 250 mL = 4 mcg/mL)
X mg diluted in 125 mL = 8 X mcg/mL (1 mg in 125 ml = 8 mcg/mL)
X mg diluted in 100 mL = 10 X mcg/mL (1 mg in 100 mL = 10 mcg/mL)
X mg diluted in 50 mL = 20 X mcg/mL (1 mg in 50 mL = 20 mcg/mL)
X mg diluted in 25 mL = 40 X mcg/mL (1 mg in 25 mL = 40 mcg/mL)

Some variation occurs from manufacturer's overfill or if the drug is in liquid form. If absolute accuracy is required, these variations can be avoided by withdrawing an amount in mL from the diluent equal to manufacturer's overfill and/or an amount equal to the amount in mL of the drug. Consult the pharmacist for specific information on manufacturer's overfill of infusion fluids used in your facility.

D1056785

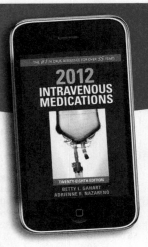

How to Use This Book

STEP 1

Refer to the index at the back of the book. You can find any drug by any name in less than 5 seconds. All drugs are cross-indexed by generic and all known trade names. The index is easily distinguished by a printed blue bar at the edge of the pages. Drugs are also indexed by pharmacologic action. With one turn of the page, all drugs included in the text with similar pharmacologic actions and their page numbers are available to you. Everything is strictly alphabetized; you will never be required to refer to additional pages to locate a drug.

STEP 2

Turn to the single page number given after the name of the drug. All information about the drug is included as continuous reading. You will rarely be required to turn to another section of the book to be completely informed. Specific breakdowns of each drug (Usual Dose, Pediatric Dose, Dose Adjustments, Dilution, Compatibility, Rate of Administration, Actions, Indications and Uses, Precautions, Contraindications, Drug/Lab Interactions, Side Effects, and Antidote) are consistent in format and printed in boldface type. Subheadings under these categories are in boldface. Scan quickly for a Usual Dose check, Dose Adjustment, Drug/Lab Interaction, Side Effect, or Antidote or carefully read all included information. The choice is yours. A quick scan will take 5 to 10 seconds. Even the most complicated drugs will take less than 2 minutes to read completely. Read each monograph carefully and completely before administering a drug to a specific patient for the first time and review it any time a new drug is added to the patient's drug profile.

That's it! A fast, complete, and accurate reference for anyone administering intravenous medications. The spiral binding is specifically designed to lie flat, leaving your hands free to secure needed supplies, prepare your medication, or even ventilate a patient while you read the needed information.

Develop the "look it up" habit. Clear, concise language and simplicity of form contribute to quick, easy use of this handbook. Before your first use, read the preface; it contains lots of helpful information.

Check out the *Intravenous Medications* website for monographs no longer included in this text and for other useful IV medication information:

http://evolve.elsevier.com/IVMeds

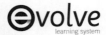
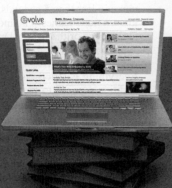

INTRAVENOUS MEDICATIONS

A Handbook for Nurses and Health Professionals

BETTY L. GAHART, RN
Nurse Consultant in Education
Napa, California
Former Director, Education and Training
Queen of the Valley Medical Center
Napa, California

ADRIENNE R. NAZARENO, PharmD
Clinical Manager, Pharmacist in Charge
Queen of the Valley Medical Center
Napa, California

TWENTY-EIGHTH EDITION

ELSEVIER
MOSBY

ELSEVIER
MOSBY

3251 Riverport Lane
St. Louis, Missouri 63043

INTRAVENOUS MEDICATIONS   ISBN: 978-0-323-05799-8

Copyright © 2012 by Mosby, Inc., an affiliate of Elsevier Inc.

NOTICES

Knowledge and best practice in this field are constantly changing. As new research and experience broaden our understanding, changes in research methods, professional practices, or medical treatment may become necessary.

Practitioners and researchers must always rely on their own experience and knowledge in evaluating and using any information, methods, compounds, or experiments described herein. In using such information or methods they should be mindful of their own safety and the safety of others, including parties for whom they have a professional responsibility.

With respect to any drug or pharmaceutical products identified, readers are advised to check the most current information provided (i) on procedures featured or (ii) by the manufacturer of each product to be administered, to verify the recommended dose or formula, the method and duration of administration, and contraindications. It is the responsibility of the practitioners, relying on their own experience and knowledge of their patients, to make diagnoses, to determine dosages and the best treatment for each individual patient, and to take all appropriate safety precautions.

To the fullest extent of the law, neither the Publisher nor the authors, contributors, or editors, assume any liability for any injury and/or damage to persons or property as a matter of products liability, negligence or otherwise, or from any use or operation of any methods, products, instructions, or ideas contained in the material herein.

Previous editions copyrighted 1973, 1977, 1981, 1984, 1988, 1989, 1990, 1991, 1993, 1994, 1995, 1996, 1997, 1998, 1999, 2000, 2001, 2002, 2003, 2004, 2005, 2006, 2007, 2008, 2009, 2010, 2011

ISBN: 978-0-323-05799-8
ISSN: 1556-7443

Managing Editor: Linda Thomas
Publishing Services Manager: Deborah L. Vogel
Senior Project Manager: Jodi M. Willard
Design Direction: Jessica Williams

Printed in the United States of America

Last digit is the print number: 9   8   7   6   5   4   3   2   1

Nursing and Pharmacology Consultants

KIM HUBER, PharmD
Clinical Pharmacist
Memorial Medical Center
1700 Coffee Rd.
Modesto, California

MEGHAN McELWAIN, RN, BSN
Continuum Pediatric Nursing
Schaumburg, Illinois

GREGORY D. NAZARENO, PharmD
Staff Pharmacist
John Muir Medical Center
Walnut Creek, California

MERRILEE NEWTON, RN, MSN
Administrative Director of Quality, Service,
   and Clinical Resource Management
Alta Bates/Summit Medical Center
Berkeley, California

Reviewers

TIMOTHY L. BRENNER, PharmD
Clinical Pharmacy Specialist
UPMC Cancer Centers
Pittsburgh, Pennsylvania

DANA H. HAMAMURA, PharmD
Clinical Pharmacist
Emergency Department
University of Colorado Hospital
Aurora, Colorado

**MICHELE MATTHEWS,
PharmD, RPh**
Assistant Professor of Pharmacy
   Practice
Massachusetts College of
   Pharmacy and Health Sciences
Brigham and Women's Hospital
Boston, Massachusetts

**CHRISTOPHER T. OWENS,
PharmD, BCPS**
Associate Professor and Chair
Pharmacy Practice and
   Administrative Sciences
Idaho State University College
   of Pharmacy
Pocatello, Idaho

**RANDOLPH E. REGAL,
BS, PharmD, RPh**
Clinical Assistant Professor
Adult Internal Medicine
Department of Pharmacy Services
University of Michigan Hospital and
   College of Pharmacy
Ann Arbor, Michigan

TRAVIS E. SONNETT, PharmD
Washington State University
College of Pharmacy
Pullman, Washington

To my husband,

Bill,

for his patience, support, and many hours of much
needed and appreciated assistance, and to our children,
Marty, Jeff, Debbie, Rick, and **Teresa;**
their spouses, **Sally, Terri, Jim,** and **Bill;**
and our grandchildren, **Meghan, Laurie, Alex, Anne,
Kathryn, Lisa, Benjamin, Matthew, Claire, Neil, Scott,** and **Alan**
for their encouragement and understanding.

BLG

To my husband,

Greg,

for his loving support and encouragement and to my children,
Danielle, Bryan, Emily, and **Mark,** for allowing me the freedom
to pursue my professional practice.

ARN

To my wife,

Sue

for his patience, support, and many hours of understanding and appreciation assistance, and to our children Marie, Jeff, Debbie, Eric, and Steven

and to my parents Hildegard Stephan, Glenda, Alex, Anne, Kathryn, Lisa, Benjamin, Matthew, Claire, Beth, Scott, and Alan for their encouragement and understanding.

REC

To my children,

and Greg

for the loving support and encouragement and to my children Danielle, Bryan, Emily, and Mark, for showing me the meaning of nurse practitioners and mothers

MBN

Preface

This Year 2012 edition marks the thirty-ninth year of publication of *Intravenous Medications.* **In this twenty-eighth edition, a total of 9 new drugs approved by the FDA for intravenous use have been incorporated.** Eight of these new drugs are presented in individual monographs and include acetaminophen (an IV form for pain and fever management), alglucosidase alfa (an enzyme replenisher for patients 8 years of age and older with late-onset [non-infantile] Pompe disease), cabazitaxel (an antineoplastic for the treatment of hormone-refractory metastatic prostate cancer), ceftaroline (a cephalosporin approved for use in acute bacterial skin and skin structure infections and community-acquired bacterial pneumonia), eribulin mesylate (an antineoplastic for the treatment of patients with metastatic breast cancer who have previously received at least two chemotherapeutic regimens), pegloticase (for the treatment of gout), belimumab (recently approved for the treatment of active, autoantibody-positive, systemic lupus erythematosus), and ipilimumab (recently approved for the treatment of unresectable or metastatic melanoma). Belimumab and ipilimumab are included in Appendix E. The ninth drug, Glassia, is a new liquid formulation of alpha-1 proteinase inhibitor and has been incorporated into the alpha-1 proteinase inhibitor monograph.

Many new uses have been approved for established drugs, and numerous safety issues have been identified by the FDA. All of these changes are incorporated so our readers have the most current information available.

We continually strive to make information in this handbook informative and easier to access. **New to this edition is identification of drugs with a Black Box Warning BBW in the main heading instead of next to the Precautions heading within the monograph.** In addition, **Black Box Warning statements are shaded** in light gray **and a different typeface is used** for instant identification wherever they appear in the text. **The compatibilities have also been updated throughout the text with the most current information.**

In the past, we have incorporated the Common Toxicity Criteria (CTC) provided by the U.S. Department of Health and Human Services, the National Institutes of Health, and the National Cancer Institute. This listing has been expanded and updated by these organizations and is too expansive to be included in an appendix. Web access to this material is available at www.cancer.gov. Search for CTCAE (Common Terminology Criteria for Adverse Events Version 3.0). Printed copies are available free of charge; call 1-800-4-CANCER (1-800-422-6237).

We are all aware that **The Joint Commission** and the **Institute for Safe Medication Practices (ISMP)** have strongly emphasized various ways to reduce errors in drug ordering and administration. One of their suggestions is to refer to a drug by both its generic and its trade name. *Intravenous Medications* **is the only reference that has consistently used both names since its first publication.** They also recommend that symbols (e.g., $<$, $>$, $\leq$, $\geq$) be spelled out. **Although we have always spelled out most of them, they are now all spelled out. The only exception is in charts, where there isn't room for the spelled out version.** The symbols are included in the Key to Abbreviations (p. xxiii) if you need a refresher. **Some**

of the other ways we assist in safe administration is to spell out the word *units;* we use Gm instead of gm so it is not confused with mg, use mcg instead of μg, and drop all trailing 0s (as in 1.0) to prevent overdoses. **The Joint Commission, ISMP, the American Pharmaceutical Association, and several other organizations have identified "High-Alert Medications" (a list of medications with the highest risk of injury when misused).** The websites of these organizations contain considerable information and identify common risk factors and suggested strategies. The top five high-alert medications are insulin, opiates and narcotics, injectable potassium chloride (or phosphate) concentrate, IV anticoagulants, and sodium chloride solutions above 0.9% (NS). Others listed are adrenergic antagonists, aminophylline-theophylline, benzodiazepines, IV calcium, cardioplegic solutions, chemotherapeutic agents, colchicine, IV digoxin, dextrose solutions greater than 10%, lidocaine, IV magnesium sulfate, neuromuscular blockers, thrombolytics, and vasoactive drugs. From the authors' viewpoint, **all drugs given by the IV route should be considered high-alert medications.** They have an immediate effect, are irretrievable, and can cause life-threatening side effects with incorrect usage.

The Joint Commission also issued a *Sentinel Event Alert* (April 2006) that urges health care organizations to pay special attention to **how tubes and catheters are connected to patients** and challenges the manufacturers of these devices to redesign them in ways that will make dangerous misconnection much less possible. Health care organizations include hospitals, ambulatory care centers, home care agencies, nursing homes, and behavioral health care facilities. Look up The Joint Commission suggestions. A preventive measure not mentioned by The Joint Commission is the **simple practice of labeling every line at the point of entry into the patient.** This should be done whenever more than a single piece of tubing (IV or other) is connected to a patient. Multiple-lumen catheters, 3-way stopcocks, chest tubes, nasogastric tubes, and any other tubing entering the patient should be labeled with its contents or use at the connection closest to the patient. In today's health care settings, patients frequently have multiple tubes inserted into their bodies. Correct labeling takes only a few seconds at the time of insertion and saves many moments of precious time every time the line needs to be accessed. Misconnection errors may be fatal; establish all of these suggestions as a standard of practice, and misconnection errors will be avoided.

Elsevier has an electronic version of *Intravenous Medications* for personal digital assistants (PDAs). This "handheld" electronic version is a convenient and portable supplement to the book. In addition, all drugs presently on the Evolve IV Meds website (http://evolve.elsevier.com/IVMeds) for *Intravenous Medications* (because of space limitations for the print version) are incorporated in this electronic version. Although the handheld version is easy to carry, keep in mind that only a few lines of text are available at any one time. It is the user's responsibility to be familiar with the complete monograph and *all* aspects of each drug before administration.

Health care today is an intense environment. The speed of change is overwhelming, but the authors and publisher of *Intravenous Medications* have a commitment to provide all health care professionals who have the responsibility to administer IV medications with annual editions that incorporate complete, accurate, and current information in a clear, concise, accessible, and reliable tool. FDA websites are monitored throughout the year and provide many important updates, such as dose changes, new pediatric doses, additional disease-specific doses, refinements in dosing applications, new indications, new drug interactions, additional precautions, updates on post-marketing side effects, and new information on antidotes. Most drugs currently approved for intravenous use are included. Exceptions are opaque dyes used in radiology, some general anesthetics used only in the OR, and a few rarely used drugs. To stay within the confines of the spiral binding, selected diagnostic agents, muscle relaxants intended for use only in the OR, and several other rarely used drugs have been moved to the Evolve IV Meds website: http://evolve.elsevier.com/IVMeds. (See p. iv for a listing.) Helpful charts for dilution and/or rate of administration are incorporated in selected monographs. A General Dilution Chart to simplify calculations is found on the inside front cover. Front matter material provides a Key to Abbreviations and Important IV Therapy Facts.

Intravenous Medications is designed for use in critical care areas, at the nursing station, in the office, in public health and home care settings, and by students and the armed services. Pertinent information can be found in a few seconds. Take advantage of its availability and quickly review every intravenous medication before administration.

The nurse is frequently placed in a variety of difficult situations. While the physician verbally requests or writes an order, the nurse must evaluate it for appropriateness, prepare it, administer it, and observe the effects. Intravenous drugs are instantly absorbed into the bloodstream, leading, it is hoped, to a prompt therapeutic action, but the risk of an inappropriate reaction is a constant threat that can easily become a frightening reality. It will be the nurse who must initiate emergency measures should adverse effects occur. This is an awesome responsibility.

If, after reviewing the information in *Intravenous Medications,* you have any questions about any order you are given, clarify it with the physician, consult the pharmacist, or consult your supervisor. The circumstances will determine whom you will approach first. If the physician thinks it is imperative to carry out an order even though you have unanswered questions, never hesitate to request that the physician administer the drug, drug combination, or dose himself or herself. In this era of constant change, the physician should be very willing to supply you, your supervisor, and/or the pharmacist with current studies documenting the validity and appropriateness of orders.

All information presented in this handbook is pertinent only to the intravenous use of the drug and not necessarily to intramuscular, subcutaneous, oral, or other means of administration.

Our sincere appreciation is extended to Gregory Nazareno, Kim Huber, and Merrilee Newton for their ongoing participation in our efforts to bring you current, accurate, and relevant information; and to Darlene Como, Linda Thomas, Deborah L. Vogel, Jodi M. Willard, and Jessica Williams at Elsevier and Joe Rekart at Graphic World, who are the editors, production staff, and design staff that make the publishing of *Intravenous Medications* happen each year. This year we have a special thank you to Betty's granddaughter Meghan, who now has her BSN and her RN. She has provided much-appreciated help with the research needed to complete this edition and is being introduced to the process of preparing updated editions.

We also wish to thank you, the users of this reference. By seeking out this information, you serve your patients' needs and contribute to the safe administration of IV meds. We will continue to strive to earn your trust and confidence as we look forward together to an exciting future for health care.

Betty L. Gahart

Adrienne R. Nazareno

Contents

Contents

Format and Content of *Intravenous Medications*

Designed to facilitate quick reference, each entry begins with the generic name of the drug in boldface type. **New to this edition is the identification of drugs with a Black Box Warning, with a symbol** `BBW` **in the main heading instead of next to the Precautions heading within the monograph.** Phonetic pronunciations appear just below the generic name. Drug categories follow. The primary category may be followed by additional ones representing the multiple uses of a drug. Associated trade names are under the generic name. Boldface type and alphabetical order enable the reader to verify correct drug names easily. The use of a Canadian maple leaf symbol (✤) preceding a trade name indicates availability in Canada only. The pH is listed in the lower right-hand corner of the title section. While this information is not consistently available, it is provided whenever possible. It represents the pH of the undiluted drug, the drug after reconstitution, or the drug after dilution for administration.

Headings within drug monographs are as follows:

Usual Dose: Doses recommended are the usual range for adults unless specifically stated otherwise. This information is presented first to enable the nurse to verify that the physician order is within acceptable parameters while checking the order and before preparation. If there are any questions, much time can be saved in clarifying them. If premedication is indicated, it will be noted here.

Pediatric Dose: Pediatric doses are specifically stated if they vary from mg/kg of body weight or M^2 dose recommended for adults. Not all drugs are recommended for use in children. See Maternal/Child for information on safety and effectiveness for use in pediatric patients.

Infant and/or Neonatal Dose: Included if available and distinct from Pediatric Dose. See Maternal/Child for information on safety and effectiveness for use in pediatric patients, including infants and neonates.

Dose Adjustments: Any situation that requires increasing or decreasing a dose is mentioned here. The range covers adjustments needed for elderly, debilitated, or hepatic or renal impairment patients; adjustments required by race or gender; or adjustments required in the presence of other medications or as physical conditions are monitored.

Dilution: Specific directions for dilution are given for all drugs if dilution is necessary or permissible. Certain medications may be available in more than one form (e.g., Advantage, Duplex); follow manufacturer's directions for reconstitution and stability. Sadly, extreme cost-consciousness has overtaken the health care system. Nurses are being requested not to dilute drugs unless specifically required by the manufacturer, in order to save the cost of a needle, a syringe, or a small vial of diluent. Always use your best judgment and keep the safety of the patient as your priority. Appropriate diluents are listed. The Solution Compatibility Chart on the inside back cover has been expanded and updated. Diluents that are not identified in Dilution will be listed in this chart. This is the only reference that provides calculation examples to simplify dilution and accurate dose measurement. Charts are available in selected monographs. If recommendations for pediatric dilutions are available, they are listed. In some situations mcg or mg/mL dilutions partially account for this variation. If there are any doubts, consult with the pharmacist and/or pediatric specialist. Generic dilution charts for grams to milligrams and milligrams to micrograms are featured on the inside front cover and facing page.

Filters: A subheading. Content here includes information included in prescribing information and information we have requested from manufacturers. Many drugs are filtered during the manufacturing process. There are numerous variations in recommendations for filtration after the manufacturing process. Filters are single-use one-way streets and are most effective when used at the last stage of mixing or dilution or in-line as administered to the patient. Most manufacturers expect that a drug distributed in an ampule will be filtered to eliminate the possibility of glass being drawn into a syringe on withdrawal of the drug. This is always a two-needle process. One process uses a standard needle to withdraw from the ampule; that needle is then replaced with a needle filter to inject the drug into the diluent. If it will not be added to a diluent, use the needle filter to withdraw from the ampule and replace it with a new standard needle to administer. When questioned, many manufacturers suggest following a specific hospital's standard, which may recommend that a drug distributed as a powder be filtered either with a needle filter on withdrawal from the vial, after reconstitution as added to the diluent, or with an in-line filter on delivery to the patient. Some acknowledge that in selected situations (e.g., open heart surgery) everything is filtered at some point before delivery to the patient. Although these responses are helpful, none of them clarify specific information about a drug. For questions, the manufacturer's pharmacist is available.

Storage: A subheading. Content here includes such items as stability, refrigeration versus room temperature, predilution versus postdilution.

COMPATIBILITIES

The focus of this section is **compatibility. Any drug not listed as compatible should be considered incompatible. *Incompatibilities are listed only when specifically identified by the manufacturer. No third-party incompatibilities are listed.***

Some monographs include only general information because that is all that is available. It may include the manufacturer's recommendation to administer separately from other drugs or the potential for reaction with some plastic infusion bags or tubing.

Other monographs include manufacturers' statements regarding the potential inactivation or inhibition of one drug on another.

Compatibilities listed by the manufacturer are listed first, followed by **compatibilities** listed by another source, which may be divided into **additive and Y-site. *Any drug not listed as compatible should be considered incompatible.*** Drugs are alphabetized by generic name for ease in locating the drugs with which you are working. To make identification easier, common trade names accompany generic names, or examples are presented for drug categories. No other reference consistently provides this helpful information.

Because compatibilities may be influenced by many factors (e.g., temperature, pH, concentration, time together in solution, a specific order of mixing), **it is imperative that you verify compatibilities with your pharmacist.** Knowledge is growing daily in this field, and your pharmacist should have current information on the pharmacy computer or access to extensive references. Many compatibility studies have been done by other parties for both additive and Y-site compatibilities. Almost all are based on specific concentrations, which may or may not relate to usual doses or recommended concentrations.

Occasionally sources disagree on compatibility. If there is conflicting information about a compatibility, you will be told that this is not recommended by the manufacturer, or *the individual drugs that may have a conflict will be underlined.*

What steps should you consider before administering any drug?

- If the drug you wish to administer is not listed in the **Compatibility** section, *consider it to be incompatible.* To administer, you must turn off the infusing IV (at the stopcock or with a clamp close to the Y-site), flush the line with a solution compatible to both drugs (and/or solutions), administer the required drug, and flush the line again before turning the previously infusing IV back on. If you are unable to discontinue the infusion IV, you must have another IV access (e.g., a multi-lumen catheter, a second, IV line, or a heparin lock). Some drugs actually require separate tubing.

- If compatibilities are included in the package insert from the manufacturer, it will be so stated. If the manufacturer lists drugs as compatible by additive or Y-site and doesn't list concentrations, this is a good assurance of compatibility. If concentrations are listed, review the concentrations of both drugs to make sure they are within the defined parameters.

- If the drug you wish to administer is listed in the **Compatibility** section of the access you wish to use (e.g., **additive or Y-site**), *you must consult with the pharmacist to confirm any specific conditions that may apply.* After your consultation, write the results of your consultation regarding the specific directions for co-administering drugs on the patient's medication record or nursing care plan so others will not need to retrace your research steps when the medication is to be given again.

- When combining drugs in a solution (additives), always consider the required rate adjustments of each drug. Can each drug produce the desired effect at the suggested rate, or is continuous adjustment necessary for one drug, making the combination impractical?

- Y-site means that the specific drug in a specific monograph is compatible at its Y-site with an injection or an infusion containing one of the drugs listed under Y-site. The reverse Y-site compatibility may not be true.

- Although some drugs may be listed as compatible at the Y-site, some drugs can be administered at the Y-site only if they are further diluted in compatible solutions and given as an infusion (e.g., potassium concentrates [e.g., acetates, chlorides, phosphates], saline solution in concentrations greater than 0.9% or NS, amino acids, and dextrose solutions greater than 10% [unless in small amounts such as 50 mL dextrose 50% in insulin-induced hypoglycemia]).

- Because today's hospital units are very specialized (e.g., cancer care, emergency room, intensive coronary care, various intensive care units, transplant units, and orthopedic units to name just a few), nursing staff in each of these areas most likely administer similar combinations of drugs to their patients. *Take the initiative and research the drug combinations that are most frequently used on your unit. Then consult with the pharmacist and make your own compatibility chart for additives and Y-site (if applicable).* By creating a chart specific to your unit, you will limit the number of consults required with the pharmacist to combinations that fall outside of the parameters you have researched. This approach will save time for every nurse on your unit and will give each of you the necessary compatibility information to administer the IV drug combinations specific to your unit.

• The Solution Compatibility Chart on the inside back cover has been expanded and updated. Diluents that are not identified in Dilution will be listed in this chart.

Rate of Administration: Accepted rates of administration are clearly stated. As a general rule, a slow rate is preferred. 25-gauge needles aid in giving a small amount of medication over time. Problems with rapid or slow injection rates are indicated here. Adjusted rates for infants, children, or the elderly are listed when available. Charts are available in selected monographs.

Actions: Clear, concise statements outline the origin of each drug, how it affects body systems, its length of action, and methods of excretion. If a drug crosses the placental barrier or is secreted in breast milk, it will be mentioned here if that information is available.

Indications and Uses: Uses recommended by the manufacturer are listed. Unlabeled uses are stated as such.

Contraindications: Contraindications are those specifically listed by the manufacturer. Consult with the physician if an ordered drug is contraindicated for the patient. The physician may have additional historical information that alters the situation or may decide that use of the drug is indicated in a critical situation.

Precautions: The section on precautions covers many areas of information needed before injecting any drug, including black-box warnings from the prescribing information. Most Black Box Warnings appear in this Precautions section; however, **all actual Black Box Warning statements are shaded** in light gray **and a different typeface is used** for instant identification wherever they appear in the text. The range of information in this category covers all facets not covered under specific headings. Each listing is as important as the next. To make it easier for spot checks (after reading the entire monograph), additional subdivisions are included.

    Monitor: A subheading that includes information such as required prerequisites for drug administration, parameters for evaluation, and patient assessments.

    Patient Education: A subheading that addresses only specific, important issues required for short-term IV use. It is expected that the health professional will always review the major points in the drug profile with any conscious patient, side effects to expect, how to cope with them, when to report them, special requirements such as the intake of extra fluids, and an overall review of what the drug does, why it is needed, and how long the patient can anticipate receiving it. Patient Medication Guides approved by the FDA are available for many drugs.

    Maternal/Child: A subheading that addresses FDA pregnancy categories (see Appendix B for a complete explanation), any known specifics affecting patients capable of conception, safety for use during lactation, safety for use in pediatric patients, and any special impact on infants and neonates.

    Elderly: A subheading that is included whenever specific information impacting this patient group is available. Always consider age-related organ impairment (e.g., cardiac, hepatic, renal, insufficient bone marrow reserve), history of previous or concomitant disease or drug therapy, and route of excretion when determining dose and evaluating side effects.

Drug/Lab Interactions: Drug/drug or drug/lab interactions are listed here. To help identify these interactions more easily, **single drugs, drug categories when there are multiple drugs, and specific tests are in boldface type.** If a conflict with the patient's drug profile is noted, consult a pharmacist immediately. Increasing or decreasing the effectiveness of a drug can be a potentially life-threatening situation. Check with the lab first on drug/lab interactions; acceptable alternatives are usually available. After this consultation, notify the physician if appropriate. To facilitate recognition, common trade names accompany generic names or examples are presented for drug categories. No other reference consistently provides this helpful information.

Side Effects: Alphabetical order simplifies confirmation that a patient's symptom could be associated with specific drug use. Specific symptoms of overdose are listed where available or distinct from usual doses.

Post-Marketing: Post-marketing side effects reported are listed.

Antidote: Specific antidotes are listed in this section. In addition, specific nursing actions to reverse undesirable side effects are clearly stated—an instant refresher course for critical situations.

Within a heading there may be references to other sections within an individual monograph (e.g., see Precautions, see Monitor, see Dose Adjustments, see Maternal/Child). These references indicate additional requirements and should be consulted before administering the drug.

Key to Abbreviations

<	less than
>	more than
$\frac{1}{4}$NS	one-fourth normal saline (0.2%)
$\frac{1}{3}$NS	one-third normal saline (0.33%)
$\frac{1}{2}$NS	one-half normal saline (0.45%)
ABGs	arterial blood gases
ACE	angiotensin converting enzyme
ACT	activated coagulation time
A/G	albumin-to-globulin ratio
AIDS	acquired immunodeficiency syndrome
ALT	(SGPT) alanine aminotransferase
AMI	acute myocardial infarction
ANC	absolute neutrophil count
aPTT	activated partial thromboplastin time
ARDS	acute respiratory distress syndrome
AST	(SGOT) aspartate aminotransferase
AUC	area under the curve
AV	atrioventricular
BMD	bone mass density
BP	blood pressure
BSA	body surface area
BUN	blood urea nitrogen
BWFI	bacteriostatic water for injection
C	Celsius
Ca	calcium
CAD	coronary artery disease
CAPD	continuous ambulatory peritoneal dialysis
CBC	complete blood cell count
CHF	congestive heart failure
Cl	chloride
CNS	central nervous system
CO_2	carbon dioxide
CPK	creatine-kinase
CrCl	creatinine clearance
CRF	chronic renal failure
CRT	controlled room temperature (20° to 25° C [68° to 77° F])
CSF	cerebrospinal fluid
C/S	culture and sensitivity
CTCAE	Common Terminology Criteria for Adverse Events
CVP	central venous pressure
D10NS	10% dextrose in normal saline
D10W	10% dextrose in water
D5/$\frac{1}{4}$NS	5% dextrose in one-quarter normal saline (0.2%)
D5/$\frac{1}{3}$NS	5% dextrose in one-third normal saline (0.33%)
D5/$\frac{1}{2}$NS	5% dextrose in one-half normal saline (0.45%)
D5LR	5% dextrose in lactated Ringer's solution
D5NS	5% dextrose in normal saline
D5R	5% dextrose in Ringer's solution
D5W	5% dextrose in water

DC	discontinued
DEHP	Diethylhexylphthalate
DIC	disseminated intravascular coagulation
dL	deciliter(s) (100 mL)
DNA	deoxyribonucleic acid
ECG	electrocardiogram
EEG	electroencephalogram
ESRD	end-stage renal disease
F	Fahrenheit
GI	gastrointestinal
GFR	glomerular filtration rate
Gm	gram(s)
gr	grain(s)
gtt	drop(s)
GU	genitourinary
Hb	hemoglobin
Hct	hematocrit
Hg	mercury
HIV	human immunodeficiency virus
hr	hour
HR	heart rate
ICU	intensive care unit
IgA	immune globulin A
ÍL	microliters, μL, mm^3
IM	intramuscular
INR	International Normalized Ratio
IP	intrapleural
IU	international unit(s)
IV	intravenously
IVIG	intravenous immune globulin
K	potassium
KCl	potassium chloride
kg	kilogram(s)
L	liter(s)
lb	pound(s)
LDH	lactic dehydrogenase
LR	lactated Ringer's injection or solution
M	molar
M^2	meter squared
MAO	monoamine oxidase
MAP	mean arterial pressure
mcg	microgram(s)
mCi	millicurie(s)
mEq	milliequivalent
Mg	magnesium
mg	milligram(s)
MI	myocardial infarction
min	minute
mL	milliliter
mmol	millimole(s)
mm^3	cubic millimeters, μL, ÍL
MDRSP	multidrug-resistant strains

MRI	magnetic resonance imaging
Na	sodium
NaCl	sodium chloride
NCI	National Cancer Institute; see CTCAE
ng	nanogram (millimicrogram)
NS	normal saline (0.9%)
NSAID	nonsteroidal anti-inflammatory drug
NSCLC	non–small-cell lung cancer
NSR	normal sinus rhythm
N/V	nausea and vomiting
OTC	over-the-counter
PAC	premature atrial contraction
PaO_2	arterial oxygen pressure
PCA	patient controlled analgesia
pg	picogram
pH	hydrogen ion concentration
PO	by mouth/orally
PSVT	paroxysmal supraventricular tachycardia
PT	prothrombin time
PTT	partial thromboplastin time
PVC	polyvinyl chloride; premature ventricular contraction
R	Ringer's injection or solution
RBC	red blood cell
refrigerate	temperature at 2° to 8° C (36° to 46° F)
RNA	ribonucleic acid
RT	room temperature
RTS	room-temperature stable
SA	sinoatrial
SC	subcutaneous
SOB	shortness of breath
SCr	serum creatinine
S/S	signs and symptoms
SW or SWI	sterile water for injection
TIA	transient ischemic attacks
TNA	3-in-1 combination of amino acids, glucose, and fat emulsion
TPN	2-in-1 combination of amino acids and glucose; total parenteral nutrition
TT	thrombin time
μL	microliters, mm^3, ÍL
ULN	upper limits of normal
URI	upper respiratory infection
UTI	urinary tract infection
VF	ventricular fibrillation
VS	vital signs
VT	ventricular tachycardia
v/v	volume-to-volume ratio
WBC	white blood cell
WBCT	whole blood clotting time
w/v	weight-to-volume ratio
w/w	weight-to-weight ratio

Important IV Therapy Facts

- Read the Preface and Format and Contents sections at least once. They'll answer many of your questions and save time.

USUAL DOSE

- Doses calculated on body weight are usually based on pretreatment weight and not on edematous weight.
- Normal renal or hepatic function is usually required for drugs metabolized by these routes.
- Formula to calculate creatinine clearance (CrCl) from serum creatinine value (Cockcroft-Gault equation):

Males: $\dfrac{\text{Weight in kg} \times (140 - \text{Age in years})}{72 \times \text{Serum creatinine (mg/dL)}} = \text{CrCl}$

Females: $0.85 \times$ Male CrCl value calculated from above formula.

Children: $K \times \dfrac{\text{Linear length or height (cm)}}{\text{SCr (mg/100 mL)}}$

   K for children >1 year of age = 0.55
   K for infants = 0.45

- Lean Body Weight (LBW)

   Males = 50 kg + 2.3 kg for each inch over 5 foot.
   Females = 45.5 kg + 2.3 kg for each inch over 5 foot.
   Children weighing 15 kg or less—Use actual body weight in kg.

- Formula to calculate body surface area (BSA):

$$\text{BSA (M}^2) = \sqrt{\dfrac{\text{Height (cm)} \times \text{Weight (kg)}}{3600}}$$

DILUTION

- Check all labels (drugs, diluents, and solutions) to confirm appropriateness for IV use.
- Sterile technique is imperative in all phases of preparation.
- Use a filter needle when withdrawing IV meds from ampules to eliminate possible pieces of glass.
- Pearls: 1 Gm in 1 Liter yields 1 mg/mL
      1 mg in 1 Liter yields 1 mcg/mL
      % of a solution equals the number of grams/100 mL
         (5% = 5 Gm/100 mL)
- Pediatric dilution: If you dilute 6.0 mg/kg in 100 mL, 1 mL/hr
            equals 1.0 mcg/kg/min
         If you dilute 0.6 mg/kg in 100 mL, 1 mL/hr
            equals 0.1 mcg/kg/min
- See charts on inside front cover.
- Do not use bacteriostatic diluents containing benzyl alcohol for neonates. May cause a fatal toxic syndrome. S/S include CNS depression, hypotension, intracranial hemorrhage, metabolic acidosis, renal failure, respiratory problems, seizures.
- Ensure adequate mixing of all drugs added to a solution.
- When combining drugs in a solution (additives), always consider the required rate adjustment of each drug.
- Examine solutions for clarity and any possible leakage.

- Frozen infusion solutions should be thawed at room temperature (25° C [77° F]) or under refrigeration. Do not force by immersion in water baths or in the microwave. All ice crystals must be melted before administration. Do not refreeze.
- Syringe prepackaging for use in specific pumps is now available for many drugs. Concentrations are often the strongest permissible, but length of delivery is accurate.
- Controlled room temperature (CRT) is considered to be 25° C (77° F). Most medications tolerate variations in temperature from 15° to 30° C (59° to 86° F).

INCOMPATIBILITIES
- Some manufacturers routinely suggest discontinuing the primary IV for intermittent infusion; usually done to avoid any possibility of incompatibility. Flushing the line before and after administration may be indicated and/or appropriate for some drugs.
- The brand of intravenous fluids or additives, concentrations, containers, rate and order of mixing, pH, and temperature all affect solubility and compatibility. Consult your pharmacist with any question, and document appropriate instructions on care plan.

TECHNIQUES
- Never hang plastic containers in a series connection; may cause air embolism.
- Confirm patency of peripheral and/or central sites. Avoid extravasation.
- Avoid accidental arterial injection; can cause gangrene.

RATE OF ADMINISTRATION
- Life-threatening reactions (time-related overdose or allergy) are frequently precipitated by a too-rapid rate of injection.

PATIENT EDUCATION
- A well-informed patient is a great asset; review all appropriate drug information with every conscious patient.

SIDE EFFECTS
- Reactions may be caused by a side effect of the drug itself, allergic response, overdose, or the underlying disease process.

Resources

PUBLICATIONS

The following publications have been used as a resource to assemble the information found in *Intravenous Medications*. Additional and more detailed information on drugs may be found in these publications:

American Heart Association: *Handbook of Emergency Cardiovascular Care for Health Care Providers, 2010.*

American Hospital Formulary Service Drug Information 2011, Bethesda, Md, 2010, American Society of Hospital Pharmacists (updated via website).

Drug facts and comparisons, St Louis, 2011, Facts and Comparisons Division, JB Lippincott.

Lexi-Comp's Drug Information Handbook, ed 19, 2010-2011, Hudson, Ohio, American Pharmacists Association.

Elsevier Guide to Oncology Drugs and Regimens, Huntington, NY, 2006, Elsevier.

The Johns Hopkins Hospital: *The Harriet Lane handbook,* ed 18, St Louis, 2009, Mosby.

Manufacturers' literature.

Merck manual of diagnosis and therapy, ed 18, Whitehouse Station, NJ, 2006, Merck Research Laboratories.

Physician's Desk Reference, ed 65, Montvale, NJ, 2011, Thomson PDR.

Tatro DS, editor: *Drug interaction facts,* St Louis, 2011, Facts and Comparisons Division, JB Lippincott.

Trissel LA: *Handbook on injectable drugs,* ed 16, 2011, American Society of Hospital Pharmacists, Inc.

WEBSITE RESOURCES

http://www.accessdata.fda.gov/scripts/cder/drugsatfda—Drug Approvals and Updates

http://www.fda.gov/safety/medwatch/default.htm—Safety Information

http://evolve.elsevier.com/IVMeds

http://www.cancer.gov—Common Terminology Criteria for Adverse Events (CTCAE)

http://www.blackboxrx.com—A listing of all drugs with a black box warning

ABATACEPT
(a-**BAY**-ta-sept)
Orencia

Anti-rheumatic agent

pH 7.2 to 7.8

USUAL DOSE
Dose is based on body weight in kilograms as shown in the following chart. After the initial dose, repeat administration at 2 and 4 weeks. Administer every 4 weeks thereafter. May be used as monotherapy or concomitantly with disease-modifying anti-rheumatic drugs (DMARDs) other than TNF antagonists; see Contraindications and Drug Interactions.

Abatacept Adult Dosing Guidelines		
Body Weight (kg)	Dose (mg)	Number of Vials
<60 kg	500 mg	2 vials
60 to 100 kg	750 mg	3 vials
>100 kg	1,000 mg	4 vials

PEDIATRIC DOSE
Pediatric patients 6 to 17 years of age who weigh less than 75 kg: 10 mg/kg/dose based on patient's body weight at each administration. After the initial dose, repeat administration at 2 and 4 weeks. Administer every 4 weeks thereafter.
Pediatric patients 6 to 17 years of age who weigh more than 75 kg: See Usual Dose and the Abatacept Adult Dosing Guidelines chart. Do not exceed a maximum dose of 1,000 mg.

DOSE ADJUSTMENTS
There is a trend toward a higher clearance with increasing body weight; see Usual Dose. No specific dose adjustments are required based on age or gender when corrected for body weight. ■ Withhold therapy in patients with severe infections. ■ The effects of renal or hepatic impairment have not been studied.

DILUTION
Using *ONLY the silicone-free disposable syringe provided* with each vial and an 18- to 21-gauge needle, reconstitute each 250-mg vial with 10 mL SW; final concentration is 25 mg/mL. (If reconstituted with a siliconized syringe, the solution must be discarded.) Direct stream of SW toward side of vial. Do not use vial if vacuum is not present. Rotate or swirl vial gently until contents have dissolved. Do not shake. After dissolution, vent vial with a needle to dissipate any foam that may be present. Solution should be clear and colorless to pale yellow. Reconstituted solution must be further diluted to 100 mL as follows: From a 100-mL infusion bag or bottle, withdraw a volume of NS equal to the volume of reconstituted abatacept solution required for the patient's dose (for 2 vials, remove 20 mL; for 3 vials, remove 30 mL; for 4 vials, remove 40 mL). Using the *same silicone-free disposable syringe provided,* slowly add the reconstituted abatacept into the infusion bag or bottle. Mix gently.

Filter: Administration through a 0.2- to 1.2-micron, non-pyrogenic, low–protein binding filter is required.

Storage: Refrigerate unopened vials at 2° to 8° C (36° to 46° F). Do not use beyond expiration date. Protect from light. Before administration, the diluted solution may be stored at CRT or refrigerated; however, infusion of the diluted solution should be completed within 24 hours of reconstitution.

COMPATIBILITY

Manufacturer states, "Should not be infused concomitantly in the same intravenous line with other agents." **Compatibility** studies have not been performed.

RATE OF ADMINISTRATION

Administration through a 0.2- to 1.2-micron, non-pyrogenic, low–protein binding filter is required.

A single dose equally distributed over 30 minutes.

ACTIONS

A soluble fusion protein that consists of the extracellular domain of human cytotoxic, T-lymphocyte–associated antigen 4 linked to the modified Fc portion of human immunoglobulin G1 (IgG1). Produced by recombinant DNA technology. Acts as a selective biologic response modulator by inhibiting T-lymphocyte activation, which is implicated in the pathogenesis of rheumatoid arthritis. Reduces pain and joint inflammation and slows the progression of structural damage to bone and cartilage. Mean half-life is 13.1 days (range 8 to 25 days).

INDICATIONS AND USES

Reduce the S/S, induce a major clinical response, inhibit the progression of structural damage, and improve the physical function in adult patients with moderately to severely active rheumatoid arthritis. May be used as monotherapy or concomitantly with DMARDs other than TNF antagonists. ▪ Reduce the S/S in pediatric patients 6 years of age and older with moderately to severely active polyarticular juvenile idiopathic arthritis. May be used as monotherapy or concomitantly with methotrexate.

CONTRAINDICATIONS

Known hypersensitivity to abatacept or any of its components (maltose, monobasic sodium phosphate). Concomitant use with TNF antagonists or other biological rheumatoid arthritis agents such as anakinra (Kineret) is not recommended; see Drug/Lab Interactions.

PRECAUTIONS

Concurrent use with a TNF antagonist (e.g., adalimumab [Humira], etanercept [Enbrel]) is associated with an increased risk of serious infections with no associated increased efficacy when compared with use of the TNF antagonist alone. Concurrent use is not recommended; see Contraindications and Drug/Lab Interactions. ▪ Hypersensitivity reactions including anaphylaxis have been reported. Emergency medical equipment and medications for treating these reactions must be readily available. ▪ Use caution in patients with a history of recurrent infections, underlying conditions that may predispose them to infections, or chronic, latent, or localized infections; see Monitor. ▪ Anti-rheumatic therapies have been associated with hepatitis B reactivation. Screening for viral hepatitis should be done before starting therapy with abatacept. Patients who screened positive for hepatitis were excluded from clinical studies. ▪ Use with caution in patients with COPD. May be at increased risk for developing respiratory adverse events (e.g., COPD exacerbation, cough, dyspnea, rhonchi). ▪ A small number of patients have developed binding antibodies to abatacept. No correlation of antibody development to clinical response or adverse events has been observed. ▪ T-cells mediate cellular immune responses. Therefore drugs that inhibit T-cell activation, including abatacept, may affect patient defenses against infection and malignancies. The impact of abatacept on the development and course of malignancies is not fully understood.

Monitor: Evaluate patients for latent tuberculosis (TB) with a TB skin test. Patients testing positive in TB screening should be treated with a standard TB regimen before initiating therapy with abatacept. ▪ Screening for viral hepatitis is recommended before initiating therapy with abatacept. ▪ Monitor for S/S of infection, especially if transitioning patient from TNF antagonist therapy to therapy with abatacept. Discontinue therapy if a serious infection develops. ▪ Monitor COPD patients for worsening of respiratory status. ▪ Monitor for S/S of hypersensitivity or infusion-related reactions; see Side Effects. ▪ Do not administer live virus vaccines. ▪ See Precautions and Drug/Lab Interactions.

Patient Education: Read manufacturer's patient information sheet prior to each infusion. ▪ Review medication list and vaccination status with physician. ▪ Report S/S of allergic reaction (e.g., rash, itching wheezing), infusion reaction (e.g., dizziness, headache), or infection promptly. Discuss previous infections, current infections, or exposure to TB.

Maternal/Child: Category C: safety for use in pregnancy has not been established. Has been shown to cross the placenta in animal studies. Use caution. ▪ Discontinue breast-feeding. ▪ A pregnancy registry has been established; contact manufacturer. ▪ Safety and effectiveness for use in pediatric patients under 6 years of age not established. ▪ Patients with juvenile idiopathic arthritis should be brought up-to-date with all immunizations before initiating therapy with abatacept.

Elderly: Specific differences in safety and efficacy not noted. Incidence of infection and malignancy is higher in the elderly. Use caution; see Precautions.

DRUG/LAB INTERACTIONS

Formal drug interaction studies have not been conducted. ▪ Has been used with methotrexate, NSAIDs (e.g., naproxen [Naprosyn, Aleve], ibuprofen [Motrin, Advil]), corticosteroids (e.g., prednisone), azathioprine (Imuran), chloroquine (Aralen), gold (Myochrysine), hydroxychloroquine (Plaquenil), leflunomide (Arava), and sulfasalazine (Azulfidine). ▪ Methotrexate, NSAIDs, corticosteroids, and TNF antagonists do not appear to influence abatacept clearance. ▪ Concurrent use with a **TNF antagonist** (e.g., adalimumab [Humira], etanercept [Enbrel], infliximab [Remicade]) is associated with an increased risk of serious infections and no significant additional efficacy over use of the TNF antagonist alone. Concurrent use is not recommended. ▪ Falsely elevated blood glucose readings may occur with **specific blood glucose monitoring systems** that react to drug products containing maltose. Abatacept contains maltose; see prescribing information. ▪ Safety and efficacy of concurrent use with **anakinra** (Kineret) has not been established. Concurrent use is not recommended. ▪ **Live virus vaccines** should not be given concurrently with or within 3 months of abatacept. ▪ May blunt the effectiveness of some **vaccinations.**

SIDE EFFECTS

In adult and pediatric patients, side effects are similar in type and frequency. The most commonly reported side effects are headache, nasopharyngitis, nausea, and upper respiratory tract infections. The most serious adverse effects are infections and malignancies. Infections are the most likely adverse event to cause interruption or discontinuation of therapy. Acute infusion-related reactions (cough, dyspnea, dizziness, flushing, headache, hypertension, hypotension, nausea, pruritus, rash, urticaria, wheezing) have been reported and usually occur within 1 hour of the infusion. Hypersensitivity reactions (anaphylaxis [rare], dyspnea, hypotension, urticaria) have been reported, usually within 24 hours of infusion. Other reactions include back or extremity pain, COPD exacerbation, dyspepsia, immunogenicity (antibody formation), and rhonchi.

ANTIDOTE

Notify physician of any side effects; most will be treated symptomatically. During clinical studies, most infusion-related reactions were mild to moderate, and therapy was discontinued in very few patients. Discontinue abatacept for any serious reaction or infection. Therapy may need to be interrupted in patients who develop infections. Treat infusion and hypersensitivity reactions as indicated (e.g., oxygen, diphenhydramine, epinephrine, corticosteroids, vasopressors, and/or fluids). Resuscitate as necessary.

# ABCIXIMAB (ab-**SIX**-ih-mab)	Platelet aggregation inhibitor Antithrombotic Monoclonal antibody
ReoPro	pH 7.2

USUAL DOSE

Premedication: In all situations, premedication with histamine H_2 antagonists (e.g., famotidine [Pepcid], ranitidine [Zantac]) may be appropriate; prophylaxis should be considered when certain conditions are present (e.g., patients with HACA antibodies, readministration of abciximab).

Percutaneous coronary intervention: 0.25 mg/kg administered 10 to 60 minutes before percutaneous coronary intervention (PCI). Follow with a continuous infusion of 0.125 mcg/kg/min (weight adjusted) to a maximum of 10 mcg/min (non–weight adjusted) for 12 hours. Used concurrently with **heparin** and **aspirin**. Establish a separate IV site for heparin. The initial bolus of **heparin** is based on the results of the baseline ACT according to low-dose weight-adjusted guidelines in the following chart, but not exceeding a total bolus dose of 7,000 units.

Guidelines for Heparin Dosing					
Low-Dose Weight-Adjusted Heparin *(Target ACT ≥200 seconds)*			Standard-Dose Weight-Adjusted Heparin *(Target ACT ≥300 seconds)*		
Initial Bolus	ACT (sec)	Heparin	Initial Bolus	ACT (sec)	Heparin
Not to exceed 7,000 units in patients >100 kg	<150	70 units/kg	Not to exceed 10,000 units in patients >100 kg	<150	100 units/kg
	150 to 199	50 units/kg		150 to 225	75 units/kg
	≥200	No heparin		226 to 299	50 units/kg
				≥300	No heparin
Additional bolus every 30 min or a 7-unit/kg/hr continuous infusion	<200	20 units/kg	Additional bolus every 30 min or a 10-unit/kg/hr continuous infusion	<275	50 units/kg
	≥200	No heparin		275 to 299	25 units/kg
				≥300	No heparin

Check ACT (Hemochron instrument used to measure) a minimum of 2 minutes after the initial and each additional heparin bolus. Give additional bolus doses of 20 units/kg until the target ACT of 200 seconds is achieved before PCI (a target ACT of up to 300 seconds using standard weight-adjusted doses of heparin has been used [see preceding chart] but may increase the risk of severe bleeding). During the procedure administer additional bolus doses every 30 minutes to maintain the target ACT. Alternately, after the target ACT is reached, a 7-unit/kg/hr continuous infusion *may be administered with no further measurement of ACT for the duration of the procedure. Unless contraindicated, administer* **aspirin,** 325 mg, 2 hours before PCI and once daily thereafter. At the completion of the procedure it is recommended that the heparin be discontinued and that removal of the sheath be accomplished within 6 hours; see Monitor for specific criteria. If prolonged therapy or later sheath removal is clinically indicated, do not discontinue heparin, but continue the 7-unit/kg/hr heparin infusion. Check the aPTT in 6 hours and adjust rate of heparin based on a target aPTT of 60 to 85 seconds. See Precautions/Monitor.

Unstable angina not responding to conventional medical therapy with planned PCI within 24 hours: *Heparin* is started before the abciximab; use a separate IV line. Maintain the aPTT between 60 and 85 seconds during the abciximab and heparin infusion period. Recent recommendations suggest that the low-dose weight-adjusted doses of heparin and anticoagulation guidelines described above are also appropriate for the planned PCI in unstable angina. The recommended dose of abciximab is 0.25 mg/kg as an IV bolus followed by a continuous infusion of 10 mcg/min for a minimum of 18 hours up to a maximum of 26 hours (PCI usually accomplished between 18 and 24 hours). Discontinue abciximab 1 hour after the PCI (i.e., removal of guidewire). Unless contraindicated, administer at least 250 mg of **aspirin** at the time heparin is begun and aspirin 50 to 500 mg daily through day 30. Oral or IV nitroglycerin may also be indicated throughout the course of treatment. The process after the completion of the procedure is the same as in percutaneous coronary intervention.

DILUTION

Available in 5-mL vials (2 mg/mL). Solution must be clear. Must be filtered with a nonpyrogenic, low–protein binding 0.2- to 0.22-micron filter before administering the bolus and the infusion. Filtering of the infusion may be done during preparation or at administration, using the appropriate in-line filter. Do not shake.

IV injection: Bolus injection may be given undiluted.

Infusion: Withdraw desired dose and further dilute with NS or D5W (5 mL [10 mg] diluted with 250 mL NS or D5W equals 40 mcg/mL).

Filters: Must be filtered with a nonpyrogenic, low–protein binding 0.2- to 0.22-micron filter before administering the bolus and the infusion. Filtering of the infusion may be done during preparation or at administration, using the appropriate in-line filter; see Dilution.

Storage: Refrigerate before use. Do not freeze. Check expiration date on vial. Contains no preservative; discard any unused portion.

COMPATIBILITY

Consider any drug NOT listed as compatible to be INCOMPATIBLE until consulting a pharmacist; specific conditions may apply.

According to the manufacturer, no **incompatibilities** have been shown with IV fluids or commonly used cardiovascular drugs; however, administration through a separate IV line and not mixing with other medications is recommended. No **incompatibilities** observed with glass bottles or polyvinyl chloride bags and administration sets.

One source suggests the following **compatibilities:**

Y-site: Adenosine (Adenocard, Adenoscan), argatroban, atropine, bivalirudin (Angiomax), diphenhydramine (Benadryl), fentanyl (Sublimaze), metoprolol (Lopressor), midazolam (Versed).

RATE OF ADMINISTRATION

IV injection: An initial dose as a bolus injection; filter at this point if not done when withdrawing from vial.

Infusion: See Usual Dose. Must be administered through an in-line, nonpyrogenic, low–protein binding filter (0.2 or 0.22 microns), if not done during preparation, and controlled by a continuous infusion pump. A 40-mcg/mL solution (10 mg in 250 mL) at a rate of 10.5 mL/hr will deliver 7 mcg/min, and 15 mL/hr will deliver 10 mcg/min. Discard unused portion at the end of the infusion.

ACTIONS

The fab fragment of the chimeric human-murine monoclonal antibody, abciximab binds to the glycoprotein GPIIb/IIIa receptor of human platelets and produces rapid dose-dependent inhibition of platelet function. It inhibits platelet aggregation by preventing the binding of fibrinogen, von Willebrand factor, and other adhesive molecules to GPIIb/IIIa receptor sites on activated platelets. Inhibition of platelet function is temporary following a bolus dose, but can be sustained at greater than 80% by continuous IV infusion. Has prevented acute thrombosis and resulted in lower rates of thrombosis as compared to aspirin and/or heparin. Initial half-life is 10 minutes. Second phase half-life is 30 minutes. A bolus dose followed by an infusion produces approximately constant free plasma concentrations throughout the infusion. Median bleeding time increases to over 30 minutes as contrasted to a baseline average of 5 minutes before administration. After the infusion is ended, free plasma concentration falls rapidly for 6 hours, then more slowly. Platelet function generally recovers gradually over 48 hours. In most patients, bleeding time returns to less than 12 minutes within 12 to 24 hours. Some abciximab remains in the circulation for 15 days or more.

INDICATIONS AND USES

An adjunct to PCI for the prevention of cardiac ischemic complications in patients undergoing PCI and in patients with unstable angina not responding to conventional medical therapy when PCI is planned within 24 hours. Abciximab use in patients not undergoing PCI has not been studied. Used concurrently with aspirin and heparin. In selected situations, clopidogrel (Plavix) or ticlopidine (Ticlid) may also be used concurrently.

Unlabeled uses: Combined with low-dose alteplase or low-dose reteplase in the early treatment of acute MI. ■ Treatment of acute ischemic stroke.

CONTRAINDICATIONS

Active internal bleeding, administration of oral anticoagulants (e.g., warfarin [Coumadin]) within 7 days unless PT is at or less than 1.2 times control, aneurysm, arteriovenous malformation, bleeding diathesis, clinically significant GI or GU bleeding within 6 weeks, history of CVA within 2 years, history of CVA with significant residual neurologic deficit, history of vasculitis (presumed or documented), hypertension (severe and uncontrolled), intracranial neoplasm, known hypersensitivity to any component of abciximab or to murine proteins, major surgery or trauma within 6 weeks, thrombocytopenia (less than $100,000/mm^3$), or the use of IV dextran before PCI or intent to use it during PCI.

PRECAUTIONS

Administered only in the hospital under the direction of a physician knowledgeable in its use and with appropriate diagnostic, laboratory, and surgical facilities available. ■ Frequently causes major bleeding complications (e.g., retroperitoneal bleeding, spontaneous GI and GU bleeding, bleeding at the arterial access site). ■ Incidence of major bleeding was reduced in clinical trials that used weight-adjusted dosing of abciximab and low-dose weight-adjusted doses of heparin, with adherence to stricter anticoagulation guidelines and early sheath removal. This was true in patients weighing less than 75 kg (165 lb) that had increased incidences of bleeding with standard weight-adjusted heparin doses. ■ Incidence of major bleeding is increased in patients with a history of prior GI disease, those over 65 years of age, and those receiving heparin, other anticoagulants, or thrombolytics (e.g., alteplase [tPA], reteplase [r-PA], streptokinase). Consider if benefits will outweigh risks, and proceed with extreme caution if use is considered necessary. ■ Incidence of major bleeding is also increased if PCI occurs within 12 hours of the onset of symptoms of an acute MI, if the PCI procedure is prolonged (lasting more than 70 minutes), or if PCI procedure fails. ■ Extreme care must be taken in accessing the femoral artery for femoral sheath placement. Only the anterior wall of the femoral artery should be punctured (use of a single-walled needle versus double-walled [Seldinger through and through technique] is important). If both walls are punctured, massive bleeding could occur. ■ Avoid concurrent sheath placement in the femoral vein if possible (sometimes used to access right coronary artery or administer large amounts of medication). ■ Use of heparin concurrently also increases the risk of bleeding. ■ Anaphylaxis can occur at any time (a protein solution). Emergency drugs and equipment must always be available. In addition, use may result in the formation of human anti-chimeric antibody (HACA). Can cause hypersensitivity reactions including anaphylaxis, thrombocytopenia, or diminished benefit if abciximab is readministered at another time or other monoclonal antibodies are administered. Consider premedication as outlined under Usual Dose. ■ See Drug/Lab Interactions.

Monitor: Before initiating, obtain results of baseline CBC, platelet count, PT, ACT, and aPTT. Type and cross-match would also be appropriate. ■ Monitor heparin anticoagulation (ACT or aPTT) and PT closely. ■ While a femoral sheath is in place, the patient must be on strict bed rest, head of the bed should be less than 30 degrees, and the appropriate limb(s) restrained in a straight position. Monitor sheath insertion site(s) and distal pulses of affected leg(s) frequently while sheath is in place and for 6 hours after removal. Measure any hematoma and monitor for enlargement. ■ Monitor platelet count 2 to 4 hours following the bolus dose and at 24 hours or before discharge, whichever is first. More frequent monitoring may be indicated. ■ Monitor patient carefully and frequently for signs of bleeding; take vital signs (avoiding automatic BP cuffs), observe any invaded sites at least every 15 minutes (e.g., sheaths, IV sites, cutdowns, punctures, Foleys, NGs); watch for hematuria, hematemesis, bloody stool, petechiae, hematoma, flank pain, muscle weakness; and do neuro checks every hour. Continue until clotting functions move toward normal. ■ Use care in handling patient; avoid arterial puncture, venipuncture, and IM injection. Use extreme precautionary methods and only compressible sites if these procedures are absolutely necessary. Apply pressure for 30 minutes to any invaded site and then apply pressure dressings. Saline or heparin locks are suggested to facilitate blood draws. ■ Discontinue heparin at least 2 to 4 hours before femoral sheath(s) are to be removed. Sheath removal should not occur until aPTT is at or less than 50 seconds or ACT is at or less than 175 seconds (approaching normal limits). Discontinue heparin after PCI, and remove sheath no sooner than 2 hours and no later than 6 hours after heparin is discontinued and while the abciximab is still infusing (aPTT must be at or less than 50 seconds or ACT at or less than 175 seconds). After removal, apply pressure to the femoral artery for at least 30 minutes. When hemostasis is confirmed, apply a pressure dressing. Maintain strict bed rest for at least 6 to 8 hours after sheath removal and/or abciximab is discontinued or 4 hours after heparin is discontinued, whichever is later. ■ Throughout process medicate as needed for back or groin pain and nausea or vomiting. ■ Remove pressure dressing before ambulation. ■ If complications arise that indicate the need for surgery within 48 to 72 hours of treatment with abciximab, an Ivy bleeding time should be obtained. Platelet function may be partly restored with platelet transfusions. ■ See Precautions, Drug/Lab Interactions, and Antidote.

Patient Education: Compliance with all measures to minimize bleeding (e.g., strict bed rest, positioning) is imperative. ■ Avoid use of razors, toothbrushes, and other sharp items. ■ Use caution while moving to avoid excessive bumping. ■ Report all episodes of bleeding and apply local pressure if indicated. ■ Expect oozing from IV sites.

Maternal/Child: Category C: use only if clearly needed and with extreme caution. ■ Safety for use during breast-feeding not established. Not known if it is secreted in breast milk; use extreme caution; probably best to postpone breast-feeding until bleeding time approaches normal. ■ Safety and effectiveness for use in pediatric patients not established. Incidence of side effects may be increased with a weight under 75 kg.

Elderly: Increased risk of major bleeding complications if weight less than 75 kg or age over 65 years; see Precautions. ■ Consider age-related organ impairment, concomitant disease, or drug therapy; may also increase risk of bleeding.

DRUG/LAB INTERACTIONS

Use with extreme caution with other drugs that affect hemostasis (e.g., **thrombolytics** [e.g., alteplase (tPA), streptokinase], **anticoagulants** [e.g., heparin, warfarin (Coumadin)], **NSAIDs** [e.g., ibuprofen (Advil, Motrin), naproxen (Aleve, Naprosyn)], **platelet aggregation inhibitors** [e.g., clopidogrel (Plavix), dipyridamole (Persantine), ticlopidine (Ticlid)] and **other glycoprotein GPIIb/IIIa receptor antagonists** [e.g., eptifibatide (Integrilin), tirofiban (Aggrastat)], **and selected antibiotics** [e.g., cefotetan]). ■ **Dextran solutions** increased the risk of major bleeding events when used concurrently with abciximab; see Contraindications. ■ **HACA titer** may precipitate an acute hypersensitivity reaction with other **diagnostic or therapeutic monoclonal antibodies** (e.g., muromonab-CD3).

SIDE EFFECTS

May cause major bleeding incidents (e.g., femoral artery or other access site, intracranial hemorrhage, spontaneous gross hematuria and other GU bleeds, spontaneous hematemesis and other GI bleeds, pulmonary hemorrhage, retroperitoneal bleeding). Decreases in hemoglobin greater than 5 Gm/dL or intracranial hemorrhage were defined as major during trials. Thrombocytopenia is common and may require platelet transfusion. Abdominal pain, back pain, bradycardia, chest pain, headache, hypotension, nausea, peripheral edema, positive HACA response, puncture site pain, and vomiting may occur. Other side effects that may occur are anemia, arrhythmias (e.g., atrial fibrillation/flutter, bradycardia, complete AV block, supraventricular tachycardia, ventricular PVCs, tachycardia, or fibrillation), confusion, hyperesthesia, intermittent claudication, leukocytosis, limb embolism, pericardial effusion, pleural effusion or pleurisy, pneumonia, pulmonary embolism, pulmonary edema, and visual disturbances. Anaphylaxis has not been reported but may occur.

ANTIDOTE

Stop the infusions of abciximab and heparin if any serious bleeding not controllable with pressure occurs. Stop infusion in patients with failed PCIs. Stop infusion if a hypersensitivity reaction occurs. Treat hypersensitivity reactions as indicated; may require epinephrine, airway management, oxygen, IV fluids, antihistamines (e.g., diphenhydramine [Benadryl]), corticosteroids (e.g., hydrocortisone sodium succinate [Solu-Cortef]), and pressor amines (e.g., dopamine). Keep physician informed. If an acute platelet decrease occurs (less than 100,000/mm^3 or a decrease of at least 25% from pretreatment value), obtain additional platelet counts in separate tubes containing ethylenediaminetetraacetic acid (EDTA), citrate, or heparin. This is to exclude pseudothrombocytopenia due to anticoagulant interaction. If true thrombocytopenia is verified, discontinue abciximab immediately. Platelet transfusions may be required. Heparin and aspirin should also be avoided if the platelet count drops below 60,000/mm^3.

ACETAMINOPHEN
(ah-**SEAT**-ah-**MIN**-oh-fen)

Ofirmev

Antipyretic
Analgesic

pH 5.5

USUAL DOSE

May be given as a single or repeated dose. Minimum dosing interval is 4 hours. No dose adjustment is necessary when converting from oral to IV dosing. The maximum daily dose of acetaminophen is based on all routes of administration (i.e., IV, oral, and rectal) and on all products containing acetaminophen.

Summary of Acetaminophen Dosing in Adults and Adolescents				
Age-Group	Dose Given q 4 hr	Dose Given q 6 hr	Maximum Single Dose	Maximum Total Daily Dose of Acetaminophen (By Any Routes)
Adults and adolescents (13 years and older) weighing ≥50 kg	650 mg	1,000 mg	1,000 mg	4,000 mg in 24 hr
Adults and adolescents (13 years and older) weighing <50 kg	12.5 mg/kg	15 mg/kg	15 mg/kg	75 mg/kg in 24 hr (up to 3,750 mg)

PEDIATRIC DOSE

Pediatric patients 2 to 12 years of age: 15 mg/kg every 6 hours or 12.5 mg/kg every 4 hours. Do not exceed a maximum single dose of 15 mg/kg or a maximum daily dose of 75 mg/kg/day. See comments under Usual Dose.

DOSE ADJUSTMENTS

A reduced total daily dose of acetaminophen may be appropriate in patients with hepatic impairment or active liver disease. ▪ A reduced total daily dose and longer dosing intervals may be appropriate in patients with a CrCl less than or equal to 30 mL/min.

DILUTION

Available in a single-use vial containing 1,000 mg/100 mL (10 mg/mL) of acetaminophen. For adults and adolescent patients weighing 50 kg or more requiring a 1,000-mg dose, administer the dose by inserting a vented intravenous set through the septum of the 100-mL vial. Doses less than 1,000 mg should be withdrawn from the vial and placed into a separate empty container before administration to avoid inadvertent administration of an overdose. Withdraw appropriate dose (650 mg or weight-based) from 100-mL vial and place in an empty container (e.g., syringe, glass bottle, plastic intravenous container) for intravenous infusion.
Filter: Information not available.
Storage: Store unopened vial at CRT. Do not refrigerate or freeze. Discard 6 hours after entry into vial or transfer into an empty container. Single-use vial. Discard any unused solution.

COMPATIBILITY

Manufacturer states, "Do not add other medications to solution. **Incompatible** with diazepam and chlorpromazine. Do not administer simultaneously."

RATE OF ADMINISTRATION

Administer as an infusion, equally distributed over 15 minutes. Pediatric doses up to 600 mg may be drawn up into a syringe and delivered via a syringe pump.

ACTIONS

A non-salicylate antipyretic and a non-opioid analgesic agent. Exact mechanism of action is unknown but is thought to act through central actions. Widely distributed into most tissues except fat. Low protein binding (10% to 25%). Half-life is approximately 2 to 3 hours. Metabolized in the liver via three different pathways. Metabolites excreted in the urine.

INDICATIONS AND USES

Management of mild to moderate pain. ▪ Management of moderate to severe pain with adjunctive opioid analgesics. ▪ Reduction of fever.

CONTRAINDICATIONS

Known hypersensitivity to acetaminophen or to any components of the IV formulation. ▪ Patients with severe hepatic impairment or severe active liver disease.

PRECAUTIONS

Administration of doses higher than recommended may result in hepatic injury, including risk of severe hepatotoxicity and death. Do not exceed maximum recommended daily dose. ▪ Use with caution in patients with hepatic impairment or active hepatic disease, alcoholism, chronic malnutrition, severe hypovolemia (e.g., due to dehydration or blood loss), or severe renal impairment (CrCl less than or equal to 30 mL/min). ▪ Hypersensitivity and anaphylactic reactions have been reported. ▪ Antipyretic effects may mask fever in patients treated for postsurgical pain. **Monitor:** Monitor for S/S of hypersensitivity reaction (e.g., respiratory distress; pruritus; rash; swelling of the face, mouth, and throat; urticaria). ▪ Baseline SCr and liver function tests may be indicated. **Maternal/Child:** Category C: epidemiologic data on oral acetaminophen use in pregnant women show no increased risk of major congenital malformations. Safety of IV formulation for use in pregnancy not established. Use only if clearly needed. ▪ Assess benefit versus risk before use during labor and delivery. ▪ Safety for use in breast-feeding not established. Acetaminophen is secreted in human milk in small quantities after oral administration. Use caution. ▪ Safety and effectiveness for treatment of acute pain or fever has not been studied in pediatric patients less than 2 years of age. **Elderly:** No overall differences in safety and efficacy were observed between older and younger patients, but greater sensitivity of some older individuals cannot be ruled out.

DRUG/LAB INTERACTIONS

Substances that induce or regulate hepatic cytochrome enzyme CYP2E1 (e.g., ethanol, isoniazid) may alter the metabolism of acetaminophen and increase its hepatotoxic potential. Effects have not been studied. ▪ Ethanol may induce hepatic cytochromes and may act as a competitive inhibitor of the metabolism of acetaminophen. ▪ Chronic acetaminophen doses of

4,000 mg/day may cause an increase in INR in patients stabilized on **warfarin**. Effect of short-term use on INR has not been studied. Monitoring of INR recommended. ■ **Many available analgesics contain acetaminophen in combination with another analgesic** (e.g., hydrocodone/acetaminophen [Vicodin, Norco], oxycodone/acetaminophen [Percocet]). Monitor total daily dose of acetaminophen coming from all possible sources.

SIDE EFFECTS

Adult patients: The most common adverse reactions were headache, insomnia, nausea, and vomiting. Less frequently reported side effects included anxiety, dyspnea, fatigue, hypersensitivity reaction, hypertension, hypokalemia, hypotension, increased aspartate aminotransferase, infusion site pain, muscle spasms, peripheral edema, and trismus.

Pediatric patients: The most common adverse reactions were agitation, atelectasis, constipation, nausea, pruritus, and vomiting. Less commonly reported side effects included abdominal pain, anemia, diarrhea, fever, headache, hypersensitivity reaction, hypertension, hypervolemia, hypoalbuminemia, hypokalemia, hypomagnesemia, hypophosphatemia, hypotension, hypoxia, increased hepatic enzymes, injection site pain, insomnia, muscle spasm, oliguria, pain in extremities, periorbital edema, peripheral edema, pleural effusion, pulmonary edema, rash, stridor, tachycardia, and wheezing.

Overdose: Hepatic necrosis, renal tubular necrosis, hypoglycemic coma, and thrombocytopenia.

Post-Marketing: Hypersensitivity and anaphylaxis (e.g., respiratory distress; pruritus; rash; swelling of the face, mouth, and throat; urticaria).

ANTIDOTE

Notify the physician of significant side effects. Discontinue immediately if symptoms associated with hypersensitivity occur. Treat as indicated (e.g., diphenhydramine, epinephrine, albuterol). Resuscitate as necessary. If an acetaminophen overdose is suspected, obtain a serum acetaminophen level and baseline liver function studies. *N*-acetylcysteine antidote may be indicated. See monograph. Contact poison control center for additional information.

ACETAZOLAMIDE SODIUM
(ah-set-ah-**ZOE**-la-myd **SO**-dee-um)

Antiglaucoma
Anticonvulsant
Diuretic
Urinary alkalinizer

Diamox   pH 9.2

USUAL DOSE
Antiglaucoma agent: 250 mg to 1 Gm/24 hr. May be given as 250-mg doses at 4- to 6-hour intervals. To rapidly lower intraocular pressure, give initial single dose of 500 mg followed by 125 to 250 mg at 4-hour intervals.
Edema of congestive heart failure or drug therapy: 250 to 375 mg or 5 mg/kg of body weight as a single dose daily; when loss of edematous fluid stops, reduce to every other day or give for 2 days followed by a day of rest.
Anticonvulsant: *Adults and pediatric patients:* Dose in epilepsy may range from 8 to 30 mg/kg/24 hr in divided doses every 6 to 12 hours (2 to 7.5 mg/kg every 6 hours or 4 to 15 mg/kg every 12 hours). Reduce initial daily dose when given with other anticonvulsants.
Urinary alkalinization: *Adults and pediatric patients:* 5 mg/kg/dose every 8 to 12 hours.

PEDIATRIC DOSE
See Maternal/Child.
Acute antiglaucoma agent: 5 to 10 mg/kg every 6 hours. Do not exceed 1,000 mg/24 hr.
Edema of congestive heart failure or drug therapy: 5 mg/kg as a single dose daily or every other day; see comment under Usual Dose. Do not exceed 1,000 mg/24 hr.
Slowly progressive hydrocephalus in infants 2 weeks to 10 months (unlabeled): 20 mg/kg/24 hr in equally divided doses every 8 hours (8.3 mg/kg every 8 hours). Up to 100 mg/kg/24 hr or a maximum dose of 2 Gm/24 hr has been used.

DOSE ADJUSTMENTS
Reduced dose required when introducing acetazolamide into a treatment regimen with other anticonvulsants. ■ Administer every 12 hours in patients with a CrCl from 10 to 50 mL/min. Avoid use in patients with a CrCl less than 10 mL/min (ineffective).

DILUTION
Each 500 mg should be diluted in 5 mL SW. May then be given by IV injection or added to standard IV fluids. IM administration not recommended.
Storage: Use within 24 hours of dilution.

COMPATIBILITY   (Underline Indicates Conflicting Compatibility Information)
Consider any drug NOT listed as compatible to be INCOMPATIBLE until consulting a pharmacist; specific conditions may apply.
One source suggests the following **compatibilities:**
Additive: Ranitidine (Zantac).
Y-site: Diltiazem (Cardizem).

RATE OF ADMINISTRATION
500 mg or fraction thereof over at least 1 minute or added to IV fluids to be given over 4 to 8 hours.

ACTIONS
A potent carbonic anhydrase inhibitor and nonbacteriostatic sulfonamide, acetazolamide depresses the tubular reabsorption of sodium, potassium, and bicarbonate. Excreted unchanged in the urine, producing diuresis, alkalinization of the urine, and a mild degree of metabolic acidosis.

INDICATIONS AND USES
Glaucoma. ■ Epilepsy. ■ Urine alkalinization to treat toxicity of weakly acidic medications (e.g., phenobarbital, lithium, salicylates). See Drug/Lab Interactions. ■ No longer the drug of choice for congestive heart failure or drug-induced edema (e.g., steroids). ■ Used orally for acute mountain sickness and hypokalemia/hyperkalemia of familial periodic paralysis.

Unlabeled uses: Prevention or treatment of alkalosis following open-heart surgery, treatment of acute pancreatitis and gastric ulcers (inhibits pancreatic and gastric secretions).

CONTRAINDICATIONS
Depressed sodium and potassium levels, hyperchloremic acidosis, marked kidney or liver disease, adrenocortical insufficiency, hypersensitivity to acetazolamide or any of its components. Long-term use contraindicated in some glaucomas.

PRECAUTIONS
Chemically related to sulfonamides; may cause serious reactions in sensitive patients. ■ May be alternated with other diuretics to achieve maximum effect. ■ Greater diuretic action is achieved by skipping a day of treatment rather than increasing dose; failure in therapy may be due to overdose or too-frequent dosage. ■ IM administration not recommended. Administration by IV injection is preferred. ■ Use with caution in impaired respiratory function (e.g., pulmonary disease, edema, infection, obstruction); may cause severe respiratory acidosis. ■ Potassium excretion is proportional to diuresis. Hypokalemia may result from diuresis or with severe cirrhosis. ■ Introduce or withdraw gradually when used as an anticonvulsant.

Monitor: Obtain baseline CBC and platelet count before use and monitor during therapy.

Patient Education: Consider birth control options.

Maternal/Child: Category D: avoid pregnancy; may cause premature delivery and congenital anomalies. ■ Discontinue breast-feeding or discontinue acetazolamide. ■ Safety for use in pediatric patients not established, but no problems are documented.

Elderly: Use caution; no documented problems, but age-related renal impairment may be a factor.

DRUG/LAB INTERACTIONS
May cause hypokalemia with concurrent use of **steroids.** ■ Hypokalemia may cause toxicity and fatal cardiac arrhythmias with **digoxin** or interfere with **insulin or oral antidiabetic agent** response, thus causing hyperglycemia. ■ Alkalinization of urine potentiates **amphetamines, ephedrine, flecainide** (Tambocor), **methenamine, procainamide, pseudoephedrine** (Sudafed), **quinidine, and tricyclic antidepressants** (e.g., amitriptyline [Elavil]) by decreasing rate of excretion. ■ May decrease response to **lithium, methotrexate, some antidepressants, phenobarbital, salicylates, and urinary antiinfectives** by increasing rate of excretion. ■ Metabolic acidosis in-

duced by acetazolamide may potentiate **salicylate** toxicity (anorexia, tachypnea, lethargy, coma, and death can occur with high-dose aspirin). ▪ Alkalinity may cause **false-positive urinary protein** and possibly **urinary steroid tests.** ▪ May depress **iodine uptake** by the thyroid.

SIDE EFFECTS

Minimal with short-term therapy. Respond to symptomatic treatment or withdrawal of drug: acidosis, anorexia, bone marrow suppression, confusion, crystalluria, drowsiness, fever, hemolytic anemia, hypokalemia (ECG changes, fatigue, muscle weakness, vomiting), paresthesias, photosensitivity, polyuria, rash, renal calculus, thrombocytopenic purpura.

ANTIDOTE

Notify physician of any adverse effects and discontinue drug if necessary. Treat hypersensitivity reactions as indicated; may require epinephrine, airway management, oxygen, IV fluids, antihistamines (e.g., diphenhydramine [Benadryl]), corticosteroids (e.g., hydrocortisone sodium succinate [Solu-Cortef]), and pressor amines (e.g., dopamine). Moderately dialyzable (20% to 40%).

ACETYLCYSTEINE INJECTION BBW *

(ah-see-till-**SIS**-tay-een in-**JEK**-shun)

Antidote

Acetadote

pH 6 to 7.5

*This drug is on the Black Box Warning list; however, a BBW is not provided in the parenteral prescribing information.

USUAL DOSE

Assess the potential risk of hepatotoxicity by determining plasma or serum acetaminophen concentrations as early as possible but no sooner than 4 hours following an acute overdose; see Precautions and Monitor. Total dose equals 300 mg/kg administered over 21 hours. Distribute dose as indicated in the following guidelines.

Loading dose (first): 150 mg/kg as an infusion over 60 minutes.

Maintenance dose (second): 50 mg/kg as an infusion over 4 hours. Follow with another **maintenance dose (third)** of 100 mg/kg as an infusion over 16 hours.

Acetylcysteine Dose Guidelines and Dilution by Weight, Patients More Than 40 kg				
Body Weight		LOADING DOSE 150 mg/kg in 200 mL diluent over 60 minutes	SECOND DOSE 50 mg/kg in 500 mL diluent over 4 hours	THIRD DOSE 100 mg/kg in 1,000 mL diluent over 16 hours
(kg)	(lb)	Acetylcysteine	Acetylcysteine	Acetylcysteine
40 kg	88 lb	30 mL	10 mL	20 mL
50 kg	110 lb	37.5 mL	12.5 mL	25 mL
60 kg	132 lb	45 mL	15 mL	30 mL
70 kg	154 lb	52.5 mL	17.5 mL	35 mL
80 kg	176 lb	60 mL	20 mL	40 mL
90 kg	198 lb	67.5 mL	22.5 mL	45 mL
100 kg	220 lb	75 mL	25 mL	50 mL

Adjust total volume administered for patients less than 40 kg and for those requiring fluid restriction according to the following chart.

Acetylcysteine Dose Guidelines and Dilution by Weight for Patients* Less Than 40 kg and/or Fluid-Restricted Patients							
Body Weight		LOADING DOSE 150 mg/kg over 60 minutes		SECOND DOSE 50 mg/kg over 4 hours		THIRD DOSE 100 mg/kg over 16 hours	
(kg)	(lb)	Acetyl-cysteine	Diluent	Acetyl-cysteine	Diluent	Acetyl-cysteine	Diluent
10 kg	22 lb	7.5 mL	30 mL	2.5 mL	70 mL	5 mL	140 mL
15 kg	33 lb	11.25 mL	45 mL	3.75 mL	105 mL	7.5 mL	210 mL
20 kg	44 lb	15 mL	60 mL	5 mL	140 mL	10 mL	280 mL
25 kg	55 lb	18.75 mL	100 mL	6.25 mL	250 mL	12.5 mL	500 mL
30 kg	66 lb	22.5 mL	100 mL	7.5 mL	250 mL	15 mL	500 mL

*For Pediatric patients; see Precautions and Maternal/Child.

Alternately, for pediatric patients weighing equal to or less than 20 kg but not exactly 10, 15, or 20 kg, the following formula is recommended:
Loading dose: 150 mg/kg. Dilute in an amount of diluent equal to 3 mL/kg of body weight (example: with a 7-kg weight, dilute 150 mg/kg [1,050 mg (5.25 mL)] of acetylcysteine in 3 × 7 mL, or 21 mL of diluent).
Maintenance dose (second): 50 mg/kg. Dilute in an amount of diluent equal to 7 mL/kg of body weight (example: with a 7-kg weight, dilute 50 mg/kg [350 mg (1.75 mL)] of acetylcysteine in 7 × 7 mL, or 49 mL of diluent).
Maintenance dose (third): 100 mg/kg. Dilute in an amount of diluent equal to 14 mL/kg of body weight (example: with a 7-kg weight, dilute 100 mg/kg [700 mg (3.5 mL)] of acetylcysteine in 14 × 7 mL, or 98 mL of diluent).

DOSE ADJUSTMENTS
Not required. Specific information and/or recommendations are not available for patients with impaired hepatic or renal function.

DILUTION
A hyperosmolar solution. Color of acetylcysteine may change from colorless to a slight pink or purple once the stopper is punctured; quality is not affected. May be diluted in D5W, ½NS, or SWFI.
Patients weighing 40 kg or more:
Loading dose (first): 150 mg/kg should be diluted in 200 mL of **compatible** diluent.
Maintenance dose (second): 50 mg/kg should be diluted in 500 mL of **compatible** diluent.
Maintenance dose (third): 100 mg/kg should be diluted in 1,000 mL of **compatible** diluent.
Patients weighing less than 40 kg or fluid-restricted patients: Total volume administered should be adjusted for patients less than 40 kg and for those requiring fluid restriction; see chart and alternate example under Usual Dose. Hyponatremia and seizures may result from large volumes in small children.
Filters: Data not available and use is not required by manufacturer. Studies on the use of filters are planned.

Storage: Store unopened vials at CRT. Diluted solution is stable for 24 hours at CRT. Do not use previously opened vials for IV administration. Discard unused portions.

COMPATIBILITY

Manufacturer states, "**Compatible** with D5W, ½NS, and SW."

RATE OF ADMINISTRATION

Usual total infusion time of all 3 doses is 21 hours. Rate reduction may be required to manage S/S of infusion reactions; see Monitor and Antidote. **Patients weighing 40 kg or more, patients weighing less than 40 kg, and fluid-restricted patients:**

Loading dose (first): An infusion evenly distributed over 60 minutes.

Maintenance dose (second): An infusion evenly distributed over 4 hours.

Maintenance dose (third): An infusion evenly distributed over 16 hours.

ACTIONS

Protects the liver by maintaining or restoring the glutathione levels (metabolites formed after an overdose of acetaminophen may deplete the hepatic stores of glutathione and cause binding of the metabolite to protein molecules within the hepatocyte, resulting in cellular necrosis). It may also act by forming an alternate compound and detoxifying the reactive metabolite. Half-life is approximately 5.6 hours. Metabolizes to various compounds. Crosses the placental barrier. Some excretion in urine.

INDICATIONS AND USES

To prevent or lessen hepatic injury after ingestion of a potentially hepatotoxic quantity of acetaminophen.

CONTRAINDICATIONS

Known hypersensitivity to acetylcysteine or any of its components.

PRECAUTIONS

Should be administered in a facility equipped to monitor the patient and respond to any medical emergency. ■ Most effective against severe hepatic injury when administered within 8 hours of ingestion. Administration before 4 hours does not allow enough time to determine an actual need for treatment with acetylcysteine; serum levels drawn before 4 hours have passed may be misleading. Effectiveness diminishes gradually after 8 hours. Should be administered if 24 hours or less has passed since ingestion, because the reported time of ingestion may not be correct and it does not appear to worsen the patient's condition. ■ Total volume administered should be adjusted for patients less than 40 kg and for patients requiring fluid restriction. If volume is not adjusted, fluid overload can occur, potentially resulting in hyponatremia, seizure, and death; see Usual Dose. ■ Use caution in patients with asthma or a history of bronchospasm. Death occurred in a patient with asthma. ■ Infusion reactions and hypersensitivity reactions have occurred. Infusion reactions usually occur within 30 to 60 minutes of beginning the infusion. ■ Clearance decreased and half-life prolonged in patients with various stages of liver damage (Child-Pugh scores of 5 to 13). ■ Rumack-Matthew nomogram does not apply to patients with repeated supratherapeutic ingestion (RSI), which is defined as ingestion of acetaminophen at doses higher than those recommended for extended periods of time. For treatment information, see prescribing information for a professional assistance line for acetaminophen overdose, or contact a regional poison control center. ■ Vial stopper does not contain natural rubber latex. ■ See Monitor and Antidote.

Monitor: Acute ingestion of 150 mg/kg or more of acetaminophen may result in hepatic toxicity. Obtain baseline hepatic function studies and monitor throughout detoxification process.
Preferred method of treatment: Estimate time of acetaminophen ingestion. If less than 24 hours since overdose, draw serum for an acetaminophen level at 4 hours post-ingestion or as soon as possible thereafter to clarify the need for intervention with acetylcysteine. The serum acetaminophen level should be evaluated on the Rumack-Matthew nomogram to determine the probability of toxicity (see package insert for copy of nomogram). ▪ If serum acetaminophen level is below the treatment line on the nomogram, discontinue the acetylcysteine if initiated as a precaution. If the plasma level is above the treatment line on the nomogram, initiate or continue treatment.
Secondary options for treatment: If serum acetaminophen levels are not available within 8 hours, initiate treatment. Do not delay treatment more than 8 hours post-ingestion. ▪ If time of ingestion is unknown or if the patient is unreliable, consider empiric initiation of acetylcysteine treatment. ▪ If a serum acetaminophen level is not available or cannot be interpreted and less than 24 hours has elapsed since ingestion, administer acetylcysteine regardless of the quantity reported to have been ingested.
All treatment options: Obtain serum acetaminophen level and baseline ALT, AST, bilirubin, blood glucose, BUN, electrolytes, PT, and SCr. Monitor as indicated by results. ▪ Monitor BP and HR before, during, and after the infusion. ▪ Evaluate serum acetaminophen level on the Rumack-Matthew nomogram. ▪ Infusion reactions may begin with acute flushing and erythema of the skin and may occur within 30 to 60 minutes of beginning the infusion. May resolve spontaneously despite continued infusion of acetylcysteine or may progress to an acute hypersensitivity reaction and/or anaphylaxis. Observe continuously for initial S/S of a hypersensitivity reaction (e.g., hypotension, rash, shortness of breath, wheezing). ▪ In suspected toxicity resulting from the extended-release acetaminophen preparation, an acetaminophen level drawn fewer than 8 hours post-ingestion may be misleading. Draw a second level at 4 to 6 hours after the initial level. If either acetaminophen level falls above the toxicity line, acetylcysteine treatment should be initiated. ▪ See Precautions and Antidote.
Patient Education: Report S/S of hypersensitivity promptly (e.g., flushing, itching, shortness of breath, feeling of faintness).
Maternal/Child: Category B: use during pregnancy only if clearly needed. ▪ Use caution; safety for use during breast-feeding not established; effects unknown. After 30 hours, acetylcysteine should be cleared from maternal blood, and breast-feeding can be resumed. ▪ No adequate or well-controlled studies in pediatric patients, but it has been used. Efficacy appears to be similar to that seen in adults; see Side Effects. ▪ Administered to a small number of preterm infants during clinical studies (a mean rate of 4.2 mg/kg/hr for 24 hours); half-life prolonged to approximately 11 hours in these newborns. ▪ Acetylcysteine was measurable in the circulation and cord blood of three newborns whose mothers were treated for acetaminophen overdose. No adverse side effects were noted, and none of the infants had evidence of acetaminophen poisoning.
Elderly: Response compared to younger adults not yet known; insufficient numbers participated in clinical studies.

DRUG/LAB INTERACTIONS
Drug-drug interaction studies have not been done.

SIDE EFFECTS
Adult and pediatric patients: Pruritus, rash, and urticaria have been reported most frequently and most commonly occur during the initial loading dose. Other reported side effects include anaphylactoid reactions, angioedema, dyspepsia, dysphoria (abnormal thinking or confusion), dyspnea, edema, erythema of the skin, eye pain, facial flushing, gait disturbances, hypotension, nausea and vomiting, palmar erythema, respiratory symptoms (e.g., bronchospasm, chest tightness, cough, respiratory distress, shortness of breath, stridor, wheezing), sweating, syncope, tachycardia, vasodilation.
Overdose: S/S of acute toxicity in animals included ataxia, convulsions, cyanosis, hypoactivity, labored respiration, and loss of righting reflex.

ANTIDOTE
Keep physician informed of all side effects. Flushing and erythema of the skin are expected. If other symptoms of a hypersensitivity reaction occur (e.g., bronchospasm, dyspnea, hypotension, wheezing), discontinue acetylcysteine and treat with diphenhydramine (Benadryl) or epinephrine as indicated. After symptoms subside, the infusion may be carefully resumed. If S/S of hypersensitivity recur, discontinue infusion permanently and consider alternate treatments. Contact Poison Control Center for possible treatment alternatives.

ACYCLOVIR
(ay-**SYE**-kloh-veer)
Zovirax

Antiviral

pH 10.5 to 11.6

USUAL DOSE
In all situations for adults, adolescents, children, and neonates, do not exceed a maximum dose of 20 mg/kg every 8 hours.
Adults and adolescents (12 years of age and older):
Herpes simplex infections; Mucosal and cutaneous HSV infections in immunocompromised patients: 5 mg/kg of body weight every 8 hours for 7 days.
Severe initial clinical episodes of herpes genitalis: 5 mg/kg every 8 hours for 5 days.
Herpes simplex encephalitis: 10 mg/kg every 8 hours for 10 days.
Herpes zoster infections (shingles) in immunocompromised patients: 10 mg/kg every 8 hours for 7 days.

PEDIATRIC DOSE
Pediatric patients under 12 years of age:
Herpes simplex infections; mucosal and cutaneous HSV infections in immunocompromised patients: 10 mg/kg every 8 hours for 7 days.
Severe initial clinical episodes of herpes genitalis: 250 mg/M^2 every 8 hours for 5 days.
Herpes simplex encephalitis: *Pediatric patients over 3 months of age:* 20 mg/kg every 8 hours for 10 days.

Herpes zoster infections (shingles) in immunocompromised patients: 20 mg/kg every 8 hours for 7 days.

NEONATAL DOSE

Neonatal herpes simplex virus infections: *Birth to 3 months:* 10 mg/kg every 8 hours for 10 days. Doses of 15 mg/kg to 20 mg/kg every 8 hours have been used for up to 14 to 21 days; safety and efficacy have not been established.

DOSE ADJUSTMENTS

Calculate dose by ideal body weight in obese individuals. ▪ Reduced dose may be indicated in the elderly based on the potential for decreased renal function and concomitant disease or drug therapy. ▪ In adults and pediatric patients with impaired renal function, reduce dose and/or adjust dosing interval based on CrCl as indicated in the following chart.

Acyclovir Dosage Adjustments for Adults and Pediatric Patients with Renal Impairment		
Creatinine Clearance (mL/min per 1.73 M^2)	Percent of Recommended Dose	Dosing Interval (hours)
>50 mL/min	100%	Every 8 hr
25-50 mL/min	100%	Every 12 hr
10-25 mL/min	100%	Every 24 hr
0-10 mL/min	50%	Every 24 hr

Plasma concentrations decrease with hemodialysis; adjustment of the dosing schedule is recommended so that an additional dose is administered after each dialysis. No supplemental dose is indicated in peritoneal dialysis after adjustment of the dosing interval.

DILUTION

Initially dissolve each 500 mg with 10 mL SW for injection (1,000 mg with 20 mL). Concentration equals 50 mg/mL. Do not use bacteriostatic water for injection (BWFI); will cause precipitation. Shake well to dissolve completely. Also available in liquid vials. Withdraw the desired dose and further dilute in an amount of solution to provide a concentration less than 7 mg/mL (70-kg adult at 5 mg/kg equals 350 mg dissolved in a total of 100 mL of solution equals 3.5 mg/mL). **Compatible** with most standard electrolyte and glucose infusion solutions.

Filters: No data available from manufacturer.

Storage: Store unopened vials at CRT. Use reconstituted solution within 12 hours; high pH may result in etching of glass vial surface after 12 hours. Use solution fully diluted for administration within 24 hours. Manufacturer will supply data showing stability for longer periods under specific conditions.

COMPATIBILITY   (Underline Indicates Conflicting Compatibility Information)

Consider any drug NOT listed as compatible to be INCOMPATIBLE until consulting a pharmacist; specific conditions may apply.

Manufacturer lists bacteriostatic water for injection (BWFI) as **incompatible.** Dilution in biologic or colloidal fluids (e.g., blood products, protein solutions) is not recommended.

One source suggests the following **compatibilities:**

Additive: Fluconazole (Diflucan), meropenem (Merrem IV).

Y-site: Allopurinol (Aloprim), amikacin (Amikin), amphotericin B cholesteryl (Amphotec), ampicillin, anidulafungin (Eraxis), caspofungin (Cancidas), cefazolin (Ancef), cefotaxime (Claforan), cefoxitin (Mefoxin), ceftazidime (Fortaz), ceftriaxone (Rocephin), cefuroxime (Zinacef), chloramphenicol (Chloromycetin), cisatracurium (Nimbex), clindamycin (Cleocin), dexamethasone (Decadron), diltiazem (Cardizem), dimenhydrinate, diphenhydramine (Benadryl), docetaxel (Taxotere), doripenem (Doribax), doxorubicin liposomal (Doxil), doxycycline, erythromycin (Erythrocin), etoposide phosphate (Etopophos), famotidine (Pepcid IV), filgrastim (Neupogen), fluconazole (Diflucan), gallium nitrate (Ganite), gentamicin, granisetron (Kytril), heparin, hydrocortisone sodium succinate (Solu-Cortef), hydromorphone (Dilaudid), imipenem-cilastatin (Primaxin), linezolid (Zyvox), lorazepam (Ativan), magnesium sulfate, melphalan (Alkeran), meperidine (Demerol), meropenem (Merrem IV), methylprednisolone (Solu-Medrol), metoclopramide (Reglan), metronidazole (Flagyl IV), milrinone (Primacor), morphine, multivitamins (M.V.I.), nafcillin (Nallpen), oxacillin (Bactocill), paclitaxel (Taxol), pemetrexed (Alimta), penicillin G potassium, pentobarbital (Nembutal), piperacillin, potassium chloride (KCl), propofol (Diprivan), ranitidine (Zantac), remifentanil (Ultiva), sodium bicarbonate, sulfamethoxazole/trimethoprim, teniposide (Vumon), theophylline, thiotepa, tobramycin, vancomycin, zidovudine (AZT, Retrovir).

RATE OF ADMINISTRATION
A single dose must be administered at a constant rate over 1 hour as an infusion. Renal tubular damage will occur with too-rapid rate of injection. Acyclovir crystals will occlude renal tubules. Use of an infusion pump or microdrip (60 gtt/mL) recommended.

ACTIONS
An antiviral agent that inhibits DNA replication in viruses (e.g., herpes simplex virus, herpes zoster virus, Epstein-Barr virus, and cytomegalovirus). Onset of action is prompt and therapeutic levels maintained for 8 hours. Widely distributed in tissues and body fluids. Metabolized to a small extent in the liver. Half-life is approximately 2.5 hours. Excreted mainly as unchanged drug in the urine. Crosses the placental and blood-brain barriers. Secreted in breast milk.

INDICATIONS AND USES
Treatment of initial and recurrent mucosal and cutaneous herpes simplex (HSV-1 and HSV-2) infections in immunosuppressed patients. ■ Severe initial clinical episodes of herpes genitalis in immunocompetent patients. ■ Herpes simplex encephalitis. ■ Neonatal herpes simplex virus infections. ■ Herpes zoster infections (shingles) in immunocompromised patients. ■ Oral acyclovir is used to treat varicella zoster (chickenpox).
Unlabeled uses: Cytomegalovirus and HSV infection after bone marrow or renal transplantation. ■ Disseminated primary eczema herpeticum. ■ Varicella pneumonia. ■ Various herpes simplex infections (e.g., erythema multiforme, ocular, proctitis). ■ Varicella zoster infections (chickenpox) in immunocompromised patients. ■ Prophylaxis of herpes simplex virus infections and herpes zoster infections in immunocompromised patients. ■ Infectious mononucleosis.

CONTRAINDICATIONS
Hypersensitivity to acyclovir or valacyclovir (Valtrex). The ganciclovir monograph indicates a contraindication for ganciclovir with acyclovir.

PRECAUTIONS

Confirm diagnosis of herpes simplex virus (HSV-1 or HSV-2) through laboratory culture. Initiate therapy as quickly as possible after symptoms identified. ▪ For IV use only; avoid IM or SC injection. ▪ Use caution in patients with underlying neurologic abnormalities, those with serious renal, hepatic, or electrolyte abnormalities, or significant hypoxia. ▪ Use caution in patients receiving interferon or intrathecal methotrexate, or with patients who have had previous neurologic reactions to cytotoxic drugs. ▪ Incidence of CNS adverse events may be more common in the elderly or in patients with decreased renal function. ▪ Isolates of herpes simplex viruses (HSV-1, HSV-2) and varicella-zoster virus (VZV) with reduced susceptibility to acyclovir have been identified. Consider the possibility of viral resistance to acyclovir in patients who show poor clinical response. ▪ Thrombotic thrombocytopenic purpura/hemolytic uremic syndrome (TTP/HUS) has been reported in immunocompromised patients receiving acyclovir. Deaths have occurred. ▪ See Contraindications.

Monitor: Maintain adequate hydration and urine flow before and during infusion. Encourage fluid intake of 2 to 3 L/day. ▪ Monitor renal function; abnormal renal function (decreased CrCl can occur), concomitant use of other nephrotoxic drugs, pre-existing renal disease, and dehydration make further renal impairment with acyclovir more likely. ▪ Confirm patency of vein; will cause thrombophlebitis. Rotate site of infusion.

Patient Education: Virus remains dormant and can still spread to others. ▪ Avoid sexual intercourse when visible herpes lesions are present. Use condoms routinely.

Maternal/Child: Category B: use during pregnancy only if benefits outweigh risk to fetus. ▪ Breast milk concentrations can be higher than maternal serum concentrations. Discontinue breast-feeding or evaluate very carefully. ▪ 10 mg/kg and 20 mg/kg doses in pediatric patients from 3 months to 16 years achieved concentrations similar to those in adults receiving 5 mg/kg to 10 mg/kg. ▪ Use with caution in neonates; they have an age-related decrease in clearance and an increase in half-life (3.8 hours).

Elderly: Effectiveness is similar to younger adults. ▪ Plasma concentrations are higher in the elderly compared to younger adults; may be due to age-related changes in renal function. ▪ Duration of pain after healing was longer in patients 65 years or older. ▪ Incidence of side effects (e.g., CNS adverse events [coma, confusion, hallucinations, somnolence], dizziness, nausea, renal adverse events, vomiting) was increased. ▪ See Dose Adjustments and Precautions.

DRUG/LAB INTERACTIONS

See Precautions. May cause neurotoxicity (e.g., severe drowsiness and lethargy) with **zidovudine.** ▪ Concurrent use with other **nephrotoxic agents** (e.g., aminoglycosides [gentamicin, tobramycin], cisplatin [Platinol]) may increase risk of nephrotoxicity, especially in patients with pre-existing renal impairment. ▪ Potentiated by **probenecid.** ▪ Synergistic effects with **ketoconazole and interferon** have been noted. Clinical importance not established. ▪ In one case report, a patient stabilized on **phenytoin and valproic acid** experienced seizures and a reduction in antiepileptic drug serum concentrations when acyclovir was added to the regimen.

SIDE EFFECTS

Acute renal failure, aggressive behavior, agitation, angioedema, ataxia, coma, confusion, delirium, diaphoresis, disseminated intravascular coagulation (DIC), dizziness, dysarthria (difficulty articulating words), elevated transaminase levels, encephalopathy, hallucinations, headache, hematuria, hemolysis, hives, hyperbilirubinemia, hypersensitivity reactions (e.g., anaphylaxis), hypotension, inflammation at injection site, lethargy, nausea, obtundation, phlebitis, rash, seizures, transient increased BUN or SCr levels, tremors, vomiting. Some patients (fewer than 1%) may have abdominal pain, anemia, anorexia, anuria, chest pain, diarrhea, edema, fatigue, fever, hemoglobinemia, hepatitis, hypokalemia, ischemia of digits, jaundice, leukocytosis, light-headedness, myalgia, neutropenia, neutrophilia, paresthesia, psychosis, pulmonary edema with cardiac tamponade, rigors, skin reactions (e.g., erythema multiforme, Stevens-Johnson syndrome, toxic epidermal necrolysis), thirst, thrombocytosis, thrombocytopenia, visual abnormalities.

ANTIDOTE

Notify physician of all side effects. Discontinue drug with onset of CNS side effects. Treatment will be symptomatic and supportive. Adequate hydration is indicated to prevent precipitation of acyclovir in the renal tubules. A 6-hour session of hemodialysis will reduce plasma acyclovir concentration by approximately 60%. Hemodialysis may be indicated in patients with acute renal failure and anuria. Treat anaphylaxis and resuscitate as necessary.

ADENOSINE
(ah-**DEN**-oh-seen)

Adenocard, Adenoscan

**Antiarrhythmic
Diagnostic agent**

pH 4.5 to 7.5

USUAL DOSE

Adenocard: Conversion of acute paroxysmal supraventricular tachycardia (PSVT): 6 mg initially. If supraventricular tachycardia not eliminated in 1 to 2 minutes, give 12 mg. The 12-mg dose may be repeated in 1 to 2 minutes if needed. Do not exceed 12 mg in any single dose.

Do not administer a repeat dose to patients who develop a high-level block on one dose of adenosine.

Adenosine is not blocked by atropine. Digitalis, quinidine, beta-adrenergic blocking agents (e.g., atenolol, esmolol), calcium channel blocking agents (e.g., verapamil), angiotensin-converting enzyme inhibitors (e.g., enalapril [Vasotec]), and other cardiac drugs can be administered without delay if indicated because of the short half-life of adenosine. Repeat episodes may be treated with adenosine or calcium channel blockers (e.g., diltiazem, verapamil).

Adenoscan: Noninvasive diagnosis of coronary artery disease with thallium tomography: 140 mcg/kg/min (0.14 mg/kg/min) as a 6-minute continuous peripheral infusion. Inject thallium at 3 minutes. May be injected directly into adenosine infusion set. Dose should be based on total body weight. ■ See Drug/Lab Interactions.

PEDIATRIC DOSE

See Maternal/Child.

Adenocard: Conversion of acute paroxysmal supraventricular tachycardia (PSVT) in pediatric patients weighing less than 50 kg: 0.05 to 0.1 mg/kg. May increase dose by 0.05 to 0.1 mg/kg increments every 2 minutes until PSVT terminated or maximum dose reached (0.3 mg/kg or 12 mg). AHA guidelines recommend 0.1 mg/kg rapid IV push. Follow each dose with a 5- to 10-mL NS flush. Double to 0.2 mg/kg if a second dose is required. Maximum first dose 6 mg. Maximum second dose and maximum single dose is 12 mg. ■ See comments in Usual Dose.

Pediatric patients weighing more than 50 kg: Same as Usual Dose.

DOSE ADJUSTMENTS

Metabolism of adenosine is independent of hepatic or renal function. No dose adjustment indicated. ■ See Drug/Lab Interactions; alternative therapy (e.g., calcium channel blockers) may be indicated.

DILUTION

Solution must be clear; do not use if discolored or particulate matter present.

Adenocard: Conversion of acute PSVT: Give undiluted directly into a vein. If given into an IV line, use the closest port to the insertion site and follow with a rapid NS flush (+/− 50 mL) to be certain the solution reaches the systemic circulation. Discard unused portion.

Adenoscan: Pharmacologic stress testing: Dilute a single dose in sufficient NS to distribute over 6 minutes.

Storage: Store at CRT 15° to 30° C (59° to 86° F); refrigeration will cause crystallization. If crystals do form, dissolve by warming to room temperature.

COMPATIBILITY

Consider any drug NOT listed as compatible to be INCOMPATIBLE until consulting a pharmacist; specific conditions may apply.

One source suggests the following **compatibilities:**

Y-site: Abciximab (ReoPro).

RATE OF ADMINISTRATION

Adenocard: Conversion of acute PSVT: Must be given as a rapid bolus IV injection over 1 to 2 seconds. Follow each dose with NS flush; see Dilution.

Adenoscan: Pharmacologic stress testing: See Usual Dose.

ACTIONS

A naturally occurring nucleoside present in all cells of the body. Has many functions. When given as a rapid IV bolus, adenosine has antiarrhythmic properties, slowing cardiac conduction (particularly at the AV node), interrupting reentry pathways through the AV node, and restoring sinus rhythm in patients with PSVT. When used as a diagnostic aid and given as a continuous infusion, adenosine acts as a vasodilator. Dilates normal coronary vessels, increasing blood flow. Has little effect on stenotic arteries. When administered with thallium-201, helps differentiate between areas of heart supplied by normal blood flow and areas supplied by stenotic coronary arteries. When larger doses are given by infusion, adenosine decreases BP and produces a reflexive increase in HR. Adenocard and Adenoscan have the same molecular structure, same solvent, diluent, and concentration. The difference in their actions is in the rate of administration; however, the FDA has approved Adenocard for converting PSVT and

Adenoscan for pharmacologic stress testing. When used for treatment of PSVT, it is effective within 1 minute. When used for diagnostic purposes, maximum effect is reached within 2 to 3 minutes of starting the infusion. Coronary blood flow velocity returns to basal levels within 1 to 2 minutes after the infusion is discontinued. Half-life is estimated to be less than 10 seconds. Adenosine is salvaged immediately by erythrocytes and blood vessel endothelial cells and metabolized for natural uses throughout the body (regulation of coronary and systemic vascular tone, platelet function, lipolysis in fat cells, intracardiac conduction).

INDICATIONS AND USES

Adenocard: To convert acute paroxysmal supraventricular tachycardia (PSVT) to normal sinus rhythm; a first-line agent according to AHA. Includes PSVT associated with accessory bypass tracts (Wolff-Parkinson-White syndrome). Does not convert atrial flutter, atrial fibrillation, or ventricular tachycardia to normal sinus rhythm (NSR).

Adenoscan: Adjunct to thallium-201 myocardial perfusion scintigraphy in patients unable to exercise adequately. (Results are similar to IV dipyridamole or exercise stress testing.)

CONTRAINDICATIONS

Known or suspected bronchospastic or bronchoconstrictive lung disease (e.g., asthma). ▪ Known hypersensitivity to adenosine. ▪ Symptomatic bradycardia, sick sinus syndrome, and second- or third-degree AV block unless a functioning artificial pacemaker is in place.

PRECAUTIONS

Both preparations: Absolutely confirm labeling for IV use. Do not use adenosine phosphate, which is for IM use in the symptomatic relief of varicose vein complications. ▪ Emergency resuscitation drugs and equipment must always be available. ▪ May produce short-lasting first-, second-, or third-degree heart block. Usually self-limiting due to short half-life. Patients who develop high-level block should not be given additional doses of adenosine. ▪ May cause bronchoconstriction. Use with caution in patients with obstructive lung disease not associated with bronchoconstriction (e.g., emphysema, bronchitis). Avoid use in patients with bronchoconstrictive or bronchospastic disease (e.g., asthma).

Adenocard: Valsalva maneuver may be used before use of adenosine in PSVTs if clinically appropriate. ▪ Transient or prolonged episodes of asystole and ventricular fibrillation have been reported. Deaths have occurred. In most instances, these cases were associated with the concomitant use of digoxin (Lanoxin) and, less frequently, with digoxin and verapamil. ▪ Some slowing of ventricular response may occur if atrial flutter or fibrillation is also present.

Adenoscan: Fatal cardiac arrest, sustained ventricular tachycardia (requiring resuscitation), and nonfatal MI have been reported. Patients with unstable angina may be at greater risk. ▪ Can cause significant hypotension. Use with caution in patients with autonomic dysfunction, stenotic valvular heart disease, pericarditis or pericardial effusion, stenotic carotid artery disease with cerebrovascular insufficiency, or uncorrected hypovolemia; may be at increased risk for hypotensive complications. ▪ Hypertension has been reported; usually resolves spontaneously. ▪ Atrial fibrillation has been reported. In reported cases, it began 1.5 to 3 minutes into the infusion, lasted for 15 seconds to 6 hours, and spontaneously converted to NSR.

Monitor: *Adenocard: Conversion of acute PSVT:* Must reach systemic circulation; see Dilution. ▪ ECG monitoring during administration recommended. Monitor BP. At the time of conversion to normal sinus rhythm, PVCs, PACs, atrial fibrillation, sinus bradycardia, sinus tachycardia, skipped beats, and varying degrees of AV nodal block are seen on the ECG in many patients. Usually last only a few seconds and resolve without intervention. ▪ Less likely to precipitate hypotension if arrhythmia does not terminate.

Adenoscan: Pharmacologic stress testing: ECG monitoring during administration recommended. Monitor HR and BP at regular intervals during infusion. ▪ Obtain images when infusion complete and redistribution images 3 to 4 hours later.

Maternal/Child: Category C: use in pregnancy only if clearly needed. Some references recommend avoiding early pregnancy. ▪ Safety for use in pediatric patients not established, but has been used for conversion of PSVT in neonates, infants, children, and adolescents. Safety for use in pharmacologic stress testing in patients under 18 years not established.

Elderly: Response similar to that seen in younger patients; however, greater sensitivity of some older patients cannot be ruled out. May have diminished cardiac function, nodal dysfunction, concomitant disease, or drug therapy that may alter hemodynamic function and produce severe bradycardia or AV block.

DRUG/LAB INTERACTIONS

Both preparations: Effects antagonized by **methylxanthines** (e.g., caffeine, theophylline); larger doses may be required or adenosine may not be effective. ▪ Potentiated by **dipyridamole** (Persantine); smaller doses of adenosine may be indicated. ▪ Cardiovascular effects increased by **nicotine;** rapid injection may induce anginal pain. ▪ May produce a higher degree of heart block with **carbamazepine** (Tegretol). ▪ Concomitant use with **digoxin alone or digoxin in combination with verapamil** has been associated with rare cases of ventricular fibrillation; see Precautions. ▪ See Usual Dose. ▪ **Adenoscan:** Before using Adenoscan for pharmacologic stress testing, avoid (or withhold for at least 5 half-lives) **adenosine antagonists** (e.g., methylxanthines) **and/or potentiators** (e.g., dipyridamole, papaverine).

SIDE EFFECTS

Both preparations: Generally predictable, short lived, and easily tolerated. Most will appear immediately and last less than 1 minute. Atrial fibrillation, bronchospasm, chest pressure, dizziness, dyspnea and/or shortness of breath, facial flushing, headache, hypertension, light-headedness, nausea, numbness, PACs, PVCs, sinus bradycardia, sinus tachycardia, skipped beats, varying degrees of AV nodal block. Less than 1% of patients complain of apprehension, blurred vision, burning, chest pain, head pressure, heavy arms, hyperventilation, hypotension, metallic taste, neck and back pain, palpitations, pressure in groin, seizures, sweating, tight throat, and tingling in arms.

Both preparations: *Major:* Arrhythmias (persistent), including VT, VF, atrial fibrillation, and torsades de pointes; bronchospasm (severe); myocardial infarction; pulmonary edema; third-degree AV block. Asystole with fatal outcome has been reported.

Post-Marketing: *Both preparations:* Seizure activity, including tonic-clonic (grand mal) seizures, and loss of consciousness. *Adenoscan:* Injection site reactions, respiratory arrest, throat tightness, vomiting. *Adenosine:* Atrial fibrillation, bradycardia, prolonged asystole, torsades de pointes, transient increase in blood pressure, VF, VT.

ANTIDOTE

Notify physician of any side effect that lasts more than 1 minute. If a side effect persists, decrease rate of infusion (Adenoscan [pharmacologic stress testing]). With either use, for progression to a major side effect discontinue adenosine. Treat symptomatically if indicated. Bradycardia may be refractory to atropine. Short half-life generally precludes overdose problems, but aminophylline 50 to 125 mg as a slow infusion is a competitive antagonist. Resuscitate as necessary.

ALBUMIN (HUMAN)
(al-**BYOO**-min **HU**-man)

Plasma volume expander
(plasma protein fraction)

Albumarc, Albuminar-5 & -25, AlbuRx 5% & 25%, Albutein 5% & 25%, Buminate 5% & 25%, Normal Serum Albumin, Plasbumin-5 & -25

pH 6.4 to 7.4

USUAL DOSE

Variable, depending on patient condition (e.g., presence of hemorrhage, hypovolemia, or shock, pulse, BP, hemoglobin and hematocrit, and amount of pulmonary or venous congestion present). Fluid and protein requirements and underlying condition determine the concentration of albumin used. 5% is usually indicated in hypovolemic or intravascularly depleted patients, and 25% is appropriate when fluid and sodium intake should be minimized (e.g., cerebral edema, hypoproteinemia, pediatric patients). The initial dose is usually 12.5 to 25 Gm. Amount of 5% given may be increased to 0.5 Gm/lb of body weight (10 mL/lb) with careful monitoring of the patient. Available as 5% solution (5 Gm/100 mL) in 50-mL, 250-mL, 500-mL, and 1,000-mL vials or as 25% solution (25 Gm/100 mL) in 20-mL, 50-mL, and 100-mL vials. The maximum dose is 6 Gm/kg/ 24 hr or 250 Gm in 48 hours (250 Gm is equal to 5 liters of 5% or 1 liter of 25%). In the absence of active hemorrhage, the total dose usually does not exceed the normal circulating mass of albumin (e.g., 2 Gm/kg of body weight).

Hypoproteinemia (hypoalbuminemia): 50 to 75 Gm as a 25% solution. Repeat doses may be required in patients who continue to lose albumin.

Hypovolemia: 25 Gm as a 5% or 25% solution. May be repeated in 15 to 30 minutes if response inadequate. If 25% solution is used, additional fluids may be needed.

Burns: Electrolyte replacement and crystalloids (e.g., IV fluids) to maintain plasma volume are required in the first 24 hours. Then begin with 25 Gm and adjust as necessary to maintain albumin level from 2 to 3 Gm/dL.

Acute nephrosis or acute nephrotic syndrome: 25 Gm of a 25% solution with a loop diuretic (e.g., furosemide [Lasix], torsemide [Demadex]) daily for 7 to 10 days.

Hemodialysis: 25 Gm of a 25% solution.

Red blood cell resuspension: 20 to 25 Gm of a 25% solution/liter of RBCs.

Cardiopulmonary bypass: Achieve a plasma albumin of 2.5 Gm/dL and hematocrit concentration of 20% with either a 5% or 25% solution. Use crystalloids (IV fluids) as a pump prime.

PEDIATRIC DOSE

0.5 to 1 Gm/kg/dose. 25% solution is usually used in infants and other pediatric patients; *do not use in preterm infants.* Monitor hemodynamic response closely. Maximum dose 6 Gm/kg/24 hr or 250 Gm/48 hr.

Hypoproteinemia (hypoalbuminemia): 1 Gm/kg/dose.

Hypovolemia: 0.5 to 1 Gm/kg/dose. May be repeated in 15 to 30 minutes if response inadequate.

Hemolytic disease of the newborn: 1 Gm/kg (4 mL/kg) of 25% albumin. One source recommends giving 1 hour before exchange transfusion. Another recommends 1 to 2 hours before blood transfusion or with transfusion (exchange 50 mL of albumin 25% for 50 mL plasma). *Do not use in preterm infants.*

Burns: See Usual Dose.

DILUTION

May be given undiluted or further diluted with NS, D5W, or D10W for infusion. NS is the preferred diluent. When sodium restriction is required, D5W may be substituted. The use of SW as a diluent is not recommended. Life-threatening hemolysis and acute renal failure can result if a sufficient volume of SW is used as a diluent. The 5% product is isotonic and osmotically approximates human plasma. One volume of 25% to four volumes of diluent is isotonic. Use only clear solutions.

Storage: Store at CRT. Use within 4 hours after opening. Discard unused portions.

COMPATIBILITY

Consider any drug NOT listed as compatible to be INCOMPATIBLE until consulting a pharmacist; specific conditions may apply.

Do not use SW as a diluent; see Dilution. Manufacturers state, "Do not mix with protein hydrolysates, amino acid mixtures, or solutions containing alcohol." Manufacturers also state, "May be administered in conjunction with or combined with other parenterals such as whole blood, plasma, glucose, saline, or sodium lactate."

One source suggests the following **compatibilities:**

Y-site: Diltiazem (Cardizem), lorazepam (Ativan).

RATE OF ADMINISTRATION

Variable, depending on indication, present blood volume, patient response, and concentration of solution. Any rate greater than 10 mL/min may cause circulatory overload and pulmonary edema. Averages are:

Normal blood volume: 5%, 2 to 4 mL/min; 25%, 1 to 2 mL/min.

Deficient blood volume (hypovolemia): A single dose as rapidly as tolerated. Repeat dose as rapidly as tolerated if indicated. As volume approaches normal, slow 5% to 2 to 4 mL/min and 25% to 1 mL/min to prevent circulatory overload and pulmonary edema.

Hypoproteinemia: 2 to 3 mL/min in adults; a single dose over 30 to 120 minutes in pediatric patients.

Infants and other pediatric patients: For uses other than hypovolemia and hypoproteinemia, the rate of administration should be about one fourth to one half the adult rate.

ACTIONS

A sterile natural plasma protein substance prepared by a specific process, which makes it free from the danger of serum hepatitis. A blood volume expander that accounts for 70% to 80% of the colloid oncotic pressure of plasma. Expands blood volume proportionately to amount of circulating blood, improves cardiac output, prevents marked hemoconcentration, aids in reduction of edema, and raises serum protein levels. Low sodium content helps to maintain electrolyte balance and should promote diuresis in presence of edema (contains 130 to 160 mEq sodium/L). Also acts as a transport protein that binds both endogenous and exogenous substances, including bilirubin and certain drugs.

INDICATIONS AND USES

Hypovolemia (with or without shock [actual or impending], with or without hemorrhage); 5% if hypovolemic, 25% if adequate hydration or edema is present. ▪ Hypoalbuminemia from inadequate production (e.g., burns, congenital analbuminemia, endocrine disorders, infection, liver disease, major injury, malignancy, malnutrition). ▪ Hypoalbuminemia from excessive catabolism (e.g., burns, major injury, nephrosis, pancreatitis, pemphigus [chronic relapsing skin disease], peritonitis, thyrotoxicosis). ▪ Hypoalbuminemia from loss from the body (e.g., hemorrhage, burn exudates, excessive renal excretion, exfoliative dermatoses, exudative enteropathy [e.g., inflammatory bowel disease]). ▪ Hypoalbuminemia from redistribution within the body (e.g., cirrhosis with ascites, inflammatory conditions, major surgery). ▪ Hypoalbuminemia secondary to pulmonary edema in adult respiratory distress syndrome (ARDS) (25%). ▪ Raising plasma oncotic pressure to treat edema of nephrosis (25%). ▪ Cardiopulmonary bypass surgery (25%). ▪ Hemolytic disease of the newborn (bilirubin binding activity) as adjunct to exchange transfusion (25%). ▪ Provide adequate volume and prevent hypoproteinemia as an adjunct to RBC resuspension.

CONTRAINDICATIONS

Anemia (severe), cardiac failure, hypersensitivity to albumin, pulmonary edema.

PRECAUTIONS

Whole blood or packed cells probably indicated if more than 1,000 mL 5% albumin required in hemorrhage; are adjunctive to use of large amounts of serum albumin to prevent anemia. Is not a substitute for whole blood in situations where both the oxygen-carrying capacity and plasma volume expansion provided by whole blood are required. ▪ May be given regardless of patient blood group. ▪ Use caution in hypertension, low cardiac reserve, hepatic or renal failure, or lack of albumin deficiency. ▪ Use caution in patients with normal or increased intravascular volume; however, patients with hypoproteinemia may have normal blood volume. ▪ Use caution in patients with burns, hypoproteinemia, or hypovolemia; an FDA-issued Dear Doctor letter identified concerns of an excess mortality rate when albumin administration was compared to NS administration in these critically ill patients. Trauma patients with concomitant traumatic brain injuries may also be at risk for increased mortality. ■ 25 Gm of albumin is the osmotic equivalent of 2 units of fresh-frozen plasma. 25 Gm of albumin provides as much plasma protein as 500 mL of plasma or 2 units of whole blood. ■ Albumin is not a source of nutrition.

Monitor: Monitor BP. ■ Hemoglobin, hematocrit, electrolyte, and serum protein evaluations are mandatory during therapy. Alkaline phosphatase may be elevated. ■ Hyponatremia may result from administration of large volumes of albumin diluted in D5W; additional monitoring of electrolytes may be required. ■ Observe patient carefully for increased bleeding resulting from more normal BP, circulatory embarrassment, pulmonary edema, or lack of diuresis. Central venous and/or pulmonary wedge pressure readings are most helpful. ■ Maintain hydration with additional fluids, especially in dehydrated patients. ■ Normal plasma albumin is 3.5 to 6 Gm/100 mL.

Maternal/Child: Category C: safety for use during pregnancy not established. ■ Do not use 25% solution in preterm infants.

Elderly: Monitor fluid intake carefully; more susceptible to circulatory overload and pulmonary edema. ■ Plasma albumin levels may be more volatile.

DRUG/LAB INTERACTIONS

Specific information not available.

SIDE EFFECTS

Chills, fever, headache, hypotension, nausea, salivation, skin rash or hives, tachycardia, vomiting.

Major: Congestive heart failure, decreased myocardial contractility, hypersensitivity reactions including anaphylaxis (rare), precipitous hypotension, pulmonary edema, salt and water retention.

ANTIDOTE

Notify the physician of all side effects. Minor side effects are generally tolerated and treated symptomatically. For major side effects, discontinue albumin and treat symptomatically. Resuscitate as necessary.

ALDESLEUKIN BBW
(al-des-**LOO**-kin)

Antineoplastic
Immunomodulator
Biologic response modifier
Recombinant interleukin-2

Interleukin-2 Recombinant, Proleukin

pH 7.2 to 7.8

USUAL DOSE
(International units [IU])

Patient selection restricted. Prescreening and baseline studies required; see Precautions/Monitor.

Standard high-dose regimen: *Intermittent IV:* 600,000 International units (IU)/kg (0.037 mg/kg) every 8 hours for 14 doses. After 9 days of rest, repeat for up to 14 more doses; this constitutes one course (two 5-day [14 or fewer doses] treatment cycles separated by a rest period of 9 days). Treat with 28 doses or until dose-limiting toxicity requiring ICU-level support occurs. Dose is based on actual patient weight.

Retreatment: Evaluate for response 4 weeks after course completion and again before scheduling start of the next course. Additional courses are considered if there is some tumor shrinkage following the previous course, a CT scan rules out disease progression, and retreatment is not contraindicated. At least 7 weeks from hospital discharge should elapse before a second course is administered.

Sometimes given in combination with other agents.

Unlabeled protocols: A low-dose regimen by intermittent IV and a continuous IV regimen have been studied; see literature. Other protocols have been used. These various protocols expressed doses of aldesleukin in Cetus, Roche, or International units. Aldesleukin is available only in International units, 1 Cetus unit = 6 IU, 1 Roche unit = 3 IU. Results from studies include stable disease or disease regression with some decreased toxicity, but efficacy not established.

DOSE ADJUSTMENTS

Information on dosing in obese and underweight patients is not available; base dose on actual patient weight. ■ Doses are frequently withheld for toxicity. Doses are actually withheld, not reduced in amount. Median number of doses actually administered in a first course is 20 for metastatic renal cell carcinoma patients and 18 for metastatic melanoma patients. Continuous infusions can be interrupted as indicated by patient symptoms.

■ Hold doses and restart based on the following chart:

Guidelines for Holding Doses of Aldesleukin	
Hold Dose for	**May Give Next Dose if**
CARDIOVASCULAR	
Atrial fibrillation, supraventricular tachycardia, bradycardia that requires treatment or is recurrent or persistent.	Patient is asymptomatic with full recovery to normal sinus rhythm.
Systolic BP <90 mm Hg with increasing requirements for pressors.	Systolic BP ≥90 mm Hg and stable or improving requirements for pressors.
Any ECG change consistent with MI or ischemia with or without chest pain; suspicion of cardiac ischemia or myocarditis.	Patient is asymptomatic, MI and myocarditis have been ruled out, clinical suspicion of angina is low, there is no incidence of ventricular hypokinesia.
PULMONARY	
O_2 saturation <90%.	O_2 saturation >90%.
CENTRAL NERVOUS SYSTEM	
Mental status changes (e.g., agitation, confusion, lethargy, somnolence). May result in coma.	Mental status changes completely resolved.
BODY AS A WHOLE	
Sepsis syndrome; patient is clinically unstable.	Sepsis syndrome has resolved, patient is clinically stable, infection is under treatment.
UROGENITAL	
SCr >4.5 mg/dL or a SCr of ≥4 mg/dL in presence of severe volume overload, acidosis, or hyperkalemia.	SCr <4 mg/dL, and fluid and electrolyte status is stable.
Persistent oliguria, urine output of <10 mL/hr for 16 to 24 hr with rising SCr.	Urine output >10 mL/hr with a decrease of SCr >1.5 mg/dL or normalization of SCr.
DIGESTIVE	
Signs of hepatic failure including encephalopathy, increasing ascites, liver pain, hypoglycemia.	Discontinue for remainder of current course. May consider a new course of treatment in 7 weeks if all signs of hepatic failure have resolved.
Stool guaiac repeatedly >3 to 4+.	Stool guaiac negative.
SKIN	
Bullous dermatitis or marked worsening of pre-existing skin condition (avoid topical steroid therapy).	Resolution of all signs of bullous dermatitis.

- After withholding a dose, no dose should be given until patient is globally assessed and specific criteria for restarting aldesleukin are met.

DILUTION (International units [IU])

Each 22,000,000 IU vial (1.3 mg) must be reconstituted with 1.2 mL of preservative-free SW (18,000,000 IU/mL [1.1 mg (1,100 mcg)/mL]).

Sterile technique imperative. Direct diluent to side of vial and gently swirl to avoid excess foaming. Do not shake. Further dilute the calculated dose in 50 mL D5W. Desired final infusion concentration is 30 to 70 mcg/mL. If the total dose is 1.5 mg or less (patient weighs less than 40 kg), the dose of aldesleukin should be diluted in a smaller volume of D5W so the final concentration remains in the acceptable range. For cases in which the volume of diluent cannot be adjusted, the addition of albumin to D5W to a concentration of 0.1% before the addition of aldesleukin provides nearly complete protein recovery (to achieve a concentration of 0.1%, add 1 mL of 5% [0.2 mL of 25%] albumin to each 50 mL of diluent [D5W]). Plastic infusion containers are preferred over glass. Do not use any filters for dilution or administration. Do not use any other diluent or infusion solution; may cause increased aggregation. Bring to room temperature before administration.

Filters: Do not use any filters for dilution or administration.

Storage: Store in refrigerator before and after reconstitution and dilution. Do not freeze. No stability problems will occur at CRT for 48 hours after dilution but has no preservatives. Do not use beyond expiration date on vial.

COMPATIBILITY   (Underline Indicates Conflicting Compatibility Information)
Consider any drug NOT listed as compatible to be INCOMPATIBLE until consulting a pharmacist; specific conditions may apply.
Manufacturer recommends not mixing with other drugs in the same container. Bacteriostatic water for injection (BWFI) or NS will increase aggregation.

One source suggests the following **compatibilities:**
Y-site: Amphotericin B (generic), calcium gluconate, diphenhydramine (Benadryl), dopamine, fluconazole (Diflucan), foscarnet (Foscavir), heparin, magnesium sulfate, metoclopramide (Reglan), ondansetron (Zofran), potassium chloride (KCl), ranitidine (Zantac), sulfamethoxazole/trimethoprim, vancomycin.

RATE OF ADMINISTRATION
Intermittent IV: A single dose as an intermittent infusion over 15 minutes. Flush main line IV with D5W before and after each use. Manufacturer recommends that any keep-open IV in place for intermittent administration be D5W.

ACTIONS
A genetically engineered recombinant protein that possesses the biologic activity of naturally occurring interleukin-2. Immunoregulatory properties include enhancement of lymphocyte mitogenesis and stimulation of long-term growth of human interleukin-2 dependent cell lines, enhancement of lymphocyte cytotoxicity, induction of killer cell (lymphokine-activated [LAK] and natural [NK]) activity, and induction of interferon-gamma production. Immunologic effects occur in a dose-dependent manner and include activation of cellular immunity with profound lymphocytosis, eosinophilia, and thrombocytopenia, as well as the production of cytokines, including tumor necrosis factor, IL-1, and gamma interferon. In vivo experiments in murine tumor models have shown inhibition of tumor growth. Following a short infusion, aldesleukin distributes rapidly into the kidneys, liver, lungs, and spleen. Half-life is approximately 85 minutes. Eliminated by metabolism in the kidney with little or no bioactive protein excreted in urine.

INDICATIONS AND USES

Prescreening mandatory. Eligibility requirements for treatment are specific and directly impact response rate and toxicity (asymptomatic preferred; symptomatic and fully ambulatory may be considered). ■ Treatment of metastatic renal cell carcinoma in adults. ■ Treatment of adults with metastatic melanoma. ■ Granted orphan designation for treatment of primary immunodeficiency disease associated with T-cell defects and non-Hodgkin's lymphoma.

Unlabeled uses: Acute myelogenous leukemia after autologous BMT. ■ Colorectal cancer. ■ In combination with highly active antiretroviral therapy in treatment of HIV patients.

CONTRAINDICATIONS

Abnormal thallium stress test or pulmonary function tests. ■ Known hypersensitivity to interleukin-2 or any component of aldesleukin. ■ Patients with organ allografts. ■ Exclude from treatment any patient with significant cardiac, pulmonary, renal, hepatic, or CNS impairment; any patient requiring treatment with steroidal agents; and any patient at higher risk for cardiovascular adverse events during periods of hypotension and fluid shifts.

Retreatment is permanently contraindicated in patients who experienced specific toxicities in a previous course of therapy (see the following chart).

Contraindications for Retreatment with Aldesleukin	
Organ System	Symptom
Cardiovascular	Sustained ventricular tachycardia ≥5 beats. Cardiac rhythm disturbances not controlled or unresponsive to management. Chest pain with ECG changes consistent with angina or myocardial infarction. Pericardial tamponade.
Pulmonary	Intubation required more than 72 hours.
Renal	Renal dysfunction requiring dialysis for more than 72 hours.
Central nervous system	Coma or toxic psychosis lasting more than 48 hours. Repetitive or difficult-to-control seizures.
Gastrointestinal	Bowel ischemia or perforation. Bleeding requiring surgery.

PRECAUTIONS

Administered in the hospital under the supervision of a qualified physician (usually a medical oncologist and/or immunologist). Intensive care facilities and specialists in cardiopulmonary and/or intensive care medicine must be available. ■ Capillary leak syndrome (CLS [extravasation of plasma proteins and fluid into the extravascular space and loss of vascular tone]) can begin immediately after aldesleukin treatment starts and results in hypotension and reduced organ perfusion that can be severe enough to result in death. CLS may be associated with angina, arrhythmias (supraventricular and ventricular), edema, GI bleed or infarction, mental status changes, myocardial infarction, renal insufficiency, and respiratory insufficiency requiring intubation. ■ Therapy should be restricted to patients with normal cardiac, pulmonary, renal (SCr less than or equal to 1.5 mg/dL), hepatic, and CNS functions as defined by appropriate tests. Patients who have had a nephrectomy are eligible for treatment if SCr is less than 1.5 mg/dL (85% of patients in one study). ▪ Withhold administration in patients who develop moderate to severe lethargy or somnolence; continued administration may result in coma. ▪ Use extreme caution in patients with normal thallium stress tests and pulmonary function tests who have a history of prior cardiac or pulmonary disease. ▪ May exacerbate disease symptoms in clinically unrecognized or untreated CNS metastases. Thoroughly evaluate and treat CNS metastases before aldesleukin therapy. Should be neurologically stable and have a negative CT scan. New neurologic signs, symptoms, and anatomic lesions following aldesleukin therapy have been reported in patients without evidence of CNS metastases. Clinical manifestations include agitation, ataxia, change in mental status, hallucinations, obtundation, speech difficulties, and coma. Cortical lesions and demyelination have been seen using MRI studies. Neurologic S/S usually resolve following discontinuation of therapy; however, there have been reports of permanent damage. ▪ Use extreme caution in patients with a history of seizures (may cause seizures), patients with fixed requirements for large volumes of fluid (e.g., hypercalcemia), those with autoimmune disorders (e.g., Crohn's disease, ulcerative colitis, psoriasis), previous cytotoxic drug therapy or radiation therapy, and patients sensitive to *Escherichia coli*–derived proteins. ▪ May cause autoimmune disease and inflammatory disorders or exacerbate pre-existing conditions (e.g., Crohn's disease, scleroderma, inflammatory arthritis, oculobulbar myasthenia gravis, glomerulonephritis, cholecystitis, cerebral vasculitis, Stevens-Johnson syndrome, bullous pemphigoid). ▪ Associated with impaired neutrophil function and an increased risk of disseminated infection, including sepsis and bacterial endocarditis. Pre-existing bacterial infections should be adequately treated before beginning therapy. Patients with indwelling central lines are at increased risk for infection with gram-positive organisms. Antibiotic prophylaxis with ciprofloxacin, nafcillin, oxacillin, or vancomycin has been associated with a reduced incidence of staphylococcal infections. ▪ Induces significant hypotension; discontinue antihypertensives during treatment. ▪ May impair thyroid function; changes may suggest autoimmunity; thyroid replacement therapy has been required in a few patients. ▪ May cause hyperglycemia and/or diabetes mellitus. ▪ See Drug/Lab Interactions.

Monitor: A central venous catheter (double or triple lumen) is frequently ordered on admission (required for continuous infusion). A minimum of two IV lines is usually required (one for the aldesleukin and its keep-open IV and one for other needed fluids and medications). One line could suffice if absolutely necessary since aldesleukin would be discontinued when colloids are administered. Flushing of line with D5W before and after aldesleukin is imperative. Ability to record CVP and draw blood samples should be available. ▪ Admission chest x-ray, ECG, CBC with differential and platelet count, blood chemistries including electrolytes and renal and liver function tests, T_3, T_4, PT, PTT, urinalysis, and body weight should be obtained. Adequate pulmonary function, normal arterial blood gases, and normal ejection fraction and unimpaired wall motion (confirmed by thallium stress test and/or a stress echocardiogram) should be documented. ▪ During drug administration obtain daily CBC with differential and platelet count, blood chemistries including electrolytes, renal and hepatic function tests, and chest x-rays. ▪ Continuous cardiac monitoring is indicated (required with BP below 90 mm Hg or any cardiac irregularity). ▪ Monitoring and flexibility in management of fluid balance and organ perfusion status is imperative. Requires constant management and balancing of effects of fluid shifts to prevent the consequences of hypovolemia (e.g., impaired organ perfusion) or fluid accumulation (e.g., edema, pulmonary edema, ascites, pulmonary effusion), which may exceed the patient's tolerance. ▪ Assess hypovolemia by central venous catheterization and frequent central venous pressure monitoring. Administer colloids (albumin, plasmanate) or crystalloids (IV fluids) as indicated for a BP drop of 20 mm Hg or greater or a systolic BP less than 90. ▪ Frequent neuro checks required (note agitation, blurred vision, confusion, depression, irritability, and persistent somnolence). ▪ Vital signs and strict I&O are required every 2 to 4 hours (much more frequently as side effects develop). ▪ Weigh daily. ▪ Assess thyroid function periodically. ▪ An ECG and cardiac enzymes are indicated for any S/S of chest pain, murmurs, gallops, irregular rhythm, or palpitations. A repeat thallium study is indicated for evidence of cardiac ischemia or CHF; may indicate ventricular hypokinesia due to myocarditis. Obtain a urinalysis as indicated. ▪ Assess pulmonary function through examination, vital signs, and pulse oximetry. Arterial blood gases are indicated for any dyspnea or respiratory impairment. ▪ Some routine medications are indicated prophylactically to reduce the incidence of side effects and to promote patient comfort. The morning of the first treatment begin acetaminophen 650 mg PO q 4 hr and indomethacin 25 mg q 6 hr (may increase nephrotoxicity) or naprosyn 500 mg q 12 hr PO for fever and arthralgia. Use an H_2 antagonist (e.g., ranitidine 150 mg PO q 12 hr) to prevent GI bleeding. Continue administration of these drugs until 12 hours after last dose of aldesleukin. Low-dose dopamine 1 to 5 mcg/kg/min can help maintain organ perfusion and urine output if given at initial onset of CLS before hypotension occurs. Antiemetics, antidiarrheals, antichill/rigors (meperidine), antihistamines, and moisturizing skin lotions will also be used throughout treatment; see Antidote for specifics. ▪ If fever occurs several days into treatment or recurs after subsiding, assume infection first, then drug. Confusion, depression, or irritability may also suggest infection. Draw cultures; administer appropriate antibiotics. ▪ Patients who have had nephrectomies may be more at risk for increases in serum BUN or creatinine, electrolyte shifts, and reduced urine output. Evaluate fluid, electrolyte, and acid-base status promptly if any of the above occur. Gradual increases without other complications (marked fluid overload, hyperkalemia, acidosis) are frequently tolerated (SCr must not exceed 4.5 mg/dL). ▪ Maintain pulmonary status as needed with O_2, diuretics (furosemide) and maintain serum bicarbonate above 15 mEq/L. Assess pulmonary status with chest x-rays. ▪ Monitor central and peripheral IV sites to reduce potential for infection. Change peripheral sites every 3 days. ▪ No restrictions on activity; use caution ambulating (orthostatic hypotension). ▪ No restrictions on diet. Encouragement may be required (anorexia and/or mouth sores). ▪ Monitor for thrombocytopenia (platelet count less than $50,000/mm^3$). Initiate precautions to prevent excessive bleeding (e.g., inspect IV sites, skin, and mucous membranes; use extreme care during invasive procedures; test urine, emesis, stool, and secretions for occult blood). ▪ Specific preparation required for discharge; refer to literature. ▪ Manufacturer supplies excellent brochures for nurses and physicians with detailed guidelines in chart form on all aspects of monitoring, toxicity, and treatment. ▪ Complete review and adequate preparation of all aspects of this therapy with the patient and family are imperative. Can reduce psychologic stress of toxicity. ▪ Tumor regression has continued for up to 12 months after one or more courses of therapy. ▪ See Dose Adjustments, Contraindications, and Antidote.

Patient Education: Many side effects will occur; report any changes you perceive so they can be evaluated and treated if needed (e.g., changes in breathing, chest or other pain, temperature, mood, light-headedness, fatigue). ▪ Request assistance for ambulation and always sit on the side of the bed first. ▪ Take only prescribed medications. ▪ Avoid alcohol. ▪ Use of effective contraceptive measures recommended for fertile men and women. ▪ Use 15 SPF sunscreen in sunlight to protect against photosensitivity. ▪ See Appendix D, p. 1434, for additional information. ▪ Manufacturer supplies a patient education booklet; review thoroughly and discuss with your physician and nurse.

Maternal/Child: Category C: animal studies not conducted; effects unknown. Benefits must outweigh risks. Contraceptive measures required before initial administration and throughout treatment. ▪ Discontinue breast-feeding. ▪ Safety for use in pediatric patients under 18 years of age not established; studies show responsiveness and toxicity similar.

Elderly: Response rates and toxicity similar to that seen in younger adults; however, some increased incidence of severe urogenital toxicities and dyspnea was noted in the elderly. ▪ Use caution, consider age-related organ impairment.

DRUG/LAB INTERACTIONS

May cause interactions with **psychotropic drugs** (e.g., analgesics, antiemetics, narcotics, sedatives, tranquilizers) because aldesleukin also affects central nervous function. ▪ Concomitant use with **cardiotoxic agents** (e.g., doxorubicin [Adriamycin]), **hepatotoxic agents** (e.g., methotrexate, asparaginase), **myelotoxic agents** (e.g., cytotoxic chemotherapy, radiation therapy), **and nephrotoxic agents** (e.g., aminoglycosides, indomethacin) may increase toxicity in these organ systems and/or delay excretion of these agents, increasing their toxicity. ▪ Effects may be potentiated by drugs that also cause blood dyscrasias **(e.g., penicillins, phenothiazines).** ▪ May cause severe hypersensitivity reactions with **iodinated contrast media.** ▪ **Glucocorticoids** (e.g., dexamethasone [Decadron]) reduce aldesleukin-induced side effects but also reduce its antitumor effectiveness. ▪ Aldesleukin-induced hypotension may be potentiated by **beta-blockers** (e.g., metoprolol, atenolol) **and antihypertensive agents** (e.g., nitroglycerin IV, nitroprusside sodium). ▪ Concurrent use with **interferon-alfa** may increase incidence of MI, myocarditis, ventricular hypokinesia, and severe rhabdomyolysis. ▪ May cause hypersensitivity reactions in patients receiving combination regimens (**high-dose aldesleukin and antineoplastics** [e.g., dacarbazine, cisplatin, tamoxifen, interferon-alfa]). ▪ Aldesleukin may decrease clearance and increase plasma levels of **indinavir** (Crixivan). ▪ Capable of altering numerous lab values; see literature.

SIDE EFFECTS

Frequent, predictable, often severe; are usually clinically manageable and frequently require intensive care management. Begin to occur shortly after therapy begins (chills, fatigue, fever, hypotension, nausea, vomiting). Frequency and severity are dose-related and schedule-dependent. Most are reversible within 2 or 3 days of discontinuation of therapy. Even with intensive management, side effects can progress to death.

Initially anorexia, arthralgia, chills, fatigue, fever, nausea, and vomiting occur. Initial symptoms of capillary leak syndrome are edema, electrolyte abnormalities, hypotension, oliguria, respiratory distress, significant weight gain, tachycardia. Effects of CLS **successively** result in *hypovolemia,* which in turn leads to hypotension→ hypoperfusion→ sinus tachycardia→ angina→ myocardial ischemia and infarction→ arrhythmias (supraventricular and ventricular)→ decreased renal perfusion→ prerenal azotemia→ oliguria→ anuria; *fluid retention/weight gain,* which in turn leads to rales→ dyspnea→ cough→ tachypnea→ hypoxia→ pleural effusion→ respiratory insufficiency requiring intubation→ diarrhea→ edema of the bowel→ refractory acidosis→ edema→ ascites; and *breakdown of blood-brain barrier* (neuropsychiatric toxicity [e.g., agitation, combativeness, confusion, hallucinations, lethargy, psychosis, somnolence]). Abdominal pain and GI bleeding may be related to diarrhea, vomiting, stomatitis, duodenal ulcer formation, bowel ischemia, infarction, or perforation. Cerebral edema and concomitant medications may impact many side effects. Lethargy and/or somnolence may lead to coma. Anemia and thrombocytopenia may occur; coagulation abnormalities (PT, PTT) reflect liver dysfunction. Hemodynamic effects similar to septic shock may be caused by tumor necrosis factor. Erythematous rash and pruritus (can progress to dry desquamation) can occur in almost all patients and are extremely uncomfortable. See Precautions and Drug/Lab Interactions.

ANTIDOTE

Temporarily discontinue aldesleukin and notify physician immediately of arrhythmias or rhythm changes, chest pain, marked changes in HR, positive neuropsychiatric check (agitation, blurred vision, persistent extreme somnolence), systolic BP below 90 mm Hg, apical HR over 120, temperature over 38° C (100.4° F), respirations over 25/min, complaints of dyspnea, decreased breath sounds, increased sputum production, urinary output less than 200 mL/4 hr, CVP reading below 3 to 4 mm H_2O, weight increase over 4 kg or 10% of baseline over 5 days, abnormal blood or urine tests (e.g., serum bicarbonate less than 15 mEq/L, SCr greater than 4 to 4.5 mg/dL [based on gradual or sudden rise and if accompanied by other complications]), severe diarrhea associated with refractory acidosis, vomiting refractory to treatment, acute changes in GI status. May be restarted based on patient response. Hold any subsequent dose for failure to maintain organ perfusion; see Dose Adjustments. Fever is routinely treated with acetaminophen and indomethacin or naprosyn; increased doses may be needed; administer rectally if nausea and vomiting are present. Suggested treatments include slow IV meperidine (Demerol) 25 to 50 mg for chills and rigidity; diphenoxylate (Lomotil), or loperamide (Imodium) PO for diarrhea (these meds may not help and diarrhea may be dose-limiting); diphenhydramine (Benadryl) 25 mg PO q 6 hr, a soothing skin cream (Eucerin), and oatmeal baths for urticaria and pruritus; temazepam (Restoril) for insomnia; ondansetron (Zofran) or prochlorperazine (Compazine) for nausea. Treat edema with furosemide (Lasix). IV fluids, albumin or plasmanate, and Trendelenburg positioning are used to maintain fluid balance and BP. If organ perfusion and BP are not sustained by dopamine 1 to

5 mcg/kg/min as a continuous infusion, increase to 6 to 10 mcg/kg/min or add phenylephrine (1 to 5 mcg/kg/min). Prolonged use of pressors at relatively high doses may cause cardiac arrhythmias. Treat arrhythmias as indicated (usually sinus or supraventricular tachycardia [adenosine, verapamil]). Use O_2 for decreased PaO_2. Use packed RBCs for anemia and to ensure maximum oxygen-carrying capacity. Platelet transfusions are indicated for thrombocytopenia or to reduce risk of GI bleeding. Use of blood modifiers to treat bone marrow toxicity may be indicated (e.g., darbepoetin alfa [Aranesp], epoetin alfa [Epogen], filgrastim [Neupogen], oprelvekin [Neumega], pegfilgrastim [Neulasta], sargramostim [Leukine]). Special precautions may be required (e.g., avoid IM injections; test urine, emesis, stool, secretions for occult blood). All treatment is supportive; recovery should begin within a few hours of cessation of aldesleukin. With normalized BP, diuretics (furosemide [Lasix]) can hasten recovery. Low-dose haloperidol (Haldol) may help severe mental status changes.

More rapid onset of dose-limiting toxicities will occur with overdose. **Dexamethasone (Decadron)** is indicated to counteract life-threatening toxicities. May result in loss of therapeutic effect.

ALEFACEPT
(ah-**LEF**-fah-sept)

Amevive

Immunosuppressant

pH 6.9

USUAL DOSE

7.5 mg as an IV bolus once each week for 12 weeks. Baseline CD4+ T-lymphocyte count must be within normal limits (e.g., 600 to 1,500/mm³ [consult lab, parameters may vary]) before the initial course of therapy begins. A repeat count is required every 2 weeks. Withhold dose if CD4+ T-lymphocyte counts are below 250 cells/mm³, and initiate weekly monitoring of CD4+ T-lymphocyte count. A second course may be considered after a 12-week waiting period if CD4+ T-lymphocyte counts are within the normal range. Data limited on retreatment with more than 2 cycles. May be given IM; however, the dose is different (larger) and is supplied in a different kit.

DOSE ADJUSTMENTS

Withhold dose if CD4+ T-lymphocyte counts are below 250 cells/mm³. ■ Discontinue alefacept if counts remain below 250 cells/mm³ for 1 month.

DILUTION

Supplied in a kit containing a single 7.5-mg vial of alefacept, SW for reconstitution, a syringe, a ¾-inch 23-gauge winged infusion set (butterfly needle), and two 23-gauge 1¼-inch needles. Using the first needle, withdraw 0.6 mL of supplied diluent (SW). Reconstitute the 7.5-mg vial by slowly injecting the diluent toward the sidewall of the vial. Do not shake or vigorously agitate; swirl gently to dissolve (should occur within 2 minutes). Some foaming will occur; avoid excessive foaming. Change to the second needle and withdraw 0.5 mL (7.5 mg of alefacept); some foam may remain in the vial. Prepare 2 additional syringes with 3 mL of NS in each one. Use the first NS syringe to prime the winged infusion set before inserting it into the vein. Confirm venous access, then attach the syringe with alefacept. The second NS syringe will be used for the postadministration flush.

Filters: Do not filter reconstituted solution during preparation or administration; see Compatibility.

Storage: Retain kit in carton until use. Store in refrigerator (2° to 8° C [36° to 46° F]), protected from light. Do not use beyond expiration date stamped on kit. Use immediately after reconstitution is preferred, but may be refrigerated in the vial for up to 4 hours if necessary. Discard reconstituted solution after 4 hours.

COMPATIBILITY

Manufacturer states, "Do not add other medications to solutions containing alefacept. Do not reconstitute with other diluents. Do not filter reconstituted solution during preparation or administration."

RATE OF ADMINISTRATION

0.5 mL (7.5 mg) as a bolus injection over no more than 5 seconds. Follow with a flush of 3 mL NS. Remove winged infusion set.

IV FORMULATION DISCONTINUED

ACTIONS

An immunosuppressive protein produced by recombinant DNA technology in a Chinese Hamster Ovary mammalian cell expression system. Selectively targets the T-cells responsible for chronic plaque psoriasis without disrupting normal immune function. Interferes with lymphocyte activation by specifically binding to the lymphocyte antigen, CD2, and inhibiting LFA-3/CD2 interaction, which plays a role in the pathophysiology of chronic plaque psoriasis. Results in a dose-dependent reduction in circulating CD4+ and CD8+ T-lymphocyte counts. May have some minor effect on cells other than T-lymphocytes. Mean half-life is 270 hours. Onset of response usually begins within 60 days after the start of therapy. Maximum response may not occur until several weeks after the 12-week regimen is complete. Median duration of response in studies was 3.5 months.

INDICATIONS AND USES

Treatment of adults with moderate to severe chronic plaque psoriasis who are candidates for systemic therapy or phototherapy (treatment of a disease by exposure to light).

CONTRAINDICATIONS

Known hypersensitivity to alefacept or any of its components (e.g., sucrose). ■ Do not initiate in patients with a CD4+ T-lymphocyte count below normal (e.g., 600 to 1,500/mm^3), patients with a history of systemic malignancy, or patients with a clinically important infection. ■ Do not administer to patients infected with HIV. May accelerate disease progression or increase complications of disease in HIV patients. ■ See Precautions and Side Effects.

PRECAUTIONS

Administer under the supervision of a physician. ■ May increase the risk of malignancies (e.g., basal or squamous cell skin cancers, lymphomas [Hodgkin's or non-Hodgkin's]). Use caution in patients who may be at high risk for malignancy. Discontinue if a malignancy develops. ■ Use caution in patients with chronic infections or a history of recurrent infection. Discontinue if a serious infection develops. ■ Do not use concurrently with other immunosuppressive agents or phototherapy. May cause excessive immunosuppression. Length of time required between alefacept therapy and initiating another immunosuppressive therapy has not been established. ■ Safety and effectiveness of concurrent administration of live or live-attenuated virus vaccines not studied; some ability to mount immunity may occur. ■ A protein substance; hypersensitivity reactions have been reported; use caution in patients with allergies. ■ Patients may develop low-titer antibodies to alefacept; no correlation with clinical response or side effects observed. ■ Hepatotoxicity has been reported (e.g., increased transaminases, fatty infiltration of the liver, hepatitis, decompensation of cirrhosis with liver failure and acute liver failure). ■ Effects in patients with impaired renal or hepatic function have not been studied. **Monitor:** Obtain CD4+ T-lymphocyte count before beginning therapy and repeat every 2 weeks before dosing. Count should be within normal limits before a regimen is initiated; see Usual Dose and Dose Adjustments. ■ Monitor for symptoms of hypersensitivity reactions; urticaria and angioedema have been reported; see Antidote. ■ Monitor for S/S of infection; see Antidote. ■ Monitor liver function tests (e.g., ALT, AST).

Patient Education: Weekly white blood cell counts required before each dose. ▪ May increase risk of developing skin cancers or lymphomas. ▪ Susceptibility to infection may be increased; report any S/S of infection (e.g., fever, chills, cold symptoms). ▪ Report S/S of hepatotoxicity (e.g., abdominal pain, anorexia, dark urine, easy bruising, jaundice, nausea or vomiting, pale stools). ▪ Female patients should notify their physician immediately if pregnancy is suspected during therapy or within 8 weeks of completing therapy. If a pregnancy occurs, enrolling in the alefacept Pregnancy Registry is encouraged. ▪ See Appendix D, p. 1434.

Maternal/Child: Category B: use during pregnancy only if clearly needed. If pregnancy occurs during therapy, assess risks of continued use. No evidence of harm to animal fetuses; see package insert and Patient Education. Crosses placental barrier in monkeys. ▪ Discontinue breast-feeding; has potential for serious harm to the infant. ▪ Safety and effectiveness for use in pediatric patients not studied; not indicated for pediatric use.

Elderly: Safety and effectiveness similar to younger patients. ▪ Incidence of infections and certain malignancies may be higher in the elderly; use caution.

DRUG/LAB INTERACTIONS

Specific drug interaction studies have not been performed. ▪ Do not use concurrently with other **immunosuppressive agents or phototherapy.** May cause excessive immunosuppression; see Precautions. ▪ Safety and effectiveness of concurrent administration of **live virus or live-attenuated virus vaccines** not studied.

SIDE EFFECTS

Treatment-limiting side effects include hypersensitivity reactions (e.g., anaphylaxis, angioedema, urticaria), lymphopenia (CD4+ T-lymphocytes below 250 cells/mm^3), headache, malignancies, and/or serious infections requiring hospitalization (e.g., appendicitis, cholecystitis, gastroenteritis, herpes simplex infection, necrotizing cellulitis, peritonsillar abscess, pneumonia, postoperative and burn wound infection, pre-septal cellulitis, toxic shock), and nausea. Most frequently reported side effects include accidental injury, chills, dizziness, increased cough, injection site inflammation, myalgia, nausea, pharyngitis, and pruritus. Cardiovascular events (e.g., coronary artery disease, MI) have also been reported.

Overdose: Arthralgia, chills, headache, sinusitis.

ANTIDOTE

Notify physician of all side effects. Most will be treated symptomatically. Discontinue alefacept if CD4+ T-lymphocyte counts remain below 250 cells/mm^3 for 1 month. Discontinue immediately if anaphylaxis or other serious hypersensitivity reaction occurs. Treat hypersensitivity reactions as indicated; may require epinephrine, airway management, oxygen, IV fluids, antihistamines (e.g., diphenhydramine [Benadryl]), corticosteroids (e.g., hydrocortisone sodium succinate [Solu-Cortef]), and pressor amines (e.g., dopamine). Discontinue if hepatotoxicity, a malignancy, or a serious infection occurs and initiate appropriate treatment. Monitor total lymphocyte count and CD4+ T-lymphocyte count closely in overdose. Resuscitate as indicated.

ALEMTUZUMAB BBW
(**ah**-lem-**TOOZ**-uh-mab)

Campath

Monoclonal Antibody
Antineoplastic

pH 6.8 to 7.4

USUAL DOSE

Premedication, dose escalation to the recommended maintenance dose, and anti-infective prophylaxis are required.

Premedication: Oral diphenhydramine (Benadryl) 50 mg and acetaminophen (Tylenol) 500 to 1,000 mg should be administered 30 minutes before the first dose, at dose escalations, and as clinically indicated. For cases in which severe infusion-related reactions have occurred, corticosteroids may be administered to help prevent or minimize subsequent reactions.

Dose escalation: Initiate at a dose of 3 mg daily. When this dose is tolerated (infusion-related toxicities are Grade 2 or less), the daily dose should be increased to 10 mg. When the 10-mg dose is tolerated, the maintenance dose of 30 mg may be initiated. In most cases, dose escalation to the maintenance dose of 30 mg can be achieved in 3 to 7 days.

Maintenance dose: 30 mg/day administered three times a week on alternate days (i.e., Monday, Wednesday, Friday). Administered for up to 12 weeks. Single doses greater than 30 mg or cumulative weekly doses greater than 90 mg have been associated with an increased incidence of pancytopenia and should *not* be administered.

Anti-infective prophylaxis: To minimize the risk of selected opportunistic infections, administer sulfamethoxazole/trimethoprim DS twice daily three times a week and famciclovir (Famvir) 250 mg or equivalent twice daily at the start of alemtuzumab therapy. Continue prophylaxis for 2 months after completion of therapy or until the CD4+ count is equal to or greater than 200 cells/mm^3, whichever occurs later.

DOSE ADJUSTMENTS

There are no dose modifications recommended for lymphopenia. ▪ Withhold alemtuzumab during serious infections or other serious adverse reactions until resolution. ▪ Discontinue alemtuzumab for autoimmune anemia or autoimmune thrombocytopenia. ▪ Recommendations for dose modification for severe neutropenia or thrombocytopenia are listed in the following chart.

Alemtuzumab Dose Modification for Neutropenia or Thrombocytopenia	
Hematologic Values	Dose Modification*
ANC less than 250/mm^3 and/or platelet count equal to or less than 25,000/mm^3	
First occurrence	Withhold alemtuzumab therapy. Resume alemtuzumab at 30 mg when ANC is equal to or greater than 500/mm^3 and platelet count is equal to or greater than 50,000/mm^3.
Second occurrence	Withhold alemtuzumab therapy. Resume alemtuzumab at 10 mg when ANC is equal to or greater than 500/mm^3 and platelet count is equal to or greater than 50,000/mm^3.

*If the delay between dosing is equal to or more than 7 days, resume alemtuzumab therapy at 3 mg and escalate to 10 mg and then to 30 mg as tolerated; see Dose and Administration.

Continued

Alemtuzumab Dose Modification for Neutropenia or Thrombocytopenia—cont'd	
Hematologic Values	Dose Modification*
Third occurrence	Discontinue alemtuzumab therapy.
Equal to or greater than 50% decrease from baseline in patients initiating therapy with a baseline ANC equal to or less than 250/mm³ and/or a baseline platelet count equal to or less than 25,000/mm³	
First occurrence	Withhold alemtuzumab therapy. Resume alemtuzumab at 30 mg upon return to baseline value(s).
Second occurrence	Withhold alemtuzumab therapy. Resume alemtuzumab at 10 mg upon return to baseline value(s).
Third occurrence	Discontinue alemtuzumab therapy.

*If the delay between dosing is equal to or more than 7 days, resume alemtuzumab therapy at 3 mg and escalate to 10 mg and then to 30 mg as tolerated; see Dose and Administration.

DILUTION
Do not shake vial before use. Withdraw the necessary amount of alemtuzumab from the ampule into a syringe. Inject into 100 mL of NS or D5W. Gently invert the bag to mix solution. Discard any unused drug.
Filters: Filtering no longer recommended by the manufacturer.
Storage: Store ampules at 2° to 8° C (36° to 46° F). Do not freeze. If accidentally frozen, thaw at 2° to 8° C before administration. Protect from direct sunlight. Prepared solution may be stored at CRT or refrigerated. Protect from light and use within 8 hours of dilution.

COMPATIBILITY
Manufacturer states, "Other drug substances should not be added or simultaneously infused through the same intravenous line." No **incompatibilities** observed with PVC bags, PVC or polyethylene-lined PVC administration sets, or low–protein binding filters.

RATE OF ADMINISTRATION
A single dose as an infusion over 2 hours. **Do not administer** as an IV push or bolus. Subcutaneous administration is unlabeled but has been used.

ACTIONS
A recombinant, DNA-derived, humanized monoclonal antibody (Campath-1H) that binds to the 21-28 kD cell surface glycoprotein, CD52. CD52 is expressed on the surface of both normal and malignant B and T lymphocytes, NK cells, most monocytes, macrophages, a subpopulation of granulocytes. Alemtuzumab binding has been observed in lymphoid tissues, the mononuclear phagocyte system, and the male reproductive tract. A proportion of bone marrow cells, including some CD34+ cells, also express variable levels of CD52. The mechanism of action is thought to be an antibody-dependent lysis of leukemic cells following cell surface binding. Exhibits nonlinear kinetics. AUC and half-life increase with repeated dosing. Mean half-life was 11 hours (range 2 to 32 hours) after the first 30-mg dose and was 6 days (range 1 to 14 days) after the last 30-mg dose. The rise in serum alemtuzumab concentration corresponds with the reduction in malignant lymphocytosis.

INDICATIONS AND USES
Treatment of B-cell chronic lymphocytic leukemia (B-CLL).

CONTRAINDICATIONS

Manufacturer states, "None."

PRECAUTIONS

Administered under the supervision of a physician experienced in the use of antineoplastic therapy in a facility equipped to monitor patient and respond to any medical emergency. ▪ Serious and, in rare instances, fatal pancytopenia/marrow hypoplasia, autoimmune idiopathic thrombocytopenia, and autoimmune hemolytic anemia have been reported. Have occurred at recommended dose. Do not exceed maximum daily or weekly recommended dose. See Usual Dose, Dose Adjustments, and Antidote. ▪ Serious and sometimes fatal bacterial, viral, fungal, and protozoan infections have been reported. Prophylaxis directed against *Pneumocystis jiroveci* pneumonia and herpes virus infections has been shown to decrease but not eliminate the occurrence of these infections. See Usual Dose, Dose Adjustments, and Antidote. ▪ Serious and sometimes fatal infusion reactions can occur; see Monitor. ▪ Use caution in patients who have had previous cytotoxic agents or radiation therapy or who have received agents that may cause blood dyscrasias; see Drug/Lab Interactions. ▪ Because of the potential for transfusion-associated graft-versus-host disease in severely lymphopenic patients, irradiation of any blood products is recommended. ▪ A small percentage of patients have developed antibodies to alemtuzumab.

Monitor: Obtain a baseline CBC, including differential and platelet count. Monitor weekly or more frequently if worsening anemia, neutropenia, or thrombocytopenia develops. ▪ Infusion reactions, including ARDS, bronchospasm, cardiac arrhythmias and/or arrest, chills, fever, hypotension, MI, N/V, pulmonary infiltrates, rash, respiratory arrest, rigors, shortness of breath, syncope, and/or urticaria may occur. Reactions may be severe. Acute infusion-related reactions were most common during the first week of therapy in clinical studies. Premedicate patient and monitor carefully during infusion. Gradual escalation to the recommended maintenance dose is required at the initiation of therapy and after interruption of therapy for 7 or more days. See Usual Dose. ▪ Monitor for CMV infection during and for 2 months after completion of therapy. Treat confirmed infection or viremia as indicated with ganciclovir (Cytovene) or equivalent. ▪ Monitor blood pressure and hypotensive symptoms carefully in patients with ischemic heart disease and in patients taking antihypertensive medications; see Drug/Lab Interactions. ▪ Monitor for thrombocytopenia (platelet count less than 50,000/mm^3). Initiate precautions to prevent excessive bleeding (e.g., inspect IV sites, skin, and mucous membranes; use extreme care during invasive procedures; test urine, emesis, stool, and secretions for occult blood). ▪ CD4+ counts should be followed after therapy until recovery to equal to or greater than 200 cells/mm^3. See Usual Dose.

Patient Education: Women of childbearing potential and men of reproductive potential should use effective contraceptive methods during treatment and for a minimum of 6 months following therapy. ▪ Promptly report any unusual side effects or signs of bleeding or bruising, infection (e.g., fever), or infusion reaction (e.g., difficulty breathing, rash). ▪ Irradiation of blood products is required until adequate lymphocyte recovery. ▪ See Appendix D, p. 1434.

Maternal/Child: Category C: avoid pregnancy. May cause fetal harm. ▪ Discontinue breast-feeding during treatment and for at least 3 months following completion of therapy. ▪ Safety and effectiveness for use in pediatric patients not established.

Elderly: Differences in safety and efficacy related to age have not been observed to date, but study numbers have been small.

DRUG/LAB INTERACTIONS

No formal drug interaction studies have been performed. ▪ May cause additive effects with **bone marrow–suppressing agents, radiation therapy, or agents that cause blood dyscrasias** (e.g., amphotericin B, antithyroid agents [Methimazole (Tapazole)], azathioprine [Imuran], chloramphenicol, ganciclovir [Cytovene], interferon, plicamycin [Mithracin], zidovudine [AZT, Retrovir]). ▪ May intensify effects of **antihypertensive medications;** see Monitor. ▪ Do not administer **chloroquine or live virus vaccines** to patients receiving antineoplastic agents.

SIDE EFFECTS

The most common serious side effects are cytopenias (anemia, lymphopenia, neutropenia, thrombocytopenia), immunosuppression/infections (CMV viremia, CMV infection, other infections), and infusion reactions (chills, dyspnea, fever, hypotension, nausea, rash, tachycardia, urticaria). GI symptoms (abdominal pain, N/V) and neurologic symptoms (insomnia, anxiety) are also reported commonly. Hypersensitivity reactions (including anaphylaxis), anorexia, arrhythmias, asthenia, autoimmune hemolytic anemia or autoimmune idiopathic thrombocytopenia, constipation, cough, depression, dizziness, dyspepsia, edema, epistaxis, febrile neutropenia, Goodpasture's syndrome, Graves disease, Guillain-Barré syndrome, headache, hypertension, infections (e.g., pneumonia, Epstein-Barr virus (EBV), progressive multifocal leukoencephalopathy (PML), and several other opportunistic infections), malaise, mucositis, myalgias, optic neuropathy, pain, purpura, rhinitis, serum sickness, somnolence, tremor, tumor lysis syndrome, and many others have been reported.

Post-Marketing: CHF, chronic inflammatory demyelinating polyradiculoneuropathy, fatal infusion reactions, fatal transfusion-associated graft-versus-host disease.

ANTIDOTE

Notify physician of all side effects. Treatment of most reactions will be supportive. Therapy should be temporarily discontinued during serious infection, serious hematologic toxicity (except lymphopenia), or other serious toxicity until the infection or adverse event resolves. Discontinue medication permanently for severe reactions, including autoimmune anemia or thrombocytopenia. Infusion reactions may be treated with acetaminophen, antihistamines (e.g., diphenhydramine), corticosteroids (e.g., hydrocortisone), and meperidine as indicated. Administration of irradiated blood products and/or blood modifiers (e.g., darbepoetin [Aransep], epoetin alfa [Epogen], filgrastim [Neupogen], pegfilgrastim [Neulasta], sargramostim [Leukine]) may be indicated to treat bone marrow toxicity. Median durations of neutropenia were 28 to 37 days, and median durations of thrombocytopenia were 9 to 21 days. Median time to recovery of CD4+ counts to equal to or greater than $200/mm^3$ is 2 to 6 months; however, full recovery of CD4+ and CD8+ counts may take more than 12 months. Discontinue alemtuzumab and provide supportive therapy in overdose. Treat hypersensitivity reactions with epinephrine, antihistamines, and corticosteroids as needed. Resuscitate as indicated.

ALFENTANIL HYDROCHLORIDE
(al-**FEN**-tah-nil hy-droh-**KLOR**-eyed)

General anesthetic
Opioid analgesic agonist
Anesthesia adjunct

Alfenta

pH 4 to 6

USUAL DOSE

Adults and pediatric patients 12 years of age and older: Dose must be individualized and titrated to the desired effect in each patient according to body weight, physical status, underlying pathologic condition, use of other drugs, and type and duration of surgical procedure and anesthesia. Usually used in conjunction with short-acting barbiturates (e.g., thiopental [Pentothal]), neuromuscular blocking agents (e.g., pancuronium, succinylcholine), and an inhalation anesthetic (e.g., nitrous oxide) to maintain balanced anesthesia. Use reduced doses of a neuromuscular blocking agent prophylactically to prevent muscle rigidity or to induce muscle relaxation after rigidity occurs. Full paralyzing doses may be used after loss of consciousness. Use of a benzodiazepine (e.g., diazepam [Valium], midazolam [Versed]) may reduce induction dose requirements, decrease time to loss of consciousness, and diminish patient recall; see Drug/Lab Interactions. See Dose Adjustments.

Alfentanil Dosing Guidelines for Use During General Anesthesia	
SPONTANEOUSLY BREATHING/ASSISTED VENTILATION	

Procedures lasting up to 30 minutes	Induction of analgesia: 8-20 mcg/kg
	Maintenance of analgesia:
	  3-5 mcg/kg q 5-20 min or
	  0.5-1 mcg/kg/min
	Total dose: 8-40 mcg/kg

ASSISTED OR CONTROLLED VENTILATION	

Incremental injection in procedures lasting longer than 30 minutes (To attenuate response to laryngoscopy and intubation)	Induction of analgesia:
	  20-50 mcg/kg
	Maintenance of analgesia:
	  5-15 mcg/kg q 5-20 min
	Total dose: Up to 75 mcg/kg

CONTINUOUS INFUSION	

In procedures lasting longer than 30 minutes (To provide attenuation of response to intubation and incision)	Infusion rates are variable and should be titrated to the desired clinical effect.
	SEE INFUSION DOSAGE GUIDELINES (NEXT PAGE)
	Induction of analgesia:
	  50-75 mcg/kg
	Maintenance of analgesia:
	  0.5-3 mcg/kg/min (average rate 1-1.5 mcg/kg/min)
	Total dose: Dependent on duration of procedure

Continued

Alfentanil Dosing Guidelines for Use During General Anesthesia—cont'd

ANESTHETIC INDUCTION	

Procedures lasting 45 minutes or longer	Induction of anesthesia:
	   130-245 mcg/kg
	Maintenance of analgesia:
	   0.5-1.5 mcg/kg/min or general anesthetic
	Total dose: Dependent on duration of procedure
	At these doses, truncal rigidity should be expected and a muscle relaxant should be utilized
	Administer slowly (over 3 minutes)
	Concentration of inhalation agents reduced by 30%-50% for initial hour

MONITORED ANESTHESIA CARE (MAC)	
For sedated and responsive, spontaneously breathing patients	Induction of MAC: 3-8 mcg/kg Maintenance of MAC: 3-5 mcg/kg q 5-20 min or 0.25-1 mcg/kg/min Total dose: 3-40 mcg/kg

INFUSION DOSAGE
Continuous infusion: 0.5-3 mcg/kg/min administered with nitrous oxide/oxygen in patients undergoing general surgery. Following an anesthetic induction dose of alfentanil, infusion rate requirements are reduced by 30%-50% for the first hour of maintenance. Changes in vital signs that indicate a response to surgical stress or lightening of anesthesia may be controlled by increasing the alfentanil to a maximum of 4 mcg/kg/min and/or administration of bolus doses of 7 mcg/kg. If changes are not controlled after three bolus doses given over a 5-minute period, a barbiturate, vasodilator, and/or inhalation agent should be used. Infusion rates should always be adjusted downward in the absence of these signs until there is some response to surgical stimulation. Rather than an increase in infusion rate, 7 mcg/kg bolus doses of alfentanil or a potent inhalation agent should be administered in response to signs of lightening of anesthesia within the last 15 minutes of surgery. Alfentanil infusion should be discontinued at least 10 to 15 minutes before the end of surgery. Discontinue 10 to 15 minutes before end of procedures in general anesthesia. Continue infusion to end of procedure during MAC, then discontinue.

PEDIATRIC DOSE

Safety for use in pediatric patients under 12 years of age not established; not recommended. Half-life and duration of action is decreased in pediatric patients; more frequent supplemental doses may be required; see Maternal/Child.

Anesthesia adjunct (unlabeled): *Loading dose:* 0.03 to 0.05 mg/kg (30 to 50 mcg/kg). Follow with supplemental single doses of 0.01 to 0.015 mg/kg (10 to 15 mcg/kg) or a continuous infusion at a rate of 0.0005 to 0.0015 mg/kg/min (0.5 to 1.5 mcg/kg/min).

DOSE ADJUSTMENTS

Reduce dose of one or both agents when given in combination with other CNS depressants (e.g., barbiturates, inhalation anesthetics, narcotic analgesics, tranquilizers). ▪ Calculate dose based on lean body weight in obese patients (more than 20% above ideal body weight). ▪ Reduced initial dose required in elderly or debilitated patients (a 40%

Continued

reduction was required in one study); reduced supplemental doses, a slower infusion rate, or longer intervals between doses may be required based on effects of initial dose. ■ Doses appropriate for general population may cause serious respiratory depression in vulnerable patients. ■ Reduced dose may be required in hypothyroidism and in impaired hepatic function. ■ See Drug/Lab Interactions.

DILUTION

IV injection: Small volumes may be given undiluted (usually by the anesthesiologist). Use of tuberculin syringe recommended (1 mL equals 500 mcg). Further dilution with 5 mL of SW or NS to facilitate titration is appropriate.

Infusion: Dilute 20 mL alfentanil with 230 mL NS, D5NS, D5W, or LR to achieve a concentration of 40 mcg/mL. Desired concentration range is 25 to 80 mcg/mL.

Storage: Store ampules at CRT; protect from light and freezing.

COMPATIBILITY

Consider any drug NOT listed as compatible to be INCOMPATIBLE until consulting a pharmacist; specific conditions may apply.

One source suggests the following **compatibilities:**

Y-site: Bivalirudin (Angiomax), cisatracurium (Nimbex), dexmedetomidine (Precedex), etomidate (Amidate), fenoldopam (Corlopam), hetastarch in electrolytes (Hextend), linezolid (Zyvox), propofol (Diprivan), remifentanil (Ultiva).

RATE OF ADMINISTRATION

IV injection: Administer over a minimum of 3 minutes. Rapid administration of lower doses or administration of full anesthetic doses will result in muscle rigidity, apnea, respiratory paralysis, loss of vascular tone, and hypotension. Titrate rate to desired patient response.

Infusion: See Usual Dose.

ACTIONS

An opioid derivative, narcotic analgesic, and descending CNS depressant. Less potent than fentanyl milligram for milligram, but achieves higher plasma concentrations. Produces hypnosis and respiratory depressant actions that outlast its analgesic effect. Onset of action is immediate. Produces analgesic effects in 1 minute. Peak effect (respiratory depression and analgesia) occurs within 1½ to 2 minutes. With induction doses, loss of consciousness occurs within 1 to 2 minutes. Provides dose-related protection against hemodynamic responses to surgical stress. Histamine release rarely occurs. May cause rigidity of chest, pharynx, and abdominal muscles, inhibiting ventilation; see Precautions/Monitor, Side Effects, Antidote. Duration of action is 5 to 10 minutes. Has a terminal half-life of 90 to 111 minutes. Cumulative effects are somewhat less than with fentanyl or sufentanil, but with repeat doses recovery may be prolonged. Recovery should occur within 10 to 15 minutes of end of procedure or 25 to 30 minutes after last incremental dose or discontinuing the infusion. Metabolized in the liver. Excreted as metabolites in urine. Crosses the placental barrier. Secreted in breast milk.

INDICATIONS AND USES

Analgesic adjunct given in incremental doses in the maintenance of anesthesia with barbiturate/nitrous oxide/oxygen. ■ Analgesic administered by continuous infusion with nitrous oxide/oxygen in the maintenance of general anesthesia. ■ Primary anesthetic agent for the induction of anesthesia in patients undergoing general surgery requiring endotracheal intubation and mechanical ventilation. ■ Analgesic component for monitored anesthesia care (MAC) during surgical or diagnostic procedures.

CONTRAINDICATIONS

Known hypersensitivity to alfentanil or known intolerance to other opioid agonists (e.g., fentanyl, sufentanil). Use during labor and delivery not recommended. In general narcotic analgesics are also contraindicated in acute or severe bronchial asthma and if an upper airway obstruction or significant respiratory depression is present.

PRECAUTIONS

For IV use only. ■ Administered by or under the direct observations of the anesthesiologist. Must have responsibility only for anesthesia and continuous observation of the patient during surgery and/or procedure. ■ Staff must be skilled in medical management of critically ill patients, cardiovascular resuscitation, and airway management. ■ Use caution; plasma clearance reduced and recovery time prolonged in the elderly and in patients with impaired liver function (half-life prolonged [up to 5.8 hours]); reduced dose may be indicated. ■ Use caution in patients with pulmonary disease, decreased respiratory reserve, or potentially compromised respiration. May cause rigidity of chest and abdominal muscles, decrease respiratory drive, and increase airway resistance; may require assisted or controlled ventilation. ■ Use caution in patients with head injury or increased intracranial pressure; risk of respiratory depression is increased. ■ Respiratory depression may cause an increased PCO_2, cerebral vasodilation, and increased intracranial pressure. Clinical course of head injury may be obscured. ■ Use caution in patients with bradyarrhythmias. ■ Use caution in patients with hypothyroidism; risk of respiratory depression and prolonged CNS depression is increased. Reduced doses may be indicated. ■ See Drug/Lab Interactions.

Monitor: Oxygen, controlled ventilation equipment, opioid antagonists (e.g., naloxone [Narcan]), and neuromuscular blocking agents (e.g., pancuronium, succinylcholine) and all emergency drugs and equipment must be immediately available. Can cause rigidity of respiratory muscles; concurrent use of a neuromuscular blocking agent can prevent or reverse muscle rigidity to permit controlled ventilation. ■ Adequate preoperative hydration is recommended to reduce incidence of hypotension. ■ Observe for hypotension, apnea, upper airway obstruction, and/or oxygen desaturation. Monitor vital signs and oxygen saturation continuously. If not unconscious, patient will appear to be asleep and forget to breathe unless commanded to do so. ■ Additional doses of alfentanil can be used to control tachycardia and hypertension during surgery. ■ Prolonged postoperative monitoring may be indicated; respiratory depression, respiratory arrest, bradycardia, asystole, arrhythmias, and hypotension may occur after initial recovery. ■ Keep patient supine; orthostatic hypotension and fainting may occur. ■ Has a short duration of action; pain medication may be required soon after initial recovery. ■ See Precautions and Drug/Lab Interactions.

Patient Education: Avoid alcohol or other CNS depressants (e.g., antihistamines, benzodiazepines [e.g., diazepam (Valium)]). ■ Blurred vision, dizziness, drowsiness, or light-headedness may occur; request assistance with ambulation. ■ Review all medications for interactions.

Maternal/Child: Category C: safety for use in pregnancy not established; has embryocidal effects in rats and rabbits. ▪ Not recommended for use during labor and delivery. ▪ Postpone breast-feeding for at least 24 hours after use of alfentanil. ▪ Muscle rigidity is more common in neonates than in older children or adults.

Elderly: See Dose Adjustments and Precautions. ▪ May markedly decrease pulmonary ventilation. ▪ Decreased protein binding, decreased clearance, and possible increased brain sensitivity may make the elderly more sensitive to effects (e.g., respiratory depression, extended recovery time, urinary retention, constipation). ▪ Lower doses may provide effective analgesia. ▪ Consider age-related organ impairment; elimination half-life is extended, postoperative recovery may be delayed.

DRUG/LAB INTERACTIONS

Use of **benzodiazepines** (e.g., diazepam [Valium], midazolam [Versed]) may decrease dose of alfentanil required and decrease patient recall, but when given immediately before or in conjunction with high doses of alfentanil, benzodiazepines may produce vasodilation, severe hypotension, and result in delayed recovery. ▪ After an anesthetic induction dose of alfentanil, requirements for **volatile inhalation anesthetics** (e.g., nitrous oxide) **and/or alfentanil infusion** are reduced by 30% to 50% for the first hour of maintenance. ▪ **Beta-adrenergic blocking agents** (e.g., metoprolol, timolol) may be used preoperatively to decrease hypertensive episodes during surgical procedures, but chronic use (including ophthalmic preparations) may also increase the risk of initial bradycardia. ▪ Respiratory depression, CNS depression, hypotensive effects, and duration of action increased with concomitant administration of other **CNS depressants** (e.g., antidepressants, antihistamines, barbiturates, benzodiazepines, haloperidol, inhalation anesthetics, narcotic analgesics, phenothiazines). Reduced doses of one or both agents usually required. ▪ Clearance decreased by **cimetidine** (Tagamet) **and erythromycin;** risk of prolonged or delayed respiratory depression may be increased. ▪ Respiratory depressant effects are additive with **neuromuscular blocking agents** (e.g., pancuronium, succinylcholine). ▪ Other opioids have caused severe hypertension with **MAO inhibitors** (e.g., selegiline [Eldepryl]). Use extreme caution; beta-blockers (e.g., propranolol) and vasodilators (e.g., nitroglycerin) should be available. ▪ Duration of action may be prolonged with other **agents that inhibit hepatic enzymes** (e.g., azole antifungals [e.g., itraconazole (Sporanox)], beta-blockers [e.g., metoprolol (Lopressor), propranolol, timolol (Novo-Timol)], calcium channel blockers [e.g., diltiazem (Cardizem), verapamil], fluoroquinolones [e.g., ciprofloxacin (Cipro), levofloxacin (Levaquin)], MAO inhibitors). ▪ Monitor closely for S/S of respiratory depression and CNS depression with concurrent use of **protease inhibitors** (e.g., saquinavir [Invirase], ritonavir [Norvir]). ▪ Use of **naltrexone** (ReVia) would require increased doses of alfentanil; may cause prolonged respiratory depression and/or circulatory collapse. Discontinue naltrexone several days before elective surgery if use of an opioid is necessary. ▪ Analgesic effects may be antagonized by **opioid agonist/antagonist analgesics;** may also cause additive CNS and respiratory depressant effects. ▪ May delay **gastric emptying** and invalidate diagnostic tests. ▪ May interfere with some **hepatobiliary imaging.** ▪ Delay **plasma amylase and lipase measurements** for at least 24 hours.

SIDE EFFECTS

Average dose: Bradycardia and hypotension may occur shortly after administration. Respiratory depression caused by alfentanil and/or muscle rigidity may progress to apnea. Agitation, arrhythmias (e.g., bradycardia, tachycardia), blurred vision, bradypnea, chest wall rigidity, dizziness, euphoria, headache, hypercapnia (increased CO_2), hypersensitivity reactions (e.g., anaphylaxis, bronchospasm, itching, laryngospasm, urticaria), hypertension, hypotension, muscle rigidity (skeletal muscles including abdomen, chest, pharynx, neck, and extremities), myoclonic movements, nausea, postoperative confusion, respiratory sedation, shivering, skeletal muscle movements, sleepiness, vomiting.

Overdose: Bradycardia; circulatory depression; cold, clammy skin; dizziness (severe); drowsiness (severe); hypotension; nervousness or restlessness (severe); pinpoint pupils of eyes; respiratory depression; weakness (severe).

ANTIDOTE

Many side effects are medical emergencies. Manage respiratory depression during surgery via endotracheal intubation and assisted or controlled ventilation; prolonged mechanical ventilation may be required. Treat postoperative respiratory depression with naloxone (Narcan); titrate dose carefully to improve respirations without reversing analgesic effects or causing other adverse effects (hypertension and tachycardia may result in left ventricular failure and pulmonary edema, especially in cardiac patients). Treat bradycardia with atropine, or alfentanil-induced bradycardia can be antagonized with the use of a neuromuscular blocking agent with vagolytic activity (e.g., pancuronium). Treat hypotension by placing the patient in a Trendelenburg position, if possible; administer IV fluids and a vasopressor (e.g., norepinephrine [Levophed], dopamine) if indicated. Naloxone may reverse hypotension postoperatively. Muscle rigidity during anesthesia induction or surgery must be controlled with neuromuscular blocking agents and controlled ventilation with oxygen. Use a neuromuscular blocking agent prophylactically to prevent muscle rigidity or to induce muscle relaxation after rigidity occurs. Neuromuscular blocking agents with vagolytic activity (e.g., pancuronium) may decrease risk of alfentanil-induced bradycardia and hypotension, but may increase the risk of hypertension or tachycardia in some patients. In patients with compromised cardiac function and/or those receiving a beta-adrenergic blocking agent preoperatively, a nonvagolytic neuromuscular blocking agent (e.g., succinylcholine) may increase the incidence and severity of bradycardia and hypotension. Respiratory depressant effects of neuromuscular blocking agents are additive with alfentanil. Postoperatively, naloxone may be used in small incremental doses to reverse skeletal muscle rigidity. Resuscitate as necessary.

ALGLUCOSIDASE ALFA BBW

(**AL**-gloo-**KOE**-si-dase **AL**-fa)

Lumizyme

Enzyme replenisher

USUAL DOSE

Premedication: Pretreatment with antihistamines (e.g., diphenhydramine [Benadryl]), antipyretics (e.g., acetaminophen [Tylenol]), and/or corticosteroids (e.g., dexamethasone [Decadron]) may be considered; see Precautions and Monitor.

Alglucosidase alfa: 20 mg/kg of body weight as an infusion every 2 weeks.

PEDIATRIC DOSE

Pediatric patients 8 years of age and older: See Usual Dose. Pediatric patients younger than 8 years were not included in clinical trials.

DOSE ADJUSTMENTS

None indicated.

DILUTION

Each vial contains 50 mg of alglucosidase alfa. Determine the number of vials needed to provide the calculated dose. Patient weight in kg multiplied by the dose in mg/kg equals the patient dose. The number of vials needed is calculated by dividing the total dose in mg by 50 (the number of mg in one vial). For example, a 68-kg patient would receive a 1,360-mg dose (68 kg × 20 mg/kg = 1,360 mg). 1,360 mg divided by 50 mg/vial equals 27.2 vials. Round up or down to the closest whole number, so 27 vials would be required (confirm with the prescribing physician). Before reconstitution, allow vials and diluent to reach room temperature (should take approximately 30 minutes). Reconstitute each vial with 10.3 mL SW. *Do not use a filter needle during any step of the alglucosidase alfa dilution process; see Filters.* Direct diluent by slowly releasing each drop down the inside wall of each vial. Avoid forceful impact of the SW on the lyophilized cake, and avoid foaming. Roll and tilt each vial gently to dissolve; *do not invert, swirl, or shake.* Protect reconstituted solution from light. Total extractable volume in each vial is 50 mg in 10 mL (5 mg/mL). A few thin white strands or translucent fibers are expected and will filter out during administration. Must be further diluted in a specific amount of NS *immediately* after reconstitution. See chart under Rate of Administration for specific volume of diluent to use based on weight in kg. Total infusion volume for a 68-kg patient equals 500 mL (270 mL of alglucosidase alfa and 230 mL NS). Remove excess volume from the infusion bag to achieve the desired volume (270 mL of NS for the preceding example). Remove air space from the infusion bag containing the desired volume for dilution to minimize particle formation resulting from the sensitivity of alglucosidase alfa to air-liquid interfaces. Next, slowly withdraw the calculated dose of drug from the reconstituted vials (a total of 270 mL in the preceding example) and add it to the NS remaining in the infusion bag (230 mL in the preceding example). *Must be added into the fluid itself and not into the air space of the infusion bag.* Use only clear solutions. Gently invert or massage the infusion bag to mix the solution. *Avoid foaming. Do not shake.*

Filters: *Do not use filter needles during reconstitution or dilution.* Filter diluted solution through an in-line, low–protein binding, 0.2-micron filter for administration.

Storage: Refrigerate unopened vials at 2° to 8° C (36° to 46° F). Do not use after the expiration date on the vial. Immediate use of reconstituted and diluted solutions is preferred but, if necessary, they may be refrigerated for up to 24 hours. Discard unused reconstituted solution. Protect from light and do not freeze or shake. For single use only; discard unused drug.

COMPATIBILITY

Manufacturer states, "Should not be infused in the same IV line with other products."

RATE OF ADMINISTRATION

Use of an infusion pump required. Diluted solution should be filtered through an in-line, low–protein binding, 0.2-micron filter for administration. Begin with an **initial infusion rate** of no more than 1 mg/kg/hr. After patient tolerance is established, the infusion may be increased by 2 mg/kg/hr every 30 minutes until a **maximum infusion rate** of 7 mg/kg/hr is reached. Obtain vital signs at the end of each step. Should an infusion reaction occur at any step, slow or temporarily discontinue the infusion until symptoms subside. Additional premedication may be indicated. If the patient remains stable, continue at 7 mg/kg/hr until the infusion is complete (approximately 4 hours). Total volume of infusion is determined by the patient's body weight. Volume and rate of infusion for given weight ranges are listed in the following chart.

Recommended Alglucosidase Alfa Infusion Volumes and Rates					
Patient Weight Range (kg)	Total Infusion Volume (mL)	Step 1 1 mg/kg/hr (mL/hr)	Step 2 3 mg/kg/hr (mL/hr)	Step 3 5 mg/kg/hr (mL/hr)	Step 4 7 mg/kg/hr (mL/hr)
20.1-30 kg	150 mL	8 mL/hr	23 mL/hr	38 mL/hr	53 mL/hr
30.1-35 kg	200 mL	10 mL/hr	30 mL/hr	50 mL/hr	70 mL/hr
35.1-50 kg	250 mL	13 mL/hr	38 mL/hr	63 mL/hr	88 mL/hr
50.1-60 kg	300 mL	15 mL/hr	45 mL/hr	75 mL/hr	105 mL/hr
60.1-100 kg	500 mL	25 mL/hr	75 mL/hr	125 mL/hr	175 mL/hr
100.1-120 kg	600 mL	30 mL/hr	90 mL/hr	150 mL/hr	210 mL/hr
120.1-140 kg	700 mL	35 mL/hr	105 mL/hr	175 mL/hr	245 mL/hr
140.1-160 kg	800 mL	40 mL/hr	120 mL/hr	200 mL/hr	280 mL/hr
160.1-180 kg	900 mL	45 mL/hr	135 mL/hr	225 mL/hr	315 mL/hr
180.1-200 kg	1,000 mL	50 mL/hr	150 mL/hr	250 mL/hr	350 mL/hr

ACTIONS

Alglucosidase consists of the human enzyme acid alpha glucosidase, which is produced by recombinant DNA technology in a Chinese hamster ovary cell line. Pompe disease is an inherited disorder of glycogen metabolism caused by the deficiency or absence of GAA. GAA is required for glycogen cleavage. Without GAA, glycogen accumulates in tissue, leading to progressive muscle weakness. Alglucosidase binds to receptors on the cell surface, where it is internalized and transported into lysosomes, resulting in increased enzymatic activity and glycogen cleavage. Half-life is 2 to 3 hours.

INDICATIONS AND USES

A lysosomal glycogen-specific enzyme indicated for patients 8 years and older with late (non-infantile) onset of Pompe disease (GAA deficiency) who do not have evidence of cardiac hypertrophy. ■ Another formulation of alglucosidase alfa (Myozyme) is indicated to improve ventilator-free survival in infantile-onset Pompe disease.

CONTRAINDICATIONS

Manufacturer states, "None;" see Precautions.

PRECAUTIONS

Administer under the direction of a physician knowledgeable in its use in a facility with adequate diagnostic and treatment facilities to monitor the patient and respond to any medical emergency. ■ Because of rapid disease progression in Pompe disease patients less than 8 years of age, alglucosidase alfa is available only through a restricted distribution program called the LUMIZYME ACE Program. Only prescribers and health care facilities enrolled can prescribe, dispense, and administer it. Patients must be enrolled in and meet all conditions of the program. ■ Infusion and/or hypersensitivity reactions may be life threatening and have included anaphylactic shock, apnea, bradycardia, dyspnea, hypotension, respiratory arrest, and tachycardia. ■ Other reactions include angioedema (including tongue or lip swelling, periorbital edema, and face edema), back pain, bronchospasm, chest discomfort/pain, convulsions, cyanosis, decreased oxygen saturation/hypoxia, dizziness, feeling hot, fever, flushing/erythema, headache, hyperhidrosis, hypertension, nausea, nervousness, pallor, paresthesia, peripheral coldness, pruritus, rash, restlessness, tachypnea, throat tightness, urticaria, and wheezing. Some reactions were IgE mediated. ■ Severe cutaneous reactions, including necrotizing skin lesions, have been reported. Systemic immune-mediated reactions have been observed. May occur several weeks to 3 years after initiation of therapy. ■ Use caution when administering a general anesthetic to patients with Pompe disease. ■ During infusions patients with acute underlying respiratory illness or compromised cardiac and/or respiratory function may be at risk for serious cardiac or respiratory compromise. ■ Use extreme care if a decision is made to readminister after a severe hypersensitivity reaction. Some patients have been rechallenged and have been able to continue therapy under close clinical supervision. **Monitor:** Obtain baseline vital signs and repeat as needed and with each increase in dosage. ■ Severe reactions may require infusion interruption, administration of antihistamines, corticosteroids, IV fluids, and/or oxygen. ■ Patients with acute underlying respiratory illness or compromised cardiac and/or respiratory function may require prolonged observation times. ■ If anaphylaxis or severe allergic reaction occurs, discontinue immediately and initiate appropriate medical treatment; epinephrine may be indicated. ■ Monitor for development of systemic immune complex–mediated reactions involving the skin and other organs. ■ Patients should be monitored every 3 months for 2 years and annually thereafter for formation of IgG antibodies. ■ Patients who develop IgG antibodies may be evaluated for inhibition of enzyme activity or cellular uptake of enzyme. ■ There is no marketed test for antibodies against alglucosidase alfa; contact the Genzyme Corporation for further information.

Patient Education: Promptly report early symptoms of a hypersensitivity or infusion reaction (e.g., chills or rigors, difficulty breathing, fever, flushing, headache, itching, rash, shortness of breath). ▪ Discuss possible delayed infusion reaction and follow-up instructions with a health care professional. ▪ Patients must be enrolled and meet all conditions in the proper registry to receive alglucosidase alfa.

Maternal/Child: Category B: use during pregnancy only if clearly needed. A pregnancy registry has been established. Enrollment is encouraged during pregnancy, labor and delivery, and breast-feeding; contact manufacturer. ▪ Effects when used during labor and delivery are not known. ▪ Effects during breast-feeding unknown; use caution. ▪ Safety and effectiveness for use in patients with infantile-onset Pompe disease or late (noninfantile) onset Pompe disease who are less than 8 years of age has not been established.

Elderly: Numbers in clinical studies insufficient to determine if the elderly respond differently from younger subjects.

DRUG/LAB INTERACTIONS
Drug interaction studies have not been conducted.

SIDE EFFECTS
The most common adverse reactions are infusion reactions (including anaphylaxis), diarrhea, dyspnea, flushing/feeling hot, loss of hearing, neck pain, pain in extremity, pharyngolaryngeal pain, pruritus, rash/erythema, urticaria, and vomiting. Serious adverse reactions include anaphylactic reactions such as angioedema, chest pain/discomfort, and throat tightness. Other serious adverse reactions include coronary artery disease, dehydration, gastroenteritis, intervertebral disk protrusion, and pneumonia. Additional infusion reactions include agitation, cough, increased lacrimation, irritability, livedo reticularis, respiratory distress, retching, rigors, and tremor. Delayed-onset infusion reactions include dizziness; epistaxis; insomnia; malaise; muscle spasms; musculoskeletal pain, stiffness, and weakness; neck pain; pharyngolaryngeal pain; and urticaria.

Post-Marketing: Deaths resulted from aortic dissection, cardiac failure, cardiorespiratory arrest, CVA, hemothorax, pneumothorax, respiratory failure, sepsis, and skin necrosis. Bronchospasm, cyanosis, hypoxia, hypertension, hypotension, lung infection, stridor, systemic and cutaneous immune-mediated reactions (including necrotizing skin lesions), and tachycardia have been reported.

ANTIDOTE
Keep physician informed of side effects; may be treated symptomatically if indicated. If an infusion reaction occurs, reduce rate or discontinue alglucosidase alfa until symptoms subside. Additional antipyretics (e.g., acetaminophen [Tylenol]), antihistamines (e.g., diphenhydramine [Benadryl]), or corticosteroids (e.g., dexamethasone [Decadron]) may be indicated. With additional premedication and/or a reduction in the rate of infusion, patients may be able to continue treatment. If a severe infusion reaction, hypersensitivity, or anaphylactic reaction occurs, discontinue alglucosidase alfa immediately and treat as indicated. Cardiopulmonary resuscitation, mechanical ventilatory support, oxygen supplementation, IV fluids, antihistamines (e.g., diphenhydramine [Benadryl]), inhaled beta-adrenergic agonists (e.g., albuterol [Ventolin]), epinephrine (Adrenalin), and IV corticosteroids (e.g., hydrocortisone sodium succinate [Solu-Cortef]) have been required.

ALLOPURINOL SODIUM
(al-oh-**PYOUR**-ih-nohl **SO**-dee-um)

Aloprim

Antigout
Antihyperuricemic
Antineoplastic adjunct

pH 10.8 to 11.8

USUAL DOSE

IV and oral doses are therapeutically equivalent. Oral dose can replace an IV dose at any time. See Monitor.

200 to 400 mg/M^2/day as a single infusion or in equally divided doses at 6-, 8-, or 12-hour intervals (50 to 100 mg/M^2 every 6 hours, 67 to 133 mg/M^2 every 8 hours, or 100 to 200 mg/M^2 every 12 hours). Total dose should not exceed 600 mg/day.

PEDIATRIC DOSE

Recommended starting dose is 200 mg/M^2/day. Usually given in equally divided doses at 6- to 8-hour intervals (50 mg/M^2 every 6 hours or 67 mg/M^2 every 8 hours). Another source says the daily dose may be given at 6-, 8-, or 12-hour intervals or as a single daily infusion. Studies found no significant difference in dose response in pediatric patients. An alternate source suggests 10 mg/kg/day with a maximum total dose of 600 mg/day (2.5 mg/M^2 every 6 hours, 3.3 mg/M^2 every 8 hours, or 5 mg/M^2 every 12 hours). See comments in Usual Dose.

DOSE ADJUSTMENTS

Dialysis patients may require the usual dose of allopurinol. In patients with impaired renal function not on dialysis, reduce dose based on CrCl according to the following chart.

Allopurinol Dosing in Impaired Renal Function	
CrCl (mL/min)	Dose
10-20 mL/min	200 mg daily
3-10 mL/min	100 mg daily
<3 mL/min	100 mg daily at extended intervals (more than 24 hr if necessary)

Treat with the lowest effective dose to minimize side effects. ▪ Dose with normal renal function may be increased or decreased based on electrolytes and serum uric acid levels. ▪ Lower doses and/or extended intervals may be required in the elderly; consider potential for decreased organ function, concomitant disease, or other drug therapy. ▪ See Drug/Lab Interactions.

DILUTION

Available as a single-dose vial containing 500 mg of allopurinol. Reconstitute with 25 mL of SW for injection (yields 20 mg/mL). Swirl until completely dissolved. Must be further diluted with NS or D5W. Maximum concentration for administration is 6 mg/mL. 19 mL of additional diluent per 20 mg (1 mL) yields 1 mg/mL, 9 mL of additional diluent yields 2 mg/mL, and 2.3 mL of additional diluent yields 6 mg/mL.

Storage: Store unopened vials at CRT. Do not refrigerate the reconstituted and/or diluted product; begin infusion within 10 hours of reconstitution.

COMPATIBILITY

Consider any drug NOT listed as compatible to be INCOMPATIBLE until consulting a pharmacist; specific conditions may apply.
Manufacturer recommends administering sequentially and flushing before and after administration. Manufacturer lists the following drugs as **incompatible:** amikacin (Amikin), amphotericin B (generic), carmustine (BiCNU), cefotaxime (Claforan), chlorpromazine (Thorazine), clindamycin (Cleocin), cytarabine (ARA-C), dacarbazine (DTIC), daunorubicin (Cerubidine), diphenhydramine (Benadryl), doxorubicin (Adriamycin), doxycycline, droperidol (Inapsine), floxuridine (FUDR), gentamicin, haloperidol (Haldol), idarubicin (Idamycin), imipenem-cilastatin (Primaxin), mechlorethamine (nitrogen mustard) (Mustargen), meperidine (Demerol), methylprednisolone (Solu-Medrol), metoclopramide (Reglan), minocycline (Minocin), nalbuphine, ondansetron (Zofran), prochlorperazine (Compazine), promethazine (Phenergan), sodium bicarbonate, streptozocin (Zanosar), tobramycin, vinorelbine (Navelbine). *Do not use solutions containing sodium bicarbonate.*

One source suggests the following **compatibilities:**
Y-site: Acyclovir (Zovirax), aminophylline, aztreonam (Azactam), bleomycin (Blenoxane), bumetanide, buprenorphine (Buprenex), butorphanol (Stadol), calcium gluconate, carboplatin (Paraplatin), cefazolin (Ancef), cefotetan, ceftazidime (Fortaz), ceftriaxone (Rocephin), cefuroxime (Zinacef), cisplatin (Platinol), cyclophosphamide (Cytoxan), dactinomycin (Cosmegen), dexamethasone (Decadron), doxorubicin liposomal (Doxil), enalaprilat (Vasotec IV), etoposide (VePesid), famotidine (Pepcid IV), filgrastim (Neupogen), fluconazole (Diflucan), fludarabine (Fludara), fluorouracil (5-FU), furosemide (Lasix), gallium nitrate (Ganite), ganciclovir (Cytovene), granisetron (Kytril), heparin, hydrocortisone sodium succinate (Solu-Cortef), hydromorphone (Dilaudid), ifosfamide (Ifex), lorazepam (Ativan), mannitol, mesna (Mesnex), methotrexate, metronidazole (Flagyl IV), mitoxantrone (Novantrone), morphine, piperacillin, potassium chloride (KCl), ranitidine (Zantac), sulfamethoxazole/trimethoprim, teniposide (Vumon), thiotepa, ticarcillin/clavulanate (Timentin), vancomycin, vinblastine, vincristine, zidovudine (AZT, Retrovir).

RATE OF ADMINISTRATION

Manufacturer's recommendation not available. A maximum dose should take at least ½ to 1 hour or more based on volume with diluent and patient comfort and/or requirements. Include in hydration fluids. See Compatibility.

ACTIONS

A xanthine oxidase inhibitor. Metabolized to oxypurinol. Acts on purine catabolism without disrupting the biosynthesis of purines. Reduces the production of uric acid by inhibiting the biochemical reactions immediately preceding its formation. Decreases uric acid concentrations in both serum and urine. Prevents or decreases urate deposition, decreasing the occurrence or progression of gout or urate nephropathy. Onset of action is within 10 minutes. Reduction of serum uric acid concentration occurs in 2 to 3 days. Peak concentrations are related to dose. Pharmacokinetic and plasma profiles of allopurinol and oxypurinol, as well as half-lives and systemic clearance, are similar with IV or oral administration. Systemic exposure to oxypurinol is also similar by both routes at each dose level. Cleared by glomerular filtration; some oxypurinol is reabsorbed in the kidney tubules. Secreted in breast milk.

INDICATIONS AND USES
Management of patients with leukemia, lymphoma, and solid tumor malignancies who are receiving cancer therapy that causes elevations of serum and urinary uric acid levels and who cannot tolerate oral therapy. Consider prophylactic use before initiation of and during chemotherapy in patients who are NPO, are nauseated and vomiting, or have malabsorption problems, dysphagia, or GI tract dysfunctions. IV route is used to attain rapid, significant blood levels; accurately dose pediatric patients; and dose patients with questionable compliance. Used prophylactically before the initiation of and during chemotherapy to prevent tumor lysis syndrome (TLS) and its sequela, acute uric acid nephropathy (AUAN).
Unlabeled uses: Preservation of cadaveric kidneys for transplantation.

CONTRAINDICATIONS
Any patient who has had a severe reaction to allopurinol (usually a hypersensitivity reaction).

PRECAUTIONS
For IV infusion only. ■ A skin rash or other beginning signs of hypersensitivity may be followed by exfoliative, urticarial, and purpuric lesions; Stevens-Johnson syndrome; generalized vasculitis; irreversible hepatotoxicity; and/or rarely death. ■ Incidence of hypersensitivity reactions may be increased in patients with decreased renal function especially in those receiving concurrent thiazides (e.g., chlorothiazide [Diuril]); use with caution. ■ See Drug/Lab Interactions.
Monitor: Whenever possible, begin allopurinol therapy 24 to 48 hours before the start of chemotherapy known to cause tumor cell lysis (including adrenocorticosteroids). ■ Monitor serum uric acid levels and electrolytes before and during therapy. Monitor serum uric acid levels to determine dose and frequency required to maintain uric acid levels within the normal range. ■ Hydration with 3,000 mL/M^2/day (twice the level of maintenance fluid replacement) is recommended to promote a high volume of urine output (more than 2 L/day in adults) with low urate concentration. ■ Maintain urine at neutral or slightly alkaline pH. To increase solubility of uric acid, alkalinity of urine may be increased with sodium bicarbonate. ■ Monitor renal and hepatic systems before and during therapy. ■ Monitoring of liver function suggested in patients with pre-existing liver disease, in patients with increases in liver function tests, and in patients who develop anorexia, pruritus, or weight loss. ■ Observe for symptoms of TLS (e.g., hyperuricemia, hyperkalemia, hyperphosphatemia, and hypocalcemia). If untreated, may develop AUAN leading to renal failure requiring hemodialysis. ■ Bone marrow suppression has been reported; monitor CBC periodically.
Patient Education: Report promptly blood in the urine, painful urination, irritation of the eyes, skin rash, or swelling of the lips or mouth. ■ Major acute toxicities may be allergic or renal. ■ May cause drowsiness; use caution in activities that require alertness. Request assistance for ambulation.
Maternal/Child: Category C: potential benefits must justify potential risks to fetus. ■ Use caution if required during breast-feeding.

Elderly: Lower-end initial doses or extended intervals may be appropriate in the elderly; see Dose Adjustments.

DRUG/LAB INTERACTIONS

May increase toxicity of **didanosine** (Videx); concurrent use not recommended. ▪ Inhibits metabolism and increases effects and toxicity of **thiopurines** (e.g., azathioprine [Imuran], mercaptopurine [Purinethol]). Reduce dose of thiopurine to one third to one fourth. ▪ **Uricosuric agents** (e.g., sulfinpyrazone [Anturane], probenecid [Benemid], colchicine) may increase elimination of active metabolites of allopurinol; may increase urinary excretions of uric acid. ▪ Prolongs half-life of **dicumarol;** monitor PT or PTT and adjust anticoagulant dose as indicated. ▪ Frequency of skin rash increased with **ampicillin/amoxicillin.** ▪ Bone marrow suppression may be increased when given concurrently with **cytotoxic agents** (e.g., cyclophosphamide [Cytoxan]); risk of bleeding or infection may be increased. ▪ May prolong half-life of **chlorpropamide** (Diabinese). ▪ Hypersensitivity reactions may be increased with **ACE inhibitors** (e.g., enalaprilat) **or thiazide diuretics** (e.g., chlorothiazide [Diuril]). ▪ Concurrent use with **cyclosporine** (Sandimmune) may increase cyclosporine serum levels. A reduced dose of cyclosporine may be indicated; monitoring of cyclosporine serum levels suggested. ▪ Larger doses (more than 600 mg/day) may decrease clearance and increase toxicity of **theophyllines** (e.g., Aminophylline).

SIDE EFFECTS

Fewer than 1% of patients have had side effects directly attributable to allopurinol. Most were hypersensitivity reactions (e.g., nausea and vomiting, rash, and renal failure/insufficiency) and of mild to moderate severity. Xanthine crystalluria has been rarely reported in long-term therapy with oral allopurinol.

ANTIDOTE

Discontinue allopurinol at the first sign of skin rash or any other allergic reaction. Do not restart. Keep physician informed of all side effects. Symptoms of TLS require immediate intervention and correction of electrolyte abnormalities to avoid kidney damage. Treat hypersensitivity reactions as indicated; may require epinephrine (Adrenalin), diphenhydramine (Benadryl), corticosteroids (hydrocortisone), and/or oxygen. Allopurinol is dialyzable, but effectiveness of hemodialysis or peritoneal dialysis in an overdose is not known.

ALPHA₁-PROTEINASE INHIBITOR (HUMAN)

Alpha₁-antitrypsin replenisher

(**AL**-fah **PRO**-teen-ayse in-**HIB**-ih-ter [**HU**-man])

Alpha₁-antitrypsin, Alpha₁-PI,
Aralast, Glassia, Prolastin, Zemaira

pH 7.2 to 7.8 (Aralast) ■
pH 6.6 to 7.4 (Prolastin)

USUAL DOSE

60 mg/kg once a week as an infusion.

Manufacturers of Prolastin recommend immunizing every patient against hepatitis B before administration. If immediate treatment is required, give a single dose of hepatitis B immune globulin (human) 0.06 mL/kg IM at the same time as the initial dose of hepatitis B vaccine.

DILUTION

All preparations: Bring components to room temperature (diluent [SW], lyophilized preparation of alpha₁-PI, or ready-to-use solution). Must be used within 3 hours of reconstitution or entry into vial. Must be filtered before or during administration.

Aralast and Prolastin: Insert one end of the double-ended transfer needle (shortest end for Prolastin) into the diluent. Invert the bottle of diluent and insert the other end of the transfer needle at a 45-degree angle into the alpha₁-PI; diluent will be drawn into the alpha₁-PI by a vacuum. Remove the diluent bottle and transfer device. Allow the reconstituted solution to stand until contents appear to be in solution, then swirl gently to completely dissolve. May take 5 to 10 minutes. *Do not shake or invert vial until ready to withdraw contents.*

Glassia: Available as a single-use vial containing 1 Gm of functional alpha₁-PI in 50 mL of ready-to-use solution. Solution should be clear and colorless to yellow-green. Do not use if product is cloudy. Infusion can be made directly from the vial, or vials may be pooled in an empty, sterile IV container. When infusing directly from the vial, use a vented spike adapter and a 5-micron in-line filter (neither is supplied). When infusing from a sterile IV container, use a vent filter (not supplied) to withdraw Glassia from the vial, and then use the supplied 5-micron filter needle to transfer Glassia into the infusion container. Attach an IV administration set and administer through a 5-micron in-line filter (not supplied).

Zemaira: Insert the white end of the double-ended transfer needle into the center of the upright diluent vial. Invert the diluent vial and insert the green end of the double-ended transfer needle into the center of the product vial. Use minimum force. Diluent will be drawn into the alpha₁-PI by a vacuum. Wet the lyophilized cake completely by gently tilting the product vial. Do not allow the air inlet filter to face downward, and use care not to lose the vacuum. Remove the diluent bottle and transfer device. Gently swirl until the powder is completely dissolved. May take 5 to 10 minutes. *Do not shake or invert vial until ready to withdraw contents.*

Aralast will yield a 0.5 Gm/25 mL vial or a 1 Gm/50 mL vial (20 mg/mL).
Glassia will yield a 1 Gm/50 mL vial (20 mg/mL).
Prolastin will yield a 0.5 Gm/20 mL vial or 1 Gm/40 mL vial (25 mg/mL).
Zemaira will yield a 1 Gm/20 mL vial (50 mg/mL).
Filters: All products must be filtered before or during administration.

Manufacturers supply either a filter needle to withdraw alpha₁-PI from the vial or an in-line filter (to be used in the IV line or for pooling). Several vials may be pooled into an empty sterile IV solution container. **Glassia** supplies only a filter needle for transfer; see Dilution for other filter requirements.

Storage: Refrigerate *Glassia* in carton until use. Contains no preservatives and no latex. *Prolastin* must be refrigerated before reconstitution. *Aralast* should be refrigerated before reconstitution, but it can be stored at temperatures up to 25° C (77° F) for up to 1 month. *Zemaira* may be refrigerated before reconstitution or stored at temperatures up to 25° C (77° F). *All Preparations:* Avoid freezing. Do not use after expiration date on vials. Must be used within 3 hours of reconstitution or entry into vial.

COMPATIBILITY
Manufacturers state, "Should be given alone, without mixing with other agents or diluting solutions."

RATE OF ADMINISTRATION
Aralast, Prolastin, Zemaira: 0.08 mL/kg/min is recommended.
Glassia: Do not exceed 0.04 mL/kg/min.

If an infusion reaction or other adverse effects occur, a reduced rate or interruption of the infusion may be indicated until symptoms subside; see Side Effects and Antidote.

ACTIONS
Aralast, Prolastin, Zemaira are sterile, stable, lyophilized preparations. **Glassia** is a ready-to-use solution. All are obtained from human plasma. Increases and maintains functional levels of alpha₁-PI in the epithelial lining of the lower respiratory tract. Provides adequate antineutrophil elastase activity in the lungs of individuals with alpha₁-antitrypsin deficiency. Weekly infusions of alpha₁-PI usually maintain serum levels above a target threshold of 11 micromoles. Numerous processes employed during manufacture to eliminate potential for viral transmission from human plasma; see Precautions.

INDICATIONS AND USES
Treatment of congenital alpha₁-antitrypsin deficiency, a potentially fatal deficiency; used for chronic replacement (augmentation and maintenance therapy) only in individuals with alpha₁-antitrypsin deficiency and selected types of clinically demonstrated emphysema.

CONTRAINDICATIONS
Individuals with selective IgA deficiencies (IgA level less than 15 mg/dL for **Aralast**) who have known antibodies against IgA (anti-IgA antibodies). IgA may be present and severe reactions, including anaphylaxis, can occur. ▪ Known hypersensitivity to any alpha₁-PI product or any product components.

PRECAUTIONS
For IV use only. Confirm diagnosis of congenital alpha₁-antitrypsin deficiency with selected clinically demonstrated emphysema. ▪ May contain trace amounts of IgA. Patients with selective or severe IgA deficiency and with known antibodies to IgA have a greater risk for developing severe hypersensitivity and anaphylactic reactions; see Contraindications. ▪ Each unit of plasma tested and found nonreactive to HIV antibody, Creutzfeldt-Jakob disease, hepatitis B surface antigen, and hepatitis C. Transmission of these viruses is still possible. ▪ Will increase plasma volume; use caution in patients at risk for circulatory overload. ▪ Long-term effects from

continued use are not known. ▪ Individuals severely deficient in endogenous alpha₁-PI are unable to maintain an adequate antiprotease defense and are subject to more rapid proteolysis of the alveolar walls leading to chronic lung disease. Pulmonary infections, including pneumonia and acute bronchitis, are common in these individuals.

Monitor: Monitor V/S and observe patient continuously throughout infusion. ▪ Blood levels of alpha₁-PI have been maintained above the functional level of 80 mg/dL with this replacement therapy. Serum levels determined by commercial immunologic assays may not reflect actual functional alpha₁-PI levels. ▪ Assess lung sounds and rate and quality of respirations before each infusion. ▪ Monitor for S/S of a hypersensitivity reaction (e.g., dyspnea, flushing, hypotension, rash, tachycardia); emergency equipment, medications, and supplies must be available.

Patient Education: Inform of risks and of safety precautions taken during manufacturing process. ▪ Note changes in breathing pattern or sputum production; avoid smoking. ▪ Report S/S of a hypersensitivity reaction promptly (e.g., dyspnea, faintness, hypotension, hives, tightness of the chest). ▪ Report S/S of parvovirus B19 (e.g., chills, drowsiness, fever, and runny nose, followed 2 weeks later by a rash and joint pain). Parvovirus B19 may be more serious in pregnant women and immune-compromised individuals.

Maternal/Child: Category C: use in pregnancy only when clearly needed. May present risk to fetus; benefits must justify risks. ▪ Safety for use during breast-feeding not established, effects unknown. ▪ Safety for use in pediatric patients not established.

Elderly: Differences in response compared to younger adults not known. As for all patients, dosing for elderly patients should be appropriate to their overall situation.

DRUG/LAB INTERACTIONS
No specific information available.

SIDE EFFECTS
All formulations: Consider risk potential for contracting AIDS, Creutzfeldt-Jakob disease, hepatitis B, or hepatitis C. Hypersensitivity reactions, including anaphylaxis, chills, dyspnea, hypotension, rash, and tachycardia, have been reported; see Contraindications.

Aralast: Cough, headache, and pharyngitis are most common. Asthma, back pain, bloating, bronchitis, dizziness, pain, peripheral edema, rash, rhinitis, sinusitis, somnolence, and viral infection may occur.

Glassia: Dizziness and headache are most common. Chest discomfort, cough, increased hepatic enzymes, sinusitis, and URI have been reported. Cholangitis, exacerbation of COPD, and severe headache may occur.

Prolastin: Mild transient leukocytosis several hours after transfusion. Dizziness, fever, or light-headedness may occur.

Zemaira: Asthenia, bronchitis, chest pain, cough, dizziness, fever, headache, injection site pain and/or hemorrhage, paresthesia, pruritus, rhinitis, sinusitis, sore throat, and upper respiratory infections may occur.

ANTIDOTE
All side effects except potential transmission of viral diseases usually subside spontaneously. Keep the physician informed. If side effects occur, interrupt or discontinue infusion until symptoms subside, then resume at a tolerated rate. Discontinue alpha₁-PI and treat anaphylaxis (antihistamines, epinephrine, corticosteroids) as indicated. Resuscitate as necessary.

ALPROSTADIL BBW

(al-**PROSS**-tah-dill)

Prostaglandin E₁, Prostin VR Pediatric

Prostaglandin
(ductus arteriosus patency adjunct)

USUAL DOSE

Pediatric patients: Begin with 0.05 to 0.1 mcg/kg of body weight/min. When therapeutic response is achieved, reduce infusion rate in increments to the lowest dose that maintains the response (e.g., reduce from 0.1 to 0.05 or from 0.025 to 0.01 mcg/kg/min). If necessary, dose may be increased gradually to a maximum of 0.4 mcg/kg/min. Generally these higher rates do not produce greater effects. May be given through infusion in a large vein or, if necessary, through an umbilical artery catheter placed at the ductal opening.

DILUTION

Each 500 mcg must be further diluted with NS or D5W. Various volumes may be used depending on infusion pump capabilities and desired infusion rate.

Guidelines for Dilution and Rate of Infusion for Desired Dose of Alprostadil			
Diluent (mL)	Concentration (mcg/mL)	Desired Dose (mcg/kg/min)	Rate of Infusion (mL/min/kg)
250 mL	2 mcg/mL	0.1 mcg/kg/min	0.05 mL/min/kg
25 mL	20 mcg/mL	0.1 mcg/kg/min	0.005 mL/min/kg

Storage: Refrigerate until dilution. Prepare fresh solution for administration every 24 hours.

COMPATIBILITY

Consider any drug NOT listed as compatible to be INCOMPATIBLE until consulting a pharmacist; specific conditions may apply.

One source suggests the following **compatibilities:**

Solutions: D5½NS, D5½NS with KCl 20 mEq/L, D10½NS, D10½NS with KCl 20 mEq/L.

Y-site: Ampicillin, cefazolin (Ancef), cefotaxime (Claforan), chlorothiazide (Diuril), dobutamine, dopamine, fentanyl (Sublimaze), gentamicin, methylprednisolone (Solu-Medrol), nitroprusside sodium, tobramycin, vancomycin, vecuronium.

RATE OF ADMINISTRATION

See Usual Dose. Infusion pump capable of delivering 0.005, 0.01, 0.02, or 0.05 mL/min/kg required. Use for the shortest time possible at the lowest rate therapeutically effective. Decrease rate of infusion *stat* if a significant fall in arterial pressure occurs.

ACTIONS

A naturally occurring acidic lipid. Smooth muscle of the ductus arteriosus is susceptible to its relaxing effect, which reduces BP and peripheral resistance and increases cardiac output and rate. In newborns it relaxes and may open the ductus. Metabolized by oxidation almost instantly (80% in one pass through the lungs). Remainder excreted as metabolites in the urine.

INDICATIONS AND USES

Temporarily maintain the patency of the ductus arteriosus until corrective or palliative surgery can be performed on infants with pulmonary atresia, pulmonary stenosis, tricuspid atresia, tetralogy of Fallot, interruption of the aortic arch, coarctation of the aorta, or transposition of the great vessels.
■ Used by intercavernosal injection to treat impotence.

CONTRAINDICATIONS

None known. Not indicated for infant respiratory distress syndrome (hyaline membrane disease).

PRECAUTIONS

Usually administered by trained personnel in pediatric intensive care facilities. ■ Establish a diagnosis of cyanotic heart disease (restricted pulmonary blood flow). ■ Response is poor in infants with Po_2 values of 40 mm Hg or those more than 4 days old. More effective with lower Po_2. ■ Apnea has been experienced in 10% to 20% of treated neonates. ■ Use caution in neonates with bleeding tendencies; inhibits platelet aggregation.

Monitor: Monitor respiratory status continuously. Ventilatory assistance must be immediately available. May cause apnea, especially in infants under 2 kg. Apnea usually appears during the first hour of infusion. ■ Monitor arterial pressure intermittently by umbilical artery catheter, auscultation, or Doppler transducer. Decrease rate of infusion *stat* if a significant fall in arterial pressure occurs. ■ Decrease or stop infusion if infant develops increased respiratory distress; bleeding, bruising, or hematoma formation; or sudden changes in cardiac status (e.g., decreased BP, bradycardia, cardiac arrest, cyanosis). ■ Measure effectiveness with increase of Po_2 in infants with restricted pulmonary blood flow and increase of BP and blood pH in infants with restricted systemic blood flow.

DRUG/LAB INTERACTIONS

Inhibits **platelet aggregation.**

SIDE EFFECTS

Cardiac arrest, cerebral bleeding, cortical proliferation of long bones, diarrhea, DIC, hyperextension of the neck, hyperirritability, hypothermia, seizures, sepsis, tachycardia. Many other side effects have occurred in 1% or less of infants receiving alprostadil.

Overdose: Apnea, bradycardia, flushing, hypotension, pyrexia.

ANTIDOTE

Notify physician of all side effects. Discontinue immediately if apnea or bradycardia occurs. Institute emergency measures. If infusion is restarted use extreme caution. Decrease or stop infusion if infant develops increased respiratory distress; bleeding, bruising, or hematoma formation; or sudden changes in cardiac status (e.g., decreased BP, bradycardia, cardiac arrest, cyanosis). Decrease rate if pyrexia, hypotension, or fall in arterial pressure occurs. Flushing is usually caused by incorrect intra-arterial catheter placement. Reposition.

ALTEPLASE, RECOMBINANT

(**AL**-teh-playz)

Activase, ✤rt-PA, Tissue Plasminogen
Activator, tPA ▪ Cathflo Activase

Thrombolytic agent
(recombinant)

pH 7.3

USUAL DOSE

Selected indications (e.g., acute ischemic stroke, weight under 65 or 67 kg in acute MI) require exact weight-adjusted dosing. To deliver an accurate dose without possibility of overdose, calculate desired dose and withdraw any amount **NOT** needed from a 50- or 100-mg vial and discard. In all situations follow total dose with at least 30 mL of NS or D5W through the IV tubing to ensure administration of total dose.

ACUTE MYOCARDIAL INFARCTION

Total dose is based on patient weight and should not exceed 100 mg. Concurrent administration of heparin, aspirin, and/or dipyridamole (Persantine) has been consistently used in MI patients receiving alteplase therapy. MI patients in the **accelerated infusion** studies received a loading dose of heparin 5,000 units, followed by 1,000 units/hr by continuous infusion for 48 hours. Dose is adjusted to raise aPTT to between 1.5 to 2 times control. Aspirin therapy was usually concurrent (e.g., 160 mg chewable aspirin on admission, followed by 160 to 325 mg/day) or followed with aspirin after 48 hours. 90% of MI patients receiving the 3-hour infusion also received heparin as a continuous infusion with or without a loading dose and either aspirin or dipyridamole; see Precautions and Monitor. The earlier intervention occurs, the better the results. Most effective if administered within 4 to 6 hours of onset of symptoms of acute myocardial infarction.

Accelerated infusion; weight greater than 67 kg: A total dose of 100 mg titrated over 90 minutes as an IV infusion. Initially give a bolus of 15 mg over 2 minutes. Follow with 50 mg evenly distributed over 30 minutes. Infuse the remaining 35-mg dose evenly distributed over 60 minutes. See comments under Usual Dose.

Accelerated infusion; weight equal to or less than 67 kg: See comments in first paragraph of Usual Dose. Initially give a bolus of 15 mg over 2 minutes. Follow with 0.75 mg/kg (not to exceed a 50-mg dose) evenly distributed over 30 minutes. Then infuse 0.5 mg/kg (not to exceed a 35-mg dose) evenly distributed over 60 minutes. Total dose not to exceed 100 mg. See comments under Usual Dose.

3-hour infusion; weight 65 kg or greater: A total dose of 100 mg titrated over 3 hours as an IV infusion. Initially, give a bolus of 6 to 10 mg over 2 minutes. Follow with 50 to 54 mg (total 60-mg dose) evenly distributed over the first hour. Follow with 20 mg/hr for 2 hours. See comments under Usual Dose.

3-hour infusion; weight less than 65 kg: Calculate total dose using 1.25 mg/kg of body weight. See comments in first paragraph of Usual Dose. Give three fifths (60%) of this total calculated dose in the first hour (10% of which should be given as an initial bolus dose). Give the remaining 40% of this total calculated dose equally distributed over 2 hours. See comments under Usual Dose. *Continued*

ACUTE ISCHEMIC STROKE

0.9 mg/kg. Do not exceed the maximum dose of 90 mg. See comments in Usual Dose. Give a bolus of 10% of the calculated dose over 1 minute followed by balance of calculated dose (90%) as an infusion evenly distributed over 60 minutes. Treatment must start within 3 hours of onset of symptoms, but after bleeding in the brain has been ruled out (usually by a non-contrast CT scan of the brain). Do not give aspirin, heparin, or warfarin for 24 hours; see Precautions.

PULMONARY EMBOLISM

100 mg titrated over 2 hours as an IV infusion. Diagnosis should be confirmed by objective means (e.g., lung scan, pulmonary angiography). Begin heparin at end of infusion or immediately after it is complete. Thrombin time (TT) or PTT should be twice normal or less.

CENTRAL VENOUS ACCESS DEVICE (CVAD) OCCLUSIONS, CATHFLO ACTIVASE

See Rate of Administration, Precautions, Monitor, and Maternal/Child.
Patient weight 30 kg or greater: Instill 2 mg in 2 mL into the occluded catheter.
Patient weight less than 30 kg: Instill 110% of the internal lumen volume of the occluded catheter into the occluded catheter. Do not exceed 2 mg in 2 mL.

Attempt to aspirate blood from the catheter after 30 minutes of dwell time. If catheter function has been restored, aspirate 4 to 5 mL of blood in patients equal to or greater than 10 kg or 3 mL of blood in patients less than 10 kg to remove Cathflo Activase and residual clot, then gently irrigate the catheter with NS.

If catheter function has not been restored (unable to aspirate blood), allow the first dose to remain in the catheter for 90 additional minutes of dwell time and then attempt to aspirate again (total elapsed time is 120 minutes). If catheter function has been restored, aspirate and irrigate as above. If function has not been restored, a second dose may be instilled and the dwell time and aspiration process repeated.

DILUTION

Myocardial infarction, stroke, and pulmonary embolism: Must be reconstituted with SWFI without preservatives (provided by manufacturer). Available in 50- and 100-mg vials (1 mg/mL). Consider patient's hemodynamic status. Use of filters or filter needles not recommended. Protein adsorption may occur with resulting drug loss. *50-mg vials:* Use a large-bore (18-gauge) needle and direct the stream of diluent into the lyophilized cake. A vacuum must be present when the diluent is added to the powder for injection. Do not use if vacuum not present. Slight foaming is expected; let stand for several minutes to dissipate large bubbles. If necessary, may be further diluted to 0.5 mg/mL immediately before administration with an equal volume of NS or D5W. Do not shake. Mix by swirling or slow inversion; avoid agitation during dilution. Dilution with less than the recommended volume to concentrations greater than 1 mg/mL will also result in a hypertonic solution. Dilution beyond 0.5 mg/mL may cause precipitation. Use balance (at least 30 mL) of 250-mL bottle of NS or D5W to clear tubing after infusion and ensure delivery of total dose; NS is preferred.

Connect NS or D5W to metriset and pump tubing. Clamp between solution and metriset. Add alteplase to metriset. Prime tubing with alteplase. Bolus dose can be given when indicated by IV injection through a med port or by IV pump. Administer balance of dose as outlined in Usual Dose section, adjusting pump rate of delivery as required. Complete by flushing tubing with IV solution.

100-mg vial: Diluent and transfer device provided (does not contain a vacuum). Insert one end of transfer device into upright vial of diluent (do not invert diluent vial yet). Hold alteplase vial upside down and push center of vial down onto piercing pin. Now invert vials and allow diluent to flow into alteplase. Small amount (0.5 mL) of diluent will not transfer. Swirl gently to dissolve. Do not shake. Process takes several minutes. An infusion set may be inserted into puncture site created by piercing pin. Hang by plastic capping on bottom of vial. Prime tubing with alteplase and administer as outlined above for 50-mg vials.

Cathflo Activase for CVAD occlusion: Supplied as a sterile lyophilized powder in 2-mg vials. Must be reconstituted with 2.2 mL of SW without preservatives. Direct diluent stream into the powder. Allow to stand undisturbed until large bubbles dissipate; may foam slightly. Mix by swirling gently; do not shake. Should be completely dissolved within 3 minutes. Final concentration is 1 mg/mL. If the 2-mg vials are not available, some pharmacies dilute 50 mg of alteplase with 50 mL of SW without preservatives (1 mg/mL). Withdraw 2.2 mL (2.2 mg) to 2- or 5-mL sterile disposable syringes. In studies these were transferred to sterile glass vials and frozen. Defrost and use as needed (22 prepared doses).

Filters: Use of filters or filter needles not recommended. Protein adsorption may occur with resulting drug loss.

Storage: *Systemic alteplase:* Protect from light in cartons. May be stored at CRT or refrigerated before and/or after reconstitution. Manufacturer recommends reconstitution immediately before use. Must be used within 8 hours of reconstitution. Discard unused solution. Stable as a 0.5 mg/mL solution in NS or D5W for 8 hours at CRT.

Cathflo Activase: Refrigerate unopened vials; protect from light during extended storage. Reconstitution immediately before use is recommended, but solution may be used up to 8 hours after reconstitution if refrigerated at 2° to 30° C. Do not use beyond expiration date on vial. Discard unused solution.

COMPATIBILITY

Consider any drug NOT listed as compatible to be INCOMPATIBLE until consulting a pharmacist; specific conditions may apply.

Manufacturer states, "No other medication should be added to infusion solutions containing alteplase. Do not use other infusion solutions (e.g., SW, bacteriostatic water for injection [BWFI] or other preservative-containing solutions) for further dilution"; see Dilution. One source suggests D5W used for reconstitution or further dilution may cause a precipitate.

One source suggests the following **compatibilities:**

Y-site: Lidocaine, metoprolol (Lopressor), and propranolol through **Y-site** of free-flowing alteplase infusion.

RATE OF ADMINISTRATION

Systemic alteplase: See specific rates for each diagnosis under Usual Dose. In all situations use an infusion pump (preferred) or a metriset with microdrip (60 gtt/mL) and IV tubing without a filter to facilitate accurate administration. Do not use any filters. Distribute final flush over 30 minutes. NS preferred for flushing of IV line.

Cathflo Activase: Avoid excessive pressure or force while attempting to clear catheters; see Usual Dose, Precautions, and Monitor.

ACTIONS

A tissue plasminogen activator and enzyme produced by recombinant DNA. It binds to fibrin in a thrombus and converts plasminogen to plasmin. Plasmin digests fibrin and dissolves the clot. With therapeutic doses, a decrease in circulating fibrinogen makes the patient susceptible to bleeding. Onset of action is prompt, effecting patency of the vessel within 1 to 2 hours in most patients. Prompt opening of arteries increases probability of improved function. Cleared from the plasma by the liver within 5 (50%) to 10 (80%) minutes after the infusion is discontinued. Some effects may linger for 45 minutes to several hours.

INDICATIONS AND USES

Systemic alteplase: Management of acute myocardial infarction in adults for the lysis of thrombi obstructing coronary arteries, the reduction of infarct size, the improvement of ventricular function, the reduction of the incidence of congestive heart failure, and the reduction of mortality associated with acute MI. Recent studies suggest alteplase or reteplase are the drugs of choice. ■ Current AHA recommendations identify thrombolytic agents as Class I therapy in patients with recent onset of chest pain (within 6 hours) consistent with acute MI and at least 0.1 mV of ST segment elevation in at least two ECG leads. Use in all other patients based on age, accurate diagnosis, and time from onset of chest pain. ■ Management of acute ischemic stroke in adults to improve neurologic recovery and reduce incidence of disability. ■ Management of acute massive pulmonary embolism in adults for the lysis of acute pulmonary emboli either obstructing blood flow to a lobe or multiple segments of the lung or accompanied by unstable hemodynamics (e.g., failure to maintain BP).

Cathflo Activase: Restoration of function to CVADs as assessed by the ability to withdraw blood.

Unlabeled uses: *Systemic alteplase:* Treatment of unstable angina pectoris and deep vein thrombosis. Has been shown to restore blood flow to frostbitten limbs (0.075 mg/kg/hr for 6 hours). Has been used to clear thrombi in central venous catheters (2 mg bolus into the blocked catheter), in the occlusion of small blood vessels by microthrombi, and in management of peripheral thromboembolism (0.5 to 1 mg/hr intra-arterially).

CONTRAINDICATIONS

Acute myocardial infarction/pulmonary embolism: Active internal bleeding, arteriovenous malformation or aneurysm, bleeding diathesis, cerebrovascular accident, intracranial or intraspinal surgery or trauma within 2 months, intracranial neoplasm, severe uncontrolled hypertension.

Acute ischemic stroke: Active internal bleeding. Evidence of intracranial hemorrhage on pretreatment evaluation. Clinical presentation suggestive of subarachnoid hemorrhage (even with normal CT). History of intracranial hemorrhage, intracranial neoplasm, arteriovenous malformation, or aneurysm. History of intracranial surgery, serious head trauma, or previous stroke within 3 months. Known bleeding diathesis (e.g., current use of oral anticoagulants [e.g., warfarin] with an INR greater than 1.7 or a PT greater than 15 seconds). Administration of heparin within 48 hours before onset of stroke with an elevated aPTT as presentation (greater than upper limit of normal for laboratory). Platelet count less than 100,000/mm^3. Seizure observed at the same time as the onset of stroke. Uncontrolled hypertension at time of treatment (e.g., systolic above 175 or diastolic above 110) and patient requires aggressive treatment to reduce BP to within these limits. **Cathflo Activase:** Known hypersensitivity to alteplase or its components.

PRECAUTIONS

All systemic indications: A 150-mg dose has caused increased intracranial bleeding; do not use. ▪ Administered under the direction of a physician knowledgeable in its use and with appropriate emergency drugs and diagnostic and laboratory facilities available. ▪ A greater alteration of hemostatic status than with heparin. Strict bed rest indicated to reduce risk of bleeding. Use extreme care with the patient; avoid any excessive or rough handling or pressure (including too-frequent BPs); avoid invasive procedures (e.g., arterial puncture, venipuncture, IM injection). If these procedures are absolutely necessary, use extreme precautionary methods (use radial artery instead of femoral; use small-gauge catheters and needles, and sites that are easily observed and compressible where bleeding can be controlled; avoid handling catheter sites; and use extended pressure application of up to 30 minutes). Minor bleeding occurs often at catheter insertion sites. Avoid use of razors and toothbrushes. ▪ Use extreme caution in the following situations: abnormal blood glucose (less than 50 or greater than 400 mg/dL), major surgery or serious trauma (excluding head trauma; see Contraindications) in the previous 14 days, GI or GU bleeding within 21 days, or puncture of noncompressible vessels (e.g., arterial puncture, spinal puncture, thoracentesis) within the previous 10 days; cerebrovascular disease; hypertension (systolic equal to or greater than 175 mm Hg or diastolic above 110 mm Hg); mitral stenosis with atrial fibrillation (likelihood of left heart thrombus); acute pericarditis; subacute bacterial endocarditis; coagulation disorders, including those secondary to severe hepatic or renal disease; severe liver dysfunction; pregnancy and first 10 days postpartum; hemorrhagic ophthalmic conditions (e.g., diabetic hemorrhagic retinopathy); septic thrombophlebitis; patients on anticoagulants; patients over 75 years of age; any situation where bleeding might be hazardous or difficult to manage because of location. ▪ Not antigenic (does not promote antibody formation). Risk of hypersensitivity reactions less than with streptokinase. A second course can be administered if reocclusion occurs. May increase risk of severe hemorrhage, especially if effects of first dose have not subsided. ▪ Onset of orolingual angioedema has been reported in patients with acute MI and acute ischemic stroke. Onset may occur during or up to 2 hours after infusion. Associated with concomitant use of angiotensin-converting enzyme inhibitors. Most resolved with prompt treatment; see Drug/Lab Interactions.

Myocardial infarction: Reperfusion arrhythmias occur frequently (e.g., sinus bradycardia, accelerated idioventricular rhythm, PVCs, ventricular tachycardia); have antiarrhythmic meds available at bedside. ▪ Simultaneous therapy with continuous infusion of heparin (with or without a loading dose and aspirin or dipyridamole) is used to reduce the risk of rethrombosis. Increases risk of bleeding; see Usual Dose. ▪ Standard treatment for myocardial infarction continues simultaneously with alteplase therapy except if temporarily contraindicated (e.g., arterial blood gases, unless absolutely necessary).

Acute ischemic stroke: Treatment facility must be able to provide evaluation and management of intracranial hemorrhage. ▪ Do not use anticoagulants (e.g., heparin, aspirin, coumadin) during the first 24 hours. If any anticoagulant is indicated after 24 hours, consider performing a non-contrast CT scan or other sensitive diagnostic imaging method to rule out any intracranial hemorrhage before starting an anticoagulant. Another source suggested that antiplatelet agents (e.g., ticlopidine [Ticlid], dipyridamole [Persantine]) and anticoagulants should not be used within the first 24 hours. ▪ Risks of alteplase therapy in the treatment of acute ischemic stroke may be increased in patients with severe neurologic deficit at presentation (increased risk of intracranial hemorrhage), patients with major early infarct signs on CT scan (e.g., substantial edema, mass effect, or midline shift). ▪ Treatment may begin before coagulation study results are known in patients without recent use of oral anticoagulants or heparin. Discontinue infusion if pretreatment INR is greater than 1.7, PT is greater than 15 seconds, or an elevated aPTT is identified. ▪ Benefits of therapy have not been studied in patients treated with alteplase more than 3 hours after the onset of symptoms; use is not recommended. Risk of intracranial hemorrhage increased; may cause cerebral edema with fatal brain herniation. ▪ Safety and efficacy in patients with minor neurologic deficit or rapidly improving symptoms before treatment is begun has not been studied; caution is recommended.

Pulmonary emboli: Begin heparin at end of infusion or immediately after it is complete. Thrombin time (TT) or PTT should be twice normal or less.

Cathflo Activase: Consider causes of catheter dysfunction other than thrombus formation (e.g., catheter malposition, mechanical failure, constriction by a suture, lipid deposits or drug precipitates within the catheter lumen). ▪ Do not apply vigorous suction during attempts to determine catheter occlusion; may risk damage to the vascular wall or collapse of soft-walled catheters. Avoid excessive pressure during instillation of Cathflo Activase into the catheter; may cause rupture of the catheter or expulsion of the clot into the circulation. ▪ Use caution with patients who have active internal bleeding, thrombocytopenia, other hemostatic defects (including those secondary to hepatic or renal disease). ▪ Use caution in patients who have conditions for which bleeding constitutes a significant hazard, who would be difficult to manage because of location, who are at high risk for embolic complication (e.g., venous thrombosis in the region of the catheter), or who have had any of the following within 48 hours: surgery, obstetrical delivery, percutaneous biopsy of viscera or deep tissues, or puncture of noncompressible vessels. ▪ Use caution in the presence of known or suspected infection in the catheter; may release a localized infection into the systemic circulation. ▪ See Monitor. ▪ Safety and effectiveness of doses greater than 2 mg has not been established.

Monitor: *All systemic indications:* Best to establish a separate IV line for alteplase. ▪ Obtain appropriate clotting studies (e.g., PT, TT, PTT, aPTT, CBC, fibrinogen levels, platelets). ▪ Diagnosis-specific baseline studies (e.g., ECG, CPK in myocardial infarction, non-contrast CT brain scan, and neurologic assessment in acute ischemic stroke, and lung scan or pulmonary angiography in pulmonary embolism) are indicated. ▪ Baseline assessment (patient condition, pain, hematomas, petechiae, or recent wounds) should be completed before administration. ▪ Type and cross-match may also be ordered. ▪ Start IV if indicated (not previously established, other medications being administered through current IV, to have a line available for additional treatment). ▪ Maintain strict bed rest; monitor the patient carefully and frequently for pain and signs of bleeding; observe catheter sites at least every 15 minutes and apply pressure dressings to any recently invaded site; watch for hematuria, hematemesis, bloody stool, petechiae, hematoma, flank pain, muscle weakness; and do neuro checks every hour (or more frequently if indicated). Continue until normal clotting function returns. ▪ Monitor BP and maintain within appropriate limits with antihypertensives or vasopressors as indicated. ▪ Monitor for signs of orolingual angioedema during and for at least 2 hours after infusion. ▪ Watch for extravasation; may cause ecchymosis and/or inflammation. Restart IV at another site. Moist compresses may be helpful. ▪ See Precautions and Drug/Lab Interactions.

Myocardial infarction: Monitor ECG continuously, and record strips with greatest ST segment elevation initially and every 15 minutes for at least 4 hours. A 12-lead ECG is indicated when therapy is complete.

Acute ischemic stroke: Printed protocol guidelines are available from manufacturer and include the following recommendations. ▪ Before the initiation of therapy, determine actual time of onset of stroke. ▪ Obtain baseline hematocrit, platelet count, and blood glucose. INR, PT, or aPTT is recommended in patients with recent use of oral anticoagulants or heparin. Obtain baseline BP, neurologic exam, and non-contrast CT brain scan. ▪ Monitor BP every 15 minutes before beginning therapy; should be below 175/110 mm Hg. If over 175/110 mm Hg, BP may be treated with nitroglycerin paste (can be wiped off if BP drops quickly) and/or one or two 10- or 20-mg doses of labetalol (Tradate) give by IV injection within 1 hour. If these measures do not reduce BP below 175/110 mm Hg and keep it down, the patient should not be treated with alteplase. ▪ During and after treatment, monitor BP every 15 minutes for 2 hours, every 30 minutes for 6 hours, then every 1 hour for 18 hours. Avoid hypotension; may decrease perfusion of alteplase; a diastolic BP around 100 mm Hg helps to maintain sufficient mean arterial pressure to reperfuse stroke area. *See Antidote for protocol to treat hypertension occurring after treatment has been started.* ▪ Hemorrhage in the brain occurs frequently during treatment with alteplase during the first 36 hours; monitor carefully. Acute neurologic deterioration, new headache, acute hypertension, or nausea and vomiting may indicate the occurrence of intracranial hemorrhage. If intracranial hemorrhage is suspected, discontinue alteplase and obtain a non-contrast CT scan. ▪ Monitor for S/S of atrial fibrillation and/or acute MI. ▪ Studies did not show an increase in mortality and did confirm that more patients had minimal or no disability at 3 months.

Cathflo Activase: Aseptic technique imperative. ▪ Avoid force while attempting to clear catheters; may rupture catheter or dislodge clot into the circulation. ▪ To prevent air from entering the open catheter and the circulatory system, instruct the patient to exhale and hold his/her breath any time the catheter is not connected to the IV tubing or a syringe. ▪ See Precautions.

Patient Education: Compliance with all measures to minimize bleeding (e.g., strict bed rest) is very important. ▪ Avoid use of razors, toothbrushes, and other sharp items. Use caution while moving to avoid excessive bumping. ▪ Report all episodes of bleeding and apply local pressure if indicated. Expect oozing from IV sites.

Maternal/Child: *Systemic alteplase:* Category C: safety for use in pregnancy, breast-feeding, and pediatric patients not established.

Cathflo Activase: Category C: use during pregnancy only if benefits justify potential risk to the fetus. ▪ Use caution during breast-feeding. ▪ Has been used in patients 2 weeks to 17 years of age. Rates of serious adverse events as well as restoration of catheter function similar to adults.

Elderly: *Systemic alteplase:* See Indications and Precautions. ▪ May have poorer prognosis following acute MI and pre-existing conditions that may increase risk of intracranial bleeding. Select patients carefully to maximize benefits.

Cathflo Activase: No incidents of intracranial hemorrhage, embolic events, or major bleeding events were observed during studies. ▪ Use caution in the elderly with conditions known to increase the risk of bleeding; see Precautions.

DRUG/LAB INTERACTIONS
Risk of bleeding may be increased by any medicine that affects blood clotting, including **anticoagulants** (e.g., heparin, lepirudin [Refludan], warfarin [Coumadin]); **any medication that may cause hypoprothrombinemia, thrombocytopenia, or GI ulceration or bleeding** (e.g., selected antibiotics [e.g., cefotetan], aspirin, NSAIDs [e.g., ibuprofen (Advil, Motrin), naproxen (Aleve, Naprosyn)]); **and/or any other medication that inhibits platelet aggregation** (e.g., clopidogrel [Plavix], dipyridamole [Persantine], glycoprotein GPIIb/IIIa receptor antagonists [e.g., abciximab (ReoPro), eptifibatide (Integrilin), tirofiban (Aggrastat)], plicamycin [Mithracin], sulfinpyrazone [Anturane], ticlopidine [Ticlid], valproic acid [Depacon]). Concurrent use not recommended with the exception of heparin and aspirin (in AMI) to reduce the risk of rethrombosis. If concurrent or subsequent use indicated (e.g., management of acute coronary syndrome, percutaneous coronary intervention), monitor PT and aPTT closely. ▪ Concurrent use with **nitroglycerin** decreases plasma concentrations of alteplase, impairing the thrombolytic effect. ▪ Orolingual angioedema has been reported with concomitant use of **angiotensin-converting enzyme inhibitors** (e.g., enalapril [Vasotec], enalaprilat [Vasotec IV], lisinopril [Zestril]). ▪ **Coagulation tests** will be unreliable; specific procedures can be used; notify the lab of alteplase use.

SIDE EFFECTS
Systemic alteplase: Bleeding is most common: internal (GI tract, GU tract, retroperitoneal, or intracranial sites), epistaxis, gingival, and superficial or surface bleeding (venous cutdowns, arterial punctures, sites of recent surgical intervention). Mild to serious hypersensitivity reactions (including anaphylaxis) have occurred. Fever, hypotension, nausea and vomiting, reperfusion arrhythmias, and stroke have occurred. Cholesterol embolization syndrome (e.g., acute renal failure, bowel infarction, cerebral infarction, gangrenous digits, hypertension, livedo reticularis, myocardial infarction, pancreatitis, purple toe, retinal artery occlusion, rhabdomyolysis, spinal cord infarction) can occur with thrombolytics but has been reported rarely.

Post-Marketing: Orolingual angioedema; rare fatalities from upper airway hemorrhage from intubation trauma.

Cathflo Activase: Gastrointestinal bleeding, sepsis, and venous thrombosis have occurred. There were no reports of intracranial hemorrhage or pulmonary emboli during clinical trials.

ANTIDOTE

Systemic alteplase: Notify physician of all side effects. Note even the most minute bleeding tendency. Oozing at IV sites is expected. Control minor bleeding by local pressure. For severe bleeding in a critical location or suspected intracranial bleeding, discontinue alteplase and any heparin therapy immediately. Obtain PT, aPTT, platelet count, and fibrinogen. Draw blood for type and cross-match. Platelets and cryoprecipitate are most commonly used but whole blood, packed RBCs, fresh-frozen plasma, desmopressin, tranexamic acid (Cyklokapron) and aminocaproic acid (Amicar) may be indicated. Topical preparations of aminocaproic acid may stop minor bleeding. Consider protamine if heparin has been used. Treat bradycardia with atropine, reperfusion arrhythmias with lidocaine or procainamide; VT or VF may require cardioversion. If hypotension occurs, reduce rate promptly. If not resolved, vasopressors (e.g., dopamine), Trendelenburg position, and suitable plasma expanders (e.g., albumin, plasma protein fraction [plasmanate], or hetastarch) may be indicated. Do not use Dextran. ▪ *Protocol for treatment of hypertension occurring during treatment for acute ischemic stroke:* Monitor BP every 15 minutes; observe for hypertension/hypotension. If diastolic BP is greater than 140 mm Hg, start an IV infusion of nitroprusside sodium (0.5 to 10 mcg/kg/min). If systolic BP greater than 230 mm Hg and/or diastolic BP is 121 to 140 mm Hg, give labetalol 20 mg IV over 1 to 2 minutes. This dose may be repeated and/or doubled every 10 minutes, up to 150 mg. Alternatively, following the first bolus of labetalol, an IV infusion of labetalol 2 to 8 mg/min may be initiated and continued until the desired BP is reached. If satisfactory response is not obtained, use nitroprusside sodium. If systolic BP is 180 to 230 mm Hg and/or diastolic BP is 105 to 120 mm Hg on two readings 5 to 10 minutes apart, give labetalol 10 mg IV over 1 to 2 minutes. The dose may be repeated or doubled every 10 to 20 minutes, up to 150 mg. Alternatively, following the first bolus of labetalol, an IV infusion of labetalol 2 to 8 mg/min may be initiated and continued until the desired BP is reached. Treat minor hypersensitivity reactions symptomatically. If angioedema occurs, treat promptly with antihistamines (e.g., diphenhydramine [Benadryl]), IV corticosteroids, or epinephrine and consider discontinuing the alteplase infusion. Discontinue drug and treat anaphylaxis as indicated; resuscitate as necessary.

Cathflo Activase: Discontinue Cathflo Activase and withdraw it from the catheter if serious bleeding in a critical location (e.g., intracranial, gastro-intestinal, retroperitoneal, pericardial) occurs. Discontinue drug and treat anaphylaxis as indicated; resuscitate as necessary. In the event of accidental administration of a 2-mg dose directly into the systemic circulation, the concentration of circulating levels of alteplase would be expected to return to exogenous levels of 5 to 10 ng/mL within 30 minutes.

AMIFOSTINE
(am-ih-**FOS**-teen)

Ethyol

Antidote
Antineoplastic adjunct
Cytoprotective agent

USUAL DOSE

PROPHYLACTIC REDUCTION OF CISPLATIN-INDUCED NEPHROTOXICITY, PROPHYLACTIC REDUCTION OF CISPLATIN INDUCED–NEUROTOXICITY (UNLABELED), AND PROPHYLACTIC REDUCTION OF ANTINEOPLASTIC AGENT BONE MARROW TOXICITY (UNLABELED)

Must be administered in conjunction with cisplatin. Adequate hydration and premedication required before administration; see Premedication below, Monitor, and cisplatin monograph.

Premedication: Premedication to prevent severe nausea and vomiting is recommended before each dose. Usual regimen includes dexamethasone 20 mg IV and a serotonin $5HT_3$ receptor antagonist (e.g., ondansetron [Zofran], granisetron [Kytril]) given before and in conjunction with amifostine infusion.

Amifostine: 910 mg/M^2. Cisplatin dose must be given within 30 minutes of starting the amifostine infusion, but only after the full dose of amifostine is administered.

REDUCTION OF MODERATE TO SEVERE XEROSTOMIA FROM RADIATION OF THE HEAD AND NECK

Premedication: Premedication to prevent nausea and vomiting is recommended before each dose. Oral $5HT_3$ receptor antagonists alone or in combination with other antiemetics are recommended. Adequate hydration required; see Monitor.

Amifostine: 200 mg/M^2 once daily as a 3-minute infusion, starting 15 to 30 minutes before standard fraction radiation therapy.

DOSE ADJUSTMENTS

Dosing should be cautious in the elderly. Consider potential for decreased organ function and concomitant disease or drug therapy.

Reduction of cumulative renal toxicity with chemotherapy: Temporarily discontinue the infusion if the systolic BP decreases significantly from the baseline value. See the following chart.

Guideline for Interrupting Amifostine Infusion due to Decrease in Systolic Blood Pressure					
	Baseline Systolic Blood Pressure (mm Hg)				
	<100	100-119	120-139	140-179	≥180
Decrease in systolic blood pressure during infusion of amifostine (mm Hg)	20	25	30	40	50

Infusion may be restarted to deliver the full dose if the BP returns to normal within 5 minutes and the patient is asymptomatic. If the BP does not return to baseline within 5 minutes and/or the patient is symptomatic (e.g., bradycardia, fainting, unconscious), the full dose cannot be delivered and subsequent doses should be reduced to 740 mg/M^2.

Reduction of moderate to severe xerostomia from radiation of the head and neck: Temporarily discontinue the infusion if the systolic BP decreases significantly from the baseline value. See the chart on the preceding page. Hypotension not as likely with this 200 mg/M^2 dose. Infusion may be restarted to deliver the full dose if the BP returns to normal within 5 minutes and the patient is asymptomatic. If the BP does not return to baseline within 5 minutes and/or the patient is symptomatic (e.g., bradycardia, fainting, unconscious), the full dose cannot be delivered.

DILUTION

Each 500-mg vial should be reconstituted with 9.7 mL of NS (50 mg/mL). May be further diluted with NS to concentrations from 5 to 40 mg/mL. An additional 2.5 mL of NS will yield 40 mg/mL; 90 mL NS will yield 5 mg/mL.

Filters: Not required by manufacturer. Additional data not available.

Storage: Store at CRT before reconstitution. Reconstituted or diluted solution prepared in PVC infusion bags is stable for 5 hours at room temperature or 24 hours if refrigerated.

COMPATIBILITY

Consider any drug NOT listed as compatible to be INCOMPATIBLE until consulting a pharmacist; specific conditions may apply.

Use of any additive, diluent, or solution other than NS is not recommended by manufacturer.

One source suggests the following **compatibilities:**

Y-site: Amikacin (Amikin), aminophylline, ampicillin, ampicillin/sulbactam (Unasyn), aztreonam (Azactam), bleomycin (Blenoxane), bumetanide, buprenorphine (Buprenex), butorphanol (Stadol), calcium gluconate, carboplatin (Paraplatin), carmustine (BiCNU), cefazolin (Ancef), cefotaxime (Claforan), cefotetan, cefoxitin (Mefoxin), ceftazidime (Fortaz), ceftriaxone (Rocephin), cefuroxime (Zinacef), ciprofloxacin (Cipro IV), clindamycin (Cleocin), cyclophosphamide (Cytoxan), cytarabine (ARA-C), dacarbazine (DTIC), dactinomycin (Cosmegen), daunorubicin (Cerubidine), dexamethasone (Decadron), diphenhydramine (Benadryl), dobutamine, docetaxel (Taxotere), dopamine, doxorubicin (Adriamycin), doxycycline, droperidol (Inapsine), enalaprilat (Vasotec IV), etoposide (VePesid), famotidine (Pepcid IV), fluconazole (Diflucan), fludarabine (Fludara), fluorouracil (5-FU), furosemide (Lasix), gallium nitrate (Ganite), gemcitabine (Gemzar), gentamicin, granisetron (Kytril), haloperidol (Haldol), heparin, hydrocortisone sodium succinate (Solu-Cortef), hydromorphone (Dilaudid), idarubicin (Idamycin), ifosfamide (Ifex), imipenem-cilastatin (Primaxin), leucovorin calcium, lorazepam (Ativan), magnesium sulfate, mannitol (Osmitrol), mechlorethamine (nitrogen mustard), meperidine (Demerol), mesna (Mesnex), methotrexate, methylprednisolone (Solu-Medrol), metoclopramide (Reglan), metronidazole (Flagyl IV), mitomycin (Mutamycin), mitoxantrone (Novantrone), morphine, nalbuphine, ondansetron (Zofran), pemetrexed (Alimta), piperacillin, potassium chloride (KCl), promethazine (Phenergan), ranitidine (Zantac), sodium bicarbonate, streptozocin (Zanosar), sulfamethoxazole/trimethoprim, teniposide (Vumon), thiotepa, ticarcillin/clavulanate (Timentin), tobramycin, vancomycin, vinblastine, vincristine, zidovudine (AZT, Retrovir).

RATE OF ADMINISTRATION

Reduction of cumulative renal toxicity with chemotherapy: A single dose evenly distributed over 15 minutes. Complete amifostine dose but begin cisplatin within 30 minutes after beginning amifostine. Amifostine must be given over 15 minutes; longer infusion times increase the risk of side effects, especially hypotension. Shorter infusion times have not been studied.

Reduction of moderate to severe xerostomia from radiation of the head and neck: A single dose evenly distributed over 3 minutes. Begin infusion 15 to 30 minutes before standard fraction radiation therapy.

ACTIONS

A cytoprotective agent. Rapidly metabolized by alkaline phosphatase in tissues to an active metabolite that can reduce the nephrotoxic effects of cisplatin and the toxic effects of radiation on normal oral tissues. This protective metabolite is generated in greater amounts in normal tissues versus tumor tissues and is available to bind to and detoxify reactive metabolites of cisplatin and/or radiation. It reduces the incidence of cisplatin toxicity including nephrotoxicity but does not cause other toxic reactions. Its protective metabolite can also scavenge reactive oxygen species generated by exposure to either cisplatin or radiation. May adversely affect antitumor effects of cisplatin. Rapidly cleared from plasma with an elimination half-life of 8 minutes. Pretreatment with antiemetics does not alter its actions. Measurable levels of the metabolite have been found in bone marrow; minimal excretion in urine.

INDICATIONS AND USES

Reduce the cumulative renal toxicity associated with repeated administration of cisplatin in patients with advanced ovarian cancer. May allow higher cumulative doses of cisplatin and cyclophosphamide. ■ Reduce the incidence of moderate to severe xerostomia (dryness of the mouth from salivary gland dysfunction) in patients undergoing postoperative radiation treatment for head and neck cancer, where the "radiation port" includes a substantial portion of the parotid glands.

Unlabeled uses: Reduce acute and cumulative hematologic toxicity associated with various chemotherapy regimens (e.g., cisplatin, cyclophosphamide, carboplatin; see literature). ■ Decrease frequency or severity of cisplatin-induced neurotoxicity. ■ Reduce the damaging effects of paclitaxel on lung fibroblasts.

CONTRAINDICATIONS

Known sensitivity to aminothiol compounds or mannitol. ■ Not recommended for patients receiving chemotherapy for malignancies if chemotherapy can produce significant survival benefit or cure; may interfere with effectiveness of chemotherapy regimen and reduce incidence of cure. ■ Not recommended for patients who are hypotensive, dehydrated, or for those receiving antihypertensive therapy that cannot be stopped for 24 hours before amifostine is administered. ■ Not recommended for patients receiving definitive radiotherapy. Tumor-protective effect in this setting has not been ruled out.

PRECAUTIONS

Use caution in the elderly and in patients with pre-existing cardiovascular or cerebrovascular conditions (e.g., arrhythmias, congestive heart failure, history of stroke, history of ischemic heart disease). ■ Hypotension and nausea and vomiting can be severe; use caution in any situation in which these side effects may have serious consequences. ▪ Discontinue antihypertensive therapy 24 hours before administering amifostine. ▪ Hypersensitivity reactions, including anaphylaxis and severe cutaneous reactions, have been reported; see Monitor and Side Effects. Deaths have occurred. ▪ Facilities for monitoring the patient and responding to any medical emergency must be available.

Monitor: *All indications:* Adequate hydration required before administration of amifostine. ▪ Monitor fluid balance carefully, especially in conjunction with highly emetogenic chemotherapy (e.g., cisplatin). ▪ See Usual Dose for premedication requirements. Additional antiemetics may be required to offset nausea and vomiting of chemotherapy drugs. ▪ Keep patient in supine position during and immediately after the infusion. ▪ Hypersensitivity and/or severe cutaneous reactions may occur during or after infusion; monitor closely before, during, and after administration. Serious cutaneous reactions may develop weeks after initiation of therapy. ▪ Monitor serum calcium. Risk of hypocalcemia increased in some patients (e.g., nephrotic syndrome or patients receiving multiple doses). Calcium supplements may be required. ▪ See Dose Adjustments, Rate of Administration, and Antidote.

Reduction of cumulative renal toxicity with chemotherapy: Discontinue antihypertensive therapy if indicated; see Contraindications, Precautions, Drug/Lab Interactions. ▪ Obtain baseline BP and monitor at least every 5 minutes during and immediately after the infusion. Continue monitoring BP as indicated. ▪ Hypertension may be exacerbated by several causes (e.g., interruption of antihypertensive therapy, IV hydration). Monitor BP closely. ▪ Hypotension can occur at any time but is more frequent toward the end of the infusion, and recovery usually begins within 5 to 6 minutes after infusion is discontinued.

Reduction of xerostomia from radiation: Monitor BP before and immediately after the infusion and as indicated by results.

Patient Education: Void before administration. ▪ May produce significant hypotension. Effects may be additive with medications currently being taken. Review all medications (prescription and nonprescription) with nurse and/or physician. ▪ Must remain in supine position until BP stabilized, then request assistance for ambulation. ▪ Report feelings of faintness or nausea promptly. ▪ Promptly report development of any rash or skin condition.

Maternal/Child: Category C: use only if potential benefits justify risk to fetus; embryotoxic in rabbits at doses lower than required for humans. ▪ Discontinue breast-feeding. ▪ Safety for use in pediatric patients not established; experience is limited.

Elderly: Response similar to younger adults; however, dosing should be cautious; see Dose Adjustments. ▪ Monitor fluid balance closely; avoid dehydration. ▪ Hypotension may be sudden and severe; monitor closely. ▪ See Contraindications and Precautions.

DRUG/LAB INTERACTIONS

Antihypertensive therapy (**e.g., ACE inhibitors** [e.g., enalaprilat], **calcium channel blocking agents** [e.g., nicardipine, verapamil], **diuretics** [e.g., furosemide, torsemide], **nitroglycerin, nitroprusside sodium**) should be discontinued 24 hours before amifostine administration; see Contraindications. ▪ Use extreme caution in any patient receiving medications with **hypotensive effects** (**antidepressants, benzodiazepines, beta-adrenergic blocking agents**

[e.g., atenolol, esmolol, metoprolol, propranolol], **lidocaine, magnesium, narcotics, nitrates, paclitaxel, procainamide**); will cause additive hypotension.

SIDE EFFECTS

Hypotension and severe nausea and vomiting occur frequently. Hypotension may be associated with apnea, arrhythmias (e.g., atrial fibrillation/flutter, bradycardia, extrasystoles, tachycardia), chest pain, dyspnea, hypoxia, myocardial ischemia, and rarely renal failure, respiratory and cardiac arrest, seizures, and unconsciousness. Dehydration, dizziness, feelings of cold or warmth, flushing, hiccups, hypocalcemia, loss of consciousness, somnolence, and/or transient hypertension or exacerbation of pre-existing hypertension may occur. Hypersensitivity reactions (e.g., anaphylaxis [rare], arrhythmias, chest tightness, chills, cutaneous eruptions, dyspnea, fever, hypoxia, laryngeal edema, pruritus, sneezing, urticaria) have occurred. Most cutaneous eruptions, pruritus, and urticaria were mild; however, serious skin reactions such as erythema multiforme, exfoliative dermatitis, rash, Stevens-Johnson syndrome (rare), toxic epidermal necrolysis, and urticaria have been reported. Serious skin reactions have been reported more frequently when amifostine is used as a radioprotectant.

Overdose: Hypotension is the most likely symptom. Anxiety and reversible urinary retention have occurred at higher doses. Up to 3 doses have been given within 24 hours without unexpected side effects.

ANTIDOTE

Keep physician informed of side effects. Treatment of nausea and vomiting is imperative to encourage patients to continue treatment with full doses of chemotherapeutic agents. Hypotension may be dose-limiting. If the systolic BP decreases significantly (see Dose Adjustments chart), temporarily discontinue the amifostine still infusing, place the patient in Trendelenburg position, and administer an infusion of NS at a separate site. Vasopressors (e.g., dopamine, norepinephrine [Levophed]) may be required. If indicated, restart infusion if BP returns to baseline within 5 minutes and patient is asymptomatic. Discontinue amifostine immediately and permanently if an acute hypersensitivity or cutaneous reaction occurs. Dermatologic consult may be required. Treat anaphylaxis and resuscitate as necessary.

AMIKACIN SULFATE BBW
(am-ih-**KAY**-sin **SUL**-fayt)

Amikin

**Antibacterial
(aminoglycoside)**

pH 3.5 to 5.5

USUAL DOSE

Up to 15 mg/kg of body weight/24 hr equally divided into 2 or 3 doses at equally divided intervals (5 mg/kg every 8 hours or 7.5 mg/kg every 12 hours). Dosage based on ideal weight of lean body mass. Do not exceed a total adult dose of 15 mg/kg/24 hr in an average weight patient or 1.5 Gm in heavier patients by all routes in 24 hours.

Studies suggest that a single daily dose of 15 to 20 mg/kg (instead of divided into 2 or 3 doses) may provide higher peak levels and enhance drug effectiveness while actually reducing or having no adverse effects on risk of toxicity. Various procedures for monitoring blood levels are in use. Some health facilities are monitoring with trough levels; others may draw levels at predetermined times and plot the concentration on nomograms. Depending on the protocol in place, doses or intervals may be adjusted. See Precautions.

Mycobacterium avium **complex:** 15 mg/kg/24 hr in equally divided doses every 8 to 12 hours (5 mg/kg every 8 hours or 7.5 mg/kg every 12 hours). Part of a 3- to 5-agent regimen.

PEDIATRIC DOSE

15 to 22.5 mg/kg/24 hr equally divided into 2 or 3 doses and given every 8 to 12 hours (5 to 7.5 mg/kg every 8 hours or 7.5 to 11.25 mg/kg every 12 hours). Do not exceed 1.5 Gm/24 hr. A single daily dose is also being used in pediatric patients. See comments under Usual Dose.

NEWBORN DOSE

See Maternal/Child.

10 mg/kg of body weight as a loading dose, then 7.5 mg/kg/dose. Intervals of 7.5 mg/kg dose adjusted based on age as follows:

Under 28 weeks' gestation and less than 7 days of age: Give every 24 hours.
Under 28 weeks' gestation and over 7 days or 28 to 34 weeks' gestation and under 7 days of age: Give every 18 hours.
28 to 34 weeks' gestation and over 7 days of age or over 34 weeks' gestation and under 7 days of age: Give every 12 hours.
Over 34 weeks' gestation and over 7 days of age: Give every 8 hours.

DOSE ADJUSTMENTS

Reduce daily dose commensurate with amount of renal impairment and/or increase intervals between injections. ▪ Reduced dose or extended intervals may be required in the elderly. ▪ See Drug/Lab Interactions.

DILUTION

Each 500 mg or fraction thereof is diluted with 100 to 200 mL D5W, D5NS, or NS. Amount of diluent may be decreased proportionately with dosage for infants and other pediatric patients. Available for pediatric injection as 50 mg/mL.

Storage: Diluted solution stable at room temperature for 24 hours.

COMPATIBILITY   (Underline Indicates Conflicting Compatibility Information)
Consider any drug NOT listed as compatible to be INCOMPATIBLE until consulting a pharmacist; specific conditions may apply.
Do not physically premix with other drugs; administer separately as recommended by manufacturer. Inactivated in solution with beta-lactam antibiotics (e.g., cephalosporins, penicillins) and vancomycin. Do not mix in the same solution. Appropriate spacing required because of physical **incompatibilities**. See Drug/Lab Interactions.

One source suggests the following **compatibilities:**
Solution: Manufacturer lists D5W, D5/¼NS, D5/½NS, NS, LR, D5 in Normosol M (Plasma-Lyte 56 in D5W), D5 in Normosol R (Plasma-Lyte 148 in D5W). Other sources list additional solutions.
Y-site: Acyclovir (Zovirax), amifostine (Ethyol), amiodarone (Nexterone), anidulafungin (Eraxis), aztreonam (Azactam), bivalirudin (Angiomax), caspofungin (Cancidas), cefepime (Maxipime), ceftazidime (Fortaz), cisatracurium (Nimbex), cyclophosphamide (Cytoxan), dexamethasone (Decadron), dexmedetomidine (Precedex), diltiazem (Cardizem), docetaxel (Taxotere), doripenem (Doribax), enalaprilat (Vasotec IV), esmolol (Brevibloc), etoposide phosphate (Etopophos), fenoldopam (Corlopam), filgrastim (Neupogen), fluconazole (Diflucan), fludarabine (Fludara), foscarnet (Foscavir), furosemide (Lasix), gemcitabine (Gemzar), granisetron (Kytril), hetastarch in electrolytes (Hextend), hydromorphone (Dilaudid), idarubicin (Idamycin), labetalol (Trandate), levofloxacin (Levaquin), linezolid (Zyvox), lorazepam (Ativan), magnesium sulfate, melphalan (Alkeran), meperidine (Demerol), midazolam (Versed), milrinone (Primacor), morphine, nicardipine (Cardene IV), ondansetron (Zofran), paclitaxel (Taxol), pemetrexed (Alimta), remifentanil (Ultiva), sargramostim (Leukine), teniposide (Vumon), thiotepa, tigecycline (Tygacil), vinorelbine (Navelbine), warfarin (Coumadin), zidovudine (AZT, Retrovir).

RATE OF ADMINISTRATION
A single dose over at least 30 to 60 minutes. Infants should receive a 1- to 2-hour infusion.

ACTIONS
An aminoglycoside antibiotic with neuromuscular blocking action. Bactericidal against many gram-negative organisms resistant to other antibiotics including other aminoglycosides such as gentamicin, kanamycin (Kantrex), and tobramycin. Well distributed through all body fluids. Usual half-life is 2 to 3 hours. Half-life is prolonged in infants, postpartum females, fever, liver disease and ascites, spinal cord injury, cystic fibrosis, and the elderly; shorter in severe burns. Crosses the placental barrier. Excreted in the kidneys. Cross-allergenicity does occur between aminoglycosides.

INDICATIONS AND USES
Short-term treatment of serious infections caused by susceptible organisms (e.g., gram-negative bacteria) generally resistant to alternate drugs that have less potential toxicity. ■ Effective in infections of the respiratory and urinary tracts, CNS (including meningitis), skin and soft tissue, intraabdominal (including peritonitis), bacterial septicemia (including neonatal sepsis), burns, and postoperative infections. ■ Considered initial therapy in suspected gram-negative infections after culture and sensitivity is drawn. ■ Penicillins may be required concomitantly in neonatal sepsis to treat possible infections from gram-positive organisms.

Unlabeled uses: Treatment of *Mycobacterium avium* complex, a common infection in AIDS (part of a multiple [3 to 5] drug regimen).

CONTRAINDICATIONS

Known amikacin or aminoglycoside sensitivity. Sulfite sensitivity may be a contraindication.

PRECAUTIONS

Sensitivity studies indicated to determine susceptibility of causative organism to amikacin. ▪ Response should occur in 24 to 48 hours. Safety for use longer than 14 days not established. ▪ Superinfection may occur from overgrowth of nonsusceptible organisms. ▪ May contain sulfites; use caution in patients with asthma. ▪ Single daily dosing has been used effectively in abdominal, pelvic inflammatory, and GU infections in patients with normal renal function. Not recommended in bacteremia caused by *Pseudomonas aeruginosa,* endocarditis, meningitis, during pregnancy or in patients less than 6 weeks postpartum. Limited data available for use in all other situations (e.g., burns, cystic fibrosis, elderly, pediatrics, renal impairment). ▪ Risk of nephrotoxicity and neurotoxicity (e.g., auditory and vestibular ototoxicity) increased in patients with pre-existing renal damage or in normal renal function with prolonged use. Partial or total irreversible deafness may continue to develop after amikacin is discontinued. ▪ *Clostridium difficile*–associated diarrhea (CDAD) has been reported. May range from mild diarrhea to fatal colitis. Consider in patients who present with diarrhea during or after treatment with amikacin.

Monitor: Maintain good hydration. ▪ Narrow range between toxic and therapeutic levels. Periodically monitor peak and trough concentrations to avoid peak serum concentrations above 30 mcg/mL and trough concentrations above 5 to 10 mcg/mL. ▪ Monitor urine protein, presence of cells and casts, and decreased specific gravity. Watch for decreased urine output, rising BUN and SCr, and declining CrCl levels. Dose adjustment may be necessary. ▪ Closely monitor patients with impaired renal function for nephrotoxicity and neurotoxicity (e.g., auditory and vestibular ototoxicity); nephrotoxicity may be reversible. ▪ Routine serum levels and hearing evaluations are recommended. ▪ Monitor serum calcium, magnesium, and sodium; levels may decline. ▪ In extended treatment, monitor serum levels, electrolytes, and renal, auditory, and vestibular functions frequently. ▪ See Drug/Lab Interactions.

Patient Education: Report promptly any changes in balance, hearing loss, weakness, or dizziness. ▪ Consider birth control options. ▪ Promptly report diarrhea or bloody stools that occur during treatment or up to several months after an antibiotic has been discontinued; may indicate CDAD and require treatment.

Maternal/Child: Category D: avoid pregnancy. Potential hazard to fetus. ▪ Safety for use during breast-feeding not established; use extreme caution. ▪ Peak concentrations are generally lower in infants and young children. ▪ Use extreme caution in premature infants and neonates; immature kidney function will result in prolonged half-life.

Elderly: Consider less toxic alternatives. ▪ Longer intervals between doses may be more important than smaller doses. ▪ Monitor renal function and drug levels carefully. Measurement of CrCl more useful than BUN or SCr to assess renal function. ▪ Half-life prolonged.

DRUG/LAB INTERACTIONS

Synergistic when used in combination with **beta-lactam antibiotics** (e.g., cephalosporins, penicillins) **and vancomycin.** Synergism may be inconsistent; see Compatibility. ■ Concurrent use topically or systemically with any other **ototoxic or nephrotoxic agents** should be avoided. May have dangerous additive effects with **anesthetics** (e.g., enflurane), **other neuromuscular blocking antibiotics** (e.g., kanamycin), **diuretics** (e.g., furosemide [Lasix]), **beta-lactam antibiotics** (e.g., cephalosporins), **vancomycin, and many others.** ■ **Neuromuscular blocking muscle relaxants** (e.g., atracurium [Tracrium], succinylcholine) are potentiated by aminoglycosides. *Apnea can occur.* ■ Aminoglycosides are potentiated by **anticholinesterases** (e.g., edrophonium), **antineoplastics** (e.g., nitrogen mustard, cisplatin). ■ May be antagonized by **bacteriostatic antibiotics** (e.g., chloramphenicol, erythromycin, and tetracyclines); bacterial action may be affected.

SIDE EFFECTS

Occur more frequently with impaired renal function, higher doses, prolonged administration, in dehydrated or elderly patients, and in patients receiving other ototoxic or nephrotoxic drugs. Fever, headache, hypotension, nausea, paresthesias, seizures, skin rash, tremor, vomiting.

Major: Albuminuria, anemia, arthralgia, azotemia, CDAD, eosinophilia, loss of balance, neuromuscular blockade, oliguria, ototoxicity, RBCs and WBCs or casts in urine, respiratory depression or arrest, rising SCr.

ANTIDOTE

Notify physician of all side effects. If minor side effects persist or any major symptom appears, discontinue drug and notify physician. Treatment is symptomatic, or a reduction in dose may be required. In overdose hemodialysis may be indicated. Monitor fluid balance, CrCl, and plasma levels carefully. Complexation with ticarcillin may be as effective as hemodialysis. Consider exchange transfusion in the newborn. Calcium salts or neostigmine may reverse neuromuscular blockade. Treat CDAD with fluids, electrolytes, protein supplements, and oral vancomycin (Vancocin) or metronidazole (Flagyl) as indicated. In severe cases, surgical evaluation may be indicated. Resuscitate as necessary.

AMINOCAPROIC ACID
(a-mee-noh-ka-**PROH**-ick **AS**-id)

Amicar

Antifibrinolytic
Antihemorrhagic

pH 6 to 7.6

USUAL DOSE
4 to 5 Gm initially over 1 hour. Follow with 1 Gm/hr for 8 hours or until bleeding is controlled. In acute bleeding syndromes, the 4- to 5-Gm dose may be given as a continuous infusion over the first hour, followed by a continuous infusion of 1 Gm/hr for 8 hours or until bleeding is controlled. Maximum dose is 30 Gm/24 hr.

Prevent recurrence of subarachnoid hemorrhage (unlabeled): 36 Gm/24 hr. One source suggests administering 18 Gm in 400 mL D5W every 12 hours for 10 days. Follow with oral therapy.

Prevention of perioperative bleeding during cardiac surgery (unlabeled): 10 Gm as an infusion over 20 to 30 minutes before skin incision. Follow with 1 to 2.5 Gm/hr (usually 2 Gm/hr) until the end of the operation. Infusion may be continued for 4 hours after protamine reversal of heparin. In addition, 10 Gm may be added to the cardiopulmonary bypass circuit priming solution. An alternate regimen is 10 Gm over 20 to 30 minutes before skin incision, followed by 10 Gm after heparin administration, then 10 Gm when cardiopulmonary bypass is discontinued and before protamine reversal of heparin. Another source suggests a loading dose of 80 mg/kg over 20 minutes followed by 30 mg/kg/hr, or a loading dose of 60 mg/kg over 20 minutes followed by 30 mg/kg/hr plus a 10-mg/kg dose in the priming solution of the cardiopulmonary bypass pump.

PEDIATRIC DOSE
Unlabeled: See Maternal/Child. 100 mg/kg of body weight or 3 Gm/M^2 during the first hour. Follow with a continuous infusion of 33.3 mg/kg/hr or 1 Gm/M^2/hr. Do not exceed 18 Gm/M^2/24 hr.

DOSE ADJUSTMENTS
May be required with impaired renal or hepatic function.

DILUTION
1 Gm equals 4 mL of prepared solution. Further dilute with **compatible** infusion solutions (NS, D5NS, D5W, DW [SW for injection], or Ringer's solution). Do not use DW in patients with subarachnoid hemorrhage. Up to 50 mL of diluent may be used for each 1 Gm.

Storage: Before use store at CRT. Do not freeze.

COMPATIBILITY
Compatible in D5W and NS. One source suggests **compatibility** at the **Y-site** with fenoldopam (Corlopam).

RATE OF ADMINISTRATION
5 Gm or fraction thereof over first hour in 250 mL of solution; then administer each succeeding 1 Gm over 1 hour in 50 to 100 mL of solution. Use of an infusion pump for accurate dose recommended. Rapid administration or insufficient dilution may cause hypotension, bradycardia, and/or arrhythmia.

ACTIONS
A monaminocarboxylic acid that acts as an inhibitor of fibrinolysis. Inhibits plasminogen activator substances; to a lesser degree inhibits

plasmin activity. Increases fibrinogen activity in clot formation by inhibiting the enzyme required for destruction of formed fibrin. Onset of action is prompt, but will last less than 3 hours. Partially metabolized. Half-life is 2 hours. Excreted in urine. Easily penetrates RBCs and tissue cells after prolonged administration.

INDICATIONS AND USES

Useful in enhancing hemostasis when fibrinolysis contributes to bleeding. ▪ Treatment of fibrinolytic bleeding, which may be associated with surgical complications following heart surgery (with or without cardiac bypass procedures) and portacaval shunt, hematologic disorders such as aplastic anemia, acute and life-threatening abruptio placentae, hepatic cirrhosis, and neoplastic disease such as carcinoma of the prostate, lung, stomach, and cervix. ▪ Urinary fibrinolysis (normal physiologic phenomenon), which may result from severe trauma, anoxia, shock, surgical hematuria complications following prostatectomy and nephrectomy, or nonsurgical hematuria resulting from polycystic or neoplastic disease of the GU system. ▪ Prophylaxis and treatment of postsurgical hemorrhage. **Unlabeled uses:** Prevent recurrence of subarachnoid hemorrhage. ▪ Control of bleeding in thrombocytopenia. ▪ Prevention of perioperative bleeding during cardiac surgery. ▪ Prophylaxis and treatment during dental surgical procedures (hemophilia and/or hemorrhage).

CONTRAINDICATIONS

Evidence of an active intravascular clotting process. ▪ Uncertainty as to whether the cause of bleeding is primary fibrinolysis (PF) or disseminated intravascular coagulation (DIC). This distinction must be made before administration; see Precautions. ▪ Do not use aminocaproic acid in the presence of DIC without concomitant heparin.

PRECAUTIONS

Should not be administered without a definite diagnosis and/or lab findings indicative of hyperfibrinolysis. ▪ The following tests are used to differentiate primary fibrinolysis (PF) from disseminated intravascular coagulation (DIC). Platelet count should be normal in PF but is usually decreased in DIC; protamine paracoagulation test is negative in PF and positive in DIC (a precipitate forms when protamine sulfate is dropped into citrated plasma); euglobulin clot lysis test is abnormal in PF but normal in DIC. ▪ In life-threatening situations, transfusion and other appropriate emergency measures may be required. ▪ Avoid use in patients with hematuria of upper urinary tract origin. Has caused glomerular capillary thrombosis in the renal pelvis and ureters, leading to intrarenal obstruction. ▪ Use with caution in patients with cardiac disease. May cause hypotension and bradycardia. Endocardial hemorrhage and fatty degeneration of the myocardium have been reported in animals. ▪ Use with caution in patients with hepatic disease. Etiology of bleeding may be multifactorial and difficult to diagnose. ▪ Use with caution in patients with renal impairment; see Dose Adjustments. Kidney stones have been reported in animal studies. ▪ Skeletal muscle weakness with necrosis of muscle fibers has been reported after prolonged use; see Monitor. ▪ An increased incidence of certain neurologic deficits (e.g., cerebral ischemia, cerebral vasospasm, hydrocephalus) associated with the use of antifibrinolytic agents in the treatment of subarachnoid hemorrhage has been reported. Relationship to drug therapy versus natural disease process or diagnostic procedures (e.g., angiography) is unclear.

Monitor: See Precautions and Contraindications. ■ Use only in conjunction with general and specific tests to determine the amount of fibrinolysis present (e.g., fibrinogen, PT, aPTT). ■ Monitor lab evaluations as appropriate for diagnosis (e.g., platelet count, clotting factors, CPK, AST). ■ Vital signs, intake and output, any signs of bleeding, and neurologic assessment should be monitored based on patient condition. ■ Observe for thromboembolic complications (e.g., chest pain, dyspnea, edema, hemoptysis, leg pain, or positive Homans' sign). ■ Monitor for S/S of skeletal muscle damage. May range from mild myalgias with weakness to severe proximal myopathy with rhabdomyolysis, myoglobinuria, and acute renal failure. ■ Monitor lab evaluations as appropriate for diagnosis (e.g., platelet count, clotting factors, CPK, AST).

Patient Education: Move slowly with help to avoid orthostatic hypotension.

Maternal/Child: Category C: safety for use in pregnancy and breast-feeding not established. ■ Safety for use in pediatric patients not established but is used. ■ Contains benzyl alcohol, which has been associated with "gasping syndrome" in neonates (sudden onset of gasping respirations, hypotension, bradycardia, and cardiovascular collapse).

Elderly: Consider age-related impaired organ function; reduced dose may be indicated.

DRUG/LAB INTERACTIONS

Potential for thrombus formation increased with concurrent use of **estrogens.** ■ Frequently used with **clotting factor complexes** (e.g., factor IX complex, anti-inhibitor coagulant complex), but risk of thrombus formation may be increased. Delay administration for 8 or more hours after clotting factor complexes. ■ Prolongation of template **bleeding time** has been reported during continuous infusions exceeding 24 Gm/day.

SIDE EFFECTS

Generally well tolerated. Abdominal pain, agranulocytosis, bradycardia, coagulation disorder, confusion, cramps, decreased vision, diarrhea, dizziness, dyspnea, edema, grand mal seizure, hallucinations, headache, hypersensitivity reactions (including anaphylaxis), hypotension, increased BUN and CPK, injection site reactions, intracranial hypertension, leukopenia, malaise, muscle weakness, myalgia, myopathy, myositis, nausea, peripheral ischemia, pruritus, pulmonary embolism, renal failure, rhabdomyolysis, rash, stuffy nose, stroke, syncope, tearing, thrombocytopenia, thrombophlebitis, thrombosis, tinnitus, vomiting.

Overdose: Acute renal failure, convulsions, death.

ANTIDOTE

Treat side effects symptomatically. Discontinue use of drug with any suspicion of thrombophlebitis, thromboembolic complications, or if CPK is elevated (myopathy). In life-threatening situations, fresh whole blood transfusions, fibrinogen infusions, and other emergency measures may be required. May be removed by hemodialysis or peritoneal dialysis.

AMINOPHYLLINE
(am-ih-**NOFF**-ih-lin)

**(79% Theophylline), Theophylline
Ethylenediamine**

Bronchodilator
Respiratory stimulant

pH 8.6 to 9

USUAL DOSE

To obtain maximum benefit with minimal risk of adverse effects, dosing must be individualized based on serum theophylline concentration and patient response. Monitor frequently to avoid toxicity. Only aminophylline premixed in solution or aminophylline containing 20 mg of theophylline for each 25 mg of aminophylline is intended for IV use (approximately 79% theophylline). *All doses are based on lean body weight;* theophylline does not distribute into fatty tissue. *All doses listed are milligrams of aminophylline to be administered.*

BRONCHODILATION IN ACUTE ASTHMA OR BRONCHOSPASM

With an average mean volume of distribution of 0.5 L/kg (range is 0.3 to 0.7 L/kg), each mg/kg of theophylline given over 30 minutes should result in an average 2 mcg/mL increase in serum theophylline concentration. **Adults, children, infants and neonates who *HAVE NOT* received a theophylline preparation in the previous 24 hours:** An *initial loading dose* of 5 to 6 mg/kg of lean body weight (5.7 mg of aminophylline is equal to 4.6 mg/kg of theophylline) should produce a serum concentration of 10 mcg/mL (range 6 to 16 mcg/mL). Measure serum theophylline concentration in 30 minutes to determine if additional loading doses are indicated. Once a serum concentration of 10 to 15 mcg/mL is obtained with loading dose(s), it should be maintained with a continuous infusion. Rate of infusion is based on the pharmacokinetic parameters (e.g., volume of distribution, clearance, concomitant disease states) of the specific patient population and should achieve a target serum concentration of 10 mcg/mL. See Dose Adjustments and Monitor for recommendations of serum theophylline testing after an infusion is started. **Adults, children, infants and neonates who *HAVE* received a theophylline preparation in the previous 24 hours:** *A serum theophylline concentration must be obtained before considering any loading dose.* Calculate the appropriate loading dose with the following formula.

$$D = (\text{Desired C} - \text{Measured C}) \times (V)$$

D is the loading dose, C is the serum theophylline concentration, and V is the volume of distribution (0.5 L/kg). Desired serum concentration in this situation should be conservative (e.g., 10 mcg/mL) to allow for variability in the volume of distribution; carefully evaluating the patient condition and risk versus benefit. It is not recommended by the manufacturer, but another source suggests that a smaller loading dose may be considered if it is not immediately possible to obtain a theophylline serum concentration. Carefully evaluate the patient's condition and risk versus benefit. The potential for theophylline toxicity must be ruled out. For example, if significant respiratory distress is present, a smaller loading dose of 2.5 mg/kg should increase the theophylline level by approximately 5 mcg/mL. In the absence of toxicity, this increase is unlikely to cause significant side effects and may improve the clinical picture. In all situations, measure serum theophylline concentration in 30 minutes to determine if additional loading doses are indicated. Once a serum concentration of 10 to 15 mcg/mL is obtained with or without loading dose(s), it should be maintained with a continuous infusion. Rate of infusion is based on the pharmacokinetic parameters (e.g., volume of distribution, clearance, concomitant disease states) of the specific patient population and should achieve a target serum concentration of 10 mcg/mL. See Dose Adjustments and Monitor for recommendations of serum theophylline testing after an infusion is started. **Maintenance infusion:** Desired theophylline serum concentration is 10 mcg/mL. Most maintenance doses can be reduced within the first 12 hours based on serum theophylline levels and depending on patient condition and response; see Dose Adjustments. Because of a large interpatient variability in theophylline clearance, each patient may differ from the mean value used to calculate these infusion rates. Another serum concentration is recommended one expected half-life after starting the continuous infusion; see Dose Adjustments.

Aminophylline Infusion Rates Following an Appropriate Loading Dose	
Patient Population	Aminophylline Infusion Rate in mg/kg/hr[a] (Actual theophylline administered in mg/kg/hr is in parentheses)
Neonates up to 24 days of age	1.25 mg/kg *every 12 hours* (1 mg/kg *every 12 hours*)[b]
Neonates over 24 days of age	1.875 mg/kg *every 12 hours* (1.5 mg/kg *every 12 hours*)[b]
Infants 6 to 52 weeks of age	mg/kg/hr = 0.01 × age in weeks + 0.21[c] (0.008 × age in weeks + 0.21)
Children 1 to 9 years	1 mg/kg/hr (0.8 mg/kg/hr)
Children 9 to 12 years	0.875 mg/kg/hr (0.7 mg/kg/hr)
Adolescent smokers 12 to 16 years	0.875 mg/kg/hr (0.7 mg/kg/hr)
Adolescent nonsmokers 12 to 16 years	0.625 mg/kg/hr (0.5 mg/kg/hr)[d]
Adults (healthy nonsmokers 16 to 60 years)	0.5 mg/kg/hr (0.4 mg/kg/hr)[d]
Elderly over 60 years	0.375 mg/kg/hr (0.3 mg/kg/hr)[e]
Cardiac decompensation, cor pulmonale, liver dysfunction, sepsis with multi-organ failure, or shock	0.25 mg/kg/hr (0.2 mg/kg/hr)[e]

[a]Lower initial dose may be required for patients receiving other drugs that decrease theophylline clearance (e.g., cimetidine [Tagamet]).
[b]To achieve a target concentration of 7.5 mcg/mL for neonatal apnea.
[c]The 0.21 factor was not adjusted from the theophylline formula because it may not have the same proportional value. See package insert or contact Abbott if additional information desired.
[d]Not to exceed 900 mg/day unless serum levels indicate need for a larger dose.
[e]Not to exceed 400 mg/day or 21 mg/hr (17 mg/hr as theophylline) unless serum levels indicate need for a larger dose.

Continued

REVERSE ADENOSINE-MEDIATED EFFECTS OF DIPYRIDAMOLE IN ADULTS (UNLABELED)
50 to 100 mg over 30 to 60 seconds. Do not exceed a rate of 50 mg/30 sec.
Maximum dose is 250 mg.

NEONATAL DOSE

Apnea and bradycardia of prematurity (unlabeled): *Loading dose:* 5 to 6 mg/kg
given over 20 to 30 minutes. See all criteria under Usual Dose.
Maintenance dose: See Maintenance Infusion under Usual Dose. Manufacturer recommends keeping serum theophylline level at 7.5 mcg/mL.
Another source recommends 1 to 2 mg/kg/dose every 6 to 8 hours.

DOSE ADJUSTMENTS

To determine if the concentration is accumulating or declining from the
post–loading dose level, a serum concentration is recommended one
expected half-life after starting the continuous infusion; see the following
chart or see literature for a complete summary. If the level is declining
(higher than average clearance) consider an additional loading dose or
increasing the infusion rate. If the level is increasing, assume accumulation
and decrease the infusion rate before the level exceeds 20 mcg/mL.

Theophylline Half-Life (Approximate)	
Age	Half-Life Mean (Range) in Hours
Premature neonates, see Maternal/Child	
3 to 15 days	30 (17 to 43) hours
25 to 57 days	20 (9.4 to 30.6) hours
Term infants, see Maternal/Child	
1 to 2 days	25.7 (25 to 26.5) hours
3 to 30 weeks	11 (6 to 29) hours
Children	
1 to 4 years	3.4 (1.2 to 5.6) hours
4 to 12 years	Not reported in studies
13 to 15 years	Not reported in studies
16 to 17 years	3.7 (1.5 to 5.9) hours
Adults (16 to 60 years) and healthy nonsmok-ing asthmatics	8.7 (6.1 to 12.8) hours
Elderly (over 60 years); nonsmokers with normal cardiac, liver, and renal function	9.8 (1.6 to 18) hours

There are huge variances in patients with concurrent illness or altered
physiologic states (e.g., acute pulmonary edema, COPD, cystic fibrosis,
fever with acute viral respiratory illness in pediatric patients [9 to 15
years], liver disease, pregnancy, sepsis with multi-organ failure, thyroid
disease); see package insert. ■ In patients with cor pulmonale, cardiac
decompensation, liver dysfunction, or in those taking drugs that markedly
reduce theophylline clearance (e.g., cimetidine [Tagamet]), the initial
aminophylline infusion rate should not exceed 21 mg/hr (17 mg/hr as
theophylline) unless serum concentrations can be monitored every 24
hours. Up to 5 days may be required before steady state is reached in these

patients; see Drug Interactions. ▪ To decrease the risk of side effects associated with unexpected large increases in serum theophylline concentration, dose adjustment recommendations should be considered as the upper limit.

Final Dose Adjustment Guided by Serum Theophylline Concentration*	
Peak Serum Concentration	Dose Adjustment
Less than 9.9 mcg/mL	If symptoms are not controlled and current dose is tolerated, increase infusion rate about 25%. Recheck serum concentration after 12 hours in pediatric patients and 24 hours in adults for further dose adjustment.
10 to 14.9 mcg/mL	If symptoms are controlled and current dose is tolerated, maintain infusion rate and recheck serum concentration at 24-hour intervals. If symptoms are not controlled and current dose is tolerated, consider adding additional medication(s) to treatment regimen.
15 to 19.9 mcg/mL	Consider 10% decrease in infusion rate to provide greater margin of safety, even if current dose is tolerated.†
20 to 24.9 mcg/mL	Decrease infusion rate by 25%, even if no side effects are present. Recheck serum concentration after 12 hours in pediatric patients and 24 hours in adults to guide further dose adjustment.
25 to 30 mcg/mL	Stop infusion for 12 hours in pediatric patients and 24 hours in adults and decrease subsequent infusion rate at least 25% even if no side effects are present. Recheck serum concentration after 12 hours in pediatric patients and 24 hours in adults to guide further dose adjustment. If symptomatic, stop infusion and consider need for overdose treatment; see Antidote.
Over 30 mcg/mL	Stop the infusion and treat overdose as indicated; see Antidote. If aminophylline is subsequently resumed, decrease infusion rate by at least 50% and recheck serum concentration after 12 hours in pediatric patients and 24 hours in adults to guide further dose adjustment.

*Dose increases should not be made in patients with an acute exacerbation of symptoms unless the steady-state serum theophylline concentration is less than 10 mcg/mL.
†Dose reduction and/or serum theophylline concentration measurement is indicated whenever side effects are present, physiologic abnormalities that can reduce theophylline clearance occur (e.g., sustained fever), or a drug that interacts with theophylline is added or discontinued; see Precautions and Drug/Lab Interactions.

DILUTION
Check vial carefully; must state, "For IV use." Warm to room temperature. Only the 25 mg/mL solution may be given by IV injection undiluted, but further dilution for infusion in at least 100 to 200 mL of D5W is preferred. NS or dextrose in saline solutions may be used. Available prediluted. Crystals will form if solution pH falls below 8.
Storage: Usually stored between 15° and 30° C (59° and 86° F). Protect from light and freezing.

COMPATIBILITY   (Underline Indicates Conflicting Compatibility Information)
Consider any drug NOT listed as compatible to be INCOMPATIBLE until consulting a pharmacist; specific conditions may apply.
Manufacturer states, "Should not be mixed in a syringe with other drugs but should be added separately to the IV solution," and recommends discontinuing other solutions infusing at the same site if there is a potential problem with admixture **incompatibility.** Manufacturer recommends avoiding admixtures with alkali labile drugs (e.g., epinephrine, norepinephrine [Levophed], isoproterenol [Isuprel], penicillin G potassium). Precipitation in acidic media may occur with the undiluted solution but not to dilute solutions in IV infusions.

One source suggests the following **compatibilities:**
Additive: Amikacin (Amikin), amobarbital, ascorbic acid, calcium gluconate, chloramphenicol (Chloromycetin), dexamethasone (Decadron), dimenhydrinate, diphenhydramine (Benadryl), dopamine, erythromycin (Erythrocin), esmolol (Brevibloc), flumazenil (Romazicon), furosemide (Lasix), heparin, hydrocortisone sodium succinate (Solu-Cortef), lidocaine, meropenem (Merrem IV), methyldopate, methylprednisolone (Solu-Medrol), midazolam (Versed), nafcillin (Nallpen), nitroglycerin IV, pentobarbital (Nembutal), phenobarbital (Luminal), potassium chloride (KCl), ranitidine (Zantac), sodium bicarbonate, vancomycin, zinc.
Y-site: Allopurinol (Aloprim), amifostine (Ethyol), amphotericin B cholesteryl (Amphotec), anidulafungin (Eraxis), aztreonam (Azactam), bivalirudin (Angiomax), ceftazidime (Fortaz), cisatracurium (Nimbex), cladribine (Leustatin), dexmedetomidine (Precedex), diltiazem (Cardizem), docetaxel (Taxotere), doripenem (Doribax), doxorubicin liposomal (Doxil), enalaprilat (Vasotec IV), esmolol (Brevibloc), etoposide phosphate (Etopophos), famotidine (Pepcid IV), filgrastim (Neupogen), fluconazole (Diflucan), fludarabine (Fludara), foscarnet (Foscavir), gallium nitrate (Ganite), gemcitabine (Gemzar), granisetron (Kytril), hetastarch in electrolytes (Hextend), inamrinone (Amrinone), labetalol (Trandate), levofloxacin (Levaquin), linezolid (Zyvox), melphalan (Alkeran), meropenem (Merrem IV), micafungin (Mycamine), morphine, nicardipine (Cardene IV), paclitaxel (Taxol), pancuronium, pemetrexed (Alimta), piperacillin/tazobactam (Zosyn), potassium chloride (KCl), propofol (Diprivan), ranitidine (Zantac), remifentanil (Ultiva), sargramostim (Leukine), tacrolimus (Prograf), teniposide (Vumon), thiotepa, vecuronium.

RATE OF ADMINISTRATION
A single dose over a minimum of 20 to 30 minutes. Most references suggest a minimum of 30 minutes. Do not exceed an average rate of 1 mL or 25 mg/min when giving by IV injection or as an infusion. Rapid administration may cause cardiac arrhythmias. Discontinue primary infusion if theophylline administered by piggyback or additive tubing and a possible **incompatibility** problem exists.
Reverse adenosine-mediated effects of dipyridamole: See Usual Dose.

ACTIONS
An alkaloid xanthine derivative. It relaxes smooth muscle in the airways (bronchodilation) and suppresses the response of the airways to stimuli (non-bronchodilator prophylactic effects). Cardiac output, urinary output, and sodium excretion are increased. Skeletal and cardiac muscles are stimulated, as is the CNS to a lesser degree. There is peripheral vasodilation. It decreases pulmonary artery pressure and lowers the threshold of

the respiratory center to CO_2. Well distributed throughout the body. In adults and pediatric patients over 1 year of age, 90% of a dose is metabolized in the liver. Because of a large interpatient variability in theophylline clearance, half-life varies extensively based on age, concurrent illness, or altered physiological state; see Dose Adjustments, Precautions, Maternal/Child, and Elderly. Excreted in a changed form in the urine. Crosses the placental barrier. Secreted in breast milk.

INDICATIONS AND USES

Adjunct to inhaled beta-2 selective agonists (e.g., albuterol) and systemic corticosteroids for the treatment of acute exacerbations of the symptoms and reversible airflow obstruction associated with asthma and other chronic lung diseases (e.g., emphysema, chronic bronchitis).

Unlabeled uses: Apnea and bradycardia of prematurity. ▪ Reduce bronchospasm in cystic fibrosis and acute descending respiratory infections. ▪ Relieve periodic apnea and increase arterial blood pH in patients with Cheyne-Stokes respirations. ▪ Reverse adenosine-mediated effects of dipyridamole (Persantine) (e.g., angina pectoris, bronchospasm, severe hypotension, ventricular arrhythmias).

CONTRAINDICATIONS

Known sensitivity to theophylline or ethylenediamine.

PRECAUTIONS

There is an increase in the volume of distribution of theophylline (primarily due to reduction in plasma protein binding) in premature neonates, patients with hepatic cirrhosis, uncorrected acidemia, the elderly, and women during the third trimester of pregnancy. Toxicity may occur in the therapeutic range. ▪ Theophylline clearance may be reduced in neonates (term and premature); children less than 1 year; elderly (over 60 years); infants less than 3 months of age with reduced renal function; patients with acute pulmonary edema, congestive heart failure, cor pulmonale, hypothyroidism, liver disease (e.g., cirrhosis, acute hepatitis), sepsis with multiorgan failure, shock; or in patients with a fever of 102° F or more for 24 hours or more, or lesser temperature elevations for longer periods. Risk of severe toxicity increased in these patient populations; dose reduction and more frequent monitoring may be required. ▪ Use with extreme caution in patients with active peptic ulcer disease, cardiac arrhythmias (not including bradyarrhythmias), or seizures; may exacerbate these conditions. ▪ Initiate oral therapy as soon as symptoms are adequately improved. Wait 4 to 6 hours after last IV dose or measure serum levels. ▪ May cause hypercalcemia at therapeutic theophylline concentrations in patients with hyperthyroid disease. ▪ See Maternal/Child and Drug/Lab Interactions.

Monitor: Monitor serum levels as directed in Usual Dose and Dose Adjustments to achieve maximum benefit with minimum risk. Each 0.5 mg/kg will increase serum theophylline by 1 mcg/mL. 10 mcg/mL to less than 20 mcg/mL is considered therapeutic. Peak serum level is best measured 20 to 30 minutes after initial loading dose, a half life after the initial infusion, or 12 to 14 hours into continuous infusion. ▪ Monitor vital signs, including lung sounds. ▪ Monitor for all signs of toxicity; see Side Effects. Serious toxicity may not be preceded by less severe side effects. ▪ Serum theophylline measurements are indicated before making a dose increase; whenever signs or symptoms of toxicity are present; whenever a new illness presents, an existing illness worsens, or a change in treatment regimen is initiated that may alter theophylline clearance (e.g., sustained fever, hepatitis [see Precautions], or drugs that may interact [see Drug/Lab Interactions]); and every 24 hours throughout the infusion. ■ Stop the IV infusion and obtain a serum theophylline concentration immediately in any patient on aminophylline who develops nausea or vomiting (particularly repetitive vomiting) or if any other signs of toxicity occur, even if another cause is suspected. ■ Dose increases should not be made in patients with an acute exacerbation of symptoms unless the steady-state serum theophylline concentration is less than 10 mcg/mL. ■ Patients with a very high initial clearance rate (low steady-state serum theophylline concentrations at above-average doses) are likely to experience large changes in serum concentration in response to dose changes. ■ Maintain hydration. ■ See Precautions, Maternal/Child, Elderly, and Drug/Lab Interactions.

Patient Education: Do not take or discontinue any prescription or over-the-counter medication, including herbal products, without physician's approval. ■ Promptly report S/S of toxicity (e.g., nausea and vomiting).

Maternal/Child: Category C: use in pregnancy only if clearly indicated. ■ Neonates may have therapeutic blood levels and may develop apnea from theophylline withdrawal. ■ Elimination of drug is prolonged in premature infants, neonates, and children up to 1 year. Use with extreme caution in pediatric patients. Has caused fatal reactions. Elimination reaches maximum values by 1 year of age, remains fairly constant to 9 years of age, and slowly decreases by approximately 50% to adult values at 16 years of age. ■ Pediatric patients under the age of 1 year, as well as neonates with decreased renal function, require careful attention to dosing and frequent monitoring of serum theophylline concentrations. ■ Secreted in breast milk; some sources recommend discontinuing breast-feeding. If the decision is made to breast-feed, monitor infant for evidence of side effects.

Elderly: Compared to healthy young adults, clearance of theophylline is decreased an average of 30% in healthy elderly. Monitor dosing carefully; frequent serum theophylline concentrations are recommended. See Dose Adjustments, Precautions, and Monitor.

DRUG/LAB INTERACTIONS

Review of patient drug profile by pharmacist is imperative at time of initiation of aminophylline and with any change in medication regimen. ■ Do not use one **xanthine derivative** concurrently with another **xanthine derivative, ephedrine, or other sympathomimetic drugs.** ■ Xanthines antagonize or potentiate or are themselves antagonized or potentiated by many drug groups. Monitor serum levels as indicated. **Theophylline clearance increased and serum levels decreased by aminoglutenide, barbiturates, carbamazepine** (Tegretol), **isoproterenol** (Isuprel), **hydantoins** (e.g., phenytoin [Dilantin]), **rifampin** (Rifadin), **smoking, sulfinpyrazone** (Anturane). **Theophylline clearance decreased and serum levels increased by alcohol, allopurinol, beta-adrenergic blockers** (e.g., propranolol), **cimetidine** (Tagamet), **ciprofloxacin** (Cipro IV), **clarithromycin, disulfiram** (Antabuse), **erythromycin, estrogen-containing oral contraceptives, fluvoxamine** (Luvox), **interferon alfa-A, methotrexate, mexiletine, pentoxifylline** (Trental), **propafenone** (Rythmol), **tacrine** (Cognex), **thiabendazole** (Mintezol), **ticlopidine** (Ticlid), **troleandomycin** (TAO), **verapamil.** ■ Inhibits **pancuronium;** increased doses of pancuronium may be required to achieve neuromuscular blockade. ■ **Carbamazepine** (Tegretol) **and loop diuretics** (e.g., furosemide [Lasix]) may increase or decrease serum levels. ■ Reduces sedative effect of **benzodiazepines** (e.g., diazepam [Valium], midazolam [Versed]) **and of propofol** (Diprivan); increased doses of sedatives may be required. To avoid respiratory depression, reduce sedative dose if aminophylline is discontinued or if dose is significantly reduced. ▪ May decrease **lithium** levels. Dose adjustment and monitoring of lithium levels may be indicated. ▪ Concurrent use with **halothane** may induce cardiac arrhythmias. ▪ Concurrent use with **ketamine** may lower aminophylline seizure level. ▪ Concurrent use with **ephedrine** may increase nausea, nervousness, and insomnia. ▪ May increase **lab values** for free fatty acids, glucose, HDL, LDL, total cholesterol, uric acid, and urinary free cortisol excretion. ▪ Caffeine and xanthine metabolites in neonates or patients with renal dysfunction may cause readings from some **immunoassay techniques** to be higher than the actual serum theophylline concentration. ▪ Interferes with **dipyridamole-assisted MI perfusion studies.**

SIDE EFFECTS

Headache, insomnia, nausea, vomiting most common when peak serum concentrations are less than 20 mcg/mL. Rarely a severe hypersensitivity reaction of the skin (e.g., exfoliative dermatitis) may occur. Toxicity resulting in death may occur suddenly at levels less than 20 mcg/mL, especially in certain populations (see Precautions); may occur more frequently with serum levels above 20 mcg/mL. Anxiety, cardiac arrest, arrhythmias (e.g., atrial fibrillation, ventricular fibrillation), convulsions, delirium, dizziness, flushing, hyperpyrexia, intractable seizures, nausea, peripheral vascular collapse, persistent vomiting, restlessness, temporary hypotension.

Overdose: *Acute:* Acid/base disturbances, arrhythmias (e.g., sinus tachycardia), hyperglycemia, hypokalemia, seizures (usually with serum concentrations over 100 mcg/mL), vomiting, and death have occurred.

Chronic: All of the above plus various arrhythmias, seizures (with serum concentration greater than 30 mcg/mL), and death.

ANTIDOTE

With onset of any side effect, discontinue drug and notify physician. ▪ Stop the IV infusion and obtain a serum theophylline concentration immediately in any patient on aminophylline who develops nausea or vomiting (particularly repetitive vomiting) or if any other signs of toxicity occur, even if another cause is suspected. ▪ For mild symptoms the physician may choose to continue the drug at a decreased dose and rate of administration. All side effects will be treated symptomatically. Maintain adequate ventilation and adequate hydration. Grand mal seizures may not respond to anticonvulsants. Diazepam (Valium) may be most effective. Treat atrial arrhythmias with verapamil, ventricular arrhythmias with lidocaine or procainamide. Use dopamine for hypotension. Do not use stimulants. Resuscitate as necessary.

Continued

MANUFACTURER'S SPECIFIC RECOMMENDATIONS FOR ACUTE AND CHRONIC OVERDOSE
Acute overdose (e.g., excessive loading dose or excessive infusion rate for less than 24 hours) or chronic overdose (e.g., excessive infusion rate for more than 24 hours): Serum concentration 20 to 30 mcg/mL: Stop the infusion, monitor the patient, and obtain a serum theophylline concentration in 2 to 4 hours to ensure that the concentration is decreasing.
Acute overdose with a serum concentration of 30 to 100 mcg/mL or chronic overdose with serum concentrations greater than 30 mcg/mL in patients less than 60 years of age: Stop the infusion. Administer multiple-dose, oral-activated charcoal and measures to control emesis. Monitor the patient and obtain serial theophylline concentrations every 2 to 4 hours to determine the effectiveness of therapy and to determine further treatment decisions. Institute extracorporeal removal if emesis, seizures, or cardiac arrhythmias cannot be adequately controlled.
Acute overdose with a serum concentration greater than 100 mcg/mL or chronic overdose with serum concentrations greater than 30 mcg/mL in patients 60 years or older: Stop the infusion. Consider prophylactic anticonvulsant therapy. Administer multiple-dose oral-activated charcoal and measures to control emesis. Consider extracorporeal removal, even if the patient has not experienced a seizure. Monitor the patient and obtain serial theophylline concentrations every 2 to 4 hours to determine the effectiveness of therapy and to determine further treatment decisions.
Extracorporeal removal: Weigh risk versus benefits. Charcoal hemoperfusion is the most effective and increases theophylline clearance up to six-fold, but hypotension, hypocalcemia, and platelet consumption and bleeding diatheses may occur. Hemodialysis is about as efficient as multiple-dose oral-activated charcoal and has a lower risk of serious complications. Consider hemodialysis when charcoal hemoperfusion is not feasible and multiple-dose oral-activated charcoal is ineffective because of intractable emesis. Serum theophylline concentrations may rebound 5 to 10 mcg/mL after either treatment is discontinued due to redistribution of theophylline from the tissue compartment. Peritoneal dialysis is ineffective, and exchange transfusions in neonates have been minimally effective.

AMIODARONE HYDROCHLORIDE
(am-ee-**OH**-dah-rohn hy-droh-**KLOR**-eyed)

Nexterone

Antiarrhythmic

pH 4.08

USUAL DOSE
TREATMENT AND PROPHYLAXIS OF VENTRICULAR TACHYCARDIA (VT) AND VENTRICULAR FIBRILLATION (VF)

1,000 mg over the first 24 hours in 3 distinct segments; two loading infusions and a maintenance infusion. Use of a dedicated central venous catheter preferred.

Rapid loading infusion: 150 mg specifically diluted solution (1.5 mg/mL) over 10 minutes. Follow immediately with the slow loading infusion.

Slow loading infusion: 360 mg specifically diluted solution (1.8 mg/mL) at 1 mg/min over the next 6 hours.

Maintenance infusion: 540 mg of 1.8 mg/mL solution at 0.5 mg/min over 18 hours. Maintenance infusion is usually continued at 0.5 mg/min for 48 to 96 hours or until ventricular arrhythmias are stabilized. May be continued with caution for up to 2 to 3 weeks. Transfer to oral therapy as soon as feasible (guidelines are in package insert).

TREATMENT OF BREAKTHROUGH VENTRICULAR FIBRILLATION (VF) OR HEMODYNAMICALLY UNSTABLE VENTRICULAR TACHYCARDIA (VT)

At any time that breakthrough VF or hemodynamically unstable VT occurs during administration, a supplemental rapid loading infusion (150 mg over 10 minutes) may be repeated. May be specifically diluted 1.5 mg/mL solution or rate of the maintenance infusion (1.8 mg/mL) may be temporarily increased to equal 150 mg (83.33 mL) over 10 minutes. During trials total doses above 1,800 to 2,100 mg (including added doses for breakthrough VF/VT) increased the risk of hypotension. In life-threatening arrhythmias, AHA guidelines state that this rapid loading infusion (150 mg over 10 minutes) may be repeated every 10 minutes as needed and recommend a maximum cumulative dose of 2.2 Gm/24 hr.

CARDIAC ARREST (UNLABELED)

300 mg (6 mL) or 5 mg/kg as a bolus injection. Flush with 10 mL D5W or NS. Should be given through a separate IV line immediately after the first dose of epinephrine (1 mg) and before the fourth electrical countershock. Supplemental doses of 150 mg (3 mL) may be given for recurrent bouts of VT/VF. AHA guidelines recommend a first dose of 300 mg IV push and a second dose, if needed, of 150 mg IV push. After return of spontaneous circulation (ROSC), initiate the slow loading infusion and maintenance infusion as above. If effective, discontinue amiodarone and reassess arrhythmia management within 6 to 24 hours.

SUPRAVENTRICULAR ARRHYTHMIAS (UNLABELED)

150 mg over 10 minutes as a loading dose. Follow with an infusion of 360 mg over 6 hours followed by a maintenance infusion of 0.5 mg/min. Other regimens used during studies to convert atrial fibrillation and atrial flutter to sinus rhythm include 5 mg/kg over 3 to 5 minutes; 5 to 7 mg/kg as a 30-minute infusion followed by a continuous infusion to a maximum total dose of 1,500 mg/24 hr; an infusion of 2 mg/kg/hr continued for up

Continued

to 2 hours after conversion to a stable sinus rhythm or a maximum dose of 2,400 mg/24 hr.

INTRAVENOUS TO ORAL TRANSITION

Guidelines for IV to oral transition are located in manufacturer's literature. See Prescribing Information or consult pharmacist.

PEDIATRIC DOSE

Safety for use in pediatric patients (particularly infants and neonates) not established and not recommended; see Contraindications and Maternal/Child.

Treatment of refractory pulseless VT, VF (unlabeled): AHA guidelines recommend 5 mg/kg by IV bolus. May repeat to a maximum of 15 mg/kg/24 hr. Total dose in adolescents is 2.2 Gm/24 hr. Maximum single dose is 300 mg.

Treatment of perfusing supraventricular and ventricular arrhythmias (unlabeled): AHA guidelines recommend 5 mg/kg as an infusion over 20 to 60 minutes (maximum single dose 300 mg). May repeat to a maximum of 15 mg/kg/24 hr. Total dose in adolescents is 2.2 Gm/24 hr.

DOSE ADJUSTMENTS

Rate of maintenance infusion may be increased to achieve effective arrhythmia suppression. ▪ Not required in renal or hepatic disease. Another source suggests a reduced dose in hepatic failure. ▪ Dose selection should be cautious in the elderly. Reduced initial doses may be indicated based on the potential for decreased organ function and concomitant disease or drug therapy.

DILUTION

Available as a premixed solution in 1.5 mg/mL and 1.8 mg/mL concentrations or as a vial that must be further diluted. To further dilute vials, do not use evacuated glass intravenous bottles. Use only commercially available D5W (D5W or NS may be used for Nexterone) solutions in polyolefin or glass containers in any prepared solution that will be given over more than 2 hours. PVC containers are suitable only for dilution of the rapid loading dose; see Compatibility and Precautions.

Rapid-loading infusion: Dilute 150 mg (3 mL) in 100 mL D5W; concentration is 1.5 mg/mL (D5W or NS may be used for Nexterone).

Slow-loading infusion and maintenance infusion: Dilute 900 mg (18 mL) in 500 mL D5W; concentration is 1.8 mg/mL (D5W or NS may be used for Nexterone). Dilutions from 1 to 6 mg/mL have been used for maintenance solutions after the first 24 hours. Use of a central venous catheter is recommended; however, concentrations over 2 mg/mL for longer than 1 hour must be administered through a central venous catheter. Higher concentrations (3 to 6 mg/mL) have caused peripheral vein phlebitis and hepatocellular necrosis; see Precautions.

Cardiac arrest (unlabeled): Loading dose (300 mg or 5 mg/kg) or supplemental boluses (150 mg) may be given undiluted. Has also been diluted in up to 20 mL D5W (D5W or NS may be used for Nexterone).

Filters: Use of a 0.2-micron in-line filter recommended by manufacturer. States "filtering does not affect potency." Another source suggests no significant loss of drug potency with the use of a 0.22-micron cellulose ester membrane filter.

Storage: Store ampules and premixed solutions in their carton at CRT. Use solutions diluted in PVC containers within 2 hours; use those diluted in glass or polyolefin containers within 24 hours. Protect from light and freezing.

COMPATIBILITY (Underline Indicates Conflicting Compatibility Information)

Consider any drug NOT listed as compatible to be INCOMPATIBLE until consulting a pharmacist; specific conditions may apply.

Manufacturer recommendations include: Do not use evacuated glass intravenous bottles. Administer through a dedicated IV line (central venous catheter preferred). Absorbs to PVC tubing but loss accounted for in specified dose; follow infusion regimen closely. Leaches out plasticizers, including DEHP, from IV tubing. The degree of leaching increases when the solution is infused at a higher concentration or a slower infusion rate than recommended. Manufacturer lists aminophylline, cefazolin (Ancef), heparin, mezlocillin (Mezlin), and sodium bicarbonate as **incompatible** at the **Y-site.**

One source suggests the following **compatibilities:**

Additive: Dobutamine, furosemide (Lasix), lidocaine, potassium chloride (KCl), procainamide (Pronestyl), quinidine, verapamil.

Y-site: Amikacin (Amikin), amphotericin B (generic), atracurium (Tracium), atropine, calcium chloride, calcium gluconate, caspofungin (Cancidas), cefazolin (Ancef), ceftriaxone (Rocephin), cefuroxime (Zinacef), ciprofloxacin (Cipro IV), clindamycin (Cleocin), dexmedetomidine (Precedex), dobutamine, dopamine, doripenem (Doribax), doxycycline, epinephrine (Adrenalin), eptifibatide (Integrilin), erythromycin (Erythrocin), esmolol (Brevibloc), famotidine (Pepcid IV), fenoldopam (Corlopam), fentanyl (Sublimaze), fluconazole (Diflucan), furosemide (Lasix), gentamicin, hetastarch in electrolytes (Hextend), insulin (regular), isoproterenol (Isuprel), labetalol (Trandate), lepirudin (Refludan), lidocaine, lorazepam (Ativan), magnesium sulfate, methylprednisolone (Solu-Medrol), midazolam (Versed), milrinone (Primacor), morphine, nesiritide (Natrecor), nitroglycerin IV, nitroprusside sodium, norepinephrine (Levophed), penicillin G potassium, phentolamine (Regitine), phenylephrine (Neo-Synephrine), potassium chloride (KCl), procainamide (Pronestyl), tirofiban (Aggrastat), tobramycin, vancomycin, vasopressin, vecuronium.

RATE OF ADMINISTRATION

Volumetric pump required for administration. Surface properties of diluted solution reduce drop size; use of a drop counter infusion set causes underdosing. Use of a 0.2-micron in-line filter is also recommended. A central venous catheter is recommended for all concentrations and is required for concentrations greater than 2 mg/mL. Adhere to prescribed rates; risk of hypotension is increased in the first hours of treatment and with increased rates; may cause secondary renal or hepatic failure; see Precautions. Avoid IV bolus doses in patients with marked cardiomegaly, a continuous infusion is preferred. Do not use plastic containers in a series; could result in air embolism.

Rapid loading infusion or breakthrough treatment of VF/VT: 150 mg over 10 minutes (15 mg/min). Do not exceed a rate of 30 mg/min.

Slow loading infusion: 1 mg/min or 33.3 mL/hr (0.556 mL/min) of 1.8 mg/mL solution for 6 hours.

Maintenance infusion: 0.5 mg/min or 16.6 mL/hr (0.278 mL/min) of 1.8 mg/mL solution for 18 hours. A continuing maintenance solution should deliver 720 mg/24 hr at 0.5 mg/min whether the concentration is

1.8 mg/mL or 6 mg/mL. May be continued at this rate for up to 2 to 3 weeks as described in Usual Dose.

Cardiac arrest (unlabeled): Loading or supplemental doses by IV bolus injection. Follow with 10 mL flush of D5W or NS through Y-tube or three-way stopcock. May be given through a free-flowing infusion of D5W (D5W or NS may be used for Nexterone). After return of spontaneous circulation (ROSC), initiate the slow loading and maintenance infusions as above.

ACTIONS

An antiarrhythmic agent. Generally considered a class III antiarrhythmic drug, but possesses characteristics of all four antiarrhythmic classes. Decreases number of VT/VF events. It prolongs the duration of action potentials in cardiac fibers, depresses conduction velocity, slows conduction and prolongs refractoriness at the AV node, and exhibits some alpha and beta blockade activity. Raises the threshold for VF and may prevent its recurrence. Also has vasodilatory effects that decrease cardiac workload and myocardial oxygen consumption. Uptake by the myocardium is rapid; antiarrhythmic effect is prompt (clinically relevant within hours); however, full effect may take days. Has an exceptionally long half-life. Metabolized in the liver by cytochrome P_{450} enzymes (specifically CYP3A4 and CYP2C8). Primarily excreted in bile. Crosses placental barrier. Secreted in breast milk.

INDICATIONS AND USES

Treatment of acute life-threatening VT/VF and prophylaxis of frequently recurring VF and hemodynamically unstable VT in patients refractory to other therapy (e.g., lidocaine, procainamide). Used until ventricular arrhythmias are stabilized; usually 48 to 96 hours, but may be given for longer periods (i.e., up to 3 weeks). ▪ Treatment of patients taking oral amiodarone who are unable to take oral medication.

Unlabeled uses: Conversion of atrial fibrillation and maintenance of a sinus rhythm. ▪ Treatment of sustained monomorphic VT in patients with acute myocardial infarction (AMI) not accompanied by chest pain, pulmonary congestion, or hypotension in patients who have failed to respond to lidocaine and synchronized DC cardioversion (ACC/AHA Committee on management of AMI). ▪ Termination and prevention of recurrence of supraventricular arrhythmias refractory to conventional treatment (e.g., paroxysmal atrial fibrillation, atrial flutter, ectopic atrial tachycardia, paroxysmal supraventricular tachycardia). ▪ Preoperative prophylaxis against AF occurring after heart surgery. ▪ Conversion of supraventricular arrhythmias to sinus rhythm in patients following cardiac surgery.

CONTRAINDICATIONS

Cardiogenic shock, corneal refractive laser surgery, known hypersensitivity to amiodarone or any of its components, including iodine; marked sinus bradycardia; second- or third-degree AV block unless a functioning pacemaker is available; sinus node dysfunction. See Drug/Lab Interactions. ▪ Not recommended for use in neonates or infants. ▪ Contraindicated with ritonavir (Norvir).

PRECAUTIONS

Usually administered by or under the direction of the physician specialist with facilities for monitoring the patient and responding to any medical emergency. ▪ Correct hypokalemia and hypomagnesemia before use; may exaggerate a prolonged QTc and cause arrhythmias (e.g., torsades de pointes). ■ May cause transient increases in liver enzymes but abnormal baseline hepatic enzymes is not a contraindication to use. ■ Use of higher than recommended loading dose concentrations and increased rates of administration have been associated with hepatocellular necrosis, hepatic coma, acute renal failure, and death. ■ May worsen existing arrhythmias or precipitate new ones, primarily torsades de pointes or new-onset VF. ■ Combination of amiodarone with other antiarrhythmics that can prolong the QTc interval should be reserved for patients with life-threatening ventricular arrhythmias who do not respond to single agent therapy; see Drug/Lab Interactions. ■ Risk of QTc prolongation is increased (with or without torsades de pointes) with other medications that can prolong the QTc (e.g., fluoroquinolones [e.g., levofloxacin (Levaquin)], macrolide antibiotics [e.g., erythromycin (Erythrocin)], azoles [e.g., fluconazole (Diflucan)]); see Drug/Lab Interactions. ■ Hypotension is the most common side effect. Usually occurs within the first several hours of therapy and appears to be rate-related. Do not exceed initial rates recommended by manufacturer. In some cases, hypotension has been refractory to treatment. Deaths have occurred. See Monitor and Antidote. ■ May cause visual impairment (e.g., optic neuropathy or optic neuritis); has progressed to permanent blindness. ■ May cause pulmonary toxicity (e.g., ARDS, bronchospasm, cough, dyspnea, hemoptysis, hypoxemia, wheezing). Usually seen with long-term use, but acute pulmonary hypersensitivity has been reported after short-term IV use and with or without IV use. Has progressed to respiratory failure and death. The elderly and patients with pre-existing lung disease may be at increased risk and have a poorer prognosis if pulmonary toxicity develops; see Side Effects. ■ Adult respiratory distress syndrome (ARDS) has been reported in patients receiving oral amiodarone following surgery. ■ Monitor patients undergoing general anesthesia closely; may increase sensitivity to myocardial depressant and conduction defects of halogenated inhalation anesthetics (hypotension and atropine-resistant bradycardia). ■ Use caution in patients with cardiomyopathy, hepatic failure, left ventricular dysfunction, or thyroid dysfunction. ■ May cause hypothyroidism or hyperthyroidism. Amiodarone-induced hyperthyroidism may result in thyrotoxicosis and/or the possibility of arrhythmia breakthrough or aggravation. Deaths have occurred. ■ Thyroid nodules and/or thyroid cancer have been reported in patients treated with amiodarone. ■ See Compatibility and Drug/Lab Interactions. *Cardiac arrest:* Incidence of hypotension and/or myocardial depression may be less than with procainamide (Pronestyl). ■ Has been used as an alternative agent in patients who have developed torsades de pointes previously with class Ia antiarrhythmic agents (e.g., disopyramide [Norpace], procainamide, quinidine).

Monitor: Continuous ECG and HR monitoring is mandatory to observe for arrhythmias. Watch for QTc prolongation; may cause proarrhythmia (torsades de pointes). ■ Monitor for bradycardia and AV block. A temporary pacemaker should be available. Consider the possibility of hyperthyroidism if new signs of arrhythmia appear. ■ Monitor BP closely to minimize hypotension (occurs frequently with initial rates); see Rate of Administration, Precautions, and Antidote. ■ Confirm patency of vein. Reduce rate or concentration for pain or redness at injection site. Incidence of phlebitis markedly increased with concentrations above 2.5 mg/mL. For infusions longer than 1 hour, do not exceed a concentration of 2 mg/mL unless a central venous line is used. ▪ Monitor serum electrolytes and acid-base balance, especially in patients with prolonged diarrhea and those receiving diuretics. ▪ Monitor liver enzymes (AST, ALT, GGT) for elevations indicating progressive injury. ▪ Monitor pulmonary status (e.g., FiO_2, SaO_2, PaO_2, chest x-ray); baseline pulmonary function tests recommended; repeat as indicated. ▪ Monitoring of SCr and BUN may be indicated. ▪ Monitor thyroid function tests before treatment and periodically thereafter. Patients with a history of thyroid nodules, goiter, or other thyroid dysfunction and the elderly should be monitored closely. Amiodarone is eliminated slowly, and abnormal function tests may persist for weeks or months after it is discontinued. ▪ Regular ophthalmic exams, including funduscopy and slit lamp exams, are recommended. Prompt ophthalmic exams recommended at first sign of visual impairment. May require discontinuation of amiodarone therapy. ▪ Serum amiodarone levels greater than 2.5 mcg/mL have been associated with a higher incidence of side effects. ▪ See Precautions and Drug/Lab Interactions.

Patient Education: Most manufacturers of corneal refractive laser surgery devices contraindicate this procedure in patients receiving amiodarone. ▪ Report promptly any feelings of faintness, difficulty breathing, or pain or stinging along injection site. Review side effect profile, including S/S of hypothyroidism or hyperthyroidism. ▪ Nonhormonal birth control recommended. ▪ Numerous drug interactions. Review all medications, including OTC medications, with physician or pharmacist. ▪ Avoid grapefruit juice if transitioned to oral amiodarone.

Maternal/Child: Category D: avoid pregnancy or use only if benefit to mother justifies risk to fetus. Has caused infrequent neonatal congenital goiter/hypothyroidism and hyperthyroidism in addition to other adverse effects. ▪ Discontinue breast-feeding. ▪ Safety for use during labor and delivery not established. ▪ Safety and effectiveness for use in pediatric patients not established. ▪ A manufacturer's warning letter has been issued citing potentially fatal or developmental side effects in infants and neonates; see Contraindications. Another source suggests amiodarone may adversely affect male reproductive tract development in infants, neonates, and toddlers. ▪ Vials contain benzyl alcohol, which has been associated with "gasping syndrome" in neonates (sudden onset of gasping respirations, hypotension, bradycardia, and cardiovascular collapse).

Elderly: Differences in response between the elderly and younger patients have not been identified; however, clearance is slower and half-life may be doubled (up to 47 days). See Dose Adjustments. ▪ May be at increased risk for pulmonary toxicity; see Precautions.

DRUG/LAB INTERACTIONS

Amiodarone has a long half-life; drug interactions may persist long after it is discontinued.

Contraindicated with ritonavir (Norvir). Should not be given concurrently with **ibutilide** (Corvert). ▪ Concurrent use with other **antiarrhythmic agents** (e.g., disopyramide [Norpace], mexiletine, procainamide [Pronestyl], quinidine) increases their serum concentrations and may result in additive increases in QT prolongation and serious arrhythmias. One source recommends reducing the dose of previously given antiarrhythmic agents by 30% to 50% several days after starting amiodarone and then gradually withdrawing them altogether. Another suggests reducing the dose of any antiarrhythmic therapy required in addition to amiodarone to one-half the recommended dose. Monitor serum levels if possible. ▪ QT prolongation has been reported with concomitant administration of amiodarone and **fluoroquinolones** (e.g., levofloxacin [Levaquin]), **macrolide antibiotics** (e.g., erythromycin [Erythrocin]), **azoles** (e.g., fluconazole [Diflucan]), **loratadine** (Claritin), **trazodone** (Desyrel), **and grapefruit juice (oral therapy);** see Precautions. ▪ May decrease metabolism and increase serum levels of **digoxin.** One source recommends reducing digoxin dose by 50% or withdrawing completely when amiodarone therapy is initiated. ▪ Use with **potassium-depleting diuretics** (e.g., chlorothiazide [Diuril], furosemide [Lasix], indapamide [Lozol]) may lead to increased risk of arrhythmias due to hypokalemia. ▪ Inhibits metabolism and increases anticoagulant effect (e.g., increased PT and INR) of **warfarin** (Coumadin). Dose reduction of the anticoagulant and careful monitoring of PT or INR recommended. Effects may persist long after amiodarone discontinued. ▪ May decrease metabolism and increase serum levels of **cyclosporine** (Sandimmune), **flecainide** (Tambocor), **hydantoins** (e.g., phenytoin [Dilantin]), **lidocaine, methotrexate, procainamide** (Pronestyl), **quinidine, and theophyllines** (Aminophylline). May cause toxicity; monitor serum levels. Reduced doses indicated. ▪ Concomitant use with **simvastatin** (Zocor) has been associated with myopathy/rhabdomyolysis. ▪ May cause bradycardia, decreased cardiac output, and hypotension with **fentanyl** (Sublimaze). ▪ Therapeutic plasma concentrations of **flecainide** (Tambocor) can be maintained with reduced doses because amiodarone interferes with flecainide metabolism. ▪ Amiodarone clearance increased and plasma levels decreased with **cholestyramine** (Questran), **phenytoin** (Dilantin), **rifampin** (Rifadin), **and St. John's wort.** ▪ **Cimetidine** (Tagamet) **and protease inhibitors** (e.g., indinavir [Crixivan]) may decrease clearance and increase plasma levels of amiodarone. ▪ May increase risk of atrioventricular block, bradycardia, and hypotension with **beta-blockers** (e.g., propranolol) **and calcium channel blockers** (e.g., diltiazem [Cardizem], verapamil). ▪ May inhibit conversion of **clopidogrel** (Plavix) to its active metabolite, resulting in ineffective inhibition of platelet aggregation. ▪ Monitor patients undergoing **general anesthesia** closely. May increase sensitivity to myocardial depressant and conduction defects of **halogenated inhalation anesthetics** (hypotension and atropine-resistant bradycardia). ▪ PO use for longer than 2 weeks may decrease metabolism and increase serum levels of **dextromethorphan** (Robitussin DM), **methotrexate, and phenytoin.** ▪ See Precautions.

SIDE EFFECTS

Hypotension or pain at the IV site are the most common side effects. Agranulocytosis, anaphylaxis, anemia (aplastic and/or hemolytic), angioedema, anorexia, arrhythmias (e.g., AV block, bradycardia, new onset VT/VF, sinus arrest, torsades de pointes), adult respiratory distress syndrome (ARDS), ataxia, cardiac arrest, cardiogenic shock, confusion, congestive heart failure, delirium, disorientation, dizziness, dry eyes, hallucinations, hepatotoxicity (liver function test abnormalities), impotence, muscle weakness, myopathy, nausea, nephrotoxicity, neutropenia, pancreatitis, pancytopenia, paresthesias, peripheral neuropathy, photosensitivity, pleuritis, pruritus, pseudotumor cerebri (swelling that resembles a tumor), pulmonary toxicity (including bronchiolitis obliterans organizing pneumonia [may be fatal]), renal impairment, respiratory disorders (including cough, dyspnea, hemoptysis, hypoxia, pulmonary infiltrates and/or mass on chest x-ray, respiratory failure), rhabdomyolysis, skin disorders (e.g., epididymitis, erythema multiforme, exfoliative dermatitis, Stevens-Johnson syndrome, toxic epidermal necrolysis [may be fatal]), syndrome of inappropriate antidiuretic hormone secretion (SIADH), thrombocytopenia, thyroid dysfunction, and visual impairment/loss of vision may occur. In addition to these side effects, overdose or extended use may cause hepatic and/or renal failure secondary to hypotension.

Overdose: AV block, bradycardia, cardiogenic shock, death, hepatotoxicity, hypotension.

ANTIDOTE

Keep physician informed of all side effects and treat promptly as appropriate; many are life threatening. Reduce rate and/or concentration for pain at IV site. Monitor hepatic enzymes closely. Reduce rate or discontinue for progressive hepatic injury. Treat hypotension and cardiogenic shock by slowing the infusion rate. Vasopressors (e.g., dopamine, norepinephrine [Levophed]), inotropic agents (e.g., digoxin), and volume expansion may be indicated. Slow infusion rate or discontinue if bradycardia and/or AV block occur; may require a temporary pacemaker. If torsades de pointes occurs, stop all cardioactive drugs (e.g., antiarrhythmics, digoxin, antidepressants, phenothiazines) and normalize electrolytes (e.g., potassium, magnesium). Atrial overdrive pacing may be required to stabilize cardiac rhythm. Dose reduction or discontinuation of amiodarone may be required if thyroid abnormalities develop. Thyroid hormone supplementation may be required in hypothyroidism. Initiation of antithyroid drugs (e.g., propylthiouracil [PTU]), beta-blockers (e.g., propranolol), and/or temporary corticosteroid therapy may be necessary for treatment of hyperthyroidism. In severe thyrotoxicosis where amiodarone cannot be discontinued, thyroidectomy may be used as treatment. Experience with surgical intervention is limited; could induce thyroid storm. Amiodarone is not dialyzable. Resuscitate as necessary.

AMPHOTERICIN B BBW * ■
AMPHOTERICIN B LIPID-BASED
PRODUCTS
(am-foe-**TER**-ih-sin)

Abelcet, AmBisome, Amphotec

Antifungal
Antiprotozoal
(AmBisome)

pH 5.7 to 8 ■ 5 to 6

*The Black Box Warning applies only to the generic formulation.

USUAL DOSE

Each product has different biochemical, pharmacokinetic, and pharmacodynamic properties. They are not interchangeable from dose to dose in a given patient between each other or traditional amphotericin.

ABELCET (AMPHOTERICIN B LIPID COMPLEX INJECTION)

Adults and pediatric patients: 5 mg/kg/24 hr as an infusion. Repeat daily until clinical response or mycologic cure.

AMPHOTEC (AMPHOTERICIN B CHOLESTERYL SULFATE COMPLEX FOR INJECTION)
Adults and pediatric patients: 3 to 4 mg/kg/24 hr as an infusion. Pretreatment with antipyretics, antihistamines, or corticosteroids may be indicated; see Precautions and Antidote. On the first day of treatment, begin with a test dose of 10 mL of the final diluted preparation and infuse over 15 to 30 minutes. Observe the patient for the next 30 minutes. If there is no adverse reaction, continue with the calculated dose. May be increased to 6 mg/kg/24 hr if there is no improvement or if the fungal infection progresses. See Indications.

AMBISOME (AMPHOTERICIN B LIPOSOME FOR INJECTION)
Adults, children, and infants over 1 month of age: All doses are by infusion.
Empirical therapy in febrile, neutropenic patients: 3 mg/kg/24 hr.
Systemic fungal infections (e.g., *Aspergillus, Candida, Cryptococcus*): 3 to 5 mg/kg/24 hr.
Treatment of cryptococcal meningitis in HIV-infected patients: 6 mg/kg/24 hr.
Visceral leishmaniasis in immunocompetent patients: 3 mg/kg/24 hr on Days 1 through 5. Repeat 3 mg/kg on Day 14 and on Day 21. A repeat course of therapy may be useful if parasitic clearance is not achieved.
Visceral leishmaniasis in immunocompromised patients: 4 mg/kg/24 hr on Days 1 through 5. Repeat 4 mg/kg on Days 10, 17, 24, 31, and 38. During clinical studies parasitic clearance was not achieved or relapse within 6 months occurred in 88.2% of patients. Usefulness of repeat courses not determined.

GENERIC (TRADITIONAL AMPHOTERICIN B)
Adults and pediatric patients: Begin with a test dose of 0.1 mg/kg up to 1 mg maximum dose in 20 to 50 mL D5W. Infuse over 10 to 30 minutes. Determine size of therapeutic dose by intensity of reaction over a 4-hour period. Usual is 0.25 mg/kg of body weight/24 hr gradually increased in 0.125 to 0.25 mg/kg increments to 1 mg/kg/24 hr or a maximum of 50 mg/day (average dose is 0.5 mg/kg) as tolerance permits. Maximum dose for pediatric patients is 1 mg/kg/day or 30 mg/M^2/day. Up to 1.5 mg/kg/24 hr may be given on alternate-day therapy. Several months of therapy are usually required and recommended for cure. Dosage must be adjusted to each specific patient. In some instances, higher doses can be used.

Mannitol 12.5 Gm immediately before and after each dose of generic amphotericin B may reduce nephrotoxic effects. See Precautions for additional suggestions.

DOSE ADJUSTMENTS
ABELCET: Full dose usually required; base on SCr and overall patient condition.
AMPHOTEC/AMBISOME: No dose adjustments suggested.
GENERIC: Full dose required even in impaired renal function, but reduce dose or discontinue drug if BUN greater than 40 mg/100 mL or SCr greater than 3 mg/100 mL. Gradual dose increases are essential. Whenever medicine is not given for 7 days or longer, restart treatment at lowest dosage level.

DILUTION
ABELCET: Available in 50-mg (10-mL) and 100-mg (20-mL) vials. The new 50-mg vial facilitates accurate dosing and reduction of waste. Shake vial until all yellow sediment is dissolved. Maintain aseptic technique. Withdraw an exact total daily dose from one or more vials using one or more

syringes and 18-gauge needles. Replace needle(s) on syringe(s) with the 5-micron filter(s) supplied with each vial. A new filter must be used for each 400 mg (80 mL) of Abelcet. Empty syringe contents through filter into an infusion of D5W. 4 mL of diluent (D5W) is required for each 1 mL (5 mg) of Abelcet to achieve a final concentration of 1 mg/mL. For *pediatric* and/or fluid-restricted patients (e.g., patients with cardiovascular disease) reduce diluent by half (approximate concentration of 2 mg/mL). pH 5.5 to 6. Use only clear solutions and discard unused portion.

AMPHOTEC: Available in 50-mg or 100-mg vials. Reconstitute by rapidly adding 10 mL of SW for each 50 mg of Amphotec (5 mg/mL). Use of a 20-gauge needle is recommended. Shake gently, rotating the vial until all solids have dissolved. May be opalescent or clear. Must be further diluted for infusion with D5W (see the following chart). Final desired concentration is approximately 0.6 mg/mL (range with recommended amounts of diluent is 0.16 mg/mL to 0.83 mg/mL). Do not filter or use an in-line filter. See Compatibility and Rate of Administration.

Guidelines for Dilution of Amphotec		
Dose of Amphotec (mg)	Volume of Reconstituted Amphotec (mL)	Infusion Bag Size for D5W for Injection (mL)
10-35 mg	2-7 mL	50 mL
35-70 mg	7-14 mL	100 mL
70-175 mg	14-35 mL	250 mL
175-350 mg	35-70 mL	500 mL
350-1,000 mg	70-200 mL	1,000 mL

AMBISOME: Reconstitute each 50-mg vial with 12 mL SW (without a bacteriostatic agent) to yield 4 mg/mL. Shake vial vigorously for 30 seconds; forms a yellow translucent suspension. Withdraw an exact total daily dose from one or more vials using one or more 20-mL syringes and needles. Replace needle(s) with the 5-micron filter(s) supplied with each vial. A new filter must be used for each 50-mg vial. Empty syringe contents through filter into an infusion of D5W. Use sufficient diluent to achieve a final concentration of 1 to 2 mg/mL, pH 5 to 6. For *pediatric patients:* may be further diluted to concentrations of 0.2 to 0.5 mg/mL for infants and small children to provide adequate volume for infusion.

GENERIC: A 50-mg vial is initially diluted with 10 mL of SW for injection (without a bacteriostatic agent); 5 mg equals 1 mL. Shake well until solution is clear. Further dilute each 1 mg in at least 10 mL of D5W. Dextrose must have a pH above 4.2. Concentration of solution must not be greater than 0.1 mg/mL. Do not use any other diluent. Use a sterile 20-gauge or larger needle at each step of the dilution. Maintain aseptic technique. Larger pore 1-micron filters may be used. Use only fresh solutions without evidence of precipitate or foreign matter. Light sensitive but protection from light not required unless solution exposed over 8 hours. pH 5.7 to 8.

Filters: *Abelcet:* 5-micron filter(s) supplied with each vial. A new filter must be used for each 400 mg (80 mL) of Abelcet. Empty syringe contents through filter into an infusion solution. Do not use an in-line filter.
Amphotec: Do not filter or use an in-line filter.
AmBisome: 5-micron filter(s) supplied with each vial. A new filter must be used for each 50-mg vial. Empty syringe contents through filter into an infusion solution. Do not use an in-line filter smaller than 1 micron.
Generic: Larger pore 1-micron filters may be used; see Dilution.
Storage: *Abelcet:* Before reconstitution, refrigerate vials and protect from light. Do not freeze. Diluted solution is stable 48 hours if refrigerated and an additional 6 hours at room temperature.
Amphotec: Store unopened vials in carton at CRT. Refrigerate reconstituted or diluted solutions; must be used within 24 hours. Do not freeze. Discard unused drug.
AmBisome: Unopened vials may be stored at temperatures up to 25° C (77° F). Vials reconstituted with SW may be refrigerated for up to 24 hours. Do not freeze. Infusion of fully diluted solution must begin within 6 hours. Discard unused drug.
Generic: Before reconstitution, refrigerate vials and protect from light. Do not freeze. Preserve concentrate in refrigerator up to 7 days or 24 hours at room temperature. Use diluted solution promptly.

COMPATIBILITY　　　　(Underline Indicates Conflicting Compatibility Information)
Consider any drug NOT listed as compatible to be INCOMPATIBLE until consulting a pharmacist; specific conditions may apply.

ALL FORMULATIONS
In all situations, use a separate infusion line or flush an existing line with D5W before and after administration.

ABELCET
Do not mix with any other diluent, drug, or solution. Use only D5W. Manufacturer states that **compatibility** with any other diluent has not been established. Another source lists **compatibility** at the **Y-site** with <u>anidulafungin (Eraxis)</u>, <u>doripenem (Doribax)</u>.

AMBISOME/AMPHOTEC/GENERIC
Do not mix with any other diluent, drug, or solution. Use only SW for reconstitution and D5W for dilution for infusion. Use of any other solution or the presence of a bacteriostatic agent (e.g., benzyl alcohol) may cause precipitation. Another source lists AmBisome as **compatible** at the **Y-site** with <u>anidulafungin (Eraxis)</u>, <u>doripenem (Doribax)</u>.

AMPHOTEC
One source suggests the following **compatibilities:**
Y-site: Acyclovir (Zovirax), aminophylline, cefoxitin (Mefoxin), clindamycin (Cleocin), dexamethasone (Decadron), <u>doripenem (Doribax)</u>, fentanyl (Sublimaze), furosemide (Lasix), ganciclovir (Cytovene), granisetron (Kytril), hydrocortisone sodium succinate (Solu-Cortef), ifosfamide (Ifex), lorazepam (Ativan), mannitol, methotrexate, methylprednisolone (Solu-Medrol), nitroglycerin IV, sulfamethoxazole/trimethoprim, sufentanil (Sufenta), vinblastine, vincristine, zidovudine (AZT, Retrovir).

GENERIC
One source suggests the following **compatibilities:**
Additive: *Not recommended by manufacturer.* Fluconazole (Diflucan), heparin, sodium bicarbonate.

Y-site: Aldesleukin (Proleukin, Interleukin-2), amiodarone (Nexterone), cisatracurium (Nimbex), diltiazem (Cardizem), doripenem (Doribax), remifentanil (Ultiva), sargramostim (Leukine), tacrolimus (Prograf), teniposide (Vumon), thiotepa, zidovudine (AZT, Retrovir).

RATE OF ADMINISTRATION
ALL AMPHOTERICINS: Rapid infusion may cause hypotension, hypokalemia, arrhythmia, and shock. Infusion reactions can occur with all amphotericin B formulations. See Precautions, Side Effects, and Antidote. With all formulations, flush existing line with D5W before and after administration or use a separate IV line.

ABELCET: Total daily dose as an infusion at 2.5 mg/kg/hr. Contents of diluted solution must be mixed by shaking at least every 2 hours. Do not use an in-line filter.

AMPHOTEC: See rate for test dose in Usual Dose. Give total daily dose as an infusion at 1 mg/kg/hr. Infusion time may be shortened to a minimum of 2 hours for patients who show no evidence of intolerance or infusion-related reactions. May be extended for acute reactions or if infusion volume is not tolerated. Do not use filters.

AMBISOME: Total daily dose as an infusion over 2 hours. Use of a controlled infusion device is recommended. Infusion time may be shortened to a minimum of 1 hour for patients who show no evidence of intolerance or infusion-related reactions. Infusion time may be extended for patient discomfort or acute reactions or if infusion volume is not tolerated. Do not use any in-line filter less than 1 micron.

GENERIC: Daily dose over 2 to 6 hours by slow IV infusion. Expected reactions usually less severe with slower rate. A minimum 1-micron filter may be used.

ACTIONS
Antifungal antibiotic agents that bind to fungal cell membranes resulting in leakage of cellular contents. May be fungistatic or fungicidal according to body fluid concentration and susceptibility of the fungus. Abelcet is amphotericin B complexed with two phospholipids in a 1:1 drug-to-lipid ratio. Amphotec is amphotericin B complexed with cholesteryl sulfate in a colloidal dispersion in a 1:1 drug-to-lipid ratio. AmBisome is amphotericin B intercalated into a liposomal membrane with several components. Assay tests cannot distinguish lipid-based amphotericin from generic amphotericin B. Modification of amphotericin to the various lipid-based products alters the drug's functional properties. It allows for increased levels of drug at the site of action (usually areas where the fungi are). Overall effect is increased effectiveness with less toxicity. Not effective against bacteria, rickettsiae, or viruses. Remains in the body at a therapeutic level up to 20 hours after each infusion (Abelcet has the longest elimination half-life [up to 173 hours]). Actual distribution to organs is somewhat selective and may help to decide which product is best to use in a given situation. Route of metabolism not known. Excreted very slowly in the urine.

INDICATIONS AND USES
Because of their high cost, some clinicians suggest that the lipid-based products should be used only in patients refractory to traditional amphotericin, patients with progressing invasive fungal infections, and patients with nephrotoxicity (SCr greater than 2.5 mg/dL) or at high risk (e.g., transplant patients on cyclosporine or tacrolimus).

ABELCET: Treatment of invasive fungal infections in patients who are refractory to or intolerant of traditional amphotericin B therapy (e.g., aspergillosis, candidiasis, cryptococcosis, cryptococcal meningitis, fusariosis, zygomycosis). Has orphan drug approval for invasive coccidioidomycosis, invasive prototothecosis, and invasive sporotrichosis.

AMPHOTEC: Treatment of invasive aspergillosis in patients refractory to or intolerant of traditional amphotericin B or in patients in whom traditional amphotericin treatment has failed.

AMBISOME: Empirical therapy for presumed fungal infection in febrile, neutropenic patients. ▪ Treatment of patients with aspergillosis, candida, and/or cryptococcus infections refractory to traditional amphotericin B or in patients in whom renal impairment or unacceptable toxicity precludes the use of traditional amphotericin B. ▪ Treatment of visceral leishmaniasis. ▪ Treatment of cryptococcal meningitis in HIV-infected patients. ▪ AmBisome is frequently used in BMT patients on cyclosporine.

GENERIC: Treatment of fungal infections that are progressive and potentially fatal, such as aspergillosis, cryptococcosis, blastomycosis, and disseminated forms of candidiasis, coccidioidomycosis, and histoplasmosis, mucormycosis, and sporotrichosis. These infections must be caused by specific organisms. Not recommended for treatment of noninvasive forms of fungal disease in patients with normal neutrophil counts.

Unlabeled uses: Abelcet is used to prevent fungal infections in bone marrow transplant patients (0.1 mg/kg/day). Lipid-based products are used to treat primary amoebic meningoencephalitis caused by *Naegleria fowleri* and for low-dose chemoprophylaxis in immunocompromised patients at risk for aspergillosis.

CONTRAINDICATIONS

All amphotericin formulations: Known sensitivity to amphotericin B or any components of its formulations unless a life-threatening situation is present.

PRECAUTIONS

ALL AMPHOTERICIN FORMULATIONS: Diagnosis should be positively established by culture or histologic study. ▪ Close clinical observation is imperative. Anaphylaxis has occurred; emergency equipment and supplies must be available. ▪ Infusion reactions are common; pretreatment with antipyretics, antihistamines (e.g., diphenhydramine [Benadryl]), and/or selective use of corticosteroids may be indicated. ▪ Use caution in patients receiving leukocyte transfusions; may cause acute pulmonary toxicity. Separate times of administration as much as possible. ▪ Diabetes must be well controlled before treatment with amphotericin is begun. ▪ Nephrotoxicity is the usual dose-limiting factor for use of traditional amphotericin B. Impairment may improve with dose reduction or alternate day therapy, but some residual dysfunction is possible. Lipid-based formulations are associated with less nephrotoxicity. Most studies show equivalent or superior effectiveness compared to traditional amphotericin. Introduction of lipid-based products to patients with increased CrCl and BUN from traditional amphotericin has decreased the CrCl and BUN. ▪ Pseudomembranous colitis has been reported. May range from mild to life threatening. Consider in patients that present with diarrhea during or after treatment with amphotericin B.

ABELCET: Renal toxicity is dose dependent but has been consistently less nephrotoxic than uncomplexed amphotericin B.

AMPHOTEC/AMBISOME: Incidence of renal toxicity significantly lower than with uncomplexed amphotericin B.

GENERIC: Should be used primarily for treatment of patients with progressive and potentially life-threatening fungal infections. It should not be used to treat non-invasive forms of fungal disease such as oral thrush, vaginal candidiasis, and esophageal candidiasis in patients with normal neutrophil counts. ▪ To prevent overdose, verify product name and dose, especially if dose exceeds 1.5 mg/kg. ▪ Hospitalization preferred to initiate therapy. ▪ A small amount of heparin added to the infusion may reduce the incidence of thrombophlebitis. ▪ Meperidine (Demerol) or nonsteroidal anti-inflammatory agents (e.g., ibuprofen) before administration or hydrocortisone 0.7 mg/kg of body weight added to the infusion may prevent febrile reactions including chills; corticosteroids not recommended for concomitant use in other situations because they exaggerate hypokalemia. ▪ Prophylactic antiemetics and antihistamines are also appropriate.

Monitor: *All amphotericin formulations:* Obtain baseline CBC, PT, serum electrolytes, renal (e.g., creatine kinase, BUN, SCr) and liver function (e.g., ALT, AST) tests. Repeat frequently during therapy; recommended weekly. Monitor creatine kinase and PT as indicated during therapy. ▪ Discontinue or reduce dose until renal function improves if increase in BUN or SCr is clinically significant (e.g., BUN greater than 40 mg/dL or SCr greater than 3 mg/dL). Side effects (e.g., hypokalemia, hypomagnesemia, impaired renal function) may be life threatening. ▪ Monitor vital signs and I&O. Record every 30 minutes for up to 4 hours after infusion is complete. ▪ Encourage fluids to maintain hydration.

Patient Education: *All amphotericin formulations:* Review all medical conditions and medications before beginning treatment. ▪ Discomfort associated with infusion. ▪ Report difficulty breathing promptly. ▪ Long-term therapy required to effect a cure. ▪ Report diarrhea, fever, increased or decreased urination, loss of appetite, stomach pain, sore throat, and any unusual bleeding or bruising, tiredness, or weakness.

Maternal/Child: *All amphotericin formulations:* Category B: has been used successfully during pregnancy but adequate studies not available. Use only if clearly needed. ▪ Safety for use in breast-feeding and pediatric patients not established. Discontinue nursing. ▪ Generic amphotericin B has been used in pediatric patients. Lipid-based preparations have been used in pediatric patients without any unexpected side effects. Safety of use of AmBisome in infants under 1 month of age not established.

Elderly: Consider age-related impaired body functions. Lipid-based preparations have been used without unexpected side effects.

DRUG/LAB INTERACTIONS
Drug interaction studies have not been done for lipid-based preparations, but interactions similar to generic amphotericin B are expected. ▪ **Corticosteroids** will increase hypokalemia and may cause arrhythmias. Use with caution only if indicated to control drug reactions or, if necessary, monitor serum electrolytes and cardiac function closely. ▪ Hypokalemic effect may be increased with **thiazides,** may potentiate **digoxin** toxicity, and/or may enhance the curariform effect of **neuromuscular blocking agents** (e.g., rocuronium [Zemuron], succinylcholine); monitor serum potassium levels. ▪ Avoid use or use extreme caution with other **nephrotoxic drugs; aminoglycosides** (e.g., gentamicin, tobramycin), **selected antibiotics** (e.g., vancomycin), **antineoplastics** (e.g., cisplatin, nitrogen mustard), **anesthetics** (e.g.,

methoxyflurane [Penthrane]), **antituberculars** (e.g., capreomycin [Capestat]), **cyclosporine** (Sandimmune), **diuretics** (e.g., furosemide [Lasix], torsemide [Demadex]), **pentamidine.** Nephrotoxic effects are additive. Frequent monitoring of renal function indicated if any other nephrotoxic drug must be used. ▪ Nephrotoxicity and myelotoxicity are both increased when given concurrently with **zidovudine** (AZT, Retrovir). ▪ Potentiates nephrotoxicity of **cyclosporine;** alternate immunosuppressive therapy recommended. ▪ Concurrent use with **antineoplastic agents** (e.g., methotrexate) **or radiation therapy** may increase renal toxicity and incidence of bronchospasm and hypotension. ▪ Enhances antifungal effects of **flucytosine** (Ancobon) **and other antiinfectives.** May increase toxicity. ▪ Antagonism between amphotericin B and **imidazole antifungals** (e.g., ketoconazole, miconazole, fluconazole) has been reported. ▪ Acute pulmonary toxicity occurred in patients receiving **leukocyte transfusion;** separate administration times as much as possible.

SIDE EFFECTS

LIPID-BASED PREPARATIONS: Most side effects similar to generic amphotericin B but occur with less frequency and intensity. Acute reactions, including fever and chills, may occur within 1 to 2 hours of starting the infusion. Infusion-related cardiorespiratory reactions may include dyspnea, hypertension, hyperventilation, hypotension, hypoxia, tachycardia, and vasodilation. More common with initial doses and subside with subsequent doses. Arrhythmia, bronchospasm, and shock can occur. Anaphylaxis and cardiac arrest from overdose have been reported.

GENERIC: Common even at doses below therapeutic; may begin to occur within 15 to 20 minutes: anorexia, chills, convulsions, diarrhea, fever, headache, phlebitis, vomiting. Anaphylactoid reactions, anemia, cardiac disturbances (including fibrillation and arrest), coagulation defects, hypertension, hypokalemia, hypotension, and numerous other side effects occur fairly frequently. Renal function impaired in 80% of patients. May reverse after treatment ends, but some permanent damage likely. Pseudomembranous colitis has been reported.

ANTIDOTE

ALL AMPHOTERICIN FORMULATIONS: Notify the physician of all side effects. Many are reversible if the drug is discontinued. Some will respond to symptomatic treatment. Acute reactions (e.g., fever, chills, hypotension, nausea, and vomiting) usually lessen with subsequent doses. These acute infusion-related reactions can be managed by pretreatment with antipyretics, antihistamines, and/or corticosteroids or reduction of the rate of infusion and prompt treatment with antihistamines and/or corticosteroids and meperidine (Demerol) for chills. If anaphylaxis or serious respiratory distress occurs, discontinue amphotericin and treat as necessary. Give no further infusions. Hemodialysis not effective in overdose. Discontinue if BUN and alkaline phosphatase are abnormal. Dantrolene has been used to prevent (50 mg PO) or treat (50 mg IV) severe, shaking chills.

GENERIC: Administration of generic amphotericin B on alternate days may decrease the incidence of some side effects. Urinary alkalinizers may minimize renal tubular acidosis.

ABELCET/AMPHOTEC: Overdose has caused cardiac arrest. Discontinue drug and treat symptomatically.

AMPICILLIN SODIUM
(am-pih-**SILL**-in **SO**-dee-um)

Antibacterial
(penicillin)

pH 8 to 10

USUAL DOSE

Range is from 1 to 12 Gm/24 hr for adults and pediatric patients weighing 20 kg or more. Larger doses may be indicated based on the seriousness of the infection. Some clinicians suggest a weight of 40 kg to receive adult dose range.

Respiratory tract or skin and skin structure infections: 250 to 500 mg every 6 hours.

GI or GU infections: 500 mg every 6 hours.

Septicemia or bacterial meningitis: 8 to 14 Gm or 150 to 200 mg/kg/24 hr in equally divided doses every 3 to 4 hours (18.75 to 25 mg/kg every 3 hours or 25 to 33.3 mg/kg every 4 hours). Administer IV a minimum of 3 days; then may be given IV or IM.

Treatment of gonorrhea: 500 mg. Repeat in 8 to 12 hours. May repeat 2-dose regimen IV or IM if indicated. Ceftriaxone (Rocephin) IV or IM is most commonly used.

Listeriosis: 50 mg/kg every 6 hours.

Prevention of bacterial endocarditis in dental or respiratory tract surgery or instrumentation: 2 Gm of ampicillin 30 minutes before procedure.

Prevention of bacterial endocarditis in GI, GU, or biliary tract surgery or instrumentation: *Low to moderate risk:* A single dose of 2 Gm of ampicillin 30 minutes before procedure. *Moderate to high risk:* 2 Gm of ampicillin in conjunction with gentamicin 1.5 mg/kg (up to 80 mg) 30 minutes before procedure. Repeat 1 Gm of ampicillin or give oral amoxicillin 1 Gm in 6 hours.

Prophylaxis in high-risk cesarean section patients: 1 to 2 Gm immediately after clamping cord.

Prophylaxis of neonatal group B *Streptococcal* disease: 2 Gm to the mother during labor. Should be given at least 4 hours before delivery to ensure amniotic fluid concentrations and placental transfer of ampicillin. May repeat 1 to 2 Gm every 4 to 6 hours until delivery. Continue treatment postpartum if active signs of maternal infection develop. Routine use of prophylaxis in neonates born to these mothers is not recommended; risk must be assessed on an individual basis for each infant.

Leptospirosis (unlabeled): 500 mg to 1 Gm every 6 hours.

Typhoid fever (unlabeled): 25 mg/kg every 6 hours.

PEDIATRIC DOSE

Range is from 25 to 400 mg/kg of body weight/24 hr for pediatric patients weighing less than 20 kg. Some clinicians suggest a weight up to 40 kg is appropriate for pediatric use. Do not exceed adult dose or 12 Gm.

Respiratory tract or skin and skin structure infections: 25 to 50 mg/kg/24 hr in equally divided doses every 4 to 6 hours (4.16 to 8.3 mg/kg every 4 hours or 6.25 to 12.5 mg/kg every 6 hours).

GI or GU infections: 50 to 100 mg/kg/24 hr in equally divided doses every 6 hours (12.5 to 25 mg/kg every 6 hours).

Septicemia or bacterial meningitis: 100 to 200 mg/kg/24 hr in equally divided doses every 3 to 4 hours (12.5 to 25 mg/kg every 3 hours or 16.6 to 33.3 mg/kg every 4 hours).

Empiric treatment of bacterial meningitis in infants and children 2 months to 12 years of age: Some clinicians recommend 200 to 400 mg/kg/24 hr in equally divided doses every 4 to 6 hours (33.3 to 66.6 mg/kg every 4 hours to 50 to 100 mg/kg every 6 hours). Given in conjunction with chloramphenicol. Satisfactory response should occur within 48 hours or initiate alternate therapy. Administer any regimen IV a minimum of 3 days, then may be given IV or IM.

Prevention of bacterial endocarditis in dental or respiratory tract surgery or instrumentation: 50 mg/kg of ampicillin 30 minutes before procedure.

Prevention of bacterial endocarditis in GI, GU, or biliary tract surgery or instrumentation: *Low to moderate risk:* A single dose of 50 mg/kg 30 minutes before procedure. *Moderate to high risk:* 50 mg/kg of ampicillin in conjunction with gentamicin 1.5 mg/kg (up to 80 mg) 30 minutes before procedure. Repeat 25 mg/kg of ampicillin or oral amoxicillin in 6 hours.

NEONATAL DOSE

Age up to 7 days: *weight less than 2,000 Gm:* 25 mg/kg every 12 hours. *2,000 Gm or more:* 25 mg/kg every 8 hours.

Over 7 days of age: *weight less than 1,200 Gm:* 25 mg/kg every 12 hours. *1,200 to 2,000 Gm:* 25 mg/kg every 8 hours. *More than 2,000 Gm:* 25 mg/kg every 6 hours.

Empiric treatment of bacterial meningitis in neonates and infants less than 2 months of age: 100 to 300 mg/kg/24 hr in equally divided doses (e.g., 33.3 to 100 mg/kg every 8 hours) in conjunction with IM gentamicin. Administer any regimen IV a minimum of 3 days, then may be given IV or IM.

Bacterial meningitis in neonates and infants less than 2 months of age: Age up to 7 days: *weight less than 2,000 Gm:* 50 to 75 mg/kg every 12 hours. *2,000 Gm or more:* 50 to 75 mg/kg every 8 hours.

Over 7 days of age: *weight less than 2,000 Gm:* 50 mg/kg every 8 hours. *2,000 Gm or more:* 50 mg/kg every 6 hours.

DOSE ADJUSTMENTS

Patients with a CrCl of 10 to 50 mL/min may require the usual dose every 6 to 12 hours. Reduce dose by increasing interval to 12 to 16 hours in severe renal impairment (CrCl less than 10 mL/min). Another source suggests no dose adjustment with a CrCl of 30 mL/min or greater and dosing every 8 hours for a CrCl of 10 mL/min or less. Administer 250 mg every 12 hours to peritoneal dialysis patients, and hemodialysis patients should receive a supplemental dose after each dialysis.

DILUTION

Each 500 mg or fraction thereof must be reconstituted with at least 5 mL of SW for injection. Use within 1 hour of reconstitution. May be further diluted in 50 mL or more of selected IV solutions. Stable for 8 hours at concentrations up to 30 mg/mL in NS, LR, sodium lactate, or SW. Stable in D5/½NS or 10% invert sugar in water for 4 hours at concentrations up to 2 mg/mL. Stable in D5W for 4 hours at concentrations up to 2 mg/mL but only for 2 hours at concentrations up to 20 mg/mL. Must be administered before stability expires.

COMPATIBILITY   (Underline Indicates Conflicting Compatibility Information)
Consider any drug NOT listed as compatible to be INCOMPATIBLE until consulting a pharmacist; specific conditions may apply.
Inactivated in solution with aminoglycosides (e.g., amikacin [Amikin], gentamicin). Do not mix in the same solution. Appropriate spacing and/or separate sites required. See Drug/Lab Interactions.

One source suggests the following **compatibilities:**

Additive: Aztreonam (Azactam), cefepime (Maxipime), clindamycin (Cleocin), erythromycin (Erythrocin), furosemide (Lasix), heparin, hydrocortisone sodium succinate (Solu-Cortef), metronidazole (Flagyl IV), ranitidine (Zantac), verapamil.

Y-site: Acyclovir (Zovirax), alprostadil, amifostine (Ethyol), anidulafungin (Eraxis), aztreonam (Azactam), bivalirudin (Angiomax), calcium gluconate, cisatracurium (Nimbex), cyclophosphamide (Cytoxan), dexmedetomidine (Precedex), diltiazem (Cardizem), docetaxel (Taxotere), doxapram (Dopram), doxorubicin liposomal (Doxil), enalaprilat (Vasotec IV), esmolol (Brevibloc), etoposide phosphate (Etopophos), famotidine (Pepcid IV), filgrastim (Neupogen), fludarabine (Fludara), foscarnet (Foscavir), gemcitabine (Gemzar), granisetron (Kytril), heparin, hetastarch in electrolytes (Hextend), hetastarch in NS (Hespan), hydromorphone (Dilaudid), insulin (regular), labetalol (Trandate), levofloxacin (Levaquin), linezolid (Zyvox), magnesium sulfate, melphalan (Alkeran), meperidine (Demerol), milrinone (Primacor), morphine, multivitamins (M.V.I.), pantoprazole (Protonix IV), pemetrexed (Alimta), phytonadione (vitamin K_1), potassium chloride (KCl), propofol (Diprivan), remifentanil (Ultiva), tacrolimus (Prograf), teniposide (Vumon), theophylline, thiotepa, vancomycin.

RATE OF ADMINISTRATION
A single dose over 10 to 15 minutes when given by IV injection. In 100 mL or more of solution, administer at prescribed infusion rate but never exceed IV injection rate. Too-rapid injection may cause seizures.

ACTIONS
A semisynthetic penicillin. Bactericidal against many gram-positive and some gram-negative organisms. Appears in all body fluids. Appears in cerebrospinal fluid only if inflammation is present. Crosses the placental barrier. Excreted in urine. Secreted in breast milk.

INDICATIONS AND USES
Highly effective against severe infections caused by gram-positive and some gram-negative organisms (e.g., respiratory tract, skin and skin structure, GI and GU, bacterial meningitis, endocarditis, listeriosis, septicemia). Not effective with penicillinase-producing staphylococci. ▪ Prevention of bacterial endocarditis in dental and respiratory tract surgery or instrumentation. ▪ Prevention of bacterial endocarditis in GI, GU, or biliary surgery or instrumentation. Used concurrently with gentamicin. ▪ Drug of choice during labor for prevention of neonatal group B streptococcal infections. **Unlabeled uses:** Prophylaxis in high-risk cesarean section patients. Treatment of leptospirosis. Treatment of typhoid fever.

CONTRAINDICATIONS
Known penicillin or cephalosporin sensitivity (not absolute); see Precautions. Infectious mononucleosis because of increased incidence of rash.

PRECAUTIONS

Hypersensitivity reactions, including fatalities, have been reported in patients undergoing penicillin therapy; most likely to occur in patients with a history of penicillin allergy or sensitivity to multiple allergens. There have been reports of individuals with a history of penicillin hypersensitivity experiencing severe reactions when treated with cephalosporins. Check history of previous hypersensitivity reactions to penicillins, cephalosporins, or other allergens. Actual incidence of cross-allergenicity not established but may be more common with first-generation cephalosporins. ■ Sensitivity studies indicated to determine susceptibility of the causative organism to ampicillin. ■ To reduce the development of drug-resistant bacteria and maintain its effectiveness, ampicillin should be used to treat or prevent only those infections proven or strongly suspected to be caused by bacteria. ■ Avoid prolonged use of this drug; superinfection caused by overgrowth of nonsusceptible organisms may result. ■ *Clostridium difficile*–associated diarrhea (CDAD) has been reported. May range from mild diarrhea to fatal colitis. Consider in patients who present with diarrhea during or after treatment with ampicillin. ■ Side effects increased in some patients; see Side Effects.

Monitor: Watch for early symptoms of hypersensitivity reactions, especially in individuals with a history of allergic problems. ■ AST may be increased. Renal, hepatic, and hematopoietic function should be checked during prolonged therapy. ■ Test all patients with syphilis for HIV. ■ Electrolyte imbalance and cardiac irregularities from sodium content are possible. Contains 2.9 mEq sodium/Gm. May aggravate CHF. Observe for hypokalemia. ■ May cause thrombophlebitis; observe carefully and rotate infusion sites.

Patient Education: May require alternate birth control. ■ Promptly report diarrhea or bloody stools that occur during treatment or up to several months after an antibiotic has been discontinued; may indicate CDAD and require treatment.

Maternal/Child: Category B: use only if clearly needed. ■ May cause diarrhea, candidiasis, or allergic response in nursing infants. ■ Elimination rate markedly reduced in neonates.

Elderly: Consider degree of age-related impaired renal function.

DRUG/LAB INTERACTIONS

Streptomycin potentiates bactericidal activity against enterococci. ■ May be used concurrently with **aminoglycosides** (e.g., gentamicin), but these drugs must never be mixed in the same infusion (mutual inactivation). If given concurrently, administer at separate sites. ■ May be antagonized by **bacteriostatic antibiotics** (e.g., chloramphenicol, erythromycin, and tetracyclines); may interfere with bactericidal action. ■ Concomitant use with **beta-adrenergic blockers** (e.g., propranolol) may increase risk of anaphylaxis and inhibit treatment. ■ Potentiated by **probenecid** (Benemid); toxicity may result. ■ Increased risk of bleeding with **heparin**. ■ May decrease clearance and increase toxicity of **methotrexate**. ■ Decreases effectiveness of **oral contraceptives;** breakthrough bleeding or pregnancy could result. ■ Ampicillin-induced skin rash potentiated by **allopurinol** (Aloprim). ■ False-positive glucose reaction with **Clinitest and Benedict's or Fehling's solution.** ■ May cause **false values** in other lab tests; see literature.

SIDE EFFECTS

Primarily hypersensitivity reactions such as anaphylaxis, exfoliative dermatitis, rashes, and urticaria. May cause CDAD. Hypersensitivity myocarditis can occur (fever, eosinophilia, rash, sinus tachycardia, ST-T changes, and cardiomegaly). Anemia, leukopenia, and thrombocytopenia have been reported. Thrombophlebitis will occur with long-term use. Higher than normal doses may cause neurologic adverse reactions including convulsions, especially with impaired renal function. Incidence of side effects increased in patients with viral infections or those taking allopurinol (Aloprim).

ANTIDOTE

Notify the physician of any side effect. For severe symptoms, discontinue the drug, treat hypersensitivity reactions (antihistamines, epinephrine, corticosteroids), and resuscitate as necessary. Hemodialysis is effective in overdose. Treat CDAD with fluids, electrolytes, protein supplements, and oral vancomycin (Vancocin) or metronidazole (Flagyl) as indicated. In severe cases, surgical evaluation may be indicated.

AMPICILLIN SODIUM AND SULBACTAM SODIUM

(am-pih-**SILL**-in **SO**-dee-um and sull-**BACK**-tam **SO**-dee-um)

Unasyn

Antibacterial
(penicillin and beta-lactamase inhibitor)

pH 8 to 10

USUAL DOSE

Adults and pediatric patients weighing 40 kg or more: 1.5 to 3 Gm every 6 hours (1 Gm ampicillin with 0.5 Gm sulbactam to 2 Gm ampicillin with 1 Gm sulbactam). All commercial preparations in the U.S. have a 2:1 ratio of ampicillin to sulbactam (e.g., 1.5 Gm = 1 Gm ampicillin plus 0.5 Gm sulbactam). Do not exceed 4 Gm **sulbactam**/24 hr. *All doses in this monograph include ampicillin and sulbactam within the recommended dose.*

PEDIATRIC DOSE

IV use for more than 14 days is not recommended. See comments under Adult Dose.

Skin and skin structure infections in pediatric patients over 1 year of age and less than 40 kg: 300 mg/kg/day (200 mg/kg ampicillin and 100 mg/kg sulbactam) in equally divided doses as an infusion every 6 hours (75 mg/kg every 6 hours).

The American Academy of Pediatrics suggests use in pediatric patients over 1 month of age in the following doses.

Mild to moderate infections: 150 to 225 mg/kg/day (100 to 150 mg/kg of ampicillin and 50 to 75 mg/kg sulbactam) in equally divided doses as an infusion every 6 hours (37.5 to 56.5 mg/kg every 6 hours).

Severe infections: 300 to 450 mg/kg/day (200 to 300 mg/kg of ampicillin and 100 to 150 mg/kg of sulbactam) in equally divided doses as an infusion every 6 hours (75 mg/kg to 112.5 mg/kg every 6 hours).

DOSE ADJUSTMENTS
May be indicated in the elderly. ▪ Reduce total daily dose in impaired renal function according to the following chart.

Ampicillin/Sulbactam Dose Guidelines in Impaired Renal Function	
Creatinine Clearance (mL/min per 1.73 M²)	Dose/Frequency
30 mL/min or more	Usual recommended dose q 6 to 8 hr
15 to 29 mL/min	Usual recommended dose q 12 hr
5 to 14 mL/min	Usual recommended dose q 24 hr
Hemodialysis patients	Usual recommended dose q 24 hr On day of dialysis, give immediately after dialysis

DILUTION
Each 1.5 Gm or fraction thereof must be initially reconstituted with at least 3.2 mL of SW for injection (375 mg/mL). Allow to stand to dissipate foaming. Solution should be clear. Must be further diluted to a final concentration of 3 to 45 mg/mL in one of the following solutions and given by slow IV injection or as an intermittent IV infusion: D5W, D5/½NS, 10% invert sugar in water, LR, ⅙ M sodium lactate solution, or NS. 3 Gm/L equals 3 mg/mL, 3 Gm/125 mL equals 24 mg/mL. Also available in piggyback vials and ADD-Vantage vials for use with ADD-Vantage infusion containers.

Storage: Store at CRT before dilution. Stable in all specifically listed solutions in any dilution for at least 2 hours. Stability in each solution varies (see literature).

COMPATIBILITY   (Underline Indicates Conflicting Compatibility Information)
Consider any drug NOT listed as compatible to be INCOMPATIBLE until consulting a pharmacist; specific conditions may apply.
May be inactivated in solution with aminoglycosides (e.g., amikacin [Amikin], gentamicin). Do not mix in the same solution. Appropriate spacing and/or separate sites required. See Drug/Lab Interactions.

One source suggests the following **compatibilities:**
Additive: Aztreonam (Azactam).
Y-site: Amifostine (Ethyol), anidulafungin (Eraxis), aztreonam (Azactam), bivalirudin (Angiomax), cefepime (Maxipime), cisatracurium (Nimbex), dexmedetomidine (Precedex), diltiazem (Cardizem), docetaxel (Taxotere), enalaprilat (Vasotec IV), etoposide phosphate (Etopophos), famotidine (Pepcid IV), fenoldopam (Corlopam), filgrastim (Neupogen), fluconazole (Diflucan), fludarabine (Fludara), gallium nitrate (Ganite), gemcitabine (Gemzar), granisetron (Kytril), heparin, hetastarch in electrolytes (Hextend), insulin (regular), linezolid (Zyvox), meperidine (Demerol), morphine, paclitaxel (Taxol), palonosetron (Aloxi), pemetrexed (Alimta), remifentanil (Ultiva), tacrolimus (Prograf), teniposide (Vumon), theophylline, thiotepa, vancomycin.

RATE OF ADMINISTRATION
IV injection: A single dose over a minimum of 10 to 15 minutes.
Intermittent IV: A single dose over 15 to 30 minutes or longer, depending on amount of solution. Too-rapid injection may cause seizures.

ACTIONS

A semisynthetic penicillin. The addition of sulbactam improves ampicillin's bactericidal activity against beta-lactamase–producing strains resistant to penicillins and cephalosporins. A broad-spectrum antibiotic and beta-lactamase inhibitor effective against selected gram-positive, gram-negative, and anaerobic organisms (see literature). Peak serum levels achieved by end of infusion. Appears in all body fluids. Half-life is 1 hour. Crosses the placental barrier. Excreted in the urine. Secreted in breast milk.

INDICATIONS AND USES

Treatment of skin and skin structure and intra-abdominal and gynecologic infections due to susceptible strains of specific organisms.

CONTRAINDICATIONS

Known penicillin, cephalosporin (not absolute [see Precautions]), or beta-lactamase inhibitor sensitivity (not absolute [see Precautions]); infectious mononucleosis because of increased incidence of rash.

PRECAUTIONS

Hypersensitivity reactions, including fatalities, have been reported in patients undergoing penicillin therapy; most likely to occur in patients with a history of penicillin allergy or sensitivity to multiple allergens. There have been reports of individuals with a history of penicillin hypersensitivity experiencing severe reactions when treated with cephalosporins. Check history of previous hypersensitivity reactions to penicillins, cephalosporins, or other allergens. Actual incidence of cross-allergenicity not established but may be more common with first-generation cephalosporins. ■ Studies indicated to determine the causative organism and susceptibility to ampicillin/sulbactam. ■ To reduce the development of drug-resistant bacteria and maintain its effectiveness, ampicillin and sulbactam should be used to treat or prevent only those infections proven or strongly suspected to be caused by bacteria. ■ Avoid prolonged use of this drug; superinfection caused by overgrowth of nonsusceptible organisms may result. ■ Elimination of sulbactam increased in cystic fibrosis patients. ■ Use caution in patients with CHF, a history of bleeding disorders, or GI disease (e.g., colitis). ■ *Clostridium difficile*–associated diarrhea (CDAD) has been reported. May range from mild diarrhea to fatal colitis. Consider in patients who present with diarrhea during or after treatment with ampicillin and sulbactam.

Monitor: Watch for early symptoms of hypersensitivity reactions, especially in individuals with a history of allergic problems. ■ AST may be increased. Renal, hepatic, and hematopoietic function should be checked during prolonged therapy. ■ Test all patients with syphilis for HIV. ■ May cause thrombophlebitis. Observe carefully and rotate infusion sites. ■ Electrolyte imbalance and cardiac irregularities from sodium content are possible. Contains 5 mEq sodium/1.5 Gm. May aggravate CHF. Observe for hypokalemia.

Patient Education: Report promptly; fever, rash, sore throat, unusual bleeding or bruising, severe stomach cramps, and/or diarrhea, seizures. ■ May require alternate birth control. ■ Promptly report diarrhea or bloody stools that occur during treatment or up to several months after an antibiotic has been discontinued; may indicate CDAD and require treatment.

Maternal/Child: Category B: studies in rabbits have not shown adverse effects on fertility or in the fetus. Use only if clearly needed. ■ May cause diarrhea, candidiasis, or allergic response in nursing infants. ■ Safety for

IV use in pediatric patients over 1 year of age has been established for skin and skin structure infections but not for other uses; however, it is in use. Elimination rate markedly reduced in neonates. ▪ Safety and effectiveness of IM use in pediatric patients not established.
Elderly: Consider degree of age-related impaired renal function. ▪ See Dose Adjustments.

DRUG/LAB INTERACTIONS

Streptomycin potentiates bactericidal activity against enterococci. ▪ Frequently used concomitantly with **aminoglycosides** (e.g., gentamicin), but these drugs must never be mixed in the same infusion (mutual inactivation). If given concurrently, administer at separate sites. ▪ May be antagonized by **bacteriostatic antibiotics** (e.g., chloramphenicol, erythromycin, tetracyclines); may interfere with bactericidal action. ▪ May decrease clearance and increase toxicity of **methotrexate.** ▪ Decreases effectiveness of **oral contraceptives;** breakthrough bleeding or pregnancy could result. ▪ Ampicillin-induced skin rash potentiated by **allopurinol** (Aloprim). ▪ False-positive glucose reaction with **Clinitest and Benedict's or Fehling's solution.** ▪ May cause **false values** in other lab tests; see literature.

SIDE EFFECTS

Full scope of hypersensitivity reactions, including anaphylaxis, are possible. Burning, discomfort, and pain at injection site; diarrhea, rash, and thrombophlebitis occur most frequently. Abdominal distention; candidiasis; chest pain; chills; decreased hemoglobin, hematocrit, RBC, WBC, lymphocytes, neutrophils, and platelets; decreased serum albumin and total protein; dysuria; edema; epistaxis; erythema; facial swelling; fatigue; flatulence; glossitis; headache; hypersensitivity myocarditis (fever, eosinophilia, rash, sinus tachycardia, ST-T changes and cardiomegaly); increased alkaline phosphatase, BUN, creatinine, LDH, AST, ALT; increased basophils, eosinophils, lymphocytes, monocytes, and platelets; itching, malaise, mucosal bleeding, nausea and vomiting, RBCs and hyaline casts in urine, substernal pain, tightness in throat, and urine retention can occur. May cause CDAD. Higher than normal doses may cause neurologic adverse reactions, including convulsions; especially with impaired renal function.

ANTIDOTE

Notify the physician of any side effect. For severe symptoms, discontinue the drug, treat hypersensitivity reactions as indicated (e.g., antihistamines, epinephrine, corticosteroids) and resuscitate as necessary. Treat CDAD with fluids, electrolytes, protein supplements, and oral vancomycin (Vancocin) or metronidazole (Flagyl) as indicated. In severe cases, surgical evaluation may be indicated. Hemodialysis may be effective in overdose.

ANIDULAFUNGIN
(a-**nid**-yoo-luh-**FUN**-jin)
Eraxis

Antifungal
(Echinocandin)

USUAL DOSE
Candidemia and other Candida infections (intra-abdominal abscess and peritonitis): Begin with a *loading dose* of 200 mg as an infusion on Day 1. Follow with a daily dose of 100 mg as an infusion beginning on Day 2. Base duration of treatment on patient's clinical response. In general, antifungal therapy should continue for at least 14 days after the last positive culture. **Esophageal candidiasis:** Begin with a *loading dose* of 100 mg as an infusion on Day 1. Follow with a daily dose of 50 mg as an infusion beginning on Day 2. Treat for a minimum of 14 days and for at least 7 days following resolution of symptoms. Relapse of esophageal candidiasis has occurred in patients with HIV infections; suppressive antifungal therapy may be considered after a course of treatment.

DOSE ADJUSTMENTS
No dose adjustment is indicated based on age, gender, or race; in patients with any degree of renal or hepatic insufficiency; or in patients using concomitant medications that are known metabolic substrates, inhibitors, or inducers of cytochrome P_{450} (CYP450) isoenzymes; see Drug/Lab Interactions. ■ No dose adjustment is required in patients with HIV who are receiving concomitant antiretroviral therapy (e.g., HIV protease inhibitors [e.g., amprenavir (Agenerase), indinavir (Crixivan), nelfinavir (Viracept), ritonavir (Norvir), saquinavir (Invirase)]).

DILUTION
Each 50-mg vial must be reconstituted with 15 mL of SW, and each 100-mg vial must be reconstituted with 30 mL of SW. The resulting concentration is 3.33 mg/mL. Aseptically transfer the reconstituted dose (50, 100, or 200 mg) into the appropriately sized IV container of D5W or NS for infusion as shown in the following chart. The final concentration of infusion solution is 0.77 mg/mL.

Dilution Requirements for Administration of Anidulafungin				
Dose (mg)	Number of Unit Packs Required	Total Reconstituted Volume (mL)	Volume of NS or D5W for Infusion	Total Infusion Volume (mL)
50 mg	1-50 mg	15 mL	50 mL	65 mL
100 mg	2-50 mg or 1-100 mg	30 mL	100 mL	130 mL
200 mg	4-50 mg or 2-100 mg	60 mL	200 mL	260 mL

Filters: No data available from manufacturer.
Storage: Store unopened vials, reconstituted vials, and fully diluted solutions at 2° to 8° C (36° to 46° F). Reconstituted solution may be refrig-

erated for up to 1 hour before dilution. Fully diluted infusion solution should be used within 24 hours. Do not freeze in any form.

COMPATIBILITY   (Underline Indicates Conflicting Compatibility Information)
Consider any drug NOT listed as compatible to be INCOMPATIBLE until consulting a pharmacist; specific conditions may apply.
Manufacturer states, "Do not mix or co-infuse with other medications or electrolytes. **Compatibility** of anidulafungin with intravenous substances, additives, or medications other than D5W or NS has not been established."
One source suggests the following **compatibilities:**
Y-site: Acyclovir (Zovirax), amikacin (Amikin), aminophylline, amphotericin B lipid complex (Abelcet), amphotericin liposomal (AmBisome), ampicillin, ampicillin/sulbactam (Unasyn), carboplatin (Paraplatin), cefazolin (Ancef), cefepime (Maxipime), cefoxitin (Mefoxin), ceftazidime (Fortaz), ceftriaxone (Rocephin), cefuroxime (Zinacef), ciprofloxacin (Cipro IV), cisplatin (Platinol), clindamycin (Cleocin), cyclophosphamide (Cytoxan), cyclosporine (Sandimmune), cytarabine (ARA-C), daunorubicin (Cerubidine), dexamethasone (Decadron), digoxin (Lanoxin), dobutamine, docetaxel (Taxotere), dopamine, doripenem (Doribax), doxorubicin (Adriamycin), epinephrine (Adrenalin), erythromycin (Erythrocin), etoposide phosphate (Etopophos), famotidine (Pepcid IV), fentanyl (Sublimaze), fluconazole (Diflucan), fluorouracil (5-FU), furosemide (Lasix), ganciclovir (Cytovene), gemcitabine (Gemzar), gentamicin, heparin, hydrocortisone sodium succinate (Solu-Cortef), ifosfamide (Ifex), imipenem-cilastatin (Primaxin), leucovorin calcium, levofloxacin (Levaquin), linezolid (Zyvox), meperidine (Demerol), meropenem (Merrem IV), methylprednisolone (Solu-Medrol), metronidazole (Flagyl IV), midazolam (Versed), morphine, mycophenolate (CellCept IV), norepinephrine (Levophed), paclitaxel (Taxol), pantoprazole (Protonix IV), phenylephrine (Neo-Synephrine), piperacillin/tazobactam (Zosyn), potassium chloride, quinupristin/dalfopristin (Synercid), ranitidine (Zantac), sulfamethoxazole/trimethoprim, tacrolimus (Prograf), ticarcillin/clavulanate (Timentin), tobramycin, vancomycin, vincristine, voriconazole (VFEND IV), zidovudine (AZT, Retrovir).

RATE OF ADMINISTRATION
Flush IV line with D5W or NS before and after infusion.
Do not exceed an infusion rate of 1.1 mg/min (equivalent to 1.4 mL/min or 84 mL/hr when diluted as directed). Infusion at a rate greater than 1.1 mg/min may cause histamine-mediated reactions (e.g., dyspnea, flushing, hypotension, pruritus, rash, urticaria).

ACTIONS
A semi-synthetic lipopeptide, anidulafungin is an echinocandin, the newest class of antifungal agents. Acts by inhibiting the synthesis of 1,3-beta-D-glucan, an integral component of the fungal cell wall not present in mammalian cells. Extensively protein bound. Steady state is achieved after a loading dose. Not metabolized, it undergoes slow chemical degradation. Hepatic metabolism has not been observed. Anidulafungin is not a clinically relevant substrate, inducer, or inhibitor of cytochrome P_{450} (CYP450) isoenzymes. Terminal half-life ranges from 40 to 50 hours. Some excretion in feces, with minimal excretion in urine.

INDICATIONS AND USES

Treatment of the following fungal infections: candidemia and other forms of *Candida* infections (intra-abdominal abscess and peritonitis) and esophageal candidiasis. ▪ Has not been studied in *Candida* infections associated with endocarditis, osteomyelitis, and meningitis. ▪ Has not been studied in sufficient numbers of neutropenic patients to determine effectiveness.

CONTRAINDICATIONS

Hypersensitivity to anidulafungin or any of its components (e.g., fructose, mannitol, polysorbate 80, tartaric acid, sodium hydroxide, and/or hydrochloric acid); or other echinocandins (e.g., micafungin [Mycamine]).

PRECAUTIONS

Do not give as an IV bolus; for IV infusion only. ▪ Abnormal liver function tests have been reported. Isolated cases of significant hepatic dysfunction, hepatitis, or worsening hepatic failure have occurred. Incidence may be increased in patients with serious underlying conditions who are receiving additional concomitant medications. Evaluate risk versus benefit of continued anidulafungin therapy. ▪ During studies, endoscopically documented relapse rates were higher in patients treated for esophageal candidiasis with anidulafungin than in patients treated with fluconazole (Diflucan). ▪ *Candida* isolates with reduced susceptibility to anidulafungin have been reported, which suggests a potential for development of drug resistance. Clinical significance unknown. Cross-resistance with other echinocandins (e.g., micafungin [Mycamine]) have not been studied. ▪ Has been shown to be active against *Candida albicans* resistant to fluconazole (Diflucan). ▪ See Monitor and Antidote.

Monitor: Specimens for fungal culture, serologic testing, and histopathologic testing should be obtained before therapy to isolate and identify causative organisms. Therapy may begin as soon as all specimens are obtained and before results are known. Reassess after test results are known. ▪ Baseline CBC with differential and platelet count, BUN, and liver function tests (e.g., ALT, AST) may be indicated. ▪ Monitor for evidence of impaired hepatic function (e.g., increased ALT, AST, serum alkaline phosphatase). ▪ Monitor for S/S of a histamine-mediated reaction (e.g., bronchospasm, dyspnea, flushing, hypotension, pruritus, rash, urticaria). ▪ Monitor for S/S of a hypersensitivity reaction (e.g., bronchospasm, dyspnea, hives, hypotension, pruritus, rash, swelling of eyelids, lips, or face); discontinue infusion if a hypersensitivity reaction occurs.

Patient Education: Promptly report shortness of breath, dizziness or fainting, itching, rash, or swelling of extremities. ▪ Report S/S of liver dysfunction (anorexia, fatigue, jaundice, nausea and vomiting, dark urine, or pale stools).

Maternal/Child: Category C: use during pregnancy only if benefits justify risk to fetus. Some abnormalities, including skeletal changes, occurred in animal studies. ▪ Use caution if required during breast-feeding. Secreted in milk of drug-treated rats; not known if anidulafungin is secreted in human milk. ▪ Safety and effectiveness for use in pediatric patients not established; however, some immunocompromised pediatric (2 through 11 years) and adolescent (12 through 17 years) patients with neutropenia were included in studies; see prescribing information.

Elderly: Differences in response compared to younger adults not identified.

DRUG/LAB INTERACTIONS

Anidulafungin is not a clinically relevant substrate, inducer, or inhibitor of cytochrome P_{450} (CYP450) isoenzymes. It is considered unlikely that it will have a clinically relevant effect on the metabolism of drugs metabolized by CYP450 isoenzymes and/or other drugs likely to be coadministered with it. ■ No dose adjustment of either drug is indicated when coadministered with **cyclosporine** (Sandimmune), **tacrolimus** (Prograf), **or voriconazole** (VFEND IV). ■ No dose adjustment of anidulafungin is indicated when it is coadministered with **liposomal amphotericin B** (AmBisome) **or rifampin** (Rifadin).

SIDE EFFECTS

Patients treated for candidemia and other *Candida* infections: Deep vein thrombosis; diarrhea; elevated ALT, AST, alkaline phosphatase, and hepatic enzymes; and hypokalemia.

Patients treated for esophageal candidiasis: Dyspepsia (aggravated); elevated ALT, AST, and gamma-glutamyl transferase; fever; headache; leukopenia; nausea; neutropenia; phlebitis; rash; and vomiting.

Histamine-mediated reactions (e.g., bronchospasm, dyspnea, flushing, hypotension, pruritus, rash, urticaria) or hypersensitivity reactions may occur. Significant hepatic dysfunction (e.g., hepatitis, hepatocellular damage, hyperbilirubinemia, or hepatic failure) has occurred. Many other side effects have been reported in small numbers of patients.

ANTIDOTE

Notify physician of all side effects; most will be treated symptomatically. Reduce rate of infusion if a histamine-mediated reaction occurs. If a hypersensitivity reaction occurs, discontinue anidulafungin and treat as indicated. Appropriate treatment may include oxygen, epinephrine, antihistamines (e.g., diphenhydramine [Benadryl]), vasopressors (e.g., dopamine), corticosteroids, IV fluids, and ventilation equipment. S/S indicative of hepatic side effects may require evaluation of benefits versus risk of continuing anidulafungin therapy. Not removed by hemodialysis. Resuscitate as indicated.

ANTIHEMOPHILIC FACTOR (HUMAN OR RECOMBINANT)

Antihemorrhagic

(an-tie-hee-moe-**FIL**-ik **FAK**-tor)

Advate, AHF, Bioclate, Factor VIII, Helixate, Helixate FS, Hemofil M, Hyate: C Porcine AHF, Koate DVI, Kogenate, Kogenate FS, Monarc-M, Monoclate-P, Recombinate, ReFacto, Xyntha

Available factor VIII products and their origins include the following:
Advate, Helixate FS, Kogenate FS, ReFacto, Xyntha: Recombinant, stabilized without human albumin. Advate is formulated with trehalose; Helixate FS, Kogenate FS, ReFacto, and Xyntha are formulated with sucrose (amount of sucrose should not affect blood glucose concentrations).
Bioclate, Helixate, Kogenate, Recombinate: Recombinant, stabilized in human albumin.
Alphanate and Humate P (see AHF and von Willebrand Factor Complex), Koate DVI: From human plasma, intermediate and high purity.
Hemofil M, Monarc-M, Monoclate-P: From human plasma, immunoaffinity purified (ultrahigh purity).
Hyate: C Porcine AHF: Reserved for patients with inhibitors to human factor VIII.

USUAL DOSE (International units [IU])

Adults and pediatric patients: Completely individualized. Based on degree of deficiency, desired antihemophilic factor level, body weight, severity of bleeding, and presence of factor VIII inhibitors. Identify factor VIII deficiency and level assays before administration. One International unit (IU) is approximately equal to the level of factor VIII activity in 1 mL of fresh pooled human plasma. Recombinant products may be substituted for plasma-derived products without disrupting treatment regimen. A plasma antihemophilic factor level of about 30% of normal is needed for effective hemostasis when hemorrhage is present; greater percentages are required for surgical procedures, and only 5% to 10% of normal may be needed to control hemarthrosis. Each preparation suggests a different formula; end results are similar. An example is:

$$AHF/IU \text{ required} =$$
$$\text{Body weight (kg)} \times \text{Desired factor VIII increase (\% of normal)} \times 0.5$$

$$\text{Expected factor VIII increase (\% of normal)} =$$
$$AHF/IU/kg \text{ dose administered} \times 2$$

Examples of doses are as follows:
Prophylactic management: (e.g., severe factor VIII deficiency with frequent hemorrhages). Raise factor VIII level to 15% of normal. Repeat every 1 to 2 days. Usually requires 250 units daily in patients weighing less than 50 kg, 500 units daily in patients weighing more than 50 kg. Increase dose until bleeding episodes are adequately controlled.
Early hemarthrosis (blood into a joint or its synovial cavity), muscle bleed, or oral bleed: Raise factor VIII level to 20% to 40%. Usually requires 5 to 10 units/kg initially. Repeat infusion every 12 to 24 hours for 1 to 3 days until the bleeding episode as indicated by pain is resolved or healing is

achieved. If early hemarthrosis is treated promptly, lowest doses may be adequate.

More extensive hemarthrosis, muscle bleed, or hematoma: Raise factor VIII level to 30% to 60%. Usually requires 10 to 25 units/kg initially. Adjust dose based on circulating AHF levels and repeat infusion every 8 or 12 to 24 hours for 3 days or more until pain and disability are resolved.

Life-threatening bleeds (e.g., head injury, throat bleed, severe abdominal pain): Raise factor VIII level to 60% to 100%. Usually requires 40 to 50 units/kg initially. Adjust dose based on circulating AHF levels and repeat infusion every 8 to 24 hours until threat is resolved.

Minor surgery, including tooth extraction: Raise factor VIII level to 60% to 80% (*Advate* 60% to 100%, *Xyntha* 30% to 60%). Usually requires 25 to 40 units/kg. A single infusion plus oral antifibrinolytic therapy within 1 hour is sufficient in 70% of patients. Additional dosing every 12 to 24 hours may be needed to control bleeding.

Major surgery: Raise factor VIII level to 80% to 100% (*Advate* 80% to 120%, *Xyntha* 60% to 100%). Usually requires 45 to 50 units/kg initially. Repeat infusion every 8 to 24 hours depending on state of healing. Reduce dose as indicated by state of healing. Increase dose if level falls below 30%.

Maintenance doses: Vary slightly with specific products; see literature.

Hyate: C Porcine AHF: *Treatment of hemorrhagic episodes:* In patients with plasma antibody levels less than 50 Bethesda units/mL, the manufacturer suggests an initial dose of 100 to 150 porcine units/kg. Other sources suggest an initial dose of 50 to 150 porcine units/kg. If a patient has plasma antibody levels greater than 50 Bethesda units/mL, further specific testing must be completed to determine if they will benefit from treatment; see literature. *Prophylaxis of hemorrhagic episodes:* 20 to 60 porcine units/kg every other day has been used for long-term prophylaxis in the home. Supplement with 40 to 50 porcine units/kg if hemarthrosis develops.

DOSE ADJUSTMENTS

If AHF does not significantly improve the PTT, factor VIII antibodies are probable; may respond to an increased dose, especially if titer is less than 10 Bethesda units/mL. Frequent determinations of circulating AHF levels indicated.

DILUTION

Consult individual product instructions in the package insert; each product has a specific process for dilution. Information may be updated frequently. All preparations provide diluent and usually provide administration equipment, including needles (single- or double-ended), filters or filter needles, syringes, and/or administration sets for each vial. Actual number of AHF units shown on each vial. Use only the diluent provided, and maintain strict aseptic technique. Use a plastic syringe to prevent binding to glass surfaces. Warm to room temperature (25° C) before dilution and maintain throughout administration to avoid precipitation of active ingredients.

Filters: Supplied by manufacturer. If more than one bottle is required for a dose, multiple bottles may be drawn into the same syringe; however, a new filter needle must be used to withdraw contents of each bottle of antihemophilic factor.

Storage: Before reconstitution, store all formulations except Hyate: C Porcine at 2° to 8° C (35° to 46° F). Do not freeze. Most formulations can be stored at CRT not to exceed 25° C (77° F) for 2 months or more before reconstitution; check individual product. Protect Xyntha from light during storage. Before reconstitution, store *Hyate: C Porcine AHF* at −15° to −20° C (5° to −4° F). Maintain at CRT after dilution. Do not use beyond expiration dates on bottles.

COMPATIBILITY

Administration through a separate line without mixing with other IV fluids or medications is recommended. If antihemophilic factor is given as a continuous IV, one source says heparin 1 to 5 units/mL of concentrate may be added to avoid thrombophlebitis.

RATE OF ADMINISTRATION

Reduce rate of infusion or temporarily discontinue if there is a significant increase in pulse rate or S/S of hypersensitivity occur. Rate is based on patient comfort.

Most preparations suggest beginning with a rate of 2 mL/min and increasing gradually up to 10 mL/min if appropriate. Administration of a single dose in 5 to 10 minutes is generally well tolerated. Consult product information. Other sources list the following information:

Advate: A single dose over 5 minutes or less. Do not exceed a rate of 10 mL/min.

Bioclate, Hemofil M, Monarc-M, and Recombinate: May be given at a rate not to exceed 10 mL/min.

Helixate, Helixate FS, Kogenate, Kogenate FS, ReFacto: A single dose over 5 to 10 minutes is usually well tolerated. Do not exceed a rate of 10 mL/min.

Monoclate-P: Begin with a rate of 2 mL/min. Do not exceed 4 mL/min.

Xyntha: A single dose over several minutes, based on patient comfort.

ACTIONS

AHF is one of nine major factors in the blood that must act in sequence to produce coagulation, or clotting. It is the specific clotting factor deficient in patients with hemophilia A (classic hemophilia) and can temporarily correct the coagulation defect in these patients. Has a half-life of 10 to 18 hours. One IU of AHF increases the plasma concentration of factor VIII by 2%. **Plasma-based AHF:** A lyophilized concentrate of coagulation factor VIII (antihemophilic factor) prepared by various processes (e.g., heat treatment, chemical inactivation, solvent detergent treatment, immunoaffinity chromatography). Obtained from fresh (less than 3 hours old) human plasma cryoprecipitate. Tested and determined free from hepatitis and HIV viruses and containing acceptable ALT concentrations. **Recombinant AHF:** Produced through genetic engineering technology. Purified using monoclonal antibody purification techniques, ion exchange chromatography, and immunoaffinity chromatography. Risk of viral transmission eliminated because it is not derived from human blood. **Porcine AHF:** No evidence of viral transmission; pigs do not harbor hepatitis or HIV.

INDICATIONS AND USES

Control or prevent bleeding episodes and for perioperative management in patients with hemophilia A. (Congenital factor VIII deficiency of classic hemophilia.) Advate is considered to be of therapeutic value in patients with Factor VIII inhibitors not exceeding 10 Bethesda units. ReFacto is recommended for short-term routine prophylaxis. Porcine products may be used in patients with plasma antibody levels against human antihemophilic factor with inhibitor titers from 10 to 50 Bethesda units. Must be tested for cross-reactivity before administration.

Unlabeled uses: Adjunct in the treatment of disseminated intravascular coagulation (DIC).

CONTRAINDICATIONS

Hypersensitivity to a specific component of a product (e.g., mouse, hamster, or bovine protein [monoclonal-antibody–derived factor VIII], various stabilizers) or a previous life-threatening hypersensitivity reaction, including anaphylaxis, to a specific product. Not effective for bleeding in patients with von Willebrand's disease.

PRECAUTIONS

Should be administered under the direction of the physician specialist. ■ Treatment of choice when volume or RBC replacement is not needed; avoids hypervolemia and hyperproteinemia. ■ Desmopressin is preferred treatment in mild to moderate hemophilia A. ■ Hepatitis B vaccination indicated in all patients with hemophilia; usually done at birth or time of diagnosis. ■ Risk of transmitting hepatitis or HIV is markedly reduced with newer plasma-based products. There are no reported instances of new seroconversions to HIV with currently marketed products. ■ No risk of any viral transmission (hepatitis or HIV) with recombinant products. ■ Intravascular hemolysis can occur when large volumes are given to individuals with blood groups A, B, or AB. Monitor for progressive anemia. ■ Type-specific cryoprecipitate has been used to maintain adequate factor VIII levels and is appropriate in selected cases; carries risk of possible delayed seroconversion after viral infection (HIV, hepatitis A, B, or C). ■ Inhibitor titers above 10 Bethesda units/mL may make hemostatic control with AHF impossible or impractical because of the large dose required. Inhibitor titer may rise after AHF infusion due to an anamnestic (immunologic memory) response to the AHF antigen. Use of an alternate product may be indicated (e.g., factor IX complex concentrates, antihemophilic factor [Porcine], or anti-inhibitor coagulant complex). ■ Not useful to treat other coagulation factor deficiencies. ■ Components of some products may contain latex; use caution to avoid a hypersensitivity reaction.

Monitor: Identification of factor VIII deficiency with determination of circulating AHF levels should be obtained before administration and during treatment. Adjust dose as indicated. ■ Monitor pulse before and during treatment. ■ Monitor for the development of factor VIII inhibitors. Should be suspected if factor VIII plasma levels are not obtained or if bleeding is not controlled with an appropriate dose. ■ Monitor patients with a known or suspected inhibitor to Factor VIII more frequently. ■ Monitor for S/S of a hypersensitivity reaction. ■ See Precautions.

Patient Education: Prophylactic hepatitis B vaccine recommended. ■ Instruction for self-administration and proper preparation may be appropriate. ■ Discontinue antihemophilic factor and immediately report S/S of a hypersensitivity reaction (e.g., hives, itching, hypotension, rash, tightness of the chest, wheezing). ■ HIV screening every 2 to 3 months; not required with recombinant products. ■ Review prescription and non-prescription medications with a health care provider.

Maternal/Child: Category C: use only if clearly needed. ■ Use caution during breast-feeding. ■ Safe for use in pediatric patients of all ages, including newborns. (**Advate** and **Xyntha** did not include newborns in clinical trials.)

DRUG/LAB INTERACTIONS
Specific information not available.

SIDE EFFECTS
Usually respond to reduced rate of administration. Massive doses may cause acute hemolytic anemia, hyperfibrinogenemia, increased bleeding tendency, or jaundice (rare).

Plasma-based AHF: Clouding or loss of consciousness, flushing, headache, hypersensitivity reactions (anaphylaxis, backache, chills, erythema, fever, hives, hypotension, nausea, stinging at infusion site, tightness of chest, urticaria, wheezing), lethargy, paresthesias, somnolence, tachycardia, or vomiting may occur. Consider risk potential of contracting AIDS or hepatitis; risk of withholding treatment outweighs any risk associated with use.

Recombinant products: Arthralgia; asthenia; burning, erythema, and pruritus at injection site; chest discomfort; chills; cold feet; cough; diarrhea; dizziness; edema of lower extremities; fever; flushing; headache; hypotension (slight); increased sweating; lethargy; nausea; rash; sore throat; or an unusual taste in the mouth may occur. Hypersensitivity reactions, including anaphylaxis, may occur.

ANTIDOTE
Most side effects usually subside spontaneously in 15 to 20 minutes and are generally related to the rate of infusion. Keep the physician informed. Slow or discontinue infusion temporarily if pulse rate increases or beginning S/S of hypersensitivity reactions occur. Discontinue immediately and treat hypersensitivity reactions (antihistamines, epinephrine, corticosteroids). Resuscitate as necessary.

ANTIHEMOPHILIC FACTOR ■ VON WILLEBRAND FACTOR COMPLEX (HUMAN)

Antihemorrhagic

(an-tie-hee-moe-**FIL**-ik **FAK**-tor)

Alphanate, Humate-P

USUAL DOSE
(International units [IU])

Completely individualized. Based on degree of deficiency, desired antihemophilic factor level, body weight, severity of bleeding, and presence of Factor VIII inhibitors. One International unit (IU) of Factor VIII or 1 IU of von Willebrand factor:Ristocetin Cofactor (vWF:RCof) is approximately equal to the level of factor VIII activity or vWF:RCof found in 1 mL of fresh pooled human plasma.

ALPHANATE
Treatment of hemophilia A (adults): Dose requirements and frequency are calculated on the basis of an expected initial response of 2% of normal FVIII:C IU/kg of body weight administered. Assess adequacy of treatment by clinical effects and monitoring of Factor VIII activity. See Precautions. The following general dosages are recommended for adult patients:

Alphanate Dose Guidelines for the Treatment of Adults with Hemophilia A	
Hemorrhagic Event	**Dosage (AHF FVIII:C IU/kg body weight)**
Minor hemorrhage: Bruises, cuts, or scrapes or uncomplicated joint hemorrhage	FVIII:C levels should be brought to 30% of normal (15 FVIII IU/kg twice daily) until hemorrhage stops and healing has been achieved (1 to 2 days).
Moderate hemorrhage: Nose, mouth, and gum bleeds; dental extractions; hematuria	FVIII:C levels should be brought to 50% (25 FVIII IU/kg twice daily). Continue until healing has been achieved (2 to 7 days on average).
Major hemorrhage: Joint or muscle hemorrhage, major trauma, hematuria, intracranial and/or intraperitoneal bleeding	FVIII:C levels should be brought to 80% to 100% of normal for at least 3 to 5 days (40 to 50 FVIII IU/kg twice daily). Then maintain at 50% (25 FVIII IU/kg twice daily) until healing has been achieved. May require treatment for up to 10 days.
Surgery	Prior to surgery, FVIII:C levels should be brought to 80% to 100% of normal (40 to 50 FVIII IU/kg twice daily). For the next 7 to 10 days or until healing has been achieved, patient should be maintained at 60% to 100% FVIII levels (25 to 50 FVIII IU/kg twice daily).

IU, International unit.

Alphanate Dose Guidelines for Prophylaxis During Surgery and Invasive Procedures of Adult and Pediatric Patients with von Willebrand Disease (Except Type 3 Patients Undergoing Surgery)	
Bleeding Prophylaxis for Surgical or Invasive Procedures	**Dosage (AHF vWF:RCof IU/kg body weight)**
Adult	Preoperative dose: 60 vWF:RCof IU/kg body weight. Subsequent infusions: 40 to 60 vWF:RCof IU/kg body weight at 8- to 12-hour intervals as clinically needed. Dosing may be reduced after the third postoperative day. Continue treatment until healing is complete.
Adult	**Minor procedure:** vWF activity of 40% to 50% for at least 1 to 3 days postoperatively.
Adult	**Major procedure:** vWF activity of 40% to 50% for at least 3 to 7 days postoperatively.
Pediatric	Initial dose: 75 vWF:RCof IU/kg body weight. Subsequent infusions: 50 to 75 vWF:RCof IU/kg body weight at 8- to 12-hour intervals as clinically needed. Dosing may be reduced after the third postoperative day. Continue treatment until healing is complete.

IU, International unit.

Continued

HUMATE-P

Treatment of hemophilia A (adults): As a general rule, 1 IU of Factor VIII activity per kg body weight will increase the circulating Factor VIII level by approximately 2 IU/dL. Assess adequacy of treatment by clinical effects and monitoring of Factor VIII activity. See Precautions. The following general dosages are recommended for adult patients:

Humate-P Dose Recommendations for the Treatment of Hemophilia A*	
Hemorrhage Event	Dosage (IU† FVIII:C/kg body weight)
Minor • Early joint or muscle bleed • Severe epistaxis	Loading dose 15 IU FVIII:C/kg to achieve FVIII:C plasma level of approximately 30% of normal; one infusion may be sufficient If needed, half of the loading dose may be given once or twice daily for 1-2 days
Moderate • Advanced joint or muscle bleed • Neck, tongue, or pharyngeal hematoma without airway compromise • Tooth extraction • Severe abdominal pain	Loading dose 25 IU FVIII:C/kg to achieve FVIII:C plasma level of approximately 50% of normal Followed by 15 IU FVIII:C/kg every 8-12 hours for first 1-2 days to maintain FVIII:C plasma level at 30% of normal Then same dose once or twice a day for up to 7 days or until adequate wound healing
Life-threatening • Major operations • Gastrointestinal bleeding • Neck, tongue, or pharyngeal hematoma with potential for airway compromise • Intracranial, intra-abdominal, or intrathoracic bleeding • Fractures	Initially 40-50 IU FVIII:C/kg Followed by 20-25 IU FVIII:C/kg every 8 hours to maintain FVIII:C plasma level at 80%-100% of normal for 7 days Then continue the same dose once or twice a day for another 7 days in order to maintain the FVIII:C level at 30%-50% of normal

*In all cases, the dose should be adjusted individually by clinical judgment of the potential for compromise of a vital structure, and by frequent monitoring of factor VIII activity in the patient's plasma.
†*IU*, International unit.

Treatment of von Willebrand Disease (vWD) (adults and pediatric patients): As a rule, 40-80 IU vWF:RCof (corresponding to 16 to 32 IU Factor VIII in Humate-P) per kg body weight given every 8 to 12 hours. Repeat doses are administered as needed based on monitoring of appropriate clinical and laboratory measures. Expected levels of vWF:RCof are based on an expected in vivo recovery of 1.5 IU/dL rise per IU/kg vWF:RCof administered. The administration of 1 IU of Factor VIII per kg body weight can be expected to lead to a rise in circulating vWF:RCof of approximately 3.5 to 4 IU/dL. The following general dosages are recommended for adult and pediatric patients:

Humate-P Dose Recommendations for Treatment of von Willebrand Disease in Adult and Pediatric Patients		
Classification	Hemorrhage	Dosage (IU* vWF:RCof/kg body weight)
TYPE 1		
Mild *(Where use of desmopressin is known or suspected to be inadequate)* Baseline vWF:RCof activity typically >30% of normal (i.e., >30 IU/dL)	**Major (examples)** • Severe or refractory epistaxis • GI bleeding • CNS trauma • Traumatic hemorrhage	Loading dose 40 to 60 IU/kg Then 40 to 50 IU/kg every 8 to 12 hours for 3 days to keep the nadir level of vWF:RCof >50% of normal (i.e., >50 IU/dL) Then 40 to 50 IU/kg daily for a total of up to 7 days of treatment
Moderate or Severe Baseline vWF:RCof activity typically <30% of normal (i.e., <30 IU/dL)	**Minor (examples)** • Epistaxis • Oral bleeding • Menorrhagia	40 to 50 IU/kg (1 or 2 doses)
	Major (examples) • Severe or refractory epistaxis • GI bleeding • CNS trauma • Hemarthrosis • Traumatic hemorrhage	Loading dose of 50 to 75 IU/kg Then 40 to 60 IU/kg every 8 to 12 hours for 3 days to keep the nadir level of vWF:RCof >50% of normal (i.e., >50 IU/dL) Then 40 to 60 IU/kg daily for a total of up to 7 days of treatment *Factor VIII:C levels should be monitored and maintained according to the guidelines for hemophilia A therapy†*
TYPE 2 (ALL VARIANTS) AND TYPE 3		
	Minor (clinical indications above)	40 to 50 IU/kg (1 or 2 doses)
	Major (clinical indications above)	Loading dose of 60 to 80 IU/kg Then 40 to 60 IU/kg every 8 to 12 hours for 3 days to keep the nadir level of vWF:RCof >50% of normal (i.e., >50 IU/dL) Then 40 to 60 IU/kg daily for a total of up to 7 days of treatment *Factor VIII:C levels should be monitored and maintained according to the guidelines for hemophilia A therapy†*

*IU, International unit.
†In instances where both FVIII and vWF levels must be monitored.

Prevention of excessive bleeding during and after surgery in vWD: In the case of emergency surgery, administer a loading dose of 50 to 60 IU/kg Humate-P and closely monitor the patient's trough coagulation factor levels. Measurement of incremental in vivo recovery (IVR) and assessment of baseline plasma vWF:RCof and FVIII:C levels is recommended in all patients prior to surgery. Calculation of the loading dose requires four values: the target peak plasma vWF:RCof level, the baseline vWF:RCof level, body weight (BW) in kilograms, and IVR. If individual recovery

Continued

values are not available, a standardized loading dose can be used based on an assumed vWF:RCof IVR of 2 IU/dL per IU/kg of vWF:RCof product administered.

vWF:RCof and FVIII:C Humate-P Loading Dose Recommendations for the Prevention of Excessive Bleeding During and After Surgery			
Type of Surgery	vWF:RCof Target Peak Plasma Level	FVIII:C Target Peak Plasma Level	Calculation of Loading Dose (to be administered 1 to 2 hours before surgery)
Major	100 IU/dL	80 to 100 IU/dL	Δ* vWF:RCof × BW (kg)/IVR† = IU vWF:RCof required. If incremental IVR is not available, assume an IVR of 2 IU/dL per IU/kg and calculate the loading dose as follows: (100 − Baseline plasma vWF:RCof) × BW (kg)/2 In the case of emergency surgery, administer a dose of 50 to 60 IU/kg.
Minor/oral‡	50 to 60 IU/dL	40 to 50 IU/dL	Δ* vWF:RCof × BW (kg)/IVR† = IU vWF:RCof required

*Δ = Target peak plasma vWF:RCof − Baseline plasma vWF:RCof.
†IVR = Incremental recovery as measured in the patient.
‡Oral surgery is defined as removal of fewer than three teeth, if the teeth are non-molars and have no bony involvement. Removal of more than one impacted wisdom tooth is considered major surgery due to the expected difficulty of the surgery and the expected blood loss, particularly in subjects with type 2A or type 3 vWD. Removal of more than two teeth is considered major surgery in all patients.

vWF:RCof and FVIII:C Target Trough Plasma Level and Minimum Duration of Treatment Recommendations for Subsequent Maintenance Doses of Humate-P for the Prevention of Excessive Bleeding During and After Surgery					
	vWF:RCof Target Trough Plasma Levels*		FVIII:C Target Trough Plasma Levels*		
Type of Surgery	Up to 3 Days Following Surgery	After Day 3	Up to 3 Days Following Surgery	After Day 3	Minimum Duration of Treatment
Major	>50 IU/dL	>30 IU/dL	>50 IU/dL	>30 IU/dL	72 hours
Minor	≥30 IU/dL	—	—	>30 IU/dL	48 hours
Oral†	≥30 IU/dL	—	—	>30 IU/dL	8 to 12 hours‡

*Trough levels for either coagulation factor should not exceed 100 IU/dL.
†See note on oral surgery in previous chart.
‡At least one maintenance dose following surgery based on individual pharmacokinetic values.

PEDIATRIC DOSE

Treatment of hemophilia A (unlabeled): For immediate control of bleeding, follow the general recommendations for dosing and administration for adults. See Usual Dose and Maternal/Child.

DOSE ADJUSTMENTS

Adjust subsequent doses based on FVIII:C plasma level achieved or as outlined in specific charts.

DILUTION

Consult individual product instructions in the package insert; each product has a specific process for dilution. Information may be updated frequently.

Alphanate provides diluent, a double-ended transfer needle, and a microaggregate filter for use in administration. **Humate-P** provides diluent and a filter transfer set.

Alphanate and Humate-P: Actual number of AHF units are shown on each vial. Use only the diluent provided and maintain strict aseptic technique. Use a plastic syringe to prevent binding to glass surfaces. Warm to room temperature (25° C) before dilution and maintain throughout administration to avoid precipitation of active ingredients.

Filters: Filters supplied by manufacturer; see Dilution.

Storage: *Alphanate:* Refrigerate before use. Avoid freezing. May be stored at CRT for up to 2 months. Label vial with date removed from refrigeration. *Humate-P:* Store up to 25° C (up to 77° F). Avoid freezing. *Alphanate and Humate-P:* Do not refrigerate after reconstitution. Confirm expiration date on vial. Administer within 3 hours of reconstitution to ensure sterility. Discard any unused solution.

COMPATIBILITY

Specific information not available. Administration through a separate line without mixing with other IV fluids or medications is generally recommended for these products.

RATE OF ADMINISTRATION

Inject solution slowly. Rapid administration may result in vasomotor reactions.

Humate-P recommends a maximum rate of 4 mL/min.

Alphanate recommends a maximum rate not to exceed 10 mL/min.

ACTIONS

A purified, sterile, lyophilized concentrate of antihemophilic factor (Factor VIII) and von Willebrand Factor (vWF). Factor VIII is an essential cofactor in the activation of Factor X, leading ultimately to the formation of thrombin and fibrin. It is the specific clotting factor deficient in patients with hemophilia A (classic hemophilia). vWF is important for correcting the coagulation defect in patients with von Willebrand disease (vWD). It promotes platelet aggregation and platelet adhesion on damaged vascular endothelium and acts as a stabilizing carrier protein for the procoagulant protein Factor VIII. vWF activity is measured with an assay that uses an agglutinating cofactor called Ristocetin (RCof). The vWF:RCof assay provides a quantitative measurement of vWF function by determining how well vWF helps platelets adhere to one another. Reduced vWF:RCof activity indicates a deficiency of vWF. Following administration of FVIII/vWF, there is a rapid increase of plasma Factor VIII activity, followed by a rapid decrease in activity and then a slower rate of decrease in activity. The mean initial half-life in hemophilic patients is 8.3 to 27.5 hours with Alphanate and 12.2 hours (range: 8.4 to 17.4 hours) with Humate-P. In patients with vWD, bleeding time decreases. Antihemophilic Factor/von Willebrand Factor Complex is obtained from pooled human fresh-frozen plasma. Multiple methods of purification are used to inactivate infectious agents, including viruses.

INDICATIONS AND USES

ALPHANATE

Prevention and control of bleeding in patients with Factor VIII deficiency due to hemophilia A or acquired Factor VIII deficiency. ▪ Prophylaxis for surgical and/or invasive procedures in adult and pediatric patients with von Willebrand disease (vWD) (type 1 or 2) in which the use of desmopressin is either ineffective or contraindicated. ▪ Not indicated for patients with severe vWD (type 3).

HUMATE-P

Treatment and prevention of bleeding in adult patients with hemophilia A. ▪ Treatment of spontaneous and trauma-induced bleeding episodes and prevention of excessive bleeding during and after surgery in adult and pediatric patients with severe vWD or with mild or moderate vWD in which the use of desmopressin is known or suspected to be inadequate. ▪ Safety and efficacy of prophylactic dosing to prevent spontaneous bleeding and to prevent excessive bleeding related to surgery have not been established in patients with vWD.

CONTRAINDICATIONS

ALPHANATE: None known when used as indicated.

HUMATE-P: History of anaphylactic or severe systemic response to AHF-vWF preparations or known hypersensitivity to any of its components.

PRECAUTIONS

ALPHANATE AND HUMATE-P: For IV use only. ▪ Health care professionals should use caution during administration; may have risk of exposure to viral infection. ▪ Important to establish that coagulation disorder is caused by Factor VIII or vWF deficiency. Not useful in treatment of other deficiencies. ▪ Manufactured from human plasma. Risk of transmitting infectious agents (e.g., HIV, hepatitis and, theoretically, Creutzfeldt-Jakob disease) has been greatly reduced by screening, testing, and manufacturing techniques. However, risk of transmission cannot be totally eliminated. ▪ Hepatitis A and B vaccines are recommended for patients receiving plasma derivatives. ▪ Thrombotic events have been reported. Use caution in patients with known risk factors for thrombosis. Incidence may be higher in females. ▪ Inhibitors may develop with large or frequent doses; see Monitor.

Monitor: Complex contains blood group isoagglutinins (anti-A and anti-B). When very large or frequently repeated doses are needed, as when inhibitors are present or when presurgical and postsurgical care is involved, patients of blood groups A, B, and AB should be monitored for signs of intravascular hemolysis and decreasing hematocrit values; see Antidote. ▪ Replacement therapy should be monitored by appropriate coagulation tests, especially in cases involving major surgery. Monitor Factor VIII and vWF:RCof as indicated in dosing guidelines.

Patient Education: Prophylactic hepatitis A and hepatitis B vaccines recommended. ▪ Report symptoms of possibly transmitted viral infections immediately. Symptoms may include anorexia, arthralgias, fatigue, jaundice, low grade fever, nausea, or vomiting. ▪ Report rash or any other sign of hypersensitivity reaction promptly.

Maternal/Child: Category C: use only if clearly needed. ▪ Adequate and well-controlled studies with long-term evaluation of joint damage have not been done in pediatric patients. Joint damage may result from suboptimal treatment of hemarthroses. ▪ Safety and effectiveness for use in neonates with vWD has not been established. Has been used safely in infants, children, and adolescents with vWD.

Elderly: Numbers insufficient to determine differences in response compared with younger adults. Consider overall status in dosing.

DRUG/LAB INTERACTIONS

Specific information not available.

SIDE EFFECTS

ALPHANATE AND HUMATE-P: Usually well tolerated. Rare cases of hypersensitivity reactions, including anaphylaxis, have been reported (symptoms may include chest tightness, edema, fever, pruritus, rash, throat tightness). Other reported side effects include chills, headache, lethargy, nausea and vomiting, paresthesia, phlebitis, somnolence, and vasodilation. Inhibitors of Factor VIII may occur.

Post-Marketing: *Alphanate:* In addition to the above, cardiac arrest, femoral venous thrombosis, flushing, itching, joint pain, pulmonary embolus, seizure, shortness of breath, swelling of the parotid gland, urticaria.

Humate-P: Hypersensitivity reactions (including anaphylaxis), development of inhibitors to Factor VIII, hemolysis, hypervolemia, thromboembolic complications.

ANTIDOTE

Keep physician informed of all side effects. If mild reactions occur (mild allergic reaction, chills, nausea, or stinging at the infusion site) and additional treatment is indicated, a product from a different lot should be considered. Discontinue immediately at first sign of a moderate to severe hypersensitivity reaction. Treat as necessary (antihistamines, epinephrine, corticosteroids). Development of acute hemolytic anemia, increased bleeding tendency, or hyperfibrinogenemia may require transfusion with Type O red blood cells. Discontinue administration of Alphanate/Humate-P and consider alternative therapy. Resuscitate as necessary.

ANTI-INHIBITOR COAGULANT COMPLEX BBW
(an-**TIE**-in-**HIH**-bih-tor coe-**AG**-you-lant **COM**-plex)
Feiba NF

Antihemorrhagic

USUAL DOSE
A unit of **Feiba NF (nanofiltered and vapor heated)** is expressed as factor VIII inhibitor bypassing activity. Identification of factor VIII inhibitor levels and PT mandatory before administration.

FEIBA NF
Range is 50 to 100 units/kg.
Specific suggested dosing regimens include:
Joint hemorrhage: 50 units/kg; repeat at 12-hour intervals if indicated. May be increased to 100 units/kg if indicated. Continue treatment until clinical improvement (e.g., mobilization of the joint, reduction of swelling, relief of pain). *Do not exceed 200 units/kg/24 hr.*
Mucous membrane bleeding: 50 units/kg; repeat at 6-hour intervals if indicated. Monitor visible bleeding sites and hematocrit closely. May be increased to 100 units/kg every 6 hours for up to 2 doses if bleeding does not stop. *Do not exceed 200 units/kg/24 hr.*
Serious soft tissue hemorrhage: 100 units/kg; repeat at 12-hour intervals if indicated.
Other severe hemorrhage (e.g., CNS bleeding): 100 units/kg; repeat at 12-hour intervals if indicated. Feiba NF may be indicated at 6-hour intervals until clear clinical improvement occurs.

DILUTION
Actual number of units shown on each vial. Use only the diluent provided and maintain strict aseptic technique. Bring to room temperature before reconstitution. Follow manufacturer's guidelines for reconstitution using the BAXJECT device. May stick to sides of glass syringes; use of plastic syringes recommended. Gently swirl. Do not shake. May be given through Y-tube or three-way stopcock of infusion set. To avoid hypotension from prekallikrein activator (PKA), give **Feiba NF** within 3 hours of reconstitution.
Filters: The manufacturer of *Feiba NF* uses a needleless transfer device and has no recommendation for use of an in-line filter.
Storage: Refrigerate before reconstitution; do not refrigerate after reconstitution. Avoid freezing. Within the indicated shelf life, may be stored at RT (not to exceed 25° C [77° F]) for up to 6 months. Do not leave at RT beyond its shelf life and do not return to refrigeration. Record date of removal from refrigeration on package before moving to RT.

COMPATIBILITY
Specific information not available. Administration through a separate line without mixing with other IV fluids or medications is generally recommended. If anti-inhibitor coagulant is given as a continuous IV, one source says heparin 5 to 10 units/mL of concentrate may be added to avoid thrombophlebitis.

RATE OF ADMINISTRATION

If symptoms of too-rapid infusion (headache, flushing, changes in BP or pulse rate) occur, discontinue until symptoms subside. Restart at a lower rate.

Feiba NF: Do not exceed 2 units/kg/min.

ACTIONS

An activated prothrombin complex prepared from pooled human plasma. Controls bleeding in patients with factor VIII inhibitors. Mechanism of action is not well understood. Onset of response is usually within 12 hours. Peak response is usually seen within 36 to 72 hours.

Feiba NF: 1 unit of activity is the amount of anti-inhibitor coagulant complex (AICC) that will shorten the aPTT of a high-titer factor VIII inhibitor reference plasma to 50% of the blank value.

INDICATIONS AND USES

Prophylaxis and treatment of hemorrhagic complications in hemophiliacs (hemophilia A or B) with factor VIII inhibitors who are bleeding or will undergo elective or emergency surgery. Anti-inhibitor coagulant complex (AICC) is most frequently indicated if presenting factor VIII inhibitor levels are above 5 to 10 Bethesda units (BU) or rise to that level following treatment with antihemophilic factor (AHF). Patients whose factor VIII inhibitor levels are between 5 and 10 BU and whose inhibitor levels remain at those levels may be treated with either AHF or AICC. Patients whose inhibitor levels are less than or equal to 5 BU and whose inhibitor levels remain at those levels may be treated with AHF.

Unlabeled uses: Feiba NF has been used in the prophylaxis and treatment of hemorrhagic complications in non-hemophiliacs with acquired inhibitors to factors VIII, XI, and XII.

CONTRAINDICATIONS

Patients with a normal coagulation mechanism; patients with significant signs of DIC; treatment of bleeding due to coagulation factor deficiencies in the absence of inhibitors to coagulation factors VIII or IX.

PRECAUTIONS

Anamnestic responses (development of antibodies, reducing effectiveness of the drug) with a rise in factor VIII inhibitor titers have been seen in up to 20% of cases. ▪ Thrombotic and thromboembolic events have been reported (e.g., DIC, venous thrombosis, pulmonary embolism, MI, and stroke). Risk of complications may be increased in surgical patients, in patients with thrombotic risk factors, and in patients receiving higher doses. Patients receiving more than 100 units/kg/dose or 200 mg/kg/day are at increased risk for DIC or acute coronary ischemia. Use high doses only as long as necessary to stop bleeding. ▪ Patients with DIC, advanced atherosclerotic disease, crush injury, septicemia, or concomitant treatment with recombinant factor VIIa (e.g., NovoSeven, NovoSeven RT) have an increased risk of developing thrombotic events due to circulating tissue factor (TF) or predisposing coagulopathy. ▪ Use with caution and only if there are no therapeutic alternatives in patients at risk for DIC or arterial or venous thrombosis or in patients with existing thrombotic conditions (e.g., MI or venous thrombosis). ▪ Use with caution in patients with a history of coronary heart disease, liver disease, or postoperative immobilization, in the elderly, and in neonates; weigh benefits versus risk. ▪ Do not use Feiba NF for the treatment of bleeding episodes resulting from coagulation factor deficiencies. ▪ Made from human plasma and may contain infectious agents (e.g., HIV, Creutzfeldt-Jakob disease, hepatitis B, or hepatitis C). Numerous steps in the manufacturing process are used to reduce the potential for infection. ■ See Drug/Lab Interactions.

Monitor: Monitor PT before and after treatment. Only accurate means of treatment evaluation; see Drug/Lab Interactions. ■ Monitor vital signs before, during, and after the infusion. ■ Monitor for S/S of acute coronary ischemia, DIC, and other thrombotic or thromboembolic events (e.g., changes in BP and HR, chest pain, cough, respiratory distress); see Antidote. ■ Laboratory indications of DIC may include decreased fibrinogen, decreased platelet count, and/or the presence of fibrin-fibrinogen degradation products (FDP) or significantly prolonged TT, PT, or PTT. ■ Monitor for S/S of a hypersensitivity reaction (e.g., rash, shortness of breath).

Patient Education: Manufactured from pooled human plasma. Possibility of viral transmission exists. Promptly report S/S of viral infections (e.g., chills, drowsiness, fever, runny nose followed by joint pain, rash or abdominal pain, dark urine, jaundice, nausea, vomiting).

Maternal/Child: Category C: use only if clearly needed. ■ Data not available for use in newborns.

Elderly: May have increased risk for thromboembolic complications.

DRUG/LAB INTERACTIONS

Not recommended for use with **antifibrinolytic products** (aminocaproic acid, tranexamic acid). Feiba NF has been used with **antifibrinolytics;** however, they should be used with caution and not administered until at least 12 hours after Feiba NF. ■ aPTT, WBCT, and other **clotting factor tests** do not correlate with clinical improvement. Attempts to normalize these values may lead to overdose and DIC.

SIDE EFFECTS

Anaphylaxis, bradycardia, chest pain, chills, cough, decreased fibrinogen concentration, decreased platelet count, DIC, fever, flushing, headache, hypertension, hypotension, myocardial infarction, prolonged PT, prolonged PTT, prolonged thrombin time, respiratory distress, tachycardia, thrombosis or thromboembolism, urticaria. Consider risk potential of contracting AIDS or hepatitis.

Overdose: Increased risk for DIC, MI, or thromboembolism.

Post-Marketing: Anaphylactic reaction, DIC, hypersensitivity, hypoaesthesia, facial hypoaesthesia, hypotension, injection site pain, thromboembolism, thrombosis.

ANTIDOTE

If side effects occur, discontinue the infusion and notify the physician. May be resumed at a slower rate or discontinued, or an alternate product may be used. Symptoms of DIC (BP and pulse rate changes, respiratory discomfort, chest pain, cough, prolonged clotting tests, cyanosis of hands and feet, persistent bleeding from puncture sites or mucous membranes) require discontinuation of the infusion and immediate treatment. Treat anaphylaxis or other hypersensitivity reactions (changes in BP or HR [may indicate prekallikrein activity]) with antihistamines, epinephrine, corticosteroids and resuscitate as necessary.

ANTITHROMBIN III
(an-tie-**THROM**-bin)

AT-III, Thrombate III

Anticoagulant
Antithrombotic

pH 6.5 to 7.5

USUAL DOSE
(International units [IU])

Loading dose, maintenance dose, and dosing intervals are completely individualized based on confirmed diagnosis (see Precautions), patient weight, clinical condition, degree of deficiency, type of surgery or procedure involved, physician judgment, desired level of antithrombin III (AT-III), and actual plasma levels achieved as verified by appropriate lab tests. One unit/kg should raise the level of AT-III by 1.4%. The desired AT-III level after the first dose should be about 120% of normal (normal is 0.1 to 0.2 Gm/L). AT-III levels must be maintained at normal or at least above 80% of normal for 2 to 8 days depending on individual patient factors. Usually achieved by administration of a maintenance dose once daily. Concomitant administration of heparin usually indicated; see Drug/Lab Interactions.

Calculate the initial loading dose using the following formula (assumes a plasma volume of 40 mL/kg):

$$\text{Dosage units} = \frac{(\text{Desired AT-III level [\%]} - \text{Baseline AT-III [\%]}) \times \text{Body weight (kg)}}{\div 1.4\%}$$

For a 70-kg patient with a baseline AT-III level of 57% the initial dose of Thrombate III would be $(120\% - 57\%) \times 70 \div 1.4 = 3,150$ International units (IU). Measurement of plasma levels is suggested preinfusion, 20 minutes postinfusion (peak), 12 hours postinfusion, and preceding next infusion (trough). If recovery differs from the anticipated rise of 1.4% for each IU/kg, modify the formula accordingly. If the above patient has a 20-minute AT-III level of 147%, the increase in AT-III measured for each 1 IU/kg administered is $(147\% - 57\%) \times 70 \text{ kg} \div 3,150 \text{ IU} = 2\%$ rise for each IU/kg administered. This in vivo recovery would be used to calculate future doses. A maintenance dose of approximately 60% of the loading dose every 24 hours is the average required to maintain plasma levels between 80% and 120%. Dose and interval based on plasma levels.

DOSE ADJUSTMENTS

See Drug/Lab Interactions.

DILUTION

Diluent, double-ended needles for dilution, and filter needle for aspiration into a syringe are provided. Warm unopened diluent and concentrate to room temperature. Enter diluent bottle first. Enter vacuum concentrate bottle with needle at an angle. Direct diluent from above to sides of vial to gently moisten all contents. Remove diluent bottle and transfer needle; swirl continuously until completely dissolved. Draw into a syringe through the filter needle. Remove filter needle; replace with an administration set (not provided). For larger doses, several bottles may be drawn into one syringe. Use a separate filter needle for each bottle.

Filters: Filter needle supplied by manufacturer; see Dilution. For larger doses, several bottles may be drawn into one syringe. Use a separate filter needle for each bottle.

Storage: Store in refrigerator before dilution; avoid freezing. Do not refrigerate after reconstitution. Use within 3 hours of reconstitution.

COMPATIBILITY

Administration through a separate line without mixing with other IV fluids or medications is recommended.

RATE OF ADMINISTRATION

Too-rapid injection may cause dyspnea.

A single dose over 10 to 20 minutes.

ACTIONS

Manufactured from human plasma, purified and heat treated through specific processes, AT-III is a plasma-based protein produced by the body to inactivate specific clotting proteins and control clot formation. Identical to heparin cofactor I, a factor in plasma necessary for heparin to exert its anticoagulant effect. It inactivates thrombin and the activated forms of factors IX, X, XI, and XII (all coagulation enzymes except factors VIIa and XIIIa). Increases AT-III levels within 30 minutes and has a half-life of up to 3 days.

INDICATIONS AND USES

Treatment of patients with hereditary AT-III deficiency to prevent thrombosis during surgical or obstetric procedures (replacement therapy) or during acute thrombotic episodes.

CONTRAINDICATIONS

None when used as indicated.

PRECAUTIONS

For IV use only. ▪ Confirm diagnosis of hereditary AT-III deficiency based on a clear family history of venous thrombosis as well as decreased plasma AT-III levels and the exclusion of acquired deficiency. Present laboratory tests may not be able to identify all cases of congenital AT-III deficiency. ▪ Every unit of plasma used to manufacture AT-III is tested and found nonreactive for HBsAg and negative for antibody to HIV by FDA-approved tests, then heat-treated by a special process. Even with these precautions, individuals who receive multiple infusions may develop viral infection, particularly non-A, non-B hepatitis. HIV infection remains a remote possibility. ▪ May reverse heparin resistance.

Monitor: See varying methods for measuring AT-III levels under Usual Dose. Should be measured at least twice daily until the patient is stabilized and peak and trough levels established, then measured daily. All blood work should be drawn immediately before the next infusion of AT-III.

Patient Education: Inform of risks of thrombosis in connection with pregnancy and surgery and the fact that AT-III deficiency is hereditary.

Maternal/Child: Neonatal AT-III levels should be measured immediately after birth if parents are known to have AT-III deficiency (fatal neonatal thromboembolism [e.g., aortic thrombi] has occurred). Treatment of the neonate should be under the direction of a physician knowledgeable about coagulation disorders. Normal full-term and premature infants have lower than adult averages of AT-III plasma levels. ▪ Category B: use only if clearly indicated. Fetal abnormalities not noted when administered in the third trimester. ▪ Safety for use in pediatric patients not established.

DRUG/LAB INTERACTIONS

Half-life of AT-III decreases with concurrent **heparin** treatment. The anticoagulant effect of heparin is enhanced and a reduced dose of heparin is indicated to avoid bleeding.

SIDE EFFECTS

Bowel fullness, chest pain, chest tightness, chills, cramps, dizziness, fever, film over eye, foul taste in mouth, hives, light-headedness, oozing and hematoma formation, and shortness of breath have occurred with Thrombate III. Some patients with acquired AT-III deficiency diagnosed with disseminated intravascular coagulation (DIC) have had diuretic and vasodilatory effects. Rapid infusion may cause dyspnea.

ANTIDOTE

Levels of 150% to 210% found in a few patients have not caused any apparent complications. Observe for bleeding. Reduce rate of infusion immediately for dyspnea. Decrease rate or interrupt infusion as indicated until side effects subside. Keep physician informed of patient's lab values and condition.

ANTITHROMBIN RECOMBINANT
(an-tie-**THROM**-bin re-**KOM**-be-nant)

Atryn

**Anticoagulant
Antithrombotic**

pH 7

USUAL DOSE

(International Units [IU])

Dose must be individualized for each patient and is based on the pretreatment level of functional antithrombin (AT) (expressed in percent of normal) and on body weight in kilograms according to the following chart. Treatment goal is to restore and maintain functional AT activity levels between 80% and 120% (0.8 to 1.2 IU/mL) of normal. Treatment should be initiated before delivery or approximately 24 hours before surgery to ensure AT level is in the target range. Different dosing formulas are used for the treatment of surgical and pregnant patients. Pregnant women being treated with antithrombin recombinant for any peripartum or perioperative event, including a cesarean section, should be treated according to the dosing formula for pregnant women.

Antithrombin Recombinant Dosing Formula for Surgical Patients and Pregnant Women	
Loading Dose (IU)	Maintenance Dose (IU/hr)
Surgical Patients	
$\dfrac{(100\text{-Baseline AT activity level})}{2.3} \times$ Body weight (kg)	$\dfrac{(100\text{-Baseline AT activity level})}{10.2} \times$ Body weight (kg)
Pregnant Women	
$\dfrac{(100\text{-Baseline AT activity level})}{1.3} \times$ Body weight (kg)	$\dfrac{(100\text{-Baseline AT activity level})}{5.4} \times$ Body weight (kg)

Check AT level just after surgery or delivery; AT activity may be rapidly decreased by surgery or delivery. If AT activity level is below 80%, administer an additional bolus dose to rapidly restore decreased AT activity level. Then restart the maintenance dose at the same rate of infusion as before the bolus. Monitor AT activity at least once or twice daily and adjust doses according to the table in Dose Adjustments. Continue treatment until adequate follow-up anticoagulation is established.

DOSE ADJUSTMENTS

Antithrombin Recombinant AT Activity Monitoring and Dose Adjustment			
Initial Monitor Time	AT Level	Dose Adjustment	Recheck AT Level
2 hr after initiation of treatment	<80%	Increase by 30%	2 hr after each dose adjustment
	80% to 100%	None	6 hr after initiation of treatment or dose adjustment
	>120%	Decrease by 30%	2 hr after each dose adjustment

DILUTION
(International Units [IU])

Bring vials to RT no more than 3 hours before reconstitution. Each vial contains approximately 1,750 IU; exact potency is stated on the carton and label. Immediately before use, each vial **must** be reconstituted with 10 mL SW. **Do not shake.** Draw the reconstituted solution from one or more vials into a sterile syringe. May administer reconstituted solution directly or may further dilute in an infusion bag containing NS (e.g., dilute to obtain a final concentration of 100 IU/mL). Administer using an infusion set with a 0.22-micron in-line filter.

Filters: Use of a 0.22-micron in-line filter required during infusion.

Storage: Before use, refrigerate vials between 2° and 8° C (36° and 46° F). Use reconstituted or diluted solution within 8 to 12 hours of preparation. Do not use beyond expiration date on vial. Discard unused product.

COMPATIBILITY
Specific information not available. Because of specific use and unique formulation, consider administering through a separate line without mixing with other IV fluids or medications.

RATE OF ADMINISTRATION
Loading dose: Administer as an infusion over 15 minutes. Follow immediately with the **maintenance dose** as a continuous infusion at the calculated IU/hr rate.

ACTIONS
(International Units [IU])

A recombinant human antithrombin produced by DNA technology. A DNA coding sequence for human antithrombin and a mammary gland–specific DNA sequence are introduced into genetically engineered goats. The goats' milk contains the antithrombin. The amino acid sequence of antithrombin recombinant is identical to that of human plasma-derived antithrombin. Purified through numerous processes to eliminate potential viruses. AT is the principal inhibitor of thrombin and Factor Xa. AT neutralizes the activity of thrombin and Factor Xa by forming a complex that is rapidly removed from the circulation. When AT is bound to heparin, the ability of antithrombin to inhibit thrombin and Factor Xa can be enhanced by greater than 300- to 1,000-fold. Half-life range based on IU/kg is 11.6 to 17.7 hours. This recombinant formulation has a shorter half-life and more rapid clearance compared with plasma-derived antithrombin (e.g., Thrombate III). Secreted in breast milk.

INDICATIONS AND USES
Prevention of perioperative and peripartum thromboembolic events in patients with hereditary antithrombin deficiency. ■ **Not indicated for treatment** of thromboembolic events in patients with hereditary antithrombin deficiency.

CONTRAINDICATIONS
Known hypersensitivity to goat and goat milk proteins.

PRECAUTIONS
For IV use only. ■ Confirm diagnosis of hereditary antithrombin deficiency. ■ Hypersensitivity reactions may occur at any time during the infusion, thus requiring discontinuation of the infusion. ■ The anticoagulant effect of drugs that use antithrombin to exert their anticoagulation (e.g., heparin, low-molecular-weight heparins such as enoxaparin [Lovenox]) may be altered when antithrombin recombinant is added or withdrawn. Avoid excessive or insufficient anticoagulation by monitoring coagulation tests suitable for the anticoagulant used (e.g., aPTT and

anti-Factor Xa activity). To avoid bleeding or thrombosis, perform these tests regularly and at close intervals, especially during the first hours after the start or withdrawal of antithrombin recombinant. ▪ See Drug/Lab Interactions.

Monitor: Specific coagulation tests are required before administration and throughout the infusion process; see Usual Dose and Precautions. ▪ Monitor throughout the infusion for S/S of a hypersensitivity reaction (e.g., hives, hypotension, generalized urticaria, tightness of the chest, wheezing, and/or anaphylaxis). ▪ Monitor for S/S of bleeding or thrombosis.

Patient Education: Inform physician of a past or present allergy to goats or goat milk. ▪ Promptly report S/S of a hypersensitivity reaction (e.g., rash, shortness of breath, wheezing). ▪ Risk of bleeding increased when used with other anticoagulants. Report bleeding from any source.

Maternal/Child: Category C: use during pregnancy only if clearly needed. Studies have not shown that antithrombin recombinant increases the risk of fetal abnormalities if administered during the third trimester of pregnancy. Adverse reactions have not been reported in neonates born to women treated with antithrombin recombinant during clinical trials. ▪ Indicated for use in women with hereditary antithrombin deficiency during labor and delivery. ▪ Levels that appear in breast milk are estimated to be the same as in normal lactating women; however, use only if clearly needed and with caution during breast-feeding. ▪ Safety and effectiveness for use in pediatric patients not established.

Elderly: Numbers in clinical studies insufficient to determine if elderly patients respond differently than younger subjects. Dosing should be cautious in the elderly. Reduced doses may be indicated based on the potential for decreased organ function and concomitant disease or drug therapy.

DRUG/LAB INTERACTIONS

The anticoagulant effect of **heparin and low-molecular-weight heparin** is enhanced by antithrombin. Concurrent use with these anticoagulants may alter the half-life of antithrombin. Concurrent use with **heparin, low-molecular-weight heparins** such as enoxaparin (Lovenox), **or other anticoagulants** that use antithrombin to exert their anticoagulant effect must be monitored clinically and biologically. To avoid excessive anticoagulation, perform regular coagulation tests (aPTT and, where appropriate, anti-Factor Xa activity) at close intervals and adjust the dose of anticoagulant as indicated.

SIDE EFFECTS

Hemorrhage and infusion site reactions were most commonly reported. Hemorrhage may be serious (intra-abdominal, hemarthrosis, and postprocedural). Less common side effects include feeling hot, hematoma, hematuria, hepatic enzyme abnormalities, hypersensitivity reactions (including anaphylaxis), and non-cardiac chest pain.

ANTIDOTE

Keep physician informed of patient's lab values and condition. Discontinue the infusion if a hypersensitivity reaction occurs. ▪ Treat anaphylaxis immediately with oxygen, epinephrine (Adrenalin), antihistamines (e.g., diphenhydramine [Benadryl]), vasopressors (e.g., dopamine), corticosteroids, albuterol (Ventolin), IV fluids, and ventilation equipment as indicated. Resuscitate as necessary.

ANTI-THYMOCYTE GLOBULIN (RABBIT) BBW
(an-tie-**THI**-mo-cite **GLOB**-you-lin)

Thymoglobulin

Immunosuppressant

pH 7 to 7.4

USUAL DOSE

Premedication: To reduce the incidence and intensity of side effects during the infusion of anti-thymocyte globulin; premedication 1 hour before the infusion with corticosteroids (e.g., dexamethasone [Decadron]), acetaminophen (e.g., Tylenol), and/or an antihistamine (e.g., diphenhydramine [Benadryl]) is recommended.

Anti-thymocyte globulin: 1.5 mg/kg of body weight daily for 7 to 14 days. Given as an infusion into a high flow vein. Used in conjunction with maintenance immunosuppression (e.g., tacrolimus [Prograf], mycophenolate [Cell-Cept]); see Drug/Lab Interactions.

DOSE ADJUSTMENTS

Reduce dose by one-half if WBC count is between 2,000 and 3,000 cells/mm^3 or if platelet count is between 50,000 and 75,000 cells/mm^3. ▪ Consider withholding dose or stopping anti-thymocyte therapy if WBC count falls below 2,000 cells/mm^3 or platelets fall below 50,000 cells/mm^3.

DILUTION

Calculate the number of vials required (25 mg/vial), 5 mL of SW as diluent per vial is supplied. Drug and diluent must be warmed to room temperature before dilution. Absolute sterile technique required throughout dilution process. For each vial required use a new syringe and needle. Withdraw 5 mL of diluent and inject into lyophilized powder. Rotate vial gently until powder is completely dissolved. Do not shake. Each reconstituted vial contains 25 mg (5 mg/mL). Must be further diluted by transferring into 50 mL of infusion solution (saline or dextrose) for each 25 mg of anti-thymocyte globulin. Total volume is usually between 50 to 500 mL. Invert the infusion bag gently once or twice to mix the solution.

Filters: Use of a 0.22-micron in-line filter recommended.

Storage: Refrigerate and protect from light until removed to prepare for reconstitution. Do not freeze. Do not use after expiration date on vial. Use reconstituted vials within 4 hours. Use infusion solutions immediately. Discard unused drug.

COMPATIBILITY   (Underline Indicates Conflicting Compatibility Information)

Consider any drug NOT listed as compatible to be INCOMPATIBLE until consulting a pharmacist; specific conditions may apply.

Administration through a separate line without mixing with other IV fluids or medications is suggested because of specific use and potential for anaphylaxis.

One source suggests the following **compatibilities:**

Y-site: <u>Heparin</u>, hydrocortisone sodium succinate (Solu-Cortef).

RATE OF ADMINISTRATION

Use of a high-flow vein and a 0.22-micron filter recommended. Well-tolerated and less likely to produce side effects (e.g., chills and fever) when administered at the recommended rate and the patient is premedicated.

Initial dose: A total daily dose equally distributed over a minimum of 6 hours.

Subsequent doses: A total daily dose equally distributed over a minimum of 4 hours.

ACTIONS

A purified, pasteurized, gamma immune globulin, obtained by immunization of rabbits with human thymocytes. Mechanism of action not fully understood. May induce immunosuppression by T-cell depletion and immune modulation. Made up of a variety of antibodies that recognize key receptors on T-cells (those cells responsible for attacking and rejecting a foreign substance within the body). Anti-thymocyte globulin antibodies can inactivate and kill these T-cells, thus reversing the rejection process. May prevent organ loss and reduce the need for retransplantation. T-cell depletion is usually observed within a day of initiating thymoglobulin therapy. Half-life averages 2 to 3 days but the drug remains active, targeting the offending immune cells for days to weeks after treatment.

INDICATIONS AND USES

Treatment of kidney transplant acute rejection in conjunction with concomitant immunosuppression.

Unlabeled uses: Compassionate use in the treatment of acute rejection in bone marrow, heart, and liver transplants. Orphan drug status for the treatment of myelodysplastic syndrome (MDS).

CONTRAINDICATIONS

Patients with a known allergy to rabbit proteins, an acute viral illness, or a history of anaphylaxis during rabbit immunoglobulin administration.

PRECAUTIONS

Administered only under the direction of a physician experienced in immunosuppressive therapy and management of renal transplant patients in a facility with adequate laboratory and supportive medical resources. ■ Not considered effective for treating antibody-mediated (humoral) rejections. ■ Prolonged use or overdose in combination with other immunosuppressive agents may cause over-immunosuppression resulting in severe infections and may increase the incidence of lymphoma or post-transplant lymphoproliferative disease (PTLD) or other malignancies. Use of appropriate antiviral, antibacterial, antiprotozoal, and/or antifungal prophylaxis is recommended. In clinical trials, viral prophylaxis with ganciclovir infusion was used. ■ In clinical trials, anti-rabbit antibodies developed in 68% of patients. Controlled studies on repeat use of anti-thymocyte globulin in patients with anti-rabbit antibodies have not been conducted. Use caution if repeat courses are indicated, monitoring of lymphocyte count is recommended to ensure that T-cell depletion is achieved. ■ If anaphylaxis occurs during or after therapy, further administration of anti-thymocyte globulin is contraindicated.

Monitor: Close clinical observation is imperative. Monitor for side effects during and after infusion. Anaphylaxis has occurred; emergency equipment, medications, and supplies must be available. ■ Obtain baseline and monitor WBC and platelet counts during therapy. Thrombocytopenia or neutropenia may occur and are reversible following dose adjustment; see Dose Adjustments. ■ Monitoring of the lymphocyte count (i.e., total lymphocyte count and T-cell counts [absolute and/or subset]) may help assess the degree of T-cell depletion. ▪ Monitor carefully for signs of infection. ▪ Prophylactic antibiotics may be indicated pending results of C/S in a febrile neutropenic patient. ▪ See Precautions and Drug/Lab Interactions. **Patient Education:** Imperative that all medications (especially immunosuppressants) be reviewed with physician. ▪ Report any previous hypersensitivity/anaphylactic reaction. ▪ Report acute viral infections immediately. ▪ Promptly report chest pain, irregular or rapid heartbeat, shortness of breath, swelling of the face or throat, or wheezing during infusion of medication. ▪ See Appendix D, p. 1434. ▪ May be associated with an increased risk of malignancy.

Maternal/Child: Category C: safety for use during pregnancy and breastfeeding not established. Safety and effectiveness for use in pediatric patients not established. Use only if clearly needed. ▪ Has been used in pediatric patients in limited European studies and in the United States for compassionate use. Response similar to adults.

Elderly: Specific information not available.

DRUG/LAB INTERACTIONS

Concurrent use with **immunosuppressants** (e.g., azathioprine [Imuran], cyclosporine [Sandimmune], mycophenolate [Cell-Cept], tacrolimus [Prograf]) may potentiate the immunosuppressive action of these agents; many transplant centers decrease maintenance immunosuppression therapy during the period of antibody therapy. ▪ May **stimulate the production of antibodies,** which cross-react with rabbit immune globulins. ▪ May interfere with **rabbit antibody-base immunoassays** and with **cross-match or panel-reactive antibody cytotoxicity assays.**

SIDE EFFECTS

Are dose-limiting. Abdominal pain, asthenia, diarrhea, dizziness, dyspnea, fever, headache, hyperkalemia, hypertension, infection, infusion reaction (e.g., chills and fever), leukopenia, malaise, nausea, pain, peripheral edema, tachycardia, and thrombocytopenia were reported frequently. Anaphylaxis has been reported.

Overdose: Leukopenia or thrombocytopenia.

ANTIDOTE

Notify physician of all side effects. Most can be managed symptomatically. Manage leukopenia or thrombocytopenia during therapy or in overdose with dose reduction. Infusion reactions are managed with premedication and reduction in the rate of infusion. Treat infections aggressively; see Precautions. May require discontinuation of therapy. Discontinue infusion and/or therapy immediately if anaphylaxis occurs. Treat anaphylaxis immediately with epinephrine (Adrenalin), diphenhydramine (Benadryl), oxygen, vasopressors (e.g., dopamine), corticosteroids, IV fluids, and ventilation equipment as indicated. Resuscitate as necessary.

ANTIVENIN CROTALIDAE POLYVALENT IMMUNE FAB (OVINE)

Antivenin

(an-tee-**VEN**-in kro-**TAL**-ih-day pol-ih-**VAY**-lent im-**MYOUN** fab)

CroFab

USUAL DOSE

Contact Poison Control Center for individual treatment advice.

Premedication: Premedication may be indicated for patients with allergies. Obtain blood work before administration; see Contraindications, Precautions, and Monitor. Initiate as soon as possible after crotalid snakebite in patients who develop signs of progressive envenomation (e.g., worsening local injury, coagulation abnormality, or systemic signs of envenomation); see Monitor. Has been effective when given within 6 hours of snakebite. **Initial dose:** Skin testing for sensitivity to serum is not required. 4 to 6 vials is the recommended initial dose based on clinical experience. Adjust based on severity of envenomation when patient is initially assessed. Observe for up to 1 hour after initial dose administered. Desired outcome is complete control of the envenomation (i.e., complete arrest of local manifestations, and return of coagulation tests and systemic signs to normal).

Repeat doses: If control of symptoms is not accomplished by the initial dose, give an additional dose of 4 to 6 vials. This dose may be repeated until initial control of the envenomation syndrome has been achieved. After initial control has been established, give additional 2-vial doses every 6 hours for up to 18 hours (3 doses). Optimal dosing following the 18-hour scheduled dose has not been determined. Additional 2-vial doses may be given as directed by the treating physician, based on the patient's clinical response. Up to 18 vials have been given without any observed direct toxic effect. Scheduled dosing/rather than PRN dosing may provide better control of envenomation symptoms caused by the continued leaking of venom from depot sites.

PEDIATRIC DOSE

Absolute venom dose following snakebite is expected to be the same in pediatric patients and adults, no dose adjustment for age is required. See Maternal/Child.

DOSE ADJUSTMENTS

No dose adjustments recommended.

DILUTION

Reconstitute each vial with 10 mL SW. Mix by continuous gentle swirling. Further dilute the contents of the reconstituted vial(s) in 250 mL NS and mix by gently swirling.

Storage: Refrigerate unopened vials, do not freeze. Reconstituted vials and diluted solution must be used within 4 hours.

COMPATIBILITY

Specific information not available. Administration through a separate line without mixing with other IV fluids or medications is suggested because of specific use and potential for anaphylaxis.

RATE OF ADMINISTRATION

Infuse at a rate of 25 to 50 mL/hr over the first 10 minutes. Carefully observe for hypersensitivity reactions. If no adverse reaction occurs, increase rate to administer 250 mL equally distributed over 1 hour. Reduce rate of administration if infusion-related reactions occur (e.g., fever, low back pain, nausea, wheezing), and monitor closely.

ACTIONS

A venom-specific Fab fragment of immunoglobulin G (IgG) obtained from the blood of healthy sheep flocks immunized with one of four snake venoms; see Indications for specific venoms. To obtain the final product, the four different monospecific antivenins are mixed. Works by binding and neutralizing venom toxins, facilitating their redistribution away from target tissues and their elimination from the body. Half-life is estimated to be 12 to 23 hours.

INDICATIONS AND USES

Management of patients with minimal or moderate North American rattlesnake envenomation (*Crotalus atrox* [Western Diamondback rattlesnake], *Crotalus adamanteus* [Eastern Diamondback rattlesnake], *Crotalus scutulatus* [Mohave rattlesnake], and *Agkistrodon piscivorus* [Cottonmouth or Water Moccasin]). Early use (within 6 hours) is advised to prevent clinical deterioration and the occurrence of systemic coagulation abnormalities. ▪ No clinical data is available supporting effectiveness in patients presenting with severe envenomation.

Unlabeled uses: May possess antigenic cross-reactivity against the venoms of some Middle Eastern and North African snakes, no clinical data available.

CONTRAINDICATIONS

Known history of hypersensitivity to sheep, papaya, or papain unless benefits outweigh risks and appropriate management for anaphylactic reactions is readily available.

PRECAUTIONS

Usually administered in the hospital by or under the direction of the physician specialist with adequate diagnostic and treatment facilities readily available. ▪ Patients with allergies to dust mites, latex, papain, chymopapain, other papaya extracts, the pineapple enzyme bromelain, or sheep protein may be at risk for a hypersensitivity reaction to this antivenin; see Contraindications, use caution. ▪ Contains 0.11 mg of mercury per vial (ethyl mercury from thimerosal). Exposure from 18-vial dose is 1.9 mg of mercury. Definitive data not available, literature suggests that information related to methyl mercury toxicities may be applicable. ▪ Recurrent coagulation abnormalities (e.g., decreased fibrinogen, decreased platelets, and elevated PT) defined as the return of a coagulation abnormality after it has been successfully treated with antivenin, were observed in patients who experienced coagulation abnormalities during their initial hospitalization and occurred in approximately one-half of patients studied. Crotalidae immune fab has a shorter persistence in the blood than crotalid venoms that can leak from depot sites over a prolonged period of time; repeat dosing to prevent or treat such recurrence may be necessary. Optimal dosing to prevent recurrent coagulopathy has not been determined. ▪ Use caution if a repeat course of treatment is required for a subsequent envenomation episode, crotalidae immune fab is a foreign protein and antibodies may develop producing sensitivity.

Monitor: Before antivenin is administered, draw adequate blood for baseline studies (e.g., type and cross-match, CBC, hematocrit, platelet count, PT, clot retraction, bleeding and coagulation times, BUN, electrolytes, and bilirubin). ▪ Severity of envenomation is based on six body categories: cardiovascular, gastrointestinal, hematologic, local wound (e.g., pain, swelling, and ecchymosis), nervous system, and pulmonary effects. Specific parameters of minimal, moderate, and severe envenomation are outlined in the following chart.

	Definition of Minimal, Moderate, and Severe Envenomation Used in Clinical Studies of Crotalidae Polyvalent Immune Fab
Envenomation Category	Definition
Minimal	*Swelling, pain, and ecchymosis* limited to the immediate bite site. *Systemic signs and symptoms* absent. *Coagulation parameters* normal with no clinical evidence of bleeding.
Moderate	*Swelling, pain, and ecchymosis* involving less than a full extremity or, if bite was sustained on the trunk, head or neck, extending less than 50 cm. *Systemic signs and symptoms* may be present but not life-threatening, including but not limited to nausea, vomiting, oral paresthesia or unusual tastes, mild hypotension (systolic BP less than 90 mm Hg), mild tachycardia (HR less than 150), and tachypnea. *Coagulation parameters* may be abnormal, but no clinical evidence of bleeding present. Minor hematuria, gum bleeding, and nose-bleeds are allowed if they are not considered severe in the investigator's judgment.
Severe	*Swelling, pain, and ecchymosis* involving more than an entire extremity or threatening the airway. *Systemic signs and symptoms* are markedly abnormal, including severe alteration of mental status, severe hypotension, severe tachycardia, tachypnea, or respiratory insufficiency. *Coagulation parameters* are abnormal, with serious bleeding or severe threat of bleeding.

▪ Anaphylactic and anaphylactoid reactions, delayed hypersensitivity reactions (late serum reaction or serum sickness), and a possible febrile response to immune complexes formed by animal antibodies and neutralized venom components may occur. Observe all patients continuously for signs and symptoms of an acute hypersensitivity reaction (e.g., angioedema, bronchospasm with wheezing or cough, erythema, hypotension, pruritus, stridor, tachycardia, urticaria). ▪ Monitor all vital signs at frequent intervals. Observe for signs of shock; treat with IV fluids, blood products, plasma expanders, vasopressors (e.g., dopamine) as indicated. ▪ Keep emergency equipment available at all times, including oxygen, epinephrine, antihistamines (e.g., IV diphenhydramine [Benadryl]), corticosteroids, albuterol, vasopressors (e.g., dopamine), and ventilation equipment. ▪ Initiate two IV lines as soon as possible; one to be used for supportive therapy, the other for antivenin and electrolytes. ▪ A decrease in platelets not responsive to whole blood transfusion can occur with rattlesnake bites, platelet count should approach normal limits within 1 hour of administering crotalidae immune fab. ▪ Follow-up monitoring is required for S/S of delayed hypersensitivity reactions or serum sickness (e.g., arthralgia, fever, myalgia, rash). ▪ Test urine specimens for microscopic erythrocytes. ▪ If coagulation abnormalities occur, consider other disease processes associated with coagulation disorders (e.g., cancer, collagen disease, CHF, diarrhea, elevated temperature, hepatic disorder, hyperthyroidism, poor nutritional state, steatorrhea, vitamin K deficiency). ▪ Monitor patients who experience coagulopathy due to snakebite during hospitalization for initial treatment for several weeks after discharge. Recurrent coagulopathy may persist for 2 weeks or more. Assess the need for retreatment and/or use of anticoagulant or antiplatelet agents. ▪ Supportive measures to treat other manifestations of the snakebite (e.g., hypotension, pain, swelling, wound infection) should be implemented. **Patient Education:** Immediately report any S/S of delayed hypersensitivity reactions or serum sickness (e.g., pruritus, rash, or urticaria occurring after discharge). ▪ Promptly report unusual bruising or bleeding (e.g., nosebleeds, excessive bleeding after toothbrushing or superficial injuries, blood in stools or urine, excessive menstrual bleeding, petechiae). May occur for up to 1 week or longer and indicate need for additional treatment. **Maternal/Child:** Category C: use during pregnancy only if clearly needed. ▪ Use caution, safety for use during breast-feeding not established. ▪ Exposure to mercury has been associated with neurological and renal toxicities. Developing fetuses and very young children are most susceptible and are at greater risk.

Elderly: No specific studies on elderly patients.

DRUG/LAB INTERACTIONS

Studies have not been conducted.

SIDE EFFECTS

Pruritus, rash, and urticaria are frequent side effects. Anorexia, back pain, cellulitis, chest pain, chills, circumoral paresthesia, cough, delayed hypersensitivity reactions (late serum reaction or serum sickness), ecchymosis, febrile response to immune complexes formed by animal antibodies and neutralized venom components, general paresthesia, hypersensitivity reactions including anaphylaxis, hypotension, increased sputum, myalgia, nausea, nervousness, recurrent coagulopathy, and wound infection have occurred.

ANTIDOTE

Keep physician informed of all side effects and extent or progression of envenomation. Reduce the rate of administration if infusion-related reactions occur (e.g., fever, low back pain, nausea, wheezing). Monitor closely and discontinue antivenin if symptoms worsen or a hypersensitivity reaction occurs. Treat hypersensitivity reactions and/or anaphylaxis immediately with oxygen, epinephrine, antihistamines (e.g., IV diphenhydramine [Benadryl]), corticosteroids, albuterol, vasopressors (e.g., dopamine), and ventilation equipment as indicated. Recurrent coagulopathy may require re-hospitalization and additional antivenin administration. Resuscitate as necessary.

ANTIVENIN *(LATRODECTUS MACTANS)* Antivenin
(an-tee-**VEN**-in **lat**-roh-**DEK**-tus **MACK**-tans)
Black Widow Spider Species Antivenin

USUAL DOSE

Testing for sensitivity to horse serum required before use. See Precautions for additional pretreatment requirements.

Entire contents of 1 vial of antivenin (2.5 mL) is recommended for adults and pediatric patients. One vial is usually enough, but a second dose may be necessary in rare instances. Best results obtained if administered within 4 hours of envenomation.

PEDIATRIC DOSE

Same as adult dose. See Maternal/Child.

DILUTION

Each single dose (6,000 antivenin units) must be initially diluted with 2.5 mL SW for injection (supplied). Keep needle in rubber stopper of antivenin and shake vial to dissolve contents completely. Must be further diluted in 10 to 50 mL NS for IV injection.

Storage: Refrigerate unopened vials; do not freeze. Refrigerate reconstituted and/or diluted solution; discard in 6 hours.

COMPATIBILITY

Specific information not available. Administration through a separate line without mixing with other IV fluids or medications is suggested because of specific use and potential for anaphylaxis.

RATE OF ADMINISTRATION

A single dose over a minimum of 15 minutes.

ACTIONS

Prepared from the blood serum of horses immunized against the venom of the black widow spider. One unit will neutralize one average mouse-lethal dose of black widow spider venom when both are injected simultaneously under lab conditions.

INDICATIONS AND USES

Treatment of patients with symptoms resulting from bites of black widow spiders *(Latrodectus mactans)* and similar spiders.

CONTRAINDICATIONS

Hypersensitivity to horse serum unless only treatment available for a life-threatening situation. Several techniques including preload of antihistamine and/or desensitization may be considered (see literature).

PRECAUTIONS

Read drug literature supplied with antivenin completely before use. Essential to evaluate symptoms and individual status of each patient. ■ Determine patient response to any previous injections of serum of any type and history of any hypersensitivity reactions. ■ Hospitalize patient if possible. ■ Muscle relaxants may be the initial treatment of choice in healthy individuals between 16 and 60. Antivenin use may be deferred while patient is observed. ■ Test every patient without exception for sensitivity to horse serum (1-mL vial of 1:10 dilution horse serum supplied). Conjunctival test and skin test recommended for maximum safety. Usually begin with the conjunctival test.

Conjunctival test: Instill 1 drop 1:10 horse serum into conjunctival sac for adults (1 drop 1:100 dilution for pediatric patients). Itching, redness, burning, and/or lacrimation within 10 minutes is a positive reaction. A drop of NS in the opposite eye is used as a control and should be asymptomatic. Reverse adverse effects of positive reaction with 1 drop epinephrine ophthalmic solution.

Skin test: Inject no more than 0.02 mL of 1:10 horse serum intradermally. In patients with a history of allergies use a 1:100 solution. A similar injection of NS can be used as a control. Compare in 10 minutes. An urticarial wheal surrounded by a zone of erythema is a positive reaction. ▪ A systemic reaction may occur even when both sensitivity tests are negative. ▪ May be given IM. IV preferred in severe cases, if patient is in shock, or in pediatric patients under 12 years of age.

Monitor: Supportive therapy is indicated. 10 mL of 10% calcium gluconate IV may control muscle pain. Morphine may be needed. Barbiturates or diazepam may be used for restlessness. Prolonged warm baths are helpful; corticosteroids have been used. ▪ Observe patient constantly for respiratory paralysis. Can occur from toxin alone, and narcotics and sedatives may precipitate respiratory depression. ▪ Observe for serum sickness for 8 to 12 days.

Patient Education: Contact physician immediately for any S/S of a delayed hypersensitivity reaction (e.g., rash, pruritus, urticaria) after hospital discharge.

Maternal/Child: Category C: use only if clearly needed. ▪ Safety for use in breast-feeding not established. ▪ Safety for use in pediatric patients not established, but there have been no adverse effects when used.

DRUG/LAB INTERACTIONS

Concomitant use of **antihistamines** may interfere with sensitivity tests. **Narcotics** and **sedatives** may precipitate respiratory depression.

SIDE EFFECTS

Acute anaphylaxis with urticaria, respiratory distress, and vascular collapse. Serum sickness may occur. Usually appears in 7 to 12 days. Local pain, local erythema, and urticaria without systemic reaction can occur.

ANTIDOTE

Discontinue the drug and notify the physician of all side effects. Treat anaphylaxis immediately. Epinephrine (Adrenalin), diphenhydramine (Benadryl), oxygen, vasopressors (dopamine), corticosteroids, H_2 antagonists (e.g., ranitidine [Zantac]), and ventilation equipment must always be available. Resuscitate as necessary.

ARGATROBAN
(ahr-**GAT**-troe-ban)

Anticoagulant
pH 3.2 to 7.5

USUAL DOSE

Discontinue all parenteral anticoagulants (e.g., heparin) and obtain baseline blood tests including an aPTT (prophylaxis or treatment) and ACT (PCI) before administration of argatroban; see Monitor.

Prophylaxis or treatment of thrombosis in patients with or at risk for heparin-induced thrombocytopenia (HIT/HITTS): Begin *argatroban* with an initial dose of 2 mcg/kg/min as a continuous infusion. Steady-state levels usually obtained within 1 to 3 hours. Check the aPTT in 2 hours. Adjust the mcg/kg/min dose (not to exceed 10 mcg/kg/min) as clinically indicated until the steady-state aPTT is 1.5 to 3 times the initial baseline value (not to exceed 100 seconds).

Anticoagulant in patients with or at risk for HIT/HITTS undergoing percutaneous coronary interventions (PCI): *Aspirin* 325 mg 2 to 24 hours before planned PCI was administered in studies. After venous or arterial sheaths are in place, begin *argatroban* with an initial infusion of 25 mcg/kg/min via a large-bore IV line. Next, administer a bolus of 350 mcg/kg over 3 to 5 minutes. 5 to 10 minutes after completion of bolus dose, check the ACT. The PCI may proceed if the ACT is greater than 300 seconds but less than 450 seconds. If ACT is less than 300 seconds, give an additional IV bolus of 150 mcg/kg, increase the infusion rate to 30 mcg/kg/min, and check the ACT in 5 to 10 minutes. If ACT is greater than 450 seconds, decrease the infusion rate to 15 mcg/kg/min and recheck the ACT in 5 to 10 minutes. When a therapeutic ACT has been achieved (between 300 and 450 seconds), the infusion dose in effect at the time the therapeutic ACT is achieved should be continued for the duration of the procedure. For situations outside these parameters, see Dose Adjustment. If anticoagulation is required after PCI, continue argatroban, but lower infusion rate to between 2.5 and 5 mcg/kg/min. Draw an aPTT in 2 hours and adjust the infusion rate as clinically indicated (not to exceed 10 mcg/kg/min) to reach an aPTT between 1.5 and 3 times baseline value (not to exceed 100 seconds); see All Situations in Monitor if transfer to oral anticoagulation is indicated.

DOSE ADJUSTMENTS

All situations: No dose adjustment indicated in patients with impaired renal function, or based on age or gender.

Prophylaxis or treatment of thrombosis in patients with or at risk for heparin-induced thrombocytopenia (HIT/HITTS): Reduce initial dose to 0.5 mcg/kg/min in patients with moderate hepatic impairment. There is a four-fold decrease in argatroban clearance in these patients, titrate dose carefully and monitor aPTT closely.

Anticoagulant in patients with or at risk for HIT/HITTS undergoing percutaneous coronary interventions (PCI): In case of dissection, impending abrupt closure, thrombus formation during the procedure, or inability to achieve or maintain an ACT over 300 seconds, additional bolus doses of 150 mcg/kg may be given and the infusion rate increased to 40 mcg/kg/min. Check the ACT after each additional bolus or change in rate of infusion. ▪ See Precautions for patients with clinically significant liver disease.

DILUTION

Each 250-mg vial must be diluted in 250 mL of NS, D5W, or LR to a concentration of 1 mg/mL. Mix by repeated inversion of the diluent bag for a minimum of 1 minute. Solution may initially be briefly hazy. Do not expose prepared solutions to direct sunlight.

Storage: Store vials in carton at CRT, protected from light and freezing. Diluted solution stable in ambient indoor light for 24 hours at 25° C (77° F), with excursions to 15° to 30° C (59° to 86° F) permitted. Light-resistant measures such as foil protection for IV lines are not necessary. Stable for up to 96 hours protected from light and stored at CRT or refrigerated.

COMPATIBILITY

Consider any drug NOT listed as compatible to be INCOMPATIBLE until consulting a pharmacist; specific conditions may apply.

Manufacturer states, "Should not be mixed with other drugs prior to dilution in a suitable IV fluid." Consider specific use and dose adjustment requirements.

One source suggests the following **compatibilities:**

Y-site: Abciximab (ReoPro), atropine, diltiazem (Cardizem), diphenhydramine (Benadryl), dobutamine, dopamine, eptifibatide (Integrilin), fenoldopam (Corlopam), fentanyl (Sublimaze), furosemide (Lasix), hydrocortisone sodium succinate (Solu-Cortef), lidocaine, metoprolol (Lopressor), midazolam (Versed), milrinone (Primacor), morphine, nesiritide (Natrecor), nitroglycerin IV, nitroprusside sodium, norepinephrine (Levophed), phenylephrine (Neo-Synephrine), tirofiban (Aggrastat), vasopressin, verapamil.

RATE OF ADMINISTRATION

Prophylaxis or treatment of thrombosis in patients with or at risk for heparin-induced thrombocytopenia (HIT/HITTS):

Argatroban Infusion Rates for 2 mcg/kg/min Dose (1 mg/mL Final Concentration)	
Body Weight (kg)	Infusion Rate (mL/hr)
50 kg	6 mL/hr
60 kg	7 mL/hr
70 kg	8 mL/hr
80 kg	10 mL/hr
90 kg	11 mL/hr
100 kg	12 mL/hr
110 kg	13 mL/hr
120 kg	14 mL/hr
130 kg	16 mL/hr
140 kg	17 mL/hr

Anticoagulant in patients with or at risk for HIT/HITTS undergoing percutaneous coronary interventions (PCI): See Usual Dose and/or Dose Adjustments for specific rates and criteria.

ACTIONS

An anticoagulant that is a highly selective synthetic direct thrombin inhibitor derived from L-arginine. It reversibly binds to the thrombin active site and exerts its anticoagulant effects by inhibiting thrombin-catalyzed or induced reactions, including fibrin formation; activation of coagulation factors V, VIII, and XIII and protein C; and platelet aggregation. Highly selective for thrombin with little or no effect on related serine proteases (trypsin, factor Xa, plasmin, and kallikrein). Inhibits both free and clot-bound thrombin. Does not require the co-factor antithrombin III for antithrombic activity, and does not interact with heparin-induced antibodies. Produces a dose-dependent increase in aPTT, ACT, INR, PT, and TT. Anticoagulant effects are immediate. Steady-state levels of both drug and anticoagulant effect are usually attained within 1 to 3 hours and are maintained until the infusion is discontinued or the dose adjusted. Distribution is primarily in the extracellular fluid. Metabolized in the liver. Half-life range is 39 to 51 minutes. Excreted primarily in feces with some excretion in urine.

INDICATIONS AND USES

An anticoagulant for prophylaxis or treatment of thrombosis in patients with heparin-induced thrombocytopenia (HIT). ▪ An anticoagulant in patients with or at risk for heparin-induced thrombocytopenia undergoing percutaneous coronary intervention (PCI). May be used in combination with aspirin.

Unlabeled uses: An alternative to heparin during hemodialysis.

CONTRAINDICATIONS

Hypersensitivity to argatroban or any of its components and patients with overt major bleeding.

PRECAUTIONS

All situations: Use with extreme caution in disease states and other circumstances in which there is an increased danger of hemorrhage, including severe hypertension; immediately following lumbar puncture; spinal anesthesia; major surgery, especially involving the brain, spinal cord, or eye; hematologic conditions associated with increased bleeding tendencies such as congenital or acquired bleeding disorders and gastrointestinal lesions such as ulcerations. ▪ Concomitant therapy with thrombolytic agents (e.g., alteplase [tPA], reteplase [Retavase], streptokinase) may increase the risk of bleeding, including life-threatening intracranial bleeding; see Drug/Lab Interactions. ▪ Safety and effectiveness of argatroban for cardiac indications other than PCI in patients with HIT not established.

Prophylaxis or treatment of thrombosis: Use caution in patients with hepatic disease, argatroban clearance is decreased four-fold and elimination half-life is increased. Full reversal of anticoagulant effect may require longer than 4 hours. See Dose Adjustments.

PCI: Avoid use of high dose of argatroban in PCI patients with clinically significant hepatic disease or AST/ALT levels greater than 3 times the upper limit of normal. These patients were not included in clinical trials.

Monitor: *All situations:* Obtain baseline and monitor platelet count, hemoglobin, hematocrit, and occult blood in stool in addition to required aPTT or ACT; see Usual Dose and specific parameters as follows. ▪ Other coagulation tests (e.g., PT, INR, and TT) are affected by argatroban but therapeutic ranges for these tests have not been identified. ▪ Observe carefully for symptoms of a hemorrhagic event (e.g., unexplained fall in hematocrit, fall in BP, or any other unexplained symptom). ■ Recovery of platelet count usually occurs by day 3. ■ HIT is a serious, immune-mediated complication of heparin therapy that may result in subsequent venous and arterial thrombosis. Initial treatment of HIT is to discontinue all heparin, but patients still require anticoagulation for prevention and treatment of thromboembolic events. ■ Initiate oral anticoagulation with warfarin (Coumadin) when appropriate. Do not use a loading dose of warfarin, use the expected daily dose. Monitor INR daily. Concurrent use with warfarin results in prolongation of the PT and INR beyond that produced by warfarin alone. With doses of argatroban up to 2 mcg/kg/min, argatroban can be discontinued when the INR is greater than 4 on combined therapy. After argatroban is discontinued, repeat the INR in 4 to 6 hours. If the INR is below the desired therapeutic range, resume the infusion of argatroban and repeat the procedure daily until the desired therapeutic range on warfarin alone is reached. See Drug/Lab Interactions. With doses of argatroban more than 2 mcg/kg/min the INR relationship is less predictable. Reduction of dose to 2 mcg/kg/min is recommended. **Prophylaxis or treatment of thrombosis:** Obtain a baseline aPTT before treatment begins. Repeat aPTT in 2 hours, after any dose adjustment, and as indicated to achieve desired target aPTT of 1.5 to 3 times baseline. ■ No enhancement of aPTT response was observed in subjects receiving repeated administration of argatroban. Repeated administration has been tolerated with no loss of anticoagulant activity and no evidence of neutralizing antibodies. No change in dose is required.

PCI: Obtain baseline ACT before dosing; repeat ACT 5 to 10 minutes after bolus dosing, after a change in infusion rate, and at the end of the PCI procedure. Draw additional ACTs every 20 to 30 minutes during a prolonged procedure. ■ Follow standard procedures for maintenance and care of venous or arterial sheaths. Remove sheaths no sooner than 2 hours after discontinuing argatroban and when ACT has decreased to less than 160 seconds. ■ See Dose Adjustments if anticoagulation is required after PCI.

Patient Education: Report all episodes of bleeding. ■ Report tarry stools. ■ Compliance with all measures to minimize bleeding is very important (e.g., avoid use of razors, toothbrushes, other sharp items). ■ Use caution while moving to avoid excess bumping.

Maternal/Child: Category B: use during pregnancy only if clearly needed. ■ Discontinue breast-feeding. ■ Safety and effectiveness for use in pediatric patients under 18 years of age not established. ■ Has been used in a small number of pediatric patients with HIT or HITTS who require an alternative to heparin therapy. See package insert for dosing recommendations and monitoring parameters. Clearance is decreased in seriously ill pediatric patients.

Elderly: Response similar to that in younger patients. See Dose Adjustments for the elderly with impaired liver function.

DRUG/LAB INTERACTIONS

If argatroban is to be initiated after cessation of **heparin** therapy, allow sufficient time for heparin's effect on the aPTT to decrease. ■ Drug interactions have not been demonstrated between argatroban and concomitantly administered **aspirin or acetaminophen.** ■ Risk of bleeding may be increased by any medicine that affects blood clotting, including **anticoagulants** (e.g., heparin, lepirudin [Refludan], warfarin [Coumadin]); **any medication that may cause hypoprothrombinemia, thrombocytopenia, or GI ulcera-**

tion or bleeding (e.g., selected antibiotics [e.g., cefotetan], aspirin, NSAIDs [e.g., ibuprofen (Advil, Motrin), naproxen (Aleve, Naprosyn)]); **and/or any other medication that inhibits platelet aggregation** (e.g., clopidogrel [Plavix], dipyridamole [Persantine], glycoprotein GPIIb/IIIa receptor antagonists [e.g., abciximab (ReoPro), eptifibatide (Integrilin), tirofiban (Aggrastat)], plicamycin [Mithracin], sulfinpyrazone [Anturane], ticlopidine [Ticlid], valproic acid [Depacon]). If concurrent or subsequent use is indicated, monitor aPTT and PT closely. ▪ In clinical testing, was not found to interact with **digoxin or erythromycin** (a potent inhibitor of CYP3A4/5). ▪ Concurrent use with **warfarin** results in prolongation of the PT and INR beyond that produced by warfarin alone; see Monitor. The combination causes no further reduction in vitamin K dependent factor Xa than that seen with warfarin alone. Relationship between INR obtained on combined therapy and INR obtained on warfarin alone is dependent on both the dose of argatroban and the thromboplastin reagent used.

SIDE EFFECTS

All situations: Bleeding is the most frequent adverse event. Hypersensitivity reactions (e.g., coughing, dyspnea, hypotension, rash) have been reported, most frequently in patients who also received streptokinase or contrast media.

Prophylaxis or treatment of thrombosis: During clinical trials, intracranial bleeding occurred only in patients with AMI receiving argatroban concurrently with thrombolytic therapy (streptokinase or TPA) and in patients who had an onset of acute stroke within 12 hours of study entry. Other bleeding included a decreased hemoglobin and hematocrit, GI bleeding, GU bleeding, hematuria, hemoptysis, limb and below-knee amputation stump, multisystem hemorrhage and DIC, venous access. Abdominal pain, abnormal renal function, arrhythmias (e.g., atrial fibrillation, ventricular tachycardia), cardiac arrest, cerebrovascular disorder, coughing, diarrhea, fever, hypotension, nausea, pain, pneumonia, sepsis, URI, and vomiting have occurred.

PCI: Retroperitoneal and GI bleeding occurred in a few patients. Other minor bleeding included coronary arteries, a decreased hemoglobin and hematocrit; GI bleeding; GU bleeding; hematuria; groin, hemoptysis, and access site (venous or arterial). Abdominal pain, back pain, bradycardia, chest pain, fever, headache, hypotension. MI and other serious coronary events, nausea, and vomiting have occurred.

Overdose: Symptoms of acute toxicity in animals included clonic convulsions, coma, loss of righting reflex, paralysis of hind limbs, and tremors.

ANTIDOTE

No specific antidote is available. Obtain aPTT, ACT, and/or other coagulation tests. Overdose with or without bleeding may be controlled by discontinuing argatroban or by decreasing the infusion dose; aPTT should return to baseline within 2 to 4 hours after discontinuation. Reversal may take longer in patients with hepatic impairment. If life-threatening bleeding develops and excessive plasma levels of argatroban are suspected, immediately stop argatroban infusion. Determine aPTT and hemoglobin and prepare for blood transfusion as appropriate. Follow current guidelines for treatment of shock as indicated (fluid, vasopressors [e.g., dopamine], Trendelenburg position, plasma expanders [e.g., albumin, hetastarch]). Approximately 20% of argatroban may be cleared through dialysis.

ARSENIC TRIOXIDE BBW

(**AR**-sen-ik try-**OKS**-ide)

Trisenox

Antineoplastic

pH 7.5 to 8.5

USUAL DOSE

12-lead ECG, serum electrolytes (calcium, magnesium, and potassium), and serum creatinine required before beginning therapy; see Monitor.

Induction schedule: 0.15 mg/kg of body weight daily as an infusion until bone marrow remission. Total induction dose should not exceed 60 doses.

Consolidation schedule: Begin 3 to 6 weeks after completion of induction therapy. 0.15 mg/kg daily for 25 doses over a period of up to 5 weeks.

PEDIATRIC DOSE

Pediatric patients from 5 to 16 years of age: See Usual Dose. See Maternal/Child.

DOSE ADJUSTMENTS

Patients with severe renal impairment (CrCl less than 30 mL/min) or severe hepatic impairment (Child-Pugh Class C) should be closely monitored for toxicity. Dose reduction may be indicated. ■ Use in dialysis has not been studied.

DILUTION

Specific techniques required; see Precautions. Ampule contains 10 mg/10 mL (1 mg/mL). Dilute each daily dose with 100 to 250 mL D5W or NS immediately after withdrawal from the ampule and give as an infusion.

Storage: Store ampules at CRT. Do not freeze. Do not use beyond expiration date. Discard unused portions of each ampule, contains no preservatives. Diluted solutions are stable for 24 hours at RT and 48 hours if refrigerated.

COMPATIBILITY

Manufacturer states, "Do not mix arsenic trioxide with other medications."

RATE OF ADMINISTRATION

A single daily dose as an infusion over 1 to 2 hours. May be extended up to 4 hours if acute vasomotor reactions are observed (e.g., flushing, hypertension, hypotension, pallor). May be given through a peripheral vein, a central venous catheter is not required.

ACTIONS

An antineoplastic agent. Mechanism of action not understood. May cause morphologic changes and DNA fragmentation in selected promyelocytic leukemia cells and damage or degrade selected fusion proteins. In clinical trials, median time to bone marrow remission was 44 days and to onset of complete remission (absence of visible leukemic cells in bone marrow and peripheral recovery of platelets and WBC with a confirmatory bone marrow about 30 days later) was 53 days. Responses were seen in all age-groups ranging from 6 to 72 years. Arsenious acid is the pharmacologically active species of arsenic trioxide. Metabolized in the liver (not by the cytochrome P_{450} family of isoenzymes). Elimination half-life is 10 to 14 hours. Arsenic is stored mainly in liver, kidney, heart, lung, hair, and nails. Excreted in urine. Crosses the placental barrier. Secreted in breast milk.

INDICATIONS AND USES

Induction of remission and consolidation in patients with acute promyelocytic leukemia (APL) who are refractory to, or have relapsed from, retinoid and anthracycline chemotherapy, and whose APL is characterized by the presence of the t(15:17) translocation or PML/RAR-alpha gene expression.

Unlabeled uses: Orphan drug status for treatment of chronic myeloid leukemia (CML), acute promyelocytic leukemia (APL), multiple myeloma (MM), malignant glioma, myelodysplastic syndrome, liver cancer, and chronic lymphocytic leukemia (CLL).

CONTRAINDICATIONS

Known hypersensitivity to arsenic.

PRECAUTIONS

Follow guidelines for handling cytotoxic agents. See Appendix A, p. 1429.

■ Administered by or under the direction of a physician experienced in the management of patients with acute leukemia, with facilities for monitoring the patient and responding to any medical emergency. ■ Symptoms similar to those associated with retinoic-acid–acute promyelocytic leukemia (RA-APL) or APL differentiation syndrome (dyspnea, fever, pleural or pericardial effusions, pulmonary infiltrates, and weight gain with or without leukocytosis) have been reported in some patients treated with arsenic trioxide and can be fatal. See Monitor and Antidote. ■ May cause QT interval prolongation and complete atrioventricular block. QT prolongation can lead to torsades de pointes, which can be fatal. Risk of torsades de pointes is increased by extent of QT prolongation, concomitant administration of QT prolonging drugs, a history of torsades de pointes, pre-existing QT interval prolongation, congestive heart failure, administration of potassium-wasting diuretics, or other conditions that result in hypokalemia or hypomagnesemia; see Drug/Lab Interactions. QT prolongation was observed between 1 and 5 weeks after infusion and returned toward baseline by the end of 8 weeks after infusions were complete. ■ Has been associated with the development of hyperleukocytosis. WBC counts during induction were higher than during consolidation. Treatment with additional chemotherapy was not required. ■ Use caution in patients with impaired renal function; exposure may be increased. Monitor patients with severe renal impairment (CrCl less than 30 mL/min) closely for toxicity; dose reduction may be required. ■ Use with caution in patients with impaired hepatic function. Data are limited. Monitor patients with severe hepatic impairment (Child-Pugh Class C) closely for toxicity.

Monitor: *Before initiating therapy:* Obtain baseline 12-lead ECG, CBC with differential, platelet count, coagulation profile (e.g., PT), serum electrolytes (e.g., calcium, magnesium, and potassium), and serum creatinine. Correct preexisting electrolyte abnormalities and, if possible, discontinue drugs that are known to prolong the QT interval; see Drug/Lab Interactions. If the QT interval is greater than 500 msec, corrective measures should be completed and the QT interval reassessed with serial ECGs before starting arsenic trioxide. *During therapy:* Monitor electrolytes, CBC (including differential), platelet count, and coagulation profile (e.g., PT) at least twice weekly during induction and weekly during consolidation. May be indicated more frequently. Keep potassium concentrations above 4 mEq/dL and magnesium concentrations above 1.8 mg/dL. ■ Monitor ECG weekly and more frequently in unstable patients. No data on the effect of arsenic trioxide on the QT interval during the infusion. If the QT interval is greater than 500 msec at any time during therapy, reassess the patient, correct concomitant risk factors, and consider risk/benefit of continuing versus suspending arsenic trioxide. If syncope or rapid or irregular heartbeat develops, the patient should be hospitalized for ECG monitoring and monitoring of serum electrolytes. Temporarily discontinue arsenic trioxide. Do not resume therapy until the QT interval is less than 460 msec, electrolyte abnormalities are corrected, and syncope and irregular heartbeat cease. ▪ Monitor for thrombocytopenia (platelet count less than 50,000/mm^3). Initiate precautions to prevent excessive bleeding (e.g., inspect IV sites, skin, and mucous membranes; use extreme care during invasive procedures; test urine, emesis, stool, and secretions for occult blood). ▪ Monitor for signs of APL differentiation syndrome (e.g., abnormal chest auscultatory findings or radiographic abnormalities, dyspnea, weight gain, and unexplained fever). If symptoms occur, irrespective of the leukocyte count, begin immediate treatment with high-dose steroids (e.g., dexamethasone 10 mg IV twice daily); continue for at least 3 days or longer until S/S resolve. Termination of arsenic trioxide treatment is not usually required. ▪ See Precautions.

Patient Education: Avoid pregnancy, may cause fetal harm. Nonhormonal birth control recommended. Notify physician immediately if a pregnancy is suspected. ▪ Report dizziness, dyspnea, fainting, fever, rapid or irregular heartbeat, and weight gain immediately. ▪ Review all prescription and nonprescription drugs with your physician. ▪ See Appendix D, p. 1434.

Maternal/Child: Category D: avoid pregnancy. May cause fetal harm. Effective birth control required. ▪ Discontinue breast-feeding. ▪ Limited clinical data for pediatric use. In one study, five patients ranging in age from 5 to 16 years were included in clinical studies, and three achieved a complete response. In another study, the toxicity profile observed in 13 pediatric patients was similar to that seen in adults. ▪ Safety and effectiveness for pediatric patients under 4 years of age not established.

Elderly: Response similar to that in younger patients. ▪ Monitor renal function closely.

DRUG/LAB INTERACTIONS

Concurrent use with **other drugs that prolong the QT interval, including antiarrhythmics** (e.g., amiodarone [Nexterone], disopyramide [Norpace], ibutilide [Corvert], mexiletine, procainamide [Pronestyl], quinidine), **antihistamines, azole antifungals** (e.g., itraconazole [Sporanox]), **fluoroquinolones** (e.g., levofloxacin [Levaquin]), **phenothiazines** (e.g., thioridazine [Mellaril]), **and tricyclic antidepressants** (e.g., amitriptyline [Elavil], imipramine [Tofranil]); may cause torsades de pointes and could be fatal. ▪ Concurrent use with drugs that may cause hypokalemia or other electrolyte abnormalities (e.g., **amphotericin B, diuretics** [e.g., furosemide (Lasix)]) may increase the risk of hypokalemia and cardiac arrhythmias.

SIDE EFFECTS

Abdominal pain, anemia, chest pain, cough, diarrhea, dizziness, dyspnea, edema, fatigue, headache, hyperglycemia, hyperkalemia, hypertension, hypokalemia, hypomagnesemia, hypotension, hypoxia, itching, leukocytosis, nausea, neutropenia (may be febrile), palpitations, pleural effusion, rash, thrombocytopenia, URI, and vomiting. Numerous other side effects have been reported (see literature).

Major: Adverse events rated Grade 3 or 4 on the Common Terminology Criteria for Adverse Events (CTCAE) were common. APL differentiation syndrome, atrial arrhythmias, hyperglycemia, hyperleukocytosis, QT interval 500 msec or more (with or without torsades de pointes) also occurred.

Overdose: Acute arsenic toxicity (e.g., confusion, convulsions, and muscle weakness).

Post-Marketing: Pancytopenia, peripheral neuropathy, ventricular extrasystoles, and tachycardia associated with QT prolongation.

ANTIDOTE

Keep physician informed of all side effects. Those classified as average will usually be treated symptomatically. Major side effects may be fatal and require aggressive treatment as well as temporarily withholding or discontinuing arsenic trioxide. In all situations, monitor electrolytes; maintain potassium and magnesium within prescribed limits. Treat APL differentiation syndrome immediately with high-dose steroids (dexamethasone [Decadron] 10 mg IV twice daily) for at least 3 days or until signs and symptoms resolve (interruption of arsenic trioxide therapy not consistently required). Temporarily discontinue arsenic trioxide for QT prolongation 500 msec or more; see Monitor for recommendations and treat any serious or symptomatic arrhythmia (e.g., conduction abnormalities, VT, torsades de pointes) promptly. Discontinue therapy and treat acute arsenic intoxication with dimercaprol (BAL) 3 mg/kg IM every 4 hours until immediate life-threatening toxicity subsides. Then treat with penicillamine 250 mg PO up to four times a day (approximately 1 Gm/day). Hyperleukocytosis was not treated with additional chemotherapy during clinical trials.

ASCORBIC ACID
(a-**SKOR**-bik **AS**-id)

Sodium Ascorbate, Vitamin C

Nutritional supplement
(vitamin)

pH 5.5 to 7

USUAL DOSE
Up to 6 Gm/24 hr has been given without toxicity.

Nutritional protection: 70 to 150 mg daily. 100 to 200 mg daily may be required during chronic dialysis.

Prevention or treatment of scurvy: 100 to 250 mg 1 to 3 times daily. Give for a minimum of several days; up to 2 to 3 weeks may be indicated.

Enhance wound healing: 300 to 500 mg daily for 7 to 10 days.

Burns: 1 to 2 Gm daily.

PEDIATRIC DOSE
Nutritional protection: 30 mg daily. *Premature infants* may require 75 to 100 mg daily.

Prevention or treatment of scurvy: 100 to 300 mg/24 hr. Give in divided doses. Give for a minimum of several days; up to 2 to 3 weeks may be indicated.

DILUTION
May be given undiluted or may be administered diluted in IV infusion solutions. Soluble in the more commonly used solutions, such as D5W, D5NS, NS, LR, Ringer's injection, or sodium lactate injection. Slight coloration does not affect the medication.

Storage: Protect from freezing and from light.

COMPATIBILITY   (Underline Indicates Conflicting Compatibility Information)
Consider any drug NOT listed as compatible to be INCOMPATIBLE until consulting a pharmacist; specific conditions may apply.

One source suggests the following **compatibilities:**

Additive: Amikacin (Amikin), aminophylline, calcium chloride, calcium gluconate, chloramphenicol (Chloromycetin), chlorpromazine (Thorazine), colistimethate (Coly-Mycin M), diphenhydramine (Benadryl), erythromycin (Erythrocin), heparin, kanamycin (Kantrex), methyldopate, penicillin G potassium, prochlorperazine (Compazine), promethazine (Phenergan), verapamil.

Y-site: Warfarin (Coumadin).

RATE OF ADMINISTRATION
IV injection: 100 mg or fraction thereof over 1 minute.

Infusion: Administer at ordered rate for standard infusion (e.g., over 4 to 8 hours).

ACTIONS
This water-soluble vitamin is necessary for the formation of collagen in all fibrous tissue, carbohydrate metabolism, connective tissue repair, maintenance of intracellular stability of blood vessels, and many other body functions. Not stored in the body. Daily requirements must be met. Completely utilized; excess is excreted unchanged in the urine. Crosses placental barrier. Secreted in breast milk.

INDICATIONS AND USES
Prevention and treatment of vitamin C deficiency, which may lead to scurvy. ▪ Give pre-op and post-op to enhance wound healing. ▪ Prolonged

IV therapy. ▪ Increased vitamin requirements or replacement therapy in severe burns, extensive injuries, and severe infections. ▪ Prematurity. ▪ Deficient intestinal absorption of water-soluble vitamins. ▪ Prolonged or wasting diseases. ▪ Hemovascular disorders and delayed fracture and wound healing require increased intake.

CONTRAINDICATIONS
There are no absolute contraindications.

PRECAUTIONS
Vitamin C is better absorbed and utilized by IM injection. ▪ Use caution in cardiac patients. Sodium or calcium content may antagonize other drugs or overall condition. ▪ Use caution in diabetics and patients prone to recurrent renal calculi or undergoing stool occult blood tests. May contain sulfites; use caution in allergic individuals.

Monitor: Increased urinary excretion is diagnostic for vitamin C saturation. ▪ Continue curative doses until clinical symptoms subside or urinary saturation occurs.

Maternal/Child: Use caution in pregnancy; high dose may adversely affect fetus.

DRUG/LAB INTERACTIONS
Potentiates **oral contraceptives, ferrous iron absorption, salicylates, and sulfonamides.** ▪ May antagonize **anticoagulants.** ▪ 2 Gm/day will lower urine pH and will cause reabsorption of **acidic drugs and** crystallization with **sulfonamides.** ▪ May inhibit **phenothiazines.** ▪ Plasma levels decreased by **smoking cigarettes;** increased doses of ascorbic acid may be required. ▪ May cause false-negative **occult blood** in stool. ▪ May cause false-positive or false-negative in **urine glucose tests.** ▪ **Can alter numerous test results;** must be individually evaluated.

SIDE EFFECTS
Occur only with too-rapid injection: temporary dizziness or faintness. Diarrhea or renal calculi may occur with large doses.

ANTIDOTE
Discontinue administration temporarily. Resume administration at a decreased rate. If side effects persist, discontinue drug and notify the physician.

ASPARAGINASE
(ah-**SPAIR**-ah-jin-ays)

Elspar, ✤Kidrolase

Antineoplastic
(enzyme)

pH 7.4

USUAL DOSE   (International units [IU])
ADULTS AND PEDIATRIC PATIENTS
Therapeutic dose may be given IV or IM.
Skin test: Required before initial dose and whenever 7 days or more elapse
between doses. See Dilution for preparation. Give 2 International units
(IU) intradermally and observe for 1 hour for the appearance of a wheal or
erythema.
Intermittent IV: Very specific amount to be given on a specific day or days in
a specific regimen of other chemotherapeutic agents, i.e., 1,000 IU/kg of
body weight/day for 10 successive days beginning on day 22 of regimen
with specific prednisone and vincristine doses. When used as a single agent
(rare unless combination therapy is not appropriate), the usual dose for
adults and pediatric patients is 200 IU/kg/day for 28 days.
Desensitization process for administration: Extensive process. See drug
literature.

DILUTION   (International units [IU])
Specific techniques required; see Precautions. Initially reconstitute each
10-mL vial (10,000 IU) with 4 mL of SW for Kidrolase and 5 mL of SW
or NS for Elspar. Both result in 2,000 IU/mL.
Skin test: Withdraw 0.1 mL from the above solution and further dilute with
9.9 mL NS (20 IU/mL). 0.1 mL of this solution equals 2 IU.
Intermittent IV: Use 2,000 IU/mL solution. May be given direct IV or further
diluted with 50 to 100 mL of D5W or NS and administered as an infusion
through Y-tube or three-way stopcock of a free-flowing infusion of D5W
or NS. Use only clear solutions.
Filters: May contain fiberlike particles; use of 5-micron in-line filter
recommended. Loss of potency has been observed with the use of a
0.2-micron filter.
Storage: Refrigerate before and after dilution. Discard Elspar after 8 hours.
Reconstituted Kidrolase may be refrigerated up to 14 days. Discard any
solution that is cloudy.

COMPATIBILITY
*Consider any drug NOT listed as compatible to be INCOMPATIBLE until consult-
ing a pharmacist; specific conditions may apply.*
One source suggests the following **compatibilities:**
Y-site: Methotrexate, sodium bicarbonate.

RATE OF ADMINISTRATION
Intermittent IV: Each dose evenly distributed over at least 30 minutes.

ACTIONS
An enzyme derived from *Escherichia coli* that rapidly depletes asparagine
from cells. Some malignant cells have a metabolic defect that makes them
dependent on exogenous asparagine for survival. They are unable to
synthesize asparagine as normal cells do. Undergoes metabolic degradation. Range of plasma half-life is 8 to 30 hours. Trace amounts excreted in
urine.

INDICATIONS AND USES
Induces remissions in pediatric and adult patients with acute lymphocytic leukemia. Primarily used in specific combinations with other chemotherapeutic agents. ■ May be useful in other leukemias and non-Hodgkin's lymphoma. ■ Not indicated for use as a single agent unless combination therapy is not appropriate.

CONTRAINDICATIONS
Hypersensitivity to asparaginase, pancreatitis, or history of pancreatitis.

PRECAUTIONS
Follow guidelines for handling cytotoxic agents. See Appendix A, p. 1429.
■ Administered by or under the direction of the physician specialist in a hospital setting with facilities for monitoring the patient and responding to any medical emergency. ■ Hypersensitivity reactions are frequent and are not completely predictable on the basis of the intradermal skin test. Desensitization procedures may be used in patients who have a positive skin test or in patients who have had previous treatment with asparaginase; however, desensitization is not without risk. ■ Rarely used as a single agent; not recommended for maintenance therapy. ■ Impairs liver function; may increase toxicity of other drugs.

Monitor: Toxicity and short-term effectiveness limit use. More toxic in adults than in pediatric patients. ■ Avoid giving at night. ■ Observe patient carefully during and after infusion. Monitor BP every 15 minutes for at least 1 hour. ■ Appropriate treatment for anaphylaxis must always be available. Risk increased if patient has received asparaginase before. ■ Allopurinol, increased fluid intake, and alkalinization of the urine may be required to reduce uric acid levels. ■ Frequent blood cell counts, bone marrow evaluation, serum amylase, blood sugar, and evaluation of liver and kidney function are necessary. ■ Nausea and vomiting can be severe. Prophylactic administration of antiemetics recommended to increase patient comfort. ■ Predisposition to infection probable. Prophylactic antibiotics may be indicated pending results of C/S in a febrile neutropenic patient. ■ Monitor for thrombocytopenia (platelet count less than 50,000/mm^3). Initiate precautions to prevent excessive bleeding (e.g., inspect IV sites, skin, and mucous membranes; use extreme care during invasive procedures; test urine, emesis, stool, and secretions for occult blood).

Patient Education: Report all symptoms promptly; verbalize all questions. ■ Assess birth control requirements. Nonhormonal contraception advised. ■ See Appendix D, p. 1434.

Maternal/Child: Category C: will have teratogenic effects on the fetus. Evaluate benefit versus risk for anyone who is pregnant or may become pregnant. ■ Discontinue breast-feeding.

Elderly: Toxicity may be more severe. ■ Consider age-related organ impairment.

DRUG/LAB INTERACTIONS
Toxicity of all agents may be increased if asparaginase is given before or concurrently with **vincristine and prednisone.** May be less pronounced if asparaginase is given 12 to 24 hours after vincristine and prednisone. ■ Blocks the effects of **methotrexate** for as long as asparagine concentrations are suppressed. Some suggest administering asparaginase 24 hours after methotrexate; others suggest these agents should not be used together

while asparagine concentrations are suppressed. ▪ May interfere with **thyroid function test interpretation.** ▪ Do not administer any **live virus vaccine** to patients receiving antineoplastic drugs. ▪ See Precautions.

SIDE EFFECTS

Occur frequently (usually within 30 minutes), even with the initial dose, and may cause death. Hypersensitivity reactions including anaphylaxis (even if skin test negative and/or hypersensitivity reactions have not occurred with previous doses), agitation, azotemia, bleeding, bone marrow suppression, coma, confusion, depression, fatigue, hallucinations, hepatitis, hyperglycemia, hyperthermia (fatal), hypofibrinogenemia and depression of other clotting factors, liver function abnormalities (increased ALT, AST, alkaline phosphatase, and bilirubin; decreased albumin), nausea and vomiting, fulminating pancreatitis (fatal).

ANTIDOTE

Notify physician of all side effects. Asparaginase may have to be discontinued until recovery or permanently discontinued. Symptomatic and supportive treatment is indicated. Treat anaphylaxis with epinephrine, corticosteroids, oxygen, and antihistamines. There is no specific antidote.

ATRACURIUM BESYLATE `BBW`
(ah-trah-**KYOUR**-ee-um **BES**-ih-layt)

Atracurium Besylate PF, Tracrium

Neuromuscular
blocking agent
(nondepolarizing)
Anesthesia adjunct

pH 3.25 to 3.65

USUAL DOSE
Adjunct to general anesthesia for adults and pediatric patients over 2 years of age: Must be individualized, depending on previous drugs administered and degree and length of muscle relaxation required. 0.4 to 0.5 mg/kg of body weight initially as an IV bolus. Must be used with adequate anesthesia and/or sedation and after unconsciousness induced. Determine need for maintenance dose based on beginning symptoms of neuromuscular blockade reversal determined by a peripheral nerve stimulator. To maintain muscle relaxation a maintenance dose may be given as a bolus injection of 0.08 to 0.1 mg/kg and is required in approximately 25 to 40 minutes and every 15 to 25 minutes. May alternately be given as a continuous IV infusion of 2 to 15 mcg/kg/min. Repeated doses have no cumulative effect if recovery is allowed to begin before administration.

Adjunct to general anesthesia for infants and children 1 month to 2 years of age: 0.3 to 0.4 mg/kg for infants and children under halothane anesthesia. See Usual Dose for maintenance dose; may be required more frequently.

Support of intubated, mechanically ventilated, or respiratory-controlled adult ICU patients (unlabeled): An initial infusion rate of 11 to 13 mcg/kg/min (range 4.5 to 29.5) provides adequate neuromuscular blockade. Published reports describe a wide interpatient variability in dosing requirements for maintenance ranging from 2.3 to 23 mcg/kg/min (0.14 to 1.38 mg/kg/hr) in adult ICU patients. Occasional adult patients have needed very high infusion rates (greater than 60 mcg/kg/min). In *pediatric* ICU patients maintenance doses ranged from 10 to 30 mcg/kg/min (0.6 to 1.8 mg/kg/hr). A specific initial dose for pediatric patients has not yet been defined.

DOSE ADJUSTMENTS
Reduce dose by one third (0.25 to 0.35 mg/kg) if isoflurane or enflurane are used as general anesthetics. ▪ Reduce dose to 0.3 to 0.4 mg/kg if using halothane anesthetic, in patients with a history of cardiovascular disease, or a history suggesting greater risk of histamine release (allergies), or following succinylcholine administration. Succinylcholine must show signs of wearing off before atracurium is given. Use caution. ▪ Reduce maintenance dose by one half where hypothermia is induced (e.g., cardiac bypass). ▪ See Drug/Lab Interactions.

DILUTION
Initial IV bolus may be given undiluted. Maintenance dose for anesthesia and mechanical ventilation support must be further diluted in NS, D5W, or D5NS and given as a continuous infusion titrated to symptoms of neuromuscular blockade reversal. 20 mg (2 mL) diluted in 98 mL yields 200 mcg/mL (0.2 mg/mL). 50 mg (5 mL) diluted in 95 mL yields 500 mcg/mL (0.5 mg/mL).

Storage: Refrigerate. Diluted solution stable for 24 hours refrigerated or at room temperature.

COMPATIBILITY   (Underline Indicates Conflicting Compatibility Information)
Consider any drug NOT listed as compatible to be INCOMPATIBLE until consulting a pharmacist; specific conditions may apply.
One source suggests the following **compatibilities:**
Additive: Ciprofloxacin (Cipro IV), dobutamine, dopamine, esmolol (Brevibloc), gentamicin, isoproterenol (Isuprel), lidocaine, morphine, potassium chloride (KCl), procainamide (Pronestyl), vancomycin.
Y-site: Amiodarone (Nexterone), cefazolin (Ancef), cefuroxime (Zinacef), dobutamine, dopamine, epinephrine (Adrenalin), esmolol (Brevibloc), etomidate (Amidate), fenoldopam (Corlopam), fentanyl (Sublimaze), gentamicin, heparin, hetastarch in electrolytes (Hextend), hydrocortisone sodium succinate (Solu-Cortef), isoproterenol (Isuprel), lorazepam (Ativan), midazolam (Versed), milrinone (Primacor), morphine, nitroglycerin IV, nitroprusside sodium, propofol (Diprivan), ranitidine (Zantac), sulfamethoxazole/trimethoprim, vancomycin.

RATE OF ADMINISTRATION
In adults or pediatric patients, adjust infusion rate according to clinical assessment of the patient's response. Use of a peripheral nerve stimulator is recommended.
Adjunct to general anesthesia: Initial IV bolus over 30 to 60 seconds.
Maintenance dose: In the 200 mcg/mL dilution, 5 mcg/kg/min will be delivered by a rate of 0.025 mL/kg/min or 1.75 mL/min for a 70-kg patient. Adjust rate to specific dose desired. Drug literature has additional rate calculations.
Mechanical ventilation support in ICU: See Usual Dose for specific rates and criteria.

ACTIONS
A nondepolarizing skeletal muscle relaxant. A less potent histamine releaser than metocurine. Causes paralysis by interfering with neural transmission at the myoneural junction. Onset of action is dose dependent. Produces maximum neuromuscular blockade within 3 to 5 minutes and lasts about 25 minutes. When infusion is discontinued, some recovery occurs within 30 minutes. Recovery to 75% averages 60 minutes (range 32 to 108 minutes). It may be several hours before complete recovery occurs. Excreted as metabolites in bile and urine. Crosses the placental barrier.

INDICATIONS AND USES
Adjunctive to general anesthesia to facilitate endotracheal intubation and to relax skeletal muscles during surgery or mechanical ventilation.
Unlabeled uses: Support of intubated, mechanically ventilated, or respiratory-controlled patients in ICU.

CONTRAINDICATIONS
Known hypersensitivity to atracurium.

PRECAUTIONS
For IV use only. ■ Administered by or under the observation of the anesthesiologist. Appropriate emergency drugs and equipment for monitoring the patient and responding to any medical emergency must be readily available. ■ Use extreme caution in patients with significant cardiovascular disease or a history of allergies or allergic reaction. ■ Severe anaphylactic reactions have been reported with neuromuscular blocking agents; some have been fatal. Use caution in patients who have had an anaphylactic reaction to another neu-

romuscular blocking agent (depolarizing or nondepolarizing); cross-reactivity has occurred. ■ Myasthenia gravis and other neuromuscular diseases increase sensitivity to drug. Can cause critical reactions. ■ Respiratory depression with propofol (Diprivan) or morphine may be preferred in some patients requiring mechanical ventilation. ■ Bradycardia is fairly common since atracurium will not counteract the bradycardia produced by many anesthetic agents or vagal stimulation. ■ Acid-base and/or electrolyte imbalance, debilitation, hypoxic episodes, and/or the use of other drugs (e.g., broad-spectrum antibiotics, narcotics, steroids) may prolong the effects of atracurium.

Monitor: This drug produces apnea. Controlled artificial ventilation with oxygen must be continuous and under direct observation at all times. Maintain a patent airway. ■ Use a peripheral nerve stimulator to monitor response to atracurium and avoid overdose. ■ Patient may be conscious and completely unable to communicate by any means. Has no analgesic or sedative properties. ■ Action potentiated by hypokalemia and some carcinomas. ■ Action is altered by dehydration, electrolyte imbalance, body temperature, and acid-base imbalance. *Mechanical ventilation support in ICU:* Physical therapy is recommended to prevent muscular weakness, atrophy, and joint contracture. Muscular weakness may be first noticed during attempts to wean patient from the ventilator.

Maternal/Child: Category C: use in pregnancy only if use justifies potential risk to fetus. Has been used during cesarean section; monitor infant carefully. ■ Use caution during breast-feeding. ■ Safety for use in infants under 1 month of age not established. ■ Contains benzyl alcohol; may cause "gasping syndrome" in premature infants.

Elderly: No adjustments identified.

DRUG/LAB INTERACTIONS

Potentiated by **general anesthetics** (e.g., enflurane, isoflurane, halothane), **many antibiotics** (e.g., lincosamides [clindamycin (Cleocin)], aminoglycosides [kanamycin (Kantrex), gentamicin], polypeptides [bacitracin, colistimethate]), **corticosteroids, diuretics, diazepam** (Valium) **and other muscle relaxants, magnesium sulfate, meperidine, morphine, procainamide** (Pronestyl), **quinidine, succinylcholine, verapamil, and others.** May need to reduce dose of atracurium; use with caution. ▪ Duration of neuromuscular block may be shorter and dose requirements may be higher during maintenance infusion in patients stabilized on **carbamazepine** (Tegretol) **and phenytoin** (Dilantin). ▪ Antagonized by **acetylcholine, anticholinesterases, azathioprine, and theophylline.** ▪ **Succinylcholine** must show signs of wearing off before atracurium is given. Use caution.

SIDE EFFECTS

Prolonged action resulting in respiratory insufficiency or apnea. Airway closure caused by relaxation of epiglottis, pharynx, and tongue muscles. Hypersensitivity reactions including anaphylaxis are possible. Bradycardia, bronchospasm, dyspnea, flushing, histamine release, hypotension, laryngospasm, reaction at injection site, shock, and tachycardia may occur. Rare reports of seizures with use of atracurium in ICU could be caused by other conditions or medications. Malignant hyperthermia is rare but may occur.

ANTIDOTE

All side effects are medical emergencies. Treat symptomatically. Controlled artificial ventilation must be continuous. Pyridostigmine (Regonol) or neostigmine given with atropine will probably reverse the muscle relaxation. Not effective in all situations; may aggravate severe overdosage. Resuscitate as necessary.

ATROPINE SULFATE
(**AH**-troh-peen **SUL**-fayt)

Anticholinergic
Antiarrhythmic
Antidote

pH 3.5 to 6.5

USUAL DOSE

Bradyarrhythmias: 0.4- to 1-mg bolus repeated every 3 to 5 minutes up to a total dose of 2 mg can be used to achieve a desired pulse rate above 60. AHA guidelines recommend 0.5 mg every 3 to 5 minutes as needed, the *total dose not to exceed 0.04 mg/kg (3 mg).* The use of shorter dosing intervals (3 minutes) and higher maximum dose range (0.04 mg/kg) is suggested in severe clinical conditions. Subsequent doses of 0.5 to 1 mg may be given at 4- to 6-hour intervals. Doses under 0.5 mg may cause paradoxical slowing of HR.

Smooth muscle relaxation and suppression of secretions: 0.4 to 0.6 mg every 4 to 6 hours.

During surgery: Above doses appropriate except during cyclopropane anesthesia. Start with 0.4 mg or less. Administer very slowly to avoid ventricular arrhythmias; see Drug/Lab Interactions.

Cardiac asystole or pulseless electrical activity: AHA guidelines state, "Routine use during pulseless electrical activity or asystole is unlikely to have a therapeutic benefit."

Antidote to reverse muscarinic effects of anticholinesterase agents: 0.6 to 1.2 mg for each 0.5 to 2.5 mg of neostigmine or 10 to 20 mg of pyridostigmine administered. Administer in a separate syringe, concurrently or a few minutes before the anticholinesterase agent. If bradycardia is present, bring pulse up to 80 by giving IV atropine first. See neostigmine, pyridostigmine, or physostigmine monographs.

Antidote for acute poisoning from exposure to anticholinesterase compounds (e.g., organophosphate pesticides, nerve gases, and mushroom poisoning): 1 to 2 mg may be given in a single dose and repeated every 5 to 60 minutes. In severe poisoning 2 to 6 mg may be given and repeated at 5- to 60-minute intervals until muscarinic signs and symptoms subside and repeated if they appear. Up to 50 mg may be required in the first 24 hours. Use oral atropine for maintenance; withdraw gradually to avoid recurrence of symptoms (e.g., pulmonary edema). A cholinase reactivator (e.g., pralidoxime) is administered concomitantly except in carbamate exposure.

PEDIATRIC DOSE

Fatal dose of atropine in pediatric patients may be as low as 10 mg. See Maternal/Child.

Bradyarrhythmias: 0.01 to 0.03 mg/kg of body weight can be used to achieve a pulse rate above 80 in a distressed infant under 6 months or above 60 in a child. Minimum dose is 0.1 mg. Maximum single dose is 0.5 mg in a child, 1 mg for an adolescent. May be repeated in 5-minute intervals two times. AHA guidelines recommend 0.02 mg/kg. May repeat dose one time. Maximum total dose for a child is 1 mg, for an adolescent 3 mg. When used for bradycardia or asystole in infants and small children, vagolytic doses are required. Doses less than 0.1 mg may cause paradoxical bradycardia.

Smooth muscle relaxation and suppression of secretions: 0.01 mg/kg. Minimum dose is 0.1 mg in the newborn; up to 0.4 mg for a 12 year old. Usually given SC. May repeat every 4 to 6 hours.
Bronchospasm: 0.05 mg/kg in 2.5 mL NS every 6 to 8 hours. Minimum dose 0.25 mg; maximum dose is 1 mg.
Antidote to reverse muscarinic effects of anticholinesterase agents: 0.02 mg/kg of atropine concomitantly with 0.04 mg/kg of neostigmine. See Usual Dose for additional information.
Antidote for acute poisoning from exposure to anticholinesterase compounds (e.g., organophosphate compounds, nerve gases, mushroom poisoning): 0.05 mg/kg; repeat every 10 to 30 minutes until muscarinic signs and symptoms subside, and repeat if they reappear. See Usual Dose for additional information.

DOSE ADJUSTMENTS
Reduced dose may be indicated in the elderly. ▪ See Drug/Lab Interactions and Pediatric Dose.

DILUTION
May be given undiluted, but may prefer to dilute desired dose in at least 10 mL of SW for injection. Do not add to IV solutions. Inject through Y-tube or three-way stopcock of infusion set. Also available in combination with edrophonium (Enlon-Plus) to reverse cholinesterase toxicity caused by reversal of nondepolarizing muscle relaxants.

COMPATIBILITY   (Underline Indicates Conflicting Compatibility Information)
Consider any drug NOT listed as compatible to be INCOMPATIBLE until consulting a pharmacist; specific conditions may apply.
One source suggests the following **compatibilities:**
Additive: Dobutamine, furosemide (Lasix), meropenem (Merrem IV), sodium bicarbonate, verapamil.
Y-site: Abciximab (ReoPro), amiodarone (Nexterone), argatroban, bivalirudin (Angiomax), doripenem (Doribax), etomidate (Amidate), famotidine (Pepcid IV), fenoldopam (Corlopam), fentanyl (Sublimaze), heparin, hydrocortisone sodium succinate (Solu-Cortef), hydromorphone (Dilaudid), inamrinone (Amrinone), meropenem (Merrem IV), methadone (Dolophine), morphine, nafcillin (Nallpen), palonosetron (Aloxi), potassium chloride (KCl), propofol (Diprivan), sufentanil (Sufenta), tirofiban (Aggrastat).

RATE OF ADMINISTRATION
1 mg or fraction thereof over 1 minute.

ACTIONS
Atropine is an anticholinergic drug and a potent belladonna alkaloid. It produces local, central, and peripheral effects on the body. The main therapeutic uses of atropine are peripheral, affecting smooth muscle, cardiac muscle, and gland cells. Reverses cholinergic-mediated decreases in HR, systemic vascular resistance, and BP. This drug can interfere with vagal stimuli. It is widely distributed in all body fluids. Metabolized by the liver and excreted in urine and bile. Crosses placental barrier. Secreted in breast milk.

INDICATIONS AND USES
Treatment of symptomatic sinus bradycardia, syncope from Stokes-Adams syndrome, and high-degree atrioventricular block with profound

bradycardia. ▪ AHA guidelines recommend as the primary drug to treat symptomatic sinus bradycardia and as the second drug (after) epinephrine for asystole or pulseless electrical activity. ▪ Suppression of salivary, gastric, pancreatic, and respiratory secretions. ▪ To relieve pylorospasm, hypertonicity of the small intestine, and hypermotility of the colon. ▪ To relieve biliary and ureteral colic. ▪ Antidote to reverse cholinesterase toxicity (muscarinic effects) caused by reversal of nondepolarizing muscle relaxants by neostigmine, physostigmine, and pyridostigmine. ▪ Antidote for specific poisons such as organophosphorus insecticides, nerve gases, and mushroom poisoning *(Amanita muscaria)*. ▪ Temporary, reversible muscarinic blockade when excessive (or sometimes normal) muscarinic effects are judged to be life threatening or are producing severe symptoms. ▪ Used in combination with many other drugs to produce a desired effect (e.g., edrophonium [Enlon, Enlon-Plus]).

CONTRAINDICATIONS
Hypersensitivity to atropine, acute glaucoma, acute hemorrhage with unstable cardiovascular status, asthma, hepatic disease, intestinal atony of the elderly or debilitated, myasthenia gravis, myocardial ischemia, obstructive disease of the GI or GU tracts, paralytic ileus, pyloric stenosis, renal disease, severe ulcerative colitis, tachycardia, toxic megacolon.

PRECAUTIONS
Use caution in prostatic hypertrophy, chronic lung disease, infants and small children, the elderly and debilitated, in urinary retention, during cyclopropane anesthesia, and in myocardial ischemia or infarction. ▪ Increases myocardial oxygen demand and can trigger tachyarrhythmias. ▪ Doses less than 0.5 mg may further slow HR. ▪ May be given endotracheally. ▪ Considered possibly harmful in AV block at the His-Purkinje level or with newly appearing wide QRS complexes.
Monitor: Vital signs and/or ECG based on specific situation.
Patient Education: Use caution if task requires alertness; may cause blurred vision, dizziness, or drowsiness. ▪ Report eye pain, flushing, or skin rash promptly. ▪ Report dry mouth, difficulty urinating, constipation, or increased light sensitivity.
Maternal/Child: Category C: safety for use in pregnancy, breast-feeding, and pediatric patients not established. ▪ Toxicity to nursing infants probable.
Elderly: May produce excitement, agitation, confusion, or drowsiness. ▪ May precipitate undiagnosed glaucoma. ▪ Potential for constipation and urinary retention increased. ▪ Has potential to increase memory impairment. ▪ See Dose Adjustments and Precautions.

DRUG/LAB INTERACTIONS
Potentiated by **other drugs with anticholinergic activity** (e.g., amantadine, [Symmetrel], glycopyrrolate, phenothiazines [e.g., prochlorperazine (Compazine)], tricyclic antidepressants [e.g., amitriptyline (Elavil), imipramine (Tofranil)]). Reduce dose of atropine. ▪ Antipsychotic effects of **phenothiazines** (e.g., prochlorperazine [Compazine]) may be decreased. ▪ Concurrent use with **cyclopropane anesthesia** may cause ventricular arrhythmias; use of **glycopyrrolate** in increments of 0.1 mg or less is preferred. ▪ Potentiates effects of many oral drugs by delaying gastric emptying and increasing rate of absorption (e.g., **atenolol, digoxin, nitrofurantoin, thiazide diuretics).** ▪ Antagonistic to many drugs (e.g., **edrophonium** [Tensilon], **pyridostigmine** [Regonol]).

SIDE EFFECTS

Anhidrosis, anticholinergic psychosis, blurred vision, bradycardia (temporary), constipation, dilation of the pupils, dryness of the mouth, flushing, gastroesophageal reflux, heat prostration from decreased sweating, nausea, paralytic ileus, postural hypotension, tachyarrhythmias, urinary hesitancy and retention (especially in males), and vomiting may occur.

Overdose: Coma, death, delirium, elevated BP, fever, paralytic ileus, rash, respiratory failure, stupor, tachycardia.

ANTIDOTE

Discontinue if side effects increase or are severe. Notify physician. Use standard treatments to manage cardiac arrhythmias. Physostigmine salicylate (Antilirium) reverses most cardiovascular and CNS effects; however, it may cause profound bradycardia, seizures, or asystole. Neostigmine methylsulfate (Prostigmin) is an alternate antidote. Sustain physiologic functions at a normal level. Use diazepam (Valium), phenobarbital (Luminal), or chloral hydrate to relieve excitement. Administer pilocarpine, 10 mg (SC), until the mouth is moist.

AZACITIDINE
(ay-za-**SYE**-ti-deen)
Vidaza

Antineoplastic

USUAL DOSE

Premedication: Prophylactic administration of antiemetics (e.g., granisetron [Kytril], ondansetron [Zofran]) is indicated before each dose.

First treatment cycle: An initial dose of 75 mg/M^2 as an IV infusion or as a SC injection once daily for 7 days is recommended for all patients regardless of baseline hematology.

Subsequent treatment cycles: Cycles should be repeated every 4 weeks. Dose may be increased to 100 mg/M^2 if no beneficial effect is seen after 2 treatment cycles and if no toxicity other than nausea and vomiting has occurred. Treatment is recommended for a minimum of 4 to 6 cycles; however, a complete or partial response may require additional treatment cycles. Repeat cycles may be administered as long as the patient continues to benefit. See Dose Adjustments for dose delay or reduction recommendations for hematologic response, renal toxicities, and/or electrolyte disturbances.

DOSE ADJUSTMENTS

Dose Adjustments of Azacitidine Based on Baseline Hematologic Responses

In any given subsequent cycle for patients with a baseline (start of treatment) WBC equal to or greater than 3 × 10^9/L (3,000 cells/mm^3), ANC equal to or greater than 1.5 × 10^9/L (1,500 cells/mm^3), and platelets equal to or greater than 75 × 10^9/L (75,000 cells/mm^3): Adjust the dose based on nadir counts according to the following chart.

Nadir Counts		% Dose in the Next Cycle
ANC (cells/mm^3)	Platelets (cells/mm^3)	
<500 cells/mm^3	<25,000 cells/mm^3	50%
500 to 1,500 cells/mm^3	25,000 to 50,000 cells/mm^3	67%
>1,500 cells/mm^3	>50,000 cells/mm^3	100%

In any given subsequent cycle for patients with a baseline (start of treatment) WBC less than 3 × 10^9/L (3,000 cells/mm^3), ANC less than 1.5 × 10^9/L (1,500 cells/mm^3), or platelets less than 75 × 10^9/L (75,000 cells/mm^3): Adjust the dose based on nadir counts and bone marrow biopsy cellularity at the time of the nadir according to the following chart. *The exception is the presence of clear improvement in differentiation (% of mature granulocytes is higher and ANC is higher than at the onset of that course) at the time of the next cycle. If this improvement occurs, the dose of the current treatment should be continued.*

WBC or Platelet Nadir (% Decrease in Counts from Baseline)	Bone Marrow Biopsy Cellularity at Time of Nadir (%)		
	30% to 60%	15% to 30%	<15%
	% Dose in the Next Course		
50% to 75%	100%	50%	33%
>75%	75%	50%	33%

If a nadir as defined in this table has occurred, the next course of treatment should be given 28 days after the start of the preceding course, provided that both the WBC and the platelet count are greater than 25% above the nadir and are rising. If a greater than 25% increase above the nadir is not seen by day 28, counts should be reassessed every 7 days. If a 25% increase is not seen by day 42, the patient should be treated with 50% of the scheduled dose.

Dose adjustments of azacitidine based on renal function and serum electrolytes: If unexplained reductions in serum bicarbonate levels to less than 20 mEq/L occur, reduce the dose by 50% on the next course. ■ If unexplained elevations of BUN or SCr occur, delay the next cycle until values return to baseline and then reduce the dose by 50% on the next course. ■ Use care in dose selection for the elderly; reduced doses may be indicated based on overall renal function.

DILUTION

Specific techniques required; see Precautions. Available as a lyophilized powder in single-use vials containing 100 mg. More than one vial may be required for a single dose. Reconstitute each vial with 10 mL SW. Vigorously shake or roll each vial until all solids are dissolved. Solution equals 10 mg/mL. Withdraw the required amount of azacitidine to deliver the desired dose and inject into a 50- or 100-mL infusion bag of NS or LR. Administration must be complete within 1 hour of reconstitution. Discard unused portions appropriately.

Filters: Specific information not available.

Storage: Store in cartons at CRT. Reconstituted solutions may be held at 25° C (77° F), but administration must be complete within 1 hour of reconstitution.

COMPATIBILITY

Consider any drug NOT listed as compatible to be INCOMPATIBLE until consulting a pharmacist; specific conditions may apply.

Manufacturer lists azacitidine as **incompatible** with D5W, hetastarch, or any solution that contains bicarbonate. These solutions have the potential to increase the rate of degradation of azacitidine.

RATE OF ADMINISTRATION

A single dose equally distributed over 10 to 40 minutes. Administration must be complete within 1 hour of reconstitution.

ACTIONS

A pyrimidine nucleoside analog of cytidine. A hypomethylating antineoplastic agent. Cytotoxic effects cause the death of rapidly dividing cells, including cancer cells that are no longer responsive to normal growth control mechanisms. Non-proliferating cells are relatively insensitive to azacitidine. This hypomethylation may restore normal function to genes that are critical for cellular differentiation and proliferation and also allow the formation of normal bone marrow cells. May be metabolized by the liver. Effect on metabolism by known microsomal enzyme inhibitors or inducers has not been studied, and its potential to inhibit cytochrome P_{450} enzymes is not known. Half-life is 4 hours. Primarily excreted in urine with minimal excretion in feces. Crosses the placental barrier.

INDICATIONS AND USES

Treatment of patients with the following French-American-British (FAB) myelodysplastic syndrome (MDS) subtypes such as refractory anemia, refractory anemia with ringed sideroblasts (if accompanied by neutropenia or thrombocytopenia or requiring transfusions), refractory anemia with excess blasts, refractory anemia with excess blasts in transformation, and chronic myelomonocytic leukemia.

CONTRAINDICATIONS
Known hypersensitivity to azacitidine or mannitol, patients with advanced malignant hepatic tumors.

PRECAUTIONS
Follow guidelines for handling cytotoxic agents; see Appendix A, p. 1429. ▪ If azacitidine comes into contact with skin, immediately wash with soap and water. If it comes into contact with mucous membranes, flush thoroughly with water. ▪ Administer by or under the direction of a physician specialist in a facility with adequate diagnostic and treatment facilities to monitor the patient and respond to any medical emergency. ▪ Use caution in patients with liver disease; potentially hepatotoxic in patients with severe pre-existing hepatic impairment; see Contraindications. Rare cases of progressive hepatic coma and death have been reported in patients with extensive tumor burden due to metastatic disease, especially when baseline albumin is less than 3 Gm/dL. ▪ Rare reports of renal abnormalities (e.g., elevated serum creatinine, renal failure, and death) have occurred in patients treated with azacitidine in combination with other chemotherapeutic agents for non-MDS conditions. ▪ Renal tubular acidosis (a fall in serum bicarbonate to less than 20 mEq/L in association with an alkaline urine and hypokalemia [serum potassium less than 3 mEq/L]) developed in 5 patients treated with azacitidine and etoposide. ▪ The effects of race or renal or hepatic impairment on the pharmacokinetics of azacitidine have not been studied. ▪ Anemia, leukopenia, neutropenia, and thrombocytopenia may be dose-limiting toxicities. ▪ Patients with MDS produce poorly functioning and immature blood cells and experience anemia, bleeding, fatigue, infection, and weakness. High-risk MDS patients may experience bone marrow failure, which may lead to death from bleeding and infection. ▪ MDS can progress to acute leukemia (AML).

Monitor: Obtain a baseline CBC with platelets and monitor before each dosing cycle and as indicated to monitor response and toxicity between cycles. ▪ Obtain baseline renal and hepatic function (BUN, SCr, bilirubin) studies; monitor during treatment as indicated. ▪ Use prophylactic antiemetics to reduce nausea and vomiting and to increase patient comfort. ▪ Monitor for S/S of infection. Prophylactic antibiotics may be indicated pending results of C/S in a febrile neutropenic patient. ▪ Monitor for thrombocytopenia (platelet count less than 50,000/mm^3). Initiate precautions to prevent excessive bleeding (e.g., inspect IV sites, skin, and mucous membranes; use extreme care during invasive procedures; test urine, emesis, stool, and secretions for occult blood). ▪ Avoid administration of live virus vaccine to immunocompromised patients. ▪ Observe for S/S of a hypersensitivity reaction; specific information not available. ▪ See Precautions and Antidote.

Patient Education: Avoid pregnancy; nonhormonal birth control recommended for both males and females. Women should report a suspected pregnancy immediately. Males should not father a child during treatment with azacitidine. ▪ Inform physician about any underlying liver or renal disease.

Maternal/Child: Category D: avoid pregnancy; may cause fetal harm. Males should not father a child while receiving treatment with azacitidine. ▪ Discontinue breast-feeding; has the potential for causing serious harm to nursing infants. ▪ Safety and effectiveness for use in pediatric patients not established.

Elderly: Safety and effectiveness similar to younger adults. ▪ Consider age-related renal impairment; dosing should be cautious; see Dose Adjustments. Monitor renal function.

DRUG/LAB INTERACTIONS

Formal drug interaction studies have not been completed. ▪ Effect on metabolism by known microsomal enzyme inhibitors or inducers has not been studied, and its potential to inhibit cytochrome P_{450} enzymes is not known. ▪ Do not administer **live virus vaccines** to patients receiving antineoplastic agents.

SIDE EFFECTS

Anemia; constipation; diarrhea; ecchymosis; fatigue; fever; hypokalemia; infection; injection site bruising, erythema, and pain; leukopenia; nausea; neutropenia; petechiae; rales; rigors; thrombocytopenia; weakness; and vomiting have been reported most commonly. Febrile neutropenia, fever, leukopenia, neutropenia, pneumonia, and thrombocytopenia were the most frequent cause of dose reduction, delay, and discontinuation. Infusion site erythema or pain and catheter site reactions such as infection, erythema, or hemorrhage were reported with IV administration. Elevated SCr, hepatic coma, hypokalemia, renal failure, and renal tubular acidosis have also been reported. Numerous other side effects may be associated with azacitidine.

ANTIDOTE

Notify physician of any side effects. Most will be treated symptomatically. Dose may be reduced or delayed for hematologic toxicity, renal toxicity, or electrolyte disturbances. See Dose Adjustments for specific criteria. Blood and blood products, antibiotics, and other adjunctive therapies must be available. No known antidote; monitor blood counts and provide supportive care in overdose. ▪ Resuscitate as necessary.

AZATHIOPRINE SODIUM BBW

(ay-zah-**THIGH**-oh-preen **SO**-dee-um)

Immunosuppressant

pH 9.6

USUAL DOSE

3 to 5 mg/kg of body weight/24 hr. Begin treatment within 24 hours of renal homotransplantation. In some cases, doses are given 1 to 3 days prior to transplantation. Maintenance dose is 1 to 3 mg/kg/24 hr. Individualized adjustment is imperative. Do not increase to toxic levels because of threatened rejection. Oral and IV doses are therapeutically equivalent; transfer to oral therapy as soon as practical.

DOSE ADJUSTMENTS

Dose reduction is recommended in patients with reduced thiopurine S-methyltransferase (TPMT) activity; see Precautions. ■ Reduce dose in impaired kidney function (especially immediately after transplant or with cadaveric kidneys) and in persistent negative nitrogen balance. ■ Dose reduction may be required if there is a rapid fall or a persistently low leukocyte count. ■ Decrease dose to one third to one fourth of the usual dose when given concomitantly with allopurinol. Consider further dose reduction or alternative therapy in patients with low or absent TPMT activity who are receiving both drugs. ■ See Drug/Lab Interactions and Precautions/Monitor.

DILUTION

Specific techniques suggested; see Precautions. Each 100 mg should be initially reconstituted with 10 mL of SW. Swirl the vial gently until completely in solution. May be further diluted in a minimum of 50 mL of NS, D5W, or D5NS and given as an infusion. See Compatibility.

Storage: Store unopened vials at 15° to 25° C (59° to 77° F). Protect from light. Use diluted solution within 24 hours.

COMPATIBILITY

Specific information not available. Listed as **incompatible** with preservatives (e.g., methylparaben, phenol, propylparaben). Administer separately. Converts to 6-mercaptopurine in alkaline solutions and sulfhydryl compounds. Flush IV line with a **compatible** IV fluid before and after administration.

RATE OF ADMINISTRATION

A single dose properly diluted and infused over 30 to 60 minutes. Actual range may be 5 minutes to 8 hours.

ACTIONS

An immunosuppressive antimetabolite. It is chemically cleaved to the antineoplastic compound 6-mercaptopurine. Exact method of action is unknown. It suppresses hypersensitivities of the cell-mediated type and causes variable alterations in antibody production. Action depends on the temporal relationship to antigenic stimulus or engraftment. Has little effect on established graft rejections or secondary responses. Metabolized readily with small amounts excreted in the urine. Crosses placental barrier. Secreted in breast milk.

INDICATIONS AND USES

Adjunct to prevent rejection in renal homotransplantation. ■ Used PO to treat rheumatoid arthritis; see package insert.

CONTRAINDICATIONS

Known hypersensitivity to azathioprine. ▪ Patients with rheumatoid arthritis who have been treated with alkylating agents (e.g., chlorambucil [Leukeran], cyclophosphamide [Cytoxan], melphalan [Alkeran]) may have a prohibitive risk of neoplasm if treated with azathioprine.

PRECAUTIONS

Follow guidelines for handling cytotoxic agents; see Appendix A, p. 1429. ▪ Usually administered in the hospital by or under the direction of a physician experienced in immunosuppressive therapy and management of organ transplant patients. ▪ Adequate laboratory and supportive medical resources must be available. ▪ Chronic immunosuppression may increase possibility of malignant tumor growth. Has mutogenic potential to both men and women and possible hematologic toxicities. Patients with Crohn's disease or inflammatory bowel disease, particularly adolescents and young adults, may have a higher risk of malignancies, including hepatosplenic T-cell lymphoma (HSTCL), with azathioprine alone or in combination therapy with TNF blockers (e.g., infliximab [Remicade]). ▪ Use caution with other myelosuppressive drugs or radiation therapy. ▪ Toxic hepatitis or biliary status may necessitate discontinuing drug. ▪ Severe leukopenia, thrombocytopenia, macrocytic anemia, and/or pancytopenia may occur. ▪ Serious infections (bacterial, fungal, protozoal, and viral) may occur and can be fatal. ▪ Rapid bone marrow suppression progressing to severe, life-threatening myelotoxicity may occur in patients with inherited intermediate, low, or absent TPMT. Genotyping or phenotyping may help identify these patients. Accurate phenotyping results are not possible in patients who have received recent blood transfusions. ▪ Hematologic toxicities are dose-related and may be more severe in renal transplant patients whose homograft is undergoing rejection. ▪ A GI hypersensitivity reaction (e.g., severe nausea and vomiting) has been reported. May also cause diarrhea, elevations of liver function tests, fever, hypotension, malaise, myalgias, and rash. Usually develops within the first several weeks of therapy and resolves when azathioprine is discontinued.

Monitor: Monitor CBC with platelets weekly for the first month, twice monthly for the second and third months, then monthly or more frequently if dose adjustments or other therapy changes are necessary. Drug should be withdrawn or dose reduced at first sign of abnormally large fall in the leukocyte count or other evidence of persistent bone marrow suppression. ▪ Observe constantly for signs of infection. Prophylactic antibiotics may be indicated pending results of C/S in a febrile neutropenic patient.▪ Monitor for S/S of malignancies such as HSTCL (e.g., abdominal pain, hepatomegaly, night sweats, persistent fever, weight loss).

Patient Education: Avoid pregnancy; nonhormonal birth control recommended. ▪ Promptly report abdominal pain, fever, unusual bruising or bleeding, and/or S/S of infection. ▪ Obtain all lab work as directed. ▪ See Appendix D, p. 1434.

Maternal/Child: Category D: avoid pregnancy. Can cause fetal harm. ▪ Discontinue breast-feeding. ▪ Safety and effectiveness for use in pediatric patients not established.

Elderly: Dose selection should be cautious; consider age-related renal impairment; see Dose Adjustments. Monitor renal function.

DRUG/LAB INTERACTIONS

Allopurinol (Aloprim) inhibits the metabolism of azathioprine, increasing its activity and toxicity. Reduce dose to one third or one fourth of usual; see Dose Adjustments. ▪ Inhibits anticoagulant effects of **warfarin** (Coumadin). ▪ Concurrent use with **bone marrow suppressants, radiation therapy, other immunosuppressants** (e.g., cyclosporine [Sandimmune]) **or other drugs that may cause blood dyscrasias** (e.g., sulfamethoxazole/ trimethoprim [Bactrim]) may increase toxicity. ▪ Concurrent use with **ACE inhibitors** (e.g., captopril [Capoten]) may induce anemia and severe leukopenia. ▪ Plasma levels of the metabolite 6-MP may be increased by **methotrexate.** ▪ **Aminosalicylates** (e.g., sulfasalazine [Azulfidine], me-salamine [Asacol, Pentasa], olsalazine [Dipentum]) may inhibit TPMT, increasing the risk of toxicity. Use caution if concomitant therapy is required. ▪ Antibody response to **vaccines** may be suppressed. Do not use **live virus vaccines** in patients receiving azathioprine.

SIDE EFFECTS

Principal and potentially serious side effects are hematologic and gastro-intestinal. Risk of infection and neoplasia are also significant. Frequency and severity of side effects depend on dose, duration of therapy, and on patient's underlying condition and concomitant therapy. Leukopenia and/or thrombocytopenia are dose-dependent and dose limiting. Other side effects include alopecia; anemia; anorexia; arthralgia; bleeding; diarrhea; fever; hepatic veno-occlusive disease; hepatosplenic T-cell lymphoma; hepatotoxicity characterized by elevation of serum alkaline phosphatase, bilirubin, and serum transaminases (e.g., ALT, AST); hypotension; infec-tion; jaundice; malaise; myalgias; nausea; neoplasia; oral lesions; pancre-atitis; skin rash; Sweet's syndrome (acute febrile neutrophilic dermatosis); vomiting. A GI hypersensitivity reaction (e.g., severe nausea and vomiting) has been reported; see Precautions.

ANTIDOTE

Notify the physician of all side effects. Most can be treated symptomati-cally and may reverse when the drug is discontinued. The GI hypersen-sitivity reactions can occur within hours of a rechallenge. Drug may be decreased or discontinued or other immunosuppressive agents utilized. Hematopoietic depression may require temporary or permanent discon-tinuation of treatment and may be indicated even if rejection of graft may occur. Dialysis may be useful in overdose (partially dialyzable).

AZITHROMYCIN
(az-**zith**-roh-**MY**-sin)

Zithromax

Antibacterial
(azalide/macrolide)

pH 6.4 to 6.6

USUAL DOSE

Community-acquired pneumonia: 500 mg as a single daily dose for a minimum of 2 days. Follow with 500 mg of oral azithromycin as a single daily dose. Total course of therapy (IV + oral) should be 7 to 10 days. **Pelvic inflammatory disease:** 500 mg as a single daily dose for 1 to 2 days. Follow with 250 mg of oral azithromycin as a single daily dose. Total course of therapy (IV + oral) should be 7 days. If anaerobic microorganisms are also suspected, concurrent administration of an antibacterial agent with anaerobic activity is recommended (e.g., metronidazole [Flagyl]).

DOSE ADJUSTMENTS

Reduced dose may be required in impaired liver or renal function; see Precautions. ▪ See Drug/Lab Interactions.

DILUTION

Each 500-mg vial must be reconstituted with 4.8 mL SW. Shake well to ensure dilution (100 mg/mL). Further dilute each 500 mg of reconstituted solution with 250 to 500 mL of one of the following solutions: D5W, NS, ½NS, D5/⅓NS, D5/½NS, D5/½NS with 20 mEq KCl, LR, D5LR, D5/Normosol M, D5/Normosol R. 500 mL diluent yields 1 mg/mL, 250 mL yields 2 mg/mL. Concentrations greater than 2 mg/mL have caused local IV site reactions and should be avoided.

Storage: Reconstituted or diluted solution stable at CRT for 24 hours. Diluted solution stable for up to 7 days if refrigerated.

COMPATIBILITY   (Underline Indicates Conflicting Compatibility Information)

Consider any drug NOT listed as compatible to be INCOMPATIBLE until consulting a pharmacist; specific conditions may apply.

Manufacturer states, "Other IV substances, additives, or medications should not be added to azithromycin, or infused simultaneously through the same IV line." Flush IV line with a **compatible** IV fluid before and after administration.

One source suggests the following **compatibilities:**

Y-site: Bivalirudin (Angiomax), caspofungin (Cancidas), dexmedetomidine (Precedex), diphenhydramine (Benadryl), dolasetron (Anzemet), doripenem (Doribax), droperidol (Inapsine), hetastarch in electrolytes (Hextend), ondansetron (Zofran), tigecycline (Tygacil).

RATE OF ADMINISTRATION

Do not give by IV bolus; must be infused over at least 1 hour.

1 mg/mL dilution: A single dose equally distributed over a minimum of 1 hour; over 3 hours is preferred.

2 mg/mL dilution: A single dose equally distributed over at least 1 hour.

ACTIONS

An azalide (subclass of macrolide) antibiotic. Active against selected organisms, including aerobic and facultative gram-positive and gram-negative organisms and other organisms, including *Chlamydia* and *Mycoplasma pneumoniae*. It is derived from erythromycin but is chemically different. Interferes with microbial protein synthesis by binding a ribosomal subunit of a susceptible microorganism. Concentration in phagocytes may contribute to distribution in inflamed tissues. Activity not affected by beta-lactamase production. Trough levels increase with successive doses. Has a long tissue half-life permitting once-a-day dosing. Eliminated by the liver. Primarily excreted as unchanged drug in bile. Up to 14% excreted in urine within 24 hours.

INDICATIONS AND USES

Treatment of community-acquired pneumonia and pelvic inflammatory disease caused by specific organisms (e.g., *Staphylococcus aureus, Streptococcus pneumoniae, Haemophilus influenzae, Neisseria gonorrhoeae, Chlamydia trachomatis.* See product insert for complete list). Many other indications for oral use.

CONTRAINDICATIONS

Hypersensitivity to azithromycin, erythromycin, or any macrolide antibiotic or ketolide antibiotic (e.g., telithromycin [Ketek]). ▪ Patients with a history of cholestatic jaundice/hepatic dysfunction associated with prior use of azithromycin.

PRECAUTIONS

For IV use only. ▪ Specific sensitivity studies are indicated to determine susceptibility of the causative organism to azithromycin. ▪ To reduce the development of drug-resistant bacteria and maintain its effectiveness, azithromycin should be used only to treat or prevent infections proven or strongly suspected to be caused by bacteria. ▪ Has demonstrated cross-resistance with erythromycin-resistant gram-positive organisms. Most strains of *Enterococcus faecalis* and methicillin-resistant staphylococci are resistant to azithromycin. ▪ Use extreme caution; hypersensitivity reactions have recurred even after azithromycin was discontinued and hypersensitivity reactions treated. Anaphylaxis resulting in fatalities has been reported rarely. ▪ Principally eliminated in the liver; use caution in patients with impaired hepatic function. Hepatotoxicity, including abnormal liver function, hepatitis, cholestatic jaundice, hepatic necrosis, and hepatic failure have been reported; deaths have occurred. ▪ Use caution in patients with impaired renal function; no data available on effects of IV azithromycin. ▪ Use caution in patients with prolonged QT intervals; macrolide antibiotics have caused ventricular arrhythmias, including ventricular tachycardia and torsades de pointes. ▪ Timing of transfer to oral therapy should be based on clinical response. ▪ Avoid prolonged use; superinfection caused by overgrowth of nonsusceptible organisms may result. ▪ *Clostridium difficile*–associated diarrhea (CDAD) has been reported. May range from mild diarrhea to fatal colitis. Consider in patients who present with diarrhea during or after treatment with azithromycin. ▪ May cause exacerbations of symptoms of myasthenia gravis or new onset of myasthenia syndrome.

Monitor: Monitor vital signs. ▪ Observe closely for signs of a hypersensitivity reaction; see Antidote. ▪ Monitoring of liver function may be indicated; see Precautions. ▪ Monitor infusion site for inflammation and/or extravasation. ▪ Contains 4.96 mEq of sodium/vial. Observe for electrolyte imbalance and cardiac irregularities. May aggravate CHF. ▪ See Drug/Lab Interactions and Antidote.

Patient Education: Discontinue azithromycin and report any signs of an allergic reaction immediately (difficulty breathing, itching, rash, swelling). ▪ Discontinue azithromycin and report S/S of hepatitis (e.g., dark urine, jaundice, loss of appetite, malaise, nausea and vomiting). ▪ Promptly report diarrhea or bloody stools that occur during treatment or up to several months after an antibiotic has been discontinued; may indicate CDAD and require treatment.

Maternal/Child: Category B: safety for use during pregnancy and breast-feeding not established; use with caution and only if clearly needed. ▪ Safety and effectiveness for use in pediatric patients under 16 years of age not established. ▪ Has been administered to pediatric patients age 6 months to 16 years by the oral route. The most common side effects in this age-group included abdominal pain, diarrhea, headache, nausea, rash, and vomiting.

Elderly: Response similar to that seen in younger adults. ▪ Consider age-related organ impairment.

DRUG/LAB INTERACTIONS

May have a modest effect on the pharmacokinetics of **atorvastatin** (Lipitor), **carbamazepine** (Tegretol), **cetirizine** (Zyrtec), **didanosine** (Videx), **efavirenz** (Sustiva), **fluconazole** (Diflucan), **indinavir** (Crixivan), **midazolam** (Versed), **rifabutin** (Mycobutin), **sildenafil** (Viagra), **theophylline, sulfamethoxazole/trimethoprim** (Bactrim, Septra), or **zidovudine** (AZT, Retrovir). ▪ **Efavirenz and fluconazole** may have a modest effect on the pharmacokinetics of azithromycin. No dose adjustment is necessary with coadministration of these drugs. ▪ May increase the anticoagulant effects of **warfarin** (Coumadin); monitoring of PT is indicated. ▪ *Other macrolide antibiotics cause interactions when given concomitantly with the following drugs; azithromycin has not been studied.* ▪ May inhibit metabolism and increase serum levels and effects of **cyclosporine** (Sandimmune), **phenytoin** (Dilantin), **and terfenadine;** reduced doses of these drugs may be indicated. ▪ May increase **digoxin levels;** monitoring of digoxin levels is indicated. ▪ May cause acute ergot toxicity (severe peripheral vasospasm and dysesthesia) with **ergotamine or dihydroergotamine.**

SIDE EFFECTS

Usually mild to moderate in severity and reversible after azithromycin discontinued. Abdominal pain; anemia; anorexia; arrhythmias; cough; diarrhea; dizziness; dyspnea; facial edema; fatigue; fungal infections; hypotension; increase in AST, ALT, and/or alkaline phosphatase levels; injection site pain or local inflammation; leukopenia; malaise; nausea; oral candidiasis; pancreatitis; pharyngitis; pleural effusion; rashes; rhinitis; stomatitis; vaginitis; vomiting. Serious abnormal liver function, including hepatitis and cholestatic jaundice, cases of hepatic necrosis, and hepatic failure (some resulting in death) have occurred. Acute interstitial nephritis (fever, joint pain, skin rash) is rare but may cause acute renal failure. Allergic reactions (e.g., angioedema, anaphylaxis, and dermatologic reactions including Stevens-Johnson syndrome and toxic epidermal necrolysis) have been reported rarely and may be fatal; see Precautions. Rare reports of QT prolongation and torsades de pointes have been reported. CDAD has been reported.

ANTIDOTE

Notify physician of any side effects. Discontinue azithromycin for hypersensitivity reactions and S/S of hepatitis. Treat hypersensitivity reactions as indicated and resuscitate as necessary. Additional hypersensitivity reactions have recurred after azithromycin has been discontinued and initial treatment completed. Prolonged observation is required. Mild cases of CDAD may respond to discontinuation of azithromycin. Treat CDAD with fluids, electrolytes, protein supplements, and oral vancomycin (Vancocin) or metronidazole (Flagyl) as indicated. In severe cases, surgical evaluation may be indicated.

AZTREONAM
(az-**TREE**-oh-nam)

Azactam

**Antibacterial
(monobactam)**

pH 4.5 to 7.5

USUAL DOSE

Urinary tract infection: 500 mg to 1 Gm every 8 or 12 hours.

Moderately severe systemic infections: 1 or 2 Gm every 8 to 12 hours.

Severe systemic, or life-threatening infections: 2 Gm every 6 or 8 hours. Use the full suggested dose. Do not exceed 8 Gm/24 hr.

Normal renal function required. Duration of therapy depends on the severity of the infection. Continue for at least 2 days after all symptoms of infection subside. Can produce therapeutic serum levels given intraperitoneally in dialysis fluid.

PEDIATRIC DOSE

See Maternal/Child.

Mild to moderate infections: 30 mg/kg every 8 hours.

Moderate to severe infections: 30 mg/kg every 6 or 8 hours. Maximum recommended dose is 120 mg/kg/24 hr.

Cystic fibrosis: 50 mg/kg every 6 to 8 hours. Maximum dose is 8 Gm/24 hr.

NEONATAL DOSE

Neonatal doses are **unlabeled;** see Maternal/Child.

30 mg/kg/dose. Interval between doses based on age and weight as follows:

Less than 1,200 Gm and 0 to 4 weeks of age: Give every 12 hours.

Less than 2,000 Gm and 0 to 7 days of age: Give every 12 hours.

1,200 to 2,000 Gm and over 7 days of age: Give every 8 hours.

More than 2,000 Gm and 0 to 7 days of age: Give every 8 hours.

More than 2,000 Gm and over 7 days of age: Give every 6 hours.

DOSE ADJUSTMENTS

Dosing in the elderly should be cautious and reduced based on CrCl; consider potential for decreased organ function and concomitant disease or drug therapy. ▪ Prolonged serum levels may occur in patients with renal insufficiency. After an initial loading dose of 1 or 2 Gm, reduce succeeding doses by 50% in patients with CrCl between 10 and 30 mL/min/1.73 M^2. ▪ After an initial loading dose of 500 mg, 1 Gm, or 2 Gm, reduce succeeding doses by 75% in patients with CrCl less than 10 mL/min/1.73 M^2 or in patients supported by dialysis. In addition 12.5% of the maintenance dose may be given after a dialysis session in serious or life-threatening situations.

DILUTION

Usually light yellow, may become slightly pink on standing; does not affect potency.

IV injection: Reconstitute a single dose with 6 to 10 mL of SW for injection. Shake immediately and vigorously. Use immediately and discard any unused solution.

Intermittent IV: Initially reconstitute each single dose with a minimum of 3 mL of SW for injection. Shake immediately and vigorously. Must be further diluted in at least 50 mL of D5W, NS, or other **compatible** infusion solutions for each 1 Gm of aztreonam (see chart on inside back cover or literature). Concentration should not exceed 20 mg/mL or 2% w/v. Available in vials and premixed Galaxy infusion bags.

Storage: Concentrations exceeding 2% should be used promptly unless prepared with SW or NS. Other reconstituted or diluted solutions are stable for 48 hours at room temperature or up to 7 days if refrigerated. Vials are for single use only; discard unused amounts. When specific diluents are used, may be frozen for up to 3 months. Thaw at room temperature (see literature); do not refreeze.

COMPATIBILITY (Underline Indicates Conflicting Compatibility Information)
Consider any drug NOT listed as compatible to be INCOMPATIBLE until consulting a pharmacist; specific conditions may apply.
Manufacturer lists as **incompatible** with metronidazole (Flagyl IV), nafcillin (Nallpen).

One source suggests the following **compatibilities:**
Solution: See chart on inside back cover. Others listed by manufacturer include D5/Ionosol B, Isolyte E, D5/Isolyte E, D5/Isolyte M, Normosol-R, D5/Normosol-R, D5/Normosol-M, Mannitol 5% and 10%, D5/Plasma-Lyte, Travert injection 10%, Travert injection 10% and Electrolytes (multiple).

Additive: Manufacturer lists ampicillin, cefazolin (Ancef), clindamycin (Cleocin), gentamicin, tobramycin, and vancomycin diluted in specific concentrations and in specific solutions and states, "Other admixtures are not recommended."

Other sources list ampicillin/sulbactam (Unasyn), cefoxitin (Mefoxin), ciprofloxacin (Cipro IV), linezolid (Zyvox), vancomycin.

Y-site: Allopurinol (Aloprim), amifostine (Ethyol), amikacin (Amikin), aminophylline, ampicillin, ampicillin/sulbactam (Unasyn), bivalirudin (Angiomax), bleomycin (Blenoxane), bumetanide, buprenorphine (Buprenex), butorphanol (Stadol), calcium gluconate, carboplatin (Paraplatin), carmustine (BiCNU), caspofungin (Cancidas), cefazolin (Ancef), cefepime (Maxipime), cefotaxime (Claforan), cefotetan, cefoxitin (Mefoxin), ceftazidime (Fortaz), ceftriaxone (Rocephin), cefuroxime (Zinacef), ciprofloxacin (Cipro IV), cisatracurium (Nimbex), cisplatin (Platinol), clindamycin (Cleocin), cyclophosphamide (Cytoxan), cytarabine (ARA-C), dacarbazine (DTIC), dactinomycin (Cosmegen), daptomycin (Cubicin), dexamethasone (Decadron), dexmedetomidine (Precedex), diltiazem (Cardizem), diphenhydramine (Benadryl), dobutamine, docetaxel (Taxotere), dopamine, doxorubicin (Adriamycin), doxorubicin liposomal (Doxil), doxycycline, droperidol (Inapsine), enalaprilat (Vasotec IV), etoposide (VePesid), etoposide phosphate (Etopophos), famotidine (Pepcid IV), fenoldopam (Corlopam), filgrastim (Neupogen), fluconazole (Diflucan), fludarabine (Fludara), fluorouracil (5-FU), foscarnet (Foscavir), furosemide (Lasix), gallium nitrate (Ganite), gemcitabine (Gemzar), gentamicin, granisetron (Kytril), haloperidol (Haldol), heparin, hetastarch in electrolytes (Hextend), hydrocortisone sodium succinate (Solu-Cortef), hydromorphone (Dilaudid), idarubicin (Idamycin), ifosfamide (Ifex), imipenem-cilastatin (Primaxin), insulin (regular), leucovorin calcium, linezolid (Zyvox), magnesium sulfate, mannitol, mechlorethamine (nitrogen mustard), melphalan (Alkeran), meperidine (Demerol), mesna (Mesnex), methotrexate, methylprednisolone (Solu-Medrol), metoclopramide (Reglan), morphine, nalbuphine, nicardipine (Cardene IV), ondansetron (Zofran), pemetrexed (Alimta), piperacillin, piperacillin/

tazobactam (Zosyn), potassium chloride (KCl), promethazine (Phenergan), propofol (Diprivan), quinupristin/dalfopristin (Synercid 20 mg/mL), ranitidine (Zantac), remifentanil (Ultiva), sargramostim (Leukine), sodium bicarbonate, sulfamethoxazole/trimethoprim, teniposide (Vumon), theophylline, thiotepa, ticarcillin/clavulanate (Timentin), tigecycline (Tygacil), tobramycin, <u>vancomycin</u>, vinblastine, vincristine, vinorelbine (Navelbine), zidovudine (AZT, Retrovir).

RATE OF ADMINISTRATION
IV injection: A single dose equally distributed over 3 to 5 minutes.
Intermittent IV: A single dose over 20 to 60 minutes. May be given through Y-tube or three-way stopcock of infusion set. Do not infuse simultaneously with other drugs or solutions except in proven **compatibility**. Flush common IV tubing before and after administration.

ACTIONS
A synthetic monobactam antibiotic. Bactericidal through inhibition of bacterial cell wall synthesis to a wide spectrum of specific gram-negative aerobic organisms including *Pseudomonas aeruginosa*. Effective against many otherwise resistant organisms. Therapeutic levels widely distributed into many body fluids and tissues. Peak serum levels reached in 1 hour. Serum half-life averages 1.7 hours; range is 1.5 to 2 hours. Primarily excreted in the urine with some excretion through feces. Crosses placental barrier. Secreted in breast milk.

INDICATIONS AND USES
Treatment of serious lower respiratory tract, urinary tract, skin and skin structure, gynecologic, and intra-abdominal infections and bacterial septicemia. Most effective against specific gram-negative organisms (see literature). ▪ Adjunctive therapy to surgery for the management of infections.

CONTRAINDICATIONS
Known hypersensitivity to aztreonam or its components.

PRECAUTIONS
Specific studies are indicated to identify the causative organism and susceptibility to aztreonam. ▪ To reduce the development of drug-resistant bacteria and maintain its effectiveness, aztreonam should be used to treat or prevent only those infections proven or strongly suspected to be caused by bacteria. ▪ Before C/S data are available, antimicrobial therapy with agents to cover gram-positive and/or anaerobic microorganisms may be indicated. ▪ Avoid prolonged use of drug; superinfection caused by overgrowth of nonsusceptible organisms may result. ▪ Cross-reactivity with other beta-lactam antibiotics (e.g., penicillins, cephalosporins, and/or carbapenems) is rare but can occur with or without prior exposure. Use with caution in patients with a history of hypersensitivity reactions to beta-lactam antibiotics. ▪ *Clostridium difficile*–associated diarrhea (CDAD) has been reported. May range from mild diarrhea to fatal colitis. Consider in patients who present with diarrhea during or after treatment with aztreonam. ▪ Epidermal necrolysis has been reported rarely in patients receiving aztreonam who have undergone BMT and have other risk factors (e.g., graft-versus-host disease, radiation therapy, sepsis).
Monitor: Watch for early symptoms of a hypersensitivity reaction. Use caution in patients with known sensitivity to penicillins, cephalosporins, or carbapenems. ▪ Monitor renal and hepatic function, especially in the elderly. ▪ Monitor renal function with concurrent administration of higher doses or prolonged administration of aminoglycosides (e.g., gentamicin).

■ May cause thrombophlebitis. Use small needles and large veins and rotate infusion sites.

Patient Education: Report pain or burning at injection site or S/S of a hypersensitivity reaction (e.g., difficulty breathing, flushing, itching, rash). ■ Promptly report diarrhea or bloody stools that occur during treatment or up to several months after an antibiotic has been discontinued; may indicate CDAD and require treatment.

Maternal/Child: Category B: use in pregnancy and breast-feeding only if clearly needed. ■ Consider discontinuing breast-feeding. ■ Safety for use in infants under 9 months of age not established. ■ Limited data are available for treatment of infants and pediatric patients with septicemia or skin and skin-structure infections (caused by *H. influenzae* type b). ■ Higher doses of aztreonam may be indicated in pediatric patients with cystic fibrosis. ■ IV route is suggested for pediatric patients; data are limited for IM injection and impaired renal function.

Elderly: Reduced doses may be indicated. Monitor renal function; see Dose Adjustments. ■ Response is similar to that seen in younger patients; however, clearance is decreased and half-life is prolonged.

DRUG/LAB INTERACTIONS

Adverse interaction may occur with **beta-lactamase–inducing antibiotics** (e.g., cefoxitin, imipenem); do not use concurrently. ■ May be used concomitantly with **aminoglycosides** in severe infections. Nephrotoxicity and ototoxicity can be markedly increased when both drugs are utilized. ■ **Probenecid and furosemide** do increase blood levels; not clinically significant. ■ Bactericidal activity of aztreonam may be antagonized by **chloramphenicol** (Chloromycetin). ■ See Side Effects.

SIDE EFFECTS

Full scope of allergic reactions, including anaphylaxis, angioedema, bronchospasm. Burning, discomfort, and pain at injection site; diarrhea; nausea and vomiting; and rash occur most frequently. Abdominal cramps; altered taste; CDAD; confusion; diaphoresis; diplopia; dizziness; dyspnea; elevated alkaline phosphatase, AST, ALT, and SCr; eosinophilia; erythema multiforme; exfoliative dermatitis; fever; halitosis; headache; hematologic changes (e.g., anemia, neutropenia); hepatitis; hypotension; insomnia; jaundice; mouth ulcer; nasal congestion; numb tongue; paresthesia; petechiae; phlebitis/thrombophlebitis; positive Coombs' test; prolonged PT and PTT; pruritus; purpura; seizures; sneezing; tinnitus; transient ECG changes (ventricular bigeminy and PVCs); urticaria; vaginitis; vertigo can occur.

ANTIDOTE

Notify physician of any side effects. Discontinue the drug if indicated. Treat hypersensitivity reactions as indicated and resuscitate as necessary. Mild cases of CDAD may respond to discontinuation of drug. Treat CDAD with fluids, electrolytes, protein supplements, and oral vancomycin (Vancocin) or metronidazole (Flagyl) as indicated. In severe cases, surgical evaluation may be indicated. Hemodialysis or peritoneal dialysis may be useful in overdose.

BASILIXIMAB BBW
(bah-zih-**LIX**-ih-mab)
Simulect

Recombinant monoclonal antibody
Immunosuppressant

USUAL DOSE
Basiliximab should only be administered once it has been determined that the patient will receive the graft and concomitant immunosuppression. Patients who have received a previous course of basiliximab should only be re-exposed to a subsequent course of therapy with extreme caution. Used concurrently with cyclosporine (Sandimmune) and corticosteroids. **Organ rejection prophylaxis in renal transplant:** 2 doses of 20 mg each as an infusion. Administer the first dose within 2 hours before transplantation. Give the second dose 4 days after transplantation. Withhold the second dose if complications such as severe hypersensitivity reactions to basiliximab or graft loss occurs.

PEDIATRIC DOSE
Less than 35 kg: 2 doses of 10 mg each (discard remaining product after each dose).
35 kg or more: 2 doses of 20 mg each.
In all pediatric patients, administer the first dose within 2 hours before transplantation. Give the second dose 4 days after transplantation. See Actions and Maternal/Child. Withhold second dose if complications occur (e.g., hypersensitivity reactions or graft loss).

DOSE ADJUSTMENTS
No dose adjustments indicated.

DILUTION
Reconstitute each single dose with 5 mL of SW. Shake gently to dissolve powder. After reconstitutions may be given as an IV injection or may be further diluted to 50 mL with NS or D5W. When mixing, gently invert to avoid foaming; do not shake.
Storage: Store unopened vials in the refrigerator (2° to 8° C [36° to 46° F]). Should be used within 4 hours of reconstitution. If necessary, may be refrigerated for up to 24 hours. Discard prepared solution after 24 hours.

COMPATIBILITY
Manufacturer states, "Other drug substances should not be added or infused simultaneously through the same IV line." No **incompatibilities** observed with polyvinyl chloride bags and administration sets.

RATE OF ADMINISTRATION
May be given through a peripheral or central vein.
IV injection: May be given as a bolus injection over 30 to 60 seconds. Incidence of N/V and local reaction including pain increased.
Infusion: A single dose properly diluted over 20 to 30 minutes.

ACTIONS
A chimeric (murine/human) monoclonal antibody produced by recombinant DNA technology. Functions as an immunosuppressant. Specifically binds to and blocks the interleukin-2 receptor alpha chain (IL-2Rα, also known as CD25 antigen), thereby inhibiting IL-2 driven proliferation of activated T cells which play a key role in organ rejection. Reduces/minimizes acute rejection. IL-2Rα is expressed selec-

tively on activated, but not resting, T cells. This selectivity prevents the profound generalized immunosuppression seen with other immunosuppressants used in organ transplantation and may decrease the risk of infection and development of lymphoproliferative disorders. Two 20-mg doses block the receptor for 4 to 6 weeks post-transplantation, the critical risk period for acute organ rejection. Has reduced the incidence of biopsy-confirmed acute rejections while minimizing side effects seen with other immunosuppressants. Clinical benefit demonstrated in a broad range of patients, regardless of age, gender, race, donor type, or history of diabetes mellitus as long as serum levels exceed 0.2 mg/mL (by ELISA). Mean half-life is 4 to 10.4 days. Half-life is increased (5.2 to 17.8 days) and distribution volume and clearance are decreased by about 50% in pediatric patients 2 to 11 years of age. Crosses the placental barrier. May be secreted in breast milk.

INDICATIONS AND USES
Prophylaxis of acute organ rejection in patients receiving renal transplants. Used as part of an immunosuppressive regimen that includes cyclosporine and corticosteroids. Dosing regimen may also include either azathioprine (Imuran) or mycophenolate (CellCept IV).

CONTRAINDICATIONS
Known hypersensitivity to basiliximab or any of its components (composite of human and murine antibodies).

PRECAUTIONS
Usually administered by or under the direction of a physician experienced in immunosuppressive therapy and management of organ transplant patients. Adequate laboratory and supportive medical resources must be available. ▪ Severe acute (onset within 24 hours) hypersensitivity reactions including anaphylaxis have been reported both with initial exposure and/or following re-exposure after several months. Emergency equipment and drugs for the treatment of severe hypersensitivity reactions must be readily available. Withhold the second dose of basiliximab if a hypersensitivity reaction occurs. ▪ Re-administration after an initial course of therapy has not been studied in humans, but other monoclonal antibodies have precipitated anaphylactoid reactions. ▪ Potential for causing lymphoproliferative disorders, CMV, and other opportunistic infections is unknown. ▪ Use with caution in patients with infections or malignancies. ▪ It is not known whether basiliximab use will have a long-term effect on the ability of the immune system to respond to antigens first encountered during induced immunosuppression. ▪ Low titers of anti-idiotype antibodies and human antimurine antibodies (HAMA) to basiliximab have been detected in some patients during treatment; no adverse effects have been noted.

Monitor: Obtain baseline CBC with differential and platelets and baseline renal and liver tests if not already completed for other immunosuppressant agents. ▪ Monitor vital signs. ▪ Observe closely for signs of infection (fever, sore throat, tiredness) or unusual bleeding or bruising. ▪ Prophylactic antibiotics may be indicated pending results of C/S in a febrile immunosuppressed patient. ▪ Symptoms of cytokine release syndrome (e.g., chills, fever, dyspnea, and malaise) have not been reported but may occur; observe carefully. ▪ See Drug/Lab Interactions.

Patient Education: Report difficulty in breathing or swallowing, rapid heartbeat, rash, or itching immediately. ▪ Report swelling of lower extremities and weakness. ▪ Avoid pregnancy; nonhormonal birth control preferred.

Women with childbearing potential should use effective contraception before beginning basiliximab therapy, during therapy, and for 2 months after completion. ■ See Appendix D, p. 1434.

Maternal/Child: Category B: use during pregnancy only if benefits justify the potential risk to the fetus. Avoid pregnancy; effective contraception required; see Patient Education. ■ Discontinue breast-feeding. ■ Has been used in pediatric patients from 2 to 15 years of age. No adequate or well-controlled studies completed. See differences in Actions. Most frequent side effects were fever and urinary infections.

Elderly: Age-related dosing not required. Adverse events similar to younger adults. Use caution when giving immunosuppressive drugs to the elderly.

DRUG/LAB INTERACTIONS

Has been administered concurrently with **antilymphocyte globulin** (ALG), **antithymocyte globulin** (ATG), **azathioprine** (Imuran), **corticosteroids, cyclosporine** (Sandimmune), **muromonab CD3** (Orthoclone), **and mycophenolate** (CellCept); no additional adverse reactions noted. ■ **May increase or decrease numerous lab values,** including serum calcium and potassium and fasting blood glucose.

SIDE EFFECTS

Basiliximab did not appear to alter the pattern, frequency, or severity of known side effects associated with the use of immunosuppressive drugs. Abdominal pain, anemia, constipation, diarrhea, edema, fever, headache, hyperkalemia, hypersensitivity reactions (including anaphylaxis, bronchospasm, capillary leak syndrome, cardiac failure, cytokine release syndrome, dyspnea, hypotension, pulmonary edema, pruritus, rash, respiratory failure, sneezing, tachycardia, urticaria, wheezing), hypertension, hypokalemia, insomnia, nausea, pain, peripheral edema, upper respiratory infections, urinary tract infections. Incidence of N/V and local reaction including pain increased with bolus injection. Severe hypersensitivity reactions (including anaphylaxis), capillary leak syndrome, and cytokine release syndrome have been reported. Incidence of infections, lymphomas, or other malignancies similar to placebo groups in studies.

ANTIDOTE

Notify physician of all side effects. Most will be treated symptomatically. Basiliximab may be discontinued or alternate immunosuppressive agents substituted. Discontinue immediately if anaphylaxis occurs, and treat with oxygen, epinephrine, corticosteroids, and/or antihistamines (e.g., diphenhydramine [Benadryl]). Resuscitate as necessary.

BENDAMUSTINE HYDROCHLORIDE
(ben-deh-**MUS**-teen)

Treanda

Antineoplastic
Alkylating agent

pH 2.5 to 3.5

USUAL DOSE

Chronic lymphocytic leukemia (CLL): 100 mg/M^2 as an IV infusion on Days 1 and 2 of a 28-day cycle. May be repeated for up to 6 cycles. Premedication with antihistamines (e.g., diphenhydramine [Benadryl]), antipyretics (e.g., acetaminophen [Tylenol]), and corticosteroids may be indicated; see Monitor and Antidote.

Non-Hodgkin's lymphoma (NHL): 120 mg/M^2 as an IV infusion on Days 1 and 2 of a 21-day cycle. May be repeated for up to 8 cycles.

DOSE ADJUSTMENTS

Chronic lymphocytic leukemia (CLL) and non-Hodgkin's lymphoma (NHL): Delay treatment for Grade 4 hematologic toxicity or clinically significant nonhematologic toxicity equal to or greater than Grade 2. In addition, dose reduction may be indicated; see specific indication. Reinitiate treatment, if indicated, when nonhematologic toxicity has recovered to equal to or less than Grade 1 and/or the ANC has recovered to equal to or greater than 1,000 cells/mm^3 and platelets have recovered to equal to or greater than 75,000 cells/mm^3. ▪ No dose adjustment indicated based on age, gender, or race; see Precautions.

Chronic lymphocytic leukemia (CLL): Reduce dose to 50 mg/M^2 on Days 1 and 2 of each cycle for Grade 3 or greater hematologic toxicity. If Grade 3 or greater toxicity recurs, reduce dose to 25 mg/M^2 on Days 1 and 2 of each cycle. ▪ Reduce dose to 50 mg/M^2 on Days 1 and 2 of each cycle for clinically significant Grade 3 or greater nonhematologic toxicity. ▪ Dose re-escalation in subsequent cycles may be considered by the treating physician.

Non-Hodgkin's lymphoma (NHL): Reduce dose to 90 mg/M^2 on Days 1 and 2 of each cycle for Grade 4 hematologic toxicity. If Grade 4 toxicity recurs, reduce the dose to 60 mg/M^2 on Days 1 and 2 of each cycle. ▪ Reduce dose to 90 mg/M^2 on Days 1 and 2 of each cycle for Grade 3 or greater nonhematologic toxicity. If Grade 3 or greater toxicity recurs, reduce the dose to 60 mg/M^2 on Days 1 and 2 of each cycle.

DILUTION

Specific techniques required; see Precautions: Reconstitute each 25-mg vial with 5 mL of SWI and each 100-mg vial with 20 mL of SWI; concentration is 5 mg/mL. Shake well. Should completely dissolve within 5 minutes. Do not use if particulate matter is observed. Within 30 minutes of reconstitution, withdraw the desired dose from the vial(s) and further dilute in 500 mL NS or D2.5/½ NS. Final concentration of infusion solution should be 0.2 to 0.6 mg/mL. Mix thoroughly; solution should be clear and colorless to slightly yellow.

Filters: Specific information not available.

Storage: Protect unopened vials from light in original package and store at CRT. Solution diluted in NS or D2.5/½ NS is stable for 3 hours at CRT and room light or for 24 hours refrigerated at 2° to 8° C (36° to 47° F).

Administration must be completed within these times (e.g., 3 or 24 hours based on type of storage). Discard any unused solution.

COMPATIBILITY

Manufacturer states, "**Compatibility** with other diluents has not been determined."

RATE OF ADMINISTRATION

Chronic lymphocytic leukemia (CLL): Total daily dose as an infusion equally distributed over 30 minutes.

Non-Hodgkin's lymphoma (NHL): Total daily dose as an infusion equally distributed over 60 minutes.

ACTIONS

A bifunctional mechlorethamine derivative. An alkylating agent. Active against both quiescent and dividing cells. Exact mode of action unknown. May lead to cell death by damaging the DNA in cancer cells as well as by disrupting normal cell division. Highly protein bound. Distributes freely in human red blood cells. Primarily metabolized via hydrolysis to metabolites with low cytotoxic activity and excreted in feces.

INDICATIONS AND USES

Treatment of patients with chronic lymphocytic leukemia (CLL). Has resulted in a delay in disease progression, and some patients had no signs of disease in their blood after treatment. Effectiveness compared with first-line therapies other than chlorambucil (Leukeran) has not been studied. ▪ Treatment of patients with indolent B-cell non-Hodgkin's lymphoma that has progressed during or within 6 months of treatment with rituximab (Rituxan) or a rituximab-containing regimen.

CONTRAINDICATIONS

Known hypersensitivity to bendamustine or mannitol.

PRECAUTIONS

Follow guidelines for handling cytotoxic agents. See Appendix A, p. 1429. ▪ Administered by or under the direction of the physician specialist in a facility equipped to monitor the patient and respond to any medical emergency. ▪ Do not use in patients with a CrCl less than 40 mL/min. Use with caution in patients with mild or moderate renal impairment; no formal studies conducted. ▪ Use with caution in patients with mild hepatic impairment. Do not use in patients with moderate hepatic impairment (AST or ALT 2.5 to 10 times the ULN and total bilirubin 1.5 to 3 times the ULN) or severe hepatic impairment (total bilirubin greater than 3 times the ULN). No formal studies conducted. ▪ Myelosuppression may be severe and require a dose delay. Deaths from myelosuppression-related adverse reactions have occurred. ▪ Infections, including pneumonia and sepsis, have been reported. Has been associated with septic shock and death. ▪ Infusion and/or hypersensitivity reactions are common and have resulted in anaphylaxis (rare). Usually occur in the second and/or subsequent cycles of therapy. ▪ Tumor lysis syndrome (TLS) has been reported and may occur in the first treatment cycle. S/S are rapid reduction in tumor volume, renal insufficiency, hyperkalemia, hypocalcemia, hyperuricemia, or hyperphosphatemia. May lead to acute renal failure and death. ▪ Skin reactions, including rash, toxic skin reactions, and bullous exanthema, have been reported; see Drug/Lab Interactions and Antidote. ▪ Premalignant and malignant diseases, including myelodysplastic syndrome, myeloproliferative disorders, acute myeloid leukemia, and bronchial carcinoma have been reported. Causal relationship has not been determined.

Monitor: Obtain baseline CBC with differential and platelet count. Monitor CBC with differential weekly, and monitor platelet count each cycle. Hematologic nadir usually occurs in the third week. If recovery to recommended values does not occur before Day 28, delay dose until recovery occurs. ▪ Obtain baseline CrCl, AST, ALT, and total bilirubin; repeat as indicated. ▪ Monitor closely for S/S of infusion or hypersensitivity reactions (e.g., chills, fever, pruritus, rash). Discontinue bendamustine if a severe reaction occurs. Inquire about possible symptoms that suggest a minor reaction after the first infusion. Consider premedication with antihistamines (e.g., diphenhydramine [Benadryl]), antipyretics (e.g., acetaminophen [Tylenol]), and corticosteroids in patients who have experienced a Grade 1 or 2 infusion reaction; see Antidote. ▪ Monitor for S/S of TLS. In patients at risk for TLS, prevention and treatment of hyperuricemia may be accomplished with adequate hydration. Allopurinol has been used during the beginning of bendamustine therapy; see Drug/Lab Interactions. Monitor uric acid levels. Monitor electrolytes, particularly potassium, and treat as indicated. ▪ Monitor patients with skin reactions closely. Withhold or discontinue bendamustine if skin reactions are severe or progressive. ▪ Use prophylactic antiemetics to reduce nausea and vomiting and increase patient comfort. ▪ Observe for S/S of infection (e.g., fever). Prophylactic antibiotics may be indicated pending results of C/S in a febrile neutropenic patient. ▪ Monitor for thrombocytopenia (platelet count less than 50,000 cells/mm^3). Initiate precautions to prevent excessive bleeding (e.g., inspect IV sites, skin, and mucous membranes; use extreme care during invasive procedures; test urine, emesis, stool, and secretions for occult blood). ▪ Monitor IV site for signs of extravasation during and after administration (e.g., infection, pain, redness, swelling, necrosis); extravasation has resulted in hospitalization.

Patient Education: Avoid pregnancy; nonhormonal birth control is recommended for both men and women throughout treatment and for 3 months after treatment is complete; report a suspected pregnancy immediately. May pose a risk to reproductive capacity in both males and females. ▪ Promptly report signs of infection (e.g., chills, fever) or allergic reaction (e.g., dyspnea, itching, rash). ▪ Report IV site burning or stinging promptly. ▪ See Appendix D, p. 1434.

Maternal/Child: Category D: avoid pregnancy; can cause fetal harm. May also cause impaired spermatogenesis, azoospermia, and total germinal aplasia in males. Males and females of childbearing age must use birth control. ▪ If the drug is used during pregnancy or if the patient becomes pregnant during therapy, inform the patient of the potential hazard to the fetus. ▪ Has the potential for serious side effects; discontinue breast-feeding. ▪ Safety and effectiveness for use in pediatric patients not established.

Elderly: Side effect profile similar for all age-groups studied.

Chronic lymphocytic leukemia (CLL): Response to bendamustine was improved in all age-groups over the response to chlorambucil; however, response in the elderly was less than in younger adults. The progression-free survival time was somewhat longer for younger adults compared with those 65 years of age or older.

Non-Hodgkin's lymphoma (NHL): Effectiveness and duration of response similar for all age-groups.

DRUG/LAB INTERACTIONS

No formal drug interaction studies have been conducted. ▪ Active metabolites of bendamustine are formed via cytochrome P_{450} CYP1A2. **Inhibitors of CYP1A2** (e.g., ciprofloxacin [Cipro], fluvoxamine [Luvox]) may increase plasma concentrations of bendamustine and decrease plasma concentrations of active metabolites. **Inducers of CYP1A2** (e.g., omeprazole [Prilosec], smoking) may decrease plasma concentrations of bendamustine and increase plasma concentrations of its active metabolites. Use caution or consider alternative treatments if concomitant treatment with CYP1A2 inhibitors or inducers is indicated. ▪ Not likely to inhibit metabolism via other selected CYP isoenzymes or to induce the metabolism of substrates of cytochrome P_{450} enzymes. ▪ Cases of Stevens-Johnson syndrome (SJS) and toxic epidermal necrolysis (TEN) have been reported with concomitant administration of **allopurinol and other medications known to cause these syndromes** (e.g., rituximab [Rituxan]). ▪ *In vitro* data suggest that the breast cancer resistance protein (BCRP) and/or other efflux transporters may have a role in bendamustine transport.

SIDE EFFECTS

Anorexia, constipation, cough, diarrhea, dyspnea, fatigue, fever, headache, myelosuppression (anemia, febrile neutropenia, leukopenia, neutropenia, thrombocytopenia), nausea, rash, stomatitis, and vomiting were most common. Other side effects reported include asthenia; chills; decreased CrCl; dry mouth; elevated AST, ALT, and bilirubin levels; herpes simplex; hypersensitivity and/or infusion reactions (e.g., anaphylaxis [rare], pruritus, rash); hypertension; hyperuricemia; infections; lymphopenia; malaise; malignancies; mucosal inflammation; nasopharyngitis; pneumonia; sepsis; somnolence; stomatitis; TLS; and weakness. Hypersensitivity reactions and fever required study withdrawal in some patients.
Post-Marketing: Anaphylaxis, extravasation resulting in hospitalization, infusion site reactions (irritation, pain, phlebitis, pruritus, swelling), Stevens-Johnson syndrome, and toxic epidermal necrolysis.
Overdose: Ataxia, cardiac arrhythmias, convulsions, respiratory distress, sedation, tremor.

ANTIDOTE

Keep physician informed of all side effects and hematologic parameters. Side effects may decrease in severity with reduced dose. Bone marrow depression may require withholding bendamustine until recovery occurs. Administration of whole blood products (e.g., packed RBCs, platelets, leukocytes) may be required. Selected blood modifiers (e.g., erythropoiesis-stimulating agents [ESAs (Aranesp, Epogen, Mircera)], filgrastim [Neupogen], oprelvekin [Neumega], pegfilgrastim [Neulasta], sargramostim [Leukine]) may be indicated to treat bone marrow toxicity. Discontinue the infusion immediately for any life-threatening side effect (e.g., clinically significant bronchospasm, cardiac arrhythmias, severe hypotension). Consider premedication with antihistamines (e.g., diphenhydramine [Benadryl]), antipyretics (e.g., acetaminophen [Tylenol]), and corticosteroids in subsequent cycles in patients who have experienced a Grade 1 or 2 hypersensitivity and/or infusion reaction. Grade 3 or 4 reactions have not typically been re-challenged, consider discontinuing bendamustine. Withhold or discontinue bendamustine if skin reactions are severe or progressive. There is no specific antidote. Supportive therapy as indicated will help sustain the patient in toxicity.

BEVACIZUMAB BBW
(beh-vah-**SIZZ**-ih-mab)

Avastin

Recombinant monoclonal antibody
Angiogenesis inhibitor
Antineoplastic

pH 6.2

USUAL DOSE
Do not begin therapy until at least 28 days after major surgery. Surgical incisions should be fully healed. May be used in combination with other antineoplastic agents or as a single agent. See Dose Adjustments, Monitor, and Precautions. Continue treatment until disease progression or unacceptable toxicity occurs.

Metastatic carcinoma of the colon or rectum: Administered as an infusion once every 2 weeks. 5 mg/kg when used in combination with bolus IFL (irinotecan [Camptosar], fluorouracil [5-FU], leucovorin calcium). 10 mg/kg when used in combination with FOLFOX4 (fluorouracil [5-FU], leucovorin calcium, and oxaliplatin [Eloxatin]).

Nonsquamous, non–small cell lung cancer: 15 mg/kg as an infusion every 3 weeks in combination with carboplatin (Paraplatin) and paclitaxel (Taxol).

Metastatic breast cancer: 10 mg/kg every 2 weeks in combination with paclitaxel (Taxol).

Glioblastoma: 10 mg/kg every 2 weeks.

Metastatic renal cell carcinoma: 10 mg/kg every 2 weeks in combination with interferon alfa.

DOSE ADJUSTMENTS
No dose adjustments are recommended based on age, gender, or race. ▪ No dose adjustments are recommended for patients with impaired hepatic or renal function; bevacizumab was not studied in these patients. ▪ Permanently discontinue if GI perforation, fistula formation in the GI tract (e.g., enterocutaneous, esophageal, duodenal, rectal), intra-abdominal abscess, fistula formation involving an internal organ, wound dehiscence (parting of the sutured lips of a surgical wound) or wound healing complications requiring medical intervention, serious bleeding, a severe arterial thromboembolic event, nephrotic syndrome, hypertensive crisis or hypertensive encephalopathy, or reversible posterior leukoencephalopathy syndrome (RPLS) develops; see Monitor and Precautions. ▪ Temporarily discontinue if moderate to severe proteinuria (equal to or greater than 2 Gm), severe hypertension not controlled with medical management, and/or a severe infusion reaction occurs; see Monitor and Precautions. ▪ Withhold bevacizumab for at least 4 weeks before elective surgery (half-life is approximately 20 days but has a wide range). Incision must be fully healed before therapy is resumed.

DILUTION
Available in single-use vials containing 100 mg in 4 mL or 400 mg in 16 mL (25 mg/mL). Calculate desired dose and choose the appropriate vial or combination of vials. Must be further diluted to a total volume of 100 mL with NS. Withdraw and discard a volume of NS equal to the volume of the dose of bevacizumab from an infusion container of 100 mL

NS. Then withdraw the desired volume of bevacizumab and add to the NS to achieve a total volume of 100 mL for infusion.

Filters: Not required by manufacturer; however, studies using a 0.2-micron in-line filter were done, and drug potency appeared to be maintained.

Storage: Store in original carton in refrigerator at 2° to 8° C (36° to 46° F). Protect from light. ***Do not shake or freeze.*** Diluted solutions may be refrigerated for up to 8 hours. Contains no preservatives; unused portions must be discarded.

COMPATIBILITY

Manufacturer states, "Should not be administered with or mixed with dextrose solutions." **Incompatibilities** with polyvinylchloride or polyolefin bags have not been observed.

RATE OF ADMINISTRATION

Do not administer as an IV push or bolus. Must be given as an infusion. Administer following concurrent chemotherapy. Infusion reactions are not common but may occur; see Monitor.

Initial infusion: A single dose equally distributed over 90 minutes.

Second infusion: If the initial infusion is well tolerated, the second infusion may be administered equally distributed over 60 minutes.

Subsequent infusions: If the 60-minute infusion is well tolerated, subsequent infusions may be administered equally distributed over 30 minutes.

ACTIONS

A humanized IgG$_1$ monoclonal antibody produced by recombinant DNA technology. Has anti-angiogenesis properties; it binds to and inhibits the biologic activity of human vascular endothelial growth factor (VEGF). The interaction of VEGF with its receptors leads to endothelial cell proliferation and new blood vessel formation. By binding VEGF, bevacizumab prevents the interaction of VEGF with its receptors on the surface of endothelial cells, thus inhibiting the development of new blood vessels around tumors (a tumor-starving mechanism) and resulting in a reduction of microvascular growth and an inhibition of metastatic disease progression. Predicted time to steady-state was 100 days. Half-life is approximately 20 days (range is 11 to 50 days). IgG antibodies may cross the placental barrier and be secreted in breast milk.

INDICATIONS AND USES

First-line or second-line treatment of metastatic carcinoma of the colon or rectum. Used in combination with intravenous 5-fluorouracil–based chemotherapy (e.g., IFL, FOLFOX4). Effectiveness as a single agent has not been established. ■ First-line treatment of patients with unresectable, locally advanced, recurrent, or metastatic nonsquamous, non–small cell lung cancer. Given in combination with carboplatin and paclitaxel. ■ Treatment of metastatic breast cancer in patients who have not received chemotherapy for metastatic Her-2–negative breast cancer. Given in combination with paclitaxel. Not indicated for disease progression following anthracycline and taxane chemotherapy administered for metastatic disease. ■ Treatment of glioblastoma as a single agent for patients with progressive disease following prior therapy. ■ Treatment of metastatic renal cell cancer. Given in combination with interferon alfa.

CONTRAINDICATIONS

Manufacturer states, "No known contraindications." However, bevacizumab must be discontinued if GI perforation, wound dehiscence requiring medical intervention, serious bleeding, nephrotic syndrome, or hypertensive crisis develops. ▪ Use with caution in patients with known hypersensitivity to murine proteins, bevacizumab, or any of its components. ▪ Not recommended for use in patients with recent hemoptysis (greater than or equal to ½ teaspoon of red blood).

PRECAUTIONS

Do not administer as an IV push or bolus. Must be given as an infusion. ▪ Should be administered by or under the direction of a physician specialist in a facility equipped to monitor the patient and respond to any medical emergency. ▪ Has been shown to impair wound healing; withhold bevacizumab for a minimum of 28 days after major surgery; surgical incision must be fully healed. Withhold at least 28 days before elective surgery (half-life is approximately 20 days but has a wide range). Appropriate intervals between surgery and the beginning of bevacizumab therapy and/or the end of bevacizumab therapy and subsequent elective surgery have not been determined. ▪ GI perforation with or without fistula formation and/or intra-abdominal abscesses have occurred at various times during treatment; deaths have been reported. Consider GI perforation in any patient with complaints of abdominal pain associated with constipation, fever, nausea, and vomiting. ▪ Nongastrointestinal fistula formation has been reported, in some cases with a fatal outcome. Fistula formations involving tracheo-esophageal, bronchopleural, biliary, vaginal, renal, and bladder areas have been reported. ▪ Severe or fatal hemorrhage, including CNS hemorrhage, epistaxis, GI bleed, hemoptysis, and vaginal bleeding occurred up to five times more frequently in patients receiving bevacizumab. Do not administer bevacizumab to patients with serious bleeding or hemoptysis. ▪ Permanently discontinue bevacizumab in patients with gastrointestinal perforation, wound dehiscence requiring medical intervention, and recent hemoptysis of equal to or greater than ½ teaspoon of red blood; see Antidote. ▪ May cause severe hypertension that may be persistent. Treatment is required. Complications can include hypertensive encephalopathy and CNS hemorrhage; see Monitor and Antidote. ▪ Reversible posterior leukoencephalopathy syndrome (RPLS) has been reported. May present with blindness and other visual and neurologic disturbances, confusion, headache, lethargy, and seizures. Mild to severe hypertension may be present. MRI is required to confirm diagnosis. Symptoms usually resolve gradually with discontinuation of bevacizumab and treatment of hypertension. ▪ Severe neutropenia, febrile neutropenia, and infection with neutropenia have been reported in patients treated with myelosuppressive chemotherapy plus bevacizumab. ▪ Proteinuria occurred during studies and progressed to nephrotic syndrome in some patients. Findings consistent with thrombotic microangiopathy have been found on kidney biopsy in some patients. In other patients, proteinuria decreased within several months after therapy was discontinued. ▪ CHF has been reported. Incidence is higher in patients receiving bevacizumab who have received prior or concurrent anthracyclines (e.g., doxorubicin [Adriamycin], idarubicin [Idamycin]) and/or left chest wall irradiation. ▪ Infusion reactions are infrequent but have occurred. S/S may include chest pain, diaphoresis, Grade 3 hypersensitivity, headache, hypertension, hypertensive crisis associated with neurologic S/S, oxygen desaturation, rigors, and wheezing. ▪ Serious and sometimes fatal arterial thromboembolic events (e.g., CVA [stroke], MI, TIA, angina) and venous thromboembolic events (e.g., deep vein thrombosis, intra-abdominal thrombosis) have been reported. Incidence is greater with bevacizumab given in combination with chemotherapy as compared to those receiving chemotherapy alone. Risk increased in patients with a history of arterial thromboembolism and in patients greater than 65 years of age. ▪ A protein substance, it has the potential for producing immunogenicity; however, high-titer human anti-bevacizumab antibodies were not detected in studies. ▪ See Drug/Lab Interactions and Antidote.

Monitor: Obtain baseline BP, CBC with differential and platelets, electrolytes, and urinalysis. ▪ Monitor for S/S of an infusion reaction (e.g., bronchospasm, chills, dyspnea, fever, hypotension, itching, rash, stridor, wheezing). ▪ Monitor V/S and BP at least every 2 weeks; monitor more frequently in patients with hypertension. ACE inhibitors, beta-blockers, calcium channel blockers, and diuretics may be used to manage hypertension. Continue to monitor BP at regular intervals after therapy is discontinued. ▪ Repeat CBC with differential and platelets and electrolytes as indicated. ▪ Use of prophylactic antibiotics may be indicated pending C/S in a febrile, neutropenic patient. ▪ Obtain serial urinalyses in patients with 1+ proteinuria. Obtain 24-hour urine collections in patients with new-onset, worsening proteinuria or 2+ proteinuria. Monitor patients with moderate to severe proteinuria until improvement and/or resolution is observed. Repeat urinalyses and/or 24-hour urine collections as indicated. ▪ Monitor for S/S of CHF (e.g., cyanosis, dyspnea on mild exertion, edema, fatigue on exertion, hypoxemia, intolerance to cold, jugular venous distention, orthopnea, pulmonary rales, tachycardia, third heart sound). ▪ Check surgical wounds for wound dehiscence and monitor for S/S of bleeding or GI perforation (e.g., abdominal pain, constipation, epistaxis, fever, hypotension, nausea and vomiting). ▪ See Dose Adjustments, Rate of Administration, Precautions, and Antidote.

Patient Education: Avoid pregnancy during treatment and for an extended period after completion of therapy (some drug could remain in the system for up to 6 months or more). Nonhormonal birth control recommended; see Maternal/Child. Women should report a suspected pregnancy immediately. ▪ Full disclosure of health history is imperative. ▪ Report any unusual or unexpected symptoms or side effects promptly (e.g., abdominal pain, bleeding from any source, constipation, dyspnea, persistent cough, sudden onset of worsening neurologic function, vomiting, wound separation). ▪ See Appendix D, p. 1434.

Maternal/Child: Category C: use during pregnancy or in any woman not using adequate contraception only if potential benefit justifies potential risk to fetus. Adverse fetal outcomes have been observed in rabbits. Angiogenesis is critical to fetal development. Inhibition of angiogenesis by bevacizumab is likely to harm a fetus. ▪ Discontinue breast-feeding during treatment with bevacizumab and for a prolonged period following treatment (half-life may be up to 50 days). ▪ Safety and effectiveness for use in pediatric patients not established. ▪ Dose-related physeal dysplasia (variations in the growth plate) occurred in tested juvenile monkeys; partially reversible after therapy is discontinued. ▪ See Pediatric Dose.

Elderly: Overall survival was similar compared to younger adults; however, the incidence of some side effects was increased (e.g., anemia, anorexia, arterial thromboembolic events [e.g., CVA (stroke), MI, TIA, angina], asthenia, CHF, constipation, deep thrombophlebitis, dehydration, diarrhea, dyspepsia, edema, epistaxis, fatigue, GI hemorrhage, hypertension, hypokalemia, hyponatremia, hypotension, ileus, increased cough, leukopenia, nausea and vomiting, proteinuria, sepsis, venous thromboembolic events [e.g., deep vein thrombosis, intra-abdominal thrombosis, pulmonary embolism], voice alteration).

DRUG/LAB INTERACTIONS

Drug interaction studies have not been completed. ▪ Has been administered concurrently with a regimen of **irinotecan, 5-fluorouracil, and leucovorin.** Studies indicate no significant effect of bevacizumab on the pharmacokinetics of irinotecan or its active metabolite SN-38. ▪ Has been administered with **carboplatin, paclitaxel, and interferon alfa.** ▪ Several cases of microangiopathic hemolytic anemia (MAHA) have been reported in patients with solid tumors who are receiving concomitant therapy with bevacizumab and **sunitinib malate** (Sutent). This combination therapy is not approved and not recommended. ▪ **ACE inhibitors, beta-blockers, calcium channel blockers, and diuretics** have been coadministered to control hypertension.

SIDE EFFECTS

The most common side effects include back pain, dry skin, epistaxis, exfoliative dermatitis, headache, hypertension, lacrimation (excess), proteinuria, rectal hemorrhage, rhinitis, and taste alteration. Major, dose-limiting, and potentially life-threatening side effects include arterial thromboembolic events (e.g., angina, cerebral infarction, MI, TIA), bleeding episodes (e.g., CNS hemorrhage, epistaxis [severe], GI hemorrhage, hemoptysis, vaginal bleeding), GI perforations, hypertensive crises, nongastric intestinal fistula formation, proteinuria and/or nephrotic syndrome, reversible posterior leukoencephalopathy syndrome (RPLS), and surgery and wound healing complications. Other reported side effects included abdominal pain, abnormal gait, alopecia, anorexia, asthenia, bilirubinemia, CHF, colitis, confusion, constipation, cough, dehydration, diarrhea, dizziness, dry mouth, dyspepsia, dysphonia, dyspnea, edema, fatigue, flatulence, hematologic toxicity (e.g., anemia, leukopenia, neutropenia, thrombocytopenia), hypokalemia, hyponatremia, hypotension, ileus, infection, myalgia, nail disorder, nausea, pain, pneumonitis, renal thrombotic microangiopathy (manifested as severe proteinuria), sensory neuropathy, sepsis, skin discoloration, skin ulcer, stomatitis, syncope, venous thromboembolic events (e.g., deep vein thrombosis, intra-abdominal thrombosis, pulmonary embolism), voice alteration, vomiting, urinary frequency and urgency, weight loss.

Post-Marketing: Anastomotic ulceration, acute hypertensive episodes, GI fistula formation (e.g., gastrointestinal, enterocutaneous, esophageal, duodenal, rectal), GI perforation, intestinal necrosis, intra-abdominal abscess, mesenteric venous occlusion, nasal septum perforation, pancytopenia, polyserositis, pulmonary hypertension.

ANTIDOTE

Keep physician informed of all side effects. May constitute a medical emergency or will be treated symptomatically as indicated. Permanently discontinue if any of the following develop: GI perforation, fistula formation in the GI tract (e.g., enterocutaneous, esophageal, duodenal, rectal), intra-abdominal abscess, fistula formation involving an internal organ, wound dehiscence requiring medical intervention, serious bleeding requiring medical intervention, nephrotic syndrome, a severe arterial thromboembolic event, reversible posterior leukoencephalopathy syndrome, hypertensive crisis, or hypertensive encephalopathy. Treat these side effects aggressively; see Precautions and Monitor. Discontinue bevacizumab for severe infusion reactions and treat as indicated (e.g., epinephrine, diphenhydramine [Benadryl], IV fluids, oxygen). Data on rechallenge not available. Temporarily discontinue if moderate to severe proteinuria (equal to or greater than 2 Gm) occurs. Resume therapy when proteinuria is less than 2 Gm/24hr; see Monitor and Precautions. Temporarily discontinue if severe hypertension not controlled with medical management occurs; see Monitor and Precautions. Thromboembolic events (e.g., deep vein thrombosis, intra-abdominal thrombosis, pulmonary embolism) were treated with full-dose warfarin (Coumadin) during clinical trials. Monitor INR closely. Bleeding occurred in patients with elevated INRs; relationship to bevacizumab not determined. Withhold bevacizumab for at least 28 days before elective surgery (half-life is approximately 20 days but has a wide range). Incision must be fully healed before therapy is resumed.

BIVALIRUDIN

(**by**-val-ih-**ROO**-din)

Angiomax

Anticoagulant

pH 5 to 6

USUAL DOSE

Obtain baseline blood tests before administration; see Monitor and Drug/Lab Interactions. Initiate just prior to percutaneous coronary intervention (PCI). Given in combination with aspirin.

Aspirin: 300 to 325 mg before PCI and daily thereafter.

Bivalirudin: Begin with an IV bolus dose of 0.75 mg/kg. Follow with an infusion at 1.75 mg/kg/hr for the duration of the PCI procedure. Perform an ACT 5 minutes after the bolus dose has been administered. An additional bolus dose of 0.3 mg/kg should be given if needed (e.g., ACT less than 225 seconds). The infusion may be continued for 4 hours postprocedure at the discretion of the treating physician. After 4 hours a reduced infusion rate of 0.2 mg/kg/hr may be administered for up to 20 hours if indicated. Administration with glycoprotein GPIIb/IIIa inhibitors (e.g., abciximab [ReoPro], eptifibatide [Integrilin], tirofiban [Aggrastat]) should be considered in any of the following circumstances:

- Decreased flow or reflow
- Dissection with decreased flow
- New or suspected thrombus
- Persistent residual stenosis
- Distal embolization
- Unplanned stent placement
- Suboptimal stenting
- Side branch closure
- Abrupt closure, clinical instability
- Prolonged ischemia

DOSE ADJUSTMENTS

Reduce infusion rate in impaired renal function as indicated in the following chart. No reduction in the bolus dose is needed.

Guidelines for Bivalirudin Dose Adjustments in Impaired Renal Function*	
Renal Function (GFR)	Infusion Rate (mg/kg/hr)
GFR >30 mL/min	1.75 mg/kg/hr
GFR 10 to 29 mL/min	1 mg/kg/hr
Patients on hemodialysis	0.25 mg/kg/hr

*The ACT should be monitored in renally impaired patients.

DILUTION

Bolus and initial infusion: Reconstitute each 250-mg vial with 5 mL SW. Gently swirl to dissolve. Each 250-mg vial must be further diluted in 50 mL of D5W or NS to yield a final concentration of 5 mg/mL (e.g., 1 vial in 50 mL, 2 vials in 100 mL, and 5 vials in 250 mL).

Low rate or subsequent infusion: After reconstitution as above, the 250-mg vial should be further diluted in 500 mL of D5W or NS to yield a final concentration of 0.5 mg/mL.
Storage: Store unopened vials at RT. Do not freeze reconstituted or diluted solution. Reconstituted solution stable for 24 hours refrigerated. Concentrations between 0.5 mg/mL and 5 mg/mL are stable at CRT for up to 24 hours. Discard unused portion of reconstituted solution.

COMPATIBILITY   (Underline Indicates Conflicting Compatibility Information)
Consider any drug NOT listed as compatible to be INCOMPATIBLE until consulting a pharmacist; specific conditions may apply.
Manufacturer lists alteplase (Activase, tPA), amiodarone (Nexterone), amphotericin B (generic), chlorpromazine (Thorazine), diazepam (Valium), <u>dobutamine</u>, prochlorperazine (Compazine), reteplase (Retavase, r-PA), streptokinase, and vancomycin as **incompatible** through the same IV line (**Y-site** or piggyback). No **incompatibilities** observed with glass bottles or polyvinyl chloride bags and administration sets.

One source suggests the following **compatibilities:**
Y-site: Abciximab (ReoPro), alfentanil (Alfenta), amikacin (Amikin), aminophylline, ampicillin, ampicillin/sulbactam (Unasyn), atropine, azithromycin (Zithromax), aztreonam (Azactam), bumetanide, butorphanol (Stadol), calcium gluconate, cefazolin (Ancef), cefepime (Maxipime), cefotaxime (Claforan), cefotetan, cefoxitin (Mefoxin), ceftazidime (Fortaz), ceftriaxone (Rocephin), cefuroxime (Zinacef), ciprofloxacin (Cipro IV), clindamycin (Cleocin), dexamethasone (Decadron), digoxin (Lanoxin), diltiazem (Cardizem), diphenhydramine (Benadryl), <u>dobutamine</u>, dopamine, doxycycline, droperidol (Inapsine), enalaprilat (Vasotec IV), ephedrine, epinephrine (Adrenalin), epoprostenol (Flolan), eptifibatide (Integrilin), erythromycin (Erythrocin), esmolol (Brevibloc), famotidine (Pepcid IV), fentanyl (Sublimaze), fluconazole (Diflucan), furosemide (Lasix), gentamicin, haloperidol (Haldol), heparin, hydrocortisone sodium succinate (Solu-Cortef), hydromorphone (Dilaudid), inamrinone (Amrinone), isoproterenol (Isuprel), labetalol (Trandate), levofloxacin (Levaquin), lidocaine, lorazepam (Ativan), magnesium, mannitol (Osmitrol), meperidine (Demerol), methylprednisolone (Solu-Medrol), metoclopramide (Reglan), metoprolol (Lopressor), metronidazole (Flagyl IV), midazolam (Versed), milrinone (Primacor), morphine, nalbuphine, nitroglycerin IV, nitroprusside sodium, norepinephrine (Levophed), phenylephrine (Neo-Synephrine), piperacillin, piperacillin/tazobactam (Zosyn), potassium chloride, procainamide (Pronestyl), promethazine (Phenergan), ranitidine (Zantac), sodium bicarbonate, sufentanil (Sufenta), sulfamethoxazole/trimethoprim, theophylline, thiopental (Pentothal), ticarcillin/clavulanate (Timentin), tirofiban (Aggrastat), tobramycin, verapamil, warfarin (Coumadin).

RATE OF ADMINISTRATION
The following chart details by patient weight in kilograms, the amount of the bolus dose, the rate in mL/hr of the initial infusion, and the rate in mL/hr of the subsequent infusion.

Bivalirudin Dosing Guidelines

Weight (kg)	Using 5 mg/mL Concentration		Using 0.5 mg/mL Concentration
	Bolus (0.75 mg/kg) (mL)	Infusion (1.75 mg/kg/hr) (mL/hr)	Subsequent Low-rate Infusion (0.2 mg/kg/hr) (mL/hr)
43-47	7 mL	16 mL/hr	18 mL/hr
48-52	7.5 mL	17.5 mL/hr	20 mL/hr
53-57	8 mL	19 mL/hr	22 mL/hr
58-62	9 mL	21 mL/hr	24 mL/hr
63-67	10 mL	23 mL/hr	26 mL/hr
68-72	10.5 mL	24.5 mL/hr	28 mL/hr
73-77	11 mL	26 mL/hr	30 mL/hr
78-82	12 mL	28 mL/hr	32 mL/hr
83-87	13 mL	30 mL/hr	34 mL/hr
88-92	13.5 mL	31.5 mL/hr	36 mL/hr
93-97	14 mL	33 mL/hr	38 mL/hr
98-102	15 mL	35 mL/hr	40 mL/hr
103-107	16 mL	37 mL/hr	42 mL/hr
108-112	16.5 mL	38.5 mL/hr	44 mL/hr
113-117	17 mL	40 mL/hr	46 mL/hr
118-122	18 mL	42 mL/hr	48 mL/hr
123-127	19 mL	44 mL/hr	50 mL/hr
128-132	19.5 mL	45.5 mL/hr	52 mL/hr
133-137	20 mL	47 mL/hr	54 mL/hr
138-142	21 mL	49 mL/hr	56 mL/hr
143-147	22 mL	51 mL/hr	58 mL/hr
148-152	22.5 mL	52.5 mL/hr	60 mL/hr

ACTIONS

An anticoagulant that is a specific and reversible direct thrombin inhibitor. It directly inhibits thrombin by specifically binding both to the catalytic site and to the anion-binding exosite of circulating and clot-bound thrombin. Inhibits both free and clot-bound thrombin without requiring endogenous cofactors (i.e., mode of action is independent of antithrombin III and is not inhibited by components of the platelet release reaction [e.g., platelet factor 4]). Produces a dose-dependent increase in aPTT, PT, TT, and ACT. Anticoagulant effect is immediate. Cleared from plasma by a combination of renal mechanisms and proteolytic cleavage. The binding of bivalirudin to thrombin is reversible resulting in recovery of thrombin active site functions. Coagulation times return to baseline approximately 1 hour after completion of infusion. Half-life averages 25 minutes. 20% of unchanged drug excreted in urine.

INDICATIONS AND USES
An anticoagulant for use in patients with unstable angina undergoing percutaneous transluminal coronary angioplasty (PTCA). (Used in place of heparin.) Used concurrently with aspirin. ▪ As an anticoagulant for use in patients undergoing PCI. Used in combination with aspirin and may be used in combination with glycoprotein GPIIb/IIIa antagonists (e.g., abciximab [ReoPro], eptifibatide [Integrilin]) as medically indicated. ▪ Patients with, or at risk for, heparin-induced thrombocytopenia (HIT) or heparin-induced thrombocytopenia and thrombosis syndrome (HITTS) undergoing percutaneous coronary intervention (PCI).

Unlabeled uses: Has been used in place of heparin in cardiac catheterization, AMI, and unstable angina; safety and effectiveness not established.

CONTRAINDICATIONS
Hypersensitivity to bivalirudin or its components; active major bleeding.

PRECAUTIONS
For IV use only. ▪ Most bleeding associated with the use of bivalirudin in PCI/PTCA occurs at the site of arterial puncture, however, hemorrhage can occur at any site. Consider a hemorrhagic event if there is an unexplained fall in BP or hematocrit or other unexplained symptom and discontinue bivalirudin. ▪ Has been associated with an increased risk of thrombus formation when used in gamma brachytherapy (percutaneous intracoronary brachytherapy). Fatalities have occurred. Imperative to maintain meticulous catheter technique, with frequent aspiration and flushing to minimize conditions of stasis within the catheter and vessels. ▪ Use with caution in disease states and other circumstances in which there is an increased danger of hemorrhage including severe hypertension; immediately following lumbar puncture; spinal anesthesia; major surgery, especially involving the brain, spinal cord, or eye; hematologic conditions associated with increased bleeding tendencies such as congenital or acquired bleeding disorders and gastrointestinal lesions such as ulcerations. ▪ Safety for use in combination with thrombolytic agents (e.g., alteplase [tPA], reteplase [Retavase], streptokinase) has not been established; see Drug/Lab Interactions. ▪ Safety for use in patients with unstable angina who are not undergoing PCI or in patients with other acute coronary syndromes has not been established. ▪ Half-life extended in patients with impaired renal function; see Dose Adjustments. ▪ Limited data regarding reexposure to bivalirudin; positive antibodies developed in 2 patients and neither developed clinical evidence of a hypersensitivity reaction.

Monitor: Discontinue low-molecular-weight heparin at least 8 hours prior to the procedure and administration of bivalirudin. ▪ Before therapy, obtain platelet count, hemoglobin and hematocrit, SCr, ACT, aPTT, TT, and PT. ▪ Dose is not titrated to ACT; however the ACT was checked at 5 minutes and again in 45 minutes during original clinical studies. ▪ Monitor anticoagulation status in patients with impaired renal function receiving reduced doses. ▪ Observe carefully for symptoms of a hemorrhagic event (e.g., unexplained fall in hematocrit, fall in BP, or any other unexplained symptom).

Patient Education: Risk of bleeding may be increased; discuss medical history and list of all medications (prescription and over-the-counter) with your health care provider; see Drug Interactions. ▪ Report all episodes of bleeding. ▪ Report tarry stools. ▪ Compliance with all measures to minimize bleeding is very important (e.g., avoid use of razors, toothbrushes, other sharp items). ▪ Use caution while moving to avoid excess bumping. **Maternal/Child:** Category B: safety for use during pregnancy not established. May have adverse effects on the fetus and the potential for maternal bleeding is increased, particularly during the third trimester. Use only if clearly needed. ▪ Not known if bivalirudin is secreted in human milk, use caution if required during breast-feeding. ▪ Safety and effectiveness for use in pediatric patients not established.

Elderly: Response similar to younger adults. ▪ See Dose Adjustments for the elderly with impaired renal function. ▪ Bleeding events are more common in the elderly. Puncture site hemorrhage and hematoma were observed more frequently in patients over 65 years of age.

DRUG/LAB INTERACTIONS

Discontinue **low-molecular-weight heparin** at least 8 hours prior to the procedure and administration of bivalirudin. ▪ Risk of bleeding may be increased by any medicine that affects blood clotting, including **anticoagulants** (e.g., heparin, lepirudin [Refludan], warfarin [Coumadin]); **any medication that may cause hypoprothrombinemia, thrombocytopenia, or GI ulceration or bleeding** (e.g., selected antibiotics [e.g., cefotetan], aspirin, NSAIDs [e.g., ibuprofen (Advil, Motrin), naproxen (Aleve, Naprosyn)]); **and/or any other medication that inhibits platelet aggregation** (e.g., clopidogrel [Plavix], dipyridamole [Persantine], glycoprotein GPIIb/IIIa receptor antagonists [e.g., abciximab (ReoPro), eptifibatide (Integrilin), tirofiban (Aggrastat)], plicamycin [Mithracin], sulfinpyrazone [Anturane], ticlopidine [Ticlid], valproic acid [Depacon]). If concurrent or subsequent use is indicated, monitor closely.

SIDE EFFECTS

Bleeding is the most frequent adverse event; incidence in clinical studies was less than with heparin. Abdominal pain, anxiety, back pain, bradycardia, dyspepsia, fever, headache, hypersensitivity reactions including anaphylaxis, hypertension, hypotension, injection site pain, insomnia, nausea, nervousness, pain, pelvic pain, thrombus formation (with fatalities), urinary retention, and vomiting have occurred.

ANTIDOTE

No specific antidote is available. Overdose with or without bleeding may be controlled by discontinuing bivalirudin. Discontinuation leads to a gradual reduction in anticoagulant effects due to metabolism of the drug depending on dose/overdose and concentration achieved. ACT or aPTT should return to normal within 1 to 4 hours after discontinuation. Reversal may take longer in patients with renal impairment. If life-threatening bleeding develops and excessive plasma levels of bivalirudin are suspected, immediately stop infusion. Determine aPTT, ACT, and hemoglobin and prepare for blood transfusion as appropriate. Follow current guidelines for treatment of shock as indicated (fluid, vasopressors [e.g., dopamine], Trendelenburg position, plasma expanders [e.g., albumin, hetastarch]). Treat hypersensitivity reactions as indicated; may require epinephrine, airway management, oxygen, IV fluids, antihistamines (e.g., diphenhydramine [Benadryl]), corticosteroids (e.g., hydrocortisone sodium succinate [Solu-Cortef]), and pressor amines (e.g., dopamine). Bivalirudin is removed by hemodialysis.

BLEOMYCIN SULFATE BBW

(blee-oh-**MY**-sin **SUL**-fayt)

Blenoxane

Antineoplastic
(antibiotic)

pH 4.5 to 6

USUAL DOSE

Squamous cell carcinoma, non-Hodgkin's lymphoma, testicular carcinoma: 0.25 to 0.5 units/kg of body weight/dose (10 to 20 units/M^2), once or twice weekly (1 unit equals 1 mg). The first two doses in lymphoma patients should not exceed 2 units in order to rule out hypersensitivity.

Hodgkin's disease: Dosage as above. After a 50% response, a maintenance dose of 1 unit daily or 5 units weekly is recommended.

DOSE ADJUSTMENTS

Unit/kg dose based on average weight in presence of edema or ascites. ▪ Dose selection in the elderly should be cautious; consider decreased renal function and concomitant disease or drug therapy. ▪ Reduce dose in impaired renal function as indicated in the following table.

CrCl (mL/min)	Bleomycin Dose
50 mL/min and above	100%
40-50 mL/min	70%
30-40 mL/min	60%
20-30 mL/min	55%
10-20 mL/min	45%
5-10 mL/min	40%

DILUTION

Specific techniques required; see Precautions. Each 15 units or fraction thereof must be reconstituted with 5 mL or more of NS. For IV injection, further dilution is not necessary, but has been further diluted in 50 to 100 mL NS and given as an intermittent infusion. May be given through Y-tube or three-way stopcock of a free-flowing IV.

Filters: No data available from manufacturer. Another source indicates no significant drug loss with the use of a 0.22-micron filter.

Storage: Refrigerate powder. Diluted solution stable at room temperature for 24 hours.

COMPATIBILITY

Consider any drug NOT listed as compatible to be INCOMPATIBLE until consulting a pharmacist; specific conditions may apply.

Manufacturer states, "Should not be reconstituted or diluted with D5W or other dextrose-containing diluents."

One source suggests the following **compatibilities:**

Additive: Amikacin (Amikin), dexamethasone (Decadron), diphenhydramine (Benadryl), fluorouracil (5-FU), gentamicin, heparin, streptomycin, tobramycin, vinblastine, vincristine.

Y-site: Allopurinol (Aloprim), amifostine (Ethyol), aztreonam (Azactam), cefepime (Maxipime), cisplatin (Platinol), cyclophosphamide (Cytoxan), doxorubicin (Adriamycin), doxorubicin liposomal (Doxil), droperidol (Inapsine), etoposide phosphate (Etopophos), filgrastim (Neupogen), fludarabine (Fludara), fluorouracil (5-FU), furosemide (Lasix), gemcitabine (Gemzar), granisetron (Kytril), heparin, leucovorin calcium, melphalan (Alkeran), methotrexate, metoclopramide (Reglan), mitomycin (Mutamycin), ondansetron (Zofran), paclitaxel (Taxol), piperacillin/tazobactam (Zosyn), sargramostim (Leukine), teniposide (Vumon), thiotepa, vinblastine, vincristine, vinorelbine (Navelbine).

RATE OF ADMINISTRATION
IV injection: Each 15 to 30 unit dose over 10 minutes.
Intermittent infusion: A single dose over 15 to 30 minutes or 1 unit/minute.

ACTIONS
An antibiotic antineoplastic agent, cell cycle phase-specific, that seems to act by splitting and fragmentation of double-stranded DNA. Inhibits DNA synthesis and, to a lesser extent, RNA and protein synthesis. It localizes in tumors. Improvement usually noted within 2 to 3 weeks. Widely distributed throughout the body. Inactivated by an enzyme that is widely distributed in normal tissue with the exception of the skin and lungs. Half-life is approximately 2 hours. About 60% to 70% excreted in urine.

INDICATIONS AND USES
Testicular carcinoma; may induce complete remission with vinblastine and cisplatin. ▪ Palliative treatment, adjunct to surgery or radiation, in patients not responsive to other chemotherapeutic agents or those with squamous cell carcinoma of the skin, head, esophagus, neck, or GU tract, including the cervix, vulva, scrotum, and penis; in Hodgkin's disease and other lymphomas. ▪ Injected into pleural cavity to treat malignant pleural effusion.

CONTRAINDICATIONS
Patients who have demonstrated a hypersensitive or idiosyncratic reaction to it.

PRECAUTIONS
Follow guidelines for handling cytotoxic agents. See Appendix A, p. 1429. ▪ May be given by the IM, IV, SC, or IP routes. ▪ Administered by or under the direction of the physician specialist. ▪ Administer in a facility with adequate diagnostic and treatment facilities to monitor the patient and respond to any medical emergency. ▪ May be used with other antineoplastic drugs to achieve tumor remission. ▪ Pulmonary toxicity may progress from nonspecific pneumonitis to pulmonary fibrosis and death. Pulmonary toxicity increases markedly with advancing age or with total doses greater than 400 units but has been seen in younger patients and in patients treated with lower doses. It may occur at lower doses when bleomycin is used in combination with other antineoplastic agents. Risk of developing pulmonary toxicity is greater when O_2 is administered in surgery. To prevent this side effect, it has been recommended that the FiO_2 be maintained at concentrations approximating that of room air during surgery and in the postoperative period. Additionally, fluid replacement should be closely monitored and focus more on colloid (e.g., albumin) administration rather than on crystalloid (e.g., NS, LR) administration. ▪ A severe idiosyncratic reaction (similar to anaphylaxis) has been reported in approximately 1% of lymphoma patients. S/S include hypotension, mental confusion, fever, chills, and wheezing; may be immediate or delayed for several hours. More common after the first or

second doses. ■ Use with extreme caution in patients with significant renal impairment or compromised pulmonary function.

Monitor: Obtain a baseline chest x-ray, and recheck every 1 to 2 weeks to detect pulmonary changes. ■ To identify subclinical pulmonary toxicity, monitor pulmonary diffusion capacity for carbon monoxide monthly. Should remain 30% to 35% above pretreatment value. Earliest signs of pulmonary toxicity are rales and dyspnea. ■ Monitor renal, hepatic, and central nervous systems and skin for symptoms of toxicity. ■ Determine patency of vein; avoid extravasation. ■ Maintain adequate hydration. ■ Prophylactic antiemetics may reduce nausea and vomiting and increase patient comfort. ■ Observe closely for all signs of infection. Prophylactic antibiotics may be indicated pending results of C/S in a febrile neutropenic patient. ■ Acetaminophen, diphenhydramine (Benadryl), and steroids (e.g., hydrocortisone) may be used prophylactically to reduce incidence of fever and anaphylaxis. ■ See Precautions.

Patient Education: Use nonhormonal contraception. ■ Report any possible side effects promptly. ■ Report stinging or burning at IV site promptly. ■ See Appendix D, p. 1434. ■ Pulmonary toxicity more likely in smokers.

Maternal/Child: Category D: avoid pregnancy. ■ Not recommended during breast-feeding. ■ Safety and effectiveness for use in pediatric patients not established. Volume of distribution and half-life is comparable to that in adults.

Elderly: Response similar to that seen in younger adults; however, pulmonary toxicity is more common in patients older than 70 years of age. ■ See Dose Adjustments; monitoring of renal function suggested.

DRUG/LAB INTERACTIONS

See Precautions. ■ Vascular toxicities (e.g., myocardial infarction, CVA, thrombotic microangiopathy, cerebral arteritis) or Raynaud's phenomenon have occurred rarely when bleomycin is used in combination with **other antineoplastic agents.** ■ May decrease GI absorption of **digoxin and hydantoins** (e.g., phenytoin). ■ Do not administer **live virus vaccines** to patients receiving antineoplastic drugs. ■ Causes sensitization of lung tissue to O_2; increases risk of pulmonary toxicity with **O_2 and general anesthetics.** ■ **Cisplatin** may inhibit renal elimination and increase toxicity.

SIDE EFFECTS

Alopecia, anorexia, chills, dyspnea, fever, hypotension, malaise, nausea, phlebitis (infrequent), rales, scleroderma-like skin changes, stomatitis, tenderness of the skin, tumor site pain, vomiting, weight loss.

Major: Severe idiosyncratic reaction similar to anaphylaxis (up to 6 hours after test dose), chest pain (acute with sudden onset suggestive of pleuropericarditis), pneumonitis, pulmonary fibrosis, skin toxicity (including nodules on hands, desquamation of skin, hyperpigmentation, and gangrene).

ANTIDOTE

Notify the physician of all side effects. Minor side effects will be treated symptomatically. Discontinue the drug immediately and notify the physician of any symptom of major side effects. Provide immediate treatment (epinephrine [Adrenalin] and diphenhydramine [Benadryl] for anaphylaxis, antibiotics and steroids for pneumonitis) or supportive therapy as indicated.

BORTEZOMIB

(bore-**TEH**-zo-mib)

Velcade

Antineoplastic

pH 2 to 6.5

USUAL DOSE

See Dose Adjustments for recommended starting dose modifications for patients with moderate to severe hepatic impairment.

Previously untreated multiple myeloma: 1.3 mg/M^2/dose as an IV bolus. Given in combination with oral melphalan (Alkeran) and oral prednisone for nine 6-week cycles as outlined in the following chart. For Cycles 1 to 4, administer twice weekly (Days 1, 4, 8, 11, 22, 25, 29, 32). For Cycles 5 to 9, administer once weekly (Days 1, 8, 22, 29). At least 72 hours should elapse between consecutive doses of bortezomib.

Dosage Regimen for Patients with Previously Untreated Multiple Myeloma Twice-Weekly Bortezomib (Cycles 1-4)											
Week	1				2		3	4		5	6
Bortezomib (1.3 mg/M^2)	Day 1	—	—	Day 4	Day 8	Day 11	Rest period	Day 22	Day 25	Day 29	Day 32	Rest period
Melphalan (9 mg/M^2) Prednisone (60 mg/M^2)	Day 1	Day 2	Day 3	Day 4	—	—	Rest period	—	—	—	—	Rest period
Once-Weekly Bortezomib (Cycles 5-9 When Used in Combination with Melphalan and Prednisone)											
Week	1				2		3	4		5	6
Bortezomib (1.3 mg/M^2)	Day 1	—	—	—	Day 8	—	Rest period	Day 22	—	Day 29	—	Rest period
Melphalan (9 mg/M^2) Prednisone (60 mg/M^2)	Day 1	Day 2	Day 3	Day 4	—	—	Rest period	—	—	—	—	Rest period

Relapsed multiple myeloma and mantle cell lymphoma: 1.3 mg/M^2/dose as an IV bolus 2 times a week for 2 weeks (Days 1, 4, 8, and 11). Follow with a 10-day rest period (Days 12 through 21). At least 72 hours should elapse between doses of bortezomib (e.g., Days 1, 4, 8, and 11). A treatment cycle is 21 days. See Dose Adjustments. For extended therapy of more than 8 cycles, bortezomib may be administered on the above standard schedule or on a maintenance schedule of once weekly for 4 weeks (Days 1, 8, 15, and 22), followed by a 13-day rest period (Days 23 to 35).

Combination therapy in multiple myeloma: *Bortezomib:* Administer 1.3 mg/M^2 as an IV bolus on Days 1, 4, 8, and 11 every 3 weeks.

Doxil: Administer 30 mg/M^2 on Day 4 following bortezomib. Continue for up to 8 cycles until disease progression or the occurrence of unacceptable toxicity. *Continued*

DOSE ADJUSTMENTS

Dose adjustments are based on clinical toxicities. ■ Dose adjustments are not required for patients with renal insufficiency, including those requiring dialysis. Bortezomib may be partially removed by dialysis. Administer after dialysis. ■ Dose adjustments based on age, gender, or race have not been evaluated; see Precautions. See the following charts for recommended starting dose modifications for patients with moderate to severe hepatic impairment, dose adjustments in combination therapy with melphalan and prednisone, and bortezomib-related neuropathic pain and/or peripheral sensory or motor neuropathy in relapsed multiple myeloma and mantle cell lymphoma.

Recommended Starting Dose Modification for Bortezomib in Patients with Hepatic Impairment			
	Bilirubin Level	SGOT (AST) Levels	Modification of Starting Dose
Mild	≤1 × ULN	>ULN	None
Mild	>1 to 1.5 × ULN	Any	None
Moderate	>1.5 to 3 × ULN	Any	Reduce bortezomib to 0.7 mg/M² in the first cycle. Consider dose escalation to 1 mg/M² or further dose reduction to 0.5 mg/M² in subsequent cycles based on patient tolerance.
Severe	>3 × ULN	Any	

Combination therapy with melphalan and prednisone in previously untreated multiple myeloma: Before each treatment cycle, platelet count should be equal to or greater than 70×10^9/L, and ANC should be equal to or greater than 1×10^9/L. Nonhematologic toxicities should have resolved to Grade 1 or baseline. Dose modifications for subsequent cycles are outlined in the following chart.

Dose Modifications During Cycles of Combination Bortezomib, Melphalan, and Prednisone Therapy	
Toxicity	Dose Modification or Delay
Hematologic toxicity during a cycle: If prolonged Grade 4 neutropenia or thrombocytopenia, or thrombocytopenia with bleeding, is observed in the previous cycle	Consider reducing the melphalan dose by 25% in the next cycle.
If platelet count is ≤30 × 10⁹/L or ANC is ≤0.75 × 10⁹/L on a bortezomib-dosing day (other than Day 1)	Bortezomib dose should be withheld.
If several bortezomib doses in consecutive cycles are withheld due to toxicity	Bortezomib dose should be reduced by 1 dose level (from 1.3 mg/M² to 1 mg/M², or from 1 mg/M² to 0.7 mg/M²).

Continued

| Dose Modifications During Cycles of Combination Bortezomib, Melphalan, and Prednisone Therapy—cont'd ||
Toxicity	Dose Modification or Delay
Grade ≥3 nonhematologic toxicities	Bortezomib therapy should be withheld until symptoms of the toxicity have resolved to Grade 1 or baseline. Bortezomib may then be reinitiated with 1 dose-level reduction (from 1.3 mg/M² to 1 mg/M², or from 1 mg/M² to 0.7 mg/M²). For bortezomib-related neuropathic pain and/or peripheral neuropathy, hold or modify bortezomib as outlined in the chart for dose modification for bortezomib-related neuropathic pain and/or peripheral neuropathy.

*Graded according to Common Terminology Criteria for Adverse Events (CTCAE).

Relapsed multiple myeloma and mantle cell lymphoma: Withhold dose if a Grade 3 nonhematologic toxicity (e.g., 6 to 10 emeses/24 hr, severe infection) or a Grade 4 hematologic toxicity (e.g., thrombocytopenia less than 25,000/mm³) occurs. When symptoms have resolved, resume treatment with a dose reduced by 25% (1.3 mg/M²/dose reduced to 1 mg/M²/dose, 1 mg/M²/dose reduced to 0.7 mg/M²/dose). ■ See Doxil monograph for additional dose adjustments required in Doxil and bortezomib combination therapy for treatment of multiple myeloma. ■ Reduce dose in patients who develop bortezomib-related neuropathic pain and/or peripheral sensory or motor neuropathy according to the following chart.

| Recommended Dose Modification for Bortezomib-Related Neuropathic Pain and/or Peripheral Sensory or Motor Neuropathy* ||
Severity of Peripheral Neuropathy Signs and Symptoms	Modification of Dose and Regimen
Grade 1 (paresthesias, weakness, and/or loss of reflexes) without pain or loss of function	No action.
Grade 1 with pain or Grade 2 (interfering with function but not with activities of daily living)	Reduce dose to 1 mg/M².
Grade 2 with pain or Grade 3 (interfering with activities of daily living)	Withhold therapy until toxicity resolves. When toxicity resolves, reinitiate with a reduced dose of 0.7 mg/M² and change treatment schedule to once per week.
Grade 4 (sensory neuropathy that is disabling or motor neuropathy that is life threatening or leads to paralysis)	Discontinue bortezomib.

*Graded according to Common Terminology Criteria for Adverse Events (CTCAE).

DILUTION

Specific techniques required; see Precautions. Reconstitute each 3.5-mg vial with 3.5 mL NS. Concentration equals 1 mg/mL.

Storage: Stable until expiration date when stored at CRT in original package and protected from light. Reconstituted solution stable at CRT for up to 8 hours in a syringe or in original vial when exposed to normal indoor lighting. Must be given within 8 hours.

COMPATIBILITY

Specific information not available. Consider specific use; consult pharmacist.

RATE OF ADMINISTRATION

A single dose as an IV bolus injection over 3 to 5 seconds. May be given into a peripheral vein. To ensure the full dose is administered, flush with NS after injection.

May also be given through an IV port if the primary IV is temporarily discontinued. Flush with NS before and after administration.

ACTIONS

A reversible inhibitor of the 26S proteasome, which is a large protein complex that degrades ubiquitinated proteins. The blocking of this proteasome disrupts numerous biologic pathways related to the growth and survival of cancer cells and can lead to cell death. Distributes widely to peripheral tissues. Over 80% is bound to plasma proteins. Mean elimination half-life after multiple doses ranges from 76 to 108 hours after the 1.3 mg/M^2 dose. Metabolized in the liver via selected cytochrome P$_{450}$ enzymes. Pathways of elimination in humans have not been determined. Median time to response was 38 days (range 30 to 127 days).

INDICATIONS

Treatment of patients with multiple myeloma. ■ Treatment of multiple myeloma in combination with doxorubicin liposomal injection (Doxil) in patients who have received one prior therapy but have not previously received bortezomib. ■ Treatment of patients with mantle cell lymphoma who have been treated with at least one prior therapy.

CONTRAINDICATIONS

Hypersensitivity to bortezomib, boron, or mannitol.

PRECAUTIONS

Follow guidelines for handling cytotoxic agents. See Appendix A, p. 1429. ■ For IV use only. ■ Administered by or under the supervision of a physician experienced in the use of antineoplastic therapy in a facility equipped to monitor the patient and respond to any medical emergency. ■ Bortezomib therapy causes peripheral neuropathy. Both sensory and motor peripheral neuropathy have been reported. Use caution in patients with pre-existing peripheral neuropathy; symptoms may worsen. Many have been treated previously with neurotoxic agents. ■ May cause orthostatic/ postural hypotension. Use with caution in patients with a history of syncope, in patients receiving concomitant medications that may cause hypotension, and in patients who are dehydrated. ■ Thrombocytopenia and neutropenia have been reported; see Monitor. ■ Gastrointestinal and intracerebral hemorrhages have been reported. ■ Acute development or exacerbation of CHF and/or new onset of decreased left ventricular ejection fraction has been reported. ■ Pulmonary disorders of unknown etiology such as pneumonitis, interstitial pneumonia, lung infiltration, and acute respiratory distress syndrome (ARDS) have been reported. ■ Pulmonary hypertension in the absence of left heart failure or significant pulmonary disease has been reported. ■ Reversible posterior leukoencephalopathy syndrome (RPLS) has been reported rarely. Patients may present with blindness, confusion, headache, hypertension, lethargy, seizure, or other visual or neurologic disturbances. MRI may be used to confirm diagnosis. ▪ Use caution in patients with moderate to severe liver impairment. Clearance decreased; see Monitor and Dose Adjustments. Use caution in patients with liver impairment who are receiving multiple concomitant medications and/or who have serious underlying medical conditions; asymptomatic increases in liver enzymes, hyperbilirubinemia, hepatitis, and rare cases of acute liver failure have been reported. May be reversible if bortezomib is discontinued. Information on rechallenging these patients is limited. ▪ Patients with a high tumor burden are at increased risk for tumor lysis syndrome. ▪ Consider antiviral prophylaxis. Herpes simplex and herpes zoster reactivation have been reported.

Monitor: Obtain baseline CBC with differential and platelet count; monitor frequently during treatment. Monitor platelet count before each dose. ▪ Obtain baseline electrolytes, including serum calcium and potassium and serum and urine M-protein. Monitor fluid and electrolyte balance and replace as indicated. Prevent dehydration. ▪ Monitor BP closely. Dehydration and/or concomitant medications may cause hypotension. Assist with ambulation. ▪ Monitor patients at risk for or with existing heart disease closely for S/S of CHF (e.g., exertional dyspnea, orthopnea, edema, tachycardia, pulmonary rales, a third heart sound, jugular venous distention) and/or for new onset of decreased left ventricular ejection fraction. ▪ Confirm patency of vein; however, tissue damage did not occur with extravasation during clinical studies. ▪ Monitor patients with impaired liver function closely for S/S of bortezomib toxicity. Baseline liver studies may be appropriate. Repeat as indicated. ▪ Use prophylactic antiemetics to reduce nausea and vomiting and increase patient comfort. ▪ Antidiarrheal medication (e.g., loperamide [Imodium]) may be indicated. ▪ Monitor for S/S of peripheral neuropathy (e.g., hyperesthesia [sensitivity of skin], hypoesthesia [impairment of any sense, especially touch], neuropathic pain or weakness, paresthesia [abnormal sensation such as burning, prickling]). Incidence may be increased in patients treated previously with neurotoxic agents (e.g., cisplatin [Platinol], thalidomide [Thalomid], vinca alkaloids [e.g., vincristine). See Dose Adjustments; may require change of dose or schedule. Improvement in or a resolution of peripheral neuropathy has been reported following dose adjustment or discontinuation of bortezomib. ▪ Monitor for neutropenia and thrombocytopenia (platelet count less than 50,000/mm^3). Occurs in a cyclical pattern with nadirs occurring after the last dose of each cycle and typically recovering before initiation of the next cycle. Initiate precautions to prevent excessive bleeding (e.g., inspect IV sites, skin, and mucous membranes; use extreme care during invasive procedures; test urine, emesis, stool, and secretions for occult blood). ▪ Monitor uric acid levels before and during therapy. Allopurinol and/or alkalinization of the urine may be indicated for serious tumor lysis syndrome. ▪ Hypoglycemia and hyperglycemia have been reported in patients taking oral diabetic agents. Monitor blood glucose levels and adjust antidiabetic medications as indicated; see Drug/Lab Interactions. ▪ Monitor respiratory status closely. Any change in condition should be evaluated promptly and treated as indicated.

Patient Education: Avoid pregnancy; use effective contraceptive measures. Should pregnancy occur, notify physician immediately and discuss potential hazards. ▪ May cause dizziness, fatigue, hypotension, or syncope; use caution when driving or operating machinery. ▪ Review all medications with your physician and/or pharmacist; effects of medications for high blood pressure and other medications that may lower blood pressure may increase hypotension. Other agents may increase peripheral neuropathy. May interfere with medications for diabetes. ▪ Review of monitoring requirements and adverse events before therapy is imperative. ▪ Avoid dehydration; promptly report diarrhea, dizziness, fainting spells, light-headedness, and vomiting. ▪ Promptly report any signs of infection (e.g., chills, fever, night sweats) or signs of bleeding (e.g., bruising, tarry stools, blood in urine, pinpoint red spots on skin). ▪ Promptly report symptoms of peripheral neuropathy (e.g., burning sensation, skin sensitivity, impairment of any sense [especially touch]). If these symptoms pre-existed, report if they seem to be worse. ▪ Promptly report shortness of breath or swelling of the ankles, feet, or legs. ▪ See Appendix D, p. 1434.

Maternal/Child: Category D: avoid pregnancy; may cause fetal harm. Use of effective contraception required. ▪ Discontinue breast-feeding. ▪ Safety and effectiveness for use in pediatric patients not established.

Elderly: Safety and effectiveness similar to other age-groups; however, greater sensitivity in the elderly cannot be ruled out. In clinical trials, patients over 65 years of age had a slightly increased incidence of Grade 3 or 4 toxicity.

DRUG/LAB INTERACTIONS

Drug interaction studies are limited. ▪ Coadministration with **ketoconazole** (Nizoral) increases bortezomib exposure. Monitor for toxicity. ▪ Coadministration with **prednisone and melphalan** (Alkeran) increases bortezomib exposure. Increase is unlikely to be significant. ▪ Has been administered with **omeprazole** (Prilosec) without effect. ▪ A poor inhibitor of selected cytochrome P_{450} enzymes; however, concomitant administration of **inhibitors or inducers of selected cytochrome P_{450} enzymes** may cause toxicity or reduce effectiveness of bortezomib. Consult pharmacist. **Inhibitors** may reduce metabolism and increase serum levels of bortezomib. Examples of inhibitors may include cimetidine (Tagamet), erythromycins, grapefruit juice, antifungal agents (e.g., itraconazole [Sporanox]), nefazodone, ritonavir (Norvir), verapamil. **Inducers** may increase metabolism and decrease serum levels and effectiveness of bortezomib. Examples of inducers may include carbamazepine (Tegretol), phenobarbital (Luminal), phenytoin (Dilantin), rifampin (Rifadin). ▪ Hypotension may be increased by **agents that induce hypotension** (e.g., alcohol, antihypertensives [e.g., ACE inhibitors (e.g., lisinopril)], beta-blockers [e.g., atenolol (Tenormin)], opioid narcotics, sildenafil [Viagra], tricyclic antidepressants [e.g., amitryptyline (Elavil), imipramine (Tofranil)]). ▪ Peripheral neuropathy may be increased by numerous agents. Some examples are **acyclovir** (Zovirax), **amiodarone** (Nexterone), **antineoplastics** (e.g., cisplatin [Platinol], **vinca alkaloids** [e.g., vincristine]), **foscarnet** (Foscavir), **isoniazid** (INH), **nitrofurantoin** (Furadantin), **thalidomide** (Thalomid), **statins** (e.g., lovastatin [Mevacor], simvastatin [Zocor]). ▪ May increase or decrease the effects of **oral antidiabetic agents** (e.g., glyburide [DiaBeta], glipizide [Glucotrol]). Monitor blood glucose levels and adjust dose of antidiabetic medication as indicated.

SIDE EFFECTS

Diarrhea, fatigue, peripheral neuropathy, excessive vomiting, and thrombocytopenia may be dose limiting. Most common side effects reported include abdominal pain, anemia, anorexia, arthralgia, asthenic conditions (fatigue, malaise, weakness), blurred vision, constipation, cough, dehydration, diarrhea, diplopia, dizziness, dysgeusia (altered taste), dyspepsia, dyspnea, edema (lower limb), fever, headache, herpes zoster, hypotension (including orthostatic/postural), ileus, injection site reactions, insomnia, leukopenia, lower respiratory and lung infections, lymphopenia, muscle cramps, myalgia, nasopharyngitis, nausea and vomiting, neutropenia, pain (abdominal, back, bone, limb), pneumonia, pruritus, psychiatric disorders (e.g., agitation, confusion, mental status change, psychotic disorder, suicidal ideation), rash, reactivation of herpes virus infections (zoster and simplex), rigors, syncope, and thrombocytopenia. Numerous other side effects have been reported that may or may not be related to bortezomib and may include hypersensitivity reactions (including anaphylaxis), and immune complex–mediated hypersensitivity), ARDS and other pulmonary disorders, bleeding (e.g., GI, intracerebral), CVA, GI disorders (serious [e.g., acute pancreatitis, ischemic colitis, paralytic ileus]), hepatic disorders (e.g., cholestasis, liver failure, portal vein thrombosis), hyperbilirubinemia, hypernatremia, hyperuricemia, hypocalcemia, hypokalemia, hyponatremia, infections (e.g., aspergillosis, bacteremia, herpes, listeriosis, oral candidiasis, septic shock, toxoplasmosis, URI), MI, pleural effusion, pulmonary embolism, pulmonary hypertension, renal disorders (e.g., acute or chronic renal failure, calculus, hemorrhagic cystitis, hydronephrosis), respiratory distress, RPLS, and tumor lysis syndrome.

Post-Marketing: Acute diffuse infiltrative pulmonary disease, acute febrile neutrophilic dermatosis (Sweet's syndrome), acute pancreatitis, cardiac arrhythmias (including complete AV block), cardiac tamponade, deafness (bilateral), DIC, dysautonomia, encephalopathy, hepatitis, herpes meningoencephalitis, ischemic colitis, ophthalmic herpes, and toxic epidermal necrolysis. 2% of patients died. Cause of death may have been related to bortezomib and included cardiac arrest, CHF, pneumonia, renal failure, respiratory failure, and sepsis.

Overdose: Profound progressive hypotension, tachycardia, and decreased cardiac contractility. Symptomatic hypotension and thrombocytopenia with fatal outcomes have been reported in patients who received more than twice the recommended dose.

ANTIDOTE

Keep physician informed of all side effects. Most will be treated symptomatically as indicated. Temporarily discontinue bortezomib if Grade 4 thrombocytopenia occurs (less than 25,000/mm^3); may be resumed at a reduced dose after thrombocytopenia is resolved. Severe thrombocytopenia may require platelet transfusions. Reduce dose, withhold dose, or discontinue based on S/S of peripheral neuropathy. Symptoms of peripheral neuropathy may improve or return to baseline if bortezomib is discontinued. Hypotension may respond to adjustment of antihypertensive medications, hydration, or administration of mineralocorticoids. Recovery from neutropenia may be spontaneous or may be treated with filgrastim (G-CSF, Neupogen) or pegfilgrastim (Neulasta). Treat anemia as indicated with whole blood products (e.g., packed RBCs) or blood modifiers (e.g., darbepoetin alfa [Aranesp], epoetin alfa [Epogen]). Discontinue bortezomib in patients who develop RPLS. In overdose, monitor V/S continuously and provide supportive care. Maintain BP with dopamine, epinephrine, or norepinephrine (Levophed) as needed. Maintain body temperature. There is no specific antidote; supportive therapy will help sustain the patient in toxicity. Resuscitate as indicated.

BOTULISM IMMUNE GLOBULIN (INTRAVENOUS HUMAN)
Immunizing Agent (Passive)
(**BOT**-yoo-lism im-**MYOUN GLOB**-you-lin, in-tra-**VEE**-nus **HU**-man)
BabyBIG

Available from the California Department of Health Services.

PEDIATRIC DOSE
Infants under 1 year of age: 1 mL/kg (50 mg/kg) as a single-dose IV infusion. Administer as soon as the diagnosis of infant botulism is made. See Maternal/Child.

DILUTION
Calculate the number of vials required for the desired dose. Each single-dose vial contains 100 mg. A 10-kg infant would require 500 mg (50 mg/kg × 10 kg = 500 mg, or 5 vials). Reconstitute the lyophilized powder with 2 mL of SW provided by the manufacturer to provide a 50 mg/mL solution. A transfer needle or large syringe may be used to add the SW. If a transfer needle is used, insert one end into the vial of SW first. Supplied in an evacuated vial; the SW should transfer by suction. Direct the stream of SW toward the side of the vial. To hasten the dissolution, release the residual vacuum after the water is transferred into the evacuated vial. Rotate the vial gently to wet all the powder. **Do not shake.** Allow approximately 30 minutes for dissolution. Solution should be clear, colorless, and free of particulate matter. Further dilution is not required.
Storage: Store lyophilized product between 2° and 8° C (35.6° and 46.4° F). Infusion should begin within 2 hours of reconstitution and should be completed within 4 hours of reconstitution.
Filter: Use of an in-line or syringe-tip, sterile, disposable filter (18 micron) is recommended.

COMPATIBILITY
Consider any drug NOT listed as compatible to be INCOMPATIBLE until consulting a pharmacist; specific conditions may apply.
Manufacturer recommends administration through a separate IV line without admixture with other drugs. May be "piggybacked" into a pre-existing line if the line contains either NS or one of the following dextrose solutions (with or without NaCl added): D2½W, D5W, D10W, or D20W. If a pre-existing line must be used, botulism immune globulin should not be diluted more than 1:2 with any of the previously named solutions.

RATE OF ADMINISTRATION
Administer intravenously using a low-volume tubing (e.g., 60 gtts/mL) and a constant infusion pump. An in-line or syringe-tip, sterile, disposable filter (18 micron) is recommended. Begin infusion at 0.5 mL/kg/hr (25 mg/kg/hr). If no untoward reactions after 15 minutes, the rate may be increased to 1 mL/kg/hr (50 mg/kg/hr) for the remainder of the infusion. **Do not exceed this rate.** Reduce rate at onset of patient discomfort, any minor side effects (e.g., flushing), or other adverse reactions. Discontinue for significant hypotension or S/S of hypersensitivity. At the recommended rate, the infusion should be completed after 67.5 minutes. See Precautions.

ACTIONS

A specialty immunoglobulin (IgG) containing neutralizing antibodies to botulinum toxin types A and B. Should provide the relevant antibodies at levels sufficient to neutralize the expected levels of circulating neurotoxins in infants who may have been exposed to botulinum toxin types A or B. Pooled from adult human plasma selected for their high titers of neutralizing antibody against botulinum neurotoxins type A and B. Purified and standardized by several specific methods (e.g., solvent-detergent viral inactivation process decreases the possibility of transmission of blood-borne pathogens [e.g., HIV, hepatitis]). Half-life is approximately 28 days. Should provide a protective level of neutralizing antibodies for 6 months.

INDICATIONS AND USES

Treatment of infants less than 1 year of age with infant botulism caused by toxin type A or B. Has been shown to decrease the average length of hospital and ICU stay, the average length of time on a mechanical ventilator, and the average number of weeks tube feeding is required in patients with infant botulism.

CONTRAINDICATIONS

Patients with a prior history of severe reaction to other human immuno-globulin preparations or any component of the formulation. Patients with selective immunoglobulin A deficiency have the potential to develop anti-bodies to immunoglobulin A and could have anaphylactic reactions to subsequent administration of blood products that contain immunoglobulin A.

PRECAUTIONS

IGIV products have been associated with renal dysfunction, acute renal failure, osmotic nephrosis, and death. IGIV products that contain sucrose as a stabilizer have demonstrated an increased risk of renal dysfunction. Botulism immune globulin contains sucrose as a stabilizer. Use extreme caution in patients with any degree of renal insufficiency or in patients who may be predisposed to acute renal failure. Predisposed patients may include patients with diabetes mellitus, paraproteinemia, sepsis, or volume depletion and/or patients receiving known nephrotoxic drugs. Consider benefit versus risk before use. Use of the minimum concentration available and the minimum rate of infusion is recommended. ■ May cause aseptic meningitis syndrome (AMS). May begin from 2 hours to 2 days after treatment. Symptoms are drowsiness, fever, headache (severe), nausea and vomiting, nuchal rigidity, painful eye movements, and photophobia. CSF studies may be positive with pleocytosis and elevated protein levels. Other causes of meningitis must be ruled out. AMS usually resolves with discontinuation of therapy. ■ With the use of botulism immune globulin, as with all plasma products, there is a slight possibility for transmission of blood-borne viral agents and, theoretically, the Creutzfeldt-Jakob disease agent. Risk is reduced by screening donors and various manufacturing processes such as viral inactivation. Risk of transmission versus benefit of treatment must be assessed for each patient.

Monitor: Obtain a baseline SCr and BUN. ■ Assess infant's volume status prior to initiating treatment. Patients must not be volume depleted. ■ Monitor vital signs and observe patient continuously during infusion. ■ Acute systemic hypersensitivity reactions were not observed in clinical trials but are possible. Epinephrine and emergency equipment should be readily available. ■ Monitor renal function (e.g., BUN, SCr) and urine output as indicated in infants at increased risk for renal failure.

Patient Education: Inform parents of possible side effects. ■ Review possible alteration of immunization schedule.

Maternal/Child: Not indicated for adult patients. ■ Safety and effectiveness for use in pediatric patients over 1 year of age not established.

Elderly: Not indicated for adult patients.

DRUG/LAB INTERACTIONS

May interfere with immune response to **live virus vaccines** (e.g., polio, measles, mumps, rubella). Defer vaccination with live virus vaccines until approximately 5 months after administration of botulism immune globulin. If such vaccinations were given shortly before or after administration of botulism immune globulin, a revaccination may be necessary.

SIDE EFFECTS

Many of the adverse events observed in studies are part of the known pathophysiology of infant botulism. The most common side effect was a mild, transient, erythematous rash of the face or trunk. Other frequent side effects included back pain, chills, fever, muscle cramps, nausea, rash, vomiting, and wheezing. Other reported reactions included abdominal distention, agitation, anemia, atelectasis, body temperature decrease, convulsions, cough, dehydration, dysphagia, edema, hypertension, hyponatremia, hypotension, injection site reaction, irritability, metabolic acidosis, nasal congestion, neurogenic bladder, oral candidiasis, otitis media, pneumonia, rales, respiratory arrest, rhonchi, stridor, tachycardia, tachypnea, urinary tract infections. Possible reactions not yet reported with botulism immune globulin but reported with other IVIG products include anaphylaxis, angioneurotic edema, renal toxicity (e.g., increased SCr and BUN, acute renal failure, acute tubular necrosis, proximal tubular nephropathy, osmotic nephrosis), and volume overload.

ANTIDOTE

Reduce rate of infusion for patient discomfort or any sign of adverse reaction and in patients at risk for renal insufficiency. Discontinue the drug immediately for any signs of hypersensitivity reaction or renal insufficiency. Notify the physician. Treat anaphylaxis immediately. Epinephrine (Adrenalin), diphenhydramine (Benadryl), oxygen, vasopressors (e.g., dopamine), corticosteroids, and ventilation equipment must always be available. Resuscitate as necessary.

BUMETANIDE `BBW`
(byou-**MET**-ah-nyd)

Diuretic (loop)
pH 6.8 to 7.8

USUAL DOSE
0.5 to 1 mg. May be repeated at 2- to 3-hour intervals. Do not exceed 10 mg/24 hr. Can be used for patients allergic to furosemide. 1:40 mg ratio (bumetanide to furosemide) is used to determine dose. Individualize dose and schedule; see Precautions/Monitor.

DOSE ADJUSTMENTS
Start at lower end of dosing range in the elderly. Consider decreased cardiac, hepatic, or renal function; concomitant disease; and other drug therapy.

DILUTION
May be given undiluted. Not usually added to IV solutions but **compatible** with D5W, NS, and LR. Usually given through Y-tube or three-way stopcock of infusion set. Use only freshly prepared solutions for infusion. Discard after 24 hours.

COMPATIBILITY   (Underline Indicates Conflicting Compatibility Information)
Consider any drug NOT listed as compatible to be INCOMPATIBLE until consulting a pharmacist; specific conditions may apply.
One source suggests the following **compatibilities:**
Additive: Furosemide (Lasix).
Y-site: Allopurinol (Aloprim), amifostine (Ethyol), aztreonam (Azactam), bivalirudin (Angiomax), caspofungin (Cancidas), cefepime (Maxipime), cisatracurium (Nimbex), cladribine (Leustatin), dexmedetomidine (Precedex), diltiazem (Cardizem), docetaxel (Taxotere), doripenem (Doribax), etoposide phosphate (Etopophos), filgrastim (Neupogen), gemcitabine (Gemzar), granisetron (Kytril), hetastarch in electrolytes (Hextend), lorazepam (Ativan), melphalan (Alkeran), meperidine (Demerol), micafungin (Mycamine), milrinone (Primacor), morphine, oxaliplatin (Eloxatin), pemetrexed (Alimta), piperacillin/tazobactam (Zosyn), propofol (Diprivan), remifentanil (Ultiva), teniposide (Vumon), thiotepa, vinorelbine (Navelbine).

RATE OF ADMINISTRATION
A single dose by IV injection over 1 to 2 minutes. Give infusion at prescribed rate.

ACTIONS
A sulfonamide diuretic, antihypertensive, and antihypercalcemic agent related to the thiazides. A loop diuretic agent. Extremely potent. Onset of action is within minutes and duration of action may last 4 to 6 hours. Apparently acts on the proximal and distal ends of the tubule and the ascending limb of the loop of Henle to excrete water, sodium, chloride, and potassium. Will produce diuresis in alkalosis or acidosis. Rapidly distributed, it is excreted primarily in the urine.

INDICATIONS AND USES
Edema associated with congestive heart failure, cirrhosis of the liver with ascites, renal diseases including nephrotic syndrome. ■ Acute pulmonary edema. ■ Edema unresponsive to other diuretic agents. ■ Diuresis in pa-

tients allergic to furosemide. ▪ Adjunct in combination with other antihypertensive agents in the treatment of hypertensive crisis.

Unlabeled uses: Treatment of hypercalcemia.

CONTRAINDICATIONS

Anuria, known hypersensitivity to bumetanide. Use caution in patients with hepatic coma or in states of severe electrolyte depletion. Do not use until condition is improved or corrected. See Precautions.

PRECAUTIONS

May be used concurrently with aldosterone antagonists (e.g., spironolactone [Aldactone]) for more effective diuresis and to prevent excessive potassium loss. ▪ May increase blood glucose; has precipitated diabetes mellitus. ▪ May lower serum calcium level, causing tetany. ▪ In rare instances may precipitate an acute attack of gout. ▪ Risk of ototoxicity increased with higher doses, rapid injection, decreased renal function, or concurrent use with other ototoxic drugs; see Drug/Lab Interactions. ▪ Patients allergic to sulfonamides may have an allergic reaction to bumetanide. ▪ Excessive doses can lead to profound diuresis with water and electrolyte depletion.

Monitor: Monitor for excessive diuresis with water and electrolyte depletion. Routine checks on electrolyte panel, CO_2, serum glucose, uric acid, and BUN are necessary during therapy. Potassium chloride replacement may be required.

Patient Education: Hypotension may cause dizziness; move slowly, and request assistance to sit on edge of bed or ambulate. ▪ May decrease potassium levels and require a supplement.

Maternal/Child: Category C: use in pregnancy only if clearly needed. ▪ Consider discontinuing breast-feeding. ▪ Safety and effectiveness for use in pediatric patients not established. ▪ Has been used in infants age 4 days to 6 months at doses ranging from 0.005 mg/kg to 0.1 mg/kg. Maximal diuretic effect seen at doses of 0.035 to 0.04 mg/kg. Elimination half-life decreases during the first month of life from approximately 6 hours at birth to 2.4 hours at 1 month.

Elderly: Response similar to that seen in younger patients; however, dose selection should be cautious; see Dose Adjustments. Consider increased sensitivity to hypotensive and electrolyte effects and increased risk of circulatory collapse or thromboembolic episodes. ▪ Monitoring of renal function suggested.

DRUG/LAB INTERACTIONS

Causes excessive potassium depletion with **corticosteroids, thiazide diuretics** (e.g., hydrochlorothiazide [Hydrodiuril]), **amphotericin B** (all formulations). ▪ Potentiates **antihypertensive drugs** (e.g., nitroglycerin, nitroprusside sodium); reduced dose of the antihypertensive agent or both drugs may be indicated. ▪ May cause transient or permanent deafness with doses exceeding the usual or when given in conjunction with **other ototoxic drugs** (e.g., aminoglycosides [e.g., gentamicin], cisplatin). ▪ **Amphotericin B** (all formulations) may increase potential for ototoxicity and nephrotoxicity; avoid concurrent use. ▪ Nephrotoxicity increased by other **nephrotoxic agents** (e.g., acyclovir [Zovirax], aminoglycocides, ciprofloxacin [Cipro], cyclosporine [Sandimmune], vancomycin); avoid concurrent use. ▪ May increase serum levels of **lithium** (may cause toxicity). ▪ May cause cardiac arrhythmias with **amiodarone** (Nexterone) **or digoxin** (potassium depletion). ■ Risk of cardiotoxicity increased with **pimozide** (Orap) **and sparfloxacin** (Zagam); concurrent use not recommended. ■ May enhance or inhibit actions of **nondepolarizing muscle relaxants** (e.g., atracurium [Tracrium]) **or theophyllines.** ■ May cause hyperglycemia with **insulin or sulfonylureas** (e.g., tolbutamide) by decreasing glucose tolerance. ■ Effects may be inhibited by **ACE inhibitors** (e.g., captopril [Capoten]), **NSAIDs** (e.g., ibuprofen [Motrin]), **probenecid, or** in patients with cirrhosis and ascites who are taking **salicylates.** ■ May cause profound diuresis and serious electrolyte abnormalities with **thiazide diuretics** (e.g., chlorothiazide [Diuril]) because of synergistic effects. ■ Do not use concomitantly with **ethacrynic acid** (Edecrin); risk of ototoxicity markedly increased. ■ Smoking may increase secretion of ADH-decreasing diuretic effects and cardiac output. ■ See Precautions.

SIDE EFFECTS
Usually occur in prolonged therapy, seriously ill patients, or following large doses.

Abdominal pain, arthritic pain, azotemia, dizziness, ECG changes, elevated SCr, encephalopathy, headache, hyperglycemia, hyperuricemia, hypocalcemia, hypochloremia, hypomagnesemia, hyponatremia, hypotension, impaired hearing, muscle cramps, nausea, pruritus, rash.

Major: Anaphylactic shock, blood volume reduction, circulatory collapse, dehydration, excessive diuresis, hypokalemia, metabolic acidosis, thrombocytopenia, vascular thrombosis, and embolism.

ANTIDOTE
If minor side effects are noted, discontinue the drug and notify the physician, who may treat the side effects symptomatically and continue the drug. If side effects are progressive or any major side effect occurs, discontinue the drug immediately and notify the physician. Treatment of major side effects is symptomatic and aggressive and includes fluid and electrolyte replacement. Resuscitate as necessary.

BUPRENORPHINE HYDROCHLORIDE
(byou-pren-**OR**-feen hy-droh-**KLOR**-eyed)

Narcotic analgesic
(agonist-antagonist)
Anesthesia adjunct

Buprenex

pH 3.5 to 5.5

USUAL DOSE
Pain control: 0.3 mg (1 mL). Repeat every 6 hours as necessary. May be repeated in 30 to 60 minutes, if indicated. These dose recommendations have been lowered because of excessive respiratory depression with doses up to 0.6 mg. 25 to 250 mcg/hr has been given as a continuous infusion to manage postoperative pain.

Reverse fentanyl-induced anesthesia (unlabeled): 0.3 to 0.8 mg 1 to 4 hours after induction of anesthesia and 30 minutes before end of surgery.

PEDIATRIC DOSE
2 to 12 years of age: Pain control: 2 to 6 mcg/kg of body weight every 4 to 8 hours. A repeat dose in 30 to 60 minutes is not recommended. Longer intervals (6 to 8 hours) are suggested and should provide sufficient pain relief. Determine appropriate interval through clinical assessment. See Maternal/Child.

DOSE ADJUSTMENTS
Reduce dose by one half in high-risk patients (e.g., elderly or debilitated, respiratory disease), when other CNS depressants have been given, and in the immediate postoperative period; see Drug/Lab Interactions. ▪ Reduced dose may be required in impaired liver function.

DILUTION
IV injection: May be given undiluted.

Infusion: May be further diluted with NS, D5W, D5NS, or LR injection and given as an infusion. 1 mg in 250 mL = 4 mcg/mL, 3 mg in 250 mL = 12 mcg/mL.

Filters: Not required by manufacturer; however, 0.2-micron filters were used during manufacturing. No loss of drug potency expected.

Storage: Before use, store at CRT. Avoid freezing and/or prolonged exposure to light.

COMPATIBILITY
Consider any drug NOT listed as compatible to be INCOMPATIBLE until consulting a pharmacist; specific conditions may apply.

One source suggests the following **compatibilities:**

Y-site: Allopurinol (Aloprim), amifostine (Ethyol), aztreonam (Azactam), cefepime (Maxipime), cisatracurium (Nimbex), cladribine (Leustatin), docetaxel (Taxotere), etoposide phosphate (Etopophos), filgrastim (Neupogen), gemcitabine (Gemzar), granisetron (Kytril), linezolid (Zyvox), melphalan (Alkeran), oxaliplatin (Eloxatin), pemetrexed (Alimta), piperacillin/tazobactam (Zosyn), propofol (Diprivan), remifentanil (Ultiva), teniposide (Vumon), thiotepa, vinorelbine (Navelbine).

RATE OF ADMINISTRATION
Titrate slowly according to symptom relief and respiratory rate.

IV injection: A single dose over 3 to 5 minutes.

Infusion: See Usual Dose. Use of a metriset (60 gtt/min) or a controlled infusion device recommended.

ACTIONS

A synthetic narcotic agonist-antagonist analgesic. Thirty times as potent as morphine in analgesic effect (0.3 mg equivalent to 10 mg morphine) and has the antagonist effect of naloxone in larger doses. Does produce respiratory depression. Pain relief is effected in 2 to 3 minutes and lasts up to 6 hours. Metabolized in the liver. Primarily excreted through feces. Crosses the placental barrier. Secreted in breast milk.

INDICATIONS AND USES

Relief of moderate to severe pain.

Unlabeled use: Reverse fentanyl-induced anesthesia.

CONTRAINDICATIONS

Hypersensitivity to buprenorphine.

PRECAUTIONS

Usually given IM. ▪ May precipitate withdrawal symptoms if stopped too quickly after prolonged use or if patient has been on opiates. ▪ Use caution in asthma, respiratory depression or difficulty from any source, impaired renal or hepatic function, the elderly or debilitated, myxedema or hypothyroidism, adrenocortical insufficiency, CNS depression or coma, toxic psychoses, prostatic hypertrophy or urethral stricture, acute alcoholism, delirium tremens, or kyphoscoliosis. ▪ May elevate cerebrospinal fluid pressure; use caution in head injury, intracranial lesions, and other situations with increased intracranial pressure.

Monitor: Naloxone (Narcan), oxygen, and controlled respiratory equipment must be available. Naloxone is only partially effective in reversing respiratory depression. ▪ Observe patient frequently and monitor vital signs. ▪ Keep patient supine to minimize side effects; orthostatic hypotension and fainting may occur. Observe closely during ambulation. ▪ Pain control usually more effective with routinely administered doses. Determine appropriate interval through clinical assessment.

Patient Education: Avoid use of alcohol or other CNS depressants (e.g., antihistamines, diazepam [Valium]). ▪ Use caution performing any task requiring alertness; may cause dizziness, euphoria, and sedation. ▪ Request assistance for ambulation. ▪ May be habit forming.

Maternal/Child: Category C: safety for use during pregnancy, labor and delivery, or breast-feeding not established. Use only when clearly needed. ▪ Not recommended in pediatric patients under 2 years of age but has been used in pediatric patients as young as 9 months of age.

Elderly: See Dose Adjustments. ▪ May be more sensitive to effects (e.g., respiratory depression, urinary retention, constipation, dizziness). ▪ Analgesia should be effective with lower doses. ▪ Consider possibility of decreased organ function.

DRUG/LAB INTERACTIONS

Respiratory and CNS effects may be additive with **barbiturate anesthetics** (e.g., thiopental [Pentothal]); reduced doses of both drugs may be indicated. ▪ May cause respiratory depression and cardiovascular collapse with **diazepam** (Valium); reduced doses of both drugs may be indicated. ▪ May decrease analgesic effects of **other narcotics;** avoid concurrent use. ▪ Clearance decreased and serum levels increased by **cytochrome P$_{450}$ inhibitors** (e.g., azole antifungal agents [e.g., itraconazole (Sporanox)], macrolide antibiotics [e.g., erythromycin], protease inhibitors [e.g., ritonavir (Norvir)]). Monitor with concurrent use; dose adjustment may be indicated. ■ Clearance increased and serum levels decreased by **cytochrome P$_{450}$ inducers** (e.g., carbamazepine [Tegretol], phenytoin [Dilantin], rifampin [Rifadin]). Use caution; dose adjustments may be indicated. ■ Manufacturer suggests caution when used in combination with **MAO inhibitors** (e.g., selegiline [Eldepryl]).

SIDE EFFECTS

Excessive sedation is a major side effect. Has caused death from respiratory depression. Acute and chronic hypersensitivity reactions (e.g., anaphylaxis, angioneurotic edema, bronchospasm, hives, pruritus, rash), bradycardia, clammy skin, constipation, cyanosis, dizziness, dyspnea, headache, hypertension, hypotension, nausea, pruritus, tachycardia, vertigo, visual disturbances, vomiting.

ANTIDOTE

With increasing severity of any side effect or onset of symptoms of overdose, discontinue the drug and notify the physician. Naloxone hydrochloride (Narcan) will help to reverse respiratory depression, but is not as effective as it is with other narcotics. A patent airway, artificial ventilation, oxygen therapy, and other symptomatic treatment must be instituted promptly. Treat anaphylaxis and resuscitate as necessary.

BUSULFAN BBW
(byou-**SUL**-fan)

Busulfex

Antineoplastic
(alkylating agent)

pH 3.4 to 3.9

USUAL DOSE

Administered in combination with cyclophosphamide as a component of a conditioning regimen prior to bone marrow or peripheral blood progenitor cell replacement support.

Premedication: Premedicate patients with phenytoin (use of other anticonvulsants not recommended) and an antiemetic (e.g., $5HT_3$ antiemetics such as ondansetron [Zofran], granisetron [Kytril]). Continue antiemetic administration on a fixed schedule throughout busulfan therapy. See Monitor, Drug Interactions, and Side Effects.

Busulfan: 0.8 mg/kg of ideal body weight (IBW) or actual body weight, whichever is lower, administered through a central venous catheter every 6 hours for 4 days (16 doses). Six hours after the 16th busulfan dose (on BMT day minus 3 [3 days prior to BMT]), begin cyclophosphamide at a dose of 60 mg/kg/day for 2 days. Before and after each infusion, flush the catheter line with 5 mL NS or D5W.

PEDIATRIC DOSE

See Maternal/Child.

Initial doses are based on a small trial and are unlabeled. Therapeutic drug monitoring and dose adjustment based on AUC determination following the first dose are recommended. See manufacturer's literature for details.

Actual body weight equal to or less than 12 kg: 1.1 mg/kg.

Actual body weight greater than 12 kg: 0.8 mg/kg.

DOSE ADJUSTMENTS

In obese or severely obese patients, dose should be based on an adjusted ideal body weight (AIBW). Calculate as follows:

$$AIBW = IBW + 0.25 \times (Actual\ weight\ [kg] - IBW)$$

■ Busulfan has not been studied in patients with renal or hepatic insufficiency. See Precautions.

DILUTION

Specific techniques required; see Precautions. Supplied in vials containing 60 mg/10 mL (6 mg/mL). Must be diluted prior to infusion with either NS or D5W. The diluent volume should be 10 times the busulfan volume to ensure a final concentration of approximately 0.5 mg/mL. Remove calculated dose of busulfan from vial. Inject the contents of the syringe into an intravenous bag or syringe that contains the calculated amount of diluent. Always add the busulfan to the diluent rather than the diluent to the busulfan. Mix thoroughly by inverting several times. The dose for a 70-kg patient would be prepared using the following steps:

1. 70 kg × 0.8 mg/kg = 56 mg.
2. 56 mg ÷ 6 mg/mL = 9.3 mL busulfan needed.
3. 9.3 × 10 = 93 mL.
4. Add 9.3 mL of busulfan to 93 mL of NS or D5W.
5. Final concentration = 56 mg ÷ 102.3 mL = 0.54 mg/mL.

Filters: 5-micron Nylon filter has been used; see Compatibility.

Storage: Refrigerate. Busulfan diluted with NS or D5W is stable for 8 hours at room temperature, but infusion must be completed within that time. When diluted with NS and refrigerated, it is stable for 12 hours, but infusion must be completed within that time.

COMPATIBILITY

Do not use polycarbonate syringes or polycarbonate filter needles. Manufacturer states, "Do not infuse concomitantly with another intravenous solution of unknown **compatibility.** Flush central venous catheter line before and after administration with at least 5 mL of NS or D5W."

RATE OF ADMINISTRATION

Before and after each infusion, flush the catheter line with 5 mL NS or D5W.

Busulfan: Infuse over 2 hours using an infusion pump.

Cyclophosphamide: Infuse over 1 hour.

ACTIONS

A bifunctional alkylating agent. Cell cycle phase–nonspecific. Interferes with DNA replication, leading to cytotoxicity and cell death. Distributes equally into plasma and CSF. Metabolized in the liver. Excreted partially in the urine, primarily as metabolites.

INDICATIONS AND USES

For use in combination with cyclophosphamide as a conditioning regimen prior to allogeneic hematopoietic progenitor cell transplantation for chronic myelogenous leukemia. ■ Has orphan drug approval as preparative therapy for treatment of malignancies with BMT and treatment of brain cancer.

CONTRAINDICATIONS

Previous hypersensitivity to busulfan or any of its components (polyethylene glycol and dimethylacetamide).

PRECAUTIONS

Follow guidelines for handling cytotoxic agents. See Appendix A, p. 1429. ■ Administered by or under the direction of a physician who is experienced in allogeneic hematopoietic stem cell transplantation, the use of cancer chemotherapeutic drugs, and the management of patients with severe pancytopenia. ■ Adequate diagnostic and treatment facilities must be readily available to manage therapy and any complications that arise. ■ Profound myelosuppression, including granulocytopenia, thrombocytopenia, anemia, or any combination of these will occur. ■ Seizures have been reported. Use caution when administering to patients with a history of seizures or head trauma or patients who are receiving other potentially epileptogenic drugs (e.g., imipenem-cilastatin [Primaxin], meperidine [Demerol]). ■ Anticonvulsant prophylactic therapy should be initiated with phenytoin before busulfan treatment. ■ High busulfan AUC values (greater than 1,500 µM•min) may be associated with an increased risk of developing hepatic veno-occlusive disease (VOD). Patients who have received prior radiation therapy, three or more cycles of chemotherapy, or a prior progenitor cell transplant may be at an increased risk of developing hepatic VOD with the recommended busulfan dose and regimen. ■ Cardiac tamponade has been reported in pediatric patients with thalassemia who received high doses of oral busulfan and cyclophosphamide. No patients treated in the busulfan injection trials experienced cardiac tamponade. ■ Bronchopulmonary dysplasia with pulmonary fibrosis is a rare but serious complication following chronic busulfan therapy. Average onset of symptoms is 4 years after therapy (range: 4 months to 10 years). ▪ May cause cellular dysplasia in many organs. Dysplasia may be severe enough to cause difficulty in interpretation of exfoliative cytologic examinations of the lungs, bladder, breast, and the uterine cervix. ▪ Secondary malignancies, including acute nonlymphocytic leukemia, myeloproliferation syndrome, and carcinoma have been reported in patients treated with alkylating agents.

Monitor: Obtain a baseline and a daily CBC, including differential and platelet count, during treatment and until engraftment is demonstrated. Absolute neutrophil count (ANC) dropped below 0.5×10^9/L at a median of 4 days posttransplant and recovered at a median of 13 days when prophylactic G-CSF was used. Thrombocytopenia (platelets less than 25,000/mm^3 or platelet transfusion required) occurred at a median of 5-6 days. ▪ Monitor for signs of local or systemic infection or bleeding. Antibiotic therapy and platelet and RBC support should be used when medically indicated. ▪ Monitor for thrombocytopenia (platelet count less than 50,000/mm^3). Initiate precautions to prevent excessive bleeding (e.g., inspect IV sites, skin, and mucous membranes; use extreme care during invasive procedures; test urine, emesis, stool, and secretions for occult blood). ▪ Serum transaminases, alkaline phosphatase, and bilirubin should be obtained daily through transplant day 28 to monitor for signs of hepatotoxicity, and the onset of hepatic VOD. Jones' criteria may be used to diagnose VOD (hyperbilirubinemia, and two of the following three findings: painful hepatomegaly, weight gain more than 5%, or ascites). ▪ Obtain baseline and periodic uric acid concentrations. ▪ Use of anticonvulsants other than phenytoin may result in higher busulfan plasma AUCs and an increased risk of VOD or seizures. When other anticonvulsants are used, plasma busulfan AUC should be monitored; see Drug/Lab Interactions.

Patient Education: Nonhormonal birth control recommended. ▪ May be at increased risk of developing a secondary malignancy. ▪ See Appendix D, p. 1434.

Maternal/Child: Category D: avoid pregnancy. Can cause fetal harm. Has mutagenic potential. ▪ Discontinue breast-feeding. ▪ Safety and efficacy for use in pediatric patients not established. Clearance has been shown to be higher in pediatric patients than in adults, necessitating the development of alternative dosing regimens for oral busulfan in pediatric patients. A recent small pharmacokinetic study suggests an unlabeled dosing regimen; see Pediatric Dose and manufacturer's literature.

Elderly: Has been used in a small number of patients over 55 years of age. All achieved myeloablation and engraftment.

DRUG/LAB INTERACTIONS

Itraconazole (Sporanox), **metronidazole** (Flagyl), **and cyclophosphamide** (Cytoxan) decrease busulfan clearance, increasing the AUC and risk of toxicity. ▪ **Phenytoin** increases the clearance of busulfan. Because the pharmacokinetics of busulfan were studied in patients treated with phenytoin, the clearance of busulfan at the recommended dose may be lower and the AUC higher in patients not treated with phenytoin. ▪ **Acetaminophen** (Tylenol) may decrease clearance of busulfan. Avoid administration of acetaminophen 72 hours prior to or with busulfan therapy. ▪ Do not administer **live virus vaccines** to patients receiving antineoplastic drugs. ▪ Busulfan has been used with **fluconazole** (Diflucan), **ondansetron** (Zofran),

and granisetron (Kytril). ▪ May cause additive effects with **bone marrow–suppressing agents or agents that cause blood dyscrasias** (e.g., amphotercin B, antithyroid agents, azathioprine [Imuran], chloramphenicol, ganciclovir [Cytovene], interferon, plicamycin [Mithracin], zidovudine) **and radiation therapy.** Adjust busulfan dose based on blood cell counts. ▪ Risk of uric acid nephropathy increased with **sulfinpyrazone** (Anturan); allopurinol may be preferred to prevent or treat hyperuricemia. ▪ See Precautions.

SIDE EFFECTS

Profound myelosuppression, including granulocytopenia, thrombocytopenia, anemia, or a combination of these, will occur in 100% of patients. ▪ Other nonhematologic adverse events occurring in more than 20% of patients include abdominal pain or enlargement, ALT elevation, anorexia, anxiety, asthenia, back pain, chest pain, chills, constipation, cough, creatinine elevation, depression, diarrhea, dizziness, dry mouth, dyspepsia, dyspnea, edema, epistaxis, fever, headache, hyperbilirubinemia, hyperglycemia, hypersensitivity reactions, hypertension, hypervolemia, hypocalcemia, hypokalemia, hypomagnesemia, infection, inflammation or pain at injection site, insomnia, lung disorders, nausea, pain, pruritus, rash, rectal disorder, rhinitis, seizures, stomatitis (mucositis), tachycardia, third-degree heart block, thrombosis, vasodilation (flushing or hot flashes), vomiting, weight gain secondary to edema. ▪ Graft-versus-host disease, hepatic veno-occlusive disease and death have also been reported. ▪ Dimethylacetamide (DMA), the solvent used in busulfan formulation, has been associated with adverse reactions such as confusion, hallucinations, hepatotoxicity, lethargy, and somnolence. The relative contribution of DMA to neurologic and hepatic toxicities observed with busulfan is difficult to determine. ▪ Numerous other side effects have occurred.

ANTIDOTE

Treat minor side effects symptomatically. In the absence of hematopoietic progenitor cell transplantation, the normal dosage of busulfan injection constitutes an overdose. Monitor hematologic status closely, and institute supportive measures as indicated. Administration of whole blood products (e.g., packed RBCs, platelets, leukocytes) and/or blood modifiers (e.g., darbepoetin alfa [Aranesp], epoetin alfa [Epogen], filgrastim [Neupogen], oprelvekin [Neumega], pegfilgrastim [Neulasta], sargramostim [Leukine]) may be indicated to treat bone marrow toxicity. Dialysis and administration of glutathione may be considered in an overdose (busulfan is metabolized by conjugation with glutathione).

BUTORPHANOL TARTRATE
(byou-**TOR**-fah-nohl **TAHR**-trayt)

Narcotic analgesic
(agonist-antagonist)
Anesthesia adjunct

Butorphanol Tartrate PF, Stadol, Stadol PF

pH 3 to 5.5

USUAL DOSE

Pain control: 1 mg. Repeat every 3 to 4 hours as necessary. Range is 0.5 to 2 mg.

Preoperative or preanesthetic: 2 mg 60 to 90 minutes before surgery. Individualize dose. Usually given IM.

Labor: 1 to 2 mg at full term in early labor; may be repeated after 4 hours. Use alternate analgesia if delivery is expected to occur within 4 hours.

Adjunct to balanced anesthesia: 2 mg just before induction or 0.5 to 1 mg in increments during anesthesia. Increments may be up to 0.06 mg/kg and should be based on previous sedative, analgesic, and hypnotic drugs. Patients seldom require less than 4 mg or more than 12.5 mg. Administered only under the direction of the anesthesiologist.

DOSE ADJUSTMENTS

Reduce dose to one half of the recommended dose and increase the interval between doses to at least 6 hours for impaired liver or renal function and in the elderly; adjust as indicated by patient response. ▪ Another source suggests that patients with a glomerular filtration rate (GFR) of 10 to 50 mL/min receive 75% of the usual dose given at the normal dosage interval and that patients with a GFR less than 10 mL/min receive 50% of the usual dose given at the normal dosage interval. No dose adjustment is necessary for patients with a GFR greater than 50 mL/min. ▪ Reduce dose when other CNS depressants have been given and in the immediate postoperative period. Use the smallest effective dose and extend intervals between doses. ▪ See Drug/Lab Interactions.

DILUTION

May be given undiluted. Avoid aerosol spray while preparing a syringe for use. Rinse with cool water following skin contact. Available preservative free.

Storage: Store at CRT. Protect from light and freezing.

COMPATIBILITY

Consider any drug NOT listed as compatible to be INCOMPATIBLE until consulting a pharmacist; specific conditions may apply.

One source suggests the following **compatibilities:**

Y-site: Allopurinol (Aloprim), amifostine (Ethyol), aztreonam (Azactam), bivalirudin (Angiomax), cefepime (Maxipime), cisatracurium (Nimbex), cladribine (Leustatin), dexmedetomidine (Precedex), docetaxel (Taxotere), doxorubicin liposomal (Doxil), enalaprilat (Vasotec IV), esmolol (Brevibloc), etoposide phosphate (Etopophos), fenoldopam (Corlopam), filgrastim (Neupogen), fludarabine (Fludara), gemcitabine (Gemzar), granisetron (Kytril), hetastarch in electrolytes (Hextend), labetalol (Trandate), linezolid (Zyvox), melphalan (Alkeran), nicardipine (Cardine IV), oxaliplatin (Eloxatin), paclitaxel (Taxol), pemetrexed (Alimta), piperacillin/tazobactam (Zosyn), propofol (Diprivan), remifentanil (Ultiva), sargramostim (Leukine), teniposide (Vumon), thiotepa, vinorelbine (Navelbine).

RATE OF ADMINISTRATION
Each 2 mg or fraction thereof over 3 to 5 minutes. Frequently titrated according to symptom relief and respiratory rate.

ACTIONS
A potent narcotic analgesic with some narcotic agonist-antagonist effects. Exact mechanism of action is unknown. Analgesia similar to morphine is produced. Does produce respiratory depression, but this does not increase markedly with larger doses. Pain relief is effected almost immediately, peaks at 30 minutes, and lasts about 2 to 4 hours. Causes some hemodynamic changes that increase the workload of the heart. Metabolized in the liver. Excreted in urine and feces. Crosses the blood-brain barrier and placental barrier. Secreted in breast milk.

INDICATIONS AND USES
Relief of moderate to severe pain. ▪ Preoperative or preanesthetic medication, as a supplement to anesthesia. ▪ Relief of pain during early labor.

CONTRAINDICATIONS
Hypersensitivity to butorphanol or its components (some products contain benzethonium chloride).

PRECAUTIONS
Not used for narcotic-dependent patients because of antagonist activity. ▪ May increase cardiac workload; use in myocardial infarction, ventricular dysfunction, and coronary insufficiency only if benefits outweigh risks. ▪ Use caution in respiratory depression or difficulty from any source, obstructive respiratory conditions, head injury, and impaired liver or kidney function. ▪ May elevate cerebrospinal pressure. ▪ Prolonged continuous use may result in physical dependence or tolerance. ▪ In overdose situations, always consider the possibility of multiple drug ingestion. **Monitor:** Naloxone (Narcan), oxygen, and controlled respiratory equipment must be available. Duration of action of butorphanol usually exceeds that of naloxone; repeated dosing may be necessary. ▪ Observe patient frequently and monitor vital signs. ▪ Keep patient supine to minimize side effects; orthostatic hypotension and fainting may occur. Observe closely during ambulation. ▪ Pain control usually more effective with routinely administered doses. Determine appropriate interval through clinical assessment.
Patient Education: Avoid use of alcohol or other CNS depressants (e.g., antihistamines, diazepam [Valium]). ▪ Use caution performing any task requiring alertness; may cause dizziness, euphoria, and sedation. ▪ Request assistance for ambulation. ▪ May be habit forming.
Maternal/Child: Category C: safety for use in pregnant women before 37 weeks' gestation not established; use only if benefit justifies potential risk to fetus. ▪ Has been used safely during labor of term infants. Has been associated with transient (10 to 90 minutes) sinusoidal fetal heart rate patterns. Use caution if abnormal fetal heart rate is present; manufacturer states "was not associated with adverse outcomes." Alternative analgesia suggested if delivery is expected to occur within 4 hours. ▪ Use caution in breast-feeding; an estimated 4 mcg/L has been found in breast milk; may be clinically insignificant. ▪ Safety and effectiveness for use in pediatric patients under 18 years of age not established.
Elderly: Mean half-life may be extended by 25%, may be more sensitive to effects (e.g., respiratory depression, constipation, dizziness, urinary retention). ▪ Analgesia should be effective with lower doses; see Dose

Adjustments. ■ Consider decreased organ function, concomitant disease, or other drug therapy.

DRUG/LAB INTERACTIONS

Potentiated by **cimetidine** (Tagamet), **phenothiazines** (e.g., chlorpromazine [Thorazine]), **droperidol** (Inapsine), **and CNS depressants** such as narcotic analgesics, general anesthetics, alcohol, anticholinergics, antihistamines, barbiturates, benzodiazepines (e.g., diazepam [Valium]), hypnotics, MAO inhibitors, neuromuscular blocking agents (e.g., atracurium [Tracrium]), psychotropic agents, and sedatives. Reduced doses of both drugs may be indicated; use the smallest effective dose of butorphanol and/or extend intervals between doses. ■ Effects may be altered by other **medications that affect hepatic metabolism of drugs** (e.g., aminophylline, erythromycin). Reduced doses of butorphanol and/or longer intervals between doses may be indicated. ■ May decrease analgesic effects of **other narcotics;** avoid concurrent use. ■ Will cause an increase in conjunctival changes with **pancuronium.**

SIDE EFFECTS

Dizziness, nausea and/or vomiting, and somnolence occur most frequently. Abdominal pain, anorexia, anxiety, asthenia, bronchitis, clammy skin, confusion, constipation, cough, diplopia, dizziness, drug dependence, dry mouth, dyspnea, euphoria, floating feeling, flushing, hallucinations, headache, hypersensitivity reactions (e.g., pruritis), hypotension, insomnia, lethargy, nervousness, palpitations, paresthesia, respiratory depression, sweating, tremor, unusual dreams, vasodilation, vertigo, warmth. May cause increased pulmonary artery pressure, pulmonary wedge pressure, left ventricular end-diastolic pressure, systemic arterial pressure, pulmonary vascular resistance, and cardiac workload.

Overdose: Cardiovascular insufficiency, hypoventilation, coma, and death. May be associated with ingestion of multiple drugs.

ANTIDOTE

With increasing severity of any side effect or onset of symptoms of overdose, discontinue the drug and notify the physician. Most side effects will be treated symptomatically. Treat hypertension with antihypertensives (e.g., nitroglycerin, nitroprusside sodium). Naloxone hydrochloride (Narcan) will reverse respiratory depression. Duration of action of butorphanol usually exceeds that of naloxone; repeated dosing may be necessary. A patent airway, adequate ventilation, oxygen therapy, and other symptomatic treatment must be instituted promptly. Vasodilation may cause hypotension.

C1 ESTERASE INHIBITOR (HUMAN)

(C 1 **ES**-ter-ase in-**HIB**-it-or)

Berinert

Protein C1 Inhibitor

pH 4.5 to 8.5

USUAL DOSE

20 units/kg as an IV injection.

DILUTION

Available in a kit containing one 500-unit vial of C1 esterase inhibitor, one 10-mL vial of SW, one Mix2Vial filtered transfer set, and one alcohol swab. Bring components to room temperature. C1 esterase inhibitor is a lyophilized concentrate and requires reconstitution. The Mix2Vial transfer set provided requires a specific technique to accomplish reconstitution; see manufacturer's literature for instructions. Alternately, for each vial of C1 esterase inhibitor and provided diluent, place all components on a flat surface, remove the flip caps from the drug and diluent vials, swab the vials with alcohol, and allow them to dry. Insert one end of a double-ended transfer needle into the diluent. Invert the diluent bottle and insert the other end of the transfer needle into the drug vial. Diluent will be drawn into the drug vial by a vacuum. Remove the transfer device and diluent vial. Gently swirl the drug vial to fully dissolve. Solution should be colorless, clear, and free from visible particles. Concentration equals 50 units/mL. Do not use if cloudy, discolored, or contains particulates. Attach a vented filter spike to a 10-mL (or larger) syringe and withdraw the contents. Contents of multiple vials may be pooled in a single administration device (e.g., syringe). Use a double-ended transfer needle and a new vented filter spike for each vial requiring reconstitution.

Filters: A Mix2Vial filtered transfer set is provided for each single-use dose or, alternately, a double-ended needle and a vented filter spike are required.

Storage: Store in carton at 2° to 25° C (36° to 77° F) until ready for use. Do not freeze. Protect from light. Do not use beyond expiration date. Reconstituted solution must be used within 8 hours; do not refrigerate or freeze. Discard unused drug.

COMPATIBILITY

Manufacturer states, "Do not mix C1 esterase inhibitor with other medicinal products, and administer by a separate infusion line."

RATE OF ADMINISTRATION

A single dose at a rate of approximately 4 mL/min.

ACTIONS

C1 esterase inhibitor is a normal constituent of human blood and is a serine proteinase inhibitor. It has an important inhibiting potential on several of the major cascade systems, including the complement system, the intrinsic coagulation (contact) system, the fibrinolytic system, and the coagulation cascade. Hereditary angioedema (HAE) patients have low levels of endogenous or functional C1 esterase inhibitor. It is thought that increased vascular permeability and the clinical manifestation of HAE attacks (e.g., local tissue swelling of hands, feet, limbs, face, intestinal tract, and airway [larynx or trachea]) are primarily mediated through contact system activation. Suppression of contact system activation by C1 esterase inhibitor through the inactivation of plasma kallikrein and factor XIIa is thought to modulate vascular permeability by preventing the generation of bradykinin. Supplying additional C1 esterase inhibitor activity by IV injection facilitates the normal process. One unit of C1 inhibitor corresponds to the amount of C1 esterase inhibitor present in 1 mL of fresh citrated plasma. Plasma levels of C1 inhibitor increase within 1 hour or less of IV administration. The half-life range is 7.4 to 22.8 hours.

INDICATIONS AND USES

Treatment of acute abdominal or facial attacks of hereditary angioedema (HAE) in adult and adolescent patients. ▪ Safety and effectiveness for use as prophylactic therapy not established. An alternate C1 inhibitor product, Cinryze, is approved for routine prophylaxis.

CONTRAINDICATIONS

Known life-threatening hypersensitivity reactions, including anaphylaxis to C1 esterase inhibitor preparations.

PRECAUTIONS

Severe hypersensitivity reactions, including anaphylaxis, may occur. Administer in a facility capable of monitoring the patient and responding to any medical emergency. Epinephrine should be immediately available. ▪ Thrombotic events (e.g., myocardial infarction, pulmonary embolism, arterial thrombosis, deep vein thrombosis) have occurred in patients receiving off-label high-dose C1 esterase inhibitor therapy. ▪ Made from human plasma and may contain infectious agents (e.g., HIV, Creutzfeldt-Jakob disease, hepatitis B, or hepatitis C). Numerous steps in the manufacturing process are used to reduce the potential for infection.

Monitor: Observe for symptoms of a hypersensitivity reaction (e.g., anaphylaxis, generalized urticaria, hives, hypotension, tightness in the chest, wheezing). Reaction may occur during injection or after injection is complete. ▪ Symptoms of an HAE attack may be similar to S/S of hypersensitivity reactions. Evaluate carefully to initiate the correct treatment. There is usually no itching or hives with an HAE attack. ▪ Monitor patients with known risk factors for thrombotic events; see Precautions.

Patient Education: Inform patients of the risks for infectious agent transmission and of safety precautions taken during manufacturing process. ▪ Promptly report symptoms of a hypersensitivity reaction (e.g., difficulty breathing, feeling faint, hives, itching, tightness in the chest, wheezing). ▪ Promptly report symptoms of a possible thrombosis (e.g., altered consciousness or speech; loss of sensation or motor power; new-onset swelling and pain in the abdomen, chest, or limbs; shortness of breath). ▪ Discuss all medications used (e.g., prescription, nonprescription, over-the-counter, herbal, supplements) with the physician. ▪ Consult a health care professional before travel.

Maternal/Child: Category C: safety and effectiveness for use during pregnancy, labor, and delivery has not been established; use only if clearly needed. ▪ Not known if C1 esterase inhibitor is secreted in human milk; use only if clearly needed during breast-feeding. ▪ Safety and effectiveness for use in pediatric patients less than 12 years of age not established.

Elderly: Numbers in clinical studies insufficient to determine if the elderly respond differently than do younger subjects.

DRUG/LAB INTERACTIONS

No drug interaction studies have been conducted.

SIDE EFFECTS

The most common side effects observed include abdominal pain, diarrhea, headache, muscle spasms, pain, subsequent HAE attack, and vomiting. An increase in the severity of pain associated with HAE was the most serious side effect during clinical trials. Other reported side effects include back pain, dysgeusia, facial pain, and hereditary angioedema.

Post-Marketing: Reported side effects from use outside the United States include hypersensitivity/anaphylactic reactions, viral transmission (e.g., acute hepatitis C), chills, fever, and injection site pain or redness.

ANTIDOTE

Keep the physician informed of side effects. Interrupt or discontinue injection if indicated (e.g., hypersensitivity reaction, HAE attack, thrombotic event). If appropriate and if symptoms subside, infusion may be resumed at a tolerated rate. ▪ Discontinue C1 esterase inhibitor and treat anaphylaxis immediately with oxygen, epinephrine (Adrenalin), antihistamines (e.g., diphenhydramine [Benadryl]), vasopressors (e.g., dopamine), corticosteroids, albuterol (Ventolin), IV fluids, and ventilation equipment as indicated. Resuscitate as necessary.

C1 INHIBITOR (HUMAN)   Protein C1 inhibitor
(C 1 in-**HIB**-a-tor)
Cinryze   pH 6.6 to 7.4

USUAL DOSE

1,000 units as an IV injection over 10 minutes (1 mL/min). May be repeated every 3 or 4 days as necessary for routine prophylaxis against angioedema attacks in patients with hereditary angioedema (HAE).

DILUTION   (International units [IU])

If refrigerated, bring components to RT (two 500-unit vials of C1 inhibitor and two 5-mL vials of SW [not supplied by manufacturer]). For each 500-unit vial, insert one end of a double-ended transfer needle into the SW diluent. Invert the bottle of diluent and rapidly insert the other end of the transfer needle into the slightly angled C1 inhibitor vial. Diluent will be drawn into the C1 inhibitor vial by a vacuum. Do not use if there is no vacuum. Remove the transfer device and diluent vial. Gently swirl the C1 inhibitor vial until the powder is completely dissolved. Do not use if turbid or discolored (should be colorless to slightly blue and clear). Attach a filter needle to a 10-mL syringe and withdraw 500 units (5 mL) from each vial (total dose 1,000 units in 10 mL [100 units/mL]).

Filters: Use of a filter needle is required to withdraw reconstituted solution into a syringe; may be used for both 500-IU vials (a single dose).

Storage: Store in carton between 2° and 25° C (36° and 77° F). Protect from light. Do not freeze. Reconstituted solution must be administered at RT within 3 hours of preparation. Do not use beyond expiration date on vial. Discard unused product.

COMPATIBILITY

Manufacturer states, "Do not mix with other materials."

RATE OF ADMINISTRATION
A single dose equally distributed over 10 minutes (1 mL/min).

ACTIONS
C1 inhibitor is a normal constituent of human blood; a serine proteinase inhibitor. It regulates activation of the complement and intrinsic coagulation (contact system) pathway and regulates the fibrinolytic system. Patients with HAE have low levels of endogenous or functional C1 inhibitor. It is thought that increased vascular permeability and the clinical manifestation of HAE attacks are mediated primarily through contact system activation. Suppression of contact system activation by C1 inhibitor through the inactivation of plasma kallikrein and factor XIIa is thought to modulate vascular permeability by preventing the generation of bradykinin. Supplying additional C1 inhibitor activity by IV injection facilitates the normal process. One unit of C1 inhibitor corresponds to the amount of C1 inhibitor present in 1 mL of normal fresh plasma. Plasma levels of C1 inhibitor increase within 1 hour or less of IV administration. Half-life is 56 hours (range 11 to 108 hours).

INDICATIONS AND USES
Routine prophylaxis against angioedema attacks in adolescent and adult patients with hereditary angioedema (HAE). HAE is caused by low levels or improper functioning of a protein called C1 inhibitor. Blood vessels are affected, and people with HAE can develop rapid swelling of the hands, feet, limbs, face, intestinal tract, or airway (larynx or trachea). Has caused death by suffocation.

CONTRAINDICATIONS
Known life-threatening hypersensitivity to C1 inhibitor or its components.

PRECAUTIONS
Severe hypersensitivity reactions, including anaphylaxis, may occur. Administer in a facility capable of monitoring the patient and responding to any medical emergency. Epinephrine should be immediately available. ■ Thrombotic events (e.g., myocardial infarction, pulmonary embolism, arterial thrombosis, deep vein thrombosis) have occurred in patients receiving off-label high-dose C1 inhibitor therapy. ■ Made from human plasma and may contain infectious agents (e.g., HIV, Creutzfeldt-Jakob disease, hepatitis B, or hepatitis C). Numerous steps in the manufacturing process are used to reduce the potential for infection.
Monitor: Observe for symptoms of a hypersensitivity reaction (e.g., chest pain, dizziness, dyspnea, fever, flushing, hypotension, nausea, pruritus, rash, rigors, urticaria). ■ Symptoms of an HAE attack may be similar to S/S of hypersensitivity reactions. Evaluate carefully to initiate the correct treatment. There is usually no itching or hives with an HAE attack. ■ Monitor patients with known risk factors for thrombotic events; see Precautions.
Patient Education: Inform patient of risks for infectious agent transmission and of safety precautions taken during the manufacturing process. ■ Promptly report symptoms of a hypersensitivity reaction (e.g., difficulty breathing, feeling faint, hives, itching, tightness in the chest, wheezing). ■ Promptly report symptoms of a possible thrombosis (e.g., altered consciousness or speech; loss of sensation or motor power; new-onset swelling and pain in the abdomen, chest, or limbs; shortness of breath).

Maternal/Child: Category C: safety and effectiveness for use during pregnancy, labor, and delivery not established; use only if clearly needed. ▪ Not known if C1 inhibitor is secreted in human milk; use caution if required during breast-feeding. ▪ Safety and effectiveness for use in neonates, infants, or other pediatric patients not established. Clinical studies included patients 9, 14, and 16 years of age.

Elderly: Numbers in clinical studies insufficient to determine if elderly patients respond differently than younger subjects.

DRUG/LAB INTERACTIONS
No drug interaction studies have been conducted.

SIDE EFFECTS
The most common side effects reported include headache, rash, sinusitis, and upper respiratory tract infections. Back pain, bronchitis, limb injury, pain in extremity, pruritus, and viral URIs also occurred. Hypersensitivity reactions, including anaphylaxis, hives, hypotension, tightness of the chest, urticaria, and wheezing, have occurred. Serious events not considered drug related have occurred and include death due to foreign body embolus, exacerbation of HAE attacks, pre-eclampsia resulting in an emergency cesarean section, and stroke.

ANTIDOTE
Keep the physician informed of any side effects. Interrupt or discontinue injection if indicated until symptoms subside, then resume at a tolerated rate. ▪ Discontinue C1 inhibitor and treat anaphylaxis immediately with oxygen, epinephrine (Adrenalin), antihistamines (e.g., diphenhydramine [Benadryl]), vasopressors (e.g., dopamine), corticosteroids, albuterol (Ventolin), IV fluids, and ventilation equipment as indicated. Resuscitate as necessary.

CABAZITAXEL BBW
(ka-**BAZ**-i-**TAX**-el)
Jevtana

Antineoplastic agent
(taxane)

USUAL DOSE
Premedication: Must be premedicated at least 30 minutes before each dose to prevent severe hypersensitivity reactions. Usual regimen includes IV administration of an antihistamine (diphenhydramine [Benadryl] 25 mg or equivalent), a corticosteroid (dexamethasone [Decadron] 8 mg or equivalent steroid), and an H_2 antagonist (ranitidine [Zantac] 50 mg or equivalent H_2 antagonist).

Antiemetic prophylaxis is recommended and may be given orally or IV as needed.

Cabazitaxel: 25 mg/M^2 as a 1-hour infusion every 3 weeks. Given in combination with oral prednisone 10 mg administered daily throughout cabazitaxel treatment.

DOSE ADJUSTMENTS
Recommendations for dose adjustment for adverse reactions are listed in the following chart.

| Recommended Cabazitaxel Dose Modifications for Adverse Reactions ||
Toxicity*	Dose Modification
Prolonged Grade ≥3 neutropenia (greater than 1 week) despite appropriate medication, including G-CSF	Delay treatment until neutrophil count is >1,500 cells/mm^3, then reduce dose of cabazitaxel to 20 mg/M^2. Use G-CSF for secondary prophylaxis.
Febrile neutropenia	Delay treatment until improvement or resolution and until neutrophil count is >1,500 cells/mm^3, then reduce dose of cabazitaxel to 20 mg/M^2. Use G-CSF for secondary prophylaxis.
Grade ≥3 diarrhea or persisting diarrhea despite appropriate medication and fluid and electrolytes replacement.	Delay treatment until improvement or resolution, then reduce dose of cabazitaxel to 20 mg/M^2.

*Toxicities graded in accordance with National Cancer Institute (NCI) Common Terminology Criteria for Adverse Events (CTCAE), version 3.0.

Discontinue if any of these reactions continue at a cabazitaxel dose of 20 mg/M^2.

DILUTION

Specific techniques required; see Precautions. Must be diluted by a specific 2-step process and given as an infusion. Do not use PVC infusion containers and polyurethane infusion sets for preparation or administration. A clear yellow to brownish-yellow viscous solution.

Step 1: Initially withdraw the entire contents of the provided diluent and insert into the vial of cabazitaxel (60 mg/1.5 mL). When transferring the diluent, direct the needle onto the inside wall of the cabazitaxel vial to limit foaming. Gently mix by repeated inversions for at least 45 seconds to ensure full mixing of drug and diluent. Do not shake. Allow to stand for a few minutes to allow most of the foam to dissipate. Should not contain visible particulate matter. Concentration of the resultant dilution is 10 mg/mL. This initially diluted solution should be used immediately but must be used within 30 minutes of entry into the vial.

Step 2: Withdraw the recommended dose from the 10-mg/mL vial of cabazitaxel. Further dilute into a sterile 250-mL PVC-free container of either NS or D5W for infusion. If a dose greater than 65 mg is required, use a larger volume of NS or D5W infusion so a concentration of 0.26 mg/mL is not exceeded. Concentration of the final solution should be between 0.10 and 0.26 mg/mL. Thoroughly mix by gently inverting the bag or bottle.

Filters: Use of a 0.22-micron in-line filter is required for administration (not supplied).

Storage: Before use, store at 25° C (77° F), with excursions permitted between 15° to 30° C (59° to 86° F). Do not refrigerate. Initial diluted solution should be used immediately but must be used within 30 minutes; discard any unused portion. Final infusion solution should be used within 8 hours (including infusion time) at RT or within 24 hours (including infusion time) if refrigerated. Both solutions are supersaturated and may crystallize over time. Discard if crystallization occurs. Discard if either the initial diluted solution or final solution is not clear or appears to have precipitation.

COMPATIBILITY

Manufacturer states, "Do not use PVC infusion containers and polyurethane infusion sets for preparation or administration. Should not be mixed with any other drugs."

RATE OF ADMINISTRATION

A single dose properly diluted as an infusion over 1 hour. Use of a 0.22-micron in-line filter required for administration. See Dilution and Compatibility.

ACTIONS

An antineoplastic belonging to the taxane class. Prepared by semi-synthesis with a precursor extracted from yew needles. A microtubule inhibitor, it binds to tubulin and promotes its assembly into microtubules while simultaneously inhibiting disassembly. This leads to the stabilization of microtubules, which results in the inhibition of mitotic and interphase cellular functions. It is active in docetaxel-sensitive tumors and has demonstrated activity in tumor models insensitive to chemotherapy, including docetaxel. Highly protein bound (89% to 92%). Equally distributed between blood and plasma. Extensively metabolized in the liver, mainly by the CYP3A4/5 isoenzyme and to a lesser extent by CYP2C8. Terminal half-life is approximately 95 hours. Mainly excreted in feces as numerous metabolites with minimal excretion of unchanged drug in urine.

INDICATIONS AND USES

Treatment of patients with hormone-refractory metastatic prostate cancer previously treated with a docetaxel-containing treatment regimen. Used in combination with oral prednisone.

CONTRAINDICATIONS

Patients with neutrophil counts of equal to or less than 1,500/mm^3. ■ Patients with a history of severe hypersensitivity reactions to cabazitaxel or other drugs formulated with polysorbate 80. ■ Not recommended for patients with impaired hepatic function (total bilirubin equal to or greater than the ULN, or AST and/or ALT equal to or greater than 1.5 times the ULN).

PRECAUTIONS

Follow guidelines for handling cytotoxic agents. See Appendix A, p. 1429. ■ Usually administered by or under the direction of the physician specialist in a facility with adequate diagnostic and treatment facilities to monitor the patient and respond to any medical emergency. ■ If initial or fully diluted solution should come in contact with the skin, immediately and thoroughly wash with soap and water. If contact with mucosa occurs, immediately and thoroughly wash with water. ■ Neutropenia resulting in fatal infections (sepsis or septic shock) has occurred. Primary prophylaxis with G-CSF should be considered in high-risk patients (e.g., extensive prior radiation ports, over 65 years of age, poor nutritional status, poor performance status, previous episodes of febrile neutropenia, or other serious co-morbidities that may result in increased complications from prolonged neutropenia). Therapeutic use of G-CSF and secondary prophylaxis should be considered in all patients considered to be at increased risk for neutropenia complications. ■ Severe hypersensitivity reactions have occurred; all patients are premedicated to lessen the intensity of a hypersensitivity reaction. Patients with a history of severe hypersensitivity reactions should not be

rechallenged with cabazitaxel. ▪ Nausea, vomiting, and severe diarrhea may occur. Deaths related to diarrhea and electrolyte imbalance have occurred. ▪ Deaths due to renal failure have occurred, and most occurred in association with sepsis, dehydration, or obstructive uropathy. ▪ Use with caution in patients with severe renal impairment (CrCl less than 30 mL/min) or in patients with ESRD. ▪ Patients with impaired hepatic function (total bilirubin equal to or greater than the ULN, or AST and/or ALT equal to or greater than 1.5 times the ULN) were excluded from clinical trials. Hepatic impairment increases the risk of severe and life-threatening complications with cabazitaxel and other drugs belonging to the same class that are metabolized in the liver; see Drug/Lab Interactions. **Monitor:** Obtain baseline CBC with differential and platelets. Monitor weekly during Cycle 1 and before each treatment cycle thereafter. ▪ If febrile neutropenia or prolonged neutropenia (greater than 1 week) occur despite appropriate medications (e.g., G-CSF), dose reduction is indicated. May not be restarted until the neutrophil count recovers to a level greater than 1,500 cells/mm^3; see Contraindications and Dose Adjustments. ▪ G-CSF may be administered to reduce the risks of neutropenia complications; see Precautions. ▪ Monitor closely for hypersensitivity reactions, especially during the first and second infusions. May occur within the first few minutes, and beginning symptoms may include bronchospasm, generalized rash/erythema, and hypotension. ▪ Monitor for nausea, vomiting, and diarrhea. Use prophylactic antiemetics to reduce nausea and vomiting and increase patient comfort. Rehydrate and use antidiarrheal medications as indicated. ▪ Monitor for S/S of impending renal failure (dehydration, reduced urine output). Monitoring of CrCl or SCr may be indicated. ▪ Observe closely for signs of infection. Prophylactic antibiotics may be indicated pending results of C/S in a febrile neutropenic patient. ▪ Monitor for thrombocytopenia (platelet count less than 50,000/mm^3). Initiate precautions to prevent excessive bleeding (e.g., inspect IV sites, skin, and mucous membranes; use extreme care during invasive procedures; test urine, emesis, stool, and secretions for occult blood).
Patient Education: Avoid pregnancy; nonhormonal birth control recommended. ▪ Routine monitoring of blood counts imperative. ▪ Oral prednisone must be taken as prescribed. ▪ Promptly report S/S of a hypersensitivity reaction (e.g., hives, rash, shortness of breath or trouble breathing, swelling of eyelids, lips, or face). ▪ May cause severe and/or fatal infections, dehydration, and renal failure. Take your temperature often and promptly report a fever. ▪ Promptly report burning on urination, cough, decreased urine output, hematuria, muscle aches, and/or significant diarrhea or vomiting. ▪ Drug interactions may occur, review prescription and non-prescription drugs with your physician. ▪ Certain side effects may be more frequent or severe in the elderly. ▪ See Appendix D, p. 1434.
Maternal/Child: Category D: avoid pregnancy. Can cause fetal harm. ▪ Discontinue breast-feeding. ▪ Safety and effectiveness for use in pediatric patients not established.
Elderly: Patients over 65 years of age are more likely to experience fatal outcomes not related to disease progression and certain serious adverse reactions, including neutropenia and febrile neutropenia. The incidence of asthenia, dehydration, dizziness, fatigue, fever, and urinary tract infections was also increased in the elderly.

DRUG/LAB INTERACTIONS

Formal drug interaction studies have not been conducted. ▪ Prednisone administered at 10 mg daily did not affect the pharmacokinetics of cabazitaxel. ▪ Primarily metabolized through CYP3A. Concomitant administration with **strong CYP3A4 inhibitors** (e.g., atazanavir [Reyataz], clarithromycin [Biaxin], indinavir [Crixivan], itraconazole [Sporanox], ketoconazole [Nizoral], nefazodone, nelfinavir [Viracept], ritonavir [Norvir], saquinavir [Invirase], telithromycin [Ketek], and voriconazole [VFEND]) should be avoided. Serum concentration of cabazitaxel is expected to increase. ▪ Use caution when administered concomitantly with **moderate CYP3A inhibitors.** ▪ Concomitant administration with **strong CYP3A4 inducers** (e.g., carbamazepine [Tegretol], phenytoin [Dilantin], phenobarbital [Luminal], rifabutin [Mycobutin], rifampin [Rifadin], and rifapentine [Priftin]) should be avoided. Serum concentration of cabazitaxel is expected to decrease. ▪ Avoid use of **St. John's Wort;** may also decrease concentration of cabazitaxel.

SIDE EFFECTS

Abdominal pain, alopecia, anorexia, arthralgia, asthenia, back pain, bone marrow suppression (e.g., anemia, leukopenia, neutropenia, thrombocytopenia), constipation, cough, diarrhea, dysgeusia, dyspnea, fatigue, fever, hematuria, nausea, peripheral neuropathy, and vomiting are most common. Serious side effects include gastrointestinal symptoms, hypersensitivity reactions, neutropenia, febrile neutropenia, and renal failure. Cardiac arrhythmia, dehydration, dizziness, dyspepsia, dysuria, headache, hypotension, mucosal inflammation, muscle spasms, pain, peripheral edema, UTI, and weight loss have also occurred.

Overdose: Exacerbation of adverse reactions such as bone marrow suppression and GI disorders.

ANTIDOTE

Keep physician informed of all side effects. Most will be treated symptomatically as indicated. Minor hypersensitivity reactions may subside with temporary discontinuation of cabazitaxel and additional antihistamines, corticosteroids, or H_2 antagonists. Reduction in rate of administration may allow continued treatment. Discontinue immediately if severe reactions occur; may require epinephrine (Adrenalin), antihistamines (e.g., diphenhydramine [Benadryl]), corticosteroids (e.g., dexamethasone [Decadron]), or bronchodilators (e.g., albuterol [Ventolin], theophylline [Aminophylline]). Neutropenia can be profound but may be treated with filgrastim (G-CSF, Neupogen). Severe thrombocytopenia may require platelet transfusions. Severe anemia (less than 8 Gm/dL) may require packed cell transfusions; moderate anemia (less than 11 Gm/dL) may be treated with darbepoetin alfa (Aranesp) or epoetin alfa (Epogen). Discontinue cabazitaxel if adverse reactions continue after the dose adjustment to 20 mg/M². There is no specific antidote for overdose. Administer G-CSF as soon as possible and closely monitor chemistry, vital signs and other functions. Resuscitate if indicated.

CAFFEINE CITRATE
(**KAF**-feen **SIT**-rayt)

Cafcit

CNS stimulant
Respiratory stimulant adjunct

pH 4.7

PEDIATRIC DOSE

The dose expressed as caffeine base is one half the dose when expressed as caffeine citrate. The recommended loading dose and maintenance dose are listed in the following chart.

Guidelines for Loading and Maintenance Doses of Caffeine Citrate		
	Dose of Cafcit (volume)	Dose Expressed as Caffeine Citrate
Loading dose	1 mL/kg	20 mg/kg for 1 dose
Maintenance dose	0.25 mL/kg	5 mg/kg every 24 hours

Begin maintenance dose 24 hours after loading dose. Maintenance dose may be given IV or orally. Duration of treatment beyond 10 to 12 days has not been studied. See Precautions.

DOSE ADJUSTMENTS

May adjust maintenance dose using serum concentrations of caffeine. ■ To avoid toxicity in neonates with impaired renal or hepatic function, use with caution and monitor serum concentrations.

DILUTION

Both the IV and the oral doses are supplied in vials containing 60 mg/3 mL of caffeine citrate (30 mg/3 mL of caffeine base). Confirm vial is for IV use. Withdraw calculated dose and dilute with sufficient D5W to administer at the recommended rate of administration.

Storage: Store at CRT. Single-use vial. Discard any unused solution. Stable for 24 hours at room temperature when mixed with any of the solutions listed in Compatibility.

COMPATIBILITY

Consider any drug NOT listed as compatible to be INCOMPATIBLE until consulting a pharmacist; specific conditions may apply.

Solution: Manufacturer lists D5W; another source adds D5/¼NS, D5/¼NS with 20 mEq KCL/L.

Additive: Manufacturer lists amino acid solution 8.5% (Aminosyn 8.5%), calcium gluconate 10%, D5W, dextrose 50%, dopamine 40 mg/mL diluted to 0.6 mg/mL with D5W, fentanyl diluted to 10 mcg/mL with D5W, heparin sodium diluted to 1 unit/mL with D5W, IV fat emulsion 20% (Intralipid 20%).

One source suggests the following **compatibilities:**

Y-site: Doxapram (Dopram), levofloxacin (Levaquin).

RATE OF ADMINISTRATION

Use of a syringe pump infuser is recommended.

Loading dose: Infuse over 30 minutes.

Maintenance dose: Infuse over 10 minutes.

ACTIONS

A bronchial smooth muscle relaxant, a CNS and cardiac stimulant, and a diuretic. Structurally related to other methylxanthines (e.g., theophylline and theobromine). Exact mechanism of action in apnea of prematurity is not known. Postulated mechanisms include stimulation of the respiratory center, increased minute ventilation, decreased threshold to hypercapnia, increased response to hypercapnia, increased skeletal muscle tone, decreased diaphragmatic fatigue, increased metabolic rate, increased oxygen consumption, blood vessel dilatation, central vessel vasoconstriction, and smooth muscle relaxation. Readily distributes into the brain. Caffeine levels in the CSF of preterm neonates approximate plasma levels. Metabolized in the liver by the cytochrome P_{450} system. Metabolism and elimination in the preterm neonate are much slower than in adults due to immature hepatic and/or renal function. Mean half-life and fraction excreted unchanged in the urine is inversely related to gestational/postconceptual age. In neonates, the half-life is approximately 3 to 4 days and the fraction excreted unchanged in the urine is approximately 86% (within 6 days). By 9 months of age, the metabolism of caffeine approximates that seen in adults (half-life is 5 hours and amount excreted unchanged is 1%). Interconversion between caffeine and theophylline have been reported in preterm neonates. After theophylline administration, caffeine levels are approximately 25% of theophylline levels. After caffeine administration, 3% to 5% of caffeine administered converts to theophylline.

INDICATIONS AND USES

Short-term treatment of apnea of prematurity in infants more than 28 but less than 33 weeks' gestational age. In one study apnea of prematurity was defined as having at least 6 apnea episodes of more than 20 seconds duration in a 24-hour period with no other identifiable cause of apnea. **Unlabeled uses:** Prevention of postoperative apnea in former preterm infants.

CONTRAINDICATIONS

Hypersensitivity to any of its components.

PRECAUTIONS

Reports in the literature suggest a possible association between the use of methylxanthines and the development of necrotizing enterocolitis. Necrotizing enterocolitis, resulting in death in some cases, has been reported in neonates receiving caffeine citrate. ■ Apnea of prematurity is a diagnosis of exclusion. Other causes of apnea (e.g., CNS disorders, primary lung disease, anemia, sepsis, metabolic disturbances, cardiovascular abnormalities, or obstructive apnea) should be ruled out or properly treated prior to initiating therapy with caffeine citrate. ■ Is a CNS stimulant. Use with caution in infants with seizure disorders. ■ May increase heart rate, left ventricular output, and stroke volume. Use with caution in infants with cardiovascular disease. ■ Duration of treatment of apnea of prematurity in trials has been limited to 10 to 12 days. Safety and efficacy of therapy beyond this time have not been established. ■ Safety and efficacy for use in prophylactic treatment of sudden infant death syndrome (SIDS) or before extubation in mechanically ventilated infants have not been established. ■ Use with caution in infants with impaired renal or hepatic function; see Dose Adjustments and Monitor. ■ Patients sensitive to other xanthines (e.g., aminophylline) may also be sensitive to caffeine.

Monitor: Obtain baseline serum caffeine levels in infants previously treated with theophylline, since preterm infants metabolize theophylline to caffeine; see Actions. Levels should also be obtained in infants born to mothers who ingested caffeine before delivery, as caffeine readily crosses the placenta. Caffeine levels ranged from 8 to 40 mg/L in clinical trials. A therapeutic plasma concentration range has not been determined, but one source suggests 5 to 25 mcg/mL. Serious toxicity has been reported at levels exceeding 50 mg/L. Monitor levels periodically during treatment to avoid toxicity. Monitoring is especially important in infants with impaired renal or hepatic function; see Dose Adjustments. ▪ Monitor serum glucose periodically. Hypoglycemia and hyperglycemia have been reported. ▪ Monitor for S/S of necrotizing enterocolitis (e.g., gastric distention, vomiting, bloody stools). Screening stools for occult blood may be helpful in identifying early-onset necrotizing enterocolitis.

Patient Education: Caregivers should be instructed to consult physician if infant continues to have apnea events and to not increase the dose of caffeine citrate without consulting a physician. ▪ Contact physician at the first sign of lethargy or GI intolerance (e.g., abdominal distention, vomiting, or bloody stools). ▪ Dose must be accurately measured, and any unused solution must be discarded.

Maternal/Child: Category C: no controlled studies; benefits should outweigh risks. ▪ Half-life is increased in pregnant women. ▪ Half-life may be in excess of 100 hours in infants under 6 months of age due to immature liver function.

DRUG/LAB INTERACTIONS

Metabolized by the cytochrome P_{450} system. Lower caffeine doses may be required with coadministration of medications that **inhibit the P_{450} system,** decreasing the elimination of caffeine (e.g., cimetidine [Tagamet] and ketoconazole [Nizoral]). Higher caffeine doses may be needed with coadministration of medications that **induce the P_{450} system,** increasing the elimination of caffeine (e.g., phenobarbital and phenytoin). ▪ Interconversion between caffeine and **theophylline** has been reported. Concurrent use of these drugs is not recommended; see Actions.

SIDE EFFECTS

Cardiovascular effects (e.g., tachycardia, increased left ventricular output, and increased stroke volume), CNS stimulation (e.g., irritability, jitteriness, restlessness), GI effects (e.g., feeding intolerance, gastritis, increased gastric aspirate, and necrotizing enterocolitis), hyperglycemia, hypoglycemia, renal effects (e.g., increased urine output, increased CrCl, and increased sodium and calcium excretion).

Overdose: Signs and symptoms of caffeine overdose in the preterm infant may include: elevated BUN, elevated total leukocyte concentration, fever, fine tremor of extremities, hyperglycemia, hypertonia, insomnia, jitteriness, nonpurposeful jaw and lip movements, opisthotonos, seizures, tachypnea, tonic-clonic movements, or vomiting.

ANTIDOTE

Notify the physician of any side effects. Treatment of overdose is primarily symptomatic and supportive. Seizures may be treated with intravenous administration of diazepam (Valium) or a barbiturate such as pentobarbital (Nembutal). Caffeine levels have been shown to decrease after exchange transfusions. Resuscitate as necessary.

CALCITRIOL

(kal-si-TRYE-ole)

Calcijex

Vitamin D

pH 5.9 to 7

USUAL DOSE

Effectiveness of calcitriol therapy is dependent on adequate daily intake of calcium. The RDA of calcium in adults is 800 mg. Calcium supplementation or proper dietary measures must be initiated and maintained.

Hypocalcemia and/or secondary hyperparathyroidism: Recommended initial dose, depending on the severity of hypocalcemia and/or secondary hyperparathyroidism, is 1 mcg (0.02 mcg/kg) to 2 mcg administered at each hemodialysis treatment (three times weekly, approximately every other day). Initial doses have ranged from 0.5 to 4 mcg three times weekly.

Information supplied by the manufacturer suggests that the relative dosing of paricalcitol to calcitriol is 4:1. When converting a patient from calcitriol to paricalcitol, the initial dose of paricalcitol should be four times greater than the patient's dose of calcitriol.

PEDIATRIC DOSE

Hypocalcemia in end stage renal disease (ESRD) (unlabeled): 0.01 to 0.05 mcg/kg/dose given 3 times a week; see Maternal/Child. See all comments under Usual Dose.

DOSE ADJUSTMENTS

Adjust dosing based on patient response. Begin dosing at lower end of dose range in the elderly; see Elderly. If a satisfactory response is not observed, dose may be increased by 0.5 to 1 mcg at 2- to 4-week intervals. Monitor serum calcium, phosphorus, and calcium × phosphorus product (Ca × P) frequently during any dose adjustment period; see Monitor. ■ Discontinue therapy if elevated calcium level or a Ca × P product of greater than 70 is noted. Reinitiate therapy at a lower dose when parameters normalize. ■ Calcitriol dose may need to be reduced as the parathyroid hormone (PTH) levels decrease in response to therapy. The currently accepted target range for intact parathyroid hormone (iPTH) in chronic renal failure (CRF) patients is no more than 1.5 to 3 times the non-uremic upper limit of normal. Incremental dosing must be individualized and commensurate with PTH, serum calcium, and phosphorus levels. The following chart is a suggested approach to dose titration.

Calcitriol Suggested Dosing Guidelines	
PTH Levels	Calcitriol Dose
The same or increasing	Increase
Decreasing by <30%	Increase
Decreasing by >30% but <60%	Maintain
Decreasing by >60%	Decrease
One and one-half to three times the upper limit of normal	Maintain

DILUTION
May be given undiluted. Available in 1-mcg/mL ampules.
Storage: Store ampules at CRT. Protect from light. Calcitriol may be drawn up into a syringe up to 8 hours prior to administration but must be protected from direct sunlight.

COMPATIBILITY
Specific information not available; consult pharmacist.

RATE OF ADMINISTRATION
Administer as a bolus dose into the venous line at the end of hemodialysis.

ACTIONS
The active form of vitamin D_3 (cholecalciferol). Must be metabolically activated in liver and kidney before it is fully active on its target tissues. In bone, acts with PTH to stimulate resorption of calcium. In kidneys, increases tubular reabsorption of calcium. Stimulates intestinal calcium transport, and directly suppresses synthesis and release of PTH from the parathyroid gland. A vitamin D–resistant state may exist in uremic patients because of the failure of the kidney to adequately convert precursors to the active compound, calcitriol. Duration of action is 3 to 5 days.

INDICATIONS AND USES
Management of hypocalcemia in patients undergoing chronic renal dialysis. Has been shown to significantly reduce elevated PTH levels, which results in improvement in renal osteodystrophy.

CONTRAINDICATIONS
Patients with hypercalcemia or evidence of vitamin D toxicity.

PRECAUTIONS
Since calcitriol is the most potent form of vitamin D available, oral vitamin D supplements should be discontinued during treatment. ■ Dietary phosphorus should be restricted and a non–aluminum phosphate–binding compound (e.g., calcium acetate [PhosLo], sevelamer [Renagel]) should be administered to control serum phosphorus levels in patients undergoing dialysis.
Monitor: Obtain baseline serum calcium, phosphorus, aluminum, albumin, and PTH assays. ■ Serum calcium levels should be corrected for serum albumin using the following equation: Corrected Ca = observed Ca + 0.8 × (normal albumin − observed albumin). For example: If serum calcium is 7 mg/dL and observed albumin is 2.5 Gm/dL, Corrected Ca = 7 + 0.8 × (4 − 2.5) = 8.2 mg/dL. All decisions regarding therapy should be based on corrected calcium values. ■ Monitor magnesium, alkaline phosphatase, and 24-hour urinary calcium and phosphorus periodically. ■ Criteria used to determine if calcitriol should be administered include: serum calcium less than 11.5 mg/dL, Ca × P less than 70, serum albumin less than 60 mcg/L (within normal limits), and PTH more than 3 times the upper limit of normal. ■ Serum calcium, phosphorus, and the Ca × P product should be monitored twice weekly during dose titration. Once stable, decrease monitoring to once monthly. See Dose Adjustments. ■ PTH levels, once stable, should be monitored every 3 months. Adynamic bone lesions may develop if PTH levels are suppressed to abnormal levels. If PTH levels fall below the target range (1.5 to 3 times the upper limit of normal), the calcitriol dose should be reduced. Discontinuation may result in rebound effect. Therefore, gradual titration downward to a new maintenance dose is recommended; see Dose Adjustments. ■ Overdosage of vitamin D is dangerous. May induce hypercalcemia

and/or hypercalciuria. If clinically significant hypercalcemia develops, dose should be reduced or held. Chronic hypercalcemia can lead to generalized vascular calcification, nephrocalcinosis, and other soft-tissue calcification. The serum Ca × P product should not be allowed to exceed 70. Radiographic evaluation of suspect anatomical regions may be useful in early detection of this condition; see Side Effects and Antidote. ▪ Use with caution in patients receiving digoxin. Hypercalcemia may precipitate cardiac arrhythmias; see Drug/Lab Interactions.

Patient Education: Report symptoms of hypercalcemia promptly. Dose adjustment or treatment may be required. Strict adherence to dietary supplementation of calcium and restriction of phosphorus is required to ensure optimal effectiveness of therapy. Phosphate-binding compounds (e.g., calcium acetate [PhosLo]) may be needed to control serum phosphorus levels in patients with CRF, but excessive use of aluminum-containing products (e.g., aluminum hydroxide gel [Alternagel]) should be avoided. ▪ Avoid use of unapproved nonprescription medications, including magnesium-containing antacids.

Maternal/Child: Category C: safety for use in pregnancy not established. Benefits must outweigh risks. ▪ Safety for use in breast-feeding not established. A decision should be made whether to discontinue nursing or to discontinue the drug. ▪ Safety and effectiveness have been studied in a small number of pediatric patients, ages 13 to 18 years, with ESRD on hemodialysis. The mean weekly dose ranged from 1 to 1.4 mcg. Use in this study program appeared to be safe and effective. See package insert for study information.

Elderly: Begin dosing at lower end of dose range. Consider age-related organ impairment, concomitant disease, and/or drug therapy; see Dose Adjustments.

DRUG/LAB INTERACTIONS

Specific interaction studies have not been performed. ▪ **Digoxin** toxicity is potentiated by hypercalcemia. Use caution when calcitriol is prescribed concomitantly with digoxin compounds. ▪ **Phosphate or vitamin D–related compounds** should not be taken concomitantly with calcitriol. ▪ **Magnesium-containing antacids** and calcitriol should not be used concomitantly. Hypermagnesemia may result.

SIDE EFFECTS

Overdose or chronic administration may lead to hypercalcemia, hypercalciuria, and hyperphosphatemia. High intake of calcium and phosphate concomitant with calcitriol therapy may lead to similar abnormalities. Signs and symptoms of vitamin D intoxication associated with hypercalcemia include *Early:* bone pain, constipation, dry mouth, headache, metallic taste, muscle pain, nausea, somnolence, vomiting, and weakness. *Late:* albuminuria, anorexia, cardiac arrhythmias, conjunctivitis (calcific), decreased libido, ectopic calcification, elevated BUN, elevated AST and ALT, hypercholesterolemia, hypertension, hyperthermia, nocturia, overt psychosis (rare), pain at injection site, pancreatitis, photophobia, polydipsia, polyuria, pruritus, rhinorrhea, and weight loss. Rare cases of hypersensitivity reactions, including anaphylaxis, have been reported.

ANTIDOTE

Notify physician of any side effects. Treatment of patients with clinically significant hypercalcemia (more than 1 mg/dL above the upper limit of normal range) consists of supportive measures, immediate dose reduction or interruption of therapy, initiation of a low-calcium diet, withdrawal of calcium supplements, patient mobilization, attention to fluid and electrolyte imbalances, assessment of electrocardiographic abnormalities (critical in patients receiving digoxin), and hemodialysis or peritoneal dialysis against a calcium-free dialysate, as warranted. Hypercalcemia usually resolves in 2 to 7 days. Monitor serum calcium levels frequently until calcium levels return to within normal limits. May reinitiate calcitriol therapy at a dose 0.5 mcg less than prior dose. See Dose Adjustments.

CALCIUM CHLORIDE
(**KAL**-see-um **KLOR**-eyed)

Electrolyte replenisher
Antihypocalcemic
Cardiotonic
Antihyperkalemic
Antihypermagnesemic

pH 5.5 to 7.5

USUAL DOSE

*In a 10% solution, 10 mL (1 Gm) contains 13.6 mEq (272 mg) of calcium; 1 mL (100 mg), 1.36 mEq (27.2 mg). **All doses based on a 10% solution.***

Hypocalcemic disorders (prophylaxis, treatment, electrolyte replacement, maintenance): 5 to 10 mL (500 mg to 1 Gm) at intervals of 1 to 3 days. Repeat doses may be required and are based on patient response or serum calcium levels. May be given as part of a TPN program.

Magnesium intoxication: 5 mL (500 mg). Observe for signs of recovery before giving any additional calcium.

Hyperkalemia ECG disturbances of cardiac function: 1 to 10 mL (100 mg to 1 Gm); titrate dose by monitoring ECG changes. AHA guidelines recommend 5 to 10 mL of a 10% solution (500 mg to 1 Gm). Repeat as needed.

Cardiac resuscitation (see Indications for specific uses): 0.02 to 0.04 mL/kg (2 to 4 mg/kg); repeat at 10-minute intervals as indicated or as measured by serum deficits of calcium. Consider need for calcium (usually gluconate or gluceptate) for every 500 mL of whole blood if arrest occurs in a situation requiring copious blood replacement.

Overdose of calcium channel blockers or beta adrenergic blockers (unlabeled): AHA guidelines recommend 5 to 10 mL of a 10% solution (500 mg to 1 Gm). May repeat as needed.

PEDIATRIC DOSE

Do not administer into a scalp vein in pediatric patients; see Precautions, Monitor, and Maternal/Child.

Hypocalcemic disorders: 0.027 to 0.05 mL/kg of body weight (2.7 to 5 mg/kg) of a 10% solution. Up to 10 mL (1 Gm)/day may be required. No data from clinical trials is available regarding repeat doses. Sources suggest repeat doses every 4 to 6 hours based on patient response or serum calcium levels.

Cardiac resuscitation (see Indications for specific uses): 0.2 mL/kg of a 10% solution (20 mg/kg). Repeat as indicated at 10-minute intervals. AHA guidelines recommend consideration of this dose for documented or suspected hypocalcemia or hyperkalemia as well as for hypomagnesemia and calcium channel blocker overdose.

DILUTION

May be given undiluted, but preferably diluted with an equal amount of SW or NS for injection to make a 5% solution. Solution should be warmed to body temperature. May be further diluted with most common infusion solutions and given as an intermittent or continuous infusion.

COMPATIBILITY   (Underline Indicates Conflicting Compatibility Information)

Consider any drug NOT listed as compatible to be INCOMPATIBLE until consulting a pharmacist; specific conditions may apply.
Calcium salts not generally mixed with carbonates, phosphates, sulfates, or tartrates. *Extreme caution and a specific multi-step process are required when calcium and phosphates are combined in parenteral nutrition solutions. Consult pharmacist.*

One source suggests the following **compatibilities:**
Additive: Amikacin (Amikin), ascorbic acid, chloramphenicol (Chloromycetin), <u>dobutamine</u>, dopamine, hydrocortisone sodium succinate (Solu-Cortef), isoproterenol (Isuprel), lidocaine, <u>magnesium sulfate</u>, norepinephrine (Levophed), penicillin G potassium and sodium, pentobarbital (Nembutal), phenobarbital (Luminal), <u>sodium bicarbonate</u>, verapamil.
Y-site: Amiodarone (Nexterone), dobutamine, doxapram (Dopram), epinephrine (Adrenalin), esmolol (Brevibloc), inamrinone (Amrinone), <u>micafungin (Mycamine)</u>, milrinone (Primacor), morphine, nitroprusside sodium (Nitropress), paclitaxel (Taxol).

RATE OF ADMINISTRATION
0.5 to 1 mL of solution over 1 minute. Administration into a central or deep vein is preferred; see Monitor. Stop or slow infusion rate if patient complains of discomfort. Do not exceed the equivalent of 1 mL calcium chloride/minute by IV injection or infusion. Rapid administration may cause bradycardia; heat waves; local burning sensation; metallic, calcium, or chalky taste; moderate drop in BP; peripheral vasodilation; or a sense of oppression.

ACTIONS
Calcium is a basic element prevalent in the human body. It affects bones, nerves, muscles, glands, cardiac and vascular tone, and normal coagulation of the blood. It is excreted in the urine and feces.

INDICATIONS AND USES
Calcium preparations other than calcium chloride are often preferred except in cardiac resuscitation or calcium channel blocker toxicity. ▪ Increase plasma calcium levels in hypocalcemic disorders (e.g., tetany [neonatal, parathyroid deficiency], vitamin D deficiency, alkalosis, conditions associated with intestinal malabsorption). ▪ Treat ECG disturbances caused by hyperkalemia. ▪ Adjunctive therapy in sensitivity reactions (especially with urticaria), insect bites or stings (relieve muscle cramping), acute symptoms of lead colic, rickets, or osteomalacia. ▪ Cardiac resuscitation only to treat hypocalcemia, hyperkalemia, or calcium-channel blocker toxicity (verapamil, diltiazem), or after open heart surgery if epinephrine does not produce effective myocardial contractions. ▪ Antidote for cardiac and respiratory depression of magnesium sulfate toxicity.
Unlabeled uses: Treatment of arrhythmias and/or hypotension caused by an overdose of calcium channel blockers (e.g., diltiazem [Cardizem], verapamil or beta-adrenergic blockers (e.g., atenolol [Tenormin], metoprolol [Lopressor], propranolol). ▪ Prevention of hypotension caused by calcium channel blockers.

CONTRAINDICATIONS
Digitalized patients, hypercalcemia, ventricular fibrillation. Not recommended in the treatment of asystole and electromechanical dissociation.

PRECAUTIONS

Three times more potent than calcium gluconate. ▪ For IV use only. ▪ See Drug/Lab Interactions.
Monitor: Confirm patency of vein; select a large vein and use a small needle to reduce vein irritation. Administration into a central or deep vein is preferred. Necrosis and sloughing will occur with IM or SC injection or extravasation. ▪ Keep patient recumbent after injection to prevent postural hypotension. ▪ Monitor vital signs carefully. ▪ Monitor serum calcium levels as indicated. May cause hyperchloremic acidosis.
Maternal/Child: Category C: safety for use in pregnancy and breast-feeding not established. Use only when clearly needed. ▪ Rarely used IV in pediatric patients. Use of a less irritating salt preferred because of small vein size.

DRUG/LAB INTERACTIONS

Will increase **digoxin** toxicity and may cause arrhythmias. If necessary, give small amounts very slowly. ▪ Potentiated by **thiazide diuretics** (e.g., chlorothiazide [Diuril]); may cause hypercalcemia or calcium toxicity. ▪ May reduce plasma levels of **atenolol** (Tenormin). ▪ Can reduce neuromuscular paralysis and respiratory depression produced by **antibiotics such as kanamycin** (Kantrex). ▪ Antagonizes **verapamil;** can reverse clinical effects. ▪ May cause metabolic alkalosis and inhibit binding of potassium with **sodium polystyrene sulfonate.**

SIDE EFFECTS

Usual doses will produce a local burning sensation, moderate drop in BP, and peripheral vasodilation. May cause bradycardia, cardiac arrest, heat waves; metallic, calcium, or chalky taste; prolonged state of cardiac contraction, sense of oppression, or tingling sensation, especially with a too-rapid rate of administration.
Overdose: Coma, intractable nausea and vomiting, lethargy, markedly elevated plasma calcium level, weakness, and sudden death.

ANTIDOTE

If side effects occur, further dilution and decrease in the rate of administration may be necessary. If side effects persist, discontinue the drug and notify the physician. IV infusion of sodium chloride (to maintain normovolemia) and furosemide (Lasix) 80 to 100 mg IV every 2 to 4 hours (with caution) is recommended in overdose. Sodium chloride competes with calcium for reabsorption in the renal tubules; furosemide enhances the activity. Together they will reduce hypercalcemia by causing a marked increase in calcium excretion. Monitoring of fluid, electrolytes, and cardiac and respiratory status is imperative. Disodium edetate may be used with extreme caution as a calcium chelating agent if overdose is critical. For extravasation inject affected area with 1% procaine hydrochloride and hyaluronidase to reduce venospasm and dilute calcium. Use a 27- or 25-gauge needle. Warm, moist compresses may be helpful. Resuscitate as necessary.

CALCIUM GLUCONATE
(**KAL**-see-um **GLOO**-koh-nayt)

Electrolyte replenisher
Antihypocalcemic
Cardiotonic
Antihyperkalemic
Antihypermagnesemic

pH 6 to 8.2

USUAL DOSE
All doses based on a 10% solution.
Hypocalcemia disorders/maintenance: 5 to 20 mL (2.3 to 9.3 mEq). Repeat as required. Daily dose ranges from 4.65 to 70 mEq. Larger amounts may be given as an intermittent or continuous IV infusion. 10 mL (1 Gm in a 10% solution) contains 4.65 mEq (93 mg) of calcium.
Emergency elevation of serum calcium: 15 to 30.1 mL (7 to 14 mEq). Repeat every 1 to 3 days based on patient response.
Cardiac resuscitation (see Indications for specific uses): 5 to 8 mL (2.3 to 3.6 mEq). Repeat at 10-minute intervals as indicated by clinical condition or serum calcium level.
Hyperkalemia with secondary cardiac toxicity: 4.8 to 30.1 mL (2.25 to 14 mEq). ECG monitoring required; observe results and repeat in 1 to 2 minutes if indicated.
Hypocalcemic tetany: 9.7 to 34.4 mL (4.5 to 16 mEq). Repeat as indicated to control tetany.
Magnesium intoxication: 9.7 to 19.4 mL (4.5 to 9 mEq). Repeat as indicated by patient response; observe for signs of recovery before giving additional calcium.
Exchange transfusion: Approximately 2.9 mL (1.35 mEq) with each 100 mL of citrated blood.

PEDIATRIC DOSE
Do not administer into a scalp vein in pediatric patients; see Precautions/ Monitor. *All doses based on a 10% solution.*
Hypocalcemia disorders/maintenance: 5 mL/kg/day (2.3 mEq/kg/day) or 120 mL/M^2/day (56 mEq/M^2/day) in divided doses.
Emergency elevation of serum calcium: 2.2 to 15 mL (1 to 7 mEq). Repeat every 1 to 3 days based on patient response.
Hypocalcemic tetany: 1.1 to 1.5 mL/kg (0.5 to 0.7 mEq/kg) 3 or 4 times daily until tetany is controlled.
Cardiac resuscitation (see Indications for specific uses): 0.6 to 1 mL/kg of a 10% solution (60 to 100 mg/kg). Repeat if indicated. AHA guidelines recommend consideration of this dose for documented or suspected hypocalcemia or hyperkalemia as well as for hypomagnesemia and calcium channel blocker overdose.

NEONATAL DOSE
Do not administer into a scalp vein in neonates; see Precautions/Monitor.
Hypocalcemia disorders/maintenance: Not more than 2 mL (0.93 mEq).
Emergency elevation of serum calcium: Up to 2.2 mL (1 mEq). Repeat every 1 to 3 days based on patient response.

Continued

Hypocalcemic tetany: 5.2 mL/kg/24 hr (2.4 mEq/kg/24 hr) in divided doses.

Exchange transfusion: 1 mL (0.45 mEq) with each 100 mL citrated blood.

DILUTION

May be given undiluted or may be further diluted in up to 1,000 mL of NS for infusion. Solution should be warmed to body temperature. Solution must be clear and free of crystals. Crystals can be dissolved by heating to 80° C (146° F) in a dry heat oven for at least 1 hour. Shake vigorously; cool to room temperature. Discard if crystals persist.

Pediatric and neonatal dilution: Must be further diluted with NS.

COMPATIBILITY (Underline Indicates Conflicting Compatibility Information)

Consider any drug NOT listed as compatible to be INCOMPATIBLE until consulting a pharmacist; specific conditions may apply.

Calcium salts not generally mixed with carbonates, phosphates, sulfates, or tartrates. *Extreme caution and a specific multi-step process are required when calcium and phosphates are combined in parenteral nutrition solutions. Consult pharmacist.*

One source suggests the following **compatibilities:**

Additive: Amikacin (Amikin), aminophylline, ascorbic acid, chloramphenicol (Chloromycetin), furosemide (Lasix), heparin, hydrocortisone sodium succinate (Solu-Cortef), lidocaine, magnesium sulfate, norepinephrine (Levophed), penicillin G potassium and sodium, phenobarbital (Luminal), potassium chloride (KCl), prochlorperazine (Compazine), tobramycin, vancomycin, verapamil.

Y-site: Aldesleukin (Proleukin), allopurinol (Aloprim), amifostine (Ethyol), amiodarone (Nexterone), ampicillin, aztreonam (Azactam), bivalirudin (Angiomax), cefazolin (Ancef), cefepime (Maxipime), ciprofloxacin (Cipro IV), cisatracurium (Nimbex), cladribine (Leustatin), dexmedetomidine (Precedex), dobutamine, docetaxel (Taxotere), doripenem (Doribax), doxapram (Dopram), doxorubicin liposomal (Doxil), enalaprilat (Vasotec IV), epinephrine (Adrenalin), etoposide phosphate (Etopophos), famotidine (Pepcid IV), fenoldopam (Corlopam), filgrastim (Neupogen), gemcitabine (Gemzar), granisetron (Kytril), hetastarch in electrolytes (Hextend), labetalol (Trandate), linezolid (Zyvox), melphalan (Alkeran), meropenem (Merrem IV), micafungin (Mycamine), midazolam (Versed), milrinone (Primacor), nicardipine (Cardene IV), oxaliplatin (Eloxatin), piperacillin/tazobactam (Zosyn), potassium chloride (KCl), prochlorperazine (Compazine), propofol (Diprivan), remifentanil (Ultiva), sargramostim (Leukine), tacrolimus (Prograf), teniposide (Vumon), thiotepa, vinorelbine (Navelbine).

RATE OF ADMINISTRATION

In all situations stop or slow infusion rate if patient complains of discomfort. Rapid administration may cause vasodilation, decreased BP, cardiac arrhythmias, syncope, and cardiac arrest.

IV injection: Undiluted, each 0.5 mL or fraction thereof over 1 minute. Do not exceed 2 mL/min (200 mg).

Intermittent IV: Do not exceed a rate of 200 mg/min (IV injection rate).

Infusion: Diluted in 1,000 mL of NS, it may be given over 12 to 24 hours. Do not exceed 200 mg/min.

Pediatric and neonatal rate of administration: Slow rate of administration considerably. Observe continuously.

ACTIONS

Calcium is a basic element prevalent in the human body. It affects bones, nerves, glands, cardiac and vascular tone, and normal coagulation of the blood. It crosses the placental barrier and is secreted in breast milk. It is excreted in the urine and feces.

INDICATIONS AND USES

Increase plasma calcium levels in hypocalcemic disorders (e.g., tetany [neonatal, parathyroid deficiency], vitamin D deficiency, alkalosis, conditions associated with intestinal malabsorption). ▪ Adjunctive therapy in sensitivity reactions (especially with urticaria), insect bites or stings (relieve muscle cramping), acute symptoms of lead colic, rickets, or osteomalacia. ▪ Cardiac resuscitation only to treat hypocalcemia, hyperkalemia, or calcium-channel blocker overdose (verapamil, diltiazem). ▪ Antidote for cardiac and respiratory depression of magnesium sulfate toxicity. ▪ Prevention of hypocalcemia during exchange transfusions. ▪ Decrease capillary permeability in allergic conditions, nonthrombocytopenic purpura and exudative dermatoses (e.g., dermatitis herpetiformis). ▪ Treat pruritus of eruptions caused by drugs. ▪ Treat ECG disturbances caused by hyperkalemia or verapamil-induced hypotension.

Unlabeled uses: Treatment of verapamil overdose, acute hypotension from verapamil, and prevention of initial hypotension when it could be detrimental to a specific patient and verapamil is required.

CONTRAINDICATIONS

IM use in infants and small children. Digitalized patients, hypercalcemia, ventricular fibrillation.

PRECAUTIONS

Has only one third the potency of calcium chloride. ▪ For IV use only; IM use permitted in adults only if IV administration cannot be accomplished; see Monitor.

Monitor: Confirm patency of vein; select a large vein and use a small needle to reduce vein irritation. Local necrosis and abscess formation can occur with IM or SC injection or extravasation. ▪ Keep patient recumbent after injection to prevent postural hypotension. ▪ Monitor vital signs carefully.

Maternal/Child: Category C: safety for use in pregnancy not established; benefits must outweigh risk. ▪ See Contraindications.

DRUG/LAB INTERACTIONS

Will increase **digoxin** toxicity and may cause arrhythmias. If necessary, give small amounts very slowly. ▪ Potentiated by **thiazide diuretics** (e.g., chlorothiazide [Diuril]); may cause hypercalcemia or calcium toxicity. ▪ May reduce plasma levels of **atenolol** (Tenormin). ▪ Antagonizes **verapamil**; can reverse clinical effects. ▪ May cause metabolic alkalosis and inhibit binding of potassium with **sodium polystyrene sulfonate.**

SIDE EFFECTS

Rare when given as recommended: bradycardia, cardiac arrhythmias, cardiac arrest, heat waves, hypotension; metallic, calcium, or chalky taste; sense of oppression, syncope, tingling, and vasodilation can occur with too-rapid rate of administration. Depression of neuromuscular function, flushing, prolonged state of cardiac contraction can occur.

Overdose: Coma, intractable nausea and vomiting, lethargy, markedly elevated plasma calcium level, weakness, and sudden death.

ANTIDOTE

If side effects occur, further dilution and decrease in the rate of administration may be necessary. If side effects persist, discontinue the drug and notify the physician. IV infusion of sodium chloride (to maintain normovolemia) and furosemide (Lasix) 80 to 100 mg IV every 2 to 4 hours (with caution) are recommended in overdose. Sodium chloride competes with calcium for reabsorption in the renal tubules; furosemide enhances the activity. Together they will reduce hypercalcemia by causing a marked increase in calcium excretion. Monitoring of fluid, electrolytes, and cardiac and respiratory status is imperative. Disodium edetate may be used with extreme caution as a calcium chelating agent if overdosage is critical. For extravasation inject affected area with 1% procaine hydrochloride and hyaluronidase to reduce venospasm and dilute calcium. Use a 27- or 25-gauge needle. Warm, moist compresses may be helpful. Resuscitate as necessary.

CAPREOMYCIN BBW

(kap-ree-oh-**MYE**-sin)

Capastat

Antibacterial
(antituberculosis)

USUAL DOSE

1 Gm daily, not to exceed 20 mg/kg/day. Give for 60 to 120 days, followed by 1 Gm two or three times weekly. Therapy for tuberculosis should be maintained for 12 to 24 months. Administered in combination with at least one other antituberculosis agent to which the patient's strain of tubercle bacilli is susceptible.

DOSE ADJUSTMENTS

The elderly and patients with reduced renal function should have dosage reduction based on CrCl using the guidelines in the following chart. These dosages are designed to achieve a mean steady-state capreomycin level of 10 mcg/mL. Elevation of BUN above 30 mg/dL or any other evidence of decreasing renal function warrants evaluation of patient. Dose reduction or discontinuation of therapy may be required.

Estimated Dosages to Attain Mean Steady-State Serum Capreomycin Concentration of 10 mcg/mL Based on CrCl			
	Dose* (mg/kg) Based on Dosing Intervals		
CrCl (mL/min)	**24 hr**	**48 hr**	**72 hr**
0 mL/min	1.29 mg/kg	2.58 mg/kg	3.87 mg/kg
10 mL/min	2.43 mg/kg	4.87 mg/kg	7.30 mg/kg
20 mL/min	3.58 mg/kg	7.16 mg/kg	10.7 mg/kg
30 mL/min	4.72 mg/kg	9.45 mg/kg	14.2 mg/kg
40 mL/min	5.87 mg/kg	11.7 mg/kg	
50 mL/min	7.01 mg/kg	14.0 mg/kg	
60 mL/min	8.16 mg/kg		
80 mL/min	10.4 mg/kg†		
100 mL/min	12.7 mg/kg†		
110 mL/min	13.9 mg/kg†		

*Optional dosing intervals are given. Longer intervals are expected to provide greater peaks and lower trough serum levels than shorter intervals.
†See Usual Dose.

DILUTION

Reconstitute each 1-Gm vial with 2 mL of NS or SW. Allow 2 to 3 minutes for complete dissolution. Withdraw calculated dose and further dilute in 100 mL NS.

Filters: No data available from manufacturer.

Storage: Store at CRT before reconstitution. After reconstitution, stable for 24 hours if refrigerated.

COMPATIBILITY
Specific information not available; consult pharmacist.

RATE OF ADMINISTRATION
A single dose as an infusion over 60 minutes. Neuromuscular blockade or respiratory paralysis may occur following rapid intravenous infusion. See Precautions and Side Effects.

ACTIONS
A polypeptide antibiotic isolated from *Streptomyces capreolus.* Active against strains of *Mycobacterium tuberculosis.* Half-life is 4 to 6 hours in patients with normal renal function. Excreted primarily unchanged in urine. Small amounts excreted in bile. Crosses the placenta. Does not penetrate into CSF.

INDICATIONS AND USES
Used concomitantly with other appropriate antituberculosis agents to treat pulmonary infections caused by capreomycin-susceptible strains of *M. tuberculosis* when the primary agents (isoniazid, rifampin, ethambutol, aminosalicylic acid, and streptomycin) have been ineffective or cannot be used because of toxicity or the presence of resistant tubercle bacilli.

CONTRAINDICATIONS
Hypersensitivity to capreomycin.

PRECAUTIONS
Usually given IM; IV used in patients with limited muscle mass. ▪ Sensitivity studies necessary to determine susceptibility of causative organism to capreomycin. ▪ To reduce the development of drug-resistant bacteria and maintain its effectiveness, capreomycin should be used to treat or prevent only those infections proven or strongly suspected to be caused by bacteria. ▪ Use with caution in patients with pre-existing auditory impairment, dehydration, or renal insufficiency or when used concomitantly with other potentially ototoxic or nephrotoxic drugs (e.g., aminoglycosides [e.g., amikacin (Amikin), gentamicin, tobramycin], colistin sulfate, polymyxin A, vancomycin). Must weigh risk of additional cranial nerve VIII (auditory and vestibular) damage or renal injury against benefit of therapy. ▪ Coadministration with other parenteral antituberculosis agents (e.g., streptomycin) is not recommended. Toxicity is additive. ▪ Renal injury, with tubular necrosis, elevation of BUN or SCr, and abnormal urinary sediment (casts, RBCs, WBCs), has been reported. Elderly patients, patients with abnormal renal function or dehydration, and patients receiving other nephrotoxic drugs are at increased risk for developing acute tubular necrosis. ▪ Elevation of BUN above 30 mg/dL or other evidence of decreasing renal function warrants evaluation of patient. Dose reduction or discontinuation of drug may be necessary; see Dose Adjustments. Clinical significance of abnormal urine sediment and slight increase in BUN or SCr during long-term therapy is not known. ▪ The peripheral neuromuscular blocking action seen with other polypeptide antibiotics (colistin sulfate, polymyxin A sulfate) and aminoglycosides (e.g., kanamycin, neomycin, streptomycin) has been reported with capreomycin. ▪ Cross-resistance between capreomycin and kanamycin, neomycin and viomycin reported. No cross-resistance observed between capreomycin and aminosalicylic acid, cycloserine, ethambutol, ethionamide, isoniazid, and streptomycin. ▪ Use with caution in patients with allergies (especially drug allergies).

Monitor: Audiometric measurements and assessment of vestibular function should be performed before initiation of therapy and at regular intervals during treatment. ▪ Obtain baseline SCr, BUN, liver function tests, and electrolytes before initiating therapy. Reduced dosage required for patients with impaired renal function; see Dose Adjustments. Weekly monitoring of renal function and periodic monitoring of electrolytes and liver function tests are recommended. ▪ Obtain serum calcium, potassium, and magnesium levels frequently; hypocalcemia, hypokalemia, and hypomagnesemia may occur during therapy. ▪ Monitor for S/S of hypersensitivity.

Patient Education: Compliance with full course of therapy is imperative. Report any side effects promptly.

Maternal/Child: Category C: safety for use during pregnancy and breast-feeding not established. Benefits must outweigh risks. Crosses the placenta. ▪ Safety and effectiveness for use in pediatric patients not established.

Elderly: Response similar to younger adults; however, dosing should be cautious; see Dose Adjustments. ▪ May be at increased risk of toxicity because of age-related decrease in renal function; monitor renal function. ▪ More likely to have impaired hearing at baseline. Initial and periodic audiometric measurement and assessment of vestibular function is recommended. See Precautions.

DRUG/LAB INTERACTIONS

Neuromuscular blockade of **nondepolarizing neuromuscular blocking agents** (e.g., vecuronium) may be enhanced with concurrent use of capreomycin because of synergistic effects and may be further enhanced by **ether or methoxyflurane anesthesia.** ▪ Risk of neuromuscular blockade increased when administered concurrently or sequentially with **polymyxins or aminoglycosides** (e.g., kanamycin, neomycin, streptomycin); see Precautions. ▪ Neuromuscular blockade antagonized by **neostigmine.** ▪ Risk of ototoxicity, nephrotoxicity, and respiratory paralysis increased when administered concurrently or sequentially with **other potentially ototoxic or nephrotoxic medications** (e.g., aminoglycosides [e.g., amikacin (Amikin), gentamicin, streptomycin, tobramycin], colistin sulfate, polymyxin A, vancomycin); see Precautions.

SIDE EFFECTS

Abnormal liver function tests, abnormal urine sediment, dizziness, electrolyte disturbances resembling Bartter's syndrome, as well as hypocalcemia, hypokalemia, and hypomagnesemia, elevated BUN or SCr, eosinophilia, febrile reactions, hypersensitivity, leukocytosis, leukopenia, maculopapular skin rash, pain and induration at injection site, subclinical auditory loss (high-tone acuity), thrombocytopenia, tinnitus, toxic nephritis, urticaria, vertigo.

ANTIDOTE

Protect airway and support ventilation and perfusion. Hydrate patient to maintain urine output of 3 to 5 mL/kg/hr. Monitor fluid balance, electrolytes, renal function, vital signs, and blood gases; treat abnormalities as indicated. Hemodialysis may be useful. Resuscitate as necessary.

CARBOPLATIN BBW
(**KAR**-boh-plah-tin)
Paraplatin

Antineoplastic
(alkylating agent)
pH 5 to 7

USUAL DOSE

Before giving a dose in a cycle, it is recommended that platelets be above 100,000/mm^3 and neutrophils above 2,000/mm^3; see Dose Adjustments. The Calvert formula for carboplatin dosing based on pre-existing renal function and/or desired platelet nadir determines the patient's dose.

$$\text{Total dose (mg)} = (\text{Target AUC}) \times (\text{GFR} + 25)$$

Dose is calculated in milligrams, not mg/M^2. The ordering physician determines the target AUC (area under the curve) and supplies the required information on the GFR (glomerular filtration rate) or CrCl, as well as the desired response. The pharmacist calculates the correct dose. See package insert for additional information.

Initial treatment of advanced ovarian cancer in combination with cyclophosphamide: Carboplatin 300 mg/M^2 plus cyclophosphamide 600 mg/M^2 on Day 1 every 4 weeks for 6 cycles or carboplatin dose targeted by Calvert equation to an AUC of 6 to 7 plus cyclophosphamide 600 mg/M^2 on Day 1 every 4 weeks.

Palliative treatment of recurrent ovarian cancer after prior chemotherapy: *As a single agent:* With normal renal function (CrCl greater than 60 mL/min), give 360 mg/M^2 on Day 1 every 4 weeks or a dose targeted by Calvert equation to an AUC of 4 to 6 appears to provide an appropriate dose range in these patients.

Treatment of brain tumor (unlabeled): *As a single agent:* 560 mg/M^2 every 4 weeks.

Treatment of unresectable non–small-cell lung cancer (NSCLC [unlabeled]): Given in combination with paclitaxel (Taxol). Many dosage regimens are being used. Examples are: paclitaxel 135 to 175 mg/M^2 as either a continuous infusion over 24 hours or an intermittent IV over 3 hours on Day 1. Follow on Day 2 with carboplatin 300 mg/M^2 or dose targeted by Calvert equation to an AUC of 6. Repeat this cycle every 4 weeks for up to 6 cycles. Another source suggests paclitaxel 135 mg/M^2 as a continuous infusion over 24 hours on Day 1 or 175 mg/M^2 IV over 3 hours on Day 1. Follow either of these doses with carboplatin dose targeted by Calvert equation to an AUC of 7.5. Repeat cycle every 21 days.

DOSE ADJUSTMENTS

Single agent or combination therapy. Dose adjustment is based on nadir after prior dose according to the chart on the next page.

Carboplatin Dose Based on Bone Marrow Suppression		
Platelets/mm^3	Neutrophils/mm^3	Adjusted Dose (from Prior Course)
>100,000	>2,000	Increase to 125%
50,000-100,000	500-2,000	No adjustment
<50,000	<500	Decrease to 75%

Once the dose has been increased to 125% of the starting dose, no further dose increases are indicated. ▪ With impaired renal function (CrCl 16 to 40 mL/min), give 200 mg/M^2; CrCl 41 to 59 mL/min, give 250 mg/M^2. Discontinue if the CrCl is less than 16 mL/min. Adjust dose by percentages and criteria as indicated for normal renal function. ▪ Bone marrow suppression is more severe in patients who have had prior therapy, especially with cisplatin and when carboplatin is used with other bone marrow–suppressing therapies or radiation, and may be more severe in the elderly. Reduced dose may be indicated. Monitor carefully and manage dose and timing to reduce additive effects.

DILUTION
Specific techniques required; see Precautions. Immediately before use dilute each 10 mg of carboplatin with 1 mL of SW for injection, D5W, or NS (50 mg with 5 mL, 150 mg with 15 mL, 450 mg with 45 mL). All yield 10 mg/mL. Should be further diluted with NS or D5W to 1 to 4 mg/mL (add 10 mL additional diluent to each 10 mg to obtain 1 mg/mL and 2.5 mL to each 10 mg to obtain 4 mg/mL). Do not use needles or IV tubing with aluminum parts to mix or administer; a precipitate will form and decrease potency. Best to mix immediately before use. Discard solution 8 hours after dilution at room temperature, 24 hours if refrigerated.
Storage: Store unopened vials at 15° to 30° C (59° to 86° F). Protect from light.

COMPATIBILITY   (Underline Indicates Conflicting Compatibility Information)
Consider any drug NOT listed as compatible to be INCOMPATIBLE until consulting a pharmacist; specific conditions may apply.
Forms a precipitate if in contact with aluminum (e.g., needles, syringes, catheters).
One source suggests the following **compatibilities:**
Additive: Cisplatin (Platinol), etoposide (VePesid), ifosfamide (Ifex), ifosfamide with etoposide, paclitaxel (Taxol).
Y-site: Allopurinol (Aloprim), amifostine (Ethyol), anidulafungin (Eraxis), aztreonam (Azactam), caspofungin (Cancidas), cefepime (Maxipime), cladribine (Leustatin), doripenem (Doribax), doxorubicin liposomal (Doxil), etoposide phosphate (Etopophos), filgrastim (Neupogen), fludarabine (Fludara), gemcitabine (Gemzar), granisetron (Kytril), linezolid (Zyvox), melphalan (Alkeran), micafungin (Mycamine), ondansetron (Zofran), oxaliplatin (Eloxatin), paclitaxel (Taxol), palonosetron (Aloxi), pemetrexed (Alimta), piperacillin/tazobactam (Zosyn), propofol (Diprivan), sargramostim (Leukine), teniposide (Vumon), thiotepa, topotecan (Hycamtin), vinorelbine (Navelbine).

RATE OF ADMINISTRATION
A single dose as an infusion over a minimum of 15 minutes. Extend administration time based on amount of diluent and patient condition.

ACTIONS

An alkylating agent. An improved platinum-based compound similar to cisplatin but with improved therapeutic effects. Better tolerated by patients, carboplatin causes less nausea and vomiting, less neurotoxicity, and less nephrotoxicity than cisplatin. Myelosuppression is generally reversible and manageable with antibiotics and transfusions. Produces interstrand DNA cross-links and is cell-cycle nonspecific. Not as heavily protein bound as cisplatin. Majority of carboplatin is excreted in the urine within 24 hours.

INDICATIONS AND USES

Initial treatment of advanced ovarian cancer in combination with other approved chemotherapeutic agents (e.g., cyclophosphamide). ▪ Palliative treatment of recurrent ovarian cancer after prior chemotherapy, including patients treated with cisplatin.

Unlabeled uses: In combination with paclitaxel (Taxol) to treat unresectable non–small-cell lung cancer (NSCLC) and fallopian tube and peritoneal cancers of ovarian origin. ▪ Treatment of brain tumors. ▪ Treatment of breast and bladder cancers, lymphomas (Hodgkin's and non-Hodgkin's), malignant melanoma, small-cell lung cancer, and retinoblastoma; and to replace cisplatin in treatment of endometrial, esophageal, head and neck, lung, and testicular cancers and relapsed and refractory acute leukemia. May be used as a single agent but most effective in protocols.

CONTRAINDICATIONS

Hypersensitivity to cisplatin or other platinum-containing compounds or mannitol; severe bone marrow suppression; significant bleeding.

PRECAUTIONS

Follow guidelines for handling cytotoxic agents. See Appendix A, p. 1429. ▪ Usually administered by or under the direction of the physician specialist. ▪ Bone marrow suppression is dose related and may be severe, resulting in infection and/or bleeding. Anemia may be cumulative and may require transfusion support. ▪ Anaphylaxis has been reported and may occur within minutes of administration. ▪ Risk of hypersensitivity increased in patients previously exposed to platinum therapy. Patients sensitive to other platinum compounds (e.g., cisplatin) may be sensitive to carboplatin. ▪ Peripheral neurotoxicity is uncommon, but risk may be increased in patients over 65 years of age and in patients previously treated with cisplatin. ▪ Secondary malignancies, including acute nonlymphocytic leukemia, myeloproliferation syndrome, and carcinoma have been reported in patients treated with alkylating agents.

Monitor: BUN and SCr should be done before each dose. CrCl, WBC, platelet count, and hemoglobin are recommended before each dose and weekly thereafter. Platelet count recommended to be 100,000/mm^3 and neutrophils 2,000/mm^3 before a dose can be repeated; see Dose Adjustments. Anemia is frequent and cumulative. Transfusion is often indicated. ▪ Excessive hydration or forced diuresis not required, but maintain adequate hydration and urinary output. ▪ Nausea and vomiting are frequently severe but less than with cisplatin; generally last 24 hours. Prophylactic administration of antiemetics is indicated. Various protocols, including metoclopramide (Reglan) and ondansetron (Zofran), dexamethasone (Decadron) and lorazepam (Ativan), droperidol (Inapsine) or haloperidol (Haldol) and dexamethasone, or prochlorperazine (Compazine) are used. ▪ Observe for symptoms of hypersensitivity reactions during administration; epinephrine, corticosteroids, and antihistamines should be available. ▪ Observe closely for symptoms of infection. Prophylactic antibiotics may be indicated pending results of C/S in a febrile neutropenic patient. ▪ Monitor for thrombocytopenia (platelet count less than 50,000/mm^3). Initiate precautions to prevent excessive bleeding (e.g., inspect IV sites, skin, and mucous membranes; use extreme care during invasive procedures; test urine, emesis, stool, and secretions for occult blood).

Patient Education: Nonhormonal birth control recommended. Manufacturer provides a patient information booklet. ▪ See Appendix D, p. 1434.

Maternal/Child: Category D: avoid pregnancy. ▪ Discontinue breastfeeding. ▪ Significant hearing loss has been reported in pediatric patients; occurred with higher-than-recommended doses of carboplatin in combination with other ototoxic agents. ▪ Safety and effectiveness for use in pediatric patients not established.

Elderly: Neurotoxicity and myelotoxicity may be more severe. ▪ Consider possibility of decreased renal function. ▪ See Dose Adjustments and Precautions.

DRUG/LAB INTERACTIONS

Nephrotoxicity and ototoxicity is additive when used with other **ototoxic or nephrotoxic agents** (e.g., acyclovir [Zovirax], aminoglycosides [e.g., gentamicin], cisplatin [Platinol], rifampin [Rifadin], quinidine). Use with caution. ▪ Bone marrow toxicity increased with other **antineoplastic agents, radiation therapy, and/or other agents that may cause blood dyscrasias** (e.g., anticonvulsants [e.g., phenytoin (Dilantin)], cephalosporins, mycophenolate [CellCept], rituximab [Rituxan]). Dose adjustment of either or both drugs may be indicated. ▪ Do not administer **live virus vaccines** to patients receiving antineoplastic drugs. ▪ See Dose Adjustments.

SIDE EFFECTS

Allergic reactions, including anaphylaxis, can occur during administration. Alopecia (rare), anemia, anorexia, bleeding, bone marrow suppression (usually reversible), bronchospasm, bruising, changes in taste, constipation, death, decreased urine output, decreased serum electrolytes, dehydration, diarrhea, erythema, fatigue, fever, hemolytic uremic syndrome (rare, cancer associated), hypotension, infection, laboratory test abnormalities (alkaline phosphatase, aspartate aminotransferase [AST], BUN, SCr, total bilirubin), nausea and vomiting (severe), neutropenia, ototoxicity, peripheral neuropathies, pruritus, rash, stomatitis, thrombocytopenia, urticaria, visual disturbances, weakness.

ANTIDOTE

Notify physician of all side effects. Symptomatic and supportive treatment is indicated. Withhold carboplatin until myelosuppression is reversed. Administration of whole blood products (e.g., packed RBCs, platelets, leukocytes) may be required. Blood modifiers (e.g., darbepoetin alfa [Aranesp], epoetin alfa [Epogen], filgrastim [Neupogen], oprelvekin [Neumega], pegfilgrastim [Neulasta], sargramostim [Leukine]) may be indicated to treat bone marrow toxicity. Treat anaphylaxis with epinephrine, corticosteroids, oxygen, and antihistamines. There is no specific antidote.

CARMUSTINE (BCNU) BBW
(kar-**MUS**-teen)

BiCNU

Antineoplastic
(alkylating agent/nitrosourea)

pH 5.6 to 6

USUAL DOSE

Initial dose is 150 to 200 mg/M². May be given as a single dose, or one half of the calculated dose may be given initially and repeated the next day. Repeat every 6 weeks if bone marrow is sufficiently recovered. Repeat course should not be administered until leukocytes are above 4,000/mm³ and platelets are above 100,000/mm³. Repeat doses adjusted according to hematologic response of previous dose (see Dose Adjustments).

DOSE ADJUSTMENTS

Bone marrow toxicity is cumulative. Dose adjustments must be considered *based on the nadir blood counts from the prior dose* according to the following chart.

Carmustine Dose Adjustment Based on Bone Marrow Suppression		
Nadir After Prior Dose		Percentage of Prior Dose to Be Given
Leukocytes/mm³	Platelets/mm³	%
≥4,000	≥100,000	100%
3,000-3,999	75,000-99,999	100%
2,000-2,999	25,000-74,999	70%
<2,000	<25,000	50%

Adjust doses accordingly when carmustine is used in combination with other myelosuppressive drugs or in patients with depleted bone marrow reserve. ▪ Dosing should be cautious in the elderly. Lower-end initial doses may be indicated. Consider decrease in cardiac, hepatic, and renal function; concomitant disease; or other drug therapy; see Elderly.

DILUTION

Specific techniques required; see Precautions. Initially dilute 100-mg vial with supplied sterile diluent (3 mL of dehydrated alcohol injection). Further dilute with 27 mL of SW for injection. Each mL will contain 3.3 mg carmustine. Withdraw desired dose and further dilute in 100 mL or more of D5W and give as an infusion. Use glass containers; loss of potency occurs in PVC containers and IV tubing.

Filters: No significant loss of potency with any size cellular ester membrane filter when reconstituted or diluted as recommended.

Storage: Must be protected from light in all forms. Store unopened vials of the dry drug (carmustine) in refrigerator (2° to 8° C [35° to 46° F]). Supplied diluent may be stored at CRT or refrigerated. After reconstitution and after further dilution to a concentration of 0.2 mg/mL in D5W, may be stored at RT but must be used within 8 hours. Temperatures above 27° C (80° F) will cause liquefaction of the drug powder; discard immediately.

COMPATIBILITY

Consider any drug NOT listed as compatible to be INCOMPATIBLE until consulting a pharmacist; specific conditions may apply.

Manufacturer lists as **incompatible** with polyvinyl chloride infusion bags; use only glass containers.

One source suggests the following **compatibilities:**

Y-site: Amifostine (Ethyol), aztreonam (Azactam), cefepime (Maxipime), etoposide phosphate (Etopophos), filgrastim (Neupogen), fludarabine (Fludara), gemcitabine (Gemzar), granisetron (Kytril), melphalan (Alkeran), ondansetron (Zofran), piperacillin/tazobactam (Zosyn), sargramostim (Leukine), teniposide (Vumon), thiotepa, vinorelbine (Navelbine).

RATE OF ADMINISTRATION

Each single dose must be given as an infusion over a minimum of 1 and up to 2 hours. Reduce rate for pain or burning at injection site, flushing of the skin, or suffusion of the conjunctiva.

ACTIONS

An alkylating agent of the nitrosourea group with antitumor activity, cell cycle phase nonspecific. Degraded to metabolites within 15 minutes of administration. Effectively crosses the blood-brain barrier; levels of radioactivity in the CSF are equal to or more than 50% of those measured concurrently in plasma. Excreted in changed form in urine. Small amounts excreted as respiratory CO_2.

INDICATIONS AND USES

Palliative therapy as a single agent or in established combination therapies in the treatment of brain tumors; multiple myeloma; Hodgkin's disease; and some non-Hodgkin's lymphomas.

CONTRAINDICATIONS

Hypersensitivity to carmustine.

PRECAUTIONS

Follow guidelines for handling cytotoxic agents. See Appendix A, p. 1429. ▪ Administered by or under the direction of the physician specialist. ▪ Delayed bone marrow suppression may be severe, especially in an already compromised patient, and result in infection and/or bleeding. Anemia may be cumulative and may require transfusion support. ▪ Pulmonary toxicity is dose related. Risk is increased with a cumulative dose greater than 1,400 mg/M^2. Delayed-onset pulmonary fibrosis has occurred up to 17 years after treatment with injectable carmustine in patients who received it in childhood or early adolescence. ▪ Often used with other antineoplastic drugs in reduced doses to achieve tumor remission. ▪ Secondary malignancies, including acute nonlymphocytic leukemia, myeloproliferation syndrome, and carcinoma have been reported in patients treated with alkylating agents.

Monitor: Determine absolute patency and quality of vein and adequate circulation of extremity. Severe cellulitis may result from extravasation. ▪ Delayed toxicity probable in 4 to 6 weeks; wait at least 6 weeks between doses; obtain baseline CBC, including leukocyte and platelet counts, and monitor weekly. ▪ Obtain baseline pulmonary function studies and monitor pulmonary function frequently during treatment. Risk of pulmonary toxicity is increased in patients with a baseline below 70% of the predicted forced vital capacity (FVC) or carbon monoxide diffusing capacity (DLco). ▪ Periodic monitoring of liver and renal function tests is recommended. ▪ Nausea and vomiting can be severe. Prophylactic administration of antiemetics recommended. ▪ Avoid contact of carmustine solution with the skin. ▪ Observe for any signs of infection. Prophylactic antibiotics may be indicated pending results of C/S in a febrile neutropenic patient. ▪ Maintain hydration. ▪ Monitor for thrombocytopenia (platelet count less than 50,000/mm^3). Initiate precautions to prevent excessive bleeding (e.g., inspect IV sites, skin, and mucous membranes; use extreme care during invasive procedures; test urine, emesis, stool, and secretions for occult blood).

Patient Education: Nonhormonal birth control recommended. ▪ Report stinging or burning at IV site promptly. ▪ See Appendix D, p. 1434.

Maternal/Child: Category D: avoid pregnancy; embryotoxic and teratogenic in rats; has mutagenic potential. ▪ Discontinue breast-feeding. ▪ Safety and effectiveness for use in pediatric patients not established. Risk versus benefit must be carefully considered due to a high risk of pulmonary toxicity occurring years after treatment and resulting in death.

Elderly: Dose selection should be cautious; see Dose Adjustments. ▪ Toxicity may be increased. ▪ Monitoring of renal function is suggested.

DRUG/LAB INTERACTIONS

Potentiated by **cimetidine** (Tagamet); increased myelosuppression (e.g., leukopenia and neutropenia) have been reported with concurrent use. ▪ Inhibits **digoxin and phenytoin** (Dilantin); may reduce serum levels. ▪ Do not administer **vaccines or chloroquine** to patients receiving antineoplastic drugs. ▪ See Dose Adjustments.

SIDE EFFECTS

Most are dose related and can be reversed. Bone marrow toxicity (especially leukopenia and thrombocytopenia) is most pronounced at 4 to 6 weeks; can be severe and cumulative with repeated dosage. Anemia, chest pain, elevated liver function test results, flushing of skin and suffusion of conjunctiva from too-rapid infusion rate, headache, hyperpigmentation and burning of skin (from actual contact with solution), hypersensitivity reactions, hypotension, nausea and vomiting, neuroretinitis, pulmonary infiltrates or fibrosis with long-term therapy, renal abnormalities, retinal hemorrhage, and tachycardia.

ANTIDOTE

Notify physician of all side effects. Most will decrease in severity with reduced dosage, increased time span between doses, or symptomatic treatment. May reduce therapeutic effectiveness. Bone marrow suppression may require withholding carmustine until recovery occurs. Administration of whole blood products (e.g., packed RBCs, platelets, leukocytes) may be required. Blood modifiers (e.g., darbepoetin alfa [Aranesp], epoetin alfa [Epogen], filgrastim [Neupogen], oprelvekin [Neumega], pegfilgrastim [Neulasta], sargramostim [Leukine]) may be indicated to treat bone marrow toxicity. There is no specific antidote. Supportive therapy as indicated will help sustain the patient in toxicity. For extravasation, elevate extremity; consider injection of long-acting dexamethasone (Decadron LA) or hyaluronidase (Wydase) throughout extravasated tissue. Use a 27- or 25-gauge needle. Apply warm, moist compresses.

CASPOFUNGIN ACETATE
(**kas**-po-**FUN**-jin **AS**-ah-tayt)
Cancidas

Antifungal

pH 6.6

USUAL DOSE

Empirical therapy: 70 mg as an infusion on Day 1. Beginning on Day 2, reduce subsequent doses to 50 mg/day. Duration of empiric therapy is based on clinical response and should continue at least until resolution of neutropenia. Patients found to have a fungal infection should be treated for a minimum of 14 days; treatment should continue for at least 7 days after both neutropenia and clinical symptoms have resolved.

Candidemia and other *Candida* infections: 70 mg as an infusion on Day 1. Beginning on Day 2, reduce subsequent doses to 50 mg/day. Duration of treatment is based on clinical and microbiologic response. Usually continued for at least 14 days after the last positive culture. Persistently neutropenic patients may require a longer course of therapy pending resolution of the neutropenia. A 150-mg dose has been studied in a small number of adult patients. Efficacy of this higher dose was not significantly better than the 50-mg dose.

Esophageal candidiasis: 50 mg daily as an infusion. Continue for 7 to 14 days after symptom resolution. A 70-mg loading dose has not been studied for this indication. Suppressive oral therapy following treatment with caspofungin may be considered to decrease the risk of relapse of oropharyngeal candidiasis in patients with HIV infections.

Invasive aspergillosis: 70 mg as an infusion on Day 1. Beginning on Day 2, reduce subsequent doses to 50 mg/day. Duration of treatment is based on severity of the underlying disease, recovery from immunosuppression, and clinical response.

PEDIATRIC DOSE

Pediatric patients 3 months to 17 years of age: 70 mg/M^2 as an infusion on Day 1. Beginning on Day 2, reduce subsequent doses to 50 mg/M^2/day. Regardless of the patient's calculated dose, the loading dose and/or the daily maintenance dose should not exceed a maximum of 70 mg. Duration of therapy for each indication should be individualized as outlined in Usual Dose.

DOSE ADJUSTMENTS

All diagnoses: *Adult and pediatric patients:* Dose adjustment is not indicated based on age, gender, or race. ■ See Drug/Lab Interactions.

Adults: Dose adjustment is not indicated in patients with impaired renal function or in patients with mild impaired hepatic function (Child-Pugh score 5 to 6). ■ In patients with moderate hepatic insufficiency (Child-Pugh score 7 to 9), reduce daily doses to 35 mg after the initial dose of 50 or 70 mg. ■ Dose may be increased from 50 to 70 mg daily in patients not clinically responding to the 50-mg dose; experience limited. ■ In patients receiving concurrent administration of rifampin (Rifadin), increase the daily dose to 70 mg. An increase in the daily dose to 70 mg/day should be considered in patients who are not clinically responding and are taking

Continued

other inducers and/or mixed inducers/inhibitors of caspofungin clearance, specifically carbamazepine (Tegretol), dexamethasone (Decadron), efavirenz (Sustiva), nevirapine (Viramune), and phenytoin (Dilantin).

Pediatric patients: If the 50-mg/M^2 daily dose is well tolerated but does not provide adequate clinical response, it may be increased to 70 mg/M^2 (not to exceed a total dose of 70 mg). ▪ There is no experience in pediatric patients with any degree of hepatic insufficiency. ▪ Consider a dose of 70 mg/M^2 (not to exceed a total dose of 70 mg) in pediatric patients receiving inducers of caspofungin clearance, specifically carbamazepine (Tegretol), dexamethasone (Decadron), efavirenz (Sustiva), nevirapine (Viramune), phenytoin (Dilantin), and rifampin (Rifadin).

DILUTION
Available in 70-mg and 50-mg vials. Select appropriate dose and allow vial of caspofungin to come to room temperature. Reconstitute selected dose with 10.8 mL of NS, SW, or BWFI. Mix gently to achieve a clear solution; should dissolve completely. The 70-mg vial will yield 7 mg/mL, and the 50-mg vial will yield 5 mg/mL.

Adults: Withdraw 10 mL of reconstituted solution and add to 250 mL of NS, ½NS, ¼NS, or LR for infusion. If a 70-mg vial is not available, reconstitute two 50-mg vials and withdraw a total of 14 mL to be further diluted in 250 mL of the above solutions. When preparing a 35-mg dose, withdraw 7 mL from the reconstituted 50-mg vial and further dilute in 250 mL of the previously listed solutions. In fluid-restricted or pediatric patients, the appropriate volume of caspofungin may be added to reduced volumes of the above solutions, not to exceed a final concentration of 0.5 mg/mL.

Pediatric patients: The choice of vial used should be based on the total dose to be administered. Pediatric doses less than 50 mg should be withdrawn from a 50-mg vial to ensure accuracy. After reconstitution, withdraw the volume required to provide the correct dose, and add to a volume of NS, ½NS, ¼NS, or LR for infusion to achieve a final concentration not to exceed 0.5 mg/mL.

Storage: Refrigerate unopened vials. Reconstituted vials may be kept at CRT for 1 hour before preparing as an infusion solution. Fully diluted solutions may be stored at less than or equal to 25° C (77° F) for 24 hours or refrigerated for 48 hours.

COMPATIBILITY   (Underline Indicates Conflicting Compatibility Information)
Manufacturer states, "Do not mix or co-infuse caspofungin with other medications. Do not use diluents containing dextrose."

One source suggests the following **compatibilities:**

Y-site: Acyclovir (Zovirax), amikacin (Amikin), amiodarone (Nexterone), azithromycin (Zithromax), aztreonam (Azactam), bumetanide, carboplatin (Paraplatin), ciprofloxacin (Cipro IV), cisplatin (Platinol), cyclosporine (Sandimmune), daptomycin (Cubicin), daunorubicin (Cerubidine), diltiazem (Cardizem), diphenhydramine (Benadryl), dobutamine, dolasetron (Anzemet), dopamine, doripenem (Doribax), doxorubicin (Adriamycin), epinephrine (Adrenalin), etoposide phosphate (Etopophos), famotidine (Pepcid IV), fentanyl (Sublimaze), fluconazole (Diflucan), ganciclovir (Cytovene), gentamicin, hydralazine, hydrocortisone sodium succinate (Solu-Cortef), hydromorphone (Dilaudid), ifosfamide (Ifex), imipenem-cilastatin (Primaxin), insulin (regular), levofloxacin (Levaquin), linezolid (Zyvox), lorazepam (Ativan), magnesium sulfate, melphalan (Alkeran), meperidine (Demerol), meropenem (Merrem IV), metronidazole (Flagyl IV), midazolam (Versed), milrinone (Primacor), mitomycin (Mutamycin), morphine, mycophenolate (CellCept IV), norepinephrine (Levophed), ondansetron (Zofran), pantoprazole (Protonix IV), phenylephrine (Neo-Synephrine), potassium chloride, quinupristin/dalfopristin (Synercid), tacrolimus (Prograf), tobramycin, vancomycin, vasopressin, vincristine, voriconazole (VFEND IV).

RATE OF ADMINISTRATION
A single dose as an infusion evenly distributed over 1 hour.

ACTIONS
An antifungal. An echinocandin or glucan synthesis inhibitor. It attacks the fungal cell wall and inhibits the synthesis of beta (1,3)-D-glucan, an essential component of the cell wall of susceptible *Aspergillus* and *Candida* species. Beta (1,3)-D-glucan is not found in human cells. Extensively bound to albumin (97%). After completion of an IV infusion, plasma concentrations decline in several phases, each with its own half-life (e.g., 9 to 11 hours, 40 to 50 hours). Distribution, rather than excretion or biotransformation, is the primary mechanism influencing plasma clearance. Slowly metabolized by hydrolysis and *N*-acetylation, eventually breaking down to amino acids and their degradates. Excreted in urine and feces.

INDICATIONS AND USES
Empirical therapy for presumed fungal infections in febrile, neutropenic patients. ▪ Treatment of invasive aspergillosis in patients who are refractory to or intolerant of other therapies (i.e., amphotericin B [generic], lipid formulations of amphotericin B [e.g., Abelcet, AmBisome, Amphotec], and/or itraconazole [Sporanox]). Has not been studied for initial therapy for invasive aspergillosis. ▪ Treatment of esophageal candidiasis. ▪ Treatment of candidemia and the following *Candida* infections: intraabdominal abscesses, peritonitis, and pleural space infections. Has not been studied in endocarditis, osteomyelitis, and meningitis due to *Candida*.

CONTRAINDICATIONS
Known hypersensitivity to caspofungin or any of its components.

PRECAUTIONS
Concomitant use with cyclosporine is not recommended unless the potential benefit outweighs the risk; see Monitor and Drug/Lab Interactions. ▪ Hepatic abnormalities, including elevated liver function tests (LFTs), clinically significant hepatic dysfunction, hepatitis, and hepatic failure have been reported. Abnormal LFTs have been seen in healthy volunteers and in adult and pediatric patients treated with caspofungin. ▪ There is no clinical experience in adult patients with severe hepatic insufficiency (Child-Pugh score greater than 9) or in pediatric patients with any degree of hepatic impairment. ▪ Drug resistance in patients with invasive aspergillosis has not been observed. ▪ Mutants of *Candida* with reduced susceptibility to caspofungin have been identified in some patients.

Monitor: Most patients have serious underlying medical conditions (e.g., bone marrow transplant, HIV, malignancies) requiring multiple concomitant medications. Obtain baseline studies as required and repeat as indicated. ▪ Monitor vital signs. ▪ Observe for S/S of a hypersensitivity reaction. ▪ Encourage fluids to maintain hydration. ▪ Effects of severe hepatic impairment unknown; monitor liver function tests (e.g., AST, ALT) in patients with pre-existing impaired hepatic function and any time S/S suggestive of liver dysfunction develop (e.g., jaundice, lethargy). ▪ Monitor liver function in patients receiving therapy with both caspofungin and cyclosporine. Monitor closely in patients who develop abnormal liver function tests. The risk/benefit of continued therapy should be evaluated. ▪ See Drug/Lab Interactions.

Patient Education: Review all medical conditions and medications before beginning treatment. ▪ Promptly report pain at infusion site, symptoms of histamine reactions (e.g., facial swelling, pruritus, rash, sensation of warmth), hypersensitivity reactions (e.g., chills, difficulty breathing, hypotension, rash), or hepatic toxicity (e.g., jaundice).

Maternal/Child: Category C: use during pregnancy only if benefits outweigh potential risks to fetus. Based on animal studies, may cause fetal harm. ▪ Has been found in the milk of lactating, drug-treated rats; use caution if required during breast-feeding or discontinue breast-feeding. ▪ Safety and effectiveness for use in neonates and infants under 3 months of age not studied.

Elderly: Response similar to that in younger patients. Dose adjustment is not recommended; however, use caution; may have greater sensitivity to its effects.

DRUG/LAB INTERACTIONS

Concomitant use with **cyclosporine** (Sandimmune) is not recommended unless benefit outweighs risk. By Day 10 of concomitant administration some patients had a transient ALT 2 to 3 times the upper limit of normal, and the AUC of caspofungin had increased by about 35%. ▪ Pharmacokinetics of caspofungin are not altered by **amphotericin B, itraconazole,** (Sporanox), **mycophenolate** (CellCept), **nelfinavir** (Viracept), **or tacrolimus** (Prograf). ▪ Serum concentrations of tacrolimus may be somewhat decreased with concomitant administration; monitor tacrolimus concentrations and adjust dose as indicated. ▪ **Inducers and/or mixed inducers/ inhibitors of caspofungin clearance** (e.g., carbamazepine [Tegretol], dexamethasone [Decadron], efavirenz [Sustiva], nevirapine [Viramune], phenytoin [Dilantin], rifampin [Rifadin]) may significantly increase caspofungin clearance and require an increase in dose; see Dose Adjustments. ▪ Although its clearance may be affected by the enzyme inducers previously mentioned, caspofungin is not an inhibitor or inducer of any enzyme in the cytochrome P_{450} (CPY) system. It is not a substrate (a substance on which an enzyme acts) for P-glycoprotein and is a poor substrate for cytochrome P_{450} enzymes. It is not expected to interact with drugs metabolized by this system (e.g., amiodarone [Nexterone], calcium channel blockers [e.g., diltiazem (Cardizem), verapamil], cimetidine [Tagamet], MAO inhibitors [e.g., selegiline (Eldepryl)]).

SIDE EFFECTS

Side effect profile is similar in both adult and pediatric patients. Incidence difficult to assess because of multiple medical conditions and multiple medications. Most commonly reported side effects include chills, diarrhea, elevated liver function tests (e.g., alkaline phosphatase, ALT, AST), fever, hypokalemia, and rash. Other side effects reported include abdominal pain, ARDS, cough, diaphoresis, flushing, headache, hyperbilirubinemia, hypercalcemia, hyperglycemia, hypertension, hypomagnesemia, hypotension, increased RBCs and protein in urine, infusion-related reactions, injection site reactions, nausea, peripheral edema, phlebitis, pneumonia, pulmonary edema, radiographic infiltrates, tachycardia, and vomiting. Possible histamine-mediated symptoms (e.g., angioedema, bronchospasm, facial swelling, pruritus, rash, sensation of warmth) and anaphylaxis with dyspnea, stridor, and worsening of rash have been reported.

Post-Marketing: Erythema multiforme, hepatic necrosis, hepatobiliary adverse reactions (e.g., clinically significant hepatic dysfunction, hepatitis, hepatic failure) in adult and pediatric patients with serious underlying medical conditions, pancreatitis, renal dysfunction (clinically significant), skin exfoliation, and Stevens-Johnson syndrome.

ANTIDOTE

Notify physician of all side effects; most will be treated symptomatically. Discontinue caspofungin and notify physician of abnormal liver function tests progressing to clinical S/S of liver disease. Rash may be the first sign of an exfoliative skin disorder in immunocompromised patients; discontinue caspofungin and notify physician. Not removed by hemodialysis. Treat anaphylaxis as indicated and/or resuscitate as necessary.

CEFAZOLIN SODIUM
(sef-**AYZ**-oh-lin **SO**-dee-um)

Ancef, Kefzol

Antibacterial (cephalosporin)

pH 4.5 to 7

USUAL DOSE

250 mg to 1.5 Gm every 6 to 8 hours. Up to 6 Gm is usual, but 12 Gm in 24 hours has been used, depending on severity of infection.

Mild infections: 250 to 500 mg every 8 hours.

Moderate to severe infections: 500 mg to 1 Gm every 6 to 8 hours.

Life-threatening infections (e.g., endocarditis, septicemia): 1 to 1.5 Gm every 6 hours.

Pneumococcal pneumonia: 500 mg every 12 hours.

Uncomplicated GU infections: 1 Gm every 12 hours.

Perioperative prophylaxis: 1 Gm 30 minutes to 1 hour before incision. For lengthy procedures (e.g., 2 hours or more), 0.5 to 1 Gm may be repeated in the OR. Administer every 6 to 8 hours for 24 hours.

Endocarditis prophylaxis (unlabeled): 1 Gm 30 minutes before surgery.

PEDIATRIC DOSE

Over 1 month of age: 6.25 to 25 mg/kg of body weight every 6 hours, or 8.3 to 33.3 mg/kg every 8 hours. Do not exceed adult dose.

Endocarditis prophylaxis (unlabeled): 25 mg/kg 30 minutes before start of surgery. Do not exceed 1 Gm.

NEONATAL DOSE

See Maternal/Child.

Less than 7 days of age or over 7 days but under 2,000 Gm (unlabeled): 20 mg/kg every 12 hours.

7 days to 1 month of age and 2,000 Gm or more (unlabeled): 20 mg/kg every 8 hours.   *Continued*

DOSE ADJUSTMENTS

Reduced doses or extended intervals may be indicated in the elderly; consider age-related impaired organ function, nutritional status, and concomitant disease or drug therapy. In impaired renal function, the initial dose in adults and pediatric patients should be as above. Reduce all subsequent doses according to the following charts.

Cefazolin Dose Guidelines in Impaired Renal Function for Adults		
CrCl or SCr	Dose	Frequency
CrCl >55 mL/min or SCr ≤1.5 mg%	Full	Normal
CrCl 35-54 mL/min or SCr 1.6 to 3 mg%	Full	q 8 hr or less frequently
CrCl 11-34 mL/min or SCr 3.1 to 4.5 mg%	½ Usual dose	q 12 hr
CrCl 10 mL/min or less or SCr ≥4.6 mg%	½ Usual dose	q 18-24 hr

Cefazolin Dose Guidelines in Impaired Renal Function for Pediatric Patients		
Creatinine Clearance (mL/min)	Dose	Frequency
>70 mL/min	Full	Normal
40-70 mL/min	60% of normal daily dose*	q 12 hr
20-40 mL/min	25% of normal daily dose*	q 12 hr
5-20 mL/min	10% of normal daily dose*	q 24 hr

*In equally divided doses.

DILUTION

Each 1 Gm or fraction thereof must be reconstituted with at least 2.5 mL of SW for injection. Shake well. To reduce the incidence of thrombophlebitis, may be further diluted in 50 to 100 mL of D5W, NS, or other **compatible** infusion solutions (see chart on inside back cover or literature) and given as an intermittent infusion. Available premixed and in piggyback vials (vent bottle before adding diluent, dilute to 50 to 100 mg, and shake well). 10-mg pharmacy bulk vials may be reconstituted with SW or with NS 45 mL (1 Gm/5 mL) or 96 mL (1 Gm/10 mL). May be administered through Y-tube, three-way stopcock, or additive infusion set. **Storage:** Before reconstitution, protect from light and store at CRT. Give within 24 hours of preparation if stored at CRT or within 10 days if under refrigeration. Discard pharmacy bulk vials within 4 hours after initial entry.

COMPATIBILITY   (Underline Indicates Conflicting Compatibility Information)

Consider any drug NOT listed as compatible to be INCOMPATIBLE until consulting a pharmacist; specific conditions may apply.

May be used concomitantly with aminoglycosides (e.g., amikacin [Amikin], gentamicin), but these drugs must never be mixed in the same infusion (mutual inactivation). If given concurrently, administer at separate sites.

One source suggests the following **compatibilities:**

Additive: Aztreonam (Azactam), clindamycin (Cleocin), famotidine (Pepcid IV), fluconazole (Diflucan), linezolid (Zyvox), meperidine (Demerol), metronidazole (Flagyl IV), verapamil.

Y-site: Acyclovir (Zovirax), allopurinol (Aloprim), alprostadil, amifostine (Ethyol), amiodarone (Nexterone), anidulafungin (Eraxis), atracurium (Tracrium), aztreonam (Azactam), bivalirudin (Angiomax), calcium gluconate, cisatracurium (Nimbex), cyclophosphamide (Cytoxan), dexmedetomidine (Precedex), diltiazem (Cardizem), docetaxel (Taxotere), doxapram (Dopram), doxorubicin liposomal (Doxil), enalaprilat (Vasotec IV), esmolol (Brevibloc), etoposide phosphate (Etopophos), famotidine (Pepcid IV), fenoldopam (Corlopam), filgrastim (Neupogen), fluconazole (Diflucan), fludarabine (Fludara), foscarnet (Foscavir), gallium nitrate (Ganite), gemcitabine (Gemzar), granisetron (Kytril), heparin, hetastarch in electrolytes (Hextend), hetastarch in NS (Hespan), hydromorphone (Dilaudid), insulin (regular), labetalol (Trandate), lidocaine, linezolid (Zyvox), magnesium sulfate, melphalan (Alkeran), meperidine (Demerol), midazolam (Versed), milrinone (Primacor), morphine, multivitamins (M.V.I.), nicardipine (Cardene IV), ondansetron (Zofran), palonosetron (Aloxi), pancuronium, pantoprazole (Protonix IV), propofol (Diprivan), ranitidine (Zantac), remifentanil (Ultiva), sargramostim (Leukine), tacrolimus (Prograf), teniposide (Vumon), theophylline, thiotepa, vancomycin, vecuronium, warfarin (Coumadin).

RATE OF ADMINISTRATION

IV injection: Each 1 Gm or fraction thereof over 3 to 5 minutes. Extend administration time as indicated by amount of solution and condition of patient.

ACTIONS

A semisynthetic, first-generation, broad-spectrum cephalosporin antibiotic that is bactericidal through inhibition of cell wall synthesis to some gram-positive and gram-negative organisms, including staphylococci and streptococci. A number of organisms are resistant to this cephalosporin. Peak serum levels achieved by end of infusion. Widely distributed in most tissues, body fluids (CSF minimal), bone, gallbladder, myocardium, and skin and soft tissue. Serum half-life is 1.8 hours. Excreted rapidly in the urine. Crosses the placental barrier. Secreted in breast milk.

INDICATIONS AND USES

Treatment of serious infections of the bone, joints, skin, soft tissue, respiratory tract, biliary tract, and GU tract; septicemia and endocarditis. Effective only if the causative organism is susceptible. ■ Perioperative prophylaxis. ■ Biliary tract infections. ■ Not recommended for prophylaxis in GU procedures.

Unlabeled uses: Prophylaxis of bacterial endocarditis.

CONTRAINDICATIONS

Previous hypersensitivity reaction to cephalosporins; see Precautions.

PRECAUTIONS

Hypersensitivity reactions, including fatalities, have been reported and include reports of individuals with a history of penicillin hypersensitivity or sensitivity to multiple allergens experiencing severe reactions when treated with cephalosporins. Check history of previous hypersensitivity reactions to penicillins, cephalosporins, or other allergens. Actual incidence of cross-allergenicity not established but may be more common with first-generation cephalosporins. ▪ Sensitivity studies indicated to determine susceptibility of the causative organisms to cefazolin. ▪ To reduce the development of drug-resistant bacteria and maintain its effectiveness, cefazolin should be used to treat or prevent only those infections proven or strongly suspected to be caused by bacteria. ▪ Continue for at least 2 to 3 days after all symptoms of infection subside. ▪ Avoid prolonged use of drug; superinfection caused by overgrowth of nonsusceptible organisms may result. ▪ Use caution in patients with impaired renal function, allergies, or a history of GI disease (especially colitis). ▪ With inappropriately high doses, seizures may occur in patients with impaired renal function. ▪ May decrease prothrombin activity, especially in patients with impaired renal or hepatic function, those with a poor nutritional state, and those receiving extended courses of antimicrobial therapy. ▪ *Clostridium difficile*–associated diarrhea (CDAD) has been reported. May range from mild diarrhea to fatal colitis. Consider in patients who present with diarrhea during or after treatment with cefazolin.

Monitor: Watch for early symptoms of hypersensitivity reactions. ▪ Obtain baseline PT and monitor, especially in at-risk patients (see Precautions); vitamin K may be indicated. ▪ Observe for electrolyte imbalance and cardiac irregularities. Contains 2.1 mEq sodium per Gm. ▪ See Drug/Lab Interactions; additional monitoring may be indicated (e.g., renal function, drug serum levels, PT).

Patient Education: Report promptly any bleeding or bruising, diarrhea, or symptoms of allergy (e.g., difficulty breathing, hives, itching, rash). ▪ Promptly report diarrhea or bloody stools that occur during treatment or up to several months after an antibiotic has been discontinued; may indicate CDAD and require treatment.

Maternal/Child: Category B: safety for use during pregnancy and breast-feeding not established. No problems documented. ▪ Safety for use in premature infants and neonates under 1 month of age not established; immature renal function will increase blood levels.

Elderly: No specific problems documented. ▪ See Usual Dose and Dose Adjustments.

DRUG/LAB INTERACTIONS

Risk of nephrotoxicity may be increased with **aminoglycosides and other nephrotoxic agents** (e.g., loop diuretics [e.g., furosemide (Lasix)]). ▪ **Probenecid** inhibits excretion, resulting in elevated cefazolin levels. Dose reduction of cefazolin may be necessary. ▪ May be antagonized by **bacteriostatic antibiotics** (e.g., chloramphenicol, erythromycin, tetracyclines); may interfere with bactericidal action. ▪ Large amounts of **cephalosporins and/or salicylates** may induce hypoprothrombinemia (deficiency of prothrombin [Factor II]). The addition of **agents that may affect platelet aggregation and/or may have GI ulcerative potential** (e.g., NSAIDs [ibuprofen (Advil, Motrin), naproxen (Aleve, Naprosyn)] or sulfinpyrazone [Anturane]) may increase risk of hemorrhage. ▪ False-positive reaction for **urine glucose** except with enzyme-based tests (e.g., Chemstix). ▪ See Compatibility and Side Effects.

SIDE EFFECTS

Anorexia; CDAD; diarrhea; elevated BUN and creatinine levels; hypersensitivity reactions including anaphylaxis; leukopenia; local site pain; nausea and vomiting; neutropenia; oral thrush; phlebitis; positive direct and indirect Coombs' test; prolonged PT; transient elevation of AST, ALT, and alkaline phosphatase; seizures (large doses); thrombophlebitis; vaginal itching or discharge. Hypoprothrombinemia (rare) and hemolytic anemia may occur. Serum sickness–like reactions have occurred (e.g., arthralgia, fever, polyarthritis, skin rashes), usually after a second course of therapy. Usually resolve after cephalosporins are discontinued. Hepatitis and renal failure have been reported.

ANTIDOTE

Notify the physician of any side effects. Discontinue the drug if indicated. Mild cases of CDAD may respond to discontinuation of cefazolin. Treat CDAD with fluids, electrolytes, protein supplements, and oral vancomycin (Vancocin) or metronidazole (Flagyl) as indicated. In severe cases, surgical evaluation may be indicated. Antihistamines and corticosteroids may be indicated to manage symptoms of serum sickness. Discontinue cefazolin and treat hypersensitivity reaction as indicated (airway, oxygen, IV fluids, antihistamines [e.g., diphenhydramine], corticosteroids [e.g., hydrocortisone sodium succinate (Solu-Cortef)], epinephrine, pressor-amines [e.g., dopamine]) and resuscitate as necessary. Hemodialysis may be useful in overdose.

CEFEPIME HYDROCHLORIDE
(**SEF**-eh-pim hy-droh-**KLOR**-eyed)

Maxipime

Antibacterial
(cephalosporin)

pH 4 to 6

USUAL DOSE

Adults: Range is from 0.5 Gm to 2 Gm. Usually given every 12 hours. Dose based on severity of disease and/or specific susceptibility of the causative organism according to the following chart.

Cefepime Dose Guidelines			
Site and Type of Infection	Dose	Frequency	Duration (days)
Mild to Moderate Uncomplicated or complicated urinary tract infections, including pyelonephritis	0.5-1 Gm IV/IM	q 12 hr	7-10
Severe Uncomplicated or complicated urinary tract infections, including pyelonephritis	2 Gm IV	q 12 hr	10
Moderate to Severe Pneumonia	1-2 Gm IV	q 12 hr	10
Moderate to Severe Uncomplicated skin and skin structure infections	2 Gm IV	q 12 hr	10
Empiric Therapy For febrile neutropenic patients	2 Gm IV	q 8 hr	7 or until neutropenia resolves
Complicated Intra-abdominal infections	Cefepime 2 Gm IV q 12 hr in combination with metronidazole 500 mg or 7.5 mg/kg q 6 hr, not to exceed 4 Gm/24 hr of metronidazole		7-10

PEDIATRIC DOSE

Pediatric patients 2 months to 16 years; weight up to 40 kg: 50 mg/kg every 12 hours for 7 to 10 days. Increase frequency to every 8 hours for empiric monotherapy in febrile neutropenia. Do not exceed adult dose.

DOSE ADJUSTMENTS

In impaired renal function, the initial dose should be as above, but all remaining doses should be reduced based on CrCl according to the following chart (e.g., if the normal dose is 1 Gm every 12 hours with a CrCl greater than 60, the maintenance dose would be reduced to 1 Gm every 24 hours with a CrCl between 30 and 60 mL/min). Dose reductions should be comparable in *pediatric patients.*

Cefepime Dose Guidelines in Impaired Renal Function				
Creatinine Clearance (mL/min)	Recommended Maintenance Schedule (relative to normal dosing schedule)			
Normal Recommended Dosing Schedule (>60 mL/min)	500 mg q 12 hr	1 Gm q 12 hr	2 Gm q 12 hr	2 Gm q 8 hr
30-60 mL/min	500 mg q 24 hr	1 Gm q 24 hr	2 Gm q 24 hr	2 Gm q 12 hr
11-29 mL/min	500 mg q 24 hr	500 mg q 24 hr	1 Gm q 24 hr	2 Gm q 24 hr
<11 mL/min	250 mg q 24 hr	250 mg q 24 hr	500 mg q 24 hr	1 Gm q 24 hr
CAPD	500 mg q 48 hr	1 Gm q 48 hr	2 Gm q 48 hr	2 Gm q 48 hr
*Hemodialysis	1 Gm on Day 1, then 500 mg q 24 hr			1 Gm q 24 hr

*On hemodialysis days, cefepime should be administered following hemodialysis. Whenever possible, administer at the same time each day.

Consult literature or Important IV Therapy Facts, p. xxvii, for conversion formula if dose is to be based on SCr. ▪ Reduced dose may be required in the elderly based on renal function. ▪ Dose adjustment not required in impaired hepatic function.

DILUTION

Available in vials (IM/IV), ADD-Vantage preparations, and as Galaxy frozen premixed solutions containing 1 Gm/50 mL or 2 Gm/100 mL. *Vials* may be reconstituted (see the following chart) and then further diluted with NS, D5W, D10W, D5NS, D5LR, ⅙ M sodium lactate, Normosol-R, or D5/Normosol M. Concentrations between 1 mg/mL and 40 mg/mL are acceptable. (500 mg reconstituted with 5 mL = 100 mg/mL, further diluted with 95 mL = 5 mg/mL, with 45 mL = 10 mg/mL.)

ADD-Vantage vials must only be diluted with 50 to 100 mL of NS or D5W in ADD-Vantage infusion containers.

Galaxy frozen premixed solutions: Thaw at RT or under refrigeration. Do not force thaw by immersion in water baths or by microwave irradiation. Solution components may precipitate when frozen; should dissolve at RT. After reaching RT, shake solution. Discard if remains cloudy or a leak is detected by squeezing the container.

Cefepime Dilution Guidelines			
Single-Dose Vials for Intravenous/ Intramuscular Administration	Amount of Diluent to Be Added (mL)	Approximate Available Volume (mL)	Approximate Cefepime Concentration (mg/mL)
CEFEPIME VIAL CONTENT			
500 mg (IV)	5 mL	5.6 mL	100 mg/mL
500 mg (IM)	1.3 mL	1.8 mL	280 mg/mL
1 Gm (IV)	10 mL	11.3 mL	100 mg/mL
1 Gm (IM)	2.4 mL	3.6 mL	280 mg/mL
2 Gm (IV)	10 mL	12.5 mL	160 mg/mL
ADD-VANTAGE			
1 Gm vial	50 mL	50 mL	20 mg/mL
1 Gm vial	100 mL	100 mL	10 mg/mL
2 Gm vial	50 mL	50 mL	40 mg/mL
2 Gm vial	100 mL	100 mL	20 mg/mL

Filters: Specific information from studies not available; contact manufacturer for further information.

Storage: Store cefepime in the dry state between 2° to 25° C (36° to 77° F); protect from light. Reconstituted or diluted solutions are stable for 24 hours at CRT and 7 days if refrigerated. Store Galaxy containers at or below −20° C (−4° F). Once thawed, do not refreeze.

COMPATIBILITY   (Underline Indicates Conflicting Compatibility Information)
Consider any drug NOT listed as compatible to be INCOMPATIBLE until consulting a pharmacist; specific conditions may apply.
Manufacturer recommends temporarily discontinuing other solutions infusing at the same site during intermittent infusion. May be used concomitantly with aminoglycosides (e.g., gentamicin, tobramycin), aminophylline, metronidazole (Flagyl IV), and vancomycin, but these drugs must never be mixed in the same infusion (mutual inactivation or other potential interactions). If given concurrently, administer at separate sites.
   Sources suggest the following **compatibilities:**
Additive: Manufacturer lists specific concentrations of amikacin (Amikin), ampicillin, clindamycin (Cleocin), heparin, potassium chloride (KCl), and theophylline. Other sources add metronidazole (Flagyl IV) and vancomycin.
Y-site: Ampicillin/sulbactam (Unasyn), anidulafungin (Eraxis), aztreonam (Azactam), bivalirudin (Angiomax), bleomycin (Blenoxane), bumetanide, buprenorphine (Buprenex), butorphanol (Stadol), calcium gluconate, carboplatin (Paraplatin), carmustine (BiCNU), cyclophosphamide (Cytoxan), cytarabine (ARA-C), dactinomycin (Cosmegen), dexamethasone (Decadron), dexmedetomidine (Precedex), dobutamine, docetaxel (Taxotere), dopamine, doxorubicin liposomal (Doxil), fenoldopam (Corlopam), fluconazole (Diflucan), fludarabine (Fludara), fluorouracil (5-FU), furose-

mide (Lasix), granisetron (Kytril), hetastarch in electrolytes (Hextend), hydrocortisone sodium succinate (Solu-Cortef), hydromorphone (Dilaudid), imipenem-cilastatin (Primaxin), insulin (regular), ketamine (Ketalar), leucovorin calcium, lorazepam (Ativan), melphalan (Alkeran), mesna (Mesnex), methotrexate, methylprednisolone (Solu-Medrol), metronidazole (Flagyl IV), milrinone (Primacor), <u>morphine</u>, mycophenolate (CellCept IV), paclitaxel (Taxol), piperacillin/tazobactam (Zosyn), <u>propofol (Diprivan)</u>, ranitidine (Zantac), remefentanil (Ultiva), sargramostim (Leukine), sodium bicarbonate, sufentanil (Sufenta), sulfamethoxazole/trimethoprim, thiotepa, ticarcillin/clavulanate (Timentin), tigecycline (Tygacil), valproate (Depacon), <u>vancomycin</u>, zidovudine (AZT, Retrovir).

RATE OF ADMINISTRATION

Do not use plastic containers in a series connection; could result in air embolism. May be given through Y-tube or three-way stopcock of infusion set; see Compatibility.

Intermittent infusion: A single dose equally distributed over 30 minutes.

ACTIONS

A semisynthetic, extended-spectrum, fourth-generation cephalosporin antibiotic. Bactericidal to both gram-positive and gram-negative organisms, including many strains resistant to third-generation cephalosporins and aminoglycosides. Acts by inhibition of bacterial wall synthesis. Has a well-balanced spectrum with good antistaphylococcal activity, enhanced activity against gram-negative organisms, and good antipseudomonal activity. Peak serum levels achieved by end of infusion; half-life is 1.7 to 2.3 hours. Therapeutic levels last for 12 hours, allowing for twice-daily dosing. Well distributed into many body fluids and tissues. Crosses inflamed meninges to enter CSF. Partially metabolized; 85% excreted unchanged in urine. Secreted in breast milk.

INDICATIONS AND USES

Treatment of moderate to severe pneumonia caused by susceptible organisms, including cases associated with concurrent bacteremia. ■ Treatment of uncomplicated and complicated urinary tract infections caused by susceptible organisms, including pyelonephritis and cases associated with concurrent bacteremia. ■ Treatment of uncomplicated skin and skin structure infections caused by susceptible organisms. ■ Empiric monotherapy in the treatment of febrile neutropenic patients. ■ Treatment of complicated intra-abdominal infections in adults; used in combination with metronidazole (Flagyl). ■ See literature for list of susceptible organisms.

CONTRAINDICATIONS

Patients who have shown immediate hypersensitivity reactions to cefepime, any cephalosporin, penicillins, or other beta-lactam antibiotics; see Precautions. ■ Solutions containing dextrose may be contraindicated in patients with known allergies to corn or corn products.

PRECAUTIONS

Hypersensitivity reactions, including fatalities, have been reported and include reports of individuals with a history of penicillin hypersensitivity or sensitivity to multiple allergens experiencing severe reactions when treated with cephalosporins. Check history of previous hypersensitivity reactions to penicillins, cephalosporins, or other allergens. Actual incidence of cross-allergenicity not established but may be more common with first-generation cephalosporins. ■ Specific sensitivity studies are indicated to determine susceptibility of the causative organism to cefepime. ■ To reduce the development of drug-resistant bacteria and maintain its effectiveness, cefepime should be used to treat or prevent only those infections proven or strongly suspected to be caused by bacteria. ■ Generally more resistant to hydrolysis by beta-lactamases than third-generation cephalosporins are. ■ IM injection is used only for mild to moderate urinary tract infections. ■ Avoid prolonged use of drug; superinfection caused by overgrowth of nonsusceptible organisms may result. ■ Continue for at least 2 days after all symptoms of infection subside. ■ May decrease prothrombin activity, especially in patients with impaired renal or hepatic function, those in a poor nutritional state, and those receiving extended courses of antimicrobial therapy. ■ Use caution in patients with a history of GI disease (especially colitis). ■ Serious adverse events, including encephalopathy (changes in consciousness, including confusion, hallucinations, stupor, and coma), myoclonus, seizures, and other life-threatening or fatal events have occurred. Patients with impaired renal function may be at greater risk, especially if doses are not properly adjusted; see Dose Adjustments and monitor closely. In most cases, neurotoxicity was reversible and resolved after cefepime was discontinued and/or after hemodialysis. ■ *Clostridium difficile*–associated diarrhea (CDAD) has been reported. May range from mild diarrhea to fatal colitis. Consider in patients who present with diarrhea during or after treatment with cefepime. ■ Contains arginine, which may alter glucose metabolism and elevate serum potassium. ■ Higher-end doses may increase incidence and severity of rash and require cefepime to be discontinued. ■ Insufficient data exist for monotherapy of febrile neutropenia in patients at high risk for severe infection (e.g., history of recent bone marrow transplant, hypotension on presentation, underlying hematologic malignancy, severe or prolonged neutropenia). No data are available for patients with septic shock. ■ If meningitis is suspected or documented, an alternate agent with demonstrated clinical effectiveness should be used.

Monitor: Watch for early symptoms of a hypersensitivity reaction. ■ Obtain baseline CBC with differential and platelets and SCr. ■ Obtain baseline PT and monitor, especially in at-risk patients (see Precautions); vitamin K may be indicated. ■ Monitoring of serum glucose and electrolytes (e.g., potassium, calcium) may be indicated. ■ May cause thrombophlebitis. ■ Monitor and re-evaluate frequently the need for continued antimicrobial treatment in patients whose fever resolves but who remain neutropenic for more than 7 days. ■ See Drug/Lab Interactions.

Patient Education: Promptly report any bleeding or bruising or symptoms of hypersensitivity (e.g., difficulty breathing, hives, itching, rash). ■ Promptly report diarrhea or bloody stools that occur during treatment or up to several months after an antibiotic has been discontinued; may indicate CDAD and require treatment. ■ Promptly report neurologic S/S (e.g., change in consciousness, confusion, hallucinations, seizures, stupor).

Maternal/Child: Category B: safety for use during pregnancy, labor and delivery, and breast-feeding not established; use only if clearly needed. ■ Safety and effectiveness not established for infants under 2 months of age or for treatment of serious infections in pediatric patients in whom the suspected or proven pathogen is *Haemophilus influenzae type b*. ■ Pharmacokinetics in pediatric patients and adults are similar. Dose modification similar to adults is indicated in impaired renal function; see Dose

Adjustments. ■ Immature renal function of infants and small children will increase blood levels of all cephalosporins.

Elderly: No specific problems documented. Consider age-related impaired organ function, nutritional status, and concomitant disease or drug therapy; reduced dose or extended intervals may be indicated; see Dose Adjustments. Monitor for hypocalcemia.

DRUG/LAB INTERACTIONS

Risk of nephrotoxicity may be increased with **aminoglycosides and other nephrotoxic agents** (e.g., loop diuretics [e.g., furosemide (Lasix)]); monitor renal function closely. ■ Risk of ototoxicity may be increased when administered with aminoglycosides (e.g., gentamicin). ■ May cause a false-positive **direct Coombs' test.** ■ May have a false-positive reaction for **urine glucose** except with enzyme-based tests (e.g., Clinistix). ■ See Side Effects. ■ Although it has not been specifically studied with cefepime, other cephalosporins have the following drug interactions. May be antagonized by **bacteriostatic antibiotics** (e.g., chloramphenicol, erythromycin, tetracyclines); may interfere with bactericidal action. ■ Large amounts of **cephalosporins and/or salicylates** may induce hypoprothrombinemia (deficiency of prothrombin [Factor II]). The addition of **agents that affect platelet aggregation and/or may have GI ulcerative potential** (e.g., NSAIDs [ibuprofen (Advil, Motrin), naproxen (Aleve, Naprosyn)] or sulfinpyrazone [Anturane]) may increase risk of hemorrhage. ■ See Compatibility.

SIDE EFFECTS

Local reactions (including phlebitis), pain and/or inflammation, and rash are most common. Full scope of hypersensitivity reactions (e.g., anaphylaxis, itching, rash, shock, urticaria). Bone marrow suppression (e.g., agranulocytosis, leukopenia, neutropenia, thrombocytopenia); CDAD; diarrhea; elevated alkaline phosphatase, AST, ALT, BUN; fever; headache; nausea and vomiting; oral moniliasis; prolonged PT; seizures (large doses or standard doses in renally impaired); vaginitis. Serum sickness–like reactions have occurred (e.g., arthralgia, fever, polyarthritis, skin rashes), usually after a second course of therapy. Usually resolve after cephalosporins are discontinued. Hypoprothrombinemia (rare) and hemolytic anemia may occur.

Overdose: Encephalopathy (disturbances of consciousness, including confusion, hallucinations, stupor, and coma), myoclonus, neuromuscular excitability, seizures.

Post-Marketing: Agranulocytosis, anaphylaxis, encephalopathy, myoclonus, seizures.

ANTIDOTE

Notify physician of any side effects. Discontinue cefepime and treat hypersensitivity reactions as indicated (airway, oxygen, IV fluids, epinephrine, corticosteroids, pressor amines [e.g., dopamine], antihistamines [e.g., diphenhydramine]). Resuscitate as necessary. Discontinue cefepime if seizures occur and treat with anticonvulsants (e.g., diazepam [Valium]). Mild cases of CDAD may respond to discontinuation of cefepime. Treat CDAD with fluids, electrolytes, protein supplements, and oral vancomycin (Vancocin) or metronidazole (Flagyl) as indicated. In severe cases, surgical evaluation may be indicated. Antihistamines and corticosteroids may be indicated to manage symptoms of serum sickness. Hemodialysis may be useful in overdose.

CEFOTAXIME SODIUM
(sef-oh-**TAX**-eem **SO**-dee-um)

**Antibacterial
(cephalosporin)**

Claforan

pH 5 to 7.5

USUAL DOSE

Range is 2 to 12 Gm/24 hr. Depends on seriousness of infection. Maximum daily dose is 12 Gm. Duration of treatment depends on the organism and infection being treated. A minimum of 10 days is recommended for infections caused by *group A beta-hemolytic streptococci* to guard against the risk of rheumatic fever or glomerulonephritis.

Uncomplicated infections: 1 Gm every 12 hours.

Moderate to severe infections: 1 to 2 Gm every 8 hours.

Serious infections and septicemia: 2 Gm every 6 to 8 hours.

Life-threatening infections: 2 Gm every 4 hours.

Higher doses often reduced with positive clinical response.

Disseminated gonococcal infections: 1 Gm every 8 hours; continue for 24 to 48 hours after symptoms improve. Transfer to oral cefixime to complete a minimum of 1 week of treatment.

Perioperative prophylaxis: 1 Gm 30 to 90 minutes before incision. Equal to or less than 60 minutes is recommended. May be repeated in a lengthy procedure. In *cesarean section* give initial dose after cord is clamped, then 1 Gm at 6 and 12 hours postoperatively.

PEDIATRIC DOSE

Maximum daily dose 12 Gm/24 hr. Differentiation between premature and normal gestational age is not necessary.

0 to 1 week of age: 50 mg/kg/dose every 12 hours.

1 to 4 weeks of age: 50 mg/kg/dose every 8 hours. One source increases the interval to every 12 hours in infants weighing less than 1,200 Gm.

1 month to 12 years, weight less than 50 kg: 50 to 180 mg/kg/24 hr equally divided into 4 to 6 doses (8.3 to 30 mg/kg/dose every 4 hours or 12.5 to 45 mg/kg/dose every 6 hours). Use higher-end doses for serious infections, including meningitis.

Weight 50 kg or more: See Usual Dose.

DOSE ADJUSTMENTS

In impaired renal function with a CrCl less than 20 mL/min/1.73 M^2, reduce dose by one half and maintain same dosing interval. ▪ Reduced doses or extended intervals may be indicated in the elderly. Consider age-related impaired organ function, nutritional status, and concomitant disease or drug therapy. ▪ See Usual Dose and Drug/Lab Interactions.

DILUTION

Each dose (500 mg, 1 Gm, 2 Gm) must be reconstituted with 10 mL SW, D5W, NS, or other **compatible** infusion solution (see chart on inside back cover or literature). Do not prepare with diluents having a pH above 7.5; see Compatibility. Solution color ranges from pale yellow to light amber. Available premixed and in ADD-Vantage vials for use with ADD-Vantage infusion containers. May be further diluted with 50 to 100 mL of **compatible** solutions and given as an intermittent infusion or added to larger volumes and given as a continuous infusion. (1 Gm in 14 mL of SW is isotonic.)

Storage: Store unopened cartons at CRT. Protect from excessive light. Stability ranges from 12 hours at RT to 10 days refrigerated depending on concentration and infusion container; see prescribing information.

COMPATIBILITY   (Underline Indicates Conflicting Compatibility Information)

Consider any drug NOT listed as compatible to be INCOMPATIBLE until consulting a pharmacist; specific conditions may apply.

May be used concomitantly with aminoglycosides (e.g., amikacin [Amikin], gentamicin), but these drugs must never be mixed in the same infusion (mutual inactivation). If given concurrently, administer at separate sites. Manufacturer recommends temporarily discontinuing other solutions infusing at the same site during intermittent infusion and states, "Do not add supplementary medications to premixed plastic IV containers." Manufacturer also states, "Should not be prepared with solutions having a pH above 7.5, such as sodium bicarbonate."

One source suggests the following **compatibilities:**

Additive: Clindamycin (Cleocin), metronidazole (Flagyl IV), verapamil.

Y-site: Acyclovir (Zovirax), alprostadil, amifostine (Ethyol), aztreonam (Azactam), bivalirudin (Angiomax), cisatracurium (Nimbex), cyclophosphamide (Cytoxan), dexmedetomidine (Precedex), diltiazem (Cardizem), docetaxel (Taxotere), etoposide phosphate (Etopophos), famotidine (Pepcid IV), fenoldopam (Corlopam), fludarabine (Fludara), granisetron (Kytril), hetastarch in electrolytes (Hextend), hydromorphone (Dilaudid), levofloxacin (Levaquin), lorazepam (Ativan), magnesium sulfate, melphalan (Alkeran), meperidine (Demerol), midazolam (Versed), milrinone (Primacor), morphine, ondansetron (Zofran), propofol (Diprivan), remifentanil (Ultiva), sargramostim (Leukine), teniposide (Vumon), thiotepa, tigecycline (Tygacil), vancomycin, vinorelbine (Navelbine).

RATE OF ADMINISTRATION

See Compatibility. Injection and intermittent infusion may be given through Y-tube or three-way stopcock of infusion set.

IV injection: A single dose equally distributed over a minimum of 3 to 5 minutes. Rapid bolus injections (less than 60 seconds) have caused life-threatening arrhythmias.

Intermittent IV: A single dose over 30 minutes.

Continuous infusion: 500 to 1,000 mL over 6 to 24 hours, depending on total dose and concentration.

ACTIONS

A broad-spectrum, third-generation cephalosporin antibiotic. Bactericidal to many gram-negative, gram-positive, and anaerobic organisms. Effective against many otherwise resistant organisms. Inhibits bacterial cell wall synthesis. Distributed into most body tissues and fluids, including inflamed meninges. Some metabolites formed. Half-life is approximately 1 hour. Excreted in the urine. Crosses placental barrier. Secreted in breast milk.

INDICATIONS AND USES

Treatment of serious lower respiratory tract, urinary tract, skin and skin structure, intra-abdominal, bone and joint, CNS, gynecologic infections, and bacteremia/septicemia. Most effective against specific organisms (see literature). ■ Perioperative prophylaxis.

Unlabeled uses: Treatment of disseminated gonococcal infections and Lyme disease.

CONTRAINDICATIONS

Previous hypersensitivity reaction to cephalosporins; see Precautions.

PRECAUTIONS

Hypersensitivity reactions, including fatalities, have been reported and include reports of individuals with a history of penicillin hypersensitivity or sensitivity to multiple allergens experiencing severe reactions when treated with cephalosporins. Check history of previous hypersensitivity reactions to penicillins, cephalosporins, or other allergens. Actual incidence of cross-allergenicity not established but may be more common with first-generation cephalosporins. ■ Sensitivity studies indicated to determine susceptibility of the causative organism to cefotaxime. ■ To reduce the development of drug-resistant bacteria and maintain its effectiveness, cefotaxime should be used to treat or prevent only those infections proven or strongly suspected to be caused by bacteria. ■ Continue for 2 to 3 days after all symptoms of infection subside. ■ Avoid prolonged use of drug; superinfection caused by overgrowth of nonsusceptible organisms may result. ■ Use caution in patients with impaired renal function, allergies, or a history of GI disease (especially colitis). ■ *Clostridium difficile*–associated diarrhea (CDAD) has been reported. May range from mild diarrhea to fatal colitis. Consider in patients who present with diarrhea during or after treatment with cefotaxime. ■ Granulocytopenia and, rarely, agranulocytosis can occur, especially during prolonged therapy; see Monitor.

Monitor: Watch for early symptoms of a hypersensitivity reaction. ■ Monitor CBC if duration of treatment is more than 10 days. ■ May cause thrombophlebitis. Use small needles and large veins, and rotate infusion sites. ■ Observe for electrolyte imbalance or cardiac irregularities. Contains 2.2 mEq sodium per Gm. ■ See Drug/Lab Interactions; additional monitoring may be indicated (e.g., renal function, drug serum levels, PT).

Patient Education: Report promptly any bleeding or bruising or symptoms of hypersensitivity (e.g., difficulty breathing, hives, itching, rash). ■ Promptly report diarrhea or bloody stools that occur during treatment or up to several months after an antibiotic has been discontinued; may indicate CDAD and require treatment.

Maternal/Child: Category B: safety for use during pregnancy and breast-feeding not established. No problems documented. ■ Immature renal function of infants and small children will increase blood levels of all cephalosporins.

Elderly: No specific problems documented; see Dose Adjustments.

DRUG/LAB INTERACTIONS

Risk of nephrotoxicity may be increased with **aminoglycosides and other nephrotoxic agents** (e.g., loop diuretics [such as furosemide (Lasix)]). ■ **Probenecid** inhibits excretion. Reduced dose of cefotaxime may be required with concomitant use. ■ May be antagonized by **bacteriostatic antibiotics** (e.g., chloramphenicol, erythromycin, tetracyclines); may interfere with bactericidal action. ■ Large amounts of **cephalosporins and/or salicylates** may induce hypoprothrombinemia (deficiency of prothrombin [Factor II]). The addition of **agents that affect platelet aggregation and/or may have GI ulcerative potential** (e.g., NSAIDs [ibuprofen (Advil, Motrin), naproxen (Aleve, Naprosyn)] or sulfinpyrazone [Anturane]) may increase risk of hemorrhage. ■ See Compatibility and Side Effects. ■ May cause a positive direct **Coombs' test.** ■ May produce a false-positive reaction for **urine glucose** except with enzyme-based tests (e.g., Chemstix).

SIDE EFFECTS

Generally well tolerated. Most common side effect is a local reaction at the injection site. Less frequent reactions include full scope of hypersensitivity reactions, including anaphylaxis; CDAD; colitis; decreased hemoglobin or decreased hematocrit; decreased platelet functions; diarrhea; dyspnea; elevation of AST, ALT, total bilirubin, alkaline phosphatase, LDH, and BUN (transient); eosinophilia; fever; leukopenia; local site pain; nausea; oral thrush; positive direct Coombs' test; prolonged PT; seizures (large doses); thrombophlebitis; transient neutropenia; vaginitis; vomiting. Serum sicknesslike reactions have occurred (e.g., arthralgia, fever, poly-arthritis, skin rashes), usually after a second course of therapy. Generally resolve after cephalosporins are discontinued.

Post-Marketing: Arrhythmia (with rapid injection), cutaneous reactions (e.g., isolated cases of erythema multiforme, Stevens-Johnson syndrome, toxic epidermal necrolysis), encephalopathy (e.g., impairment of consciousness, abnormal movements and seizures), hematologic reactions (e.g., agranulocytosis, hemolytic anemia, thrombocytopenia), hepatic reactions (e.g., cholestasis, elevated gamma-glutamyl transferase (GGT) and bilirubin, hepatitis, jaundice), renal reactions (e.g., interstitial nephritis and transient elevations in SCr.

ANTIDOTE

Notify the physician of any side effects. Discontinue the drug if indicated. Mild cases of CDAD may respond to discontinuation of cefotaxime. Treat CDAD with fluids, electrolytes, protein supplements, and oral vancomycin (Vancocin) or metronidazole (Flagyl) as indicated. In severe cases, surgical evaluation may be indicated. Antihistamines and corticosteroids may be indicated to manage symptoms of serum sickness. Treat hypersensitivity reactions as indicated and resuscitate as necessary. Hemodialysis may be useful in overdose.

CEFOXITIN SODIUM
(seh-**FOX**-ih-tin **SO**-dee-um)

Mefoxin

Antibacterial (cephalosporin)

pH 4.2 to 8

USUAL DOSE

Cefoxitin Dosing Guidelines		
Type of Infection	Dose and Frequency	Total Daily Dose
Uncomplicated forms* of infections such as pneumonia, urinary tract infection, cutaneous infection	1 Gm every 6 to 8 hr	3 to 4 Gm
Moderately severe or severe infections	1 Gm every 4 hr or 2 Gm every 6 to 8 hr	6 to 8 Gm
Infections commonly needing antibiotics in higher doses (e.g., gas gangrene)	2 Gm every 4 hr or 3 Gm every 6 hr	12 Gm

*Including patients in whom bacteremia is absent or unlikely.

Perioperative prophylaxis: 2 Gm 30 minutes to 1 hour before incision. Follow with 2 Gm every 6 hours for 24 hours.

Prophylaxis during cesarean section: 2 Gm after clamping the umbilical cord. May repeat in 4 hours and again in 8 hours.

Prophylaxis during transurethral prostatectomy (unlabeled): 1 Gm before surgery. May be repeated every 8 hours for up to 5 days.

PEDIATRIC DOSE

Pediatric patients over 3 months of age: *Mild to moderate infections:* 20 to 25 mg/kg every 6 hours or 26.66 to 33.33 mg/kg every 8 hours (80 to 100 mg/kg/24 hr). *Severe infections:* 16.66 to 26.66 mg/kg every 4 hours or 25 to 40 mg/kg every 6 hours (100 to 160 mg/kg/24 hr). Do not exceed adult dose and/or 12 Gm.

Perioperative prophylaxis in pediatric patients over 3 months of age: 30 to 40 mg/kg 30 minutes to 1 hour before incision and every 6 hours for 24 hours.

NEONATAL DOSE

Use sterile cefoxitin sodium USP only. Other formulations may contain benzyl alcohol.

30 to 33.3 mg/kg every 8 hours (90 to 100 mg/kg/24 hr).

DOSE ADJUSTMENTS

Reduced dose or extended intervals may be indicated in the elderly; consider age-related impaired organ function, nutritional status, and concomitant disease or drug therapy. ■ In impaired renal function, the initial dose should be as previously listed, but all remaining doses should be based on CrCl according to the following chart. See Drug/Lab Interactions.

Cefoxitin Maintenance Dose in Adults with Impaired Renal Function		
Creatinine Clearance (mL/min)	Dose (Gm)	Frequency
30-50 mL/min	1-2 Gm	q 8-12 hr
10-29 mL/min	1-2 Gm	q 12-24 hr
5-9 mL/min	0.5-1 Gm	q 12-24 hr
<5 mL/min	0.5-1 Gm	q 24-48 hr

Hemodialysis patients should receive a loading dose of 1 to 2 Gm after each dialysis in addition to the maintenance dose listed in the previous chart.

In pediatric patients, one source recommends reducing the dose and frequency consistent with the recommendations for adults. Another source recommends increasing the dosing interval based on CrCl according to the following chart.

Cefoxitin Maintenance Dose in Pediatric Patients with Impaired Renal Function	
Creatinine Clearance (mL/min)	Frequency
>50 mL/min	q 8 hr
10-50 mL/min	q 8-12 hr
<10 mL/min	q 24-48 hr

DILUTION

Each 1 Gm or fraction thereof must be reconstituted with at least 10 mL of SW, D5W, or NS. A single dose may be further diluted in 50 to 100 mL of most common infusion solutions (see chart on inside back cover and literature). The use of butterfly needles and dilution in up to 1,000 mL of D5W, D5NS, or NS are preferred when administering larger doses as a continuous infusion. Available premixed and in piggyback vials. May be given through a Y-tube, three-way stopcock, additive infusion set, or as a continuous infusion.

Storage: Reconstituted solutions are stable at CRT for 6 hours and 7 days if refrigerated. Solutions diluted in 50 to 1,000 mL diluent are stable for 18 to 24 hours at CRT and up to 48 hours if refrigerated. Thaw frozen containers at CRT or under refrigeration. Do not force thaw. Stable for 21 days if refrigerated. Do not refreeze.

COMPATIBILITY   (Underline Indicates Conflicting Compatibility Information)

Consider any drug NOT listed as compatible to be INCOMPATIBLE until consulting a pharmacist; specific conditions may apply.

May be used concomitantly with aminoglycosides (e.g., amikacin [Amikin], gentamicin), but these drugs must never be mixed in the same infusion (mutual inactivation). If given concurrently, administer at separate sites. Manufacturer recommends temporarily discontinuing other solutions infusing at the same site during intermittent infusion.

One source suggests the following **compatibilities:**

Additive: Aztreonam (Azactam), clindamycin (Cleocin), metronidazole (Flagyl IV), multivitamins (M.V.I.), sodium bicarbonate (Neut), verapamil.

Y-site: Acyclovir (Zovirax), amifostine (Ethyol), amphotericin B cholesteryl (Amphotec), anidulafungin (Eraxis), aztreonam (Azactam), bivalirudin (Angiomax), cisatracurium (Nimbex), cyclophosphamide (Cytoxan), dexmedetomidine (Precedex), diltiazem (Cardizem), docetaxel (Taxotere), doxorubicin liposomal (Doxil), etoposide phosphate (Etopophos), famotidine (Pepcid IV), fluconazole (Diflucan), foscarnet (Foscavir), gemcitabine (Gemzar), granisetron (Kytril), hetastarch in electrolytes (Hextend), hydromorphone (Dilaudid), linezolid (Zyvox), magnesium sulfate, meperidine (Demerol), morphine, ondansetron (Zofran), propofol (Diprivan), ranitidine (Zantac), remifentanil (Ultiva), teniposide (Vumon), thiotepa, vancomycin.

RATE OF ADMINISTRATION

See Compatibility. Each 1 Gm or fraction thereof over 3 to 5 minutes or longer as indicated by amount of solution and condition of the patient. Rate of continuous infusion should be by physician order.

ACTIONS

A semisynthetic, second-generation cephalosporin antibiotic that is bactericidal to many gram-positive, gram-negative, and anaerobic organisms. Inhibits cell wall synthesis. Peak serum levels achieved by end of infusion. Widely distributed into most body tissues and fluids (CSF minimal), bone, gallbladder, myocardium, and skin and soft tissues. Half-life is 41 to 59 minutes. Excreted rapidly in the urine. Crosses the placental barrier. Secreted in breast milk.

INDICATIONS AND USES

Treatment of serious respiratory, GU, intra-abdominal, gynecologic, bone and joint, skin and skin structure infections and septicemia. Effective only if the causative organism is susceptible. If *C. trachomatis* is a suspected pathogen, antichlamydial coverage is indicated. ▪ Perioperative prophylaxis.

Unlabeled uses: Treatment of acute pelvic inflammatory disease (CDC recommendation). ▪ Treatment of oral bacterial *Eikenella corrodens*. ▪ Prophylaxis during transurethral prostatectomy.

CONTRAINDICATIONS

Previous hypersensitivity reaction to cephalosporins; see Precautions.

PRECAUTIONS

Hypersensitivity reactions, including fatalities, have been reported and include reports of individuals with a history of penicillin hypersensitivity or sensitivity to multiple allergens experiencing severe reactions when treated with cephalosporins. Check history of previous hypersensitivity reactions to penicillins, cephalosporins, or other allergens. Actual incidence of cross-allergenicity not established but may be more common with first-generation cephalosporins. ▪ Sensitivity studies indicated to determine susceptibility of the causative organism to cefoxitin. ▪ To reduce the development of drug-resistant bacteria and maintain its effectiveness, cefoxitin should be used to treat or prevent only those infections proven or strongly suspected to be caused by bacteria. ▪ Continue for at least 2 to 3 days after all symptoms of infection subside. ▪ Avoid prolonged use of drug; superinfection caused by overgrowth of nonsusceptible organisms may result. ▪ Use caution in patients with impaired renal function, allergies, or a history of GI disease (especially colitis). ▪ *Clostridium difficile*–associated diarrhea (CDAD) has been reported. May range from mild diarrhea to fatal colitis. Consider in patients who present with diarrhea during or after treatment with cefoxitin. ▪ Continue treatment for group A beta-hemolytic streptococcal infections for 10 days or more to decrease the risk of rheumatic fever or glomerulonephritis.

Monitor: Watch for early symptoms of a hypersensitivity reaction. ▪ Use extreme caution in the penicillin-sensitive patient; incidence of cross-sensitivity may be up to 10%. ▪ Thrombophlebitis may result from prolonged or high dosage; use small needles, larger veins, and rotate infusion sites. ▪ Observe for electrolyte imbalance or cardiac irregularities. Contains 2.3 mEq sodium/Gm. ▪ Periodic monitoring of CBC, SCr, and liver function tests is recommended during prolonged therapy. ▪ See Drug/Lab Interactions; additional monitoring may be indicated (e.g., renal function, drug serum levels, PT).

Patient Education: Report promptly any bleeding or bruising or symptoms of allergy (e.g., difficulty breathing, hives, itching, rash). ▪ Promptly report diarrhea or bloody stools that occur during treatment or up to several months after an antibiotic has been discontinued; may indicate CDAD and require treatment.

Maternal/Child: Category B: safety for use during pregnancy and breast-feeding not established. No problems documented. ▪ Do not use formulations containing benzyl alcohol in infants and children under 3 months. ▪ Immature renal function will increase blood levels. ▪ Eosinophilia and elevated AST associated with higher doses in infants and children.

Elderly: Response similar to that seen in younger adults. Dose selection should be cautious; see Dose Adjustments. Monitoring of renal function suggested.

DRUG/LAB INTERACTIONS

Risk of nephrotoxicity may be increased with **aminoglycosides and other nephrotoxic agents** (e.g., loop diuretics such as furosemide [Lasix]). ▪ **Probenecid** inhibits excretion. Reduced dose of cefoxitin may be required with concomitant use. ▪ May be antagonized by **bacteriostatic antibiotics** (e.g., chloramphenicol, erythromycin, tetracyclines); may interfere with bactericidal action. ▪ Large doses of **cephalosporins and/or salicylates** may induce hypoprothrombinemia (deficiency of prothrombin [Factor II]). The addition of **agents that affect platelet aggregation and/or may have GI ulcerative potential** (e.g., NSAIDs [ibuprofen (Advil, Motrin), naproxen (Aleve, Naprosyn)] or sulfinpyrazone [Anturane]) may increase risk of hemorrhage. ▪ False-positive reaction for **urine glucose** except with enzyme-based tests (e.g., Chemstix). ▪ Positive **Coombs' test**. ▪ False increases in **creatinine levels** with Jaffe method. ▪ See Compatibility and Side Effects.

SIDE EFFECTS

Local site reactions are most common. Anorexia; CDAD; colitis; flushing; hypersensitivity reactions, including anaphylaxis; eosinophilia; leukopenia; nausea and vomiting; neutropenia; oral thrush; phlebitis; prolonged

PT; proteinuria; seizures (large doses); thrombophlebitis; transient elevation of AST, ALT, BUN, and alkaline phosphatase; and urticaria have occurred. Hypoprothrombinemia (rare) and hemolytic anemia may occur. Serum sickness–like reactions have occurred (e.g., arthralgia, fever, polyarthritis, skin rashes), usually after a second course of therapy. Generally resolve after cephalosporins are discontinued.

ANTIDOTE

Notify physician of any side effects. Discontinue the drug if indicated. Treat CDAD with fluids, electrolytes, protein supplements, and oral vancomycin (Vancocin) or metronidazole (Flagyl) as indicated. In severe cases, surgical evaluation may be indicated. Treat hypersensitivity reactions as indicated and resuscitate as necessary. Hemodialysis may be useful in overdose. Antihistamines and corticosteroids may be indicated to manage symptoms of serum sickness.

CEFTAROLINE FOSAMIL
(cef-**TAR**-oh-leen **FOS**-a-mil)

Teflaro

Antibacterial
(cephalosporin)

pH 4.8 to 6.5

USUAL DOSE
600 mg every 12 hours as an IV infusion. Duration of therapy should be guided by the severity and the site of infection and the patient's clinical and bacteriologic progress as shown in the following table.

Dosage of Ceftaroline				
Infection	Dosage	Frequency	Infusion Time (hours)	Recommended Duration of Total Antimicrobial Therapy
Acute bacterial skin and skin structure infection (ABSSSI)	600 mg	q 12 hr	1 hr	5-14 days
Community-acquired bacterial pneumonia (CABP)	600 mg	q 12 hr	1 hr	5-7 days

DOSE ADJUSTMENTS
Dose adjustment required with renal impairment as outlined in the following table.

Dosage of Ceftaroline in Patients with Renal Impairment	
Estimated CrCl* (mL/min)	Recommended Dosage Regimen
>50 mL/min	600 mg q 12 hr
>30 to ≤50 mL/min	400 mg q 12 hr
≥15 to ≤30 mL/min	300 mg q 12 hr
End-stage renal disease, including hemodialysis†	200 mg q 12 hr‡

*CrCl as calculated by Cockcroft-Gault formula.
†End-stage renal disease is defined as CrCl <15 mL/min.
‡Ceftaroline is hemodialyzable; administer after hemodialysis on hemodialysis days.

■ Dose adjustment is not indicated based on gender, race, or hepatic function. ■ Reduced dose may be indicated in the elderly based on age-related renal impairment.

DILUTION
Reconstitute with SWFI as shown in the following table. Mix gently. Time to dissolution is less than 2 minutes.

Preparation of Ceftaroline for Intravenous Use			
Dosage Strength (mg)	Volume of Diluent to Be Added (mL)	Approximate Ceftaroline Concentration (mg/mL)	Amount to Be Withdrawn
400	20 mL	20 mg/mL	Total volume
600	20 mL	30 mg/mL	Total volume

Further dilute the reconstituted solution in 250 mL of NS, D5W, D2.5W, ½NS, or LR. Infusion solution ranges from clear to light yellow to dark yellow depending on the concentration and the storage conditions.

Filter: Data not available

Storage: Store unopened vials in the refrigerator at 2° to 8° C (36° to 46° F). Diluted solution should be used within 6 hours when stored at RT or within 24 hours when refrigerated.

COMPATIBILITY
Manufacturer states, "Should not be mixed with or physically added to solutions containing other drugs." **Compatibility** with other drugs has not been established.

RATE OF ADMINISTRATION
A single dose equally distributed over 1 hour.

ACTIONS
A semi-synthetic, broad-spectrum cephalosporin. Ceftaroline fosamil, a prodrug, is converted into the bioactive ceftaroline in plasma by a phosphatase enzyme. Bactericidal to many gram-negative and gram-positive organisms. Inhibits bacterial cell wall synthesis. Protein binding is minimal (20%). Ceftaroline undergoes hydrolysis, forming an inactive metabolite. Half-life is approximately 2.2 to 3 hours. Both ceftaroline and its metabolites are primarily eliminated by the kidneys.

INDICATIONS AND USES
Treatment of adults with infections caused by susceptible strains of microorganisms in conditions, including acute bacterial skin and skin structure infections (ABSSSI) and community-acquired bacterial pneumonia (CABP).

CONTRAINDICATIONS
Known serious hypersensitivity to ceftaroline or other members of the cephalosporin class.

PRECAUTIONS
Hypersensitivity reactions and serious skin reactions, including fatalities, have been reported and include reports of individuals with a history of penicillin hypersensitivity or sensitivity to multiple allergens experiencing severe reactions when treated with cephalosporins. Check history of previous hypersensitivity reactions to penicillins, cephalosporins, carbapenems, or other allergens. Actual incidence of cross-allergenicity not established but may be more common with first-generation cephalosporins. ■ Specific sensitivity studies are indicated to determine susceptibility of the causative organism to ceftaroline. ■ To reduce the development of drug-resistant bacteria and maintain its effectiveness, ceftaroline should be used to treat only those infections proven or strongly suspected

to be caused by bacteria. ▪ *Clostridium difficile*–associated diarrhea (CDAD) has been reported. May range from mild diarrhea to fatal colitis. Consider in patients who present with diarrhea during or after treatment with ceftaroline. ▪ Seroconversion from a negative to a positive direct Coombs' test occurred in approximately 10% of patients in Phase 3 trials. No adverse reactions representing hemolytic anemia were reported. If anemia develops during or after treatment with ceftaroline, drug-induced hemolytic anemia should be considered and diagnostic studies, including a direct Coombs' test, should be performed.

Monitor: Watch for early symptoms of a hypersensitivity reaction. ▪ Obtain baseline CBC with differential and platelet count and SCr.

Patient Education: Promptly report S/S of a hypersensitivity reaction (e.g., rash, hives, wheezing, shortness of breath). ▪ Promptly report diarrhea or bloody stools that occur during treatment or up to several months after an antibiotic has been discontinued; may indicate CDAD and require treatment.

Maternal/Child: Category B: safety for use during pregnancy and breast-feeding not established; use only if clearly needed. ▪ Safety and effectiveness for use in pediatric patients not established.

Elderly: No specific problems documented. Efficacy and safety appear similar to that seen in younger patients. Consider age-related renal impairment; see Dose Adjustments.

DRUG/LAB INTERACTIONS
No clinical drug-drug interaction studies have been conducted. There is minimal potential for drug-drug interactions between ceftaroline and CYP450 substrates, inhibitors, or inducers; drugs known to undergo active renal secretion; and drugs that may alter renal blood flow.

SIDE EFFECTS
The most common side effects were diarrhea, nausea, and rash. Hypersensitivity reactions were the most frequently reported serious side effects leading to discontinuation of therapy. Other less frequently reported side effects included constipation, hypokalemia, increased transaminases (ALT, AST), phlebitis, and vomiting. Several other side effects were reported in less than 2% of the population studied.

ANTIDOTE
Notify physician of any side effects. Discontinue the drug if indicated. Treat hypersensitivity reactions as indicated (e.g., diphenhydramine [Benadryl], epinephrine [Adrenolin], albuterol [Ventolin]) and resuscitate as necessary. Discontinue ceftaroline for suspected drug-induced hemolytic anemia and initiate supportive therapy as indicated (e.g., transfusion). Mild cases of CDAD may respond to discontinuation of ceftaroline. Treat CDAD with fluids, electrolytes, protein supplements, and oral vancomycin (Vancocin) or metronidazole (Flagyl) as indicated. In severe cases, surgical evaluation may be indicated. Ceftaroline is removed by hemodialysis.

CEFTAZIDIME
(sef-**TAY**-zih-deem)

Fortaz, Tazicef

Antibacterial
(cephalosporin)

pH 5 to 8

USUAL DOSE

Range is from 250 mg to 2 Gm every 8 to 12 hours. Dosage based on severity of disease, condition of the patient, and susceptibility of the causative organism.

Uncomplicated GU infections: 250 mg every 12 hours.

Complicated GU infections: 500 mg every 8 to 12 hours.

Uncomplicated pneumonia and skin and skin structure infections: 500 mg to 1 Gm every 8 hours.

Bone and joint infections: 2 Gm every 12 hours.

Severe or life-threatening infections (especially in immunocompromised patients), meningitis, serious gynecologic and intra-abdominal infections: 2 Gm every 8 hours.

Pseudomonal lung infections in cystic fibrosis patients (must have normal renal function): 30 to 50 mg/kg of body weight every 8 hours. Do not exceed 6 Gm/24 hr.

Melioidosis (unlabeled): 40 mg/kg every 8 hours.

PEDIATRIC DOSE

Use sodium carbonate formulation (Fortaz, Tazicef) only for infants and children under 12 years. Components of other formulations may be harmful. Reserve higher doses for immunocompromised pediatric patients or those with cystic fibrosis or meningitis. Do not exceed 6 Gm/24 hr.

Pediatric patients 1 month to 12 years of age: 30 to 50 mg/kg of body weight every 8 hours.

NEONATAL DOSE

Use sodium carbonate formulation only (Fortaz, Tazicef); components of other formulations may be harmful.

Neonates up to 4 weeks of age: 30 mg/kg every 12 hours.

The American Academy of Pediatrics suggests the following doses:

Less than 1 week of age weighing 2 kg or less: 50 mg/kg every 12 hours.

Less than 1 week of age weighing more than 2 kg: 50 mg/kg every 8 or 12 hours.

Neonates from 1 to 4 weeks of age: 50 mg/kg every 8 hours.

DOSE ADJUSTMENTS

Reduced dose or extended intervals may be indicated in the elderly; consider age-related impaired organ function, nutritional status, and concomitant disease or drug therapy. ■ In impaired renal function, the initial dose should be as above, but all remaining doses should be based on CrCl according to the following chart. If the normal dose would be lower than the doses in the chart, use the lower dose. Adjustment for pediatric patients is similar to adults; consider body surface or lean body mass and reduce dosing frequency.

Ceftazidime Maintenance Dose in Impaired Renal Function		
Creatinine Clearance (mL/min)	Dose	Frequency
31-50 mL/min	1 Gm	q 12 hr
16-30 mL/min	1 Gm	q 24 hr
6-15 mL/min	500 mg	q 24 hr
<5 mL/min	500 mg	q 48 hr
Hemodialysis patients	1 Gm	After each dialysis session
Peritoneal dialysis patients	500 mg	q 24 hr

In patients with impaired renal function who have severe infection (normally requiring a 6-Gm/24 hr dose), the dose in the previous chart may be increased by 50% or the dosing frequency may be increased. In patients undergoing hemodialysis, give a loading dose of 1 Gm followed by 1 Gm after each dialysis. ▪ In peritoneal dialysis patients (CAPD), give a loading dose of 1 Gm followed by 500 mg every 24 hours. ▪ Dose reduction not required in impaired hepatic function.

DILUTION

IV injection: Reconstitute 0.5 Gm with 5.3 mL of SW. To obtain a dose of 500 mg, withdraw 5 mL from vial. Reconstitute 1 Gm or more with 10 mL of SW for injection. Shake well. Dilution generates CO_2. Invert vial and completely depress plunger of syringe. Insert needle through stopper and keep it within the solution. Expel bubbles from solution in syringe before injection.

Intermittent IV: A single dose may be further diluted in 50 to 100 mL of D5W, NS, or other **compatible** infusion solutions for injection (see literature or chart on inside back cover). Also available premixed, in infusion packs, in piggyback vials, and in ADD-Vantage vials for use with ADD-Vantage infusion containers.

Storage: Store unopened vials in carton at CRT. Protect from light. Administer within 12 hours of preparation if stored at CRT, or refrigerate for up to 3 days. May be frozen for up to 3 months after initial dilution; thaw at room temperature (see instructions); do not refreeze. Will be light yellow to amber in color depending on concentration and diluent. Premixed infusion packs, piggyback vials, and ADD-Vantage vials have different storage requirements; consult prescribing information.

COMPATIBILITY   (Underline Indicates Conflicting Compatibility Information)

Consider any drug NOT listed as compatible to be INCOMPATIBLE until consulting a pharmacist; specific conditions may apply.

May be used concomitantly with aminoglycosides (e.g., amikacin [Amikin], gentamicin, and vancomycin), but these drugs must never be mixed in the same infusion (mutual inactivation). If given concurrently, administer at separate sites and flush IV line before and after administration. Manufacturer recommends temporarily discontinuing other solutions infusing at the same site during intermittent infusion and states, "Do not add supplementary medications to premixed plastic IV containers."

One source suggests the following **compatibilities:**

Additive: Clindamycin (Cleocin), fluconazole (Diflucan), linezolid (Zyvox), metronidazole (Flagyl IV).

Y-site: Acyclovir (Zovirax), allopurinol (Aloprim), amifostine (Ethyol), aminophylline, anidulafungin (Eraxis), aztreonam (Azactam), bivalirudin (Angiomax), ciprofloxacin (Cipro IV), cisatracurium (Nimbex), daptomycin (Cubicin), dexmedetomidine (Precedex), diltiazem (Cardizem), dobutamine, docetaxel (Taxotere), dopamine, doxapram (Dopram), enalaprilat (Vasotec IV), epinephrine (Adrenalin), esmolol (Brevibloc), etoposide phosphate (Etopophos), famotidine (Pepcid IV), fenoldopam (Corlopam), filgrastim (Neupogen), fluconazole (Diflucan), fludarabine (Fludara), foscarnet (Foscavir), furosemide (Lasix), gallium nitrate (Ganite), gemcitabine (Gemzar), granisetron (Kytril), heparin, hetastarch in electrolytes (Hextend), hydromorphone (Dilaudid), insulin (regular), ketamine (Ketalar), labetalol (Trandate), linezolid (Zyvox), melphalan (Alkeran), meperidine (Demerol), methylprednisolone (Solu-Medrol), milrinone (Primacor), morphine, nicardipine (Cardene IV), ondansetron (Zofran), paclitaxel (Taxol), propofol (Diprivan), ranitidine (Zantac), remifentanil (Ultiva), sargramostim (Leukine), sufentanil (Sufenta), tacrolimus (Prograf), teniposide (Vumon), theophylline, thiotepa, tigecycline (Tygacil), valproate (Depacon), vancomycin, vinorelbine (Navelbine), zidovudine (AZT, Retrovir).

RATE OF ADMINISTRATION

See Compatibility. May be given through Y-tube or three-way stopcock of infusion set.

IV injection: A single dose equally distributed over 3 to 5 minutes.

Intermittent IV: A single dose over 30 minutes.

ACTIONS

A broad-spectrum, third-generation cephalosporin antibiotic. Bactericidal to selected gram-negative, gram-positive, and anaerobic organisms. Effective against many otherwise resistant organisms, including *Pseudomonas aeruginosa*. Inhibits bacterial cell wall synthesis. Peak serum levels achieved by end of infusion. Therapeutic levels distributed into many body fluids and tissues including CSF and aqueous humor. Half-life is 1.9 hours. Excreted unchanged in the urine. Crosses placental barrier. Secreted in breast milk.

INDICATIONS AND USES

Treatment of serious lower respiratory tract, urinary tract, skin and skin structure, bone and joint, gynecologic, intra-abdominal, CNS infections (including meningitis), and bacterial septicemia. Most effective against specific organisms (see literature).

Unlabeled uses: Treatment of melioidosis; empiric treatment of febrile neutropenia.

CONTRAINDICATIONS

Previous hypersensitivity reaction to cephalosporins; see Precautions.

PRECAUTIONS

Hypersensitivity reactions, including fatalities, have been reported and include reports of individuals with a history of penicillin hypersensitivity or sensitivity to multiple allergens experiencing severe reactions when treated with cephalosporins. Check history of previous hypersensitivity reactions to penicillins, cephalosporins, or other allergens. Actual incidence of cross-allergenicity not established but may be more common with first-generation cephalosporins. ▪ Specific sensitivity studies indicated to determine susceptibility of causative organism to ceftazidime. ▪ To reduce the development of drug-resistant bacteria and maintain its effectiveness, ceftazidime should be used to treat or prevent only those infections proven or strongly suspected to be caused by bacteria. ▪ Continue for at least 2 days after all symptoms of infection subside. ▪ Use with caution in patients with renal impairment. Elevated levels of ceftazidime in these patients can lead to asterixis, coma, encephalopathy, myoclonia, neuromuscular excitability, and seizures; see Dose Adjustments. ▪ May be associated with a fall in prothrombin activity. Patients at risk include those with renal or hepatic impairment, those with poor nutritional status, those receiving a protracted course of antimicrobial therapy, and/or those previously stabilized on anticoagulant therapy; see Monitor. ▪ Avoid prolonged use of drug; superinfection caused by overgrowth of nonsusceptible organisms may result. ▪ Use caution in patients with allergies or a history of GI disease (especially colitis). ▪ *Clostridium difficile*–associated diarrhea (CDAD) has been reported. May range from mild diarrhea to fatal colitis. Consider in patients who present with diarrhea during or after treatment with ceftazidime.

Monitor: Watch for early symptoms of a hypersensitivity reaction. ▪ May cause thrombophlebitis. Use small needles and large veins, and rotate infusion sites. ▪ Observe for electrolyte imbalance and cardiac irregularities. Contains 2.3 mEq of sodium/Gm. Ceptaz does not contain sodium. ▪ Monitor PT and administer vitamin K as indicated; see Precautions. ▪ See Drug/Lab Interactions; additional monitoring may be indicated (e.g., renal function, drug serum levels, PT).

Patient Education: Report promptly any bleeding or bruising or symptoms of allergy (e.g., difficulty breathing, hives, itching, rash). ▪ Promptly report diarrhea or bloody stools that occur during treatment or up to several months after an antibiotic has been discontinued; may indicate CDAD and require treatment.

Maternal/Child: Category B: safety for use during pregnancy and breast-feeding not established. No problems documented. ▪ Immature renal function of infants and small children will increase blood levels of all cephalosporins. ▪ Only specific solutions can be used in pediatric patients.

Elderly: No specific problems documented. ▪ See Usual Dose and Dose Adjustments.

DRUG/LAB INTERACTIONS

Risk of nephrotoxicity may be increased with **aminoglycosides and other nephrotoxic agents** (e.g., loop diuretics such as furosemide [Lasix]). ▪ **Probenecid** does not increase blood levels as it does with other cephalosporins. ▪ May be antagonized by **bacteriostatic antibiotics** (e.g., chloramphenicol, erythromycin, tetracyclines); may interfere with bactericidal action. ▪ Large amounts of **cephalosporins and/or salicylates** may induce hypoprothrombinemia (deficiency of prothrombin [Factor II]). The addition of **agents that affect platelet aggregation and/or may have GI ulcerative potential** (e.g., NSAIDs [ibuprofen (Advil, Motrin), naproxen (Aleve, Naprosyn)] or sulfinpyrazone [Anturane]) may increase risk of hemorrhage. ▪ May reduce the effectiveness of **oral estrogen/progesterone contraceptives.** ▪ False-positive **Coombs' test.** ▪ May have a false-positive reaction for **urine glucose** except with enzyme-based tests (e.g., Chemstix). ▪ See Compatibility and Side Effects.

SIDE EFFECTS

Full scope of hypersensitivity reactions, including anaphylaxis and cardiopulmonary arrest. Aplastic anemia; burning, discomfort, and pain at injection site; CDAD; colitis; diarrhea; dizziness; elevated alkaline phosphatase, AST, ALT, GGT, and BUN; erythema multiforme; jaundice; nausea and vomiting; prolonged PT; renal impairment; seizures (large doses); Stevens-Johnson syndrome; toxic nephropathy; toxic epidermal necrolysis; urticaria. Hypoprothrombinemia (rare) and hemolytic anemia may occur. Serum sickness–like reactions have occurred (e.g., arthralgia, fever, polyarthritis, skin rashes), usually after a second course of therapy. Generally resolve after cephalosporins are discontinued.

Overdose: Asterixis, coma, encephalopathy, neuromuscular excitability, and seizures may occur in patients with renal impairment; see Precautions.

Post-Marketing: Hemorrhage, hyperbilirubinemia, jaundice, toxic nephropathy.

ANTIDOTE

Notify physician of any side effects. Discontinue the drug if indicated. Treat hypersensitivity reaction as indicated and resuscitate as necessary. Mild cases of CDAD may respond to discontinuation of ceftazidime. Treat CDAD with fluids, electrolytes, protein supplements, and oral vancomycin (Vancocin) or metronidazole (Flagyl) as indicated. In severe cases, surgical evaluation may be indicated. Hemodialysis may be useful in overdose. Antihistamines and corticosteroids may be indicated to manage symptoms of serum sickness.

CEFTRIAXONE SODIUM

(sef-try-**AX**-ohn **SO**-dee-um)

Rocephin

Antibacterial (cephalosporin)

pH 6.6 to 6.7

USUAL DOSE

Adults and pediatric patients over 12 years: 1 to 2 Gm/24 hr. May be given as a single dose every 24 hours or equally divided into 2 doses and given every 12 hours. For infections caused by *Staphylococcus aureus* (MSSA), recommended daily dose is 2 to 4 Gm. Do not exceed a total dose of 4 Gm/24 hr.

Meningitis: 2 Gm every 12 hours.

Disseminated gonococcal infections (unlabeled): 1 Gm daily. Continue for 24 to 48 hours after improvement. Transfer to oral dosing and continue for a minimum of 7 days.

Perioperative prophylaxis: 1 Gm IV 30 minutes to 2 hours before incision. Used primarily in patients undergoing coronary artery bypass surgery and in contaminated or potentially contaminated surgeries.

Lyme diseases (unlabeled): 2 Gm daily for 14 days (range 14 to 28 days).

PEDIATRIC DOSE

Pediatric patients 1 month to 12 years of age: See Maternal/Child.

Skin and soft tissue and other serious infections (other than meningitis): 50 to 75 mg/kg of body weight/24 hr as a single dose or in equally divided doses every 12 hours (25 to 37.5 mg/kg every 12 hours). Do not exceed a total dose of 2 Gm/24 hr.

Bacterial meningitis: Begin with a loading dose of 100 mg/kg on day 1 (do not exceed a total dose of 4 Gm), follow with 100 mg/kg/day (not to exceed 4 Gm) as a single dose or in equally divided doses every 12 hours (50 mg/kg every 12 hours). An alternate regimen begins with an 80- to 100-mg/kg loading dose (not over 4 Gm); follow with 80 mg/kg at 12-hour intervals for 2 doses, then 80 to 100 mg/kg every 24 hours. Continue for 7 to 14 days depending on the causative organism. Single daily doses must be given at the same time each day to maintain adequate CSF concentrations.

Lyme diseases (unlabeled): 50 to 100 mg/kg/day for 14 days (range 10 to 28 days). Maximum dose is 2 Gm.

NEONATAL DOSE

Hyperbilirubinemic neonates, especially premature neonates, should not receive ceftriaxone; see Contraindications and Maternal/Child.

Neonatal doses may also be given IM. See Maternal/Child.

The American Academy of Pediatrics (AAP) recommends the following:

Less than 7 days of age: 50 mg/kg/day as a single daily dose.

1 to 4 weeks of age and weighing less than 2 kg: 50 mg/kg day.

1 to 4 weeks of age and weighing more than 2 kg: 50 to 75 mg/kg/day.

Bacterial meningitis: Same as Pediatric Dose.

Infants born to mothers with gonococcal infections: 25 to 50 mg/kg one time only (do not exceed 125 mg).

DOSE ADJUSTMENTS

In adults with both hepatic and renal impairment, dose should not exceed 2 Gm daily unless serum concentrations of ceftriaxone are monitored. ▪ Dose adjustment not required for elderly patients with doses up to 2 Gm/day. ▪ See Drug/Lab Interactions.

DILUTION

Initially reconstitute each 250 mg with 2.4 mL (500 mg with 4.8 mL) of SW, NS, D5W, D10W, D5NS, or D5/½NS for injection (see chart on inside back cover or literature for additional diluents). Each mL will contain 100 mg. A single dose must be further diluted with 50 to 100 mL of the same solution and be given as an intermittent infusion. Shake well. Concentrations of 10 mg/mL to 40 mg/mL are recommended for intermittent infusion. Should not be reconstituted, further diluted, or simultaneously administered with calcium-containing IV solutions. A precipitate can form; see Compatibility. Available premixed and in ADD-Vantage vials for use with ADD-Vantage infusion containers.

Storage: Store vials at RT 25° C (77° F) or below and protect from light. Stable at RT for at least 24 hours in stated solutions or selected solutions up to 10 days if refrigerated. D5NS and D5/½NS should not be refrigerated. Stability and color (light yellow to amber) depend on concentration and diluent. Thaw frozen solutions at room temperature before use. Discard unused portions; do not refreeze.

COMPATIBILITY   (Underline Indicates Conflicting Compatibility Information)

Consider any drug NOT listed as compatible to be INCOMPATIBLE until consulting a pharmacist; specific conditions may apply.

Manufacturer states, "Do not use diluents containing calcium, such as Ringer's solution or Hartmann's solution, to reconstitute or further dilute ceftriaxone. Particulate formation can result. Ceftriaxone and calcium-containing solutions, including continuous calcium-containing infusions such as parenteral nutrition, should not be mixed or coadministered simultaneously via a **Y-site.**" However, in patients other than neonates, ceftriaxone and calcium-containing solutions may be administered sequentially if the infusion lines are thoroughly flushed between infusions with a **compatible** fluid; see Contraindications and Precautions. Manufacturer lists as **compatible** with metronidazole (Flagyl IV) as an additive in NS or D5W if the concentration of metronidazole does not exceed 5 to 7.5 mg/mL with ceftriaxone 10 mg/mL as an admixture. Mixture is stable at RT for 24 hours. Precipitation will occur if refrigerated or if concentration of metronidazole exceeds 8 mg/mL. No studies have been done with Flagyl IV RTU. Manufacturer lists aminoglycosides (e.g., gentamicin), amsacrine (Amsidyl), fluconazole (Diflucan), and vancomycin as **incompatible** and states, "May be given sequentially with thorough flushing of the IV line with **compatible** solution between the administrations."

One source suggests the following **compatibilities:**

Additive: Manufacturer lists metronidazole (Flagyl IV) not to exceed 5 to 7.5 mg/mL with ceftriaxone 10 mg/mL admixed in D5W or NS. Do not refrigerate; a precipitate will form.

Y-site: Acyclovir (Zovirax), allopurinol (Aloprim), amifostine (Ethyol), amiodarone (Nexterone), anidulafungin (Eraxis), aztreonam (Azactam), bivalirudin (Angiomax), cisatracurium (Nimbex), daptomycin (Cubicin), dexmedetomidine (Precedex), diltiazem (Cardizem), docetaxel (Taxotere), doxorubicin liposomal (Doxil), drotrecogin alfa (Xigris), etoposide phosphate (Etopophos), famotidine (Pepcid IV), fenoldopam (Corlopam), fludarabine (Fludara), foscarnet (Foscavir), gallium nitrate (Ganite), gemcitabine (Gemzar), granisetron (Kytril), heparin, linezolid (Zyvox), melphalan (Alkeran), meperidine (Demerol), methotrexate, morphine, paclitaxel (Taxol), pantoprazole (Protonix IV), pemetrexed (Alimta), propofol (Diprivan), remifentanil (Ultiva), sargramostim (Leukine), sodium bicarbonate, tacrolimus (Prograf), teniposide (Vumon), theophylline, thiotepa, tigecycline (Tygacil), vancomycin, warfarin (Coumadin), zidovudine (AZT, Retrovir).

RATE OF ADMINISTRATION

Intermittent IV: A single dose over 30 minutes.

ACTIONS

A broad-spectrum, third-generation cephalosporin antibiotic. Bactericidal to selected gram-negative, gram-positive, and anaerobic organisms. Effective against many otherwise resistant organisms. Inhibits bacterial cell wall synthesis. Therapeutic concentrations achieved in many body fluids and tissues, including CSF. Highly protein bound. Has a long half-life (range is 5.8 to 8.7 hours); once-a-day dosing sufficient. Peak serum levels achieved by end of infusion. Excreted through urine, bile, and feces. Crosses placental barrier. Secreted in breast milk.

INDICATIONS AND USES

Treatment of serious lower respiratory tract, urinary tract, skin and skin structure, bone and joint, and intra-abdominal infections. ▪ Bacterial septicemia. ▪ Meningitis. ▪ Most effective against specific organisms (see literature). ▪ Perioperative prophylaxis. ▪ Given IM for additional indications (e.g., acute bacterial otitis, CDC recommendations for gonorrhea, pelvic inflammatory disease [considered treatment of choice]).

Unlabeled uses: Treatment of Lyme disease and numerous other infections. ■ Disseminated gonococcal infections. ■ IM for CDC recommendation for chancroid.

CONTRAINDICATIONS

Previous hypersensitivity reaction to cephalosporins; see Precautions. ■ Hyperbilirubinemic neonates (newborn to 28 days), especially premature neonates; see Maternal/Child. ■ Coadministration with calcium-containing IV solutions, including parenteral nutrition, in infants up to 28 days of age is contraindicated because of the risk of precipitation of ceftriaxone-calcium salt. Cases of fatal reactions with precipitates in lungs and kidneys have been reported in neonates. In some cases, the infusion lines and the times of administration of the ceftriaxone and calcium-containing solution differed; see Precautions and Compatibility.

PRECAUTIONS

Hypersensitivity reactions, including fatalities, have been reported and include reports of individuals with no known hypersensitivity or previous exposure, as well as those with a history of penicillin hypersensitivity or sensitivity to multiple allergens, experiencing severe reactions when treated with cephalosporins. Check history of previous hypersensitivity reactions to penicillins, cephalosporins, or other allergens. Actual incidence of cross-allergenicity not established but may be more common with first-generation cephalosporins. ■ Sensitivity studies are indicated to determine susceptibility of the causative organism to ceftriaxone. ■ To reduce the development of drug-resistant bacteria and maintain its effectiveness, ceftriaxone should be used to treat or prevent only those infections proven or strongly suspected to be caused by bacteria. ■ Continue for at least 2 to 3 days after all symptoms of infection subside. Usual course of therapy 4 to 14 days; *S. pyogenes* requires treatment for 10 days. In serious invasive infection, continue for 5 to 7 days after cultures are negative. ■ Should not be reconstituted, further diluted, or simultaneously administered with calcium-containing IV solutions. A precipitate can form; see Compatibility. There are no data on potential interactions between ceftriaxone and oral calcium-containing products or between IM ceftriaxone and oral or IV calcium-containing products. ■ May be associated with a fall in prothrombin activity. Patients at risk include those with renal or hepatic impairment, those with poor nutritional status, those receiving a protracted course of antimicrobial therapy, and/or those previously stabilized on anticoagulant therapy; see Monitor. ■ Avoid prolonged use of drug; superinfection caused by overgrowth of nonsusceptible organisms may result. ■ Use caution in patients with both impaired renal and hepatic function, allergies, or a history of GI disease (especially colitis). ■ *Clostridium difficile*–associated diarrhea (CDAD) has been reported. May range from mild diarrhea to fatal colitis. Consider in patients who present with diarrhea during or after treatment with ceftriaxone. ■ Immune-mediated hemolytic anemia has been reported in both adults and pediatric patients. Fatalities have occurred. ■ Prolonged use may lead to gallbladder disease. Sonographic abnormalities in the gallbladder of patients treated with ceftriaxone have been reported. These abnormalities have been determined to be predominantly a ceftriaxone-calcium salt and may be misinterpreted as gallstones. The abnormalities appear to be transient and reversible with the discontinuation of ceftriaxone. ■ Pancreatitis, possibly secondary to biliary obstruction, has been reported.

Monitor: Watch for early symptoms of a hypersensitivity reaction. ▪ Single daily dose reduces incidence of thrombophlebitis. Use of small needles, large veins, and rotation of infusion sites is preferred. ▪ Monitor PT and administer vitamin K as indicated (e.g., 10 mg weekly). ▪ Monitor CBC for development of cephalosporin-induced anemia. ▪ Observe for electrolyte imbalance and cardiac irregularities. Contains 3.6 mEq sodium per Gm. ▪ See Dose Adjustments and Drug/Lab Interactions; additional monitoring may be indicated (e.g., renal function, drug serum levels, PT).

Patient Education: Report promptly any bleeding or bruising or symptoms of allergy (e.g., difficulty breathing, hives, itching, rash). ▪ Promptly report diarrhea or bloody stools that occur during treatment or up to several months after an antibiotic has been discontinued; may indicate CDAD and require treatment.

Maternal/Child: Category B: safety for use during pregnancy and breastfeeding not established. No problems documented. ▪ Immature renal function of infants and small children will increase blood levels of all cephalosporins. ▪ Use is contraindicated in hyperbilirubinemic neonates less than 28 days of age (especially premature neonates). Ceftriaxone can displace bilirubin from its binding sites on albumin. Risk of bilirubin encephalopathy exists; see Contraindications and Precautions.

Elderly: Response similar to other age-groups; however, greater sensitivity of the elderly cannot be ruled out; see Dose Adjustments.

DRUG/LAB INTERACTIONS

Risk of nephrotoxicity may be increased with **aminoglycosides and other nephrotoxic agents** (e.g., loop diuretics such as furosemide [Lasix]). ▪ **Probenecid** does not increase blood levels as it does with other cephalosporins. ▪ May be antagonized by **bacteriostatic antibiotics** (e.g., chloramphenicol, erythromycin, tetracyclines); may interfere with bactericidal action. ▪ Large amounts of **cephalosporins and/or salicylates** may induce hypoprothrombinemia (deficiency of prothrombin [Factor II]). The addition of **agents that affect platelet aggregation and/or may have GI ulcerative potential** (e.g., NSAIDs [ibuprofen (Advil, Motrin), naproxen (Aleve, Naprosyn)] or sulfinpyrazone [Anturane]) may increase risk of hemorrhage. ▪ False-positive **Coombs' test**. ▪ May produce false-positive reaction for **urine glucose** except with enzyme-based tests (e.g., Chemstix). ▪ See Compatibility and Side Effects.

SIDE EFFECTS

Full scope of hypersensitivity reactions, including anaphylaxis with fatal outcome, have been reported. Agranulocytosis, "biliary sludge" or pseudolithiasis; allergic pneumonitis; bleeding episodes; burning, discomfort, and pain at injection site; casts in urine; CDAD; colitis; diarrhea; dizziness; dysgeusia; eosinophilia; elevated alkaline phosphatase, bilirubin, BUN, creatinine, AST, and ALT; headache; leukopenia; nausea and vomiting; nephrolithiasis; pancreatitis; prolonged PT; renal precipitations; seizures; thrombophlebitis. Other hematologic reactions (e.g., anemia, hemolytic anemia, hypoprothrombinemia [rare], lymphopenia, neutropenia, thrombocytopenia) may occur. Serum sickness–like reactions have occurred (e.g., arthralgia, fever, polyarthritis, skin rashes), usually after a second course of therapy. Generally resolve after cephalosporins are discontinued.

Post-Marketing: Dermatologic reactions (e.g., allergic dermatitis, exanthema, and isolated cases of Stevens-Johnson syndrome and toxic epidermal necrolysis), oliguria, stomatitis. Fatal cases of ceftriaxone-calcium precipitates in lungs and kidneys of neonates have been reported; see Contraindications, Precautions, and Maternal/Child.

ANTIDOTE

Notify physician of any side effects. Discontinue the drug if indicated (e.g., CDAD, hypersensitivity reactions, seizures, S/S of gallbladder disease). Treat hypersensitivity reactions as indicated and resuscitate as necessary. Mild cases of CDAD may respond to discontinuation of ceftriaxone. Treat CDAD with fluids, electrolytes, protein supplements, and oral vancomycin (Vancocin) or metronidazole (Flagyl) as indicated. In severe cases, surgical evaluation may be indicated. Vitamin K may be useful in bleeding episodes, or drug may need to be discontinued. Not removed by hemodialysis. Antihistamines and corticosteroids may be indicated to manage symptoms of serum sickness.

CEFUROXIME SODIUM
(sef-your-**OX**-eem **SO**-dee-um)

Zinacef

**Antibacterial
(cephalosporin)**

pH 5 to 8.5

USUAL DOSE

Dependent on seriousness of infection. Usual dose is 750 mg to 1.5 Gm every 8 hours for 5 to 10 days. Maximum dose is 3 Gm every 8 hours. **Uncomplicated infections (gonococcal, pneumonia, skin and soft tissue, urinary tract):** 750 mg every 8 hours.

Severe or complicated infections and bone and joint infections: 1.5 Gm every 8 hours.

Life-threatening or infections due to less susceptible organisms: 1.5 Gm every 6 hours.

Bacterial meningitis: 3 Gm every 8 hours; see Precautions.

Perioperative prophylaxis: 1.5 Gm IV 30 minutes to 1 hour before incision; then 750 mg every 8 hours during prolonged procedures. 1.5 Gm at induction of anesthesia and every 12 hours to total dose of 6 Gm in open heart surgery.

PEDIATRIC DOSE

Do not exceed adult dose.

Pediatric patients 3 months of age or older: 50 to 100 mg/kg/day in equally divided doses every 6 to 8 hours (12.5 to 25 mg/kg every 6 hours or 16.7 to 33.3 mg/kg every 8 hours). Higher-end dosing used for more serious infections.

Bone and joint infections: 50 mg/kg every 8 hours. Up to 1.5 Gm/dose has been given.

Bacterial meningitis: 200 to 240 mg/kg/day in equally divided doses every 6 to 8 hours (50 to 60 mg/kg every 6 hours or 66.7 to 80 mg/kg every 8 hours); see Precautions.

NEONATAL DOSE

Neonatal doses are unlabeled; see Maternal/Child.

Infants under 3 months of age: One source recommends 10 to 30 mg/kg every 12 hours.

Bacterial meningitis: 100 mg/kg/day in equally divided doses every 8 or 12 hours (33.3 mg/kg every 8 hours or 50 mg/kg every 12 hours); see Precautions.

DOSE ADJUSTMENTS

Reduced doses or extended intervals may be indicated in the elderly; consider age-related impaired organ function, nutritional status, and concomitant disease or drug therapy.

Adults: Reduce total daily dose if renal function impaired according to the following chart. ■ See Drug/Lab Interactions.

Cefuroxime Dose Guidelines in Impaired Renal Function in Adults		
Creatinine Clearance (mL/min)	Dose	Frequency
>20 mL/min	750 mg-1.5 Gm	q 8 hr
10-20 mL/min	750 mg	q 12 hr
<10 mL/min	750 mg	q 24 hr
Hemodialysis patients	An additional dose of 750 mg at end of each dialysis session	

Pediatric patients: In pediatric patients with impaired renal function, reduce frequency as indicated in the chart for adults.

DILUTION

Reconstitute 750 mg with 8.3 mL SW for injection. Reconstitute 1.5 Gm with 16 mL SWI. Shake well. May be further diluted to 50 or 100 mL with D5W, NS, or other **compatible** infusion solution (see chart on inside back cover or literature) and given as an intermittent infusion, or added to 500 to 1,000 mL and given as a continuous infusion. Available premixed, in piggyback vials, infusion packs, and in ADD-Vantage vials for use with ADD-Vantage infusion containers.

Storage: In dry state, store between 15° and 30° C (59° to 86° F); protect from light. Reconstituted vials are stable for 24 hours at CRT or 48 hours if refrigerated. Diluted solutions may be stable for up to 7 days if refrigerated.

COMPATIBILITY   (Underline Indicates Conflicting Compatibility Information)

Consider any drug NOT listed as compatible to be INCOMPATIBLE until consulting a pharmacist; specific conditions may apply.

May be used concomitantly with aminoglycosides (e.g., amikacin [Amikin], gentamicin), but these drugs must never be mixed in the same infusion (mutual inactivation). If given concurrently, administer at separate sites. Manufacturer recommends temporarily discontinuing other solutions infusing at the same site during intermittent infusion and lists sodium bicarbonate **incompatible** as a diluent.

Sources suggest the following **compatibilities:**

Additive: Manufacturer lists heparin (10 and 50 units/mL in NS) and potassium chloride (10 and 40 mEq/L in NS). Other sources list clindamycin (Cleocin), furosemide (Lasix), metronidazole (Flagyl IV), midazolam (Versed).

Y-site: Acyclovir (Zovirax), allopurinol (Aloprim), amifostine (Ethyol), amiodarone (Nexterone), anidulafungin (Eraxis), atracurium (Tracrium), aztreonam (Azactam), bivalirudin (Angiomax), cisatracurium (Nimbex), cyclophosphamide (Cytoxan), dexmedetomidine (Precedex), diltiazem (Cardizem), docetaxel (Taxotere), etoposide phosphate (Etopophos), famotidine (Pepcid IV), fenoldopam (Corlopam), fludarabine (Fludara), foscarnet (Foscavir), gemcitabine (Gemzar), granisetron (Kytril), hetastarch in electrolytes (Hextend), hydromorphone (Dilaudid), linezolid (Zyvox), melphalan (Alkeran), meperidine (Demerol), milrinone (Primacor), morphine, ondansetron (Zofran), pancuronium, pemetrexed (Alimta), propofol (Diprivan), remifentanil (Ultiva), sargramostim (Leukine), tacrolimus (Prograf), teniposide (Vumon), thiotepa, vancomycin, vecuronium.

RATE OF ADMINISTRATION

See Compatibility. Injection or intermittent infusion may be given through Y-tube or three-way stopcock of infusion set.

IV injection: A single dose equally distributed over 3 to 5 minutes.

Intermittent IV: A single dose over 30 minutes.

Continuous infusion: 500 to 1,000 mL over 6 to 24 hours, depending on total dose and concentration.

ACTIONS

A broad-spectrum, second-generation cephalosporin antibiotic. Bactericidal to selected gram-negative, gram-positive, and anaerobic organisms. Effective against many otherwise resistant organisms. Inhibits bacterial cell wall synthesis. Peak serum levels achieved by end of infusion. Widely distributed. Therapeutic concentrations found in pleural fluid, joint fluid, bile, sputum, bone, aqueous humor, and CSF. Half-life is 80 minutes. Excreted in the urine. Crosses placental barrier. Secreted in breast milk.

INDICATIONS AND USES

Treatment of serious lower respiratory tract, urinary tract, bone and joint, skin and skin structure infections, septicemia, and meningitis. Most effective against specific organisms and when mixed organisms are present (see literature). ■ Perioperative prophylaxis. ■ Used IM to treat gonorrhea.

CONTRAINDICATIONS

Previous hypersensitivity reaction to cephalosporins; see Precautions.

PRECAUTIONS

Hypersensitivity reactions, including fatalities, have been reported and include reports of individuals with a history of penicillin hypersensitivity or sensitivity to multiple allergens experiencing severe reactions when treated with cephalosporins. Check history of previous hypersensitivity reactions to penicillins, cephalosporins, or other allergens. Actual incidence of cross-allergenicity not established but may be more common with first-generation cephalosporins. ■ Sensitivity studies indicated to determine susceptibility of the causative organism to cefuroxime. ■ To reduce the development of drug-resistant bacteria and maintain its effectiveness, cefuroxime should be used to treat or prevent only those infections proven or strongly suspected to be caused by bacteria. ■ Continue for at least 2 to 3 days after all symptoms of infection subside. ■ Continue treatment of *Streptococcus pyogenes* infections for a minimum of 10 days to decrease the risk of rheumatic fever or glomerulonephritis. ■ Avoid prolonged use of drug; superinfection caused by overgrowth of nonsusceptible organisms may result. ■ Use caution in patients with impaired renal function, allergies, or a history of GI disease (especially colitis). ■ *Clostridium difficile*–associated diarrhea (CDAD) has been reported. May range from mild diarrhea to fatal colitis. Consider in patients who present with diarrhea during or after treatment with cefuroxime. ■ May be associated with a fall in prothrombin activity. Patients at risk include those with renal or hepatic impairment, patients with poor nutritional status, patients receiving a protracted course of antimicrobial therapy, and patients previously stabilized on anticoagulant therapy; see Monitor. ■ Mild to moderate hearing loss has been reported in a few pediatric patients treated for meningitis.

Monitor: Watch for early symptoms of a hypersensitivity reaction. ■ May cause thrombophlebitis. Use small needles and large veins, and rotate infusion sites. ■ Monitor renal function periodically during therapy. ■ Observe for electrolyte imbalance and cardiac irregularities. Contains

2.4 mEq sodium/Gm. ▪ Monitor PT and administer vitamin K as indicated. ▪ See Drug/Lab Interactions; additional monitoring may be indicated (e.g., renal function, drug serum levels).

Patient Education: Report promptly any bleeding or bruising or symptoms of allergy (e.g., difficulty breathing, hives, itching, rash). ▪ Promptly report diarrhea or bloody stools that occur during treatment or up to several months after an antibiotic has been discontinued; may indicate CDAD and require treatment.

Maternal/Child: Category B: safety for use during pregnancy and breast-feeding not established. No problems documented. ▪ Is used in infants under 3 months of age, but safety not established; immature renal function will increase blood levels.

Elderly: See Dose Adjustments. ▪ Response similar to other age-groups; however, greater sensitivity of the elderly cannot be ruled out.

DRUG/LAB INTERACTIONS

Risk of nephrotoxicity may be increased with **aminoglycosides and other nephrotoxic agents** (e.g., loop diuretics such as furosemide [Lasix]). ▪ **Probenecid** inhibits excretion. Reduced dose of cefuroxime may be required with concomitant use. ▪ May be antagonized by **bacteriostatic antibiotics** (e.g., chloramphenicol, erythromycin, tetracyclines); bactericidal action may be negated. ▪ Large amounts of **cephalosporins and/or salicylates** may induce hypoprothrombinemia (deficiency of prothrombin [Factor II]). The addition of **agents that affect platelet aggregation and/or may have GI ulcerative potential** (e.g., NSAIDs [ibuprofen (Advil, Motrin), naproxen (Aleve, Naprosyn)] or sulfinpyrazone [Anturane]) may increase risk of hemorrhage. ▪ May reduce effectiveness of **estrogen/progesterone oral contraceptives.** ▪ May cause a false-negative reaction in specific **blood glucose** tests (ferricyanide). ▪ False-positive reaction for **urine glucose** except with enzyme-based tests (e.g., Chemstix). ▪ False-positive **Coombs' test.** ▪ See Compatibility and Side Effects.

SIDE EFFECTS

Full scope of hypersensitivity reactions including anaphylaxis. Angioedema, CDAD, colitis, decreased hemoglobin, hematocrit, or platelet functions; diarrhea; dyspnea; elevation of AST, ALT, total bilirubin, alkaline phosphatase, LDH, and BUN (transient); eosinophilia; fever; leukopenia; local site pain; nausea; oral thrush; prolonged PT; seizures (large doses and decreased renal function); transient neutropenia; thrombocytopenia; thrombophlebitis; vaginitis; vomiting. Hypoprothrombinemia (rare) and hemolytic anemia may occur. Serum sickness–like reactions have occurred (e.g., arthralgia, fever, polyarthritis, skin rashes), usually after a second course of therapy. Generally resolve after cephalosporins are discontinued.

ANTIDOTE

Notify physician of any side effects. Discontinue the drug if indicated. Mild cases of CDAD may respond to discontinuation of drug. Treat CDAD with fluids, electrolytes, protein supplements, and oral vancomycin (Vancocin) or metronidazole (Flagyl) as indicated. In severe cases, surgical evaluation may be indicated. Treat hypersensitivity reactions and resuscitate as necessary. Hemodialysis or peritoneal dialysis may be somewhat useful in overdose. Antihistamines and corticosteroids may be indicated to manage symptoms of serum sickness.

CETUXIMAB BBW
(seh-**TUX**-ih-mab)
Erbitux

Recombinant monoclonal antibody
Antineoplastic

pH 7 to 7.4

USUAL DOSE

Premedication: To prevent or attenuate severe infusion reactions, premedicate with diphenhydramine 50 mg IV 30 to 60 minutes before each dose.

Squamous cell carcinoma of the head and neck (SCCHN) in combination with radiation therapy:

First infusion: 400 mg/M^2 as an initial loading dose 1 week **before the initiation** of a course of radiation therapy.

Subsequent infusions: 250 mg/M^2 once each week for the duration of radiation therapy (6 to 7 weeks). Complete infusion 1 hour before radiation therapy.

Squamous cell carcinoma of the head and neck as monotherapy:

First infusion: 400 mg/M^2 as an initial loading dose.

Subsequent infusions: 250 mg/M^2 once each week as a maintenance dose. Continue until disease progression or unacceptable toxicity.

Colorectal cancer in combination with irinotecan or as monotherapy:

First infusion: 400 mg/M^2 as an initial loading dose.

Subsequent infusions: 250 mg/M^2 once each week as a maintenance dose. Continue until disease progression or unacceptable toxicity.

DOSE ADJUSTMENTS

No dose adjustment required based on age, gender, race, or hepatic or renal function. ■ No dose adjustment indicated for mild to moderate skin toxicity. ■ If a mild or moderate (Grade 1 or 2) or non-serious (Grade 3 or 4) infusion reaction occurs (e.g., chills, dyspnea, fever), reduce the infusion rate by 50% for the balance of that infusion and for all further infusions. ■ Permanently discontinue cetuximab therapy if a severe (Grade 3 or 4) infusion reaction occurs. ■ If a severe acneform rash is experienced, adjust infusion schedule according to the following chart. **Dose modification is not recommended for severe radiation dermatitis.**

Cetuximab Dose Modification Guidelines for Occurrences of Severe Acneform Rash			
Severe Acneform Rash	Cetuximab	Outcome	Cetuximab Dose Modification
1st occurrence	Delay infusion 1 to 2 weeks	Improvement	Continue at 250 mg/M^2
		No improvement	Discontinue cetuximab
2nd occurrence	Delay infusion 1 to 2 weeks	Improvement	Reduce dose to 200 mg/M^2
		No improvement	Discontinue cetuximab
3rd occurrence	Delay infusion 1 to 2 weeks	Improvement	Reduce dose to 150 mg/M^2
		No improvement	Discontinue cetuximab
4th occurrence	Discontinue cetuximab		

DILUTION

Available in 100 mg/50 mL and 200 mg/100 mL vials (2 mg/mL). Multiple vials may be needed for each dose. Solution is clear and may contain small amounts of easily visible white particulates. *Do not shake or dilute.*

To administer via an infusion pump: Using a new needle, vented spike, or transfer device for each vial, transfer the desired dose of cetuximab into a sterile evacuated container or bag. Glass containers, polyolefin bags (e.g., Baxter Intravia), ethylene vinyl acetate bags (e.g., Baxter Clintec), DEHP plasticized PVC bags (e.g., Abbott Lifecare), or PVC bags are all suitable containers. See Rate of Administration.

To administer via a syringe pump: Using a new needle or new vented spike for each vial, draw up the volume of one vial at a time into a sterile syringe. Repeat process as indicated by the volume of the syringe until desired dose is in syringe(s). See Rate of Administration.

Filters: Use of a low–protein binding, 0.22-micron in-line filter is required; see Rate of Administration.

Storage: Refrigerate vials at 2° to 8° C (36° to 46° F). Do not freeze. Preparations in infusion containers are chemically and physically stable for 12 hours if refrigerated or 8 hours at CRT. Discard remaining solution in the infusion container after 8 hours at CRT. Discard any unused portion of the vial.

COMPATIBILITY

Specific information not available; however, manufacturer states, "Cetuximab should be piggybacked to the patient's infusion line." Manufacturer recommends flushing the infusion line with NS before the infusion and at the end of the infusion to ensure delivery of the entire dose.

RATE OF ADMINISTRATION

Do not administer as an IV push or bolus. Must be given as an infusion via an infusion pump or a syringe pump. Must be administered through a low–protein binding, 0.22-micron in-line filter placed as proximal to the patient as is practical and piggybacked to the patient's infusion line. Prime infusion line with cetuximab. Flush the infusion line with NS after the infusion.

To administer with an infusion pump: Attach the infusion line, including the filter, to the infusion bag. Prime with cetuximab before piggybacking to the patient's infusion line. Set desired rate of infusion.

To administer with a syringe pump: Place the syringe into the syringe driver of the pump and set the rate. Filter must be between the syringe pump and the patient. Connect the syringe pump to an infusion line (extension), including the filter; then prime the infusion line with cetuximab, piggyback to the patients' infusion line, and start the infusion. Repeat this procedure until the calculated volume has been infused.

First infusion: The initial loading dose should be infused evenly distributed over 2 hours (120 minutes). Do not exceed a rate of 5 mL/min. In patients who have mild to moderate infusion reactions, decrease the rate of administration by 50% and continue this reduced rate for all subsequent infusions. See Dose Adjustments.

Subsequent infusions: Weekly maintenance doses should be infused evenly distributed over 1 hour (60 minutes). Do not exceed a rate of 5 mL/min. In patients who have mild to moderate infusion reactions, decrease the rate of administration by 50% and continue this reduced rate for all subsequent infusions. See Dose Adjustments.

ACTIONS

An antineoplastic agent. A humanized IgG_1 monoclonal antibody produced by recombinant DNA technology. Designed to bind to the epidermal growth factor receptor (EGFR) found on the surface of both normal cells and malignant tumor cells. It interferes with the growth and survival of cancer cells by binding to tumor cells that overexpress the EGFR so that the normal (natural) EGFR cannot bind to the tumor cells and stimulate them to grow. Anti-tumor effects were not observed in normal cells or in tumor cells that did not express the EGFR. With the recommended dose regimen, cetuximab concentrations reached steady-state levels by the third weekly infusion with a mean half-life of 112 hours (range 63 to 230 hours). IgG antibodies may cross the placental barrier and may be secreted in breast milk.

INDICATIONS AND USES

Treatment of locally or regionally advanced SCCHN in combination with radiation therapy. ■ Used as a single agent for the treatment of recurrent or metastatic SCCHN in whom platinum-based chemotherapy has failed. ■ Treatment of EGFR-expressing cancer of the colon or rectum that has spread to other parts of the body (metastatic). Used in combination with irinotecan (Camptosar) in patients who are refractory to irinotecan-based chemotherapy (combination of irinotecan, leucovorin, and fluorouracil). Used as a single agent in patients who cannot tolerate irinotecan or in those who have failed treatment with both irinotecan (Camptosar) and oxaliplatin (Eloxatin) based regimens.

CONTRAINDICATIONS

Manufacturer states, "None." However, a repeat dose is contraindicated in any patient who has a severe infusion reaction (Grade 3 or 4). ■ Use with caution in patients with known hypersensitivity to murine proteins, cetuximab, or any of its components.

PRECAUTIONS

Do not administer as an IV push or bolus. Must be given as an infusion via an infusion pump or a syringe pump. ■ Should be administered by or under the direction of the physician specialist in a facility equipped to monitor the patient and respond to any medical emergency. ■ Severe infusion reactions and hypersensitivity reactions have occurred, and some have been fatal (less than 1 in 1,000). Most severe reactions occur with the first infusion and have occurred even with the use of prophylactic antihistamines. S/S of severe reactions may include hypotension, rapid onset of airway obstruction (e.g., bronchospasm, hoarseness, stridor), urticaria, and/or cardiac arrest. Some patients experienced their first infusion reaction during later infusions. ■ Risk of cardiac arrest and/or sudden death increased in patients with SCCHN treated with radiation therapy. Use with caution in combination with radiation therapy in patients with a history of arrhythmias, coronary artery disease, or congestive heart failure. ■ Pulmonary toxicity, including interstitial lung disease (ILD), has been reported. Interstitial pneumonitis with non-cardiogenic pulmonary edema resulted in the death of a patient. Use caution in patients with pre-existing fibrotic lung disease. ■ Severe dermatologic toxicities, including acneform rash, skin drying, and fissuring, and inflammatory and infectious sequelae (e.g., blepharitis [inflammation of the eyelids], cellulitis [diffuse subcutaneous inflammation of connective tissues], cheilitis [inflammation of the lip], conjunctivitis, cyst, hypertrichosis, and keratitis) are common and may be dose limiting. Complications involving *S. aureus* sepsis and abscesses requiring incision and drainage have been reported. ■ Safety for use in combination with radiation therapy and cisplatin has not been established. Death and serious cardiotoxicity have been seen in trials. ■ A protein substance, it has the potential for producing immunogenicity. However, there does not appear to be a relationship between the appearance of antibodies to cetuximab and the safety or antitumor activity of the molecule. ■ See Monitor and Antidote.

Monitor: Expression of EGFR has been detected in nearly all patients with SCCHN. Evidence of positive EGFR expression should be confirmed before initiating treatment in patients with colorectal cancers. Testing should be performed by a laboratory with demonstrated proficiency to avoid unreliable results. The DakoCytomation test kit was used during clinical studies. ■ Monitor VS frequently. ■ Observe patient closely during every infusion and for at least 1 hour after each infusion. Infusion reactions can occur at any time, even in patients who are premedicated with diphenhydramine and/or who have not had infusion reactions with previous doses; see Precautions. S/S of Grade 1 and 2 infusion reactions include chills, fever, and dyspnea. S/S of severe reactions may include hypotension, rapid onset of airway obstruction (e.g., bronchospasm, hoarseness, stridor), loss of consciousness, MI, shock, urticaria, and/or cardiac arrest. Increase observation period for patients who experience infusion reactions. ■ Monitor magnesium, calcium, and potassium periodically during therapy and for 8 weeks following completion. Electrolyte loss may occur from days to months after initiating cetuximab. Oral or parenteral electrolyte replacement may be indicated. ■ Monitor for S/S of dermatologic toxicity such as acneform rash (e.g., multiple follicular-pustular–appearing lesions on the face, upper chest, back, and extremities), skin drying, and fissuring. Dose adjustments or termination of therapy may be indicated; see Dose Adjustments and Precautions. The first onset of acneform rash may occur within the first 2 weeks, may subside when treatment is discontinued, or may persist for longer periods. Inflammatory or infectious sequelae (e.g., blepharitis, cellulitis, cheilitis, cyst) may develop and should be treated promptly. ■ Monitor for S/S of interstitial lung disease (e.g., dyspnea on exertion, nonproductive cough, inspiratory crackles on chest examination). Worsening symptoms may require interruption or discontinuation of cetuximab therapy. ■ See Dose Adjustments, Rate of Administration, Precautions, and Antidote.

Patient Education: Avoid pregnancy; nonhormonal birth control recommended for both females and males during therapy and for 6 months following the last dose. See Maternal/Child. Women should report a suspected pregnancy immediately. ■ Review potential side effects before therapy. ■ Report any unusual or unexpected symptoms or side effects promptly, especially infusion-related reactions (e.g., dyspnea, feeling of faintness, hives, wheezing). ■ Sunlight can worsen the skin reactions that may occur. Limit exposure to the sun, and wear sunscreen, protective clothing, and hats when outdoors. ■ See Appendix D, p. 1434.

Maternal/Child: Category C: has the potential to be transferred from the mother to the developing fetus; avoid pregnancy. Use during pregnancy or in any woman not using adequate contraception methods only if benefit justifies the potential risk to the fetus. ▪ Discontinue breast-feeding during treatment with cetuximab and for 60 days following the last dose. ▪ Safety and effectiveness for use in pediatric patients not established.

Elderly: Safety and effectiveness similar to younger adults; incidence of side effects may be somewhat increased.

DRUG/LAB INTERACTIONS

No evidence of pharmacokinetic interactions between cetuximab and irinotecan. ▪ No other drug interaction studies have been completed. ▪ The safety of combination use with **cisplatin** has not been established. Death and serious cardiotoxicity have been observed when **cetuximab, cisplatin, and radiation therapy** have been used concomitantly.

SIDE EFFECTS

The most common side effects are cutaneous adverse reactions (e.g., nail changes, pruritus, rash), diarrhea, headache, and infection. The most serious side effects are cardiopulmonary arrest, dermatologic toxicity, infusion reactions, interstitial lung disease, pulmonary embolus, radiation dermatitis, renal failure, and sepsis.

SCCHN: Confusion; dehydration; diarrhea; dry mouth; elevated ALT, AST, and alkaline phosphatase; mucositis/stomatitis/pharyngitis; and radiation dermatitis/toxicities occurred with more frequency in this group and were considered serious.

Colorectal cancer: Dehydration, diarrhea, fever, kidney failure, pulmonary embolus, and sepsis occurred with more frequency in this group and were considered serious.

All diagnoses: Abdominal pain, acneform rash, asthenia, chills, constipation, dysphagia, electrolyte abnormalities (e.g., hypocalcemia, hypokalemia, hypomagnesemia), fever, malaise, nausea and vomiting, and weight loss occur frequently. Other side effects reported include alopecia, anemia, anorexia, back pain, conjunctivitis, cough (increased), depression, dyspepsia, dyspnea, headache, insomnia, leukopenia, nail disorders (paronychial inflammation of the toes and fingers), pain, peripheral edema, pruritus, skin disorders, stomatitis.

ANTIDOTE

Keep physician informed of all side effects. May constitute a medical emergency or will be treated symptomatically as indicated. Hypersensitivity or infusion-related side effects may resolve with reduction in the rate of infusion by 50% and by continued use of premedication with diphenhydramine (Benadryl). Discontinue cetuximab immediately for severe infusion reactions; *do not re-challenge.* Treat hypersensitivity or infusion reactions as indicated; may require use of epinephrine, corticosteroids, diphenhydramine, bronchodilators (e.g., albuterol [Ventolin], aminophylline), IV saline, oxygen, and/or acetaminophen. Dermatologic toxicities may be dose limiting (see Dose Adjustments) or may be treated with topical and/or oral antibiotics as appropriate. Use of topical corticosteroids is not recommended. Discontinue cetuximab with the onset of acute or worsening pulmonary symptoms. Treat as indicated; cetuximab therapy may need to be discontinued. Replace electrolytes as indicated. Resuscitate if indicated.

CHLORAMPHENICOL
SODIUM SUCCINATE BBW

(klor-am-**FEN**-ih-kohl **SO**-dee-um **SUK**-suh-nayt)

Chloromycetin

Antibacterial

pH 6.4 to 7

USUAL DOSE

For all age levels, determine baseline blood studies before administration. Avoid repeated courses of this drug if at all possible. Treatment should not be continued longer than the time required to produce a cure with little or no risk or relapse of disease.

Adults and pediatric patients with mature metabolic processes (e.g., normal kidney and liver function): 12.5 mg/kg every 6 hours. In exceptional cases, infections due to moderately resistant organisms may require up to 25 mg/kg every 6 hours. Severe infections (e.g., bacteremia or meningitis), especially when adequate cerebrospinal fluid concentrations are desired, may require up to 25 mg/kg every 6 hours. These increased doses must be reduced to 12.5 mg/kg every 6 hours as soon as possible. Maximum dose is 4 Gm/24 hr. Change to oral form as soon as practical.

NEONATAL DOSE

See Maternal/Child.

Infants under 2 weeks of age or older infants with immature metabolic processes (e.g., premature infants): 6.25 mg/kg every 6 hours. Close monitoring of blood concentrations by microtechniques is recommended (information available from manufacturer).

Another source suggests a *loading dose* followed by *maintenance doses* based on age and weight. The first maintenance dose should be given 12 hours after the loading dose.

Loading dose: 20 mg/kg.

Maintenance dose: *Under 7 days of age or 7 days of age or older and under 2 kg:* 25 mg/kg of body weight once daily.

Over 7 days of age and over 2 kg: 25 mg/kg every 12 hours.

Infants 2 weeks of age or older with mature metabolic processes: 6.25 mg/kg every 6 hours. May increase to 12.5 mg/kg every 6 hours if indicated by severity of infection. See comments under Adult Dose.

DOSE ADJUSTMENTS

Reduce dose and/or initiate oral therapy as soon as feasible. ■ Reduce dose and/or extend intervals in infants and children with immature metabolic processes. See specific dose recommendations. Close monitoring of blood concentrations by microtechniques is recommended. ■ In patients with immature or impaired hepatic or renal function, dose reduction may be required. ■ Dosing should be cautious in the elderly. Consider decreased organ function and concomitant disease or drug therapy.

DILUTION

Each 1 Gm should be reconstituted with 10 mL of SW for injection or D5W to prepare a 10% solution (100 mg/mL). May be further diluted in 50 to 100 mL of D5W for intermittent infusion. Give through Y-tube, three-way stopcock, or additive infusion set.

Storage: Store at CRT. Administer within 24 hours of preparation.

COMPATIBILITY

Consider any drug NOT listed as compatible to be INCOMPATIBLE until consulting a pharmacist; specific conditions may apply.
One source suggests the following **compatibilities:**
Solution: Most common infusion solutions.

Additive: Amikacin (Amikin), aminophylline, ascorbic acid, calcium chloride, calcium gluconate, colistimethate (Coly-Mycin M), dimenhydrinate, dopamine, ephedrine, heparin, hydrocortisone sodium succinate (Solu-Cortef), kanamycin (Kantrex), lidocaine, magnesium sulfate, methyldopate, methylprednisolone (Solu-Medrol), nafcillin (Nallpen), oxacillin (Bactocill), oxytocin (Pitocin), penicillin G potassium and sodium, pentobarbital (Nembutal), phenylephrine (Neo-Synephrine), phytonadione (vitamin K_1), potassium chloride (KCl), ranitidine (Zantac), sodium bicarbonate, thiopental (Pentothal), verapamil.

Y-site: Acyclovir (Zovirax), cyclophosphamide (Cytoxan), enalaprilat (Vasotec IV), esmolol (Brevibloc), foscarnet (Foscavir), hydromorphone (Dilaudid), labetalol (Trandate), magnesium sulfate, meperidine (Demerol), morphine, nicardipine (Cardene IV), tacrolimus (Prograf).

RATE OF ADMINISTRATION

IV injection: 1 Gm or fraction thereof over a minimum of 1 minute.
Intermittent infusion: A single dose over 10 to 30 minutes.

ACTIONS

Effective against a wide range of gram-positive and gram-negative bacteria. Primarily bacteriostatic. May be bactericidal at high concentrations or against highly susceptible organisms. Acts by inhibiting protein synthesis. Well distributed in therapeutic doses throughout the body, especially in the liver and kidneys. Lowest concentrations are found in the brain and spinal fluid; however, chloramphenicol enters cerebrospinal fluid even in the absence of meningeal inflammation, appearing in concentrations about half of those found in the blood. Partially metabolized. Excreted in urine, bile, and feces. Crosses the placental barrier. Secreted in breast milk.

INDICATIONS AND USES

Only in serious infections in which potentially less dangerous drugs are ineffective or contraindicated; acute *Salmonella typhi* infections, meningeal infections (e.g., *Hemophilus influenzae*), bacteremia, rickettsia, lymphogranuloma psittacosis, and other serious gram-negative infections. ■ Cystic fibrosis regimens.

CONTRAINDICATIONS

Known chloramphenicol sensitivity. Must not be used in the treatment of trivial infections.

PRECAUTIONS

Serious blood dyscrasias (e.g., aplastic anemia, hypoplastic anemia, thrombocytopenia, and granulocytopenia) resulting in irreversible bone marrow suppression and death are known to occur. Aplastic anemia resulting in leukemia has been reported. Blood dyscrasias have occurred after both short-term and longer-term therapy. Do not use if potentially less dangerous agents would be effective. ■ Administration in a hospital with facilities for monitoring the patient and responding to any medical emergency is preferred. ■ Sensitivity studies mandatory to determine susceptibility of the causative organism not only to chloramphenicol but also to other less dangerous drugs. ■ Superinfection caused by overgrowth of nonsusceptible organisms, including fungi,

is possible. Treatment should not be continued longer than required to produce a cure with little or no risk of relapse of the disease. ▪ For IV use only. ▪ A reversible type of bone marrow suppression characterized by vacuolization of the erythroid cells, reduction of reticulocytes, and leukopenia is dose related and usually responds to withdrawal of chloramphenicol. ▪ *Clostridium difficile*–associated diarrhea (CDAD) has been reported. May range from mild diarrhea to fatal colitis. Consider in patients who present with diarrhea during or after treatment with chloramphenicol. ▪ Use caution in patients with impaired hepatic and/or renal function. **Monitor:** Obtain blood studies (CBC) before initiating therapy and approximately every 2 days during therapy; discontinue drug if blood studies show any indication of anemia, leukopenia, reticulocytopenia, thrombocytopenia, or any blood study findings attributable to chloramphenicol. ▪ Monitor chloramphenicol serum levels at least weekly, and more often if indicated (e.g., impaired liver or kidney function, immature metabolic processes, suspicion of beginning blood dyscrasias). ▪ Therapeutic levels range between 15 and 25 mcg/mL for meningitis; 10 and 20 mcg/mL for other infections. Trough levels should range between 5 and 15 mcg/mL for meningitis; 5 and 10 mcg/mL for other infections. ▪ Monitor hepatic and renal function as indicated; see Dose Adjustments. ▪ See Drug/Lab Interactions.
Patient Education: Promptly report fever, sore throat, tiredness, unusual bleeding, or bruising. ▪ Promptly report diarrhea or bloody stools that occur during treatment or up to several months after an antibiotic has been discontinued; may indicate CDAD and require treatment.
Maternal/Child: Category C: no studies documented. Use during pregnancy with extreme caution; may have toxic effects on fetus. ▪ Discontinue breast-feeding. ▪ Blood concentration in all premature and full-term neonates under 2 weeks of age differs from that of other neonates. Use caution, lower doses, and/or extended intervals in premature infants and newborns. May cause gray syndrome (e.g., abdominal distension with or without emesis, progressive pallid cyanosis, vasomotor collapse, irregular respiration, death within a few hours of onset of symptoms); monitor serum levels; see Precautions/Monitor.
Elderly: See Dose Adjustments. ▪ Response similar to that seen in younger patients. ▪ Monitor renal function.

DRUG/LAB INTERACTIONS

May cause irreversible bone marrow suppression. Avoid concurrent therapy with **drugs that cause blood dyscrasias** (e.g., penicillins, hydantoins [phenytoin (Dilantin)]), **other bone marrow suppressants** (e.g., cytotoxic drugs, radiation therapy). ▪ Increases serum levels of **oral antidiabetics** (e.g., chlorpropamide [Diabinase]) and increases hypoglycemic effects; dose reduction may be required. ▪ May be synergistic with or antagonize effects of **aminoglycosides, cephalosporins, and penicillins.** (Is used with ampicillin in pediatric patients.) ▪ Chloramphenicol can inhibit specific P_{450} enzymes; reduced metabolism and increased serum levels may occur in agents also metabolized by that route (e.g., **chlorpropamide** [Diabinese], **phenobarbital, phenytoin** [Dilantin], **tolbutamide, warfarin** [Coumadin]). ▪ Concurrent use with **hydantoins** (e.g., phenytoin [Dilantin]) may decrease or increase the effectiveness of chloramphenicol. Hydantoin levels may be increased, resulting in toxicity. ▪ Concurrent use with **phenobarbital** may decrease chloramphenicol serum levels and increase phenobarbital serum levels, resulting in phenobarbital toxicity. Monitor serum levels of both drugs if concurrent use is indicated. ▪ Concurrent administration with **anticoagulants** (e.g., heparin, warfarin [Coumadin]) may prolong PT. ▪ May increase **serum iron** levels. ▪ May delay response to **antianemia drugs** (e.g., iron preparations, vitamin B_{12}, folic acid). Avoid concurrent use in patients with anemia if possible. ▪ **Rifampin** increases chloramphenicol metabolism and decreases its effects.

SIDE EFFECTS

Blood dyscrasias (e.g., aplastic anemia, hypoplastic anemia, granulocytopenia, thrombocytopenia) may result in irreversible bone marrow suppression and death. CDAD, confusion, depression, diarrhea, fever, gray syndrome of newborns and infants, headache, hypersensitivity reactions (e.g., angioedema, anaphylaxis, fever, rashes, urticaria), leukemia, nausea, optic and peripheral neuritis, paroxysmal nocturnal hemoglobinuria, pseudomembranous colitis, rashes, stomatitis, vomiting, and many others. *May be fatal.*

ANTIDOTE

Notify the physician immediately of any adverse symptoms. Discontinue the drug upon appearance of anemia, leukopenia, reticulocytopenia, thrombocytopenia, or any other blood study findings attributable to chloramphenicol. Discontinue the drug for symptoms of optic and peripheral neuritis. Monitoring of plasma levels is imperative in all patients and especially in neonates. Treat hypersensitivity reactions as indicated. Treat CDAD with fluids, electrolytes, protein supplements, and oral vancomycin (Vancocin) or metronidazole (Flagyl) as indicated. In severe cases, surgical evaluation may be indicated. Resuscitate as necessary.

CHLORPROMAZINE HYDROCHLORIDE BBW

(klor-**PROH**-mah-zeen hy-droh-**KLOR**-eyed)

Thorazine

Phenothiazine
Antipsychotic
Antiemetic

pH 3 to 5

USUAL DOSE

Use of the IV route is reserved for the treatment of acute nausea and vomiting in surgery, intractable hiccups, and tetanus.

Acute nausea and vomiting in surgery: 2 mg. May repeat at 2-minute intervals as indicated. Do not exceed 25 mg. Usually given as an infusion.

Intractable hiccups: 25 to 50 mg diluted in 500 to 1,000 mL of NS. Given as a slow IV infusion with patient flat in bed. Monitor BP closely.

Tetanus: 25 to 50 mg as an infusion of at least 1 mg/mL. Individualize dose to patient response and tolerance. Repeat every 6 to 8 hours. Usually given in conjunction with barbiturates.

PEDIATRIC DOSE

See Maternal/Child. IV route rarely used for pediatric patients. Not recommended for use in infants less than 6 months of age.

Acute nausea and vomiting in surgery, pediatric patients 6 months of age or older: 1 mg. May repeat at 2-minute intervals as indicated. Monitor for hypotension. Another source suggests 2.5 to 4 mg/kg/24 hr in equally divided doses every 6 to 8 hours (0.625 to 1 mg/kg every 6 hours or 0.83 to 1.33 mg/kg every 8 hours). Usual IV/IM dose does not exceed 2.5 to 4 mg/kg/24 hr or 40 mg/24 hr (whichever is less) in pediatric patients 6 months to 5 years of age or up to 50 lbs, and 75 mg/24 hr in pediatric patients 5 to 12 years of age.

Tetanus: 0.55 mg/kg of body weight (0.25 mg/lb) every 6 to 8 hours. Do not exceed 40 mg/24 hr for up to 23 kg (50 lbs) and 75 mg/24 hr for up to 50 kg (50 to 100 lbs), except in severe cases.

DOSE ADJUSTMENTS

Adjust dose to the individual and severity of condition. Reduce dose of any medication potentiated by phenothiazines by one fourth to one half. See Drug/Lab Interactions. ▪ Reduce dose by one fourth to one half in the elderly, debilitated patients, or emaciated patients, and increase very gradually by response.

DILUTION

Each 25 mg (1 mL) must be diluted with 24 mL of NS for injection. 1 mL will equal 1 mg. May be further diluted in 500 to 1,000 mL of NS and given as an infusion. Handle carefully; may cause contact dermatitis. Sensitive to light. Slightly yellow color does not alter potency. Discard if markedly discolored.

Storage: Store at CRT. Protect from light and freezing.

COMPATIBILITY   (Underline Indicates Conflicting Compatibility Information)

Consider any drug NOT listed as compatible to be INCOMPATIBLE until consulting a pharmacist; specific conditions may apply.

One source suggests the following **compatibilities:**

Additive: Ascorbic acid, ethacrynic acid (Edecrin), theophylline.

Y-site: Cisatracurium (Nimbex), cisplatin (Platinol), cladribine (Leustatin), cyclophosphamide (Cytoxan), cytarabine (ARA-C), dexmedetomidine (Precedex), docetaxel (Taxotere), doxorubicin (Adriamycin), doxorubicin liposomal (Doxil), famotidine (Pepcid IV), fenoldopam (Corlopam), filgrastim (Neupogen), fluconazole (Diflucan), gemcitabine (Gemzar), granisetron (Kytril), heparin, hetastarch in electrolytes (Hextend), hydrocortisone sodium succinate (Solu-Cortef), ondansetron (Zofran), oxaliplatin (Eloxatin), potassium chloride (KCl), propofol (Diprivan), remifentanil (Ultiva), teniposide (Vumon), thiotepa, vinorelbine (Navelbine).

RATE OF ADMINISTRATION

Titrate to symptoms and vital signs. See Precautions.

IV injection: Each 1 mg or fraction thereof over 1 minute.

Infusion: Given very slowly. Do not exceed 1 mg/min.

Pediatric rate: Do not exceed 1 mg or fraction thereof over 2 minutes.

ACTIONS

A phenothiazine derivative with effects on the central, autonomic, and peripheral nervous systems. A psychotropic agent. Decreases anxiety and tension, relaxes muscles, produces sedation, and tranquilizes. Has an antiemetic effect and potentiates CNS depressants. Has strong antiadrenergic and anticholinergic activity. Also possesses slight antihistaminic and antiserotonin activity. Onset of action is prompt and of short duration in small IV doses. Extensively metabolized in liver and kidney and excreted primarily in urine. Crosses the placental barrier. Secreted in breast milk.

INDICATIONS AND USES

The IV route is used only for the treatment of acute nausea and vomiting in surgery, the treatment of intractable hiccups, and as an adjunct in the treatment of tetanus. ▪ Used IM or PO for the treatment of schizophrenia and the management of psychotic disorders. ▪ Also indicated IM, PO, or rectally to relieve restlessness and apprehension before surgery, to manage acute intermittent porphyria, to control manic episodes in manic-depressive illness, and to treat severe behavioral problems in pediatric patients.

Unlabeled uses: Treatment of phencyclidine (PCP) psychosis. ▪ Treatment of migraine headaches (IV or IM). ▪ To reduce choreiform movements of Huntington's disease.

CONTRAINDICATIONS

Hypersensitivity to phenothiazines, comatose or severely depressed states, or the presence of large amounts of CNS depressants (e.g., alcohol, barbiturates, narcotics).

PRECAUTIONS

Not approved for dementia-related psychosis; mortality risk in elderly dementia patients taking conventional or atypical antipsychotics is increased; most deaths are due to cardiovascular or infectious events. ▪ Use of the IV route is reserved for the treatment of acute nausea and vomiting in surgery, intractable hiccups, and tetanus. IM injection preferred. ▪ Use caution in patients with bone marrow suppression; glaucoma; cardiovascular, liver, renal, and chronic respiratory diseases; and acute respiratory diseases of pediatric patients. ▪ Re-exposure of patients who have experienced jaundice, skin reactions, or blood dyscrasias with a phenothiazine is not recommended. Cross-sensitivity may occur. ▪ May produce ECG changes (e.g., prolonged QT interval, changes in T waves). ▪ Use with caution in patients with a history of seizure disorders; may lower seizure threshold. ▪ Extrapyramidal symptoms caused by chlorpromazine may be confused with CNS signs of an undiagnosed disease (e.g., Reye's syndrome or encephalopathy). ▪ May mask diagnosis of brain tumor, drug intoxication, and intestinal obstruction. ▪ Tardive dyskinesia (potentially irreversible involuntary dyskinetic movements) may develop. Use smallest doses and shortest duration of therapy to minimize risk. ▪ Neuroleptic malignant syndrome (NMS) characterized by hyperpyrexia, muscle rigidity, altered mental status, and autonomic instability has been reported; see Antidote. ▪ May cause paradoxical excitation in pediatric patients and the elderly. ▪ Use phenothiazines with extreme caution in pediatric patients with a history of sleep apnea, a family history of SIDS, or in the presence of Reye's syndrome. ▪ May contain sulfites; use caution in patients with asthma. ▪ Taper dose gradually following high dose or extended therapy to prevent possible occurrence of withdrawal symptoms (e.g., dizziness, gastritis, nausea, tremors, and vomiting).

Monitor: Keep patient in supine position throughout treatment and for at least ½ hour after treatment. Ambulate slowly and carefully; may cause postural hypotension. ▪ Monitor BP and pulse before and during administration and between doses. ▪ Cough reflex is often depressed; monitor closely if nauseated or vomiting to prevent aspiration. ▪ Anticholinergic and cardiac effects may be troublesome during anesthesia. For patients receiving phenothiazines, taper and discontinue preoperatively if they will not be continued after surgery. ▪ May discolor urine pink to reddish brown. ▪ Photosensitivity of skin is possible. ▪ See Drug/Lab Interactions. **Patient Education:** Request assistance for ambulation; may cause dizziness or fainting. ▪ Observe caution performing tasks that require alertness. ▪ Avoid use of alcohol and other CNS depressants (e.g., diazepam [Valium], narcotics). ▪ Possible eye and skin photosensitivity. Avoid unprotected exposure to sun. ▪ Urine may discolor to pink or reddish brown. **Maternal/Child:** See Precautions and Contraindications. ▪ Category C: use during pregnancy only when clearly needed. Use near term may cause maternal hypotension and adverse neonatal effects (e.g., extrapyramidal syndrome, hyperreflexia, hyporeflexia, jaundice). ▪ Fetuses and infants have a reduced capacity to metabolize and eliminate; may cause embryo toxicity, increase neonatal mortality, or cause permanent neurologic damage. May contain benzyl alcohol; use not recommended in neonates. ▪ Not recommended during breast-feeding. Increases risk of dystonia and tardive dyskinesia. ▪ Children metabolize antipsychotic agents more rapidly than adults and are at increased risk to develop extrapyramidal actions, especially during acute illness (e.g., chickenpox, CNS infections, dehydration, gastroenteritis, measles); monitor closely. **Elderly:** See Dose Adjustments and Precautions. ▪ Have a reduced capacity to metabolize and eliminate. May have increased sensitivity to postural hypotension, anticholinergic and sedative effects. ▪ Increased risk of extrapyramidal side effects (e.g., tardive dyskinesia, parkinsonism).

DRUG/LAB INTERACTIONS

Use with **epinephrine** not recommended; may cause precipitous hypotension. ▪ Use with **agents that produce hypotension** (e.g., antihypertensives, benzodiazepines, diuretics, lidocaine, paclitaxel) may produce severe hypotension. ▪ Increased CNS, respiratory depression, and hypotensive effects with **CNS depressants** (e.g., narcotics, alcohol, anesthetics, and barbiturates); reduced doses of these agents usually indicated. ▪ Chlorpromazine does not potentiate the anticonvulsant actions of **barbiturates.** Doses of **anticonvulsant barbiturates** should not be decreased if chlorpromazine is introduced. Instead begin chlorpromazine at a lower dose and titrate to effect. ▪ Chlorpromazine may lower the seizure threshold. It may also interfere with **phenytoin and valproic acid** clearance, increasing potential for toxicity. Dose adjustment of anticonvulsants may be necessary. ▪ Additive effects with **MAO inhibitors** (e.g., selegiline [Eldepryl]), **anticholinergics, antihistamines, antihypertensives, hypnotics, muscle relaxants, rauwolfia alkaloids, and thiazide diuretics;** dose adjustment may be necessary. ▪ **Barbiturates** may also increase metabolism of chlorpromazine and reduce its effects. ▪ Risk of cardiotoxicity increased with **pimozide** (Orap) **and sparfloxacin** (Zagam); concurrent use not recommended. ▪ Risk of additive QT interval prolongation, cardiac depressant effects, and cardiac arrhythmias increased with **cisapride** (Propulsid), **disopyramide** (Norpace), **erythromycin, probucol** (Lorelco), **procainamide** (Pronestyl), **and quinidine.** ▪ Concurrent use with **antidepressants** (e.g., fluoxetine [Prozac], paroxetine [Paxil]), **tricyclic antidepressants** (e.g., amitriptyline [Elavil], imipramine [Tofranil]), **or MAO inhibitors** (e.g., selegiline [Eldepryl]) may increase effects of both drugs; risk of NMS may be increased. ▪ Use with **antithyroid drugs** may increase risk of agranulocytosis. ▪ May inhibit antiparkinson effects of **levodopa.** ▪ May decrease pressor response to **ephedrine.** ▪ May increase anticholinergic effect of

orphenadrine (Norflex). ■ May decrease effects of **oral anticoagulants.** ■ Concurrent use with **haloperidol, droperidol, or metoclopramide** may cause increased extrapyramidal effects. ■ Use with **metrizamide** (Amipaque) may lower seizure threshold; discontinue chlorpromazine 48 hours before myelography and do not resume for 24 hours after test completed. ■ Metabolism and clearance of chlorpromazine is increased in cigarette **smokers;** decreased plasma levels and effectiveness may occur; dose adjustment of chlorpromazine may be indicated. ■ Decreased drowsiness may occur in cigarette **smokers.** May be offset by increased doses of chlorpromazine. ■ Use caution during anesthesia with **barbiturates** (e.g., methohexital, thiopental); may increase frequency and severity of hypotension and neuromuscular excitation. ■ Encephalopathic syndrome has been reported with concurrent use of **lithium;** monitor for S/S of neurologic toxicity. ■ Capable of innumerable other interactions. ■ May cause false-positive **pregnancy test** and false-positive **amylase, PKU, and other urine tests.**

SIDE EFFECTS
Usually transient if drug discontinued, but may require treatment if severe. Anaphylaxis, cardiac arrest, distorted Q and T waves, drowsiness, excitement, extrapyramidal symptoms (e.g., abnormal positioning, extreme restlessness, pseudoparkinsonism, weakness of extremities), fever, hematologic toxicities (e.g., agranulocytosis, aplastic anemia, leukopenia, thrombocytopenia), hypersensitivity reactions, hypertension, hypotension (occurs less frequently in smokers), melanosis, photosensitivity, tachycardia, tardive dyskinesia, and many others.
Overdose: Can cause convulsions, hallucinations, and death.

ANTIDOTE
Discontinue the drug at onset of any side effect and notify the physician. Discontinue chlorpromazine and all drugs not essential to concurrent therapy immediately if NMS occurs. Will require intensive symptomatic treatment, medical monitoring, and management of concomitant medical problems. Counteract hypotension with norepinephrine (Levophed) or phenylephrine (Neo-Synephrine) and IV fluids. Counteract extrapyramidal symptoms with benztropine (Cogentin) or diphenhydramine (Benadryl). Use diazepam (Valium) followed by phenytoin (Dilantin) for convulsions or hyperactivity. Maintain a clear airway and adequate hydration. Epinephrine is contraindicated for hypotension; further hypotension will occur. Phenytoin may be helpful in ventricular arrhythmias. Avoid analeptics such as caffeine and sodium benzoate in treating respiratory depression and unconsciousness; they may cause convulsions. Resuscitate as necessary. Not removed by dialysis.

CIDOFOVIR INJECTION BBW

(sih-**DOF**-oh-veer in-**JEK**-shun)

Vistide

Antiviral
(nucleotide analog)

pH 6.7 to 7.6

USUAL DOSE

Preliminary lab work required before each dose; see Monitor. A specific protocol is required; see the following chart. A 4-Gm course of oral probenecid is required on the day of each infusion of cidofovir to reduce the risk of renal impairment. Hydration with 1 to 2 liters of NS is required to help reduce proteinuria and prevent increases in SCr. Infrequent dosing schedule may eliminate need for an indwelling IV catheter, reducing discomfort and potential for infection.

Induction: 5 mg/kg in 100 mL NS once weekly for 2 consecutive weeks.

Maintenance: 5 mg/kg in 100 mL NS once every other week.

Overview of the Treatment Regimen for Cidofovir		
Before Cidofovir Infusion	During Cidofovir Infusion	After Cidofovir Infusion
1. Patient takes 2 Gm of probenecid* (4 × 500 mg tablets) 3 hours before cidofovir infusion	1. Begin IV infusion of cidofovir (5 mg/kg body weight in 100 mL NS) at a constant rate over 1 hour†	1. Patient takes 1 Gm of probenecid (2 × 500 mg tablets) 2 hours after the *end* of cidofovir infusion
2. Infuse first liter of NS over 1 to 2 hours immediately before starting cidofovir infusion	2. For patients who can tolerate the extra fluid load, infuse a second liter of NS. If administered, initiate either at the start of the cidofovir infusion or immediately afterward, and infuse over a 1- to 3-hour period	2. Patient takes 1 Gm of probenecid (2 × 500 mg tablets) 8 hours after the *end* of cidofovir infusion

*Patients receiving concomitant probenecid and zidovudine should temporarily discontinue zidovudine or decrease the zidovudine dose by 50% on days of combined zidovudine and probenecid administration.

†The recommended dosage, frequency, or infusion rate must not be exceeded.

DOSE ADJUSTMENTS

Reduce dose to 3 mg/kg for the remainder of therapy, if SCr increases by 0.3 to 0.4 mg/dL above baseline. ■ 5 mg/kg may be given to patients who develop a 2^+ proteinuria but have a stable SCr. Encourage oral hydration; additional IV hydration may be appropriate. ■ Discontinue cidofovir if the SCr increases by 0.5 mg/dL or more above baseline or if proteinuria 3^+ or more develops. ■ Restarting cidofovir in patients whose renal function has returned to baseline after a SCr elevation of more than 0.5 mg/dL is not recommended. ■ Discontinue cidofovir in any patient who requires therapy with a nephrotoxic agent; see Contraindications. Cidofovir may be restarted after other nephrotoxic therapy is complete, an adequate washout period of at least 7 days has passed, and adequate renal function (SCr less than 1.5 mg/dL) is confirmed.

DILUTION

Specific techniques required; see Precautions. A calculated dose must be diluted in 100 mL of NS. **Storage:** Store unopened vials at CRT. May be refrigerated but must be used within 24 hours of dilution with NS. Allow to return to room temperature before administration. Discard partially used vials.

COMPATIBILITY

Manufacturer states, "**Compatibility** with Ringer's solution, LR, or bacteriostatic IV fluids not evaluated; no data available to support the addition of other drugs or supplements for concurrent administration."

RATE OF ADMINISTRATION

A single dose as an infusion at a constant rate over 1 hour. Use of an infusion pump is recommended.

ACTIONS

A nucleotide analog antiviral. Its active intracellular metabolite selectively inhibits CMV DNA synthesis. It is incorporated into the growing viral DNA chain, resulting in reductions in the rate of viral DNA synthesis. This action is independent of virus infection (acyclovir or ganciclovir require activation by a virally encoded enzyme). Elimination half-life is short (2.6 hours), but it has a long intracellular half-life, which permits infrequent dosing. Primarily excreted in urine (70% to 85% in 24 hours with concomitant doses of probenecid).

INDICATIONS AND USES

Treatment of newly diagnosed or relapsing CMV retinitis in patients with AIDS is the only approved indication.

CONTRAINDICATIONS

Pre-existing renal dysfunction (e.g., baseline SCr more than 1.5 mg/dL, calculated CrCl equal to or less than 55 mL/min, or a urine protein equal to or greater than 100 mg/dL [equivalent to a 2^+ or more proteinuria]). ■ Patients receiving agents with nephrotoxic potential (e.g., aminoglycosides, amphotericin B, foscarnet (Foscavir), NSAIDs [ibuprofen (Advil, Motrin), naproxen (Aleve, Naprosyn)], IV pentamidine, vancomycin). No other nephrotoxic agent should be administered within 7 days of starting cidofovir or concomitantly during cidofovir therapy. ■ Hypersensitivity to cidofovir and/or a history of clinically severe hypersensitivity (e.g., hypotension, respiratory distress) to probenecid or other sulfa-containing medications (e.g., sulfamethoxazole/trimethoprim).

PRECAUTIONS

Follow guidelines for handling cytotoxic agents. See Appendix A, p. 1429. ■ Administered by or under the direction of the physician specialist, preferably in an environment where emergency treatment is available. ■ This formulation is for IV use only; **DO NOT** use for intraocular injection. ■ Safety and effectiveness have not been established for treatment of other CMV infections (e.g., pneumonitis, gastroenteritis, congenital or neonatal CMV disease) or for CMV disease in non–HIV-infected individuals. ■ Calculated CrCl may not accurately estimate renal function in emaciated (e.g., patients with AIDS) or extremely muscular patients; a 24-hour urine collection may be required. ■ CMV resistant to ganciclovir may also be resistant to cidofovir, but may be sensitive to foscarnet (Foscavir). ■ CMV resistant to foscarnet (Foscavir) may be sensitive to cidofovir. ■ Nephrotoxicity is dose limiting and is the major toxicity of cidofovir. Do not exceed recommended dose, frequency, or rate of administration; may cause increased risk of renal toxicity. Acute renal failure requiring dialysis or contributing to death has occurred with as few as 1 or 2 doses of cidofovir. ■ Renal function may not return to baseline after treatment with cidofovir. ■ Proteinuria is an early indicator of nephrotoxicity; continued administration of cidofovir may lead to additional proximal tubular cell injury resulting in glycosuria, decreased serum phosphate, uric acid, and bicarbonate; increased SCr; and/or acute renal failure, which may necessitate dialysis. ■ May cause granulocytopenia (e.g., neutropenia). ■ Although some reference sources have published doses for patients with impaired renal function, this drug is contraindicated in such patients and should be given only to those who meet specific dosing criteria; see Contraindications.

Monitor: 24 to 48 hours before each cidofovir infusion, obtain SCr, urine protein (via dipstick or quantitative urinalysis), and CBC with differential (absolute neutrophil count [ANC]). Repeat between doses if indicated. ■ Administration of probenecid as ordered and adequate hydration (oral and IV) are imperative. ■ Antiretroviral therapy may be continued with the exception of zidovudine; see Drug/Lab Interactions. ■ Probenecid frequently causes fever, flushing, headache, nausea with or without emesis, and rash. Use acetaminophen for prophylaxis or treatment of fever or headache. Encourage ingestion of food before each dose of probenecid to reduce nausea; prophylactic antiemetics (e.g., ondansetron [Zofran]) are appropriate. Consider use of antihistamines (e.g., diphenhydramine [Benadryl]) for prophylaxis or treatment in patients who develop mild hypersensitivity reactions (e.g., rash). Severe hypersensitivity reactions (e.g., laryngospasm, hypotension) have occasionally been reported with probenecid. Usually occur within several hours after patients have received probenecid even though they have received it before with no adverse reactions. Observe patient carefully for hypersensitivity reactions. Treatment for anaphylaxis (e.g., epinephrine, corticosteroids, and antihistamines) must be readily available. ■ Monitor intraocular pressure, visual acuity, and ocular symptoms with a baseline ophthalmologic exam and periodically during therapy. Uveitis or iritis has been reported; may be treated with topical steroids. Risk of increased intraocular pressure and other visual problems may be increased in patients with pre-existing diabetes mellitus. ■ Use of the Cockcroft-Gault formula is recommended if a precise estimate of CrCl measurement is indicated.

Patient Education: Not a cure for CMV retinitis. Retinitis may recur during maintenance or after treatment; regular ophthalmologic exams imperative. ■ Full compliance with regimen imperative (e.g., probenecid with food, increased IV and oral hydration, regular lab testing). ■ Report diarrhea, eye pain or change in vision, fever, headache, loss of appetite, rash, nausea, and vomiting promptly. ■ Report concomitant medication changes or additions. ■ Notify all health care personnel of treatment with probenecid to avoid interactions. ■ Consider birth control options; See Precautions/Maternal/Child.

Maternal/Child: Category C: should not be used during pregnancy; embryotoxic in animals. A potential carcinogen; knowledge of effects on women unknown. ■ Women of childbearing age should use effective contraception during cidofovir therapy and for 1 month after completion. ■ Men should use barrier contraception during cidofovir therapy and for 3 months after completion. ■ Has caused reduced testicular weight and hypospermia in animals. ■ Do not administer to nursing mothers. HIV-infected mothers are advised not to breast-feed to avoid transmission to an uninfected child. ■ Safety and effectiveness for use in pediatric patients not established. Use in pediatric patients with extreme caution and only if the benefits of treatment outweigh the risks of long-term carcinogenicity and reproductive toxicity. Consult physician specialist for adjustments in probenecid and hydration.

Elderly: Effects have not been studied; monitor renal function carefully.

DRUG/LAB INTERACTIONS

Limited information available. Drug profile review by pharmacist imperative. ■ Nephrotoxicity increased by other **nephrotoxic agents** (e.g., aminoglycosides [e.g., amikacin, gentamicin], amphotericin B [generic, Abelcet], foscarnet [Foscavir], IV pentamidine, NSAIDs [e.g., ibuprofen (Motrin)], vancomycin); see Contraindications. ■ Prior treatment with **foscarnet** (Foscavir) may also increase the risk of nephrotoxicity; monitor renal function carefully. ■ **Probenecid** decreases clearance of zidovudine; temporarily discontinue or reduce dose of zidovudine by 50% on days of combined zidovudine and probenecid administration. ■ **Probenecid** may have interactions with numerous other drugs (e.g., **acetaminophen, acyclovir** [Zovirax], **ACE inhibitors** [e.g., enalaprilat (Vasotec)], **aminosalicylic acid, barbiturates, benzodiazepines** [e.g., diazepam, lorazepam (Ativan), midazolam], **bumetamide, chlorpropamide** [Diabinese], **clofibrate, ddC, famotidine, furosemide, methotrexate, NSAIDs** [e.g., ketoprofen (Orudis), ibuprofen (Advil, Motrin), naproxen (Aleve, Naprosyn)], **theophyllines**), usually decreasing their rate of excretion and increasing toxicity. Consider withholding any drug that may interact with probenecid on the day of cidofovir administration.

SIDE EFFECTS

Nephrotoxicity is dose limiting. Metabolic acidosis (Fanconi's syndrome), neutropenia, and ocular hypotony may be dose limiting and require prompt treatment. Anorexia, asthenia, decreased intraocular pressure, decreased serum bicarbonate, chills, diarrhea, dyspnea, fever, headache, increased creatinine, infection, nausea and vomiting, ophthalmic effects (e.g., change in vision, eye pain, increased sensitivity to light, reddened eyes), pneumonia, proteinuria, rash, and unusual tiredness or weakness may occur.

ANTIDOTE

There is no specific antidote. Keep physician informed. Adequate hydration, use of probenecid, and careful monitoring will help to reduce potential for renal impairment and may minimize other side effects. Filgrastim (Neupogen) may be used to treat neutropenia. See Monitor for management of probenecid side effects. Discontinue cidofovir based on criteria in Dose Adjustments. Treat overdose for 3 to 5 days with probenecid 1 Gm three times daily and vigorous IV hydration to tolerance. Treat anaphylaxis and resuscitate as indicated. Hemodialysis may be helpful in overdose. High-flux hemodialysis has reduced serum level of cidofovir by up to 75%.

CIPROFLOXACIN BBW
(sip-row-**FLOX**-ah-sin)

Cipro IV

**Antibacterial
(fluoroquinolone)**

pH 3.3 to 4.6

USUAL DOSE
Dose based on severity and nature of the infection, susceptibility of the causative organism, integrity of host-defense mechanisms, and renal and hepatic status. Range is from 200 to 400 mg according to the following chart. Continue for 7 to 14 days (at least 2 days after all symptoms of infection subside). Bone and joint infections may require treatment for 4 to 6 weeks or more. May be transferred to oral dosing when appropriate; see Monitor.

Ciprofloxacin Dose Guidelines				
Infection	Type of Severity	Unit Dose	Frequency	Duration
Urinary tract	Mild/moderate	200 mg	q 12 hr	7-14 days
	Severe/ complicated	400 mg	q 12 hr	
Lower respiratory tract	Mild/moderate	400 mg	q 12 hr	7-14 days
	Severe/ complicated	400 mg	q 8 hr	
Nosocomial pneumonia	Mild/moderate/ severe	400 mg	q 8 hr	10-14 days
Skin and skin structure	Mild/moderate	400 mg	q 12 hr	7-14 days
	Severe/ complicated	400 mg	q 8 hr	
Bone and joint	Mild/moderate	400 mg	q 12 hr	≥4-6 weeks
	Severe/ complicated	400 mg	q 8 hr	
Septicemia (Canada)		400 mg	q 12 hr	
Acute sinusitis	Mild/moderate	400 mg	q 12 hr	10 days
Chronic bacterial prostatitis	Mild/moderate	400 mg	q 12 hr	28 days
Inhalation anthrax*	Post-exposure	400 mg	q 12 hr	60 days
Intra-abdominal, complicated	Ciprofloxacin + metronidazole	400 mg 500 mg	q 12 hr q 6 hr	7-14 days
Empirical therapy in febrile neutro- penic patients	Ciprofloxacin + piperacillin	400 mg 50 mg/kg	q 8 hr q 4 hr	7-14 days

*Begin drug administration as soon as possible after suspected or confirmed exposure.

Continued

PEDIATRIC DOSE

Used only when alternate therapy cannot be used; see Precautions and Maternal/Child. *In all situations, do not exceed an IV dose of 400 mg.*
Inhalation anthrax (post-exposure): 10 mg/kg every 12 hours. May transfer to oral therapy when appropriate. Dose is 15 mg/kg PO every 12 hours. Do not exceed a 500-mg dose PO. Administer for 60 days.

Complicated UTIs or pyelonephritis in patients from 1 to 17 years of age: Dosing and initial route (IV or PO) should be determined by severity of infection. 6 to 10 mg/kg IV every 8 hours. May transfer to oral therapy with a dose of 10 to 20 mg/kg PO every 12 hours at discretion of physician. Do not exceed a 750-mg dose PO. Total duration of treatment is 10 to 21 days.

Pulmonary exacerbations of cystic fibrosis in patients from 5 to 17 years of age (unlabeled): 10 mg/kg/dose every 8 hours for 1 week. Follow with 20 mg/kg/dose PO every 12 hours for 3 to 14 additional days to complete a 10- to 21-day regimen; see Monitor. Do not exceed 1.2 Gm/24 hr.

Another source suggests:
Other infections: *Infants and children (unlabeled):* 7.5 to 10 mg/kg of body weight every 12 hours. Do not exceed 800 mg/24 hr.
Neonates (unlabeled): 3.5 to 20 mg/kg every 12 hours.

DOSE ADJUSTMENTS

Increase interval between doses (200 to 400 mg every 18 to 24 hours) if CrCl is less than 30 mL/min (see literature for additional information). ▪ Information on dosing adjustments for pediatric patients with renal insufficiency is not available. ▪ Dose reduction not required based on age; see Elderly. ▪ See Drug/Lab Interactions.

DILUTION

Available prediluted in D5W in latex-free plastic infusion containers ready for use. A clear, colorless to slightly yellow solution. Do not hang plastic containers in a series; may cause air embolism. Also available in 20- and 40-mL vials containing 10 mg/mL (1% solution), which must be diluted with NS, D5W, SW, D10W, D5/¼NS, D5/½NS, or LR to a final concentration of 1 to 2 mg/mL.
Filters: No recommendations available from manufacturer.
Storage: Store at CRT before dilution; protect from light, excessive heat, and freezing. Stable for up to 14 days refrigerated or at room temperature in the final diluted concentration.

COMPATIBILITY   (Underline Indicates Conflicting Compatibility Information)

Consider any drug NOT listed as compatible to be INCOMPATIBLE until consulting a pharmacist; specific conditions may apply.
Manufacturer recommends temporarily discontinuing other solutions infusing at the same site during intermittent infusion through a **Y-site** or volume control and that ciprofloxacin be administered separately and the IV line be flushed before and after administration of any other drug.

One source suggests the following **compatibilities:**
Additive: Amikacin (Amikin), atracurium (Tracrium), aztreonam (Azactam), cyclosporine (Sandimmune), dobutamine, dopamine, fluconazole (Diflucan), gentamicin, lidocaine, linezolid (Zyvox), metronidazole (Flagyl IV), midazolam (Versed), norepinephrine (Levophed), pancuronium, potassium chloride (KCl), ranitidine (Zantac), tobramycin, vecuronium.
Y-site: Amifostine (Ethyol), amino acids with dextrose, amiodarone (Nexterone), <u>anidulafungin (Eraxis)</u>, aztreonam (Azactam), bivalirudin (Angi-

omax), calcium gluconate, caspofungin (Cancidas), ceftazidime (Fortaz), cisatracurium (Nimbex), dexmedetomidine (Precedex), digoxin (Lanoxin), diltiazem (Cardizem), dimenhydrinate, diphenhydramine (Benadryl), dobutamine, docetaxel (Taxotere), dopamine, doripenem (Doribax), doxorubicin liposomal (Doxil), etoposide phosphate (Etopophos), fenoldopam (Corlopam), gallium nitrate (Ganite), gemcitabine (Gemzar), gentamicin, granisetron (Kytril), hetastarch in electrolytes (Hextend), lidocaine, linezolid (Zyvox), lorazepam (Ativan), magnesium sulfate, metoclopramide (Reglan), midazolam (Versed), milrinone (Primacor), piperacillin, potassium acetate, potassium chloride (KCl), promethazine (Phenergan), quinupristin/dalfopristin (Synercid [1 mg/mL]), ranitidine (Zantac), remifentanil (Ultiva), sodium bicarbonate, sodium chloride, tacrolimus (Prograf), teniposide (Vumon), thiotepa, tigecycline (Tygacil), tobramycin, vasopressin, verapamil.

RATE OF ADMINISTRATION
A single dose must be equally distributed over 60 minutes as an infusion. Too-rapid administration and/or the use of a small vein may increase incidence of local site inflammation and other side effects. May be given through a Y-tube or three-way stopcock of infusion set. Temporarily discontinue other solutions infusing at the same site.

ACTIONS
A synthetic, broad-spectrum antimicrobial agent, a fluoroquinolone. Bactericidal to a wide range of aerobic gram-negative and gram-positive organisms through interference with the enzymes needed for synthesis of bacterial DNA. Onset of action is prompt, and serum levels are dose related. Half-life averages 5 to 6 hours. Readily distributed to body fluids (saliva, nasal and bronchial secretions, sputum, skin blister fluid, lymph, peritoneal fluid, bile and prostatic secretions). Found in lung, skin, fat, muscle, cartilage, and bone. Levels in cerebrospinal fluid and eye fluids are lower than plasma levels. Limited metabolism. Excreted primarily as unchanged drug in the urine, usually within 24 hours. A small amount is excreted in the bile and feces. Crosses placental barrier. Secreted in breast milk.

INDICATIONS AND USES
Treatment of mild, moderate, severe, and complicated infections of the urinary tract, lower respiratory tract, and skin and skin structure. ■ Treatment of mild, moderate, and severe nosocomial pneumonia. ■ Treatment of acute sinusitis, bone and joint infections, chronic bacterial prostatitis, and septicemia (Canada). ■ Treatment of complicated intra-abdominal infections in combination with metronidazole (Flagyl). ■ Empirical therapy in febrile neutropenic patients in combination with piperacillin. ■ Reduce the incidence or progression of disease in adults or pediatric patients following exposure to aerosolized *Bacillus anthracis* (Anthrax). ■ Treatment of complicated UTI and pyelonephritis due to *Escherichia coli* in pediatric patients 1 to 17 years of age; see Maternal/Child. ■ Most effective against specific organisms (see literature). ■ Additional appropriate therapy required if anaerobic organisms are suspected of contributing to the infection. ■ Oral route of administration indicated for treatment of other infections (e.g., infectious diarrhea, typhoid fever, urethral and cervical gonococcal infections).
Unlabeled uses: Treatment of tuberculosis in combination with other antituberculosis agents (e.g., rifampin). ■ Treatment of *Mycobacterium avium*

complex infection in AIDS patients. ▪ Cystic fibrosis. ▪ Prophylaxis in endocarditis.

CONTRAINDICATIONS
Known hypersensitivity to ciprofloxacin or any other quinolone antimicrobial agent (e.g., levofloxacin [Levaquin], norfloxacin [Noroxin]) or any of the product components. ▪ Concomitant administration with tizanidine (Zanaflex) is contraindicated.

PRECAUTIONS
Specific culture and sensitivity studies indicated to determine susceptibility of the causative organism to ciprofloxacin. ▪ The emergence of bacterial resistance to fluoroquinolones and the occurrence of cross-resistance with other fluoroquinolones have been observed and are of concern. Proper use of fluoroquinolones and other classes of antibiotics is encouraged to avoid the emergence of resistant bacteria from overuse. ▪ *Pseudomonas aeruginosa* may develop resistance during treatment. Ongoing culture and sensitivity studies indicated. ▪ Prolonged use may cause superinfection because of overgrowth of nonsusceptible organisms. Monitor carefully. ▪ *Clostridium difficile*–associated diarrhea (CDAD) has been reported. May range from mild diarrhea to fatal colitis. Consider in patients who present with diarrhea during or after treatment with ciprofloxacin. ▪ Convulsions, increased intracranial pressure, and toxic psychosis have been reported in patients receiving quinolones, including ciprofloxacin. Ciprofloxacin may also cause CNS events, including confusion, depression, dizziness, hallucinations, and tremors. ▪ Use caution in patients with impaired renal function and known CNS disorders (e.g., epilepsy, severe cerebral arteriosclerosis, or any other factors that predispose to seizures). ▪ Tendinitis and tendon rupture that required surgical repair or resulted in prolonged disability have been reported in patients receiving quinolones. Most frequently involves the Achilles tendon but has also been reported with the shoulder, hand, biceps, thumb, and other tendon sites. ▪ Tendon rupture may occur during or after fluoroquinolone therapy. Risk may be increased in patients over 60 years of age; in patients taking corticosteroids; in patients with heart, kidney, or lung transplants; with strenuous physical activity; and in patients with renal failure or previous tendon disorders such as rheumatoid arthritis. ▪ Fluoroquinolones have neuromuscular blocking activity. Serious adverse events, including ventilatory support and deaths, have been reported in patients with myasthenia gravis. Avoid use in patients with a known history of myasthenia gravis; may exacerbate muscle weakness. ▪ Rare cases of peripheral neuropathy (e.g., paresthesias, hypoesthesias, dysesthesias [impairment of sensitivity or touch], or weakness) have been reported. ▪ Prolongation of the QT interval on ECG and infrequent cases of arrhythmia (including torsades de pointes) have been reported with the use of some fluoroquinolones. The risk of arrhythmia may be reduced by avoiding their use in the presence of hypokalemia, significant bradycardia, cardiomyopathy, or concurrent treatment with class 1A antiarrhythmic agents (e.g., quinidine, procainamide [Pronestyl]) or with class III antiarrhythmic agents (e.g., amiodarone [Nexterone], sotalol [Betapace]). ▪ Other serious events (sometimes fatal) due to hypersensitivity or uncertain etiology have been reported with fluoroquinolones; see Side Effects, Post-Marketing. Discontinue ciprofloxacin at the first appearance of a skin rash, jaundice, or other signs of hypersensitivity. ▪ Moderate to severe photosensitivity/

phototoxicity reactions have been reported in patients receiving quinolones; see Patient Education.

Monitor: May cause anaphylaxis with the first or succeeding doses, even in patients without known hypersensitivity. Emergency equipment must always be available. ▪ Monitor for S/S of peripheral neuropathy. Discontinue ciprofloxacin at the first symptoms of neuropathy (e.g., pain, burning, tingling, numbness and/or weakness) or if patient is found to have deficits in light touch, pain, temperature, position sense, vibratory sensation, and/or motor strength. ▪ Maintain adequate hydration and acidity of urine throughout treatment. Will form crystals in alkaline urine. ▪ Monitor hematopoietic, hepatic, and renal systems during prolonged treatment. ▪ Use of large veins recommended to reduce incidence of local irritation. Symptoms of local irritation do not preclude further administration of ciprofloxacin unless they recur or worsen. Generally resolve when infusion complete. ▪ Concomitant use with theophylline may cause cardiac arrest, respiratory failure, seizures, and/or status epilepticus. If concomitant use cannot be avoided, monitor serum levels of theophylline and adjust dose as indicated. ▪ Doses will increase slightly with transfer to oral ciprofloxacin (e.g., 200 mg IV every 12 hours equals 250 mg PO every 12 hours; 400 mg IV every 12 hours equals 500 mg PO every 12 hours; 400 mg IV every 8 hours equals 750 mg PO every 12 hours). ▪ See Drug/Lab Interactions.

Patient Education: A patient medication guide is available from the manufacturer. ▪ Inform physician of any history of myasthenia gravis. Patients with a history of myasthenia gravis should promptly report breathing problems or worsening muscle weakness. ▪ Consider birth control options. ▪ Photosensitivity has occurred in a minimum number of patients, but it is best to avoid excessive sunlight or artificial ultraviolet light. May cause severe sunburn; wear protective clothing, use sunscreen, and wear dark glasses outdoors. Report a sunburn-like reaction or skin eruption promptly. ▪ Request assistance for ambulation; may cause dizziness and lightheadedness. Use caution in tasks that require alertness. ▪ Effects of caffeine- or theophylline-containing preparations may be increased. Limit or eliminate concurrent use. Monitor if concurrent use necessary. ▪ Report tendon pain or inflammation promptly; rest and refrain from exercise. ▪ Promptly report skin rash or any other hypersensitivity reaction. ▪ Promptly report pain, burning, tingling, numbness and/or weakness. ▪ Inform physician of any history of seizures. ▪ Parents should inform physician of any history of joint-related problems and should promptly report any joint-related problems that develop during or after therapy. ▪ Promptly report diarrhea or bloody stools that occur during treatment or up to several months after an antibiotic has been discontinued; may indicate CDAD and require treatment.

Maternal/Child: Category C: use during pregnancy only if benefits justify potential risk to fetus and mother. ▪ Discontinue breast-feeding. ▪ Safety for use in pediatric patients under 18 years of age not established except for use post-exposure of inhalation anthrax and UTIs or pyelonephritis. Appropriateness based on risk/benefit assessment. ▪ May erode cartilage of weight-bearing joints or cause other signs of arthropathy in infants and children. ▪ Has been used in infants and children to treat serious infections unresponsive to other antibiotic regimens.

Elderly: Safety and effectiveness similar to younger adults. ▪ May be at increased risk of experiencing side effects (e.g., CNS effects, drug-associated effects on the QT interval, tendinitis, tendon rupture); see Precautions. Half-life may be slightly extended because of age-related renal impairment; see Dose Adjustments. Monitoring of renal function may be useful.

DRUG/LAB INTERACTIONS

Ciprofloxacin is an inhibitor of the hepatic CYP1A2 enzyme pathway. Coadministration with other drugs metabolized by this route, such as **methylxanthines** (e.g., theophylline) **or tizanidine** (Zanaflex), results in increased plasma concentrations of these drugs, which may cause significant toxicity. **Concomitant administration with tizanidine (Zanaflex) is contraindicated** (hypotensive and sedative effects potentiated). ▪ May cause serious or fatal reactions with **theophylline** (e.g., cardiac arrhythmias or arrest, respiratory failure, or seizures). If must be used concomitantly, monitor serum levels of theophylline and decrease dose as appropriate. Observe closely with caffeine intake; has caused similar problems. ▪ Use with **cyclosporine** may cause an increase in SCr and nephrotoxic effects. ▪ May potentiate **oral anticoagulants** (e.g., warfarin [Coumadin]); monitor PT/INR. ▪ Potentiated by **probenicid;** may require dose adjustment based on ciprofloxacin serum levels. ▪ Serum levels may be increased with **cimetidine** (Tagamet). ▪ Severe hypoglycemia has been reported with concomitant use of **glyburide** (DiaBeta); monitor serum glucose levels. ▪ May increase or decrease serum **phenytoin** levels; monitor phenytoin levels with concomitant use. ▪ Two case reports suggest concurrent administration with **foscarnet** (Foscavir) may cause seizures; monitor patient carefully. ▪ Risk of CNS stimulation and seizures may be increased with concurrent use of **NSAIDs** (e.g., ibuprofen [Advil, Motrin], naproxen [Aleve, Naprosyn]). ▪ Concurrent use with **methotrexate** requires close monitoring. May inhibit renal tubular transport of methotrexate, thereby increasing methotrexate serum levels and the risk of toxicity. ▪ Coadministration with **antiarrhythmic agents** that may prolong the QT interval (e.g., amiodarone [Nexterone], disopyramide [Norpace], quinidine) may increase the risk of life-threatening arrhythmias. ▪ Pharmacologic effects of **selected beta-blockers** (e.g., betaxolol [Kerlone], metoprolol [Lopressor], propranolol [Inderal LA]) may be increased. Monitor cardiac function when initiating or discontinuing ciprofloxacin. ▪ **Antineoplastic agents** (e.g., cyclophosphamide [Cytoxan], cytarabine [ARA-C], doxorubicin [Adriamycin]) may decrease the effectiveness of ciprofloxacin. ▪ May increase serum concentrations of many drugs (e.g, **clozapine** [Clozaril], **duloxetine** [Cymbalta], **lidocaine, methadone** [Dolophine], **mexiletine, MAO inhibitors** [e.g., rasagiline (Azilect)], **olanzapine** [Zyprexa], **procainamide** [Pronestyl], **ropivacaine** [Naropin]). Therapeutic effects and/or side effects may be increased; dose reductions of these drugs may be indicated. ▪ May cause a false-positive when **testing urine for opiates;** more specific testing methods may be indicated. ▪ See Side Effects.

SIDE EFFECTS

Diarrhea, hepatic enzyme abnormalities (elevation of alkaline phosphatase, AST, ALT, LDH, serum bilirubin), and nausea and vomiting and rash are reported most frequently. Other less frequent reactions include allergic reactions (anaphylaxis, cardiovascular collapse, death, dyspnea, edema [facial, pharyngeal, or pulmonary], eosinophilia, fever, itching, loss of consciousness, rash, urticaria); anorexia; cardiovascular effects (e.g., cardiac arrest, palpitations, QT interval prolongation, tachycardia, torsades de pointes, vasodilation, ventricular tachyarrhythmias); CDAD; CNS stimulation (confusion, hallucinations, light-headedness, restlessness, seizures, tingling, toxic psychosis, tremors); decreased hemoglobin, hematocrit, and platelet count; elevation of eosinophil and platelet counts, blood glucose, BUN, serum creatinine, serum creatine phosphokinase, serum potassium, uric acid, and triglycerides; headache; increased intracranial pressure; local site reactions; myalgias; nausea; peripheral neuropathy (e.g., pain, burning, tingling, numbness and/or weakness [see Precautions, Monitor]); photosensitivity/phototoxicity and vision changes; postural hypotension; respiratory failure; status epilepticus; tendinitis; and tendon rupture. Capable of numerous other reactions in fewer than 1% of patients.

Post-Marketing: Allergic pneumonitis, arthralgia, hematologic abnormalities (agranulocytosis, anemia [hemolytic and aplastic], leukopenia, pancytopenia, thrombocytopenia, thrombotic thrombocytopenic purpura), interstitial nephritis, jaundice, liver abnormalities (e.g., acute hepatic necrosis or failure, hepatitis, jaundice), myalgia, rash, serum sickness, severe dermatologic reactions (e.g., toxic epidermal necrolysis [Lyell's syndrome], Stevens-Johnson syndrome), vasculitis.

ANTIDOTE

Death may result from some of these side effects. Discontinue ciprofloxacin at the first appearance of a skin rash or major side effect (hypersensitivity, CDAD, CNS symptoms, dermatologic reactions, phototoxicity, or tendon rupture). Treat hypersensitivity reactions with epinephrine (Adrenalin), airway management, oxygen, IV fluids, antihistamines (diphenhydramine [Benadryl]), corticosteroids (hydrocortisone sodium succinate [Solu-Cortef]), and pressor amines (dopamine) as indicated. Treat CNS symptoms as indicated. May require diazepam (Valium) for seizures. Mild cases of CDAD may respond to discontinuation of ciprofloxacin. Treat CDAD with fluids, electrolytes, protein supplements, and oral vancomycin (Vancocin) or metronidazole (Flagyl) as indicated. In severe cases, surgical evaluation may be indicated. Drugs that inhibit peristalsis should be avoided. Keep physician informed of all side effects. Many will require symptomatic treatment; monitor closely. In overdose, observe carefully, provide supportive treatment, maintain hydration, and monitor renal function. No specific antidote; up to 10% may be removed by hemodialysis or peritoneal dialysis. Maintain patient until drug excreted.

CISATRACURIUM BESYLATE BBW

(sis-ah-trah-**KYOU**-ree-um **BES**-ih-layt)

Nimbex, Nimbex PF

Neuromuscular
blocking agent
(nondepolarizing)
Anesthesia adjunct

pH 3.25 to 3.65

USUAL DOSE

Must be individualized based on previous drugs administered (e.g., fentanyl [Sublimaze], midazolam [Versed]), desired time to intubation, and anticipated length of surgery. Must be used with adequate anesthesia and/or sedation and after unconsciousness induced. Use of a peripheral nerve stimulator is indicated in all situations.

ADJUNCT TO PROPOFOL/N₂O/O₂ ANESTHESIA FOR ADULTS (IV BOLUS)

Initial dose: 0.15 to 0.2 mg/kg. 0.15 mg/kg should provide good to excellent conditions for intubation within 2 minutes and adequate muscle relaxation for 55 minutes (range 44 to 74 min). 0.2 mg/kg (7 mL [of a 2 mg/mL conc] for a 70-kg patient) should be effective within 1.5 minutes and last for 61 minutes (range 41 to 81 min). Up to 0.4 mg/kg has been used; has a dose-related length of effectiveness.

Maintenance dose: May be given by IV bolus or as a continuous infusion. Determine need for maintenance dose based on beginning symptoms of neuromuscular blockade reversal determined by a peripheral nerve stimulator. Usually required 40 to 60 minutes after a bolus dose. Do not administer before recovery begins. Repeated doses have no cumulative effect if recovery is allowed to begin before administration. See Dose Adjustments.

IV bolus: 0.03 mg/kg (1 mL [of a 2 mg/mL conc] for a 70-kg patient) should provide an additional 20 minutes of muscle relaxation. Smaller or larger doses may be given based on expected duration of procedure.

Continuous infusion: Begin infusion with 3 mcg/kg/min to rapidly counteract the spontaneous recovery, then decrease to 1 to 2 mcg/kg/min. Monitor maintenance infusion with a peripheral nerve stimulator.

SUPPORT OF INTUBATED, MECHANICALLY VENTILATED, OR RESPIRATORY CONTROLLED ADULT ICU PATIENTS

After intubation is accomplished (usually with succinylcholine), an initial bolus dose of 0.1 mg/kg provides adequate neuromuscular blockade. Maintain with 3 mcg/kg/min (range 0.5 to 10.2 mcg/kg/min). Published reports describe a wide interpatient variability in dosing requirements that may change from day to day. Adjust infusion rate according to clinical assessment of the patient's response. Use of a peripheral nerve stimulator is recommended. Do not increase dose until there is a definite response to nerve stimulation. If recovery from neuromuscular block has progressed, readministration of a bolus dose may be necessary. Long-term use (beyond 6 days) has not been studied.

PEDIATRIC DOSE

See all comments under Usual Dose and Maternal/Child.

ADJUNCT TO HALOTHANE OR OPIOID ANESTHESIA FOR PEDIATRIC PATIENTS 1 MONTH TO 23 MONTHS OF AGE

0.15 mg/kg. Should produce maximum block in 2 minutes and adequate muscle relaxation for 43 minutes (range is 34 to 58 minutes).

ADJUNCT TO HALOTHANE OR OPIOID ANESTHESIA FOR PEDIATRIC PATIENTS 2 TO 12 YEARS OF AGE

Initial dose: 0.1 to 0.15 mg/kg as an IV bolus. 0.1 mg/kg should provide good to excellent conditions for intubation within 2.8 minutes and adequate muscle relaxation for 28 minutes (range 21 to 38 minutes). 0.15 mg/kg should produce maximum block in 3 minutes and adequate muscle relaxation for 36 minutes (range 29 to 46 minutes).

Maintenance dose: Same as adult dosing; See all comments.

DOSE ADJUSTMENTS

Reduce initial dose to 0.02 mg/kg in any condition that may result in a prolonged neuromuscular blockade (e.g., myasthenia gravis, myasthenic syndrome, carcinomatosis, debilitation, other drugs). Use a peripheral nerve stimulator to assess the level of neuromuscular block and to monitor dose requirements. See Drug/Lab Interactions. ▪ Increased initial and maintenance doses may be required in burn patients. Duration of action may be shortened. ▪ Half-life is extended but no dose adjustment is required in patients with renal or hepatic disease or in the elderly. Time of onset may be slightly faster in patients with liver disease and slower in the elderly and patients with renal disease. Slower onset may require a delay of an additional minute before intubation. ▪ Reduce maintenance dose by 30% to 40% in the presence of isoflurane or enflurane anesthesia. Larger reductions may be indicated in prolonged anesthesia. ▪ May need to reduce maintenance dose by 50% in patients undergoing coronary artery bypass surgery with induced hypothermia.

DILUTION

IV bolus: May be given undiluted.

Infusion: Further dilute in NS, D5W, or D5NS to a 0.1 mg/mL or 0.4 mg/mL solution. Using the 2 mg/mL solution, 10 mg diluted in 95 mL yields 0.1 mg/mL; 40 mg diluted in 80 mL yields 0.4 mg/mL.

ICU infusion: A 20-mL vial (10 mg/mL concentration) is available for use in ICU (200 mg/vial). 200 mg in 1,000 mL yields 0.2 mg/mL, in 500 mL yields 0.4 mg/mL.

Storage: Refrigerate in carton before use; protect from light; do not freeze. Use within 21 days if at room temperature even if it was re-refrigerated. Most diluted solutions are stable refrigerated or at room temperature for 24 hours.

COMPATIBILITY   (Underline Indicates Conflicting Compatibility Information)

Consider any drug NOT listed as compatible to be INCOMPATIBLE until consulting a pharmacist; specific conditions may apply.

Manufacturer lists propofol (Diprivan) and ketorolac (Toradol) as **incompatible.** Has an acid pH and may be **incompatible** with alkaline solutions having a pH greater than 8.5 (e.g., aminophylline, barbiturates, sodium bicarbonate).

Manufacturer lists alfentanil (Alfenta), droperidol (Inapsine), fentanyl (Sublimaze), midazolam (Versed), and sufentanil (Sufenta) as **compatible** but does not specify **additive** or **Y-site.**

Another source suggests the following **compatibilities:**

Y-site: Other sources list <u>acyclovir (Zovirax)</u>, alfentanil (Alfenta), amikacin (Amikin), <u>aminophylline</u>, <u>amphotericin B (generic)</u>, <u>ampicillin</u>, <u>ampicillin/ sulbactam (Unasyn)</u>, aztreonam (Azactam), bumetanide, buprenorphine (Buprenex), butorphanol (Stadol), calcium gluconate, <u>cefazolin (Ancef)</u>, <u>cefotaxime (Claforan)</u>, <u>cefoxitin (Mefoxin)</u>, <u>ceftazidime (Fortaz)</u>, ceftriaxone (Rocephin), cefuroxime (Zinacef), chlorpromazine (Thorazine), ciprofloxacin (Cipro IV), clindamycin (Cleocin), dexamethasone (Decadron), dexmedetomidine (Precedex), diazepam (Valium), digoxin (Lanoxin), diphenhydramine (Benadryl), dobutamine, dopamine, doxycycline, droperidol (Inapsine), drotrecogin alfa (Xigris), enalaprilat (Vasotec IV), epinephrine (Adrenalin), esmolol (Brevibloc), famotidine (Pepcid IV), fenoldopam (Corlopam), fentanyl (Sublimaze), fluconazole (Diflucan), furosemide (Lasix), ganciclovir (Cytovene), gentamicin, haloperidol (Haldol), heparin, hetastarch in electrolytes (Hextend), hydrocortisone sodium succinate (Solu-Cortef), hydromorphone (Dilaudid), imipenem-cilastatin (Primaxin), inamrinone (Amrinone), isoproterenol (Isuprel), ketorolac (Toradol), lidocaine, linezolid (Zyvox), lorazepam (Ativan), magnesium sulfate, mannitol, meperidine (Demerol), methylprednisolone (Solu-Medrol), metoclopramide (Reglan), metronidazole (Flagyl IV), midazolam (Versed), morphine, nalbuphine, nitroglycerin IV, nitroprusside sodium, norepinephrine (Levophed), ondansetron (Zofran), palonosetron (Aloxi), phenylephrine (Neo-Synephrine), piperacillin, piperacillin/tazobactam (Zosyn), potassium chloride (KCl), procainamide (Pronestyl), prochlorperazine (Compazine), promethazine (Phenergan), propofol (Diprivan), ranitidine (Zantac), remifentanil (Ultiva), sodium bicarbonate, sufentanil (Sufenta), sulfamethoxazole/trimethoprim, theophylline, thiopental (Pentothal), ticarcillin/clavulanate (Timentin), tobramycin, vancomycin, zidovudine (AZT, Retrovir).

RATE OF ADMINISTRATION

IV bolus: A single dose over 5 to 10 seconds.

Infusion for anesthesia adjunct or ICU: Use of a microdrip (60 gtt/mL) or volume infusion pump required. Adjust rate to desired dose based on the following charts for 0.1 mg/mL and 0.4 mg/mL. For 0.2 mg/mL solution in ICU, multiply rates (mL/hr) of 0.1 mg/mL solution by 2 or divide rates (mL/hr) of 0.4 mg/mL solution in half.

Cisatracurium Infusion Rates for a Concentration of 0.1 mg/mL					
Patient Weight (kg)	**Drug Delivery Rate (mcg/kg/min)**				
	1	1.5	2	3	5
	Infusion Delivery Rate (mL/hr)				
10 kg	6 mL/hr	9 mL/hr	12 mL/hr	18 mL/hr	30 mL/hr
45 kg	27 mL/hr	41 mL/hr	54 mL/hr	81 mL/hr	135 mL/hr
70 kg	42 mL/hr	63 mL/hr	84 mL/hr	126 mL/hr	210 mL/hr
100 kg	60 mL/hr	90 mL/hr	120 mL/hr	180 mL/hr	300 mL/hr

Cisatracurium Infusion Rates for a Concentration of 0.4 mg/mL					
Patient Weight (kg)	Drug Delivery Rate (mcg/kg/min)				
	1	1.5	2	3	5
	Infusion Delivery Rate (mL/hr)				
10 kg	1.5 mL/hr	2.3 mL/hr	3 mL/hr	4.5 mL/hr	7.5 mL/hr
45 kg	6.8 mL/hr	10.1 mL/hr	13.5 mL/hr	20.3 mL/hr	33.8 mL/hr
70 kg	10.5 mL/hr	15.8 mL/hr	21 mL/hr	31.5 mL/hr	52.5 mL/hr
100 kg	15 mL/hr	22.5 mL/hr	30 mL/hr	45 mL/hr	75 mL/hr

ACTIONS

A nondepolarizing skeletal muscle relaxant with intermediate onset and duration of action. An isomer of atracurium (Tracrium) with three times its potency at a mg-for-mg dose. In contrast to most of the other neuromuscular blocking agents, cisatracurium has no clinically significant effect on HR or BP with usual doses even in patients with serious cardiovascular disease, and it also does not produce a dose-related histamine release. Causes paralysis by interfering with neural transmission at the myoneural junction. Produces maximum neuromuscular blockade within 1.5 to 3 minutes and lasts about 50 minutes in adults. Recovery to 75% usually occurs within 30 minutes. Metabolized by a process that mostly bypasses both the kidney and the liver. Forms specific metabolites (e.g., alcohol, laudanosine) that do not have neuromuscular blocking activity. Because of reduced dose requirements, laudanosine accumulation is lower than with atracurium, lowering the potential of seizures. Eliminated renally, primarily as metabolites.

INDICATIONS AND USES

Adjunctive to general anesthesia for inpatients and outpatients to facilitate endotracheal intubation and to relax skeletal muscles during surgery. ■ Relax skeletal muscles during mechanical ventilation in ICU.

CONTRAINDICATIONS

Known hypersensitivity to cisatracurium, other bis-benzylisoquinolinium compounds (e.g., atracurium), and benzyl alcohol (some preparations contain benzyl alcohol).

PRECAUTIONS

For IV use only. ■ Administered by or under the observation of the anesthesiologist. Adequate facilities, emergency resuscitation drugs and equipment, neuromuscular blocking antagonists (e.g., anticholinesterase agents [e.g., neostigmine, edrophonium]), and atropine must always be available. ■ Not recommended for rapid sequence intubation; succinylcholine is usually the drug of choice. ■ Severe anaphylactic reactions have been reported with neuromuscular blocking agents; some have been fatal. Use caution in patients who have had an anaphylactic reaction to another neuromuscular blocking agent (depolarizing or nondepolarizing); cross-reactivity has occurred. ■ Myasthenia gravis and other neuromuscular diseases increase sensitivity to cisatracurium. Can cause critical reactions. ■ Sensitivity may be decreased in patients with burns or paralysis. See Dose Adjustments and Monitor. ■ In patients with renal or hepatic disease, half-life of metabolites is longer, and concentrations may be higher with long-term administration. ■ Did not trigger malignant hypertension (MH) in susceptible pigs at doses above those required for humans, but has not been studied in MH-susceptible humans. ■ Respiratory depression with propofol (Diprivan) or morphine may be preferred in some patients requiring mechanical ventilation. ■ Will not counteract the bradycardia produced by many anesthetic agents or vagal stimulation. ■ Transient hypotension and CNS excitation (generalized muscle twitching to seizures) have been reported rarely in ICU patients undergoing prolonged therapy.

Monitor: This drug produces apnea. Controlled artificial ventilation with oxygen must be continuous and under direct observation at all times. Maintain a patent airway. ■ Use a peripheral nerve stimulator to monitor drug effect, determine the need for additional doses, confirm recovery from neuromuscular block, and avoid overdose. Place on a nonparalyzed limb in patients with paralysis. ■ Monitor vital signs and ECG continuously. ■ Has no analgesic properties or effect on consciousness. Use in conjunction with anesthesia, sedation, or analgesia as indicated. ■ Action potentiated by hypokalemia and some carcinomas. ■ Action may be potentiated or antagonized by dehydration, electrolyte imbalance, body temperature, or acid-base imbalance.

Maternal/Child: Category B: use in pregnancy only if clearly needed. Safety for use during labor and delivery not established. ■ Use caution during breast-feeding; probably best to defer breast-feeding until after full recovery. ■ Safety for use in infants under 1 month of age not established. ■ 10 mL (2 mg/mL) multiple dose vials contain benzyl alcohol; do not use in newborns. ■ In pediatric patients 2 to 12 years of age, onset is faster, duration shorter, and recovery faster than in adults. In infants 1 month to 23 months of age, onset is faster; however, duration and recovery are similar to adults. ■ For induction of anesthesia in pediatric patients 1 month to 12 years of age, intubation was facilitated more reliably when cisatracurium was used in combination with halothane anesthesia than when used in combination with opioids and nitrous oxide. ■ Rare incidences of wheezing, laryngospasm, bronchospasm, rash, and itching have been reported in pediatric patients.

Elderly: Safely administered even in patients with significant cardiac disease. ■ Response similar to that seen in younger adults; however, greater sensitivity of some older individuals cannot be ruled out. ■ Onset to complete neuromuscular block slightly slower; delay intubation until fully effective. Recovery may be slower.

DRUG/LAB INTERACTIONS

Potentiated by **general anesthetics** (e.g., enflurane, isoflurane), many **antibiotics** (e.g., aminoglycosides [kanamycin (Kantrex), gentamicin], lincosamides [clindamycin (Cleocin)], polypeptides [bacitracin, colistimethate], tetracyclines), **muscle relaxants, diuretics, lithium, local anesthetics, magnesium sulfate, procainamide** (Pronestyl), **quinidine, succinylcholine, and others.** May need to reduce initial or maintenance dose of cisatracurium; use with caution. ■ Antagonized by **acetylcholine and anticholinesterases.** ■ Duration of neuromuscular block may be shorter and dose requirements may be higher during maintenance infusion in patients stabilized on **carbamazepine** (Tegretol) **or phenytoin** (Dilantin). ■ Time to onset of maximum block is faster when **succinylcholine** is given before cisatracurium. Succinylcholine must show signs of wearing off before cisatracurium is given. Use caution.

SIDE EFFECTS

Bradycardia, bronchospasm, flushing, hypotension, and rash occurred in fewer than 1% of patients. Both inadequate and/or prolonged neuromuscular blocks have been reported. Rare reports of seizures with similar agents in ICU could be caused by accumulated laudanosine, other conditions, or medications. Excessive dosing or prolonged action may result in respiratory insufficiency or apnea. Airway closure may be caused by relaxation of epiglottis, pharynx, and tongue muscles. Hypersensitivity reactions have been reported.

ANTIDOTE

Side effects can be medical emergencies. Treat symptomatically. Maintain a patent airway and continuous controlled artificial ventilation and oxygenation until full recovery is ensured. The more profound the neuromuscular block, the longer it will take until recovery begins. Recovery from neuromuscular block must be confirmed by a peripheral nerve stimulator before anticholinesterase agents (e.g., neostigmine or edrophonium [Enlon]) can be given with an anticholinergic agent (e.g., atropine) to reverse the muscle relaxation. Neostigmine 0.04 to 0.07 mg/kg at 10% recovery in conjunction with atropine should be effective in 9 to 10 minutes. Edrophonium 1 mg/kg at 25% recovery in conjunction with atropine (Enlon-Plus is edrophonium and atropine combined) should be effective in 3 to 5 minutes. Confirm recovery by 5-second head lift and grip strength. Recovery may be inhibited by cachexia, carcinomatosis, debilitation, or the concomitant use of certain drugs; see Drug/Lab Interactions. Resuscitate as necessary.

CISPLATIN BBW
(sis-**PLAH**-tin)
CDDP, Platinol

Antineoplastic
(alkylating agent)

pH 3.5 to 6

USUAL DOSE

Prehydration required; see Precautions and Monitor. See Dose Adjustments. May be given in combination with amifostine (Ethyol) to reduce nephrotoxicity and neurotoxicity of cisplatin. See amifostine monograph. Doses greater than 100 mg/M^2 once every 3 to 4 weeks are rarely used.

Metastatic testicular tumors: Used in combination with other approved chemotherapeutic agents. 20 mg/M^2 daily for 5 days per cycle.

Metastatic ovarian tumors: 75 to 100 mg/M^2 on Day 1 every 4 weeks. Used in combination with cyclophosphamide (Cytoxan) 600 mg/M^2 IV on Day 1 every 4 weeks. Another regimen uses paclitaxel 135 mg/M^2 (as a 24-hour infusion) followed by cisplatin 75 mg/M^2. Both agents are given once every 3 weeks for 6 courses. See paclitaxel monograph; premedication required. Used as a *single agent,* the dose of cisplatin is 100 mg/M^2 every 4 weeks.

First-line treatment of ovarian cancer: Given in combination with paclitaxel as follows: give paclitaxel (Taxol) 135 mg/M^2 as an infusion over 24 hours. Follow with cisplatin 75 mg/M^2 as an infusion over 6 to 8 hours. Repeat every 3 weeks. See paclitaxel monograph; premedication required. Other dose combinations and infusion times are being used.

Advanced bladder cancer: 50 to 70 mg/M^2 once every 3 to 4 weeks. 50 mg/M^2 is recommended once every 4 weeks for patients heavily pretreated with radiation or chemotherapy. Numerous other doses and combinations are used.

Non–small-cell lung cancer: Given in combination with gemcitabine as follows: gemcitabine (Gemzar) 1,000 mg/M^2 as an infusion on Days 1, 8, and 15 of each 28-day cycle. Follow the gemcitabine infusion on Day 1 with cisplatin 100 mg/M^2. See gemcitabine monograph; other dosing schedules are in use. Another regimen uses a combination of paclitaxel and cisplatin as follows: paclitaxel 135 mg/M^2 as an infusion over 24 hours followed by cisplatin 75 mg/M^2 over 6 to 8 hours. Repeat every 3 weeks. See paclitaxel monograph; premedication required. Also used with docetaxel 75 mg/M^2 infused over 1 hour followed immediately by an infusion of cisplatin 75 mg/M^2 over 30 to 60 minutes. Repeat every 3 weeks. See docetaxel monograph; premedication required.

Fallopian tube and peritoneal cancers of ovarian origin (unlabeled): Given in combination with paclitaxel as follows. Give paclitaxel 135 to 175 mg/M^2 as an infusion over 3 hours (extend to 24 hours as indicated by toxicity). Follow with cisplatin 50 to 75 mg/M^2. Repeat every 3 to 4 weeks. See paclitaxel monograph; premedication required.

DOSE ADJUSTMENTS

All doses adjusted based on prior radiation therapy or chemotherapy. ■ Initial or repeat doses may not be given unless SCr is below 1.5 mg/100 mL and/or BUN is below 25 mg/100 mL; platelets should be 100,000/mm^3 and leukocytes 4,000/mm^3; verify auditory acuity as within normal limits. ■ Dosing should be cautious in the elderly. Lower-end initial doses may be indicated. Consider decrease in cardiac, hepatic, and renal function; concomitant disease; or other drug therapy; see Elderly.

DILUTION
Specific techniques required; see Precautions. Initially dilute each 50-mg vial with 50 mL of SW for injection (1 mg/mL). Other products are available in liquid form, 1 mg/mL. Withdraw desired dose. Immediately before use, each one half of a single dose should be diluted in 1 liter of D5/¼NS, D5/½NS, or NS containing 12.5 to 25 Gm of mannitol (optional). Do not use D5W. Will decompose if adequate chloride ion not available. Is also diluted in smaller amounts of NS (100 to 500 mL). Do not use needles or IV tubing with aluminum parts to administer; a precipitate will form, and potency will decrease. See Monitor for additional optional additives.

Storage: Cisplatin remaining in multidose vial is stable at CRT for 28 days protected from light or 7 days under fluorescent light. Do not refrigerate. Reconstituted solution is stable for 20 hours at RT. Diluted solution is stable at room temperature for at least 24 hours; protect from light if it will not be used within 6 hours. Use immediately if contains mannitol.

COMPATIBILITY   (Underline Indicates Conflicting Compatibility Information)
Consider any drug NOT listed as compatible to be INCOMPATIBLE until consulting a pharmacist; specific conditions may apply.
Manufacturer states, "Do not use needles, IV sets, or equipment containing aluminum." A black platinum precipitate will form if cisplatin comes in contact with aluminum. A precipitate will form if reconstituted solutions are refrigerated.

One source suggests the following **compatibilities:**
Additive: Carboplatin (Paraplatin), cyclophosphamide (Cytoxan), etoposide (VePesid), ifosfamide (Ifex), ifosfamide with etoposide, leucovorin calcium, magnesium sulfate, mannitol, ondansetron (Zofran), paclitaxel (Taxol). Another source adds carmustine (BiCNU) and potassium chloride (KCl).

Y-site: Allopurinol (Aloprim), anidulafungin (Eraxis), aztreonam (Azactam), bleomycin (Blenoxane), caspofungin (Cancidas), chlorpromazine (Thorazine), cladribine (Leustatin), cyclophosphamide (Cytoxan), dexamethasone (Decadron), diphenhydramine (Benadryl), doripenem (Doribax), doxorubicin (Adriamycin), doxorubicin liposomal (Doxil), droperidol (Inapsine), etoposide (VePesid), etoposide phosphate (Etopophos), famotidine (Pepcid IV), filgrastim (Neupogen), fludarabine (Fludara), fluorouracil (5-FU), furosemide (Lasix), ganciclovir (Cytovene), gemcitabine (Gemzar), granisetron (Kytril), heparin, hydromorphone (Dilaudid), leucovorin calcium, linezolid (Zyvox), lorazepam (Ativan), melphalan (Alkeran), methotrexate, methylprednisolone (Solu-Medrol), metoclopramide (Reglan), mitomycin (Mutamycin), morphine, ondansetron (Zofran), paclitaxel (Taxol), palonosetron (Aloxi), pemetrexed (Alimta), prochlorperazine (Compazine), promethazine (Phenergan), propofol (Diprivan), ranitidine (Zantac), sargramostim (Leukine), teniposide (Vumon), topotecan (Hycamtin), vinblastine, vincristine, vinorelbine (Navelbine).

RATE OF ADMINISTRATION
Rates vary based on protocol. Manufacturer suggests administering each 1 liter of infusion solution over 3 to 4 hours. Give total dose (2 liters) over 6 to 8 hours. Rate must be sufficient to maintain hydration and diuresis. Infusion times of 30 to 120 minutes are common, but infusion time has

also been extended to 24 hours/dose. One source recommends a maximum rate not to exceed 1 mg/min. Too-rapid administration increases nephrotoxicity and ototoxicity.

ACTIONS

A heavy metal complex (platinum and chloride atoms). Has properties similar to alkylating agents and is cell-cycle nonspecific. Inhibits DNA synthesis by formation of DNA cross-links. Concentration is highest in liver, prostate, and kidney; somewhat lower in bladder, muscle, testicle, pancreas, and spleen; and lowest in bowel, adrenal, heart, lung, cerebrum, and cerebellum. Heavily protein bound. Only one fourth to one half of the drug is excreted in the urine by the end of 5 days. Platinum may be present in tissues for as long as 180 days after the last administration. Secreted in breast milk.

INDICATIONS AND USES

Treatment of metastatic tumors of the testes, ovaries, and advanced bladder cancer. ■ First-line therapy for treatment of advanced cancer of the ovary in combination with paclitaxel. ■ First-line treatment of patients with inoperable, locally advanced, or metastatic non–small-cell lung cancer (NSCLC) in combination with gemcitabine, paclitaxel, or docetaxel. ■ Is used in specific combinations with other chemotherapeutic drugs.
Unlabeled uses: Treatment of cancers of the brain, adrenal cortex, breast, cervix, uterus, endometrium, head and neck, esophagus, lung, skin, prostate, and stomach; sarcomas; non-Hodgkins lymphoma; trophoblastic neoplasms; and numerous other malignancies. Treatment of fallopian tube and peritoneal cancers of ovarian origin and cancers with an unknown primary site.

CONTRAINDICATIONS

Hypersensitivity to cisplatin or other platinum-containing compounds, myelosuppressed patients, pre-existing impaired renal function, or hearing deficit.

PRECAUTIONS

Follow guidelines for handling cytotoxic agents. See Appendix A, p. 1429. ■ Administered by or under the direction of the physician specialist. ■ Adequate facilities and emergency resuscitation equipment and supplies must always be available. ■ Renal toxicity can be cumulative and may be severe. ■ Other major dose-related toxicities include myelosuppression, nausea, and vomiting. ■ Ototoxicity (tinnitus, loss of high-frequency hearing, and/or deafness) can be significant and may be more pronounced in children. ■ Anaphylaxis has been reported and may occur within minutes of cisplatin administration. ■ Labeling changed to read, "Doses greater than 100 mg/M^2/cycle once every 3 to 4 weeks are rarely used." This is an effort to eliminate serious errors resulting from confusion with carboplatin (Paraplatin). ■ Neuropathies may occur with higher doses, greater frequency of average doses, or prolonged therapy. Usually occur after prolonged therapy but have been reported after a single dose. If symptoms of neuropathy are observed, discontinue cisplatin. ■ See Elderly.
Monitor: Obtain baseline CBC, SCr, BUN, CrCl and calcium, magnesium, potassium, and sodium levels. Repeat CBC weekly and other listed labs before each subsequent cycle. ■ Hydrate patient with 1 to 2 L of infusion fluid for 8 to 12 hours before injection. Urine output should exceed 100 to 150 mL/hr. ■ Maintain adequate hydration and urine output of at least 100 to 200 mL/hr for 24 hours after each dose. ■ The greater the dose, the

more hydration is required (e.g., 20 mg/M^2, 1 L; 40 mg/M^2, 2 L). Potassium chloride (20 mEq) and magnesium sulfate (8 mEq) are frequently added to predosing fluids and/or cisplatin. ▪ In addition to mannitol, furosemide (Lasix) may be added to cisplatin if fluid overload is a concern. Avoid salt and water depletion. ▪ Nausea and vomiting are frequently severe and prolonged (up to a week). Prophylactic administration of antiemetics recommended. Ondansetron (Zofran), metoclopramide (Reglan), or dexamethasone are effective in most patients. ▪ Ototoxicity is cumulative; test hearing before administration and regularly during treatment. Ototoxicity increased in pediatric patients. ▪ Monitor uric acid levels before and during treatment and maintain hydration. Allopurinol may be indicated (preferred agent); see Drug/Lab Interactions. Alkalinization of urine may also be indicated. ▪ Monitor liver function periodically and perform neurologic exams on a regular basis. ▪ Replace depleted electrolytes as necessary. ▪ Observe closely for signs of infection. Prophylactic antibiotics may be indicated pending results of C/S in a febrile neutropenic patient. ▪ Monitor for thrombocytopenia (platelet count less than 50,000/mm^3). Initiate precautions to prevent excessive bleeding (e.g., inspect IV sites, skin, and mucous membranes; use extreme care during invasive procedures; test urine, emesis, stool, and secretions for occult blood).

Patient Education: Nonhormonal birth control recommended. ▪ See Appendix D, p. 1434.

Maternal/Child: Category D: avoid pregnancy; will produce teratogenic effects on the fetus. Has a mutagenic potential. ▪ Discontinue breastfeeding. ▪ Safety and effectiveness for use in pediatric patients not established. ▪ Ototoxicity increased in pediatric patients.

Elderly: Dose selection should be cautious; see Dose Adjustments. ▪ Response (e.g., effectiveness) is similar to younger adults, but length of survival may be shorter. ▪ Incidence of myelosuppression (e.g., severe leukopenia, neutropenia, thrombocytopenia), infectious complications, nephrotoxicity, and peripheral neuropathy may be increased.

DRUG/LAB INTERACTIONS

Ototoxicity and nephrotoxicity are potentiated with other **ototoxic or nephrotoxic agents** (e.g., aminoglycosides [e.g., gentamicin] and loop diuretics [e.g., furosemide (Lasix), ethacrynic acid (Edecrin)]). Concurrent use not recommended (Lasix is used to control fluid overload, use caution). ▪ Serum levels of **anticonvulsant agents** (e.g., phenytoin [Dilantin]) may become subtherapeutic when used concurrently with cisplatin. Monitor anticonvulsant levels; increased doses may be indicated. ▪ Bone marrow toxicity increased with **other antineoplastic agents and/or radiation therapy.** ▪ Synergistic with **etoposide** (VePesid); may be beneficial. ▪ May affect renal excretion and increase toxicity of many drugs **(e.g., bleomycin, methotrexate).** ▪ Cisplatin may increase myelosuppressive effects of **taxane derivatives** (e.g., paclitaxel). ▪ Administer taxane derivative before cisplatin to decrease myelotoxicity. ▪ Response duration may be shortened with concurrent use of **pyridoxine (vitamin B$_6$) and altretamine (Hexalen).** ▪ Do not administer **live virus vaccines** to patients receiving antineoplastic agents.

SIDE EFFECTS

Are frequent; can occur with the initial dose and will become more severe with succeeding doses. Acute leukemia, alopecia, anaphylaxis (facial edema, hypotension, tachycardia, and wheezing within minutes of administration), asthenia, cardiac abnormalities, dehydration, diarrhea, electrolyte disturbances (hypocalcemia, hypokalemia, hypomagnesemia, hyponatremia, hypophosphatemia), elevated serum amylase, hemolytic anemia, hepatotoxicity, hyperuricemia, malaise, myelosuppression, nausea and vomiting, nephrotoxicity (often noted in the second week after a dose), ocular toxicity (e.g., blurred vision, cerebral blindness, optic neuritis, papilledema), ototoxicity including tinnitus and hearing loss in the high-frequency range, peripheral neuropathy (may be irreversible), vascular toxicities (e.g., cerebral arteritis, CVA, MI, or thrombotic microangiopathy [hemolytic-uremic syndrome (HUS)]), and vestibular toxicity.

Overdose: Deafness, intractable nausea and vomiting, kidney failure, liver failure, neuritis, ocular toxicity, significant myelosuppression, and death.

ANTIDOTE

Notify physician of all side effects. Cisplatin may have to be discontinued permanently or until recovery. Symptomatic and supportive treatment is indicated. Administration of whole blood products (e.g., packed RBCs, platelets, leukocytes) and/or blood modifiers (e.g., darbepoetin alfa [Aranesp], epoetin alfa [Epogen], filgrastim [Neupogen], oprelvekin [Neumega], pegfilgrastim [Neulasta], sargramostim [Leukine]) may be indicated to treat bone marrow toxicity. Pretreatment with amifostine may reduce nephrotoxic, neurotoxic, and hematologic effects. Treat anaphylaxis with epinephrine, corticosteroids, oxygen, and antihistamines. There is no specific antidote. Hemodialysis appears to have little effect on removing platinum from the body because of the rapid and high degree of protein binding.

CLADRIBINE BBW

(**KLAD**-rih-bean)

Leustatin

Antineoplastic
(antimetabolite)

pH 6 to 6.6

USUAL DOSE

In all situations, may be administered on an outpatient basis with an appropriate pump and a central venous line in place. Administer any subsequent course with extreme caution. Hematologic recovery must be considered.

Hairy cell leukemia: 0.09 mg/kg/day equally distributed as a continuous infusion over 24 hours. Repeat daily for 7 consecutive days. Another source suggests 0.1 mg/kg/day. Usually only one course of treatment is given. Patients with a partial response may require a second dose.

Other malignancies (unlabeled): 0.1 to 0.3 mg/kg/day equally distributed as a continuous infusion over 24 hours for 7 consecutive days. May be repeated if indicated every 28 to 35 days.

DOSE ADJUSTMENTS

May be required in subsequent courses, with severe bone marrow impairment, with prior radiation or myelosuppressive agents. ■ May be required in severe renal insufficiency; effects of renal or hepatic impairment on excretion of cladribine not yet clarified for humans. ■ See Drug/Lab Interactions.

DILUTION

Specific techniques required; see Precautions. Available in single-use 10-mL vials containing 10 mg (1 mg/mL). Contains no preservatives; aseptic technique imperative. May develop a precipitate at low temperatures. Warm naturally to room temperature and shake vigorously. Do not heat or microwave.

Inpatient continuous infusion: A single daily calculated dose must be added to 500 mL of NS.

Outpatient continuous infusion: A total 7-day dose is added to a calculated amount of bacteriostatic NS to make a total volume of 100 mL. Specific equipment (i.e., a sterile medication reservoir and pump capable of delivering accurate minute amounts into a central venous line [presently using SIMS Deltec medication cassette with SIMS Deltec pump]) and a specific process including the use of a 0.22-micron syringe filter are required. Preparation of cassette usually done by pharmacist. Line of cassette remains clamped until attached to central venous line and pump is functional. See literature for details and follow all specific instructions for medication pump.

Filters: To minimize the risk of microbial contamination, a 0.22-micron hydrophilic syringe filter is required in the preparation of the outpatient continuous infusion. Manufacturer recommends passing first the cladribine and then the bacteriostatic NS through the filter into the infusion reservoir. See Dilution.

Storage: Protect from light. Refrigerate or freeze before reconstitution. Never refreeze. Discard any unused concentrate. *500 mL dilution* may be refrigerated for up to 8 hours after dilution. Immediate use preferred. *100 mL dilution* is stable in reservoir of medication cassette for 7 days if correctly diluted.

COMPATIBILITY

Consider any drug NOT listed as compatible to be INCOMPATIBLE until consulting a pharmacist; specific conditions may apply.

D5W will cause degradation of cladribine. Manufacturer states, "Adherence to the recommended diluents and infusion systems is advised."

One source suggests the following **compatibilities:**

Y-site: Aminophylline, bumetanide, buprenorphine (Buprenex), butorphanol (Stadol), calcium gluconate, carboplatin (Paraplatin), chlorpromazine (Thorazine), cisplatin (Platinol), cyclophosphamide (Cytoxan), cytarabine (ARA-C), dexamethasone (Decadron), diphenhydramine (Benadryl), dobutamine, dopamine, doxorubicin (Adriamycin), droperidol (Inapsine), enalaprilat (Vasotec IV), etoposide (VePesid), famotidine (Pepcid IV), furosemide (Lasix), gallium nitrate (Ganite), granisetron (Kytril), haloperidol (Haldol), heparin, hydrocortisone sodium succinate (Solu-Cortef), hydromorphone (Dilaudid), idarubicin (Idamycin), leucovorin calcium, lorazepam (Ativan), mannitol, meperidine (Demerol), mesna (Mesnex), methylprednisolone (Solu-Medrol), metoclopramide (Reglan), mitoxantrone (Novantrone), morphine, nalbuphine, ondansetron (Zofran), paclitaxel (Taxol), potassium chloride (KCl), prochlorperazine (Compazine), promethazine (Phenergan), ranitidine (Zantac), sodium bicarbonate, teniposide (Vumon), vincristine.

RATE OF ADMINISTRATION

Inpatient continuous infusion: A single dose properly diluted evenly distributed as an infusion over 24 hours.

Outpatient continuous infusion: Administered through a central venous line (very concentrated solution). Medication reservoir and pump required (presently using Pharmacia Deltec medication cassette and pump worn as a portable pack). Set rate for equal distribution of 100 mL over 7 days. Follow all specific instructions for pump.

ACTIONS

A synthetic antineoplastic agent. Mechanism of action is not known, but it is believed to be cytotoxic by inhibiting both DNA synthesis and repair. Affects both dividing and resting cells. The 7-day course for hairy cell leukemia has resulted in complete remissions in a majority of patients with no evidence of persistent bone marrow disease. May potentially be a cure. Improvements in neurologic symptoms are occurring in patients with multiple sclerosis. In all situations time to response is about 4 months. Has immunosuppressant activity. Lymphocyte subsets (e.g., CD4, CD8 T cells) are affected; may take 6 to 12 months for full recovery. Crosses the blood-brain barrier. Average half-life is 5.4 hours. Metabolized in all cells. Specific methods of metabolism and routes of excretion are not known. Some drug does appear in urine.

INDICATIONS AND USES

Treatment of active hairy cell leukemia (HCL) as defined by clinically significant anemia, neutropenia, thrombocytopenia, or disease-related symptoms.

Unlabeled uses: Treatment of acute myeloid leukemia, chronic lymphocytic leukemia, and non-Hodgkin's lymphoma.

CONTRAINDICATIONS

Hypersensitivity to cladribine or any of its components; neonates (7 day dilution contains benzyl alcohol).

PRECAUTIONS

Follow guidelines for handling cytotoxic agents. See Appendix A, p. 1429. ■ Administered by or under the direction of the physician specialist. ■ Anticipate severe suppression of bone marrow function, including neutropenia, anemia, and thrombocytopenia; usually reversible and appears to be dose dependent. ■ Neurologic toxicity, including paraparesis and quadriparesis, has been reported. Usually occurs with higher doses but has been seen with standard dosing regimens. ■ Because of the possibility of increased toxicity, use caution in known or suspected renal insufficiency, or any severe bone marrow impairment, or prior cytoxic or radiation therapy. ■ Acute nephrotoxicity has been observed with high doses (4 to 9 times the recommended dose for HCL). Risk of toxicity increased when given concurrently with other nephrotoxic agents and/or therapies. ■ Appears to be no relationship between serum concentrations and ultimate clinical outcome. ■ Additional courses did not improve overall response. ■ Current studies suggest that overall response rate may be decreased in patients previously treated with splenectomy, deoxycoformycin (pentostatin), and in patients refractory to alpha-interferon. ■ May cause prolonged bone marrow hypocellularity; clinical significance not known.

Monitor: Obtain baseline CBC with differential (including CD4 and CD8 T cell counts) and platelets before therapy. May be repeated as indicated, but usually not required again until 7 or 8 days after treatment begins; then monitor as indicated for at least 4 to 8 weeks (anemia, neutropenia, thrombocytopenia, infection [bacterial, fungal, or viral], and bleeding are common and must be treated promptly). Monitoring schedule facilitates outpatient treatment; keep in close contact with patient. ■ Consider possibility of infection if fever occurs; appropriate lab tests, x-rays and broad-spectrum antibiotics may be indicated in suspected infection. ■ Monitor uric acid levels before and during treatment, maintain hydration; allopurinol may be indicated (preferred agent). Alkalinization of urine may also be indicated. ■ Monitor renal and hepatic function periodically. ■ Take precautions and limit invasive procedures in any patient with thrombocytopenia. Avoid constipation, and avoid alcohol and aspirin (risk of GI bleeding). ■ Platelet count usually returns to normal in 12 days (may be delayed if severe baseline thrombocytopenia was present), absolute neutrophil count (ANC) usually returns to normal in 5 weeks, and hemoglobin in 8 weeks. All should be normal by 9 weeks. ■ Complete response is indicated by an absence of hairy cells in bone marrow and peripheral blood and normalization of peripheral blood parameters. Confirm response with bone marrow aspiration and biopsy between 9 weeks and 4 months. ■ Prophylactic antiemetics may improve patient comfort. ■ Monitor for thrombocytopenia (platelet count less than 50,000/mm^3). Initiate precautions to prevent excessive bleeding (e.g., inspect IV sites, skin, and mucous membranes; use extreme care during invasive procedures; test urine, emesis, stool, and secretions for occult blood).

Patient Education: Avoid pregnancy; consider birth control options and future fertility. ■ Report fever, bleeding, cough, edema, injection site reactions, malaise, mouth sores, rashes, shortness of breath, stomach pain, and tachycardia promptly. Maintain hydration. ■ Manufacturer supplies a patient education booklet; review thoroughly and discuss with physician and nurse. ■ Review all literature provided with pump to deliver outpatient dosing. ■ See Appendix D, p. 1434.

Maternal/Child: Category D: avoid pregnancy; has potential to cause fetal harm. Has caused suppression of testicular cells in monkeys; effect on human fertility unknown. ■ Discontinue breast-feeding. ■ Safety for use in pediatric patients not established. Investigationally used in higher doses to treat relapsed acute leukemia. Dose-limiting toxicity occurred.

Elderly: Geriatric-specific problems not encountered in studies to date. Consider age-related organ impairment.

DRUG/LAB INTERACTIONS

Increased toxicity with other **myelosuppressive agents** (e.g., methotrexate). ■ May raise concentration of blood uric acid, increased doses of **antigout agents** (e.g., allopurinol [Aloprim]) may be indicated; **avoid uricosurics** (e.g., probenicid, sulfinpyrazone [Anturane]). ■ Do not administer **live virus vaccines** to patients receiving antineoplastic agents.

SIDE EFFECTS

Fever (69%) occurs first. Onset of thrombocytopenia (12%) begins in 7 to 10 days followed by anemia (severe [37%]) and neutropenia (severe [70%]). Fatigue (45%), headache (22%), injection site reactions (19%), infection (28%), nausea (28%), and rash (27%) are common. Many other side effects may or may not be related to cladribine; abdominal pain (6%), abnormal breath sounds (11%), abnormal chest sounds (9%), anorexia (17%), arthralgia (5%), asthenia (9%), chills (9%), constipation (9%), cough (10%), diaphoresis (9%), diarrhea (10%), dizziness (9%), edema (6%), epistaxis (5%), erythema (6%), insomnia (7%), malaise (7%), myalgia (7%), pain (6%), petechiae (8%), pruritus (6%), purpura (10%), shortness of breath (7%), tachycardia (6%), trunk pain (6%), weakness (9%), vomiting (13%).

Post-Marketing: Most of these additional side effects occurred in patients who received multiple courses of cladribine and include aplastic anemia, elevated bilirubin and transaminases, hemolytic anemia, hypereosinophilia, myelodysplastic syndrome, neurologic toxicity, opportunistic infections, pulmonary interstitial infiltrates (usually with an infectious etiology), Stevens-Johnson syndrome, and toxic epidermal necrolysis.

Overdose: Acute nephrotoxicity, irreversible neurologic toxicity (paraparesis/quadriparesis), severe bone marrow suppression (anemia, neutropenia, and thrombocytopenia).

ANTIDOTE

Keep physician informed of all side effects; many will be treated symptomatically as indicated. Platelet or RBC transfusions are frequently required to treat anemia or thrombocytopenia, especially during the first month. Filgrastim (Neupogen) or pegfilgrastim (Neulasta) may be used to increase neutrophil count, although recovery is usually spontaneous. Use specific antibiotics to combat infection. Discontinue cladribine if renal toxicity, neurotoxicity, or overdose occurs. No specific antidote for overdose. Supportive therapy as indicated will help sustain the patient in toxicity. Resuscitate if indicated.

CLEVIDIPINE BUTYRATE

(klev-**ID**-i-peen **BUE**-tih-rate)

Cleviprex

Calcium channel blocker
Antihypertensive

pH 6 to 8

USUAL DOSE

Must be individualized to achieve the desired BP reduction. Titrate to patient response and BP goal.

Initial dose: 1 to 2 mg/hr (2 to 4 mL/hr) as a continuous infusion.

Dose titration: Initially, double the dose at 90-second intervals. As the BP approaches goal, increase the dose by less than doubling and lengthen the time between dose adjustments to every 5 to 10 minutes. In general, a 1- to 2-mg/hr increase in dose will produce an additional 2- to 4-mm Hg decrease in systolic pressure. The maximum dose used for most patients in studies was 16 mg/hr.

Maintenance dose: The desired therapeutic response for most patients occurs at 4 to 6 mg/hr (8 to 12 mL/hr). Doses as high as 32 mg/hr (64 mL/hr) have been administered. Data are limited. Because of lipid-load restrictions, no more than 1,000 mL or an average of 21 mg/hr (42 mL/hr) is recommended per 24-hour period. In studies, most infusions were administered for less than 24 hours. There is little experience with infusions lasting more than 72 hours at any dose.

Transition to oral therapy: Discontinue or titrate the infusion downward while establishing appropriate oral therapy. Consider the lag time of onset of oral agent's effect. See Monitor.

DOSE ADJUSTMENTS

Lower-end initial doses may be indicated in the elderly. Consider the potential for decreased organ function and concomitant disease or drug therapy. ▪ Patients with abnormal hepatic or renal function may receive the initial dose listed under Usual Dose.

DILUTION

Strict aseptic technique is imperative. Available as a single-dose, ready-to-use vial containing a 0.5-mg/mL phospholipid emulsion that can support microbial growth. Invert vial gently several times before use to ensure uniformity of emulsion.

Filter: No data available from manufacturer.

Storage: Refrigerate unopened vials at 2° to 8° C (36° to 46° F) or store at 25° C (77° F) for up to 2 months. Vials stored at RT should not be returned to the refrigerator. Do not freeze. Protect from light until administration. Once vial is punctured, use within 4 hours and discard any unused portion, including that which is currently being infused.

COMPATIBILITY

Manufacturer states, "Should not be administered in the same line as other medications. Should not be diluted, but can be administered via a Y-tube or medication port with SW, NS, D5W, D5NS, D5LR, LR, and 10% amino acid."

RATE OF ADMINISTRATION

Administer as a continuous infusion as outlined in Usual Dose. Use of an infusion device required. May be given through a central or peripheral line.

ACTIONS

A dihydropyridine calcium channel blocker. Mediates the influx of calcium during depolarization in arterial smooth muscle. Reduces mean arterial BP by decreasing systemic vascular resistance in a dose-dependent manner. Does not reduce cardiac filling pressure (preload), confirming the lack of effect on venous capacitance vessels. Vasodilation and the resulting decrease in BP may produce a reflex increase in heart rate. Onset of effects begins within 2 to 4 minutes. Evidence of tolerance or hysteresis has not been observed in patients receiving infusions of up to 72 hours' duration. Full recovery of BP is achieved 5 to 15 minutes after the infusion is stopped. Rapidly distributed. Highly protein bound. Metabolized by hydrolysis in the blood and extravascular tissues, making its elimination unlikely to be affected by hepatic or renal dysfunction. Half-life is approximately 15 minutes. Excreted primarily in urine and, to a lesser extent, in feces.

INDICATIONS AND USES

Reduction of BP when oral therapy is not feasible or not desirable.

CONTRAINDICATIONS

Allergies to soybeans, soy products, eggs, or egg products. ▪ Defective lipid metabolism such as pathologic hyperlipidemia, lipoid nephrosis, or acute pancreatitis if accompanied by hyperlipidemia. ▪ Severe aortic stenosis (afterload reduction can be expected to reduce myocardial oxygen delivery).

PRECAUTIONS

For IV use only. ▪ Strict aseptic technique required; see Dilution. ▪ May produce systemic hypotension and reflex tachycardia. Dose reduction may be indicated. ▪ Use caution in patients with lipid metabolism disorders. Contains approximately 0.2 Gm of lipid per mL. Lipid intake restrictions may be necessary in these patients. A reduction in the quantity of concurrently administered lipids (e.g., propofol, IV fat) may be necessary to compensate for the amount of lipid infused as part of the clevidipine formulation. See Usual Dose. ▪ May produce a negative inotropic effect and exacerbate heart failure. ▪ Rebound hypertension may occur in patients undergoing prolonged therapy; see Monitor. ▪ Has not been studied for the treatment of hypertension associated with pheochromocytoma.

Monitor: Monitor BP and HR during infusion and until vital signs are stable. ▪ Rebound hypertension may occur in patients who receive a prolonged infusion and are not transitioned to other antihypertensive therapies. Monitor BP for at least 8 hours after the infusion is discontinued. ▪ During transition to oral therapy, continue BP monitoring until patient is stabilized. ▪ Monitor heart failure patients closely.

Patient Education: Promptly report signs of a hypertensive emergency (e.g., neurologic symptoms, vision changes, evidence of CHF). ▪ Continued follow-up and treatment of pre-existing hypertension required.

Maternal/Child: Category C: use during pregnancy only if potential benefit justifies potential risk to the fetus. ▪ Safety in labor and delivery not established. Other calcium channel blockers suppress uterine contractions in humans. ▪ Safety for use in breast-feeding not established; effects unknown. ▪ Safety and effectiveness for use in pediatric patients not established.

Elderly: Response similar to that seen in younger adults; however, greater sensitivity in the elderly cannot be ruled out. ▪ See Dose Adjustments.

DRUG/LAB INTERACTIONS

Formal studies have not been conducted. ▪ Does not have the potential for inducing or inhibiting the cytochrome P_{450} system. ▪ Use of **beta-blockers** as treatment for clevidipine-induced reflex tachycardia is not recommended. Experience is limited. ▪ If used concomitantly with **beta-blockers** and beta-blockers are to be discontinued, withdraw beta-blocker therapy gradually. Clevidipine will not protect against the effects of abrupt beta-blocker withdrawal.

SIDE EFFECTS

Acute renal failure, atrial fibrillation, cardiac arrest, dyspnea, flushing, headache, hypotension, myocardial infarction, nausea, peripheral edema, rebound hypertension, reflex tachycardia, syncope, and vomiting.

ANTIDOTE

Notify physician of any side effects; most will be treated symptomatically. Reduce dose for systemic hypotension or reflex tachycardia. Discontinue for suspected overdose. Reduction in antihypertensive effects should be seen within 5 to 15 minutes. Monitor BP and support if needed. Resuscitate as necessary.

CLINDAMYCIN PHOSPHATE BBW
(klin-dah-**MY**-cin **FOS**-fayt)

Antibacterial
Antiprotozoal
(lincosamide)

Cleocin Phosphate

pH 5.5 to 7

USUAL DOSE

Doses based on susceptibility of specific organisms; see literature.

Serious infections: 600 to 1,200 mg/24 hr in 2, 3, or 4 equally divided doses (300 to 600 mg every 12 hours, 200 to 400 mg every 8 hours, or 150 to 300 mg every 6 hours).

More severe infections: 1,200 to 2,700 mg/24 hr in 2, 3, or 4 equally divided doses (600 to 1,350 mg every 12 hours, 400 to 900 mg every 8 hours, or 300 to 675 mg every 6 hours).

Life-threatening infections: Up to 4.8 Gm/24 hr has been given.

Acute pelvic inflammatory disease (unlabeled): 900 mg every 8 hours for at least 4 days. Concurrent administration of 2 mg/kg of gentamicin as an initial dose and 1.5 mg/kg every 8 hours thereafter is recommended. Continue both drugs for at least 48 hours after patient improves. Complete 10- to 14-day treatment program with oral doxycycline or clindamycin.

CNS toxoplasmosis in AIDS (unlabeled): 1,200 to 2,400 mg/24 hr in divided doses (e.g., 300 to 600 mg every 6 hours). Up to 4.8 Gm has been required. Used in combination with pyrimethamine (Daraprim).

***Pneumocystis jiroveci* pneumonia (unlabeled):** 600 mg every 6 hours or 900 mg every 8 hours. Used in combination with primaquine.

Babesiosis (unlabeled): 1,200 to 2,400 mg/24 hr in 4 equally divided doses (300 to 600 mg every 6 hours). Continue for 7 to 10 days. Used in combination with quinine.

Prophylaxis of bacterial endocarditis: 600 mg IV or PO 30 minutes before procedure and 150 mg IV or PO in 6 hours.

PEDIATRIC DOSE

Minimum recommended dose regardless of weight is 300 mg/24 hr for severe infections.

Pediatric patients over 1 month of age: 20 to 40 mg/kg of body weight/24 hr in 3 or 4 equally divided doses for serious infections (5 to 10 mg/kg every 6 hours or 6.66 to 13.3 mg/kg every 8 hours). Alternately 350 mg/M^2/24 hr may be used (87.5 mg/M^2 every 6 hours or 116.6 mg/M^2 every 8 hours). 450 mg/M^2/24 hr may be used for more serious infections if necessary (112.5 mg/M^2 every 6 hours or 150 mg/M^2 every 8 hours).

Bone infections: 7.5 mg/kg every 6 hours.

Babesiosis (unlabeled): A suggested dose is 20 mg/kg/24 hr. Continue for 7 to 10 days. Used in combination with 25 mg/kg/24 hr of oral quinine.

Prophylaxis of bacterial endocarditis: 10 mg/kg IV or PO 30 minutes before procedure. Give 5 mg/kg IV or PO in 6 hours.

NEONATAL DOSE

See Maternal/Child.

Under 1 month of age, full term: 3.75 to 5 mg/kg every 6 hours or 5 to 6.7 mg/kg every 8 hours. Another source suggests:

Infants under 7 days of age weighing less than 2 kg: 5 mg/kg every 12 hours.

Continued

Infants under 7 days of age weighing over 2 kg: 5 mg/kg every 8 hours.
Infants over 7 days of age weighing less than 1.2 kg: 5 mg/kg every 12 hours.
Infants over 7 days of age weighing 1.2 to 2 kg: 5 mg/kg every 8 hours.
Infants over 7 days of age weighing over 2 kg: 5 mg/kg every 6 hours.

DOSE ADJUSTMENTS
May be required in severely impaired liver or renal function.

DILUTION
Available prediluted in 300-, 600-, and 900-mg ready-to-use Galaxy bags or ADD-Vantage vials for use with ADD-Vantage infusion containers, or each 18 mg must be reconstituted with a minimum of 1 mL of D5W, NS, or other **compatible** infusion solution (300 mg with 17 mL diluent, 600 mg with 34 mL, and 900 mg with 50 mL). See chart on inside back cover or product insert for additional diluents. Additional diluent (50 to 100 mL) may be used to decrease concentration, but never exceed a concentration greater than 18 mg/mL. May be further diluted in larger amounts of **compatible** infusion solutions and given as a continuous infusion after the initial dose.

Storage: Stable at CRT for 24 hours in **compatible** diluents and infusion solutions.

COMPATIBILITY   (Underline Indicates Conflicting Compatibility Information)
Consider any drug NOT listed as compatible to be INCOMPATIBLE until consulting a pharmacist; specific conditions may apply.
Manufacturer lists as **incompatible** with aminophylline, ampicillin, barbiturates, calcium gluconate, magnesium sulfate, phenytoin (Dilantin).
   Sources suggest the following **compatibilities:**
Solution: Isolyte H, D5/Isolyte M, D5/Isolyte P, Normosol R; see chart on inside back cover.
Additive: Manufacturer states no **incompatibility** has been demonstrated with gentamicin, kanamycin (Kantrex), or penicillin. Other sources list amikacin (Amikin), ampicillin, aztreonam (Azactam), cefazolin (Ancef), cefepime (Maxipime), cefotaxime (Claforan), cefoxitin (Mefoxin), ceftazidime (Fortaz), cefuroxime (Zinacef), fluconazole (Diflucan), heparin, hydrocortisone sodium succinate (Solu-Cortef), methylprednisolone (Solu-Medrol), metoclopramide (Reglan), piperacillin, potassium chloride (KCl), ranitidine (Zantac), sodium bicarbonate, tobramycin, verapamil.
Y-site: Acyclovir (Zovirax), amifostine (Ethyol), amiodarone (Nexterone), amphotericin B cholesteryl (Amphotec), anidulafungin (Eraxis), aztreonam (Azactam), bivalirudin (Angiomax), cisatracurium (Nimbex), cyclophosphamide (Cytoxan), dexmedetomidine (Precedex), diltiazem (Cardizem), docetaxel (Taxotere), doxorubicin liposomal (Doxil), enalaprilat (Vasotec IV), esmolol (Brevibloc), etoposide phosphate (Etopophos), fenoldopam (Corlopam), fludarabine (Fludara), foscarnet (Foscavir), gemcitabine (Gemzar), granisetron (Kytril), heparin, hetastarch in electrolytes (Hextend), hydromorphone (Dilaudid), labetalol (Trandate), levofloxacin (Levaquin), linezolid (Zyvox), magnesium sulfate, melphalan (Alkeran), meperidine (Demerol), midazolam (Versed), milrinone (Primacor), morphine, multivitamins (M.V.I.), nicardipine (Cardene IV), ondansetron (Zofran), pemetrexed (Alimta), piperacillin/tazobactam (Zosyn), propofol (Diprivan), remifentanil (Ultiva), sargramostim (Leukine), tacrolimus (Prograf), teniposide (Vumon), theophylline, thiotepa, vinorelbine (Navelbine), zidovudine (AZT, Retrovir).

RATE OF ADMINISTRATION

Severe hypotension and cardiac arrest can occur with too-rapid injection. **Intermittent infusion:** 30 mg or fraction thereof over at least 1 minute (each 300 mg over a minimum of 10 minutes/1,200 mg over a minimum of 40 to 60 minutes). Do not give more than 1,200 mg in single 1-hour infusion. **Continuous infusion:** Administer initial dose at 10 (15 or 20) mg/min over 30 minutes. Will result in serum levels above 4 (5 or 6) mg/mL. To maintain these serum levels, continue infusion at 0.75 (1 or 1.25) mg/min.

ACTIONS

A semisynthetic antibiotic that quickly converts to active clindamycin. It inhibits protein synthesis in the bacterial cell, producing irreversible changes in the protein-synthesizing ribosomes. Widely distributed in most body fluids, tissues, and bones. There is no clinically effective distribution to cerebrospinal fluid. Excreted in urine and feces in small amounts. Most excreted in inactive form in the urine. Crosses placental barrier. Secreted in breast milk.

INDICATIONS AND USES

Treatment of serious infections caused by susceptible anaerobic bacteria; or susceptible aerobic bacterial infections in penicillin-allergic patients; or infections that do not respond or are resistant to other less toxic antibiotics, such as penicillins or cephalosporins. ■ Treatment of acute pelvic inflammatory disease. ■ Prophylaxis of bacterial endocarditis. **Unlabeled uses:** Alternative to sulfonamides with pyrimethamine to treat CNS toxoplasmosis in AIDS patients. ■ Treat *Pneumocystis jiroveci* pneumonia in combination with primaquine. ■ Treatment of babesiosis.

CONTRAINDICATIONS

Known hypersensitivity to clindamycin or lincomycin. Treatment of minor bacterial or viral infections.

PRECAUTIONS

To reduce the development of drug-resistant bacteria and maintain its effectiveness, clindamycin should be used to treat or prevent only those infections proven or strongly suspected to be caused by bacteria. In addition, this is a highly toxic drug and is to be used only when absolutely necessary and when an alternate drug (e.g., erythromycin) is not acceptable. ■ Sensitivity studies indicated to determine susceptibility of the causative organism to clindamycin. ■ Avoid prolonged use; superinfection caused by overgrowth of nonsusceptible organisms may result. ■ Use caution with a history of GI, severe renal, or liver disease, and in patients with a history of asthma or significant allergies. ■ *Clostridium difficile*–associated diarrhea (CDAD) has been reported. May range from mild diarrhea to fatal colitis. Consider in patients who present with diarrhea during or after treatment with clindamycin. ■ Not appropriate to treat meningitis.

Monitor: Capable of causing severe, even fatal, colitis; observe for symptoms of diarrhea. ■ Periodic blood cell counts and liver and kidney studies are indicated in prolonged therapy.

Patient Education: Promptly report diarrhea or bloody stools that occur during treatment or up to several months after an antibiotic has been discontinued; may indicate CDAD and require treatment. ■ Do not treat diarrhea without notifying physician.

Maternal/Child: Category B: use only if clearly needed. ■ Best to discontinue breast-feeding, even though considered acceptable by pediatricians.

■ Each mL contains 9.45 mg benzyl alcohol. Monitor organ system functions if used in infants.

Elderly: Monitor carefully for changes in bowel frequency; may not tolerate diarrhea well.

DRUG/LAB INTERACTIONS

May potentiate other **neuromuscular blocking agents** (e.g., atracurium [Tracrium], kanamycin, streptomycin) and cause profound respiratory depression. ■ Antagonized by **erythromycin.** ■ May decrease **cyclosporine** (Sandimmune) levels. Monitor and adjust dose if necessary.

SIDE EFFECTS

Abdominal pain, agranulocytosis, anaphylaxis, anorexia, azotemia, cardiac arrest, CDAD, diarrhea, elevated ALT, eosinophilia (transient), erythema multiforme, esophagitis, hypersensitivity reactions, hypotension, jaundice, leukopenia, metallic taste, nausea, neutropenia (transient), oliguria, polyarthritis (rare), pseudomembranous colitis, skin rashes, tenesmus (straining at stool), thrombocytopenic purpura, thrombophlebitis, urticaria, vomiting.

ANTIDOTE

Notify the physician of any side effects. Discontinue the drug if indicated (e.g., CDAD, diarrhea, hypersensitivity reactions), treat hypersensitivity reactions as indicated, and resuscitate as necessary. Do not treat diarrhea with opiates or diphenoxylate with atropine (Lomotil); condition will worsen. Mild cases may respond to discontinuation of drug. Treat CDAD with fluids, electrolytes, protein supplements, and oral vancomycin (Vancocin) or metronidazole (Flagyl) as indicated. In severe cases, surgical evaluation may be indicated. Stagger administration times to prevent inappropriate binding of vancomycin. Hemodialysis or CAPD will not decrease blood levels in toxicity.

CLOFARABINE
(kloh-**FARE**-ah-been)

Clolar

Antineoplastic (antimetabolite)

pH 4.5 to 7.5

PEDIATRIC DOSE

Premedication: Prophylactic steroids (e.g., hydrocortisone 100 mg/M^2) on Days 1 through 3 may help to prevent the development of systemic inflammatory response syndrome (SIRS)/capillary leak syndrome.

Clofarabine: 52 mg/M^2 as an infusion each day for 5 consecutive days. Dose is based on body surface area (BSA), which is calculated using the actual height and weight before the start of each cycle. Repeat every 2 to 6 weeks; see Dose Adjustments. Frequency is based on recovery or return to baseline organ function. Median time between cycles during clinical studies was 28 days (range 12 to 55 days).

DOSE ADJUSTMENTS

If the patient's ANC is greater than or equal to 0.75×10^9/L, subsequent cycles may be administered no sooner than 14 days from the starting day of the previous cycle. ▪ Reduce the dose of the next cycle by 25% in patients experiencing a Grade 4 neutropenia (ANC less than 0.5×10^9/L) that lasts 4 or more weeks. ▪ Withhold clofarabine if a clinically significant infection develops. When the infection is clinically controlled, restart therapy at full dose. ▪ Discontinue if hypotension develops at any time during the 5 days of administration. If the hypotension is transient and resolves without pharmacologic intervention, reinstitute treatment (generally at a lower dose). ▪ Discontinue drug immediately if Grade 3 or higher increases in SCr or bilirubin occur; see Monitor and Antidote. May be restarted (generally with a 25% dose reduction) when the patient is stable and organ function has returned to baseline. ▪ Discontinue drug immediately if S/S of SIRS or capillary leak syndrome occur; see Monitor and Antidote. May be restarted (generally with a 25% dose reduction) when the patient is stable. ▪ Withhold clofarabine if a Grade 3 non-infectious nonhematologic toxicity occurs (excluding transient elevations in serum transaminases and/or serum bilirubin and/or nausea and vomiting that is controlled by antiemetics). With resolution or a return to baseline, restart clofarabine at a 25% dose reduction. ▪ Discontinue therapy if a Grade 4 non-infectious nonhematologic toxicity occurs.

DILUTION

Specific techniques required; see Precautions. Available in single-use 20-mL vials containing 20 mg (1 mg/mL). Contains no preservatives; aseptic technique is imperative.

Calculate the exact number of vials needed to achieve the total dosing volume required.

Total number of vials required = Total dose (mg) ÷ 20 mg

Dosing volume (mL) = Total dose (mg)

For example, a child with a body surface area (BSA) of 0.75 M^2 would need a dose of 39 mg of clofarabine (39 ÷ 20 mg = 1.95 vials, so 2 vials of clofarabine would be needed; 39 mg equals a dosing volume of 39 mL).

Withdraw the calculated dose from the vial(s). Using a 0.2-micron syringe filter, add the calculated dose to a sufficient volume of D5W or NS to provide a final concentration between 0.15 mg/mL and 0.4 mg/mL (e.g., 39 mg [39 mL in the example above] added to 100 mL of D5W or NS will provide a final concentration of approximately 0.28 mg/mL).

Filters: Use of a 0.2-micron syringe filter is recommended for use during dilution in D5W or NS.

Storage: Store unopened vials at CRT. Diluted solutions may be stored at CRT but must be used within 24 hours.

COMPATIBILITY

Manufacturer states, "To prevent drug **incompatibilities,** no other medications should be administered through the same IV line."

RATE OF ADMINISTRATION

A single dose properly diluted and evenly distributed as an infusion over 2 hours.

ACTIONS

A second-generation purine nucleoside analog. Acts by inhibiting DNA synthesis. Also disrupts the mitochondrial membrane, causing the release of mitochondrial proteins, cytochrome C, and apoptosis-inducing factors, which leads to cell death. Results in a rapid reduction of peripheral leukemia cells. Metabolism in the liver is very limited. Pathways of nonhepatic elimination not known. Estimated half-life is 5.2 hours. Excreted primarily in the urine.

INDICATIONS AND USES

Treatment of pediatric patients 1 to 21 years of age with relapsed or refractory acute lymphoblastic leukemia (ALL) after treatment with at least two prior regimens. Induction of a complete response is desired; increased survival or other clinical benefits have not been studied.

Unlabeled uses: Treatment of highly refractory and/or relapsed adult patients with ALL. Safety and effectiveness in adults not established. In a Phase 1 study of adults with refractory and/or relapsed hematologic malignancies, the pediatric dose of 52 mg/M^2 was not tolerated.

CONTRAINDICATIONS

Manufacturer states, "None."

PRECAUTIONS

Follow guidelines for handling cytotoxic agents. See Appendix A, p. 1429.
■ Administered by or under the direction of the physician specialist in a facility with adequate diagnostic and treatment facilities to monitor the patient and respond to any medical emergency. ■ May have a pre-existing immunocompromised condition. Treatment may result in prolonged neutropenia and an increased risk of infection, including severe opportunistic infections. ■ Use with great caution in patients with impaired hepatic or renal function; use has not been studied. ■ May develop tumor lysis syndrome, cytokine release syndrome, systemic inflammatory response syndrome, capillary leak syndrome, and organ dysfunction; see Monitor. ■ Patients who have previously received a hematopoietic stem cell transplant (HSCT) may be at higher risk for hepatotoxicity suggestive of veno-occlusive disease (VOD) following treatment with clofarabine (40 mg/M^2) used in combination with etoposide (VePesid 100 mg/M^2) and cyclophosphamide (Cytoxan 440 mg/M^2). Severe hepatotoxic events have been reported in pediatric patients with relapsed or refractory acute leukemia.

Monitor: Obtain baseline CBC with differential and platelets and serum electrolytes. Bone marrow suppression is expected and is usually reversible but can be severe; monitor regularly and more frequently in patients who develop cytopenias. ▪ Obtain baseline renal and hepatic function studies (e.g., SCr, bilirubin, ALT, AST), and uric acid levels. Monitor renal and hepatic function closely during the 5 days of clofarabine administration. Discontinue drug immediately if Grade 3 or higher increases in SCr or bilirubin occur; see Antidote. ▪ Obtain baseline ECG; repeat as indicated. ▪ Monitor HR, BP, and respiratory status closely during infusion. Hypotension should be reported immediately; see Antidote. ▪ Monitor for S/S of tumor lysis syndrome (e.g., hyperkalemia, hyperphosphatemia, hyperuricemia, hypocalcemia, metabolic acidosis, urate crystalluria, and renal failure). ▪ Monitor for S/S of cytokine release (e.g., hypotension, pulmonary edema, tachycardia, tachypnea); may develop into systemic inflammatory response syndrome (SIRS)/capillary leak syndrome and organ dysfunction; see Antidote. To reduce the effects of tumor lysis and other adverse events (e.g., SIRS), the continuous administration of IV fluids throughout the 5 days of clofarabine treatment is recommended. ▪ Adequate hydration, allopurinol, and alkalinization of urine are indicated ·to prevent and/or treat hyperuricemia due to tumor lysis syndrome. ▪ Observe closely for signs of infection. Prophylactic antibiotics may be indicated pending the result of C/S in a febrile neutropenic patient. ▪ Use prophylactic antiemetics to reduce nausea and vomiting and increase patient comfort. ▪ Monitor for thrombocytopenia (platelet count less than 50,000/mm^3). Initiate precautions to prevent excessive bleeding (e.g., inspect IV sites, skin, and mucous membranes; use extreme care during invasive procedures; test urine, emesis, stool, and secretions for occult blood).

Patient Education: Avoid pregnancy; nonhormonal birth control recommended for men and women. Report a suspected pregnancy immediately. ▪ Drink plenty of fluids and avoid dehydration that may be caused by diarrhea and vomiting. ▪ Promptly report bleeding, decreased urine output, dizziness, fainting spells, infection, light-headedness, rapid respiratory rate, or a rapid heart rate. ▪ Review medications with pharmacist or physician. Avoid medications that may be hepatotoxic or nephrotoxic, including OTC or herbal medications. ▪ See Appendix D, p. 1434.

Maternal/Child: Category D: avoid pregnancy; may cause fetal harm. Also has dose-related effects on male reproductive organs. ▪ Discontinue breast-feeding.

Elderly: Not indicated in this patient population.

DRUG/LAB INTERACTIONS

Clinical drug-drug interactions have not been studied; however, the following cautions should be considered. ▪ Primarily excreted by the kidneys; avoid drugs with known renal toxicity during the 5 days of clofarabine administration (e.g., **aminoglycosides** [e.g., gentamicin], **amphotericin B, NSAIDs** [e.g., ibuprofen (Advil, Motrin), naproxen (Aleve, Naprosyn)], **rifampin** [Rifadin]). ▪ The liver is a known target organ for toxicity; avoid drugs known to induce hepatic toxicity (e.g., **amiodarone** [Nexterone], **NSAIDs** [e.g., ibuprofen (Advil, Motrin), naproxen (Aleve, Naprosyn)], **phenothiazines** [e.g., prochlorperazine (Compazine)], **zidovudine** [AZT, Retrovir]). ▪ Close monitoring is required with concomitant administration of medications affecting blood pressure or cardiac function (e.g., **diuretics** [furosemide (Lasix)], **calcium channel blockers** [diltiazem (Cardizem)], **and other antihypertensives**). ■ Cytochrome P_{450} inhibitors (e.g., cimetidine [Tagamet], erythromycins, antifungal agents [e.g., itraconazole (Sporanox)], ritonavir [Norvir], verapamil) and cytochrome P_{450} inducers (e.g., carbamazepine [Tegretol], phenobarbital, phenytoin [Dilantin], rifampin [Rifadin]) are unlikely to affect the metabolism of clofarabine. The effect on cytochrome P_{450} substrates has not been studied.

SIDE EFFECTS

Bone marrow suppression (e.g., anemia, leukopenia, neutropenia, thrombocytopenia) is anticipated, appears to be dose dependent, and is usually reversible. Anxiety, diarrhea, fatigue, febrile neutropenia, fever, flushing, headache, mucosal inflammation, nausea and vomiting, palmar-plantar erythrodysesthesia syndrome, pruritus, and rash occur most frequently. Cardiac toxicity (e.g., left ventricular systolic dysfunction, pericardial effusion, tachycardia) has been reported. SIRS/capillary leak syndrome (e.g., hypotension, multi-organ failure, pulmonary edema, shock, tachycardia, tachypnea) has occurred and can be fatal. Numerous additional side effects may occur and include abdominal pain, anorexia, arthralgia, back pain, confusion, constipation, cough, depression, dermatitis, dizziness, dyspnea, edema, elevated creatinine, epistaxis, erythema, gingival bleeding, hematuria, hepatobiliary toxicity (e.g., elevated AST, ALT, bilirubin), hepatomegaly, hypertension, hypotension, infections (e.g., bacteremia, cellulitis, herpes simplex, oral candidiasis, pneumonia, sepsis, staphylococcal), injection site pain, irritability, jaundice, lethargy, myalgia, pain, petechiae, pleural effusion, renal toxicity, respiratory distress, rigors, somnolence, sore throat, transfusion reaction, tremor, weight loss.

Post-Marketing: Bone marrow failure, Stevens-Johnson syndrome, toxic epidermal necrolysis, and veno-occlusive disease.

ANTIDOTE

Keep physician informed of all side effects; most will be treated symptomatically as indicated. Discontinue if hypotension develops at any time during the 5 days of administration. If the hypotension is transient and resolves without pharmacologic intervention, reinstitute treatment (generally at a lower dose). Discontinue clofarabine immediately if early S/S of SIRS or capillary leak (e.g., hypotension) appear. Use of albumin, diuretics, and steroids may be indicated. May consider restarting (usually at a lower dose) after the patient is stabilized and organ function has returned to baseline. Discontinue clofarabine immediately if substantial increases in SCr or bilirubin occur. May be restarted (possibly at a lower dose) when the patient is stable and organ function has returned to baseline. Bone marrow suppression must be resolved before additional doses can be given. Administration of whole blood products (e.g., packed RBCs, platelets, or leukocytes) and/or blood modifiers (e.g., darbepoetin alfa [Aranesp], epoetin alfa [Epogen], filgrastim [Neupogen], oprelvekin [Neumega], pegfilgrastim [Neulasta], sargramostim [Leukine]) may be indicated to treat bone marrow toxicity. Blood modifiers can be used at the physician's discretion; however, they are not recommended for use during the 5-day clofarabine administration cycle. Use specific antibiotics to combat infection. No specific antidote for overdose. Supportive therapy as indicated will help sustain the patient in toxicity. Should a hypersensitivity reaction occur, treat with antihistamines, corticosteroids, epinephrine, and oxygen as indicated. Resuscitate if indicated.

COAGULATION FACTOR VIIa (RECOMBINANT) ▪ COAGULATION FACTOR VIIa (RECOMBINANT) RTS

Antihemorrhagic

(ko-ag-yew-**LA**-shun **FAK**-ter 7a [re-**KOM**-be-nant])

NovoSeven ▪ NovoSeven RT

pH 5.5

USUAL DOSE

HEMOPHILIA A OR B PATIENTS WITH INHIBITORS

Bleeding episodes: 90 mcg/kg every 2 hours until hemostasis is achieved, or until the treatment has been judged to be ineffective. In clinical studies, a decision on outcome was reached for a majority of patients with joint or muscle bleeds within eight doses, although more doses were required for severe bleeds. Doses between 35 and 120 mcg/kg have been used successfully. Minimum effective dose has not been established. The dose and dosing interval may be adjusted based on the severity of the bleeding and the degree of homeostasis achieved. For severe bleeds, dosing should continue at 3- to 6-hour intervals after hemostasis is achieved to maintain the hemostatic plug. The appropriate duration of post-hemostatic dosing has not been studied and should be minimized; see Precautions. If a new bleeding episode or rebleeding occurs, return to 2-hour dosing intervals. **Surgical intervention:** 90 mcg/kg immediately before the intervention. Repeat every 2 hours during intervention. *For minor surgery,* post-surgical dosing should be administered every 2 hours for 48 hours and then every 2 to 6 hours until healing has occurred. *For major surgery,* post-surgical dosing should be administered every 2 hours for 5 days and then every 4 hours until healing has occurred. Additional doses may be given if required.

CONGENITAL FACTOR VII DEFICIENCY PATIENTS

Bleeding episodes and surgical intervention: 15 to 30 mcg/kg every 4 to 6 hours until hemostasis is achieved. Doses as low as 10 mcg/kg have been effective. Dose and dosing interval should be adjusted to each individual based on the severity of bleeding and the degree of hemostasis achieved. Minimal effective dose has not been determined.

ACQUIRED HEMOPHILIA

70 to 90 mcg/kg every 2 to 3 hours until hemostasis is achieved. Minimum effective dose has not been determined.

PEDIATRIC DOSE

See Usual Dose. Clinical studies were conducted with dosing determined according to body weight and not according to age. See Maternal/Child.

DOSE ADJUSTMENTS

Dose and administration interval may be adjusted based on the severity of the bleeding and the degree of hemostasis achieved. If patient develops intravascular coagulation or thrombosis, dosage should be reduced or treatment stopped; see Monitor.

DILUTION

NovoSeven and NovoSeven RT (room temperature stable [RTS]): Aseptic technique is imperative.

NovoSeven: Available in 1.2-, 2.4-, and 4.8-mg vials. Bring vial and SW to CRT. Inject 2.2 mL SW into 1.2-mg vial, 4.3 mL SW into 2.4-mg vial, or 8.5 mL SW into 4.8-mg vial, aiming the needle against the side so that the stream of water runs down the vial wall. Do not inject SW directly onto the powder. Gently swirl vial until powder is completely dissolved. Final concentration following reconstitution is approximately 0.6 mg/mL (600 mcg/mL). Withdraw calculated dose into a syringe for administration by IV injection.

NovoSeven RT: Available in packages that contain 1-, 2-, or 5-mg vials with a specified volume of histidine diluent. Select the appropriate vial package based on the calculated dose. Bring vial and diluent to RT. Do not exceed 37° C (98.6° F). Reconstitute powder with provided diluent, aiming the needle (20- to 26-gauge needle recommended) and the stream of diluent against the side of the vial. Do not inject the diluent directly on the powder. Do not use SW or other diluents. Gently swirl vial until powder is completely dissolved. Final concentration of reconstituted solution is 1 mg/mL (1,000 mcg/mL).

Storage: *NovoSeven:* Refrigerate before reconstitution. ***NovoSeven RT:*** Before reconstitution, refrigerate or store between 2° and 25° C (36° and 77° F). ***NovoSeven and NovoSeven RT:*** Avoid exposure to direct sunlight. After reconstitution, store at CRT or refrigerate. Should be used within 3 hours. Do not freeze reconstituted product or store in syringe. Discard unused product.

COMPATIBILITY
Manufacturer states, "Intended for IV injection only and should not be mixed with infusion solutions. Do not store reconstituted solution in syringes." If line needs to be flushed before or after NovoSeven RT administration, use NS.

RATE OF ADMINISTRATION
A single dose as a slow IV injection over 2 to 5 minutes, depending on dose administered.

ACTIONS
A vitamin K–dependent glycoprotein structurally similar to human plasma–derived Factor VIIa. Produced by recombinant DNA technology. Promotes hemostasis by activating the extrinsic pathway of the coagulation cascade. When complexed with tissue factor, can activate coagulation Factor X to Factor Xa, and coagulation Factor IX to Factor IXa. Factor Xa, in complex with other factors, then converts prothrombin to thrombin. This leads to the formation of a hemostatic plug by converting fibrinogen to fibrin. Half-life is 2.3 hours. Duration of action is 3 hours.

INDICATIONS AND USES
Treatment of bleeding episodes or prevention of bleeding in surgical interventions or invasive procedures in hemophilia A or B patients with inhibitors to Factor VIII or Factor IX and in patients with acquired hemophilia. ■ Treatment of bleeding episodes or prevention of bleeding in surgical interventions or invasive procedures in patients with congenital FVII deficiency.

CONTRAINDICATIONS
Hypersensitivity to coagulation factor VIIa (recombinant), any of its components, and in patients with known hypersensitivity to mouse, hamster, or bovine proteins.

PRECAUTIONS

Should be administered to patients only under the direct supervision of a physician experienced in the treatment of hemophilia. ▪ Concomitant use of NovoSeven RT with other formulations is not recommended due to potential dosing errors based on different concentrations. ▪ The extent of the risk of thrombotic adverse events after treatment in patients with hemophilia and inhibitors is not known but is considered to be low. Patients with disseminated intravascular coagulation (DIC), advanced atherosclerotic disease, crush injury, or septicemia may have an increased risk of developing thrombotic events due to circulating tissue factor or predisposing coagulopathy. The extent of the risk of arterial and venous thromboembolic adverse events after treatment in patients **without hemophilia** is also not known. A clinical study in elderly nonhemophilia patients with intracranial hemorrhage indicated an increased risk of arterial thromboembolic adverse events with the use of coagulation factor VIIa, including myocardial ischemia and/or infarction and cerebral ischemia and/or infarction. ▪ Biologic and clinical effects of prolonged elevated levels of Factor VIIa have not been studied; therefore, the duration of post-hemostatic dosing should be minimized, and patients should be appropriately monitored by a physician experienced in the treatment of hemophilia during this time period.

Monitor: Evaluation of hemostasis should be used to determine the effectiveness of therapy and to provide a basis for modification of the treatment schedule; coagulation parameters do not necessarily correlate with or predict the effectiveness of therapy. Coagulation parameters (e.g., PT, aPTT, plasma FVII clotting activity [FVII:C]) may be used as an adjunct to the clinical evaluation of hemostasis in monitoring the effectiveness and treatment schedule, although these parameters have shown no direct correlation to achieving hemostasis. ▪ Patients with factor VII deficiency should be monitored for PT and factor VII coagulant activity before and after treatment. If the factor VIIa activity fails to reach the expected level, if PT is not corrected, or if bleeding is not controlled after treatment with the recommended doses, antibody formation should be suspected and analysis for antibodies should be performed. ▪ Monitor patients if they develop signs or symptoms of activation of the coagulation system or thrombosis. When there is laboratory confirmation of intravascular coagulation or presence of clinical thrombosis, dosage should be reduced or the treatment stopped, depending on the patient's symptoms; see Dose Adjustments.

Patient Education: Discuss benefits versus risk of therapy and signs of hypersensitivity reactions including hives, urticaria, chest tightness, wheezing, hypotension, and anaphylaxis. ▪ Signs of bleeding may be similar to signs of thrombosis and can include new-onset swelling and pain in the limbs or abdomen, new-onset chest pain, shortness of breath, loss of sensation or motor power, or altered consciousness or speech.

Maternal/Child: Category C: safety for use during pregnancy and breastfeeding not established. Use only if clearly indicated and benefit justifies potential risk to the fetus. ▪ A decision should be made whether to discontinue nursing or to discontinue the drug. ▪ The safety and effectiveness was not determined to be different in various age-groups from infants to adolescents (0 to 16 years of age); see Pediatric Dose.

Elderly: Geriatric patients were not enrolled in clinical trials.

DRUG/LAB INTERACTIONS

The risk of potential interaction between Factor VIIa and coagulation factor concentrates has not been adequately evaluated. Simultaneous use of **activated prothrombin complex concentrates** (e.g., anti-inhibitor coagulant complex [Autoplex-T, Feiba VH]) **or prothrombin complex concentrates** (e.g., Factor IX [AlphaNine SD, Benefix]) should be avoided. ▪ Although specific drug interactions were not studied in clinical trials, coagulation factor VIIa (recombinant) has been used concomitantly with **antifibrinolytic therapies** (e.g., tranexamic acid [Cyclokapron], aminocaproic acid [Amicar]).

SIDE EFFECTS

Generally well tolerated. The majority of patients reporting side effects received more than 12 doses. Most serious adverse reactions are thrombotic events; however, the risk in patients with hemophilia and inhibitors is considered to be low. Arthralgia, arthrosis, bradycardia, coagulation disorder, DIC, edema, fever, decreased fibrinogen plasma, decreased prothrombin, decreased therapeutic response, headache, hemarthrosis, hemorrhage, hypersensitivity reactions, hypertension, hypotension, increased fibrinolysis, injection site reaction, nausea, pain, pneumonia, pruritus, purpura, rash, renal function abnormalities, shock, subdural hematoma, thrombosis, vomiting.

Post-Marketing: High D-dimer levels and consumptive coagulopathy, thromboembolic events including myocardial ischemia and/or infarction, cerebral ischemia and/or infarction, thrombophlebitis, arterial thrombosis, deep vein thrombosis and related pulmonary embolism, and isolated cases of hypersensitivity reactions including anaphylaxis have occurred following use in both labeled and unlabeled indications.

ANTIDOTE

Discontinue drug and notify physician of any major side effects. Treat hypersensitivity reactions as indicated. For thrombosis or DIC, anticoagulation with heparin may be indicated.

CONIVAPTAN HYDROCHLORIDE
(kon-ih-**VAP**-tan hy-droh-**KLOR**-eyed)
Vaprisol

Arginine vasopressin
antagonist

pH 3 to 3.8

USUAL DOSE

Loading dose: 20 mg as an IV infusion over 30 minutes. Follow with 20 mg administered as a **continuous infusion** evenly distributed over 24 hours. May be administered for an additional 1 to 3 days as a continuous infusion of 20 mg/day. The total duration of infusion (after the loading dose) should not exceed 4 days.

DOSE ADJUSTMENTS

If the serum sodium does not rise at the desired rate, the dose may be titrated up to 40 mg as a continuous infusion over 24 hours. 40 mg is the maximum daily dose. ▪ A reduced dose may be required if the patient experiences an undesirably rapid rate of rise of serum sodium; see Precautions. ▪ If hyponatremia persists or recurs (after initial interruption of therapy) and the patient has no evidence of neurologic sequelae, conivaptan may be resumed at a reduced dose; see Monitor. ▪ A reduced dose may also be required in patients who develop hypotension or hypovolemia; see Monitor. ▪ Reduced dose required in patients with hepatic impairment (Child-Pugh Class A, B, or C) or in patients with moderate renal impairment (CrCl 30 to 60 mL/min). Initiate with a loading dose of 10 mg. Follow with a continuous infusion of 10 mg over 24 hours for 2 days to a maximum of 4 days. Use in patients with severe renal impairment (CrCl less than 30 mL/min) is not recommended; see Contraindications.

DILUTION

Available in a single-use, ready-to-use (RTU) plastic container containing 20 mg conivaptan in 100 mL D5W or in an ampule containing 20 mg/vial. *The ampule must be further diluted only with D5W.* To prepare the **loading dose,** withdraw 20 mg (4 mL) from an ampule and inject into a 100-mL bag of D5W. Gently invert the bag several times. To prepare the **continuous infusion,** withdraw 20 mg (4 mL) and inject into a 250-mL bag of D5W. Gently invert the bag several times. Doses of 40 mg administered as a 24-hour continuous infusion may also be prepared in a 250-mL bag of D5W. If the RTU container is being administered as a 40-mg dose, administer two consecutive 20 mg/100 mL containers over 24 hours.

Filters: A filter needle should be used when drawing up medications from glass ampules.

Storage: Store in carton at CRT. Protect from light and freezing. When using an ampule, mix infusion immediately before administration. Complete infusion within 24 hours of mixing. Stable in D5W for 24 hours.

COMPATIBILITY

Manufacturer states, "Should not be mixed or administered with lactated Ringer's. Should not be combined with any other product in the same intravenous line or bag."

RATE OF ADMINISTRATION

Loading dose: A single dose equally distributed over 30 minutes as an infusion.

Continuous infusion: A single dose equally distributed over 24 hours.

ACTIONS

A nonpeptide, dual antagonist of arginine vasopressin (AVP) V_{1A} and V_2 receptors. The level of AVP in the blood is critical for the regulation of water and electrolyte balance and is usually elevated in both euvolemic and hypervolemic hyponatremia (in euvolemic hyponatremia there is an increase in total body water, but the sodium content remains the same; in hypervolemic hyponatremia both sodium and water content in the body increase, but the water gain is greater). AVP excess is associated with hyponatremia without edema. The AVP effect is mediated through V_2 receptors that help maintain plasma osmolality. Conivaptan blocks V_2 receptors in the renal collecting ducts, resulting in aquaresis (excretion of free water). This is generally accompanied by increased net fluid loss, increased urine output, and decreased urine osmolality. Conivaptan is highly protein bound. It is metabolized in the liver by the cytochrome P_{450} isoenzyme, CYP3A. Its half-life is 5.3 to 8.1 hours, depending on dose. Primarily excreted in the feces and, to a lesser extent, in urine. Crosses the placenta in animals.

INDICATIONS AND USES

For use in the hospitalized patient to treat euvolemic and hypervolemic hyponatremia. Euvolemic hyponatremia may occur in the syndrome of inappropriate secretion of antidiuretic hormone (SIADH, an inability of the body to excrete dilute urine) or in the setting of certain conditions, including hypothyroidism, adrenal insufficiency, and pulmonary disorders. ▪ Not indicated for the treatment of the S/S of heart failure. Raising serum sodium with conivaptan has not been shown to provide a symptomatic benefit.

CONTRAINDICATIONS

Patients with hypovolemic hyponatremia. ▪ Hypersensitivity to conivaptan or any of its components (propylene glycol, ethanol, lactic acid). ▪ Coadministration with potent CYP3A inhibitors, such as clarithromycin, indinavir, itraconazole, ketoconazole, and ritonavir; see Drug Interactions. ▪ Premixed solution contains dextrose, which may be contraindicated in patients with a known allergy to corn or corn products. ▪ Anuria (no benefit expected).

PRECAUTIONS

For IV use only. ▪ Use only in hospitalized patients. ▪ Safety for use in hypovolemic, hyponatremic patients with underlying CHF has not been established. Should be used to raise sodium in these patients only after other treatment options have been considered. ▪ An overly rapid increase in serum sodium concentration (more than 12 mEq/L/24 hr) may result in serious sequelae. Although not observed in clinical trials, osmotic demyelination syndrome (brain cell dehydration) has been reported following rapid correction of low serum sodium concentration. Osmotic demyelination results in dysarthria, lethargy, affective changes, spastic quadriparesis, seizures, coma, or death. Patients with severe malnutrition, alcoholism, or advanced liver disease may be at increased risk; use slower rates of correction; see Monitor. ▪ Reduced doses required in patients with hepatic impairment and moderate renal impairment; see Dose Adjustments. ▪ May cause significant infusion site reaction; see Monitor.

Monitor: Dilute ampule as directed; administer via a large vein. Monitor infusion site and rotate every 24 hours. ▪ Monitor serum sodium concentration and neurologic status closely during therapy. If an overly rapid increase in serum sodium concentration occurs (greater than 12 mEq/L/24 hr), administration should be discontinued. If the sodium continues to rise, administration should not be resumed. If hyponatremia persists or recurs (after initial interruption of therapy) and the patient has no evidence of neurologic sequelae, conivaptan may be resumed at a reduced dose. ■ Monitor vital signs, urine output and osmolality, and volume status of patient. Discontinue therapy in patients who develop hypotension or hypovolemia. Once the patient is again euvolemic and is no longer hypotensive, therapy may be resumed at a reduced dose; see Dose Adjustments.

Patient Education: Promptly report any burning at the infusion site or other side effects. ■ Request assistance for ambulation. ■ Review list of allergies and medications with physician or pharmacist.

Maternal/Child: Category C: use during pregnancy only if benefits justify risk to the fetus. Has been shown to cause fetal harm in animals. ■ Discontinue breast-feeding. ■ Safety and effectiveness for use in pediatric patients has not been studied.

Elderly: Response similar to that seen in the general study population.

DRUG/LAB INTERACTIONS

A substrate of CYP3A. Coadministration with inhibitors of this enzyme could lead to an increase in conivaptan concentrations, the effect of which is unknown. Concomitant use with **potent CYP3A4** inhibitors such as clarithromycin (Biaxin), indinavir (Crixivan), itraconazole (Sporanox), ketoconazole (Nizoral), and ritonavir (Norvir) is contraindicated. ■ A potent inhibitor of CYP3A. May increase plasma concentrations of drugs that are primarily metabolized by this enzyme. Coadministration with **amlodipine** (Norvasc), **midazolam** (Versed), **and simvastatin** (Zocor) resulted in increased concentrations of each of the drugs. Two cases of rhabdomyolysis occurred in patients who were receiving a **CYP3A4-metabolized HMG-CoA reductase inhibitor** (e.g., simvastatin [Zocor]). Avoid concomitant use with drugs eliminated primarily by **CYP3A4-mediated metabolism.** Do not initiate subsequent therapy with **CYP3A4 substrate drugs** until at least 1 week after an infusion of conivaptan. ■ May decrease clearance and increase serum concentration of **digoxin.** Monitor digoxin levels. ■ Captopril (Capoten) and furosemide (Lasix) do not appear to affect the pharmacokinetics of conivaptan. ■ Does not appear to affect PT/INR when coadministered with warfarin (Coumadin). ■ Does not appear to affect the QT interval.

SIDE EFFECTS

The most common adverse reactions are infusion site reactions (e.g., erythema, fever, headache, hypokalemia, orthostatic hypotension, pain, peripheral edema, phlebitis). Other reactions that occurred in more than 2% of patients include anemia, atrial fibrillation, confusion, constipation, diarrhea, hypertension, hypomagnesemia, hyponatremia, hypotension, insomnia, nausea, pharyngolaryngeal pain, pneumonia, pruritus, pyrexia, ST segment depression on ECG, thirst, urinary tract infection, and vomiting.

ANTIDOTE

Notify physician of any side effects. Most will be treated symptomatically. Discontinue therapy if there is an overly rapid increase in serum sodium concentration or if the patient experiences hypotension or hypovolemia. Discontinue therapy permanently if neurologic sequelae are present; see Precautions, Monitor, and Dose Adjustments. Resuscitate as necessary.

CONJUGATED ESTROGENS BBW
(**KON**-jyou-**gay**-ted **ES**-troh-jens)

Premarin Intravenous

Hormone
(estrogen)
Antihemorrhagic

pH 7.2 to 7.4

USUAL DOSE

25 mg in 1 injection. May be repeated in 6 to 12 hours if indicated.

DILUTION

Reconstitute with 5 mL SWI, directing the flow of diluent gently against the side of the vial. Agitate gently. Do not shake violently. Do not use if discolored or if precipitate is present. Dilution in an IV infusion is not recommended.

Storage: Refrigerate prior to use. Use immediately after reconstitution.

COMPATIBILITY

Consider any drug NOT listed as compatible to be INCOMPATIBLE until consulting a pharmacist; specific conditions may apply.

Manufacturer lists as **incompatible** with ascorbic acid, protein hydrolysate, or any solution with an acid pH.

According to the manufacturer, infusion with other agents is not generally recommended. May be given at Y-tube if **compatible** solutions are infusing (NS, dextrose, and invert sugar solutions). According to one source, it is **compatible** at the **Y-site** with potassium chloride (KCl).

RATE OF ADMINISTRATION

5 mg or fraction thereof over 1 minute. Must be given direct IV or through IV tubing close to needle site. Infusion solution must be **compatible**. Too-rapid injection may cause flushing.

ACTIONS

A mixture of conjugated estrogens obtained from natural sources. Administration provides a rapid and temporary increase in estrogen levels. Acts at several points on the clotting cascade, enhancing coagulability of the blood, especially in the capillary beds. Promptly corrects bleeding due to estrogen deficiency. Widely distributed in the body. Metabolized primarily in the liver and excreted in the urine. Secreted in breast milk.

INDICATIONS AND USES

Treatment of abnormal uterine bleeding caused by hormonal imbalance in the absence of organic pathology. Indicated for short-term use only to provide a rapid and temporary increase in estrogen levels.

Unlabeled uses: Postcoital contraception.

CONTRAINDICATIONS

Known, suspected, or history of breast cancer, deep venous thrombosis, or pulmonary embolism. ■ Estrogen-dependent neoplasia, pregnancy, undiagnosed abnormal genital bleeding, active or recent (e.g., within the past year) arterial thromboembolic disease (e.g., stroke, MI), liver dysfunction or disease. ■ Hypersensitivity to this product or its ingredients. ■ Other specific contraindications for estrogens must be considered.

PRECAUTIONS

IV therapy with conjugated estrogens is indicated for short-term use. However, warnings and precautions associated with oral therapy should be considered (e.g., changes in vaginal bleeding, headache, hypersensitivity reactions, skin reactions, and many more); see Precautions and prescribing information. ■ Estrogens with or without progestins should not be used for the prevention of cardiovascular disease or dementia. ■ Even though bleeding is controlled, the etiology of the bleeding must be determined and definitive therapy instituted. ■ May cause fluid retention. Use with caution in patients with cardiac or renal dysfunction. ■ Use with caution in asthma, diabetes, endometriosis, epilepsy, hepatic hemangiomas, hepatic or gallbladder disease, hypercalcemia or hypocalcemia, hypercholesterolemia, hypertriglyceridemia, hypertension, migraines, obesity, porphyria, systemic lupus erythematosus, or tobacco use; may exacerbate condition. ■ Retinal vascular thrombosis has been reported in patients receiving estrogen therapy. Discontinue therapy and obtain ophthalmologic exam if visual disturbances occur. ■ Patients dependent on thyroid hormone replacement therapy (e.g., levothyroxine [Synthroid]) who are also receiving estrogen may require dose adjustment of thyroid replacement medication. ■ Estrogens may increase the risk of endometrial and breast cancer. ■ May increase the risk of deep venous thrombosis, MI, pulmonary embolism, stroke, and dementia. ■ Follow immediately with oral estrogens as recommended for dysfunctional uterine bleeding.

Monitor: Monitor VS; may cause a temporary BP elevation.

Patient Education: Review health history and disease states with physician before beginning treatment with conjugated estrogens. ■ Review possible side effects with physician and report any side effects promptly.

Maternal/Child: Category X: avoid pregnancy. ■ Do not use during breast-feeding. Detectable amounts have been found in breast milk and may decrease quantity and quality of milk. ■ Safety for use in pediatric patients not established. Extended use may accelerate epiphyseal closure, which could result in short adult stature.

Elderly: Differences in response compared to younger adults not identified.

DRUG/LAB INTERACTIONS

May decrease effects of **oral antidiabetics.** ■ **Barbiturates** (e.g., phenobarbital), **carbamazepine** (Tegretol), **phenytoin** (Dilantin), **rifampin** (Rifadin), **and St. John's wort** increase metabolism and decrease serum levels and effects. ■ Plasma concentrations may be increased with coadministration of **clarithromycin** (Biaxin), **erythromycin, itraconazole** (Sporanox), **ketoconazole** (Nizoral), **ritonavir** (Norvir), **and grapefruit juice.** ■ May decrease metabolism and increase serum levels of **cyclosporine.** May increase risk of cyclosporine toxicity. ■ Increased risk of hepatotoxicity with **other hepatotoxic agents** (e.g., dantrolene [Dantrium]). ■ May increase **blood glucose** levels and **serum lipids.** ■ May reduce response to **metyrapone test.** ■ May alter numerous **coagulation tests, glucose tolerance, and thyroid and other protein-binding tests.**

SIDE EFFECTS

Rare when used as directed; flushing, nausea, vomiting. IV therapy with conjugated estrogens is indicated for short-term use. However, the numerous adverse reactions associated with oral therapy should be considered (e.g., changes in vaginal bleeding, headache, hypersensitivity reactions, skin reactions, and many more); see Precautions and prescribing information.

ANTIDOTE

No toxicity has been reported throughout years of clinical use. Discontinue if jaundice occurs.

COSYNTROPIN
(koh-**SIN**-troh-pin)

Cortrosyn

Diagnostic agent
(adrenocorticotropic)

pH 5.5 to 7.5

USUAL DOSE
250 mcg (0.25 mg). Up to 750 mcg (0.75 mg) has been used.

PEDIATRIC DOSE
Pediatric patients over 2 years of age: May use adult dose, but 125 mcg (0.125 mg) is usually adequate.

Pediatric patients 2 years of age or less: 125 mcg (0.125 mg). Usually given IM.

DILUTION
Available as a lyophilized powder (Cortrosyn) or as a solution (cosyntropin). Reconstitute powder with 1 mL NS. For IV use, both formulations should be diluted with 2 to 5 mL of NS. May be given directly IV after this initial dilution or further diluted in D5W or NS and given as an infusion (250 mcg in 250 mL equals 1 mcg/mL).

Storage: *Cortrosyn:* Store at CRT. ***Cosyntropin (liquid formulation):*** Store at 2° to 8° C (36° to 46° F); protect from light and freezing. Discard any unused drug.

COMPATIBILITY
Manufacturer states, "Should not be added to blood or plasma; may be inactivated by enzymes." Consider specific use.

RATE OF ADMINISTRATION
IV injection: A single dose over 2 minutes.

Infusion: A single dose at a rate of approximately 40 mcg/hr over 6 hours.

ACTIONS
A synthetic form of adrenocorticotropic hormone (ACTH). Stimulates the adrenal cortex to secrete adrenocortical hormone. Does not increase cortisol secretion in patients with primary adrenocortical insufficiency. Peak plasma cortisol levels occur in 1 to 2 hours depending on formulation used.

INDICATIONS AND USES
Diagnostic aid for adrenocortical insufficiency.

CONTRAINDICATIONS
Hypersensitivity to cosyntropin.

PRECAUTIONS
The liquid formulation of cosyntropin is for IV use only. Cortrosyn may be used IV or IM. ▪ Preferable to ACTH because it is less likely to cause hypersensitivity reactions; however, hypersensitivity reactions have occurred. Administer in a facility equipped to monitor the patient and respond to any medical emergency. ▪ May be used in patients who have had a hypersensitivity reaction to ACTH.

Monitor: Continuous observation for at least the first 30 minutes is mandatory. Observe frequently thereafter. ▪ Check BP frequently; may cause elevated BP and salt and water retention. ▪ Monitor correct collection of specimens; see prescribing information for specific details. ▪ See Drug/Lab Interactions.

Patient Education: May mask signs of infection. ▪ May decrease resistance. ▪ Avoid immunization with live virus vaccines.
Maternal/Child: Category C: use during pregnancy only if benefits outweigh risks. ▪ Use with caution during breast-feeding; potential exists for serious reactions in nursing infants.

DRUG/LAB INTERACTIONS
Plasma cortisol may be falsely elevated with **cortisone, hydrocortisone, or spironolactone.** Patients receiving cortisone, hydrocortisone, or spironolactone should omit their pre-test doses on the day of testing. ▪ Abnormally high basal plasma cortisol levels may also occur in patients taking inadvertent doses of **cortisone or hydrocortisone** on the test day and in women taking drugs that contain **estrogen.** ▪ Many drug reactions are possible with corticosteroids, but usually not a concern with specific diagnostic use. ▪ May accentuate electrolyte loss associated with **diuretic therapy.**

SIDE EFFECTS
Bradycardia, hypertension, peripheral edema, rash, tachycardia are most common. Hypersensitivity reactions, including anaphylaxis (rare), have occurred.

ANTIDOTE
Notify the physician of any side effect. Keep epinephrine and diphenhydramine available to treat anaphylaxis. Resuscitate as necessary.

CYCLOPHOSPHAMIDE
(sye-kloh-**FOS**-fah-myd)

Lyophilized Cytoxan, Neosar, ✤Procytox

Antineoplastic
(alkylating agent/
nitrogen mustard)

pH 3 to 7.5

USUAL DOSE

Although effective alone in susceptible malignancies, cyclophosphamide is more frequently used concurrently or sequentially with other antineoplastic agents. See Monitor.

Malignant diseases (adult and pediatric patients): *As a single agent:* The initial dose may be 40 to 50 mg/kg of body weight, usually given in divided doses over 2 to 5 days. Induction doses may range as high as 100 mg/kg. Alternate dosing schedules are: 3 to 5 mg/kg twice weekly, or 10 to 15 mg/kg every 7 to 10 days, or 1.5 to 3 mg/kg/24 hr. Higher doses have been used, based on the condition being treated. With doses over 1 Gm/M^2, consider the use of mesna to attenuate or reduce the incidence of hemorrhagic cystitis. *Combination protocols:* Numerous combination therapies are in use. Has been used with bleomycin, busulfan, carboplatin, carmustine, cisplatin, cytarabine, dacarbazine, dexamethasone, doxorubicin, etoposide, fluorouracil, methotrexate, mitoxantrone, prednisone, and vincristine.

Adjuvant treatment of operable node-positive breast cancer: Treatment protocol includes cyclophosphamide, doxorubicin, and docetaxel. Administer cyclophosphamide 500 mg/M^2 and doxorubicin 50 mg/M^2. One hour later, give docetaxel 75 mg/M^2. Repeat every 3 weeks for 6 cycles. See docetaxel (Taxotere) and doxorubicin (Adriamycin) monographs.

Polymyositis (unlabeled): 500 mg every 1 to 3 weeks as an IV infusion over 1 hour.

Polyarteritis nodosa (unlabeled): Begin with 4 mg/kg/24 hr. Adjust dose based on patient response.

PEDIATRIC DOSE

Malignant diseases: See Usual Dose.

DOSE ADJUSTMENTS

Dose based on average weight in presence of edema or ascites. ■ Dose is reduced by one third to one half if hematologic disease is present or there has been extensive radiation therapy. ■ Reduced dose may be required in the adrenalectomized patient and in impaired hepatic function. ■ Dosing should be cautious in the elderly. Lower-end initial doses may be indicated. Consider decrease in cardiac, hepatic, and renal function; concomitant disease; or other drug therapy; see Elderly. ■ Often used with other antineoplastic drugs in reduced doses to achieve tumor remission.

DILUTION

Specific techniques required; see Precautions. Each 100 mg must be diluted with 5 mL of SW or bacteriostatic water for injection (paraben preserved only); yields 20 mg/mL. Shake solution gently and allow to stand until clear. Further dilution with up to 250 mL D5W, NS, D5NS, ½NS, LR, or D5R is recommended to reduce side effects. Do not use heat to facilitate dilution. See Monitor.

Filters: May be filtered through available micron sizes of cellulose ester membrane filters.

Storage: Diluted solution must be used within 24 hours when stored at RT. Stable up to 6 days if refrigerated. Do not store cyclophosphamide in temperatures over 37° C (90° F).

COMPATIBILITY   (Underline Indicates Conflicting Compatibility Information)
Consider any drug NOT listed as compatible to be INCOMPATIBLE until consulting a pharmacist; specific conditions may apply.

One source suggests the following **compatibilities:**

Additive: Bleomycin (Blenoxane), cisplatin (Platinol), fluorouracil (5-FU), mesna (Mesnex), methotrexate, mitoxantrone (Novantrone), ondansetron (Zofran).

Y-site: Allopurinol (Aloprim), amifostine (Ethyol), amikacin (Amikin), ampicillin, anidulafungin (Eraxis), aztreonam (Azactam), bleomycin (Blenoxane), cefazolin (Ancef), cefepime (Maxipime), cefotaxime (Claforan), cefoxitin (Mefoxin), cefuroxime (Zinacef), chloramphenicol (Chloromycetin), chlorpromazine (Thorazine), cisplatin (Platinol), cladribine (Leustatin), clindamycin (Cleocin), dexamethasone (Decadron), diphenhydramine (Benadryl), doripenem (Doribax), doxorubicin (Adriamycin), doxorubicin liposomal (Doxil), doxycycline, droperidol (Inapsine), erythromycin (Erythrocin), etoposide phosphate (Etopophos), famotidine (Pepcid IV), filgrastim (Neupogen), fludarabine (Fludara), fluorouracil (5-FU), furosemide (Lasix), gallium nitrate (Ganite), ganciclovir (Cytovene), gemcitabine (Gemzar), gentamicin, granisetron (Kytril), heparin, hydromorphone (Dilaudid), idarubicin (Idamycin), kanamycin (Kantrex), leucovorin calcium, linezolid (Zyvox), lorazepam (Ativan), melphalan (Alkeran), methotrexate, methylprednisolone (Solu-Medrol), metoclopramide (Reglan), metronidazole (Flagyl IV), mitomycin (Mutamycin), morphine, nafcillin (Nallpen), ondansetron (Zofran), oxacillin (Bactocill), oxaliplatin (Eloxatin), paclitaxel (Taxol), palonosetron (Aloxi), pemetrexed (Alimta), penicillin G potassium, piperacillin, piperacillin/tazobactam (Zosyn), prochlorperazine (Compazine), promethazine (Phenergan), propofol (Diprivan), ranitidine (Zantac), sargramostim (Leukine), sodium bicarbonate, sulfamethoxazole/trimethoprim, teniposide (Vumon), thiotepa, ticarcillin/clavulanate (Timentin), tobramycin, topotecan (Hycamtin), vancomycin, vinblastine, vincristine, vinorelbine (Navelbine).

RATE OF ADMINISTRATION

May be given by IV push, as an intermittent infusion, or through the Y-tube or three-way stopcock if the IV solution is dextrose or saline.

Injection: Each 100 mg or fraction thereof of properly diluted solution (20 mg/mL) over 1 minute. May be given through Y-tube or three-way stopcock of a free-flowing IV or as a direct IV injection followed with an NS flush. One source suggests doses up to 500 mg may be given by injection.

Intermittent infusion: Infuse doses over 500 mg diluted in 100 to 250 mL over 20 to 60 minutes. One source suggests extending administration time to 2 hours in bone marrow transplantation. Another source suggests doses equal to or less than 1,000 mg diluted in 50 mL NS may be given over 10 to 15 minutes, and doses greater than 1,000 mg diluted in 100 mL NS or doses greater than 2,000 mg diluted in 250 mL NS may be given over 20 to 30 minutes. See Monitor.

ACTIONS

An alkylating agent of the nitrogen mustard group with antitumor activity; cell cycle phase nonspecific, but most effective in S phase. It is an inert compound but is activated by hepatic microsomal enzymes to produce regression in the size of malignant tumors. Elimination half-life is 3 to 10 hours. Metabolized in the liver, it or its metabolites are excreted in the urine. Secreted in breast milk.

INDICATIONS AND USES

To suppress or retard neoplastic growth. Has been used in lymphomas such as Hodgkin's disease, non-Hodgkin's, leukemias, and multiple myeloma; in mycosis fungoides and in numerous other malignancies (e.g., bladder, breast, neuroblastoma, ovarian, retinoblastoma, sarcomas [bony and soft tissue], small-cell lung cancer). Used in pediatric patients for acute and chronic leukemias, Hodgkin's or non-Hodgkin's lymphomas, neuroblastoma, and retinoblastoma. ▪ Adjuvant treatment of operable node-positive breast cancer in combination with doxorubicin and docetaxel. Used orally to treat many other indications including biopsy-proven nephrotic syndrome in pediatric patients when disease fails to respond to primary therapy or primary therapy causes intolerable side effects.
Unlabeled uses: Severe rheumatologic conditions. ▪ Polyarteritis nodosa. ▪ Alone or in combination with corticosteroids to treat polymyositis.

CONTRAINDICATIONS

Previous hypersensitivity, severely depressed bone marrow function.

PRECAUTIONS

Follow guidelines for handling cytotoxic agents. See Appendix A, p. 1429. ▪ Administered by or under the direction of the physician specialist. ▪ Use caution in cases of leukopenia, thrombocytopenia, bone marrow infiltrated with malignant cells, previous radiation therapy, previous cytotoxic therapy, and severe hepatic or renal disease. ▪ Wait 5 to 7 days after a major surgical procedure before beginning treatment. May interfere with normal wound healing. ▪ Do not administer any live virus vaccine to patients receiving antineoplastic drugs. ▪ May cause syndrome of inappropriate antidiuretic hormone (SIADH) with normal doses because of fluid loading. ▪ May result in reversible hemorrhagic ureteritis or renal tubular necrosis. ▪ One incident of cross-sensitivity with other alkylating agents has been reported. ▪ Anaphylaxis resulting in death has been reported. ▪ Pseudomembranous colitis has been reported. May range from mild to life threatening. Consider in patients that present with diarrhea during or after treatment with cyclophosphamide. ▪ Stevens-Johnson syndrome and toxic epidermal necrolysis have occurred rarely.
Monitor: Prehydration with 500 to 1,000 mL NS recommended, especially with higher doses. ▪ Marked leukopenia will occur after the initial dose. Recovery should begin in 7 to 10 days. ▪ Monitor neutrophils and platelets and examine urine for RBCs on a regular basis. ▪ Maintenance doses are regulated by an acceptable leukocyte count (2,500 to 4,000 cells/mm³) and the absence of serious side effects. The maximum effective maintenance dose should be used. ▪ Observe continuously for infection. Prophylactic antibiotics may be indicated pending results of C/S in a febrile neutropenic patient. ▪ Use antiemetics for patient comfort. ▪ Acute hemorrhagic cystitis occurs in 7% to 12% of patients; administer before 4 PM to decrease amount of drug remaining in bladder overnight. Encourage fluid intake (2 or 3 L of fluids per day [PO or IV] are recommended, especially with

doses over 1,000 mg). Encourage frequent voiding to prevent cystitis. ▪ Monitor for thrombocytopenia (platelet count less than 50,000/mm^3). Initiate precautions to prevent excessive bleeding (e.g., inspect IV sites, skin, and mucous membranes; use extreme care during invasive procedures; test urine, emesis, stool, and secretions for occult blood).

Patient Education: Nonhormonal birth control recommended. ▪ Increase fluid intake and void frequently. ▪ See Appendix D, p. 1434.

Maternal/Child: Category D: may produce teratogenic effects on the fetus. Has a mutagenic potential. ▪ Discontinue breast-feeding. ▪ When given in remission, has been effective in prolonging the duration of the remission in pediatric patients with acute lymphoblastic (stem-cell) leukemia. ▪ Safety profile in pediatric patients similar to that of adults.

Elderly: Consider age-related organ impairment. Dose selection should be cautious; see Dose Adjustments. Toxicity may be increased. Monitoring of renal function is suggested.

DRUG/LAB INTERACTIONS

Half-life increased and metabolic concentrations decreased with **chloramphenicol.** ▪ **Thiazide diuretics** (e.g., chlorothiazide [Diuril]) may prolong leukopenia. ▪ Increased risk of bleeding with **anticoagulants** (e.g., warfarin [Coumadin]); dose reduction of anticoagulant may be indicated. ▪ May reduce serum **digoxin** levels. ▪ Can potentiate **doxorubicin**-induced cardiotoxicity. ▪ May prolong neuromuscular blockade and prolonged respiratory depression caused by **succinylcholine.** These effects are dose dependent and may occur up to several days after cyclophosphamide is discontinued. ▪ May decrease effectiveness of **quinolone antibiotics** (e.g., ciprofloxacin [Cipro]). ▪ Risk of bleeding or infection may be increased with **allopurinol** (Aloprim). ▪ Chronic administration of high doses of **phenobarbital** may increase metabolism of cyclophosphamide and decrease its effectiveness. ▪ Capable of many other interactions.

SIDE EFFECTS

Alopecia (regrowth may be slightly darker), amenorrhea, asthenia, gonadal suppression, leukopenia (see Precautions), malaise, mucosal ulcerations, nausea and vomiting, darkening of skin and fingernails, susceptibility to infection.

Major: Anaphylaxis (death), bone marrow suppression, hemorrhagic ureteritis (reversible), interstitial pneumonitis, pulmonary fibrosis, pseudomembranous colitis, renal tubular necrosis (reversible), secondary neoplasia, SIADH, sterile hemorrhagic cystitis (which can be fatal).

ANTIDOTE

Minor side effects will be treated symptomatically if necessary. Discontinue the drug and notify the physician of hematuria immediately. Formalin bladder instillation may control cystitis. Mesna has decreased incidence of cystitis. Administration of whole blood products (e.g., packed RBCs, platelets, leukocytes) and/or blood modifiers (e.g., darbepoetin alfa [Aranesp], epoetin alfa [Epogen], filgrastim [Neupogen], oprelvekin [Neumega], pegfilgrastim [Neulasta], sargramostim [Leukine]) may be indicated to treat bone marrow toxicity. There is no specific antidote. Supportive therapy as indicated will help sustain the patient in toxicity. Approximately 36% can be removed by hemodialysis.

CYCLOSPORINE BBW
(sye-kloh-**SPOR**-een)

Sandimmune

Immunosuppressant

USUAL DOSE
5 to 6 mg/kg of body weight as a single dose 4 to 12 hours before transplantation. Repeat once each day until oral dosage form can be tolerated. Individualized adjustment is imperative and may be required on a daily basis. Administered at ⅓ of the oral dose in patients temporarily unable to take oral cyclosporine. Administered in conjunction with adrenal corticosteroids; different regimens used; see prescribing information.

PEDIATRIC DOSE
Same as adult dose; however, higher doses may be required. See Maternal/Child.

DOSE ADJUSTMENTS
Reduced dose may be required in impaired renal function. ■ Higher doses may be required in pediatric patients. ■ Lower-end doses may be indicated in the elderly. Consider impaired organ function and concomitant disease or other drug therapy. ■ See Monitor and Drug/Lab Interactions.

DILUTION
Each 50 mg should be diluted immediately before use with 20 to 100 mL of NS or D5W and given as an infusion. May leach phthalate from polyvinylchloride containers; use diluents in glass infusion bottles. Dilute immediately before use and discard unused portion.

Filters: Filtered through a 0.45-micron polyprolene filter during manufacturing. Has a high ethanol content, which the filter must accommodate. A large-bore needle filter may be used when withdrawing cyclosporine from an ampule. Adsorption should be negligible, but if there is concern, draw diluent through the same filter. In-line filtering is acceptable. Manufacturer indicates that cyclosporine molecules are small enough to pass through an in-line filter as small as 0.22 microns. Loss of potency is not expected. Another source used 0.22- and 0.45-micron filters and indicates an initial loss of potency that recovered to full concentration.

Storage: Before use, store ampules at CRT. Protect from light. Discard diluted solution after 24 hours.

COMPATIBILITY
(Underline Indicates Conflicting Compatibility Information)

Consider any drug NOT listed as compatible to be INCOMPATIBLE until consulting a pharmacist; specific conditions may apply.

Leaches out plasticizers, including DEHP from PVC infusion bags and IV tubing; use of non-PVC containers and IV tubing recommended.

One source suggests the following **compatibilities:**

Additive: Ciprofloxacin (Cipro IV).

Y-site: Anidulafungin (Eraxis), caspofungin (Cancidas), doripenem (Doribax), linezolid (Zyvox), micafungin (Mycamine), propofol (Diprivan), sargramostim (Leukine).

RATE OF ADMINISTRATION
A single dose properly diluted as a slow IV infusion equally distributed over 2 to 6 hours.

ACTIONS

A potent immunosuppressive agent. Interferes with IL-2 production and blocks T-cell proliferative signals during early T-cell activation. Prolongs survival of kidney, liver, and heart allogeneic transplants in the human. Measured by specific or nonspecific assays. Extensively metabolized by the cytochrome P_{450} hepatic enzyme system. Half-life is 19 hours (range 10 to 27 hours). Primarily excreted in bile and to a small extent in urine. Crosses the placental barrier. Secreted in breast milk.

INDICATIONS AND USES

Prophylaxis of organ rejection in kidney, liver, and heart allogeneic transplants in conjunction with adrenocortical steroids. ■ Treatment of chronic rejection in patients previously treated with other immunosuppressive agents. Reserve parenteral formulation for when oral administration not feasible.

Unlabeled uses: Prophylaxis of organ rejection in pancreas, bone marrow, and heart/lung transplantation. ■ Severe ulcerative colitis.

CONTRAINDICATIONS

Hypersensitivity cyclosporine or polyoxyethylated castor oil.

PRECAUTIONS

Anaphylactic reactions have been reported with the IV formulation. These reactions may be related to the IV vehicle Cremophor EL; patients who experienced these reactions have subsequently been treated with the oral formulation of cyclosporine without incident. Because of the risk of anaphylaxis, IV cyclosporine should be reserved for patients who are unable to take oral therapy. ■ Usually administered in the hospital by or under the direction of a physician experienced in immunosuppressive therapy and management of organ transplant patients. ■ Adequate laboratory and supportive medical resources must be available. ■ All formulations may be given concomitantly with adrenocortical steroids. Manufacturer has a Black Box Warning. *Do not administer cyclosporine with any other immunosuppressive agent except adrenocortical steroids.* ■ Can cause hepatotoxicity and nephrotoxicity; see Monitor. In impaired renal function, if rejection is severe, try other immunosuppressive therapy or allow rejection and removal of the kidney rather than increase dose of cyclosporine. ■ May cause lymphomas and other malignancies, particularly those of the skin. Increased risk of developing a malignancy appears to be related to the intensity and duration of immunosuppression. Some malignancies may be fatal. ■ Patients receiving immunosuppressive therapies, including cyclosporine and cyclosporine-containing regimens, are at increased risk for infections (viral, bacterial, fungal, parasitic). Both generalized and localized infections can occur. Pre-existing infections may be aggravated. Latent infections may be reactivated, including BK virus–associated nephropathy. Fatal outcomes have been reported. ■ Encephalopathy has been reported. May be manifest as impaired consciousness, convulsions, visual disturbances, loss of motor function, movement disorders, and psychiatric disturbances. Predisposing factors may include hypertension, hypomagnesemia, hypocholesterolemia, high-dose corticosteroids, high cyclosporine blood levels, and graft-versus-host disease. Patients receiving liver transplants may be more susceptible to encephalopathy than patients receiving kidney transplants. Reversal of encephalopathy has occurred after discontinuation or dose reduction of cyclosporine. ■ Convulsions have been reported, particularly in patients receiving concomitant therapy with high-dose methylprednisolone. ▪ Significant hyperkalemia (sometimes associated with hyperchloremic acidosis) and hyperuricemia has been reported. ▪ A syndrome of thrombocytopenia and microangiopathic hemolytic anemia that may result in graft failure has been reported. ▪ Optic disc edema, including papilledema, with possible visual impairment secondary to benign intracranial hypertension has been reported. ▪ See Drug/Lab Interactions.

Monitor: Observe for S/S of an anaphylactic reaction (e.g., blood pressure changes; bronchospasm; dyspnea; edema of face, tongue, or throat; itching; rash; tachycardia; wheezing). Monitor continuously for the first 30 minutes of the infusion and frequently thereafter. ▪ Can cause hepatotoxicity and nephrotoxicity. Monitor BUN, SCr, serum bilirubin, and liver enzymes frequently. Timing and amount of rise in BUN and creatinine and degree of nephrotoxicity or hepatotoxicity distinguish between need for dose reduction or symptoms of organ rejection. ▪ May be difficult to distinguish between nephrotoxicity and rejection. Up to 20% of patients may have simultaneous nephrotoxicity and rejection. See package insert for a table discussing differential diagnoses for each. ▪ Monitor cyclosporine blood levels. Measured by specific or nonspecific assay. 24-hour specific trough values of 100 to 200 ng/mL of whole blood or 24-hour nonspecific trough values of 250 to 800 ng/mL of whole blood minimize side effects and rejection events. Nonspecific assays trough values are higher because they include metabolites. Plasma levels may range from ½ to ⅓ of whole blood levels. Consistent use of one assay is recommended. Confirm assay method to evaluate appropriately. ▪ Observe constantly for signs of infection (fever, sore throat, tiredness) or unusual bleeding or bruising. ▪ Prophylactic antibiotics may be indicated pending results of C/S. ▪ Monitor for development of BK virus–associated nephropathy. Dose reduction may be indicated. ▪ Monitor BP. Hypertension is a common side effect. Initiation or modification of antihypertensive therapy may be indicated; do not use potassium-sparing diuretics (e.g., spironolactone [Aldactone]); may increase risk of hyperkalemia. ▪ See Precautions and Drug/Lab Interactions.

Patient Education: Use nonhormonal birth control. Do not use oral contraceptives. See Appendix D, p. 1434. ▪ Do not make any changes in formulation (e.g., IV, capsules, oral solution) without physician direction; products are not equivalent. May require dose adjustment. ▪ Review side effects with a health care professional and report all side effects promptly. ▪ Capable of multiple drug-drug interactions; obtain physician approval before adding or stopping medications. ▪ Compliance with frequent laboratory tests is imperative.

Maternal/Child: Category C: safety for use in pregnancy not established. Should not be used unless benefit to the mother justifies potential risk to the fetus. Use in men and women capable of conception not established. Reported outcomes of pregnancies in women who received cyclosporine are difficult to evaluate. It is not possible to separate the effects of cyclosporine from the effects of other medications, underlying maternal disorders, or other aspects of the transplantation process. Negative outcomes included prematurity, low birth weight, fetal loss, and various malformations. ▪ Discontinue breast-feeding. ▪ Safety for use in pediatric patients not established but has been used in patients as young as 6 months.

Accidental parenteral overdose in premature neonates has caused serious symptoms of intoxication.

Elderly: Dose selection should be cautious; see Dose Adjustments. ▪ Differences in response compared to younger adults not identified.

DRUG/LAB INTERACTIONS

Interactions are numerous and potentially life threatening. Review of drug profile by pharmacist imperative. ▪ Risk of nephrotoxicity increased when given with other drugs that may potentiate renal dysfunction. Use extreme caution and monitor renal function closely. Manufacturer lists **antibiotics** (e.g., ciprofloxacin [Cipro], gentamicin, tobramycin, sulfamethoxazole/trimethoprim, vancomycin), **antifungals** (e.g., amphotericin B, caspofungin [Cancidas], ketoconazole [Nizoral]), **anti-inflammatory drugs** (e.g., azapropazon [Rheumox], colchicine, diclofenac [Voltaren, Cataflam], naproxen [Aleve, Naprosyn], sulindac [Clinoril]), **H₂ antagonists** (e.g., cimetidine [Tagamet], ranitidine [Zantac]), **immunosuppressives** (e.g., tacrolimus [Prograf]), **antineoplastics** (e.g., melphalan [Alkeran]), **and fibric acid derivatives** (e.g., fenofibrate [Tricor]). Other sources list **acyclovir** (Zovirax), **foscarnet** (Foscavir), **selected quinolones** (e.g., norfloxacin [Noroxin]), **and numerous other nephrotoxic drugs.** ▪ Concurrent administration with **colchicine** may cause cyclosporine toxicity (e.g., GI, hepatic, renal, and neuromuscular toxicity). Cyclosporine may decrease the clearance and increase the toxic effects of colchicine (e.g., myopathy, neuropathy), especially in patients with renal impairment. With concurrent use, close clinical observation is required. Reduce colchicine dose, or discontinue as indicated. ▪ May increase **diclofenac** (Voltaren) serum levels with concomitant administration; initiate diclofenac dose at the lower end of the therapeutic range. ▪ Cyclosporine is extensively metabolized by CYP3A4 and is a substrate of the multidrug efflux transporter P-glycoprotein. **Drugs that inhibit or induce CYP3A4, P-glycoprotein transporter, or both** will result in an alteration of cyclosporine concentrations. Toxicity or allograft rejection may occur. ▪ Cyclosporine plasma levels may be increased with concurrent use of **protease inhibitors** (e.g., indinavir [Crixivan], nelfinavir [Viracept], ritonavir [Norvir], saquinavir [Invirase]), which are metabolized by cytochrome P_{450} 3A; use caution. ▪ Drugs that inhibit the cytochrome P_{450} system may decrease the metabolism of cyclosporine and increase its serum concentrations. Manufacturer lists **allopurinol** (Aloprim), **amiodarone** (Nexterone), **antibiotics** (e.g., azithromycin [Zithromax], clarithromycin, erythromycin, quinupristin/dalfopristin [Synercid]), **antifungals** (e.g., fluconazole [Diflucan], itraconazole [Sporanox], ketoconazole [Nizoral], voriconazole [VFEND]), **bromocriptine** (Parlodel), **calcium channel blockers** (e.g., diltiazem [Cardizem], nicardipine [Cardene], verapamil), **colchicine, danazol** (Danocrine), **glucocorticoids** (e.g., methylprednisolone [Solu-Medrol]), **imatinib** (Gleevec), **metoclopramide** (Reglan), **nefazodone, and oral contraceptives.** Monitor blood levels with concurrent use to avoid cyclosporine toxicity. ▪ Drugs that decrease cyclosporine absorption should be avoided. Manufacturer lists **antibiotics** (e.g., nafcillin [Nallpen], rifampin [Rifadin]), **anticonvulsants** (e.g., carbamazepine [Tegretol], oxcarbazepine [Trileptal], phenobarbital [Luminal], phenytoin [Dilantin]), **bosentan** (Tracleer), **octreotide** (Sandostatin), **orlistat** (Alli), **terbinafine** (Lamisil), **ticlopidine** (Ticlid), **St. John's wort, and sulfinpyrazone** (Anturane). Other sources list **probucol** (Panavir), **sulfamethoxazole/trimethoprim;** monitor levels to avoid transplant rejection. ▪ **Rifabutin** (Mycobutin) may increase metabolism of cyclosporine; use care with concomitant use. ▪ Cyclosporine inhibits CYP3A4 and the multidrug efflux transporter P-glycoprotein and may increase plasma concentrations of co-medications that are substrates of CYP3A4, P-glycoprotein, or both. Cyclosporine reduces clearance and may increase blood levels of **colchicine, digoxin, etoposide, methotrexate, and prednisolone;** in addition it may decrease the volume distribution of digoxin and cause toxicity rather quickly. With concurrent use, monitor digoxin levels, reduce digoxin dose, or discontinue as indicated. Cyclosporine may decrease the clearance of **HMG-CoA reductase inhibitors (statins)** such as atorvastatin (Lipitor), lovastatin (Mevacor), pravastatin (Pravachol), simvastatin (Zocor) and, rarely, fluvastatin (Lescol). Cases of myotoxicity (including muscle pain and weakness, myositis, and rhabdomyolysis) have been reported with concomitant use. Dose reduction of statins is indicated. Statins may be temporarily withheld or discontinued in patients with S/S of myopathy or potential for renal injury, including renal failure, secondary to rhabdomyolysis. ▪ May decrease **mycophenolate** (CellCept) levels. Monitor levels closely when cyclosporine is added or removed from a drug regimen containing mycophenolate. ▪ Concurrent use of cyclosporine with **imipenem-cilastatin** (Primaxin) may increase CNS toxicity of both agents. ▪ Potentiates **nondepolarizing muscle relaxants** (e.g., atracurium [Tracrium]); will prolong neuromuscular blockade. ▪ Do not use **potassium-sparing diuretics** (e.g., spironolactone [Aldactone]); may increase risk of hyperkalemia. Use caution when coadministered with **other potassium-sparing drugs** (e.g., angiotensin-converting inhibitors [e.g., enalaprilat (Vasotec IV), lisinopril (Prinivil)], angiotensin II receptor antagonists [e.g., losartan (Cozaar), valsartan (Diovan)]), **potassium-containing drugs,** and/or in patients on a **potassium-rich diet.** Hyperkalemia can occur. ▪ May cause convulsions with **methylprednisolone.** ▪ May be given in combination with **steroids** but has additive effects with other **immunosuppressive agents;** may increase risk of lymphoma. ▪ Concurrent administration with **sirolimus** (Rapamune) increases blood levels of sirolimus. To minimize the effect on blood levels, administer sirolimus 4 hours after cyclosporine dose. ▪ Elevations in SCr have been reported with coadministration of **sirolimus** and cyclosporine. Effect is usually reversible with cyclosporine dose reduction. ▪ Serum levels may increase with **chloroquine** (Aralen). ▪ Avoid use in psoriasis patients receiving **other immunosuppressive agents or radiation therapy, including PUVA and UVB.** Immunosuppression may be excessive. ▪ May increase the plasma concentrations of **repaglinide** (Prandin), which increases the risk for hypoglycemia. Monitor blood glucose levels closely. ▪ Vaccinations may be less effective. Do not use **live virus vaccines** in patients receiving cyclosporine. ▪ **Grapefruit juice** may affect certain enzymes of the P_{450} enzyme system and should be avoided.

SIDE EFFECTS
The most common side effects include gum hyperplasia, hirsutism, hypertension, renal dysfunction, and tremor. Other side effects include acne, convulsions, cramps, diarrhea, encephalopathy, glomerular capillary thrombosis, headache, hepatotoxicity, hyperkalemia, hyperuricemia, hypomagnesemia, infection, leukopenia, lymphoma, microangiopathic hemolytic anemia, nausea and vomiting, paresthesia, skin rash, and throm-

bocytopenia. Hypersensitivity reactions including anaphylaxis have occurred. Stevens-Johnson syndrome and toxic epidermal necrolysis have occurred rarely.

Post-Marketing: BK virus–associated nephropathy.

ANTIDOTE
Notify physician of all side effects. Most can be treated symptomatically. Drug may be decreased or discontinued or other immunosuppressive agents utilized. Discontinue infusion at the first sign of a severe hypersensitivity reaction. Treat hypersensitivity as indicated; may require oxygen, epinephrine (Adrenalin), antihistamines (e.g., diphenhydramine [Benadryl]), vasopressors (e.g., dopamine), corticosteroids, albuterol, IV fluids, and/or ventilation equipment. Nephrotoxicity, hepatotoxicity, encephalopathy, or hematopoietic depression may require temporary reduction of dosage or permanent withholding of treatment. Dialysis is not effective in overdose.

CYTARABINE BBW

(sye-**TAIR**-ah-bean)

ARA-C, ✤Cytosar, Cytosar-U

Antineoplastic (antimetabolite)

pH 5

USUAL DOSE
Acute nonlymphocytic leukemia in adult and pediatric patients: *Single agent:* 200 mg/M^2/24 hr as a continuous infusion for 5 days. Repeat every 2 weeks. *Combination chemotherapy:* Dose is variable depending on specific regimen or protocol. Examples are 100 mg/M^2/24 hr as a continuous infusion or 100 mg/M^2 as an IV injection every 12 hours. Repeat daily on days 1 through 7. Another regimen uses 100 to 200 mg/M^2 or 2 to 6 mg/kg/24 hr as a continuous infusion or equally divided into 2 or 3 doses and given by IV injection or intermittent infusion. Given for 5 to 10 days. Maintain treatment until therapeutic effect or toxicity occurs. Modify on a day-to-day basis for maximum individualized effectiveness.

Acute myelocytic leukemia or erythroleukemia in adult and pediatric patients: As a single agent, 100 to 200 mg/M^2/24 hr or 3 mg/kg/24 hr for 5 to 10 days as a continuous infusion or in divided doses by IV injection. Total dose is 1,000 mg/M^2. Repeat every 2 weeks.

DOSE ADJUSTMENTS
Dose (mg/kg) based on average weight in presence of edema or ascites. ▪ Dose reduction may be indicated in impaired hepatic or renal function. ▪ See Precautions/Monitor. ▪ Usually used with other antineoplastic drugs in specific doses to achieve tumor remission. ▪ Withhold or modify dose based on degree of bone marrow suppression; see Monitor.

DILUTION
Specific techniques required; see Precautions. Some preparations are liquid and do not require reconstitution or each 100 mg must be reconstituted with 5 mL (500 mg with 10 mL) of SW for injection with benzyl alcohol 0.9%. Solution pH about 5. May be given by IV injection as is or further

diluted in NS or D5W and given as an infusion. IV injection should be through a free-flowing IV tubing. Use only clear solutions.
Storage: Stable at room temperature for 48 hours.

COMPATIBILITY   (Underline Indicates Conflicting Compatibility Information)
Consider any drug NOT listed as compatible to be INCOMPATIBLE until consulting a pharmacist; specific conditions may apply.
One source suggests the following **compatibilities:**
Additive: Daunorubicin (Cerubidine), gentamicin, hydrocortisone sodium succinate (Solu-Cortef), lincomycin (Lincocin), methotrexate, methylprednisolone (Solu-Medrol), mitoxantrone (Novantrone), ondansetron (Zofran), potassium chloride (KCl), sodium bicarbonate, vincristine.
Y-site: Amifostine (Ethyol), anidulafungin (Eraxis), aztreonam (Azactam), cefepime (Maxipime), chlorpromazine (Thorazine), cladribine (Leustatin), dexamethasone (Decadron), diphenhydramine (Benadryl), doxorubicin liposomal (Doxil), droperidol (Inapsine), etoposide phosphate (Etopophos), famotidine (Pepcid IV), filgrastim (Neupogen), fludarabine (Fludara), furosemide (Lasix), gemcitabine (Gemzar), gentamicin, granisetron (Kytril), heparin, hydrocortisone sodium succinate (Solu-Cortef), hydromorphone (Dilaudid), idarubicin (Idamycin), linezolid (Zyvox), lorazepam (Ativan), melphalan (Alkeran), methotrexate, methylprednisolone (Solu-Medrol), metoclopramide (Reglan), morphine, ondansetron (Zofran), paclitaxel (Taxol), pemetrexed (Alimta), piperacillin/tazobactam (Zosyn), prochlorperazine (Compazine), promethazine (Phenergan), propofol (Diprivan), ranitidine (Zantac), sargramostim (Leukine), sodium bicarbonate, teniposide (Vumon), thiotepa, vinorelbine (Navelbine).

RATE OF ADMINISTRATION
IV injection: Each 100 mg or fraction thereof over 1 to 3 minutes.
IV infusion: Single daily dose properly diluted over 30 minutes to 24 hours, depending on amount of infusion solution and dosage regimen.

ACTIONS
An antimetabolite and pyrimidine antagonist that interferes with the synthesis of DNA. Cell cycle specific for S phase. Through various chemical processes this deprivation acts more quickly on rapidly growing cells and causes their death. Cytotoxic and cytostatic. A potent bone marrow suppressant. Crosses the blood-brain barrier. Serum half-life averages 1 to 3 hours. Metabolized in the liver and excreted in the urine.

INDICATIONS AND USES
Induction and maintenance of remission in acute nonlymphocytic leukemia in adults and pediatric patients. Also used for treatment of acute lymphocytic leukemia (ALL), the blast phase of chronic myelocytic leukemia, and acute myelocytic leukemia (AML). ▪ Is used intrathecally in the treatment of meningeal leukemia. A liposomal formulation (DepoCyt) is available for intrathecal use only, lipofoam molecules contained in this product are much too large for IV use.

CONTRAINDICATIONS
Hypersensitivity to cytarabine, pre-existing drug-induced bone marrow suppression.

PRECAUTIONS
Follow guidelines for handling cytotoxic agents. See Appendix A, p. 1429.
▪ Administered by or under the direction of a physician specialist in a facility with adequate diagnostic and treatment facilities to monitor the patient and respond to any medical emergency. ▪ Remissions induced by cytarabine are

brief unless followed by maintenance therapy. ▪ Use caution with impaired liver or renal function. ▪ Severe GI, pulmonary, or CNS toxicity has occurred with experimental cytarabine regimens. Toxicities are different (e.g., reversible corneal toxicity, hemorrhagic conjunctivitis, cerebral and cerebellar dysfunction, severe GI ulceration) from those seen with conventional therapy. Deaths have been reported. ▪ Benzyl alcohol may cause a fatal "gasping syndrome" in premature infants.

Monitor: Leukocyte and platelet counts should be monitored daily. ▪ During induction therapy, WBC depression is biphasic with the first nadir occurring at days 7 to 9 and a deeper fall at days 15 to 24. Platelet depression begins around day 5 and reaches a nadir at days 12 to 15. ▪ Hold or modify therapy for platelet count less than 50,000 or polymorphonuclear granulocytes less than 1,000 cells/mm^3. Restart therapy when bone marrow recovery is confirmed. ▪ Monitor bone marrow, liver, and renal function at regular intervals during therapy. ▪ Higher doses tolerated by IV injection compared with IV infusion, but the incidence and intensity of nausea and vomiting are increased. ▪ Prophylactic administration of antiemetics recommended. ▪ Be alert for signs of bone marrow suppression, bleeding, infection, or neurotoxicity. These side effects are dose- and schedule-dependent. ▪ Monitor for thrombocytopenia (platelet count less than 50,000/mm^3). Initiate precautions to prevent excessive bleeding (e.g., inspect IV sites, skin, and mucous membranes; use extreme care during invasive procedures; test urine, emesis, stool, and secretions for occult blood). ▪ Prophylactic antibiotics may be indicated pending results of C/S in a febrile neutropenic patient. ▪ Monitor uric acid levels; maintain hydration; allopurinol may be indicated.

Patient Education: Nonhormonal birth control recommended. ▪ See Appendix D, p. 1434. ▪ Promptly report early signs of neurotoxicity (e.g., ataxia, confusion, lethargy).

Maternal/Child: Category D: avoid pregnancy. May produce teratogenic effects on the fetus, especially during the first trimester. ▪ Discontinue breast-feeding. ▪ See Drug/Lab Interactions.

Elderly: Consider age-related organ impairment; toxicity may be increased.

DRUG/LAB INTERACTIONS

May inhibit **digoxin** absorption. ▪ Do not administer any **live virus vaccines** to patients receiving antineoplastic drugs. ▪ May cause acute pancreatitis in patients who previously received **L-asparaginase.** ▪ May antagonize action of **gentamicin** against *Klebsiella.* ▪ May antagonize antifungal actions of **flucytosine** (Ancobon). ▪ Clearance decreased and toxicity increased with **nephrotoxic agents** (e.g., aminoglycosides [gentamicin]); may cause neurotoxic symptoms (e.g., ataxia, confusion, lethargy). ▪ Concurrent use of high doses of **cytarabine** with cisplatin may increase ototoxicity.

SIDE EFFECTS

Abdominal pain, bone marrow suppression (e.g., anemia, leukopenia, thrombocytopenia), bone pain, cardiomyopathy, chest pain, conjunctivitis, diarrhea, esophagitis, fever, hepatic dysfunction, hypersensitivity reactions, hyperuricemia, malaise, megaloblastosis, mucosal bleeding, myalgia, nausea, oral ulceration, pancreatitis, peripheral motor and sensory neuropathies, rash, stomatitis, thrombophlebitis, vomiting. Higher than usual dose regimens may cause severe coma, GI ulcerations and peritonitis, personality changes, pulmonary toxicity, somnolence, or death.

ANTIDOTE

Notify the physician of all side effects. Most will be treated symptomatically. Some toxicity is necessary to produce remission. Discontinue the drug for serious bone marrow suppression. Administration of whole blood products (e.g., packed RBCs, platelets, leukocytes), and/or blood modifiers (e.g., darbepoetin alfa [Aranesp], epoetin alfa [Epogen], filgrastim [Neupogen], oprelvekin [Neumega], pegfilgrastim [Neulasta], sargramostim [Leukine]) may be indicated to treat bone marrow toxicity. Drug must be restarted as soon as signs of bone marrow recovery occur, or its effectiveness will be lost. Use corticosteroids for cytarabine syndrome (fever, myalgia, bone pain, occasional chest pain, maculopapular rash, conjunctivitis, malaise). Usually occurs in 6 to 12 hours after administration. Continue cytarabine if patient responds to corticosteriods. There is no specific antidote; supportive therapy as indicated will help to sustain the patient in toxicity.

CYTOMEGALOVIRUS IMMUNE GLOBULIN INTRAVENOUS (HUMAN) BBW *
(sigh-toh-**meg**-ah-lo-**VIGH**-rus ih-**MUNE** **GLAW**-byoo-lin)

CMV-IGIV, CytoGam

Passive immunizing agent
Antibacterial
Antiviral

*This drug is on the Black Box Warning list; however, a BBW is not provided in the parenteral prescribing information.

USUAL DOSE

150 mg/kg is the maximum recommended dose per infusion.

Kidney transplant: 150 mg/kg of body weight as an IV infusion. This initial dose must be given within 72 hours of transplant. Additional infusions of 100 mg/kg are given at 2, 4, 6, and 8 weeks post-transplant, then reduced to 50 mg/kg at 12 and 16 weeks post-transplant.

Heart, liver, lung, and pancreas transplants: 150 mg/kg of body weight as an IV infusion. This initial dose must be given within 72 hours of transplant. Consider use in combination with ganciclovir (Cytovene) 10 mg/kg/day for 14 days. Additional infusions of cytomegalovirus IGIV containing 150 mg/kg are given at 2, 4, 6, and 8 weeks post-transplant, then reduced to 100 mg/kg at 12 and 16 weeks post-transplant.

DILUTION

Absolute sterile technique required; contains no preservatives. Available in 20- and 50-mL vials (50 mg/mL); multiple vials may be required. Use only if clear and colorless. Enter vial only once and initiate infusion within 6 hours. Must be completely infused within 12 hours of dilution. See Rate of Administration.

Filters: Use of an in-line filter (pore size 15 microns [0.2 microns acceptable]) is required; see Rate of Administration.

Storage: Store dry powder in refrigerator between 2° and 8° C (35° to 46° F).

COMPATIBILITY

Administration through a separate infusion line recommended. If absolutely necessary, may be piggybacked in a pre-existing line containing NS, ½NS, dextrose 2.5%, 5%, 10%, or 20% in water or saline. Do not dilute CMV-IGIV more than one part to two parts of any of these solutions.

RATE OF ADMINISTRATION

Use of an in-line filter (pore size 15 microns [0.2 microns acceptable]) and a constant infusion pump (e.g., IVAC) is required. Begin with a rate of 15 mg/kg/hr. May be increased to 30 mg/kg/hr in 30 minutes if no discomfort or adverse effects. May be increased in another 30 minutes to 60 mg/kg/hr if no discomfort or adverse effects. Do not exceed the 60 mg/kg/hr rate or allow the volume infused to exceed 75 mL/hr regardless of mg/kg/hr dose. Slow rate of infusion at onset of patient discomfort or any adverse reactions. Infusion must be complete within 12 hours of dilution. Subsequent doses may be increased at 15-minute intervals using the same mg/kg/hr rates and adhering to the volume maximum of 75 mL/hr.

ACTIONS

A sterile solution of immunoglobulin Gm (IgG). Derived from pooled adult human plasma selected for high titers of antibody for cytomegalovirus (CMV). Purified by a specific process. Can raise the relevant antibody levels sufficiently to attenuate or reduce the incidence of serious CMV disease. Antibody levels will last 2 to 3 weeks. Recent studies of combined prophylaxis with CMV-IGIV and ganciclovir have shown reductions in the incidence of serious CMV-associated disease in CMV-seronegative recipients of CMV-seropositive organs below that expected from one drug alone.

INDICATIONS AND USES

Prophylaxis of CMV disease associated with transplantation of kidney, heart, liver, lung, and pancreas. In transplants of these organs other than kidney from CMV-seropositive donors to seronegative recipients, prophylactic CMV-IGIV should be considered in combination with ganciclovir.

CONTRAINDICATIONS

History of a prior severe reaction associated with any human immunoglobulin preparations. Individuals with selective immunoglobulin A deficiency may develop antibodies to IgA and are at risk for anaphylaxis.

PRECAUTIONS

75% of untreated recipients would be expected to develop CMV disease. Use of CMV-IGIV has effected a 50% reduction in this disease rate. Effective results have been obtained with a variety of immunosuppressive regimens (e.g., combinations of azathioprine, cyclosporine, prednisone). ▪ A fatal CMV infection occurred even with ganciclovir treatment in one patient, who inadvertently missed a single injection.

Monitor: Continuous monitoring of vital signs is preferred. Must be monitored before infusion, at every rate change, the midpoint, at the conclusion, and several times after completion. ▪ All supplies for emergency treatment of acute anaphylactic reaction must be available; see Antidote.

Patient Education: Adherence to the prescribed regimen is imperative.

Maternal/Child: Category C: safety for use during pregnancy or breastfeeding not established. Use only if clearly needed.

DRUG/LAB INTERACTIONS

Defer vaccination with any **live virus vaccine** (e.g., measles, mumps, rubella) until 3 months after CMV-IGIV administration.

SIDE EFFECTS

Incidence related to rate of administration; back pain, chills, fever, flushing, hypotension, muscle cramps, nausea, vomiting, wheezing. Hypersensitivity reactions, including anaphylaxis, are possible.

ANTIDOTE

With onset of any minor side effect, reduce rate of infusion immediately or discontinue temporarily. Discontinue CMV-IGIV if symptoms persist and notify the physician. May be treated symptomatically and infusion resumed at a slower rate if symptoms subside. Discontinue CMV-IGIV if hypotension or anaphylaxis occur and treat immediately. Epinephrine (Adrenalin), diphenhydramine (Benadryl), oxygen, vasopressors (e.g., dopamine), corticosteroids, and ventilation equipment must always be available. Resuscitate as necessary.

DACARBAZINE BBW

(dah-**KAR**-bah-zeen)

DTIC, DTIC-Dome

Antineoplastic
(alkylating agent)

pH 3 to 4

USUAL DOSE

Malignant melanoma: 2 to 4.5 mg/kg of body weight/24 hr for 10 days. May be repeated at 4-week intervals. May administer 250 mg/M^2 daily for 5 days. Repeat in 3 weeks. Has proved as effective in lesser doses as in larger doses. Individualized response determines dosage of subsequent treatments.

Hodgkin's disease: 150 mg/M^2/24 hr for 5 days. Repeat every 4 weeks. Used in combination with other drugs in a specific regimen. An alternate regimen is 375 mg/M^2 on Days 1 and 15 every 4 weeks or 100 mg/M^2/day for 5 days. Given as part of a specific protocol.

DOSE ADJUSTMENTS

Dose (mg/kg) based on average weight in presence of edema or ascites. ■ Used with other antineoplastic drugs and radiation therapy in reduced doses to achieve tumor remission. ■ Dose reduction may be required in impaired liver and renal function.

DILUTION

Specific techniques required; see Precautions. Each 100-mg vial is diluted with 9.9 mL (200 mg with 19.7 mL) of SW for injection (10 mg/mL). Further dilution in 50 to 250 mL of D5W or NS for infusion is preferred. May be given through Y-tube or three-way stopcock of infusion set through a free-flowing IV.

Storage: Discard in 6 to 8 hours if kept at room temperature. Reconstituted solution stable for 72 hours, diluted solution for 24 hours if refrigerated at 4° C (39° F).

COMPATIBILITY   (Underline Indicates Conflicting Compatibility Information)
Consider any drug NOT listed as compatible to be INCOMPATIBLE until consulting a pharmacist; specific conditions may apply.
One source suggests the following **compatibilities:**
Additive: Ondansetron (Zofran).

Y-site: Amifostine (Ethyol), aztreonam (Azactam), doxorubicin liposomal (Doxil), etoposide phosphate (Etopophos), filgrastim (Neupogen), fludarabine (Fludara), granisetron (Kytril), heparin, melphalan (Alkeran), ondansetron (Zofran), paclitaxel (Taxol), palonosetron (Aloxi), sargramostim (Leukine), teniposide (Vumon), thiotepa, vinorelbine (Navelbine).

RATE OF ADMINISTRATION
Total dose over 30 to 60 minutes. More rapid rate may cause severe venous irritation.

ACTIONS
An antineoplastic agent. Exact mechanism of action is not known; may inhibit DNA and RNA synthesis. It is an alkylating agent, cell cycle phase nonspecific. Probably localizes in the liver and is excreted in the urine.

INDICATIONS AND USES
Metastatic malignant melanoma. ▪ Hodgkin's disease. ▪ Soft-tissue sarcomas.

Unlabeled uses: Treatment of malignant pheochromocytoma with cyclophosphamide and vincristine. ▪ Treatment of metastatic malignant melanoma with tamoxifen.

CONTRAINDICATIONS
Known hypersensitivity to dacarbazine.

PRECAUTIONS
Follow guidelines for handling cytotoxic agents. See Appendix A, p. 1429. ▪ Administered by or under the direction of the physician specialist. ▪ Bone marrow suppression is the most common toxicity. ▪ Hepatic necrosis has been reported. ▪ Consider potential for therapeutic benefit versus risk for toxicity. ▪ Use caution in impaired liver and renal function.
Monitor: Determine absolute patency of vein; a stinging or burning sensation indicates extravasation; severe cellulitis and tissue necrosis will result. Discontinue injection; use another vein. ▪ Monitor bone marrow function, white and RBC count, and platelet count frequently. ▪ Nausea and vomiting may be reduced by restricting oral intake of fluid and foods for 4 to 6 hours before administration. Use prophylactic antiemetics. ▪ Be alert for signs of bone marrow suppression, bleeding, or infection. ▪ Monitor for thrombocytopenia (platelet count less than 50,000/mm³). Initiate precautions to prevent excessive bleeding (e.g., inspect IV sites, skin, and mucous membranes; use extreme care during invasive procedures; test urine, emesis, stool, and secretions for occult blood). ▪ Prophylactic antibiotics may be indicated pending results of C/S in a febrile neutropenic patient.
Patient Education: Protect skin surfaces; may cause photosensitive skin reactions. ▪ Nonhormonal birth control recommended. ▪ Report burning or stinging at IV site promptly. ▪ See Appendix D, p. 1434.
Maternal/Child: Category C: safety for use in pregnancy or breast-feeding and in men and women capable of conception not established. ▪ Carcinogenic and teratogenic in animals. ▪ Discontinue breast-feeding.
Elderly: Consider age-related organ impairment; toxicity may be increased.

DRUG/LAB INTERACTIONS

Do not administer any **live virus vaccines** to patients receiving antineoplastic drugs. ▪ Inhibited by **phenobarbital and phenytoin** (Dilantin). ▪ Potentiates **allopurinol.** ▪ Effects of dacarbazine may be increased with **ciprofloxacin** (Cipro), **isoniazid** (INH), **fluvoxamine** (Luvox), **ketoconazole** (Nizoral), **miconazole** (Monistat), **and norfloxacin** (Noroxin). Effects may be decreased with **carbamazepine** (Tegretol), **phenobarbital, and rifampin** (Rifadin).

SIDE EFFECTS

Leukopenia and thrombocytopenia may be serious enough to cause death. Alopecia, anaphylaxis, anorexia, facial flushing, facial paresthesias, fever, hepatotoxicity, malaise, myalgia, nausea, skin necrosis, vomiting.

ANTIDOTE

Notify physician of all side effects. Most will be treated symptomatically. Bone marrow suppression may require temporary or permanent withholding of treatment. Administration of whole blood products (e.g., packed RBCs, platelets, leukocytes) and/or blood modifiers (e.g., darbepoetin alfa [Aranesp], epoetin alfa [Epogen], filgrastim [Neupogen], oprelvekin [Neumega], pegfilgrastim [Neulasta], sargramostim [Leukine]) may be indicated to treat bone marrow toxicity. There is no specific antidote. Supportive therapy as indicated will help sustain the patient in toxicity. For extravasation, elevate extremity; consider injection of long-acting dexamethasone (Decadron LA) throughout extravasated tissue. Use a 27- or 25-gauge needle. Apply moist, warm compresses.

DACTINOMYCIN BBW

(dack-tin-oh-**MY**-sin)

Cosmegen

Antineoplastic
(antibiotic)

pH 5.5 to 7

USUAL DOSE

Dose will depend on tolerance of the patient, the size and location of the tumor, and the use of other forms of therapy. Calculate each dose carefully before administration. Calculation of the dose for obese or edematous patients should be based on body surface area. The dose intensity per 2-week cycle for adult and pediatric patients should not exceed 15 mcg/kg/day (0.015 mg/kg/day) or 400 to 600 mcg/M^2/day (0.4 to 0.6 mg/M^2/day) for 5 days.

Wilms' tumor, childhood rhabdomyosarcoma, and Ewing's sarcoma: 15 mcg/ kg/day for 5 days. May be administered in various combinations and schedules with other chemotherapeutic agents.

Metastatic nonseminomatous testicular cancer: 1,000 mcg/M^2 (1 mg/M^2) on Day 1 as part of a combination regimen.

Gestational trophoblastic neoplasia: 12 mcg/kg/day for 5 days as a single agent or 500 mcg on Days 1 and 2 as part of a combination regimen.

PEDIATRIC DOSE

Same as Usual Dose for adults; see Contraindications.

DOSE ADJUSTMENTS

Calculate dose based on body surface area in presence of edema or ascites. ■ Used with other antineoplastic drugs in reduced doses to achieve tumor remission. ■ Reduce dose of dactinomycin and radiation therapy when used concurrently, if either has been used previously, or if previous chemotherapy has been employed. ■ Dose selection should be cautious in the elderly. Consider potential for decreased cardiac, hepatic, and renal function, and concomitant disease or drug therapy; see Elderly.

DILUTION

Specific techniques required; see Precautions. Highly toxic. Both powder and solution must be handled with care. Dilute each 0.5-mg vial with 1.1 mL of preservative-free SW for injection (0.5 mg/mL). SW with preservative (benzyl alcohol or paraben) will cause precipitation. Use 2.2 mL to yield 0.25 mg/mL (vent vial to relieve pressure). Very corrosive to soft tissue. Use sterile two-needle technique if given by IV injection; one needle to dilute and withdraw and one needle to inject into the vein (rinse with blood or IV solution before removing). May be given by IV injection, through the Y-tube or three-way stopcock of a free-flowing infusion of D5W or NS, or further diluted in 50 mL of the above solutions for infusion.

Filters: Manufacturer states, "Use of some in-line cellulose ester membrane filters have resulted in loss of potency." Another source suggests no loss of drug potency with a 5-micron stainless steel depth filter.

Storage: Store at 25° C (77° F); excursion permitted to 15° to 30° C (59° to 86° F). Protect from light and humidity. Discard any unused portion.

COMPATIBILITY

Consider any drug NOT listed as compatible to be INCOMPATIBLE until consulting a pharmacist; specific conditions may apply.

Forms a precipitate with SW that contains preservatives. Cellulose ester membrane filters may reduce dose by partial removal of dactinomycin.

One source suggests the following **compatibilities:**

Y-site: Allopurinol (Aloprim), amifostine (Ethyol), aztreonam (Azactam), cefepime (Maxipime), etoposide phosphate (Etopophos), fludarabine (Fludara), gemcitabine (Gemzar), granisetron (Kytril), melphalan (Alkeran), ondansetron (Zofran), sargramostim (Leukine), teniposide (Vumon), thiotepa, vinorelbine (Navelbine).

RATE OF ADMINISTRATION

IV injection: A single dose over 2 to 3 minutes.

IV infusion: A single dose over 10 to 15 minutes.

ACTIONS

A highly toxic antibiotic antineoplastic agent, cell cycle phase nonspecific. Cytotoxic, it interferes with cell division by binding DNA to slow production of RNA. Found in high concentrations in the kidney, liver, and spleen. Does not penetrate the blood-brain barrier. Minimally metabolized. Elimination half-life is approximately 36 hours. Excreted as unchanged drug in bile and urine.

INDICATIONS AND USES

As part of a combination chemotherapy and/or multi-modality regimen for treatment of Wilms' tumor, childhood rhabdomyosarcoma, Ewing's sarcoma, and metastatic nonseminomatous testicular cancer. ■ Alone or in combination with other chemotherapeutic agents for the treatment of gestational trophoblastic neoplasia.

Unlabeled uses: Kaposi's sarcoma, osteosarcoma.

CONTRAINDICATIONS

Exposure to chickenpox, herpes zoster, known sensitivity to dactinomycin, infants under 6 to 12 months of age.

PRECAUTIONS

Follow guidelines for handling cytotoxic agents. Review before handling and follow diligently. See Appendix A, p. 1429. ▪ For IV use only. Do not administer IM or SC. ▪ Highly toxic; both the powder and solution must be handled and administered with care. Inhalation of dust or vapors and contact with skin or mucous membranes, especially those of the eyes, must be avoided. If eye contact occurs, rinse for at least 15 minutes with water, saline or a balanced salt ophthalmic solution and then seek immediate ophthalmologic consultation. If skin contact occurs, remove contaminated clothing and rinse area for 15 minutes. Medical attention should be sought immediately and clothes should be destroyed. ▪ Administered by or under the direction of a physician specialist. ▪ In general, dactinomycin should not be administered concomitantly with radiation therapy in the treatment of Wilms' tumor unless the benefit outweighs the risk. Hepatomegaly and elevated AST levels have been reported. ▪ Hepatic veno-occlusive disease that may be associated with intravascular clotting disorder and multi-organ failure has been reported. Pediatric patients younger than 48 months of age may be at increased risk. ▪ May have increased incidence of second primary tumors following treatment with dactinomycin and radiation. Long-term follow-up of cancer survivors is indicated.

Monitor: Very corrosive to soft tissue; determine absolute patency of vein. A stinging or burning sensation indicates extravasation; severe cellulitis and tissue necrosis will result. Discontinue injection; use another vein. Close observation and reconstructive surgery consultation are recommended. ▪ Monitor renal, hepatic, and bone marrow function frequently. ▪ Except for immediate nausea and vomiting, side effects may not appear for 2 to 4 days and may not peak for 1 to 2 weeks. Always observe closely. Use prophylactic antiemetics. ▪ If stomatitis, diarrhea, or severe hematopoietic depression appears, discontinue therapy until the patient has recovered. ▪ An increased incidence of GI toxicity, bone marrow suppression, and skin and mucosal reactions has been reported when dactinomycin is administered in combination with radiation therapy. ▪ Monitor for thrombocytopenia (platelet count less than 50,000/mm^3). Initiate precautions to prevent excessive bleeding (e.g., inspect IV sites, skin, and mucous membranes; use extreme care during invasive procedures; test urine, emesis, stool, and secretions for occult blood). ▪ Allopurinol, increased fluid intake, and alkalinization of urine may be required to reduce uric acid levels. ▪ Observe closely for signs of infection. Prophylactic antibiotics may be indicated pending results of C/S in a febrile neutropenic patient.

Patient Education: Nonhormonal birth control recommended. ▪ Report burning or stinging at IV site promptly. ▪ See Appendix D, p. 1434.

Maternal/Child: Category D: avoid pregnancy. May produce teratogenic effects on the fetus; use caution in men and women capable of conception. ▪ Discontinue breast-feeding. ▪ See Contraindications and Precautions.

Elderly: Response similar to that in younger adults; however, recent studies suggest elderly may be at increased risk for myelosuppression; see Dose Adjustments.

DRUG/LAB INTERACTIONS

Radiation therapy potentiates dactinomycin. ▪ Dactinomycin alone may reactivate erythema from **previous radiation therapy.** ▪ Do not administer **live virus vaccines** to patients receiving antineoplastic drugs. ▪ Inhibits action of **penicillin.** ▪ See Dose Adjustments. ▪ May interfere with **bioassay procedures** used in determining antibacterial drug levels.

SIDE EFFECTS

Toxic reactions are frequent, may be severe, and may be dose limiting; however, the severity of toxicity varies markedly and is only partly dependent on the dose administered. Abdominal pain, acne, alopecia, anaphylaxis, anorexia, bone marrow suppression (e.g., anemia, aplastic anemia, agranulocytosis, febrile neutropenia, leukopenia, neutropenia, thrombocytopenia), cheilitis, diarrhea, dysphagia, erythema flare-up, esophagitis, fatigue, fever, GI ulceration, hypocalcemia, lethargy, liver toxicity (ascites, hepatitis, hepatic failure with reports of death, hepatic veno-occlusive disease, hepatomegaly, and liver function test abnormalities), malaise, myalgia, nausea, pharyngitis, pneumonitis, proctitis, skin eruptions, ulcerative stomatitis, vomiting.

ANTIDOTE

Any side effect can result in death. Notify the physician of all side effects. Most will be treated symptomatically. Bone marrow suppression may require withholding dactinomycin until recovery occurs. No specific antidote. Supportive therapy as indicated will help sustain the patient in toxicity. Administration of whole blood products (e.g., packed RBCs, platelets, leukocytes) and/or blood modifiers (e.g., darbepoetin alfa [Aranesp], epoetin alfa [Epogen], filgrastim [Neupogen], oprelvekin [Neumega], pegfilgrastim [Neulasta], sargramostim [Leukine]) may be indicated to treat bone marrow toxicity. For extravasation, discontinue immediately and elevate extremity. Apply ice to site four times daily for 3 days. Close observation and reconstructive surgery consultation recommended.

DANTROLENE SODIUM
(**DAN**-troh-leen **SO**-dee-um)

Dantrium

Skeletal muscle relaxant
(direct acting)

pH 9.5

USUAL DOSE

In patients known to be susceptible to malignant hyperthermia, oral dantrolene is indicated prophylactically preoperatively and postoperatively for 1 to 3 days following therapeutic IV treatment. Postoperative dosing is indicated after emergency treatment.

Prophylactic dose: 2.5 mg/kg as an infusion. Begin administration 1¼ hours before anesthesia, and administer over 1 hour. Oral dantrolene may be used.

Therapeutic or emergency dose: 1 mg/kg of body weight as an initial dose. Repeat as necessary until symptoms subside or a cumulative dose of 10 mg/kg is reached. Entire regimen may be repeated if symptoms reappear. Dose required depends on degree of susceptibility to malignant hyperthermia, length of time of exposure to triggering agent, and time lapse between onset of crisis and beginning of treatment. Discontinue all anesthetic agents at the first sign of a malignant hyperthermia reaction. Administration of 100% oxygen is recommended.

Post-crisis follow-up: An oral dose of 4 to 8 mg/kg/day for 1 to 3 days to prevent recurrences. If oral dosing not feasible, begin IV dose at 1 mg/kg and individualize by increasing based on patient response.

PEDIATRIC DOSE

Prophylactic, therapeutic, and post-crisis follow-up doses are the same as for adults; see Maternal/Child.

DOSE ADJUSTMENTS

Dose selection should be cautious in the elderly. Reduced doses may be indicated based on the potential for decreased organ function and concomitant disease or drug therapy.

DILUTION

Each 20 mg must be diluted with 60 mL SW for injection without a bacteriostatic agent. Shake until solution is clear. May be administered through a Y-tube or three-way stopcock of infusion tubing. If large volumes will be used, transfer to plastic infusion bags; do not use glass bottles; see Compatibility.

Storage: Store undiluted vials at CRT and protect from light. Protect diluted solution from direct light and discard after 6 hours.

COMPATIBILITY

Manufacturer states, "D5W, NS, and acidic solutions are **not compatible** and should not be used." May form a precipitate with glass bottles; use of plastic IV bags recommended.

RATE OF ADMINISTRATION

Prophylactic dose: A single dose as an infusion distributed over 1 hour.

Therapeutic or emergency dose: Each single dose should be given by rapid continuous IV push. Follow immediately with subsequent doses as indicated.

Follow-up dose: Each single dose over 2 to 3 minutes.

ACTIONS

A direct-acting skeletal muscle relaxant. Inhibits excitation-contraction coupling by interfering with the release of the calcium ion from the sarcoplasmic reticulum to reverse the physiologic cause of malignant hyperthermia. Has no appreciable effect on cardiovascular or respiratory function. Onset of action is prompt and lasts about 5 hours. Half-life is 4 to 8 hours. Metabolized in the liver and excreted in urine. Readily crosses the placental barrier. Secreted in breast milk.

INDICATIONS AND USES

Management of the fulminant hypermetabolism of skeletal muscle characteristics of malignant hyperthermic crises in patients of all ages. ▪ Perioperatively to prevent, treat, or minimize the severity of clinical and laboratory signs of malignant hyperthermia in individuals who may be or are known to be susceptible.

CONTRAINDICATIONS

None when used as indicated for malignant hyperthermia crisis.

PRECAUTIONS

Use caution in patients with impaired pulmonary or cardiac function or history of liver disease. ▪ Discontinue all anesthetic agents immediately when onset of malignant hyperthermia is recognized. S/S of the fulminant hypermetabolism of skeletal muscle characteristic of malignant hyperthermia crisis are tachycardia, tachypnea, central venous desaturation, hypercapnia, metabolic acidosis, skeletal muscle rigidity, cyanosis, mottling of skin, fever, increased use of anesthesia circuit CO_2 absorber. ▪ Hepatotoxicity has been reported.

Monitor: Monitor ECG, vital signs, electrolytes, and urine output continuously. ▪ Oxygen needs are increased. ▪ Manage metabolic acidosis. ▪ Institute cooling measures. ▪ Confirm absolute patency of vein; avoid extravasation. ▪ Monitor hepatic function frequently, including ALT, AST. ▪ S/S of malignant hyperthermia crises include central venous desaturation, cyanosis and mottling of the skin, hypercarbia, increased utilization of anesthesia circuit carbon dioxide absorber, metabolic acidosis, skeletal muscle rigidity, tachycardia, tachypnea and, in many cases, fever.

Patient Education: May experience decreased grip strength, weakness in leg muscles, and light-headedness postoperatively. May persist for 48 hours. ▪ Request assistance for ambulation. ▪ Use caution when eating; choking and difficulty swallowing has been reported on day of administration. ▪ Avoid alcohol and other CNS depressants (e.g., diazepam [Valium]). ▪ Avoid tasks that require alertness. ▪ Promptly report bloody or tarry stools, itching, jaundice (yellow color) of eyes and skin, or skin rash.

Maternal/Child: Category C: embryocidal with larger doses in rats. Benefits must outweigh risks. ▪ Discontinue breast-feeding. ▪ Use caution in pediatric patients under 5 years; safety not established.

Elderly: Dose selection should be cautious; see Dose Adjustments.

DRUG/LAB INTERACTIONS

Ability to bind to plasma proteins inhibited by **warfarin and clofibrate;** increased by **tolbutamide.** ▪ Avoid concurrent use of **calcium channel blockers** (e.g., diltiazem [Cardizem]) **and dantrolene.** Myocardial depression, arrhythmias, and hyperkalemia have been reported. ▪ May potentiate **vecuronium**-induced neuromuscular blockade. ▪ May cause hepatotoxicity with **estrogens,** especially in women over 35 years of age.

SIDE EFFECTS

Dizziness, drowsiness, erythema, injection site reactions, loss of grip strength, pulmonary edema, thrombophlebitis, urticaria, and weakness. Anaphylaxis has been reported.

ANTIDOTE

No specific antidote is available or needed when used correctly. Notify physician and initiate supportive measures (adequate airway and ventilation, monitor ECG) in overdosage. Discontinue all anesthetic agents at the first sign of a malignant hyperthermia reaction. Administration of 100% oxygen is recommended. Large amounts of IV fluids may be needed to prevent crystalluria. Treat anaphylaxis and resuscitate as necessary.

DAPTOMYCIN
(dap-toe-**MY**-sin)

Cubicin

Antibacterial
(cyclic lipopeptide)

USUAL DOSE

Complicated skin and skin structure infections: 4 mg/kg once every 24 hours for 7 to 14 days. Do not administer more frequently than once daily.

***Staphylococcus aureus* bloodstream infections (bacteremia), including those with right-sided endocarditis:** 6 mg/kg once every 24 hours for 2 to 6 weeks. Duration of treatment is dependent on diagnosis. Safety data for use more than 28 days is limited. Do not administer more frequently than once daily.

DOSE ADJUSTMENTS

Dose adjustment required in patients with severe renal impairment. In patients with CrCl less than 30 mL/min, including patients undergoing hemodialysis or CAPD, administer a single dose (4 or 6 mg/kg) every 48 hours. If possible, administer dose following completion of hemodialysis on hemodialysis days. ■ No specific dose adjustments required based on age, gender, obesity, or mild to moderate hepatic impairment. Has not been studied in patients with severe hepatic impairment.

DILUTION

Available in 500-mg vials. Reconstitute each 500-mg vial by slowly directing 10 mL of NS to vial sides (50 mg/mL). Ensure wetting of entire daptomycin product. Allow vial to stand for 10 minutes, then gently rotate to ensure complete dilution. *To minimize foaming, avoid vigorous agitation or shaking during or after reconstitution.* Freshly reconstituted solutions range in color from pale yellow to light brown. May be administered as a 50 mg/mL reconstituted solution or may be further diluted with 50 to 100 mL of NS before administration and given as an infusion.

Filters: No data available from manufacturer.

Storage: Refrigerate unopened vials at 2° to 8° C (36° to 46° F). Both reconstituted and diluted solutions are stable for 12 hours at RT or up to 48 hours refrigerated. The combined time (vial and infusion bag) at RT should not exceed 12 hours. Combined refrigeration time (vial and infusion bag) should not exceed 48 hours. Recent studies by the manufacturer suggest that solutions diluted in NS and stored in PVC infusion bags may be stable for up to 10 days refrigerated at 5° C (40° F).

COMPATIBILITY (Underline Indicates Conflicting Compatibility Information)
Consider any drug NOT listed as compatible to be INCOMPATIBLE until consulting a pharmacist; specific conditions may apply.
Manufacturer states, "Additives or other medications should not be added to daptomycin single-use vials or infused simultaneously through the same intravenous line. If the same intravenous line is used for sequential infusion of several different drugs, the line should be flushed with a **compatible** infusion solution before and after infusion with daptomycin."

■ Manufacturer states, "Daptomycin is **compatible** with NS and LR but is **incompatible** with dextrose-containing diluents." ■ Do not use in conjunction with ReadyMED® elastomeric infusion pumps (Cardinal Health, Inc.); an **incompatibility** occurs because of an impurity leaking from this pump system into the daptomycin solution.

One source suggests the following **compatibilities:**
Y-site: Aztreonam (Azactam), caspofungin (Cancidas), ceftazidime (Fortaz), ceftriaxone (Rocephin), dopamine, doripenem (Doribax), fluconazole (Diflucan), gentamicin, heparin, levofloxacin (Levaquin), lidocaine.

RATE OF ADMINISTRATION
See Compatibility. Flushing of the IV line before and after infusion may be indicated.
Injection: A single dose properly reconstituted over 2 minutes.
Infusion: A single dose properly diluted over 30 minutes.

ACTIONS
A cyclic lipopeptide antibacterial agent. Binds to bacterial membranes and causes a rapid depolarization of the membrane potential. Loss of the membrane potential leads to inhibition of protein, DNA and RNA synthesis, which results in bacterial cell death. Exhibits bactericidal activity against aerobic gram-positive bacteria and has been shown to retain potency against antibiotic-resistant, gram-positive bacteria, including isolates resistant to methicillin, vancomycin, and linezolid. Cross-resistance between daptomycin and other antibacterial agents has not been reported. Highly protein bound, primarily to albumin. Site of metabolism has not been identified. Half-life is approximately 7 to 9 hours. Is excreted primarily by the kidney. A small fraction is excreted through the feces.

INDICATIONS AND USES
Treatment of complicated skin and skin structure infections caused by susceptible strains of several aerobic gram-positive microorganisms and *Staphylococcus aureus* bloodstream infections (bacteremia), including those with right-sided infective endocarditis caused by methicillin-susceptible and methicillin-resistant isolates. The effectiveness of daptomycin in patients with left-sided endocarditis due to *S. aureus* has not been demonstrated. See manufacturer's literature.

CONTRAINDICATIONS
Known hypersensitivity to daptomycin. ■ **Not** indicated for treatment of pneumonia. In phase 3 studies of community-acquired pneumonia, the death rate and rates of serious cardiorespiratory adverse events were higher in the daptomycin-treated patients than in the comparator-treated patients. These differences were due to lack of therapeutic effectiveness of daptomycin in the treatment of community-acquired pneumonia.

PRECAUTIONS

C/S indicated to determine susceptibility of causative organism to daptomycin. ▪ To reduce the development of drug-resistant bacteria and maintain its effectiveness, daptomycin should be used to treat or prevent only those infections that are proven or strongly suspected to be caused by susceptible bacteria. ▪ Combination therapy may be clinically indicated if the documented or presumed pathogens include Gram-negative or anaerobic organisms. ▪ Eosinophilic pneumonia has been reported. Onset is usually 2 to 4 weeks after initiation of daptomycin and improves when therapy is discontinued. Patient may present with fever, dyspnea with hypoxic respiratory insufficiency, and diffuse pulmonary infiltrates. ▪ Superinfection caused by the overgrowth of nonsusceptible organisms may occur with antibiotic use. Treat as indicated. ▪ *Clostridium difficile*–associated diarrhea (CDAD) has been reported. May range from mild diarrhea to fatal colitis. Consider in patients who present with diarrhea during or after treatment with daptomycin. ▪ Skeletal muscle effects associated with daptomycin have been observed. Elevations in serum creatine phosphokinase (CPK) and rhabdomyolysis have been reported. Some cases involved patients treated concurrently with daptomycin and HMG-CoA reductase inhibitors; see Drug/Lab Interactions. ▪ Adverse events, possibly reflective of peripheral or cranial neuropathy (e.g., paresthesias, Bell's palsy), have been reported rarely. ▪ Hypersensitivity reactions, including anaphylaxis, have been reported. ▪ In clinical trials, decreased efficacy was observed in patients with moderate baseline renal impairment (CrCl less than 50 mL/min).

Monitor: Obtain baseline and weekly SCr, BUN, and CPK levels. Patients who received recent, prior, or concomitant therapy with an HMG-CoA reductase inhibitor (e.g., simvastatin [Zocor], lovastatin [Mevacor]), patients with renal insufficiency, and patients who develop unexplained elevations in CPK while receiving daptomycin should be monitored more frequently. See Precautions and Antidote. ▪ Monitor for S/S of hypersensitivity reactions (e.g., dyspnea, fever, flushing, hypotension, nausea, pruritus, rash, urticaria). ▪ Monitor for the development of muscle pain or weakness, particularly in the distal extremities. ▪ Monitor for S/S of neuropathy. ▪ Repeat blood cultures indicated in patients with persisting or relapsing *S. aureus* infection or poor clinical response. MIC (minimum inhibitory concentration) susceptibility testing and diagnostic evaluation to rule out sequestered foci of infection may be indicated. Surgical intervention (e.g., débridement, removal of prosthetic device) may be required. ▪ Monitor for S/S of eosinophilic pneumonia (e.g., cough, fever, difficulty breathing, shortness of breath). Treatment with systemic steroids is recommended.

Patient Education: Review side effects with physician. Promptly report muscle pain or weakness, S/S of neuropathy, or new or worsening cough, fever, difficulty breathing, or shortness of breath. ▪ Review medications (prescription and non-prescription) with health care provider. ▪ Promptly report diarrhea or bloody stools that occur during treatment or up to several months after an antibiotic has been discontinued; may indicate CDAD and require treatment.

Maternal/Child: Category B: use during pregnancy only if clearly needed. ▪ Safety for use during breast-feeding not established; effects unknown. Use caution. ▪ Safety and effectiveness for use in pediatric patients under 18 years of age not established.

Elderly: Lower clinical success rates were seen in patients 65 years of age or older. In addition, adverse events were more common in this age-group. Consider age-related renal impairment. See Dose Adjustment.

DRUG/LAB INTERACTIONS

Daptomycin does not appear to inhibit or induce the activities of the cytochrome P_{450} isoforms: 1A2, 2A6, 2C9, 2C19, 2D6, 2E1, and 3A4. It is unlikely that it will inhibit or induce the metabolism of drugs metabolized by this system. ▪ *In vitro* synergistic interactions occurred with **aminoglycosides, beta-lactam antibiotics, and rifampin** (Rifadin) against some isolates of staphylococci and enterococci, including some methicillin-resistant *Staphylococcus aureus* (MRSA) isolates and some vancomycin-resistant enterococci isolates. ▪ Has been administered with **warfarin.** Does not appear to affect the pharmacokinetics of either drug. However, daptomycin can cause a significant concentration-dependent false prolongation of PT and elevation of INR when certain recombinant thromboplastin reagents are used for the assay. This drug-lab interaction can be minimized by drawing specimens for PT/INR near the time of trough plasma concentrations of daptomycin. Evaluation of PT/INR using an alternative method may be required. ▪ Inhibitors of **HMG-CoA reductase** (e.g., simvastatin [Zocor], atorvastatin [Lipitor]) may cause myopathy, which is manifested as muscle pain or weakness associated with elevated levels of CPK and possible rhabdomyolysis. Consider temporarily suspending the use of HMG-CoA reductase inhibitors in patients receiving daptomycin. ▪ Has been used concomitantly with aztreonam (Azactam). No dose adjustment for either antibiotic was required. ▪ No dose adjustment is required when given concomitantly with probenecid.

SIDE EFFECTS

Most side effects are mild to moderate in intensity. Side effects occurring in 2% or more of patients include abnormal liver function tests, anemia, anxiety, arthralgia, asthenia, back pain, constipation, diarrhea, dizziness, dyspepsia, dyspnea, edema, elevated CPK, fever, fungal infections, gram-negative infections, headache, hyperkalemia, hypertension, hypokalemia, hypotension, injection site pain, insomnia, limb pain, nausea and vomiting, pruritus, rash, renal failure, sweating, and urinary tract infections. Less frequently reported side effects include abdominal pain, anxiety, back pain, *Candida* infections, cardiac failure, CDAD, cellulitis, chest pain, confusion, cough, decreased appetite, edema, elevated alkaline phosphatase, hyperglycemia, hypoglycemia, hypokalemia, and sore throat. Muscle pain or weakness, rhabdomyolysis, and peripheral neuropathy have been reported rarely. See Precautions. Hypersensitivity reactions including anaphylaxis, difficulty swallowing, hives, pruritus, shortness of breath, and truncal erythema have been reported. Other reactions have been reported in fewer than 1% of study patients. See manufacturer's literature.

Post-Marketing: Pulmonary eosinophilia.

ANTIDOTE

Notify physician of any side effects. Discontinue drug in patients with unexplained S/S of myopathy in conjunction with CPK elevation greater than 1,000 units/L (approximately 5 times the upper limit of normal) or in patients without reported symptoms who have marked elevation in CPK (equal to or greater than 10 times the upper limit of normal). In animal studies, skeletal muscle effects and neuropathies were reversible with discontinuation of the drug. Discontinue daptomycin at the first sign of eosinophilic pneumonia. Treatment with systemic steroids is recommended. Treat CDAD with fluids, electrolytes, protein supplements, and oral vancomycin (Vancocin) or metronidazole (Flagyl) as indicated. In severe cases, surgical evaluation may be indicated. Treat hypersensitivity reactions as indicated (e.g., oxygen, diphenhydramine, epinephrine, corticosteroids, vasopressors, and/or fluids). Approximately 15% of daptomycin is removed during a 4-hour hemodialysis run. Approximately 11% is recovered over 48 hours with peritoneal dialysis. Use of a high-flux dialysis membrane may increase the amount of drug removal. Resuscitate as necessary.

DARBEPOETIN ALFA BBW

(**DAR**-beh-**poh**-eh-tin **AL**-fah)

Aranesp

Antianemic agent

pH 5.7 to 6.4

USUAL DOSE

Adult and pediatric patients: Rate of hemoglobin increase is dose dependent and varies among patients. Availability of iron stores, baseline hemoglobin, and concurrent medical problems affect the rate and extent of response. Use the lowest dose for each patient that will gradually increase the hemoglobin concentration to avoid the need for RBC transfusion and achieve and maintain a hemoglobin within the range of 10 to 12 Gm/dL. If a patient fails to respond or maintain a response, other etiologies should be considered and evaluated. See Monitor, Precautions, and Maternal/Child.

Anemia associated with chronic renal failure (CRF): *Starting dose:* 0.45 mcg/kg of body weight once per week. May be given by IV or SC injection. The IV route is recommended for patients on hemodialysis; see Precautions. See Dose Adjustments and Maternal/Child.

Anemia associated with chemotherapy in cancer patients: 2.25 mcg/kg once a week. SC injection recommended. Alternately, give a dose of 500 mcg once every 3 weeks. See Dose Adjustments, Precautions, and Maternal/Child. *Darbepoetin alfa should not be initiated at hemoglobin levels equal to or greater than 10 Gm/dL.* Discontinue darbepoetin after completion of a chemotherapy course.

Conversion from epoetin alfa to darbepoetin alfa: Estimate starting dose of darbepoetin based on the weekly dose of epoetin alfa at the time of substitution as shown in the following chart. Administer darbepoetin once per week in patients who were receiving epoetin alfa 2 to 3 times a week and once every 2 weeks in patients who were receiving epoetin alfa once per week. Titrate to achieve and maintain the lowest hemoglobin level sufficient to avoid the need for RBC transfusion and to maintain within the range of 10 to 12 Gm/dL. The route of administration (IV or SC) should remain the same.

Darbepoetin Alfa Starting Dose Based on Previous Epoetin Alfa Dose		
Previous Weekly Epoetin Alfa Dose (units/week)	Weekly Darbepoetin Alfa Dose (mcg/week)	
	Adult	Pediatric
<1,500 units/week	6.25 mcg/week	See *
1,500 to 2,499 units/week	6.25 mcg/week	6.25 mcg/week
2,500 to 4,999 units/week	12.5 mcg/week	10 mcg/week
5,000 to 10,999 units/week	25 mcg/week	20 mcg/week
11,000 to 17,999 units/week	40 mcg/week	40 mcg/week
18,000 to 33,999 units/week	60 mcg/week	60 mcg/week
34,000 to 89,999 units/week	100 mcg/week	100 mcg/week
≥90,000 units/week	200 mcg/week	200 mcg/week

*Data insufficient to determine a darbepoetin alfa conversion dose in pediatric patients receiving a weekly epoetin alfa dose of less than 1,500 units/week.

DOSE ADJUSTMENTS

Based on hemoglobin. Dose should be started slowly and adjusted for each patient to achieve and maintain the lowest hemoglobin level sufficient to avoid the need for RBC transfusion and to maintain hemoglobin levels within the range of 10 to 12 Gm/dL. If hemoglobin excursions outside the recommended range occur, the dose must be adjusted. Allow sufficient time before adjusting a dose; increased hemoglobin levels may not be observed for 2 to 6 weeks. Dose adjustments should not be made more frequently than once a month.

Anemia associated with chronic renal failure (CRF):
Reduce dose by 25%

If the hemoglobin is increasing and approaching 12 Gm/dL.

If the hemoglobin continues to increase after dose reduction by 25%, *withhold doses* until hemoglobin begins to decrease, then resume dosing at 25% below the previous dose.

If the hemoglobin increases by more than 1 Gm/dL in any 2-week period.

Increase dose by 25%

If the hemoglobin increases by less than 1 Gm/dL in a 4-week period. Further increases may be made at 4-week intervals until the specified hemoglobin is obtained.

For patients whose hemoglobin does not attain a level within the desired range of 10 to 12 Gm/dL after appropriate dose titration over a 12-week period, evaluate and treat other causes of anemia; see Precautions. Do not administer higher doses. Use lowest dose that will maintain a hemoglobin level sufficient to avoid the need for recurrent RBC transfusions. Continue monitoring and adjust dose if responsiveness improves. If responsiveness does not improve and recurrent RBC transfusions continue to be required, discontinue darbepoetin therapy. Many patients may be maintained on a dose that is lower than the starting dose. Predialysis patients, in particular, may require lower doses. Some patients may be adequately maintained with an SC dose administered once every 2 weeks. *Continued*

Anemia associated with chemotherapy in cancer patients:
Reduce dose by 40%

If the hemoglobin exceeds 12 Gm/dL, **withhold doses** until the hemoglobin approaches a level at which a transfusion might be required, then resume dosing at 40% below the previous dose.

If the hemoglobin increases by more than 1 Gm/dL in any 2-week period or if the hemoglobin reaches a level needed to avoid transfusion, reduce dose by 40% of the previous dose.

Increase dose to 4.5 mcg/kg

In patients receiving weekly administration, if the hemoglobin increases by less than 1 Gm/dL after 6 weeks of therapy.

Discontinue if there is no response as measured by hemoglobin levels or if transfusions are still required after 8 weeks of therapy.

DILUTION

Available in numerous concentrations and in two formulations (polysorbate or albumin solutions). Supplied in vials or pre-filled syringes with needle guards (needle cover contains a derivative of latex). Check labeling carefully to confirm IV use. Must be given undiluted as an IV injection. Do not administer in conjunction with other drug solutions. **Do not shake** and keep covered to protect from room light until administration. Vigorous shaking or exposure to light will render solution biologically inactive. Single-dose vial contains no preservatives. Use only 1 dose per vial, then discard.

Filters: Not required; however, it was filtered during manufacturing with 0.2-micron millipore filters. No significant loss of potency expected with use of non–protein binding filters of a similar size or larger.

Storage: Store at 2° to 8° C. Do not freeze or shake. Protect from light.

COMPATIBILITY

Manufacturer states, "Do not administer in conjunction with other drug solutions."

RATE OF ADMINISTRATION

A single dose over at least 1 minute.

ACTIONS

An erythropoiesis-stimulating protein produced by recombinant DNA technology. Closely related to human erythropoietin. Production of endogenous erythropoietin is impaired in patients with chronic renal failure, and erythropoietin deficiency is the primary cause of their anemia. Darbepoetin has the same biologic effects as erythropoietin produced naturally by the kidneys. Stimulates bone marrow to produce RBCs, increasing the reticulocyte count within 10 days and the red cell count, hemoglobin, and hematocrit within 2 to 6 weeks. Normal iron stores are necessary because it steps up RBC production to a rate above what the body usually makes. New cells need iron, which is quickly depleted. Distribution is confined to the vascular space. Half-life is approximately 21 hours. Continued therapy will maintain improved RBC levels and decrease the need for transfusions.

INDICATIONS AND USES

Treatment of anemia associated with chronic renal failure, including patients receiving dialysis and patients not receiving dialysis. ■ As a SC injection to treat chemotherapy-induced anemia in adult cancer patients who have non-myeloid malignancies. Studies to determine whether darbepoetin increases mortality or decreases progression-free/recurrence-free survival are ongoing. ■ Not indicated for use in patients receiving hormonal agents, therapeutic biologic products, or radiotherapy unless receiving concomitant myelosuppressive chemotherapy. ▪ Not indicated for patients receiving myelosuppressive therapy when the anticipated outcome is cure; see Precautions. ▪ Has not been shown to improve symptoms of anemia, quality of life, fatigue, or patient well-being; see Precautions. ▪ Not indicated for reduction in allogeneic RBC transfusions in patients scheduled for surgical procedures.

CONTRAINDICATIONS

Known hypersensitivity to albumin, polysorbate, or darbepoetin. Uncontrolled hypertension.

PRECAUTIONS

May be given IV or SC to patients not receiving dialysis. ▪ May increase risk of serious and life-threatening cardiovascular events and death. Higher risk may be associated with a higher hemoglobin and/or a higher rate of rise of hemoglobin. Individualize dosing to achieve and maintain a hemoglobin level within the range of 10 to 12 Gm/dL and to avoid a rate of rise of more than 1 Gm/dL in a 2-week period. ▪ Increases in hemoglobin of greater than 1 Gm/dL during any 2-week period have been associated with an increased incidence of cardiac arrest, neurologic events (e.g., seizures, stroke), exacerbations of hypertension, congestive heart failure (CHF), vascular thrombosis/ischemia/infarction, acute MI, deep vein thrombosis (DVT), pulmonary embolus, hemodialysis graft occlusion, and fluid overload/edema. See Dose Adjustments. ▪ Administration of erythropoiesis-stimulating agents (ESAs) to cancer patients shortened the overall survival time and/or increased the risk of tumor progression or recurrence in clinical studies of some patients with breast, cervical, head and neck, lymphoid, and non–small cell lung malignancies. To minimize these risks, as well as the risks of serious cardiovascular and thrombovascular events, use the lowest dose needed to avoid a red blood cell transfusion. Use only to treat anemia due to concomitant myelosuppressive chemotherapy and discontinue after completion of a chemotherapy course. Prescribers and hospitals are now required to enroll in and comply with the ESA APPRISE Oncology Program to prescribe and/or dispense ESAs to patients with cancer. See prescribing information Black Box Warning. ▪ BP may increase during therapy with darbepoetin. Hypertensive encephalopathy and seizures have been observed. ▪ Patients with uncontrolled hypertension should not be treated with darbepoetin until BP has been adequately controlled. ▪ In addition to low baseline hemoglobin and inadequate iron stores, delayed or diminished response may result from concurrent medical problems (e.g., infections, inflammatory or malignant processes, occult blood loss, underlying hematologic disease, folic acid or vitamin B_{12} deficiency, hemolysis, aluminum intoxication, osteofibrosis cystica, bone marrow fibrosis, pure red cell aplasia [PRCA], or anti-erythropoietin antibody-associated anemia). ▪ Safety and efficacy have not been established in patients with underlying hematologic diseases (e.g., hemolytic anemia, sickle cell anemia, thalassemia, porphyria). ▪ Therapy results in an increase in RBCs and a decrease in plasma volume, which could reduce dialysis efficiency; adjustment of dialysis prescription may be necessary. ▪ Not intended for use in anemias caused by iron or folate deficiencies, hemolysis, or GI bleeding or for use in treating symptoms of anemia, including dizziness, fatigue, low energy, poor quality of life, or shortness of breath. ▪ Use with caution in patients with epilepsy. ▪ Not a substitute for emergency transfusion in patients requiring immediate correction of severe anemia. ▪ As with all proteins, there is a potential for immunogenicity. The incidence of antibody development in patients receiving darbepoetin has not been determined. Use caution; hypersensitivity reactions and/or anaphylaxis can occur. ▪ Pure red cell aplasia (PRCA) and severe anemia, with or without other cytopenias, in association with neutralizing antibodies to erythropoietin has been observed. Most often reported in CRF patients receiving epoetin alfa by SC injection. Evaluate any patient who develops a sudden loss of response to darbepoetin alfa accompanied by severe anemia and low reticulocyte count. Physicians may contact the manufacturer (Amgen) for help with evaluation of these patients. ▪ The formulation containing albumin carries a risk for transmission of viral diseases or Creutzfeldt-Jakob disease. Donor screening and manufacturing processes make this risk extremely remote. ▪ Darbepoetin is a growth factor that stimulates RBC production. Erythropoetin receptors are also found on the surfaces of normal, nonhematopoietic tissue and some malignant cell lines. The possibility that darbepoetin can act as a growth factor for any tumor type cannot be ruled out.

Monitor: Monitor hemoglobin weekly in patients who are initiating therapy. Continue until stable and the maintenance dose has been established, then monitor at regular intervals. ▪ Monitor hemoglobin weekly for at least 4 weeks following adjustment of therapy. Once stabilized, continue to monitor at regular intervals. ▪ Monitor BP routinely. Initiation or intensification of antihypertensive therapy and dietary restrictions may be necessary. If BP is difficult to control by pharmacologic or dietary measures, the dose of darbepoetin should be reduced or withheld. ▪ Monitor for the presence of premonitory neurologic symptoms during initiation of therapy or when dose is adjusted. Seizures have been reported; see Precautions. ▪ Predialysis patients may be more responsive to the effects of therapy. Monitor BP, hemoglobin, renal function, and fluid and electrolyte balance. During the transition period onto dialysis, hemoglobin and BP should be monitored carefully; see Dose Adjustments. ▪ Normal iron stores required to support epoetin-stimulated erythropoiesis. Transferrin saturation should be at least 20% and ferritin at least 100 ng/mL (100 mcg/L). Monitor before and during therapy. Supplemental iron (ferrous sulfate 325 mg PO 3 times a day) is usually required to increase and maintain transferrin saturation. Administration of parenteral iron may be necessary in some patients.

Patient Education: Risk of seizures, especially for first several months of therapy. Do not drive or operate heavy equipment. ▪ Stress the importance of compliance with diet, iron and vitamin (e.g., folic acid, B_{12}) supplementation, and dialysis regimen. ▪ Close monitoring of BP and hemoglobin is imperative. ▪ Promptly report S/S of a hypersensitivity reaction, pain or swelling in the legs, shortness of breath (SOB), increase in BP, dizziness, or loss of consciousness. ▪ Menses may resume; possibility of pregnancy. Contraception may be indicated. ▪ Additional instruction (e.g., equipment, techniques) will be required in patients who will self-administer (manufacturer supplies brochure). ▪ Increased risk of mortality, serious cardiovascular events, thromboembolic events, and tumor progression or recurrence. ▪ All patients should (but patients with cancer must) discuss the risks of using an ESA with a health care professional.

Maternal/Child: Category C: may present risk to fetus; benefits must justify risk. ▪ Use caution in nursing mothers. ▪ Safety and effectiveness for use in the initial treatment of anemic pediatric CRF patients less than 1 year of age or in the conversion from epoetin alfa to darbepoetin in these patients not established. Safety and effectiveness similar to adult conversion studies in pediatric CRF patients over 1 year of age. ▪ Safety and effectiveness for use in pediatric cancer patients not established. ▪ Half-life and plasma concentrations in pediatric patients 3 years of age and older are similar to those seen in adults. See package insert.

Elderly: Response similar to that found in younger patients; however, the elderly may have a greater sensitivity to its effects. ▪ Monitor blood chemistry and BP carefully due to increased risk of renal and/or cardio-vascular complications.

DRUG/LAB INTERACTIONS
Specific information not available.

SIDE EFFECTS
Chronic renal failure patients: Commonly reported *serious* adverse reactions include angina, cardiac arrhythmia, CHF, sepsis, vascular access thrombosis. Other commonly reported side effects were diarrhea, fever, headache, hypertension, hypotension, infection (e.g., abscess, bacteremia, peritonitis, pneumonia, sepsis), myalgia, nausea. Less commonly reported side effects include abdominal pain, angina, arthralgia, asthenia, back pain, constipation, cough, dizziness, fatigue, flu-like symptoms, fluid overload, hypersensitivity reactions (e.g., rash, urticaria), injection site reactions (infection, hemorrhage), limb pain, peripheral edema, upper respiratory tract infection, vomiting. PRCA and severe anemia, with or without other cytopenias, in association with neutralizing antibodies has been reported; see Precautions. Cardiac arrest and death have been reported.

Cancer patients receiving chemotherapy: The most frequently reported *serious* adverse events include death, dehydration, dyspnea, fever, pneumonia, and vomiting. Other commonly reported side effects include diarrhea, edema, fatigue, and nausea. Arthralgia, constipation, dizziness, headache, hypertension, myalgia, rash, seizures, and thrombotic events (e.g., pulmonary embolism, thrombosis) are less commonly reported.

ANTIDOTE
Notify physician of all side effects; most will be treated symptomatically. Excessive hypertension may require discontinuation of darbepoetin until BP is controlled or may respond to a reduction in dose of darbepoetin or to an increase in antihypertensive therapy. Reduce dose of darbepoetin in patients with an increase in hemoglobin of more than 1 Gm/dL in 2 weeks or in patients with hemoglobin over 12 Gm/dL. May need to withhold darbepoetin until hemoglobin falls to desired goal. Consider phlebotomy in the event of overdose or polycythemia. If overdose or polycythemia does occur, monitor closely for cardiovascular events and hematologic abnormalities. When resuming therapy, monitor closely for evidence of rapid increases in hemoglobin concentration (greater than 1 Gm/dL within 14 days) and reduce dose as indicated. Adjustments in dialysis prescription may be required during dialysis to prevent clotting. Permanently discontinue therapy in patients with antibody-mediated anemia. Patients should not be switched to other erythropoietic proteins, because antibodies may cross-react. Treat minor hypersensitivity reactions symptomatically. Discontinue drug and treat anaphylaxis as indicated; resuscitate as necessary.

DAUNORUBICIN HYDROCHLORIDE BBW ▪
DAUNORUBICIN CITRATE
LIPOSOMAL INJECTION BBW

(daw-noh-**ROO**-bih-sin hy-droh-**KLOR**-eyed)
(daw-noh-**ROO**-bih-sin **SIH**-trate **LIP**-oh-sohm-ul)

Cerubidine ▪ **DaunoXome**

**Antineoplastic
(anthracycline)**

pH 4.5 to 6.5 ▪ 4.9 to 6

USUAL DOSE

CONVENTIONAL DAUNORUBICIN

Adult acute nonlymphocytic leukemia: 45 mg/M^2/day on Days 1, 2, and 3 in adults under age 60 (adults over age 60 may require reduction to 30 mg/M^2/day). Used in specific protocol combination therapy (e.g., cytarabine 100 mg/M^2/day for 7 days). Regimen repeated every 3 to 4 weeks. In these subsequent courses, repeat daunorubicin, 30 to 45 mg/M^2/day (depending on age) for only 2 days and cytarabine for only 5 days. To obtain a normal-appearing bone marrow may require up to 3 courses.

Adult acute lymphocytic leukemia: 45 mg/M^2/day on Days 1, 2, and 3. Used in combination therapy (e.g., vincristine, prednisone, and L-asparaginase).

In all situations, when remission is complete, an individual maintenance program should be established.

DAUNOXOME (LIPOSOMAL INJECTION)

Advanced, HIV-associated Kaposi's sarcoma: 40 mg/M^2 as an IV infusion. Repeat every 2 weeks. Continue treatment until there is evidence of disease progression (specifics outlined in package insert).

PEDIATRIC DOSE

CONVENTIONAL DAUNORUBICIN

See Maternal/Child.

Acute lymphocytic leukemia in pediatric patients 2 years of age and older: 25 mg/M^2/day on Day 1 each week, vincristine 1.5 mg/M^2 on Day 1 each week, and prednisone 40 mg/M^2 PO daily. Remission should be obtained in 4 weeks. If a partial remission is obtained after 4 weeks, 1 or 2 more weeks of treatment may produce a complete remission.

Acute lymphocytic leukemia in infants and children less than 2 years of age or less than 0.5 M^2 body surface: Calculate dose based on weight instead of body surface area: 1 mg/kg.

DAUNOXOME: Safety for use in pediatric patients not established.

DOSE ADJUSTMENTS

ALL DAUNORUBICINS: See Precautions/Monitor.

CONVENTIONAL DAUNORUBICIN: Profound bone marrow suppression is usually required to eradicate the leukemic cells and induce a complete remission. Evaluate bone marrow and peripheral blood to determine need for additional courses. ▪ See Usual Dose for adults over 60 years of age. ▪ Reduce dose in impaired hepatic or renal function according to the following chart.

Daunorubicin Dosing in Impaired Hepatic or Renal Function		
Serum Bilirubin	Serum Creatinine	Dose Reduction
1.2 to 3.0 mg	—	25%
>3 mg	—	50%
—	>3 mg	50%

DAUNOXOME: Reduce dose to 75% of normal (30 mg/M^2) if serum bilirubin is 1.2 to 3 mg/dL. Reduce dose to 50% of normal (20 mg/M^2) if serum bilirubin or creatinine is greater than 3 mg/dL. ▪ Withhold dose if absolute granulocyte count is less than 750 cells/mm^3.

DILUTION

Specific techniques required; see Precautions.

CONVENTIONAL DAUNORUBICIN: Each 20 mg must be diluted with 4 mL of SW for injection (5 mg/mL). Agitate gently to dissolve completely. Further dilute each dose with 10 to 15 mL of NS. Must be given through Y-tube or three-way stopcock of a free-flowing infusion of D5W or NS. May be added to 100 mL NS and given as an infusion. Use extreme caution.

DAUNOXOME: Dilute each single dose with an equal amount of D5W. Available as a 2 mg/mL preservative-free solution. Withdraw calculated volume (dose of DaunoXome) from vial; transfer to a sterile infusion bag that contains an equal volume of D5W. Desired concentration is 1 mg/mL. Do not use any other diluent. A translucent red liposomal dispersion; do not use if opaque. Do not use in-line filters for infusion. See Compatibility.

Filters: *DaunoXome:* Manufacturer states, "Do not use in-line filters for infusion."

Storage: *Conventional daunorubicin:* Protect from sunlight. Diluted solution stable 24 hours at room temperature, 48 hours if refrigerated; then discard. *DaunoXome:* Refrigerate unopened vials; avoid freezing. Protect from light. Discard unused drug. Reconstituted solutions may be refrigerated for a maximum of 6 hours.

COMPATIBILITY   (Underline Indicates Conflicting Compatibility Information)

Consider any drug NOT listed as compatible to be INCOMPATIBLE until consulting a pharmacist; specific conditions may apply.

CONVENTIONAL DAUNORUBICIN

Manufacturer states, "Should not be administered mixed with other drugs or heparin."

One source suggests the following **compatibilities:**

Additive: *Not recommended by manufacturer.* Cytarabine (ARA-C), etoposide (VePesid), hydrocortisone sodium succinate (Solu-Cortef).

Y-site: Amifostine (Ethyol), anidulafungin (Eraxis), caspofungin (Cancidas), etoposide phosphate (Etopophos), filgrastim (Neupogen), gemcitabine (Gemzar), granisetron (Kytril), melphalan (Alkeran), methotrexate, ondansetron (Zofran), sodium bicarbonate, teniposide (Vumon), thiotepa, vinorelbine (Navelbine).

DAUNOXOME

Manufacturer states, "The only fluid that may be mixed with daunoxome is D5W. Must not be mixed with saline, bacteriostatic agents such as benzyl alcohol, or any other solution."

RATE OF ADMINISTRATION

CONVENTIONAL DAUNORUBICIN

IV injection: A single dose of properly diluted medication over 3 to 5 minutes.

IV infusion: A single dose evenly distributed over 30 to 45 minutes.

DAUNOXOME

A single dose as an infusion evenly distributed over 60 minutes. Do not use an in-line filter. Back pain, flushing, and chest tightness may occur. Usually subsides if infusion is stopped, and usually does not recur if infusion is restarted at a slower rate after symptoms subside.

ACTIONS

CONVENTIONAL DAUNORUBICIN: A highly toxic antibiotic antineoplastic agent. Rapidly cleared from plasma, it inhibits synthesis of DNA. Cell cycle specific for S phase; exact method of action is unknown; antimitotic, cytotoxic, and immunosuppressive. Widely distributed in tissues, with the highest concentrations occurring in the spleen, kidneys, liver, lungs, and heart. Does not cross blood-brain barrier. Metabolized in the liver and other tissues. Elimination half-life is 18 to 30 hours. Slowly excreted in bile and urine.

DAUNOXOME: A liposomal preparation of daunorubicin formulated to maximize selectivity for solid tumors. In the circulation, the liposomal preparation protects the entrapped daunorubicin from chemical and enzymatic degradation, minimizes protein binding, and generally decreases uptake by normal (non–reticuloendothelial system) tissues. The mechanism of delivery is not known, but may be through the often altered and/or compromised vasculature of tumors. In animals, it has been shown to accumulate in tumors to a greater extent than conventional daunorubicin. Released over time within the cells of the solid tumor. Persists at high levels within tumor tissue for several days. It differs from conventional daunorubicin because it mostly confines itself to vascular fluid volume. Plasma clearance is slower and the AUC (area under the curve) is larger.

INDICATIONS AND USES

CONVENTIONAL DAUNORUBICIN: Treatment of acute nonlymphocytic leukemia in adults (myelogenous, monocytic, erythroid). ▪ Combination therapy for induction of remission in acute lymphocytic leukemia in adults and pediatric patients.

DAUNOXOME: Currently approved only for first-line cytotoxic therapy for advanced HIV-associated Kaposi's sarcoma.

CONTRAINDICATIONS

CONVENTIONAL DAUNORUBICIN: Hypersensitivity to daunorubicin or any of its components. **Not absolute;** pre-existing bone marrow suppression, impaired cardiac function, pre-existing infection; see Precautions.

DAUNOXOME: History of hypersensitivity reaction to previous treatment with DaunoXome or any of its components (includes conventional daunorubicin). Not recommended in patients with less than advanced HIV-related Kaposi's sarcoma.

PRECAUTIONS

ALL DAUNORUBICINS: Follow guidelines for handling cytotoxic agents. See Appendix A, p. 1429. ▪ Administered by or under the direction of the physician specialist with facilities for monitoring the patient and responding to any medical emergency. ▪ For IV use only; do not give IM or SC. ▪ Severe myelosuppression may occur and may lead to infection or hemorrhage. ▪ Use extreme caution in pre-existing drug-induced bone marrow suppression, existing heart disease, previous treatment with other anthracyclines (e.g., doxorubicin [Adriamycin]), or radiation therapy encompassing the heart. ▪ Incidence of myocardial toxicity increases after a total cumulative dose that exceeds 400 to 550 mg/M^2 in adults, 300 mg/M^2 in pediatric patients more than 2 years of age, or 10 mg/kg in pediatric patients less than 2 years of age. Potentially fatal congestive heart failure may occur either during therapy or months to years after therapy is complete. ▪ Urine may be reddish color (from dye, not hematuria).

Monitor: ALL DAUNORUBICINS: Monitor CBC including differential and platelet count before each dose. ▪ Monitoring of liver function, kidney function, ECG, chest x-ray, echocardiography, and systolic ejection fraction indicated before and during therapy; recommended before each course. ▪ Evaluation of cardiac function by medical history and physical exam is recommended before each dose; see Precautions. ▪ Monitor closely for S/S of hemorrhage or infection; may be life threatening. ▪ Prophylactic antibiotics may be indicated pending results of C/S in a febrile neutropenic patient. ▪ Determine absolute patency of vein. A stinging or burning sensation indicates extravasation; discontinue injection and use another vein. Severe cellulitis and tissue necrosis will result from extravasation with conventional daunorubicins; has not been observed with DaunoXome. ▪ Prophylactic antiemetics may reduce nausea and vomiting and increase patient comfort. ▪ Monitor uric acid levels; maintain hydration; alkalinization of urine or allopurinol may be indicated. ▪ Monitor for thrombocytopenia (platelet count less than 50,000/mm^3). Initiate precautions to prevent excessive bleeding (e.g., inspect IV sites, skin, and mucous membranes; use extreme care during invasive procedures; test urine, emesis, stool, and secretions for occult blood).

CONVENTIONAL DAUNORUBICIN: May cause acute congestive heart failure with total cumulative doses over 550 mg/M^2 in adults (400 mg/M^2 if previous treatment with doxorubicin or radiation therapy in area of heart), 300 mg/M^2 in pediatric patients over 2 years, and 10 mg/kg in pediatric patients under 2 years.

DAUNOXOME: May also cause cardiomyopathy. Monitoring of LVEF recommended at total cumulative doses of 320 mg/M^2, 480 mg/M^2, and every 240 mg/M^2 thereafter.

Patient Education: Nonhormonal birth control recommended. ▪ Report IV site burning or stinging promptly. ▪ Secondary leukemias have been reported. ▪ See Appendix D, p. 1434.

Maternal/Child: ALL DAUNORUBICINS: Category D: can cause fetal harm. Avoid pregnancy. ▪ Safety for use in breast-feeding not established; discontinue breast-feeding. ▪ Cardiotoxicity may be more frequent and occur at lower cumulative doses in pediatric patients. ▪ See Monitor.

DAUNOXOME: Safety for use in pediatric patients not established.

Elderly: Cardiotoxicity and myelotoxicity may be more severe. Consider age-related renal impairment. Safety of DaunoXome for use in the elderly has not been established.

DRUG/LAB INTERACTIONS

Concurrent use with **cyclophosphamide** (Cytoxan) may increase cardiotoxicity. ▪ Dose reduction may be required with concurrent use of **other myelosuppressive agents**. ▪ Concurrent use with **hepatotoxic agents** (e.g., high-dose methotrexate) may increase risk of toxicity. ▪ Risk of cardiotoxicity increased in patients previously treated with maximum cumulative doses of **other anthracyclines** (e.g., doxorubicin [Adriamycin], idarubicin [Idamycin]) **and/or radiation encompassing the heart.** ▪ Do not administer **vaccines or chloroquine** to patients receiving antineoplastic drugs. ▪ See Precautions.

SIDE EFFECTS

ALL DAUNORUBICINS: Bone marrow suppression and cardiotoxicity are dose related and dose limiting.

CONVENTIONAL DAUNORUBICIN: Acute congestive heart failure, alopecia (reversible), bone marrow suppression (marked with average doses), chills, decrease in systolic ejection fraction, depressed QRS voltage, diarrhea, fever, gonadal suppression, mucositis, myocarditis, nausea, pericarditis, skin rash, vomiting.

DAUNOXOME: Granulocytopenia is most common. Symptoms common to conventional daunorubicin may also occur. Infusion related back pain, chest tightness, and flushing may be related to liposomal formulation.

Overdose: Will cause increased severity of myelosuppression, fatigue, nausea, and vomiting.

ANTIDOTE

Most side effects will be tolerated or treated symptomatically. Keep physician informed. Close monitoring of cumulative dosage, bone marrow, ECG, chest x-ray, echocardiography, and systolic ejection fraction may prevent most serious and potentially fatal side effects. There is no specific antidote. Supportive therapy as indicated will help sustain the patient in toxicity. Administration of whole blood products (e.g., packed RBCs, platelets, leukocytes) and/or blood modifiers (e.g., darbepoetin alfa [Aranesp], epoetin alfa [Epogen], filgrastim [Neupogen], oprelvekin [Neumega], pegfilgrastim [Neulasta], sargramostim [Leukine]) may be indicated to treat bone marrow toxicity. For extravasation, aspirate as much infiltrated drug as possible, flood site with normal saline, and inject hydrocortisone sodium succinate (Solu-Cortef) or hyaluronidase (Wydase) throughout extravasated tissue. Use a 27- or 25-gauge needle. Cold, moist compresses may be helpful; elevate extremity. Site should be observed promptly by a reconstructive surgeon.

DECITABINE FOR INJECTION
(deh-**SIGHT**-ah-been for in-**JEK**-shun)

**Antineoplastic
(miscellaneous)**

Dacogen

pH 6.7 to 7.3

USUAL DOSE

There are two treatment options. With either regimen, treatment for a minimum of 4 cycles is recommended. A complete or partial response may take longer than 4 cycles.

Premedication: Standard anti-emetic therapy is indicated.

Option 1: 15 mg/M^2 as an infusion over 3 hours. Repeat every 8 hours for 3 days. Repeat this complete cycle every 6 weeks. See Dose Adjustments and Monitor.

Option 2: 20 mg/M^2 as an infusion over 1 hour. Repeat once each day for 5 days. Repeat this complete cycle every 4 weeks. See Dose Adjustments and Monitor.

DOSE ADJUSTMENTS

Option 1 and Option 2: Hematologic recovery to at least an ANC equal to or greater than 1,000 cells/mm^3 and platelets equal to or greater than 50,000 cells/mm^3 is required before subsequent cycles are administered. ▪ If a SCr equal to or greater than 2 mg/dL, an ALT or a total bilirubin equal to or greater than 2 times the ULN, and/or an active or uncontrolled infection occur, do not restart decitabine therapy until the toxicity is resolved. ▪ No additional dose reductions are indicated based on age, gender, or race; see Precautions and Elderly.

Option 1: If hematologic recovery requires more than 6 weeks but less than 8 weeks, delay repeat cycle of decitabine for up to 2 weeks. When therapy is restarted, reduce dose for that cycle to 11 mg/M^2 every 8 hours (33 mg/M^2/day, 99 mg/M^2/cycle). ▪ If hematologic recovery requires more than 8 weeks but less than 10 weeks, assess the patient for disease progression (by bone marrow aspirates). If disease progression has not occurred, delay repeat cycle of decitabine for up to 2 more weeks to allow for hematologic recovery. When therapy is restarted, reduce dose for that cycle to 11 mg/M^2 every 8 hours (33 mg/M^2/day, 99 mg/M^2/cycle). In subsequent cycles, maintain or increase dose based on hematologic recovery.

DILUTION

Specific techniques required; see Precautions. Reconstitute a single vial (50 mg) with 10 mL SW (each mL contains 5 mg of decitabine at a pH of 6.7 to 7.3). Further dilute immediately with NS, D5W, or LR to a final concentration of 0.1 to 1 mg/mL (further dilute each mL with 4 mL additional diluent for a 1 mg/mL concentration or 49 mL for a 0.1 mg/mL concentration). Must be used within 15 minutes of reconstitution. If decitabine will not be used within 15 minutes of reconstitution, it must be diluted using cold (2° C to 8° C) infusion fluids and stored at 2° C to 8° C (36° F to 46° F) for up to a maximum of 7 hours.

Filters: Specific information not available.

Storage: Store unopened vials at 25° C (77° F); excursions permitted to 15° to 30° C (59° to 86° F). Use of reconstituted and/or diluted solution within

15 minutes of reconstitution is preferred or a specific process is required; see Dilution.

COMPATIBILITY

Specific information not available. Consider specific use; consult pharmacist.

RATE OF ADMINISTRATION

Option 1: A single dose as an infusion equally distributed over 3 hours.

Option 2: A single dose as an infusion equally distributed over 1 hour.

ACTIONS

A hypomethylating antineoplastic agent. Cytotoxic to proliferating cells through a process that incorporates it into DNA, inhibits the enzyme DNA methyltransferase, and causes hypomethylation of DNA, leading to cell disintegration and/or death. This hypomethylation in neoplastic cells may restore normal function to genes that are critical for the control of cellular differentiation and proliferation and allow the formation of normal RBCs and platelets. Patients with myelodysplastic syndromes who have responded to decitabine have become transfusion independent. Terminal half-life range is 0.21 to 0.82 hours. Extensively metabolized by an unknown route(s). Protein binding is negligible.

INDICATIONS AND USES

Treatment of patients with myelodysplastic syndromes (MDS), including previously treated and untreated *de novo* and secondary MDS of all French-American-British subtypes (refractory anemia, refractory anemia with ringed sideroblasts, refractory anemia with excess blasts, refractory anemia with excess blasts in transformation, and chronic myelomonocytic leukemia) and intermediate-1, intermediate-2, and high-risk International Prognostic Scoring System groups.

CONTRAINDICATIONS

Manufacturer states, "None."

PRECAUTIONS

Follow guidelines for handling cytotoxic agents. See Appendix A, p. 1429. ▪ Administered by or under the direction of a physician specialist in a facility with adequate diagnostic and treatment facilities to monitor the patient and respond to any medical emergency. ▪ The effects of age, gender, race, or renal or hepatic impairment on the pharmacokinetics of decitabine have not been studied. ▪ Myelosuppression and worsening neutropenia may occur more frequently in the first or second treatment cycles and may not indicate progression of underlying MDS. Neutropenia and thrombocytopenia may be dose-limiting toxicities. ▪ Patients with MDS produce poorly functioning and immature blood cells and experience anemia, bleeding, fatigue, infection, and weakness. High-risk MDS patients may experience bone marrow failure, which may lead to death from bleeding and infection. ▪ MDS can progress to acute leukemia (AML). ▪ Use caution in patients with renal or hepatic impairment. Use has not been studied.

Monitor: Obtain a baseline CBC with platelets and monitor before each dosing cycle and as indicated between cycles. ▪ Consider early institution of growth factors as indicated. ▪ Obtain a baseline and monitor renal and hepatic function (BUN, SCr, bilirubin) as indicated. ▪ Use prophylactic antiemetics to reduce nausea and vomiting and increase patient comfort. ▪ Monitor for S/S of infection. Prophylactic antibiotics may be indicated pending results of C/S in a febrile neutropenic patient. ▪ Monitor for thrombocytopenia (platelet count less than 50,000/mm^3). Initiate precautions to prevent excessive bleeding (e.g., inspect IV sites, skin, and mucous membranes; use extreme care during invasive procedures; test urine, emesis, stool, and secretions for occult blood). ▪ Avoid administration of live virus vaccine to immunocompromised patients. ▪ Observe for S/S of a hypersensitivity reaction; specific information not available. ▪ See Precautions and Antidote.

Patient Education: Avoid pregnancy; nonhormonal birth control recommended for both males and females; see Maternal/Child. Women should report a suspected pregnancy immediately. ▪ Discuss possible liver or kidney disease with a health care professional. ▪ Report S/S of infection (e.g., fever, sore throat), bruising, bleeding, or other suspected side effects.

Maternal/Child: Category D: avoid pregnancy; may cause fetal harm. Females should use birth control until at least 1 month after treatment with decitabine is discontinued. Males should not father a child until at least 2 months after treatment with decitabine is discontinued. ▪ Discontinue breast-feeding; has potential for serious harm to nursing infants. ▪ Safety and effectiveness for use in pediatric patients not established.

Elderly: The majority of patients in clinical trials were over 65 years of age. Safety and effectiveness similar to younger adults; however, greater sensitivity of some older individuals should be considered.

DRUG/LAB INTERACTIONS

Formal drug interactions studies have not been completed. In vitro studies suggest that decitabine is unlikely to inhibit or induce the activities of human hepatic cytochrome P$_{450}$ isoenzymes. ▪ Plasma protein binding is negligible; interactions due to displacement of more highly protein bound drugs from plasma proteins are not expected. ▪ Do not administer **live virus vaccines** to immunocompromised patients who are receiving antineoplastic agents.

SIDE EFFECTS

Cough, constipation, diarrhea, fatigue, fever, hyperglycemia, nausea, and petechiae have been reported most commonly. Bone marrow suppression (anemia, neutropenia, thrombocytopenia) was the most frequent cause of dose reduction, delay, and discontinuation. Grade 3 or 4 adverse events included febrile neutropenia, leukopenia, neutropenia, and thrombocytopenia. During clinical trials, therapy was also discontinued because of abnormal liver function tests, cardiopulmonary arrest, intracranial hemorrhage, *Mycobacterium avium* complex infection, and pneumonia. Atrial fibrillation, central line infection, febrile neutropenia, neutropenia, and pulmonary edema also resulted in delayed doses; bone marrow suppression (anemia, neutropenia, thrombocytopenia), depression, edema, lethargy, pharyngitis, and tachycardia resulted in reduced doses. Numerous other side effects may occur.

Post-Marketing: Acute febrile neutrophilic dermatosis (Sweet's syndrome) has been reported.

Overdose: Increased myelosuppression, including prolonged neutropenia and thrombocytopenia.

ANTIDOTE

Notify physician of any side effects. Most will be treated symptomatically. Dosage may be delayed for hematologic toxicity. Hematologic recovery to at least an ANC equal to or greater than 1,000 cells/mm^3 and platelets equal to or greater than 50,000 cells/mm^3 between cycles is required; see

Dose Adjustments. If a SCr equal to or greater than 2 mg/dL, an ALT or a total bilirubin equal to or greater than 2 times the ULN, and/or an uncontrolled infection occur, discontinue decitabine therapy until the toxicity is resolved. Blood and blood products, antibiotics, and other adjunctive therapies must be available. Blood modifiers (e.g., darbepoetin alfa [Aranesp], epoetin alfa [Epogen], filgrastim [Neupogen], oprelvekin [Neumega], pegfilgrastim [Neulasta], sargramostim [Leukine]) may be indicated to treat bone marrow toxicity. No known antidote; provide supportive care in overdose. ▪ Resuscitate as necessary.

DEFEROXAMINE MESYLATE

(deh-fer-**OX**-ah-meen **MES**-ih-layt)

Desferal

Antidote
Chelating agent

pH 4 to 6

USUAL DOSE

Acute iron intoxication in adults and pediatric patients over 3 years of age: IM use preferred for all patients not in shock; see Precautions. Administer an initial dose of 1,000 mg at a rate not to exceed 15 mg/kg/hr. May be followed with 500 mg every 4 hours for 2 doses at a rate not to exceed 125 mg/hr (adults) or 15 mg/kg/hr (pediatric patients). Depending on clinical response, subsequent doses of 500 mg every 4 to 12 hours may be administered. *Do not exceed 6 Gm in 24 hours by way of any or all routes—IV, IM, clysis, or oral.* As soon as clinical condition permits, IV route should be changed to IM.

Chronic iron overload: 500 to 1,000 mg daily as an IM injection. In addition, administer 2,000 mg IV with each unit of blood transfused at a rate not to exceed 15 mg/kg/hr. Administer separately from blood. Do not exceed 6 Gm in 24 hours.

Aluminum toxicity (unlabeled): Dose must be individualized. One source recommends 5 to 10 mg/kg 4 to 6 hours before dialysis. May repeat every 7 to 10 days as needed. 100 mg can bind 4.1 mg of aluminum.

PEDIATRIC DOSE

Acute iron intoxication in pediatric patients over 3 years of age: See Usual Dose. *Do not exceed a rate of 15 mg/kg/hr or a total dose of 6 Gm in 24 hours.*
Chronic iron overload: *Do not exceed a rate of 15 mg/kg/hr or a total dose of 6 Gm in 24 hours.*

DOSE ADJUSTMENTS

Dose selection should be cautious in the elderly based on the potential for decreased organ function and concomitant disease or drug therapy.

DILUTION

Each 500 mg must be diluted in 5 mL of SW for injection. When completely dissolved, deferoxamine must be further diluted in an IV solution; ½NS, NS, D5W, D10W, and LR are **compatible.** Dissolve completely before use.

Storage: Store unopened vial at room temperature. Reconstituted solution may be stored at room temperature for 24 hours if it has been prepared in a sterile laminar flow hood. Do not refrigerate reconstituted solution. Single-dose vial. Discard unused portion of vial.

COMPATIBILITY

Manufacturer states, "Reconstituting in solvents or under conditions other than indicated may result in precipitation. Turbid solutions should not be used."

RATE OF ADMINISTRATION

Initial 1,000 mg may be administered at a rate not to exceed 15 mg/kg/hr. Follow with 500 mg over 4 hours for 2 doses. Depending on clinical response, subsequent 500-mg doses may be given over 4 to 12 hours. In these subsequent doses, do not exceed a rate of 125 mg/hr (adults) or 15 mg/kg/hr (pediatric patients); see Precautions, Side Effects, Overdose.

ACTIONS

A heavy metal antagonist that chelates iron and aluminum. As an iron-chelating agent, deferoxamine complexes with iron to form ferrioxamine, a stable chelate that prevents the iron from entering into further chemical reactions. Chelates iron from ferritin and hemosiderin but not readily from transferrin, hemoglobin, or cytochromes. 1 Gm of deferoxamine can theoretically sequester 85 mg of iron (as the ferric ion); however, the rate of complex formation is pH dependent. Metabolized by plasma enzymes via unknown pathways. Chelate is readily soluble in water and passes easily through the kidneys, giving the urine a characteristic reddish color. Also excreted in feces through the bile.

INDICATIONS AND USES

To facilitate the removal of iron in the treatment of acute iron intoxication. Is an adjunct to, not a substitute for, standard measures used to treat acute iron intoxication. Such measures may include induction of emesis and/or gastric lavage; suction and maintenance of a clear airway; control of shock with IV fluids, blood, oxygen, and vasopressors; and correction of acidosis. ■ Treatment of chronic iron overload due to transfusion-dependent anemias.

Unlabeled uses: Diagnosis and management of aluminum accumulation in bone of renal failure patients. ■ Treatment of aluminum toxicity in hemodialysis patients; see Contraindications. ■ In conjunction with hemodialysis for treatment of acute aluminum encephalopathy.

CONTRAINDICATIONS

Severe renal disease or anuria. ■ Hypersensitivity to deferoxamine.

PRECAUTIONS

IM administration is preferred. May be given SC by hypodermoclysis. IV administration should be used only in a state of cardiovascular shock or chronic iron overload and then only by slow IV infusion. Flushing, urticaria, hypotension, and shock have occurred with rapid infusion. ■ Ocular and auditory disturbances have been reported with high doses, in patients with low ferritin levels, or when the drug is administered over a prolonged period of time. Disturbances may be reversible with early detection and immediate cessation of therapy. ■ Increases in SCr, renal tubular disorders, and acute renal failure have been reported. ■ High doses in patients with concomitant low ferritin levels have been associated with growth retardation. Growth velocity may partially resume to pretreatment rates with dose reduction; see Maternal/Child. ■ Acute respiratory distress syndrome (ARDS) has been reported following treatment with excessively high intravenous doses in patients with acute iron intoxication or thalassemia. ▪ Rare cases of mucormycosis (some fatal) and generalized infections with *Yersinia enterocolitica* and *Yersinia pseudotuberculosis* have been reported. Discontinue therapy, obtain cultures, and institute proper therapy at first sign of infection. ▪ Impairment of cardiac function has been reported following concomitant treatment with deferoxamine and vitamin C (more than 500 mg daily). However, patients with chronic iron overload may become vitamin C deficient. Cautious vitamin C supplementation may be required. Begin supplementation only after initial month of deferoxamine therapy. Limit daily dose to 200 mg given in divided doses. Avoid concomitant use of vitamin C and deferoxamine in patients with pre-existing cardiac failure. ▪ Treatment with deferoxamine in the presence of aluminum overload may result in decreased serum calcium and aggravation of hyperparathyroidism. In patients with aluminum-related encephalopathy who are undergoing dialysis, deferoxamine may cause neurologic dysfunction (seizures). May precipitate onset of dialysis dementia. ▪ See Drug/Lab Interactions.

Monitor: Deferoxamine is adjunctive therapy; see Precautions for standard measures for treating acute iron intoxication. ▪ Monitor for development of ocular disturbances. May include blurred vision; development of cataracts after prolonged administration in chronic iron overload; decreased visual acuity (including vision loss; vision defects; scotoma; impaired peripheral, color, and night vision; optic neuritis; cataracts; corneal opacities; and retinal pigmentary abnormalities). Periodic visual acuity tests, slit-lamp examinations, and funduscopy are recommended with prolonged therapy. ▪ Monitor for development of auditory disturbances. May include tinnitus and hearing loss, including high-frequency sensorineural hearing loss. Periodic audiometry is recommended with prolonged therapy. ▪ Monitor cardiac function in patients receiving concomitant therapy with vitamin C and deferoxamine. Cardiac dysfunction may be reversible with discontinuation of vitamin C. ▪ Monitor serum ferritin and serum iron. ▪ In acute iron intoxication, larger-than-normal amounts of IV fluids are required to maintain intravascular volume and prevent kidney damage. Monitor renal function. ▪ Monitor blood gases, central venous pressure (CVP), and cardiac output as indicated to assess the effects of absorbed iron.

Patient Education: Report any hearing or vision changes. ▪ Do not take vitamin C unless prescribed by physician. ▪ Do not drive or operate hazardous machinery if dizziness, visual or auditory impairment, or other nervous system disturbances are experienced. ▪ May cause reddish discoloration of urine.

Maternal/Child: Category C: use only if potential benefit justifies potential risk to fetus. ▪ Use caution during breast-feeding. ▪ Safety and effectiveness for use in pediatric patients under 3 years of age not established. ▪ Monitor body weight and growth every 3 months in pediatric patients; see Precautions. ▪ Supplementation may be required in pediatric patients who become vitamin C deficient. In general, 50 mg daily is sufficient for pediatric patients under 10 years of age. 100 mg is sufficient in older pediatric patients; see Precautions and Drug/Lab Interactions.

Elderly: See Dose Adjustments and Drug/Lab Interactions. ▪ Risk of cardiac decompensation increased. ▪ Post-marketing reports suggest a possible increased risk of eye disorders (color blindness, maculopathy, and scotoma) and an increased risk of hearing loss or deafness.

DRUG/LAB INTERACTIONS

Risk of cardiac decompensation is increased when given concurrently with large doses (greater than 200 mg) of **vitamin C** (ascorbic acid). However, vitamin C increases the availability of iron for chelation. Small doses of a vitamin C supplement may be required. ▪ Concurrent treatment with **prochlorperazine** (Compazine) may lead to a temporary impairment in consciousness. ▪ Discontinue deferoxamine 48 hours before **scintigraphy with gallium-67.** Imaging results may be distorted because of rapid urinary excretion of deferoxamine-bound gallium-67.

SIDE EFFECTS

Occur more frequently with too-rapid administration; abdominal discomfort, adult respiratory distress syndrome (ARDS), arthralgia, diarrhea, dysuria, fever, flushing of the skin, growth retardation and bone changes, headache, high-frequency sensorineural hearing loss and/or tinnitus, hypersensitivity reactions (anaphylaxis, angioedema, generalized rash, urticaria), hypotension, impaired hepatic and/or renal function, increased ALT and AST, infection (mucormycosis, *Yersinia*), injection site reactions, muscle spasms, myalgia, nausea, neurologic disturbances (dizziness; peripheral sensory, motor, or mixed neuropathy; paresthesias; exacerbation or precipitation of aluminum-related dialysis encephalopathy), seizures, shock, tachycardia, visual disturbances (blurred vision, decreased acuity or loss of vision, retinopathy, scotoma, and others). Blood dyscrasias (e.g., leukopenia, thrombocytopenia) have been reported. See Precautions.

Overdose: Acute transient loss of vision, acute renal failure, agitation, aphasia, bradycardia, CNS depression including coma, headache, hypotension, GI disturbances, nausea, and tachycardia may occur with too rapid administration, inadvertent IV bolus, or overdose.

Post-Marketing: Renal dysfunction (e.g., increased SCr, renal tubular disorders, acute renal failure).

ANTIDOTE

At first sign of side effects, decrease rate of administration. If side effects persist, discontinue drug and notify physician. Further dilution and decrease in rate of administration may be necessary. Readily dialyzable. Resuscitate as indicated.

DENILEUKIN DIFTITOX **BBW**
(den-ih-**LOO**-kin **DIF**-tih-tox)

Ontak

Antineoplastic
Biological response modifier

pH 6.9 to 7.2

USUAL DOSE

Pretesting indicated; see Monitor.

Premedication: Premedicate with an antihistamine (e.g., diphenhydramine [Benadryl]) and acetaminophen (Tylenol) before each infusion.

Denileukin diftitox: 9 or 18 mcg/kg/day administered as an IV infusion for 5 consecutive days. Repeat course every 21 days for 8 cycles.

DOSE ADJUSTMENTS

In patients with hypoalbuminemia, administration of denileukin diftitox should be delayed until serum albumin levels are at least 3 Gm/dL; see Monitor.

DILUTION

Each 2-mL vial contains 300 mcg (150 mcg/mL) of frozen recombinant denileukin diftitox. Thaw in refrigerator (2° to 8° C) for not more than 24 hours or at CRT for 1 to 2 hours. Bring to CRT before preparing dose. Do not heat. Gently swirl contents of vial. Do not shake. Solution may be hazy initially. Haze should clear as solution reaches CRT. The concentration of denileukin diftitox must be at least 15 mcg/mL during all steps in the preparation of the infusion solution. This is best accomplished by aseptically withdrawing the calculated dose of denileukin diftitox and injecting it into an empty infusion bag. For each 1 mL of denileukin diftitox from the vial(s), no more than 9 mL of sterile NS without preservative should then be added to the bag. For example: A 70-kg patient receiving a 9-mcg/kg dose would require 630 mcg of denileukin diftitox (or 4.2 mL). Withdraw 4.2 mL of denileukin diftitox from vials and inject into an empty infusion bag. Add no more than 37.8 mL (9 × 4.2 mL) of preservative-free NS to infusion bag. The final solution will be 630 mcg in 42 mL of solution, which equals the desired concentration of 15 mcg/mL. Diluted denileukin diftitox must be prepared and stored in a plastic syringe or soft plastic IV infusion bag. Do not use a glass container; see Compatibility.

Filters: Manufacturer states, "Do not administer through an in-line filter."

Storage: Store unopened vials in freezer at −10° C (14° F). Prepared solutions should be administered within 6 hours. Discard unused solution. Do not refreeze.

COMPATIBILITY

Manufacturer states, "Do not physically mix denileukin diftitox with other drugs." Do not mix in glass. Adsorption to glass may occur in the dilute state.

RATE OF ADMINISTRATION

A single dose evenly distributed over 30 to 60 minutes. Administer via peripheral or central vein by a pump device or IV infusion bag. Do not administer as a bolus injection. Do not administer through an in-line filter. If adverse reactions occur during the infusion, the infusion should be discontinued or the rate should be reduced depending on the severity of the reaction. There is no clinical experience with infusion times lasting more than 80 minutes.

ACTIONS

A recombinant DNA–derived cytotoxic protein. A fusion protein that utilizes both the cytotoxic action of diphtheria toxin and the cell-targeting ability of human interleukin-2 (IL-2) to kill certain leukemia and lymphoma cells. Targets specific receptors (IL-2 receptors) on malignant cells while minimizing damage to normal cells that do not express the receptor. Ex vivo studies suggest that denileukin diftitox interacts with the high-affinity IL-2 receptor on the cell surface and inhibits cellular protein synthesis, resulting in cell death within hours. No differences in pharmacologic action noted based on age, gender, and/or race. Half-life in lymphoma patients is 70 to 80 minutes. Development of antibodies to denileukin diftitox has been shown to increase clearance; see Precautions.

INDICATIONS AND USES

Treatment of patients with persistent or recurrent cutaneous T-cell lymphoma whose malignant cells express the CD25 component of the IL-2 receptor. The safety and efficacy of denileukin diftitox in patients with CTCL whose malignant cells do not express the CD25 component of the IL-2 receptor have not been examined.

CONTRAINDICATIONS

Hypersensitivity to denileukin diftitox, any of its components, diphtheria toxin, or interleukin-2.

PRECAUTIONS

Administered under the supervision of a physician experienced in the use of antineoplastic therapy and the management of patients with cancer. Administer in a facility equipped and staffed for cardiopulmonary resuscitation and in which the patient can be properly monitored. ▪ Infusion and/or hypersensitivity reactions, defined as symptoms occurring within 24 hours of infusion and resolving within 48 hours of the last infusion in that course, have been reported and may be serious or life threatening. Deaths have occurred. Incidence of infusion reactions appears to decrease after the first 2 courses of therapy. ▪ Capillary leak syndrome (CLS) has resulted in death. CLS characterized by at least two of the following three symptoms (edema, hypoalbuminemia [3 Gm/dL or less], hypotension), has been reported. Symptoms are not required to occur simultaneously to be described as capillary leak syndrome. Onset can occur at any time. Usually occurs within 2 weeks of the infusion but may be delayed. Patients with edema or pre-existing low serum albumin levels may be predisposed to this syndrome. Symptoms may persist or worsen after denileukin diftitox is discontinued; treatment and/or hospitalization may be required; deaths have been reported. Use special caution in patients with pre-existing cardiovascular disease. ▪ A significant percentage of patients treated with denileukin diftitox tested positive for antibodies at baseline, probably due to a prior exposure to diphtheria toxin or its vaccine. With each subsequent course, the percent of patients who tested positive increased, C_{max} and AUC decreased, and clearance increased with increasing antibody formation. The formation of neutralizing antibodies was assessed in a number of patients. Evidence of inhibited functional activity in the cellular assay was seen. ▪ Loss of visual acuity (usually with loss of color vision, with or without retinal pigment mottling) has been reported. Some patients recover; however, most report persistent visual impairment.

Monitor: Before administration of denileukin diftitox, the patient's malignant cells should be tested for CD25 expression. A testing service for the assay of CD25 on skin biopsy samples is available; see manufacturer's prescribing information. ▪ Monitor CBC and a blood chemistry panel, including liver and renal function, before therapy and weekly during therapy. ▪ Monitor serum albumin levels before each course of therapy. Nadir occurs 1 to 2 weeks after administration. Delay administration if necessary until serum albumin levels are at least 3 Gm/dL. Note Dose Adjustments. ▪ Observe for capillary leak syndrome. Monitor weight, edema, BP, and serum albumin levels on an outpatient basis. ▪ Monitor for signs and symptoms of infection. Patients with CTCL have a predisposition to cutaneous infections, and binding of denileukin diftitox to activated lymphocytes and macrophages may lead to cell death and may impair patient's immune system. ▪ Monitor for thrombocytopenia (platelet count less than 50,000/mm^3). Initiate precautions to prevent excessive bleeding (e.g., inspect IV sites, skin, and mucous membranes; use extreme care during invasive procedures; test urine, emesis, stool, and secretions for occult blood). ▪ Monitor injection site. To minimize occurrence or phlebitis, change the injection site frequently. ▪ See Precautions, Side Effects, and Antidote.

Patient Education: Promptly report orthostatic hypotension (dizziness), weight gain, or edema following infusion. ▪ Weigh self daily. ▪ Report breathing problems, chest pain, chills, fever, tachycardia, and/or urticaria following infusion. ▪ Report vision changes. ▪ Keep physician informed of all side effects.

Maternal/Child: Category C: safety for use in pregnancy not established. Use only if clearly needed. ▪ Discontinue breast-feeding. ▪ Safety and effectiveness in pediatric patients not established.

Elderly: Numbers in clinical studies insufficient to determine if the elderly respond differently than do younger adults.

DRUG/LAB INTERACTIONS

Drug interaction studies have not been conducted.

SIDE EFFECTS

All patients experienced at least one adverse event. The occurrence of side effects tended to diminish in frequency and severity after the first two courses of therapy. ▪ The most common side effects were cough, diarrhea, dyspnea, edema, fatigue, fever, headache, nausea, peripheral edema, pruritus, and rigors. The most common serious side effects were capillary leak syndrome, infusion reactions, and vision changes, including loss of visual acuity. During initial studies the most common reasons for discontinuation of therapy were systemic flu-like symptoms (e.g., anorexia, asthenia, chills, fever, malaise, nausea, and vomiting), hypoalbuminemia, infection, rash, respiratory events (e.g., dyspnea, apnea, pulmonary edema, or pneumonia), and capillary leak syndrome. The most common reasons for therapy-related hospitalization were evaluation of fever, management of capillary leak syndrome, or dehydration secondary to gastrointestinal toxicity. ▪ Other reported side effects include anorexia, arthralgia, asthenia, back pain, chest pain, dizziness, dysgeusia, hypotension, myalgia, pain, rash, upper respiratory tract infection, and vomiting.

Post-Marketing: Visual acuity loss.

ANTIDOTE

Notify physician of any side effects. If adverse reactions occur during administration, the infusion should be discontinued or the rate should be reduced depending on the severity of the reaction. If a serious infusion reaction occurs, immediately stop and permanently discontinue denileukin diftitox. IV antihistamines, corticosteroids, and/or epinephrine may be required. Most symptoms of the flu-like syndrome will respond to treatment with antipyretics and/or antiemetics (e.g., promethazine [Phenergan] or prochlorperazine [Compazine]). Premedication with acetaminophen and an antihistamine 30 to 60 minutes before each infusion may help reduce the frequency and/or severity of symptoms. While on therapy, patients may continue to receive acetaminophen every 4 to 6 hours while awake. Fever, chills, and/or pain not controlled with acetaminophen alone may be treated with an NSAID. Rigors may be treated with meperidine. Skin rashes may require treatment with topical and/or oral corticosteroids. Treatment of capillary leak syndrome depends on whether edema or hypotension is the primary clinical problem. Patients who present with dehydration should be considered for IV fluid replacement therapy. If BP is still not adequate after replacement therapy, pressor agents (e.g., dopamine) should be considered. Use of diuretics should be avoided in patients whose intravascular depletion has not been corrected. However, patients who present primarily with edema may benefit from diuretic therapy. Continuous monitoring of fluid status, weight, and BP is essential. If overdose occurs, hepatic and renal function and overall fluid status should be closely monitored. Resuscitate as necessary.

DESMOPRESSIN ACETATE

(des-moh-**PRESS**-in **AS**-ah-tayt)

DDAVP, 1-Deamino-8-D-Arginine Vasopressin

Hormone
Antidiuretic
Antihemorrhagic

pH 3.5 to 4

USUAL DOSE

Diabetes insipidus: 2 to 4 mcg daily in 2 divided doses. Adjust each dose individually for an adequate diurnal rhythm of water turnover. IV dose has 10 times the antidiuretic effect of intranasal desmopressin. Available as a tablet to manage cranial central diabetes insipidus.

Hemophilia A and von Willebrand's disease (type 1): 0.3 mcg/kg of body weight. Administer 30 minutes preoperatively.

DOSE ADJUSTMENTS

Many specific requirements depending on diagnosis; see Precautions, Monitor. ▪ Dosing should be cautious in the elderly. Consider potential for decreased organ function and concomitant disease or drug therapy. See Elderly and Contraindications. ▪ Reduce dose accordingly when transferring from intranasal to IV administration.

DILUTION

Diabetes insipidus: May be given undiluted.

Hemophilia A and von Willebrand's disease (type 1): Dilute a single dose in 10 mL of NS for pediatric patients under 10 kg; 50 mL for adults and pediatric patients over 10 kg. Must be given as an infusion.

Storage: Refrigerate at 2° to 8° C (36° to 46° F). Use diluted product promptly.

COMPATIBILITY

Specific information not available. Consider specific use; consult pharmacist.

RATE OF ADMINISTRATION

Diabetes insipidus: A single dose by IV injection over 1 minute.

Hemophilia A and von Willebrand's disease (type 1): A single dose as an infusion over 15 to 30 minutes.

ACTIONS

A synthetic analog of the natural hormone arginine vasopressin (human antidiuretic hormone—ADH). It is more potent than arginine vasopressin in increasing plasma levels of factor VIII activity in patients with hemophilia A and von Willebrand's disease (Type 1). Produces dose-related increase in factor VIII levels within 30 minutes and peaks in 90 to 120 minutes. Duration of anti-hemorrhagic action is 4 to 24 hours in mild hemophilia A and 3 hours in von Willebrand's disease. Onset of action as an antidiuretic is prompt. Half-life is biphasic (7.8 minutes for fast phase and 75.5 minutes for slow phase). Increases water resorption in the kidney, increases urine osmolality, and decreases urine output. Clinically effective antidiuretic doses are usually below the levels needed to affect vascular or visceral smooth muscle. Excreted in urine.

INDICATIONS AND USES

Antidiuretic replacement therapy in the management of central (cranial) diabetes insipidus. ■ Management of the temporary polyuria and polydipsia following head trauma or surgery in the pituitary region. ■ Maintenance of hemostasis in patients with hemophilia A or von Willebrand's disease during surgical procedures and postoperatively. ■ To stop bleeding in patients with hemophilia A or von Willebrand's disease with episodes of spontaneous or trauma-induced injuries.

CONTRAINDICATIONS

Infants under 3 months in hemophilia A or von Willebrand's disease, known hypersensitivity to desmopressin, patients with moderate to severe renal impairment (CrCl less than 50 mL/min), and patients with hyponatremia or a history of hyponatremia.

PRECAUTIONS

Use caution in patients with coronary artery insufficiency or hypertension. ■ When administered to patients who do not have a need for the antidiuretic effect, fluid intake should be adjusted downward to decrease the potential occurrence of water intoxication and hyponatremia. S/S may include headache, nausea and vomiting, decreased serum sodium, weight gain, restlessness, fatigue, lethargy, disorientation, depressed reflexes, loss of appetite, irritability, muscle weakness, muscle spasms, and abnormal mental status (e.g., confusion, decreased consciousness, hallucinations). Pediatric and elderly patients may be at increased risk. ■ Use with caution in patients with habitual or psychogenic polydipsia. May be more likely to drink excessive amounts of water, increasing their risk of hyponatremia. ■ Excessive fluid intake may result in an extreme decrease in plasma osmolality. May lead to seizures, coma, and respiratory arrest. ■ Use with caution in patients predisposed to thrombus formation. ■ Use with caution in patients with conditions associated with fluid and electrolyte imbalance (e.g., cystic fibrosis, CHF, renal disorders). ■ Severe hypersensitivity reactions, including anaphylaxis, have been reported. ■ See Drug Interactions.

Monitor: *Diabetes insipidus:* Not effective for the treatment of nephrogenic diabetes insipidus. ▪ Confirm diagnosis of diabetes insipidus by the water deprivation test, the hypertonic saline infusion test, and the response to ADH. ▪ Monitor continued response by measuring urine volume and osmolality. ▪ Plasma osmolality may be needed. Monitor serum electrolytes in therapy lasting longer than 7 days. ▪ Accuracy and effectiveness of dose measured by duration of sleep and adequate, not excessive, water turnover.

Hemophilia A: May be considered for use in patients with factor VIII activity levels from 2% to 5% with careful monitoring. Generally used only when the factor VIII activity level is above 5%. ▪ Not indicated in patients with hemophilia B or those with factor VIII antibodies. ▪ Monitor factor VIII coagulant, factor VIII antigen, factor VIII ristocetin cofactor, and aPTT.

von Willebrand's disease (type 1): Most effective when factor VIII activity level above 5%. ▪ Monitor bleeding time, factor VIII activity levels, ristocetin cofactor activity, and von Willebrand factor antigen during therapy to ensure adequate levels. ▪ Not indicated for treatment of severe classic von Willebrand's disease (Type 1), Type IIB von Willebrand's disease (will induce platelet aggregation), or if there is evidence of an abnormal molecular form of factor VIII antigen.

Hemophilia and von Willebrand's disease: Sometimes used with aminocaproic acid. ▪ Monitor BP and pulse during infusion. ▪ Determine need for repeat administration of desmopressin or use of blood products by laboratory response as well as the clinical condition of the patient. Tachyphylaxis (lessening of response; i.e., a gradual diminution of the factor VIII activity increase) has been seen when given more frequently than every 48 hours.

Patient Education: When antidiuretic effect is not needed, caution patients (especially the young and the elderly) to limit fluid intake to satisfy thirst needs only; this decreases potential occurrence of water intoxication and hyponatremia.

Maternal/Child: Category B: use only when clearly indicated in pregnancy and breast-feeding. ▪ Risk of hyponatremia and water intoxication increased in pediatric patients. Restrict fluid intake. ▪ Safety for use in pediatric patients under 12 years of age with diabetes insipidus not established. ▪ See Contraindications.

Elderly: Risk of hyponatremia and water intoxication increased. Use caution and careful fluid intake restriction. ▪ Response similar to that seen in younger adults. Dosing should be cautious in the elderly. Monitor renal function; see Dose Adjustments.

DRUG/LAB INTERACTIONS

May produce hypertension with other **vasopressors** (e.g., dopamine). ▪ Antidiuretic effect may be potentiated by **chlorpropamide** (Diabinese) **or carbamazepine** (Tegretol). ▪ Use caution when administered concurrently with other medications that can increase the risk of water intoxication with hyponatremia (e.g., **carbamazepine** [Tegretol], **chlorpromazine** [Thorazine], **lamotrigine** [Lamictal], **NSAIDs** [e.g., ibuprofen (Advil, Motrin), naproxen (Aleve, Naprosyn)], **opiate analgesics, selective serotonin reuptake inhibitors** [e.g., sertraline (Zoloft)], **tricyclic antidepressants** [e.g., imipramine (Tofranil)]). ▪ Hyponatremic convulsions have been reported with concomitant use with **oxybutynin** (Ditropan) **and imipramine** (Tofranil-PM).

SIDE EFFECTS
Are infrequent. High doses may produce facial flushing, headache, hypertension (slight), hypotension with a compensatory tachycardia, mild abdominal cramps, nausea, thrombotic events (cerebrovascular thrombosis, MI), and vulval pain. May cause burning, local erythema, and swelling at site of injection; hyponatremia with resultant sequelae (see Precautions); and water intoxication. Anaphylaxis has been reported.

ANTIDOTE
Notify physician of all side effects. Most will respond to reduction of dose or rate of administration, or symptomatic treatment. May need to discontinue drug. Resuscitate as necessary.

DEXAMETHASONE SODIUM PHOSPHATE
(dex-ah-**METH**-ah-zohn **SO**-dee-um **FOS**-fayt)

Hormone (adrenocorticoid/ glucocorticoid)
Anti-inflammatory, Antiemetic
Immunosuppressant, Diagnostic agent

Decadron, Decadron Phosphate   pH 7 to 8.5

USUAL DOSE
Average dose range is 0.5 to 24 mg daily. May be divided into 2 to 4 doses. IV dexamethasone is usually given in an emergency situation or when oral dosing is not feasible. Larger doses may be justified by patient condition. Repeat until adequate response, then decrease dose as indicated. Total dose usually does not exceed 80 mg/24 hr. Dosage must be individualized. High-dose treatment is utilized until patient condition stabilizes, usually no longer than 48 to 72 hours. Doses similar by IV or oral route.

Anti-inflammatory: See average dose range above.

Shock: Several regimens have been suggested:
1 to 6 mg/kg as a single injection; *or*
40 mg. Repeat every 2 to 6 hours as needed; *or*
20 mg as a *loading dose,* followed by a continuous infusion of 3 mg/kg equally distributed over 24 hours.

Cerebral edema: *Loading dose:* 10 mg. ***Maintenance dose:*** 4 mg every 6 hours (usually given IM). Reduce dose after 2 to 4 days. Discontinue gradually over 5 to 7 days. A brain tumor requiring treatment before dexamethasone can be discontinued is the exception.

Cerebral edema (ICP) in recurrent or inoperable brain tumors: 2 mg every 8 to 12 hours (usually given IM). Adjust based on patient response.

Antiemetic in management of emesis-inducing chemotherapy: Several regimens have been used:
10 to 20 mg before chemotherapy. Lower doses may be given over the next 24 to 72 hours if necessary; *or*
Give a loading dose of 4 to 8 mg/M^2. May repeat 2 to 4 mg/M^2 every 6 hours; *or*
20 mg combined with 8 mg of ondansetron (Zofran) in 50 mL D5W before chemotherapy; *or*

20 mg 40 minutes before administration of chemotherapeutic agent. Given concurrently with metoclopramide and lorazepam or diphenhydramine; *or*

10 mg 30 minutes before administration of chemotherapeutic agent. Given concurrently with oral dexamethasone 8 mg beginning prior evening, 4 mg every 4 to 6 hours continuing through treatment day, with droperidol or haloperidol.

Airway edema: *Adult and pediatric patients:* 0.25 to 0.5 mg/kg every 6 hours for croup or beginning 24 hours before elective extubation. Repeat for 4 to 6 doses. Up to 1 mg/kg/24 hr may be given in divided doses before and after extubation.

Allergic conditions: (Usually given IM or PO) 4 to 8 mg on the first day, then PO in decreasing doses (1.5 mg every 12 hours on Days 2 and 3; 0.75 mg every 12 hours on Day 4; and 0.75 mg on Days 5 and 6).

Meningitis: *Adult and pediatric patients:* 0.15 mg/kg/dose every 6 hours for 4 days.

Primary or secondary adrenocortical insufficiency (physiologic replacement): 0.03 to 0.15 mg/kg/24 hr or 0.6 to 0.75 mg/M^2/24 hr given in divided doses every 6 to 12 hours (0.015 to 0.075 mg/kg every 12 hours, or 0.0075 to 0.0375 mg/kg every 6 hours, or 0.3 to 0.375 mg/M^2 every 12 hours, or 0.15 to 0.1875 mg/M^2 every 6 hours). Usually given IM. Dexamethasone has minimal mineralocorticoid properties; may require a concomitant mineralocorticoid (e.g., hydrocortisone IV or PO). Hydrocortisone is the drug of choice for this indication.

PEDIATRIC DOSE

See Maternal/Child.

Cerebral edema: *Loading dose:* 0.5 to 1.5 mg/kg of body weight. *Maintenance dose:* 0.2 to 0.5 mg/kg/24 hr in equally divided doses every 6 hours (0.05 to 0.125 mg/kg every 6 hours) for 5 days, then gradually decrease.

Airway edema: See Usual Dose.

Antiemetic: *Loading dose:* 4 to 8 mg/M^2. May repeat 2 to 4 mg/M^2 every 6 hours.

Anti-inflammatory: 0.03 to 0.15 mg/kg/24 hr in equally divided doses every 6 to 12 hours (0.015 to 0.075 mg/kg every 12 hours or 0.0075 to 0.0375 mg/kg every 6 hours).

Meningitis: See Usual Dose.

DOSE ADJUSTMENTS

Reduced dose may be required in the elderly and with cyclophosphamide.
■ See Drug/Lab Interactions.

DILUTION

May be given undiluted or added to IV glucose or saline solutions and given as an infusion. 24 mg/mL product for IV use only; 4 mg/mL may be used IM/IV.

Storage: Use diluted solutions within 24 hours. Sensitive to heat. Protect from freezing.

COMPATIBILITY   (Underline Indicates Conflicting Compatibility Information)

Consider any drug NOT listed as compatible to be INCOMPATIBLE until consulting a pharmacist; specific conditions may apply.

One source suggests the following **compatibilities:**

Additive: <u>Amikacin (Amikin)</u>, aminophylline, bleomycin (Blenoxane), furosemide (Lasix), granisetron (Kytril), lidocaine, meropenem (Merrem

IV), mitomycin (Mutamycin), nafcillin (Nallpen), ondansetron (Zofran), palonosetron (Aloxi), prochlorperazine (Compazine), ranitidine (Zantac), verapamil.

Y-site: Acyclovir (Zovirax), allopurinol (Aloprim), amifostine (Ethyol), amikacin (Amikin), amphotericin B cholesteryl (Amphotec), anidulafungin (Eraxis), aztreonam (Azactam), bivalirudin (Angiomax), cefepime (Maxipime), cisatracurium (Nimbex), cisplatin (Platinol), cladribine (Leustatin), cyclophosphamide (Cytoxan), cytarabine (ARA-C), dexmedetomidine (Precedex), docetaxel (Taxotere), doripenem (Doribax), doxorubicin (Adriamycin), doxorubicin liposomal (Doxil), etoposide phosphate (Etopophos), famotidine (Pepcid IV), fentanyl (Sublimaze), filgrastim (Neupogen), fluconazole (Diflucan), fludarabine (Fludara), foscarnet (Foscavir), gallium nitrate (Ganite), gemcitabine (Gemzar), granisetron (Kytril), heparin, hetastarch in electrolytes (Hextend), hydromorphone (Dilaudid), levofloxacin (Levaquin), linezolid (Zyvox), lorazepam (Ativan), melphalan (Alkeran), meperidine (Demerol), meropenem (Merrem IV), methadone (Dolophine), methotrexate, milrinone (Primacor), morphine, ondansetron (Zofran), oxaliplatin (Eloxatin), paclitaxel (Taxol), pemetrexed (Alimta), piperacillin/tazobactam (Zosyn), potassium chloride (KCl), propofol (Diprivan), remifentanil (Ultiva), sargramostim (Leukine), sodium bicarbonate, sufentanil (Sufenta), tacrolimus (Prograf), teniposide (Vumon), theophylline, thiotepa, vinorelbine (Navelbine), zidovudine (AZT, Retrovir).

RATE OF ADMINISTRATION
A single dose over 1 minute or less if necessary. As an IV infusion, give at prescribed rate.

ACTIONS
An anti-inflammatory glucocorticoid. A synthetic adrenocortical steroid with little sodium retention. Very soluble in water. Seven times as potent as prednisolone and 20 to 30 times as potent as hydrocortisone. Has minimal mineralocorticoid activity. Primarily used for anti-inflammatory and immunosuppressive effects. May be used in conjunction with other forms of therapy, such as epinephrine for acute hypersensitivity reactions or antibiotics for acute infections. Metabolized primarily in the liver and excreted as inactive metabolites in urine. Crosses the placental barrier. Excreted in urine and breast milk.

INDICATIONS AND USES
Supplementary therapy for severe allergic/hypersensitivity reactions. ▪ Reduction of acute edematous states (cerebral edema, airway edema). ▪ Shock unresponsive to conventional therapy. ▪ Acute exacerbations of disease for patients receiving steroid therapy. ▪ Adrenocortical insufficiency; total, relative, and operative. ▪ Antiemetic for chemotherapy-induced vomiting (e.g., cisplatin). Has numerous other uses by other routes of administration (e.g., IM, intra-articular, intralesional, intrasynovial, soft-tissue injection, oral inhalant).

Unlabeled uses: Adjunct to treatment of meningitis with antibiotics (to reduce incidence of ototoxicity). ▪ Dexamethasone or betamethasone are given IM to the mother to accelerate the production of lung surfactant in utero in the prevention of respiratory distress syndrome of premature infants.

CONTRAINDICATIONS

Hypersensitivity to any product component including sulfites, systemic fungal infections. **Relative contraindications:** Active or latent peptic ulcer, acute or healed tuberculosis, acute or chronic infections (especially chickenpox), acute psychoses, diabetes mellitus, diverticulitis, fresh intestinal anastomoses, myasthenia gravis, ocular herpes simplex, osteoporosis, pregnancy, psychotic tendencies, renal insufficiency, thromboembolic tendencies.

PRECAUTIONS

Withdrawal from therapy should be gradual to avoid precipitation of symptoms of adrenal insufficiency. The patient is observed, especially under stress, for up to 2 years. ▪ Prophylactic antacids may prevent peptic ulcer complications. ▪ Use with caution in hypothyroidism and cirrhosis. **Monitor:** May increase insulin needs in diabetes. ▪ Monitor electrolytes periodically. May cause sodium retention and potassium and calcium excretion. May cause hypertension secondary to fluid and electrolyte disturbances. ▪ May mask signs of infection. ▪ Administer a single dose before 9 AM to reduce suppression of individual's adrenocortical activity. ▪ Periodic ophthalmic exams may be necessary with prolonged treatment. ▪ See Drug/Lab Interactions. **Patient Education:** Report edema, tarry stools, or weight gain promptly. Anorexia, diarrhea, dizziness, fatigue, low blood sugar, nausea, weakness, weight loss, and vomiting promptly. May indicate adrenal insufficiency after dose reduction or discontinuing therapy; report any of these symptoms. ▪ May mask signs of infection and/or decrease resistance. ▪ Diabetics may have an increased requirement for insulin or oral hypoglycemics. ▪ Avoid immunization with live virus vaccines. ▪ Carry ID stating steroid dependent if receiving prolonged therapy. **Maternal/Child:** Category C: has caused birth defects; benefits must outweigh risks. ▪ Observe newborn for hypoadrenalism if mother has received large doses. ▪ Monitor growth and development of pediatric patients receiving prolonged treatment. ▪ Use of a preservative-free solution recommended for neonates. **Elderly:** Reduced muscle mass and plasma volume may necessitate a reduced dose. Monitor BP, blood glucose, and electrolytes carefully. ▪ Increased risk of hypertension. ▪ Higher risk of glucocorticoid-induced osteoporosis. ▪ Avoid aluminum-based antacids (risk of Alzheimer's disease).

DRUG/LAB INTERACTIONS

Aminoglutethimide (Cytadren) **and mitotane** (Lysodren) suppress adrenal function and increase metabolism of dexamethasone two-fold. Not recommended for concurrent use, or dexamethasone dose may require doubling to be effective. Use of hydrocortisone suggested. ▪ Metabolism increased and effects reduced by **hepatic enzyme–inducing agents** (e.g., alcohol, barbiturates [e.g., phenobarbital], hydantoins [e.g., phenytoin (Dilantin)], rifampin [Rifadin]); dose adjustments may be required when adding or deleting from drug profile. ▪ Risk of hypokalemia increased with **amphotericin B or potassium-depleting diuretics** (e.g., thiazides, furosemide, ethacrynic acid). Monitor potassium levels and cardiac function. ▪ Increased risk of **digoxin** toxicity secondary to hypokalemia. ▪ May also decrease effectiveness of **potassium supplements;** monitor serum potassium. ▪ **Diuretics** decrease sodium and fluid retention effects of corticosteroids; corticosteroids decrease sodium excretion and diuretic effects of diuretics. ■ Clearance increased and effects decreased with **ephedrine.** ■ May antagonize effects of **anticholinesterases** (e.g., neostigmine), **isoniazid, salicylates, and somatrem;** dose adjustments may be required. ■ Clearance decreased and effects increased with **estrogens, oral contraceptives, and ketoconazole** (Nizoral). ■ May interact with **anticoagulants, nondepolarizing muscle relaxants** (e.g., atracurium [Tracrium]), **or theophyllines;** may inhibit or potentiate action; monitor carefully. ■ Monitor patients receiving **insulin or thyroid hormones** carefully; dose adjustments of either or both agents may be required. ■ Do not vaccinate with **attenuated virus vaccines** (e.g., smallpox) during therapy. ■ **Altered protein-binding capacity** will impact effectiveness of this drug. ■ **Smoking** may antagonize therapeutic effects. ■ See Precautions. ■ Decreases uptake of **radioactive material** in cerebral edema; will alter brain scan.

SIDE EFFECTS
Do occur but are usually reversible: burning, Cushing's syndrome, electrolyte imbalance, euphoria, glycosuria, headache, hyperglycemia, hypersensitivity reactions including anaphylaxis, hypertension, insomnia, menstrual irregularities, mood swings, peptic ulcer, perforation and hemorrhage, protein catabolism, sweating, thromboembolism, tingling, weakness, and many others.

ANTIDOTE
Notify the physician of any side effect. Treat side effects as indicated. Resuscitate as necessary for anaphylaxis and notify physician. Keep epinephrine immediately available.

DEXMEDETOMIDINE HYDROCHLORIDE
(dex-**med**-ih-**TOM**-ih-deen hy-droh-**KLOR**-eyed)

Precedex

Alpha₂-adrenoceptor agonist
Sedative-hypnotic

pH 4.5 to 7.0

USUAL DOSE

Dosing should be individualized and titrated to desired clinical response.
ICU sedation: *Loading dose:* 1 mcg/kg as an infusion over 10 minutes. A loading dose may not be necessary in patients who are being converted from alternate sedative therapy. See Dose Adjustments.

Maintenance infusion: 0.2 to 0.7 mcg/kg/hr. Adjust rate to achieve the desired level of sedation; see Monitor. Dexmedetomidine is *not* indicated for infusions lasting longer than 24 hours. Has been infused in mechanically ventilated patients before, during, and after extubation provided the infusion does not exceed 24 hours. See Dose Adjustments.

Procedural sedation: Loading dose for both adult and/or awake fiber optic intubation patients: 1 mcg/kg as an infusion over 10 minutes. For less invasive procedures (e.g., ophthalmic surgery), a loading dose of 0.5 mcg/kg as an infusion over 10 minutes may be sufficient. See Dose Adjustments.

Maintenance infusion for adult patients: Begin with 0.6 mcg/kg/hr. Titrate to achieve desired level of sedation. Usual range is 0.2 to 1 mcg/kg/hr. See Dose Adjustments.

Maintenance infusion for awake fiber optic intubation patients: A dose of 0.7 mcg/kg/hr is recommended until the endotracheal tube is secured, then titrate to achieve desired level of sedation as above. See Dose Adjustments.

DOSE ADJUSTMENTS

Reduced doses may be required in patients with hepatic impairment and in the elderly. ▪ For patients over 65 years of age, reduce the loading dose for procedural sedation to 0.5 mcg/kg/hr. ▪ Dose reduction of either or both agents may be required when coadministered with anesthetics, sedatives, hypnotics, or opioids; see Drug Interactions.

DILUTION

Supplied in single-use vials containing 200 mcg/2 mL. Must be diluted before administration. Preparation of the solution is the same, whether for loading dose or maintenance infusion. Withdraw 2 mL of dexmedetomidine and add to 48 mL of NS for a final concentration of 4 mcg/mL. Shake gently.

Storage: Store unopened vials at CRT.

COMPATIBILITY

Consider any drug NOT listed as compatible to be INCOMPATIBLE until consulting a pharmacist; specific conditions may apply.

According to the manufacturer, the **compatibility** of dexmedetomidine with blood, serum, or plasma has not been established; avoid coadministration. Manufacturer lists as **incompatible** with amphotericin B and diazepam (Valium). Adsorption of dexmedetomidine to some types of natural rubbers may occur. Although dexmedetomidine is dosed to effect, it is advisable to use administration components that are made with synthetic or coated natural rubber gaskets.

Manufacturer lists the following **compatibilities:** NS, D5W, 20% mannitol, LR, magnesium sulfate (100 mg/mL), and 0.3% potassium chloride solution.

One source suggests the following **compatibilities:**
Y-site: Alfentanil (Alfenta), amikacin (Amikin), aminophylline, amiodarone (Nexterone), ampicillin, ampicillin/sulbactam (Unasyn), atracurium (Tracrium), atropine, azithromycin (Zithromax), aztreonam (Azactam), bumetanide, butorphanol (Stadol), calcium gluconate, cefazolin (Ancef), cefepime (Maxipime), cefotaxime (Claforan), cefotetan, cefoxitin (Mefoxin), ceftazidime (Fortaz), ceftriaxone (Rocephin), cefuroxime (Zinacef), chlorpromazine (Thorazine), ciprofloxacin (Cipro IV), cisatracurium (Nimbex), clindamycin (Cleocin), D5W, dexamethasone (Decadron), digoxin (Lanoxin), diltiazem (Cardizem), diphenhydramine (Benadryl), dobutamine, dolasetron (Anzemet), dopamine, doxycycline, droperidol (Inapsine), enalaprilat (Vasotec IV), ephedrine, epinephrine (Adrenalin), erythromycin (Erythrocin), esmolol (Brevibloc), etomidate (Amidate), famotidine (Pepcid IV), fenoldopam (Corlopam), fentanyl (Sublimaze), fluconazole (Diflucan), furosemide (Lasix), gentamicin, glycopyrrolate, granisetron (Kytril), haloperidol (Haldol), heparin, hydromorphone (Dilaudid), inamrinone (Amrinone), isoproterenol (Isuprel), ketorolac (Toradol), labetalol (Trandate), levofloxacin (Levaquin), lidocaine, linezolid (Zyvox), lorazepam (Ativan), magnesium, meperidine (Demerol), methylprednisolone (Solu-Medrol), metoclopramide (Reglan), metronidazole (Flagyl IV), midazolam (Versed), milrinone (Primacor), morphine, nalbuphine, nitroglycerin IV, nitroprusside sodium, norepinephrine (Levophed), NS, ondansetron (Zofran), pancuronium, phenylephrine (Neo-Synephrine), piperacillin, piperacillin/tazobactam (Zosyn), potassium chloride, procainamide (Pronestyl), prochlorperazine (Compazine), promethazine (Phenergan), propofol (Diprivan), ranitidine (Zantac), remifentanil (Ultiva), rocuronium (Zemuron), sodium bicarbonate, succinylcholine (Anectine), sufentanil (Sufenta), sulfamethoxazole/trimethoprim, theophylline, thiopental (Pentothal), ticarcillin/clavulanate (Timentin), tobramycin, vancomycin, vecuronium, verapamil.

RATE OF ADMINISTRATION
Administer using a controlled infusion device. Rapid IV or bolus administration may result in bradycardia and sinus arrest.
Loading dose: Infuse over 10 minutes. Increase infusion time (decrease infusion rate) if transient hypertension develops; see Monitor and Antidote.
Maintenance infusion: See Usual Dose. Titrate to desired clinical effect.

ACTIONS
A relatively selective alpha$_2$-adrenoceptor agonist with sedative properties. In animal studies, the desired alpha$_2$ selectivity is seen following slow IV infusions of low and medium doses (10 to 300 mcg/kg), but both alpha$_1$ and alpha$_2$ activity are seen following slow IV infusion of high doses (equal to or greater than 1,000 mcg/kg) or with rapid IV administration. Appears to have both sedative and moderate analgesic activity and may decrease the requirement for concomitant sedation and analgesia when used as a short-term infusion in the ICU setting. Other actions include reduced BP, HR, and reduced salivation. Highly protein bound. Almost completely metabolized in the liver via direct glucuronidation and cytochrome P$_{450}$-mediated metabolism. Metabolites excreted primarily in

urine and to a small extent in feces. Half-life is approximately 2 hours. Pharmacokinetics not altered by age or gender.

INDICATIONS AND USES
Sedation of initially intubated and mechanically ventilated patients during treatment in an intensive care setting. Should be administered by continuous infusion not to exceed 24 hours. ▪ Sedation of non-intubated patients before and/or during surgical and other procedures.

CONTRAINDICATIONS
None noted.

PRECAUTIONS
Administered by persons skilled in the management of patients in the intensive care or operating room setting. ▪ Clinically significant episodes of bradycardia and sinus arrest have been reported in young, healthy volunteers with high vagal tone or with different routes of administration, including rapid intravenous or bolus administration; see Rate of Administration. ▪ Hypotension and bradycardia have been reported. Decreases sympathetic nervous system activity. Use caution in patients with advanced heart block, severe ventricular dysfunction, diabetes mellitus, chronic hypertension, hypovolemia, and the elderly; hypotension and/or bradycardia may be more pronounced. Clinical intervention may be required; see Antidote. ▪ Patients may be arousable and alert when stimulated. This alone should not be considered as evidence of lack of effectiveness in the absence of other clinical signs and symptoms. ▪ Dexmedetomidine should not be administered for longer than 24 hours. Adverse events related to withdrawal (e.g., agitation, hypertension, nausea and vomiting, tachycardia) have been reported with prolonged infusions. Most withdrawal-related events were seen 24 to 48 hours following discontinuation of the infusion. Withdrawal symptoms have not been seen with discontinuation of short-term infusions (less than 6 hours). ▪ Use beyond 24 hours has been associated with tolerance and tachyphylaxis and a dose-related increase in adverse reactions. ▪ Use with caution in patients with hepatic impairment. Clearance of dexmedetomidine is decreased; see Dose Adjustments.

Monitor: Continuous monitoring of VS, oxygenation, and cardiac and fluid status imperative. ▪ Hypovolemia may increase risk of hypotension. ▪ Use of a sedation scale (e.g., Ramsay) recommended for monitoring of sedative effect. ▪ Transient hypertension has been observed primarily during the loading dose in association with initial peripheral vasoconstrictive effects. Treatment is generally not required; see Antidote. ▪ See Precautions.

Patient Education: Report abdominal pain, agitation, confusion, constipation, diarrhea, dizziness, excessive sweating, headache, nervousness, salt cravings, weakness, or weight loss that occur within 48 hours.

Maternal/Child: Category C: safety for use in pregnancy not established. Studies suggest fetal exposure should be expected. ▪ Safety for use during labor and delivery and with breast-feeding not established. Use only when clearly indicated. ▪ Safety and effectiveness in pediatric patients under 18 years of age not established.

Elderly: In patients older than 65 years, a higher incidence of bradycardia and hypotension was observed following administration of dexmedetomidine. ▪ Consider age-related organ impairment and history of previous or concomitant disease or drug therapy. ▪ See Dose Adjustments.

DRUG/LAB INTERACTIONS

In vitro studies showed no evidence of cytochrome P_{450}-mediated drug interactions that are likely to be of clinical significance. ▪ Potentiated by **anesthetics** (e.g., enflurane, isoflurane, sevoflurane), **sedatives or hypnotics** (e.g., barbiturates, benzodiazepines [e.g., diazepam (Valium), midazolam (Versed)], propofol [Diprivan]), **and opioids** (e.g., alfentanil, meperidine, morphine). Reduced doses of both drugs may be indicated. See Dose Adjustments. ▪ Concurrent use with other **vasodilators** (e.g., nitroglycerin, nitroprusside sodium) **or negative chronotropic agents** (e.g., beta blockers [e.g., metoprolol (Lopressor)], calcium channel blockers [e.g., diltiazem (Cardizem)]) may have an additive effect; use with caution.

SIDE EFFECTS

The most common treatment-emergent side effects, occurring in more than 2% of patients in both ICU and procedural sedation studies, included bradycardia, dry mouth, and hypotension. Other frequently reported side effects requiring treatment were anemia, fever, hypertension, hypoxia, nausea, tachycardia, and vomiting. Less frequently reported side effects include abnormal vision, acidosis, agitation, apnea, arrhythmia (e.g., atrial fibrillation), bronchospasm, confusion, delirium, dizziness, dyspnea, hallucination, headache, heart block, hypercapnia, hyperkalemia, hypoventilation, increased alkaline phosphatase, increased GGT (gamma glutamyltransferase), increased ALT, increased AST, increased sweating, infection, light anesthesia, neuralgia, neuritis, pain, pleural effusion, pulmonary edema, rigors, sinus arrest, somnolence, and speech disorder.

Overdose: Bradycardia, cardiac arrest, first-degree AV block, hypotension, second-degree heart block.

ANTIDOTE

Keep physician informed of all side effects. Hypotension and bradycardia may be treated by slowing or stopping the dexmedetomidine infusion, increasing the rate of IV fluid administration, elevation of the lower extremities, or use of pressor amines (e.g., dopamine). Administration of anticholinergic agents (e.g., atropine or glycopyrrolate) may be considered to modify vagal tone. Transient hypertension during loading dose may be treated by decreasing the rate of the infusion. Resuscitate as necessary.

DEXRAZOXANE
(dex-rah-**ZOX**-ayn)

Totect, Zinecard

Antidote
Antineoplastic adjunct
Chelating agent

pH 3.5 to 5.5

USUAL DOSE

TOTECT

Administer once daily for 3 consecutive days. Initiate treatment as soon as possible and within 6 hours of extravasation. Doses should be given 24 hours apart (+ or − 3 hours); see Precautions. Recommended regimen is:
Day 1 and Day 2: 1,000 mg/M^2 not to exceed 2,000 mg.
Day 3: 500 mg/M^2 not to exceed 1,000 mg.

ZINECARD

Administered in conjunction with doxorubicin. Dose ratio of dexrazoxane to doxorubicin (Adriamycin) is 10:1 (e.g., 500 mg/M^2 dexrazoxane to 50 mg/M^2 doxorubicin). Doxorubicin dose must be given within 30 minutes of starting the dexrazoxane injection, but only after the full dose of dexrazoxane is administered.

PEDIATRIC DOSE

TOTECT AND ZINECARD

Safety for use in pediatric patients not established.

ZINECARD

One source indicates that 3,500 mg/M^2/24 hr for 3 days is the maximum tolerated dose based on coagulation parameters.

DOSE ADJUSTMENTS

TOTECT AND ZINECARD

Decrease the recommended dose of dexrazoxane by 50% in patients with moderate to severe renal impairment (CrCl less than 40 mL/min). Ratio of Zinecard to doxorubicin will be 5:1 (e.g., 250 mg/M^2 dexrazoxane to 50 mg/M^2 doxorubicin). ▪ Consider age-related impaired organ function and concomitant disease or drug therapy in the elderly; see Elderly. ▪ See Antidote. ▪ Has not been evaluated in hepatic insufficiency.

ZINECARD

When administering Zinecard, the dose of dexrazoxane is dependent on the dose of doxorubicin. When the dose of doxorubicin is reduced (e.g., patients with hyperbilirubinemia), adjust the dexrazoxane dose accordingly. Maintain a 10:1 ratio (dexrazoxane to doxorubicin) except in patients with CrCl less than 40 mL/min.

DILUTION

Specific techniques required; see Precautions.

TOTECT

Reconstitute each 500-mg vial with 50 mL of provided diluent (10 mg/mL). Further dilute the calculated dose in 1,000 mL of NS.

ZINECARD

Initially reconstitute each 250 mg (500 mg) with 25 mL (50 mL) of ⅙ M sodium lactate diluent provided by manufacturer (10 mg/mL). May be further diluted with D5W or NS. Concentration should range from 1.3 to 5 mg/mL. An additional 25 mL (50 mL) of diluent would yield 5 mg/mL; 75 mL (150 mL) would yield 2.5 mg/mL.

Storage: *Totect and Zinecard:* Store unopened vials at CRT. Protect from light. *Totect:* Reconstituted solution should be used immediately (within 2 hours). Diluted product stable for 4 hours from time of reconstitution and dilution when stored below 25° C (77° F). *Zinecard:* Reconstituted or diluted solution stable for 6 hours at CRT or refrigerated. Discard unused solutions.

COMPATIBILITY

Consider any drug NOT listed as compatible to be INCOMPATIBLE until consulting a pharmacist; specific conditions may apply.

Manufacturer states, "Should not be mixed or administered with other drugs"; degrades rapidly at a pH above 7.

One source suggests the following **compatibilities:**

Y-site: Gemcitabine (Gemzar) and pemetrexed (Alimta).

RATE OF ADMINISTRATION

Totect

Administer a single dose as an IV infusion equally distributed over 1 to 2 hours. Infuse at RT with normal lighting.

Zinecard

A single dose may be given by slow IV push or rapid infusion (given over 10 to 15 minutes in one study). Complete dexrazoxane dose but begin doxorubicin within 30 minutes of beginning dexrazoxane.

ACTIONS

Dexrazoxane

Rapidly distributed, at least partly metabolized. Elimination half-life is 2.5 hours. Primarily excreted in urine. See Drug/Lab Interactions.

Totect

Diminishes tissue damage resulting from extravasation of anthracycline drugs. Exact mode of action unknown. May inhibit topoisomerase II reversibly.

Zinecard

A cardioprotective agent. A potent intracellular chelating agent that readily penetrates cell membranes and interferes with iron-mediated free radical generation thought to be, in part, responsible for anthracycline-induced cardiomyopathy. Reduces the incidence of doxorubicin cardiomyopathy.

INDICATIONS AND USES

Totect

Treatment of extravasation resulting from IV anthracycline chemotherapy.

Zinecard

Reduce the incidence and severity of cardiomyopathy associated with cumulative doses of doxorubicin exceeding 300 mg/M^2. May allow higher doses of doxorubicin and improved response rates and duration. Currently approved only for use in women with metastatic breast cancer who would benefit from continuing doxorubicin therapy above this cumulative dose.

■ *Not recommended for use with the initiation of doxorubicin therapy.*

CONTRAINDICATIONS

Totect

None known.

Zinecard

Do not use with chemotherapy regimens that do not contain an anthracycline or in the initiation of doxorubicin therapy.

PRECAUTIONS

TOTECT AND ZINECARD

Follow guidelines for handling cytotoxic agents. See Appendix A, p. 1429. ▪ Usually administered by or under the direction of the physician specialist. ▪ Use with caution in patients with renal or hepatic impairment; see Dose Adjustments.

TOTECT

Cytotoxic when administered to patients receiving anthracycline-containing chemotherapy; additive myelosuppression (leukopenia, neutropenia, thrombocytopenia) may occur. ▪ Administer in a large vein in an extremity/area other than the one affected by extravasation. Cooling procedures such as ice packs, if used, should be removed from the area at least 15 minutes before administration to allow sufficient blood flow to the extravasated area.

ZINECARD

Evidence indicates that the use of dexrazoxane with the initiation of fluorouracil, doxorubicin, and cyclophosphamide (FAC) therapy interferes with the antitumor efficacy of the regimen. In one breast cancer trial, a lower response rate and a shorter time to progression were seen in patients who received dexrazoxane with their first cycle of FAC therapy. This use is not recommended; see Indications and Contraindications.

Monitor: TOTECT AND ZINECARD: Use of prophylactic antiemetics may be indicated.

TOTECT: Monitor CBC and differential and platelet count for increased bone marrow suppression. ▪ Obtain baseline and periodic renal and liver function tests as indicated.

ZINECARD: Obtain baseline ECG, serum levels of iron and zinc, and liver and renal function tests. Monitor at intervals. Baseline left ventricular ejection fraction (LVEF) helpful. ▪ Obtain baseline CBC and differential and platelet count. Monitor for increased bone marrow suppression. ▪ Reduces but does not eliminate the risk of doxorubicin-induced cardiotoxicity. Monitor for signs of congestive heart failure (e.g., basilar rales, S_3 gallop, paroxysmal nocturnal dyspnea, significant dyspnea on exertion, cardiomegaly by x-ray, or progressive decline from baseline of LVEF). A decline in QRS voltage on a 6-lead ECG of more than 30% may indicate cardiomyopathy.

Patient Education: Nonhormonal birth control recommended. ▪ Report pain at injection site promptly.

Maternal/Child: TOTECT: Category D: avoid pregnancy. Can cause fetal harm. ZINECARD: Category C: safety for use in pregnancy not established. TOTECT AND ZINECARD: Embryotoxic and teratogenic in rats at doses lower than required for humans. May cause testicular atrophy. ▪ Discontinue breast-feeding. ▪ Safety for use in pediatric patients not established.

Elderly: Response similar to that seen in younger patients. ▪ Monitor renal function; see Dose Adjustments.

DRUG/LAB INTERACTIONS
TOTECT AND ZINECARD
May have additive bone marrow suppressant effects with **other bone marrow suppressants** (e.g., fluorouracil [5-FU], cyclophosphamide [Cytoxan]).

■ Does not affect pharmacokinetics of **doxorubicin.**

TOTECT
Dimethylsulfoxide (DMSO) should not be used in patients who are receiving dexrazoxane for treatment of anthracycline-induced extravasation.

ZINECARD
Not indicated for use in initiation of doxorubicin therapy; may interfere with antitumor effects of combination regimens.

SIDE EFFECTS
Administered to patients receiving chemotherapeutic agents; side effect profile reflects a combination of dexrazoxane, underlying disease, and chemotherapy. Most common side effects are fever, injection site pain, nausea, and vomiting. Increased myelosuppression (e.g., granulocytopenia, leukopenia, and thrombocytopenia); may be dose limiting. Coagulation abnormalities, decreased serum zinc, increased serum iron, increased AST and ALT, and increased serum triglycerides do occur. Alopecia, anorexia, diarrhea, and stomatitis, as well as other side effects, may occur.

ANTIDOTE
Keep physician informed of side effects; most will be treated symptomatically. Recovery from myelosuppression similar with or without dexrazoxane. A reduced dose may be indicated if coagulation abnormalities develop. Hemodialysis or peritoneal dialysis may be useful in overdose.

DEXTRAN HIGH MOLECULAR WEIGHT

Plasma volume expander

(**DEX**-tran hi mo-**LEK**-u-ler)

Dextran 70, Dextran 75, Gentran 75

pH 3 to 7

USUAL DOSE

Variable, depending on amount of fluid loss and resultant hemoconcentration. Initially 30 Gm (500 mL). Total dose should not exceed 1.2 Gm/kg (20 mL/kg) of body weight in the first 24 hours for adult and pediatric patients. May give 0.6 Gm/kg (10 mL/kg) every 24 hours thereafter if indicated. *Use of Dextran 1 is indicated for prophylaxis of serious anaphylactic reactions.*

DILUTION

Available as a 6% solution in 500-mL bottles properly diluted in NS or D5W and ready for use. Dextran 70 (Cutter) is available in a 250-mL bottle. Use only clear solution. Crystallization of dextran can occur at low temperatures. Submerge in warm water and dissolve all crystals before administration.

Storage: Store at constant temperature not above 25° C (76° F). Discard partially used solution; no preservative added.

COMPATIBILITY

One source suggests that drugs should not be added to a dextran solution.

RATE OF ADMINISTRATION

Variable, depending on indication, present blood volume, and patient response. Initial 500 mL may be given at 20 to 40 mL/min if hypovolemic. If additional high molecular weight dextran is required, reduce flow to lowest rate possible to maintain hemodynamic status desired. In normovolemic patients, rate should not exceed 4 mL/min.

ACTIONS

A glucose polymer that approximates colloidal properties of human albumin. Provides hemodynamically significant plasma volume expansion in excess of the amount infused for about 24 hours. Dilutes total serum proteins and hematocrit values. Smaller dextran molecules are eliminated in urine; larger molecules are degraded to glucose.

INDICATIONS AND USES

Adjunct in treatment of shock or impending shock caused by burns, hemorrhage, surgery, or trauma.

Unlabeled uses: Treatment of nephrosis, toxemia of late pregnancy, and prevention of postoperative deep vein thrombosis.

CONTRAINDICATIONS

Severe bleeding disorders; marked hemostatic defects (e.g., thrombocytopenia, hypofibrinogenemia), even if drug-induced (e.g., heparin, warfarin); known hypersensitivity to dextran; breast-feeding and pregnancy unless a lifesaving measure; severe congestive cardiac failure; renal failure.

PRECAUTIONS

For IV use only. ■ Used when whole blood or blood products are not available. Not a substitute for whole blood or plasma proteins. ■ Use extreme caution in heart disease, impaired hepatic or renal function, congestive heart failure, pulmonary edema, in patients with edema and sodium retention of pathologic abdominal conditions, and in patients receiving anticoagulants or corticosteroids.

Monitor: Monitor pulse, BP, central venous pressure, and urine output every 5 to 15 minutes for the first hour and hourly thereafter while indicated. ▪ Maintain hydration of patient with additional IV fluids; dextran promotes tissue dehydration. Avoid overhydration with dilution of electrolyte balance. ▪ Change IV tubing or flush well with normal saline before infusing blood. Dextran will promote coagulation of blood in the tubing (glucose content). ▪ May reduce coagulability of the circulating blood. Observe patient for increased bleeding; maintain hematocrit above 30%. ▪ Hemoglobin, hematocrit, electrolyte, and serum protein evaluations are necessary during therapy. ▪ 500 mL contains 77 mEq of sodium and chloride. ▪ See Drug/Lab Interactions.

Maternal/Child: Category C: safety for use in pregnancy and breast-feeding not established.

DRUG/LAB INTERACTIONS

Draw blood for **laboratory tests and type and cross-match** before giving dextran, or notify laboratory of its use. May alter type and cross-match, blood sugar, total protein, and total bilirubin evaluation. ▪ May produce elevated **urine specific gravity** (also symptom of dehydration) and increase **AST and ALT.** ▪ See Monitor for interaction with blood.

SIDE EFFECTS

Bleeding, dehydration, fever, hypotension, joint pain, nausea, overhydration, tightness of the chest, urticaria, vomiting, wheezing. Severe anaphylaxis and death have occurred. Excessive doses have caused wound hematoma, seroma, and bleeding; distant bleeding (hematuria, melena); and pulmonary edema.

ANTIDOTE

Notify physician of any side effect. Discontinue the drug immediately at the first sign of a hypersensitivity reaction, provided other means of sustaining the circulation are available. Use epinephrine (Adrenalin) and/or antihistamines (diphenhydramine [Benadryl]) as indicated. Factor VIII infusion may reverse excessive bleeding. Resuscitate as necessary.

DEXTRAN LOW MOLECULAR WEIGHT

Plasma volume expander

(**DEX**-tran lo mo-**LEK**-u-ler)

Dextran 40, Gentran 40,
L.M.D. 10%, Rheomacrodex

pH 3 to 7

USUAL DOSE

Adjunct in shock: Variable, depending on amount of fluid loss and resultant hemoconcentration. Do not exceed 2 Gm/kg (20 mL) of body weight total over first 24 hours and 1 Gm/kg (10 mL) total over each succeeding 24 hours. Discontinue infusion after 5 days of therapy. *Dextran 1 is indicated for prophylaxis of serious anaphylactic reactions.*

Prophylaxis of venous thrombosis and/or pulmonary embolism: 10 mg/kg of body weight on day of surgery. 500 mL daily for 2 to 3 days, then 500 mL every 2 to 3 days up to 2 weeks. Length of treatment based on risk of thromboembolic complication. *Note previous comment on use of dextran 1.*

As priming fluid: 10 to 20 mL/kg of body weight. Do not exceed this dose. May be used in conjunction with other priming fluids.

DILUTION

Available as a 10% solution in 500-mL bottles properly diluted in NS or D5W and ready for use. Use only clear solution. Crystallization of dextran can occur at low temperatures. Submerge in warm water and dissolve all crystals before administration.

Storage: Store at constant temperature not above 25° C (76° F). Discard partially used solution; no preservative added.

COMPATIBILITY

Consider any drug NOT listed as compatible to be INCOMPATIBLE until consulting a pharmacist; specific conditions may apply.

One source suggests that drugs should not be added to a dextran solution. Another source suggests the following **compatibilities:**

Y-site: Enalaprilat (Vasotec IV), famotidine (Pepcid IV), and nicardipine (Cardene IV).

RATE OF ADMINISTRATION

Initial 500 mL may be given rapidly. Remainder of any desired daily dose should be evenly distributed over 8 to 24 hours depending on use. Slow rate or discontinue dextran for rapid increase of central venous pressure.

ACTIONS

A low-molecular-weight, rapid, but short-acting plasma volume expander. A colloid hypertonic solution, it increases plasma volume by once or twice its own volume. Helps to restore normal circulatory dynamics, increasing arterial and pulse pressure, central venous pressure, and cardiac output. Improves microcirculatory flow and prevents sludging in venous channels. Mobilizes water from body tissues and increases urine output.

INDICATIONS AND USES

Adjunctive therapy in the treatment of shock caused by hemorrhage, burns, trauma, or surgery. ■ Prophylaxis during surgical procedures with a high incidence of venous thrombosis and pulmonary embolism. ■ Pump priming during extracorporeal circulation.

CONTRAINDICATIONS

Severe bleeding disorders, marked hemostatic defects (e.g., thrombocytopenia, hypofibrinogenemia) even if drug-induced (e.g., heparin, warfarin), known hypersensitivity to dextran, breast-feeding and pregnancy unless a lifesaving measure, severe congestive cardiac failure, renal failure.

PRECAUTIONS

For IV use only. ■ Use caution in heart disease, renal shutdown, congestive heart failure, pulmonary edema, patients with edema and sodium retention, and patients taking corticosteroids.

Monitor: Monitor pulse, BP, central venous pressure (if possible), and urine output every 5 to 15 minutes for the first hour and hourly thereafter while indicated. ■ Slow rate or discontinue dextran for rapid increase of central venous pressure (normal 7 to 14 mm H_2O pressure). ■ If anuric or oliguric after 500 mL of dextran, discontinue the dextran. Mannitol may help increase urine flow. ■ Maintain hydration of patient with additional IV fluids; dextran promotes tissue dehydration. Avoid overhydration and dilution of serum electrolytes. ■ Change IV tubing or flush well with normal saline before superimposing blood. Dextran will promote coagulation of blood in the tubing (glucose content). ■ May reduce coagulability of the circulating blood slightly. Observe for bleeding complications, particularly following surgery or if patient is being anticoagulated. Maintain hematocrit above 30%. ■ 500 mL contains 77 mEq of sodium and chloride. ■ See Drug/Lab Interactions.

Maternal/Child: Category C: safety for use in pregnancy and breast-feeding not established.

DRUG/LAB INTERACTIONS

Draw blood for **laboratory tests and type and cross-match** before giving dextran, or notify laboratory of its use. May alter type and cross-match, blood sugar, total protein, and total bilirubin evaluation. ■ May produce elevated **urine specific gravity** (also a symptom of dehydration) and increase **AST and ALT.** ■ See Monitor for interaction with blood.

SIDE EFFECTS

Bleeding, dehydration, fever, hypotension, joint pain, nausea, overhydration, tightness of chest, urticaria, vomiting, wheezing. Severe anaphylaxis and death can occur. Excessive doses have caused wound hematoma, wound seroma, wound bleeding, distant bleeding (hematuria, melena), and pulmonary edema.

ANTIDOTE

Notify the physician of any side effect. Discontinue the drug immediately at the first sign of a hypersensitivity reaction, provided other means of sustaining the circulation are available. Use epinephrine (Adrenalin) and/or antihistamines (diphenhydramine [Benadryl]) as indicated. Factor VIII infusion may reverse excessive bleeding. Resuscitate as necessary.

DEXTROSE
(**DEX**-trohs)

Glucose

**Nutritional
(carbohydrate)**

pH 3.5 to 6.5

USUAL DOSE

Depends on use and age, weight, and clinical condition of the patient. The average normal adult requires 2 to 3 L of fluid daily to replace water loss through perspiration and urine.

2½% (25 Gm/L) or 5% (50 Gm/L) dextrose: 50 to 1,000 mL. May be repeated as indicated. Consider total amount of fluid.

10% dextrose (100 Gm/L): 5 mL. May repeat as necessary or 500 to 1,000 mL once or twice every 24 hours as indicated.

20% dextrose (200 Gm/L): 500 mL once or twice every 24 hours as indicated.

50% dextrose (500 Gm/L): 20 mL (10 Gm) to 50 mL (25 Gm). May repeat if indicated in *insulin-induced hypoglycemia.*

10% (100 Gm/L), 20% (200 Gm/L), 30% (300 Gm/L), 38.5% (385 Gm/L), 40% (400 Gm/L), 50% (500 Gm/L), 60% (600 Gm/L), 70% (700 Gm/L): 500 to 1,500 mL/24 hr as an infusion after admixture with other solutions such as amino acids or fat emulsion. Used for nutritional support.

PEDIATRIC DOSE

Dose is dependent on use, weight, clinical condition, and laboratory results. See Rate of Administration, Precautions, Monitor, and Maternal/Child.

NEONATAL DOSE

Dose is dependent on use, weight, clinical condition, and laboratory results. See Rate of Administration, Precautions, Monitor, and Maternal/Child.

Acute symptomatic hypoglycemia: 250 to 500 mg/kg of body weight of 10% to 25% dextrose.

DOSE ADJUSTMENTS

Dosing should be cautious in the elderly. Lower-end initial doses may be indicated. Consider decrease in organ function, concomitant disease, or other drug therapy. See Rate of Administration and Precautions.

DILUTION

May be given undiluted in prepared solutions or further diluted to achieve desired final concentration. Check label for aluminum content; see Precautions. Dextrose solutions are excellent media for bacterial growth. Do not use unless the solution is entirely clear and the vial is sterile. Do not store after adding additives.

Storage: Store at 20° to 25° C (68° to 77° F). Protect from freezing.

COMPATIBILITY

Will cause pseudoagglutination of red blood cells if administered simultaneously with whole blood. Consult pharmacist or refer to individual drug monograph before admixing with other drugs or solutions. Mix thoroughly.

RATE OF ADMINISTRATION

2½% and 5% solution, rate dependent on amount.

10% solution, 5 mL over 10 to 15 seconds.

10% solution, 1,000 mL over at least 3 hours.

20% solution, 500 mL over 30 to 60 minutes.

50% solution, 3 mL over 1 minute.

500 mL of 30% to 70% solution over 4 to 12 hours, depending on body weight. A rate of 0.5 Gm/kg/hr will not cause glycosuria. At 0.8 Gm/kg/hr 95% is retained and will cause glycosuria. May cause hyperosmolar syndrome.

Excessive or rapid administration in very-low-birth-weight infants may cause hyperglycemia, hypoglycemia, or increased serum osmolality and possible intracerebral hemorrhage.

ACTIONS

A parenteral fluid and nutrient replenisher. A monosaccharide, it provides glucose calories for metabolic needs. Metabolized to CO_2 and water. Its oxidation provides water to sustain volume and may help lower excess ketone production. Restores blood glucose levels. May help minimize liver glycogen depletion and may exert a protein-sparing action. Hypertonic solutions (20% to 50%) act as diuretics and reduce CNS edema. Readily excreted by the kidneys, producing diuresis.

INDICATIONS AND USES

Provide calories and fluid by peripheral infusion when calories and fluid are required (2½%, 5%, 10%). ■ Provide calories by central IV infusion in conditions requiring a minimum volume of fluid (20%). ■ Provide calories by central IV infusion in combination with other amino acid solutions as total parenteral nutrition (10% to 70%). ■ Treatment of insulin-induced hypoglycemia (50%). ■ Treatment of acute symptomatic episodes of hypoglycemia in the neonate and infant (25%). ■ Shock (sustain blood volume). ■ Diuresis (20% to 50% solution). ■ Hyperkalemia (20% solution). ■ As a diluent for IV administration of medications (2½% to 10% solutions usually). A sclerosing solution (25% to 50% solution, 3 to 20 mL).

CONTRAINDICATIONS

Delirium tremens with dehydration; diabetic coma while blood sugar is excessive; hepatic coma intracranial or intraspinal hemorrhage; glucose-galactose malabsorption syndrome. Solutions containing dextrose may be contraindicated in patients with known allergies to corn or corn products.

PRECAUTIONS

Use caution in severe kidney damage. ■ 50% dextrose can be used as a sclerosing agent and will cause thrombosis. ■ Use caution in infants of diabetic mothers, in patients with carbohydrate intolerance or subclinical or overt diabetes, and in patients receiving corticosteroids. ■ Use dextrose with extreme caution in low-birth-weight or septic infants. May cause severe hyperglycemia, may increase serum osmolality, and may cause intracerebral hemorrhage. ■ To prevent hypokalemia, fasting patients with good renal function (especially patients undergoing digoxin therapy) should have adequate amounts of potassium added to hypertonic dextrose solutions. ■ Some solutions may contain aluminum. In impaired kidney function, aluminum may reach toxic levels. Premature neonates are particularly at risk because of their immature kidneys and requirement for calcium and phosphate, which also contain aluminum. Research indicates that patients with impaired renal function who receive greater than 4 to 5 mcg/kg/day of parenteral aluminum are at risk for developing CNS or bone toxicity associated with aluminum accumulation. ■ Concentrated dextrose solutions, if administered too rapidly, may result in significant hyperglycemia and possible hyperosmolar syndrome characterized by mental confusion and loss of consciousness. Fatty infiltration of the liver, acute respiratory failure, and difficulty in weaning hypermetabolic patients from the respirator may be caused by excessive carbohydrate calories.

Monitor: *Adult and pediatric patients:* Do not use as a diluent for blood or administer simultaneously through the same infusion set; dextrose in any dilution causes clumping of RBCs unless sodium chloride is added. ■ For concentrations over 12.5% (hypertonic) very large (central) veins and slow administration are absolutely necessary. ■ Confirm patency of vein; avoid extravasation. ■ Use with caution in patients with known subclinical or overt diabetes. Insulin requirements may be increased. Monitor blood glucose. ■ Monitor changes in fluid balance, electrolyte concentrations, and acid-base balance during prolonged therapy or as indicated by patient condition. ■ Potassium and vitamins are readily depleted. Watch for any signs of beginning deficiency and replace as needed. Add other electrolytes and minerals as required by fluid and electrolyte status. ■ Can cause fluid or solute overload. May result in dilution of serum electrolyte concentrations, overhydration, congested states, or pulmonary edema. ■ Rapid administration of hypertonic solutions will cause hyperglycemia (over 0.5 Gm/kg/hr) and may cause hyperosmolar syndrome. ■ Concentrated dextrose solutions must not be withdrawn abruptly. Will cause reactive hypoglycemia. Reduce rate of administration gradually and then follow with administration of 5% or 10% dextrose solution. ■ See Rate of Administration and Precautions.

Pediatric patients: Monitor serum glucose frequently, especially in infants, neonates, and low-birth-weight infants. ■ Small volumes of fluid may affect fluid and electrolyte balance in very small infants and neonates. Renal function may be immature and the ability to excrete fluid and solute loads limited. Monitor fluid intake, urine output, and serum electrolytes closely in infants, neonates, and low-birth-weight infants.

Maternal/Child: Category C: safety for use in pregnancy and breast-feeding not established. Benefits must outweigh risks. Use caution and monitor fluid balance, glucose and electrolyte concentrations, and acid-base balance of both mother and fetus as indicated by their conditions. ■ See Precautions.

Elderly: Lower-end initial doses may be indicated; see Dose Adjustments. Monitoring of renal function may be useful. Specific age-related differences in response have not been identified.

DRUG/LAB INTERACTIONS
See Monitor.

SIDE EFFECTS
Rare in small doses administered slowly: acidosis, alkalosis, febrile reactions, fluid overload (congested states, pulmonary edema, overhydration, dilution of serum electrolyte concentrations), hyperglycemia (during infusion), hyperosmolar syndrome (mental confusion, loss of consciousness), hypersensitivity reactions (e.g., anaphylaxis; coughing; difficulty breathing; periorbital, facial, and/or laryngeal edema; pruritus; sneezing; and uticaria), hypokalemia, hypovitaminosis, infection at injection site, reactive hypoglycemia (after infusion), venous thrombosis or phlebitis.

ANTIDOTE
Discontinue the drug and notify the physician of the side effect. Symptomatic treatment is probable.

DIAZEPAM
(dye-**AYZ**-eh-pam)

Benzodiazepine
Sedative-hypnotic
Antianxiety agent
Anticonvulsant
Amnestic
Skeletal muscle relaxant (adjunct)

Valium ■ ✤Diazemuls   pH 6.2 to 6.9 ■ pH 8

USUAL DOSE

Maximum dose except in status epilepticus is 30 mg in 8 hours. Note some changes in times of administration between conventional diazepam (Valium) and emulsified forms (e.g., Diazemuls). The emulsified form is no longer available in the United States.

PREOPERATIVE MEDICATION
Conventional diazepam (Valium): 5 to 10 mg before surgery.
Emulsified diazepam (Diazemuls): 10 mg 1 to 2 hours before surgery.

MODERATE ANXIETY DISORDERS AND SYMPTOMS OF ANXIETY
All formulations: 2 to 5 mg. Repeat in 3 to 4 hours if necessary.

SEVERE ANXIETY DISORDERS AND SYMPTOMS OF ANXIETY
All formulations: 5 to 10 mg. Repeat in 3 to 4 hours if necessary.

ACUTE ALCOHOL WITHDRAWAL
All formulations: 10 mg initially, then 5 to 10 mg in 3 to 4 hours if necessary.

STATUS EPILEPTICUS
All formulations: 5 to 10 mg. May be repeated at intervals of 10 to 15 minutes up to a total dose of 30 mg. May repeat in 2 to 4 hours. Another source suggests 0.2 to 0.5 mg/kg every 15 to 30 minutes for 2 or 3 doses. Some specialists start with 20 mg and titrate the total dose over 10 minutes or until seizures stop. Maximum dose in 24 hours is 100 mg.

CARDIOVERSION
Conventional diazepam (Valium): 5 to 15 mg 5 to 10 minutes before procedure begins.
Emulsified diazepam (Diazemuls): 5 to 15 mg 10 to 20 minutes before procedure begins.

ENDOSCOPY
Conventional diazepam (Valium): 10 mg or less is usually effective given immediately before procedure begins; titrate to desired sedation (e.g., slurred speech). Up to 20 mg may be indicated if a narcotic is not used.
Emulsified diazepam (Diazemuls): 5 to 10 mg 30 minutes before the procedure begins; titrate to desired sedation (e.g., slurred speech). Up to 20 mg may be indicated if a narcotic is not used.

MUSCLE SPASM
All formulations: 5 to 10 mg. Repeat in 3 to 4 hours if necessary. Larger doses may be required in tetanus.

PEDIATRIC DOSE

Safety for use in neonates not established but is used. Neonates have reduced or immature organ function; may be susceptible to prolonged CNS depression. Avoid small veins (e.g., dorsum of hand or wrist); see Monitor. Use in infants and children is most frequent in tetany, status epilepticus, or hypersensitivity reactions. Use of longer-acting anticonvulsants (e.g., phenobarbital, phenytoin) following diazepam may be indicated. Not recommended but is used for other general indications.

SEDATIVE/MUSCLE RELAXANT
All formulations: 0.04 to 0.2 mg/kg every 2 to 4 hours. Maximum dose 0.6 mg/kg in 8 hours.

TETANUS IN PEDIATRIC PATIENTS FROM 30 DAYS OF AGE TO 5 YEARS OF AGE
Respiratory assistance must be available.

All formulations: 1 to 2 mg every 3 to 4 hours.

Conventional diazepam (Valium): One source suggests a maximum single dose not to exceed 0.25 mg/kg; repeat in 15 to 30 minutes if necessary. A third dose may be given, but if it does not relieve symptoms, consider alternative therapy.

TETANUS IN PEDIATRIC PATIENTS 5 YEARS OF AGE OR OLDER
Respiratory assistance must be available.

All formulations: 5 to 10 mg every 3 to 4 hours.

Conventional diazepam (Valium): One source suggests a maximum single dose not to exceed 0.25 mg/kg; repeat in 15 to 30 minutes if necessary. A third dose may be given, but if it does not relieve symptoms, consider alternative therapy.

STATUS EPILEPTICUS IN NEONATES (UNLABELED)
All formulations: 0.3 to 0.75 mg/kg every 15 to 30 minutes for 2 to 3 doses. Maximum total dose is 5 mg.

STATUS EPILEPTICUS IN PEDIATRIC PATIENTS FROM 30 DAYS OF AGE TO 5 YEARS OF AGE
All formulations: 0.2 to 0.5 mg every 2 to 5 minutes to a maximum 5-mg dose. May repeat in 2 to 4 hours. Another source suggests 0.2 to 0.5 mg/kg every 15 to 30 minutes to a maximum 5-mg dose.

STATUS EPILEPTICUS IN PEDIATRIC PATIENTS 5 YEARS OF AGE OR OLDER
All formulations: 1 mg every 2 to 5 minutes to a maximum 10-mg dose. May repeat in 2 to 4 hours. Another source suggests 0.2 to 0.5 mg/kg every 15 to 30 minutes to a maximum 10-mg dose.

DOSE ADJUSTMENTS
Reduce dose by one half for the elderly or debilitated, in impaired liver or renal function, in patients with limited pulmonary reserve, and in the presence of other CNS depressants. Begin with a small dose and increase in gradual increments. ■ See Drug/Lab Interactions.

DILUTION
All formulations: Do not dilute or mix with any other drug. Should be given directly into the vein. Inject into IV tubing close to vein site only when direct IV injection is not feasible. Consider heparin lock for frequent injection. Change site every 2 to 3 days. Some precipitation or adsorption into plastic tubing may occur.

Conventional diazepam: *Not soluble in any solution.* If dilution is imperative, add dilution solution to diazepam, not diazepam to solution; consult pharmacist. Direct IV administration is preferred but can be administered at a Y-tube injection site.

Emulsified diazepam: May be diluted with their emulsion base [Intralipid or Nutralipid]). Mixture should be used within 6 hours. In any other solution, *emulsion may be destabilized and may not be visually apparent.* **Incompatible** with polyvinylchloride infusion sets. If a filter is used for emulsified forms, it must have a pore size of 5 microns or more so as not to break down the emulsion. Emulsified forms eliminate the use of nonphysiologic, potentially irritating solvents.

Filters: *Emulsified diazepam:* If a filter is used for emulsified forms, it must have a pore size of 5 microns or more to prevent breakdown of the emulsion.

Storage: *Conventional diazepam (Valium):* Store at CRT in cartons to protect from light. Do not freeze.

Emulsified diazepam (Diazemuls): Store below 25° C (77° F) unless manufacturer suggests refrigeration. Do not freeze. Protect from light. Note expiration date.

COMPATIBILITY   (Underline Indicates Conflicting Compatibility Information)
Consider any drug NOT listed as compatible to be INCOMPATIBLE until consulting a pharmacist; specific conditions may apply.

Manufacturers for all preparations recommend not mixing with any other drug or solution in syringe or solution. Precipitation can occur. Emulsified forms are **incompatible** with polyvinylchloride infusion sets. *Emulsion may be destabilized and may not be visually apparent.* See Dilution.

One source suggests the following **compatibilities:**

CONVENTIONAL DIAZEPAM
Additive: Verapamil.

Y-site: Cisatracurium (Nimbex), dobutamine, fentanyl (Sublimaze), hydromorphone (Dilaudid), methadone (Dolophine), morphine, nafcillin (Nallpen), quinidine gluconate, remifentanil (Ultiva), sufentanil (Sufenta).

EMULSIFIED DIAZEPAM
Additive: Intralipid, Nutralipid; see Dilution.

RATE OF ADMINISTRATION
If a filter is used for emulsified forms, it must have a pore size of 5 microns or more so as not to break down the emulsion.

Adults: 5 mg (1 mL) or fraction thereof over 1 minute.

Infants and other pediatric patients: Give total dose over a minimum of 3 minutes, but do not exceed a rate of 0.25 mg/kg over 3 minutes.

ACTIONS
A benzodiazepine that depresses the central, autonomic, and peripheral nervous systems in an undetermined manner. Exerts antianxiety, sedative/hypnotic, amnesic, anticonvulsant, skeletal muscle relaxant, and antitremor effects. Diminishes patient recall. Metabolized in the liver; stays in the body in appreciable amounts for several days and is excreted very slowly in the urine. Crosses the placental barrier. Secreted in breast milk.

INDICATIONS AND USES
Management of moderate to severe anxiety disorders or short-term relief of symptoms of anxiety. ▪ Acute alcohol withdrawal. ▪ Acute stress reactions. ▪ Muscle spasm. ▪ Status epilepticus and severe recurrent convulsive seizures, including tetany. ▪ Preoperative medication, including endoscopic procedures. ▪ Cardioversion.

Unlabeled uses: Conscious sedation in dental procedures, treatment of panic disorders.

CONTRAINDICATIONS
Known hypersensitivity, open-angle glaucoma unless receiving appropriate therapy, shock, coma, acute alcoholic intoxication with depression of vital signs. Emulsion in Dizac contains soybean oil; do not use in patients with known hypersensitivity to soy protein.

PRECAUTIONS
Check label carefully. Some preparations are for IV use only (e.g., Diazemuls); others can be given IM/IV (e.g., Valium). ▪ Drug of choice for

initial treatment of status epilepticus or seizures resulting from drug overdose or poisoning. Some specialists administer phenytoin simultaneously to facilitate long-term control (onset of action is not as immediate as diazepam). Oral phenytoin or phenobarbital may be used for maintenance. ▪ May not be effective if seizures are due to acute brain lesions. ▪ Not recommended for treatment of petit mal or petit mal variant seizures; may cause tonic state epilepticus. ▪ Use caution in the elderly, those who are very ill, and those with limited pulmonary reserve (e.g., chronic lung disease) or unstable cardiac status. ▪ Withdrawal symptoms will occur for several weeks after extended or large doses. ▪ Hypoalbuminemia may increase the incidence of side effects. ▪ Intended for short-term use only. ▪ Available PO and as a rectal gel.

Monitor: See Dilution. ▪ To reduce the incidence of thrombophlebitis, avoid smaller veins. Extravasation or arterial administration hazardous. ▪ Oxygen, respiratory assistance, and flumazenil (Romazicon) must always be available. ▪ Bed rest required for a minimum of 3 hours after IV injection.

Patient Education: May produce drowsiness or dizziness. Request assistance with ambulation and use caution performing tasks that require alertness. Do not drive or operate hazardous machinery until all effects have subsided. ▪ Avoid use of alcohol or other CNS depressants (e.g., antihistamines, barbiturates). ▪ May be habit-forming with long-term use or high-dose therapy. ▪ Has amnestic potential; may impair memory. ▪ Consider birth control options.

Maternal/Child: Category D: has caused birth deformities, especially in the first trimester. ▪ Not recommended during pregnancy, childbirth, or while breast-feeding.

Elderly: See Dose Adjustments. Start with a small dose and increase gradually based on response. ▪ More sensitive to therapeutic and adverse effects (e.g., ataxia, dizziness, oversedation). ▪ IV injection may be more likely to cause apnea, bradycardia, hypotension, and cardiac arrest. ▪ See Precautions and Drug/Lab Interactions.

DRUG/LAB INTERACTIONS

Concurrent use with other **CNS depressants** (e.g., alcohol, antihistamines, barbiturates, MAO inhibitors [e.g., selegiline (Eldepryl)], narcotics [e.g., morphine, meperidine (Demerol), fentanyl], phenothiazines [e.g., prochlorperazine (Compazine)], tricyclic antidepressants [e.g., imipramine (Tofranil-PM)]) may result in additive effects for up to 48 hours. Reduced doses of both drugs may be indicated. ▪ May increase serum concentrations of **digoxin and phenytoin** (Dilantin); monitor digoxin and phenytoin serum levels. ▪ **Ritonavir** (Norvir) may increase risk of prolonged sedation and respiratory depression. Concurrent use not recommended. Benzodiazepines metabolized by alternate routes may be safer (e.g., lorazepam [Ativan], oxazepam [Serax], temazepam [Restoril]). ▪ Concurrent use with **beta-blockers** (e.g., metoprolol [Lopressor], propranolol [Inderal]), **cimetidine** (Tagamet), **disulfiram** (Antabuse), **estrogen-containing oral contraceptives, fluoxetine** (Prozac), **isoniazid** (Nydrazid), **itraconazole** (Sporanox), **ketoconazole** (Nizoral), **omeprazole** (Prilosec), **probenecid, and valproic acid** (Depakene) may inhibit hepatic metabolism, resulting in increased plasma concentrations of benzodiazepines. ▪ Diazepam decreases clearance and increases toxicity of **zidovudine** (AZT, Retrovir). ▪ May increase clearance and decrease effectiveness of **levodopa**. ▪

Hypotensive effects of benzodiazepines may be increased by **any agent that induces hypotension** (e.g., antihypertensives, CNS depressants, diuretics, lidocaine, paclitaxel). ▪ Use with **rifampin** (Rifadin) increases clearance and reduces effects of diazepam. ▪ **Theophyllines** (e.g., Aminophylline) antagonize sedative effects of benzodiazepines. ▪ **Smoking** increases metabolism and clearance of diazepam, decreasing plasma levels and sedative effects. ▪ **Clozapine** (Leponex) has caused respiratory distress or cardiac arrest in a few patients; use concurrently with extreme caution. ▪ Decreased drowsiness may occur in cigarette **smokers**, especially if elderly. ▪ **Grapefruit juice** may affect certain enzymes of the P_{450} enzyme system and should be avoided.

SIDE EFFECTS

Apnea, ataxia, blurred vision, bradycardia, cardiac arrest, cardiovascular collapse, coma, confusion, coughing, depressed respiration, depression, diminished reflexes, drowsiness, dyspnea, headache, hiccups, hyperexcited states, hyperventilation, laryngospasm, neutropenia, nystagmus, somnolence, syncope, venous thrombosis and phlebitis at injection site, vertigo.

ANTIDOTE

Notify the physician of all side effects. Reduction of dosage may be required. Discontinue the drug for major side effects or paradoxical reactions, including hyperexcitability, hallucinations, and acute rage. Flumazenil (Romazicon) will reverse all sedative effects of benzodiazepines. A patent airway, artificial ventilation, oxygen therapy, and other symptomatic treatment must be instituted promptly. May cause emesis; observe closely. Treat hypersensitivity reaction, or resuscitate as necessary.

DIGOXIN IMMUNE FAB (OVINE)
(dih-**JOX**-in im-**MYOUN** fab)

Digibind, DigiFab

Antidote
(digoxin intoxication)

pH 6 to 8

USUAL DOSE

Testing for sensitivity to sheep serum and/or premedication may be indicated; see Contraindications and Monitor.

Acute toxicity in adults and pediatric patients: Determine dose by symptoms and clinical findings. Serum concentration may not reflect actual toxicity for 6 to 12 hours. Symptoms of life-threatening toxicity due to digoxin overdose include severe arrhythmias (e.g., VT, VF), progressive bradycardia, second- or third-degree heart block not responsive to atropine, and/or serum potassium levels exceeding 5 to 5.5 mEq/L in adults and 6 mEq/L in pediatric patients.

Dose in numbers of vials based on ingested dose is calculated by dividing the body load of digoxin in milligrams by 0.5. Each vial of *Digibind* contains 38 mg/vial and will bind 0.5 mg digoxin. Each vial of *DigiFab* contains 40 mg/vial and will bind 0.5 mg of digoxin. Dose may also be based on serum digoxin levels (see package insert; has charts for adults and pediatric patients).

An initial dose of up to 20 vials has been used. 20 vials will bind approximately 50 (0.25 mg) tablets of Lanoxin and should provide adequate treatment of most life-threatening ingestions in adult and pediatric patients. If ingested substance is unknown, if serum digoxin level is not available, or if there is concern about sensitivity to the serum, consider giving 10 vials. Observe clinical response and repeat if indicated. In clinical trials of Digibind the average dose was 10 vials. A single dose may be repeated in several hours if toxicity has not reversed or appears to recur. Febrile reactions are dose related.

Toxicity in chronic therapy: *Adults:* 6 vials should be adequate to reverse most cases of toxicity in adults in acute distress or if a serum digoxin concentration is not available.

Pediatric patients: less than 20 kg: 1 vial should be adequate if signs of toxicity are present.

DILUTION

Each vial must be diluted with 4 mL of SW for injection (results in 9.5 mg/mL for Digibind and 10 mg/mL for DigiFab). Mix gently. May be given in this initial dilution or may be further diluted with any desired amount of NS (with *Digibind,* 34 mL NS/vial yields 1 mg/mL; with *DigiFab,* 36 mL NS/vial yields 1 mg/mL). Consider volume overload in pediatric patients when further diluting in NS. Administer to infants after initial dilution using a tuberculin syringe to deliver an accurate dose with less volume; for extremely small doses, dilute to 1 mg/mL before administration.

Filters: *Digibind:* Must be given through a 0.22-micron membrane filter.

Storage: Refrigerate unreconstituted vials. Use reconstituted solution promptly or store in refrigerator for up to 4 hours.

COMPATIBILITY

Specific information not available. Consider specific use; consult pharmacist.

RATE OF ADMINISTRATION

Decrease the rate of infusion or discontinue temporarily if an infusion reaction occurs. Do not give as an IV bolus injection unless cardiac arrest is imminent. Be prepared to treat anaphylaxis.

Digibind: Must be given through a 0.22-micron membrane filter. A single dose as an IV infusion equally distributed over 15 to 30 minutes.

DigiFab: A single dose as an infusion over 30 minutes.

ACTIONS

Antigen-binding fragments (Fab) prepared from specific antidigoxin antibodies produced in sheep are isolated and purified. Fab fragments bind molecules of digoxin and make them unavailable for binding at their site of action. Freely distributed in extracellular space. Reduces the level of free digoxin in the serum. Onset of action is prompt, with improvement in symptoms of toxicity within 30 minutes. Fab-digoxin complexes are cleared by the kidney. DigiFab is also cleared in the reticuloendothelial system.

INDICATIONS AND USES

Digibind: Treatment of patients with life-threatening digoxin intoxication or overdose (digoxin).

DigiFab: Treatment of patients with life-threatening or potentially life-threatening digoxin toxicity or overdose. Not indicated for milder cases of digoxin toxicity.

All formulations: Indicated for known suicidal or accidental consumption of fatal doses of digoxin, including ingestion of 10 mg or more of digoxin in previously healthy adults, 4 mg (or more than 0.1 mg/kg) in previously healthy pediatric patients, or ingestion causing steady-state serum concentrations greater than 10 ng/mL. ▪ Indicated for chronic ingestions causing steady-state serum digoxin concentrations exceeding 6 ng/mL in adults or 4 ng/mL in pediatric patients. ▪ Indicated for manifestations of life-threatening toxicity due to digoxin overdose, including severe ventricular arrhythmias (such as VT or VF), progressive bradycardia, or third-degree heart block not responsive to atropine. ▪ Also indicated when potassium concentrations are above 5 to 5.5 mEq/L in adults or 6 mEq/L in pediatric patients with rapidly progressive S/S of digoxin toxicity. ▪ See Precautions and Maternal/Child.

CONTRAINDICATIONS

None known when used for specific indications. If hypersensitivity exists and treatment is necessary, premedicate with corticosteroids and diphenhydramine and prepare to treat anaphylaxis.

PRECAUTIONS

Administered under the direction of the physician specialist with facilities for monitoring the patient and responding to any medical emergency. Cardiac arrest can result from ingestion of more than 10 mg digoxin by healthy adults, 4 mg digoxin by healthy pediatric patients, or serum digoxin levels above 10 ng/mL. ▪ Larger doses of digoxin immune Fab act more quickly but increase the possibility of febrile or hypersensitivity reactions. ▪ Use caution in impaired cardiac function. Inability to use cardiac glycosides may endanger patient. Support with dopamine or vasodilators. ▪ The clinical problem may not be caused by digoxin toxicity if the patient fails to respond to digoxin immune Fab. ▪ Consider that multiple drugs may have been used and are producing toxicity in suicide attempts. ▪ See Monitor and Drug/Lab Interactions.

Monitor: Although allergy testing is not required before treating life-threatening digoxin toxicity, patients allergic to ovine proteins or those who have previously received antibodies or Fab fragments produced from sheep are at risk. Determine patient response to any previous injections of serum of any type and history of any allergic-type reactions. In addition, **DigiFab** considers that patients with allergies to papain, chymopapain, other papaya extracts, or the pineapple enzyme bromelain may be at risk. **Digibind** provides the information below on sensitivity testing; that information is not included in the package insert for **DigiFab**. ▪ Test for sensitivity if indicated. Make a 1 : 100 solution by diluting 0.1 mL of reconstituted solution (10 mg/mL) with 9.9 mL sterile NS (100 mcg/mL).

Scratch test: Make a ¼-inch skin scratch through a drop of 1 : 100 dilution in NS. Inspect the site in 20 minutes. An urticarial wheal surrounded by a zone of erythema is a positive reaction.

Skin test: Inject 0.1 mL (10 mcg) of 1 : 100 dilution intradermally. Inspect the site in 20 minutes. A urticarial wheal surrounded by a zone of erythema is a positive reaction. Concomitant use of antihistamines may interfere with sensitivity tests. If skin testing causes a systemic reaction, place a tourniquet above the testing site and treat anaphylaxis.

▪ Standard treatment of digoxin intoxication includes withdrawal of the intoxicating agent, correction of electrolyte disturbances (especially hyperkalemia), acid-base imbalances, hypoxia, and treatment of cardiac arrhythmias. ■ Monitor VS, ECG, and potassium concentration frequently during and after drug administration. ■ Monitor for S/S of an acute hypersensitivity reaction (e.g., angioedema, bronchospasm with wheezing or cough, erythema, hypotension, laryngeal edema, pruritus, stridor, tachycardia, urticaria). ■ Obtain serum digoxin concentrations if possible. High margin of error will occur if drawn soon after ingestion. 6 to 8 hours are required after the last digoxin dose to obtain an accurate serum concentration. ■ Potassium may be shifted from inside to outside the cell, causing increased renal excretion. May appear to have hyperkalemia while there is a total body deficit of potassium. When the digoxin effect is reversed, hypokalemia may develop rapidly. ■ Do not redigitalize until all Fab fragments have been eliminated from the body. May take several days. May take longer in severe renal impairment, and reintoxication may occur by release of newly unbound digoxin into the blood. ■ See Precautions and Drug/Lab Interactions.

Maternal/Child: Category C: use only when clearly indicated and benefits outweigh risks in pregnancy, breast-feeding, and infants. ■ *Digibind* indicates that it should be used in infants and children if more than 0.3 mg of digoxin is ingested, if serum digoxin levels equal to or greater than 6.4 nmol/L, or if there is underlying heart disease.

Patient Education: Contact the physician immediately if S/S of a delayed hypersensitivity reaction or serum sickness occur (e.g., rash, pruritus, urticaria).

Elderly: Consider age-related impaired renal function; monitor closely for recurrent toxicity; see Monitor.

DRUG/LAB INTERACTIONS

Will cause a precipitous rise in **total serum digoxin,** but most will be bound to the Fab fragment. Will interfere with digoxin immunoassay measurements until Fab fragment is completely eliminated. ■ **Catecholamines** (e.g., epinephrine) may aggravate digoxin arrhythmias. ■ See skin test in Monitor.

SIDE EFFECTS

Acute anaphylaxis with urticaria, respiratory distress, and vascular collapse are possible. Exacerbation of congestive heart failure and low cardiac output states and increased ventricular response in atrial fibrillation may occur due to withdrawal of digoxin effects. Hypokalemia may be life threatening.

ANTIDOTE

Notify the physician of all side effects. Discontinue the drug and treat anaphylaxis immediately. Corticosteroids, epinephrine (Adrenalin [see Drug/Lab Interactions]), diphenhydramine (Benadryl), oxygen, IV fluids, vasopressors (dopamine), and ventilation equipment must always be available. Resuscitate as necessary. Treat hypokalemia cautiously when necessary. Support exacerbated cardiac conditions as necessary.

DIGOXIN INJECTION
(dih-**JOX**-in in-**JEK**-shun)

Cardiac glycoside
Antiarrhythmic
Inotropic agent

Digoxin Pediatric, Lanoxin, Lanoxin Pediatric

pH 6.8 to 7.2

USUAL DOSE

Calculate dose based on lean body weight (LBW), CrCl, age, as well as concomitant disease states, concurrent medications, and other factors that may alter the effects of digoxin. In general, the dose of digoxin used should be determined on clinical grounds. An example of a usual dose is 0.25 to 0.5 mg (1 to 2 mL) as the **initial dose,** followed by 0.25 to 0.5 mg (1 to 2 mL) at 4- to 6-hour intervals until digitalized (approximately 4 to 6 hours). Assess clinical response (e.g., serum digoxin levels) before each additional dose. 0.5 to 1 mg (2 to 4 mL) is usually required for digitalization; see Monitor.

Slow ventricular response in atrial fibrillation/atrial flutter or alternative drug for re-entry SVT (AHA states, "May be of limited use"): AHA guidelines recommend a loading dose of 4 to 6 mcg/kg over 5 minutes. Second and third boluses of 2 to 3 mcg/kg to follow at 4- to 8-hour intervals (total loading dose of 8 to 12 mcg/kg is divided over 8 to 16 hours). Monitor HR and ECG. Check digoxin levels no sooner than 4 hours after an IV dose.

PEDIATRIC DOSE

Use 0.1 mg/mL pediatric injection (100 mcg/mL).

Digitalizing dose: Give one half of total daily dose initially, then two doses of one fourth total daily dose at 8-hour intervals. Assess clinical response before each additional dose. If using a tuberculin syringe to measure a pediatric dose, do not flush syringe with parenteral solution after contents are injected, may result in an overdose.

Usual Digitalizing and Maintenance Dosages of Digoxin in Pediatric Patients		
Age	Digitalizing Dose (mcg/kg)*	Daily IV Maintenance Dose (mcg/kg)†
Premature	15-25 mcg/kg	20%-30% of IV loading dose‡ divided and given every 12 hours
Full-term	20-30 mcg/kg	
1-24 months	30-50 mcg/kg	
2-5 years	25-35 mcg/kg	25%-35% of IV loading dose‡
5-10 years	15-30 mcg/kg	
Over 10 years	8-12 mcg/kg	

*IV digitalizing doses are 80% of oral digitalizing doses; see Pediatric Dose for correct division of digitalizing dose.
†Divided daily dosing is recommended for pediatric patients under 10 years of age.
‡Projected or actual digitalizing dose providing clinical response.

DOSE ADJUSTMENTS

Reduce dose in partially digitalized patients, in patients with impaired renal function, and in the elderly. ■ Dose reduction may be required before cardioversion. ■ See Drug/Lab Interactions; adjustments may be required with numerous drugs. ■ Reduced doses may be indicated in advanced heart failure, myocardial infarction, severe carditis, or severe pulmonary disease. ■ See Precautions.

DILUTION

May be given undiluted or each 1 mL may be diluted in 4 mL SW, NS, D5W, or LR for injection. Less diluent will cause precipitation. Use diluted solution immediately. Give through Y-tube or three-way stopcock of IV infusion set. See Pediatric Dose.

Storage: Store unopened vials at CRT protected from light.

COMPATIBILITY   (Underline Indicates Conflicting Compatibility Information)

Consider any drug NOT listed as compatible to be INCOMPATIBLE until consulting a pharmacist; specific conditions may apply.

Manufacturer recommends not mixing with other drugs in the same container and not administering simultaneously via the same IV line.

One source suggests the following **compatibilities** *(not recommended by manufacturer):*

Additive: Furosemide (Lasix), lidocaine, ranitidine (Zantac), verapamil.

Y-site: <u>Anidulafungin (Eraxis)</u>, bivalirudin (Angiomax), ciprofloxacin (Cipro IV), cisatracurium (Nimbex), dexmedetomidine (Precedex), diltiazem (Cardizem), doripenem (Doribax), famotidine (Pepcid IV), fenoldopam (Corlopam), hetastarch in electrolytes (Hextend), inamrinone (Amrinone), <u>insulin (regular)</u>, linezolid (Zyvox), meperidine (Demerol), meropenem (Merrem IV), midazolam (Versed), milrinone (Primacor), morphine, nesiritide (Natrecor), potassium chloride (KCl), remifentanil (Ultiva), tacrolimus (Prograf).

RATE OF ADMINISTRATION

Each single dose over a minimum of 5 minutes.

ACTIONS

A crystalline cardiac glycoside obtained from *Digitalis lanata;* this is a fast-acting hydrolytic product of lanatoside C. Onset of action is within 5 to 30 minutes and lasts 2 to 3 days. It has positive inotropic action, increasing the strength of myocardial contraction. It also alters the electric behavior of heart muscle through actions on myocardial automaticity, conduction velocity, and refraction. Results are a slower, stronger beat with increased cardiac output. Venous pressure falls, coronary circulation is increased, and heart size may become more normal. Widely distributed throughout the body and rapidly excreted in the urine. Secreted in breast milk.

INDICATIONS AND USES

Treatment of mild to moderate heart failure. ■ Control of ventricular response rates in patients with chronic atrial fibrillation; see Precautions.

CONTRAINDICATIONS

Ventricular fibrillation and known hypersensitivity to digoxin or other digitalis preparations.

PRECAUTIONS

IV administration is the preferred parenteral route. Used only when oral therapy is not feasible or rapid therapeutic effect is necessary. ■ Diltiazem (Cardizem) or verapamil generally preferred to treat atrial fibrillation; adenosine (Adenocard, Adenoscan) preferred to treat PSVT. ■ Commonly prolongs the PR interval; may cause severe sinus bradycardia or sinoatrial block in patients with pre-existing sinus node disease and may cause

advanced or complete heart block in patients with pre-existing incomplete AV block. Consider insertion of a pacemaker before treatment with digoxin in these patients. ▪ Use in patients with an accessory AV pathway (Wolff-Parkinson-White syndrome) is not recommended unless the conduction down the accessory pathway has been blocked either pharmacologically or by surgery. Cardioversion is usually used to treat PSVT in these patients. ▪ Avoid use in patients with heart failure associated with preserved left ventricular systolic function (e.g., acute cor pulmonale, amyloid heart disease, constrictive pericarditis, idiopathic hypertrophic subaortic stenosis, restrictive cardiomyopathy). Has been used in select patients with these diagnoses to treat chronic atrial fibrillation. ▪ Avoid use in patients with myocarditis; may precipitate vasoconstriction. ▪ Use caution in patients with electrolyte disorders because potassium or magnesium depletion sensitizes the myocardium to digoxin; toxicity may occur with serum digoxin concentrations below 2 ng/mL. ▪ Patients with beriberi heart disease may fail to respond adequately to digoxin if the underlying thiamine deficiency is not treated concomitantly. ▪ Some clinicians suggest stopping digoxin 12 hours before surgery to reduce risk of perioperative arrhythmias in digitalized patients. The exception is patients with supraventricular tachyarrhythmias; they should receive a dose the morning of surgery. ▪ Use with caution in patients with hypercalcemia or liver or kidney disease; see Dose Adjustments. ▪ Hypocalcemia may nullify effect of digoxin. If calcium levels need to be restored to normal, give calcium slowly and in small amounts. Death has occurred in digitalized patients receiving calcium. ▪ Hypothyroidism may reduce requirements for digoxin. Addressing the underlying condition is suggested in patients with heart failure and/or atrial arrhythmias resulting from hypermetabolic or hyperdynamic states (e.g., hyperthyroidism, hypoxia, or arteriovenous shunt). ▪ Use caution in patients with myocardial infarction. May cause an increase in myocardial oxygen demand and ischemia. ▪ Some clinicians suggest reducing the dose of digoxin for 1 to 2 days before an elective cardioversion. If countershock is necessary (last-resort treatment of life-threatening arrhythmias), begin with low voltage levels and increase gradually to avoid ventricular arrhythmias. ▪ See Drug/Lab Interactions.
Monitor: Hypomagnesemia, hypokalemia, and hypercalcemia may predispose patient to digoxin toxicity. Monitor electrolytes frequently during therapy. Avoid rapid changes. Supplements indicated to maintain normal serum electrolyte levels. ▪ Monitor HR and BP. ▪ Baseline and periodic ECG monitoring suggested. May prolong the PR interval and cause depression of the ST segment on ECG. ▪ ECG monitoring recommended in pediatric patients to avoid intoxication. ▪ Monitor digoxin levels. Draw at least 6 to 8 hours after last dose, preferably just before next dose. Therapeutic effects usually achieved with serum levels in a range from 0.8 to 1.5 ng/mL. Toxic threshold is equal to or greater than 2 ng/mL. ▪ Monitor renal function. ▪ See Precautions and Drug/Lab Interactions.
Maternal/Child: Category C: use only if clearly needed. ▪ Has been used to treat fetal tachycardia. ▪ Use caution during breast-feeding.
Elderly: Monitor carefully. Reduced dose may be indicated. Consider reduced body mass and reduced kidney function.
DRUG/LAB INTERACTIONS
Monitor serum levels carefully and adjust doses as indicated. ▪ **Potassium-depleting diuretics** (e.g., furosemide [Lasix], chlorothiazide [Diuril]) are a

major contributing factor to digitalis toxicity. ■ **Calcium** may produce serious arrhythmias in digitalized patients, particularly with too-rapid IV administration. ■ **Alprazolam** (Xanax), **amiodarone** (Nexterone), **indomethacin** (Indocin), **itraconazole** (Sporanox), **propafenone** (Rythmol), **quinidine,** and **spironolactone** (Aldactone) may raise serum digoxin concentration due to a reduction in clearance and/or in volume of distribution of digoxin. AHA states, "Reduce digoxin dose by 50% when used with **amiodarone** (Nexterone)." ■ Synergistic with **beta-blockers** (e.g., atenolol [Tenormin], metoprolol [Lopressor]) and **calcium channel blockers** (e.g., verapamil, diltiazem [Cardizem]). Additive effects on AV node conduction may result in advanced or complete heart block. ■ Both **digitalis glycosides and beta-blockers** slow AV conduction and decrease heart rate; concomitant use may increase risk of bradycardia. ■ Concurrent administration with **carvedilol** (Coreg) increases digoxin concentrations. Monitor digoxin with changes in carvedilol dosing. ■ **Succinylcholine** may cause a sudden extrusion of potassium from muscle cells; may cause arrhythmias in digitalized patients. ■ Increased risk of arrhythmias with **sympathomimetic amines** (e.g., epinephrine). ■ Initiation of **thyroid treatment** may require an increase in digoxin dose. ■ Serum levels and therapeutic effects may be reduced by **rifampin** (Rifadin). Impact may be increased in impaired renal function because nonrenal clearance of digoxin is increased. ■ See Precautions and Monitor.

SIDE EFFECTS

Seldom last more than 3 days after drug is discontinued. Any form of digoxin may cause partial or AV block and almost any arrhythmia, including paroxysmal tachycardia, atrial tachycardia, fibrillation, or standstill. *First ECG signs of toxicity* are ST segment sagging, PR prolongation, and possible bigeminal rhythm. *Clinical signs of toxicity* are mostly anorexia, blurred vision, confusion, diarrhea, disturbed color (yellow) vision, dizziness, headache, mental disturbances (e.g., anxiety, delirium, depression, hallucination), nausea, photopsia (points of light in peripheral vision), rash, vomiting, and weakness. Toxicity can cause death.

ANTIDOTE

Discontinue the drug at the first sign of toxicity and notify the physician. Dosage may be decreased or discontinued. For severe toxicity, digoxin immune Fab is a specific antidote. Consider causes of toxicity (electrolyte disturbances, thyroid, concurrent medications) and treat as indicated. Serum potassium must be obtained before administering potassium salts. See Precautions. Peritoneal dialysis or hemodialysis not effective in overdose.

DIHYDROERGOTAMINE MESYLATE **BBW** Ergot alkaloid
(dye-hy-droh-er-**GOT**-ah-meen **MES**-ih-layt)   Migraine agent

D.H.E. 45   pH 3.2 to 4

USUAL DOSE

Abort or prevent headaches: 1 mg (1 mL). May be repeated in 1 hour. No more than 2 doses (2 mg total) may be given IV in 24 hours. Do not exceed 6 mg in 1 week; see Precautions. Administration of an antiemetic (e.g., metoclopramide [Reglan] 10 mg) PO 1 hour before dihydroergotamine is recommended.

Chronic intractable headache: 0.5 mg (0.5 mL). Administer an antiemetic IV (e.g., metoclopramide) about 10 minutes before injection.

Prevention of orthostatic hypotension associated with spinal or epidural anesthesia (unlabeled): 0.5 mg (0.5 mL). Give a few minutes before anesthetic.

PEDIATRIC DOSE

See Maternal/Child. Administration of an antiemetic (e.g., metoclopramide, prochlorperazine), usually PO, 1 hour before dihydroergotamine is recommended.

Pediatric patients 6 to 9 years of age: 100 to 150 mcg (0.1 to 0.15 mg).

Pediatric patients 9 to 12 years of age: 200 mcg (0.2 mg).

Pediatric patients 12 to 16 years of age: 250 to 500 mcg (0.25 to 0.5 mg).

For all age ranges, repeat up to 2 doses at 20-minute intervals if necessary. Another source suggests 250 mcg (0.25 mg) at the start of the attack. Repeat in 1 hour if necessary.

DILUTION

May be given undiluted.

Storage: Protect ampules from light and heat.

COMPATIBILITY

Specific information not available. Consider specific use; consult pharmacist.

RATE OF ADMINISTRATION

1 mg or fraction thereof over 1 minute.

ACTIONS

An alpha-adrenergic blocking agent that causes constriction of both peripheral and cerebral blood vessels and produces depression of central vasomotor centers. Metabolized by the liver. Metabolites eliminated primarily in feces. Secreted in breast milk.

INDICATIONS AND USES

To abort or prevent vascular headaches (migraine, histamine cephalalgia). Used when rapid control is desired or other routes not feasible. ■ Treatment of chronic intractable headache.

Unlabeled uses: To prevent orthostatic hypotension associated with spinal or epidural anesthesia. Use SC to enhance heparin effects in preventing postoperative deep vein thrombosis after abdominal, thoracic, or pelvic surgeries or total hip replacement and IM or SC to treat orthostatic hypotension.

CONTRAINDICATIONS

Breast-feeding, coronary artery disease, hepatic or renal disease, hypersensitivity, uncontrolled hypertension, peripheral vascular disease, pregnancy or women who may become pregnant, sepsis. ■ Coadministration with potent CYP3A4 inhibitors, including protease inhibitors and macrolide antibiotics, is contraindicated; see Drug/Lab Interactions.

PRECAUTIONS

IM or SC use is preferred but may be given IV to obtain a more rapid effect. ■ Coadministration with potent CYP3A4 inhibitors, including protease inhibitors and macrolide antibiotics, increases the risk of vasospasm, leading to cerebral ischemia and/or ischemia of the extremities (peripheral). May be serious and/or life threatening; see Contraindications and Drug/Lab Interactions. ■ Use only when a clear diagnosis of migraine has been established. Do not exceed dosing guidelines or use for chronic daily administration; see Usual Dose.

Monitor: Monitor vital signs; observe closely. ■ See Drug/Lab Interactions.
Patient Education: Consider birth control options. ■ Take only as directed. ■ Report ineffectiveness or an increase in frequency or severity of headaches. ■ Report chest pain, increased HR, itching, muscle pain or weakness of arms or legs, numbness or tingling of extremities, or swelling.
Maternal/Child: Category X: avoid pregnancy. See Contraindications. ■ Safety for use in pediatric patients not established. Severe side effects (e.g., extrapyramidal reactions may occur). Pretreatment with an antiemetic may be helpful. Limit pediatric use to patients who have not responded to less toxic treatment.
Elderly: Increased risk of hypothermia and ischemic complications (e.g., cardiac, peripheral). ■ Consider age-related renal impairment.

DRUG/LAB INTERACTIONS

Contraindicated with potent CYP3A4 inhibitors, including **antifungals** (itraconazole [Sporanox], ketoconazole [Nizoral]), **protease inhibitors** (ritonavir [Norvir], nelfinavir [Viracept], and indinavir [Crixivan]), **and macrolide antibiotics** (clarithromycin [Biaxin], erythromycin, and troleandomycin [TAO]); see Contraindications and Precautions. ■ Administer less potent CYP3A4 inhibitors with caution as vasospasm may occur. **Less potent inhibitors** include, but are not limited to, saquinavir (Invirase), nefazodone, fluconazole (Diflucan), grapefruit juice, fluoxetine (Prozac), fluvoxamine (Luvox), zileuton (Zyflo), and clotrimazole (Gyne-Lotrimin, Mycelex). ■ Opposes vasodilating effects of **nitrates** (e.g., nitroglycerin), decreasing their effectiveness. ■ May cause hypertensive crisis in combination with other **vasopressors** (e.g., epinephrine). ■ May cause peripheral vasoconstriction with ischemia and/or cyanosis with **beta-adrenergic blockers** (e.g., propranolol [Inderal]) and **nicotine.**

SIDE EFFECTS

Rare in therapeutic doses, but may include angina pectoris, blindness, gangrene, muscle pains, muscle weakness, nausea, numbness and tingling of the fingers and toes, pleural and retroperitoneal fibrosis, thirst, uterine bleeding, and vomiting.

ANTIDOTE

Discontinue the drug and notify the physician of any side effects. Another drug will probably be chosen if further treatment is indicated. Vasodilators (nitroprusside sodium) and CNS stimulants (e.g., caffeine and sodium benzoate) are indicated as an antidote. Heparin and low-molecular-weight dextran may be used to reduce thrombosis due to excessive vasoconstriction. Hemodialysis may be indicated. Resuscitate as necessary.

DILTIAZEM HYDROCHLORIDE
(dill-**TYE**-a-zem hy-droh-**KLOR**-eyed)

Cardizem

Calcium channel blocker
Antiarrhythmic

pH 3.7 to 4.1

USUAL DOSE

0.25 mg/kg of body weight initially (20 mg for the average patient). Some patients may respond to an initial dose of 0.15 mg/kg. A second dose of 0.35 mg/kg may be given in 15 minutes if needed to achieve HR reduction (25 mg for the average patient). Any additional bolus doses used to achieve an appropriate response must be individualized to each patient. Patients with PSVT will probably respond to bolus doses and may not require an infusion, but to maintain reduction in HR in patients with atrial fibrillation or atrial flutter, immediately follow with an intravenous infusion at an initial rate of 10 mg/hr. May only be used for up to 24 hours. Some patients may maintain response with an initial rate of 5 mg/hr. Infusion may be increased by 5 mg/hr increments to a maximum dose of 15 mg/hr. Discontinue infusion within 24 hours. Oral antiarrhythmic agents (e.g., digoxin, quinidine, procainamide, calcium channel blockers [e.g., diltiazem, verapamil], beta blockers [e.g., atenolol, metoprolol, propranolol]) to maintain reduced HR are usually started within 3 hours of initial bolus of diltiazem.

DOSE ADJUSTMENTS

Specific mg/kg dose must be used for patients with low body weights. ■ Reduced dose may be indicated in impaired hepatic or renal function. ■ Dose selection should be cautious in the elderly. Reduced doses may be indicated based on potential for decreased organ function and concomitant disease or drug therapy. ■ See Drug/Lab Interactions.

DILUTION

Available as a solution in 25- or 50-mg vials (5 mg/mL), as a powder with supplied diluent (Lyo-ject syringe 25 mg [5 mg/mL]), and in a piggyback monovial containing 100 mg (with transfer needle set to facilitate preparation of an infusion). Dilute according to the following charts.

Cardizem Injectable or Cardizem Lyo-Ject Syringe				
Diluent Volume	Quantity of Cardizem (Diltiazem) Injection	Final Concentration	Administration	
			Dose	Infusion Rate
100 mL	125 mg (25 mL)	1 mg/mL	5 mg/hr 10 mg/hr 15 mg/hr	5 mL/hr 10 mL/hr 15 mL/hr
250 mL	250 mg (50 mL)	0.83 mg/mL	5 mg/hr 10 mg/hr 15 mg/hr	6 mL/hr 12 mL/hr 18 mL/hr
500 mL	250 mg (50 mL)	0.45 mg/mL	5 mg/hr 10 mg/hr 15 mg/hr	11 mL/hr 22 mL/hr 33 mL/hr

Continued

Cardizem Injectable or Cardizem Lyo-Ject Syringe—cont'd				
Diluent Volume	Quantity of Cardizem (Diltiazem) Injection	Final Concentration	Administration	
			Dose	Infusion Rate
100 mL	100 mg (1 monovial)	1 mg/mL	5 mg/hr 10 mg/hr 15 mg/hr	5 mL/hr 10 mL/hr 15 mL/hr
250 mL	200 mg (2 monovials)	0.8 mg/mL	5 mg/hr 10 mg/hr 15 mg/hr	6.25 mL/hr 12.5 mL/hr 18.8 mL/hr
500 mL	200 mg (2 monovials)	0.4 mg/mL	5 mg/hr 10 mg/hr 15 mg/hr	12.5 mL/hr 25 mL/hr 37.5 mL/hr

IV injection: May be given undiluted through Y-tube or three-way stopcock of tubing containing NS, D5W, or D5/½NS.

Infusion: May be further diluted for infusion in any of the above solutions.

Filters: No data available from manufacturer.

Storage: Vials may be stored at room temperature for up to 1 month, then discarded. Refrigeration before and after dilution preferred. Use within 24 hours of dilution. Discard unused medication and/or solution. Do not freeze.

COMPATIBILITY   (Underline Indicates Conflicting Compatibility Information)
Consider any drug NOT listed as compatible to be INCOMPATIBLE until consulting a pharmacist; specific conditions may apply.

Manufacturer recommends that **all formulations** not be mixed with any other drugs in the same container and, if possible, that they not be co-infused in the same IV line.

Cardizem Lyo-Ject Syringe is listed by the manufacturer as **incompatible** at the **Y-site** with acetazolamide (Diamox), acyclovir (Zovirax), aminophylline, ampicillin, ampicillin/sulbactam (Unasyn), diazepam (Valium), furosemide (Lasix), hydrocortisone sodium succinate (Solu-Cortef), methylprednisolone (Solu-Medrol), mezlocillin (Mezlin), nafcillin (Nallpen), phenytoin (Dilantin), rifampin (Rifadin), sodium bicarbonate. **Cardizem** is listed as **incompatible** with all of the above and insulin (regular).

Cardizem Monovial is listed by the manufacturer as **incompatible** at the **Y-site** with acetazolamide (Diamox), acyclovir (Zovirax), diazepam (Valium), furosemide (Lasix), phenytoin (Dilantin), rifampin (Rifadin).

Manufacturer lists **Cardizem Lyo-Ject Syringe** as **compatible** at the **Y-site** with insulin (regular) and lists the **Cardizem Monovial** (1 mg/mL) in NS as **compatible** at the **Y-site** with aminophylline, ampicillin, ampicillin/sulbactam (Unasyn), hydrocortisone sodium succinate (Solu-Cortef), insulin (regular), methylprednisolone (Solu-Medrol), mezlocillin (Mezlin), nafcillin (Nallpen), sodium bicarbonate.

One source lists the following **compatibilities** but does not differentiate formulations:

Y-site: <u>Acetazolamide (Diamox)</u>, <u>acyclovir (Zovirax)</u>, albumin, amikacin (Amikin), <u>aminophylline</u>, amphotericin B (generic), <u>ampicillin</u>, <u>ampicillin/sulbactam (Unasyn)</u>, argatroban, aztreonam (Azactam), bivalirudin (Angiomax), bumetanide, <u>caspofungin (Cancidas)</u>, cefazolin (Ancef), cefotaxime (Claforan), cefotetan, cefoxitin (Mefoxin), ceftazidime (Fortaz), ceftriaxone (Rocephin), cefuroxime (Zinacef), ciprofloxacin (Cipro IV), clindamycin (Cleocin), dexmedetomidine (Precedex), digoxin (Lanoxin), dobutamine, dopamine, doripenem (Doribax), doxycycline, epinephrine (Adrenalin), erythromycin (Erythrocin), esmolol (Brevibloc), fenoldopam (Corlopam), fentanyl (Sublimaze), fluconazole (Diflucan), gentamicin, heparin, hetastarch in electrolytes (Hextend), hetastarch in NS (Hespan), hydrocortisone sodium succinate (Solu-Cortef), hydromorphone (Dilaudid), imipenem-cilastatin (Primaxin), insulin (regular), labetalol (Trandate), lidocaine, lorazepam (Ativan), meperidine (Demerol), methylprednisolone (Solu-Medrol), metoclopramide (Reglan), metronidazole (Flagyl IV), midazolam (Versed), milrinone (Primacor), morphine, multivitamins (M.V.I.), nafcillin (Nallpen), nesiritide (Natrecor), nicardipine (Cardene IV), nitroglycerin IV, nitroprusside sodium, norepinephrine (Levophed), oxacillin (Bactocill), penicillin G potassium, pentamidine, piperacillin, potassium chloride (KCl), potassium phosphates, procainamide (Pronestyl), ranitidine (Zantac), sodium bicarbonate, sulfamethoxazole/trimethoprim, theophylline, ticarcillin/clavulanate (Timentin), tobramycin, vancomycin, vasopressin, vecuronium.

RATE OF ADMINISTRATION
IV injection: Each single dose equally distributed over 2 minutes.
Infusion: 5 mg to 15 mg/hr based on patient response. See charts under Dilution for diluent, dose, and infusion rate information. Use of a metriset (60 gtt/min) required; volumetric infusion pump preferred.

ACTIONS
Directly inhibits the influx of calcium ions through slow channels during membrane depolarization of cardiac and vascular smooth muscle. Effective in supraventricular tachycardias because it slows conduction through the AV node, prolongs the effective refractory period, reduces ventricular rates, and helps to prevent embolic complications. Also slows conduction through the SA node. Prevents reentry phenomena through the AV node. Reduces HR (10% with a single dose, 20% at peak effectiveness), systolic and diastolic BP, systemic vascular resistance, pulmonary artery systolic and diastolic BPs, and coronary vascular resistance with no significant effect on contractility, left ventricular end diastolic pressure, right atrial pressure, or pulmonary capillary wedge pressure. Increases cardiac output and stroke volume. Has little or no effect on normal AV nodal conduction at normal HRs. Produces less myocardial depression than verapamil. Effective within 3 minutes; maximum effect should occur within 2 to 7 minutes and last for 1 to 3 hours. 70% to 80% bound to plasma proteins. Metabolized in the liver. Half-life is approximately 3.4 hours following a bolus injection and increases to 4.1 to 4.9 hours with continuous infusion. Excreted in urine and bile. Secreted in breast milk.

INDICATIONS AND USES
Temporary control of rapid ventricular rate in atrial fibrillation or atrial flutter unless associated with an accessory bypass tract (e.g., Wolff-Parkinson-White syndrome or short PR syndrome). ■ Rapid conversion of paroxysmal supraventricular tachycardia (PSVT) to normal sinus rhythm including AV nodal reentrant tachycardias and reciprocating tachycardias associated with an extranodal accessory pathway (e.g., Wolff-Parkinson-White syndrome or short PR syndrome).

CONTRAINDICATIONS
Atrial fibrillation or flutter when associated with an accessory bypass tract (e.g., Wolff-Parkinson-White or short PR syndrome), cardiogenic shock, congestive heart failure (severe) unless secondary to supraventricular tachyarrhythmia treatable with diltiazem, known sensitivity to diltiazem, second- or third-degree AV block or sick sinus syndrome (unless functioning ventricular pacemaker in place), severe hypotension, patients receiving IV beta-adrenergic blocking agents (e.g., atenolol [Tenormin], propranolol [Inderal]) within 2 to 4 hours, ventricular tachycardia. Not recommended for wide QRS tachycardias of uncertain origin or for tachycardias induced by drugs or poisons.

PRECAUTIONS
For short-term use only. ■ Initial administration of IV diltiazem should take place in a facility with adequate personnel, equipment, and supplies to monitor the patient and respond to any medical emergency. ■ While diltiazem will effectively decrease HR, cardioversion will probably be required to convert atrial fibrillation or atrial flutter to a normal sinus rhythm. ■ Valsalva maneuver recommended before use of diltiazem in all paroxysmal supraventricular tachycardias if clinically appropriate. ■ Use IV diltiazem with caution in patients with pre-existing impaired ventricular function (e.g., congestive heart failure, acute myocardial infarction or pulmonary congestion documented by x-ray); may exacerbate disease. Use of oral diltiazem in these patients is contraindicated. ■ May cause second- or third-degree AV block in sinus rhythm; discontinue diltiazem if AV block occurs. ■ Can cause life-threatening tachycardia with severe hypotension in atrial fibrillation or flutter in patients with an accessory bypass tract and periods of asystole in patients with sick sinus syndrome. ■ Use with caution in impaired renal or hepatic function. ■ Ventricular premature beats (VPBs) may occur on conversion of PSVT to sinus rhythm; considered to have no clinical significance. ■ Continue regular dosing on day of OR and thereafter unless otherwise specified by physician. If discontinued, may cause severe angina or MI.

Monitor: Accurate pretreatment diagnosis differentiating wide-complex QRS tachycardia of supraventricular origin from ventricular origin is imperative. ■ ECG monitoring during administration preferred; must be available. ■ Monitor BP and HR closely. ■ Emergency resuscitation drugs and equipment must always be available. ■ See Drug/Lab Interactions.

Maternal/Child: Category C: large doses (5 to 10 times mg/kg dose) have resulted in embryo and fetal death and skeletal abnormalities in animals. ■ Discontinue breast-feeding. ■ Safety and effectiveness for use in pediatric patients not established.

Elderly: See Dose Adjustments. ■ Half-life may be prolonged. ■ May cause tinnitus.

DRUG/LAB INTERACTIONS
Do not give concomitantly (within a few hours) with IV **beta-adrenergic blocking agents** (e.g., atenolol [Tenormin], propranolol [Inderal]); see Contraindications. May result in bradycardia, AV block, and/or depression of contractility. Use extreme caution if these drugs are administered orally or if patient has received before admission; usually tolerated. ■ May result in additive effects with **any agent known to affect cardiac contractility and/or SA or AV node conduction** (e.g., digoxin [Lanoxin], disopyramide [Norpace],

procainamide [Pronestyl], beta-blockers [e.g., propranolol], quinidine). ▪ Is used with **digoxin,** but monitor for excessive slowing of HR and/or AV block. ▪ Coadministration with **amiodarone** (Nexterone) may result in bradycardia and decreased cardiac output. Monitor closely. ▪ May increase effects of certain **benzodiazepines** (e.g., midazolam [Versed], triazolam [Halcion]), **buspirone** (BuSpar), **methylprednisolone** (Solu-Medrol). ▪ May increase serum concentrations of **digoxin, HMG-CoA reductase inhibitors** (e.g., atorvastatin [Lipitor], simvastatin [Zocor]), **imipramine** (Tofranil), **sirolimus** (Rapamune), **and tacrolimus** (Prograf). Monitor serum levels and/or monitor for S/S of toxicity. ▪ May potentiate **anesthetics;** titrate both drugs carefully. ▪ May decrease metabolism and increase serum concentrations and toxicity of **drugs metabolized by the cytochrome P$_{450}$ enzyme system** (e.g., amlodipine [Norvasc], carbamazepine [Tegretol], cyclosporine [Sandimmune], quinidine, theophylline, valproate [Depacon]). ▪ Metabolism may be decreased and serum concentrations increased by **cimetidine** (Tagamet) **and ranitidine** (Zantac). ▪ Metabolism may be increased and serum concentrations decreased by **rifampin** (Rifadin). Adjust dose as needed. ▪ May increase **moricizine** (Ethmozine) serum concentrations. Moricizine may decrease diltiazem concentrations. ▪ May increase **nifedipine** (Procardia) serum concentrations; nifedipine may increase diltiazem serum concentrations. ▪ Variable effects when administered with **lithium.** Has caused decreased effectiveness of lithium and may cause neurotoxicity. ▪ **Any drug metabolized in the liver** may cause competitive inhibition of metabolism (e.g., insulin).

SIDE EFFECTS
Arrhythmia (junctional rhythm or isorhythmic dissociation), flushing, hypotension (asymptomatic and symptomatic), and injection site reactions (burning, itching) occurred most frequently and were most often mild and transient but could have serious potential. Amblyopia, asthenia, atrial flutter, AV block (first- or second-degree), bradycardia, chest pain, congestive heart failure, constipation, dizziness, dry mouth, dyspnea, edema, elevated alkaline phosphatase and AST, headache, hyperuricemia, nausea, paresthesia, pruritus, sinus node dysfunction, sinus pause, skin eruptions (including rare reports of exfoliative dermatitis or Stevens-Johnson syndrome), sweating, syncope, ventricular arrhythmias, ventricular fibrillation, ventricular tachycardia, and vomiting have occurred.

ANTIDOTE
Discontinue diltiazem if a high-degree AV block occurs in sinus rhythm. Notify physician promptly of all side effects. Treatment will depend on clinical situation; maintain IV fluids as indicated. Rapid ventricular response in atrial flutter/fibrillation should respond to cardioversion, procainamide, and/or lidocaine. Treat bradycardia, AV block, and asystole with standard AHA protocol (atropine, isoproterenol, pacing). Treat cardiac failure with inotropic agents (isoproterenol, dopamaine, or dobutamine) and diuretics. Calcium chloride will reverse effects of verapamil; may be useful with diltiazem. Dopamine or norepinephrine (levarterenol) and Trendelenburg position should reverse hypotension. Treat hypersensitivity reactions or resuscitate as necessary. Not removed by hemodialysis.

DIPHENHYDRAMINE HYDROCHLORIDE
(dye-fen-**HY**-drah-meen
hy-droh-**KLOR**-eyed)

**Antihistamine
Antidyskinetic/antiparkinsonism
Antiemetic
Antivertigo agent
Sedative-hypnotic**

Benadryl, Benadryl PF, Diphenhydramine PF

pH 5 to 6

USUAL DOSE
10 to 50 mg. Up to 100 mg may be given. Individualize dose based on patient symptoms and response. Total dosage should not exceed 400 mg/24 hr.

PEDIATRIC DOSE
See Contraindications and Maternal/Child.
Pediatric patients after neonatal period: 1.25 mg/kg/dose every 6 hours as needed or 150 mg/M^2/24 hr in equally divided doses given every 6 hours (37.5 mg/M^2 every 6 hours). Never exceed a total dosage of 300 mg/24 hr.
Anaphylaxis or phenothiazine overdose: 1 to 2 mg/kg IV slowly.

DOSE ADJUSTMENTS
Reduce dose for the elderly or debilitated. ▪ See Drug/Lab Interactions.

DILUTION
May be given undiluted.
Filters: No data available from manufacturer.
Storage: Store below 40° C (104° F), preferably between 15° and 30° C (59° and 86° F). Protect from light and freezing.

COMPATIBILITY (Underline Indicates Conflicting Compatibility Information)
Consider any drug NOT listed as compatible to be INCOMPATIBLE until consulting a pharmacist; specific conditions may apply.
One source suggests the following **compatibilities:**
Additive: Amikacin (Amikin), aminophylline, ascorbic acid, bleomycin (Blenoxane), colistimethate (Coly-Mycin M), erythromycin (Erythrocin), hydrocortisone sodium succinate (Solu-Cortef), lidocaine, methyldopa, nafcillin (Nallpen), penicillin G potassium and sodium.
Y-site: Abciximab (ReoPro), acyclovir (Zovirax), aldesleukin (Proleukin), amifostine (Ethyol), argatroban, azithromycin (Zithromax), aztreonam (Azactam), bivalirudin (Angiomax), buprenorphine (Buprenex), caspofungin (Cancidas), ciprofloxacin (Cipro IV), cisatracurium (Nimbex), cisplatin (Platinol), cladribine (Leustatin), cyclophosphamide (Cytoxan), cytarabine (ARA-C), dexmedetomidine (Precedex), docetaxel (Taxotere), doripenem (Doribax), doxorubicin (Adriamycin), doxorubicin liposomal (Doxil), etoposide phosphate (Etopophos), famotidine (Pepcid IV), fenoldopam (Corlopam), fentanyl (Sublimaze), filgrastim (Neupogen), fluconazole (Diflucan), fludarabine (Fludara), gallium nitrate (Ganite), gemcitabine (Gemzar), granisetron (Kytril), heparin, hetastarch in electrolytes (Hextend), hydrocortisone sodium succinate (Solu-Cortef), hydromorphone (Dilaudid), idarubicin (Idamycin), linezolid (Zyvox), melphalan (Alkeran), meperidine (Demerol), meropenem (Merrem IV), methadone (Dolophine), methotrexate, morphine, ondansetron (Zofran), oxaliplatin (Eloxatin), paclitaxel (Taxol), pemetrexed (Alimta),

piperacillin/tazobactam (Zosyn), potassium chloride (KCl), propofol (Diprivan), remifentanil (Ultiva), sargramostim (Leukine), sufentanil (Sufenta), tacrolimus (Prograf), teniposide (Vumon), thiotepa, vinorelbine (Navelbine).

RATE OF ADMINISTRATION
25 mg or fraction thereof over 1 minute. Extend injection time in non-emergency situations and pediatric patients. See Maternal/Child.

ACTIONS
A potent antihistamine, it is capable of blocking the effects of histamine at various receptor sites, either eliminating a hypersensitivity reaction or greatly modifying it. It also has anticholinergic (antispasmodic), antiemetic, antivertigo, and sedative effects. It has rapid onset of action and is widely distributed throughout the body, including the CNS. A portion of this drug is metabolized in the liver; the rest is excreted unchanged in the urine. Half-life is 1 to 4 hours. Some secretion may occur in breast milk.

INDICATIONS AND USES
Allergic reactions to blood or plasma. ■ Supplemental therapy to epinephrine in anaphylaxis and other uncomplicated allergic/hypersensitivity reactions requiring prompt treatment (e.g., angioedema, pruritus, urticaria). ■ Preoperative or generalized sedation. ■ Management of parkinsonism, including drug-induced (e.g., phenothiazines [e.g., prochlorperazine (Compazine)]). ■ Severe nausea and vomiting. ■ Motion sickness. ■ To replace oral therapy when it is impractical or contraindicated.

CONTRAINDICATIONS
Breast-feeding, hypersensitivity to antihistamines, newborn or premature infants.

PRECAUTIONS
IV route used only in emergency situations. ■ Avoid SC or perivascular injection. ■ Use with extreme caution in infants, children, elderly or debilitated individuals, asthmatic attack, bladder neck obstruction, narrow-angle glaucoma, lower respiratory tract infections, prostatic hypertrophy, pyloroduodenal obstruction, and stenosing peptic ulcer.
Monitor: Will induce drowsiness. ■ Monitor vital signs; observe closely. ■ See Drug/Lab Interactions.
Patient Education: Do not drive or operate hazardous equipment until effects wear off. ■ May cause drowsiness and dizziness; request help to ambulate. ■ Avoid alcohol and other CNS depressants (e.g., diazepam [Valium], narcotics).
Maternal/Child: See Contraindications, Precautions, Monitor, and Side Effects. ■ Category B: use only when clearly needed. May increase risk of abnormalities during the first trimester. ■ Not recommended during breast-feeding. Small amounts may be distributed into breast milk, causing irritability or excitement in infants. ■ Use extreme caution in infants and children; may cause hallucinations, convulsions, or death. May also reduce mental alertness and cause paradoxical excitation.
Elderly: See Dose Adjustments, Precautions, Monitor, and Side Effects. ■ May cause confusion, dizziness, hyperexcitability, hypotension and/or sedation. ■ Sensitivity to anticholinergic effects is increased (e.g., blurred vision, constipation, dry mouth, urinary retention).

DRUG/LAB INTERACTIONS

Increases effectiveness of **epinephrine** and is often used in conjunction with it. ▪ Potentiates **anticholinergics** (e.g., atropine); **alcohol, beta-blockers** (e.g., metoprolol [Lopressor], propranolol [Inderal]), **hypnotics, itraconazole (Sporanox), sedatives, tranquilizers, and other CNS depressants** (e.g., reserpine, antipyretics); **thioridazine** (Mellaril); **procarbazine** (Matulane); **and others.** Reduced dose of potentiated drug may be indicated. ▪ Anticholinergic and CNS sedative effects prolonged by **MAO inhibitors** (e.g., selegiline [Eldepryl]). Concurrent use not recommended. ▪ Effectiveness of many drugs is reduced in combination with diphenhydramine because of increased metabolism. ▪ May inhibit the wheal and flare reaction to **antigen skin tests.**

SIDE EFFECTS

Rare when used as indicated: anaphylaxis; blurring of vision; confusion; constipation; diarrhea; difficulty in urination; diplopia; drowsiness; drug rash; dryness of mouth, nose, and throat; epigastric distress; headache; hemolytic anemia; hypotension; insomnia; nasal stuffiness; nausea; nervousness; palpitations; photosensitivity; rapid pulse; restlessness; thickening of bronchial secretions; tightness of the chest and wheezing; tingling, heaviness, weakness of hands; urticaria; vertigo; vomiting. Overdose may cause convulsions, hallucinations, and death in pediatric patients.

ANTIDOTE

For exaggerated drowsiness or other disturbing side effects, discontinue the drug and notify the physician. Side effects will usually subside within a few hours or may be treated symptomatically. Treat hypotension promptly; may lead to cardiovascular collapse. Use dopamine, norepinephrine, or phenylephrine. Epinephrine is contraindicated for hypotension; further hypotension will occur. Propranolol (Inderal) is the drug of choice for ventricular arrhythmias. Treat convulsions with diazepam (Valium) 0.1 mg/kg IV slowly. Some central anticholinergic effects may require physostigmine. Avoid analeptics (e.g., caffeine); may cause convulsions. Epinephrine must be available to treat anaphylaxis. Resuscitate as necessary.

DIPYRIDAMOLE
(dye-peer-**ID**-ah-mohl)

Coronary vasodilator
Diagnostic agent
Platelet aggregation inhibitor

Persantine

pH 2.2 to 3.2

USUAL DOSE

Myocardial perfusion imaging: 0.57 mg/kg of body weight equally distributed over 4 minutes (0.142 mg/kg/min). A 70-kg adult would receive a total dose of 39.9 mg (10 mg/min). Never exceed 0.57 mg/kg dose. Thallium should be injected within 5 minutes following the 4-minute infusion of dipyridamole.

Platelet aggregation inhibitor (unlabeled): 250 mg/24 hr as an infusion.

DILUTION

Each 1 mL (5 mg) must be diluted with a minimum of 2 mL D5W, D5/½NS, or D5NS. Total volume should range from a minimum of 20 mL to 50 mL (39.9 mg [8 mL] would be diluted in a minimum of 16 mL for a total infusion of 24 mL; additional diluent can be used to facilitate titration). May not be given undiluted; will cause local irritation.

Platelet aggregation inhibitor: Each 250-mg dose should be diluted with 250 mL D5W (1 mg/mL). Concentration may be increased if larger doses required.

Storage: Undiluted drug should be stored at CRT and protected from direct light; avoid freezing.

COMPATIBILITY

Specific information not available. Consider specific use; consult pharmacist.

RATE OF ADMINISTRATION

A single dose must be equally distributed over 4 minutes (0.142 mg/kg/min).

Platelet aggregation inhibitor: 10 mg/hr as a continuous infusion. Use of a microdrip (60 gtt/mL) or infusion pump recommended.

ACTIONS

A coronary vasodilator that will cause an increase in coronary blood flow velocity of from 3.8 to 7 times greater than resting velocity. Action may result from the inhibition of adenosine uptake. Peak velocity is reached in 2.5 to 8.7 minutes. Will cause a 20% increase in HR and a mild but significant decrease in systolic and diastolic BP in the supine position. Vital signs may take up to 30 minutes to return to baseline measurements. Used in combination with thallium, visualization shows dilation with sustained enhanced flow of intact vessels, leaving reduced pressure and flow across areas of hemodynamically important coronary vascular constriction. Results achieved are comparable to exercise-induced thallium imaging. Metabolized in the liver. Excreted in bile. Secreted in breast milk.

INDICATIONS AND USES

An alternative to exercise in thallium myocardial perfusion imaging for the evaluation of coronary artery disease in patients who cannot exercise adequately.

Unlabeled uses: Prophylactic inhibition of platelet aggregation in thromboembolism and myocardial infarction.

CONTRAINDICATIONS
Hypersensitivity to dipyridamole.

PRECAUTIONS
Administered by or under the direction of the cardiologist. ■ Full facilities for treatment of any airway, cardiac emergency, or hypersensitivity, including laboratory analysis, must be available. ■ Theophylline (Aminophylline) and other emergency drugs must be immediately available. ■ Patients with a history of unstable angina or a history of asthma may be at greater risk; use extreme caution. ■ This drug has caused two fatal myocardial infarctions as well as other serious side effects in a small percentage of patients; clinical information to be gained must be weighed against risk to the patient.

Monitor: An IV line with a Y-tube or three-way stopcock must be in place. ■ Monitor vital signs continuously during infusion and for at least 15 minutes after or until return to baseline. ■ ECG monitoring using at least 1 chest lead should be continuous. ■ Patient is usually in a supine position, but tests have been conducted in a sitting position. Lower to supine with head tilted down (Trendelenburg) if hypotension occurs.

Maternal/Child: Category B: safety for use during pregnancy not established. Use only if clearly needed. ■ Temporarily discontinue breastfeeding. ■ Safety for use in pediatric patients not established.

DRUG/LAB INTERACTIONS
Theophylline bronchodilators (e.g., aminophylline, oxtriphylline [Choledyl], theophylline) reverse the effect of dipyridamole on myocardial blood flow. Interferes with dipyridamole-assisted **myocardial perfusion studies.** Withhold bronchodilators for 36 hours before testing.

SIDE EFFECTS
BP lability, chest pain/angina pectoris, dizziness, dyspnea, ECG abnormalities (e.g., extrasystoles, ST-T changes, tachycardia), fatigue, flushing, headache, hypertension, hypotension, nausea, pain (unspecified), paresthesia. Numerous other side effects occur in less than 1% of patients.

Major: Bronchospasm, cerebral ischemia (transient), fatal and nonfatal myocardial infarction, ventricular fibrillation, ventricular tachycardia (symptomatic) occurred in 0.3% of patients.

ANTIDOTE
Physician will be present throughout test administration. Theophylline (Aminophylline) is an adenosine receptor antagonist and will reverse the adenosine-mediated effects of dipyridamole (e.g., angina pectoris, bronchospasm, severe hypotension, ventricular arrhythmias). If bronchospasm or chest pain occur, administer 50 to 250 mg of theophylline at a rate not to exceed 50 mg over 30 seconds. If symptoms are not relieved by 250 mg of theophylline, sublingual nitroglycerin may be helpful. Persistent chest pain may indicate impending potentially fatal myocardial infarction. If patient condition permits, thallium may be injected and allowed to circulate for 1 minute before injection of theophylline; this will permit initial thallium perfusion imaging before reversal of vasodilatory effects of dipyridamole on coronary circulation. Use head-down supine position for hypotension before administering theophylline. After reversal of vasodilatory action, treat arrhythmias as indicated. Resuscitate as necessary.

DOBUTAMINE HYDROCHLORIDE
(doh-**BYOU**-tah-meen hy-droh-**KLOR**-eyed)

Inotropic agent
Cardiac stimulant

pH 2.5 to 5.5

USUAL DOSE
0.5 to 1 mcg/kg/min initially in patients likely to respond to minimum treatment. The usual effective initial dose ranges from 2.5 to 15 mcg/kg of body weight/min. AHA guidelines suggest 2 to 20 mcg/kg/min. Gradually adjust rate at 2- to 10-minute intervals to effect desired response. AHA guidelines recommend titrating so HR does not increase by more than 10% of baseline. Up to 40 mcg/kg/min has been used in some instances; increases potential for toxicity (e.g., myocardial ischemia). U.S. experience in controlled trials does not extend beyond 48 hours of therapy.

PEDIATRIC DOSE
2 to 20 mcg/kg/min. Initial dose usually 5 to 10 mcg/kg/min. Adjust rate to effect desired response; see Maternal/Child.

DOSE ADJUSTMENTS
Lower-end initial doses may be appropriate in the elderly based on potential for decreased organ function, concomitant disease, or other drug therapy. See Drug/Lab Interactions.

DILUTION
Available prediluted in D5W, or each 250-mg (20-mL) vial must be further diluted to at least 50 mL. Any amount of infusion solution desired above 50 mL may be used (250 mg in 1 L equals 250 mcg/mL; 250 mg in 500 mL equals 500 mcg/mL; 250 mg in 250 mL equals 1,000 mcg/mL). Adjust to fluid requirements of the patient. **Compatible** with D5W, D10W, D5/½NS, D5NS, D5/Isolyte M, LR, D5LR, Normosol-M in D5W, 20% Osmitrol in water, NS, or sodium lactate.
Pediatric dilution: 6 mg/kg in 100 mL diluent. 1 mL/hr equals 1 mcg/kg/min.
Filters: No data available from manufacturer. Another source suggests no significant drug loss through a 0.22-micron cellulose ester membrane filter.
Storage: When mixed in infusion solution, use within 24 hours. Pink coloring of solution does not affect potency; will crystallize if frozen.

COMPATIBILITY
(Underline Indicates Conflicting Compatibility Information)
Consider any drug NOT listed as compatible to be INCOMPATIBLE until consulting a pharmacist; specific conditions may apply.
Manufacturer states, "Do not add to sodium bicarbonate or any other strongly alkaline solution" (e.g., aminophylline, barbiturates [e.g., thiopental (Pentothal)]). Manufacturer recommends not using other drugs as additives, not using in conjunction with other agents, and not using with diluents containing both sodium bisulfate and ethanol.

One source suggests the following **compatibilities:**
Additive: *Not recommended by manufacturer.* Amiodarone (Nexterone), atracurium (Tracrium), atropine, <u>calcium chloride</u>, ciprofloxacin (Cipro IV), dopamine, enalaprilat (Vasotec IV), epinephrine (Adrenalin), flumazenil (Romazicon), <u>heparin</u>, hydralazine, isoproterenol (Isuprel), lidocaine, meperidine (Demerol), meropenem (Merrem IV), morphine, nitroglycerin IV, norepinephrine (Levophed), phentolamine (Regitine), phenylephrine

(Neo-Synephrine), potassium chloride (KCl), procainamide (Pronestyl), propranolol (Inderal), ranitidine (Zantac), verapamil, zidovudine (AZT, Retrovir).

Y-site: *Not recommended by manufacturer.* Alprostadil, amifostine (Ethyol), amiodarone (Nexterone), anidulafungin (Eraxis), argatroban, atracurium (Tracrium), aztreonam (Azactam), bivalirudin (Angiomax), calcium chloride, calcium gluconate, caspofungin (Cancidas), cefepime (Maxipime), ceftazidime (Fortaz), ciprofloxacin (Cipro IV), cisatracurium (Nimbex), cladribine (Leustatin), dexmedetomidine (Precedex), diazepam (Valium), diltiazem (Cardizem), docetaxel (Taxotere), dopamine, doripenem (Doribax), doxorubicin liposomal (Doxil), enalaprilat (Vasotec IV), epinephrine (Adrenalin), etoposide phosphate (Etopophos), famotidine (Pepcid IV), fenoldopam (Corlopam), fentanyl (Sublimaze), fluconazole (Diflucan), furosemide (Lasix), gemcitabine (Gemzar), granisetron (Kytril), haloperidol (Haldol), heparin, hetastarch in electrolytes (Hextend), hydromorphone (Dilaudid), inamrinone (Amrinone), insulin (regular), labetalol (Trandate), levofloxacin (Levaquin), lidocaine, linezolid (Zyvox), lorazepam (Ativan), magnesium sulfate, meperidine (Demerol), midazolam (Versed), milrinone (Primacor), morphine, nicardipine (Cardene IV), nitroglycerin IV, nitroprusside sodium, norepinephrine (Levophed), oxaliplatin (Eloxatin), pancuronium, potassium chloride (KCl), propofol (Diprivan), ranitidine (Zantac), remifentanil (Ultiva), streptokinase, tacrolimus (Prograf), theophylline, thiotepa, tigecycline (Tygacil), tirofiban (Aggrastat), vasopressin, vecuronium, verapamil, zidovudine (AZT, Retrovir).

RATE OF ADMINISTRATION

Begin with recommended dose for body weight and seriousness of condition. Gradually increase to effect desired response. May take up to 10 minutes to achieve peak effect of a specific dose. Maintain at correct therapeutic level with microdrip (60 gtt/mL) or infusion pump. Half-life of dobutamine is only about 2 minutes. See Maternal/Child.

Infusion Rate (mL/hr) for Dobutamine 500 mcg/mL												
	Patient's Weight (kg)											
Drug Delivery Rate (mcg/kg/min)	5	10	20	30	40	50	60	70	80	90	100	110
0.5	0.3	0.6	1.2	1.8	2.4	3	3.6	4.2	4.8	5.4	6	6.6
1	0.6	1.2	2.4	3.6	4.8	6	7.2	8.4	9.6	10.8	12	13.2
2.5	1.5	3	6	9	12	15	18	21	24	27	30	33
5	3	6	12	18	24	30	36	42	48	54	60	66
7.5	4.5	9	18	27	36	45	54	63	72	81	90	99
10	6	12	24	36	48	60	72	84	96	108	120	132
12.5	7.5	15	30	45	60	75	90	105	120	135	150	165
15	9	18	36	54	72	90	108	126	144	162	180	198
17.5	10.5	21	42	63	84	105	126	147	168	189	210	231
20	12	24	48	72	96	120	144	168	192	216	240	264

Infusion Rate (mL/hr) for Dobutamine 1,000 mcg/mL											
	Patient's Weight (kg)										
Drug Delivery Rate (mcg/kg/min)	5	10	20	30	40	50	60	70	80	90	100	110
0.5	0.15	0.3	0.6	0.9	1.2	1.5	1.8	2.1	2.4	2.7	3	3.3
1	0.3	0.6	1.2	1.8	2.4	3	3.6	4.2	4.8	5.4	6	6.6
2.5	0.75	1.5	3	4.5	6	7.5	9	10.5	12	13.5	15	16.5
5	1.5	3	6	9	12	15	18	21	24	27	30	33
7.5	2.25	4.5	9	13.5	18	22.5	27	31.5	36	40.5	45	49.5
10	3	6	12	18	24	30	36	42	48	54	60	66
12.5	3.75	7.5	15	22.5	30	37.5	45	52.5	60	67.5	75	82.5
15	4.5	9	18	27	36	45	54	63	72	81	90	99
17.5	5.25	10.5	21	31.5	42	52.5	63	73.5	84	94.5	105	115.5
20	6	12	24	36	48	60	72	84	96	108	120	132

Infusion Rate (mL/hr) for Dobutamine 2,000 mcg/mL											
	Patient's Weight (kg)										
Drug Delivery Rate (mcg/kg/min)	5	10	20	30	40	50	60	70	80	90	100	110
0.5	0.08	0.15	0.3	0.45	0.6	0.75	0.9	1.05	1.2	1.35	1.5	1.65
1	0.15	0.3	0.6	0.9	1.2	1.5	1.8	2.1	2.4	2.7	3	3.3
2.5	0.38	0.75	1.5	2	3	4	4.5	5	6	7	7.5	8
5	0.75	1.5	3	4.5	6	7.5	9	10.5	12	13.5	15	16.5
7.5	1.13	2.25	4.5	7	9	11	13.5	16	18	20	22.5	25
10	1.5	3	6	9	12	15	18	21	24	27	30	33
12.5	1.88	3.75	7.5	11	15	19	22.5	26	30	34	37.5	41
15	2.25	4.5	9	13.5	18	22.5	27	31.5	36	40.5	45	49.5
17.5	2.63	5.25	10.5	15.75	21	26.25	31.5	36.75	42	47.25	52.50	57.75
20	3	6	12	18	24	30	36	42	48	54	60	66

ACTIONS

A synthetic catecholamine chemically related to dopamine, it is a direct-acting inotropic agent possessing beta-stimulator activity. Induces short-term increases in cardiac output by improving stroke volume with minimum increases in rate and BP, minimum rhythm disturbances, and decreased peripheral vascular resistance. Usually most effective for only a few hours. May improve atrioventricular conduction. Peak effect obtained in 2 to 10 minutes. Has a very short duration of action. Half-life is 2 minutes; may be up to 5 minutes in preterm infants. Metabolized in the liver and other tissues. Metabolites are primarily excreted in the urine.

INDICATIONS AND USES

Short-term inotropic support in cardiac decompensation resulting from depressed contractility (organic heart disease or cardiac surgical procedures). **Unlabeled uses:** Increase cardiac output in pediatric patients with congenital heart disease undergoing cardiac catheterization.

CONTRAINDICATIONS

Hypersensitivity to any components (contains sulfites), idiopathic hypertrophic subaortic stenosis, shock without adequate fluid replacement.

PRECAUTIONS

Use extreme caution in myocardial infarction; increases in HR of more than 10% may increase myocardial ischemia and size of infarction. ▪ Contains sulfites; use caution in patients with allergies. ▪ Precipitous hypotension occurs rarely; usually reverses with a decrease in rate of administration; see Antidote. ▪ Ineffective if marked mechanical obstruction (e.g., severe valvular aortic stenosis) is present. ▪ Use for long-term treatment of CHF has been associated with increased risks of hospitalization and death.

Monitor: Correct hypovolemia and acidosis as indicated before initiating treatment. ▪ Observe patient's response continuously; monitor HR, ectopic activity, BP, and urine flow. Measure pulmonary wedge pressure, central venous pressure, and cardiac output if possible. ▪ May cause significant increase in BP or HR, especially systolic pressure. Patients with pre-existing hypertension may be at increased risk of developing an increased pressor response. ▪ Monitor for changes in fluid balance, electrolytes, and acid-base balance. ▪ Use digoxin preparation before starting dobutamine in patients with atrial fibrillation with rapid ventricular response. ▪ See Drug/Lab Interactions.

Maternal/Child: Category B: use only if benefits outweigh risks. Safety for use in pregnancy, breast-feeding, and pediatric patients not established. ▪ Increases cardiac output and systemic BP in pediatric patients of every age-group, usually at infusion rates that are lower than those that cause significant tachycardia. Less effective than dopamine in premature neonates.

Elderly: Lower-end initial doses may be indicated; see Dose Adjustments. ▪ Differences in response compared to younger adults not identified, but greater sensitivity of some elderly cannot be ruled out.

DRUG/LAB INTERACTIONS

May be ineffective if **beta-blocking drugs** (e.g., propranolol [Inderal]) have been given. ▪ Produces higher cardiac output and lower pulmonary wedge pressure when given concomitantly with **nitroprusside sodium.** ▪ May cause serious arrhythmias in presence of **cyclopropane or halogen anesthetics,** severe hypertension with **oxytocic drugs, or guanethidine** (Ismelin). ▪ Pressor response increased with **tricyclic antidepressants** (e.g., amitriptyline [Elavil], imipramine [Tofranil]) and **rauwolfia alkaloids** (e.g., reserpine [Serpasil]); may cause hypertension. ▪ Has been given concurrently without evidence of drug interaction with acetaminophen (Tylenol), atropine, digoxin preparations, folic acid, furosemide, glyceryl trinitrate (nitroglycerin), heparin, isosorbide dinitrate (Iso-Bid), lidocaine, morphine, potassium chloride, protamine, and spironolactone (Aldactone).

SIDE EFFECTS

Anginal pain, chest pain, headache, hypertension, hypokalemia, increased ventricular ectopic activity, myocardial ischemia, nausea, palpitations, shortness of breath, tachycardia. Hypersensitivity reactions (e.g., broncho-spasm, eosinophilia, fever, skin rash) have been reported. Local inflam-matory changes may occur with infiltration.

Overdose: In addition to all of the above, overdose may cause anorexia, anxiety, excessive hypertension or hypotension, myocardial ischemia, tremor, ventricular tachycardia, and/or fibrillation.

ANTIDOTE

Notify physician of all side effects. Decrease infusion rate and notify physician immediately if number of PVCs increases or there is a marked increase in pulse rate (30 or more beats) or BP (50 or more mm Hg systolic). For accidental overdose, reduce rate or temporarily discontinue until condition stabilizes. Maintain a patent airway with adequate oxygen-ation and ventilation. Treat ventricular tachyarrhythmias with propranolol (Inderal) or lidocaine. Hypertension usually responds to a reduced rate or temporarily discontinuing dobutamine. Reduce rate or discontinue do-butamine if hypotension occurs. May require treatment with vasopressors (e.g., dopamine, norepinephrine). See Precautions.

DOCETAXEL BBW

(doh-seh-**TAX**-ell)

Taxotere

**Antineoplastic agent
(taxane)**

USUAL DOSE

Premedication for all patients except those with hormone-refractory prostate cancer: Must be pretreated with oral corticosteroids to reduce the incidence and severity of fluid retention and hypersensitivity reactions. Usual regimen is dexamethasone (Decadron) 8 mg PO twice a day for 3 days. Begin 1 day before each docetaxel infusion.

Premedication for hormone-refractory prostate cancer: Administer oral dexamethasone 8 mg at 12 hours, 3 hours, and 1 hour before each docetaxel infusion (another steroid, prednisone, is part of the combination therapy).

One source suggests that pretreatment with diphenhydramine (Benadryl) and/or an H_2 antagonist (e.g., famotidine [Pepcid], ranitidine [Zantac]) given IV 30 minutes before docetaxel infusion may help reduce hypersensitivity reactions and cutaneous toxicity.

Breast cancer: 60 to 100 mg/M^2 as an infusion. Repeat every 3 weeks.

Adjuvant treatment of operable node-positive breast cancer: 75 mg/M^2 as an infusion. Administer 1 hour after doxorubicin 50 mg/M^2 and cyclophosphamide 500 mg/M^2. Repeat every 3 weeks for 6 cycles. Prophylactic G-CSF (e.g., filgrastim [Neupogen]) may be used to mitigate the risk of hematologic toxicity. See doxorubicin and cyclophosphamide monographs.

Prostate cancer (hormone refractory): 75 mg/M^2 as an infusion. Repeat every 3 weeks. Prednisone 5 mg PO twice daily is administered continuously throughout treatment. See Premedication.

First-line treatment of non–small-cell lung cancer (NSCLC): 75 mg/M^2 as an infusion over 1 hour. Follow immediately with cisplatin 75 mg/M^2 as an infusion over 30 to 60 minutes. *Premedicate* with antiemetics and hydration as required for cisplatin administration; see cisplatin monograph. Repeat regimen every 3 weeks.

NSCLC after failure of prior chemotherapy: 75 mg/M^2 as an infusion. Repeat every 3 weeks. Larger doses increased toxicity, infection, and treatment-related mortality.

Gastric adenocarcinoma: 75 mg/M^2 as an infusion over 1 hour. Follow immediately with cisplatin 75 mg/M^2 as an infusion over 1 to 3 hours (both on Day 1 only). *Premedicate* with antiemetics and hydration as required for cisplatin administration; see cisplatin and fluorouracil monographs. Follow the cisplatin infusion with fluorouracil 750 mg/M^2 as an infusion equally distributed over 24 hours. Repeat fluorouracil dose for 4 more 24-hour infusions (total of 5 days). Repeat regimen every 3 weeks. In the study, G-CSF (filgrastim [Neupogen]) was recommended during the second and/or subsequent cycles to prevent or attenuate febrile neutropenia, documented infection with neutropenia, or neutropenia lasting more than 7 days.

Continued

Induction chemotherapy followed by radiotherapy for treatment of inoperable, locally advanced squamous cell cancer of the head and neck (SCCHN): 75 mg/M^2 as an infusion over 1 hour. Follow immediately with cisplatin 75 mg/M^2 as an infusion over 1 hour (both on Day 1 only). *Premedicate* with antiemetics and hydration as required for cisplatin administration; see cisplatin monograph. Follow the cisplatin infusion with fluorouracil 750 mg/M^2 as an infusion equally distributed over 24 hours. Repeat fluorouracil for four more 24-hour infusions (total of 5 days). See fluorouracil monograph. Repeat regimen every 3 weeks for a total of four cycles. Prophylactic antibiotics were used in clinical studies. Following chemotherapy, patients should receive radiotherapy.

Induction chemotherapy followed by chemoradiotherapy for treatment of locally advanced (unresectable, low surgical cure, or organ preservation) SCCHN: 75 mg/M^2 as an infusion over 1 hour. Follow with cisplatin 100 mg/M^2 as a 30-minute to 3-hour infusion (both on Day 1 only). *Premedicate* with antiemetics and hydration as required for cisplatin administration; see cisplatin monograph. Follow the cisplatin infusion with fluorouracil 1,000 mg/M^2 as an infusion equally distributed over 24 hours. Repeat fluorouracil for three more 24-hour infusions (total of 4 days). See fluorouracil monograph. Repeat regimen every 3 weeks for 3 cycles.

Treatment of small-cell lung cancer and ovarian cancer (unlabeled): 100 mg/M^2 as an infusion. Repeat every 3 weeks.

Bladder cancer (unlabeled): 75 to 100 mg/M^2 as an infusion. Repeat every 3 weeks for up to 6 treatment cycles.

Treatment of esophageal cancer (unlabeled): *Used as a single agent:* 75 to 100 mg/M^2 as a 1-hour infusion every 21 days. *Used in combination with other agents (e.g., gemcitabine, cisplatin, 5-FU, leucovorin calcium, and radiation therapy):* 60 to 85 mg/M^2 as a 1-hour infusion every 21 to 28 days.

DOSE ADJUSTMENTS

All diagnoses: Withhold therapy if neutrophils below 1,500/mm^3 or platelets below 100,000 cells/mm^3. A 25% reduction in the dose of docetaxel is recommended during subsequent cycles following severe neutropenia (less than 500/mm^3) lasting 7 days or more, febrile neutropenia, or a Grade 4 infection. ■ Withhold therapy if bilirubin is greater than the ULN or if AST and/or ALT is greater than 1.5 times the ULN concomitant with alkaline phosphatase greater than 2.5 times the ULN. ■ Discontinue therapy in patients who develop Grade 3 or higher peripheral neuropathy. ■ Dose selection should be cautious in the elderly. Reduced doses may be indicated based on the potential for decreased organ function and concomitant disease or drug therapy. ■ Consider additional dose adjustments when docetaxel is given in combination with other chemotherapeutic agents. ■ See Precautions.

Breast cancer: Reduce dose to 75 mg/M^2 for patients initially dosed at 100 mg/M^2 who experience febrile neutropenia, severe neutropenia (neutrophils below 500/mm^3 for more than 1 week), severe or cumulative cutaneous reaction, severe (Grade 4) infection, or severe peripheral neuropathy. Further reduce to 55 mg/M^2 or discontinue docetaxel if any of the previously listed reactions persist. ■ Patients receiving the lower dose of docetaxel (60 mg/M^2) may have the dose increased gradually if lower dose was well tolerated. ■ Discontinue therapy in patients who develop Grade 3 or greater peripheral neuropathy.

Adjuvant treatment of operable node-positive breast cancer: Patients who experience febrile neutropenia should receive G-CSF (e.g., filgrastim

[Neupogen]) in all subsequent cycles. Patients who continue to experience this reaction should remain on G-CSF and have their docetaxel dose decreased to 60 mg/M^2. ▪ Reduce docetaxel dose to 60 mg/M^2 in patients who experience Grade 3 or 4 stomatitis. ▪ Reduce docetaxel dose from 75 to 60 mg/M^2 in patients who experience severe or cumulative cutaneous reactions or moderate neurosensory signs and/or symptoms. If side effects persist at the lower dose, discontinue therapy.

Prostate cancer: Reduce taxotere dose from 75 to 60 mg/M^2 in patients who experience dose-limiting toxicities (e.g., febrile neutropenia, neutrophils less than 500 cells/mm^3 for more than 1 week, severe or cumulative cutaneous reactions, or moderate neurosensory signs and/or symptoms). If side effects persist at the lower dose, discontinue therapy.

Non–small-cell lung cancer after failure of prior chemotherapy: In NSCLC patients who experience either febrile neutropenia, neutrophils less than 500 cells/mm^3 for more than 1 week, severe or cumulative cutaneous reactions, or other Grade 3 or 4 nonhematologic toxicities, withhold docetaxel until resolution of toxicity, then resume at 55 mg/M^2. ▪ Discontinue therapy in patients who develop Grade 3 or greater peripheral neuropathy.

First-line treatment of NSCLC: Reduce dose to 65 mg/M^2 in patients whose nadir of platelet count during the previous course of therapy was less than 25,000 cells/mm^3, in patients who experienced febrile neutropenia, and in patients with serious nonhematologic toxicities. Dose may be further reduced to 50 mg/M^2 as indicated. See cisplatin monograph for cisplatin dose adjustments.

Gastric adenocarcinoma and head and neck cancer: Patients who experience febrile neutropenia, documented infection with neutropenia, or neutropenia lasting more than 7 days should receive G-CSF (e.g., filgrastim [Neupogen]) in all subsequent cycles. Patients who continue to experience this reaction should remain on G-CSF and have their taxotere dose decreased to 60 mg/M^2. Reduce dose further to 45 mg/M^2 if subsequent episodes of complicated neutropenia occur. ▪ Reduce taxotere dose from 75 to 60 mg/M^2 in patients who experience Grade 4 thrombocytopenia. ▪ If the previously mentioned toxicities persist, discontinue therapy. Additional dose adjustments are outlined in the following chart.

Continued

Additional Recommended Dose Adjustments for Toxicities in Gastric Adenocarcinoma or Head and Neck Cancer Patients Treated with Docetaxel in Combination with Cisplatin and Fluorouracil	
Toxicity	**Dose Adjustment**
Diarrhea Grade 3	**First episode:** Reduce 5-FU dose by 20%. **Second episode:** Reduce docetaxel dose by 20%.
Diarrhea Grade 4	**First episode:** Reduce docetaxel and 5-FU doses by 20%. **Second episode:** Discontinue treatment.
Stomatitis Grade 3	**First episode:** Reduce 5-FU dose by 20%. **Second episode:** Stop 5-FU only at all subsequent cycles. **Third episode:** Reduce docetaxel dose by 20%.
Stomatitis Grade 4	**First episode:** Stop 5-FU only at all subsequent cycles. **Second episode:** Reduce docetaxel dose by 20%.
AST/ALT >2.5 to ≤5 × ULN and AP ≤2.5 × ULN, or AST/ALT >1.5 to ≤5 × ULN and AP >2.5 to ≤5 × ULN	Reduce docetaxel dose by 20%.
AST/ALT >5 × ULN and/or AP >5 × ULN	Discontinue docetaxel.
Peripheral neuropathy Grade 2	Reduce cisplatin dose by 20%.
Peripheral neuropathy Grade 3	Discontinue cisplatin treatment.
Ototoxicity Grade 3	Discontinue cisplatin treatment.
Rise in SCr ≥ Grade 2 (>1.5 × normal value) despite adequate rehydration	Determine CrCl before each subsequent cycle and consider the following dose reductions as outlined below.
CrCl ≥60 mL/min	Full dose of cisplatin given. Repeat CrCl before each treatment cycle.
CrCl >40 and <60 mL/min	Reduce dose of cisplatin by 50% at subsequent cycle. If CrCl was >60 mL/min at end of cycle, give full dose at the next cycle. If no recovery observed, omit cisplatin from the next treatment cycle.
CrCl <40 mL/min	Omit dose of cisplatin for **that treatment cycle only.** Discontinue cisplatin if CrCl remains at <40 mL/min. Reduce cisplatin dose by 50% if CrCl was >40 and <60 mL/min at end of cycle. Give full cisplatin dose if CrCl is >60 mL/min at end of cycle.
Plantar-palmar toxicity Grade 2 or greater	Discontinue fluorouracil until recovery, then reduce fluorouracil dose by 20%.
Other greater than Grade 3 toxicities except alopecia and anemia	Delay 5-FU chemotherapy (for a maximum of 2 weeks from the planned date of infusion) until resolution to ≤Grade 1. If medically appropriate, resume treatment.

DILUTION

Specific techniques required; see Precautions. Available in a new formulation and in several concentrations; *read label carefully.* Requires no initial dilution and is ready to add to an infusion solution; *read label carefully* to avoid overdose. Allow required number of vials to stand at room temperature for 5 minutes if refrigerated. Withdraw required amount of concentrate (20 mg/mL or 10 mg/mL) and inject into a 250-mL infusion bag or bottle of NS or D5W. Manually rotate to mix thoroughly. Should be administered through polyethylene-lined administration sets. Desired concentration should be between 0.3 and 0.74 mg/mL (100 mg in 250 mL = 0.4 mg/mL). If a dose greater than 200 mg is required, use a larger volume of NS or D5W so that a final concentration of 0.74 mg/mL is not exceeded. Solution should be clear.

Filters: Not required. Manufacturer indicates that studies show no loss of potency with in-line filtration through a 0.22-micron filter.

Storage: *Taxotere (20 mg/mL):* Unopened vials of docetaxel in cartons may be stored at 2° C (36° F) to 25° C (77° F). Protect from light. Freezing does not adversely affect unopened vials. Fully diluted infusion solutions should be used within 4 hours (including the 1-hour infusion time). *Generic 10 mg/mL solution:* Store unopened vials in original carton at 25° C (77° F); excursions permitted to 15° to 30° C (59° to 86° F). After first use, refrigerate multi-use vials at 2° to 8° C (36° to 46 ° F) for up to 28 days; protect from light.

COMPATIBILITY (Underline Indicates Conflicting Compatibility Information)

Consider any drug NOT listed as compatible to be INCOMPATIBLE until consulting a pharmacist; specific conditions may apply.

Leaches out plasticizers, including DEHP, from PVC infusion bags and administration sets. Use glass or polypropylene bottles or plastic (polypropylene or polyolefin) bags and polyethylene-lined administration sets to minimize patient exposure to leached DEHP. Do not allow concentrate to come into contact with plasticized PVC equipment or devices used to prepare solutions.

One source suggests the following **compatibilities:**

Y-site: Acyclovir (Zovirax), amifostine (Ethyol), amikacin (Amikin), aminophylline, ampicillin, ampicillin/sulbactam (Unasyn), anidulafungin (Eraxis), aztreonam (Azactam), bumetanide, buprenorphine (Buprenex), butorphanol (Stadol), calcium gluconate, cefazolin (Ancef), cefepime (Maxipime), cefotaxime (Claforan), cefotetan, cefoxitin (Mefoxin), ceftazidime (Fortaz), ceftriaxone (Rocephin), cefuroxime (Zinacef), chlorpromazine (Thorazine), ciprofloxacin (Cipro IV), clindamycin (Cleocin), dexamethasone (Decadron), diphenhydramine (Benadryl), dobutamine, dopamine, doripenem (Doribax), doxycycline, droperidol (Inapsine), enalaprilat (Vasotec IV), famotidine (Pepcid IV), fluconazole (Diflucan), furosemide (Lasix), ganciclovir (Cytovene), gemcitabine (Gemzar), gentamicin, granisetron (Kytril), haloperidol (Haldol), heparin, hydrocortisone sodium succinate (Solu-Cortef), hydromorphone (Dilaudid), imipenem-cilastatin (Primaxin), leucovorin calcium, lorazepam (Ativan), magnesium sulfate, mannitol, meperidine (Demerol), meropenem (Merrem IV), mesna (Mesnex), metoclopramide (Reglan), metronidazole (Flagyl IV), morphine, ondansetron (Zofran), oxaliplatin (Eloxatin), palonosetron (Aloxi), pemetrexed (Alimta), piperacillin, piperacillin/tazobactam (Zosyn), potassium chloride (KCl), prochlorperazine (Compazine), promethazine (Phenergan), ranitidine (Zantac), sodium bicarbonate, sulfamethoxazole/trimethoprim, ticarcillin/clavulanate (Timentin), tobramycin, vancomycin, zidovudine (AZT, Retrovir).

RATE OF ADMINISTRATION

A single dose, properly diluted, equally distributed over 1 hour. Room temperature should be cool and lighting should be low. Extended infusion times (e.g., 6 to 24 hours) or frequently repeated infusions (e.g., several days in a row) seem to increase the risk of dose-limiting mucositis.

ACTIONS

An antineoplastic. A novel, semisynthetic, antimicrotubule agent derived from the needles of the yew plant. It inhibits cancer cell division. Microtubules assemble and disassemble during the cell cycle. Docetaxel promotes assembly and blocks disassembly of microtubules, preventing the cancer cells from dividing. The end result is cancer cell death. May be up to twice as potent as paclitaxel; cross-resistance between docetaxel and paclitaxel does not occur consistently. Highly protein bound. Probably metabolized in the liver by isoenzymes of the P_{450} family. Half-life is 11.1 hours. Eliminated primarily through feces and, to a lesser extent, urine and bile.

INDICATIONS AND USES

Treatment of locally advanced or metastatic breast cancer after failure of prior chemotherapy. ■ In combination with doxorubicin and cyclophosphamide for adjuvant treatment of operable node-positive breast cancer. ■ As a single agent in the treatment of locally advanced or metastatic NSCLC after failure of platinum-based chemotherapy (e.g., cisplatin). ■ In combination with cisplatin for treatment of patients with unresectable, locally advanced, or metastatic NSCLC who have not previously received chemotherapy for this condition. ■ In combination with prednisone for the treatment of androgen-independent (hormone refractory) metastatic prostate cancer. ■ In combination with cisplatin and fluorouracil for the treatment of advanced gastric adenocarcinoma, including adenocarcinoma of the gastroesophageal junction, in patients who have not received prior chemotherapy for advanced disease. ■ In combination with cisplatin and fluorouracil for induction therapy of locally advanced SCCHN. Following chemotherapy, patients should receive radiotherapy.

Unlabeled uses: Treatment of small-cell lung cancer and ovarian cancer after first-line or platinum-based chemotherapy has failed. ■ Treatment of bladder cancer and esophageal cancer.

CONTRAINDICATIONS

Baseline neutropenia less than 1,500 cells/mm³, history of hypersensitivity reactions to docetaxel or other drugs formulated with polysorbate 80, severe impaired liver function. In the United States, docetaxel is not recommended for patients with a bilirubin above the ULN or in patients with ALT and/or AST greater than 1.5 times the ULN range and increases in alkaline phosphatase greater than 2.5 times the ULN range; see Precautions.

PRECAUTIONS

Follow guidelines for handling cytotoxic agents. See Appendix A, p. 1429. ■ Usually administered by or under direction of the physician specialist. ■ Adequate diagnostic and treatment facilities must be readily available. ■ Myelosuppression may be more frequent and more severe in patients who have received prior cytotoxic drug therapy or radiation therapy. ■ Incidence of febrile neutropenia and/or neutropenic infection increased in patients receiving docetaxel (Taxotere) in combination with cisplatin and fluorouracil (5-FU). ▪ Incidence of mortality increased in patients with abnormal liver function, in patients receiving higher doses, and in patients with NSCLC and a history of prior treatment with platinum-based chemotherapy who receive docetaxel as a single agent at a dose of 100 mg/M^2. ▪ Not recommended for patients with hepatic impairment; see Contraindications. If docetaxel is considered essential for a patient with mild hepatic impairment, initial doses of 60 to 75 mg/M^2 should be used. Risk of toxicity and death is significant. Patients with isolated elevations of transaminases greater than 1.5 times the ULN have a higher rate of adverse events but not of death. ▪ In addition to myelosuppression and hypersensitivity reactions, localized erythema of the extremities with edema followed by desquamation, severe fluid retention, severe neurosensory symptoms (e.g., dysesthesia, pain, paresthesia), and severe asthenia (usually in metastatic breast cancer patients) have been reported. Severe fluid retention may occur despite premedication with dexamethasone. ▪ Use with caution in patients with pleural effusion; may be exacerbated by docetaxel-induced fluid retention. ▪ Treatment-related acute myeloid leukemia (AML) or myelodysplasia has occurred in patients given docetaxel in combination with other chemotherapy agents and/or radiotherapy. ▪ When administering combination therapy, consult all appropriate drug monographs for relevant information. ▪ See Drug/Lab Interactions.

Monitor: Obtain baseline CBC with differential and platelets; monitor frequently during therapy and before each dose. See Dose Adjustments. ▪ Obtain baseline bilirubin, AST, ALT, and alkaline phosphatase; monitor as indicated during therapy (recommended before each dose). ▪ Determine absolute patency of vein. A stinging or burning sensation indicates extravasation; severe cellulitis and tissue necrosis may result. Discontinue injection; use another vein. ▪ Obtain baseline vital signs, monitor during and for at least 1 hour following infusion. ▪ Monitor for hypersensitivity reactions; may occur within minutes. Discontinue docetaxel if reaction is severe (e.g., bronchospasm, hypotension, generalized rash/erythema). Hypersensitivity reactions may occur even in patients premedicated with dexamethasone. Continue monitoring for a minimum of 1 hour following the infusion, especially during the first two treatment cycles. ▪ Monitor for localized erythema of the palms of the hands and soles of the feet with or without desquamation. A reduced dose may be indicated if severe. ▪ Monitor for fluid retention. Severe salt restriction and treatment with oral diuretics may be indicated. S/S of severe fluid retention include abdominal distention (severe), cardiac tamponade, dyspnea at rest, peripheral or generalized edema, pleural effusion. ▪ Observe for signs of peripheral neurotoxicity (e.g., dysesthesia, pain, paresthesia, weakness); docetaxel may need to be discontinued; see Dose Adjustments. In patients with gastric adenocarcinoma or SCCHN, a baseline neurologic exam is recommended. Repeat every 2 cycles and at the end of treatment; see Dose Adjustments. ▪ Observe for signs of infection. Use of prophylactic antibiotics may be indicated pending C/S in a febrile, neutropenic patient. Monitor patients receiving docetaxel (Taxotere), cisplatin, fluorouracil (5-FU) combination therapy closely for febrile neutropenia and/or neutropenic infection. ▪ Not highly emetogenic; routine prophylaxis with antiemetics may not be required. ▪ Monitor for thrombocytopenia (platelet count less than 50,000/mm^3); see Dose Adjustments. Initiate precautions to prevent excessive bleeding (e.g., inspect IV sites, skin, and mucous membranes; use extreme care during invasive procedures; test urine, emesis, stool, and secretions for occult blood).

Patient Education: Avoid pregnancy; nonhormonal birth control recommended. ▪ Review of monitoring requirements (e.g., CBCs, liver function tests) and adverse events before therapy imperative. ▪ Pretreatment with dexamethasone as prescribed is imperative. ▪ Report pain or burning at injection site and any unusual or unexpected symptoms or side effects as soon as possible (e.g., constipation, fever, hypersensitivity reaction [e.g., difficulty breathing, itching, rash], nausea and vomiting, shortness of breath, swelling of feet and legs, weight gain). ▪ May produce significant hypotension. Effects may be additive with current medications. Review all medications (prescription and nonprescription) with nurse and/or physician. ▪ See Appendix D, p. 1434. ▪ Obtain name and telephone number of a contact person for emergencies, questions, or problems. ▪ Seek resources for counseling or supportive therapy. ▪ Risk of delayed myelodysplasia or myeloid leukemia requires hematologic follow-up. Changes in blood counts due to leukemia and other blood disorders may occur years after treatment.

Maternal/Child: Category D: avoid pregnancy, may cause fetal harm. ▪ Discontinue breast-feeding. ▪ Safety for use in pediatric patients under 16 years of age not established. A colony-stimulating factor (e.g., filgrastim, sargramostim) has been used to reduce neutropenia and increase tolerance of the maximum dose.

Elderly: Dose selection should be cautious; see Dose Adjustments. ▪ May be at increased risk for developing side effects such as anemia, anorexia, diarrhea, dizziness, febrile neutropenia, infections, lethargy, peripheral edema, stomatitis, and weight loss. ▪ Monitor hepatic function carefully.

DRUG/LAB INTERACTIONS

Metabolism inhibited and serum levels increased with **strong CYP3A4 inhibitors** (e.g., imidazole antifungals [e.g., itraconazole (Sporanox), ketoconazole (Nizoral), voriconazole (VFEND)], protease inhibitors [e.g., atazanavir (Reyataz), indinavir (Crixivan), nelfinavir (Viracept), ritonavir (Norvir), saquinavir (Invirase)], clarithromycin [Biaxin], nefazodone, and telithromycin [Ketek]). Avoid use. A pharmacokinetic study suggests considering a 50% dose reduction of docetaxel if coadministration of a strong CYP3A4 inhibitor is required; monitor closely for toxicity. ▪ Metabolism of docetaxel may be modified by **other agents that induce, inhibit, or are metabolized by CYP3A4** (e.g., cyclosporine [Sandimmune], phenytoin [Dilantin], phenobarbital [Luminal], tacrolimus [Prograf], and many others). ▪ Additive bone marrow suppression may occur with **radiation therapy and/or other bone marrow–suppressing agents** (e.g., azathioprine [Imuran], chloramphenicol, melphalan [Alkeran]). Dose reduction may be required. ▪ Leukopenic and/or thrombocytopenic effects may be increased with **drugs that cause blood dyscrasias** (e.g., anticonvulsants [e.g., carbamazepine (Tegretol), phenytoin (Dilantin)], NSAIDs [e.g., ibuprofen (Advil, Motrin), naproxen (Aleve, Naprosyn)]). Adjust dose based on differential and platelet count. ▪ Risk of infection is increased with concurrent use of **other immunosuppressants** (e.g., azathioprine, chlorambucil [Leukeran], cyclophosphamide [Cytoxan], cyclosporine [Sandimmune], glucocorticoid corticosteroids [e.g., dexamethasone], muromonab CD-3 [Orthoclone], tacrolimus [Prograf]). ▪ Do not administer **live virus vaccines** to patients receiving antineoplastic agents.

SIDE EFFECTS

Generally reversible but can be fatal. Most common side effects across all indications are alopecia, anemia, anorexia, asthenia, constipation, diarrhea, dysgeusia, dyspnea, febrile neutropenia, fluid retention (e.g., ascites, edema, pericardial effusion, pleural effusion), hypersensitivity reactions (e.g., back pain, chest tightness, chills, drug fever, dyspnea, flushing, hypotension, pruritus, rash), infection, mucositis, myalgia, nail disorders, nausea, neuropathy, neutropenia, pain, skin reactions, thrombocytopenia, and vomiting. Increased incidence of bone marrow suppression (anemia, leukopenia, neutropenia, thrombocytopenia) and/or severity of side effects is dose dependent and can be dose limiting. Abdominal pain; acute myeloid leukemia and myelodysplasic syndrome; acute pulmonary edema; acute respiratory distress syndrome; altered hearing; amenorrhea; arthralgia; bleeding episodes; cardiac arrhythmias; CHF; colitis; confusion; conjunctivitis; cough; cutaneous reactions (e.g., localized rash on hands, feet, arms, face, thorax; erythema multiforme; severe hand and foot syndrome; Stevens-Johnson syndrome; toxic epidermal necrolysis); diarrhea; DIC (often in association with sepsis or multi-organ failure); dizziness; enteritis; esophagitis/dysphagia/odynophagia; fatigue; fever with or without infection; gastrointestinal pain and cramping; heartburn; hepatitis (sometimes fatal, primarily in patients with pre-existing liver disease); hypotension; increased ALT, AST, and bilirubin; infusion site reactions; interstitial pneumonia; lethargy; lymphedema; myocardial ischemia; neurosensory symptoms (e.g., dysesthesia, pain, paresthesia); neutropenic infection; paresthesias (e.g., pain, burning sensation); perforation of the large intestine; renal insufficiency; seizures or transient loss of consciousness; stomatitis; taste perversion; tearing; vasodilation.

Overdose: Bone marrow suppression, mucositis, peripheral neurotoxicity.

Post-Marketing: Deep vein thrombosis, dehydration, duodenal ulcer, dyspnea, esophagitis, GI hemorrhage, ileus, intestinal obstruction, ischemic colitis, MI, neutropenic enterocolitis, pulmonary embolism, pulmonary fibrosis, radiation pneumonitis, radiation recall phenomenon, renal failure (most commonly associated with concomitant nephrotoxic drugs), scleroderma-like changes (usually preceded by peripheral lymphedema), thrombophlebitis, transient visual disturbances.

ANTIDOTE

Keep physician informed of all side effects. Most will be treated symptomatically as indicated. Most hypersensitivity reactions will subside with temporary discontinuation of docetaxel, and incidence seems to decrease with subsequent doses. Severe reactions may require epinephrine (Adrenalin), antihistamines (e.g., diphenhydramine [Benadryl]), corticosteroids (e.g., dexamethasone [Decadron]), or bronchodilators (e.g., albuterol [Ventolin], theophylline [Aminophylline]). Rechallenge may be considered if there is objective tumor response and no other options. Aggressive premedication (adding cromolyn 400 mg PO four times daily has helped some patients) and reduction in rate of administration may allow continued treatment. Neutropenia can be profound and the nadir usually occurs about day 8. Recovery is generally rapid and spontaneous but may be treated with filgrastim (G-CSF, Neupogen) or pegfilgrastim (Neulasta). Severe thrombocytopenia may require platelet transfusions or treatment with oprelvekin (Neumega) may be indicated. Severe anemia (less than 8 Gm/dL) may require packed cell transfusions; moderate anemia (less than 11 Gm/dL) may be treated with darbepoetin alfa [Aranesp] or epoetin alfa (Epogen). Hypotension and bradycardia do not usually occur at the same time except in hypersensitivity. Treat only if symptomatic. Treat any serious or symptomatic arrhythmia (e.g., conduction abnormalities, ventricular tachycardia) promptly and monitor continuously during subsequent doses. Serious cutaneous reactions with desquamation (rare), serious fluid retention (more frequent with cumulative doses of 1,300 mg/M^2), persistent febrile neutropenia, severe peripheral neuropathy, or severe liver impairment may require discontinuation of docetaxel. Cutaneous reactions (palmar-plantar erythrodysesthesia) that occur despite prophylaxis may respond to pyridoxine 50 mg three times daily. There is no specific antidote for overdose. Supportive therapy will help sustain the patient in toxicity. Resuscitate if indicated.

DOLASETRON MESYLATE
(dohl-**AH**-seh-tron **MES**-ih-layt)

Anzemet

Antiemetic
(5HT$_3$ receptor antagonist)

pH 3.2 to 3.8

USUAL DOSE
Prevention of postoperative nausea and/or vomiting: 12.5 mg as a single dose 15 minutes before cessation of anesthesia.

Treatment of postoperative nausea and/or vomiting: 12.5 mg as a single dose as soon as nausea or vomiting presents.

PEDIATRIC DOSE
Doses are those recommended for *pediatric patients 2 to 16 years of age.* Safety and effectiveness in pediatric patients under 2 years of age not established; see Contraindications and Maternal/Child. Dolasetron solution for injection may be mixed with apple or apple-grape juice for oral administration to pediatric patients. See prescribing information for oral doses.

Prevention of postoperative nausea and/or vomiting: 0.35 mg/kg up to a maximum dose of 12.5 mg as a single dose 15 minutes before cessation of anesthesia.

Treatment of postoperative nausea and/or vomiting: 0.35 mg/kg up to a maximum dose of 12.5 mg as a single dose as soon as nausea or vomiting presents.

DOSE ADJUSTMENTS
No dose adjustments required for the elderly, renal failure, or impaired hepatic function; however, caution and lower-end dosing is suggested in elderly patients. Consider decreased organ function and concomitant disease or drug therapy.

DILUTION
IV injection: A single dose may be given undiluted.

IV infusion: A single dose may be further diluted up to 50 mL in NS, D5W, D5/½NS, D5LR, LR, or 10% mannitol.

Storage: Store vials at CRT; protect from light. Stable after dilution at CRT for 24 hours or 48 hours if refrigerated.

COMPATIBILITY   (Underline Indicates Conflicting Compatibility Information)

Consider any drug NOT listed as compatible to be INCOMPATIBLE until consulting a pharmacist; specific conditions may apply.

Manufacturer states, "Should not be mixed with other drugs. Flush the infusion line with a **compatible** IV solution before and after administration."

One source suggests the following **compatibilities:**

Y-site: Azithromycin (Zithromax), caspofungin (Cancidas), dexmedetomidine (Precedex), fenoldopam (Corlopam), hetastarch in electrolytes (Hextend), and oxaliplatin (Eloxatin).

RATE OF ADMINISTRATION

Flush infusion line before and after administration. May cause bradycardia, severe hypotension, and syncope during or shortly after administration.

IV injection: A single dose over 30 seconds.

IV infusion: Administer a single dose over 15 minutes.

ACTIONS

An antinauseant and antiemetic agent. A selective antagonist of specific serotonin (5-HT$_3$) receptors, similar to granisetron and ondansetron. Chemotherapeutic agents such as cisplatin increase the release of serotonin from specific cells in the GI tract, causing emesis. By antagonizing these receptors, chemotherapy-induced nausea and vomiting are prevented. Rapidly and completely metabolized to its active metabolite, hydrodolasetron. Hydrodolasetron is widely distributed throughout the body. Maximum concentration occurs 0.6 hours after injection or infusion. Average half-life is 7.3 hours. Plasma clearance increased and half-life reduced in pediatric patients, more so in younger pediatric patients. Excreted in urine and feces. Not known if dolasetron is secreted in breast milk.

INDICATIONS AND USES

Prevention of postoperative nausea and vomiting when indicated. ▪ Treatment of postoperative nausea and/or vomiting. Also available in tablet form.

Unlabeled uses: Prophylaxis and treatment of radiotherapy-induced nausea and vomiting.

CONTRAINDICATIONS

Known hypersensitivity to dolasetron. ▪ Contraindicated in adult and pediatric patients for the prevention of nausea and vomiting associated with initial and repeat courses of emetogenic cancer chemotherapy because of risk for dose-dependent QTc prolongation.

PRECAUTIONS

Prolongs the QT interval in a dose-dependent fashion. Torsades de pointes has been reported. Avoid use in patients with congenital long QT syndrome, hypokalemia, or hypomagnesemia. ▪ Has been shown to cause dose-dependent prolongation of the PR and QRS interval. Second- or third-degree atrioventricular block, cardiac arrest, and serious ventricular arrhythmias, including fatalities in both adult and pediatric patients, have been reported. At particular risk are patients with underlying structural heart disease, pre-existing conduction system abnormalities, sick sinus syndrome, atrial fibrillation with slow ventricular response, or myocardial ischemia, elderly patients, or patients receiving drugs known to prolong the PR interval (such as verapamil) and QRS interval (e.g., flecainide [Tambocor] or quinidine); use with caution and monitor ECG. Avoid use in patients with or at risk for complete heart block unless they have an implanted pacemaker. ▪ Use with caution in patients who have or may develop prolongation of cardiac conduction intervals, particularly QT intervals (e.g., patients with hypokalemia, hypomagnesemia, congenital QT syndrome, cumulative high-dose anthracycline therapy [e.g., doxorubicin (Adriamycin)], patients taking diuretics with potential for inducing electrolyte abnormalities [e.g., furosemide (Lasix), hydrochlorothiazide] or antiarrhythmic drugs or other drugs that lead to QT prolongation [amiodarone (Nexterone), procainamide (Pronestyl), quinidine]). ▪ Cross-sensitivity has been reported in patients who received other selective $5HT_3$-receptor agonists (e.g., granisetron [Kytril], ondansetron [Zofran]). These reactions have not been seen with dolasetron. ▪ Available in tablet form. ▪ See Contraindications, Maternal/Child, Drug/Lab Interactions, and Side Effects.

Monitor: Observe closely. Monitor VS. Any patient found to have a second-degree or higher AV conduction block should be monitored continuously. ▪ Correct hypokalemia and hypomagnesemia before administration of dolasetron. Monitor after administration as clinically indicated. ▪ Monitor ECG in patients with CHF and bradycardia and in all patients at risk for prolongation of the PR and QRS interval; see Precautions. ▪ Ambulate slowly to avoid orthostatic hypotension.

Patient Education: Request assistance for ambulation. ▪ May cause serious cardiac arrhythmias; discuss medical history with physician and promptly report a perceived change in heart rate, fainting, or light-headedness. ▪ Report promptly if nausea persists. ▪ Maintain adequate hydration. ▪ Review prescription medications with health care provider.

Maternal/Child: Category B: no evidence of impaired fertility or harm to fetus. Use during pregnancy only if clearly needed. ▪ Use caution if required during breast-feeding. ▪ See Contraindications. ▪ Safety and effectiveness for use in pediatric patients under 2 years of age not established. ▪ Plasma clearance increased and half-life reduced in pediatric patients, more so in younger pediatric patients. ▪ Use caution in pediatric patients who have or may develop prolongation of cardiac conduction intervals, particularly QTc. Rare cases of sustained supraventricular and ventricular arrhythmias, MI, and cardiac arrest leading to death have been reported in pediatric and adolescent patients.

Elderly: Use with caution and continuous ECG monitoring in the elderly; they are at paricular risk for prolongation of the PR, QRS, and QT interval. ▪ See Dose Adjustments and Contraindications.

DRUG/LAB INTERACTIONS

Does not induce or inhibit the cytochrome P_{450} drug metabolizing system, but metabolism of its active metabolite, hydrodolasetron, is mediated by enzymes in the P_{450} system. Plasma levels increased when given concurrently with **cimetidine** (Tagamet [inhibitor of cytochrome P_{450}]), and decreased when given concurrently with **rifampin** (Rifadin [inducer of cytochrome P_{450}]); clinical significance not known. ▪ Clearance decreased when given concurrently with **atenolol.** ▪ See Precautions and use extreme caution with **diuretics** with potential for inducing electrolyte abnormalities (e.g., furosemide [Lasix], hydrochlorothiazide [Hydrodiuril]) **or antiarrhythmic drugs or other drugs that lead to prolonged QT intervals** (e.g., amiodarone [Nexterone], procainamide [Pronestyl], quinidine). ▪ Clearance not affected by **ACE inhibitors** (e.g., enalaprilat), **calcium channel blockers** (e.g., diltiazem [Cardizem], nifedipine [Procardia], verapamil), **glyburide**

(DiaBeta), and **propranolol** (Inderal). ▪ Does not influence anesthesia recovery time.

SIDE EFFECTS

May cause bradycardia, severe hypotension, and syncope during or shortly after administration. Can cause ECG interval changes (PR, QT, JT prolongation, and QRS widening). These changes may lead to cardiovascular consequences (e.g., cardiac arrhythmias, heart block). Usually self-limiting with declining blood levels, but may last as long as 24 hours.

Dizziness, drowsiness, headache, pain, and urinary retention are most common. Sinus arrhythmia, hypotension, orthostatic hypotension, and numerous other side effects may occur in fewer than 2% of patients.

Overdose: Severe hypotension and dizziness.

Post-Marketing: Wide complex tachycardia, VT, VF, and cardiac arrest have been reported rarely.

ANTIDOTE

Most side effects will be treated symptomatically. Keep physician informed. Overdose in one patient was treated with plasma expanders (e.g., albumin, dextran), dopamine, atropine, and continuous BP and ECG monitoring. Epinephrine, atropine, and/or cardiac pacing may be required to treat ECG interval changes. Prolonged QT interval may lead to VT or other ventricular arrhythmias; telemetry monitoring may be indicated. There is no specific antidote. Treat anaphylaxis and resuscitate as necessary. Not known if dolasetron is removed by hemodialysis.

DOPAMINE HYDROCHLORIDE [BBW]
(**DOH**-pah-meen hy-droh-**KLOR**-eyed)

Inotropic agent
Cardiac stimulant
Vasopressor

pH 2.5 to 5

USUAL DOSE

Adults: 2 to 5 mcg/kg of body weight/min initially in patients likely to respond to minimum treatment. 5 to 10 mcg/kg/min may be required initially to correct hypotension in the seriously ill patient. Gradually increase by 5 to 10 mcg/kg/min at 10- to 30-minute intervals until optimum response occurs. Average dose is 20 mcg/kg/min; over 50 mcg/kg/min has been required in some instances but is not recommended. If more than 20 mcg/kg/min is required to maintain BP, consider use of norepinephrine (Levophed) in addition. Doses over 20 mcg/kg/min decrease renal perfusion.

PEDIATRIC DOSE

See Maternal/Child. Note comments in Usual Dose and those under another source below. Usual starting dose is 1 to 5 mcg/kg/min. Dose increments range from 2.5 to 5 mcg/kg/min. Usual maximum dose is 15 to 20 mcg/kg/min. Doses up to 50 mcg/kg/min have been administered. Titrate dose gradually to desired effect.

Continued

Another source suggests:
Low dose: 2 to 5 mcg/kg/min; increases renal blood flow with minimal effect on HR and cardiac output.
Intermediate dose: 5 to 15 mcg/kg/min; increases HR, cardiac contractility, cardiac output and, to a lesser extent, renal blood flow.
High dose: Doses equal to or greater than 20 mcg/kg/min; alpha adrenergic effects are prominent; decreases renal perfusion. Maximum dose recommended is 50 mcg/kg/min.

DOSE ADJUSTMENTS
Reduce dose to one tenth of the calculated amount for individuals being treated with MAO inhibitors (e.g., selegiline [Eldepryl]) and drugs with MAO-inhibiting effects (e.g., furazolidone [Furoxone]). ▪ Lower-end initial doses may be appropriate in the elderly based on potential for decreased organ function and concomitant disease or drug therapy. ▪ See Drug/Lab Interactions.

DILUTION
Each 5- or 10-mL (200-mg, 400-mg, or 800-mg) ampule must be diluted in 250 to 500 mL of the following IV solutions and given as an infusion: NS, D5W, D5NS, D5/½NS, D5LR, ⅙ M sodium lactate, or LR injection. See the following chart.

mcg/mL of Dopamine Concentrations of 40 mg/mL and 80 mg/mL in Various Volumes of Diluent		
Concentration of Dopamine	**40 mg/mL**	**80 mg/mL**
Volume of Dopamine	**5 mL (200 mg)** **10 mL (400 mg)**	**10 mL (800 mg)**
250 mL diluent	800 mcg/mL 1,600 mcg/mL	3,200 mcg/mL
500 mL diluent	400 mcg/mL 800 mcg/mL	1,600 mcg/mL
1,000 mL diluent	200 mcg/mL 400 mcg/mL	800 mcg/mL

Available prediluted in 250 mL or 500 mL of D5W. Dopamine content varies. More concentrated solutions may be used if absolutely necessary to reduce fluid volume. Also available as 160 mg/mL to be added to 100 mL of diluent (1,600 mcg/mL); may be used in patients with fluid retention or those requiring a very slow rate of infusion.
Pediatric dilution: 6 mg/kg in 100 mL D5W. 1 mL/hr equals 1 mcg/kg/min.
Storage: Discard diluted solution after 24 hours.

COMPATIBILITY   (Underline Indicates Conflicting Compatibility Information)
Consider any drug NOT listed as compatible to be INCOMPATIBLE until consulting a pharmacist; specific conditions may apply.
Manufacturer states, "Do not add to sodium bicarbonate or any other strongly alkaline solution (e.g., aminophylline, barbiturates [e.g., thiopental (Pentothal)]), oxidizing agents, or iron salts. Dopamine is inactivated in alkaline solution."
    One source suggests the following **compatibilities:**
Additive: Aminophylline, atracurium (Tracrium), calcium chloride, chloramphenicol (Chloromycetin), ciprofloxacin (Cipro IV), dobutamine, enalaprilat (Vasotec IV), flumazenil (Romazicon), gentamicin, heparin, hydrocortisone sodium succinate (Solu-Cortef), kanamycin (Kantrex), lidocaine, meropenem (Merrem IV), methylprednisolone (Solu-Medrol),

nitroglycerin IV, oxacillin (Bactocill), potassium chloride (KCl), ranitidine (Zantac), verapamil.

Y-site: Aldesleukin (Proleukin), alprostadil, amifostine (Ethyol), amiodarone (Nexterone), anidulafungin (Eraxis), argatroban, atracurium (Tracrium), aztreonam (Azactam), bivalirudin (Angiomax), caspofungin (Cancidas), cefepime (Maxipime), ceftazidime (Fortaz), ciprofloxacin (Cipro IV), cisatracurium (Nimbex), cladribine (Leustatin), daptomycin (Cubicin), dexmedetomidine (Precedex), diltiazem (Cardizem), dobutamine, docetaxel (Taxotere), doxorubicin liposomal (Doxil), enalaprilat (Vasotec IV), epinephrine (Adrenalin), esmolol (Brevibloc), etoposide phosphate (Etopophos), famotidine (Pepcid IV), fenoldopam (Corlopam), fentanyl (Sublimaze), fluconazole (Diflucan), foscarnet (Foscavir), furosemide (Lasix), gemcitabine (Gemzar), granisetron (Kytril), haloperidol (Haldol), heparin, hetastarch in electrolytes (Hextend), hydrocortisone sodium succinate (Solu-Cortef), hydromorphone (Dilaudid), inamrinone (Amrinone), labetalol (Trandate), levofloxacin (Levaquin), lidocaine, linezolid (Zyvox), lorazepam (Ativan), meperidine (Demerol), methylprednisolone (Solu-Medrol), metronidazole (Flagyl IV), micafungin (Mycamine), midazolam (Versed), milrinone (Primacor), morphine, mycophenolate (CellCept IV), nicardipine (Cardene IV), nitroglycerin IV, nitroprusside sodium, norepinephrine (Levophed), ondansetron (Zofran), oxaliplatin (Eloxatin), pancuronium, pantoprazole (Protonix IV), pemetrexed (Alimta), piperacillin/tazobactam (Zosyn), potassium chloride (KCl), propofol (Diprivan), ranitidine (Zantac), remifentanil (Ultiva), sargramostim (Leukine), tacrolimus (Prograf), theophylline, thiotepa, tigecycline (Tygacil), tirofiban (Aggrastat), vasopressin, vecuronium, verapamil, warfarin (Coumadin), zidovudine (AZT, Retrovir).

RATE OF ADMINISTRATION
Begin with recommended dose for body weight and seriousness of condition. Gradually increase by 5 to 10 mcg/kg of body weight/min to effect desired response. Use slowest possible rate to maintain adequate or preset systolic BP. Use a microdrip (60 gtt/mL) or an infusion pump for accuracy. Optimum urine flow determines correct evaluation of dosage. Decrease dose gradually; may cause marked hypotension if discontinued suddenly. Expansion of blood volume with IV fluids may be indicated.

Dopamine Infusion Rate (mL/hr) 400 mcg/mL Concentration						
Desired Dose	Weight in Kilograms					
	50 kg	60 kg	70 kg	80 kg	90 kg	100 kg
	(mL/hr)	(mL/hr)	(mL/hr)	(mL/hr)	(mL/hr)	(mL/hr)
5 mcg/kg/min	37.5	45	52.5	60	67.5	75
10 mcg/kg/min	75	90	105	120	135	150
20 mcg/kg/min	150	180	210	240	270	300
30 mcg/kg/min	225	270	315	360	405	450
40 mcg/kg/min	300	360	420	480	540	600

Dopamine Infusion Rate (mL/hr) 800 mcg/mL Concentration						
Desired Dose	Weight in Kilograms					
	50 kg	60 kg	70 kg	80 kg	90 kg	100 kg
	(mL/hr)	(mL/hr)	(mL/hr)	(mL/hr)	(mL/hr)	(mL/hr)
5 mcg/kg/min	18.75	22.5	26.25	30	33.75	37.5
10 mcg/kg/min	37.5	45	52.5	60	67.5	75
20 mcg/kg/min	75	90	105	120	135	150
30 mcg/kg/min	112.5	135	157.5	180	202.5	225
40 mcg/kg/min	150	180	210	240	270	300

ACTIONS

Dopamine is a chemical precursor of norepinephrine, possessing alpha, beta, and dopaminergic receptor–stimulating actions. Increases cardiac output with minimum increase in myocardial oxygen consumption. Dilates renal and mesenteric blood vessels at doses lower than those required to elevate systolic BP. Therapeutic doses effect little change on diastolic BP. Doses over 10 mcg/kg/min may cause peripheral vasoconstriction and marked increases in pulmonary occlusive pressure. Has short duration of action. Metabolized by monoamine oxidase (MAO) catechol O-methyltransferase (COMT) to inactive metabolites and is promptly excreted in the urine.

INDICATIONS AND USES

To correct hemodynamic imbalances, including hypotension resulting from shock syndrome of myocardial infarction, trauma, endotoxic septicemia, open heart surgery, renal failure, and chronic cardiac decompensation. ▪ Drug of choice for hypotension and shock. ▪ AHA guidelines recommend dopamine as the second drug of choice after atropine to treat symptomatic bradycardia.

Unlabeled uses: Chronic obstructive pulmonary disease (4 mcg/kg/min), congestive heart failure (2 to 5 mcg/kg/min), infant respiratory distress syndrome (begin at 5 mcg/kg/min). Low-dose dopamine has been used postoperatively to protect the kidneys of surgical patients from inflammatory insults, ischemia, and nephrotoxicity.

CONTRAINDICATIONS

Hypersensitivity to any components (contains sulfites), pheochromocytoma, uncorrected tachyarrhythmias, ventricular fibrillation.

PRECAUTIONS

Some preparations contain sulfites; use caution in patients with allergies. ▪ Use caution in patients with a history of occlusive vascular disease.

Monitor: Recognition of signs and symptoms and prompt treatment with dopamine will improve prognosis. ▪ Check BP every 2 minutes until stabilized at the desired level. Check every 5 minutes thereafter during therapy. Avoid hypertension. If possible, check central venous pressure or pulmonary wedge pressure before administration and as ordered thereafter. ▪ Use larger veins (antecubital fossa) and avoid extravasation; may cause necrosis and sloughing of tissue. Central vein preferred for continuous infusions; see Antidote. ▪ If possible, correct hypovolemia with IV fluids, whole blood or plasma as indicated; correct acidosis if present. ■ Monitor for decreased urine output, increased tachycardia, or new arrhythmias. ■ With high-dose administration, palpate pulses and monitor extremities for signs of peripheral vasoconstriction (e.g., coldness, paresthesias). ■ Therapy may be continued until the patient can maintain hemodynamic and renal functions. ■ See Maternal/Child and Drug/Lab Interactions.

Maternal/Child: Category C: safety for use in pregnancy and breast-feeding not established. If used benefits must outweigh risks. ■ Safety for use in pediatric patients not established. Has been used, but experience is limited. ■ Clearance is affected by age, renal and hepatic function. In younger children, particularly neonates, clearance is highly variable. Newborn infants may be more sensitive to the vasoconstrictive effects of dopamine. Close hemodynamic monitoring required. ■ Do not administer into an umbilical arterial catheter. Vasospastic events have been reported when dopamine is infused through an umbilical vessel.

Elderly: Lower-end initial doses may be appropriate; see Dose Adjustments. ■ Differences in response compared to younger adults not identified.

DRUG/LAB INTERACTIONS

Alkaline solutions, including sodium bicarbonate, inactivate dopamine. ■ May cause serious arrhythmias in presence of **cyclopropane or halogen anesthetics,** severe hypertension with **oxytocic drugs** (e.g., methylergonovine [Methergine] or oxytocin). ■ May cause hypertensive crisis with **MAO inhibitors** (e.g., selegiline [Eldepryl]). ■ Antagonizes effects of **guanethidine** (Ismelin). ■ Some effects may be antagonized by **alpha- or beta-blocking agents** (e.g., labetalol [Trandate], propranolol [Inderal]). ■ Pressor response may be decreased by **tricyclic antidepressants;** increased doses of dopamine may be required. ■ Will cause severe bradycardia and hypotension with **phenytoin** (Dilantin). ■ See Dose Adjustments.

SIDE EFFECTS

Aberrant conduction, anginal pain, azotemia, bradycardia, dyspnea, ectopic beats, headache, hypertension, hypotension, nausea, palpitation, piloerection, tachycardia, vasoconstriction, vomiting, widened QRS complex.

ANTIDOTE

Notify the physician of all side effects. Decrease infusion rate and notify the physician immediately for decrease in established urine flow rate, disproportionate rise in diastolic BP, increasing tachycardia, or new arrhythmias. For accidental overdosage with hypertension, reduce rate or temporarily discontinue until condition stabilizes. Phentolamine may be required. To prevent sloughing and necrosis in areas where extravasation has occurred, use a fine hypodermic needle to inject 5 to 10 mg of phentolamine (Regitine) diluted in 10 to 15 mL normal saline liberally throughout the tissue in the extravasated area. Begin as soon as extravasation is recognized.

DORIPENEM
(**DOR**-i-**PEN**-em)
Doribax

Antibacterial
(carbapenem)
pH 4.5 to 5.5

USUAL DOSE

500 mg every 8 hours. Duration of therapy is based on diagnosis as listed in the following chart.

Doripenem Dosing Guidelines			
Infection	Dosage	Frequency	Duration
Complicated intra-abdominal infection	500 mg	q 8 hr	5-14 days*
Complicated UTI, including pyelonephritis	500 mg	q 8 hr	10 days†

*Duration includes a possible switch to an appropriate oral therapy after at least 3 days of parenteral therapy and once clinical improvement has been demonstrated.
†Duration can be extended up to 14 days for patients with concurrent bacteremia.

DOSE ADJUSTMENTS

Reduced doses are indicated based on degree of renal insufficiency as noted in the following chart.

Dosage of Doripenem in Patients with Renal Impairment	
Estimated CrCl (mL/min)	Recommended Dosage Regimen
>50 mL/min	No dosage adjustment necessary
≥30 to ≤50 mL/min	250 mg q 8 hr
>10 to <30 mL/min	250 mg q 12 hr

No dose adjustment indicated based on age, gender, race, or impaired hepatic function. ▪ Dosing should be cautious in the elderly, and reduced doses may be indicated based on the potential for decreased renal function. ▪ There is insufficient information to make dose adjustment recommendations for patients undergoing hemodialysis.

DILUTION

Reconstitute a 500-mg vial with 10 mL of SW or NS. Shake gently to form a suspension with a resultant concentration of 50 mg/mL. **Caution: The reconstituted suspension is not for direct injection.** Withdraw the suspension using a syringe with a 21-gauge needle and add it to an infusion bag containing 100 mL of NS or D5W. Shake gently until clear. The final infusion solution concentration is 4.5 mg/mL. To prepare a 250-mg dose, follow the directions above. Remove 55 mL from the infusion bag that contains the 500-mg dose of doripenem diluted in NS or D5W and discard. The remaining solution will contain 250 mg of doripenem at a concentration of 4.5 mg/mL. According to the manufacturer, this is the way the 250-mg dose was prepared in clinical trials. Alternately to prevent waste, you could prepare 2 doses (one for immediate use and one for use in 8 hours) by dividing the 10 mL of reconstituted solution in half and adding each 5 mL of reconstituted solution to 50 mL of NS or D5W. Refrigerate the unused dose; see Storage.

Storage: Store unopened vial at CRT. Reconstituted vials are stable for 1 hour prior to transfer to an infusion bag. Infusion solutions diluted in NS are stable for 12 hours at RT and 72 hours refrigerated. Infusion solutions diluted in D5W are stable for 4 hours at RT and 24 hours refrigerated. (Times noted above reflect storage and infusion time.) Do not freeze infusion solutions.

COMPATIBILITY   (Underline Indicates Conflicting Compatibility Information)
Consider any drug NOT listed as compatible to be INCOMPATIBLE until consulting a pharmacist; specific conditions may apply.
Manufacturer states, "Should not be mixed with or physically added to solutions containing other drugs."

One source suggests the following **compatibilities:**
Y-site: Acyclovir (Zovirax), amikacin (Amikin), aminophylline, amiodarone (Nexterone), amphotericin B (generic), amphotericin B cholesteryl (Amphotec), amphotericin B lipid complex (Abelcet), amphotericin B liposomal (AmBisone), anidulafungin (Eraxis), atropine, azithromycin (Zithromax), bumetanide, calcium gluconate, carboplatin (Paraplatin), caspofungin (Cancidas), ciprofloxacin (Cipro IV), cisplatin (Platinol), cyclophosphamide (Cytoxan), cyclosporine (Sandimmune), daptomycin (Cubicin), dexamethasone (Decadron), digoxin (Lanoxin), diltiazem (Cardizem), diphenhydramine (Benadryl), dobutamine, docetaxel (Taxotere), dopamine, doxorubicin (Adriamycin), enalprilat (Vasotec IV), esmolol (Brevibloc), esomeprazole (Nexium IV), etoposide phosphate (Etopophos), famotidine (Pepcid IV), fentanyl (Sublimaze), fluconazole (Diflucan), fluorouracil (5-FU), foscarnet (Foscavir), furosemide (Lasix), gemcitabine (Gemzar), gentamicin, granisetron (Kytril), heparin, hydrocortisone sodium succinate (Solu-Cortef), hydromorphone (Dilaudid), ifosfamide (Ifex), insulin, labetalol (Trandate), levofloxacin (Levaquin), linezolid (Zyvox), lorazepam (Ativan), magnesium sulfate, mannitol (Osmitrol), meperidine (Demerol), methotrexate, methylprednisolone (Solu-Medrol), metoclopramide (Reglan), metronidazole (Flagyl IV), micafungin (Mycamine), midazolam (Versed), milrinone (Primacor), morphine, moxifloxacin (Avelox), norepinephrine (Levophed), ondansetron (Zofran), paclitaxel (Taxol), pantoprazole (Protonix IV), phenobarbital (Luminal), phenylephrine (Neo-Synephrine), potassium chloride, ranitidine (Zantac), sodium bicarbonate, sodium phosphate, tacrolimus (Prograf), tigecycline (Tygacil), tobramycin, vancomycin, voriconazole (VFEND IV), zidovudine (AZT, Retrovir).

RATE OF ADMINISTRATION
A single dose as an infusion equally distributed over 1 hour.

ACTIONS
A synthetic, broad-spectrum, carbapenem antibiotic. Bactericidal to selected aerobic and anaerobic gram-positive and gram-negative bacteria. Bactericidal activity results from the inhibition of bacterial cell wall synthesis. Stable to hydrolysis by most beta-lactamases, including penicillinases and cephalosporinases produced by gram-positive and gram-negative bacteria, with the exception of carbapenem-hydrolyzing beta-lactamases. Less than 10% bound to plasma proteins. Penetrates into

several body fluids and tissues, including those at the site of infection for the approved indications. Metabolized via dehydropeptidase-I. Elimination half-life is approximately 1 hour. Primarily eliminated unchanged by the kidneys.

INDICATIONS AND USES

As a single agent for treatment of complicated intra-abdominal infections and complicated urinary tract infections, including pyelonephritis caused by susceptible strains of microorganisms.

CONTRAINDICATIONS

Known hypersensitivity to doripenem or to other carbapenems (e.g., ertapenem [Invanz], imipenem-cilastatin [Primaxin]). ▪ Anaphylactic reactions to beta-lactams (e.g., penicillins and cephalosporins); see Precautions.

PRECAUTIONS

To reduce the development of drug-resistant bacteria and maintain its effectiveness, doripenem should be used to treat or prevent only those infections proven or strongly suspected to be caused by bacteria. ▪ Culture and sensitivity studies are indicated to determine susceptibility of the causative organism to doripenem. ▪ Serious and occasionally fatal hypersensitivity reactions have been reported in patients receiving therapy with beta-lactams. More likely in patients with a history of sensitivity to multiple allergens; obtain a careful history. Cross-sensitivity is possible. ▪ Prolonged use may cause superinfection because of overgrowth of nonsusceptible organisms. ▪ *Clostridium difficile*–associated diarrhea (CDAD) has been reported. May range from mild diarrhea to fatal colitis. Consider in patients who present with diarrhea during or after treatment with doripenem. ▪ Although cross-resistance may occur, some isolates resistant to other carbapenems may be susceptible to doripenem. ▪ Pneumonitis has been reported when doripenem was used investigationally via inhalation. Do not administer doripenem by this route. ▪ See Drug/Lab Interactions.

Monitor: Baseline and periodic monitoring of renal function and CBC with differential may be beneficial. ▪ Monitor for early symptoms or hypersensitivity reactions. Emergency equipment must be readily available. ▪ Monitor IV site carefully and rotate as indicated. ▪ See Drug/Lab Interactions.

Patient Education: Promptly report S/S of hypersensitivity reaction or pain at injection site. ▪ Promptly report diarrhea or bloody stools that occur during treatment or up to several months after an antibiotic has been discontinued; may indicate CDAD and require treatment. ▪ Patients with a history of seizures should review medication profile with physician before taking doripenem; see Drug/Lab Interactions.

Maternal/Child: Category B: should be used during pregnancy and breast-feeding only if clearly needed. ▪ Safety and effectiveness for use in pediatric patients not established.

Elderly: Response similar to that seen in younger patients, but greater sensitivity of some older individuals cannot be ruled out. ▪ Dosing should be cautious in the elderly; see Dose Adjustments. ▪ Monitoring of renal function may be indicated.

DRUG/LAB INTERACTIONS

Carbapenems may reduce serum **valproic acid** concentrations to subtherapeutic levels, resulting in loss of seizure control. Monitor valproic acid levels. Consider alternative antibacterial therapy. If administration of doripenem is necessary, supplemental anticonvulsant therapy should be considered. ▪ Concurrent use with **probenecid** results in elevated doripenem plasma concentrations. Concurrent use is not recommended. ▪ Does not appear to induce or inhibit the major cytochrome P_{450} isoenzymes, so it should not affect the clearance of drugs that are metabolized by these pathways.

SIDE EFFECTS

The most common adverse reactions are diarrhea, headache, nausea, phlebitis, and rash (allergic rash, bullous dermatitis, erythema, erythema multiforme, macular/papular eruptions, urticaria). Other reactions may include anemia, CDAD, hepatic enzyme elevations, hypersensitivity reactions (including anaphylaxis), oral candidiasis, pruritus, renal impairment or failure, and vulvomycotic infection.

Post-Marketing: Anaphylaxis, interstitial pneumonia, leukopenia, neutropenia, seizures, Stevens-Johnson syndrome, and toxic epidermal necrolysis.

ANTIDOTE

Keep physician informed of all side effects. Most minor side effects will be treated symptomatically. Discontinue doripenem at the first sign of hypersensitivity. Treat hypersensitivity reactions as indicated; may require epinephrine, airway management, oxygen, IV fluids, antihistamines (e.g., diphenhydramine [Benadryl]), corticosteroids, (e.g., hydrocortisone sodium succinate [Solu-Cortef]) and pressor amines (e.g., dopamine). Treat CDAD with fluids, electrolytes, protein supplements, and oral vancomycin (Vancocin) or metronidazole (Flagyl) as indicated. In severe cases, surgical evaluation may be indicated. Doripenem is partially removed by hemodialysis.

DOXERCALCIFEROL

(**DOX**-err-kal-**sif**-er-ol)

Hectorol Injection

Vitamin D analog

USUAL DOSE

Optimal dose of doxercalciferol must be individualized. The dose is adjusted in an attempt to achieve intact parathyroid hormone (iPTH) levels within a targeted range of 150 to 300 pg/mL. See Precautions and Monitor. Recommended initial dose for a patient with an iPTH level greater than 400 pg/mL is 4 mcg administered as a bolus dose three times weekly at the end of dialysis (approximately every other day). Total weekly dose is 12 mcg/week. Maximum dose was limited to 18 mcg/week in clinical studies.

DOSE ADJUSTMENTS

Adjust dosing based on patient response in order to lower blood iPTH into the range of 150 to 300 pg/mL. The following chart is a suggested approach to dose titration. Doses higher than 18 mcg weekly have not been studied. During titration monitor iPTH, serum calcium, phophorus, and calcium × phosphorus product (Ca × P) weekly. Maximize iPTH suppression while maintaining serum calcium and phosphorous levels in prescribed ranges; see Monitor. ■ Immediately suspend dosing if hypercalcemia, hyperphosphatemia, or a Ca × P product of greater than 55 mg^2/dL^2 is noted. Reinitiate therapy at a dose that is 1 mcg lower when parameters have normalized. ■ Patients with impaired hepatic function may not metabolize doxercalciferol appropriately, see Precautions.

Suggested Dose Adjustment Guidelines for Doxercalciferol	
iPTH Level	Doxercalciferol Dose Guidelines
Decreased by <50% and above 300 pg/mL	Increase by 1 to 2 mcg at 8-week intervals as necessary
Decreased by >50% and above 300 pg/mL	Maintain
150-300 pg/mL	Maintain
<100 pg/mL	Suspend for 1 week, then resume at a dose that is at least 1 mcg lower

DILUTION

May be given undiluted. Available as 2 mcg/mL solution in 2-mL vials. **Storage:** Store unopened vials at 25° C (77° F); range: 15° to 30° C (59° to 86° F). Protect from light. Discard unused portion.

COMPATIBILITY

Specific information not available. Consider specific use; consult pharmacist.

RATE OF ADMINISTRATION

Administer as a bolus dose at the end of dialysis.

ACTIONS

A synthetic vitamin D analog. Metabolizes to a naturally occurring, biologically active form of vitamin D_2 that regulates blood calcium at levels required for essential body functions (i.e., intestinal absorption of dietary calcium, tubular reabsorption of calcium by the kidney and, in conjunction with the parathyroid hormone [PTH], the mobilization of calcium from the skeleton). Acts directly on bone cells (osteoblasts) to stimulate skeletal growth, and on the parathyroid glands to suppress PTH synthesis and secretion. In uremic patients, deficient production of biologically active vitamin D metabolites leads to secondary hyperparathyroidism, which contributes to the development of metabolic bone disease. Doxercalciferol is activated in the liver. Peak blood levels are reached in 2.1 to 13.9 hours. Mean half-life range is 32 to 96 hours.

INDICATIONS AND USES

Reduction of elevated iPTH levels in the management of secondary hyperparathyroidism in patients undergoing chronic renal dialysis.

CONTRAINDICATIONS

Evidence of vitamin D toxicity, hypercalcemia, hyperphosphatemia, or known hypersensitivity to any ingredient in this product; see Precautions.

PRECAUTIONS

Overdose of any form of vitamin D, including doxercalciferol, is dangerous. Progressive hypercalcemia due to overdose of vitamin D and its metabolites may require emergency attention. Acute hypercalcemia may exacerbate tendencies for cardiac arrhythmias and seizures and may potentiate the action of digoxin drugs. Chronic administration may place patient at risk of hypercalcemia, elevated $Ca \times P$ product, and generalized vascular and other soft-tissue calcification. If clinically significant hypercalcemia develops, dose should be reduced or held. Do not allow the $Ca \times P$ product to exceed 55 mg^2/dL^2. See Side Effects and Antidote. ▪ To avoid possible additive effects and hypercalcemia, phosphate or vitamin D-related compounds should not be taken concomitantly with doxercalciferol. ▪ Oversuppression of iPTH levels may lead to adynamic bone syndrome. ▪ Hyperphosphatemia can exacerbate hyperparathyroidism. ▪ Use caution in patients with impaired hepatic function. More frequent monitoring of iPTH, calcium, and phosphorus levels is recommended. ▪ Patients with higher pretreatment serum levels of calcium (more than 10.5 mg/dL) or phosphorus (more than 6.9 mg/dL) may be more likely to experience hypercalcemia or hyperphosphatemia; see Contraindications.

Monitor: During initiation of therapy, obtain baseline serum iPTH, calcium and phosphorus levels and determine levels weekly during the early phase of treatment (i.e., first 12 weeks). For dialysis patients, serum or plasma iPTH and serum calcium, phosphorus, and alkaline phosphatase should be determined periodically. See Dose Adjustments. ▪ Calculate $Ca \times P$ (should be less than 55 mg^2/dL^2). ▪ Monitor serum calcium levels weekly after all dose changes and during subsequent dose titration. ▪ Monitor for signs and symptoms of hypercalcemia. See Side Effects. Radiographic evaluation of suspect anatomical regions may be useful in the early detection of generalized vascular or other soft-tissue calcification. ▪ Oral calcium-based or other non–aluminum-containing phosphate binders and a low phosphate diet are indicated to control serum phosphorus levels in dialysis patients. Hyperphosphatemia can lessen the effectiveness of doxercalciferol in reducing blood PTH levels. After initiating doxercalciferol therapy, the dose of calcium-containing phosphate binders should be decreased to correct persistent mild hypercalcemia (10.6 to 11.2 mg/dL for 3 consecutive determinations), or increased to correct persistent mild hyperphosphatemia (7 to 8 mg/dL for 3 consecutive determinations). ■ Persistent or markedly elevated serum calcium levels may be corrected by dialysis against a reduced calcium or calcium-free dialysate. ■ See Precautions and Drug/Lab Interactions.

Patient Education: Report symptoms of hypercalcemia promptly. Dose adjustment or treatment may be required. Strict adherence to dietary supplementation of calcium and restriction of phosphorus is required to ensure optimal effectiveness of therapy. Phosphate-binding compounds (e.g., calcium acetate [Phos-lo]) may be needed to control serum phosphorus levels in patients with CRF, but excessive use of aluminum-containing products (e.g., aluminum hydroxide gel [Alternagel]) should be avoided. ■ Review all non-prescription drugs with physician.

Maternal/Child: Category B: safety for use in pregnancy not established, use only if clearly needed. ■ Discontinue breast-feeding. ■ Safety and effectiveness for use in pediatric patients not established.

Elderly: No overall differences in effectiveness or safety observed.

DRUG/LAB INTERACTIONS

Specific interaction studies have not been performed. ■ **Digoxin** toxicity is potentiated by hypercalcemia. Use caution when doxercalciferol is prescribed concomitantly with digoxin compounds. ■ **Phosphate or vitamin D–**related compounds should not be taken concomitantly with doxercalciferol. ■ May reduce serum total **alkaline phosphatase levels.** ■ **Magnesium-containing antacids** may cause hypermagnesemia; concomitant use is not recommended. ■ Concomitant use with **cytochrome P$_{450}$ enzyme inducers** (e.g., glutethimide, phenobarbital [Luminal], phenytoin [Dilantin], rifampin [Rifadin]) may affect hydroxylation of doxercalciferol and require dose adjustments. ■ Concomitant use with **cytochrome P$_{450}$ enzyme inhibitors** (e.g., erythromycin, ketoconazole [Nizoral]) may inhibit metabolism of the active form of vitamin D, decreasing effectiveness.

SIDE EFFECTS

Dose-limiting side effects are hypercalcemia, hyperphosphatemia, and oversuppression of iPTH (less than 150 pg/mL). Overdose or chronic administration may lead to hypercalcemia. Signs and symptoms of vitamin D intoxication associated with hypercalcemia include: *Early:* anorexia, bone pain, constipation, dry mouth, headache, metallic taste, muscle pain, nausea, somnolence, vomiting, and weakness. *Late:* albuminuria, anorexia, apathy, arrested growth, cardiac arrhythmias, conjunctivitis (calcific), death, decreased libido, dehydration, ectopic calcification, elevated AST and ALT, elevated BUN, hypercholesterolemia, hypertension, hyperthermia, nocturia, overt psychosis (rare), pancreatitis, photophobia, polydipsia, polyuria, pruritus, rhinorrhea, sensory disturbances, somnolence, urinary tract infections, and weight loss.

Overdose: Hypercalcemia, hypercalciuria, hyperphosphatemia, and oversuppression of PTH secretion leading in certain cases to adynamic bone disease. High intake of calcium and phosphate concomitant with doxercalciferol may lead to similar abnormalities. High levels of calcium in the dialysate bath may contribute to hypercalcemia.

ANTIDOTE

Notify physician of any side effects. Treatment of patients with clinically significant hypercalcemia (more than 1 mg/dL above the upper limit of normal range) consists of immediate dose reduction or interruption of the therapy and includes a low-calcium diet, withdrawal of calcium supplements, patient mobilization, attention to fluid and electrolyte imbalances, assessment of electrocardiographic abnormalities (critical in patients receiving digoxin), forced diuresis, and hemodialysis or peritoneal dialysis against a calcium-free dialysate, as warranted. Monitor serum calcium levels frequently until calcium levels return to within normal limits. Not removed from blood during hemodialysis. When serum calcium levels return to within normal limits (usually 2 to 7 days), therapy may be restarted at a dose that is at least 1 mcg lower than prior therapy.

DOXORUBICIN HYDROCHLORIDE BBW ■
DOXORUBICIN HYDROCHLORIDE
LIPOSOMAL INJECTION BBW

(dox-oh-**ROO**-bih-sin hy-droh-**KLOR**-eyed)
(dox-oh-**ROO**-bih-sin hy-droh-**KLOR**-eyed
LIP-oh-sohm-ul)

Antineoplastic
(anthracycline antibiotic)

ADR, Adriamycin ■ **Doxil**

pH 3.8 to 6.5 ■ pH 6.5

USUAL DOSE

Assessment required before dosing; see Precautions and Monitor.

CONVENTIONAL DOXORUBICIN

60 to 75 mg/M^2 once every 21 days as a *single agent.* An alternate dose schedule is 30 mg/M^2 once each day for 3 days. Repeat every 4 weeks. When used in *combination* with other agents, the most common dose of doxorubicin is 40 to 60 mg/M^2 every 21 to 28 days. Recent studies suggest that cardiotoxicity may be reduced and doses may be increased by administration of 20 mg/M^2 on a weekly basis or by giving larger doses (60 to 75 mg/M^2) as a prolonged infusion (48 to 96 hours). A central venous catheter or infuse-a-port would be necessary. Dexrazoxane (Zinecard) is now available to reduce the incidence and severity of cardiomyopathy for women with metastatic breast cancer who have received 300 mg/M^2 of doxorubicin (see product insert).

Breast cancer with lymph node involvement after resection: Doxorubicin 60 mg/M^2 in combination with cyclophosphamide 600 mg/M^2 given IV sequentially on Day 1 of each 21-day treatment cycle. Four cycles have been administered.

Adjuvant treatment of operable node-positive breast cancer: Treatment protocol includes doxorubicin, cyclophosphamide, and docetaxel. Administer doxorubicin 50 mg/M^2 and cyclophosphamide 500 mg/M^2. One hour later, give docetaxel 75 mg/M^2. Repeat every 3 weeks for 6 cycles. See docetaxel and cyclophosphamide monographs.

DOXIL (LIPOSOMAL DOXORUBICIN)

AIDS-related Kaposi's sarcoma: 20 mg/M^2 once every 3 weeks. Continue as long as response is satisfactory and treatment is tolerated.

Ovarian cancer: 50 mg/M^2 as an infusion every 4 weeks for as long as the patient does not progress, shows no evidence of cardiotoxicity, and continues to tolerate treatment. A minimum of four courses is recommended.

Multiple myeloma: Given in combination with bortezomib (Velcade).

Bortezomib: Administer 1.3 mg/M^2 as an IV bolus on Days 1, 4, 8, and 11 every 3 weeks; see bortezomib monograph. *Doxil:* Administer 30 mg/M^2 on Day 4 following bortezomib. Continue regimen for up to 8 cycles until disease progression or the occurrence of unacceptable toxicity.

Breast cancer (unlabeled): 45 to 60 mg/M^2 once every 3 to 4 weeks as monotherapy. Other combination protocols are in use.

PEDIATRIC DOSE

CONVENTIONAL DOXORUBICIN: 30 mg/M^2 once each day for 3 days. Repeat every 4 weeks. See Maternal/Child.

DOXIL: Safety for use in pediatric patients not established.

DOSE ADJUSTMENTS

ALL DOXORUBICINS: *Elevated serum bilirubin:* Give 50% of above doses for serum bilirubin from 1.2 to 3 mg/mL and 25% for serum bilirubin above 3 mg/mL. ▪ See Precautions.

CONVENTIONAL DOXORUBICIN: Reduce dose in impaired liver and kidney function. ▪ Lower-end doses are appropriate for the elderly (inadequate marrow reserves) and those with prior therapy or neoplastic marrow infiltration. **Breast cancer with lymph node involvement after resection:** Reduce dose to 75% of the starting dose for neutropenic fever/infection. If necessary, delay the next cycle of treatment until the ANC is 1,000 cells/mm^3 or more and the platelet count is 100,000 cells/mm^3 or more and nonhematologic toxicities have resolved.

DOXIL: Dose adjustments are required in hematologic toxicity (see the following chart) and in patients with stomatitis or palmar-plantar erythrodysesthesia (see product literature for guidelines). Adjust or delay a dose as described in the product literature at the first sign of a Grade 2 or higher adverse event. Once the dose has been decreased, it should not be increased at a later time.

Doxil Dosing Based on Hematologic Toxicity			
Grade	ANC (cells/mm^3)	Platelets (cells/mm^3)	Modification
1	1,500-1,900 cells/mm^3	75,000-150,000 cells/mm^3	Resume treatment with no dose reduction
2	1,000-<1,500 cells/mm^3	50,000-<75,000 cells/mm^3	Wait until ANC ≥1,500 and platelets ≥75,000; redose with no dose reduction
3	500-999 cells/mm^3	25,000-<50,000 cells/mm^3	Wait until ANC ≥1,500 and/or platelets ≥75,000; redose with no dose reduction
4	<500 cells/mm^3	<25,000 cells/mm^3	Wait until ANC ≥1,500 and/or platelets ≥75,000; redose at 25% dose reduction or continue full dose with cytokine support

Dose adjustments for doxil and bortezomib combination therapy for treatment of multiple myeloma are listed in the following chart. See bortezomib monograph for additional dose adjustments.

Continued

Dose Adjustments for Doxil and Bortezomib Combination Therapy		
Patient Status	Doxil	Bortezomib
Fever ≥ 38° C ANC <1,000/mm³	Do not dose this cycle if before Day 4; if after Day 4, reduce next dose by 25%.	Reduce next dose by 25%.
On any day of drug administration after Day 1 of each cycle: Platelet count <25,000/ mm³ Hemoglobin <8 Gm/dL ANC <500/mm³	Do not dose this cycle if before Day 4; if after Day 4, reduce next dose by 25% in the following cycles if bortezomib is reduced for hematologic toxicity.	Do not dose; if 2 or more doses are not given in a cycle, reduce dose by 25% in the following cycles.
Grade 3 or 4 nonhematologic drug-related toxicity	Do not dose until recovered to Grade <2, and reduce dose by 25% for all subsequent doses.	Do not dose until recovered to Grade <2, and reduce dose by 25% for all subsequent doses.
Neuropathic pain or peripheral neuropathy	No dose adjustments.	See bortezomib manufacturer's prescribing information for dose adjustments in patients with neuropathic pain.

DILUTION

Specific techniques required; see Precautions.

CONVENTIONAL DOXORUBICIN: Each 10 mg must be diluted with 5 mL of NS. Do not use bacteriostatic diluent. An additional 5 mL of diluent for each 10 mg is recommended (2 mg/mL). Shake to dissolve completely. Also available in preservative-free solutions. May be further diluted in 50 mL or more D5W or NS and given as a continuous infusion through a central venous line.

DOXIL: Each dose must be diluted in 250 mL D5W. Not a clear solution, but a translucent red liposomal dispersion. Do not use filters. Maximum dose for dilution in 250 mL is 90 mg. Doses over 90 mg should be diluted in 500 mL D5W. See Compatibility.

Filters: *Conventional doxorubicin:* Data not available from manufacturer; however, one source indicates no evidence of drug loss when administered through a 0.2-micron in-line nylon filter, and another source indicates no significant drug loss using various types of 0.2-micron filters.

Doxil: Do not use filters during preparation or administration.

Storage: *Conventional doxorubicin:* Refrigerate unopened vials; protect from light. Reconstituted solution stable for 7 days at CRT and 15 days refrigerated. Diluted solution stable 24 hours at room temperature, 48 hours if refrigerated; then discard. Protect from sunlight.

Doxil: Refrigerate unopened vials; avoid freezing for longer than 1 month. Refrigerate diluted solution and use within 24 hours.

COMPATIBILITY (Underline Indicates Conflicting Compatibility Information)
Consider any drug NOT listed as compatible to be INCOMPATIBLE until consulting a pharmacist; specific conditions may apply.

CONVENTIONAL DOXORUBICIN

Manufacturer lists fluorouracil and heparin as **incompatible** and states mixing with other drugs is not recommended unless specific **compatibility** data available.

One source suggests the following **compatibilities:**

Additive: Bleomycin (Blenoxane), cyclophosphamide (Cytoxan), dacarbazine (DTIC), ondansetron (Zofran), paclitaxel (Taxol), vinblastine, vincristine.

Y-site: Amifostine (Ethyol), anidulafungin (Eraxis), aztreonam (Azactam), bleomycin (Blenoxane), caspofungin (Cancidas), chlorpromazine (Thorazine), cisplatin (Platinol), cladribine (Leustatin), cyclophosphamide (Cytoxan), dexamethasone (Decadron), diphenhydramine (Benadryl), doripenem (Doribax), droperidol (Inapsine), etoposide phosphate (Etopophos), famotidine (Pepcid IV), filgrastim (Neupogen), fludarabine (Fludara), fluorouracil (5-FU), furosemide (Lasix), gemcitabine (Gemzar), granisetron (Kytril), heparin, hydromorphone (Dilaudid), leucovorin calcium, linezolid (Zyvox), lorazepam (Ativan), melphalan (Alkeran), methotrexate, methylprednisolone (Solu-Medrol), metoclopramide (Reglan), mitomycin (Mutamycin), morphine, ondansetron (Zofran), oxaliplatin (Eloxatin), paclitaxel (Taxol), prochlorperazine (Compazine), promethazine (Phenergan), ranitidine (Zantac), sargramostim (Leukine), sodium bicarbonate, teniposide (Vumon), thiotepa, topotecan (Hycamtin), vinblastine, vincristine, vinorelbine (Navelbine).

DOXIL

Specific information not available. Manufacturer states, "Do not mix with other drugs unless specific **compatibility** data available. Do not use any other diluent (use D5W only). Do not use any bacteriostatic agents (e.g., benzyl alcohol)."

One source suggests the following **compatibilities:**

Y-site: Acyclovir (Zovirax), allopurinol (Aloprim), aminophylline, ampicillin, aztreonam (Azactam), bleomycin (Blenoxane), butorphanol (Stadol), calcium gluconate, carboplatin (Paraplatin), cefazolin (Ancef), cefepime (Maxipime), cefoxitin (Mefoxin), ceftriaxone (Rocephin), chlorpromazine (Thorazine), ciprofloxacin (Cipro IV), cisplatin (Platinol), clindamycin (Cleocin), cyclophosphamide (Cytoxan), cytarabine (ARA-C), dacarbazine (DTIC), dexamethasone (Decadron), diphenhydramine (Benadryl), dobutamine, dopamine, droperidol (Inapsine), enalaprilat (Vasotec IV), etoposide (VePesid), famotidine (Pepcid IV), fluconazole (Diflucan), fluorouracil (5-FU), furosemide (Lasix), ganciclovir (Cytovene), gentamicin, granisetron (Kytril), haloperidol (Haldol), heparin, hydrocortisone sodium succinate (Solu-Cortef), hydromorphone (Dilaudid), ifosfamide (Ifex), leucovorin calcium, lorazepam (Ativan), magnesium sulfate, mesna (Mesnex), methotrexate, methylprednisolone (Solu-Medrol), metronidazole (Flagyl IV), ondansetron (Zofran), piperacillin, potassium chloride (KCl), prochlorperazine (Compazine), ranitidine (Zantac), sulfamethoxazole/trimethoprim, ticarcillin/clavulanate (Timentin), tobramycin, vancomycin, vinblastine, vincristine, vinorelbine (Navelbine), zidovudine (AZT, Retrovir).

RATE OF ADMINISTRATION
CONVENTIONAL DOXORUBICIN
IV injection: A single dose of properly diluted medication over a minimum of 3 to 5 minutes. Should be given through Y-tube or three-way stopcock of a free-flowing infusion of NS or D5W. Slow injection rate further for erythematous streaking along the vein or facial flushing.

Continuous infusion: Central venous line required. Equally distributed over 24 hours.

DOXIL
Rapid infusion may increase risk of acute infusion-related reactions (e.g., apnea, asthma, back pain, bronchospasm, chills, cyanosis, facial swelling, fever, flushing, headache, hypotension, pruritus, rash, shortness of breath, syncope, tachycardia, tightness in the chest or throat). Primarily occurs during the first infusion; may resolve with a reduced rate or may take up to a day after infusion completed to resolve. Avoid rapid flushing of the infusion line.

Begin with an initial rate of 1 mg/minute to minimize the risk of infusion reactions. If no adverse infusion-related effects, the rate may be increased from the initial rate of 1 mg/min to evenly distribute and complete infusion over 1 hour.

ACTIONS
CONVENTIONAL DOXORUBICIN: A highly toxic antibiotic antineoplastic agent that is cell cycle specific for the S phase. Widely distributed and rapidly cleared from plasma, it interferes with cell division by binding with DNA to slow production of nucleic acid synthesis. Tissue levels remain constant for 7 to 10 days. Metabolized in the liver. Elimination half-life is 18 to 30 hours. Does not cross blood-brain barrier. Slowly excreted in bile and urine. Secreted in breast milk.

DOXIL: Doxorubicin encapsulated in long-circulating STEALTH liposomes (phospholipids). The small size of these liposomes and their persistence in the circulation enable them to evade immune system detection and penetrate the often altered and/or compromised vasculature of tumors. Once distributed to tumor tissue, the doxorubicin is released by an unknown mechanism. It differs from conventional doxorubicin because it mostly confines itself to vascular fluid volume. Metabolized and eliminated renally. Plasma clearance is slower. Half-life is extended to 55 hours. Concentration in Kaposi's sarcoma lesions is much higher than in normal skin (range is 3 to 53 times higher).

INDICATIONS AND USES
CONVENTIONAL DOXORUBICIN: To suppress or retard neoplastic growth. Regression has been produced in soft tissue and bone sarcomas; Hodgkin's disease; non-Hodgkin's lymphomas; acute leukemias; breast, GU, thyroid, lung, ovarian, and stomach carcinoma and transitional cell bladder carcinoma; neuroblastoma; Wilms' tumor; and many other carcinomas. ▪ Adjuvant therapy in women with evidence of axillary lymph node involvement following resection of primary breast cancer. ▪ Adjuvant treatment of operable node-positive breast cancer in combination with cyclophosphamide and docetaxel.

DOXIL: Treatment of AIDS-related Kaposi's sarcoma in patients whose disease has progressed on prior combination chemotherapy or who are intolerant to combination chemotherapy. ▪ Treatment of metastatic carcinoma of the ovary in patients with disease that is refractory to both paclitaxel and platinum-based chemotherapy regimens (e.g., cisplatin [Platinol], carboplatin [Paraplatin]). ▪ Treatment of multiple myeloma in combination with bortezomib (Velcade) in patients who have received one prior therapy but have not previously received bortezomib.

Unlabeled uses: DOXIL: Treatment of locally advanced and metastatic breast cancer.

CONTRAINDICATIONS

CONVENTIONAL DOXORUBICIN: Myelosuppression resulting from treatment with other antineoplastic agents, radiotherapy, impaired cardiac function, or previous treatment with complete cumulative doses of doxorubicin, daunorubicin, idarubicin, and/or other anthracyclines and anthracenes.

DOXIL: Breast-feeding mothers.

ALL DOXORUBICINS: History of hypersensitivity to conventional or liposomal formulations of doxorubicin or to their components.

PRECAUTIONS

ALL DOXORUBICINS: Follow guidelines for handling cytotoxic agents and patient excreta. Precautions recommended for up to 5 days after a dose. See Appendix A, p. 1429. ▪ Usually administered by or under the direction of a physician specialist, with facilities for monitoring the patient and responding to any medical emergency. ▪ For IV use only. Do not give IM or SC. ▪ **Do Not Substitute** Doxil for conventional doxorubicin on a mg/mg basis. Severe side effects have resulted. Differences in liposomal products as well as conventional products can substantially affect the functional properties of these agents; do not substitute one agent for another. ▪ Use extreme caution in pre-existing drug-induced bone marrow suppression, existing heart disease, hepatic impairment, previous treatment with other anthracyclines (e.g., daunorubicin), other cardiotoxic agents (e.g., bleomycin), concurrent cyclophosphamide therapy, or radiation therapy encompassing the heart; risk of cardiotoxicity increased and may occur at lower doses. ▪ All forms of doxorubicin may cause cardiotoxicity. Life-threatening or fatal congestive heart failure may occur during therapy or months after therapy is completed. Cardiotoxicity occurs with increasing frequency as cumulative doses increase above 300 mg/M^2. The risk of developing CHF increases rapidly with increasing total cumulative doses above 400 mg/M^2; see Antidote. Patients with active or dormant cardiovascular disease or patients who have received radiotherapy to the mediastinal area or concomitant therapy with other anthracyclines (e.g., daunorubicin, idarubicin), anthracenediones, or other cardiotoxic agents (e.g., bleomycin, cyclophosphamide, mitoxantrone, mitomycin C) may be at greater risk. These recommendations may change in specific situations now that dexrazoxane is available to reduce the incidence and severity of cardiomyopathy; however, cardiac toxicity may occur at lower cumulative doses even if cardiac risk factors are not present. ▪ May cause severe myelosuppression. ▪ May have cross-sensitivity with lincomycin. ▪ Not considered effective in the treatment of brain tumors, cancers of the kidney or large bowel, CNS metastasis, or malignant melanoma. ▪ See Maternal/Child and Side Effects.

CONVENTIONAL DOXORUBICIN: Used cautiously with other antineoplastic drugs to achieve tumor remission. ▪ Secondary acute myelogenous leukemia (AML) and myelodysplastic syndrome (MDS) have been reported in adult and pediatric patients; the occurrence of refractory secondary AML or MDS is more common when doxorubicin is given in combination with DNA-damaging antineoplastic agents or radiotherapy, in patients heavily pretreated with cytotoxic drugs, or when doses of doxorubicin have been escalated.

DOXIL: Benefits must outweigh risks if Doxil is used in patients with a history of cardiovascular disease. ▪ Has caused palmar-plantar erythrodysesthesia. Incidence may be increased with higher doses or increased frequency. Generally seen after 2 or 3 cycles, but may occur earlier. May be severe and require a dose adjustment or discontinuation of Doxil. ▪ Severe, additive myelosuppression may occur in Kaposi's sarcoma patients and may be dose limiting.

Monitor: ALL DOXORUBICINS: Monitoring of CBC including differential and platelet count, uric acid levels, electrolytes, liver function (AST, ALT, alkaline phosphatase, and bilirubin), kidney function, ECG, chest x-ray, echocardiogram, and left ventricular ejection fraction (LVEF) is necessary before and during therapy. At a minimum, CBC with platelets should be monitored before each dose. Testing for renal and hepatic function may also be indicated; see Dose Adjustments. ▪ Observe for S/S of cardiotoxicity (e.g., fast or irregular HR, shortness of breath, swelling of the feet or lower legs). Endomyocardial biopsy or gated radionuclide scans have been used to monitor potential cardiac toxicity. ▪ Maintain adequate hydration and urine alkalinization. ▪ Allopurinol may prevent formation of uric acid crystals. ▪ Be alert for signs of bone marrow suppression, bleeding, or infection. ▪ Monitor for thrombocytopenia (platelet count less than 50,000/mm^3). Initiate precautions to prevent excessive bleeding (e.g., inspect IV sites, skin, and mucous membranes; use extreme care during invasive procedures; test urine, emesis, stool, and secretions for occult blood). ▪ Use of prophylactic antibiotics may be indicated pending C/S in a febrile, neutropenic patient. Sepsis in a neutropenic patient has resulted in discontinuation of treatment and in rare cases, death. ▪ Prophylactic antiemetics are indicated. ▪ See Drug/Lab Interactions.

CONVENTIONAL DOXORUBICIN: Use only large veins. Avoid veins over joints or in extremities with compromised venous or lymphatic drainage. Determine absolute patency of vein. A stinging or burning sensation indicates extravasation; severe cellulitis and tissue necrosis will result. *Extravasation may occur with or without stinging or burning and even if blood returns well on aspiration of infusion needle.* Observe and touch site frequently to feel air and/or liquid under the skin. If extravasation occurs discontinue injection; use another vein.

DOXIL: Monitor for S/S of acute infusion reactions and/or hypersensitivity (e.g., apnea, asthma, back pain, bronchospasm, chills, cyanosis, facial swelling, fever, flushing, headache, hypotension, pruritus, rash, shortness of breath, syncope, tachycardia, tightness in the chest or throat). The majority of infusion-related reactions occur during the first infusion. ▪ Extravasation may cause irritation at infusion site. Discontinue, use another vein.

Patient Education: ALL DOXORUBICINS: Urine and other body fluids will be reddish for several days (from dye, not hematuria). ▪ Nonhormonal birth control recommended. May induce chromosomal damage in sperm. Effective contraceptive method for men required. ▪ Effects may be additive with current medications. Review all medications (prescription and nonprescription) with nurse and/or physician. ▪ Report promptly shortness of breath and/or swelling of the feet or lower legs. ▪ Report S/S of infection (e.g., chills, fever, painful urination), stomatitis, bothersome side effects, or any unusual bleeding (e.g., bruising, tarry stools). ▪ Report IV site burning, stinging, puffiness, or the feeling of liquid under the skin and any other side effects promptly. ▪ Report tingling, burning, redness, flaking, swelling, blisters or small sores on the palms of hands or soles of feet. ▪ See Precautions. ▪ See Appendix D, p. 1434.

Maternal/Child: ALL DOXORUBICINS: Category D: avoid pregnancy; can cause fetal harm. ▪ Has been used only when benefits outweigh risks. ▪ Discontinue breast-feeding. ▪ Treatment during childhood may result in abnormal cardiac function, especially in females. ▪ Infants and children are at increased risk for developing delayed cardiotoxicity; follow-up cardiac evaluation is recommended; see Precautions. ▪ Infants and children may be at greater risk for developing acute myelogenous leukemia (AML) and other neoplasms. ▪ Infants and children may develop S/S of acute "recall" pneumonitis with concomitant use of doxorubicin and dactinomycin (Cosmegen) after local radiation therapy. ▪ In infants under 2 years of age, doxorubicin clearance is similar to adults, but clearance may be increased in pediatric patients over 2 years of age. ▪ May contribute to prepubertal growth failure and/or gonadal impairment (which is usually temporary). ▪ See Precautions, extended recommendations for handling patient excreta. **DOXIL:** Safety for use in pediatric patients not established.

Elderly: ALL DOXORUBICINS: Response similar to that seen in younger adults, but greater sensitivity of some older individuals cannot be ruled out. ▪ Cardiotoxicity and myelotoxicity may be more severe in patients over 70 years of age. ▪ Consider age-related organ impairment and concomitant disease and/or drug therapy; see Dose Adjustments.

DRUG/LAB INTERACTIONS

Studies not yet completed for Doxil; interactions may be similar to conventional doxorubicins. ▪ May exacerbate **cyclophosphamide**-induced hemorrhagic cystitis or increase hepatotoxicity of **6-mercaptopurine.** ▪ May increase bone marrow toxicity of **other chemotherapeutic agents and radiation.** ▪ **Barbiturates** increase clearance and decrease effects. ▪ May decrease serum levels of **digoxin.** ▪ May decrease serum levels of **anticonvulsants** (e.g., phenytoin [Dilantin], carbamazepine [Tegretol], valproate [Depacon]) when given concurrently with **cisplatin.** ▪ Risk of cardiotoxicity increased in patients previously treated with maximum cumulative doses of **other anthracyclines** (e.g., idarubicin [Idamycin]) **and/or radiation encompassing the heart.** ▪ Concurrent use with **hepatotoxic agents** (e.g., methotrexate) may increase risk of toxicity. ▪ **Cyclosporine** (Sandimmune) **and streptozocin** (Zanosar) may decrease clearance and increase toxicity of doxorubicin. ▪ **Paclitaxel** (Taxol) appears to decrease the clearance of doxorubicin. Administration of doxorubicin before paclitaxel is recommended to prevent increased toxicity. ▪ Coadministration with high-dose **progesterone** may increase doxorubicin toxicity. ▪ Many drug interactions possible; observe patient closely. ▪ Do not administer **live virus vaccines** to patients receiving antineoplastic drugs. ▪ Increased toxicity to mucosa, myocardium, skin (including redness and exfoliative changes), and liver possible when given concurrently **with or after radiation.** ▪ Necrotizing colitis (e.g., bloody stools, cecal inflammation, severe and sometimes fatal infections) has been reported with the combination of doxorubicin by IV push daily for 3 days and **cytarabine** as a continuous infusion daily for 7 or more days. ▪ **Dexrazoxane** is given with doxorubicin to reduce cardiotoxic effects. May also decrease antitumor effectiveness if given before a cumulative dose of doxorubicin 300 mg/M^2 is reached or other chemotherapeutic agents are included in the protocol (e.g., fluorouracil). ▪ See Precautions.

SIDE EFFECTS

ALL DOXORUBICINS: Abdominal pain; alopecia (complete); anorexia; asthenia; bone marrow suppression (e.g., anemia, hypochromic anemia, leukopenia, neutropenia [ANC less than 1,000/mm^3], thrombocytopenia may be dose-limiting); cardiac toxicity (e.g., CHF); constipation; decreased serum calcium; depressed QRS voltage; diarrhea; dry skin; esophagitis; fatigue; fever; gonadal suppression; headache; hyperpigmentation of nail beds and dermal creases; hypersensitivity reactions (including life-threatening or fatal anaphylaxis); hyperuricemia; increase in alkaline phosphatase, ALT, AST, bilirubin, BUN, glucose, SCr; mucositis; nausea; oral moniliasis; paresthesia; prolonged PT; rash; recall of skin reactions due to prior radiotherapy; stomatitis; weakness; vomiting.

DOXIL: In addition to all of the above, acute infusion reactions, palmar-plantar erythrodysesthesia. *Kaposi's sarcoma* patients may be taking numerous other drugs that may confuse the overall side effect picture (e.g., didanosine [ddl], stavudine [D4T], sulfamethoxazole/trimethoprim, zalcitabine [ddC], zidovudine [AZT, Retrovir]).

Post-Marketing: Muscle spasms, myelogenous leukemia, pulmonary embolism, and skin and subcutaneous tissue disorders (e.g., erythema multiforme, Stevens-Johnson syndrome, and toxic epidermal necrolysis).

Overdose: ALL DOXORUBICINS: Increase in bone marrow suppression and mucositis.

ANTIDOTE

ALL DOXORUBICINS: Most side effects will either be tolerated or treated symptomatically. Keep the physician informed. Bone marrow toxicity may require cessation of therapy. Administration of whole blood products (e.g., packed RBCs, platelets, leukocytes) and/or blood modifiers (e.g., darbepoetin alfa [Aranesp], epoetin alfa [Epogen], filgrastim [Neupogen], oprelvekin [Neumega], pegfilgrastim [Neulasta], sargramostim [Leukine]) may be indicated to treat bone marrow toxicity. Acute cardiac failure occurs suddenly (most common when total cumulative dosage approaches 550 mg/M^2) and frequently does not respond to currently available treatment (digoxin, diuretics [e.g., furosemide (Lasix)], ACE inhibitors [e.g., enalaprilat]). Close monitoring of accumulated dosage, bone marrow, ECG, chest x-ray, echocardiography, and systolic ejection fraction may prevent most serious and potentially fatal cardiac side effects. There is no specific antidote. Supportive therapy as indicated will help sustain the patient in toxicity. Treat hypersensitivity reactions as required; discontinue therapy if severe.

CONVENTIONAL DOXORUBICIN: For extravasation flood the area with normal saline. Use a 27- or 25-gauge needle. Elevate the extremity, apply cold compresses, and ice for 30 minutes four times a day for 3 days. Site should be observed promptly by a reconstructive surgeon.

DOXIL: In addition to all of the above, treatment may have to be interrupted or discontinued for severe palmar-plantar erythrodysesthesia or acute infusion reactions. Infusion reactions may resolve with slowing of infusion rate. May be able to control palmar-plantar erythrodysesthesia by allowing it to resolve and by increasing intervals between subsequent cycles. For extravasation, discontinue infusion and apply ice over site for 30 minutes to alleviate local reaction.

DOXYCYCLINE HYCLATE
(dox-ih-**SYE**-kleen **HI**-klayt)

**Antibacterial
(tetracycline)
Antiprotozoal
Antimalarial**

Doxy 100, Doxy 200

pH 1.8 to 3.3

USUAL DOSE
ADULTS AND PEDIATRIC PATIENTS OVER 45 KG

200 mg the first day in one or two infusions followed by 100 to 200 mg/24 hr on subsequent days in one or two infusions. Depends on severity of the infection.

Primary and secondary syphilis: 150 mg every 12 hours for at least 10 days.

Acute pelvic inflammatory disease: 100 mg every 12 hours. Used in combination with cefoxitin 2 Gm every 6 hours.

Prevention and/or treatment of anthrax post-exposure: 100 mg every 12 hours.

PEDIATRIC DOSE
PEDIATRIC PATIENTS 45 KG OR LESS (BUT OVER 8 YEARS)

4.4 mg/kg of body weight/24 hr in one or two equally divided doses (2.2 mg/kg every 12 hours). Follow on subsequent days with 2.2 to 4.4 mg/kg/24 hr given once daily or in two equally divided doses (1.1 to 2.2 mg/kg every 12 hours). Do not exceed adult dose. See Maternal/Child.

Prevention and/or treatment of anthrax post-exposure: 2.2 mg/kg every 12 hours.

DOSE ADJUSTMENTS
Reduction may be indicated in impaired liver function. ▪ See Drug/Lab Interactions.

DILUTION
Check expiration date. Outdated ampules may cause nephrotoxicity. Each 100 mg or fraction thereof is diluted with 10 mL of SW or NS. Further dilute each 10 mL with 100 to 1,000 mL of a **compatible** infusion solution such as NS, D5W, R, LR, D5LR, 10% invert sugar in water, Normosol-M or Normosol-R in 5% dextrose in water, or other **compatible** solutions (see literature). Recommended concentrations 0.1 to 1 mg/mL. 1,000 mL diluent equals 0.1 mg/mL, 100 mL equals 1 mg/mL. Protect from direct sunlight during infusion.

Storage: Store at CRT; protect from light. After reconstitution, must be refrigerated and used within 72 hours.

COMPATIBILITY　　　(Underline Indicates Conflicting Compatibility Information)
Consider any drug NOT listed as compatible to be INCOMPATIBLE until consulting a pharmacist; specific conditions may apply.

One source suggests the following **compatibilities:**

Additive: <u>Meropenem (Merrem IV)</u>, ranitidine (Zantac).

Y-site: Acyclovir (Zovirax), amifostine (Ethyol), amiodarone (Nexterone), aztreonam (Azactam), bivalirudin (Angiomax), cisatracurium (Nimbex), cyclophosphamide (Cytoxan), dexmedetomidine (Precedex), diltiazem (Cardizem), docetaxel (Taxotere), etoposide phosphate (Etopophos), fenoldopam (Corlopam), filgrastim (Neupogen), fludarabine (Fludara), gemcitabine (Gemzar), granisetron (Kytril), hetastarch in electrolytes

(Hextend), hetastarch in NS (Hespan), hydromorphone (Dilaudid), linezolid (Zyvox), magnesium sulfate, melphalan (Alkeran), meperidine (Demerol), meropenem (Merrem IV), morphine, ondansetron (Zofran), propofol (Diprivan), remifentanil (Ultiva), sargramostim (Leukine), tacrolimus (Prograf), teniposide (Vumon), theophylline, thiotepa, vinorelbine (Navelbine).

RATE OF ADMINISTRATION

Each 100 mg or fraction thereof, properly diluted, over a minimum of 1 to 4 hours. 100 mg diluted in 100 mL equals 1 mg/mL and must be given over a minimum of 2 hours. 100 mg diluted in 200 mL equals 0.5 mg/mL and can be given in 1 hour if absolutely necessary. Infusion must be completed in 6 hours when diluted in LR injection with or without dextrose 5% and in 12 hours when diluted in other **compatible** solutions.

ACTIONS

A broad-spectrum tetracycline antibiotic, bacteriostatic against many gram-positive and gram-negative organisms and protozoa. Thought to interfere with the protein synthesis of microorganisms. Doxycycline is well distributed in most body tissues and is highly bound to plasma protein. Doxycycline may penetrate normal meninges, the eye, and the prostate more easily than most tetracyclines. Half-life is 12 to 22 hours. Partially metabolized in the liver and excreted in bile, urine, and feces. Crosses the placental barrier. Secreted in breast milk.

INDICATIONS AND USES

Infections caused by susceptible strains or organisms, such as rickettsiae, spirochetal agents, and many other gram-negative and gram-positive bacteria. Types of infections treated may include GU infections, including those caused by *Chlamydia trachomatis* and *Neisseria gonorrhoeae;* respiratory tract infections, including mycoplasmal pneumonia, skin and soft tissue infections, and others. ■ To substitute for contraindicated penicillin or sulfonamide therapy. ■ Drug of choice when a tetracycline is indicated for treatment of an extrarenal infection in patients with renal impairment. ■ Adjunct to amebicides in acute intestinal amebiasis. ■ Prevention and/or treatment of anthrax in all its forms, including cutaneous and inhalation anthrax post-exposure.

CONTRAINDICATIONS

Known hypersensitivity to tetracyclines; pregnancy, breast-feeding. Not recommended in pediatric patients under 8 years.

PRECAUTIONS

Sensitivity studies indicated to determine susceptibility of the causative organism to doxycycline. ■ To reduce the development of drug-resistant bacteria and maintain its effectiveness, doxycycline should be used to treat or prevent only those infections proven or strongly suspected to be caused by bacteria. ■ Continue for at least 2 to 3 days after all symptoms of infection subside. ■ Avoid prolonged use of drug; superinfection caused by overgrowth of nonsusceptible organisms may result. ■ Use caution in impaired liver function. Doxycycline serum concentrations and liver function tests are indicated. ■ Pseudomembranous colitis has been reported. May range from mild to life threatening. Consider in patients that present with diarrhea during or after treatment with doxycycline. ■ Initiate oral therapy as soon as possible. ■ Organisms resistant to one tetracycline are usually resistant to others. ■ If syphilis is suspected, perform a darkfield examination before initiating tetracyclines.

Monitor: Determine absolute patency of vein and avoid extravasation; thrombophlebitis may occur. ■ Monitor blood glucose; may reduce insulin requirements. ■ See Drug/Lab Interactions.

Patient Education: May cause dizziness or light-headedness; request assistance for ambulation. ■ Alert patient to photosensitive skin reaction. ■ Consider birth control options.

Maternal/Child: Category D: avoid pregnancy; see Contraindications. ■ May cause skeletal retardation in the fetus and infants and permanent tooth discoloration in pediatric patients under 8 years, including in utero or through mother's milk. ■ Discontinue breast-feeding.

DRUG/LAB INTERACTIONS

Inhibits **oral contraceptives;** may result in pregnancy or breakthrough bleeding. ■ May alter **lithium** levels. ■ Interferes with bactericidal action of **all penicillins** (e.g., ampicillin, oxacillin). May be toxic with **sulfonamides.** ■ Serum levels decreased by **barbiturates, carbamazepine** (Tegretol), **hydantoins** (e.g., phenytoin), and others. ■ May depress **plasma prothrombin activity;** a reduction in anticoagulant dose may be indicated.

SIDE EFFECTS

Relatively nontoxic in average doses. More toxic in large doses or if given too rapidly. Anogenital lesions, anorexia, blood dyscrasias, CNS toxicity (e.g., dizziness, light-headedness), diarrhea, dysphagia, enterocolitis, nausea, skin rashes, vomiting.

Major: Hypersensitivity reactions including anaphylaxis; blurred vision and headache (benign intracranial hypertension); bulging fontanels in infants; hepatotoxicity; pancreatitis; photosensitivity, pseudomembranous colitis, systemic candidiasis; thrombophlebitis.

ANTIDOTE

Notify the physician of all side effects. If minor side effects are progressive or any major side effect occurs, discontinue the drug, treat hypersensitivity reactions as indicated or resuscitate as necessary. Mild cases of colitis may respond to discontinuation of doxycycline. Treat antibiotic-related pseudomembranous colitis with fluid, electrolytes, protein supplements, and oral vancomycin (Vancocin) or metronidazole (Flagyl). Not removed by hemodialysis.

DROPERIDOL BBW

(droh-**PER**-ih-dohl)

Inapsine

Antiemetic
Anesthesia adjunct

pH 3 to 3.8

USUAL DOSE

May cause serious proarrhythmic effects and death; reserve use to patients for whom other treatments are ineffective or inappropriate. Dose should be individualized and initiated at a low dose. Adjust upward, with caution, to achieve the desired effect. Consider age, body weight, physical status, underlying pathological conditions, use of other drugs, type of anesthesia to be used, and surgical procedure involved; see Precautions. Maximum recommended initial dose is 2.5 mg. Additional 1.25-mg doses may be given to achieve the desired effect but should be used only if the potential benefit outweighs the potential risk.

Prevention of perioperative nausea and vomiting: 2.5 mg by slow IV injection. Additional 1.25-mg doses may be given with caution to achieve desired effect only if benefits outweigh potential risk. 0.625 to 1.25 mg has been shown to have an effect similar to ondansetron (Zofran) 4 mg.

PEDIATRIC DOSE

Prevention of perioperative nausea and vomiting, pediatric patients 2 to 12 years: The maximum recommended dose is 0.1 mg/kg (100 mcg/kg). Another source suggests 0.03 to 0.07 mg/kg/dose (30 to 70 mcg/kg/dose) over 2 minutes or up to 0.1 mg/kg/dose with caution to achieve desired effect only if benefits outweigh potential risk and total dose does not exceed 2.5 mg. May be given IM or IV. See Maternal/Child.

DOSE ADJUSTMENTS

Initiate at a low dose and adjust upward with caution to achieve the desired effect. ■ Reduce dose of narcotics and all CNS depressants to one fourth or one third of usual dose before, during, and for 24 hours after injection of droperidol. ■ If other CNS depressants (e.g., narcotics) have been given previously, reduce dose of droperidol. ■ Reduce dose for elderly, debilitated, and poor-risk patients and those with impaired kidney or liver function.

DILUTION

May be given undiluted. Give through Y-tube or three-way stopcock of the infusion set. May be added to a convenient volume of selected infusion solutions (D5W, NS, or LR).

Filters: No data available from manufacturer.

Storage: Store vials at CRT; protect from light. Diluted solutions stable at CRT for at least 48 hours (up to 7 days in selected solutions; see literature).

COMPATIBILITY

(Underline Indicates Conflicting Compatibility Information)

Consider any drug NOT listed as compatible to be INCOMPATIBLE until consulting a pharmacist; specific conditions may apply.

Manufacturer states, "Will precipitate if mixed with barbiturates" (e.g., phenobarbital [Luminal], thiopental [Pentothal]).

One source suggests the following **compatibilities:**

Y-site: Amifostine (Ethyol), azithromycin (Zithromax), aztreonam (Azactam), bivalirudin (Angiomax), bleomycin (Blenoxane), buprenorphine (Buprenex), cisatracurium (Nimbex), cisplatin (Platinol), cladribine

(Leustatin), cyclophosphamide (Cytoxan), cytarabine (ARA-C), dexmedetomidine (Precedex), docetaxel (Taxotere), doxorubicin (Adriamycin), doxorubicin liposomal (Doxil), etoposide phosphate (Etopophos), famotidine (Pepcid IV), fenoldopam (Corlopam), filgrastim (Neupogen), fluconazole (Diflucan), fludarabine (Fludara), gemcitabine (Gemzar), granisetron (Kytril), heparin, hetastarch in electrolytes (Hextend), hydrocortisone sodium succinate (Solu-Cortef), idarubicin (Idamycin), linezolid (Zyvox), melphalan (Alkeran), meperidine (Demerol), methotrexate, metoclopramide (Reglan), mitomycin (Mutamycin), ondansetron (Zofran), oxaliplatin (Eloxatin), paclitaxel (Taxol), potassium chloride (KCl), propofol (Diprivan), remifentanil (Ultiva), sargramostim (Leukine), teniposide (Vumon), thiotepa, vinblastine, vincristine, vinorelbine (Navelbine).

RATE OF ADMINISTRATION

IV injection: *Adults:* 2.5 mg or fraction thereof over 1 to 2 minutes. *Pediatric patients:* A single dose or fraction thereof over a minimum of 2 minutes. **Infusion:** Titrate by dose and desired patient response. Do not exceed rate for IV injection.

ACTIONS

An antianxiety agent that produces marked tranquilization and sedation. Has an antiemetic action also. It produces mild alpha-adrenergic blockade and produces peripheral vascular dilation. May decrease an abnormally high pulmonary arterial pressure. A dose-dependent and significant QT prolongation at all dose levels (0.1, 0.175, and 0.25 mg/kg) has been observed within 10 minutes of administration in patients without known cardiac disease. Effective in 3 to 10 minutes with maximum results in 30 minutes. Lasts 2 to 4 hours. Some effects persist for 12 hours. Metabolized in the liver. Excreted in urine and feces. Crosses placental barrier very slowly. Secreted in breast milk.

INDICATIONS AND USES

To reduce the incidence of nausea and vomiting associated with surgical and diagnostic procedures.
Unlabeled uses: Antiemetic in cancer chemotherapy including potent emetic agents (e.g., cisplatin). ■ Treatment of acute psychotic episodes manifested by severe agitation and combativeness. ■ Adjunct to local or general anesthesia.

CONTRAINDICATIONS

Known hypersensitivity to droperidol or other butyrophenones (e.g., haloperidol [Haldol]) and patients with known or suspected QT prolongation, including those with congenital long QT syndrome.

PRECAUTIONS

Use of agents other than droperidol is recommended. ■ QT prolongation and torsades de pointes have been reported with doses at or below those recommended. Some cases have occurred in patients with no known risk factors for QT prolongation, and some cases have been fatal. ■ Use with extreme caution in patients who may be at risk for development of prolonged QT syndrome (e.g., clinically significant bradycardia [less than 50 bpm]; CHF or any clinically significant cardiac disease; use of a diuretic; treatment with class IA antiarrhythmics and/or class III antiarrhythmics; treatment with MAO inhibitors [e.g., selegiline (Eldepryl)]; concomitant treatment with other drug products known to prolong the QT interval; electrolyte imbalance, in particular hypokalemia or hypomagnesemia; alcoholism; or concomitant treatment with drugs that may cause electrolyte imbalance or hypovolemia). See Drug Interactions. ■ Other risk factors may include patients over 65 years of age, alcohol abuse, pheochromocytoma, and the use of agents such as benzodiazepines, volatile anesthetics, and IV opiates. ▪ Correct hypokalemia and/or hypomagnesemia before administration. ▪ When used without a general anesthetic, topical anesthesia is still required when appropriate (e.g., bronchoscopy). ▪ May worsen symptoms of Parkinson's disease.

Monitor: A potent drug. Obtain a baseline ECG on all patients. Do not administer droperidol if a prolonged QT interval exists (QTc greater than 440 msec for males or 450 msec for females). ▪ Monitor VS and ECG closely. Monitor for palpitations, syncope, and/or other symptoms of irregular cardiac rhythm and evaluate promptly. ▪ Resuscitation equipment, a narcotic antagonist (if a narcotic has been used concurrently), IV infusion line, IV fluids, and equipment and drugs to manage emergency situations must be readily available. ▪ In patients for whom the benefit is believed to outweigh the risks of potentially serious arrhythmias, monitor for arrhythmias during the treatment and for 2 to 3 hours after treatment. ▪ Orthostatic hypotension is common; move and position patients with care. ▪ EEG pattern may be slow in returning to normal postoperatively. See Precautions.

Patient Education: Avoid activities that require alertness for 24 hours after receiving droperidol. ▪ Do not drink alcoholic beverages or take other CNS depressants (e.g., antihistamines, pain meds, sleeping pills) for 24 hours after receiving droperidol.

Maternal/Child: Category C: safety for use during pregnancy not established; is rarely used. Exceptions are selected use during cesarean section; it has also been used to treat hyperemesis gravidarum (no longer recommended). ▪ Is secreted in breast milk; avoid breast-feeding. ▪ Pediatric patients may be more susceptible to extrapyramidal side effects, especially acute dystonic reactions. ▪ Safety for use in pediatric patients under 2 years not established.

Elderly: See Dose Adjustments. ▪ More likely to experience hypotension, excessive sedation, and prolonged QT syndrome.

DRUG/LAB INTERACTIONS
Concurrent use with **fentanyl** (Sublimaze) may cause hypotension and decrease pulmonary arterial pressure. ▪ May cause precipitous hypotension with **epinephrine.** ▪ Use caution with **other CNS depressant drugs** (e.g., barbiturates, tranquilizers, opioids, and general anesthetics); may have additive or potentiating effects **with droperidol;** see Dose Adjustments. ▪ Increased risk of QT prolongation and torsades de pointes with **other drugs known to increase the QT interval** (e.g., **class IA antiarrhythmics** [e.g., disopyramide (Norpace), procainamide (Pronestyl), quinidine] **and/or class III antiarrhythmics** [e.g., amiodarone (Nexterone), dofetilide (Tikosyn), ibutilide (Corvert), sotalol (Betapace)], **anticonvulsants** [e.g., fosphenytoin (Cerebyx)], **antidepressants** [e.g., amitriptyline (Elavil), imipramine (Tofranil)], **antihistamines** [e.g., diphenhydramine (Benadryl)], **antimalarials** [e.g., chloroquine], **antineoplastics** [e.g., doxorubicin (Adriamycin)], **azole antifungal agents** [e.g., itraconazole (Sporanox)], **calcium channel blockers** [e.g., nicardipine (Cardene)], **fluoroquinolones, other neuroleptics** [e.g., haloperidol, lithium], **and many others**); see Precautions. ▪ Concurrent administration with **volatile anesthetics, benzodiazepines** (e.g., diazepam [Valium], midazolam [Versed]), or **IV opiates** (e.g., morphine) may produce prolonged QT syndrome. Initiate therapy at a low dose and adjust with caution. ▪ Concomitant treatment with **diuretics** (e.g., furosemide

[Lasix)]), **laxatives, steroids with mineralocorticoid potential** (e.g., hydrocortisone) may cause electrolyte imbalance, hypovolemia, and/or induce hypokalemia or hypomagnesemia. ▪ Concurrent use with **other agents that produce hypotension** may cause orthostatic hypotension; risk is increased with **agents that produce vasodilation** (e.g., amiodarone (Nexterone), milrinone [Primacor], nitroprusside sodium [Nitropress], nicardipine [Cardene]). ▪ See Dose Adjustments and Precautions.

SIDE EFFECTS
Common: Abnormal EEG, chills, dizziness, hallucinations, hypotension, restlessness, shivering, tachycardia.

Major/overdose: Apnea; cardiac arrest; extrapyramidal symptoms; hypotension (severe); neuroleptic malignant syndrome (altered consciousness, muscle rigidity, and autonomic instability); palpitations, syncope, or other symptoms of irregular cardiac rhythm; QT prolongation and torsades de pointes; respiratory depression; ventricular tachycardia; death.

ANTIDOTE
Notify the physician of any side effect. Minor side effects will probably be transient; for major side effects discontinue the drug, treat symptomatically, and notify the physician. Treat hypotension with fluid therapy (rule out hypovolemia) and vasopressors such as dopamine or levarterenol (Levophed). Phenylephrine may help to counteract the alpha-blocking effects of droperidol. Epinephrine is contraindicated for hypotension. Further hypotension will occur. Treat extrapyramidal symptoms with benztropine mesylate (Cogentin) or diphenhydramine (Benadryl). Treat cardiac arrhythmias as indicated (e.g., magnesium sulfate for torsades de pointes, lidocaine, for ventricular tachycardia). An increase in temperature, HR, or CO_2 production may be symptoms of neuroleptic malignant syndrome or malignant hyperpyrexia. Consider prompt treatment with dantrolene (Dantrium). Resuscitate as necessary.

DROTRECOGIN ALFA (ACTIVATED)　　Antithrombotic
(droh-treh-**KOH**-jin **AL**-fah)
Xigris

USUAL DOSE
24 mcg/kg/hr (based on actual body weight) as an infusion for a total duration of 96 hours. Dose adjustment based on clinical or laboratory parameters not recommended. If infusion is interrupted, it should be restarted at 24 mcg/kg/hr. Dose escalation or bolus doses not recommended.

DOSE ADJUSTMENTS
Dose adjustments are not indicated based on age, gender, hepatic dysfunction, or renal dysfunction. ▪ Patients with end-stage renal disease (ESRD) were excluded from the study, but clearance rates did not meaningfully differ from those in normal healthy subjects.

DILUTION
Available in 5-mg and 20-mg vials. Calculate the number of vials needed. Infusion must be complete within 12 hours of preparation. A 70-kg patient

would require 20.16 mg over 12 hours. Reconstitute each 5-mg vial with 2.5 mL of SW (10 mL SW for the 20-mg vial). Add diluent slowly and avoid inverting or shaking the vial. Swirl gently until completely dissolved. Yields a 2 mg/mL concentration. Must be further diluted in NS. Slowly withdraw the desired reconstituted dose of drotrecogin alfa. When further diluting in NS, minimize agitation of the solution by directing the stream to the side of the IV bag or bottle. Gently invert this diluted solution several times to ensure mixing without agitation. Manufacturer states "Do not transport the diluted solution between locations using mechanical delivery systems." Dilution of 20 mg in 200 mL yields 100 mcg/mL (0.1 mg/mL), in 100 mL yields 200 mcg/mL (0.2 mg/mL), and in 20 mL yields 1,000 mcg/mL (1 mg/mL). Dilution for use in an *IV infusion pump* is usually between 100 and 200 mcg/mL. Dilution for use in a *syringe pump* is usually between 100 and 1,000 mcg/mL; see Rate of Administration. **Filters:** Manufacturer's data indicate that no significant drug loss occurs with filtration through either a 0.2- or 1.2-micron in-line filter.

Storage: Vials should be refrigerated in the carton until use. Protect from light. Do not freeze or use beyond the expiration date on the vial. Contains no preservatives; use immediately after reconstitution and dilution preferred. Reconstituted solutions are considered stable for 3 hours at CRT but must be used within the 3 hours. Infusion bags may be refrigerated for up to 12 hours; maximum time limit for use (including preparation, refrigeration, and administration) is 24 hours. Prepared for use in a syringe pump; maximum time limit (including preparation/administration) is 12 hours.

COMPATIBILITY   (Underline Indicates Conflicting Compatibility Information)
Consider any drug NOT listed as compatible to be INCOMPATIBLE until consulting a pharmacist; specific conditions may apply.

Manufacturer states, "Administer via a dedicated IV line or a dedicated lumen of a multilumen central venous catheter. The only solutions that can be administered through the same line are NS, LR, dextrose, or dextrose and saline mixtures." No **incompatibilities** have been observed with glass infusion bottles or infusion bags and syringes made of polyvinylchloride, polyethylene, polypropylene, or polyolefin.

One source suggests the following **compatibilities:**
Y-site: Ceftriaxone (Rocephin), cisatracurium (Nimbex), epinephrine (Adrenalin), fluconazole (Diflucan), furosemide (Lasix), heparin, nitroglycerin IV, potassium chloride, and vasopressin.

RATE OF ADMINISTRATION
Avoid exposure of diluted solution to heat and/or direct sunlight.
Infusion: 24 mcg/kg/hr for a total duration of 96 hours. *When using low concentrations (less than approximately 200 mcg/mL) at low flow rates (less than approximately 5 mL/hr), the infusion set must be primed for approximately 15 minutes at a flow rate of approximately 5 mL/hr to reduce the amount of adsorption of drotrecogin alfa by the IV tubing.*

ACTIONS
A recombinant form of human Activated Protein C. Has the same amino acid sequence as human plasma–derived Activated Protein C, which exerts an antithrombotic effect by inhibiting factors Va and VIIIa. It inhibits plasminogen activator inhibitor-1 (PAI-1) and limits the generation of activated thrombin–activatable fibrinolysis inhibitor. May exert an antiinflammatory effect by inhibiting human tumor necrosis factor production, blocking leukocyte adhesion, and limiting thrombin-induced inflammatory

responses. Mechanisms of effect on survival in patients with severe sepsis are not completely understood. Produces dose-dependent declines in D-dimer and IL-6. Also produces declines in thrombin-antithrombin levels, prothrombin F1.2, and IL-6, more rapid increases in protein C and antithrombin levels, and normalization of plasminogen. Rapidly produces steady-state concentrations proportional to infusion rates, with maximum effects on D-dimer levels occurring at the end of the 96-hour infusion. Inactivated by endogenous plasma protease inhibitors. Plasma clearance is 50% higher in patients with severe sepsis than in healthy subjects. During clinical studies, mortality rates were significantly lower for patients receiving drotrecogin than for patients receiving a placebo. Mortality reduction was greater in patients with severe physiologic disturbances, those with serious underlying disease predating sepsis, and in older patients.

INDICATIONS AND USES

Reduction of mortality in adult patients with severe sepsis (sepsis associated with acute organ dysfunction) who have a high risk of death (as determined by APACHE II criteria). Organ dysfunction has been defined as one of the following: cardiovascular dysfunction (shock, hypotension, or need for vasopressor support despite adequate fluid resuscitation); respiratory dysfunction (relative hypoxemia [PaO_2/FiO_2 ratio less than 250]); renal dysfunction (oliguria despite adequate fluid resuscitation); thrombocytopenia (platelet count less than 80,000/mm^3 or a 50% decrease from the highest value during the previous 3 days); or metabolic acidosis with elevated lactic acid concentrations. Effectiveness in adult patients with severe sepsis and lower risk of death not established; see Precautions.

CONTRAINDICATIONS

Conditions in which bleeding could be associated with a high risk of death or significant morbidity, such as active internal bleeding, intracranial neoplasm or mass lesion or evidence of cerebral herniation, presence of an epidural catheter, recent (within 3 months) hemorrhagic stroke, recent (within 2 months) intracranial or intraspinal surgery or severe head trauma, trauma with an increased risk of life-threatening bleeding, and known hypersensitivity to drotrecogin alfa or any of its components.

PRECAUTIONS

Safety and effectiveness for use longer than 96 hours not established. ■ Administered by or under the direction of a physician experienced in its use and in a facility equipped to monitor the patient and respond to any medical emergency. ■ Bleeding is the most common serious adverse effect; evaluate each patient carefully and weigh the anticipated benefits against the potential risks. Risk of bleeding may be increased in patients with severe sepsis who have one or more of the following conditions:

- Concurrent therapeutic heparin (equal to/greater than 15 units/kg/hr).
- Platelet count less than 30,000/mm^3, even if the platelet count is increased after transfusions
- Prothrombin time-INR more than 3
- Recent (within 6 weeks) gastrointestinal bleeding
- Recent (within 3 days) thrombolytic therapy
- Recent (within 7 days) oral anticoagulants (e.g., warfarin [Coumadin]) or glycoprotein GPIIb/IIIa inhibitors (e.g., abciximab [ReoPro], eptifibatide [Integrilin], tirofiban [Aggrastat])
- Recent (within 7 days) aspirin more than 650 mg/day or other platelet inhibitors (e.g., clopidogrel [Plavix], dipyridamole [Persantine], pli-

camycin [Mithracin], sulfinpyrazone [Anturane], ticlopidine [Ticlid], valproic acid [e.g., Depakene, Depacon])
• Recent (within 3 months) ischemic stroke, intracranial arteriovenous malformation, or aneurysm
• Known bleeding diathesis
• Chronic severe hepatic disease
• Any condition in which bleeding constitutes a significant hazard or would be particularly difficult to manage because of its location
▪ Use caution and weigh risk versus benefit in patients with single organ dysfunction and recent surgery; may be at high risk of death. ▪ As with all proteins, there is a potential for immunogenicity. Antibody development has been reported rarely. Drotrecogin has not been readministered to patients with severe sepsis. ▪ Use caution; allergic reactions and/or anaphylaxis can occur. ▪ Risk of intracranial bleeding may be increased in patients with severe coagulopathy and/or severe thrombocytopenia. ▪ May prolong the aPTT so it is not a reliable test to assess the status of coagulopathy. Has minimal effect on PT, and PT can be used to monitor status of coagulopathy. ▪ The FDA is investigating the possible increased risk of serious bleeding events and death in patients with sepsis and baseline bleeding risk factors. ▪ See Drug/Lab Interactions.

Monitor: Patients with severe sepsis and organ failure require intensive and diagnosis-specific monitoring. ▪ Obtain appropriate baseline clotting studies (e.g., PT, TT, PTT, aPTT, CBC, fibrinogen levels, platelets). ▪ Baseline assessment (patient condition, pain, hematomas, petechiae, or recent wounds) should be completed. ▪ Type and cross-match may also be ordered. ▪ Monitor PT as indicated. ▪ Maintain strict bed rest; monitor the patient carefully and frequently for pain and signs of bleeding; observe catheter sites and apply pressure dressings to any recently invaded site; watch for hematuria, hematemesis, bloody stool, petechiae, hematoma, flank pain, muscle weakness; and do neuro checks as indicated. ▪ Discontinue drotrecogin alfa 2 hours before patient undergoes an invasive surgical procedure or procedures with an inherent risk of bleeding. When hemostasis is achieved, use may be reconsidered 12 hours after major invasive procedures or surgery or restarted immediately after uncomplicated, less invasive procedures. ▪ See Precautions and Drug/Lab Interactions.

Maternal/Child: Category C: use during pregnancy only if clearly needed. ▪ Discontinue breast-feeding. ▪ Safety and effectiveness for use in pediatric patients not established. Enrollment in clinical studies has been discontinued in pediatric patients with severe sepsis. Improvement compared to placebo not noted, and incidence of CNS bleeding is increased.

Elderly: Safety and effectiveness similar to younger adults; however, in clinical studies a greater reduction in mortality occurred in patients with more severe physiologic disturbances, in patients with serious underlying disease predating sepsis, and in older patients.

DRUG/LAB INTERACTIONS
Specific drug interactions not studied. ▪ Concomitant use of prophylactic **low-dose heparin** or prophylactic doses of **low-molecular-weight heparin** (e.g., enoxaparin [Lovenox]) did not appear to affect safety; effect on efficacy not evaluated. ▪ Use caution; risk of bleeding may be increased by **any medicine that affects blood clotting,** including anticoagulants (e.g., heparin, lepirudin [Refludan], warfarin [Coumadin]); **any medication that may cause hypoprothrombinemia, thrombocytopenia, or GI ulceration or bleeding**

(e.g., selected antibiotics [e.g., cefotetan], aspirin, NSAIDs [e.g., ibuprofen (Advil, Motrin), naproxen (Aleve)]); **and/or any other medication that inhibits platelet aggregation** (e.g., clopidogrel [Plavix], dipyridamole [Persantine], glycoprotein GPIIb/IIIa receptor antagonists [e.g., abciximab (ReoPro), eptifibatide (Integrilin), tirofiban (Aggrastat)], plicamycin [Mithracin], sulfinpyrazone [Anturane], ticlopidine [Ticlid], valproic acid [e.g., Depakene, Depacon]); see Precautions. ■ May interfere with **coagulation assays** based on aPTT (e.g., factor VIII, IX, and XI assays); factor concentration will be lower than true concentration. Does not interfere with assays based on PT (e.g., factor II, V, VII, X assays).

SIDE EFFECTS
Bleeding is most common. The majority of bleeding events were ecchymoses or GI tract bleeding, but intra-abdominal, intra-thoracic, retroperitoneal, intracranial, GU, and skin and soft tissue bleeding have been reported. Hypersensitivity reactions and anaphylaxis may occur.

ANTIDOTE
Notify physician of all side effects. Note even the most minute bleeding tendency. Oozing at IV sites may occur. Control minor bleeding by local pressure. If clinically important bleeding occurs, discontinue the infusion of drotrecogin alfa. Carefully assess other agents that may contribute to the bleeding. Continued use of drotrecogin alfa may be reconsidered when adequate hemostasis is achieved. For severe bleeding in a critical location or suspected intracranial bleeding, discontinue drotrecogin alfa and any heparin therapy immediately. Obtain PT, platelet count, and fibrinogen level. Draw blood for type and cross-match. Platelets, cryoprecipitate, whole blood, packed RBCs, fresh-frozen plasma, desmopressin, tranexamic acid (Cyklokapron), and aminocaproic acid (Amicar) may be indicated. Topical preparations of aminocaproic acid may stop minor bleeding. Consider protamine if heparin has been used. No known antidote; if overdose occurs, stop the infusion and monitor for signs of hemorrhagic complications. Treat minor hypersensitivity reactions symptomatically. Discontinue drug and treat anaphylaxis as indicated; resuscitate as necessary.

ECULIZUMAB BBW
(eck-you-**LIZ**-you-mab)

Soliris

Monoclonal antibody
Complement inhibitor

pH 7

USUAL DOSE
A meningococcal vaccine must be administered at least 2 weeks before initial dosing with eculizumab to all patients who have not been previously vaccinated. A booster dose may be required for patients previously vaccinated. Revaccinate according to current medical guidelines. Quadrivalent, conjugated meningococcal vaccines are strongly recommended.

Initial dose: Administer 600 mg as an infusion. Repeat once each week (every 7 days) for 3 more doses (a total of 4 weeks). Seven days after the fourth dose, administer a 900-mg dose.

Maintenance dose: 14 days after the fifth dose, begin a maintenance program of 900 mg administered every 14 days.

DOSE ADJUSTMENTS
A variance of 1 to 2 days in the scheduled administration time points is allowed if indicated. The prescribing information mentions only the administration at 12 instead of 14 days in select patients to achieve a reduction in lactic dehydrogenase (LDH) levels.

DILUTION
Available in 300 mg/30 mL single-use vials (10 mg/mL). Withdraw the required dose of eculizumab (2 vials are required for the 600-mg dose, and 3 vials are required for the 900-mg dose) and transfer it to an infusion bag. Must be further diluted to a 5 mg/mL concentration by adding an amount of NS, ½NS, D5W, or Ringer's lactate to the infusion bag equal to the total volume of the eculizumab (60 mL diluent for the 600-mg dose, and 90 mL diluent for the 900-mg dose). Total volume will be 120 mL for the 600-mg dose and 180 mL for the 900-mg dose. Invert gently to ensure thorough mixing. Allow the diluted solution to reach room temperature before infusion. Do not use an artificial heat source (e.g., microwave). Discard unused portions; contains no preservatives.

Filters: Specific information not available.

Storage: Refrigerate vials in original carton at 2° to 8° C (36° to 46° F) and protect from light. Do not use beyond the expiration date on the vial. Diluted solution is stable for 24 hours refrigerated or at CRT. Do not freeze or shake.

COMPATIBILITY
Specific information not available.

RATE OF ADMINISTRATION
Do not administer as an IV push or a bolus injection. For infusion via gravity feed, syringe-type pump, or infusion pump. A single dose as an infusion over 35 minutes. If infusion is slowed or stopped for any reason, the total infusion time should not exceed 2 hours.

ACTIONS
A recombinant, DNA-derived, humanized IgG monoclonal antibody. A genetic mutation in patients with paroxysmal nocturnal hemoglobinuria (PNH) leads to the generation of abnormal RBCs (known as PNH cells) that are deficient in terminal complement inhibitors; this deficiency makes

these RBCs sensitive to persistent terminal complement-mediated destruction. Ongoing destruction of these RBCs is called hemolysis. Eculizumab specifically binds to the complement protein and prevents complement-mediated intravascular hemolysis. It improves the lives of patients suffering from this disease by directly targeting the underlying disease process and markedly decreasing the ongoing RBC destruction that causes the hemolysis responsible for the S/S of PNH. Half-life is 190-354 hours.

INDICATIONS AND USES

A complement inhibitor for the treatment of patients with paroxysmal nocturnal hemoglobinuria (PNH) to reduce hemolysis. PNH is a rare, disabling, and life-threatening genetic mutation blood disorder defined by chronic RBC destruction (hemolysis). Symptoms may include anemia; disabling fatigue; dysphagia; dyspnea; erectile dysfunction; hemoglobinuria; jaundice; recurrent pain in the abdomen, back, or head; renal dysfunction; and thromboses. Average age of onset is the early 30s, with survival between 10 and 15 years from the time of diagnosis.

CONTRAINDICATIONS

Do not use in patients with unresolved serious *Neisseria meningitidis* infection or in patients not currently vaccinated against *N. meningitidis*.

PRECAUTIONS

For IV infusion only; do not administer by IV push or bolus injection. ■ Susceptibility to serious meningococcal infections (septicemia and/or meningitis) is increased. Meningococcal infections may become rapidly life threatening or fatal if not recognized and treated early. A meningococcal vaccine must be administered at least 2 weeks before initial dosing with eculizumab to all patients who have not been previously vaccinated. A booster dose may be required for patients previously vaccinated. Revaccinate according to current medical guidelines; see Usual Dose. Vaccination may not prevent meningococcal infections. ■ Use caution in patients with any systemic infection. Patients may have increased susceptibility to infection. ■ Serious hemolysis may occur in patients who discontinue eculizumab therapy; see Monitor. ■ A protein product; infusion reactions may occur. Hypersensitivity reactions, including anaphylaxis, are possible; however, infusion reactions severe enough to discontinue eculizumab did not occur during clinical trials. ■ Has a potential for immunogenicity. Low titers of antibodies to eculizumab have been detected but did not appear to correlate to clinical response. ■ Continue established anticoagulant therapy during eculizumab treatment; the effect of withdrawal of anticoagulant therapy during eculizumab therapy has not been established.

Monitor: Obtain baseline CBC with differential and platelets, lactic dehydrogenase (LDH), SCr, and bilirubin. ■ LDH levels increase during hemolysis. Monitoring may assist in determining the effectiveness of eculizumab therapy. ■ Monitor for early S/S of meningococcal infections (moderate to severe headache with nausea or vomiting, fever, or a stiff neck or stiff back; fever of 103° F [39.4° C] or higher; fever and a rash; confusion; and/or severe muscle aches with flu-like symptoms and light sensitivity). Evaluate immediately and treat with antibiotics if indicated. Consider discontinuing eculizumab during treatment of serious meningococcal infections. ■ Monitor for S/S of an infusion reaction (e.g., chills, dyspnea, pruritus) during infusion and for at least 1 hour post-infusion. Slow or temporarily discontinue the infusion as indicated. ■ Monitor patients who discontinue eculizumab for a minimum of 8 weeks to detect serious hemolysis and other reactions. Serious hemolysis is identified by serum LDH levels greater than pretreatment levels along with a greater than 25% decrease in PNH clone size (in the absence of dilution by transfusion) in 1 week or less, a hemoglobin level of less than 5 Gm/dL or a decrease of more than 4 Gm/dL in 1 week or less, angina, a change in mental status, a 50% increase in SCr, or thromboses (e.g., blood clots).

Patient Education: Read the patient medication guide before initiating eculizumab and before each dose. ▪ Meningococcal vaccination is required before initiating therapy. Previously vaccinated individuals may require a booster dose. Important to receive and stay up-to-date on all recommended immunizations. Discuss immunization status with physician. ▪ Eculizumab affects the immune system and can lower the ability to fight infections. Immediately report S/S of a meningococcal infection (moderate to severe headache with nausea or vomiting, fever, or a stiff neck or stiff back; fever of 103° F [39.4° C] or higher; fever and a rash; confusion; and/or severe muscle aches with flu-like symptoms and light sensitivity). Manufacturer supplies a patient safety card that lists these symptoms and is to be carried at all times and shown to all health care providers treating you. ▪ Promptly report other S/S of an infection. ▪ Promptly report chills, dyspnea, and/or itching during or soon after an infusion. ▪ Report a suspected pregnancy and/or tell your doctor if you are breast-feeding. ▪ Stopping the infusions may have serious side effects and requires prolonged monitoring.

Maternal/Child: Category C: use during pregnancy only if the benefits justify the potential risk to the fetus. Pregnant women with PNH and their fetuses have high rates of morbidity and mortality during pregnancy and postpartum. ▪ Effects of eculizumab therapy during labor and delivery are unknown. ▪ Use caution if breast-feeding; IgG is secreted in breast milk, but antibodies may not enter the neonatal and infant circulation in substantial amounts. Consider risks to infant versus benefits of breast-feeding. ▪ Safety and effectiveness for use in pediatric patients less than 18 years of age not established.

Elderly: Limited experience did not identify age-related differences in safety and effectiveness.

DRUG/LAB INTERACTIONS

Formal drug interaction studies have not been completed. ▪ Continue established anticoagulant therapy during eculizumab treatment; the effect of withdrawal of anticoagulant therapy during eculizumab therapy has not been established.

SIDE EFFECTS

Meningococcal infections (meningitis and/or septicemia) and the progression of PNH are the most serious side effects reported; may be life threatening and may occur in patients who have been vaccinated. The most commonly reported side effects are back pain, headache, nasopharyngitis, and nausea. Other reported side effects include anemia, constipation, cough, extremity pain, fatigue, fever, herpes simplex infections, influenza-like illness, myalgia, respiratory infections, and sinusitis.

Post-Marketing: Cases of serious or fatal meningococcal infections have been reported.

ANTIDOTE

Keep physician informed of all side effects. Some will be treated symptomatically. Potential meningococcal infections must be evaluated immediately and treated with antibiotics promptly; may be life threatening. Treat hypersensitivity or infusion reactions as indicated; may respond to slowing or temporarily discontinuing the infusion or may require the use of epinephrine, corticosteroids, diphenhydramine bronchodilators (e.g., albuterol [Ventolin], aminophylline), IV saline, oxygen, and/or acetaminophen. Total infusion time should not exceed 2 hours. If serious hemolysis occurs after eculizumab is discontinued, the following treatments may be indicated: transfusion with packed RBCs (or an exchange transfusion if the PNH RBCs are more than 50% of the total RBCs by flow cytometry), anticoagulation, corticosteroids, or reinstitution of eculizumab. Resuscitate as necessary.

EDETATE CALCIUM DISODIUM BBW

(**ED**-eh-tayt **KAL**-see-um **DYE**-so-dee-um)

Calcium Disodium Edetate, Calcium
Disodium Versenate, Calcium EDTA

Antidote
Chelating agent
Lead mobilization

pH 6.5 to 8

USUAL DOSE

Specific fluid requirements indicated; see Monitor and Maternal/Child. Do not exceed recommended daily dose.

Asymptomatic adults and pediatric patients with blood lead levels over 20 mcg/dL but under 70 mcg/dL: 1,000 mg/M^2/24 hr (50 mg/kg/24 hr) for 3 to 5 days. After a rest period of 2 to 4 days (preferably up to 2 weeks) to allow for redistribution of lead, repeat the process, if indicated, based on severity of lead toxicity and patient tolerance.

Symptomatic adults and pediatric patients with blood levels over 70 mcg/dL: Dimercaprol (BAL) will be given IM in divided doses every 4 hours for a minimum of 3 or up to 5 days. 4 hours after the first dose of BAL begin edetate calcium disodium 1,000 mg/M^2/24 hr (50 mg/kg/24 hr) for 5 days. If blood lead concentrations rebound to above 45 mcg/dL within 5 to 7 days after the initial course, repeat the edetate calcium disodium. Do not repeat the dimercaprol regimen.

DOSE ADJUSTMENTS

Reduce dose in pre-existing renal disease and/or adults with lead nephropathy. In adults with lead nephropathy dose is based on serum creatinine levels and repeated monthly until lead excretion is reduced toward normal according to the following chart.

Dose Adjustments in Impaired Renal Function and/or Adults with Lead Nephropathy	
Serum Creatinine Level	Dose
<2 mg/dL	1,000 mg/M^2/24 hr for 5 days
2-3 mg/dL	500 mg/M^2/24 hr for 5 days
3-4 mg/dL	500 mg/M^2/48 hr for 3 doses
>4 mg/dL	500 mg/M^2/week

DILUTION

Add total daily dose to 250 to 500 mL of D5W or NS for infusion.
Storage: Before use, store at CRT.

COMPATIBILITY

Consider any drug NOT listed as compatible to be INCOMPATIBLE until consulting a pharmacist; specific conditions may apply.

Manufacturer lists amphotericin B (generic), hydralazine, D10W, 10% invert sugar in NS, LR, Ringer's solution, ⅙ M lactate as **incompatible.** Must be diluted in specific IV solutions; see Dilution.

RATE OF ADMINISTRATION

References vary greatly. Manufacturer recommends the total daily dose be evenly distributed over 8 to 12 hours. May cause an increase in intracranial pressure with too-rapid injection in patients with lead encephalopathy and cerebral edema.

ACTIONS

A chelating agent. Helps to remove metals, especially lead, from the body. Will form a stable chelate with metals that have the ability to displace calcium from the molecule (e.g., lead, zinc, cadmium). Distributed primarily in the extracellular fluid. Half-life is 20 to 60 minutes. Chelated compounds are excreted in urine; up to 50% in 1 hour and 95% in 24 hours. The primary source of lead chelated by edetate calcium disodium is from bone. Following administration, urinary lead output increases and blood lead concentration decreases, but brain lead is significantly increased due to internal redistribution of lead.

INDICATIONS AND USES

Reduction of blood levels and depot stores of lead in lead poisoning (acute and chronic) and lead encephalopathy in both pediatric and adult patients. **Unlabeled uses:** Treatment of poisoning by radioactive and nuclear fission products such as plutonium, thorium, uranium, and yttrium. ▪ Treatment of poisoning from other heavy metals such as chromium, manganese, nickel, zinc, and possibly vanadium.

CONTRAINDICATIONS

Anuria, active renal disease, or hepatitis.

PRECAUTIONS

Do not confuse with edetate disodium, which does not chelate lead but actually removes calcium from the body and can be very dangerous. ▪ Patients with lead encephalopathy and cerebral edema may have a lethal increase in intracranial pressure with IV infusion; IM injection preferred; see Maternal/Child. ▪ Equally effective with IM or IV administration. IM route is used for all patients with overt lead encephalopathy and has been suggested as the preferred route by some for young pediatric patients. ▪ Usually given IM in pediatric patients, unless given concurrently with BAL (insufficient IM injection sites); see Maternal/Child. ▪ May produce toxic and fatal effects. ▪ Produces the same renal damage as lead poisoning (e.g., proteinuria and microscopic hematuria). ▪ Nephrotoxicity is dose dependent and may be reduced by ensuring adequate diuresis before treatment begins. ▪ Use with caution in mild renal disease; see Dose Adjustments. ▪ Patients must be removed from the source of contamination promptly. ▪ Use for diagnosis of lead poisoning as a lead mobilization test is controversial; see literature. Edetate calcium disodium mobilization test should not be used in symptomatic patients or in patients with blood levels above 55 mcg/dL for whom appropriate therapy is indicated. ▪ Not effective in mercury, gold, or arsenic poisoning.

Monitor: Urine flow must be established before dimercaprol (BAL) or edetate calcium disodium is administered. IV fluids may be used. Avoid excessive fluid in patients with cerebral edema or lead encephalopathy. Once urine flow is established, further IV fluid is restricted in all patients to basal water and electrolyte requirements. ▪ Monitor urinalysis, urine sediment, renal and hepatic function, and electrolyte levels before treatment; repeat daily in serious cases and on the second and fifth day in less serious cases. Daily urine specimens are recommended to determine status of renal function. ▪ Monitor ECG and vital signs. ▪ Elevated erythrocyte protoporphyrin levels (greater than 35 mcg/dL) indicate the need to perform a venous blood lead determination. ▪ An elevation of urinary coproporphyrin (greater than 250 mcg/day in adults and greater than 75 mcg/day in pediatric patients under 80 lbs) and an elevation of urinary delta-aminolevulinic acid (greater than 4 mg/day in adults and greater than 3 mg/M^2/day in pediatric patients) are associated with blood lead levels greater than 40 mcg/dL. ▪ Excretion of calcium is not increased, but excretion of zinc and other essential metals is; monitor and replace as indicated. ▪ Obtain specific fluid orders from the physician.

Patient Education: If no urine output for 12 hours, report immediately.

Maternal/Child: Category B: safety for use during pregnancy not established; benefits must outweigh risks. ▪ Use caution in nursing mothers. ▪ Lead poisoning is often more severe in pediatric patients compared with adult patients. Lead encephalopathy occurs more often in pediatric patients. May be incipient and thus overlooked. Mortality rate in pediatric patients has been high; see Precautions. ▪ IV injection has been associated with fatality in some young children, and IM injection is considered to be the preferred route by some clinicians.

Elderly: Consider age-related organ damage.

DRUG/LAB INTERACTIONS

Steroids will increase renal toxicity. ▪ Inhibits the action of **zinc insulin** preparations by chelating the zinc.

SIDE EFFECTS

Acute renal tubular necrosis, anemia, anorexia, arthralgia, cardiac rhythm irregularities, chills, excessive thirst, fatigue, fever, headache, hematuria, hypercalcemia, hypersensitivity (e.g., sneezing, nasal congestion), hypotension, increases in liver function tests (mild), leg and other muscle cramps, malaise, myalgia, nausea, numbness, proteinuria, tetany, tingling, transient bone marrow suppression, tremors, vomiting, weakness, zinc deficiency.

ANTIDOTE

Notify the physician of any side effects. Most will improve with a decrease in rate of the infusion or will be treated symptomatically. Discontinue if urine flow stops to avoid high tissue levels of the drug. Discontinue at the first sign of renal toxicity (e.g., presence of large renal epithelial cells or increasing numbers of RBCs). Treat cerebral edema with repeated doses of mannitol. Not known if edetate calcium disodium is dialyzable.

EDETATE DISODIUM BBW

(**ED**-eh-tayt **DYE**-so-dee-um)

EDTA Disodium, Endrate

Antihypercalcemic agent
Calcium chelating agent

pH 6.5 to 7.5

USUAL DOSE

50 mg/kg of body weight/24 hr or in equally divided doses every 12 hours (25 mg/kg every 12 hours). Total dose should not exceed 3 Gm/24 hr. Usually given for 5 days, held for 2 days. Regimen may be repeated to a total of 15 doses.

PEDIATRIC DOSE

40 mg/kg of body weight/24 hr in equally divided doses every 6 to 12 hours (20 mg/kg every 12 hours, 10 mg/kg every 6 hours). Do not exceed 70 mg/kg/24 hr or adult dose, whichever is less. See instructions in Usual Dose.

DOSE ADJUSTMENTS

Dose selection should be cautious in the elderly. Reduced doses may be indicated based on potential for decreased organ function and concomitant disease or drug therapy.

DILUTION

Recommended dose must be diluted in 500 mL D5W or NS and given as an infusion. A 0.5% solution will reduce the risk of thrombophlebitis. Do not exceed cardiac reserve in any patient. Use less diluent if necessary in pediatric patients. Must be diluted to at least a 3% solution.

Storage: Store at room temperature.

COMPATIBILITY

Specific information not available. Consider specific use; consult pharmacist.

RATE OF ADMINISTRATION

Must not exceed more than 15 mg of actual medication over 1 minute. Total dose usually given over 3 to 4 hours. Rapid IV infusion may cause a sudden drop in serum calcium, resulting in tetany, convulsions, arrhythmias, and death. Reduce rate and further dilute solution for pain at injection site.

ACTIONS

A calcium-chelating agent. Also forms chelates with other polyvalent metals (e.g., magnesium, zinc). Attracts calcium ions immediately on injection and becomes calcium disodium edetate. Capable of severely depleting the body of calcium stores. Exerts a negative inotropic effect on the heart. It is well distributed in extracellular fluids and rapidly excreted in the urine.

INDICATIONS AND USES

Treatment of cardiac arrhythmias (atrial and ventricular, especially when caused by digoxin toxicity). ▪ Hypercalcemia.

CONTRAINDICATIONS

Anuria, known sensitivity to edetate disodium, renal disease.

PRECAUTIONS

Read label carefully. Deaths have been caused when edetate disodium was administered mistakenly for edetate calcium disodium. ▪ Used only when the severity of disease indicates necessity. ▪ May produce hypocalcemia quickly, especially if used for purposes other than chelating calcium. ▪ Use

repeatedly with caution because of potential for nephrotoxicity and mobilization of extracirculatory calcium stores. ▪ Use caution in cardiac disease (may adversely affect myocardial contractility), diabetes (lower blood sugar may require less insulin), severe renal disease, liver disease, congestive heart failure (1 Gm of sodium in each 5 Gm), limited cardiac reserve and patients with a history of seizures or intracranial lesions. **Monitor:** Monitor vital signs and ECG before and during therapy. ▪ Confirm patency of vein, avoid extravasation; can cause tissue necrosis. ▪ Routine electroiyte panel (potassium deficiency) and urine specimens for casts and cells necessary during therapy. Magnesium, zinc, and other trace element deficiencies can occur. ▪ Keep patient in supine position during and after administration (15 to 30 minutes) to avoid postural hypotension. ▪ Obtain blood for serum calcium levels just before beginning a new infusion; specific lab methods required. ▪ Inhibits coagulation of blood (transient). Liver function tests may be indicated. ▪ See Drug/Lab Interactions.
Maternal/Child: Category C: safety for use in pregnancy or breast-feeding not established. Use with extreme caution and only if clearly needed.
Elderly: Reduced doses may be indicated; see Dose Adjustments. Monitoring of renal function is suggested.

DRUG/LAB INTERACTIONS

Inhibits **mannitol.** ▪ Potentiates **neuromuscular blocking antibiotics** (e.g., gentamicin). ▪ Inhibits coagulation of **blood** (transient). ▪ A sudden drop in calcium levels may decrease effects of **digoxin.** ▪ Obtain blood for **serum calcium levels** just before beginning a new infusion. Specific laboratory methods must be used for accurate evaluation.

SIDE EFFECTS

Anorexia, arthralgia, circumoral paresthesias, diarrhea, fatigue, fever, glycosuria, headache, hyperuricemia, hypotension, malaise, nasal congestion, nausea, numbness, sneezing, tearing, thirst, thrombophlebitis, urinary urgency, vomiting.
Major: Anaphylaxis, anemia, cardiac arrhythmias, dermatitis, hemorrhage, hypocalcemic tetany, prolonged QT interval, renal tubular destruction (reversible), seizures, death.

ANTIDOTE

Notify the physician of any side effect. For progression of minor side effects or any major side effect, discontinue drug immediately and notify the physician. Calcium gluconate is the antidote of choice and should be available for infusion at all times (use extreme caution if patient is digitalized). Treat mild hypotension by maintaining in supine position until recovery. Additional hydration indicated with S/S of nephrotoxicity. Treat anaphylaxis and resuscitate as necessary.

520

EDROPHONIUM CHLORIDE
(ed-roh-**FOH**-nee-um **KLOR**-eyed)

Cholinergic
Cholinesterase inhibitor
Antidote
Diagnostic agent

Enlon, Tensilon, Tensilon PF   pH 5.4

USUAL DOSE
1 to 10 mg (0.1 to 1 mL) at specified intervals depending on usage. Maximum dose should never exceed 40 mg (4 doses of 10 mg each).
Myasthenia gravis diagnosis: 10 mg (1 mL) in tuberculin syringe. Give 2 mg (0.2 mL). If no reaction occurs in 45 seconds, give remaining 8 mg (0.8 mL). Test may be repeated after 30 minutes.
Myasthenia treatment evaluation: 1 to 2 mg (0.1 to 0.2 mL) 1 hour after oral intake of drug being used for treatment. Package insert has a chart differentiating myasthenic and nonmyasthenic responses.
Myasthenia crisis evaluation: 2 mg (0.2 mL) in tuberculin syringe. Give 1 mg (0.1 mL). If the patient's condition does not deteriorate, give 1 mg (0.1 mL) after 60 seconds. Improvement in cardiac status and respiration should occur.
Antagonist to curare and other nondepolarizing muscle relaxants: 10 mg (1 mL). May be repeated as necessary up to 4 doses. (Available in combination with atropine [Enlon-Plus] for use in reversal of nondepolarizing muscle relaxants.)
Terminate paroxysmal atrial tachycardia (unlabeled): 5 to 10 mg as a bolus injection. See Dose Adjustments. Repeat once in 10 minutes if necessary.
Slow supraventricular tachycardias (unlabeled): 2 mg as a test dose. Repeat 2 mg every 1 minute until arrhythmia controlled or total dose of 10 mg is given. If HR decreases, may begin an infusion of 0.25 mg/min. May be increased to 2 mg/min if necessary.

PEDIATRIC DOSE
May be given IM if the IV route is not available; however, doses are different; check literature. See Maternal/Child.
Myasthenia gravis diagnosis: *Neonates:* 0.1 mg (0.01 mL). *Infants:* 0.5 mg (0.05 mL).
Pediatric patients less than 34 kg: 1 mg (0.1 mL); if no response in 30 to 45 seconds, give 1 mg (0.1 mL) every 30 to 45 seconds up to 5 mg (0.5 mL). *34 kg or more,* give 2 mg (0.2 mL); if no response in 30 to 45 seconds, give 1 mg (0.1 mL) every 30 to 45 seconds up to 10 mg. Another source has the same dose for neonates but recommends 0.2 mg/kg/dose (0.02 mL/kg/dose) for *infants and other pediatric patients* with 20% of a dose given as a test dose slowly. If no response in 1 minute, give in 1-mg increments to a maximum calculated dose or 10 mg, whichever is less.

DOSE ADJUSTMENTS
Reduce antiarrhythmic dose to 5 to 7 mg in the elderly.

DILUTION
May be given undiluted. In the treatment of myasthenia crisis, this drug may be diluted in D5W or NS and given as a continuous IV. Use an infusion pump or microdrip (60 gtt/mL).
Filters: No data available from manufacturer.

COMPATIBILITY

Consider any drug NOT listed as compatible to be INCOMPATIBLE until consulting a pharmacist; specific conditions may apply.

One source suggests the following **compatibilities:**

Y-site: Heparin, hydrocortisone sodium succinate (Solu-Cortef), potassium chloride (KCl).

RATE OF ADMINISTRATION

2 mg (0.2 mL) or fraction thereof over 15 to 30 seconds.

Curare antagonist: A single dose over 30 to 45 seconds.

Antiarrhythmic: See Usual Dose.

ACTIONS

An anticholinesterase and antagonist of nondepolarizing neuromuscular-blocking agents. Inhibits the enzyme acetylcholinesterase, allowing acetylcholine to accumulate at the myoneural junction. Restores normal transmission of nerve impulses. Acts within 30 to 60 seconds and has an extremely short duration of action, seldom exceeding 10 minutes. Produces vagal stimulation, shortens refractory period of atrial muscle, and slows conduction through the AV node.

INDICATIONS AND USES

Diagnosis of myasthenia gravis. ▪ Evaluation of adequate treatment of myasthenia gravis. ▪ Evaluation of emergency treatment of myasthenia crisis. ▪ An antagonist to nondepolarizing muscle relaxants (e.g., atracurium [Tracrium]). ▪ Adjunct in treatment of respiratory depression caused by Curare overdosage.

Unlabeled uses: Termination of supraventricular tachycardia unresponsive to cardiac glycosides. Adenosine is the drug of choice. ▪ Diagnosis of supraventricular tachycardia. ▪ Evaluate function of a demand pacemaker.

CONTRAINDICATIONS

Apnea, known hypersensitivity to anticholinesterase agents, mechanical intestinal and urinary obstructions of mechanical type.

PRECAUTIONS

A physician should be present when this drug is used. ▪ The term *crisis* is used when severe respiratory distress with ventilatory inadequacy occurs. The crisis may be secondary to a sudden increase in severity of myasthenia gravis (myasthenic crisis) or to overtreatment with anticholinesterase drugs (cholinergic crisis). If apnea is present, controlled ventilation must be secured before any testing with edrophonium. ▪ Use caution when administering to patients being treated with anticholinesterase drugs (e.g., neostigmine). S/S of cholinergic crisis may mimic those of myasthenic weakness, and the patient's condition may worsen with administration of edrophonium. ▪ Use caution in patients with bronchial asthma, cardiac arrhythmias, or myasthenia gravis treated with anticholinesterase drugs. ▪ Isolated cases of respiratory or cardiac arrests have been reported. ▪ Contains sulfites; use caution in patients with allergies.

Monitor: Atropine 1 mg must be available and ready for injection at all times. ▪ Continuously observe patient reactions. ▪ Anticholinesterase insensitivity may develop; withhold drugs and support respiration as necessary. ▪ See Drug/Lab Interactions.

Maternal/Child: Safety for use during pregnancy and breast-feeding not established. Use during pregnancy only if benefit justifies potential risk to mother and fetus. ▪ Discontinue breast-feeding. ▪ Safety and effectiveness in reversing neuromuscular blockade in pediatric patients not established.

However, doses of 0.1 to 1.43 mg/kg have been used; effects (antagonism) were more rapid than in adults.

DRUG/LAB INTERACTIONS
Muscarinic effects antagonized by **atropine;** see Antidote. ▪ May be inhibited by **corticosteroids and magnesium.** ▪ May cause bradycardia with **digoxin glycosides.** ▪ Briefly antagonizes the effects of **nondepolarizing neuromuscular blocking agents** (e.g., atracurium, pancuronium, vecuronium). ▪ Prolongs muscle relaxant effect of **succinylcholine.**

SIDE EFFECTS
Abdominal cramps, anorexia, anxiety, bradycardia, bronchiolar spasm, cardiac arrhythmias and arrest, cold moist skin, contraction of the pupils, convulsions, diarrhea, dysphagia, fainting, increased lacrimation, increased pulmonary secretion, increased salivation, insomnia, irritability, laryngospasm, muscle weakness, nausea, perspiration, ptosis, respiratory arrest (either muscular or central), urinary frequency and incontinence, vomiting.

ANTIDOTE
If side effects occur, discontinue the drug and notify the physician. Atropine sulfate in doses of 0.4 to 0.5 mg IV will counteract most side effects and may be repeated every 3 to 10 minutes. Endotracheal intubation or tracheostomy is considered prophylactic in anesthesia or crises. Artificial ventilation, oxygen therapy, cardiac monitoring, adequate suctioning, and treatment of shock or convulsions must be instituted and maintained as necessary. Treat hypersensitivity reactions as indicated.

EDROPHONIUM CHLORIDE AND ATROPINE SULFATE
(ed-roh-**FOH**-nee-um and **AH**-troh-peen)

Enlon-Plus

Cholinergic
Cholinesterase inhibitor
Antidote

pH 4 to 5

USUAL DOSE
0.05 to 0.1 mL/kg (0.5 to 1 mg/kg of edrophonium with 0.007 to 0.014 mg/kg of atropine). Each 1 mL of prepared solution contains 10 mg edrophonium and 0.14 mg atropine. Must be administered at a point of at least 5% recovery of twitch response to neuromuscular stimulation. Use of peripheral nerve stimulator recommended. A total dose of 1 mg/kg of edrophonium is rarely exceeded. Length of action is usually sufficient to cover effects of commonly used short- and medium-acting nondepolarizing muscle relaxants (e.g., atracurium [Tracrium], vecuronium).

DOSE ADJUSTMENTS
None required; however, caution and lower-end dosing is suggested in elderly patients. Consider decreased organ function and concomitant disease or drug therapy. ▪ Elderly patients and those with impaired renal or hepatic function may have a prolonged half-life and reduced clearance.

DILUTION

May be given undiluted through Y-tube or three-way stopcock of infusion set.

Storage: Available in vials containing 5 mL or 15 mL. Store at room temperature 15° to 26° C (59° to 78° F).

COMPATIBILITY

Specific information not available. Consider specific use; consult pharmacist.

RATE OF ADMINISTRATION

A single dose over 45 to 60 seconds.

ACTIONS

A combination of an acetylcholinesterase inhibitor and a parasympatholytic (anticholinergic) drug. Edrophonium antagonizes the effect of nondepolarizing neuromuscular blocking agents by inhibiting or inactivating acetylcholinesterase. Acetylcholine is not hydrolyzed as rapidly by acetylcholinesterase and accumulates, improving transmission of impulses across the myoneural junction. Unavoidable accumulation of acetylcholine at muscarinic cholinergic sites may cause bradycardia, bronchoconstriction, increased secretions, and other parasympathomimetic effects. Magnitude of effects varies depending on vagal nerve activity present. Atropine counteracts these side effects. Edrophonium is effective immediately with maximum antagonism within 1 to 2 minutes and lasts for 70 minutes. Atropine affects HR immediately, peaks in 2 to 16 minutes, and lasts for over 2 hours. With this combination agent, full reversal is usually accomplished before patient leaves recovery, muscarinic effects are minimized, and patient evaluation can be accomplished in OR. Some hepatic metabolism. Primarily excreted in urine, with some excretion in bile.

INDICATIONS AND USES

Reversal agent or antagonist of nondepolarizing neuromuscular blocking agents. Not effective against depolarizing neuromuscular blocking agents (e.g., succinylcholine). ▪ Adjunctive treatment of respiratory depression of curare overdose.

CONTRAINDICATIONS

Acute glaucoma, adhesions between the iris and lens of the eye, known hypersensitivity to either component or sulfites, mechanical intestinal and urinary obstructions, and pyloric stenosis.

PRECAUTIONS

Administer only by or under the direct observation of the anesthesiologist. ▪ May contain sulfites, and the stopper contains latex; use caution in patients with allergies. ▪ Use caution in patients with bronchial asthma, cardiac arrhythmias, cardiovascular disease, myasthenia gravis (or symptoms of myasthenic weakness) treated with anticholinesterase drugs, prostatic hypertrophy, and debilitated patients with chronic lung disease. ▪ Recurarization has not been reported after satisfactory reversal obtained. ▪ See Drug/Lab Interactions.

Monitor: An additional supply of atropine 1 mg must be available and ready for injection at all times. ▪ Continuously observe patient reactions and monitor responses. Monitor ECG, vital signs, and reversal with a peripheral nerve stimulator. Ventilation (assisted or controlled) must be secured. ▪ Anticholinesterase insensitivity may develop; reduce or withhold drugs and support respiration as necessary until sensitivity returns. ▪ Confirm patency of vein; will cause tissue irritation. ▪ See Drug/ Lab Interactions.

Maternal/Child: Category C: use during pregnancy only if benefits outweigh risks. ▪ Safety for use during breast-feeding or in pediatric patients not established. ▪ Pediatric patients may have increased vagal tone with greater variance in effects. ▪ Atropine rate of clearance decreased in pediatric patients less than 2 years of age, but dose adjustment not indicated.

Elderly: Differences in response have not been identified; see Dose Adjustments. ▪ Half-life is prolonged and clearance is reduced in the elderly; elimination of nondepolarizing muscle relaxants is similarly decreased.

DRUG/LAB INTERACTIONS

Never administer before any **nondepolarizing muscle relaxant** (e.g., atracurium [Tracrium]). ▪ May cause symptoms of anticholinesterase overdose (cholinergic crisis) with **anticholinesterase drugs.** ▪ Frequency and duration of bradycardia increased with **narcotic analgesics** unless given with a potent inhalant anesthetic. ▪ Excessive bradycardia may develop with **beta-adrenergic blocking agents** (e.g., atenolol [Tenormin], esmolol [Brevibloc], timolol [Timpotic]); atropine alone should be given before Enlon-Plus in these patients. ▪ Bradycardia and first-degree heart block may be increased when **muscle relaxants** with no vagolytic effects (e.g., vecuronium) are reversed. ▪ Cardiac arrest has occurred in digitalized patients and jaundiced patients receiving **anticholinesterase drugs.** ▪ Prolongs muscle relaxant effect of **succinylcholine.** ▪ Actions of **atropine** may interfere with absorption of other medications. ▪ Concomitant use of atropine with other **cholinergic drugs** (e.g., antihistamines, antiparkinson agents, antipsychotics, tricyclic antidepressants) will increase mouth dryness and other side effects (e.g., decreased GI motility).

SIDE EFFECTS

Hypersensitivity reactions including anaphylaxis; arrhythmias in up to 10% of patients (e.g., bradycardia, first-, second-, and third-degree AV block, junctional rhythms, PACs, prolonged R-R interval, PVCs, P wave changes, tachycardia). All side effects of atropine and edrophonium can occur; refer to individual monographs.

Overdose: Cholinergic crisis due to overdose or concomitant use of other anticholinesterase drugs (bradycardia, diarrhea, increased bronchial and salivary secretions, nausea, sweating, vomiting), convulsions, delirium, fever, shock, tachycardia. In atropine poisoning (delirium, fever, tachycardia), death is usually due to medullary center paralysis.

ANTIDOTE

If side effects occur, discontinue drug and notify physician. Atropine sulfate in doses of 0.4 to 0.5 mg IV will counteract most side effects of edrophonium and may be repeated every 3 to 10 minutes. Endotracheal intubation or tracheostomy is considered prophylactic in anesthesia or crisis. In all situations treatment is symptomatic and includes artificial ventilation, oxygen therapy, cardiac monitoring, adequate suctioning, and treatment of fever, shock, or convulsions. Institute and maintain as necessary. Treat hypersensitivity reactions as indicated.

ENALAPRILAT BBW
(en-**AL**-ah-prill-at)

Vasotec IV

ACE inhibitor
Antihypertensive
Vasodilator

pH 6.5 to 7.5

USUAL DOSE
1.25 mg every 6 hours. Doses up to 5 mg every 6 hours have been tolerated for up to 36 hours, but clinical studies have not shown a need for dosage over 1.25 mg. Additional doses of 1.25 mg may be given every 6 hours except in dialysis patients. Dosage is the same when converting from oral to IV therapy. Resume oral therapy as soon as tolerated. See Precautions.

PEDIATRIC DOSE
0.625 to 1.25 mg every 6 hours. See Maternal/Child.

DOSE ADJUSTMENTS
Reduce initial dose to 0.625 mg in patients taking diuretics, patients with CHF, hyponatremia, severe volume or salt depletion, a CrCl less than 30 mL/min (SCr greater than 3 mg/dL), and dialysis patients; see Rate of Administration. If the 0.625 dose is not clinically effective after 1 hour, it may be repeated. Reduce additional dose of 1.25 mg by one half for dialysis patients. ■ Blood levels markedly increased in the elderly; dose selection should be cautious. Consider decreased cardiac, hepatic, and renal function; concomitant disease; or other drug therapy. ■ See Drug/Lab Interactions and Precautions.

DILUTION
May be given undiluted through the port of a free-flowing infusion of NS, D5W, D5NS, D5LR, or Isolyte E. May also be diluted in up to 50 mL of any of the same solutions and given as an infusion.
Storage: Store at CRT. Stable for up to 24 hours after dilution.

COMPATIBILITY   (Underline Indicates Conflicting Compatibility Information)
Consider any drug NOT listed as compatible to be INCOMPATIBLE until consulting a pharmacist; specific conditions may apply.
One source suggests the following **compatibilities:**
Additive: Dobutamine, dopamine, heparin, meropenem (Merrem IV), nitroglycerin IV, nitroprusside sodium, potassium chloride (KCl).
Y-site: Allopurinol (Aloprim), amifostine (Ethyol), amikacin (Amikin), aminophylline, ampicillin, ampicillin/sulbactam (Unasyn), aztreonam (Azactam), bivalirudin (Angiomax), butorphanol (Stadol), calcium gluconate, cefazolin (Ancef), ceftazidime (Fortaz), chloramphenicol (Chloromycetin), cisatracurium (Nimbex), cladribine (Leustatin), clindamycin (Cleocin), dexmedetomidine (Precedex), dextran 40, dobutamine, docetaxel (Taxotere), dopamine, doripenem (Doribax), doxorubicin liposomal (Doxil), erythromycin (Erythrocin), esmolol (Brevibloc), etoposide phosphate (Etopophos), famotidine (Pepcid IV), fenoldopam (Corlopam), fentanyl (Sublimaze), filgrastim (Neupogen), ganciclovir (Cytovene), gemcitabine (Gemzar), gentamicin, granisetron (Kytril), heparin, hetastarch in electrolytes (Hextend), hetastarch in NS (Hespan), hydrocortisone sodium succinate (Solu-Cortef), labetalol (Trandate), lidocaine, linezolid (Zyvox), magnesium sulfate, melphalan (Alkeran), meropenem (Merrem IV), methylprednisolone (Solu-Medrol), metronidazole (Flagyl IV), morphine, naf-

cillin (Nallpen), nicardipine (Cardene IV), nitroprusside sodium, oxaliplatin (Eloxatin), pemetrexed (Alimta), penicillin G potassium, phenobarbital (Luminal), piperacillin, piperacillin/tazobactam (Zosyn), potassium chloride (KCl), potassium phosphates, propofol (Diprivan), ranitidine (Zantac), remifentanil (Ultiva), sodium acetate, sulfamethoxazole/trimethoprim, teniposide (Vumon), thiotepa, tobramycin, vancomycin, vinorelbine (Navelbine).

RATE OF ADMINISTRATION

A single dose must be evenly distributed over 5 minutes. Extend rate of infusion up to 1 hour in patients at risk for severe hypotension (e.g., heart failure, hyponatremia, high-dose diuretic therapy, recent intensive diuresis or increase in diuretic dose, renal dialysis, or severe volume and/or salt depletion of any etiology).

ACTIONS

An antihypertensive agent. An angiotensin-converting enzyme inhibitor that prevents conversion of angiotensin I to angiotensin II. Peripheral arterial resistance is reduced in hypertensive patients. In patients with heart failure, significant reduction in pulmonary capillary wedge pressure (preload), peripheral vascular resistance (afterload), BP, and heart size occurs, as well as an increase in cardiac output (stroke index) and exercise tolerance time. Initial response may take 15 minutes to 1 hour. Peak BP reduction occurs in 1 to 4 hours, and effects last up to 6 hours. Peak effects of subsequent doses may be greater than the initial dose. Excreted in urine. Crosses placental barrier. Secreted in breast milk.

INDICATIONS AND USES

Treatment of hypertension when oral therapy is not practical. ■ Heart failure not adequately responsive to diuretics and digoxin. Enalaprilat is used in addition to digoxin and diuretics. ■ Hypertensive emergencies (effects are variable).

Unlabeled uses: Treatment of hypertension or renal crisis in scleroderma.

CONTRAINDICATIONS

Hypersensitivity to enalaprilat or its components, a history of angioedema related to previous treatment with an ACE inhibitor, or hereditary or idiopathic angioedema.

PRECAUTIONS

Has been used IV for up to 7 days. ■ Use caution in patients with a history of angioedema (see Contraindications), aortic stenosis, or hypertrophic cardiomyopathy. ■ Use caution in patients with collagen vascular disease and renal disease; neutropenia and/or agranulocytosis have been reported. Monitoring of WBC may be indicated. ■ Use caution in surgery, with anesthesia, or with agents that produce hypotension. ■ May rarely cause a syndrome that starts with cholestatic jaundice, progresses to hepatic necrosis, and may progress to death. Discontinue in patients who develop elevated liver enzymes or jaundice. ■ ACE inhibitors often cause a persistent, non-productive cough, which should resolve when drug is discontinued. ■ Average dose for conversion to oral therapy is 5 mg/day as a single dose. When a reduced dose of enalaprilat IV has been indicated (e.g., diuretics, impaired renal function, dialysis), reduce initial oral dose to 2.5 mg/day as a single dose. Adjust either by patient response. ■ Patients sensitive to one ACE inhibitor may be sensitive to another. ■ See Monitor and Drug/Lab Interactions.

Monitor: Monitor vital signs very frequently. May cause precipitous drop in BP following the first dose. ▪ Use extreme caution in fluid-depleted patients. Patients with congestive heart failure may become hypotensive at any time. Arrhythmias or conduction defects may occur. ▪ Monitor BUN and SCr. An increase in either may require a decrease in dose of enalaprilat or discontinuation of a diuretic. ▪ Diuretics given concomitantly may cause a precipitous drop in BP within the first hour of the initial dose; observe the patient closely. Severe dietary salt restriction or dialysis will aggravate this effect. ▪ May cause oliguria or progressive azotemia in patients with severe congestive heart failure whose renal function is dependent on the activity of the renin-angiotensin-aldosterone system. Acute renal failure and death are possible. ▪ May cause hyperkalemia. May cause a significant increase in serum potassium with potassium-sparing diuretics or potassium supplements. Use with caution and only in documented hypokalemia. Use salt substitutes with caution. Monitor serum potassium levels. ▪ Monitoring of WBC may be indicated in patients with collagen vascular disease or renal disease. ▪ See Drug/Lab Interactions.

Patient Education: Consider birth control options. ▪ May cause dizziness; avoid sudden changes in posture and request assistance for ambulation if necessary.

Maternal/Child: Avoid pregnancy; Category C (first trimester) and Category D (second and third trimester). Can cause fetal and neonatal morbidity and death. Infants exposed to ACE inhibitors during the first trimester of pregnancy may have an increased risk of major congenital malformations. If pregnancy occurs, discontinue immediately; many alternate antihypertensive agents. ▪ Observe any infant with in utero exposure for hypotension, oliguria, and hyperkalemia. ▪ Has caused reversible acute renal failure in a premature infant whose mother received enalaprilat. ▪ Safety for use in breastfeeding not established. ▪ Safety for use in pediatric patients not established but has been used. ▪ May contain benzyl alcohol, which has been associated with a fatal "gasping syndrome" in neonates.

Elderly: Dose selection should be cautious; see Dose Adjustments and Precautions/Monitor. ▪ May be less sensitive to effects due to a decrease in plasma renin activity or more sensitive to hypotensive effects due to increased blood levels (decreased renal excretion).

DRUG/LAB INTERACTIONS

Use caution in surgery, with **anesthesia,** or with any **agents that produce hypotension.** ▪ May be used concomitantly with other **antihypertensive agents** (e.g., thiazide diuretics [chlorothiazide (Diuril)]). Effects are additive. ▪ **Diuretics** given concomitantly may cause a precipitous drop in BP. ▪ May cause hyperkalemia with **potassium-sparing diuretics** (e.g., spironolactone [Aldactone], triamterene [Dyrenium], amiloride [Midamor]), **potassium supplements, potassium-containing salt substitutes, or low-salt milk.** ▪ Use caution and consider lower doses when administering **nitroglycerin, nitroprusside sodium, other nitrates, or other vasodilators** (e.g., hydralazine). ▪ In patients with compromised renal function, concurrent use with **NSAIDs** (e.g., ibuprofen [Advil, Motrin], naproxen [Aleve, Naprosyn]) may result in further deterioration of renal function. ▪ Concurrent use with **NSAIDs** may also decrease the hypotensive effects of enalaprilat by inhibiting the renal prostaglandin synthesis and/or by causing sodium and fluid retention. ▪ May increase **lithium** concentration, resulting in lithium toxicity. ▪

Interaction with some **imaging agents** (e.g., iodohippurate, technetium) may render diagnostic renal function tests inconclusive. ▪ May decrease **hemoglobin and hematocrit** slightly. ▪ See Precautions and Monitor.

SIDE EFFECTS

Abdominal pain, angioedema, anosmia (absence of sense of smell), atrial fibrillation, bradycardia, chest pain, conjunctivitis, cough (persistent dry), diarrhea, dizziness, dry eyes, dyspnea, eosinophilic pneumonitis, fatigue, flank pain, gynecomastia, headache, hepatotoxicity, herpes zoster, hoarseness, hyperkalemia, hypotension (severe), impotence, insomnia, muscle cramps, nausea, palpitations, paresthesias, photosensitivity, pneumonia, pruritus, pulmonary edema, pulmonary embolism and infarction, pulmonary infiltrates, rash, Raynaud's phenomenon, renal failure (reversible), rhinorrhea, somnolence, sore throat, taste disturbances, tearing, toxic epidermal necrolysis, vomiting. Anaphylaxis has been reported.

ANTIDOTE

For minor side effects, notify the physician. Most will be tolerated or treated symptomatically. If symptoms progress or any major side effect occurs (angioedema, precipitous hypotension, hyperkalemia), discontinue drug and notify the physician immediately. Hypotension should respond to IV fluids if the patient's condition allows their use. Other drugs in the regimen may need to be discontinued or the dosage reduced. Epinephrine, diphenhydramine (Benadryl), and hydrocortisone may be used to treat angioedema. Maintain the patient as indicated. If cardiac arrhythmias occur, treat appropriately. Hemodialysis may be useful in toxicity.

EPINEPHRINE HYDROCHLORIDE
(ep-ih-**NEF**-rin hy-droh-**KLOR**-eyed)

Cardiac stimulant
Bronchodilator
Antiallergic
Vasopressor

Adrenalin Chloride

pH 2.5 to 5

USUAL DOSE

Hypersensitivity reactions or bronchospasm: 0.1 to 0.25 mg (1 to 2.5 mL of a 1:10,000 concentration). Start with a small dose, giving only as much as required to alleviate undesirable symptoms, and repeat as necessary (usually every 20 to 30 minutes), gradually increasing dose depending on need. Another source suggests 0.2 to 0.5 mg of 1:10,000 concentration. May be repeated as necessary.

Cardiac arrest: AHA guidelines recommend 1 mg (10 mL of a 1:10,000 concentration) IV; may repeat every 3 to 5 minutes. Follow each dose with a 20-mL IV flush to ensure delivery to systemic circulation. See Compatibility. Doses up to 0.2 mg/kg have been used for specific indications (beta-blocker or calcium channel blocker overdose). May also be given as a continuous infusion by adding 1 mg of epinephrine (1 mL of a 1:1,000 solution) to 500 mL NS or D5W. Begin with an infusion rate of 0.1 to 0.5 mcg/kg/min and titrate to response. The dose for a 70-kg patient would be 7 to 35 mcg/min. Higher doses of epinephrine are controversial.

Endotracheal: A diluted solution may be given through the endotracheal tube before an IV is established. AHA guidelines recommend 2 to 2.5 mg (of a 1:1,000 solution) diluted in 10 mL NS. Another source suggests administering the IV dose through the endotracheal tube if an IV line has not been established.

Vasopressor or maintenance dose: 1 to 10 mcg/min titrated to desired response. AHA guidelines recommend that epinephrine be used to treat symptomatic bradycardia after atropine as an alternative infusion to dopamine or to treat severe hypotension when atropine and transcutaneous pacing fail to correct the arrhythmia. For profound bradycardia or hypotension, 2 to 10 mcg/min may be given as an infusion (1 mg of 1:1,000 concentration in 500 mL NS or D5W) at a rate of 0.1 to 0.5 mcg/kg/min titrated to response.

PEDIATRIC DOSE
See Maternal/Child.

Hypersensitivity reactions or bronchospasm in infants and children: 0.01 mg/kg (0.1 mL/kg of a 1:10,000 concentration). May repeat at 20-minute to 4-hour intervals. One source suggests a maximum dose of 0.3 mg, another 0.5 mg. Usually given SC as a 1:1,000 concentration.

Severe anaphylactic shock in infants and children: One source suggests 0.1 mg IV of a 1:100,000 concentration (0.1 mL of 1:1,000 concentration diluted in 10 mL NS) given over 5 to 10 minutes. Another source suggests 0.01 mL/kg of a 1:1,000 concentration SC. Maximum 0.3 mL/dose. Repeat every 15 minutes as needed.

Bradycardia in infants and children: AHA guidelines recommend 0.01 mg/kg (0.1 mL/kg of 1:10,000 concentration) to treat symptomatic bradycardia. If IV access is not readily available, AHA guidelines recommend 0.1 mg/kg (0.1 mL/kg) of a 1:1,000 concentration via ET.

Asystolic or pulseless arrest in infants and children: AHA guidelines recommend 0.01 mg/kg (0.1 mL/kg of a 1:10,000 concentration). Another source recommends 0.01 mg/kg of a 1:10,000 concentration and suggests that the first dose should not exceed 1 mg (10 mL of a 1:10,000 concentration). Repeat every 3 to 5 minutes during arrest. Up to 0.1 to 0.2 mg/kg may be used if initial doses are ineffective. May be given via ET (0.1 mg/kg [0.1 mL/kg of a 1:1,000 concentration]) every 3 to 5 minutes until IV established, then begin with first IV dose. A third source suggests 0.01 to 0.03 mg/kg (0.1 to 0.3 mL/kg) of 1:10,000 concentration initially. May repeat every 3 to 5 minutes in neonates. In infants and children subsequent doses of 0.1 mg/kg every 3 to 5 minutes may be given if needed. Prepare an infusion and titrate from 0.1 to 1 mcg/kg/min to desired effect. Use upper dosing range if asystole present. With higher dose, be aware of preservative content to avoid toxicity.

DOSE ADJUSTMENTS
See Drug/Lab Interactions. ■ Doses larger than 1 mg may not be indicated in patients over 65 years of age and patients in ventricular fibrillation.

DILUTION
Check label. Not all epinephrine solutions can be given IV. The 1:1,000 strength is for SC or IM use only. It must be further diluted with at least 10 mL of NS to prepare a 1:10,000 solution before IV use.

IV Injection: Available prediluted (0.1 mg/mL [1:10,000 solution]) in 10-mL syringes. Available in a 30-mL vial (30 mg [1:1,000 solution]) to facilitate larger doses or continuous infusion. Each 1 mg (1 mL) of 1:1,000 solution must be diluted in at least 10 mL of NS to prepare a 1:10,000 solution.

Infusion: For occasional use as a vasopressor or for maintenance, epinephrine may be further diluted in 250 to 500 mL D5W; see the following chart. Give through Y-tube or three-way stopcock of infusion set. See chart on inside back cover for additional **compatible** solutions.

Epinephrine HCl Infusion Rates*						
Desired Dose	1 mg in 500 mL D5W (2 mcg/mL)			1 mg in 250 mL D5W 2 mg in 500 mL D5W (4 mcg/mL)		
mcg/min	mcg/hr	mL/min	mL/hr	mcg/hr	mL/min	mL/hr
1	60	0.5	30	60	0.25	15
2	120	1	60	120	0.5	30
3	180	1.5	90	180	0.75	45
4	240	2	120	240	1	60
5	300	2.5	150	300	1.25	75
6	360	3	180	360	1.5	90
7	420	3.5	210	420	1.75	105
8	480	4	240	480	2	120

*Pediatric infusion: 0.6 mg/kg in 100 mL D5W − 1 mL/hr = 0.1 mcg/kg/min

In *cardiac arrest,* 1 mg is sometimes added to 500 mL of NS or D5W.
Filters: No data available from manufacturer.
Storage: Store at CRT unless otherwise specified by manufacturer. Do not use if brown or if a sediment is present. Deteriorates rapidly. Protect from light and freezing.

COMPATIBILITY   (Underline Indicates Conflicting Compatibility Information)
Consider any drug NOT listed as compatible to be INCOMPATIBLE until consulting a pharmacist; specific conditions may apply.
Manufacturer states, "Readily destroyed and precipitate forms with alkalis, alkaline solutions (e.g., sodium bicarbonate and oxidizing agents)." *If coadministration with sodium bicarbonate is indicated, give at separate sites.* Unstable in any solution with a pH over 5.5 (e.g., aminophylline, ampicillin, lidocaine, thiopental [Pentothal], warfarin [Coumadin]).
   One source suggests the following **compatibilities:**
Additive: Amikacin (Amikin), dobutamine, furosemide (Lasix), ranitidine (Zantac), verapamil.
Y-site: Amiodarone (Nexterone), anidulafungin (Eraxis), atracurium (Tracrium), bivalirudin (Angiomax), calcium chloride, calcium gluconate, caspofungin (Cancidas), ceftazidime (Fortaz), cisatracurium (Nimbex), dexmedetomidine (Precedex), diltiazem (Cardizem), dobutamine, dopamine, drotrecogin alfa (Xigris), famotidine (Pepcid IV), fenoldopam (Corlopam), fentanyl (Sublimaze), furosemide (Lasix), heparin, hetastarch in electrolytes (Hextend), hydrocortisone sodium succinate (Solu-Cortef), hydromorphone (Dilaudid), inamrinone (Amrinone), labetalol (Trandate), levofloxacin (Levaquin), lorazepam (Ativan), midazolam (Versed), mil-

rinone (Primacor), morphine, nicardipine (Cardene IV), nitroglycerin IV, nitroprusside sodium, norepinephrine (Levophed), pancuronium, pantoprazole (Protonix IV), phytonadione (vitamin K_1), potassium chloride (KCl), propofol (Diprivan), ranitidine (Zantac), remifentanil (Ultiva), tigecycline (Tygacil), tirofiban (Aggrastat), vasopressin, vecuronium, warfarin (Coumadin).

RATE OF ADMINISTRATION

IV injection: Each 1 mg or fraction thereof over 1 minute or longer. May be given more rapidly in cardiac resuscitation; follow with 20-mL IV flush.

Infusion: Vasopressor or maintenance: 1 to 10 mcg/min titrated to desired patient response.

Cardiac arrest: Titrated to deliver a single dose over 3 to 5 minutes based on patient response. Must be delivered by central venous access. Use an infusion pump to control rate.

ACTIONS

A naturally occurring hormone secreted by the adrenal glands. A sympathomimetic drug, it imitates almost all actions of the sympathetic nervous system. Stimulates both alpha- and beta-adrenergic receptors. It is a vasoconstrictor and delays the absorption of many drugs; a potent cardiac stimulant, it strengthens the myocardial contraction (positive inotropic effect) and increases cardiac rate (positive chronotropic effect). Increases myocardial and cerebral blood flow during CPR. A potent dilator or relaxant of smooth muscle, especially bronchial muscle. Decreases blood supply to the abdomen and increases blood supply to skeletal muscles. Elevates systolic BP, lowers diastolic BP, and increases pulse pressure. Seldom used as a vasopressor because of its short duration of action. High-dose infusions (greater than 0.2 mcg/min) may produce profound vasoconstriction, compromising perfusion and possibly compromising renal and splanchnic blood flow. It is rapidly inactivated in the body by the liver and various enzymes and is excreted in changed form in the urine. Crosses placental barrier. Secreted in breast milk.

INDICATIONS AND USES

Cardiac resuscitation. First-line drug of choice when initial CPR, intubation, ventilation, and initial defibrillation have failed to achieve response in ventricular fibrillation, pulseless ventricular tachycardia, asystole, or pulseless electrical activity. ■ Drug of choice for anaphylactic shock. ■ Antidote of choice for histamine overdose and hypersensitivity reactions including bronchial asthma, urticaria, and angioneurotic edema. ■ Stokes-Adams syndrome. ■ Occasionally used as a vasopressor (e.g., symptomatic bradycardia).

CONTRAINDICATIONS

Anesthesia with halogenated hydrocarbons or cyclopropane; cerebral arteriosclerosis, hypertension, labor and delivery if maternal BP exceeds 130/80 mm Hg (may cause prolonged uterine atony with hemorrhage), hyperthyroidism, narrow-angle glaucoma, nervous instability, organic brain damage, patients receiving high doses of digoxin, shock. Do not use to treat overdosage of phenothiazines (e.g., chlorpromazine [Thorazine]); a further drop in BP will occur and irreversible shock may result. Do not use concurrently with esmolol (Brevibloc).

PRECAUTIONS

Usual route is SC except in cardiac resuscitation or as a vasopressor infusion. ■ Use caution in the elderly, in diabetics, in hypotension (except in anaphylactic shock), in patients receiving thyroid preparations, and in patients with cardiac disease, a history of seizures, or long-term emphysema or bronchial asthma with degenerative heart disease. ■ Often used with corticosteroids in treatment of anaphylactic shock. ■ Increasing BP and HR may cause myocardial ischemia, angina, and increased myocardial oxygen demand. ■ Larger doses in cardiac arrest are based on optimal response range of epinephrine (0.045 to 0.2 mg/kg). May not improve survival or neurologic outcome and may cause postresuscitation myocardial dysfunction. ■ Higher doses may be required to treat poison-induced shock.

Monitor: Check BP and HR every 5 minutes. ■ Monitoring of ECG and serum potassium and glucose concentrations may be indicated. ■ Vasoconstriction-induced tissue sloughing can occur. Avoid administering in areas of limited blood supply (e.g., fingers, toes) or if peripheral vascular disease is present. ■ Infusion during cardiac arrest must be administered by central venous access to ensure delivery to systemic circulation and to avoid extravasation. ■ Intracardiac injection or IV injection in cardiac arrest must be accompanied by cardiac massage to perfuse drug into the myocardium and permit effective defibrillation. ■ Correct acidosis, hypoxemia. ■ See Drug/Lab Interactions.

Maternal/Child: Category C: may cause anoxia in fetus. ■ Discontinue breast-feeding. May produce tachyarrhythmias in pediatric patients. ■ High doses in animals have caused increased hypertension with lower cardiac output. Risk of intracranial hemorrhage may be increased in infants and children (especially preterm infants) if hypotension is followed by hypertension. ■ See Contraindications.

Elderly: May be more sensitive to the effects of beta-adrenergic receptor agonists (e.g., hypertension, hypokalemia, tachycardia, tremor). Patients with cardiac disease may be at increased risk for adverse effects. ■ See Dose Adjustments and Precautions.

DRUG/LAB INTERACTIONS

May be used alternately with isoproterenol (Isuprel), but they may not be used together. Both are direct cardiac stimulants and death may result. Adequate interval between doses must be maintained. ■ Do not use concomitantly with **other sympathomimetic agents** (e.g., ephedrine, dopamine). Additive effects may cause toxicity. ■ Simultaneous use with **oxytocics** (e.g., methylergonovine), **MAO inhibitors** (e.g., isocarboxazid [Marplan]), **furazolidone** (Furoxone), **or guanethidine** (Ismelin) may result in hypertension or cause hypertensive crisis. ■ Pressor response increased by **tricyclic antidepressants** (e.g., amitriptyline [Elavil], imipramine [Tofranil]), **antihistamines** (e.g., diphenhydramine [Benadryl]), **rauwolfia alkaloids** (e.g., reserpine [Serpasil]), **sodium levothyroxine, and urinary alkalizers;** may cause hypertension. ■ May cause hypertension with **nonselective beta-adrenergic blockers** (e.g., propranolol). ■ Inhibited by **ergot alkaloids and phenothiazines** (e.g., prochlorperazine [Compazine]). ■ Inhibits **insulin and oral hypoglycemic agents;** increased dose may be required. ■ **Hydrocarbon anesthetics** (e.g., enflurane, halothane) **and digoxin** may sensitize the myocardium and increase the risk of arrhythmias. ■ Use with **theophylline** may increase cardiac, CNS, or GI side effects. ■ Concurrent use with **alpha-adrenergic blocking agents** (e.g., doxazosin [Cardura], labetalol [Trandate], prazosin [Minipress], terazosin [Hytrin]) may antagonize the hypertensive effects of epinephrine. ■ Interacts with many other drugs. ■ See Contraindications for additional drug interactions.

SIDE EFFECTS

Often transitory; sometimes occur with average doses.

Anxiety, dizziness, dyspnea, glycosuria, pallor, palpitations.

Overdose (frequently caused by too-rapid injection): Bradycardia (transient followed by tachycardia), cerebrovascular hemorrhage, collapse (rapid), fibrillation, headache (severe), hypertension, hypotension (irreversible), pulmonary edema, pupillary dilation, renal failure, restlessness, tachycardia, weakness, death.

ANTIDOTE

Treatment is primarily supportive. If side effects from the average dose become progressively worse, discontinue the drug and notify the physician. IM or SC route may be preferable. For a severe reaction caused by toxicity, treat the patient for shock and administer an antihypertensive agent such as phentolamine (Regitine) or nitroprusside sodium. Treat cardiac arrhythmias with a beta-adrenergic blocker (propranolol). Resuscitate as necessary.

EPIRUBICIN HYDROCHLORIDE BBW
(ep-ee-**ROO**-bih-sin hy-droh-**KLOR**-eyed)

**Antineoplastic
(anthracycline antibiotic)**

Ellence ▪ ❧Pharmorubicin PFS

pH 3 ▪ pH 4 to 5.5

USUAL DOSE

In combination therapies, epirubicin is used instead of doxorubicin in the combination regimen. Usually given on the same days and at the same intervals as the doxorubicin it replaces.

ELLENCE

Recommended starting dose is 100 to 120 mg/M^2. Patients receiving the 120-mg/M^2 dose should also receive prophylactic antibiotic therapy with sulfamethoxazole/trimethoprim or a fluoroquinolone (e.g., ciprofloxacin [Cipro]). Ellence is usually given in repeated 3- to 4-week cycles. Total dose may be given on Day 1 of each cycle or equally divided and given on Days 1 and 8 of each cycle.

One regimen used is 60 mg/M^2 of epirubicin as an infusion on Days 1 and 8 given in a regimen with oral cyclophosphamide 75 mg/M^2 on Days 1 to 14 and fluorouracil 500 mg/M^2 on Days 1 and 8. Repeat every 28 days for six cycles. Another regimen used is 100 mg/M^2 of epirubicin as an infusion together with fluorouracil 500 mg/M^2 and cyclophosphamide 500 mg/M^2. All three agents are given on Day 1 and are repeated every 21 days for 6 cycles. In either regimen the total dose of epirubicin may be given on Day 1 of each cycle or equally divided and given on Days 1 and 8 of each cycle.

❧PHARMORUBICIN PFS

Metastatic breast cancer: *Single agent:* 75 to 90 mg/M^2 once every 21 days. This dose may be divided and given on Day 1 and Day 2. An alternative weekly dose schedule of 12.5 to 25 mg/M^2 has been used and has been reported to produce less clinical toxicity than higher doses given every 3 weeks. *Combination therapy:* 50 mg/M^2. Used in combination with cyclophosphamide and fluorouracil.

Early-stage breast cancer (Stage II-IIIA): 50 to 60 mg/M^2 given on Days 1 and 8 every 4 weeks. Used in combination with cyclophosphamide and fluorouracil.

Small-cell lung cancer: *Single agent:* 90 to 120 mg/M^2 once every 3 weeks. *Combination therapy:* 50 to 90 mg/M^2. Several combinations have been used (e.g., with either cisplatin or ifosfamide; with cyclophosphamide and vincristine; with cyclophosphamide and etoposide, or with cisplatin and etoposide).

Non–small-cell lung cancer: *Single agent:* 120 to 150 mg/M^2 on Day 1 every 3 to 4 weeks. *Combination therapy:* 90 to 120 mg/M^2 on Day 1 every 3 to 4 weeks. Used in combination with cisplatin, etoposide, mitomycin, and vinblastine.

Non-Hodgkin's lymphoma: *Single agent:* 75 to 90 mg/M^2 once every 3 weeks. *Combination therapy:* 60 to 75 mg/M^2. Used in combination with cyclophosphamide, prednisone, and vincristine with or without bleomycin for the treatment of newly diagnosed non-Hodgkin's lymphoma.

Hodgkin's disease: *Combination therapy:* 35 mg/M^2 once every 2 weeks or 70 mg/M^2 once every 3 to 4 weeks. Used in combination with bleomycin, dacarbazine, and vinblastine.

Ovarian cancer: *Single agent:* 50 to 90 mg/M^2 once every 3 or 4 weeks in patients who have had prior therapy. *Combination therapy:* 50 to 90 mg/M^2 once every 3 or 4 weeks can be added to their regimen in patients who have had prior therapy; or the same dose in combination with cisplatin and cyclophosphamide is used for initial therapy of ovarian cancer.

Locally unresectable or metastatic gastric cancer: *Single agent:* 75 to 100 mg/M^2 once every 3 weeks. *Combination therapy:* 80 mg/M^2 once every 3 to 4 weeks. Used in combination with fluorouracil.

ALL FORMULATIONS

Soft tissue sarcoma (unlabeled): 45 to 60 mg/M^2/day for 2 to 3 days of a 21- or 28-day treatment cycle. Up to 150 to 180 mg/M^2 has been given on Day 1 of a 21-day treatment cycle for 8 cycles. This higher dose has not proven to be more effective but is more toxic; G-CSF support required.

Esophageal and esophagogastric junction cancers (unlabeled): 50 mg/M^2 on Day 1 of a 21-day treatment cycle. Use in conjunction with cisplatin on Day 1 and a continuous infusion of fluorouracil for up to 8 cycles. An alternate regimen uses epirubicin 50 to 60 mg/M^2 on Day 1 or 20 mg/M^2 on Days 1 to 3 of a 28-day treatment cycle in conjunction with cisplatin and fluorouracil for up to 6 cycles.

DOSE ADJUSTMENTS

ALL FORMULATIONS: Reduced dose required with elevated serum bilirubin. Give 50% of a dose for serum bilirubin from 1.2 to 3 mg/dL or AST 2 to 4 times upper limit of normal. Give 25% of a dose for serum bilirubin greater than 3 mg/mL or AST greater than 4 times upper limit of normal.

ELLENCE: Reduce dose to 75 to 90 mg/M^2 in heavily pretreated patients, those with pre-existing bone marrow suppression, or in the presence of neoplastic bone marrow infiltration. ■ Consider reduced dose in patients with severe renal impairment (SCr greater than 5 mg/dL). ■ Base dose adjustments after the first treatment cycle on hematologic response during treatment cycle nadir and nonhematologic toxicities. In patients who received the full dose on Day 1, reduce dose to 75% of initial first dose in subsequent cycles for platelet count less than 50,000/mm^3, absolute neutrophil count (ANC) less than 250/mm^3, neutropenic fever, or Grade 3 or 4 nonhematologic toxicity. Delay dose in subsequent treatment cycles until platelet count recovers to at least 100,000/mm^3, ANC recovers to at least 1,500/mm^3, and nonhematologic toxicities have recovered to equal to or less than Grade 1. For patients receiving a divided dose, reduce the Day-8 dose to 75% of the Day-1 dose if platelet counts are 75,000 to 100,000/mm^3 and ANC is 1,000 to 1,499/mm^3. Omit the Day-8 dose if platelet counts are less than 75,000/mm^3, ANC less than 1,000/mm^3, or Grade 3 or 4 nonhematologic toxicity has occurred.

✤PHARMORUBICIN PFS: Use lower dose in range for patients with inadequate marrow reserves due to old age, prior therapy, or neoplastic marrow infiltration. ■ Reduced dose, delay, or suspension of epirubicin may be required based on hematologic toxicity; manufacturer provides no specific recommendations. ■ No dose adjustment required in impaired renal function.

DILUTION

Specific techniques required; see Precautions.

ELLENCE: Available as 2 mg/mL in 25-mL and 100-mL vials. A ready-to-use, preservative-free solution; further dilution not required. Must be given through Y-tube or three-way stopcock of a free-flowing infusion of NS or D5W.

PHARMORUBICIN PFS: Available as 2 mg/mL in 5-mL, 25-mL, and 100-mL vials. Use of the 100-mL vial should be restricted to a pharmacy admixture program using a sterile transfer or dispensing device. Enter any vial only once and withdraw desired dose into a syringe. No further dilution is required.

Filters: Manufacturer indicates that studies show some initial potency loss in the first few minutes with the use of cellulose ester membrane or nylon filters; however, the total amount of drug loss is negligible. A second source has a similar statement.

Storage: *Ellence:* Refrigerate vials at 2° to 8° C (34° to 46° F); protect from light. Do not freeze. Must be used within 24 hours of first penetration of vial. Discard unused solution.

Pharmorubicin: Store unopened PFS vials in refrigerator; keep in original cartons to protect from light. Use any filled syringe within 24 hours if stored at room temperature and within 48 hours if refrigerated. Syringes prepared from the pharmacy bulk vial must be used within 24 or 48 hours of the initial puncture of that vial based on method of storage. Once the transfer set has been inserted in the bulk vial, any remaining undispensed drug must be discarded in 8 hours.

COMPATIBILITY

Consider any drug NOT listed as compatible to be INCOMPATIBLE until consulting a pharmacist; specific conditions may apply.

Manufacturers recommend not mixing with other drugs in the same syringe. Avoid prolonged contact with alkaline solutions; will result in hydrolysis of all forms of epirubicin. Do not mix with heparin or fluorouracil (5-FU); may precipitate. **Incompatible** with ifosfamide (Ifex) when combined in syringe or solution with mesna (Mesnex).

One source suggests the following **compatibilities:**

Additive: Ifosfamide (Ifex).

Y-site: Oxaliplatin (Eloxatin).

RATE OF ADMINISTRATION

IV injection: *All formulations:* A single dose over 3 to 20 minutes. Must be given through Y-tube or three-way stopcock of a free-flowing infusion of NS or D5W. Slow injection rate further for erythematous streaking along the vein or facial flushing.

ACTIONS

A semisynthetic, anthracycline, antineoplastic antibiotic agent. Exact method of action is unknown. Rapidly penetrates cell and interferes with cell division by binding with DNA to slow production of nucleic acid (RNA and DNA) and protein synthesis. Free radicals cause further cytotoxic activity. Metabolized in the liver and by other organs and cells, including RBCs. The process of glucuronidation distinguishes epirubicin from doxorubicin and may account for its faster elimination and reduced toxicity. It is less toxic and in particular less cardiotoxic than doxorubicin. Has the same antitumor effect at equal doses. WBC nadir is reached in 10 to 14 days and should return to normal by Day 21. Elimination half-life is 30 to 40 hours. Does not cross blood-brain barrier. Primarily excreted in bile; some excretion in urine.

INDICATIONS AND USES

ELLENCE: Used in combination with other agents in the treatment of patients with evidence of axillary-node tumor involvement following resection in primary breast cancer. **PHARMORUBICIN:** Treatment of metastatic as well as early stage breast cancer, small-cell lung cancer (both limited and extensive disease), advanced non–small-cell lung cancer, non-Hodgkin's lymphoma, Hodgkin's disease, Stage III and IV ovarian cancer, and metastatic and locally unresectable gastric cancers. May be used as a single agent or in combination with other chemotherapeutic agents.

Unlabeled uses: ALL FORMULATIONS: Treatment of soft-tissue sarcomas in combination with other agents. Treatment of esophageal and esophagogastric junction cancers in combination with other agents. Ellence has been used in place of Pharmorubicin for various indications.

CONTRAINDICATIONS

History of severe cardiac disease, myocardial insufficiency, recent MI, severe arrhythmias, or severe hepatic disease. Baseline neutrophil count less than 1,500 cells/mm^3 or myelosuppression resulting from treatment with other antineoplastic agents or radiation therapy. Contraindicated in patients who have received previous treatment with maximum recommended cumulative doses of daunorubicin (Cerubidine), doxorubicin (Adriamycin), idarubicin (Idamycin), mitoxantrone (Novantrone), or mitomycin C. Hypersensitivity to epirubicin, other anthracyclines, or anthracenediones.

PRECAUTIONS

Follow guidelines for handling cytotoxic agents. See Appendix A, p. 1429. In addition to standard precautions, treat spills or leakage with 1% sodium hypochlorite. For accidental contact with eyes or skin, flush with copious amounts of water, soap and water, or sodium bicarbonate. ▪ Administered by or under the direction of the physician specialist, with facilities for monitoring the patient and responding to any medical emergency. ▪ For IV use only. Do not give IM or SC. ▪ May cause severe myelosuppression. ▪ May cause serious, irreversible myocardial toxicity with congestive heart failure and/or cardiomyopathy as the cumulative dose approaches 900 mg/M^2. Cardiotoxicity may be acute or delayed, occurring months to years after treatment. Exceeding 900 mg/M^2 is not recommended; the maximum cumulative dose used in clinical trials was 720 mg/M^2. ▪ Cardiotoxicity may occur at lower cumulative doses whether or not cardiac risk factors are present. ▪ Use extreme caution in pre-existing drug-induced bone marrow suppression, existing heart disease, previous treatment with other anthracyclines (e.g., daunorubicin, doxorubicin, idarubicin), other cardiotoxic agents (e.g., bleomycin), or radiation therapy encompassing the heart; toxicity may occur at lower cumulative doses and may be additive. ▪ Administration of epirubicin after previous radiation therapy may induce an inflammatory recall reaction at the irradiation site. ▪ Incidence of secondary leukemia may be increased. Risk of developing acute myelogenous leukemia and/or myelodysplastic syndrome (AML/MDS) increases when epirubicin is given in combination with DNA-damaging antineoplastic agents, when patients have been heavily pretreated with cytotoxic drugs, or when doses of anthracyclines have been escalated. The cumulative prob-

ability of developing AML/MDS is particularly increased in patients who have received more than 720 mg/M^2 of epirubicin or more than 6,300 mg/M^2 of cyclophosphamide.
Monitor: Before beginning treatment with epirubicin, patients should recover from acute toxicities (e.g., stomatitis, neutropenia, thrombocytopenia, and infections) resulting from previous chemotherapy. ▪ Obtain baseline CBC, including differential and platelet count; serum calcium, phosphate, and potassium; SCr; uric acid level; liver function tests (AST, ALT, alkaline phosphatase, and serum bilirubin); ECG; chest x-ray; echocardiogram; and cardiac function as measured by left ventricular ejection fraction (LVEF). Monitor lab values during therapy, especially before each dose. Monitor ECG, chest x-ray, echocardiogram, and/or radionuclide angiography in patients who have had mediastinal radiation, other anthracycline or anthracene therapy, those with pre-existing cardiac disease, or S/S of impending heart disease, or those who have received prior epirubicin cumulative doses exceeding 550 mg/M^2. ▪ Monitor for signs of cardiac toxicity (e.g., rapid or irregular HR, shortness of breath, swelling of abdomen, feet, and lower legs); early signs usually include sinus tachycardia and non-specific ST-T wave changes in the ECG. ▪ Use only large veins. Avoid veins over joints or in extremities with compromised venous or lymphatic drainage. Determine absolute patency of vein. Extravasation may occur with or without stinging or burning along the injection site even if blood returns well on aspiration of the infusion needle. Observe site frequently. Extravasation can result in severe cellulitis and tissue necrosis; if it occurs, discontinue injection; use another vein. ▪ Prevention and treatment of hyperuricemia due to tumor lysis syndrome may be accomplished with adequate hydration, and if necessary, allopurinol and alkalinization of urine. ▪ Be alert for signs of bone marrow suppression, bleeding, or infection. ▪ Use of prophylactic antibiotics may be indicated pending C/S in a febrile, neutropenic patient. ▪ Monitor for thrombocytopenia (platelet count less than 50,000/mm^3). Initiate precautions to prevent excessive bleeding (e.g., inspect IV sites, skin, and mucous membranes; use extreme care during invasive procedures; test urine, emesis, stool, and secretions for occult blood). ▪ Prophylactic antiemetics are indicated. ▪ See Drug/Lab Interactions.
Patient Education: Urine will be reddish for several days (from drug, not hematuria). ▪ Nonhormonal birth control recommended. May induce chromosomal damage in sperm. Effective contraception suggested for men receiving epirubicin. ▪ Report IV site burning, stinging, or puffiness promptly. ▪ Report rapid or irregular HR, shortness of breath, and swelling of the abdomen, feet, or lower legs. ▪ Review side effects; may be severe (e.g., nausea and vomiting, cardiotoxicity). ▪ See Appendix D, p. 1434.
Maternal/Child: Category D: can cause fetal harm. Avoid pregnancy. May cause testicular atrophy. ▪ Discontinue breast-feeding. ▪ Information on safety for use in pediatric patients not available. Some studies suggest that pediatric patients may be at greater risk for anthracycline-induced acute cardiotoxicity and/or chronic CHF.
Elderly: Cardiotoxicity and myelotoxicity may be more severe; monitor closely for dose-related toxicities. ▪ See Dose Adjustments. ▪ There is a major decrease in plasma clearance of epirubicin in women over 70 years of age; monitor closely for signs of toxicity. ▪ See Dose Adjustments.

DRUG/LAB INTERACTIONS

May increase bone marrow and GI toxicity of other **chemotherapeutic agents.** ■ Increased toxicity including skin redness and exfoliative changes possible when given concurrently with or after **radiation.** ■ Monitoring of cardiac function may be indicated in patients taking **medications that may cause heart failure** (e.g., calcium channel blockers such as verapamil), beta-blockers (e.g., propranolol). ■ Plasma clearance decreased and serum levels increased by **cimetidine** (Tagamet); discontinue cimetidine. ■ Hepatic toxicity may be increased with concurrent use of **other hepatotoxic agents** (e.g., methotrexate, isoniazid [INH]). ■ Risk of cardiotoxicity increased in patients previously treated with maximum cumulative doses of **other anthracyclines** (e.g., doxorubicin [Adriamycin], idarubicin [Idamycin]) **and/or radiation encompassing the heart.** ■ Leukopenic and/or thrombocytopenic effects may be increased with **drugs that cause blood dyscrasias** (e.g., anticonvulsants [e.g., carbamazepine (Tegretol), phenytoin (Dilantin)], NSAIDs [e.g., ibuprofen (Advil, Motrin), naproxen (Aleve, Naprosyn)]). Adjust dose based on differential and platelet count. ■ Coadministration of **taxanes** (docetaxel [Taxotere] or paclitaxel [Taxol]) does not appear to affect the pharmacokinetics of epirubicin if epirubicin is given immediately following the taxane. ■ Do not administer **live virus vaccines** to patients receiving antineoplastic agents. ■ See Precautions.

SIDE EFFECTS

Dose-limiting toxicities are infection, myelosuppression (anemia, leukopenia, neutropenia, thrombocytopenia), and cardiotoxicity (usually delayed manifested by reduced LVEF and/or S/S of CHF [e.g., ascites, dependent edema, dyspnea, gallop rhythm, hepatomegaly, pleural effusion, pulmonary edema, tachycardia]). Severe cellulitis, vesication, local pain, and tissue necrosis can occur with extravasation. Venous sclerosis may result from injection into small veins or repeated injection into the same vein. Other side effects are alopecia, amenorrhea, anorexia, arrhythmias (transient), conjunctivitis, diarrhea, febrile neutropenia, fever, hot flashes, itching, keratosis, malaise, mucositis (esophagitis, stomatitis), nausea and vomiting, phlebitis, rash, recall of skin reaction associated with prior radiation. Hypersensitivity reactions have been reported.

Overdose: May cause an acute myocardial dysfunction within 24 hours. Pronounced mucositis, leukopenia, and thrombocytopenia may occur within 7 to 14 days.

ANTIDOTE

Most side effects will either be tolerated or treated symptomatically. Keep the physician informed. Hematopoietic toxicity (leukopenia, thrombocytopenia) may require dose reduction or cessation of therapy, antibiotics, platelet and granulocyte transfusions, oprelvekin (Neumega), darbepoetin alfa (Aranesp), epoetin alfa (Epogen), filgrastim (Neupogen), pegfilgrastim (Neulasta), or sargramostim (Leukine). Acute cardiac failure occurs suddenly (most common when total cumulative doses approach 900 mg/M^2) and frequently does not respond to currently available treatment. Close monitoring of accumulated dose, bone marrow, ECG, chest x-ray, echocardiography, and systolic ejection fraction may prevent most serious and potentially fatal cardiac side effects. There is no specific antidote. Supportive therapy as indicated will help sustain the patient in toxicity. Dexrazoxane is currently available to prevent cardiotoxicity of doxorubicin in specific situations; in the future it may be considered with epirubicin. If extravasation occurs, attempt aspiration of the infiltrated epirubicin. Elevate the extremity and apply local intermittent ice compresses for up to 3 days. Observe the site frequently. Should be seen by a reconstructive surgeon if local pain persists or skin changes progress after 3 to 4 days. Ulceration may require early wide excision of the involved area. Treat hypersensitivity reactions as indicated.

EPOETIN ALFA   BBW
(ee-**POH**-ee-tin **AL**-fah)

EPO, Epogen, ✤Eprex, Erythropoietin, Procrit

Recombinant human erythropoietin
Antianemic agent

pH 5.8 to 7.2

USUAL DOSE

In all situations, rate of hematocrit increase is dose dependent and varies among patients. Availability of iron stores, baseline hematocrit, and concurrent medical problems affect the rate and extent of response. Use the lowest dose for each patient that will gradually increase the hemoglobin concentration to avoid the need for RBC transfusion and to achieve and maintain a hemoglobin within the range of 10 to 12 Gm/dL; see Precautions and Monitor.

Anemia of chronic renal failure in adults: May be given by IV or SC injection or into the venous line at the end of a dialysis session. The IV route is recommended in patients on hemodialysis; see Precautions. 50 to 100 units/kg of body weight 3 times a week initially. A 55-kg (120-lb) individual would receive 2,750 units at 50 units/kg, 4,125 units at 75 units/kg, and 5,500 units at 100 units/kg. Entire contents of a vial (2,000, 3,000, or 4,000 units) has been used instead of an exact calculated dose. Predialysis patients usually require doses in the average range, peritoneal dialysis patients respond rapidly to lower doses, and higher-end doses may be required, especially in dialysis patients (see literature). Increase dose by 25% if the hemoglobin is less than 10 Gm/dL and has not increased by 1 Gm/dL after 4 weeks of therapy or if the hemoglobin decreases below 10 Gm/dL. Dose increases should not be made more frequently than once a month.

Maintenance dose: Individually titrate to achieve and maintain the lowest hemoglobin level sufficient to avoid the need for RBC transfusion and not to exceed the upper safety limit of 12 Gm/dL. Median maintenance dose is 75 units/kg 3 times/week; range is 12.5 to 525 units/kg 3 times weekly. Evaluate iron stores if hematocrit falls; see Monitor.

Anemia in zidovudine-treated, HIV-infected patients: May be given IV or SC. 100 units/kg 3 times a week for 8 weeks. Obtain endogenous serum erythropoietin level (before transfusion) before initiating therapy; see Monitor. Serum erythropoietin levels in adults should be equal to or less than 500 mUnits/mL, and the zidovudine dose should be equal to or less than 4,200 mg/week. After 8 weeks of therapy, the dose may be increased by 50 to 100 units/kg 3 times a week (total dose of 150 to 200 units/kg). Evaluate response every 4 to 8 weeks and adjust dose accordingly by 50 to 100 units/kg (total dose of 200 to 300 units/kg) to achieve and maintain the lowest hemoglobin level sufficient to avoid the need for RBC transfusion and not to exceed the upper safety limit of 12 Gm/dL. Not likely to be effective if doses of 300 units/kg 3 times a week have not corrected the anemia.

Maintenance dose: When desired response is attained (i.e., reduced transfusion requirements or increased hemoglobin), titrate dose to maintain the response and to achieve and maintain the lowest hemoglobin level sufficient to avoid the need for RBC transfusion and not to exceed the upper safety limit of 12 Gm/dL; see Dose Adjustments. Evaluate response every 4 to 8 weeks and adjust dose accordingly. Consider variations in zidovudine (AZT, Retrovir) dose and presence of infectious or inflammatory episodes.

Anemia associated with cancer patients on chemotherapy: SC injection recommended.

Regimen One: 150 units/kg 3 times a week. Obtain endogenous serum erythropoietin level (before transfusion) before initiating therapy; see Monitor. If adequate response (no reduction in transfusion requirements or rise in hemoglobin) has not occurred after 4 weeks, increase the dose up to 300 units/kg 3 times a week. Not likely to be effective if doses of 300 units/kg 3 times a week have not corrected the anemia. Adjust dose to achieve and maintain the lowest hemoglobin level sufficient to avoid the need for RBC transfusion; see Dose Adjustments. Discontinue if there is no response as measured by hemoglobin levels or if transfusions are still required after 8 weeks. Discontinue epoetin alfa after completion of a chemotherapy course.

Regimen Two: 40,000 units SC weekly. If hemoglobin does not increase 1 Gm/dL within 4 weeks (in the absence of a RBC transfusion), may increase dose to 60,000 units weekly. Doses greater than 60,000 units are not likely to be effective. Adjust dose to achieve and maintain the lowest hemoglobin level sufficient to avoid the need for RBC transfusion; see Dose Adjustments. Discontinue if there is no response as measured by hemoglobin levels or if transfusions are still required after 8 weeks. Discontinue epoetin alfa after completion of a chemotherapy course.

Reduction of allogeneic blood transfusions in surgery patients: SC injection recommended. Obtain hemoglobin before initiating therapy. Should be greater than 10 Gm/dL but less than or equal to 13 Gm/dL. 300 units/kg/ day for 10 days before surgery, on the day of surgery, and for 4 days after surgery. Has been given concurrently with anticoagulant prophylaxis. An alternate dose schedule is 600 units/kg once each week on Days 21, 14, and 7 before surgery and again on the day of surgery. Begin iron supplementation no later than the beginning of treatment with epoetin alfa and continue throughout the course of therapy. Strongly consider use of antithrombotic prophylaxis (e.g., enoxaparin [Lovenox]); see Precautions.

PEDIATRIC DOSE

May be given by IV or SC injection. The IV route is recommended in patients on hemodialysis; see Precautions. Use the lowest dose for each patient that will gradually increase the hemoglobin concentration to avoid the need for RBC transfusion and to achieve and maintain a hemoglobin within the range of 10 to 12 Gm/dL; see Precautions and Monitor.

Anemia of chronic renal failure requiring dialysis in pediatric patients 1 month to 16 years of age: *Initial:* 50 units/kg of body weight 3 times a week. May also be given into the venous line at the end of the dialysis session. Increase

Continued

dose as described in a similar section under Usual Dose. Safety and effectiveness for use in infants under 1 month of age not established.

Maintenance: Individually titrate to achieve and maintain the lowest hemoglobin level sufficient to avoid the need for RBC transfusion and not to exceed the upper safety limit of 12 Gm/dL; see Dose Adjustments. See all comments in the similar section under Usual Dose and Dose Adjustments.

Anemia of chronic renal failure not requiring dialysis in pediatric patients ages 3 months to 20 years (unlabeled): Doses of 50 to 250 units/kg 1 to 3 times a week have been reported. Increase dose as described under anemia of chronic renal failure requiring dialysis, including maintenance dose and comments in the similar section under Usual Dose and Dose Adjustments.

Anemia in zidovudine-treated, HIV-infected pediatric patients 8 months to 17 years (unlabeled): Doses of 50 to 400 units/kg 2 to 3 times a week have been reported. See all comments under the similar section in Usual Dose. Adjust dose to achieve and maintain the lowest hemoglobin level sufficient to avoid the need for RBC transfusion; see Dose Adjustments.

Anemia in pediatric cancer patients on chemotherapy, ages 6 months to 18 years: 600 units/kg IV weekly. Do not exceed 40,000 units. If hemoglobin does not increase by 1 Gm/dL within 4 weeks, may increase dose to 900 units/kg IV. Do not exceed 60,000 units. See all comments under the similar section in Usual Dose. Adjust dose to achieve and maintain the lowest hemoglobin level sufficient to avoid the need for RBC transfusion; see Dose Adjustments.

NEONATAL DOSE

Anemia of prematurity (unlabeled): 25 to 100 units/kg/dose SC 3 times a week or 200 to 400 units/kg/dose IV/SC 3 to 5 times a week for 2 to 6 weeks. Total dose per week is 600 to 1,400 units/kg. Use the lowest dose that will gradually increase the hemoglobin concentration to avoid the need for RBC transfusion and to achieve and maintain a hemoglobin not to exceed the upper safety limit of 12 Gm/dL; see Precautions, Monitor, and Dose Adjustments.

DOSE ADJUSTMENTS

All indications except reduction of allogeneic blood transfusion in surgery patients: See Usual Dose and each specific indication for dose escalation. Dose adjustment is based on hemoglobin. Adjust dose to achieve and maintain the lowest hemoglobin level sufficient to avoid the need for RBC transfusion and not to exceed the upper safety limit of 12 Gm/dL. ▪ Dose based on average weight if edema is present. ▪ For patients whose hemoglobin does not attain a level within the desired range of 10 to 12 Gm/dL after appropriate dose titration over a 12-week period, evaluate and treat other causes of anemia; see Precautions. Do not administer higher doses. Use the lowest dose that will maintain a hemoglobin level sufficient to avoid the need for recurrent RBC transfusions. Continue monitoring and adjust dose if responsiveness improves. If responsiveness does not improve and recurrent RBC transfusions continue to be required, discontinue epoetin alfa therapy. ▪ An increase in dose may be necessary in patients with aluminum toxicity. ▪ Decrease dose if hemoglobin increase exceeds 1 Gm/dL in any 2-week period or if any of the following occur: cardiac arrest, neurologic events (e.g., seizures, stroke), exacerbations of hypertension, congestive heart failure (CHF), vascular thrombosis/ischemia/infarction, acute MI, deep vein thrombosis (DVT), pulmonary embolus, or fluid overload/edema. ▪ See Precautions and Monitor.

Chronic renal failure patients: Reduce dose by 25% as the hemoglobin approaches 12 Gm/dL or if the hemoglobin increases more than 1 Gm/dL in any 2-week period.

Zidovudine-treated, HIV-infected patients and cancer patients on chemotherapy: Withhold dose if the hemoglobin exceeds 12 Gm/dL until the hemoglobin falls to 11 Gm/dL. Then restart dose at 25% below previous dose.

Cancer patients on chemotherapy: *Reduce dose* by 25% when the hemoglobin reaches a level needed to avoid transfusion or increases more than 1 Gm/dL in any 2-week period. *Withhold dose* if the hemoglobin exceeds a level needed to avoid transfusion, and restart at 25% below the previous dose when the hemoglobin approaches a level at which transfusions may be required.

DILUTION

Available in numerous concentrations; check dose on vial carefully. May be given undiluted as an IV injection. Do not shake during preparation; will render it biologically inactive. Single-dose vial contains no preservatives. Use only 1 dose per vial, then discard. Never reenter vial. Now available in multidose vial with preservative; sterile technique imperative.

Storage: Refrigerate single and multidose vials before use, multidose vial after initial use. Discard in 21 days. Do not freeze or shake. Protect from light.

Filters: Not required; however, it was filtered during manufacturing with 0.2-micron millipore filters. No significant loss of potency expected with the use of non–protein binding filters of a similar size or larger.

COMPATIBILITY

Manufacturers state, "Do not dilute or administer in conjunction with other drug solutions." One source indicates there may be protein loss from adsorption to PVC containers and tubing. Manufacturer suggests it may be mixed 1-to-1 with bacteriostatic NS in a syringe when prepared from a single-dose vial for SC injection; see literature.

RATE OF ADMINISTRATION

A single dose over at least 1 minute.

ACTIONS

An amino acid glycoprotein manufactured by recombinant DNA technology. Has the same biologic effects as erythropoietin produced naturally by the kidneys. Stimulates bone marrow to produce RBCs, increasing the reticulocyte count within 10 days and the red cell count, hemoglobin, and hematocrit within 2 to 6 weeks. Normal iron stores are necessary because it steps up RBC production to a rate above what the body usually makes. New cells need iron, which is quickly depleted. Half-life is 4 to 13 hours. Continued therapy will maintain improved RBC levels and decrease need for transfusions.

INDICATIONS AND USES

To treat anemia associated with chronic renal failure in adults and pediatric patients and decrease the need for transfusions in patients receiving dialysis (end-stage renal disease) and those not receiving dialysis. Non-dialysis patients with symptomatic anemia considered for therapy should have a hemoglobin less than 10 Gm/dL. ■ Treatment of anemias related to zidovudine (AZT, Retrovir) therapy in HIV-infected patients. ■ Treatment of anemic patients scheduled to undergo non-cardiac, non-vascular surgery to reduce the need for allogeneic blood transfusions, especially in patients at high risk for perioperative transfusions with significant anticipated blood loss (not indicated for anemic patients who are willing to donate autologous blood). ▪ Treatment of anemia resulting from chemotherapy in patients with non-myeloid malignancies. Studies to determine whether epoetin alfa increases mortality or decreases progression-free/recurrence-free survival are ongoing. ▪ Not indicated for cancer patients for the treatment of anemias resulting from other factors such as iron or folate deficiencies, hemolysis, or gastrointestinal bleeding. ▪ Not indicated for use in patients receiving hormonal agents, therapeutic biologic products, or radiotherapy unless receiving concomitant myelosuppressive chemotherapy. ▪ Not indicated for patients receiving myelosuppressive therapy when the anticipated outcome is cure; see Precautions. ▪ Has not been shown to improve symptoms of anemia, quality of life, fatigue, or patient well-being.

Unlabeled uses: Anemia of prematurity.

CONTRAINDICATIONS
Known hypersensitivity to albumin (human) or to mammalian cell-derived products, uncontrolled hypertension.

PRECAUTIONS
All patients: May be given IV or SC in patients not receiving dialysis. May be given to dialysis patients into the venous line at the end of the dialysis procedure to eliminate additional venous access. ▪ May increase the risk of serious and life-threatening cardiovascular events and death. Higher risk may be associated with a higher hemoglobin and/or a higher rate of rise of hemoglobin. Individualize dosing to achieve and maintain a hemoglobin level within the range of 10 to 12 Gm/dL and to avoid a rate of rise of more than 1 Gm/dL in a 2-week period. ▪ Increases in hemoglobin of greater than 1 Gm/dL during any 2-week period have been associated with an increased incidence of cardiac arrest, exacerbations of hypertension, congestive heart failure (CHF), vascular thrombosis/ischemia/infarction, acute MI, deep vein thrombosis (DVT), pulmonary embolus, and fluid overload/edema and may be associated with neurologic events (e.g., seizures, stroke). See Dose Adjustments. Risks are increased in patients with cancer who are not receiving chemotherapy. Risks are increased in patients receiving erythropoiesis-stimulating agents (ESAs) to reduce blood transfusions during and after orthopedic surgery; strongly consider the use of antithrombotic prophylaxis (e.g., enoxaparin [Lovenox]) in these patients. ▪ In addition to low baseline hematocrit and inadequate iron stores, delayed or diminished response may result from concurrent medical problems (infections, inflammatory or malignant processes, occult blood loss, underlying hematologic disease, folic acid or vitamin B_{12} deficiency, hemolysis, aluminum intoxication, osteitis fibrosa cystica, pure red cell aplasia [PRCA], anti-erythropoietin antibody-associated anemia). ▪ Not intended for use in anemias caused by iron or folate deficiencies, hemolysis, or GI bleeding or for use in treating symptoms of anemia, including dizziness, fatigue, low energy, poor quality of life, or shortness of breath. ▪ Use caution in patients with porphyria; may exacerbate disease. ▪ Not a substitute for emergency transfusion in patients requiring immediate correction of severe anemia. ▪ Administration of erythropoiesis-stimulating agents (ESAs) to cancer patients shortened the overall survival time and/or increased the risk of tumor progression or recurrence in clinical studies of some patients with breast, cervical, head and neck, lymphoid, and non–small-cell lung malignancies. The risks of shortened survival time and tumor progression have not

been excluded when ESAs are dosed to achieve a hemoglobin of less than 12 Gm/dL. To minimize these risks, as well as the risks of serious cardiovascular and thrombovascular events, use the lowest dose needed to avoid a red blood cell transfusion. Use only to treat anemia due to concomitant myelosuppressive chemotherapy, and discontinue after completion of a chemotherapy course. Prescribers and hospitals are now required to enroll in and comply with the ESA APPRISE Oncology Program to prescribe and/or dispense ESAs to patients with cancer. See prescribing information Black Box Warning. ▪ Pure red cell aplasia (PRCA) and severe anemia, with or without other cytopenias, in association with neutralizing antibodies to native erythropoietin has been observed. Most often reported in CRF patients receiving epoetin alfa by SC injection. Any patient who develops a sudden loss of response to epoetin alfa accompanied by severe anemia and low reticulocyte count should be evaluated. Physicians may contact manufacturer (Amgen) for help with the evaluation of these patients. ▪ Safety and efficacy not established in patients with a known history of seizure disorder or underlying hematologic disorders (e.g., sickle cell anemia, myelodysplastic syndrome, or hypercoagulable disorders). ▪ The formulation containing albumin carries a risk for transmission of viral diseases or Creutzfeldt-Jakob disease. However, donor screening and manufacturing processes make this risk extremely remote. *Chronic renal failure:* 98% of previously transfusion-dependent patients are able to maintain a stable hematocrit greater than 30% with epoetin alfa therapy. ▪ Epoetin alfa, with or without phlebotomy, has reduced iron and ferritin stores in hemodialysis patients with iron overload and associated hemosiderosis secondary to multiple RBC transfusions. ▪ Some authorities believe epoetin should be discontinued 2 weeks before planned renal engraftment to prevent risk of excessive erythrocytosis and resultant adverse effects (renal artery thrombosis with loss of graft occurred in one patient). ▪ Epoetin alfa reduces need for blood transfusions and decreases exposure to foreign histocompatibility; potential for finding a compatible graft may be increased. *HIV infection:* Epoetin has no effect on HIV disease process; primarily improves quality of life. ▪ Used concomitantly with filgrastim (G-CSF, Neupogen) to control granulocytopenia; filgrastim increases the neutrophil count while epoetin alfa increases the hemoglobin concentration. Helps maintain somewhat more normal counts in zidovudine therapy, but additional blood transfusions will probably be required.

Cancer patients on chemotherapy: Treatment of patients with grossly elevated serum erythropoietin levels (e.g., greater than 200 mU/mL) is not recommended. *Surgery patients:* Safety established only for patients receiving anticoagulation prophylaxis.

Monitor: *All patients:* A biologic product. Monitor for S/S of hypersensitivity reactions. ▪ Hypertension must be controlled before initiation of therapy. Monitor BP frequently and control aggressively; generally rises when hemoglobin or hematocrit is increasing rapidly. 25% of renal patients require an increase in antihypertensive therapy and dietary restrictions. Exacerbation of hypertension has not been observed in patients being treated with epoetin alfa for other indicated anemias; however, any indication may require a decrease in dose of epoetin if BP difficult to control or withhold epoetin until BP is controlled. ▪ CBC with differential and platelet counts; BUN; uric acid; creatinine; phosphorus; sodium; and potassium are required before treatment is initiated and at regular intervals during therapy. Modest increases are expected. Changes in dialysis treatment may be required. Monitor hemoglobin twice weekly until it stabilizes. ■ Normal iron stores required to support epoetin-stimulated erythropoiesis. Transferrin saturation should be at least 20% and ferritin at least 100 ng/mL. Monitor before and during therapy. Supplemental iron (ferrous sulfate 325 mg PO 3 times daily) is usually required to increase and maintain transferrin saturation. Administration of IV parenteral iron may be necessary in some patients. ■ Seizures rare, but more occur in the first 90 days. Observe BP and neurologic symptoms. Caution against driving or operating heavy machinery. ■ Monitor patients with pre-existing vascular disease carefully (especially those with chronic renal failure); increase in hematocrit may precipitate a cerebrovascular accident, transient ischemic attack, or myocardial infarction. ■ As anemia is corrected, elevated bleeding time decreases toward normal with epoetin treatment as it does with transfusion. Monitor hemoglobin until stable. *Chronic renal failure:* Can cause polycythemia. Baseline hemoglobin and hematocrit required. Repeat twice weekly until stabilization in the target range (hemoglobin of 10 to 12 Gm/dL, not to exceed 12 Gm/dL). Continue monitoring at regular intervals. After any dose adjustment, twice-weekly hemoglobin and hematocrit is required for 2 to 6 weeks to evaluate outcome and make further dose adjustments. See Usual Dose and Dose Adjustments. ■ Dialysis patients may require additional anticoagulation with heparin to prevent clotting of artificial kidney or clotting of the vascular access (AV shunt) and to maintain efficiency of the dialysis procedure. ■ Compliance with dialysis and/or dietary restrictions is mandatory. ■ Monitor fluid and electrolyte balance carefully in patients not receiving dialysis. Improved sense of well-being may mask need for dialysis. *HIV infection:* Effectiveness in HIV-infected patients seems to be dependent on an endogenous serum erythropoietin level less than or equal to 500 mU/mL (normal levels are 4 to 26 mU/mL) and a dose of zidovudine (AZT, Retrovir) of less than or equal to 4,200 mg/wk. Monitor hemoglobin weekly until stable. *Cancer patients on chemotherapy:* Monitor hemoglobin and hematocrit weekly until stable. *Surgery patients:* Monitor iron supplementation and anticoagulant therapy.

Patient Education: Risk of seizures, especially during first 90 days of therapy. Do not drive or operate heavy equipment. ■ Menses may resume; possibility of pregnancy. Contraception may be indicated. ■ Additional instruction (e.g., equipment, techniques) will be required in patients who will self-administer (manufacturer supplies brochure). ■ Stress importance of compliance with diet, iron, and vitamin (e.g., folic acid, B_{12}) supplementation. Close monitoring of BP and Hgb is imperative. ■ Promptly report pain or swelling in legs, SOB, increase in BP, dizziness, or loss of consciousness. ■ Increased risk of mortality, serious cardiovascular events, thromboembolic events, and tumor progression or recurrence. ■ All patients should (and patients with cancer must) discuss the risks of using an ESA with a health care professional.

Maternal/Child: Category C: may present risk to fetus; benefits must justify risk. ■ Use caution in nursing mothers. ■ Pharmacokinetics (absorption, distribution, metabolism, and excretion) in children and adolescents similar to adults. ■ Safety for use in pediatric patients not established for diagnoses other than anemia of renal disease. However, has been used in both pediatric cancer patients and pediatric HIV-infected patients with positive results. See prescribing information and published literature. ▪ Limited data available for use in neonates. It suggests that clearance may be increased compared to adults. ▪ Multidose vials contain benzyl alcohol; do not use in neonates.

Elderly: Monitor blood chemistry and BP carefully due to increased risk of renal and/or cardiovascular complications.

DRUG/LAB INTERACTIONS
Specific information not available.

SIDE EFFECTS
Generally well tolerated. Occur most frequently in patients with chronic renal failure. Increased hypertension is common, and hypertensive encephalopathy and seizures can occur. Clotted vascular access (AV shunt) and clotting of the artificial kidney may occur during dialysis. Allergic reactions have been reported. Other reported side effects are those common to the underlying disease and not necessarily attributable to epoetin and include arthralgias, asthenia, bone marrow fibrosis, cerebrovascular accident or transient ischemic attack, chest pain, cough, CVA/TIA, diarrhea, dizziness, edema, fatigue, fever, headache, hyperkalemia, myocardial infarction, nausea, polycythemia, rash, respiratory congestion, shortness of breath, tachycardia, and vomiting. PRCA and severe anemia, with or without other cytopenias, in association with neutralizing antibodies has been reported; see Precautions.

ANTIDOTE
Notify physician of all side effects; most will be treated symptomatically. Excessive hypertension may require discontinuation of epoetin until BP is controlled or may respond to reduction in dose of epoetin or to an increase in antihypertensive therapy. Reduce dose of epoetin in patients with an increase in hemoglobin over 1 Gm/dL in any 2-week period or if hemoglobin increases to greater than 12 Gm/dL. May need to withhold dose until hemoglobin falls below 13 Gm/dL. Consider phlebotomy in toxicity. Additional heparin may be required during dialysis to prevent clotting. If overdose or polycythemia does occur, monitor closely for cardiovascular events and hematologic abnormalities. When resuming therapy, monitor closely for evidence of rapid increases in hemoglobin concentration (greater than 1 Gm/dL within 14 days) and reduce dose as indicated. Permanently discontinue therapy in patients with antibody-mediated anemia. Patients should not be switched to other erythropoietic proteins because antibodies may cross-react. Treat minor hypersensitivity reactions symptomatically. Discontinue drug and treat anaphylaxis as indicated; resuscitate as necessary.

EPOPROSTENOL SODIUM

(eh-poh-**PROST**-en-ohl **SO**-dee-um)

Flolan

Vasodilating agent
Antihypertensive (pulmonary)

pH 10.2 to 10.8

USUAL DOSE

Acute dose initiation and chronic continuous infusion: May be given through a peripheral line on a temporary basis until a central venous line is established. A central venous catheter should be put in place as soon as possible and must be used for continuous long-term 24-hour administration with an ambulatory infusion pump. Begin infusion at 2 ng/kg/min. Increase in increments of 2 ng/kg/min every 15 minutes or longer until dose-limiting pharmacologic effects occur or until a tolerance limit to the drug is established and further increases in the infusion rate are not clinically warranted; see Dose Adjustments. Most common S/S of dose-limiting effects include abdominal pain, flushing, headache, hypotension, nausea, respiratory disorders, sepsis, and vomiting. If dose-limiting pharmacologic effects occur, decrease infusion rate slowly until pharmacologic effects are tolerated; see Dose Adjustments. If the initial dose of 2 ng/kg/min is not tolerated, use a lower dose. During the first 7 days of treatment in clinical trials, the dose was increased daily to a mean dose of 4.1 ng/kg/min on Day 7 of treatment. At the end of Week 12, the mean dose was 11.2 ng/kg/min. The mean incremental increase was 2 to 3 ng/kg/min every 3 weeks. Usually given concomitantly with anticoagulant therapy; see Monitor.

DOSE ADJUSTMENTS

Changes in the chronic infusion rate are to be expected. If symptoms of primary pulmonary hypertension (PPH) persist, recur, or worsen, increase infusion rate promptly by 1 to 2 ng/kg/min. Wait at least 15 minutes to assess clinical response. Observe patient for several hours to confirm patient tolerance and take BP and HR in supine and standing positions. In trials most patients progressed to a dose a little less than their acute dose-initiation intolerable dose within 12 weeks. ▪ Occurrence of dose-related side effects that do not resolve may require a decrease in the chronic infusion rate. Reduce dose gradually in 2-ng/kg/min increments and wait at least 15 minutes to assess clinical response. Use extreme caution if decreasing the dose; abrupt withdrawal or sudden large reductions may cause a rapid return of PPH symptoms and may precipitate death. ▪ In patients receiving lung transplants, doses were tapered after the initiation of cardiopulmonary bypass. ▪ Dose selection for the elderly should be cautious. ▪ Asymptomatic increases in pulmonary artery pressure with increases in cardiac output may occur during acute dose initiation; consider dose adjustment. ▪ See Precautions.

DILUTION

Infusion pump required. It must be small and lightweight; able to adjust infusion rates in 2-ng/kg/min increments; have occlusion, end of infusion, and low battery alarms; be accurate to ±6% of the programmed rate; be positive-pressure driven (continuous or pulsatile) with intervals between pulses not exceeding 3 minutes at rates required to deliver drug; and have a disposable reservoir cassette made of polyvinyl chloride, polypropylene, or glass with a capacity of at least 100 mL. Pumps used during trials were manufactured by Pharmacia Deltec, Medfusion, Inc., and Baxter Health Care. The infusion pump used in the most recent clinical trials was the CADD-1 HFX 5100 (SIMS Deltec).

Sterile diluent for epoprostenol is provided by the manufacturer. Do not use any other diluent. Concentration will be determined by desired dose/kg/min and parameters of ambulatory infusion pump to be used. See Rate of Administration. Two vials of provided sterile diluent will be required to prepare each 24-hour dose in each of the concentrations in the following chart.

Guidelines for Dilution of Epoprostenol to Various Concentrations	
To Make 100 mL of Solution with Final Concentration (ng/mL) of:	**Directions**
3,000 ng/mL	Dissolve contents of one 0.5-mg vial with 5 mL of STERILE DILUENT for epoprostenol. Withdraw 3 mL and add to sufficient STERILE DILUENT for epoprostenol to make a total of 100 mL.
5,000 ng/mL	Dissolve contents of one 0.5-mg vial with 5 mL of STERILE DILUENT for epoprostenol. Withdraw entire vial contents and add sufficient STERILE DILUENT for epoprostenol to make a total of 100 mL.
10,000 ng/mL	Dissolve contents of two 0.5-mg vials each with 5 mL of STERILE DILUENT for epoprostenol. Withdraw entire vial contents and add sufficient STERILE DILUENT for epoprostenol to make a total of 100 mL.
15,000 ng/mL	Dissolve contents of one 1.5-mg vial with 5 mL of STERILE DILUENT for epoprostenol. Withdraw entire vial contents and add sufficient STERILE DILUENT for epoprostenol to make a total of 100 mL.

Acute dose initiation may require more than one solution strength. 3,000 ng/mL and 10,000 ng/mL concentrations should be satisfactory to deliver between 2 and 16 ng/kg/min in adults. A maximum 2-day supply can be diluted at one time (200 mL). For use at room temperature, withdraw 33.3 mL and deposit in pump reservoir cassette or sterile infusion bag for each 8-hour period. If used with cold pouches and frozen gel packs, 100 mL can be placed in the pump reservoir cassette or a 100-mL sterile infusion bag for each 24-hour period. Frozen gel packs must be changed every 12 hours. Reservoir cassettes are disposable. Most patients prepare a 24-hour dose in a new reservoir cassette before a new dose is required and use cold pouches to maintain temperature.

Filters: An in-line 0.22-micron filter was used during clinical trials.

Storage: Unopened vials of epoprostenol may be stored at 15° to 25° C (59° to 77° F) in the carton to protect from light. Diluent may be stored at

15° to 25° C (59° to 77° F). Protection from light not required. See expiration dates on both. Before use, reconstituted solutions must be refrigerated and protected from light. Do not freeze. Reconstituted solution must be discarded after 48 hours or if accidentally frozen. While in use, must not be exposed to direct sunlight or temperatures above 25° C (77° F) or below 0° C (32° F). Stable in pump reservoir for only 8 hours at RT. Use of cold pouches with frozen gel packs can extend reservoir life to 24 hours. Time stored in refrigerator and in reservoir of pump must be included in maximum 48-hour time frame.

COMPATIBILITY
Manufacturer states, "Stable only when reconstituted with the provided diluent. Must not be reconstituted or mixed with any other parenteral medications or solutions prior to or during administration." One source suggests **compatibility** at the **Y-site** with bivalirudin (Angiomax).

RATE OF ADMINISTRATION
Administered by a continuous IV infusion through a central venous catheter. Peripheral access may be used temporarily until a central line can be placed. Titrate dose as outlined in Usual Dose and Dose Adjustments. Flow must not be interrupted for longer than 2 to 3 minutes. Time to completion of administration must never exceed more than 8 hours at room temperature, more than 24 hours with use of cold pouches and changing frozen gel packs every 12 hours, or more than 48 hours from time of initial reconstitution. If dose-limiting pharmacologic effects occur, decrease infusion rate slowly until pharmacologic effects are tolerated; see Dose Adjustments. The infusion rate may be calculated using the following formula:

$$\text{Infusion rate (mL/hr)} = \frac{\text{Dose (ng/kg/min)} \times \text{Weight in kg} \times 60 \text{ min/hr}}{\text{Final concentration (ng/mL)}}$$

The following charts may be used for infusion rates at a final concentration of 3,000 ng/mL or 15,000 ng/mL. See package insert for tables at additional concentrations.

Infusion Rates for Epoprostenol at a Concentration of 3,000 ng/mL							
	Dose or Drug Delivery Rate (ng/kg/min)						
Patient Weight	2	4	6	8	10	12	14	16
	Infusion Delivery Rate (mL/hr)						
10 kg	—	—	1.2	1.6	2	2.4	2.8	3.2
20 kg	—	1.6	2.4	3.2	4	4.8	5.6	6.4
30 kg	1.2	2.4	3.6	4.8	6	7.2	8.4	9.6
40 kg	1.6	3.2	4.8	6.4	8	9.6	11.2	12.8
50 kg	2	4	6	8	10	12	14	16
60 kg	2.4	4.8	7.2	9.6	12	14.4	16.8	19.2
70 kg	2.8	5.6	8.4	11.2	14	16.8	19.6	22.4
80 kg	3.2	6.4	9.6	12.8	16	19.2	22.4	25.6
90 kg	3.6	7.2	10.8	14.4	18	21.6	25.2	28.8
100 kg	4	8	12	16	20	24	28	32

Infusion Rates for Epoprostenol at a Concentration of 15,000 ng/mL						
	Dose or Drug Delivery Rate (ng/kg/min)					
Patient Weight	4	6	8	10	12	14	16
	Infusion Delivery Rate (mL/hr)					
20 kg	—	—	—	—	1	1.1	1.3
30 kg	—	—	1	1.2	1.4	1.7	1.9
40 kg	—	1	1.3	1.6	1.9	2.2	2.6
50 kg	—	1.2	1.6	2	2.4	2.8	3.2
60 kg	1	1.4	1.9	2.4	2.9	3.4	3.8
70 kg	1.1	1.7	2.2	2.8	3.4	3.9	4.5
80 kg	1.3	1.9	2.6	3.2	3.8	4.5	5.1
90 kg	1.4	2.2	2.9	3.6	4.3	5	5.8
100 kg	1.6	2.4	3.2	4	4.8	5.6	6.4

ACTIONS

A naturally occurring prostaglandin. It directly vasodilates pulmonary and systemic arterial vascular beds and inhibits platelet aggregation. Right and left ventricle afterload is reduced, and cardiac output and stroke volume are increased. Effect on HR is dose related. Produces dose-related increases in cardiac index and stroke volume and dose-related decreases in pulmonary vascular resistance, total pulmonary resistance, and mean systemic arterial pressure. Has been shown to increase exercise capacity, improve hemodynamic status, and extend survival. Onset of action is immediate. Half-life is approximately 6 minutes at body pH of 7.4. Metabolized to two primary metabolites by rapid hydrolyzation and enzymatic degradation.

INDICATIONS AND USES

Treatment of pulmonary arterial hypertension (PAH [WHO Group 1]) to improve exercise capacity. Effectiveness established predominantly in patients with NYHA Functional Class III-IV symptoms and etiologies of idiopathic or heritable PAH or PAH associated with connective tissue diseases.

CONTRAINDICATIONS

Congestive heart failure due to severe left ventricular systolic dysfunction, known hypersensitivity to epoprostenol or related compounds (e.g., alprostadil [prostaglandin E_1, Prostin VR Pediatric]).

PRECAUTIONS

Administered by or under the direction of the physician specialist. ■ During dose initiation, facilities for monitoring the patient and responding to any medical emergency must be available. ■ Causes of secondary pulmonary hypertension should be eliminated and diagnosis of PPH carefully established. ■ Abrupt withdrawal, interruptions in drug delivery, or sudden large reductions in dose may result in rebound pulmonary hypertension, including dyspnea, dizziness, and weakness. Death of one patient was attributed to these causes. Backup medication and equipment must always be available. ■ Use of a multilumen catheter should be considered if other

IV therapy is used. ■ Not recommended for patients who develop pulmonary edema during acute dose initiation; may develop pulmonary venoocclusive disease. ■ Asymptomatic increases in pulmonary artery pressure with increases in cardiac output may occur during acute dose initiation; consider dose adjustment. ■ Cardiac catheterization is used during trials for acute dose initiation but is not necessary; consider benefit versus risk. In patients undergoing lung transplants, it is recommended that the dose of epoprostenol be tapered after initiation of cardiopulmonary bypass. ■ A potent inhibitor of platelet aggregation; an increased risk for hemorrhagic complications may occur, particularly in patients with other risk factors for bleeding. ■ See Monitor, Patient Education, Drug/Lab Interactions.

Monitor: ECG monitoring and frequent monitoring of vital signs recommended during acute dose initiation. ■ Observe for dose-limiting side effects. ■ Thrombocytopenia has been reported; periodic platelet counts may be indicated. ■ To reduce the risk of pulmonary thromboembolism or systemic embolism, anticoagulant therapy is recommended concomitantly unless contraindicated. ■ Therapy may be required for months or years; consideration must be given to the ability of the patient and family to manage this care. ■ Monitor standing and supine HR and BP for several hours after any adjustment. ■ Thorough patient teaching and continued support services are imperative to facilitate a good clinical outcome. ■ See Precautions, Patient Education, Drug/Lab Interactions.

Patient Education: After initial dose titration and training, this is a self-administered drug. Must assume responsibility for drug reconstitution, drug administration, and care of the permanent central venous catheter. ■ Aseptic technique during reconstitution and with routine care of permanent indwelling central venous catheter is imperative to prevent infection. ■ Report fever or any sign of infection at catheter site (e.g., redness, warmth). ■ Delivery of medication cannot be interrupted. Interruption will cause a rapid return of PPH symptoms. ■ Should have access to a backup infusion pump and intravenous infusion sets to avoid potential interruption in drug delivery. ■ Dose adjustments should be made only under the direction of the physician except in an emergency situation (e.g., unconsciousness, collapse).

Maternal/Child: Category B: use only if clearly needed. No evidence of fetal harm in animal studies to date. ■ Safety for use during labor and delivery not established. ■ Use caution in nursing mothers; safety not established. ■ Safety for use in pediatric patients not established. ■ Some studies suggest pediatric patients may tolerate higher doses than adults.

Elderly: See Dose Adjustments. Decreased organ function (cardiac, hepatic, renal), concomitant disease, and other drug therapy may cause concern. Response of younger patients versus the elderly not documented.

DRUG/LAB INTERACTIONS

Has been used with digoxin, diuretics, anticoagulants, oral vasodilators, and oxygen. ■ Hypotension may be increased with **diuretics, antihypertensive agents, or other vasodilators.** ■ Risk of bleeding may be increased with **antiplatelet agents, anticoagulants, or NSAIDs** (e.g., ibuprofen [Advil, Motrin], naproxen [Aleve, Naprosyn]). ■ Epoprostenol may increase the bioavailability of oral **digoxin.** May decrease clearance of **furosemide** (Lasix), and **digoxin;** monitor digoxin levels.

SIDE EFFECTS

Acute dose initiation: Most common S/S of dose-limiting effects include flushing, headache, hypotension, nausea, and vomiting. Abdominal pain, agitation, anxiety/nervousness, back pain, bradycardia, chest pain, constipation, dizziness, dyspnea, dyspepsia, hyperesthesia, musculoskeletal pain, paresthesia, respiratory disorders, sepsis, sweating, tachycardia, and many other side effects may occur.

Chronic continuous infusion: Any of the above and arthralgia, bleeding at various sites, chills, diarrhea, fatigue, fever, flu-like symptoms, infection (may be local at site of catheter insertion), jaw pain, pallor, pulmonary edema, rash, sepsis, splenomegaly, thrombocytopenia.

Overdose: Hypotension, hypoxemia, respiratory arrest, and death may occur.

Post-Marketing: Anemia, hypersplenism, hyperthyroidism, pancytopenia, splenomegaly.

ANTIDOTE

Continuous maintenance of drug flow imperative. Keep physician informed of all side effects. Most will be treated with dose reduction; some may require symptomatic treatment. Call 1-800-9-FLOLAN for drug or pump problems.

EPTIFIBATIDE
(ep-tih-**FY**-beh-tide)

Integrilin

Platelet aggregation inhibitor

pH 5.35

USUAL DOSE

Used in combination with heparin and aspirin. A calculated CrCl greater than or equal to 50 mL/min is required in patients receiving the following doses. Use of the Cockroft-Gault equation is recommended for calculating CrCl. Discontinue eptifibatide infusion before CABG surgery and in patients requiring thrombolytic therapy.

ACUTE CORONARY SYNDROME

Eptifibatide: 180 mcg/kg as an IV bolus as soon as possible following diagnosis. Follow with a continuous infusion of 2 mcg/kg/min until hospital discharge or initiation of coronary artery bypass graft (CABG) surgery for up to 72 hours. Alternately, if a patient is to undergo a percutaneous coronary intervention (PCI) while receiving eptifibatide, the infusion should be continued up to hospital discharge, or for 18 to 24 hours after the procedure, whichever comes first. Patient may receive up to 96 hours of therapy. See Dosing Chart by Weight on the following page and Dose Adjustments. Dose in patients with a calculated CrCl greater than or equal to 50 mL/min weighing more than 121 kg should not exceed a bolus of 22.6 mg or an infusion rate of 15 mg/hr.

Aspirin: 160 to 325 mg PO initially and daily thereafter.

Heparin: *Medical management:* Suggested heparin dose to achieve the target aPTT of 50 to 70 seconds during medical management is *Weight 70 kg or more,* 5,000 units as an IV bolus followed by an infusion of 1,000 units/hr. *Weight less than 70 kg,* 60 units/kg as an IV bolus followed by an infusion of 12 units/kg/hr.

Patients undergoing PCI: Target ACT is 200 to 300 seconds during PCI. If heparin is initiated before PCI, give additional boluses during PCI as needed to keep ACT in range. Heparin infusion after PCI is discouraged.

PERCUTANEOUS CORONARY INTERVENTION (PCI)

Eptifibatide: 180 mcg/kg as an IV bolus immediately before initiation of PCI followed by a continuous infusion of 2 mcg/kg/min. Repeat bolus of 180 mcg/kg 10 minutes after the first bolus. Continue infusion until hospital discharge or for up to 18 to 24 hours, whichever comes first. A minimum of 12 hours of infusion is recommended. See the following chart and Dose Adjustments. Dose in patients with a calculated CrCl greater than or equal to 50 mL/min weighing more than 121 kg should not exceed a bolus of 22.6 mg or an infusion rate of 15 mg/hr.

Aspirin: 160 to 325 mg PO 1 to 24 hours before PCI and daily thereafter.

Heparin: Target ACT is 200 to 300 seconds during PCI. In patients not treated with heparin within 6 hours of PCI, give 60 units/kg as a bolus. Give additional boluses as needed during PCI to keep ACT in range. Heparin infusion is discouraged after PCI.

FOR BOTH INDICATIONS

Refer to the following Eptifibatide Dosing Chart by Weight.

Eptifibatide Dosing Chart by Weight				
	180 mcg/kg Bolus Volume	2 mcg/kg/min Infusion Rate		1 mcg/kg/min Infusion Rate	
Patient Weight	From 2 mg/mL Vial	From 2 mg/mL 100-mL Vial	From 0.75 mg/mL 100-mL Vial	From 2 mg/mL 100-mL Vial	From 0.75 mg/mL 100-mL Vial
37-41 kg	3.4 mL	2 mL/hr	6 mL/hr	1 mL/hr	3 mL/hr
42-46 kg	4 mL	2.5 mL/hr	7 mL/hr	1.3 mL/hr	3.5 mL/hr
47-53 kg	4.5 mL	3 mL/hr	8 mL/hr	1.5 mL/hr	4 mL/hr
54-59 kg	5 mL	3.5 mL/hr	9 mL/hr	1.8 mL/hr	4.5 mL/hr
60-65 kg	5.6 mL	3.8 mL/hr	10 mL/hr	1.9 mL/hr	5 mL/hr
66-71 kg	6.2 mL	4 mL/hr	11 mL/hr	2 mL/hr	5.5 mL/hr
72-78 kg	6.8 mL	4.5 mL/hr	12 mL/hr	2.3 mL/hr	6 mL/hr
79-84 kg	7.3 mL	5 mL/hr	13 mL/hr	2.5 mL/hr	6.5 mL/hr
85-90 kg	7.9 mL	5.3 mL/hr	14 mL/hr	2.7 mL/hr	7 mL/hr
91-96 kg	8.5 mL	5.6 mL/hr	15 mL/hr	2.8 mL/hr	7.5 mL/hr
97-103 kg	9 mL	6 mL/hr	16 mL/hr	3 mL/hr	8 mL/hr
104-109 kg	9.5 mL	6.4 mL/hr	17 mL/hr	3.2 mL/hr	8.5 mL/hr
110-115 kg	10.2 mL	6.8 mL/hr	18 mL/hr	3.4 mL/hr	9 mL/hr
116-121 kg	10.7 mL	7 mL/hr	19 mL/hr	3.5 mL/hr	9.5 mL/hr
>121 kg	11.3 mL	7.5 mL/hr	20 mL/hr	3.7 mL/hr	10 mL/hr

DOSE ADJUSTMENTS

ACUTE CORONARY SYNDROME

In patients with a calculated CrCl less than 50 mL/min, give a bolus of 180 mcg/kg. Decrease rate of the continuous infusion to 1 mcg/kg/min. In patients with a calculated CrCl less than 50 mL/min or a SCr greater than 2 mg/dL and weighing more than 121 kg, a maximum bolus of 22.6 mg followed by a maximum infusion rate of 7.5 mg/hr should be administered.

PCI

In patients with a calculated CrCl less than 50 mL/min, give a bolus of 180 mcg/kg. Decrease rate of the continuous infusion to 1 mcg/kg/min. Repeat bolus of 180 mcg/kg 10 minutes after the first bolus. In patients with a calculated CrCl less than 50 mL/min or a SCr greater than 2 mg/dL and weighing more than 121 kg, a maximum bolus of 22.6 mg followed by a maximum infusion rate of 7.5 mg/hr should be administered.

ALL DIAGNOSES

Dose adjustments are not required in patients with SCr between 1 and 2 mg/dL. ▪ Dose reduction may be indicated in patients over 75 years of
Continued

age weighing less than 50 kg. ▪ See Dosing Chart by Weight in Usual Dose. ▪ See Contraindications.

DILUTION

The 10-mL vial contains 20 mg of eptifibatide; the 100-mL vials contain 75 mg or 200 mg of eptifibatide.

IV bolus: Given undiluted. Withdraw total bolus dose (usually from the 10-mL vial) into a syringe.

Infusion: Usually given undiluted directly from the 75 mg/100 mL (0.75 mg/mL) or the 200 mg/100 mL (2 mg/mL) vials using an IV infusion pump. The 100-mL vial should be spiked with a vented infusion set. Center the spike within the circle on the stopper top. May be diluted with NS or D5NS. Use of a metriset or infusion pump appropriate.

Storage: Refrigerate vials at 2° to 8° C (36° to 46° F) or they may be kept at CRT for up to 2 months. Protect from light until administration. Do not use beyond the expiration or discard date. Discard any unused portion left in the vial.

COMPATIBILITY

Consider any drug NOT listed as compatible to be INCOMPATIBLE until consulting a pharmacist; specific conditions may apply.

Manufacturer lists furosemide (Lasix) as **incompatible** and states "is **incompatible** with any solution or drug not specifically listed as **compatible.**"

Manufacturer lists as **compatible** at **Y-site** with NS or D5NS with or without up to 60 mEq/L of potassium chloride as well as with alteplase (t-PA), atropine sulfate, dobutamine, heparin, lidocaine, meperidine (Demerol), metoprolol (Lopressor), midazolam (Versed), morphine, nitroglycerin IV, verapamil.

Another source adds the following **compatibilities:**

Y-site: Amiodarone (Nexterone), argatroban, bivalirudin (Angiomax), and micafungin (Mycamine).

RATE OF ADMINISTRATION

IV bolus: A single dose IV push over 1 to 2 minutes.

Infusion: See Dosing Charts by Weight under Usual Dose.

ACTIONS

A cyclic heptapeptide (amino acid) that reversibly binds to the platelet receptor glycoprotein GP IIb/IIIa of human platelets and inhibits platelet aggregation by preventing the binding of fibrinogen, von Willebrand factor, and other adhesive ligands to GP IIb/IIIa. Inhibits platelet aggregation in a dose- and concentration-dependent manner. Recovery of platelet function after termination of the eptifibatide infusion is rapid. Administered alone, eptifibatide has no measurable effect on PT or aPTT. Does not exert a pharmacologic effect on other integrins. Recommended regimens of a bolus followed by an infusion produce immediate inhibition of platelet aggregation and an early peak level, followed by a small decline, with steady state achieved within 4 to 6 hours. This decline can be prevented by administering a second bolus. Plasma elimination half-life is approximately 2.5 hours. 50% cleared from plasma by the kidneys. Balance of clearance is by nonrenal mechanisms. Has been shown to reduce clinical events (e.g., acute MI, need for urgent intervention) in patients undergoing PCI during drug administration and in those receiving medical management alone.

INDICATIONS AND USES

Used in combination with heparin, aspirin and, in selected situations, a thienopyridine (ticlopidine [Ticlid] or clopidogrel [Plavix]). ■ Treatment of patients with acute coronary syndrome (unstable angina or non–ST-segment elevation MI), including those who are to be managed medically and those undergoing PCI. In this setting, has been shown to decrease the rate of a combined endpoint of death or new MI. ■ Treatment of patients undergoing PCI, including those undergoing intracoronary stenting. In this setting has been shown to decrease the rate of a combined endpoint of death, new MI, or need for urgent intervention.

CONTRAINDICATIONS

Known hypersensitivity to any component of the product. ■ Current or planned administration of another parenteral glycoprotein GPIIb/IIIa inhibitor (e.g., abciximab [ReoPro], tirofiban [Aggrastat]). ■ Dependency on renal dialysis. ■ History of bleeding diathesis or evidence of active abnormal bleeding within the previous 30 days. ■ History of stroke within 30 days or any history of hemorrhagic stroke. ■ Major surgery within the preceding 6 weeks. ■ Severe hypertension (systolic BP greater than 200 mm Hg or diastolic BP greater than 110 mm Hg) not adequately controlled on antihypertensive therapy.

PRECAUTIONS

Use with caution in patients with platelet count less than 100,000/mm^3. ■ Use caution when given with drugs that affect hemostasis (e.g., NSAIDs [e.g., ibuprofen (Advil, Motrin), naproxen (Aleve, Naprosyn)], clopidogrel [Plavix], dipyridamole [Persantine], ticlopidine [Ticlid], warfarin [Coumadin]). Safety when used in combination with thrombolytic agents (e.g., alteplase [t-PA, Activase]), reteplase [Retavase], streptokinase [Streptase]) has not been established. See Drug/Lab Interactions. ■ Use with caution in patients with renal insufficiency; clearance is reduced and plasma levels are elevated; see Dose Adjustments. There is no experience in patients dependent on dialysis. ■ Bleeding is the most common complication encountered during therapy. ■ Risk of major bleeding increased inversely with patient weight, especially for patients weighing less than 70 kg. ■ Most major bleeding occurs at the arterial access site for cardiac catheterization or from the GI or GU tracts. ■ Acute profound thrombocytopenia has been reported; see Monitor. ■ In all studies, eptifibatide was less beneficial in women than in men. The reason is unclear. Differences in race have not been studied. ■ Because eptifibatide is readily reversible, procedures such as emergency CABG may be performed safely shortly after discontinuation of an infusion without the need for platelet transfusions. ■ Development of antibodies to eptifibatide and immune-mediated thrombocytopenia have been reported; may be associated with hypotension and/or other signs of hypersensitivity. ■ No clinical experience in patients with a baseline platelet count less than 100,000/mm^3. Monitor closely if use is indicated.

Monitor: Before therapy obtain platelet count, hemoglobin or hematocrit, SCr, and PT/aPTT. Obtain ACT in patients undergoing PCI. ■ Maintain target aPTT between 50 and 70 seconds unless PCI is to be performed. During PCI, the ACT should be maintained between 200 and 300 seconds. ■ The aPTT or ACT should be checked before sheath removal. The sheath should not be removed unless the aPTT is less than 45 seconds or the ACT is less than 150 seconds. In patients treated with heparin, bleeding can be minimized by close monitoring of the aPTT. ■ If acute profound thrombocytopenia occurs or the platelet count drops to less than 100,000/mm^3, heparin and eptifibatide should be discontinued. Monitor serial platelet counts, assess the presence of drug-dependent antibodies, and initiate appropriate therapy as indicated. ■ Monitor the patient for signs of bleeding; take vital signs (avoiding automatic BP cuffs); observe any invaded sites at least every 15 minutes (e.g., sheaths, IV sites, cutdowns, punctures, Foleys, NGs); watch for hematuria, hematemesis, bloody stool, petechiae, hematoma, flank pain, muscle weakness. Perform neuro checks frequently. If during therapy, bleeding cannot be controlled with pressure, heparin and eptifibatide should be discontinued. ■ Use care in handling patient; minimize use of urinary catheters, nasotracheal intubation, and nasogastric tubes. Avoid arterial puncture, venipuncture, and IM injection. Use extreme precautionary methods and only compressible sites if these procedures are absolutely necessary (i.e., avoid subclavian or jugular veins). Apply pressure for 30 minutes to any invaded site and then apply pressure dressings. Saline or heparin locks suggested to facilitate blood draws. ■ See Precautions.

Additional monitoring for patients receiving PCI: After PCI, eptifibatide should be continued until hospital discharge or for up to 18 to 24 hours, whichever comes first. See suggested time frames under each dose. Heparin use is discouraged after the PCI procedure. The femoral artery sheath may be removed during eptifibatide infusion, but only after heparin has been discontinued and its effects largely reversed. Heparin should be discontinued 3 to 4 hours before pulling the sheath, and an aPTT less than 45 seconds or an ACT of less than 150 seconds should be documented. ■ Care should be taken to obtain proper hemostasis after removal of the sheath using standard compressive techniques followed by close observation. Sheath hemostasis should be achieved at least 2 to 4 hours before hospital discharge.

Patient Education: Compliance with all measures to minimize bleeding (e.g., strict bed rest, positioning) is imperative. ■ Avoid use of razors, toothbrushes, and other sharp items. ■ Use caution while moving to avoid excessive bumping. ■ Report all episodes of bleeding and apply local pressure if indicated. ■ Expect oozing from IV sites.

Maternal/Child: Category B: safety for use in pregnancy not established; use only if clearly needed. ■ It is not known whether eptifibatide is excreted in breast milk; use caution if administered to a nursing mother. ■ Safety and effectiveness for use in pediatric patients not established.

Elderly: Dose adjusted by weight; see Dosing Charts by Weight in Usual Dose. ■ Clearance decreased and plasma levels increased in older patients; incidence of bleeding complications was higher and eptifibatide-associated bleeding was greater in the elderly during studies. ■ No apparent difference in effectiveness between older and younger patients.

DRUG/LAB INTERACTIONS

All studies with eptifibatide included the use of **aspirin and heparin.** In the ESPRIT study, **clopidogrel** (Plavix) **or ticlopidine** (Ticlid) were administered routinely, starting the day of PCI. Concomitant use, although indicated, increases the risk of bleeding. ■ Use caution when given with **drugs that affect hemostasis** such as **thrombolytics** (e.g., alteplase [t-PA, Activase], reteplase [Retavase], streptokinase [Streptase]), **oral anticoagulants** (e.g., warfarin [Coumadin]), **NSAIDs** (e.g., ibuprofen [Advil, Motrin], naproxen

[Aleve, Naprosyn]), **dipyridamole** (Persantine), **ticlopidine** (Ticlid), **clopidogrel** (Plavix), **selected antibiotics** (e.g., cefotetan). ■ Avoid concomitant treatment with **other inhibitors of platelet receptor glycoprotein GPIIb/IIIa** (e.g., abciximab [ReoPro], tirofiban [Aggrastat]); may have potentially serious additive effects. See Contraindications. ■ **Enoxaparin** (Lovenox) 1 mg/kg SC every 12 hours for 4 doses has been administered without altering the effects of eptifibatide.

SIDE EFFECTS

Bleeding is the most frequent adverse event; may occur more frequently in patients undergoing CABG or PCI, or in the elderly or those weighing less than 70 kg. Bleeding is usually reported as mild oozing, but major bleeding (e.g., GI bleeding, pulmonary hemorrhage, intracranial hemorrhage, and stroke) may occur. Fatal bleeding events have been reported. Laboratory findings related to bleeding include decrease in hemoglobin, hematocrit, and platelet count and occult blood in urine and feces. Other side effects that have been reported include hypersensitivity reactions, hypotension, and thrombocytopenia (acute and profound). Incidence in studies similar to that seen with placebo.

Acute toxicity: Specific information not available for humans, but decreased muscle tone, dyspnea, loss of righting reflex, petechial hemorrhages in the femoral and abdominal areas, and ptosis occurred in animals.

Post-Marketing: Immune-mediated thrombocytopenia.

ANTIDOTE

Keep physician informed of laboratory values and side effects. Discontinue the infusion of eptifibatide and heparin if any serious bleeding not controllable with pressure occurs, if CABG surgery is initiated, and/or if patient requires thrombolytic therapy. If acute profound thrombocytopenia occurs or the platelet count drops to less than 100,000/mm^3, heparin and eptifibatide should be discontinued. Monitor serial platelet counts, assess the presence of drug-dependent antibodies, and initiate appropriate therapy as indicated. Monitor closely; platelet transfusion may be required. If a hypersensitivity reaction should occur, discontinue the infusion and treat as indicated by severity (e.g., epinephrine, dopamine, theophylline, antihistamines such as diphenhydramine [Benadryl]) and/or corticosteroids as necessary. No specific antidote is available. Platelet inhibition reverses rapidly when infusion is discontinued. Hemodialysis may be useful in an overdose situation.

ERIBULIN MESYLATE
(**ER**-ih-**BUE**-lin **MES**-ih-late)
Halaven

Antineoplastic

USUAL DOSE

1.4 mg/M^2 IV over 2 to 5 minutes on Days 1 and 8 of a 21-day cycle.

DOSE ADJUSTMENTS

Dose adjustment not required based on age, gender, or race. ■ Reduce dose in patients with mild hepatic impairment (Child-Pugh Class A) to 1.1 mg/M^2 IV. ■ Patients with moderate hepatic impairment (Child-Pugh Class B) should receive 0.7 mg/M^2 IV. ■ Patients with moderate renal impairment (CrCl 30 to 50 mL/min) should receive 1.1 mg/M^2 IV. ■ Do not administer dose on Day 1 or Day 8 in patients with an ANC less than 1,000/mm^3, platelets less than 75,000/ mm^3, or Grade 3 or 4 nonhemato-logic toxicities. ■ The Day 8 dose may be delayed for a maximum of 1 week. If toxicities do not resolve or improve to Grade 2 or less by Day 15, omit the dose. If toxicities resolve or improve to Grade 2 or less by Day 15, administer at a reduced dose as outlined in the following table and initiate the next cycle no sooner than 2 weeks later. ■ If a dose has been delayed for toxicity and the toxicities have recovered to Grade 2 severity or less, resume eribulin as outlined in the following table. ■ Do not re-escalate eribulin dose after it has been reduced.

Recommended Dose Reductions for Eribulin Mesylate	
Event Description	Recommended Eribulin Dose
Permanently reduce the 1.4 mg/M^2 eribulin dose for any of the following: • ANC <500/mm^3 for >7 days • ANC <1,000/mm^3 with fever or infection • Platelets <25,000/mm^3 • Platelets <50,000/mm^3 requiring transfusion • Nonhematologic Grade 3 or 4 toxicities* • Omission or delay of Day 8 eribulin dose in previous cycle for toxicity	1.1 mg/M^2
Occurrence of any event requiring permanent dose reduction while receiving 1.1 mg/M^2	0.7 mg/M^2
Occurrence of any event requiring permanent dose reduction while receiving 0.7 mg/M^2	Discontinue eribulin

*Toxicities graded in accordance with National Cancer Institute (NCI) Common Terminology Criteria for Adverse Events (CTCAE) version 3.0.

DILUTION

Available in a single-use vial containing 1 mg/2 mL (0.5 mg/1 mL). Withdraw calculated dose and administer undiluted or may dilute in 100 mL NS.

Filter: Information not available.

Storage: Store unopened vials in carton at CRT. Store undiluted solution drawn up into a syringe for up to 4 hours at RT or 24 hours under refrigeration (4° C [40° F]). Store diluted solution for up to 4 hours at RT or 24 hours under refrigeration (4° C [40° F]). Discard unused portion of vial.

COMPATIBILITY

Manufacturer states, "Do not dilute in or administer through an IV line containing solutions with dextrose. Do not administer in the same intravenous line concurrent with other medicinal products."

RATE OF ADMINISTRATION

An IV injection evenly distributed over 2 to 5 minutes.

ACTIONS

A synthetic analog of halichondrin B, a product isolated from a marine sponge. Eribulin is a non-taxane microtubule inhibitor. Inhibits the growth phase of microtubules without affecting the shortening phase and sequesters tubulin into nonproductive aggregates. Exerts its effects via a tubulin-based antimitotic mechanism leading to G_2/M cell-cycle block, disruption of mitotic spindles and, ultimately, apoptotic cell death after prolonged mitotic blockage. Plasma protein binding is 49% to 65%. Mean elimination half-life is approximately 40 hours. There are no major human metabolites. Is eliminated primarily in feces unchanged. Small amount excreted as unchanged drug in urine.

INDICATIONS AND USES

Treatment of patients with metastatic breast cancer who have previously received at least two chemotherapeutic regimens for the treatment of metastatic disease. Prior therapy should have included an anthracycline and a taxane in either the adjuvant or metastatic setting.

CONTRAINDICATIONS

Manufacturer states, "None." ▪ Do not administer in patients with an ANC less than 1,000/mm³, platelets less than 75,000/mm³, or Grade 3 or 4 nonhematologic toxicities. ▪ Should be avoided in patients with congenital long QT syndrome.

PRECAUTIONS

May cause severe neutropenia (ANC less than 500/mm³) lasting more than 1 week. Higher incidence of Grade 4 neutropenia and febrile neutropenia seen in patients with ALT or AST greater than 3 times the ULN and in patients with a bilirubin greater than 1.5 times the ULN. ▪ Grades 3 and 4 peripheral neuropathy have been reported. Peripheral neuropathy was the most common toxicity leading to discontinuation of therapy. Neuropathy may not be reversible. ▪ QT prolongation, independent of eribulin concentration, was observed on Day 8 in an uncontrolled, open-label ECG study. ▪ Has not been studied in patients with severe hepatic impairment (Child-Pugh Class C) or renal impairment (CrCl less than 30 mL/min). ▪ See Dose Adjustments.

Monitor: Obtain baseline CBC with platelets, bilirubin, liver function tests, SCr, and electrolytes. ▪ Obtain CBC with platelets before each dose. Increase frequency of hematologic monitoring in patients who develop severe cytopenias (Grade 3 or 4); see Dose Adjustments. ▪ Assess for peripheral motor and sensory neuropathy before each dose; see Dose Adjustments. ▪ ECG monitoring is recommended in patients with CHF; bradyarrhythmias; drugs that prolong the QT interval, such as Class Ia and III antiarrhythmics (e.g., amiodarone [Nexterone], disopyramide [Norpace], dofetilide [Tikosyn], ibutilide [Corvert], N-acetylprocainamide, procainamide [Pronestyl], quinidine, sotalol [Betapace]); and electrolyte abnormalities. Correct hypokalemia or hypomagnesemia before initiating therapy and monitor electrolytes periodically during therapy. ▪ Monitor for nausea and vomiting. Use prophylactic antiemetics to reduce nausea and vomiting and increase patient comfort. ▪ Observe closely for signs of infection. Prophylactic antibiotics may be indicated pending results of C/S in a febrile neutropenic patient. ▪ In patients with thrombocytopenia (platelet count less than 50,000/mm^3), initiate precautions to prevent excessive bleeding (e.g., inspect IV sites, skin, and mucous membranes; use extreme care during invasive procedures; test urine, emesis, stool, and secretions for occult blood).

Patient Education: Avoid pregnancy. Nonhormonal birth control recommended. ▪ Promptly report S/S of infection (e.g., fever, chills, cough, burning or pain on urination). ▪ Report symptoms of peripheral neuropathy (e.g., numbness, tingling, or burning in hands or feet.)

Maternal/Child: Category D: expected to cause fetal harm. ▪ Discontinue breast-feeding. ▪ Safety and effectiveness for use in pediatric patients not established.

Elderly: No overall differences in safety were observed between older and younger patients. ▪ Consider age-related cardiac, hepatic, or renal dysfunction.

DRUG/LAB INTERACTIONS

No drug-drug interactions are expected with CYP3A4 inhibitors or P-gp inhibitors. ▪ Does not inhibit CYP1A2, CYP2C9, CYP2C19, CYP2D6, CYP2E1, or CYP3A4 enzymes or induce CYP1A2, CYP2C9, CYP2C19, or CYP3A4 enzymes at relevant clinical concentrations. Is therefore not expected to alter the plasma concentrations of drugs that are substrates of these enzymes.

SIDE EFFECTS

The most common side effects were alopecia, anemia, asthenia, constipation, fatigue, nausea, neutropenia, and peripheral neuropathy. The most common serious side effects were febrile neutropenia and neutropenia. The most common side effect resulting in discontinuation of eribulin was peripheral neuropathy. Less frequently reported side effects included anorexia, arthralgia, cough, diarrhea, dyspnea, fever, headache, liver function test abnormalities, mucosal inflammation, myalgia, pain (back, bone, extremity), UTI, vomiting, and weight loss.

ANTIDOTE

Keep physician informed of all side effects. Most will be treated symptomatically as indicated. Neutropenia can be profound. Severe peripheral neuropathies may necessitate discontinuation of eribulin. There is no specific antidote for overdose. Supportive therapy will help sustain the patient in toxicity. Resuscitate if indicated.

ERTAPENEM
(er-tah-**PEN**-em)

Invanz

USUAL DOSE
Duration of therapy is based on diagnosis as listed in the following chart.
May be given IV for up to 14 days or IM for up to 7 days.

Ertapenem Dosing Guidelines			
Infection*	Daily Dose (IV or IM) in Adults and Pediatric Patients 13 Years of Age and Older	Daily Dose (IV or IM) in Pediatric Patients 3 Months to 12 Years of Age	Duration
Complicated intra-abdominal infections	1 Gm	15 mg/kg q 12 hr†	5-14 days
Complicated skin and skin structure infections, including diabetic foot infections‡	1 Gm	15 mg/kg q 12 hr†	7-14 days§
Community-acquired pneumonia	1 Gm	15 mg/kg q 12 hr†	10-14 days‖
Complicated urinary tract infections, including pyelone-phritis	1 Gm	15 mg/kg q 12 hr†	10-14 days‖
Acute pelvic infections, including postpartum endomyometritis, septic abortion, and post-surgical gyneco-logic infections.	1 Gm	15 mg/kg q 12 hr†	3-10 days
Prophylaxis of surgical site infection in adults for elective colorectal surgery	1 Gm		Single intravenous dose given 1 hour before surgical incision

*Due to designated pathogens.
†Not to exceed 1 Gm/24 hr.
‡Has not been studied in diabetic foot infections with concomitant osteomyelitis.
§Adult patients with diabetic foot infections received up to 28 days of treatment (parenteral or parenteral plus oral switch therapy).
‖Duration includes a possible switch to an appropriate oral therapy, after at least 3 days of parenteral therapy, once clinical improvement has been demonstrated.

Continued

DOSE ADJUSTMENTS

Reduce dose to 0.5 Gm (500 mg) daily in adults with a CrCl at or less than 30 mL/min/1.73 M^2, including adults with end-stage renal insufficiency (CrCl ≤10 mL/min/1.73 M^2). No dose adjustment indicated in adults with a CrCl at or more than 31 mL/min/1.73 M^2. No data are available for pediatric patients with renal insufficiency or pediatric patients on hemodialysis. Give a supplementary dose of 150 mg to a patient who received the daily dose within 6 hours of a dialysis session. ▪ No dose adjustment indicated based on age, gender, or impaired hepatic function. ▪ Dosing should be cautious in the elderly, and reduced doses may be indicated based on potential for decreased organ function.

DILUTION

Reconstitute each 1 Gm of ertapenem with 10 mL SW, NS, BWFI. Shake well to dissolve.

Adults and pediatric patients 13 years of age and older: Further dilute in 50 mL of NS.

Pediatric patients 3 months to 12 years of age: Withdraw the volume equal to the 15 mg/kg dose and dilute in NS to a final concentration of 20 mg/mL or less.

Storage: Store unopened vials at or below 25° C (77° F). Use reconstituted and diluted solution within 6 hours when stored at RT. May refrigerate for up to 24 hours and use within 4 hours after removal. Do not freeze.

COMPATIBILITY

Consider any drug NOT listed as compatible to be INCOMPATIBLE until consulting a pharmacist; specific conditions may apply.

Manufacturer states, "Do not mix or co-infuse ertapenem with other medications. Do not use diluents containing dextrose."

One source suggests the following **compatibilities:**

Y-site: Heparin, hetastarch in NS (Hespan), potassium chloride (KCl), tigecycline (Tygacil).

RATE OF ADMINISTRATION

A single dose as an infusion equally distributed over 30 minutes.

ACTIONS

A unique, synthetic 1-beta-methyl-carbapenem structurally related to beta-lactam antibiotics. Effective against gram-positive and gram-negative aerobic and anaerobic bacteria. May effectively replace some combination therapies. Does not cover *Pseudomonas* and *Acinetobacter* species. Bactericidal activity results from inhibition of bacterial cell wall synthesis. Stable against hydrolysis by a variety of beta-lactamases, including penicillinases, cephalosporinases, and extended spectrum beta-lactamases. Hydrolyzed by metallo-beta-lactamases. Widely distributed throughout the body into many body tissues and fluids. Highly protein bound. Average half-life is 4 hours. Primarily excreted in urine (some as unchanged drug). Some excretion in feces. May cross the placental barrier. Secreted in breast milk.

INDICATIONS AND USES

Treatment of moderate to severe infections caused by susceptible strains of microorganisms in conditions that include complicated intra-abdominal infections; complicated skin and skin structure infections, including diabetic foot infections **without** osteomyelitis; community-acquired pneumonia; complicated urinary tract infections, including pyelonephritis; and acute pelvic infections, including postpartum endomyometritis, septic abortion, and post-surgical gynecologic infections. ▪ Prophylaxis of surgical site infections following elective colorectal surgery. ▪ Not recommended for use in the treatment of meningitis in pediatric patients (lack of sufficient CSF penetration).

CONTRAINDICATIONS

Known hypersensitivity to any component of ertapenem or other drugs in the same class (e.g., imipenem-cilastatin), or in patients who have had anaphylactic reactions to beta-lactams (e.g., penicillins and cephalosporins); see Precautions. ▪ The IM preparation is reconstituted with 1% lidocaine and is contraindicated for IV use and in patients with a known hypersensitivity to amide-type local anesthetics.

PRECAUTIONS

Confirm proper dilution for IV use; see Contraindications. ▪ To reduce the development of drug-resistant bacteria and maintain its effectiveness, ertapenem should be used to treat or prevent only those infections proven or strongly suspected to be caused by bacteria. ▪ Culture and sensitivity studies indicated to determine susceptibility of the causative organism to ertapenem. ▪ Serious and occasionally fatal hypersensitivity reactions have been reported in patients receiving therapy with beta-lactams. More likely in patients with a history of sensitivity to multiple allergens; obtain a careful history and watch for early symptoms of hypersensitivity reactions. Emergency equipment must be readily available; cross-sensitivity is possible. ▪ Prolonged use may cause superinfection because of overgrowth of nonsusceptible organisms. ▪ CNS stimulation and seizures have been reported. Use with caution in patients with CNS disorders (e.g., brain lesions or history of seizures) and/or compromised renal function. ▪ *Clostridium difficile*–associated diarrhea (CDAD) has been reported. May range from mild diarrhea to fatal colitis. Consider in patients who present with diarrhea during or after treatment with ertapenem. ▪ See Monitor and Drug/Lab Interactions.

Monitor: Monitor closely for S/S of hypersensitivity reactions (e.g., difficulty breathing, itching, rash, swelling of eyelids, lips, or face). ▪ Obtain baseline CBC with differential and platelets, and baseline kidney and liver studies (e.g., CrCl, serum creatinine, ALT, AST, serum bilirubin). Monitor periodically during prolonged therapy. ▪ Monitor patients who are at risk for CNS stimulation or are receiving anticonvulsant therapy for focal tremors, myoclonus, or seizures. If these symptoms occur, neurologic evaluation is indicated and dose reduction or discontinuation of ertapenem may be indicated. ▪ Monitor IV site carefully and rotate as indicated. ▪ See Precautions.

Patient Education: Report promptly: fever, rash, sore throat, unusual bleeding or bruising, severe stomach cramps and/or seizures, and pain or discomfort at the injection site. ▪ Promptly report diarrhea or bloody stools that occur during treatment or up to several months after an antibiotic has been discontinued; may indicate CDAD and require treatment. ▪ Patients with a history of seizures should review medication profile with physician before taking ertapenem; see Drug/Lab Interactions.

Maternal/Child: Category B: use during pregnancy only if clearly needed. ▪ Safety for use during breast-feeding not established; is found in breast milk. Benefits must outweigh risks to infant (e.g., diarrhea, candidiasis, or allergic response). Undetectable in breast milk 5 days after ertapenem is discontinued. ▪ Following a 1-Gm daily IV dose, plasma concentrations and half-life of ertapenem in pediatric patients 13 to 17 years of age are comparable to those in adults. ■ Compared to plasma clearance in adults, plasma clearance (mL/min/kg) in pediatric patients 3 months to 12 years of age is approximately two-fold higher. 30 mg/kg/24 hr (15 mg/kg every 12 hours) is comparable to a 1-Gm dose daily in adults. Half-life in pediatric patients 3 months to 12 years of age is 2.5 hours compared to 4 hours for adults and pediatric patients 13 years of age or older. ■ Not recommended for use in infants under 3 months; no data available.

Elderly: Dosing should be cautious in the elderly; see Dose Adjustments. ■ Response similar to that seen in younger patients, but may be more sensitive to side effects. ■ Monitoring of renal function may be indicated.

DRUG/LAB INTERACTIONS
Carbapenems may reduce serum **valproic acid** concentrations to subtherapeutic levels, resulting in a loss of seizure control. Monitor valproic acid levels. Consider alternative antibacterial therapy. If administration of ertapenem is necessary, supplemental anticonvulsant therapy should be considered. ■ **Probenicid** reduces the renal clearance of ertapenem, but this is not clinically significant. ■ Probably does not inhibit the action of **digoxin or vinblastine.** ■ Probably does not inhibit metabolism mediated by most of the cytochrome P_{450} isoenzyme system. ■ No other drug interaction studies have been conducted.

SIDE EFFECTS
Adults: CDAD, diarrhea, headache, pain at the injection site, nausea, phlebitis/thrombophlebitis, vaginitis in females and vomiting were most common and described as mild to moderate. The most commonly reported laboratory abnormalities were elevated ALT, AST, and alkaline phosphatase; increased platelets and eosinophils; and decreased neutrophils. Numerous other side effects occurred in less than 1% of patients.
Pediatric patients: Side effects similar to adults. CDAD, diarrhea, infusion site pain, erythema, and vomiting were most common.
Major: CDAD, CNS stimulation (e.g., anxiety, confusion, depression, insomnia, nightmares, paranoia, restlessness, seizures, tremor), hypersensitivity reactions (e.g., anaphylaxis, cardiovascular collapse, death, dyspnea, edema [facial, laryngeal, or pharyngeal], hypotension, itching, shock, urticaria), and pseudomembranous colitis.
Post-Marketing: Altered mental status (including aggression, delirium, and hallucinations), anaphylaxis, drug rash with eosinophilia and systemic symptoms (DRESS syndrome), dyskinesia, myoclonus, tremor.

ANTIDOTE
Keep physician informed of all side effects. Most minor side effects will be treated symptomatically. Discontinue ertapenem at the first sign of hypersensitivity (e.g., skin rash). Treat hypersensitivity reactions as indicated; may require epinephrine, airway management, oxygen, IV fluids, antihistamines (e.g., diphenhydramine [Benadryl]), corticosteroids (e.g., hydrocortisone sodium succinate [Solu-Cortef]), and pressor amines (e.g., dopamine). Treat CNS symptoms as indicated; may require dose reduction and/or anticonvulsants (e.g., phenytoin [Dilantin], diazepam [Valium]) for seizures. Mild cases of CDAD may respond to discontinuation of the drug. Treat CDAD with fluids, electrolytes, protein supplements, and oral vancomycin (Vancocin) or metronidazole (Flagyl) as indicated. In severe cases, surgical evaluation may be indicated. Ertapenem is partially removed by hemodialysis.

ERYTHROMYCIN LACTOBIONATE
(eh-**rih**-throw-**MY**-sin **LAK**-to-**bye**-oh-nayt)

Erythrocin

Antibacterial
(macrolide)

pH 6.5 to 7.7

USUAL DOSE

Antibacterial: 15 to 20 mg/kg of body weight/24 hr in equally divided doses every 6 hours (3.75 to 5 mg/kg every 6 hours). Range is 350 to 500 mg every 6 hours. Continuous infusion over 24 hours is preferred. Up to 4 Gm/24 hr has been given. See Elderly.

Legionnaires' disease: 1 Gm every 6 hours as an intermittent infusion.

Pelvic inflammatory disease: 500 mg every 6 hours as a continuous infusion for 3 days. Follow with oral erythromycin 250 mg every 6 hours for 7 days.

Diabetic gastroparesis (unlabeled): 200 mg immediately before each meal. When practical, continue treatment with oral erythromycin 3 times daily, 30 minutes before meals, for 4 weeks.

PEDIATRIC DOSE

15 to 20 mg/kg of body weight/24 hr in equally divided doses every 6 hours is recommended (3.75 to 5 mg/kg every 6 hours). Another source recommends 20 to 50 mg/kg/24 hr in equally divided doses every 6 hours (5 to 12.5 mg/kg every 6 hours). See Maternal/Child.

DOSE ADJUSTMENTS

Reduced dose may be required in impaired liver function.

DILUTION

Each 500 mg or fraction thereof must be reconstituted with 10 mL of SW without preservatives to avoid precipitation. Forms a 5% solution. Shake well to ensure dilution.

Continuous infusion (preferred): Further dilute to a 1 mg/mL solution (e.g., each 1 Gm in 1,000 mL of NS, Normosol, or LR). If a dextrose solution is used, add sodium bicarbonate (Neut) 1 mL for each 100 mL of solution.

Intermittent infusion: Dilute to a final concentration of 1 to 5 mg/mL. No less than 100 mL of IV diluent should be used (1 Gm in 1,000 mL equals 1 mg/mL; 1 Gm in 200 mL equals 5 mg/mL). Available in ADD-Vantage vials for use with ADD-Vantage infusion containers.

Storage: Store unopened vials at CRT. Reconstituted solution stable for 14 days if refrigerated or for 24 hours at room temperature. Diluted and/or buffered solution stable for 8 hours at CRT or 24 hours if refrigerated.

COMPATIBILITY   (Underline Indicates Conflicting Compatibility Information)

Consider any drug NOT listed as compatible to be INCOMPATIBLE until consulting a pharmacist; specific conditions may apply.

One source suggests the following **compatibilities:**

Additive: Aminophylline, ampicillin, ascorbic acid, diphenhydramine (Benadryl), hydrocortisone sodium succinate (Solu-Cortef), lidocaine, penicillin G potassium and sodium, pentobarbital (Nembutal), potassium chloride (KCl), prochlorperazine (Compazine), ranitidine (Zantac), sodium bicarbonate, verapamil.

Y-site: Acyclovir (Zovirax), amiodarone (Nexterone), anidulafungin (Eraxis), bivalirudin (Angiomax), cyclophosphamide (Cytoxan), dexmedetomidine (Precedex), diltiazem (Cardizem), doxapram (Dopram), enalaprilat

(Vasotec IV), esmolol (Brevibloc), famotidine (Pepcid IV), fenoldopam (Corlopam), foscarnet (Foscavir), heparin, hetastarch in electrolytes (Hextend), hydromorphone (Dilaudid), idarubicin (Idamycin), labetalol (Trandate), lorazepam (Ativan), magnesium sulfate, meperidine (Demerol), midazolam (Versed), morphine, multivitamins (M.V.I.), nicardipine (Cardene IV), tacrolimus (Prograf), theophylline, zidovudine (AZT, Retrovir).

RATE OF ADMINISTRATION

Administer with a volume control set. A slow infusion rate is recommended to reduce pain along the injection site.

Continuous infusion (preferred): A 0.1% to 0.2% solution equally distributed over 6 to 24 hours.

Intermittent infusion: 1 Gm or fraction thereof in at least 100 mL over 20 to 60 minutes.

Diabetic gastroparesis (unlabeled): 1 to 3 mg/kg/hr, usually approximately over 15 minutes.

ACTIONS

Macrolide antibiotic, bactericidal and bacteriostatic, used as a substitute for penicillin or tetracyclines. Effective against a number of gram-positive and some gram-negative organisms as well as *Chlamydia trachomatis*, mycoplasmas, and spirochetes. Inhibits protein synthesis by binding to ribosomal subunits of susceptible organisms. Diffuses readily into most bodily fluids. Metabolized by the liver and excreted in urine and bile. Crosses placental barrier. Secreted in breast milk.

INDICATIONS AND USES

Treatment of mild to moderate infections of the upper and lower respiratory tract, skin and skin structures, and gynecologic infections caused by susceptible organisms. ■ Alternative treatment in several sexually transmitted diseases in females with a history of penicillin sensitivity. ■ Legionnaires' disease. ■ Additional indications listed for oral formulation. **Unlabeled uses:** Diabetic gastroparesis.

CONTRAINDICATIONS

Known erythromycin sensitivity. See Drug/Lab Interactions. ■ Coadministration with ritonavir (Norvir) and cisapride is contraindicated. Contraindicated with astemizole and terfenadine (both have been removed from the market).

PRECAUTIONS

Sensitivity studies indicated to determine susceptibility of the causative organism to erythromycin. ■ To reduce the development of drug-resistant bacteria and maintain its effectiveness, erythromycin should be used to treat or prevent only those infections proven or strongly suspected to be caused by bacteria. ■ Begin oral therapy as soon as practical. ■ Superinfection caused by overgrowth of nonsusceptible organisms is rare unless this drug is given in combination with other antibacterial agents. ■ Use caution in impaired liver function; hepatic dysfunction, with or without jaundice, has been reported. ■ Use caution in patients with a history of cardiac disease (may induce torsades de pointes). ■ Use caution in patients with myasthenia gravis; weakness may be aggravated. ■ *Clostridium difficile*–associated diarrhea (CDAD) has been reported. May range from mild diarrhea to fatal colitis. Consider in patients who present with diarrhea during or after treatment with erythromycin.

Monitor: Monitor vital signs. ■ Monitor IV site for redness and inflammation. ■ See Drug/Lab Interactions.

Patient Education: Promptly report diarrhea or bloody stools that occur during treatment or up to several months after an antibiotic has been discontinued; may indicate CDAD and require treatment.

Maternal/Child: Category B: use only if clearly needed. ■ Considered safe for use in breast-feeding; use caution. ■ Some products contain benzyl alcohol; not recommended for use in neonates.

Elderly: When doses of 4 Gm/day or higher are used, the risk of developing erythromycin-induced hearing loss is increased in elderly patients, particularly those with impaired renal or hepatic function. ■ May be more susceptible to development of torsades de pointes. ■ May experience increased effects of oral anticoagulation; see Drug/Lab Interactions.

DRUG/LAB INTERACTIONS

Contraindicated with **ritonavir.** ■ Antibacterial activity is antagonized by coadministration of **clindamycin, lincomycin, and chloramphenicol.** ■ May inhibit **penicillins.** ■ Will increase serum levels and potentiate the effects of **alfentanil, anticoagulants** (e.g., warfarin [Coumadin]), **astemizole** (see Contraindications), **bromocriptine** (Parlodel), **carbamazepine** (Tegretol), **cisapride** (Propulsid), **cyclosporine** (Sandimmune), **digoxin, disopyramide** (Norpace), **ergot alkaloids** (e.g., Hydergine), **itraconazole** (Sporanox), **lovastatin** (Mevacor), **methylprednisolone, midazolam** (Versed), **phenytoin** (Dilantin), **terfenadine** (see Contraindications), **theophyllines, triazolam** (Halcion), **and valproate;** serious toxicity may result. ■ Concomitant administration with **cisapride** is contraindicated. May cause serious cardiotoxicity. ■ Severe **vinblastine** toxicity has been reported in conjunction with erythromycin. ■ May increase serum levels of **sildenafil** (Viagra). ■ Coadministration with **HMG-CoA reductase inhibitors** (e.g., simvastatin [Zocor]) results in increased serum levels of the antihyperlipidemic agent and increases the risk of severe myopathy and rhabdomyolysis. ■ Concurrent use with **theophylline** (aminophylline) may decrease plasma levels of erythromycin. ■ Serotonin syndrome has been reported with coadministration of erythromycin and **serotonin-uptake inhibitors** (e.g., sertraline [Zoloft], fluoxetine [Prozac]). ■ May interfere with fluorometric determination of **urinary catecholamines.**

SIDE EFFECTS

Relatively free from side effects when given as directed. Nausea and vomiting, urticaria, and mild local venous discomfort. Increased incidence of usually reversible ototoxicity with larger doses. CDAD has been reported. Torsades de pointes has been reported; see Elderly. Anaphylaxis may occur.

ANTIDOTE

Notify the physician of early or mild symptoms. For severe symptoms, discontinue the drug, treat hypersensitivity reactions, or resuscitate as necessary and notify physician. Treat CDAD with fluids, electrolytes, protein supplements, and oral vancomycin (Vancocin) or metronidazole (Flagyl) as indicated. In severe cases, surgical evaluation may be indicated. Not removed by peritoneal dialysis or hemodialysis.

ESMOLOL HYDROCHLORIDE
(**EZ**-moh-lohl hy-droh-**KLOR**-eyed)

Beta-adrenergic blocking agent
Antiarrhythmic

Brevibloc

pH 4.5 to 5.5

USUAL DOSE

Supraventricular tachycardia (SVT): 100 mcg/kg (0.1 mg/kg) of body weight/min is an average dose. Range is 50 to 200 mcg/kg/min (0.05 to 0.2 mg/kg/min). Dosage must be individualized by titration. Each step in the process consists of a loading dose followed by a maintenance dose. Begin with a *loading dose* of 500 mcg/kg/min (0.5 mg/kg/min) for 1 minute only. Follow with a *maintenance infusion* of 50 mcg/kg/min (0.05 mg/kg/min) for 4 minutes. If desired therapeutic effect has not occurred, repeat the loading dose and increase the maintenance infusion to 100 mcg/kg/min (0.1 mg/kg/min). Continue this two-step process by repeating the same loading dose while increasing the maintenance infusion by 50 mcg/kg/min (0.05 mg/kg/min). As the desired HR is approached or a safety endpoint (decreasing BP) occurs, omit the loading dose and titrate the maintenance dose up or down in 25- to 50-mcg/kg/min (0.025 to 0.05 mg/kg/min) increments to desired HR. Interval between titration steps may be increased from 5 to 10 minutes if desired. Hypotension is common and is dose related. Doses greater than 200 mcg/kg/min (0.2 mg/kg/min) are not recommended. AHA guidelines recommend a loading dose of 0.5 mg/kg over 1 minute followed by a maintenance infusion at 0.05 mg/kg/min to a maximum rate of 0.3 mg/kg/min. Titrate to effect. If response is not adequate, repeat 0.5 mg/kg bolus. Titrate infusion up to 200 mcg/kg/min (0.2 mg/kg/min); AHA states, "Higher doses unlikely to be beneficial." May be used for up to 48 hours as needed; see Precautions/Monitor.

Intraoperative and postoperative tachycardia and/or hypertension: For immediate control 80 mg (approximately 1 mg/kg) over 30 seconds. Follow with an infusion of 150 mcg/kg/minute (0.15 mg/kg/min) if necessary. Adjust as required up to 300 mcg/kg/min (0.3 mg/kg/min) to maintain desired HR and/or BP. For gradual control, use procedure listed for SVT. Higher doses (250 to 300 mcg/kg/min [0.25 to 0.3 mg/kg/min]) may be required to control BP. Another source recommends 250 to 500 mcg (0.25 to 0.5 mg) over 1 minute as a loading dose, followed with a maintenance dose of 50 mcg/kg/min (0.05 mg/kg/min) for 4 minutes. Repeat loading dose and increase maintenance dose by 50 mcg/kg/min (0.05 mg/kg/min).

PEDIATRIC DOSE

See Maternal/Child.

Antiarrhythmic (unlabeled): 50 mcg/kg/min (0.05 mg/kg/min), titrate every 10 minutes in 25- to 50-mcg/kg/min (0.025 to 0.05 mg/kg/min) increments up to 300 mcg/kg/min (0.3 mg/kg/min).

Antihypertensive (perioperative [unlabeled]): A loading dose of 100 to 500 mcg/kg (0.1 to 0.5 mg/kg) administered over 1 minute. Follow with a maintenance infusion of 25 to 100 mcg/kg/min (0.025 to 0.1 mg/kg/min). If inadequate response, repeat loading dose and/or increase maintenance dose in 25- to 50-mcg/kg/min (0.025 to 0.05 mg/kg/min) increments every 5 to 10 minutes. Titrate to individual desired response. Usual range may be from 50 to 500 mcg/kg/min (0.05 to 0.5 mg/kg/min).

DOSE ADJUSTMENTS
Reduced dose may be required in impaired renal function. ■ Reduction required with transfer to alternate agent; see Monitor. ■ See Drug/Lab Interactions.

DILUTION
Available premixed as 10 mg/mL in 100 mL NS or as 20 mg/mL in 100 mL NS (double strength). Single-dose vials are available as 100 mg/10 mL or 100 mg/5 mL (double strength) and may be given by IV injection without further dilution or may be further diluted in D5W, D5R, D5LR, D5NS, D5/½NS, NS, LR, or ½NS. Premixed solutions have a delivery port and a medication port (for withdrawing the initial bolus only). Subsequent boluses must be administered using the ready-to-use vials. **Storage:** Store vials and premix at CRT; diluted solution stable at room temperature for 24 hours.

COMPATIBILITY
Consider any drug NOT listed as compatible to be INCOMPATIBLE until consulting a pharmacist; specific conditions may apply.
Manufacturer lists as **incompatible** with sodium bicarbonate and states, "Should not be admixed with other drugs prior to dilution in suitable IV fluid, and do not introduce additives to Brevibloc premixed injection."
   One source suggests the following **compatibilities:**
Solution: D5W with 40 mEq KCl; see Dilution.
Additive: *Not recommended by manufacturer.* Aminophylline, atracurium (Tracrium), heparin.
Y-site: Amikacin (Amikin), aminophylline, amiodarone (Nexterone), ampicillin, atracurium (Tracrium), bivalirudin (Angiomax), butorphanol (Stadol), calcium chloride, cefazolin (Ancef), ceftazidime (Fortaz), chloramphenicol (Chloromycetin), cisatracurium (Nimbex), clindamycin (Cleocin), dexmedetomidine (Precedex), diltiazem (Cardizem), dopamine, doripenem (Doribax), enalaprilat (Vasotec IV), erythromycin (Erythrocin), famotidine (Pepcid IV), fenoldopam (Corlopam), fentanyl (Sublimaze), gentamicin, heparin, hetastarch in electrolytes (Hextend), hydrocortisone sodium succinate (Solu-Cortef), insulin (regular), labetalol (Trandate), linezolid (Zyvox), magnesium sulfate, methyldopa, metronidazole (Flagyl IV), micafungin (Mycamine), midazolam (Versed), morphine, nafcillin (Nallpen), nicardipine (Cardene IV), nitroglycerin IV, nitroprusside sodium, norepinephrine (Levophed), pancuronium, penicillin G potassium, phenytoin (Dilantin), piperacillin, potassium chloride (KCl), potassium phosphate, propofol (Diprivan), ranitidine (Zantac), remifentanil (Ultiva), sodium acetate, streptomycin, sulfamethoxazole/trimethoprim, tacrolimus (Prograf), tobramycin, vancomycin, vecuronium.

RATE OF ADMINISTRATION
IV injection: See Usual Dose.
Infusion: Titrate infusion according to procedure outlined in Usual Dose.

ACTIONS
A short-acting, B_1-selective adrenergic blocking agent with antiarrhythmic effects. Decreases HR and BP in a dose-related titratable manner. Hemodynamically similar to propranolol, but vascular resistance is not increased. Onset of action occurs within 1 to 2 minutes. Half-life is approx-

imately 9 minutes, and the effects last about 20 to 30 minutes. Metabolized via esterases in RBCs and excreted in urine.

INDICATIONS AND USES

Management of supraventricular tachycardia (atrial fibrillation or atrial flutter) in situations requiring short-term control of ventricular rate with a short-acting agent (perioperative, postoperative, or other emergent circumstances). ▪ Management of noncompensatory tachycardia when HR requires specific intervention. ▪ Management of intraoperative and postoperative tachycardia and/or hypertension.

Unlabeled uses: Has been used in the perioperative period to reduce cardiac morbidity and mortality in patients at risk.

CONTRAINDICATIONS

Not intended for use in chronic settings when transfer to another agent is anticipated. ▪ Do not use concurrently with epinephrine. ▪ Bradycardia, cardiogenic shock, congestive heart failure not secondary to a tachycardia responsive to beta-adrenergic blockers, overt cardiac failure, second- or third-degree heart block.

PRECAUTIONS

For IV use only. ▪ Use with extreme caution in patients with asthma, diabetes, impaired renal function, or a history of hypoglycemia. ▪ May cause hypotension at any dose; however, risk is increased with doses above 200 mcg/kg/min. ▪ May further depress cardiac contractility and precipitate heart failure. ▪ Use caution when treating patients with supraventricular arrhythmias who are hemodynamically compromised or are taking other drugs that decrease any or all of the following: peripheral resistance, myocardial filling, myocardial contractility, or electrical impulse propagation in the myocardium. Deaths have occurred. ▪ Although it has not been a problem with esmolol, it is recommended that the dose of beta-adrenergic blockers be reduced gradually to avoid rebound angina, MI, or ventricular arrhythmias. Use caution, especially in patients with coronary artery disease. See Drug/Lab Interactions.

Monitor: Continuous observation of the patient and ECG and BP monitoring are mandatory during administration. Hypotension should reverse within 30 minutes after decreasing the infusion rate or discontinuing the drug. ▪ Well tolerated if administered through a central vein. Incidence of infusion site inflammation. Incidence of inflammation or thrombophlebitis increases with dilutions greater than 10 mg/mL. ▪ Intended for short-term use only. Transfer to an alternative antiarrhythmic agent (e.g., propranolol, digoxin [Lanoxin], verapamil) is required after stable clinical status and HR control are obtained. Thirty minutes after first dose of alternative agent, reduce dose of esmolol by 50%. Monitor patient carefully. One hour after the second dose of alternative agent, discontinue esmolol infusion if condition remains satisfactory. ▪ May cause hypoglycemia and mask the symptoms. ▪ See Drug/Lab Interactions and Contraindications.

Maternal/Child: Category C: safety for use in pregnancy and breast-feeding not established. Use only when clearly indicated. Has caused fetal problems during delivery. ▪ Safety for use in pediatric patients not established.

Elderly: Potential risk of increased cardiac depression; monitor and reduce dose if indicated.

DRUG/LAB INTERACTIONS

Epinephrine concurrently is contraindicated. ▪ Use with **calcium channel blockers** (e.g., diltiazem [Cardizem], verapamil) may potentiate both drugs and result in severe depression of myocardium and AV conduction and severe hypotension. ▪ Increases **digoxin** blood levels, synergistic with digoxin; both drugs slow AV conduction. ▪ **IV morphine** increases esmolol steady-state levels by 50%. ▪ Esmolol should not be used in patients receiving **vasoconstrictive or inotropic drugs** (e.g., dopamine, epinephrine, norepinephrine [Levophed], digoxin) because of the potential for blocked cardiac contractility when the supraventricular rate is high. ▪ Concomitant use with **catecholamine-depleting drugs** (e.g., reserpine [Serpasil]) may produce additive effects. Monitor for hypotension and bradycardia. ▪ May prolong neuromuscular blockade produced by **succinylcholine.** ▪ **Warfarin** (Coumadin) may increase esmolol concentrations. Warfarin is not affected. ▪ May mask S/S of developing hypoglycemia in patients on **insulin or oral antidiabetic agents.** ▪ Concurrent use with **xanthines** (e.g., aminophylline, theophyllines) may result in mutual inhibition of therapeutic effect. ▪ Patients taking **beta-blockers** who are exposed to a potential allergen may be unresponsive to the usual dose of epinephrine used to treat a hypersensitivity reaction. ▪ See Contraindications.

SIDE EFFECTS

Hypotension and inflammation or induration of the infusion site are the major side effects. Asthenia, bronchospasm, congestive heart failure, confusion, fever, flushing, light-headedness, midscapular pain, nausea and vomiting, pallor, paresthesia, rhonchi, somnolence, speech disorders, taste disorders, and urinary retention have occurred. One grand mal seizure has been reported.

ANTIDOTE

Notify the physician of all side effects. Decrease rate or discontinue drug if hypotension occurs, and notify physician immediately. Hypotension should reverse within 30 minutes. Trendelenburg position may be appropriate. May require treatment with IV fluids or vasopressors (e.g., dobutamine, dopamine), but protracted severe hypotension may result. Unresponsive hypotension and bradycardia may be reversed by glucagon 5 to 10 mg over 30 seconds followed by a continuous infusion of 5 mg/hr. Reduce rate as condition improves. Use atropine for bradycardia, digoxin and diuretics for cardiac failure, and a beta$_2$-stimulating agent (e.g., epinephrine, albuterol) and/or a theophylline derivative for bronchospasm. Treat other side effects symptomatically and resuscitate as necessary.

ESOMEPRAZOLE SODIUM
(es-oh-**MEP**-rah-zohl **SO**-dee-um)

Nexium IV

Proton pump inhibitor
(Gastric acid inhibitor)

pH 9 to 11

USUAL DOSE
Given as an alternative to oral therapy. Resume oral therapy as soon as practical. Safety and efficacy of IV use for more than 10 days not established. Dose and serum levels similar by IV or oral route.
Adults: 20 or 40 mg as an IV injection or infusion once daily for up to 10 days.

PEDIATRIC DOSE
Administered as an infusion over 10 to 30 minutes. See comments under Usual Dose.
1 to 17 years of age: *Weight less than 55 kg:* 10 mg. *Weight 55 kg or more:* 20 mg.
1 month to less than 1 year of age: 0.5 mg/kg.

DOSE ADJUSTMENTS
No dose adjustment is required based on age or gender, in the elderly, in patients with renal insufficiency, or in patients with mild to moderate liver impairment (Child-Pugh classes A and B). ▪ Do not exceed a dose of 20 mg in patients with severe liver impairment (Child-Pugh class C [10 or over]).

DILUTION
Injection (adults): Each 20- or 40-mg dose must be reconstituted with 5 mL of NS. A single dose equals 5 mL. Mix gently until powder is dissolved.
Infusion (adults): Each 20- or 40-mg dose must be reconstituted with 5 mL of NS, LR, or D5W. A single dose equals 5 mL. Further dilute for infusion with NS, LR, or D5W to a final volume of 50 mL.
Infusion (pediatric patients 1 month to less than 1 year of age): Reconstitute a 20- or 40-mg vial with 5 mL of NS. Further dilute to a final volume of 50 mL with NS, LR, or D5W. Concentration of 20-mg vial equals 0.4 mg/mL; concentration of 40-mg vial equals 0.8 mg/mL. Withdraw desired dose (0.5 mg/kg) to administer as an infusion.
Infusion (pediatric patients 1 to 17 years of age): Reconstitute and further dilute as above. *40-mg vial:* Concentration is 0.8 mg/mL. For a 20-mg dose, withdraw 25 mL (for a 10-mg dose, withdraw 12.5 mL). *20-mg vial:* Concentration is 0.4 mg/mL. For a 20-mg dose, administer 50 mL as an infusion. For a 10-mg dose, withdraw 25 mL and administer as an infusion.
Filters: Not required or recommended; no additional data available from manufacturer.
Storage: Before use, store in carton at CRT and protect from light. Reconstituted and diluted solutions may be stored at CRT. Administer reconstituted solutions within 12 hours of reconstitution. Administer diluted solutions within 6 hours if diluted in D5W and within 12 hours if diluted in NS or LR.

COMPATIBILITY
Consider any drug NOT listed as compatible to be INCOMPATIBLE until consulting a pharmacist; specific conditions may apply.
Manufacturer states, "Should not be administered concomitantly with any other medications through the same IV site and/or tubing." Flush the IV line with a **compatible** IV solution (NS, LR, or D5W) before and after administration of esomeprazole.

One source suggests the following **compatibilities** *(not recommended by manufacturer):*
Y-site: Doripenem (Doribax).

RATE OF ADMINISTRATION
Flush the IV line with a **compatible** IV solution (NS, LR, or D5W) before and after administration of esomeprazole.

Injection (adults): A single 20- or 40-mg dose evenly distributed over no less than 3 minutes.

Infusion (adults and pediatric patients): A single dose properly diluted as an infusion and evenly distributed over 10 to 30 minutes.

ACTIONS
A proton pump inhibitor. It suppresses gastric acid secretion by specific inhibition of the H^+/K^+-ATPase in the gastric parietal cell. It blocks the final step in acid production, thus reducing gastric acidity. Effect is dose-related. Highly bound by serum protein. Extensively metabolized in the liver by the cytochrome P_{450} isoenzyme system (CYP2C19 and CYP3A4 isozymes). Half-life is 1.1 to 1.4 hours and is prolonged with increasing doses. Primarily excreted as metabolites in urine with some excretion in feces. Secreted in breast milk.

INDICATIONS AND USES
Short-term treatment of GERD with erosive esophagitis in adults and pediatric patients 1 month to 17 years of age. Used as an alternative to oral therapy when oral esomeprazole is not possible or appropriate. Safety and effectiveness for use in the initial treatment of erosive esophagitis has not been demonstrated.

CONTRAINDICATIONS
Known hypersensitivity to esomeprazole or its components (edetate disodium, sodium hydroxide) or to substituted benzimidazoles (e.g., lansoprazole [Prevacid], pantoprazole [Protonix]).

PRECAUTIONS
For IV use only; do not give IM or SC. ■ Gastric malignancy may be present even though patient's symptoms improve. ■ Discontinue as soon as the patient is able to resume oral therapy. ■ Decreased gastric acidity may increase bacterial count in GI tract. Risk of GI infections (e.g., *Campylobacter, Clostridium difficile, Salmonella*) in hospitalized patients may be slightly increased. ■ May be associated with an increased risk for osteoporosis-related fractures of the hip, wrist, or spine. Risk increased in patients receiving high-dose (multiple daily doses) and long-term therapy (a year or longer). Use lowest dose and shortest duration of therapy appropriate for the condition being treated.
Monitor: Observe for S/S of allergic reaction; anaphylaxis has been reported in post-marketing reports. ■ Monitor vital signs, pain levels, and injection site.

Patient Education: Review prescription and non-prescription drugs with physician. ▪ Oral route preferred.

Maternal/Child: Category B: use during pregnancy only if clearly needed. Animal studies did not show harm to the fetus. ▪ If the drug is indicated for the mother, breast-feeding should be discontinued. May have serious reactions in the infant and has a potential for tumorigenicity. ▪ Safety and effectiveness for use of IV formulation in pediatric patients established for ages 1 month to 17 years.

Elderly: Safety and effectiveness similar to that seen in younger adults. ▪ Consider potential for impaired liver function; see Dose Adjustments.

DRUG/LAB INTERACTIONS

Because of profound and long-lasting inhibition of gastric acid secretion, esomeprazole may interfere with the absorption of drugs in which gastric pH is an important determinant of their bioavailability (e.g., **digoxin** [Lanoxin], **iron salts** [ferrous sulfate], **ketoconazole** [Nizoral]). ▪ Increases in INR and PT have been reported when administered concurrently with **warfarin;** monitoring of INR and PT indicated. ▪ Concurrent use with **selected protease inhibitors** such as atazanavir (Reyataz) and nelfinavir (Viracept) is not recommended. Coadministration of proton pump inhibitors (e.g., esomeprazole [Nexium], pantoprazole [Protonix]) results in a significant reduction in plasma concentrations of atazanavir and nelfinavir, thus inhibiting their therapeutic effect. In contrast, elevated plasma concentrations have been reported with **other protease inhibitors** (e.g., saquinavir [Invirase], ritonavir [Norvir]); monitoring of serum levels is recommended to avoid toxicity of the antiviral agent, and dose reduction should be considered. Unchanged serum levels have been reported with some other antiretroviral drugs. ▪ The metabolism of **diazepam** (Valium) may be decreased and serum levels increased by esomeprazole; not considered clinically significant. ▪ Administration with a **combined inhibitor of CYP2C19 and CYP3A4** (e.g., voriconazole [VFEND]) may more than double the exposure (concentration) of esomeprazole. With recommended doses of esomeprazole, a dose adjustment is not normally required; however, it may be indicated in patients who require higher doses. ▪ Concurrent administration of **oral contraceptives, diazepam, phenytoin, or quinidine** did not change the pharmacokinetic profile of esomeprazole. ▪ Concurrent administration with **naproxen** (Aleve) did not appear to alter pharmacokinetics in either drug. ▪ Studies suggest no clinically significant interactions with other drugs metabolized by the cytochrome P_{450} system (e.g., amoxicillin, clarithromycin [Biaxin], phenytoin [Dilantin], quinidine). ▪ Avoid concurrent use with **clopidogrel** (Plavix); esomeprazole may interfere with the conversion of clopidogrel into its active form and decrease its effectiveness. ▪ Coadministration with cilostazol (Pletal) may increase concentrations of cilostazol and its metabolite. Consider a dose reduction of cilostazol from 100 mg to 50 mg twice daily.

SIDE EFFECTS

Generally well tolerated. Most commonly reported side effects include abdominal pain, constipation, diarrhea, dizziness, dry mouth, dyspepsia, flatulence, headache, injection site pain or reaction, nausea, respiratory infection, and sinusitis. Numerous other side effects may occur in fewer than 1% of patients.

Post-Marketing: Agranulocytosis, alopecia, anaphylaxis (rare), blurred vision, bone fracture, depression, hypomagnesemia, myalgia, pancreatitis, pancytopenia, hepatitis with or without jaundice (rare), serious dermatologic reactions (including erythema multiforme, Stevens-Johnson syndrome, and toxic epidermal necrolysis [some fatal]), and shock.

Overdose: Ataxia, changes in respiratory frequency, decreased motor activity, intermittent clonic convulsions. Consider possibility of multiple drug ingestion.

ANTIDOTE
Keep physician informed of all side effects. May be treated symptomatically. Discontinue and initiate appropriate treatment if S/S associated with post-marketing reports or overdose occur; see Side Effects. Not removed by hemodialysis.

ETOMIDATE
(eh-**TOM**-ih-dayt)

Amidate

**Anesthetic, general
Anesthesia adjunct**

USUAL DOSE
Rapid sequence intubation and/or induction of anesthesia: Dose must be individualized. 0.3 mg/kg IV (range: 0.2 to 0.6 mg/kg). Titrate to effect. Smaller, incremental doses may be administered to adult patients during short operative procedures to supplement subpotent anesthetic agents, such as nitrous oxide.

Anesthesia induction for short outpatient or ER procedures (unlabeled): 0.1 mg/kg has been used effectively. If analgesia is required, concurrent administration of fentanyl (Sublimaze) may be used.

PEDIATRIC DOSE
Rapid sequence intubation and/or induction of anesthesia: *Pediatric patients up to 10 years of age:* Safety and effectiveness have not been established.
Pediatric patients 10 years of age and older: See Usual Dose.

Anesthesia induction for short outpatient or emergency department procedures (unlabeled): 0.1 mg/kg. 0.2 mg/kg has been used in pediatric patients for fractures or major joint reduction. If analgesia is required, concurrent administration of fentanyl (Sublimaze) may be used.

DOSE ADJUSTMENTS
Dose must be individualized for each patient. ▪ Caution and lower-end dosing suggested in the elderly; consider decreased organ function and concomitant disease or drug therapy. ▪ See Drug/Lab Interactions.

DILUTION
May be given undiluted. Solution must be clear.
Filters: No data available from manufacturer.
Storage: Store at CRT. Discard unused portion.

COMPATIBILITY
Consider any drug NOT listed as compatible to be INCOMPATIBLE until consulting a pharmacist; specific conditions may apply.
One source suggests the following **compatibilities:**
Y-site: Alfentanil (Alfenta), atracurium (Tracrium), atropine, ephedrine, fentanyl (Sublimaze), lidocaine, lorazepam (Ativan), midazolam (Versed),

morphine, pancuronium, phenylephrine (Neo-Synephrine), succinylcholine, sufentanil (Sufenta).

RATE OF ADMINISTRATION

A single dose equally distributed over 30 to 60 seconds. More rapid injections may produce hypotension.

ACTIONS

A short-acting, non-barbiturate hypnotic without analgesic activity. Depending on the dose administered, it can produce all levels of CNS depression, from light sleep to coma. Anesthetic doses can induce loss of consciousness within 60 seconds. Does not cause significant cardiovascular or respiratory depression. Incidence of respiratory depression may be less than with propofol (Diprivan) or barbiturates (e.g., thiopental [Pentothal]). Has little or no effect on myocardial metabolism, cardiac output, peripheral circulation, or pulmonary circulation. Produces a slight increase in $PaCO_2$. Does not elevate plasma histamine or cause signs of histamine release. Decreases cerebral blood flow and lowers intracranial pressure. Usually lowers intraocular pressure moderately. Onset of action is within 1 minute. Duration of action is dose dependent, usually 3 to 5 minutes at a dose of 0.3 mg/kg. Metabolized in the liver and excreted primarily in the urine. Half-life is approximately 75 minutes.

INDICATIONS AND USES

Induction of general anesthesia. Useful for short outpatient, dental, and short diagnostic procedures and in high-risk patients. Usefulness of its hemodynamic properties should be weighed against the high frequency of transient skeletal muscle movements. (May be beneficial in patients with cardiopulmonary impairment because of minimal depressant effects and lack of histamine release.) One source suggests it is the intubation agent of choice in trauma and CHF. ■ Supplementation of subpotent anesthetic agents (such as nitrous oxide in oxygen) during maintenance of anesthesia for short operative procedures such as dilation and curettage or cervical conization.

Unlabeled uses: Emergency department treatment of painful procedures such as abscess drainage, cardioversion, chest tube replacement, dislocation reduction, fracture reduction, foreign body removal.

CONTRAINDICATIONS

Hypersensitivity to etomidate. ■ Not recommended for use during labor and delivery.

PRECAUTIONS

For IV use only. ■ Should be administered by or under the direct supervision of persons trained in the administration of general anesthetics and in the management of complications encountered during general anesthesia (e.g., anesthesiologists, emergency department physicians) in a facility with adequate diagnostic and treatment facilities to monitor the patient and respond to any medical emergency. ■ Induction doses of etomidate have been associated with the reduction of plasma cortisol and aldosterone concentrations that may last for 6 to 8 hours. Because of the hazards of prolonged suppression, etomidate is not intended for administration by prolonged infusion. Exogenous replacement (e.g., methylprednisolone [Solu-Medrol]) should be considered if concern exists for patients undergoing severe stress or for patients undergoing chronic oral corticosteroid therapy (e.g., prednisone).

Monitor: Monitor airway and vital signs. ■ Monitor injection site. Use of larger, more proximal arm veins is recommended to lessen incidence and severity of pain on injection. Avoid use of wrist or hand veins if possible. ■ See Precautions and Drug/Lab Interactions.

Patient Education: Avoid alcohol or other CNS depressants (e.g., antihistamines, benzodiazepines) for 24 hours following administration. ■ Do not perform tasks requiring mental alertness (e.g., driving, operating hazardous machinery) for 24 hours following administration.

Maternal/Child: Category C: safety for use in pregnancy not established; benefit must justify potential risks to fetus; see Contraindications. ■ Safety for use during breast-feeding not established; effects unknown. Use caution. ■ Safety and effectiveness for use in pediatric patients under 10 years of age not established.

Elderly: See Dose Adjustments. ■ May be more sensitive to effects (e.g., decreases in heart rate, cardiac index, and mean arterial BP).

DRUG/LAB INTERACTIONS

Administration of **fentanyl** 0.1 mg before induction with etomidate may shorten immediate recovery period. ■ May have additive effects with concomitant **anesthetics, sedatives, hypnotics, and/or opiates** (e.g., fentanyl [Sublimaze]); reduced doses of etomidate may be indicated. ■ Does not significantly alter the usual dosage requirements of **neuromuscular blocking agents** (e.g., vecuronium, pancuronium). ■ Administration of **fentanyl or diazepam** before induction with etomidate may help decrease transient skeletal muscle movements. ■ Succinylcholine-induced arrhythmias may still occur if **succinylcholine** is used in combination with etomidate.

SIDE EFFECTS

The most common adverse reactions are transient venous pain on injection and transient skeletal muscle movements, including myoclonus, averting movements, and eye movements. Less frequently reported side effects include apnea of short duration (5 to 90 seconds with spontaneous recovery), arrhythmia, bradycardia, hypertension, hyperventilation, hypotension, hypoventilation, hiccups and/or snoring (may indicate partial airway obstruction), laryngospasm, postoperative nausea and vomiting, and tachycardia.

ANTIDOTE

Discontinue drug if significant side effects or overdose occur. Support patient. Establish and maintain an airway; administer oxygen with assisted ventilation if needed. Resuscitate as necessary.

ETOPOSIDE BBW
(eh-**TOH**-poh-syd)

Etopophos PF, Etoposide Phosphate, VePesid, VP-16-213

Antineoplastic
(mitotic inhibitor)

pH 2.9 to 4

USUAL DOSE
Testicular cancer: 50 to 100 mg/M^2 daily for 5 days or 100 mg/M^2/day on Days 1, 3, and 5. Repeat at 3- to 4-week intervals. Used in combination with other chemotherapy agents.

Small-cell lung cancer: 35 mg/M^2/day for 4 days to 50 mg/M^2/day for 5 days. Repeat at 3- to 4-week intervals. Used in combination with other chemotherapy agents.

Kaposi's sarcoma (unlabeled): 150 mg/M^2/day for 3 consecutive days every 4 weeks. Repeat cycles based on patient response.

Treatment of advanced malignancies in conjunction with autogenous bone marrow transplantation (unlabeled): High-dose regimens of 400 to 800 mg/M^2/day for 3 days have been given for one or two courses.

DOSE ADJUSTMENTS
Modify dose if indicated based on myelosuppressive effects of other drugs administered in combination and any previous radiation therapy or chemotherapy (compromised bone marrow reserve). Frequently given in combination with cisplatin, bleomycin, and doxorubicin. ■ Withhold dose if platelets less than 50,000/mm^3 or absolute neutrophil count less than 500/mm^3. Do not restart until adequate recovery. ■ Dose selection should be cautious in the elderly. Reduced doses may be indicated based on potential for decreased organ function and concomitant disease or drug therapy; see Elderly. ■ Reduce dose by 25% if CrCl is 15 to 50 mL/min. Further reduction may be indicated if the CrCl is less than 15 mL/min. One source recommends decreasing dose by 50% if CrCl is less than 10 mL/min. ■ Dose reduction may be required in impaired hepatic function. One source recommends a dose reduction of 50% with a bilirubin of 1.5 to 3 or an AST of 60 to 180 units and recommends omitting the dose in patients with a bilirubin of 3.1 or greater or an AST greater than 180 units.

DILUTION
Specific techniques required; see Precautions.
NONPHOSPHATE PRODUCTS (E.G., VEPESID): Each 100 mg (5 mL) must be diluted in at least 250 mL of D5W or NS and given as an infusion (0.4 mg/mL). 500 mL of solution will yield 0.2 mg/mL. Maximum concentration to prevent precipitation is 0.4 mg/mL. Monitor closely for precipitation from dilution to completion of infusion. One source suggests dilution with LR or 10% mannitol, but cautions that crystals may form. Discard crystallized solution. Undiluted etoposide has caused acrylic or ABS plastic devices to crack and leak; handle carefully during dilution process.

PHOSPHATE PRODUCT (E.G., ETOPOPHOS): Reconstitute each 100-mg vial with 5 or 10 mL of SW, D5W, or NS (with or without benzyl alcohol). 5 mL of diluent will yield 20 mg/mL, 10 mL will yield 10 mg/mL. Further dilute to concentrations as low as 0.1 mg/mL with D5W or NS for administration. A 1-mg/mL solution has a pH of 2.9. The water solubility of Etopophos decreases the potential for precipitation following dilution and during administration.

Storage: *Nonphosphate Products (e.g., VePesid):* May be stored at CRT before dilution. Stable after dilution at CRT for 96 hours (0.2 mg/mL solution) or 24 hours (0.4 mg/mL) in D5W or NS. Stability reduced to 8 hours in LR or 10% mannitol. ***Phosphate Products (e.g., Etopophos):*** Refrigerate in carton until use. Store reconstituted solutions in glass or plastic containers under refrigeration at 2° to 8° C (36° to 46° F) for 7 days. Solutions reconstituted with non-bacteriostatic diluents may be stored at CRT for up to 24 hours. Solutions reconstituted with bacteriostatic diluents may be stored at CRT for up to 48 hours. Store fully diluted solutions under refrigeration or at CRT for up to 24 hours.

COMPATIBILITY   (Underline Indicates Conflicting Compatibility Information)
Consider any drug NOT listed as compatible to be INCOMPATIBLE until consulting a pharmacist; specific conditions may apply.

NONPHOSPHATE PRODUCTS (E.G., VEPESID)
Hydrolysis may occur in alkaline solutions.

One source suggests the following **compatibilities:**

Additive: Carboplatin (Paraplatin), cisplatin (Platinol), cytarabine (ARA-C), daunorubicin (Cerubidine), fluorouracil (5-FU), ifosfamide (Ifex), mitoxantrone (Novantrone), ondansetron (Zofran); another source adds mesna (Mesnex).

Y-site: Allopurinol (Aloprim), amifostine (Ethyol), aztreonam (Azactam), cladribine (Leustatin), doxorubicin liposomal (Doxil), fludarabine (Fludara), gemcitabine (Gemzar), granisetron (Kytril), melphalan (Alkeran), methotrexate, micafungin (Mycamine), mitoxantrone (Novantrone), ondansetron (Zofran), paclitaxel (Taxol), piperacillin/tazobactam (Zosyn), sargramostim (Leukine), sodium bicarbonate, teniposide (Vumon), thiotepa, topotecan (Hycamtin), vinorelbine (Navelbine).

PHOSPHATE PRODUCTS (E.G., ETOPOPHOS)
One source suggests the following **compatibilities:**

Additive: Specific information not available; consult pharmacist.

Y-site: Acyclovir (Zovirax), amikacin (Amikin), aminophylline, ampicillin, ampicillin/sulbactam (Unasyn), anidulafungin (Eraxis), aztreonam (Azactam), bleomycin (Blenoxane), bumetanide, buprenorphine (Buprenex), butorphanol (Stadol), calcium gluconate, carboplatin (Paraplatin), carmustine (BiCNU), caspofungin (Cancidas), cefazolin (Ancef), cefotaxime (Claforan), cefotetan (Cefotan), cefoxitin (Mefoxin), ceftazidime (Fortaz), ceftriaxone (Rocephin), cefuroxime (Zinacef), ciprofloxacin (Cipro IV), cisplatin (Platinol), clindamycin (Cleocin), cyclophosphamide (Cytoxan), cytarabine (ARA-C), dacarbazine (DTIC), dactinomycin (Cosmegen), daunorubicin (Cerubidine), dexamethasone (Decadron), diphenhydramine (Benadryl), dobutamine, dopamine, doripenem (Doribax), doxorubicin (Adriamycin), doxycycline, droperidol (Inapsine), enalaprilat (Vasotec IV), famotidine (Pepcid IV), fluconazole (Diflucan), fludarabine (Fludara), fluorouracil (5-FU), furosemide (Lasix), ganciclovir (Cytovene), gemcitabine (Gemzar), gentamicin, granisetron (Kytril), haloperidol (Haldol), heparin, hydrocortisone sodium succinate (Solu-Cortef), hydromorphone (Dilaudid), idarubicin (Idamycin), ifosfamide (Ifex), leucovorin calcium, linezolid (Zyvox), lorazepam (Ativan), magnesium sulfate, mannitol, meperidine (Demerol), mesna (Mesnex), methotrexate, metoclopramide (Reglan), metronidazole (Flagyl IV), mitoxantrone (Novantrone), morphine, nalbuphine, ondansetron (Zofran), oxaliplatin (Eloxatin), paclitaxel (Taxol), piperacillin, piperacillin/tazobactam (Zosyn), potassium chloride (KCl), promethazine (Phenergan), ranitidine (Zantac), sodium bicarbonate, streptozocin (Zanosar), sulfamethoxazole/trimethoprim, teniposide (Vumon), thiotepa, ticarcillin/clavulanate (Timentin), tobramycin, vancomycin, vinblastine, vincristine, zidovudine (AZT, Retrovir).

RATE OF ADMINISTRATION

NONPHOSPHATE PRODUCTS (E.G., VEPESID): Total desired dose, properly diluted (0.2 to 0.4 mg/mL) and evenly distributed over at least 30 to 60 minutes. Rapid infusion may cause marked hypotension. May be extended if fluid volume is a concern.

PHOSPHATE PRODUCTS (E.G., ETOPOPHOS): Total desired dose, properly reconstituted and diluted, may be given evenly distributed over as little as 5 minutes or up to 210 minutes. Do not give as a bolus injection.

ACTIONS

A semisynthetic derivative of podophyllotoxin. Cell cycle–specific for the G_2 phase, it inhibits DNA synthesis. Etopophos (phosphate) is a water-soluble ester of etoposide that promptly converts to etoposide in plasma. Half-life is from 3 to 12 hours (average is 7 hours). Highly protein-bound to human plasma proteins. Metabolized in the liver. Primarily excreted as unchanged drug or metabolites through urine and bile (feces). Secreted in breast milk.

INDICATIONS AND USES

To suppress or retard neoplastic growth in refractory testicular tumors (used in combination with other agents after previous surgery, chemotherapy, and radiotherapy). ■ Suppress or retard small-cell lung cancer (used in combination with other chemotherapeutic agents as first-line treatment). **Unlabeled uses:** High-dose regimens before bone marrow transplantation. Treatment of acute nonlymphocytic leukemias, Hodgkin's disease, non-Hodgkin's lymphomas, carcinoma of the breast, Kaposi's sarcoma, and neuroblastoma. Additional tumors have shown up to 20% response. Used alone or in combination with other agents.

CONTRAINDICATIONS

Hypersensitivity to etoposide, etoposide phosphate, or any other component of the formulations.

PRECAUTIONS

Follow guidelines for handling cytotoxic agents. See Appendix A, p. 1429. Always wear impervious gloves when handling vials containing etoposide. If a solution of etoposide contacts the skin, wash the skin immediately and thoroughly with soap and water. If there is contact with mucous membranes, flush thoroughly with water. For IV infusion only; do not give as a bolus injection. ■ Usually administered by or under the direction of the physician specialist. ■ Severe myelosuppression with resulting infection or bleeding may occur. Deaths have been reported. ■ A low serum albumin may result in an increase of free (active) etoposide, resulting in an increased risk of toxicity. Occurs more frequently in pediatric patients. ■ Hypersensitivity reactions have been reported. ■ A potential carcinogen;

acute leukemia with or without a preleukemic phase has been rarely reported. ▪ Oral dose of nonphosphate product (e.g., etoposide) is usually twice the IV dose.

Monitor: Determine absolute patency and quality of vein and adequate circulation of extremity. Avoid extravasation; may result in cellulitis, pain, swelling, and necrosis. ▪ Use caution to prevent bone marrow suppression. Obtain baseline CBC with differential and platelets. Monitor before each dose and between courses. See Dose Adjustments. ▪ Examine patient's mouth for ulceration before each dose. ▪ Monitor hepatic and renal function before and during therapy. ▪ Bone marrow recovery from a course is usually complete within 20 days. No cumulative toxicity has been reported as yet. ▪ Be alert for signs of bone marrow suppression or infection. ▪ Monitor for S/S of hypersensitivity reactions (e.g., bronchospasm, chills, dyspnea, fever, hypotension, pruritus, rash, tachycardia, urticaria). ▪ Monitor for thrombocytopenia (platelet count less than 50,000/mm^3). Initiate precautions to prevent excessive bleeding (e.g., inspect IV sites, skin, and mucous membranes; use extreme care during invasive procedures; test urine, emesis, stool, and secretions for occult blood). ▪ Prophylactic antibiotics may be indicated pending results of C/S in a febrile neutropenic patient. ▪ Maintain adequate hydration. ▪ Prophylactic antiemetics may increase patient comfort.

Patient Education: Nonhormonal birth control recommended. ▪ Report IV site burning or stinging promptly. ▪ Report chills, difficult breathing, fever, and rapid heartbeat promptly. See Appendix D, p. 1434.

Maternal/Child: Category D: avoid pregnancy. Can cause fetal harm. ▪ Discontinue breast-feeding. ▪ Has been used in pediatric patients, but safety and effectiveness not established. Anaphylactic reactions have been reported. See Precautions. ▪ Depending on the preparation, VePesid may contain benzyl alcohol or polysorbate 80; do not use in neonates or premature infants.

Elderly: Monitor renal, hepatic, and hematologic function closely. ▪ See Dose Adjustments. ▪ Incidence of anorexia, asthenia, dehydration, elevated BUN levels, granulocytopenia, leukopenia (Grade III or IV), mucositis, and somnolence occur more frequently in the elderly. ▪ May also be more sensitive to expected side effects (e.g., alopecia, gastrointestinal effects, infectious complications, and myelosuppression). Potential for greater sensitivity increased if renal function impaired.

DRUG/LAB INTERACTIONS

All products: Concurrent or consecutive use with other **bone marrow suppressants** (e.g., bleomycin, cisplatin, doxorubicin) **and/or radiation therapy** may produce additive bone marrow suppression. See Dose Adjustments. ▪ Do not administer **live virus vaccines** to patients receiving antineoplastic drugs. ▪ Clearance decreased and toxicity increased by **cyclosporine.**

NONPHOSPHATE PRODUCTS (E.G., VEPESID): May potentiate **warfarin;** monitor PT.

PHOSPHATE PRODUCT (E.G., ETOPOPHOS): Use caution with drugs that are **known to inhibit phosphatase activities** (e.g., levamisole [Ergamisol]).

SIDE EFFECTS

Bone marrow toxicity (e.g., leukopenia, neutropenia, thrombocytopenia) can be severe, is dose related, and may be dose limiting. Side effects are usually reversible: abdominal pain, alopecia, anaphylactic reactions (bronchospasm, chills, dyspnea, fever, hypotension), anemia, anorexia, constipation, diarrhea, dizziness, elevated liver function tests (e.g., AST, ALT), hepatic toxicity, hypotension, interstitial pneumonitis/pulmonary fibrosis, local soft tissue toxicity following extravasation, malaise, mucositis, nausea, neuritic pain, paralytic ileus, peripheral neurotoxicity, radiation recall dermatitis, seizures, Stevens-Johnson syndrome, stomatitis, thrombophlebitis, toxic epidermal necrolysis, vomiting. Hepatic toxicity and metabolic acidosis have occurred with higher-than-recommended doses.

ANTIDOTE

Notify the physician of all side effects; symptomatic treatment is often indicated, dose reduction may be necessary. For extravasation, discontinue the drug immediately and administer into another vein. Consider injection of long-acting dexamethasone (Decadron LA) throughout extravasated tissue. Use a 27- or 25-gauge needle. Elevate extremity; moist heat may be helpful. Hypotension is usually due to a rapid infusion rate. Discontinue infusion. Trendelenburg position and IV fluids should reverse the hypotension; vasopressors (e.g., dopamine) may be required. After recovery, restart at slower rate. Administration of whole blood products (e.g., packed RBCs, platelets, leukocytes) and/or blood modifiers (e.g., darbepoetin alfa [Aranesp], epoetin alfa [Epogen], filgrastim [Neupogen], pegfilgrastim [Neulasta], sargramostim [Leukine]) may be indicated to treat bone marrow toxicity. Discontinue infusion at the first sign of a hypersensitivity reaction; antihistamines, corticosteroids, pressor agents, or volume expanders may be indicated. Resuscitate as necessary.

FACTOR IX (HUMAN) ▪
FACTOR IX COMPLEX (HUMAN)
(**FAK**-tor 9)

Antihemorrhagic

AlphaNine SD, Mononine ▪ **Bebulin VH,**
Profilnine SD, Proplex T

pH 7 to 7.4 ▪ pH 7 to 7.4

USUAL DOSE
(International units [IU])

ALL FORMULATIONS

Completely individualized based on patient's circumstances, condition, degree of deficiency, and desired blood level percentage. Specific products may be indicated or preferred in some situations; see Indications and Uses. Range is 10 to 75 International units (IU)/kg of body weight. May be repeated every 12 hours in some situations, required only every 2 or 3 days in others. Actual number of International units contained shown on each bottle or vial. Units required to raise blood level percentages can be calculated as follows:

Body weight (kg) × Desired increase (% of normal) × 1 Unit/kg

(70 kg × 40% increase × 1 IU/kg = 2,800 IU). To maintain levels above 25%, calculate each dose to raise level to 40% to 60% of normal.

Minor hemorrhage: A single injection calculated to increase plasma level to 20% to 30%. May be repeated in 24 hours if indicated.

Major trauma or surgery: Increase plasma level to 25% to 50% and maintain at that level for a minimum of 1 week or as indicated. May require daily injections (every 18 to 30 hours).

Dental extraction: Increase plasma level to 50% before procedure; repeat if indicated.

Prophylaxis: 10 to 20 IU/kg once or twice a week or increase plasma level to 20% to 30%.

FACTOR IX COMPLEX

Reversal of coumarin effect: 15 IU/kg.

DILUTION

Diluent usually provided. Some preparations also supply double-ended needles for dilution and filter needle for aspiration into a syringe. Sterile technique imperative. Confirm expiration date. Use plastic syringes to prevent binding to glass surfaces. Factor IX and diluent should be at room temperature. Direct diluent from above to side of vial to gently moisten all contents. Swirl gently to dissolve; avoid foaming. Do not shake. May take 1 to 5 minutes. Should be clear and colorless. Must be used within 3 hours to avoid bacterial contamination. The addition of 2 to 3 units of heparin/mL factor IX complex may reduce the incidence of thrombosis. May be given through an IV administration set (often provided) if multiple vials are required. Discard any unused contents. Discard all administration equipment after single use; do not attempt to resterilize.

AlphaNine SD: Follow general directions above. After diluent is drawn through double-ended needle, remove diluent bottle first; then remove double-ended needle. ***Do not invert concentrate vial until ready to withdraw contents!*** Air from syringe into vial required to withdraw contents. Withdraw through filter.

Mononine: Follow general directions listed previously. After diluent is drawn through double-ended needle, remove diluent bottle first; then remove double-ended needle. *Use only the provided self-venting filter spike to transfer Mononine to a syringe! Do not inject any air into Mononine vial; could cause product loss.* Discard filter and use only provided wing needle and micropore tubing to administer.

Filters: Usually supplied by manufacturer. If more than one vial is required for a dose, multiple vials may be drawn into the same syringe; however, a new filter needle must be used to withdraw the contents of each vial of factor IX and/or factor IX complex (Human). Manufacturers of *AlphaNine SD* and *Mononine* provide a filter needle, which is to be used to withdraw reconstituted solution into a syringe. Discard filter needle after aspiration into the syringe. No further filtering is required for administration.

Storage: Store lyophilized powder at 2° to 8° C (36° to 46° F); do not freeze. Do not refrigerate after dilution. *Mononine* may be stored at room temperature before dilution for up to 30 days.

COMPATIBILITY

Specific information not available. Consider specific use; consult pharmacist.

RATE OF ADMINISTRATION

Average rate is 2 to 3 mL or 100 units/min. Completely individualized according to patient's condition. Decrease rate of administration for side effects such as burning or pain at injection site, chills, fever, flushing, headache, tingling, or changes in BP or pulse. Never exceed 10 mL/min.

ACTIONS

A lyophilized concentrate of human coagulation factors: IX (plasma thromboplastin and antihemophilic factor B), II (prothrombin), VII (proconvertin), and X (Stuart-Prower factor). In contrast to other products, AlphaNine SD and Mononine are highly purified factor IX and contain only minimal amounts of the other factors. All products are obtained from fresh human plasma and prepared, irradiated, and dried by specific processes. Additional processes are used to prepare AlphaNine SD and Mononine that markedly reduce the possibility of viral contamination. Concentration of 25 units/mL is 25 times greater than normal plasma. Preparations contain varying amounts of total protein in each vial. Half-life is approximately 24 hours (range 18 to 36 hours).

INDICATIONS AND USES

All factor IX products: Prevention/control of bleeding in patients with Factor IX deficiency due to hemophilia B. Indicated to correct or prevent a dangerous bleeding episode or to perform surgery. ▪ Prophylaxis to prevent spontaneous bleeding in patients with proven specific congenital deficiency (hemophilia B). **Factor IX (human):** Preferred for surgical coverage; treatment of crush injuries and/or large IM hemorrhages requiring several days of replacement therapy; and treatment in neonates, individuals with severe hepatocellular dysfunction, or those with a history of thrombotic complications associated with factor IX complex. **Factor IX complex:** Prevention/control of bleeding in patients with hemophilia A who have inhibitors to Factor VIII. ▪ Reversal of coumarin effect (fresh-frozen plasma preferred unless risk of hepatitis transfer would be life threatening). ▪ Hemorrhage caused by hepatitis-induced lack of production of liver-dependent coagulation factors. ▪ Proplex T is used for prevention or control of bleeding episodes in patients with Factor VII deficiency.

CONTRAINDICATIONS

Factor IX complex: Known liver disease with suspicion of intravascular coagulation or fibrinolysis. ▪ Factor VII deficiency except for Proplex T. **Mononine:** Known hypersensitivity to mouse protein. ▪ No other known contraindications for **AlphaNine SD** or **Bebulin VH**. ▪ **AlphaNine SD, Bebulin VH,** and **Mononine** are not indicated for replacement of any other coagulation factors.

PRECAUTIONS

Used when plasma infusions would result in hypervolemia and/or proteinemia or when blood volume or RBC replacement is not indicated. ▪ Use extreme caution in newborns, infants, postoperative patients, and patients with liver disease. Factor IX (human) (e.g., AlphaNine SD, Mononine) would be preferred because studies show no incidence of thrombin generation. ▪ Fresh-frozen plasma may be required in addition to factor IX complex when prompt reversal is required. ▪ Danger of thromboembolic episodes (DIC, myocardial infarction, pulmonary embolism, venous thrombosis) increases with plasma levels over 50%. ▪ Large or frequently repeated doses of factor IX complex may cause intravascular hemolysis in patients with type A, B, or AB blood.

Monitor: Monitor the patient's levels of coagulation factors before, after, and between administrations. *Do not overdose;* see Side Effects. ▪ AIDS or hepatitis is possible for the recipient. Health care professionals should exercise caution in handling. Possibility markedly reduced with additional preparation process of AlphaNine SD and Mononine. ▪ Observe for signs and symptoms of postoperative thrombosis or disseminated intravascular coagulation (DIC). Risk multiplies with repeated administrations except for AlphaNine, AlphaNine SD, and Mononine.

Patient Education: Alert to possible risk of HIV virus and hepatitis. ▪ Report early signs of hypersensitivity promptly (burning or pain along injection site, hives, rash, tightness of chest, wheezing). ▪ Notify physician if medication seems less effective. May be developing antibodies to factor IX. ▪ Carry identification card. ▪ Proper preparation and administration imperative if given in home.

Maternal/Child: Category C: safety for use during pregnancy not established; use only if clearly indicated; see Precautions. ▪ Use extreme caution in neonates with hepatitis; high rate of morbidity.

DRUG/LAB INTERACTIONS

Concurrent use of **aminocaproic acid** (Amicar) may increase risk of thrombosis.

SIDE EFFECTS

Burning or pain along injection site, changes in BP, chills, fever, flushing, headache, nausea, tingling, urticaria, vomiting.

Major: Anaphylaxis, DIC, hepatitis, myocardial infarction, postoperative thrombosis (rare with pure factor IX [Human] products), pulmonary embolism. Consider risk potential of contracting AIDS and hepatitis; markedly reduced with pure factor IX (Human) products (AlphaNine, AlphaNine SD, and Mononine).

ANTIDOTE

Temporarily discontinue or decrease rate of administration for minor side effects. For major symptoms, discontinue, and notify physician. Treat hypersensitivity reactions as indicated; a different lot may not cause reaction. For thrombosis or DIC, anticoagulation with heparin may be indicated.

FACTOR IX (RECOMBINANT)
(**FAK**-tor 9 [re-**KOM**-be-nant])

BeneFIX

Antihemorrhagic

USUAL DOSE

(International units [IU])

Adults and pediatric patients: Completely individualized based on the degree of deficiency, location and extent of bleeding, and the patient's clinical condition, age, and recovery of factor IX. All doses should be titrated to the patient's clinical response. Actual number of International units contained shown on each bottle or vial. Units required to raise blood level percentages are somewhat increased with this recombinant product compared to other factor IX products and can be calculated as follows:

Number of Factor IX IU Required =
Body Weight (in kg) × Desired Factor IX Increase (%) × 1.2 IU/kg

In the presence of an inhibitor, higher doses may be required.

The following chart may be used to guide dosing in bleeding episodes and surgery.

Factor IX (Recombinant) Dosing Guidelines			
Type of Hemorrhage	Circulating Factor IX Activity Required (%)	Frequency of Doses (hours)	Duration of Therapy (days)
Minor Uncomplicated hemarthroses, superficial muscle, or soft tissue	20%-30%	12-24 hours	1-2 days
Moderate Intramuscle or soft tissue with dissection, mucous membranes, dental extractions, or hematuria	25%-50%	12-24 hours	Treat until bleeding stops and healing begins, about 2 to 7 days
Major Pharynx, retropharynx, retroperitoneum, CNS, surgery	50%-100%	12-24 hours	7-10 days

Source: Roberts and Eberst.

DILUTION

Sterile diluent, double-ended needle, filter spike, and infusion set provided. Sterile technique imperative. Confirm expiration date. Use plastic syringes to prevent binding to glass surfaces. Factor IX and diluent should be at room temperature. After removing the vial caps on Factor IX and diluent, wipe with antiseptic and allow to dry. Insert short end of the double-ended needle in the diluent vial. Insert long end in the Factor IX vial with the tip directed to the side of the wall to prevent excessive foaming. Fully invert the diluent vial to a vertical position and allow the diluent to run completely into the Factor IX vial. If the diluent does not transfer completely, *do not use* (a very small amount remaining is permissible). Remove transfer needle. Gently rotate the vial to dissolve. Should be clear and colorless. Attach filter spike to the plastic syringe and insert in the reconstituted solution; invert and withdraw contents. *Do not* inject air into the vial; may cause partial loss of product. Multiple vials may be drawn in the same syringe, but a new sterile filter spike must be used for each vial. Must be used within 3 hours of reconstitution.

Filters: Supplied by manufacturer. If more than one vial is required for a dose, multiple vials may be drawn into the same syringe; however, a new filter needle must be used to withdraw the contents of each vial of factor IX (recombinant).

Storage: Refrigerate packaged product (2° to 8° C [36° to 46° F]). Packaged product may be stored at room temperature not exceeding 25° C (77° F) for up to 6 months (mark date removed from refrigerator on carton). Avoid freezing. Do not use after the expiration date.

COMPATIBILITY
Specific information not available. Consider specific use; consult pharmacist.

RATE OF ADMINISTRATION
A single dose over several minutes. Average rate during studies was 50 units/kg infused over 10 minutes. Individualized according to patient's condition and comfort level. Decrease rate for side effects such as burning or pain at injection site, chills, fever, flushing, headache, tingling, or changes in BP or pulse.

ACTIONS
An antihemorrhagic. A purified protein produced by recombinant DNA technology for use in the treatment of factor IX deficiency. Its primary amino acid sequence is identical to a form of plasma-derived factor IX, and it has structural and functional characteristics similar to those of endogenous factor IX. Inherently free from the risk of transmission of human bloodborne pathogens such as HIV, hepatitis viruses, and parvovirus. Factor IX is the specific clotting factor deficient in patients with hemophilia B and in patients with acquired factor IX deficiencies. Factor IX (Recombinant) increases plasma levels of factor IX and can temporarily correct the coagulation defect in these patients. Half-life ranges from 11 to 26 hours.

INDICATIONS AND USES
Control and prevention of hemorrhagic episodes in patients with hemophilia B (congenital factor IX deficiency or Christmas disease), including control and prevention of bleeding in surgical settings.

CONTRAINDICATIONS
Known history of hypersensitivity to hamster protein. ▪ Not indicated for the treatment of other factor deficiencies (e.g., factors II, VII, and X). ▪ Not indicated for the treatment of hemophilia A patients with inhibitors to factor VIII. ▪ Not indicated for the reversal of coumarin-induced anticoagulation. ▪ Not indicated for the treatment of bleeding due to low levels of liver-dependent coagulation factors.

PRECAUTIONS
Usually administered under the supervision of a physician experienced in the treatment of hemophilia B. ▪ Hypersensitivity reactions are possible. ▪ BeneFIX contains only coagulation factor IX, but thromboembolic episodes (e.g., disseminated intravascular coagulation [DIC], myocardial

infarction, pulmonary embolism, venous thrombosis) have been reported with other factor IX concentrates. These episodes increase with plasma levels over 50%. May be hazardous in patients with signs of fibrinolysis or DIC. ■ Because of potential thromboembolic problems, use caution in patients with liver disease, patients in the postoperative period, neonates, or in patients at risk of thromboembolic phenomena or DIC. Benefit must be weighed against risk.

Monitor: To ensure desired factor IX activity levels, precise monitoring using the factor IX activity assay is recommended, especially during surgical intervention. *Do not overdose;* see Side Effects. ■ Monitor for development of factor IX inhibitors. Patients dosed with high-purity factor IX products who develop inhibitors are at increased risk of anaphylaxis with repeat doses.

Patient Education: Hypersensitivity reactions can occur. Report difficulty breathing, hives, itching, tightness of the chest, and/or wheezing promptly. If self-administering, discontinue use and contact physician immediately.

Maternal/Child: Category C: use during pregnancy or during breast-feeding only if clearly indicated. ■ To this date, no adverse reactions related to treatment have been reported in pediatric patients.

Elderly: Response similar to other age-groups.

DRUG/LAB INTERACTIONS

Specific information not available.

SIDE EFFECTS

Allergic rhinitis, altered taste, burning or pain along injection site, burning sensation in jaw and skull, changes in BP, chills, dizziness, drowsiness, dry cough, fever, flushing, headache, lethargy, light-headedness, nausea, phlebitis at injection site, rash, tightness in the chest, tingling, urticaria, vomiting.

Major: Anaphylaxis, DIC, myocardial infarction, postoperative thrombosis (rare with pure factor IX products), pulmonary embolism.

ANTIDOTE

Temporarily discontinue or decrease rate of administration for minor side effects. If any major symptoms appear, discontinue drug and notify physician. Treat hypersensitivity reactions as indicated. For thrombosis or DIC, anticoagulation with heparin may be indicated.

FAMOTIDINE
(fah-**MOH**-tih-deen)

**Antiulcer agent
(H₂ antagonist)
Gastric acid inhibitor**

Famotidine PF, Pepcid

pH 5.7 to 6.4

USUAL DOSE

20 mg (2 mL) every 12 hours. Increase frequency of dose, not amount, if necessary for pain relief. In hypersecretory states (e.g., Zollinger-Ellison syndrome), higher doses may be required. Adjust dose to individual patient needs.

PEDIATRIC DOSE

Age 1 to 16 years: Starting dose is 0.25 mg/kg every 12 hours. Treatment duration and dose must be individualized based on clinical response, pH determination, and/or endoscopy. Doses up to 0.5 mg/kg every 12 hours may be required for gastric acid suppression. Another source suggests 0.6 to 0.8 mg/kg/24 hr (0.3 to 0.4 mg/kg every 12 hours or 0.2 to 0.27 mg/kg every 8 hours). May need to reduce interval to every 8 hours because of increased elimination. Maximum dose is 40 to 80 mg/24 hr based on diagnosis.

Neonate (unlabeled): 0.5 mg/kg/dose/24 hr.

DOSE ADJUSTMENTS

Reduce dose by one-half or increase the dosing interval to 36 to 48 hours in patients with moderate or severe renal dysfunction (CrCl less than 50 mL/min). Adjust based on patient response. Half-life may exceed 20 hours if CrCl less than 10 mL/min.

DILUTION

IV injection: Available in vials containing 10 mg/mL and as premixed solution 20 mg/50 mL. Each 20-mg vial must be diluted with 5 to 10 mL of NS or other **compatible** infusion solutions for injection (e.g., D5W, D10W, LR, SW).

Intermittent infusion: Each 20 mg may be diluted in 100 mL of D5W or other **compatible** infusion solution and given piggyback.

Storage: Refrigerate vials before dilution. Manufacturer recommends use of diluted solutions within 48 hours. However, studies suggest diluted solutions are physically and chemically stable at RT for 7 days. Store premixed Galaxy containers at CRT; avoid excessive heat.

COMPATIBILITY

(Underline Indicates Conflicting Compatibility Information)

Consider any drug NOT listed as compatible to be INCOMPATIBLE until consulting a pharmacist; specific conditions may apply.

May form a precipitate with sodium bicarbonate in concentrations greater than 0.2 mg/mL.

One source suggests the following **compatibilities:**

Solutions: Selected TNA and TPN solutions.

Additive: Cefazolin (Ancef), flumazenil (Romazicon), vancomycin.

Y-site: Acyclovir (Zovirax), allopurinol (Aloprim), amifostine (Ethyol), aminophylline, amiodarone (Nexterone), ampicillin, ampicillin/sulbactam (Unasyn), anidulafungin (Eraxis), atropine, aztreonam (Azactam), bivalirudin (Angiomax), calcium gluconate, caspofungin (Cancidas), cefazolin

(Ancef), cefotaxime (Claforan), cefotetan (Cefotan), cefoxitin (Mefoxin), ceftazidime (Fortaz), ceftriaxone (Rocephin), cefuroxime (Zinacef), chlorpromazine (Thorazine), cisatracurium (Nimbex), cisplatin (Platinol), cladribine (Leustatin), cyclophosphamide (Cytoxan), cytarabine (ARA-C), dexamethasone (Decadron), dexmedetomidine (Precedex), dextran 40, digoxin (Lanoxin), diphenhydramine (Benadryl), dobutamine, docetaxel (Taxotere), dopamine, doripenem (Doribax), doxorubicin (Adriamycin), doxorubicin liposomal (Doxil), droperidol (Inapsine), enalaprilat (Vasotec IV), epinephrine (Adrenalin), erythromycin (Erythrocin), esmolol (Brevibloc), etoposide phosphate (Etopophos), fenoldopam (Corlopam), filgrastim (Neupogen), fluconazole (Diflucan), fludarabine (Fludara), folic acid, <u>furosemide (Lasix)</u>, gemcitabine (Gemzar), gentamicin, granisetron (Kytril), haloperidol (Haldol), heparin, hetastarch in electrolytes (Hextend), hydrocortisone sodium succinate (Solu-Cortef), hydromorphone (Dilaudid), imipenem-cilastatin (Primaxin), inamrinone (Amrinone), insulin (regular), isoproterenol (Isuprel), labetalol (Trandate), lidocaine, linezolid (Zyvox), lorazepam (Ativan), magnesium sulfate, melphalan (Alkeran), meperidine (Demerol), methotrexate, methylprednisolone (Solu-Medrol), metoclopramide (Reglan), midazolam (Versed), morphine, nafcillin (Nallpen), nicardipine (Cardene IV), nitroglycerin IV, nitroprusside sodium, norepinephrine (Levophed), ondansetron (Zofran), oxacillin (Bactocill), oxaliplatin (Eloxatin), paclitaxel (Taxol), <u>palonosetron (Aloxi)</u>, pemetrexed (Alimta), phenylephrine (Neo-Synephrine), <u>phenytoin (Dilantin)</u>, phytonadione (vitamin K_1), piperacillin, potassium chloride (KCl), potassium phosphate, procainamide (Pronestyl), propofol (Diprivan), remifentanil (Ultiva), sargramostim (Leukine), sodium bicarbonate, teniposide (Vumon), theophylline, thiamine (vitamin B_1), thiotepa, ticarcillin/clavulanate (Timentin), tirofiban (Aggrastat), verapamil, vinorelbine (Navelbine).

RATE OF ADMINISTRATION
IV injection: Each 20 mg or fraction thereof over at least 2 minutes.
Intermittent infusion: Each 20-mg dose over 15 to 30 minutes.

ACTIONS
A histamine H_2 antagonist, it inhibits both daytime and nocturnal basal gastric acid secretion. It also inhibits gastric acid secretion stimulated by food and pentagastrin. Onset of action occurs within 30 minutes and lasts for 10 to 12 hours. No cumulative effect with repeated doses. 30 to 60 times more potent than cimetidine. Elimination half-life is 2.5 to 3.5 hours. Eliminated by renal and other metabolic routes. Crosses placental barrier. Secreted in breast milk.

INDICATIONS AND USES
Short-term treatment of active duodenal ulcers, benign gastric ulcers, and pathologic hypersecretory conditions in hospitalized patients or in patients unable to take oral medication. ■ Used orally for short-term treatment of gastroesophageal reflux disease (GERD) including erosive or ulcerative esophagitis. IV dose recommendations not yet available.
Unlabeled uses: GI bleeding. ■ Stress ulcer prophylaxis.

CONTRAINDICATIONS
Known hypersensitivity to H_2 receptor antagonists (e.g., cimetidine [Tagamet], famotidine [Pepcid IV], ranitidine [Zantac]) or their components; cross-sensitivity has occurred.

PRECAUTIONS

Use with caution in patients with moderate or severe renal dysfunction; see Dose Adjustments. ▪ CNS adverse effects have been reported in patients with impaired renal function. ▪ Gastric malignancy may be present even though patient is asymptomatic. ▪ Effects maintained with oral dosage. Total treatment usually discontinued after 4 to 8 weeks.

Monitor: Use antacids concomitantly to relieve pain. ▪ See Precautions.

Patient Education: Stop smoking or at least avoid smoking after last dose of the day. ▪ Gastric pain and ulceration may recur after medication is stopped.

Maternal/Child: Category B: use during pregnancy only when clearly needed. ▪ Advisable to discontinue breast-feeding. ▪ Plasma clearance is reduced and half-life is increased in pediatric patients under 3 months of age compared to older pediatric patients with pharmacokinetic parameters similar to adults.

Elderly: Response similar to that seen in younger patients; however, greater sensitivity in the elderly cannot be ruled out. ▪ Consider risk of renal dysfunction; reduced doses and monitoring of renal function may be indicated; see Dose Adjustments.

DRUG/LAB INTERACTIONS

May inhibit gastric absorption of **ketoconazole** (Nizoral). ▪ May decrease **cyclosporine** serum levels when famotidine is given concurrently with ketoconazole and cyclosporine.

SIDE EFFECTS

Constipation, diarrhea, dizziness, and headache are the most common side effects. Hypersensitivity reactions (bronchospasm, fever, pruritus, rash, eosinophilia) can occur. Abdominal discomfort, agitation, alopecia, anorexia, anxiety, arthralgias, confusion, decreased libido, depression, dry mouth, dry skin, elevated ALT, flushing, grand mal seizure, hallucinations, insomnia, interstitial pneumonia, malaise, muscular pain, nausea and vomiting, orbital edema, palpitations, paresthesias, somnolence, taste disorder, thrombocytopenia, tinnitus, and toxic epidermal necrolysis/Stevens-Johnson syndrome (very rare) have been reported. Convulsions in patients with impaired renal function have been reported rarely.

ANTIDOTE

Notify physician of all side effects. May be treated symptomatically or may respond to decrease in frequency of dosage. Resuscitate as necessary for overdosage.

FAT EMULSION, INTRAVENOUS BBW *

Nutritional
supplement
(fatty acid)

**Intralipid 10%, 20%, & 30%, Liposyn II
10% & 20%, Liposyn III 10%, 20%, & 30%**

pH 6 to 9

*This drug is on the Black Box Warning list; however, a BBW is not provided in the parenteral prescribing information.

USUAL DOSE

Some solutions may contain aluminum; see Precautions.

Total parenteral nutrition component: 500 mL of 10% or 20% on the first day. Increase dose gradually each day. Do not exceed 60% of the patient's total caloric intake or 2.5 Gm/kg of body weight. Amino acids and carbohydrates should account for the remaining caloric input.

Prevention of fatty acid deficiency: 500 mL of 10% or 250 mL of 20% twice a week should supply the recommended 4% of caloric intake as linoleate.

PEDIATRIC DOSE

Some solutions may contain aluminum; see Precautions.

Total parenteral nutrition component: 0.5 to 1 Gm/kg of body weight. Increase dose gradually each day. Do not exceed 60% of total caloric intake. Amino acids and carbohydrates should account for the remaining caloric input. Maximum dose recommended by the American Academy of Pediatrics is 3 Gm fat/kg/24 hr. Another source suggests maximum may be as high as 4 Gm fat/kg/24 hr.

Premature infants: Begin with 0.5 Gm fat/kg/24 hr (5 mL/kg/24 hr of 10% solution). See comments under Pediatric Dose and Maternal/Child.

Prevention of fatty acid deficiency: 5 to 10 mL/kg/day of a 10% solution or 2.5 to 5 mL/kg/day of a 20% solution. 8% to 10% of caloric input should be supplied by IV fat emulsion. Essential fatty acid deficiency accompanied by stress may require an increased dose to correct the deficiency.

DOSE ADJUSTMENTS

Normal renal function required. Reduced dose may be indicated.

DILUTION

Follow manufacturer's specific instructions for preparation of each individual brand. Must be given as prepared by manufacturer; check labels for aluminum content; see Precautions. Use only freshly opened solutions; discard remainder of partial dose. Do not use if there appears to be an oiling out of the emulsion. **Intralipid 30% is not to be given by direct IV infusion.** Packaged for bulk use in a pharmacy admixture program. Must be specifically combined with dextrose solutions and amino acids (TPN) so total fat content does not exceed 20%. Prepared for an individual patient in the pharmacy. Lipids may extract phthalates from phthalate-plasticized PVC. Non-phthalate infusion sets recommended; available with most commercial products.

Filters: Do not use filters; will disturb emulsion. FDA suggests the use of a 1.2-micron filter for admixtures containing lipids (e.g., 3 in 1).

Storage: Must be stored at temperatures not exceeding 25° C (77° F). Specific storage conditions required (see literature). Do not freeze. Manufacturer recommends admixtures (3 in 1) be refrigerated for no more than

24 hours after mixing and completely infused within 24 hours after removal from refrigeration.

COMPATIBILITY   (Underline Indicates Conflicting Compatibility Information) *Consider any drug NOT listed as compatible to be INCOMPATIBLE until consulting a pharmacist; specific conditions may apply.* Manufacturer recommends not mixing with any electrolyte or other nutrient solution. Infuse separately; do not disturb emulsion; no additives or medications are to be placed in bottle or tubing with the exception of heparin 1 to 2 units/mL (may be added before administration [activates lipoprotein lipase]). In actual practice, carbohydrates, amino acids, and fat emulsion are mixed in specific percentages and in a specific order to meet individual total parenteral nutritional needs but should be prepared in the pharmacy. Any addition of supplemental vitamins, minerals, or electrolytes (e.g., calcium, magnesium, phosphates) may cause a precipitate unless a specific order is followed. Precipitates are difficult to detect in lipids.

One source suggests the following **compatibilities** *(not recommended by manufacturer):*

Y-site: Specific TNA solutions may be **compatible** at the **Y-site** with specific concentrations of amikacin (Amikin), aminophylline, ampicillin, ampicillin/sulbactam (Unasyn), aztreonam (Azactam), bumetanide, buprenorphine (Buprenex), butorphanol (Stadol), calcium gluconate, carboplatin (Paraplatin), cefazolin (Ancef), cefotaxime (Claforan), cefotetan (Cefotan), cefoxitin (Mefoxin), ceftazidime (Fortaz), ceftriaxone (Rocephin), cefuroxime (Zinacef), chlorpromazine (Thorazine), ciprofloxacin (Cipro IV), cisplatin (Platinol), clindamycin (Cleocin), cyclophosphamide (Cytoxan), cyclosporine (Sandimmune), cytarabine (ARA-C), dexamethasone (Decadron), digoxin, diphenhydramine (Benadryl), dobutamine, dopamine, enalaprilat (Vasotec IV), erythromycin (Erythrocin), famotidine (Pepcid IV), fentanyl (Sublimaze), fluconazole (Diflucan), fluorouracil (5-FU), furosemide (Lasix), gentamicin, granisetron (Kytril), hydrocortisone sodium succinate (Solu-Cortef), hydromorphone (Dilaudid), ifosfamide (Ifex), imipenem-cilastatin (Primaxin), insulin (regular), isoproterenol (Isuprel), kanamycin (Kantrex), leucovorin calcium, lidocaine, magnesium sulfate, mannitol, meperidine (Demerol), meropenem (Merrem IV), mesna (Mesnex), methotrexate, methyldopate, methylprednisolone (Solu-Medrol), metoclopramide (Reglan), metronidazole (Flagyl IV), mitoxantrone (Novantrone), morphine, nafcillin (Nallpen), nitroglycerin IV, nitroprusside sodium, norepinephrine (Levophed), octreotide (Sandostatin), oxacillin (Bactocill), paclitaxel (Taxol), penicillin G potassium, piperacillin, piperacillin/tazobactam (Zosyn), potassium chloride (KCl), prochlorperazine (Compazine), promethazine (Phenergan), ranitidine (Zantac), sodium bicarbonate, sulfamethoxazole/trimethoprim, tacrolimus (Prograf), ticarcillin/clavulanate (Timentin), tobramycin, vancomycin, zidovudine (AZT, Retrovir).

RATE OF ADMINISTRATION
May be administered via a Y-tube or three-way stopcock near the infusion site. Rates of both solutions (fat emulsion and amino acid products) should be controlled by infusion pumps. Keep fat emulsion line higher than all other lines (has low specific gravity and could run up into other lines). Do not use filters; will disturb emulsion. FDA suggests use of at least a

1.2-micron filter for admixtures containing lipids (e.g., 3 in 1); precipitates difficult to detect in lipids.

Adult: *10%:* 1 mL/min or 0.1 Gm fat/min for the first 15 to 30 minutes. If no untoward effects, the dose may be increased to 2 mL/min. The daily dose should not exceed 2.5 Gm fat/kg (25 mL of 10% solution per kg). On the first day of therapy, a maximum of 500 mL of 10% solution is recommended.

20%: 0.5 mL/min or 0.1 Gm fat/min for the first 15 to 30 minutes. If no untoward effects, the rate may be increased to 1 mL/min. The daily dose should not exceed 2.5 Gm fat/kg (12.5 mL of 20% solution per kg). On the first day of therapy, a maximum of 500 mL of 20% solution is recommended.

Premature infants: 0.5 Gm fat/kg/24 hr (5 mL of 10% or 2.5 mL of 20% per 24 hours). Adjust rate and/or increase amount based on the infant's ability to eliminate fat. See comments under Usual Dose and Maternal/Child.

Pediatric: *10%:* 0.1 mL/min for the first 10 to 15 minutes. Reduce initial rate to 0.05 mL/min for a *20%* solution. If no untoward effects, rate may be increased to administer 1 mL/kg/hr of *10%* solution or 0.5 mL/kg/hr of *20%*. One source suggests a maximum rate of 0.17 Gm/kg/hr. An infusion pump is recommended. Do not exceed a rate of 50 mL/hr (20%) or 100 mL/hr (10%).

ACTIONS

An isotonic nutrient. Used as a source of calories and essential fatty acids. Contains emulsified fat particles about 0.4 to 0.5 micron in size. Total caloric value (fat, phospholipid, and glycerol) is 1.1 cal/mL for the 10% emulsion and 2 cal/mL for the 20% emulsion. Metabolized and used as a source of energy. Increases heat production and oxygen consumption. Decreases respiratory quotient. Cleared from the bloodstream by a process not fully understood.

INDICATIONS AND USES

To provide additional calories and essential fatty acids for patients requiring parenteral nutrition whose caloric requirements cannot be met by glucose or who will be receiving parenteral nutrition over extended periods (over 5 days usually). ▪ Prevent essential fatty acid deficiency.

CONTRAINDICATIONS

Any condition that disturbs normal fat metabolism, such as pathologic hyperlipemia, lipoid nephrosis, and acute pancreatitis with hyperlipemia. ▪ Severe egg allergies.

PRECAUTIONS

Isotonic; may be administered by a peripheral vein or central venous infusion. ▪ Fatty acids displace bilirubin bound to albumin. Use caution in jaundiced or premature infants. ▪ Use caution in pulmonary disease, liver disease, anemia, or blood coagulation disorders, or when there is any danger of fat embolism. ▪ Some solutions may contain aluminum. In impaired kidney function, aluminum may reach toxic levels. Premature neonates are particularly at risk because of their immature kidneys and requirement for calcium and phosphate, which also contain aluminum. Research indicates that patients with impaired renal function who receive more than 4 to 5 mcg/kg/day of parenteral aluminum are at risk for developing CNS or bone toxicity associated with aluminum accumulation. ▪ See Maternal/Child.

Monitor: Monitor lipids routinely; lipemia should clear daily. ▪ Monitor hemogram, blood coagulation, liver function tests, triglycerides, and platelet count, especially in neonates. Discontinue use for significant abnormality. ▪ See Maternal/Child.

Maternal/Child: Category C: use in pregnancy only when clearly needed; safety not established. ▪ Use caution if emulsion is administered to a woman who is breast-feeding. ▪ Use extreme caution in neonates; death from intravascular fat accumulation in the lungs has occurred. Strict adherence to dose and rate of administration is imperative. Premature and small-for-gestational-age infants have poor clearance. Administration of less than the maximum recommended dose should be considered in these patients. Monitor serum triglycerides and/or plasma free fatty acid levels to assess infant's ability to eliminate infused fat from the circulation. Frequent, even daily, platelet counts are recommended in neonatal patients receiving TPN with IV fat emulsion.

DRUG/LAB INTERACTIONS

No specific information available; see Dilution.

SIDE EFFECTS

Anaphylaxis, back pain, chest pain, cyanosis, a delayed overloading syndrome (focal seizures, fever, leukocytosis, splenomegaly, shock), dizziness, dyspnea, elevated temperature, flushing, headache, hypercoagulability, hyperlipemia, nausea and vomiting, pressure over eyes, sepsis (from contamination of IV catheter), sleepiness, sweating, thrombophlebitis (from concurrent hyperalimentation fluids), thrombocytopenia in neonates (rare), and many others.

ANTIDOTE

Notify physician of all side effects. Many will be treated symptomatically. Treat hypersensitivity reactions promptly and resuscitate as necessary. For accidental overdose, stop the infusion. Obtain blood sample for inspection of plasma, triglyceride concentration, or measurement of plasma light-scattering activity by nephelometry. Repeat blood samples until the lipid has cleared. Stop infusion immediately for any signs of acute respiratory distress. May represent pulmonary embolus or interstitial pneumonitis, which may be caused by an unseen precipitate of electrolytes (e.g., calcium and phosphates) in the solution.

FENOLDOPAM MESYLATE
(feh-**NOL**-doh-pam **MES**-ih-layt)
Corlopam

Antihypertensive
Vasodilator

USUAL DOSE

Must be given as a continuous infusion. Avoid hypotension and rapid decreases in BP. Doses ranging from 0.01 to 1.6 mcg/kg/min were studied in clinical trials. Most references suggest an initial dose of 0.1 mcg/kg/min. Doses below 0.1 mcg/kg/min have modest effects and may have minimal use. Initial doses of 0.03 to 0.1 mcg/kg/min have been associated with less reflex tachycardia than initial doses of more than 0.3 mcg/kg/min. As the dose increases, there is a greater and more rapid reduction in BP. To achieve the desired reduction in BP, titrate initial dose upward or downward in increments of 0.05 to 0.1 mcg/kg/min, no more frequently than every 15 minutes. Extend duration of intervals as desired BP goal is approached. Maximum effect of each range usually attained within 15 minutes. When the desired response is achieved, fenoldopam may be discontinued gradually or abruptly; rebound elevation of BP has not been observed. See Precautions and Drug/Lab Interactions.

See product insert for doses used in clinical trials for mild to moderate hypertension and hypertensive emergency. Manufacturer provides extensive charts documenting effects of a wide range of doses but does not suggest a standard initial dose. The manufacturer states that the initial dose may be chosen from the appropriate table and suggests selecting a dose that corresponds to the desired magnitude and rate of BP reduction.

PEDIATRIC DOSE

See comments under Usual Dose. Usual starting dose in trials was 0.2 mcg/kg/min, with an effect on mean arterial pressure (MAP) seen in 5 minutes and a maximal effect seen after 20 to 25 minutes. Increased doses of up to 0.3 to 0.5 mcg/kg/min every 20 to 30 minutes were well tolerated. Tachycardia without further decrease in MAP occurred at doses greater than 0.8 mcg/kg/min. See Maternal/Child.

DOSE ADJUSTMENTS

Dose adjustment is not required in end-stage renal disease; in patients on continuous ambulatory peritoneal dialysis (CAPD); in severe hepatic failure; or by age, gender, or race. Effects of hemodialysis have not been evaluated. ■ Caution and lower-end dosing suggested in elderly patients. Consider decreased organ function and concomitant disease or drug therapy.

DILUTION

Each 10 mg (1 mL) must be diluted with 250 mL of NS or D5W and given as a continuous infusion. (10 mg in 250 mL, 20 mg in 500 mL, or 40 mg in 1,000 mL all yield 40 mcg/mL.) Use of an infusion pump is recommended. For fluid-restricted patients, concentrations of 100 mcg/mL administered through a syringe pump have been used. 10 mg in 100 mL NS or D5W yields 100 mcg/mL.

Pediatric dilution: Mix to yield a final concentration of 60 mcg/mL (6 mg in 100 mL, 15 mg in 250 mL, or 30 mg in 500 mL of D5W or NS). Use of an infusion pump capable of delivering low infusion rates is required.

Storage: Store unopened ampules at CRT. Diluted solution is stable at CRT and normal light conditions for 24 hours. Discard any solution not used within 24 hours of preparation.

COMPATIBILITY

Consider any drug NOT listed as compatible to be INCOMPATIBLE until consulting a pharmacist; specific conditions may apply. Consider specific use and need for continuous adjustment.

One source suggests the following **compatibilities:**

Y-site: Alfentanil (Alfenta), amikacin (Amikin), aminocaproic acid (Amicar), amiodarone (Nexterone), ampicillin/sulbactam (Unasyn), argatroban, atracurium (Tracrium), atropine, aztreonam (Azactam), butorphanol (Stadol), calcium gluconate, cefazolin (Ancef), cefepime (Maxipime), cefotaxime (Claforan), cefotetan (Cefotan), ceftazidime (Fortaz), ceftriaxone (Rocephin), cefuroxime (Zinacef), chlorpromazine (Thorazine), ciprofloxacin (Cipro IV), cisatracurium (Nimbex), clindamycin (Cleocin), dexmedetomidine (Precedex), digoxin (Lanoxin), diltiazem (Cardizem), diphenhydramine (Benadryl), dobutamine, dolasetron (Anzemet), dopamine, doxycycline, droperidol (Inapsine), enalaprilat (Vasotec IV), ephedrine, epinephrine (Adrenalin), erythromycin (Erythrocin), esmolol (Brevibloc), famotidine (Pepcid IV), fentanyl (Sublimaze), fluconazole (Diflucan), gentamicin, granisetron (Kytril), haloperidol (Haldol), heparin, hetastarch in electrolytes (Hextend), hydrocortisone sodium succinate (Solu-Cortef), hydromorphone (Dilaudid), inamrinone (Amrinone), isoproterenol (Isuprel), labetalol (Trandate), levofloxacin (Levaquin), lidocaine, linezolid (Zyvox), lorazepam (Ativan), magnesium, mannitol (Osmitrol), meperidine (Demerol), metoclopramide (Reglan), metronidazole (Flagyl IV), micafungin (Mycamine), midazolam (Versed), milrinone (Primacor), morphine, nalbuphine, naloxone (Narcan), nicardipine (Cardene IV), nitroglycerin (Levophed), norepinephrine (Levophed), ondansetron (Zofran), pancuronium, phenylephrine (Neo-Synephrine), piperacillin, piperacillin/tazobactam (Zosyn), potassium chloride, procainamide (Pronestyl), promethazine (Phenergan), propofol (Diprivan), propranolol, quinupristin/dalfopristin (Synercid), ranitidine (Zantac), remifentanil (Ultiva), rocuronium (Zemuron), sufentanil (Sufenta), sulfamethoxazole/trimethoprim, theophylline, ticarcillin/clavulanate (Timentin), tobramycin, vancomycin, vecuronium, verapamil.

RATE OF ADMINISTRATION

Do not give as a bolus injection; must be given as an infusion. Use of a calibrated, mechanical infusion pump is recommended for accurate, reliable delivery of desired infusion rate. Avoid hypotension and rapid decreases in BP. Infusion may be abruptly discontinued or gradually tapered as indicated by patient condition and/or use of other antihypertensive agents. See the following chart for desired infusion rates.

Fenoldopam Adult Infusion Rate Guidelines (40 mcg/mL dilution)
Note: Concentration is different from Pediatric Patients (See Pediatric chart on next page)

Body Weight (kg)	Desired Fenoldopam Dose				
	0.025 mcg/kg/min	0.05 mcg/kg/min	0.1 mcg/kg/min	0.2 mcg/kg/min	0.3 mcg/kg/min
	Infusion Rates (mL/hr) of 40 mcg/mL solution				
40 kg	1.5 mL/hr	3 mL/hr	6 mL/hr	12 mL/hr	18 mL/hr
50 kg	1.9 mL/hr	3.8 mL/hr	7.5 mL/hr	15 mL/hr	22.5 mL/hr
60 kg	2.3 mL/hr	4.5 mL/hr	9.0 mL/hr	18 mL/hr	27 mL/hr
70 kg	2.6 mL/hr	5.3 mL/hr	10.5 mL/hr	21 mL/hr	31.5 mL/hr
80 kg	3 mL/hr	6 mL/hr	12 mL/hr	24 mL/hr	36 mL/hr
90 kg	3.4 mL/hr	6.8 mL/hr	13.5 mL/hr	27 mL/hr	40.5 mL/hr
100 kg	3.8 mL/hr	7.5 mL/hr	15 mL/hr	30 mL/hr	45 mL/hr
110 kg	4.1 mL/hr	8.3 mL/hr	16.5 mL/hr	33 mL/hr	49.5 mL/hr
120 kg	4.5 mL/hr	9 mL/hr	18 mL/hr	36 mL/hr	54 mL/hr
130 kg	4.9 mL/hr	9.8 mL/hr	19.5 mL/hr	39 mL/hr	58.5 mL/hr
140 kg	5.3 mL/hr	10.5 mL/hr	21 mL/hr	42 mL/hr	63 mL/hr
150 kg	5.6 mL/hr	11.3 mL/hr	22.5 mL/hr	45 mL/hr	67.5 mL/hr

Fenoldopam Adult Infusion Rate Guidelines (40 mcg/mL dilution) (continued)
Note: Concentration is different from Pediatric Patients (See Pediatric chart on next page)

Body Weight (kg)	Desired Fenoldopam Dose					
	0.5 mcg/kg/min	0.8 mcg/kg/min	1 mcg/kg/min	1.2 mcg/kg/min	1.4 mcg/kg/min	1.6 mcg/kg/min
	Infusion Rates (mL/hr) of 40 mcg/mL solution					
40 kg	30 mL/hr	48 mL/hr	60 mL/hr	72 mL/hr	84 mL/hr	96 mL/hr
50 kg	37.5 mL/hr	60 mL/hr	75 mL/hr	90 mL/hr	105 mL/hr	120 mL/hr
60 kg	45 mL/hr	72 mL/hr	90 mL/hr	108 mL/hr	126 mL/hr	144 mL/hr
70 kg	52.5 mL/hr	84 mL/hr	105 mL/hr	126 mL/hr	147 mL/hr	168 mL/hr
80 kg	60 mL/hr	96 mL/hr	120 mL/hr	144 mL/hr	168 mL/hr	192 mL/hr
90 kg	67.5 mL/hr	108 mL/hr	135 mL/hr	162 mL/hr	189 mL/hr	216 mL/hr
100 kg	75 mL/hr	120 mL/hr	150 mL/hr	180 mL/hr	210 mL/hr	240 mL/hr
110 kg	82.5 mL/hr	132 mL/hr	165 mL/hr	198 mL/hr	231 mL/hr	264 mL/hr
120 kg	90 mL/hr	144 mL/hr	180 mL/hr	216 mL/hr	252 mL/hr	288 mL/hr
130 kg	97.5 mL/hr	156 mL/hr	195 mL/hr	234 mL/hr	273 mL/hr	312 mL/hr
140 kg	105 mL/hr	168 mL/hr	210 mL/hr	252 mL/hr	294 mL/hr	336 mL/hr
150 kg	112.5 mL/hr	180 mL/hr	225 mL/hr	270 mL/hr	315 mL/hr	360 mL/hr

	Fenoldopam Pediatric Infusion Rate Guidelines for Pediatric Patients Between 5 and 70 kg (60 mcg/mL dilution) Note: Concentration is Different from Adult Patients				
Body Weight (kg)	**Desired Fenoldopam Dose**				
	0.2 mcg/kg/min	**0.5 mcg/kg/min**	**0.8 mcg/kg/min**	**1 mcg/kg/min**	**1.2 mcg/kg/min**
	Infusion Rates (mL/hr) of 60 mcg/mL solution				
5 kg	1 mL/hr	2.5 mL/hr	4 mL/hr	5 mL/hr	6 mL/hr
10 kg	2 mL/hr	5 mL/hr	8 mL/hr	10 mL/hr	12 mL/hr
20 kg	4 mL/hr	10 mL/hr	16 mL/hr	20 mL/hr	24 mL/hr
30 kg	6 mL/hr	15 mL/hr	24 mL/hr	30 mL/hr	36 mL/hr
40 kg	8 mL/hr	20 mL/hr	32 mL/hr	40 mL/hr	48 mL/hr
50 kg	10 mL/hr	25 mL/hr	40 mL/hr	50 mL/hr	60 mL/hr
60 kg	12 mL/hr	30 mL/hr	48 mL/hr	60 mL/hr	72 mL/hr
70 kg	14 mL/hr	35 mL/hr	56 mL/hr	70 mL/hr	84 mL/hr

ACTIONS

A peripherally acting rapid-acting vasodilator. Is an agonist at the D_1 receptor and binds with moderate affinity to the alpha$_2$ adrenoreceptor. Causes a dose-dependent fall in systolic and diastolic BP. May cause a reflex increase in HR. Onset of action begins within 5 minutes, and with continuous infusion, steady state concentrations (peak effects) are reached in 15 to 20 minutes. Increases renal blood flow by dilating both afferent and efferent arterioles. Maintains or increases glomerular filtration rate (GFR) in normotensive or hypertensive patients with or without renal insufficiency. Beneficial effects have not been seen in patients with heart failure, hepatic disease, or severe renal disease. Increases sodium excretion and decreases sodium reabsorption. Increases potassium, calcium, and phosphate excretion, with or without an increase in GFR. Elimination half-life is about 5 minutes. Metabolized in the liver primarily by conjugation (without cytochrome P_{450} enzymes). Primarily eliminated in urine; some excretion in feces.

INDICATIONS AND USES

Adult patients: In-hospital, short-term (up to 48 hours) management of severe hypertension when rapid, but quickly reversible, emergency reduction of BP is indicated, including malignant hypertension with deteriorating end-organ function.

Pediatric patients: In-hospital, short-term (up to 4 hours) for reduction in BP.

Unlabeled uses: Renal protection before study with contrast dye.

CONTRAINDICATIONS

Manufacturer states, "None known."

PRECAUTIONS

Use limited to the hospital. Adequate personnel and appropriate equipment must be available for continuous monitoring. ■ Use extreme caution in patients with glaucoma or intraocular hypertension. Has caused a dose-dependent increase in intraocular pressure. ■ Causes a dose-related tachycardia with infusion rates above 0.1 mcg/kg. May diminish over time in adults but is consistent at higher doses. Has not been reported, but could lead to ischemic cardiac events or worsened heart failure. ■ Tachycardia occurred in pediatric patients at doses greater than or equal to 0.8 mcg/kg/min. ■ May produce symptomatic hypotension. ■ Although hypotension should be avoided in all patients, use extreme caution in patients with an acute cerebral infarction or hemorrhage. ■ The effect of fenoldopam in the presence of increased intracranial pressure has not been studied. ■ Rapidly decreases serum potassium leading to hypokalemia; see Monitor. ■ Use caution; contains sulfites. Sulfite sensitivity is seen more frequently in asthmatic individuals. ■ See Drug/Lab Interactions.

Monitor: Determine patency of vein; avoid extravasation. In adults, monitor BP and HR at least every 15 minutes. Avoid hypotension. More frequent monitoring may be required, but intra-arterial BP monitoring has not been required. ■ In pediatric patients, monitoring of BP and HR should be continuous. In studies, intra-arterial monitoring was utilized. ■ Monitor serum electrolytes frequently; monitoring of serum potassium is recommended every 6 hours. Has reduced serum potassium values to less than 3 mEq/L in less than 6 hours. Oral or intravenous supplements are required. ■ Transfer to oral antihypertensive agents when BP is stable. May be added during fenoldopam infusion or following its discontinuation; monitor effects carefully. ■ See Precautions and Drug/Lab Interactions.

Patient Education: Report IV site burning or stinging promptly. ■ Request assistance to ambulate.

Maternal/Child: Category B: use only if clearly needed. ■ Use caution during breast-feeding; not known if fenoldopam is secreted in breast milk (is secreted in milk of rats). ■ Antihypertensive effects have been studied in pediatric patients under 1 month of age (at least 2 kg or full term) to 12 years of age. Pharmacokinetics are independent of age when corrected for body weight. Clinical studies did not include adolescents (12 to 16 years of age). Dose selection for this group should consider clinical condition and concomitant drug therapy.

Elderly: Dose selection should be cautious; see Dose Adjustments. ■ Response similar to other age-groups.

DRUG/LAB INTERACTIONS

No specific drug interaction studies have been conducted. ■ Concurrent use not recommended with **beta-adrenergic blocking agents** (e.g., atenolol [Tenormin], esmolol [Brevibloc], metoprolol [Lopressor], propranolol). May cause unexpected hypotension from beta-blocker inhibition of the reflex response to fenoldopam (e.g., tachycardia). ■ Has been given safely with digoxin and sublingual nitroglycerin. ■ Limited experience with concomitant use of **other antihypertensive agents** (e.g., ACE inhibitors [e.g., enalaprilat (Vasotec)], alpha$_1$-adrenergic blockers [e.g., phentolamine (Regitine), prazosin (Minipress)], calcium channel blockers [e.g., diltiazem (Cardizem), verapamil], **or thiazide or loop diuretics** [e.g., chlorothiazide (Diuril), furosemide (Lasix), torsemide (Demadex)]).

SIDE EFFECTS

Dose-dependent side effects may include hypotension with resulting tachycardia, flushing, headache, and nausea. Additional side effects unrelated to dose include abdominal pain or fullness, anxiety, back pain, constipation, diaphoresis, diarrhea, dizziness, increased SCr, injection site reaction, insomnia, nasal congestion, postural hypotension, urinary infection, and vomiting occurred in up to 5% of patients. Additional side effects have been reported in 0.5% to 5% of patients (see literature).

Major: Cardiac arrhythmias (e.g., bradycardia, extrasystoles, ST-T wave abnormalities, tachycardia), hypotension, hypokalemia, and myocardial infarction can occur with average doses.

ANTIDOTE

Keep physician informed of all side effects. Most will be treated symptomatically. Use oral and/or intravenous potassium to treat hypokalemia. Reduce dose gradually as desired BP is reached. Discontinue fenoldopam immediately for excessive hypotension. Half-life is short. Recovery should begin within 5 to 15 minutes; support patient as indicated (e.g., Trendelenburg position, IV fluids if appropriate). With short half-life the need for vasopressors is unlikely. Discontinue fenoldopam and treat life-threatening arrhythmias as indicated.

FENTANYL CITRATE
(**FEN**-tah-nil **SIT**-rayt)

Opioid analgesic
(agonist)
Anesthesia adjunct

Fentanyl, Fentanyl Citrate PF, Sublimaze   pH 4 to 7.5

USUAL DOSE

In all situations, use smallest effective dose at maximum intervals.

Adjunct to regional anesthesia: 50 to 100 mcg (0.05 to 0.1 mg).

Adjunct to general anesthesia: *Low dose:* 2 mcg/kg of body weight.

Moderate dose: 2 to 20 mcg/kg of body weight. Additional doses of 25 to 100 mcg may be administered as needed.

High dose: 20 to 50 mcg/kg of body weight. Additional doses of 25 mcg to one half the initial loading dose may be administered as needed.

General anesthetic: 50 to 100 mcg/kg of body weight administered with oxygen and a muscle relaxant.

Pain management (unlabeled): An initial dose of 25 to 100 mcg (0.025 to 0.1 mg). Follow with a continuous infusion of 1 to 2 mcg/kg/hr. Titrate to effect.

PEDIATRIC DOSE

Adjunct to general anesthesia in pediatric patients over 2 years of age: 1 to 3 mcg/kg/dose over 3 to 5 minutes. May repeat in 30 to 60 minutes. To give as an infusion, begin with 1 mcg/kg/hr and titrate to effect. Maximum dose is 3 mcg/kg/hr. See Maternal/Child.

Pain management (unlabeled): 0.5 to 2 mcg/kg/dose every 1 to 2 hours as needed or 0.5 to 2 mcg/kg/hr as a continuous infusion. Titrate to effect.

DOSE ADJUSTMENTS

Reduce dose in patients receiving other CNS depressants, such as general anesthetics, alcohol, anticholinergics, antihistamines, barbiturates, cimetidine (Tagamet), hypnotics, sedatives, psychotropic agents, and narcotic analgesics. When administered with narcotics, reduce initial narcotic dose to one fourth to one third of normal. ■ Reduce dose or increase intervals for elderly, debilitated, and poor-risk patients or those with impaired pulmonary, hepatic, or renal function. ■ See Drug/Lab Interactions.

DILUTION

Small volumes may be given undiluted (usually by the anesthesiologist). Further dilution with at least 5 mL of SW or NS for injection to facilitate titration is appropriate. Other IV solutions may be used. May be given through Y-tube or three-way stopcock of infusion set.

Storage: Store at room temperature and protect from light before dilution. Use promptly.

COMPATIBILITY (Underline Indicates Conflicting Compatibility Information)

Consider any drug NOT listed as compatible to be INCOMPATIBLE until consulting a pharmacist; specific conditions may apply.

One source suggests the following **compatibilities:**

Y-site: Abciximab (ReoPro), alprostadil, amiodarone (Nexterone), amphotericin B cholesteryl (Amphotec), anidulafungin (Eraxis), argatroban, atracurium (Tracrium), atropine, bivalirudin (Angiomax), caspofungin (Cancidas), cisatracurium (Nimbex), dexamethasone (Decadron), dexmedetomidine (Precedex), diazepam (Valium), diltiazem (Cardizem), diphenhydramine (Benadryl), dobutamine, dopamine, doripenem (Doribax), doxapram (Dopram), enalaprilat (Vasotec IV), epinephrine (Adrenalin), esmolol (Brevibloc), etomidate (Amidate), fenoldopam (Corlopam), furosemide (Lasix), haloperidol (Haldol), heparin, hetastarch in electrolytes (Hextend), hydrocortisone sodium succinate (Solu-Cortef), hydromorphone (Dilaudid), ketorolac (Toradol), labetalol (Trandate), levofloxacin (Levaquin), linezolid (Zyvox), lorazepam (Ativan), metoclopramide (Reglan), midazolam (Versed), milrinone (Primacor), morphine, nafcillin (Nallpen), nesiritide (Natrecor), nicardipine (Cardene IV), nitroglycerin IV, norepinephrine (Levophed), oxaliplatin (Eloxatin), palonosetron (Aloxi), pancuronium, phenobarbital (Luminal), potassium chloride (KCl), propofol (Diprivan), ranitidine (Zantac), remifentanil (Ultiva), sargramostim (Leukine), thiopental (Pentothal), vecuronium.

RATE OF ADMINISTRATION

Administer over 1 to 5 minutes. Too-rapid administration may result in apnea or respiratory paralysis. Rate must be titrated by desired dose and patient response.

ACTIONS

An opium derivative, narcotic analgesic, which is a descending CNS depressant. Approximately 100 times more potent than morphine milligram for milligram. It has definite respiratory-depressant actions that outlast its analgesic effect. In healthy individuals, respiratory rate returns to normal more quickly than with other opiates. Effective within one circulation time and lasts about 30 minutes. Effects are cumulative with repeat doses. Has little hypnotic activity, and histamine release rarely occurs. Cardiovascular system remains stable. Depresses many other senses or reflexes. Half-life is approximately 3.6 hours. Metabolized in the liver and excreted in the urine. Crosses the placental barrier. May be secreted in breast milk.

INDICATIONS AND USES

Adjunct to general and regional anesthesia. ▪ Short-term analgesia during perioperative period. ▪ Useful in short-duration minor surgery in outpatients and in diagnostic procedures or treatments that require the patient to be awake or very lightly anesthetized (e.g., bronchoscopy, radiologic studies, burn dressings, cystoscopy). ▪ For administration with a neuroleptic such as droperidol as an anesthetic premedication, for the induction of anesthesia, and as an adjunct in the maintenance of general and regional anesthesia. ▪ For use as an anesthetic agent with oxygen in selected high-risk patients, such as those undergoing open heart surgery or certain complicated neurologic or orthopedic procedures.

CONTRAINDICATIONS

Patients with known intolerance to fentanyl. In general, narcotic analgesics are also contraindicated in acute or severe bronchial asthma and if an upper airway obstruction or significant respiratory depression is present. Fentanyl is not recommended for use in labor and delivery.

PRECAUTIONS

Schedule II opioid agonists, including hydromorphone, morphine, oxymorphone, oxycodone, fentanyl, and methadone, have the highest potential for abuse and risk of producing respiratory depression. Alcohol, CNS depressants, and other opioids potentiate the respiratory depressant effects of hydromorphone, increasing the risk of respiratory depression that might result in death; see Drug/Lab Interactions. ▪ Primarily used by or under the direct observation of the anesthesiologist. ▪ Use caution in the elderly, in patients with impaired hepatic or renal function, and in patients with pulmonary disease; reduced dose may be indicated. ▪ Use extreme caution in craniotomy, head injury, and increased intracranial pressure. ▪ Respiratory depression may cause an increased Pco_2, cerebral vasodilation, and increased intracranial pressure. Clinical course of head injury may be obscured. ▪ Symptoms of acute abdominal conditions may be masked. ▪ Use caution in patients with bradyarrhythmias. ▪ Cough reflex is suppressed. ▪ Use caution in patients with benign prostatic hypertrophy, diarrhea resulting from poisoning until toxic material is eliminated, hypersensitivity to opiates, and in premature infants or labor and delivery of premature infants.

Monitor: Oxygen, controlled respiratory equipment, naloxone (Narcan), and neuromuscular blocking agents (e.g., succinylcholine) must always be available. May cause rigidity of respiratory muscles; may require a muscle relaxant to permit artificial ventilation. ▪ Observe patient frequently, monitor vital signs and oxygenation. Patient will appear to be asleep and may forget to breathe unless commanded to do so. ▪ Keep patient supine; orthostatic hypotension and fainting may occur. ▪ See Precautions.

Patient Education: Avoid alcohol or other CNS depressants (e.g., antihistamines, diazepam [Valium]). ▪ Blurred vision, dizziness, drowsiness, or light-headedness may occur; request assistance with ambulation. ▪ Review all medications for interactions.

Maternal/Child: Category C: safety for use in pregnancy not established; has impaired fertility and had embryocidal effects in rats. ▪ Postpone breastfeeding for at least 4 to 6 hours after use of fentanyl. ▪ Safety for use in pediatric patients under 2 years of age not established; has caused chest wall rigidity in neonates and may be associated with methemoglobinemia and hypotension in premature neonates; see Precautions.

Elderly: See Dose Adjustments and Precautions. ▪ May markedly decrease pulmonary ventilation. ▪ May be more sensitive to effects (e.g., respiratory depression, urinary retention, constipation). ▪ Lower doses may provide effective analgesia. ▪ Consider age-related organ impairment; may delay postoperative recovery.

DRUG/LAB INTERACTIONS
Concurrent use of **diazepam** (Valium) with higher doses of fentanyl may produce vasodilation, prolonged hypotension, and result in delayed recovery. ▪ CNS toxicity increased by **antidepressants** (e.g., amitriptyline [Elavil], imipramine [Tofranil], nortriptyline [Aventyl]), **beta-adrenergic blocking agents** (e.g., propranolol), **MAO inhibitors** (e.g., selegiline [Eldepryl]), **neuromuscular blocking agents** (e.g., atracurium [Tracrium]), **and phenothiazines** (e.g., chlorpromazine [Thorazine]). Reduced dose of both drugs may be indicated. ▪ Cardiovascular depression may result from concurrent use of **nitrous oxide and high-dose fentanyl.** ▪ Monitor closely for S/S of respiratory depression and CNS depression with concurrent use of **protease inhibitors** (e.g., saquinavir [Invirase], ritonavir [Norvir]). ▪ Concurrent use with **droperidol** (Inapsine) may cause hypotension and decrease pulmonary arterial pressure. ▪ CNS and cardiovascular effects may be additive with concurrent use of tranquilizing agents (**anti-anxiety agents** [e.g., diazepam (Valium), midazolam (Versed)]). Consider differences in the duration of action of each drug and use caution.

SIDE EFFECTS
Bradycardia, constipation, diaphoresis, hypersensitivity reactions, hypertension, hypotension, hypothermia, increased intracranial pressure, nausea, orthostatic hypotension, respiratory depression (slight), respiratory muscle rigidity, urinary retention, vomiting.
Overdose: Anaphylaxis, apnea, cardiac arrest, circulatory collapse, coma, excitation, hypotension (severe), inverted T wave on ECG, myocardial depression (severe), pinpoint pupils, respiratory depression (severe), tachycardia, death.

ANTIDOTE
Buprenorphine is sometimes used before the end of surgery to reverse fentanyl-induced anesthesia. With increasing severity of any side effect or onset of symptoms of overdose, discontinue the drug and notify the physician. Naloxone (Narcan) will reverse serious respiratory depression. A patent airway, artificial ventilation, oxygen therapy, and other symptomatic treatment must be instituted promptly. Treat hypotension with a Trendelenburg position and IV fluids or vasopressors (e.g., dopamine, norepinephrine [Levophed]) as needed. A fast-acting muscle relaxant (e.g., succinylcholine) may be required to facilitate ventilation. Use atropine to treat bradycardia. Muscle rigidity during anesthesia induction or surgery must be controlled with neuromuscular blocking agents (e.g., atracurium [Tracrium], vecuronium) and controlled ventilation with oxygen. Use a neuromuscular blocking agent prophylactically to prevent muscle rigidity or to induce muscle relaxation after rigidity occurs. Resuscitate as necessary.

FERUMOXYTOL
(**FER**-ue-**MOX**-i-tol)

Feraheme

Antianemic
Iron Supplement

pH 6 to 8

USUAL DOSE
An initial IV injection of 510 mg followed by a second IV injection of 510 mg 3 to 8 days later. After 1 month and an evaluation of the hematologic response, the recommended dose may be repeated in patients with persistent or recurrent iron deficiency anemia. Administer to hemodialysis patients at least 1 hour into dialysis session, after blood pressure has stabilized.

DOSE ADJUSTMENTS
No dose adjustment is required and no gender differences have been observed.

DILUTION
Available in a single-use vial containing 510 mg of elemental iron in 17 mL (30 mg/mL of elemental iron). Black to reddish brown in color. Administer as an undiluted IV injection.

Filters: Specific information not available.

Storage: Store unopened vials at CRT.

COMPATIBILITY
Specific information not available. Given as an IV injection. Consider flushing the IV line with NS before and after injection.

RATE OF ADMINISTRATION
May be administered at a rate up to 30 mg/sec (1 mL/sec). At this rate, a dose of 510 mg would be administered over a minimum of 17 seconds.

ACTIONS
An iron replacement product. A superparamagnetic iron oxide that is coated with a carbohydrate shell. The shell helps to isolate the bioactive iron from plasma components until the iron-carbohydrate complex enters the reticuloendothelial system macrophages of the liver, spleen, and bone marrow. The iron is released from the complex within the macrophages and then either enters the intracellular storage iron pool (e.g., ferritin) or is transferred to plasma transferrin for transport to erythroid precursor cells for incorporation into hemoglobin. Exhibits dose-dependent, capacity-limited elimination from plasma with a half-life of approximately 15 hours.

INDICATIONS AND USES
Treatment of iron deficiency anemia in adult patients with chronic kidney disease (CKD).

CONTRAINDICATIONS
Evidence of iron overload. ▪ Known hypersensitivity to ferumoxytol or any of its components. ▪ Anemia not caused by iron deficiency.

PRECAUTIONS
Use only when truly indicated to avoid excess storage of iron. Excessive therapy with parenteral iron can lead to excess storage of iron with the possibility of iatrogenic hemosiderosis. One source recommends discontinuing oral iron before administering parental iron. ▪ Life-threatening

hypersensitivity reactions, including anaphylaxis, have been reported. Reactions have occurred after the first dose or subsequent doses of ferumoxytol. Facilities for monitoring the patient and responding to any medical emergency must be available. ■ Clinically significant hypotension may occur following injection. ■ May transiently affect the diagnostic ability of MRI studies. Anticipated MRI studies should be conducted before administration of ferumoxytol. Alteration of MRI studies may last for up to 3 months. See manufacturer's prescribing information if MRI studies must be obtained after ferumoxytol administration. Ferumoxytol does not interfere with x-ray, computed tomography (CT), positron emission tomography (PET), single photon emission computed tomography (SPECT), ultrasound, or nuclear medicine imaging.

Monitor: Keep patient lying down after injection to prevent postural hypotension. BP should be stable in patients receiving hemodialysis before dose is administered. Continue to monitor BP for at least 60 minutes following dose administration. ■ Observe for hypersensitivity reactions (e.g., anaphylaxis, cardiac or cardiopulmonary arrest, clinically significant hypotension, pruritus, rash, syncope, unresponsiveness, urticaria, or wheezing) for at least 30 minutes after the injection. ■ Evaluate hematologic response (hemoglobin, hematocrit, ferritin, iron, and transferrin saturation) at least 1 month after the second injection. Regularly monitor response during parenteral iron therapy. Avoid evaluation of therapy immediately after therapy. In the 24 hours following administration, laboratory assays may overestimate serum iron and transferrin-bound iron by also measuring the iron in the ferumoxytol complex.

Patient Education: Review any possible reactions to past parenteral iron therapy. ■ Promptly report S/S of a hypersensitivity reaction (e.g., hives, itching, rash, shortness of breath, wheezing).

Maternal/Child: Category C: use during pregnancy only if potential benefit to the mother justifies the potential risk to the fetus. ■ Discontinue breast-feeding. ■ Safety and effectiveness for use in pediatric patients not established.

Elderly: No overall difference in safety and efficacy were observed between older and younger patients. However, greater sensitivity of older patients cannot be ruled out.

DRUG/LAB INTERACTIONS
Drug-drug interaction studies have not been conducted. ■ May reduce the absorption of concomitantly administered **oral iron** preparations.

SIDE EFFECTS
The most common side effects are constipation, diarrhea, dizziness, hypotension, nausea, and peripheral edema. Serious side effects may include hypersensitivity reactions (e.g., anaphylaxis, pruritus, rash, urticaria, or wheezing) and hypotension. Other reported side effects are abdominal pain, back pain, chest pain, cough, dyspnea, ecchymosis, edema, fever, headache, infusion site swelling, muscle spasm, vomiting.

Post-Marketing: Anaphylactic/anaphylactoid reactions, angioedema, cardiac/cardiopulmonary arrest, CHF, cyanosis, hypotension (clinically significant), ischemic myocardial events, loss of consciousness, syncope, tachycardia/rhythm abnormalities, and unresponsiveness.

ANTIDOTE

Notify the physician of significant side effects. Treat hypersensitivity reactions, or resuscitate as necessary. Epinephrine (Adrenalin) and diphenhydramine (Benadryl) should always be available. In overdose, monitor CBC, iron studies, vital signs, blood gases, glucose, and electrolytes. Maintain fluid and electrolyte balance. Correct acidosis with sodium bicarbonate. Deferoxamine is an iron chelating agent and may be useful in iron toxicity or overdose. Dialysis will not remove iron alone but will remove the iron deferoxamine complex and is indicated if oliguria or anuria is present.

FIBRINOGEN CONCENTRATE (HUMAN)
Coagulation Factor 1

(fi-**BRIN**-oh-gen **KON**-sen-trayt)

RiaSTAP

USUAL DOSE

Individualize dosing, duration of dosing, and frequency of administration based on the extent of bleeding, laboratory values, and clinical condition. A target fibrinogen level of 100 mg/dL should be maintained until hemostasis is obtained.

Dose when baseline fibrinogen level IS known: Calculate individually for each patient based on the target plasma fibrinogen level, which is based on the type of bleeding, actual measured plasma fibrinogen level, and body weight using the following formula:

$$\text{Dose (mg/kg)} = \frac{\text{(Target level [mg/dL]} - \text{Measured level [mg/dL])}}{1.7 \text{ (mg/dL per mg/kg body weight)}}$$

Dose when baseline fibrinogen level IS NOT known: 70 mg/kg.

DILUTION

Available as a single-use vial containing 900 to 1,300 mg lyophilized fibrinogen concentrate powder. Fibrinogen potency for each lot is printed on the vial label and carton. Bring fibrinogen concentrate to room temperature. Reconstitute with 50 mL SWI. Gently swirl until the powder is completely dissolved. Solution should be colorless and may be clear or slightly opalescent. Do not shake. Administer within 24 hours of reconstitution.

Filters: Specific information not available.

Storage: Store in carton between 2° and 25° C (36° and 77° F). Protect from light. Do not freeze in powder or reconstituted form. Do not use beyond expiration date on vial. Reconstituted solution is stable for 24 hours at CRT. Discard partially used vials.

COMPATIBILITY

Manufacturer states, "Do not mix with other medicinal products or intravenous solutions, and should be administered through a separate injection site."

RATE OF ADMINISTRATION

A single dose is to be given at a rate not to exceed 5 mL/min.

ACTIONS

Fibrinogen (factor 1) is a soluble plasma glycoprotein made from cryo-precipitate derived from pooled human plasma. It is a physiologic substrate of three enzymes—thrombin, factor XIIIa, and plasmin—and is an essential part of the coagulation cascade required for forming blood clots and preventing bleeding. In patients with congenital fibrinogen deficiency, it replaces the missing or low coagulation factor (normal levels range from 200 to 400 mg/dL). Less than 100 mg/dL can be associated with spontaneous bleeding; without treatment, these patients are at risk for potentially life-threatening bleeding. Half-life is 78.7 ± 18.13 hours (range 55.73 to 117.26 hours).

INDICATIONS AND USES

Treatment of acute bleeding episodes in patients with congenital fibrinogen deficiency, including afibrinogenemia and hypofibrinogenemia. ▪ Not indicated for use in dysfibrinogenemia (malfunction of fibrinogen in the blood).

CONTRAINDICATIONS

Known hypersensitivity to fibrinogen concentrate or its components.

PRECAUTIONS

For IV use only. ▪ Administration under the supervision of a physician is recommended. ▪ Severe hypersensitivity reactions, including anaphylaxis, may occur. Administer in a facility capable of monitoring the patient and responding to any medical emergency. Epinephrine should be immediately available. ▪ Thrombotic events (e.g., myocardial infarction, pulmonary embolism, arterial thrombosis, deep vein thrombosis) have occurred in patients with congenital fibrinogen deficiency with or without the use of fibrinogen concentrate therapy. Consider benefit versus risk. ▪ Made from human plasma and may contain infectious agents (e.g., HIV, Creutzfeldt-Jakob disease, hepatitis B, or hepatitis C). Numerous steps in the manufacturing process are used to reduce the potential for infection.

Monitor: Monitor fibrinogen levels during treatment. A target fibrinogen level of 100 mg/dL should be maintained until hemostasis is obtained. ▪ Observe for symptoms of a hypersensitivity reaction (e.g., chest pain, dizziness, dyspnea, fever, flushing, hypotension, nausea, pruritus, rash, rigors, urticaria). ▪ Monitor patients for S/S of thrombotic events.

Patient Education: Inform patient of risks for infectious agent transmission and of safety precautions taken during the manufacturing process. ▪ Promptly report symptoms of a hypersensitivity reaction (e.g., difficulty breathing, feeling faint, hives, itching, tightness in the chest, wheezing). ▪ Promptly report symptoms of a possible thrombosis (e.g., altered consciousness or speech; loss of sensation or motor power; new-onset swelling and pain in abdomen, chest, or limbs; shortness of breath).

Maternal/Child: Category C: safety and effectiveness for use during pregnancy, labor and delivery, and breast-feeding not studied; use only if clearly needed. ▪ Clinical studies included 5 patients between 8 and 16 years of age; a shorter half-life and faster clearance was noted in these patients.

Elderly: Numbers in clinical studies are insufficient to determine if the elderly respond differently than younger subjects.

DRUG/LAB INTERACTIONS
No drug interaction studies have been conducted.

SIDE EFFECTS
The most common side effects reported include chills, fever, headache, hypersensitivity reactions, nausea, and vomiting. The most serious side effects include hypersensitivity reactions (e.g., anaphylaxis, dyspnea, hives, hypotension, rash, tightness of the chest, urticaria, and wheezing) and thrombotic events (e.g., myocardial infarction, pulmonary embolism, arterial thrombosis, deep vein thrombosis).

ANTIDOTE
Keep the physician informed of all side effects. Interrupt or discontinue injection, if indicated, until symptoms subside; then resume at a tolerated rate. ▪ Discontinue fibrinogen concentrate if anaphylaxis or thrombotic events occur. Treat thrombotic events as indicated. Treat anaphylaxis with oxygen, epinephrine (Adrenalin), antihistamines (e.g., diphenhydramine [Benadryl]), vasopressors (e.g., dopamine), corticosteroids, albuterol (Ventolin), IV fluids, and ventilation equipment as indicated. Resuscitate as necessary.

FILGRASTIM
(fill-**GRASS**-tim)

G-CSF, Human Granulocyte Colony-Stimulating Factor, Neupogen

Colony-stimulating factor
Antineutropenic

pH 4

USUAL DOSE
Should not be used 24 hours before to 24 hours after the administration of cytotoxic chemotherapy because of the potential sensitivity of rapidly dividing myeloid cells to cytotoxic chemotherapy. Safety and effectiveness for use with concurrent radiation therapy has not been evaluated; simultaneous use should be avoided.

Cancer patients receiving myelosuppressive chemotherapy: 5 mcg/kg/24 hr as a single daily dose for 2 to 4 weeks based on specific chemotherapy protocol and post-nadir absolute neutrophil count (ANC). May be given IV by intermittent or continuous infusion, by SC injection, or as a 24-hour SC infusion. May be increased by 5 mcg/kg/24 hr increments for each chemotherapy cycle. Expect a transient increase in neutrophil counts in the first several days after initiation of therapy. Neutrophil response may not be adequate and dose increases as outlined may be required in heavily pretreated patients, those who have received prior radiation therapy to a significant portion of their medullary bone marrow (e.g., pelvis), bone marrow transplant patients, and/or those receiving dose-intensified chemotherapy. Maximum tolerated dose not identified. Up to 115 mcg/kg/24 hr has been used. In clinical trials, efficacy was observed at doses of 4 to 8 mcg/kg/day. For a sustained therapeutic response, therapy must be continued until the post-nadir ANC is 10,000/mm^3 after the expected chemotherapy nadir (lowest

Continued

point) has passed. Usually discontinued when this point is reached. (Average is 2 weeks or less.) In patients receiving dose-intensified chemotherapy, continue filgrastim until 2 consecutive ANCs equal to or greater than 10,000 cells/mm^3 are documented. (Range is 6 to 28 days.) See Monitor.

Patients with acute myeloid leukemia (AML) receiving induction or consolidation chemotherapy: Suggested dose is based on clinical studies: 5 mcg/kg/24 hr. Begin 24 hours after completion of induction or consolidation chemotherapy and continue daily until the ANC is equal to or greater than 1,000/mm^3 for 3 consecutive days. May be given IV by intermittent or continuous infusion, by SC injection, or as a 24-hour SC infusion.

Bone marrow transplant (BMT): 10 mcg/kg/24 hr as an IV infusion over 4 or 24 hours or as a continuous 24-hour SC infusion. Give the first dose at least 24 hours after cytotoxic chemotherapy and 24 hours after bone marrow infusion.

DOSE ADJUSTMENTS

Reduce dose or discontinue filgrastim if ANC greater than 10,000/mm^3 for 3 days. ■ During neutrophil recovery after BMT titrate the daily dose as shown in the following chart based on daily or three consecutive-day evaluations.

Guidelines for Filgrastim Dose Adjustments Following a Bone Marrow Transplant	
Absolute Neutrophil Count (ANC)	Filgrastim Dose
When ANC >1,000/mm^3 for 3 consecutive days	Reduce to 5 mcg/kg/day*
Then: If ANC remains >1,000/mm^3 for 3 more consecutive days	DC filgrastim*
Then: If ANC decreases to <1,000/mm^3	Resume at 5 mcg/kg/day

*If ANC decreases to less than 1,000/mm^3 at any time during the 5 mcg/kg/day administration, increase filgrastim to 10 mcg/kg/day; the above steps should then be followed.

DILUTION

Available as a single-dose vial with either 300 mcg/mL or 480 mcg/1.6 mL and as a prefilled syringe with 300 mcg/0.5 mL or 480 mcg/0.8 mL. Remove from refrigerator to allow to warm to room temperature (never longer than 24 hours). Confirm expiration date to ensure valid product. Avoid shaking. Contains no preservatives; use sterile technique, entering vial only once to withdraw a single dose. Dilute with 10 to 50 mL D5W to concentrations of 15 mcg/mL or greater. With concentrations from 5 to 15 mcg/mL, filgrastim must be combined with albumin to a final concentration of 2 mg/mL to prevent adsorption to plastic (e.g., add 2 mL of 5% albumin to each 50 mL of D5W). Discard any unused portion. Should be clear and colorless. Do not dilute to less than 5 mcg/mL.

Storage: Store in refrigerator before use. Do not allow to freeze. Do not expose to direct sunlight. Refrigerate diluted solutions and use within 24 hours. Avoid shaking. Discard any vial or prefilled syringe left at RT for more than 24 hours.

COMPATIBILITY   (Underline Indicates Conflicting Compatibility Information)
Consider any drug NOT listed as compatible to be INCOMPATIBLE until consulting a pharmacist; specific conditions may apply.
Manufacturer states, "Do not dilute with saline at any time; product may precipitate."
One source suggests the following **compatibilities:**
Solution: Diluted in D5W or D5W plus Albumin (human), filgrastim is **compatible** with glass bottles, PVC and polyolefin IV bags, and polypropylene syringes; see Dilution.
Y-site: Acyclovir (Zovirax), allopurinol (Aloprim), amikacin (Amikin), aminophylline, ampicillin, ampicillin/sulbactam (Unasyn), aztreonam (Azactam), bleomycin (Blenoxane), bumetanide, buprenorphine (Buprenex), butorphanol (Stadol), calcium gluconate, carboplatin (Paraplatin), carmustine (BiCNU), cefazolin (Ancef), cefotetan (Cefotan), ceftazidime (Fortaz), chlorpromazine (Thorazine), cisplatin (Platinol), cyclophosphamide (Cytoxan), cytarabine (ARA-C), dacarbazine (DTIC), daunorubicin (Cerubidine), dexamethasone (Decadron), diphenhydramine (Benadryl), doxorubicin (Adriamycin), doxycycline, droperidol (Inapsine), enalaprilat (Vasotec IV), famotidine (Pepcid IV), fluconazole (Diflucan), fludarabine (Fludara), gallium nitrate (Ganite), ganciclovir (Cytovene), gentamicin, granisetron (Kytril), haloperidol (Haldol), hydrocortisone sodium succinate (Solu-Cortef), hydromorphone (Dilaudid), idarubicin (Idamycin), ifosfamide (Ifex), imipenem-cilastatin (Primaxin), leucovorin calcium, lorazepam (Ativan), mechlorethamine (nitrogen mustard), melphalan (Alkeran), meperidine (Demerol), mesna (Mesnex), methotrexate, metoclopramide (Reglan), mitoxantrone (Novantrone), morphine, nalbuphine, ondansetron (Zofran), potassium chloride (KCl), promethazine (Phenergan), ranitidine (Zantac), sodium bicarbonate, streptozocin (Zanosar), sulfamethoxazole/trimethoprim, ticarcillin/clavulanate (Timentin), tobramycin, vancomycin, vinblastine, vincristine, vinorelbine (Navelbine), zidovudine (AZT, Retrovir).
RATE OF ADMINISTRATION
Recent studies suggest that an extended infusion time (intermittent or continuous) promotes increased recovery of neutrophils.
Intermittent infusion: A single dose over 15 to 30 minutes.
Continuous infusion: A single dose over 4 or 24 hours. In all situations flush IV line with D5W before and after administration.
ACTIONS
A human granulocyte colony-stimulating factor (G-CSF). Colony-stimulating factors are glycoproteins that bind to specific hematopoietic cell surface receptors and stimulate proliferation, differentiation commitment, and some end-cell functional activation. Endogenous granulocyte colony-stimulating factors are produced by monocytes, fibroblasts, and endothelial cells. They are lineage-specific with selectivity for the neutrophil lineage. With recombinant DNA technology, filgrastim is produced by specifically prepared *Escherichia coli* bacteria inserted with the human G-CSF gene. It regulates the production of neutrophils within the bone marrow. Although not species specific, it mimics the actions of endogenous glycoprotein. By accelerating the recovery of neutrophil counts following a variety of chemotherapy regimens, it decreases infections manifested by febrile neutropenia, need for hospitalization, and IV antibiotic usage. May also cause some increase in lymphocyte and monocyte

counts. Increase in circulating neutrophils is dose-dependent, and a return to baseline occurs shortly after discontinuation (50% of baseline in 1 to 2 days and to pretreatment levels in 1 to 7 days). Half-life is approximately 3.5 hours.

INDICATIONS AND USES

Decrease the incidence of infection (febrile neutropenia) in patients with non-myeloid malignancies receiving myelosuppressive anticancer drugs associated with a significant incidence of severe neutropenia with fever. ■ Reduce the time to neutrophil recovery and the duration of fever, following induction or consolidation chemotherapy treatment of adults with AML. ■ Decrease duration of neutropenia and related clinical problems (e.g., febrile neutropenia) in patients with non-myeloid malignancies receiving myeloablative chemotherapy followed by BMT. ■ Used SC to treat severe chronic neutropenia (e.g., congenital, cyclic, or idiopathic) after all diseases associated with neutropenia have been ruled out. ■ Used SC or as a 24-hour SC infusion to mobilize hematopoietic progenitor cells into the peripheral blood for collection by leukapheresis with transplantation after myeloablative chemotherapy.

Unlabeled uses: Treat drug-induced neutropenia. ■ Treat neutropenia caused by HIV disease, opportunistic infections (e.g., cytomegalovirus), or antiretroviral drugs (e.g., ganciclovir, zidovudine) in HIV-infected patients.

CONTRAINDICATIONS

Hypersensitivity to *E. coli*–derived proteins, filgrastim, or any of its components (e.g., sorbitol, tween 80).

PRECAUTIONS

Should be administered under the direction of a physician knowledgeable about appropriate use for each indication (e.g., expert in bone marrow transplantation). ■ Frequently given by SC injection or SC continuous infusion. ■ Effective in patients receiving chemotherapy with protocols containing cisplatin, cyclophosphamide, doxorubicin, etoposide, ifosfamide, mesna, methotrexate, vinblastine, and similar antineoplastic agents. ■ Effectiveness has not been evaluated in patients receiving chemotherapy associated with delayed myelosuppression (e.g., nitrosoureas [carmustine]), with mitomycin C, or with myelosuppressive doses of antimetabolites (e.g., fluorouracil or cytosine arabinoside). ■ Use extreme caution in any malignancy with myeloid characteristics; can act as a growth factor for any tumor type, particularly myeloid malignancies. ■ Acute respiratory distress syndrome (ARDS) may occur in septic patients. Evaluate for ARDS if fever, lung infiltrates, or respiratory distress develop. ■ Hypersensitivity reactions have been reported. May occur with first or subsequent doses; see Monitor. ■ Splenic rupture has been reported; fatalities have occurred. ■ Only physicians qualified to treat sickle cell patients should prescribe filgrastim to them; severe sickle cell crises have been reported and fatalities have occurred. Consider risk versus benefit. ■ Use caution in patients with congenital severe chronic neutropenia (SCN); risk of developing cytogenetic abnormalities, myelodysplastic syndromes (MDS), and acute myelogenous leukemia (AML) may be increased. ■ Chronic use at varying doses over several years may cause subclinical splenomegaly in adults and pediatric patients. ■ Alveolar hemorrhage manifesting as pulmonary infiltrates and hemoptysis and requiring hospitalization has been reported in healthy donors undergoing peripheral blood progenitor cell (PBPC) mobilization. Hemoptysis resolved when filgrastim was discontinued.

Monitor: Obtain a CBC and platelet count before chemotherapy begins and twice weekly thereafter to monitor the neutrophil count and to avoid leukocytosis. Following cytotoxic chemotherapy, the neutrophil nadir occurs earlier during cycles when filgrastim is used, duration of severe neutropenia is reduced, and WBC differentials may have a left shift. ■ Increase monitoring of CBC and platelet count to 3 times a week after bone marrow infusion. ■ In patients with SCN, obtain CBC with differential and platelet count twice a week for the first 4 weeks of therapy and during the 2 weeks following any dose adjustment. Once the patient is clinically stable, obtain labs monthly during the first year of therapy and quarterly or as indicated thereafter. ■ Perform annual bone marrow and cytogenic evaluations in patients with congenital neutropenia throughout the duration of treatment. ■ Because higher doses of chemotherapy may be tolerated, side effects associated with the chemotherapeutic drug may be more pronounced; observe carefully. ■ Observe for S/S of hypersensitivity reactions. Symptoms usually occur within 30 minutes of administration, are more common with the IV route, and usually involve at least two body systems (e.g., skin [facial edema, rash, urticaria], respiratory [dyspnea, wheezing], and cardiovascular [hypotension, tachycardia]). ■ Evaluate patients complaining of left upper abdominal pain and/or shoulder tip pain for an enlarged spleen or splenic rupture. ■ Monitor respiratory status. ■ Use caution with any additional drugs known to lower the platelet count. ■ See Precautions.

Patient Education: Promptly report any symptoms of infection (e.g., fever), abdominal or shoulder tip pain, or hypersensitivity reaction (itching, redness, swelling at the injection site). ■ May be self-injected SC by the patient at home; requires instruction. Literature includes a patient handout.

Maternal/Child: Category C: safety for use during pregnancy not established. Very large doses have caused fetal damage and death in rabbits. Use only if benefit justifies the potential risk to the fetus. Women who become pregnant during filgrastim therapy are encouraged to enroll in Amgen's Pregnancy Surveillance Program. ■ Secretion through breast milk not established; use caution during breast-feeding. ■ Safety and effectiveness for use in pediatric patients not established. Has been used in pediatric patients from 1 month to 18 years of age. Experience similar to adult population in patients with cancer. May cause bone pain, fever, or rash. ■ The relationship is unclear; however, pediatric patients with congenital neutropenia have developed cytogenic abnormalities and have undergone transformation to MDS and AML while receiving filgrastim.

Elderly: Age-related differences in safety and efficacy have not been observed.

DRUG/LAB INTERACTIONS

Interaction with other drugs has not been evaluated. ■ Use with caution **any drug that may potentiate the release of neutrophils** (e.g., lithium). Concurrent use with **vincristine** may cause a severe atypical neuropathy (foot pain, severe motor weakness). ■ Increased hematopoietic activity of the bone marrow in response to growth factor therapy has been associated with transient positive bone-imaging changes. Consider when interpreting **bone-imaging results.** ■ Increases in **LDH, serum alkaline phosphatase, and serum uric acid** have been seen.

SIDE EFFECTS

Diarrhea, fever, mucositis, nausea, and vomiting. No serious adverse reactions that would limit the use of the product have been reported. Hypersensitivity reactions (itching, redness, swelling at the injection site) have occurred; anaphylaxis has not occurred but is possible. Complaints of dose-related bone pain are common and may require analgesics. With doses above 5 mcg/kg/day, leukocytosis (WBC counts greater than 100,000/mm^3) has occurred in 5% of patients with no adverse effects reported. Cutaneous vasculitis has occurred in a few patients. Reduced dose may be indicated with subsequent treatment.

Post-Marketing: Sweet's syndrome (acute febrile neutrophilic dermatosis).

ANTIDOTE

Notify physician promptly if any signs of infection (fever) or other potential side effects occur. Monitor potential leukocytosis with twice-weekly CBCs. Discontinue therapy after ANC surpasses 10,000/mm^3 and the chemotherapy nadir has occurred. Discontinue filgrastim and notify physician immediately if a generalized hypersensitivity reaction should occur. Treat hypersensitivity reactions as indicated. Withhold or discontinue for other side effects (e.g., ARDS, hemoptysis).

FLUCONAZOLE

(flew-**KON**-ah-zohl)

Diflucan

Antifungal

pH 3.5 to 8

USUAL DOSE

IV dose has been used for a maximum of 14 days. Plasma levels are similar with IV or oral, so oral dose can replace IV dose at any time. See Monitor.

Oropharyngeal candidiasis: Initial dose of 200 mg followed by 100 mg/day for a minimum of 14 days. PO maintenance therapy usually required in patients with AIDS to prevent relapse.

Esophageal candidiasis: Initial dose of 200 mg followed by 100 mg/day for a minimum of 21 days and for at least 2 weeks after symptoms subside. Up to 400 mg/24 hr may be used.

Urinary tract or peritoneal candidiasis: 50 to 200 mg/day has been used.

Systemic candidiasis: Optimum therapeutic dose and duration of therapy not established. Doses up to 400 mg/day have been used. Initial dose of 400 mg followed by 200 mg/day for a minimum of 28 days and for at least 2 weeks after symptoms subside.

Treatment of acute cryptococcal meningitis: Initial dose of 400 mg followed by 200 mg/day for a minimum of 10 to 12 weeks after CSF culture becomes negative. Another source suggests a loading dose of 400 mg twice a day for 2 days followed by 400 mg/day for the same duration.

Suppression of cryptococcal meningitis: 200 mg/day. Usually required in patients with AIDS to prevent relapse.

Prevention of candidiasis in bone marrow transplant: 400 mg/day. If severe neutropenia (less than 500/mm^3) is expected, begin fluconazole prophylaxis several days ahead of expected neutropenia. Continue for 7 days after neutrophils reach 1,000/mm^3.

PEDIATRIC DOSE

Experience with pediatric patients is limited; see Maternal/Child.

In pediatric patients, 3 mg/kg is equivalent to an adult dose of 100 mg, 6 mg/kg to 200 mg, and 12 mg/kg to 400 mg. Some older pediatric patients may have clearance similar to an adult. Do not exceed 600 mg/day.

Oropharyngeal candidiasis: Initial dose of 6 mg/kg of body weight followed by 3 mg/kg/day for a minimum of 14 days.

Esophageal candidiasis: Initial dose of 6 mg/kg of body weight followed by 3 mg/kg/day for a minimum of 21 days and for at least 2 weeks after symptoms subside. Up to 12 mg/kg has been used.

Systemic candidiasis: 6 to 12 mg/kg/day. See Comments in Adult Dose.

Treatment of acute cryptococcal meningitis: Initial dose of 12 mg/kg of body weight followed by 6 mg/kg/day for a minimum of 10 to 12 weeks after CSF culture becomes negative. Up to 12 mg/kg/day has been used.

Suppression of cryptococcal meningitis: 6 mg/kg/day.

NEONATAL DOSE

Experience is limited; see Maternal/Child.

2 weeks to 3 months of age with meningitis or septicemia: 5 to 6 mg/kg/day PO or by IV infusion over 1 hour, or 10 mg/kg as a *loading dose* followed by 5 mg/kg.

Birth to 2 weeks of age with meningitis or septicemia: Manufacturer suggests using pediatric doses and extending the intervals to once every 72 hours. Prolonged half-life is seen in premature newborns (gestational age 26 to 29 weeks). After 2 weeks, dose may be given every 24 hours.

DOSE ADJUSTMENTS

In all adult situations the infecting organism and response to therapy may justify increased doses up to 400 mg daily. ■ Reduce each dose by 50% in patients with a CrCl at or less than 50 mL/min. ■ Give 100% of the recommended dose after each dialysis in patients receiving regular dialysis. ■ See Drug/Lab Interactions.

DILUTION

Packaged prediluted and ready for use as an iso-osmotic solution containing 2 mg/mL in both glass bottles and Viaflex Plus plastic containers. Do not remove moisture barrier overwrap of plastic container until ready for use. Tear overwrap down side at slit to open, and remove sterile inner bag. Plastic may appear somewhat opaque due to sterilization process but will clear. Squeeze inner bag firmly to check for leaks. Discard if leakage noted; sterility is impaired. Do not use if cloudy or precipitated.

Storage: Store glass bottles between 5° C (41° F) and 30° C (86° F); store plastic containers between 5° C (41° F) and 25° C (77° F). Protect both from freezing.

COMPATIBILITY   (Underline Indicates Conflicting Compatibility Information)

Consider any drug NOT listed as compatible to be INCOMPATIBLE until consulting a pharmacist; specific conditions may apply.

Manufacturer states, "Do not add supplementary medication."

One source suggests the following **compatibilities** *(not recommended by manufacturer):*

Additive: Acyclovir (Zovirax), amikacin (Amikin), amphotericin B (generic), cefazolin (Ancef), ceftazidime (Fortaz), ciprofloxacin (Cipro IV), clindamycin (Cleocin), gentamicin, heparin, meropenem (Merrem IV), metronidazole (Flagyl IV), morphine, piperacillin, potassium chloride (KCl), theophylline.

Y-site: Acyclovir (Zovirax), aldesleukin (Proleukin), allopurinol (Aloprim), amifostine (Ethyol), amikacin (Amikin), aminophylline, amiodarone (Nexterone), ampicillin/sulbactam (Unasyn), anidulafungin (Eraxis), aztreonam (Azactam), benztropine (Cogentin), bivalirudin (Angiomax), caspofungin (Cancidas), cefazolin (Ancef), cefepime (Maxipime), cefotetan (Cefotan), cefoxitin (Mefoxin), ceftazidime (Fortaz), chlorpromazine (Thorazine), cisatracurium (Nimbex), daptomycin (Cubicin), dexamethasone (Decadron), dexmedetomidine (Precedex), diltiazem (Cardizem), dimenhydrinate, diphenhydramine (Benadryl), dobutamine, docetaxel (Taxotere), dopamine, doripenem (Doribax), doxorubicin liposomal (Doxil), droperidol (Inapsine), drotrecogin alfa (Xigris), etoposide phosphate (Etopophos), famotidine (Pepcid IV), fenoldopam (Corlopam), filgrastim (Neupogen), fludarabine (Fludara), foscarnet (Foscavir), gallium nitrate (Ganite), ganciclovir (Cytovene), gemcitabine (Gemzar), gentamicin, granisetron (Kytril), heparin, hetastarch in electrolytes (Hextend), immune globulin intravenous (Gamunex), leucovorin calcium, linezolid (Zyvox), lorazepam (Ativan), melphalan (Alkeran), meperidine (Demerol), meropenem (Merrem IV), metoclopramide (Reglan), metronidazole (Flagyl IV), midazolam (Versed), morphine, nafcillin (Nallpen), nitroglycerin IV, ondansetron (Zofran), oxacillin (Bactocill), paclitaxel (Taxol), pancuronium, pemetrexed (Alimta), penicillin G potassium, phenytoin (Dilantin), piperacillin/tazobactam (Zosyn), prochlorperazine (Compazine), promethazine (Phenergan), propofol (Diprivan), quinupristin/dalfopristin (Synercid 2 mg/mL), ranitidine (Zantac), remifentanil (Ultiva), sargramostim (Leukine), tacrolimus (Prograf), teniposide (Vumon), theophylline, thiotepa, ticarcillin/clavulanate (Timentin), tigecycline (Tygacil), tobramycin, vancomycin, vasopressin, vecuronium, vinorelbine (Navelbine), zidovudine (AZT, Retrovir).

RATE OF ADMINISTRATION
A single dose as a continuous infusion at a rate not to exceed 200 mg/hr. Do not use plastic containers in series connections; air embolism could result.

ACTIONS
A synthetic, broad-spectrum, bis-Triazole antifungal agent. Inhibits fungal growth of *Candida* and *Cryptococcus neoformans* by acting on a key enzyme and depriving the fungus of ergosterol; the cell membrane becomes unstable and can no longer function normally. Human sterol synthesis is not affected. Peak plasma concentrations achieved in 1 to 2 hours; half-life extends for 30 hours (range 20 to 50 hours). Administration of a loading dose (on day 1) of twice the usual daily dose results in a plasma concentration close to steady state by day 2 when given IV or PO. Penetrates into all body fluids in similar and effective concentrations and remains constant with daily single-dose administration. 80% excreted as unchanged drug and about 11% excreted as metabolites in the urine. Secreted in breast milk.

INDICATIONS AND USES

Oropharyngeal and esophageal candidiasis. ▪ Serious candidal infections, including GU tract infections, peritonitis, and systemic Candida infections including candidemia, disseminate candidiasis, and pneumonia. May be an appropriate and less toxic alternative to amphotericin B. ▪ Cryptococcal meningitis, including suppressive therapy to prevent relapse. ▪ Prevention of candidiasis in bone marrow transplant patients. ▪ Used orally for additional indications (e.g., candidiasis prophylaxis).

Unlabeled uses: Has been used in many other fungal or parasitic infections.

CONTRAINDICATIONS

Concurrent use with cisapride (Propulsid), hypersensitivity to fluconazole or any of its components. Use caution in patients hypersensitive to other azoles (e.g., ketoconazole).

PRECAUTIONS

For IV use only; do not give IM. ▪ Specimens for fungal culture and serologic and histopathologic testing should be obtained before therapy to isolate and identify causative organisms. Therapy may begin as soon as all specimens are obtained and before results are known. ▪ Inadequate treatment may lead to a recurrence of active infection; continue treatment until clinical parameters or laboratory tests indicate that active fungal infection has subsided. See specific recommendations in Usual Dose. ▪ Use caution in patients with pre-existing liver disease. ▪ Serious hepatotoxicity may occur. Causal relationship uncertain, but many patients are taking hepatotoxic drugs for treatment of malignancies and AIDS. Note any abnormal liver function tests (e.g., AST). If any clinical signs and symptoms consistent with liver disease develop, discontinue drug. Has caused deaths. ▪ Associated with prolongation of the QT interval. Rare cases of torsades de pointes have been reported. More common in seriously ill patients with multiple confounding factors, such as heart disease, electrolyte abnormalities, and concomitant medications that may have been contributory (e.g., class IA antiarrhythmic agents [e.g., quinidine, procainamide (Pronestyl)] and class III antiarrhythmic agents [e.g., amiodarone (Nexterone), sotalol]). ▪ Exfoliative skin disorders have been reported.

Monitor: Obtain baseline liver function tests and monitor periodically during treatment. ▪ Observe for S/S of hypersensitivity or skin reactions. ▪ Consider ECG monitoring in patients at risk for QT prolongation. ▪ See Drug/Lab Interactions.

Patient Education: May cause serious problems with selected medications; review prescription and nonprescription drugs with physician or pharmacist.

Maternal/Child: Category C: safety for use in pregnancy and breast-feeding not established. Use in pregnancy only if potential benefits outweigh risk to fetus. ▪ Use in nursing mothers is not recommended. ▪ Safety profile has been studied in pediatric patients ages 1 day to 17 years. Efficacy in pediatric patients under 6 months of age has not been established. However, a small number of patients ranging from age 1 day to 6 months have been treated safely (unlabeled).

Elderly: Differences in response compared to younger adults not identified; however, may be at increased risk for side effects (e.g., acute renal failure, anemia, diarrhea, rash, and vomiting). ▪ Use caution, consider decreased cardiac, hepatic, or renal function and effects of concomitant disease or other drug therapy. ▪ See Dose Adjustments and Drug/Lab Interactions.

DRUG/LAB INTERACTIONS

Potentiated by **hydrochlorothiazide** (HydroDIURIL); decreases renal clearance of fluconazole. ▪ Inhibits metabolism and increases serum levels of **cyclosporine, phenytoin, tacrolimus** (Prograf), **and theophyllines;** careful monitoring of their plasma levels is required; nephrotoxicity has been reported with tacrolimus. ▪ Potentiates **coumarin-type anticoagulants** (e.g., warfarin); monitor PT and INR frequently. ▪ Potentiates **sulfonylureas** (oral hypoglycemic agents [e.g., glimepiride (Amaryl), glipizide (Glucotrol XL), glyburide (DiaBeta), tolbutamide]); monitor blood glucose levels. Adjust the dose of the oral hypoglycemic agent as indicated. ▪ **Rifampin** increases metabolism; fluconazole dose may need to be increased. One source recommends avoiding concurrent use. ▪ Increases serum levels of **zidovudine** (AZT, Retrovir). ▪ Increases serum levels of **rifabutin** (Mycobutin). Uveitis has been reported in patients receiving rifabutin and fluconazole concomitantly. Monitoring is recommended. ▪ Risk of cardiac arrhythmias increased with **cisapride** (Propulsid); concurrent use not recommended; see Contraindications. ▪ Fluconazole may inhibit metabolism and increase plasma concentrations of **carbamazepine** (Tegretol); monitor carbamazepine concentrations. ▪ Avoid concomitant use with **voriconazole** (VFEND). Potential for voriconazole toxicity remains if voriconazole is initiated within 24 hours of the last dose of fluconazole. ▪ May decrease metabolism and increase serum concentrations of **celecoxib** (Celebrex). ▪ May decrease metabolism and increase serum concentrations of **selected benzodiazepines** that are metabolized by the cytochrome P_{450} system (e.g., diazepam [Valium], midazolam [Versed]); a decrease in benzodiazepine dose should be considered. ▪ May increase serum concentrations and adverse effects of **alfentanil** (Alfenta), **buspirone** (BuSpar), **corticosteroids, haloperidol** (Haldol), **losartan** (Cozaar), **nisoldipine** (Sular), **sirolimus** (Rapamune), **tolterodine** (Detrol), **tricyclic antidepressants** (e.g., amitriptyline [Elavil], imipramine [Tofranil]), **and vinca alkaloids** (e.g., vincristine). Reduce doses of the above drugs as indicated to avoid toxicity. Dose may need to be increased when fluconazole is discontinued. **Tolterodine** dose should be limited to no more than 1 mg twice daily when coadministered with fluconazole. ▪ Coadministration may increase plasma levels of **protease inhibitors** (e.g., nelfinavir [Viracept], ritonavir [Norvir]), increasing the risk of toxicity. ▪ Increases serum levels of **HMG-CoA reductase inhibitors** (e.g., atorvastatin [Lipitor], lovastatin [Mevacor], simvastatin [Zocor]); rhabdomyolysis has been reported. If coadministration is necessary, reduced doses of the HMG-CoA reductase inhibitor are indicated. **Pravastatin** (Pravachol) levels may be the least affected. ▪ May increase the plasma concentrations and therapeutic effects of **zolpidem** (Ambien). ▪ May **elevate liver function tests** (e.g., ALT, AST, alkaline phosphatase, and bilirubin).

SIDE EFFECTS

More common in HIV-infected patients.

Abdominal pain, diarrhea, dizziness, dry mouth, dyspepsia, exfoliative skin disorders, headache, hepatic reactions, hypercholesterolemia, hypersensitivity reactions (including anaphylaxis with angioedema, face edema, and pruritus), hypertriglyceridemia, hypokalemia, increased appetite, increased sweating, leukopenia (including neutropenia and agranulocytosis), nausea, pallor, QT prolongation, rash, seizures, taste perversion, thrombocytopenia, torsades de pointes, tremor, vomiting.

Overdose: Cyanosis, decreased motility, decreased respirations, hallucinations, lacrimation, loss of balance, salivation, urinary incontinence. Clonic convulsions preceded death in experimental animals.

ANTIDOTE

Notify physician of all side effects; most will be treated symptomatically. Discontinue drug and notify physician of abnormal liver function tests progressing to clinical signs and symptoms of liver disease. Rash may be the first sign of an exfoliative skin disorder in immunocompromised patients; discontinue drug and notify physician. In overdose a 3-hour dialysis session will decrease plasma levels by 50%. Treat anaphylaxis or resuscitate if indicated.

FLUDARABINE PHOSPHATE BBW
(floo-**DAIR**-ah-bean **FOS**-fayt)

Fludara

Antineoplastic
(antimetabolite)

pH 7.2 to 8.2 (lyophilized)
pH 7.3 to 7.7 (liquid)

USUAL DOSE

25 mg/M^2/day for 5 consecutive days. Repeat every 4 weeks. Optimum duration of treatment not established. If there is no major toxicity, treat until maximum response achieved, then administer three additional complete cycles.

PEDIATRIC DOSE

Safety and effectiveness for use in pediatric patients not established; see Maternal/Child.

Pediatric acute lymphocytic leukemia (ALL) patients (unlabeled): Give an initial loading bolus of 10.5 mg/M^2 on Day 1 followed by a continuous infusion of 30.5 mg/M^2/day on Days 1 through 5.

Pediatric patients with solid tumors (unlabeled): Dose-limiting myelosuppression was observed with a loading dose of 8 mg/M^2 on Day 1 followed by a continuous infusion of 23.5 mg/M^2/day on Days 1 through 5. Maximum tolerated dose in solid tumor pediatric patients was a loading dose of 7 mg/M^2/day followed by a continuous infusion of 20 mg/M^2/day for 5 days.

DOSE ADJUSTMENTS

Decrease or delay dose based on evidence of hematologic or nonhematologic toxicity. Increased toxicity may occur in the elderly and in patients with renal insufficiency or bone marrow impairment. Monitor closely and adjust dose as indicated. ■ Adjust initial starting doses for patients with renal impairment as indicated in the following table.

Fludarabine Starting Dose Adjustment for Renal Impairment	
Creatinine Clearance	Starting Dose
≥80 mL/min	25 mg/M^2 (full dose)
50-79 mL/min	20 mg/M^2
30-49 mL/min	15 mg/M^2
<30 mL/min	Do not administer

DILUTION
Specific techniques required; see Precautions. Available as a sterile solution 50 mg/2 mL (25 mg/mL) or as a lyophilized solid cake (50 mg) requiring reconstitution with 2 mL of SW for injection (25 mg/mL). Should dissolve within 15 seconds. In clinical studies, each single dose was further diluted in 100 to 125 mL of NS or D5W and given as an infusion over 30 minutes.
Filters: Specific information from studies not available; contact manufacturer for further information.
Storage: Refrigerate between 2° and 8° C (36° to 46° F) before dilution. No preservative; use within 8 hours of dilution.

COMPATIBILITY
Consider any drug NOT listed as compatible to be INCOMPATIBLE until consulting a pharmacist; specific conditions may apply.
Manufacturer states, "Should not be mixed with other drugs."
One source suggests the following **compatibilities** *(not recommended by manufacturer):*
Y-site: Allopurinol (Aloprim), amifostine (Ethyol), amikacin (Amikin), aminophylline, ampicillin, ampicillin/sulbactam (Unasyn), aztreonam (Azactam), bleomycin (Blenoxane), butorphanol (Stadol), carboplatin (Paraplatin), carmustine (BiCNU), cefazolin (Ancef), cefepime (Maxipime), cefotaxime (Claforan), cefotetan (Cefotan), ceftazidime (Fortaz), ceftriaxone (Rocephin), cefuroxime (Zinacef), cisplatin (Platinol), clindamycin (Cleocin), cyclophosphamide (Cytoxan), cytarabine (ARA-C), dacarbazine (DTIC), dactinomycin (Cosmegen), dexamethasone (Decadron), diphenhydramine (Benadryl), doxorubicin (Adriamycin), doxycycline, droperidol (Inapsine), etoposide (VePesid), etoposide phosphate (Etopophos), famotidine (Pepcid IV), filgrastim (Neupogen), fluconazole (Diflucan), fluorouracil (5-FU), furosemide (Lasix), gemcitabine (Gemzar), gentamicin, granisetron (Kytril), haloperidol (Haldol), heparin, hydrocortisone sodium succinate (Solu-Cortef), hydromorphone (Dilaudid), ifosfamide (Ifex), imipenem-cilastatin (Primaxin), lorazepam (Ativan), magnesium sulfate, mannitol, mechlorethamine (nitrogen mustard), melphalan (Alkeran), meperidine (Demerol), mesna (Mesnex), methotrexate, methylprednisolone (Solu-Medrol), metoclopramide (Reglan), mitoxantrone (Novantrone), morphine, multivitamins (M.V.I.), nalbuphine, ondansetron (Zofran), pentostatin (Nipent), piperacillin, piperacillin/tazobactam (Zosyn), potassium chloride (KCl), promethazine (Phenergan), ranitidine (Zantac), sodium bicarbonate, sulfamethoxazole/trimethoprim, teniposide (Vumon), thiotepa, ticarcillin/clavulanate (Timentin), tobramycin, vancomycin, vinblastine, vincristine, vinorelbine (Navelbine), zidovudine (AZT, Retrovir).

RATE OF ADMINISTRATION
Single daily dose properly diluted for infusion over 30 minutes.

ACTIONS
A potent antineoplastic agent. A fluorinated nucleotide analog of the antiviral agent vidarabine. Rapidly converts to the active metabolite 2-fluoro-ara-ATP and interferes with the synthesis of DNA. Actual mechanism of action unknown and may be multifaceted. Median time to response in studies of patients with refractory chronic lymphocytic leukemia (CLL) was 7 to 21 weeks (range 1 to 68 weeks). Elimination half-life is approximately 20 hours. Total body clearance of the active metabolite is

correlated with the CrCl, indicating the importance of renal excretion for drug elimination.

INDICATIONS AND USES
Treatment of patients with B-cell CLL who have not responded to or progressed during treatment with at least one standard alkylating agent–containing regimen. ▪ Safety and effectiveness in previously untreated or nonrefractory patients with CLL not established.

Unlabeled uses: Treatment of non-Hodgkin's lymphoma, acute lymphocytic leukemia, acute myeloid leukemia, prolymphocytic leukemia or prolymphocytoid variant of CLL, mycosis fungoides, hairy-cell leukemia, and Waldenström's macroglobulinemia. Dose and/or efficacy not established.

CONTRAINDICATIONS
Hypersensitivity to fludarabine or its components (e.g., mannitol and sodium hydroxide). ▪ Not recommended for use in patients with severely impaired renal function (CrCl less than 30 mL/min). ▪ Not recommended for use in combination with pentostatin (Nipent); see Drug/Lab Interactions.

PRECAUTIONS
Follow guidelines for handling cytotoxic agents. See Appendix A, p. 1429. ▪ Administered by or under the direction of the physician specialist. ▪ Use with caution in advanced age, renal insufficiency, or bone marrow impairment, or in patients with immunodeficiency or a history of opportunistic infection. ▪ Severe myelosuppression (anemia, neutropenia, and thrombocytopenia) is common. Median time to nadir counts was 13 days for granulocytes and 16 days for platelets. ▪ Most patients have hematologic impairment at baseline because of disease or prior myelosuppressive therapy. Myelosuppression may be severe and cumulative. ▪ Several instances of trilineage bone marrow hypoplasia or aplasia resulting in pancytopenia, sometimes resulting in death, have been reported. Clinically significant cytopenias lasted from 2 months to 1 year and occurred in untreated and previously treated patients. ▪ Use of irradiated blood product is recommended for patients requiring transfusions during fludarabine therapy because transfusion-associated graft-versus-host disease has been reported. ▪ Use caution in patients with large tumor burdens; may cause tumor lysis syndrome. Response can occur within 1 week. ▪ Life-threatening and sometimes fatal cases of autoimmune phenomena, such as hemolytic anemia, autoimmune thrombocytopenia/thrombocytopenic purpura (ITP), Evan's syndrome, and acquired hemophilia, have been reported; see Antidote. ▪ Serious, sometimes fatal infections, including opportunistic infections and reactivations of latent viral infections (e.g., varicella zoster virus [VZV], Epstein-Barr virus, and JC virus [progressive multifocal leukoencephalopathy]), as well as disease progression and transformation (e.g., Richter's syndrome) have been reported. ▪ Severe neurotoxicity characterized by delayed blindness, coma, and death has been reported in patients who received doses that were approximately 4 times greater than the recommended dose. Significant neurotoxicity has also been reported in patients receiving doses in the recommended range. Symptoms may appear 7 to 225 days after the last dose. ▪ See Side Effects.

Monitor: Observe closely for signs of toxicity, both hematologic and nonhematologic. ▪ Obtain baseline CBC, including differential and platelet count. Repeat regularly to monitor hematopoietic suppression (especially neutrophils and platelets) and hemolysis. ▪ Obtain baseline CrCl. ▪ Observe closely for all signs of infection and any fever of unknown origin. ▪ Prophylactic antibiotics may be indicated pending results of C/S in a febrile neutropenic patient. ▪ Consider prophylactic therapy in patients at risk for developing opportunistic infections. ▪ Nausea and vomiting usually less severe than many antineoplastics; prophylactic administration of antiemetics may be indicated. ▪ Monitor for early signs of tumor lysis syndrome (e.g., flank pain, hematuria). Prevention and treatment of hyperuricemia due to tumor lysis syndrome may be accomplished with adequate hydration and, if necessary, allopurinol (Aloprim) and alkalinization of urine. ▪ Monitor for evidence of hemolysis. ▪ Monitor for S/S of neurotoxicity (e.g., agitation, coma, confusion, seizures). ▪ Monitor for thrombocytopenia (platelet count less than $50,000/mm^3$). Initiate precautions to prevent excessive bleeding (e.g., inspect IV sites, skin, and mucous membranes; use extreme care during invasive procedures; test urine, emesis, stool, and secretions for occult blood).

Patient Education: Avoid pregnancy; birth control recommended for both males and females during therapy and for at least 6 months after fludarabine regimen has been completed. ▪ Use caution while driving or operating machinery. Agitation, confusion, fatigue, seizures, visual disturbances, and weakness have been reported. ▪ Adherence to periodic blood count regimen is imperative. ▪ See Appendix D, p. 1434.

Maternal/Child: Category D: both males and females should use contraception and avoid pregnancy; may cause fetal harm; see Patient Education. ▪ Discontinue breast-feeding. ▪ Safety and effectiveness for use in pediatric patients not established; however, data have been submitted to the FDA using the doses described under Pediatric Dose. In pediatric patients, platelet counts appeared to be more sensitive than hemoglobin and WBCs to the effects of fludarabine.

Elderly: See Precautions and Dose Adjustments.

DRUG/LAB INTERACTIONS

Do not use with **pentostatin** (Nipent); may increase risk of fatal pulmonary toxicity. ▪ Do not administer **live virus vaccines** during or after treatment with fludarabine.

SIDE EFFECTS

Are frequent, may be dose limiting, and may cause death. Most common side effects include myelosuppression (anemia, neutropenia, thrombocytopenia), chills, cough, diarrhea, fatigue, fever, infection (including opportunistic and pneumonia), mucositis, nausea and vomiting, and weakness. The most serious side effects include CNS toxicity, hemolytic anemia, pulmonary toxicity, and severe bone marrow suppression. Other reported side effects include agitation, anorexia, arrhythmia, bone marrow aplasia or hypoplasia (may result in pancytopenia), cerebral hemorrhage, coma, confusion, dyspnea, dysuria, edema, elevated hepatic enzymes, esophagitis, GI bleeding/hemorrhage, headache, heart failure, hemorrhagic cystitis, infection, malaise, myalgia, pain, paresthesia, peripheral neuropathy, pulmonary toxicity (ARDS, dyspnea, interstitial pulmonary infiltrate, pulmonary fibrosis, pulmonary hemorrhage, respiratory distress and failure), rashes, seizures, sinusitis, stomatitis, visual disturbances. Onset of flank pain and hematuria may indicate tumor lysis syndrome (hyperkalemia, hyperphosphatemia, hyperuricemia, hypocalcemia, metabolic acidosis, urate crystalluria, and renal failure); one reported.

Overdose: Severe bone marrow suppression (neutropenia and thrombocytopenia). Severe neurologic toxicity including delayed blindness, coma, and death occurred from 21 to 60 days after the last dose in 36% of patients treated with doses only 4 times greater than the recommended dose. Has occurred (in no more than 0.2% of patients) with average doses.

Post-Marketing: Erythema multiforme, Stevens-Johnson syndrome, toxic epidermal necrolysis, and pemphigus (some with fatal outcomes); rare cases of myelodysplastic syndrome and acute myeloid leukemia associated with prior, concomitant, or subsequent treatment with alkylating agents, topoisomerase inhibitors (e.g., irinotecan [Camptosar]), or irradiation; progressive multifocal leukoencephalopathy (PML) within a few weeks to a year (most with a fatal outcome; some patients had prior and/or concurrent chemotherapy); trilineage bone marrow hypoplasia or aplasia resulting in pancytopenia and death; and worsening or flare-up of pre-existing skin cancer lesions and/or new onset of skin cancer during or after treatment with fludarabine.

ANTIDOTE

Notify physician of all side effects. Most will be treated symptomatically. Some toxicity is necessary to produce remission. Delay or discontinue the drug for serious hematologic depression. Administration of whole blood products (e.g., packed RBCs, platelets, leukocytes) and/or blood modifiers (e.g., darbepoetin alfa [Aranesp], epoetin alfa [Epogen], filgrastim [Neupogen], pegfilgrastim [Neulasta], sargramostim [Leukine], oprelvekin [Neumega]) may be indicated to treat bone marrow toxicity. Restart as soon as signs of bone marrow recovery occur. Delay or discontinue if neurotoxicity occurs. There is no specific antidote; supportive therapy as indicated will help sustain the patient in toxicity. Symptoms of pulmonary toxicity may improve with the use of corticosteroids; rule out an infectious origin before use. Steroids may or may not be useful in controlling hemolytic episodes.

FLUMAZENIL BBW

(floo-**MAZ**-eh-nill)

Romazicon

Benzodiazepine antagonist
Antidote

pH 4

USUAL DOSE

Reversal of conscious sedation or in general anesthesia: 0.2 mg (2 mL) as an initial dose. Assess level of consciousness. May be repeated at 1-minute intervals, assessing level of consciousness between each dose, until desired level of consciousness achieved or a total cumulative dose of 1 mg (10 mL) has been given (average dose to awakening is 0.6 mg to 1 mg). If resedation occurs (may occur if flumazenil wears off before the benzodiazepine) the above process may be repeated at 20-minute intervals as indicated. Do not give more than a cumulative dose of 1 mg in a 20-minute period or 3 mg in any 1 hour.

Management of suspected benzodiazepine overdose: 0.2 mg (2 mL) as an initial dose. Assess level of consciousness. If results inadequate, give an additional dose of 0.3 mg (3 mL) in 1 minute. If results are still inadequate, 0.5 mg (5 mL) may be repeated at 1-minute intervals. Assess level of consciousness between each dose until desired level of consciousness achieved or a total cumulative dose of 3 mg (30 mL) has been given (average dose to awakening is 1 mg to 3 mg). If a partial response is achieved with 3 mg, continue dosing in 0.5-mg increments until awakening or a cumulative dose of 5 mg is reached (rarely required). If patient has not responded to a cumulative dose of 5 mg within 5 minutes, benzodiazepines are not the major cause of sedation; discontinue use. If desired results are achieved and resedation occurs (expected), no more than 1 mg given in 0.5-mg increments may be given in any 20-minute period and no more than a cumulative total dose of 3 mg in any 1 hour.

PEDIATRIC DOSE

Reversal of conscious sedation: 0.01 mg/kg (up to 0.2 mg). Assess level of consciousness. May repeat at 1 minute intervals, assessing level of consciousness between each dose until desired level of consciousness achieved or a maximum total dose of 0.05 mg/kg (or 1 mg) has been given. Mean total dose administered in trials was 0.65 mg. See Maternal/Child.

DOSE ADJUSTMENTS

Not required for the elderly. ▪ Reduce dose and extend intervals after the initial dose in impaired liver function. ▪ Individualize dose in high-risk patients. Administer the smallest amount that is effective and wait for peak effect (6 to 10 minutes). Slower titration rates and lower total doses may be especially important in these patients (see Precautions) to reduce emergent confusion and agitation, to prevent seizures, and to evaluate effect.

DILUTION

May be given undiluted through a free-flowing IV into a large vein (to minimize pain at injection site). **Compatible** with D5W, D2½W, LR, ½NS, and NS if further dilution required by a specific situation.

Storage: Store unopened vials at CRT. Discard in 24 hours if drawn undiluted into a syringe or diluted in any solution.

COMPATIBILITY
Consider any drug NOT listed as compatible to be INCOMPATIBLE until consulting a pharmacist; specific conditions may apply.
One source suggests the following **compatibilities:**
Additive: Aminophylline, dobutamine, dopamine, famotidine (Pepcid IV), heparin, lidocaine, procainamide (Pronestyl), ranitidine (Zantac).

RATE OF ADMINISTRATION
Series of small injections allows control of the reversal of sedation to desired endpoint, avoids abrupt awakening, and minimizes the possibility of adverse effects. Rapid injection may cause withdrawal symptoms in patients with long-term exposure to benzodiazepines.
Reversal of conscious sedation or in general anesthesia: Each single dose over 15 seconds.
Management of suspected benzodiazepine overdose: Each single dose (0.2 mg [2 mL], 0.3 mg [3 mL], 0.5 mg [5 mL], respectively) is given over 30 seconds.

ACTIONS
A benzodiazepine antagonist. Competes with benzodiazepines, inhibiting their effect at benzodiazepine receptor sites. Action is very specific and reverses the effects of benzodiazepines only. Antagonizes (reverses) the sedation, impairment of recall, psychomotor impairment, and ventilatory depression produced by benzodiazepines. Duration and degree of reversal are related to dose and plasma concentration (both for amount of benzodiazepine and amount of flumazenil). Onset of action usually occurs within 1 to 2 minutes of reaching the appropriate dose, with peak effect at 6 to 10 minutes. Enables the physician to control the duration of action of benzodiazepines and to evaluate the patient's postoperative condition earlier and may facilitate the postprocedural course. In overdose, it allows the physician to communicate sooner with patients who have taken an excessive dose. Extensively metabolized in the liver. Half-life is 40 to 80 minutes. Excreted in changed form in urine and to a small extent in feces.

INDICATIONS AND USES
Adults: Complete or partial reversal of the effects of general anesthesia induced and/or maintained with benzodiazepines (e.g., diazepam [Valium], midazolam [Versed]). ■ Complete or partial reversal of the sedative effects of benzodiazepines used to produce and/or maintain conscious sedation (e.g., diagnostic and therapeutic procedures). ■ Adjunct to conventional treatment in managing benzodiazepine overdose (e.g., chlordiazepoxide [Librium], diazepam [Valium], lorazepam [Ativan], midazolam [Versed]).
Pediatric patients 1 to 17 years of age: Reversal of conscious sedation induced with benzodiazepines; see Maternal/Child. ■ Not approved for other indications but has been used at doses similar to those used for reversal of conscious sedation; see Maternal/Child.

CONTRAINDICATIONS
Known hypersensitivity to flumazenil or any benzodiazepine, patients who are on benzodiazepine therapy for control of potentially life-threatening conditions (e.g., control of intracranial pressure, status epilepticus), and patients showing signs of serious cyclic antidepressant overdose. ■ Use in treatment of benzodiazepine dependence is not recommended.

PRECAUTIONS
Excess administration increases risk of side effects and decreases desired therapeutics of benzodiazepines. ■ Will not reverse the central nervous

system (CNS) effects of drugs such as alcohol, analgesics, antidepressants, barbiturates, and narcotics. In overdose, will bring the patient to a conscious state only if a benzodiazepine is responsible for the sedation. Has reversed benzodiazepine-induced hypotension and bradycardia unresponsive to other measures (e.g., IV fluids, atropine, dopamine). ▪ Convulsions may occur, especially in patients who rely on benzodiazepines to control seizures or are physically dependent on benzodiazepines for long-term sedation, in overdose cases in which patients are showing signs of serious cyclic antidepressant overdose (some clinicians recommend a diagnostic ECG or quantitative analytical testing before use—see Contraindications), or in ICU patients who may have an unrecognized dependence on benzodiazepines because of frequent use as a sedative (can occur with only 3 to 5 days of benzodiazepine administration). Intubation with ventilatory and circulatory support may be the treatment of choice for these high-risk patients; see Dose Adjustments. ▪ Risk of adverse reactions increased in patients with a history of alcohol, benzodiazepine, or sedative use (increased frequency of benzodiazepine tolerance and dependence). Can precipitate benzodiazepine withdrawal (also high-risk; see Dose Adjustments). ▪ Use extreme caution in head injury (may alter cerebral blood flow or cause convulsions). ▪ Do not use until effects of neuromuscular blockade have been fully reversed. ▪ May cause panic attacks in patients with a history of panic disorder. ▪ Flumazenil may not completely reverse respiratory depression due to benzodiazepines in patients with serious lung disease. Additional ventilatory support may be required. ▪ Half-life prolonged based on amount of hepatic impairment. ▪ Ingestion of food increases clearance of flumazenil.

Monitor: Confirm secure airway, ventilation, and IV access before administration as indicated. ▪ Monitor BP, HR, and respirations closely. ECG monitoring and oxygenation determination by pulse oximetry is recommended. ▪ Emergency equipment and supplies, including drugs for seizure control (see Antidote), must always be available. ▪ Observe continuously for resedation, respiratory depression, preseizure activity, or other residual benzodiazepine effects for an appropriate period (2 or more hours). ▪ Extend observation time for larger doses, in presence of long-acting benzodiazepines (e.g., diazepam [Valium]), or large doses of short-acting benzodiazepines (e.g., more than 10 mg of midazolam [Versed]). ▪ Observe ambulatory patients for a minimum of 2 hours after a 1-mg dose; resedation after 2 hours is unlikely. Extend observation time as above. ▪ Awake patients may require pain medication sooner than those without benzodiazepine reversal. ▪ All postprocedural instructions must be given to the patient verbally and in writing; does not reverse benzodiazepine amnesia. ▪ See Drug/Lab Interactions.

Patient Education: Review medication use, especially benzodiazepine, alcohol, and sedative use prior to surgery or procedure. ▪ Effects of benzodiazepines may recur; for 24 to 48 hours memory and judgment may be impaired. ▪ All instructions should be in writing. ▪ Do not drive, operate hazardous machinery, or engage in activities that require alertness. ▪ Do not take alcohol, other CNS depressants (e.g., antihistamines, barbiturates), or nonprescription drugs for 24 hours.

Maternal/Child: Category C: use only if benefit justifies risk. ▪ Not recommended during labor and delivery because effect on newborn unknown. ▪ Safety for use in breast-feeding not established. ▪ Safety and effectiveness for reversal of conscious sedation induced with benzodiazepines have been established in pediatric patients 1 to 17 years of age. Resedation may occur, especially in pediatric patients 1 to 5 years of age. Safety and effectiveness of repeated flumazenil doses in pediatric patients experiencing resedation have not been established. ▪ Safety and effectiveness for other uses listed under adult indications have not been established. However, published anecdotal reports have cited safety profiles and dosing guidelines similar to those used in reversal of conscious sedation. ▪ Half-life appears to be shorter and more variable in pediatric patients.

Elderly: See Dose Adjustments. Age-related differences in safety and effectiveness have not been observed; however, a greater sensitivity of some older patients cannot be ruled out. ▪ Monitor carefully; benzodiazepine-induced sedation may be deeper and more prolonged.

DRUG/LAB INTERACTIONS

May cause cardiac arrhythmias or convulsions in cases of mixed drug overdose. These toxic effects may emerge (especially with **cyclic antidepressants** [e.g., amitriptyline (Elavil), imipramine (Tofranil)]) with reversal of benzodiazepine effect; see Precautions. May reverse sedative and anticonvulsant effects. ▪ May precipitate withdrawal symptoms if given to chronic **benzodiazepine** users. ▪ No specific deleterious interactions noted when flumazenil administered after **narcotics, inhalational anesthetics, muscle relaxants, and muscle relaxant antagonists** administered in conjunction with sedation or anesthesia. ▪ Not recommended for use in **epileptic patients** who have been receiving benzodiazepines for a prolonged period. ▪ Lab test interactions have not been evaluated.

SIDE EFFECTS

Most common at doses above 1 mg and/or with abrupt reversal.

Abnormal vision, agitation, anxiety, dizziness, dry mouth, dyspnea, emotional lability, fatigue, flushing, headache, hot flashes, hypertension, hyperventilation, insomnia, involuntary movements, irritability, muscle tension, nausea, pain or reaction (rash, thrombophlebitis) at the injection site, palpitations, panic, paresthesia, sweating, tachycardia, tinnitus, tremors, and vomiting. Convulsions, fear, and panic attacks may occur; see Precautions. Deaths have been reported. Risk increased in patients with serious underlying disease or in patients who overdose on non-benzodiazepine drugs (usually cyclic antidepressants).

Overdose: Agitation, anxiety, arrhythmias, convulsions, hyperesthesia, increased muscle tone.

ANTIDOTE

Notify the physician of any side effect. Treat symptoms of benzodiazepine withdrawal (agitation, confusion, dizziness, emotional lability, or sensory distortions) with a barbiturate, benzodiazepine, or other sedative. Larger doses may be required because of presence of flumazenil. Treat convulsions from overdose with barbiturates, benzodiazepines, and phenytoin (Dilantin). Maintain an adequate airway, adequate ventilation, and IV access at all times. Hemodialysis not effective in overdose if 1 hour has passed since administration.

FLUOROURACIL BBW

(flew-roh-**YOUR**-ah-sill)

Adrucil, 5-Fluorouracil, 5-FU

**Antineoplastic
(antimetabolite)**

pH 9.2

USUAL DOSE

Many dosing regimens are in use. Manufacturer recommends 12 mg/kg of body weight/24 hr for 4 days. Total dose should not exceed 800 mg/24 hr. If no toxicity is observed, one half dose (6 mg/kg) is given on Days 6, 8, 10, and 12 unless toxicity occurs. No medication is given on Days 5, 7, 9, or 11. Discontinue therapy on Day 12, even if no toxicity is apparent. See Precautions/Monitor. The most common form of maintenance therapy is to repeat the entire course of therapy beginning 30 days after the previous course is completed and any toxicity has subsided or to give a single dose of 10 to 15 mg/kg/week, not to exceed 1 Gm/week. Dose adjustments of subsequent doses are made depending on side effects and tolerance.

Advanced colorectal cancer (unlabeled): Various protocols have been used. Examples are leucovorin calcium 20 mg/M^2 followed by fluorouracil 425 mg/M^2, or leucovorin calcium 200 mg/M^2 followed by fluorouracil 370 mg/M^2 daily for 5 days. Repeat at 4-week intervals twice, then repeat every 28 to 35 days based on complete recovery from toxic effects. Do not initiate or continue in any patient with GI toxicity until completely subsided. Reduce fluorouracil dose based on tolerance to previous course; reduce 20% for moderate hematologic or GI toxicity, 30% for severe toxicity. Increase fluorouracil dose 10% if no toxicity. Leucovorin calcium dose is not adjusted. Alternatively, fluorouracil may also be used in combination with levoleucovorin; dose is different; see levoleucovorin monograph. Fluorouracil and leucovorin calcium are also used in combination with irinotecan (Camptosar); see irinotecan monograph.

Breast cancer (unlabeled): Various protocols have been used. An example is fluorouracil 600 mg/M^2 on Days 1 and 8 of each cycle combined with cyclophosphamide (Cytoxan) 100 mg/M^2 on Days 1 through 14 of each cycle and methotrexate 40 mg/M^2 on Days 1 and 8 of each cycle. Repeat cycles monthly (allowing a 2-week rest between cycles). Repeat for 6 to 12 cycles (6 to 12 months). Doxorubicin (Adriamycin) has also been included in this regimen. In patients older than 60 years, reduce the fluorouracil dose to 400 mg/M^2 and the initial methotrexate dose to 30 mg/M^2.

DOSE ADJUSTMENTS

For poor-risk patients or those in a poor nutritional state, either reduce dose by one half or more throughout a course of therapy or give 6 mg/kg/day for 3 days. If no toxicity observed, give 3 mg/kg on Days 5, 7, and 9. Give nothing on Days 4, 6, or 8. Do not exceed 400 mg/day. ■ Dose based on ideal body weight in presence of edema, ascites, or obesity. ■ Reduce dose in patients who have received high-dose pelvic irradiation or other cytotoxic drug therapy with alkylating agents (e.g., cisplatin, ifosfamide [Ifex]). ■ One source recommends a dose adjustment in patients with impaired hepatic function. Give the full dose if the bilirubin is 5 or less on the day of administration; omit the dose if the bilirubin is greater than 5. ■ Used with other antineoplastic drugs in reduced doses to achieve tumor remission. ■ See Usual Dose.

DILUTION
Specific techniques required; see Precautions. May be slightly discolored without affecting safety and potency. Dissolve any precipitate by heating to 60° C (140° F) and shaking vigorously. Cool to body temperature before using.

IV injection: May be given undiluted. May inject through Y-tube or three-way stopcock of a free-flowing infusion.

Infusion: May be further diluted with D5W or NS and given as an infusion. Doses up to 2 Gm are being given with extreme caution under the specific supervision of experienced specialists. Leucovorin calcium has been mixed into the solution with fluorouracil.

Storage: Store at room temperature; protect from light.

COMPATIBILITY   (Underline Indicates Conflicting Compatibility Information)
Consider any drug NOT listed as compatible to be INCOMPATIBLE until consulting a pharmacist; specific conditions may apply.
One source suggests the following **compatibilities:**

Additive: Bleomycin (Blenoxane), cyclophosphamide (Cytoxan), etoposide (VePesid), hydromorphone (Dilaudid), ifosfamide (Ifex), methotrexate, mitoxantrone (Novantrone), vincristine.

Y-site: Allopurinol (Aloprim), amifostine (Ethyol), anidulafungin (Eraxis), aztreonam (Azactam), bleomycin (Blenoxane), cefepime (Maxipime), cisplatin (Platinol), cyclophosphamide (Cytoxan), doripenem (Doribax), doxorubicin (Adriamycin), doxorubicin liposomal (Doxil), etoposide phosphate (Etopophos), fludarabine (Fludara), furosemide (Lasix), gemcitabine (Gemzar), granisetron (Kytril), heparin, hydrocortisone sodium succinate (Solu-Cortef), leucovorin calcium, linezolid (Zyvox), mannitol, melphalan (Alkeran), methotrexate, metoclopramide (Reglan), mitomycin (Mutamycin), ondansetron (Zofran), paclitaxel (Taxol), palonosetron (Aloxi), pemetrexed (Alimta), piperacillin/tazobactam (Zosyn), potassium chloride (KCl), propofol (Diprivan), sargramostim (Leukine), teniposide (Vumon), thiotepa, vinblastine, vincristine.

RATE OF ADMINISTRATION
IV injection: A single dose over 1 to 15 minutes.

Infusion: A single dose is usually administered over 24 hours. Toxicity may be lessened by extended administration.

ACTIONS
An antimetabolite. A fluorinated pyrimidine antagonist, cell cycle specific, that interferes with the synthesis of DNA and RNA. Through various chemical processes this deprivation acts more quickly on rapidly growing cells and causes their death. Distributes into tumors, intestinal mucosa, bone marrow, liver, and readily crosses the blood-brain barrier into cerebrospinal fluid and brain tissue. Metabolized by the liver within 3 hours. Half-life is approximately 16 minutes. Excretion is through the urine and as respiratory CO_2.

INDICATIONS AND USES
To suppress or slow neoplastic growth. Palliative treatment of cancers of the breast, colon, pancreas, rectum, and stomach. May be used alone or in combination with other agents.

Unlabeled uses: Has been used for the treatment of bladder, cervical, endometrial, esophageal, head and neck, ovarian, prostatic, skin (topical), and other cancers.

CONTRAINDICATIONS

Potentially serious infections, depressed bone marrow function, poor nutritional state, hypersensitivity, major surgery within the previous month.

PRECAUTIONS

Follow guidelines for handling cytotoxic agents. See Appendix A, p. 1429. ▪ Administered by or under the direction of the physician specialist with facilities for monitoring the patient and responding to any medical emergency. Hospitalization, at least during the initial course of therapy, is recommended. ▪ Use caution in patients who have had high-dose pelvic irradiation, previous alkylating agents (e.g., cisplatin), other antimetabolic drugs (e.g., methotrexate), metastatic tumor involvement of the bone marrow, impaired hepatic or renal function, or dihydropyrimidine dehydrogenase deficiency. ▪ Pseudomembranous colitis has been reported. May range from mild to life threatening. Consider in patients that present with diarrhea during or after treatment with fluorouracil.

Monitor: Confirm patency of vein. Avoid extravasation. Change peripheral injection site every 48 hours. ▪ Obtain a CBC with differential and platelet count before each dose. When given with leucovorin calcium, repeat weekly the first two courses and then at the time of anticipated WBC nadir in following courses. Electrolytes and liver function tests should be done before the first three courses, then every other course. ▪ Be alert for signs of bone marrow suppression or infection. Prophylactic antibiotics may be indicated pending results of C/S in a febrile neutropenic patient. ▪ Examine mouth and lips daily for sores or other signs of stomatitis. ▪ Prophylactic antiemetics may reduce nausea and vomiting and increase patient comfort. ▪ Toxicity increased by any form of therapy that adds to stress, poor nutrition, and bone marrow suppression. ▪ Monitor for thrombocytopenia (platelet count less than 50,000/mm^3). Initiate precautions to prevent excessive bleeding (e.g., inspect IV sites, skin, and mucous membranes; use extreme care during invasive procedures; test urine, emesis, stool, and secretions for occult blood). ▪ See Drug/Lab Interactions.

Patient Education: Nonhormonal birth control recommended. ▪ See Appendix D, p. 1434. ▪ Report IV site burning and stinging promptly. ▪ Drink at least 2 liters of fluid each day.

Maternal/Child: Category D: avoid pregnancy; can cause fetal harm. ▪ Discontinue breast-feeding. ▪ Safety for use in pediatric patients not established.

Elderly: May be more sensitive to toxic effects of the drug. Consider age-related organ impairment. ▪ See Dose Adjustments.

DRUG/LAB INTERACTIONS

Potentiates **anticoagulants.** ▪ Do not administer **live virus vaccines** to patients receiving antineoplastic drugs. ▪ **Cimetidine** (Tagamet), **interferon alfa, and leucovorin calcium** may increase toxicity. ▪ Additive bone marrow suppression may occur with **radiation therapy, other bone marrow–suppressing agents** (e.g., azathioprine [Imuran], chloramphenicol, irinotecan [Camptosar], melphalan [Alkeran], vinorelbine [Navelbine]), **and/or agents that cause blood dyscrasias** (e.g., metronidazole [Flagyl IV]). ▪ **Thiazide diuretics** (e.g., chlorothiazide [Diuril]) may prolong antineoplastic-induced leukopenia. ▪ May decrease metabolism and increase serum levels of **phenytoin** (Dilantin).

SIDE EFFECTS

Abnormal bromsulphalein (BSP), prothrombin, total protein, sedimentation rate; alopecia (reversible), anaphylaxis, bleeding, bone marrow suppression (agranulocytosis, anemia, leukopenia, pancytopenia, thrombocytopenia), cerebellar syndrome, cramps, dermatitis, diarrhea, disorientation, dry lips, erythema, esophagopharyngitis and stomatitis (may lead to sloughing and ulceration), euphoria, frequent stools, GI ulceration and bleeding, headache, hemorrhage from any site, increased skin pigmentation, infection, lacrimal duct stenosis, mouth soreness and ulceration, myocardial ischemia, nail changes, nausea, palmar-plantar erythrodysesthesia syndrome (tingling of hands and feet followed by pain, redness, and swelling), photophobia, photosensitivity, pneumopathy (cough, shortness of breath), thrombophlebitis, visual changes, vomiting (intractable). Diarrhea and stomatitis are most common and may be more severe with a prolonged duration in patients on combination therapy. Pseudomembranous colitis has been reported.

ANTIDOTE

Keep physician informed of any side effects. Discontinue the drug and notify physician promptly at the first sign of toxicity (e.g., bleeding, diarrhea, esophagopharyngitis, gastritis, intractable vomiting, rapidly falling white count, sores in or around the lips or mouth, stomatitis). Nadir of leukocyte count occurs around days 9 to 14. Recovery should be by day 30. Discontinue the drug if the WBC count is less than $3,500/mm^3$ or platelets are less than $100,000/mm^3$; should reach $4,000/mm^3$ and $130,000/mm^3$ respectively in 2 weeks; if they do not, discontinue treatment. Administration of whole blood products (e.g., packed RBCs, platelets, leukocytes, and/or blood modifiers (e.g., darbepoetin alfa [Aranesp], epoetin alfa [Epogen], filgrastim [Neupogen], pegfilgrastim [Neulasta], sargramostim [Leukine], oprelvekin [Neumega]) may be indicated to treat bone marrow toxicity. Continue to monitor for 4 weeks. Palmar-plantar erythrodysesthesia syndrome has been treated with oral pyridoxine (vitamin B_6), 100 to 150 mg daily. Death may occur from the progression of many side effects. There is no specific antidote; supportive therapy as indicated will help sustain the patient in toxicity.

FOLIC ACID
(**FOH**-lik **AS**-id)

Nutritional supplement
(vitamin)
Antianemic

pH 8 to 11

USUAL DOSE

Therapeutic dose: 0.1 to 1 mg daily (never give less than 0.1 mg). Larger doses may be required.

Maintenance dose: 0.4 mg daily. *Pregnant or lactating females:* 0.8 mg daily.

PEDIATRIC DOSE

See Maternal/Child.

Therapeutic dose: 0.1 to 1 mg daily (never give less than 0.1 mg).

Maintenance dose: *Infants:* 0.1 mg daily. *Under 4 years:* Up to 0.3 mg daily. *Over 4 years:* Same as adult.

DOSE ADJUSTMENTS

Increased initial and maintenance doses may be required in alcoholism, hemolytic, anemia, anticonvulsant therapy, or chronic infection.

DILUTION

Each dose (up to 5 mg) should be diluted in at least 50 mL of SW, D5W, or NS. May be added to most IV solutions and given as an infusion.

Storage: Protect from light and freezing.

COMPATIBILITY

Consider any drug NOT listed as compatible to be INCOMPATIBLE until consulting a pharmacist; specific conditions may apply.

Manufacturer lists as **incompatible** with calcium gluconate (even though a precipitate cannot be seen), doxapram (Dopram), heavy metal ions, iron sulfate, oxidizing agents, reducing agents, solutions with a pH less than 5.

One source suggests the following **compatibilities:**

Y-site: Famotidine (Pepcid IV).

RATE OF ADMINISTRATION

5 mg or fraction thereof over a minimum of 1 minute; usually given over 30 minutes or more in an infusion.

ACTIONS

Folic acid (pteroylglutamic acid) is part of the vitamin B complex. In humans, exogenous folate is required for nucleoprotein synthesis and the maintenance of normal erythropoiesis. It is the precursor of tetrahydrofolic acid, an important cofactor involved in the synthesis of amino acids and DNA. Stimulates the production of RBCs, WBCs, and platelets. Metabolized in the liver and excreted in the urine. Crosses the placental barrier. Secreted in breast milk.

INDICATIONS AND USES

For prevention and treatment of folic acid deficiency. Megaloblastic anemias resulting from folic acid deficiency may be seen in sprue, anemias of malnutrition, pregnancy, infancy, and childhood, developmental or surgical anomalies of the GI tract, as well as other conditions.

CONTRAINDICATIONS

Pernicious anemia unless used in combination with diagnostic testing.

PRECAUTIONS

Folic acid is not commonly administered by the IV route. Oral or IM administration provides adequate absorption in most cases. ▪ Obscures the peripheral blood picture and prevents the diagnosis of pernicious anemia. May actually aggravate the neurologic symptoms.

Monitor: Obtain CBC before and during therapy.

Maternal/Child: Category A: an important vitamin before and during pregnancy. Folate-deficient mothers have a higher incidence of fetal anomalies and complications of pregnancy. ▪ Safe for use during breast-feeding; infant may require supplementation if mother is folate deficient. ▪ Some products contain benzyl alcohol as a preservative. Avoid use in neonates. **Elderly:** More likely to have folate deficiency.

DRUG/LAB INTERACTIONS

Toxic effects of antineoplastic folic acid antagonists are blocked by **folinic acid** (leucovorin calcium) but not by folic acid IV. ▪ Increases **hydantoin** metabolism (e.g., phenytoin [Dilantin]); seizures may result. ▪ Inhibited by **dihydrofolate reductase inhibitors** (e.g., methotrexate, trimethoprim), **pyrimethamine, and triamterene** and by depressed **hematopoiesis, alcoholism,** and deficiencies of **vitamins B$_6$, B$_{12}$, C, and E.** ▪ **Aminosalicylic acid** (Pamisyl) or **sulfasalazine** (Azulfidine) may decrease serum folate levels. ▪ **Oral contraceptives** may inhibit folate metabolism.

SIDE EFFECTS

Almost nonexistent. Confusion, some slight flushing or feeling of warmth, nausea; anaphylaxis can occur.

ANTIDOTE

If anaphylaxis occurs, discontinue drug, treat anaphylaxis, and notify physician. Resuscitate as necessary.

FOMEPIZOLE INJECTION
(foh-**MEP**-ih-zoll in-**JEK**-shun)
Antizol

Antidote

USUAL DOSE

Ethylene glycol is the main component of antifreeze and coolants. Methanol is the main component of windshield washer fluid and a component of products such as Sternol (for fondue pots), Heet (gasoline antifreeze), and various paint products. Begin fomepizole treatment immediately upon suspicion of ethylene glycol or methanol ingestion based on patient history and/or anion gap metabolic acidosis, increased osmolar gap, visual disturbances, or oxalate crystals in the urine, or a documented serum ethylene glycol or methanol concentration greater than 20 mg/dL.

Adults with blood concentrations over 20 mg/dL but less than 50 mg/dL: Administer a loading dose of 15 mg/kg as a slow intravenous infusion. Follow with 10 mg/kg every 12 hours times 4 doses, then 15 mg/kg every 12 hours until ethylene glycol or methanol concentrations are undetectable or have been reduced below 20 mg/dL, and the patient is asymptomatic with normal pH.

Adults with blood concentrations of 50 mg/dL or higher, renal failure, or significant or worsening metabolic acidosis: In addition to dosing as above, dialysis should be considered to correct metabolic abnormalities and to lower the ethylene glycol or methanol concentrations below 50 mg/dL.

Dosage with renal dialysis: Amount of loading dose and following doses (mg/kg) remains the same, but fomepizole is dialyzable and the frequency of dosing should be increased to every 4 hours during hemodialysis. Base frequency on the following chart.

Fomepizole Dosing in Patients Requiring Dialysis	
DOSE AT THE BEGINNING OF HEMODIALYSIS	
If <6 hours since last fomepizole dose	If ≥6 hours since last fomepizole dose
Do not administer dose	Administer next scheduled dose
DOSING DURING HEMODIALYSIS	
Dose every 4 hours	
DOSING AT THE TIME HEMODIALYSIS IS COMPLETED	
Time between last dose and the end of the hemodialysis	
<1 hour	Do not administer dose at the end of hemodialysis
1-3 hours	Administer ½ of next scheduled dose
>3 hours	Administer next scheduled dose
MAINTENANCE DOSING OFF HEMODIALYSIS	
Give next scheduled dose 12 hours from last dose administered	

DOSE ADJUSTMENTS

Fomepizole has not been studied sufficiently to determine whether the pharmacokinetics differ for the elderly (see Elderly), pediatric patients, between genders, in renal insufficiency (excreted renally), or in hepatic insufficiency (metabolized by the liver).

DILUTION

Fomepizole solidifies at temperatures less than 25° C (77° F). If it is solidified, liquefy by running the vial under warm water or by holding in the hand. Solidification does not affect the efficacy, safety, or stability. Withdraw the appropriate dose. Each single dose *must be diluted* in at least 100 mL of NS or D5W and given as an infusion. Mix well.

Storage: Store vials at CRT 20° to 25° C (68° to 77° F). Diluted solutions are stable refrigerated or at CRT for 48 hours; however, manufacturer states should be used within 24 hours of dilution.

COMPATIBILITY

Specific information not available. Consider specific use; consult pharmacist.

RATE OF ADMINISTRATION

Each single dose must be given as a slow intravenous infusion equally distributed over 30 minutes. *Do not give undiluted or by bolus injection;* has caused serious venous irritation and phlebosclerosis.

ACTIONS

A synthetic competitive alcohol dehydrogenase inhibitor. Effectively blocks formation of toxic metabolites (glycolic and oxalic acids [ethylene glycol]) and (formic acid [methanol]). These toxins can induce metabolic acidosis, nausea and vomiting, seizures, stupor, coma, calcium oxaluria, acute tubular necrosis, blindness, and death. Has shown minimal CNS depressant effects. Plasma half-life varies with dose and has not been calculated. Rapidly distributes into total body water. Metabolized in the liver by the P_{450} mixed-function oxidase system. Significant increases in the elimination rate occur after 30 to 40 hours. Excreted in urine.

INDICATIONS AND USES

An antidote for ethylene glycol (antifreeze) or methanol (windshield wiper fluid) poisoning, or for use in suspected ethylene glycol or methanol ingestion either alone or in combination with hemodialysis.

CONTRAINDICATIONS

Known serious hypersensitivity to fomepizole or other pyrazoles (e.g., sulfinpyrazone [Anturane]).

PRECAUTIONS

Acute ethylene glycol or methanol poisoning is a medical emergency that is characterized by a syndrome that can include CNS depression, severe metabolic acidosis, renal failure, and coma. Can be lethal if left untreated or when treatment is delayed due to delayed diagnosis. The lethal dose of ethylene glycol is approximately 1.4 mL/kg. The lethal dose of methanol is approximately 1.2 mL/kg. ■ If ethylene glycol or methanol poisoning is left untreated, the natural progression of the poisoning leads to accumulation of toxic metabolites, including glycolic and oxalic acids (ethylene glycol) and formic acid (methanol). These metabolites can induce metabolic acidosis, nausea and vomiting, seizures, stupor, coma, calcium oxaluria, acute tubular necrosis, and death. ■ The diagnosis of these poisonings may be difficult because ethylene glycol and methanol levels diminish in the blood as they are metabolized. ▪ The ethylene glycol or methanol concentrations and the acid-base balance, as determined by serum electrolyte (anion gap) and/or arterial blood gas analysis, should be frequently monitored and used to guide treatment. ▪ Fomepizole has caused minor hypersensitivity reactions (mild rash, eosinophilia).

Monitor: Maintain a patent airway and support ventilation as indicated; CNS and respiratory distress may occur suddenly. ▪ Gastric lavage may be indicated if performed soon after ingestion or in patients who are comatose or at risk for seizures. ▪ Patients must be managed for metabolic acidosis, acute renal failure (ethylene glycol), adult respiratory distress syndrome, visual disturbances (methanol), and hypocalcemia which may result in tetany. Sodium bicarbonate may be required to treat metabolic acidosis. Correct electrolyte imbalance and maintain adequate urine output with IV fluids. A decrease in the amount of fluids will be required in impending renal failure to prevent fluid overload; monitor closely. ▪ Potassium supplementation and oxygen administration are usually necessary. ▪ Administer IV calcium to patients with seizures or tetany that may be caused by decreased calcium, but do not attempt to correct hypocalcemia itself (may increase precipitation of calcium oxalate crystals in the tissues). ▪ Hemodialysis is necessary in the anuric patient and should be considered in patients with severe metabolic acidosis or azotemia and in any patient with high ethylene glycol or methanol concentrations (equal to or greater than 50 mg/dL). ▪ ECG should be continuous to monitor for cardiac irregularities. ▪ EEG may be required in the comatose patient. ▪ The effective inhibition of alcohol dehydrogenase requires fomepizole plasma concentrations in the range of 100 to 300 micromol/L (8.6 to 24.6 mg/L). ▪ To assess treatment success, obtain baseline and frequently monitor measurements of blood gases, pH, electrolytes, BUN, creatinine, and urinalysis in addition to other laboratory tests as indicated by each patient's condition. ▪ To assess the status of ethylene glycol or methanol and their respective metabolite clearance, obtain baseline ethylene glycol or methanol plasma and urine concentrations and presence of urinary oxalate crystals (ethylene glycol) and monitor frequently. ▪ Obtain baseline and monitor hepatic enzymes and WBC counts during treatment; transient increases in serum transaminase levels and eosinophilia have been noted with repeated fomepizole dosing. ▪ Monitor for signs of hypersensitivity reactions; see Precautions.

Patient Education: Monitoring of urine output imperative. ▪ Cooperation with adequate hydration and frequent laboratory analysis required. ▪ Request assistance with ambulation.

Maternal/Child: Category C: use during pregnancy only if clearly needed. ▪ Decreased testicular mass in rats. ▪ Use caution during breast-feeding; not known if fomepizole is secreted in breast milk. ▪ Safety and effectiveness for use in pediatric patients not established.

Elderly: Risk of toxic reactions may be greater in patients with impaired renal function; consider age-related renal impairment.

DRUG/LAB INTERACTIONS

Has not been studied, but reciprocal interactions (increasing or decreasing clearance, effects, or toxicity) may occur with concomitant use of **drugs that induce or inhibit the cytochrome P$_{450}$ system** (e.g., carbamazepine [Tegretol], cimetidine [Tagamet], ketoconazole [Nizoral], phenytoin

[Dilantin]). Oral fomepizole significantly reduced the rate of elimination of **ethanol** (by 40%) in healthy subjects. Ethanol decreased the rate of elimination of fomepizole (by 50%).

SIDE EFFECTS

Most common side effects are dizziness, headache, and nausea. Abdominal pain, abnormal smell, anemia, anorexia, arrhythmias (bradycardia, tachycardia), back pain (lower), blurred vision, decreased awareness of surroundings, diarrhea, DIC, feeling of drunkenness, fever, hangover, heartburn, hiccups, hypersensitivity reactions (e.g., mild rash, eosinophilia), hypotension, injection site reaction, light-headedness, lymphangitis, multisystem organ failure, nystagmus, pharyngitis, phlebitis, phlebosclerosis, seizure, shock, slurred speech, somnolence, taste changes (bad or metallic), vertigo, visual problems, vomiting occurred in up to 6% of patients. **Overdose:** Dizziness, nausea, and vertigo occurred in healthy volunteers given 3 to 6 times the recommended dose.

ANTIDOTE

Keep physician informed of all side effects, laboratory results, and concurrent medical problems. Dialysis may be indicated for changes in patient condition (e.g., renal failure, significant or worsening metabolic acidosis, or a measured ethylene glycol or methanol concentration of greater than 50 mg/dL) or in the treatment of overdose. Treat side effects symptomatically as indicated. Resuscitate as necessary.

FOSAPREPITANT DIMEGLUMINE
(fos-ap-**RE**-pi-tant dye-**MEG**-loo-meen)
Emend

Antiemetic
Receptor antagonist
(Substance P/NK₁)

USUAL DOSE

Administered as a single-dose regimen or as part of a 3-day antiemetic dosing regimen for chemotherapy-induced nausea and vomiting (CINV). In the 3-day dosing regimens, *fosaprepitant 115 mg IV may be substituted for aprepitant 125 mg PO 30 minutes prior to chemotherapy on Day 1 only.* The regimens are listed in the following tables.

Single-Dose Regimen for the Prevention of Nausea and Vomiting Associated with Highly Emetogenic Cancer Chemotherapy				
	Day 1	Day 2	Day 3	Day 4
Fosaprepitant IV*	150 mg IV	None	None	None
Dexamethasone†	12 mg PO	8 mg PO	8 mg PO twice daily	8 mg PO twice daily
Ondansetron‡	32 mg IV	None	None	None

*Administer fosaprepitant 30 minutes before chemotherapy.
†Administer dexamethasone (Decadron) 30 minutes before chemotherapy on Day 1 and in the morning on subsequent days. The dose was chosen to account for the drug interaction.
‡Administer ondansetron (Zofran) 30 minutes before chemotherapy on Day 1.

3-Day Dose Regimen for the Prevention of Nausea and Vomiting Associated with Highly Emetogenic Cancer Chemotherapy				
	Day 1	Day 2	Day 3	Day 4
Fosaprepitant IV* or Aprepitant PO*	115 mg IV or 125 mg PO	80 mg PO	80 mg PO	None
Dexamethasone†	12 mg PO	8 mg PO	8 mg PO	8 mg PO
Ondansetron‡	32 mg IV	None	None	None

*Administer fosaprepitant 30 minutes before chemotherapy on Day 1 and in the morning on subsequent days.
†Administer dexamethasone (Decadron) 30 minutes before chemotherapy on Day 1 and in the morning on subsequent days. The dose was chosen to account for the drug interaction.
‡Administer ondansetron (Zofran) 30 minutes before chemotherapy on Day 1.

3-Day Dose Regimen for the Prevention of Nausea and Vomiting Associated with Moderately Emetogenic Cancer Chemotherapy			
	Day 1	Day 2	Day 3
Fosaprepitant IV* or Aprepitant PO*	115 mg IV or 125 mg PO	80 mg PO	80 mg PO
Dexamethasone†	12 mg PO	None	None
Ondansetron‡	8 mg PO Twice on Day 1	None	None

*Administer fosaprepitant 30 minutes before chemotherapy on Day 1 and in the morning on subsequent days.
†Administer dexamethasone (Decadron) 30 minutes before chemotherapy on Day 1. The dose was chosen to account for the drug interaction.
‡Administer ondansetron (Zofran) 30 to 60 minutes before chemotherapy on Day 1 and repeated one time 8 hours later.

DOSE ADJUSTMENTS

No dose adjustment indicated based on age, race, gender, renal status (including patients with ESRD on dialysis), or mild to moderate hepatic insufficiency. Data in patients with severe hepatic insufficiency (Child-Pugh score >9) not available.

DILUTION

Reconstitute each 115-mg or 150-mg vial with 5 mL of NS. Direct stream of NS to side of vial to avoid foaming. Swirl gently; do not shake. Prepare an infusion bag with 110 mL of NS for the 115-mg dose and prepare an infusion bag with 145 mL of NS for the 150-mg dose. Withdraw entire volume of reconstituted vial and transfer it into the infusion bag. Gently invert the bag 2 to 3 times. Final concentration is 1 mg/mL.

Storage: Store unopened vials at 2° to 8° C (36° to 46° F). Diluted solution is stable for 24 hours at RT.

COMPATIBILITY

Manufacturer states, "Should not be mixed or reconstituted with solutions for which physical and chemical **compatibility** have not been established. Fosaprepitant (Emend) for injection is **incompatible** with any solutions containing divalent cations (e.g., calcium or magnesium), including lactated Ringer's solution and Hartmann's solution."

RATE OF ADMINISTRATION

115-mg dose: A single dose as an infusion equally distributed over 15 minutes.

150-mg dose: A single dose as an infusion equally distributed over 20 to 30 minutes.

ACTIONS

A prodrug of aprepitant, a substance P/neurokinin$_1$ (NK$_1$) receptor antagonist. Has little or no affinity for 5HT$_3$, dopamine, and corticosteroid receptors. Fosaprepitant is rapidly converted to aprepitant following IV administration. Aprepitant inhibits emesis induced by cytotoxic chemotherapeutic agents, such as cisplatin, via central actions. Crosses the blood-brain barrier and occupies brain NK$_1$ receptors. Augments the antiemetic activity of the 5HT$_3$-receptor antagonist ondansetron and the corticosteroid dexamethasone and inhibits both the acute and delayed phases of cisplatin-induced emesis. Highly protein bound. Undergoes extensive metabolism, primarily by CYP3A4 and to a lesser extent by CYP1A2 and CYP2C19. Eliminated primarily by metabolism; not renally excreted. Half-life is approximately 9 to 13 hours.

INDICATIONS AND USES

Given in combination with other antiemetics for the prevention of acute and delayed nausea and vomiting associated with initial and repeat courses of highly emetogenic cancer chemotherapy, including high-dose cisplatin. ▪ In combination with other antiemetics for the prevention of nausea and vomiting associated with initial and repeat courses of moderately emetogenic cancer chemotherapy.

CONTRAINDICATIONS

Hypersensitivity to fosaprepitant, aprepitant, or any components of the product. ▪ Concurrent use with pimozide (Orap) or cisapride (Propulsid); see Drug Interactions.

PRECAUTIONS

A moderate inhibitor of CYP3A4 when administered as a 3-day antiemetic dosing regimen for CINV. Use with caution in patients receiving concomitant medications that are primarily metabolized through CYP3A4; see Drug Interactions. ▪ Use with caution in patients with severe hepatic insufficiency (Child-Pugh score >9); see Dose Adjustments. ▪ Hypersensitivity reactions have been observed; see Monitor. ▪ Has not been studied for treatment of established nausea and vomiting. ▪ Chronic continuous administration is not recommended. Has not been adequately studied, and the drug interaction profile could change during chronic continuous use.

Monitor: Monitor for S/S of a hypersensitivity reaction during the infusion (e.g., anaphylaxis, dyspnea, erythema, flushing, hives, itching, rash). ▪ Monitor IV site. See Drug Interactions.

Patient Education: Read manufacturer-supplied patient package insert before starting therapy and with each subsequent 3-day regimen. ▪ Discontinue use of fosaprepitant and promptly report S/S of a hypersensitivity reaction (e.g., difficulty breathing or swallowing, hives, itching, rash). ▪ Efficacy of hormonal contraceptives may be reduced during and for 28 days following administration of the last dose of aprepitant; includes birth control pills, skin patches, implants, and certain IUDs. Alternative or backup methods of contraception should be used during treatment and for 1 month following the last dose of fosaprepitant or aprepitant. ▪ Numerous drug interactions possible. A complete review of all prescription, nonprescription and herbal products is required prior to each dose. ▪ Patients on chronic warfarin therapy should have their INR checked in the 2-week period, particularly at 7 to 10 days, following initiation of regimen.

Maternal/Child: Category B: should be used during pregnancy only if clearly needed. ▪ Discontinue breast-feeding. ▪ Safety and effectiveness for use in pediatric patients not established.

Elderly: Response similar to that seen in younger patients, but greater sensitivity of some older individuals cannot be ruled out; see Dose Adjustments.

DRUG/LAB INTERACTIONS

When administered as a 3-day regimen, fosaprepitant or aprepitant is **a substrate, a moderate inhibitor, and an inducer of CYP3A4.** When administered as a single 150-mg dose, it is **a weak inhibitor of CYP3A4 and does not induce CYP3A4.** ▪ It is **also an inducer of CYP2C9.** ▪ Efficacy of **hormonal contraceptives** may be reduced during and for 28 days following administration of the last dose of fosaprepitant or aprepitant; see Patient Education. ■ Patients on chronic **warfarin** therapy should be closely monitored in the 2-week period, particularly at 7 to 10 days following initiation of fosaprepitant or aprepitant. Coadministration may result in a clinically significant decrease in INR. ■ Concurrent use with **pimozide** (Orap) **or cisapride** (Propulsid) is *contraindicated.* Inhibition of CYP3A4 by fosaprepitant or aprepitant could result in elevated plasma concentrations of these medications, potentially causing serious or life-threatening reactions; see Contraindications. ■ Aprepitant can increase plasma concentrations of **dexamethasone** (Decadron) **and methylprednisolone** (Solu-Medrol). When given concurrently with fosaprepitant or aprepitant, reduce the dexamethasone and methylprednisolone PO doses by approximately 50% and the methylprednisolone IV dose by approximately 25%. (Dexamethasone doses listed in Usual Dose take drug interaction into account.) ■ **Chemotherapy agents** that are known to be metabolized by CYP3A4 include docetaxel (Taxotere), paclitaxel (Taxol), etoposide (VePesid), irinotecan (Camptosar), ifosfamide (Ifex), imatinib (Gleevec), vinorelbine (Navelbine), vinblastine, and vincristine. In clinical studies, fosaprepitant was commonly administered with etoposide, vinorelbine, paclitaxel, and docetaxel. Dose adjustments were not required. Coadministration of fosaprepitant or aprepitant with other chemotherapy agents metabolized by CYP3A4 should be done with caution and careful monitoring. ■ May increase plasma levels of **benzodiazepines** (e.g., alprazolam [Xanax], midazolam [Versed], triazolam [Halcion]). Monitor for sedation. ■ Aprepitant is a CYP2C9 inducer. Has been shown to induce metabolism of **CYP2C9 substrates** (e.g., phenytoin [Dilantin], tolbutamide, warfarin [Coumadin]), thus decreasing plasma concentrations. Monitor patients receiving CYP2C9 substrates as indicated (e.g., plasma drug concentrations, therapeutic effect/efficacy, blood sugar control). ■ Concurrent use with **CYP3A4 inhibitors** (e.g., clarithromycin [Biaxin], diltiazem [Cardizem], itraconazole [Sporanox], ketoconazole [Nizoral], nefazodone, nelfinavir [Viracept], ritonavir [Norvir], troleandomycin [TAO]) may increase aprepitant or fosaprepitant plasma concentrations. Use caution. ■ Coadministration with **CYP3A4 inducers** (e.g., carbamazepine [Tegretol], phenytoin [Dilantin], rifampin [Rifadin]) may decrease fosaprepitant or aprepitant plasma concentrations and decrease efficacy. ■ Coadministration of **paroxetine** (Paxil) and aprepitant resulted in decreased plasma concentrations of both drugs. ■ Aprepitant is a moderate **inhibitor of CYP3A4.** Use with caution in patients receiving concomitant medications that are primarily metabolized through CYP3A4. ■ Has been given with **digoxin** (Lanoxin), **dolasetron** (Anzemet), **granisetron** (Kytril), **and ondansetron** (Zofran). Clinically significant drug interactions were not observed.

SIDE EFFECTS

The most common side effects reported include anorexia, asthenia, constipation, diarrhea, dyspepsia, eructation, fatigue, headache, hiccups, increased AST/ALT, and infusion site reactions (e.g., erythema, induration, pain, pruritus). Increased BP and infusion-site thrombophlebitis have also been reported. Many other side effects occurred in fewer than 1% of patients.

Post-Marketing: Hypersensitivity reactions, including anaphylaxis, pruritus, rash, and urticaria, have been reported.

ANTIDOTE

Keep physician informed of all side effects. Most minor side effects will be treated symptomatically. Discontinue fosaprepitant at the first sign of hypersensitivity. Treat hypersensitivity reactions as indicated; may require epinephrine, airway management, oxygen, IV fluids, antihistamines (e.g., diphenhydramine [Benadryl]), corticosteroids (e.g., hydrocortisone sodium succinate [Solu-Cortef]), and pressor amines (e.g., dopamine). Reinitiation of the infusion after a hypersensitivity reaction that occurs during the first use is not recommended. Fosaprepitant is not removed by hemodialysis.

FOSCARNET SODIUM BBW

(fos-**KAR**-net **SO**-dee-um)

Foscavir

Antiviral

pH 7.4

USUAL DOSE

Adequate hydration and specific testing required; see Monitor.

CMV retinitis: 90 mg/kg every 12 hours or 60 mg/kg every 8 hours for 14 to 21 days. Length of induction treatment based on clinical response. Begin a maintenance dose of 90 mg/kg/day the next day (Day 15 to 22). If retinitis progresses during the maintenance regimen, re-treat with the induction and maintenance regimens. Maintenance dose may be increased to 120 mg/kg/day in patients who show excellent tolerance to foscarnet or those who require early reinduction because of retinitis progression. Normal renal function required. For patients who have relapsed after induction and reinduction monotherapy with either foscarnet or ganciclovir, practitioners may consider combination therapy, which adds the alternate drug to the regimen. See the Clinical Trials section of the foscarnet sodium prescribing information.

Acyclovir-resistant HSV patients: 40 mg/kg every 8 or 12 hours for 2 to 3 weeks or until healed.

Varicella-zoster virus (unlabeled): 40 mg/kg every 8 hours for 10 to 21 days or until complete healing occurs. Higher doses have been used (e.g., 60 mg/kg every 8 hours or 100 mg/kg every 12 hours).

DOSE ADJUSTMENTS

Must be reduced and individualized according to patient's renal function. Safety and efficacy data for patients with baseline SCr greater than 2.8 mg/dL or measured 24-hour CrCl less than 50 mL/min are limited. Dose adjustment may be required during treatment even if patient had normal renal function initially. Specific calculation and testing required for both induction and maintenance dose; see the following charts.

Foscarnet Dose Adjustment Guide for Induction				
	Acyclovir-Resistant HSV		CMV Retinitis	
CrCl (mL/min/kg)	Dose of 40 mg/kg q 12 hr	Dose of 40 mg/kg q 8 hr	Dose of 60 mg/kg q 8 hr	Dose of 90 mg/kg q 12 hr
>1.4 mL/min/kg	40 mg/kg q 12 hr	40 mg/kg q 8 hr	60 mg/kg q 8 hr	90 mg/kg q 12 hr
>1-1.4 mL/min/kg	30 mg/kg q 12 hr	30 mg/kg q 8 hr	45 mg/kg q 8 hr	70 mg/kg q 12 hr
>0.8-1 mL/min/kg	20 mg/kg q 12 hr	35 mg/kg q 12 hr	50 mg/kg q 12 hr	50 mg/kg q 12 hr
>0.6-0.8 mL/min/kg	35 mg/kg q 24 hr	25 mg/kg q 12 hr	40 mg/kg q 12 hr	80 mg/kg q 24 hr
>0.5-0.6 mL/min/kg	25 mg/kg q 24 hr	40 mg/kg q 24 hr	60 mg/kg q 24 hr	60 mg/kg q 24 hr
≥0.4-0.5 mL/min/kg	20 mg/kg q 24 hr	35 mg/kg q 24 hr	50 mg/kg q 24 hr	50 mg/kg q 24 hr
<0.4 mL/min/kg	Not recommended	Not recommended	Not recommended	Not recommended

Foscarnet Dose Adjustment Guide for Maintenance in CMV Retinitis		
CrCl (mL/min/kg)	90 mg/kg/day (once daily)	120 mg/kg/day (once daily)
>1.4 mL/min/kg	90 mg/kg q 24 hr	120 mg/kg q 24 hr
>1-1.4 mL/min/kg	70 mg/kg q 24 hr	90 mg/kg q 24 hr
>0.8-1 mL/min/kg	50 mg/kg q 24 hr	65 mg/kg q 24 hr
>0.6-0.8 mL/min/kg	80 mg/kg q 48 hr	105 mg/kg q 48 hr
>0.5-0.6 mL/min/kg	60 mg/kg q 48 hr	80 mg/kg q 48 hr
≥0.4-0.5 mL/min/kg	50 mg/kg q 48 hr	65 mg/kg q 48 hr
<0.4 mL/min/kg	Not recommended	Not recommended

DILUTION

Calculate required dose. Remove any excess quantity of medication from the infusion bottle using aseptic technique. To avoid any possibility of overdose in either situation, only the calculated dose should be in the infusion bottle. Discard any excess before administration.

Central venous catheter: Standard 24-mg/mL solution may be given undiluted.

Peripheral vein: Each 1 mL of a calculated dose must be diluted with 1 mL of D5W or NS (yields a 12-mg/mL solution).

Storage: Store at CRT. Avoid excessive heat and freezing. Use only if vacuum is present and solution is clear and colorless. Use solution within 24 hours of entry into bottle.

COMPATIBILITY   (Underline Indicates Conflicting Compatibility Information)
Consider any drug NOT listed as compatible to be INCOMPATIBLE until consulting a pharmacist; specific conditions may apply.

Manufacturer states, "Administer only with NS or D5W solutions; no other drug or supplement should be administered concurrently via the same catheter." Because of chelating properties, a precipitate can occur. Manufacturer specifically lists as **incompatible** with 30% dextrose, solutions containing calcium (e.g., LR, TPN), acyclovir (Zovirax), amphotericin B (generic), diazepam (Valium), digoxin (Lanoxin), *ganciclovir (Cytovene),* leucovorin calcium, midazolam (Versed), pentamidine, phenytoin (Dilantin), prochlorperazine (Compazine), sulfamethoxazole/trimethoprim, vancomycin.

One source suggests the following **compatibilities:**

Additive: *Not recommended by manufacturer.* Potassium chloride (KCl).

Y-site: *Not recommended by manufacturer.* Aldesleukin (Proleukin), amikacin (Amikin), aminophylline, ampicillin, aztreonam (Azactam), cefazolin (Ancef), cefoxitin (Mefoxin), ceftazidime (Fortaz), ceftriaxone (Rocephin), cefuroxime (Zinacef), chloramphenicol (Chloromycetin), clindamycin (Cleocin), dexamethasone (Decadron), dopamine, doripenem (Doribax), erythromycin (Erythrocin), fluconazole (Diflucan), furosemide (Lasix), gentamicin, heparin, hydrocortisone sodium succinate (Solu-Cortef), hydromorphone (Dilaudid), imipenem-cilastatin (Primaxin), lorazepam (Ativan), metoclopramide (Reglan), metronidazole (Flagyl IV), morphine, nafcillin (Nallpen), oxacillin (Bactocill), penicillin G potassium, phenytoin (Dilantin), piperacillin, ranitidine (Zantac), sulfamethoxazole/trimethoprim, ticarcillin/clavulanate (Timentin), tobramycin, vancomycin.

RATE OF ADMINISTRATION

Infusion pump required to deliver accurate dose evenly distributed over specific time frame. Excessive plasma levels and toxicity (including hypocalcemia) will occur with too-rapid rate of infusion. Advisable to clear tubing with NS if possible before and after administration through Y-tube or three-way stopcock. Never exceed 1 mg/kg/min.

CMV Retinitis: *Induction doses:* Each 60-mg/kg dose equally distributed over a minimum of 1 hour. Increase to 1½ to 2 hours for 90-mg/kg dose. *Maintenance dose:* Each dose equally distributed over a minimum of 2 hours.

Acyclovir-resistant HSV: Each dose equally distributed over a minimum of 1 hour.

ACTIONS

An antiviral agent capable of inhibiting replication of all known herpesviruses, including cytomegalovirus (CMV), herpes simplex virus types 1 and 2 (HSV-1, HSV-2), and varicella-zoster virus (VZV [unlabeled]). Does not destroy existing viruses but stops them from reproducing and invading healthy cells. Also capable of chelating metal ions (e.g., calcium, magnesium). CMV strains resistant to ganciclovir and HSV strains resistant to acyclovir may be sensitive to foscarnet. Half-life ranges from 2 to 6 hours and increases markedly with renal impairment. Some penetration into bone and cerebrospinal fluid. Excreted unchanged in urine.

INDICATIONS AND USES

Treatment of CMV retinitis in patients with AIDS. Most frequently used in patients who do not tolerate or are resistant to ganciclovir. Combination therapy with ganciclovir is indicated for patients who have relapsed after monotherapy with either drug. ▪ Treatment of acyclovir-resistant mucocutaneous HSV infections in immunocompromised patients.

Unlabeled uses: Treatment of varicella-zoster virus (VZV) infections suspected or known to be caused by acyclovir-resistant strains in immunocompromised patients.

CONTRAINDICATIONS

Hypersensitivity to foscarnet.

PRECAUTIONS

For IV use only. ▪ Safety and efficacy of foscarnet have not been established for treatment of other CMV infections (e.g., pneumonitis, gastroenteritis), congenital or neonatal CMV disease, other HSV infections (e.g., retinitis, encephalitis), congenital or neonatal HSV disease, or CMV or HSV in nonimmunocompromised individuals. Use should be limited to treatment of conditions listed in Indications and Uses above. ▪ May cause potentially life-threatening changes in renal function with cumulative exposure. Careful monitoring of renal function and dose adjustment is imperative. Changes can occur at any time, most likely during second week of therapy. Elevations in SCr are usually reversible following dose adjustment or discontinuation of therapy. ▪ Confirm diagnosis of CMV retinitis by indirect ophthalmoscopy. Diagnosis may be supported by cultures of CMV from the throat and body fluids such as urine and blood; negative culture does not rule out CMV retinitis. ▪ Use caution in patients with a history of impaired renal function, altered calcium or other electrolyte levels, neurologic or cardiac abnormalities, a low baseline absolute neutrophil count (ANC), and those receiving other drugs known to influence minerals and electrolytes; see Drug/Lab Interactions. Has caused hyperphosphatemia, hypocalcemia, hypokalemia, hypomagnesemia, and hypophosphatemia, resulting in cardiac disturbances, seizures, and tetany. Seizures related to alterations in plasma minerals and electrolytes have been reported. ▪ Resistance has been reported to develop. May be higher in patients treated for a prolonged period. Consider the possibility of resistance in patients who show poor clinical response or who experience persistent viral excretion during treatment. ▪ Sensitivity testing for viral isolate is recommended before repeat treatment and/or to evaluate sensitivity versus development of resistance.

Monitor: Baseline 24-hour CrCl verified by creatinine index; baseline SCr, calcium, magnesium, potassium, phosphorus, and electrolytes required before treatment begins. Correct any deficiencies. ▪ Repeat entire testing process 2 to 3 times a week during induction therapy and a minimum of every 1 to 2 weeks during maintenance therapy. Foscarnet dose must be adjusted as indicated by test results. More frequent testing may be indicated in specific patients. Supplementation of minerals and electrolytes may be required during treatment. ▪ To minimize renal toxicity, hydration adequate to establish diuresis is recommended before and during treatment unless contraindicated. Give 750 to 1,000 mL NS or D5W before the first foscarnet infusion to establish diuresis. With subsequent infusions, give 750 to 1,000 mL concurrently with 90 to 120 mg/kg foscarnet and a minimum of 500 mL concurrently with 40 to 60 mg/kg. ▪ Discontinue foscarnet if CrCl drops below 0.4 mL/min/kg or serum creatinine is greater than 2.8 mg/100 mL (1 dL). Monitor patient daily until resolution of renal impairment is ensured. Safety for use in these patients has not been studied. ▪ Anemia may be severe enough to require transfusion. ▪ Phlebitis or pain may occur at site of infusion; confirm patency of vein and use large veins to ensure adequate blood flow for rapid dilution and distribution. ▪ See Drug/Lab Interactions.

Patient Education: Not a cure. Retinitis may recur during maintenance or after treatment; regular ophthalmologic exams imperative. ▪ Complete healing of HSV infections may occur, but most relapse. ▪ Perioral tingling, numbness in the extremities or paresthesias indicate electrolyte abnormalities; report immediately. ▪ Close monitoring of renal function and electrolyte balance during treatment is imperative. ▪ Cases of male and female genital irritation/ulceration have been reported. Adequate hydration and increased personal hygiene may minimize some side effects. ▪ Dose modification or discontinuation may be required for major side effects.

Maternal/Child: Category C: use only if clearly needed; has caused skeletal anomalies in animals. ▪ Excreted in maternal milk of lactating rats at three times maternal blood concentrations; human data not available. ▪ Safety for use in pediatric patients not established; deposited in teeth and bones, and deposition greater in young animals. Use only if benefits outweigh risks.

Elderly: Safety and effectiveness not established, however, foscarnet has been used in patients over 65 years of age. Side effects seen are similar to other age-groups. Consider age-related renal impairment in dose selection and monitor renal function; see Dose Adjustments.

DRUG/LAB INTERACTIONS

Because of physical **incompatibilities,** foscarnet sodium and **ganciclovir sodium** must never be mixed. ▪ Has caused hypocalcemia with parenteral **pentamidine;** deaths have been reported. ▪ Capable of causing calcium or electrolyte disorders. Use particular caution when administering **any drug known to influence serum calcium concentrations, other minerals, or electrolytes** (e.g., hypocalcemic agents [gallium nitrate (Ganite)], diuretics [furosemide (Lasix), mannitol], adrenocortical steroids). ▪ Elimination of foscarnet may be impaired and toxicity increased by **drugs that inhibit renal tubular secretion** (e.g., probenecid). ▪ Avoid concomitant use with other **nephrotoxic drugs** (e.g., aminoglycosides [e.g., gentamicin], amphotericin B [generic], cyclosporine [Sandimmune], pentamidine) unless benefits outweigh risks. ▪ Use with **fluoroquinolones** (e.g., ciprofloxacin [Cipro]) may cause seizures; monitor patient carefully. ▪ Abnormal renal function has been reported in patients receiving foscarnet and **ritonavir** (Norvir) or foscarnet and **ritonavir and saquinavir** (Invirase).

SIDE EFFECTS

Impaired renal function, alterations in plasma minerals and electrolytes, and seizures are major side effects and are dose limiting. Abnormal renal function, including acute renal failure, decreased CrCl, and increased SCr (27%); anemia (33%); bone marrow suppression (10%); diarrhea (30%); fatigue; fever (65%); headache (26%); hyperphosphatemia; hypocalcemia (perioral tingling, numbness in extremities, paresthesias, tetany); hypokalemia;

hypomagnesemia; hypophosphatemia; irritation at injection site; irritation and ulcerations of penile and vaginal epithelium; nausea (47%); rigors; seizure (10%); vomiting (26%); and death (14%) have occurred. All deaths could not be directly related to foscarnet. Abdominal pain, anorexia, anxiety, asthenia, confusion, coughing, depression, dizziness, dyspnea, granulocytopenia, hypoesthesia, infection, involuntary muscle contractions, leukopenia, malaise, neuropathy, pain, rash, sweating, and vision abnormalities have occurred in 5% of patients. Numerous other side effects have occurred in less than 5% of patients.

ANTIDOTE

There is no specific antidote. Keep physician informed. Adequate hydration and careful monitoring will help reduce potential for renal impairment and may minimize other side effects. Elevations in SCr are usually reversible (within 1 week) with dose adjustment or discontinuation but have caused death. Discontinue foscarnet if CrCl falls below 0.4 mL/min/kg or SCr is greater than 2.8 mg/100 mL. Monitor daily until resolution of renal impairment is ensured. Discontinue foscarnet if perioral tingling, numbness in the extremities, or paresthesias occur during or after infusion; evaluate calcium and electrolyte levels (decrease in ionized serum calcium may not be reflected in total serum calcium); notify physician. Administration of foscarnet can be resumed following seizures or cardiac disturbances after treatment of underlying disease, electrolyte disturbance, or after dose adjustment. Overdose can occur with too-rapid rate of infusion. Hemodialysis and hydration may be useful in overdose. Treat anaphylaxis and resuscitate as indicated.

FOSPHENYTOIN SODIUM
(**FOS**-fen-ih-toyn **SO**-dee-um)

Cerebyx

Anticonvulsant
(hydantoin)

pH 8.6 to 9

USUAL DOSE

In all situations, dose of fosphenytoin is expressed as phenytoin sodium equivalents (PE).

Status epilepticus: *Adult loading dose:* 15 to 20 mg PE/kg. Full effect is not immediate; concomitant administration of an IV benzodiazepine (e.g., diazepam [Valium]) is usually necessary to control status epilepticus. If seizures are not controlled, consider other anticonvulsants and other measures as needed (e.g., barbiturates or anesthesia). *Maintenance dose:* 4 to 6 mg PE/kg/24 hr.

Another source adds: *Elderly loading dose:* 14 mg PE/kg. See all comments under Usual Dose. See Elderly.

Nonemergent indications: *Loading dose:* 10 to 20 mg PE/kg. *Maintenance dose:* 4 to 6 mg PE/kg/24 hr. *Substitute for oral phenytoin:* May be substituted at the same total daily dose (due to a 10% increase in bioavailability [IV/IM to oral], plasma levels with the IV/IM product may be increased slightly).

PEDIATRIC DOSE

Status epilepticus loading dose (unlabeled): 15 to 20 mg PE/kg at a rate of 3 mg PE/kg/min up to 150 mg PE/min.

Nonemergent loading dose: 10 to 20 mg PE/kg.

Maintenance dose: 4 to 6 mg PE/kg initially. Safety for use in pediatric patients not established. Limited data available; no significant differences apparent to this date; see Maternal/Child.

DOSE ADJUSTMENTS

Reduced doses may be required in the elderly (see Usual Dose), in impaired renal or hepatic function, or in patients with hypoalbuminemia. ■ See Precautions, Monitor, Drug/Lab Interactions, and Antidote.

DILUTION

Use only clear solutions. Should be diluted in D5W or NS to a concentration of 1.5 to 25 mg PE/mL. Supplied solution is 50 mg PE/mL. Dilute each milliliter of fosphenytoin with 1 mL of diluent to equal 25 mg PE/mL. Dilute a 1,000-mg PE dose in 100 mL diluent to equal 10 mg PE/mL. **Storage:** Keep refrigerated; do not store at room temperature for more than 48 hours.

COMPATIBILITY

Consider any drug NOT listed as compatible to be INCOMPATIBLE until consulting a pharmacist; specific conditions may apply.

One source suggests the following **compatibilities:**

Additive: Potassium chloride (KCl).

Y-site: Lorazepam (Ativan), phenobarbital (Luminal).

RATE OF ADMINISTRATION

Each 100 to 150 mg PE or fraction thereof over a minimum of 1 minute. Risk of hypotension increased if this rate is exceeded. Slow or temporar-

ily stop rate of infusion for burning, itching, numbness, or pain along injection site.
Pediatric rate: Manufacturer recommends 1 to 3 mg PE/kg/min for pediatric patients. Another source suggests a rate of 1.6 mg PE/kg/min.
ACTIONS
A water-soluble prodrug of phenytoin. Converts to phenytoin, phosphate, and formate within 15 minutes of IV/IM administration. An anticonvulsant, chemically related to barbiturates. Selectively stabilizes seizure threshold and depresses seizure activity in the motor cortex. Modulation of voltage-dependent sodium channels of neurons thought to be the primary cellular mechanism responsible for anticonvulsant activity. Also exerts a depressant effect on the myocardium by selectively elevating the excitability threshold of the cell, reducing the cell's response to stimuli. Peak levels of fosphenytoin are achieved by the end of an infusion, but conversion to therapeutic serum levels of phenytoin takes longer. The conversion half-life of fosphenytoin to phenytoin is approximately 15 minutes. Extensively bound to protein, fosphenytoin displaces phenytoin from protein binding sites and increases free phenytoin (dose and rate dependent). Phenytoin's half-life is 12 to 28.9 hours. It is metabolized in the liver by hepatic cytochrome P_{450} enzymes and excreted in urine. Crosses the placental barrier. Secreted in breast milk.
INDICATIONS AND USES
Treatment and control of generalized convulsive status epilepticus. ▪ Treatment or prophylaxis of seizures in neurosurgical patients. ▪ Substitute for oral phenytoin when oral administration is not feasible or prompt increases in antiepileptic drug levels are needed.
CONTRAINDICATIONS
Hypersensitivity to fosphenytoin, any of its components, phenytoin, or other hydantoins. ▪ Sinus bradycardia, sinoatrial block, second- and third-degree AV block, and Adams-Stokes syndrome.
PRECAUTIONS
Doses of fosphenytoin are expressed as phenytoin equivalents; no adjustment required when substituting fosphenytoin or vice versa. Labeling of fosphenytoin has been updated by the manufacturer to reduce the incidence of dosing errors. To ensure accuracy, confirm actual dose, dilution, and amount of injection with pharmacist or another RN. ▪ Advantages of fosphenytoin over present phenytoin products include solubility in IV solutions, improved infusion site tolerance, more rapid rate of injection, and well-tolerated IM option. ▪ IV route indicated in emergency situations (e.g., status epilepticus). May be given IM in nonemergency situations. ▪ Intended for short-term parenteral use (up to 5 days). ▪ Transfer to oral phenytoin therapy as soon as feasible. ▪ Abrupt withdrawal may cause increased seizure activity. Gradually reduce dose, discontinue, or substitute alternative antiepileptic agents. ▪ Discontinue immediately for hypersensitivity reactions; with caution substitute a nonhydantoin anticonvulsant (e.g., phenobarbital [Luminal], valproate sodium [Depacon]). ▪ May cause severe cardiovascular depression (e.g., bradycardia, various degrees of AV block, ventricular fibrillation [VF]); use extreme caution in elderly or seriously ill patients. ▪ Use with caution in patients with hypotension or severe myocardial insufficiency. Risk of hypotension increased by higher

IV doses and/or rapid administration. ▪ May exacerbate porphyria. ▪ May cause acute phenytoin hepatotoxicity (e.g., elevated liver function tests, fever, jaundice, lymphadenopathy, skin eruptions). Discontinue immediately and substitute alternate anticonvulsant therapy. ▪ Has caused lymphadenopathy and hemopoietic complications (e.g., agranulocytosis, granulocytopenia, leukopenia, thrombocytopenia, or pancytopenia with or without bone marrow suppression). If lymphadenopathy occurs with or without signs of serum sickness (e.g., fever, rash, hepatotoxicity), substitute alternate anticonvulsant therapy. ▪ Sensory disturbances including severe burning, itching, and paresthesia have been reported; more common with higher doses and/or rates. ▪ Use caution with low serum albumin levels, and adjust dose as indicated. Phenytoin is highly bound to serum protein, and a reduced albumin causes an increase in free drug availability and may increase toxicity. ▪ Not effective for absence seizures; combined therapy required if both conditions present. ▪ Inhibits insulin release and may increase serum glucose; monitoring indicated in diabetics. ▪ May lower serum folate levels. ▪ Psychotic symptoms and other behavioral changes have been reported with antiepileptic drugs and may include aggression, agitation, anger, anxiety, apathy, depersonalization, depression, emotional lability, hallucinations, hostility, irritability, and suicidal tendencies. Some resolved without intervention. Others required dose reduction or discontinuation of the antiepileptic agent.

Monitor: Monitor ECG, BP, and respirations continuously during loading dose and for at least 10 to 20 minutes after infusion complete. ▪ Allow fosphenytoin time to convert to phenytoin; accurate serum levels are not available until 2 hours after the end of an IV infusion or 4 hours after IM injection. Narrow margin of error between therapeutic and toxic dose. Plasma levels above 10 mcg/mL usually control seizure activity. The acceptable range is 5 to 20 mcg/mL. Toxicity begins with nystagmus at levels exceeding 20 mcg/mL. ▪ Observe for rash and discontinue if one appears. If rash is mild, fosphenytoin may be resumed when the rash has completely disappeared. If the mild rash occurs again or the initial rash is serious in nature (e.g., exfoliative, purpuric, bullous) or lupus erythematous, Stevens-Johnson syndrome, or toxic epidermal necrolysis is suspected, discontinue fosphenytoin. Do not resume; consider alternative therapy. ▪ Phosphate is produced as a metabolite; monitor in patients who require phosphate restriction (e.g., renal impairment). ▪ Monitor closely patients who are gravely ill, have impaired liver function, or are elderly. May show early signs of toxicity. ▪ Determine absolute patency of vein; avoid extravasation. Not as alkaline as phenytoin. ▪ Observe patient closely for signs of CNS side effects; see Precautions.

Patient Education: Report burning, itching, numbness, pain, or rash. ▪ Consider birth control options; nonhormonal birth control recommended. ▪ May cause alterations in mood (e.g., aggression, agitation, anger, anxiety, apathy, decreased ability to cope, depression, hostility, irritability, thoughts of suicide); report these changes promptly. ▪ Women who are pregnant or who become pregnant should be encouraged to enroll in the North American Antiepileptic Drug (NAAED) Pregnancy Registry.

Maternal/Child: Category D: avoid pregnancy. Consider risk versus benefit. Risk of serious congenital malformations triple that of the general

population. ▪ An increase in seizure frequency may occur during pregnancy; if phenytoin is required, monitoring of plasma phenytoin levels may be helpful. ▪ Newborns whose mothers received phenytoin during pregnancy may develop a life-threatening bleeding disorder that can be prevented by giving vitamin K to the mother before delivery and to the neonate after birth. ▪ Discontinue breast-feeding. ▪ Safety for use in pediatric patients not established. ▪ See Patient Education.
Elderly: See Dose Adjustments. ▪ Sensitivity and/or toxicity may be increased because serum concentrations may be elevated due to reduced clearance, or low serum albumin may cause a decrease in protein binding and an increase in free phenytoin.

DRUG/LAB INTERACTIONS
No drugs are known to interfere with the conversion of fosphenytoin to phenytoin, although phosphatase activity may have an impact. ▪ *Capable of innumerable catastrophic drug interactions; review of drug profile by pharmacist imperative.* In all situations, monitoring of phenytoin serum levels may be indicated. ▪ Serum levels and toxicity of phenytoin may be increased by **alcohol (acute intake), amiodarone** (Nexterone), **anticonvulsants** (e.g., succinimides [ethosuximide (Zarontin)]), **antidepressants** (e.g., fluoxetine [Prozac], trazodone [Deseryl]), **chloramphenicol, chlordiazepoxide** (Librium), **H_2 antagonists** (e.g., cimetidine [Tagamet]), **diazepam** (Valium), **dicumarol, disulfiram** (Antabuse), **estrogens, fluorouracil, halothane, isoniazid** (Nydrazid), **methylphenidate** (Ritalin), **phenothiazines** (e.g., prochlorperazine [Compazine]), **salicylates** (aspirin), **sulfonamides** (e.g., sulfisoxazole), **tolbutamide, voriconazole** (VFEND). ▪ Serum levels and effectiveness of phenytoin may be decreased by **carbamazepine** (Tegretol), **chronic alcohol abuse, cisplatin, and reserpine** (Serpasil). ▪ Serum levels of phenytoin may be increased or decreased by **phenobarbital** (Luminal), **valproate sodium** (Depacon), **valproic acid** (Depakene). Similarly, phenytoin may unpredictably affect the levels and efficacy of these drugs. ▪ **Tricyclic antidepressants** (e.g., amitriptyline [Elavil], imipramine [Tofranil]) may precipitate seizures in susceptible patients. Dose adjustment of fosphenytoin may be indicated. ▪ Phenytoin will inhibit the effects of **anticoagulants** (e.g., warfarin [Coumadin]), **corticosteroids, cardiac glycosides** (e.g., digoxin), **doxycycline, estrogens, furosemide** (Lasix), **itraconazole** (Sporanox), **oral contraceptives, rifampin** (Rifadin), **quinidine, theophylline, vitamin D.** ▪ Alters some **clinical laboratory tests** (e.g., may decrease T_4, increase glucose, alkaline phosphatase, and GGT may produce low results in dexamethasone or metyrapone tests).

SIDE EFFECTS
Transient ataxia, dizziness, headache, nystagmus, paresthesia, pruritus, and somnolence are the most common side effects; are dose and rate related; occur within several minutes of the start of the infusion; and usually resolve within 10 minutes of completion. Risks of side effects increased with upper-end doses given at upper-end rates. Coma, hyperreflexia, hypotension, lethargy, nausea, slurred speech, tremor, and vomiting are also signs of increased toxicity. Confusional states (e.g., delirium, encephalopathy, psychosis) and, rarely, irreversible cerebellar dysfunction can occur with high plasma concentrations. Fosphenytoin breaks down into formate and phosphate metabolites that may cause formate toxicity in

overdose situations (hypocalcemia, metabolic acidosis, muscle spasms, paresthesia, and seizures). Psychotic symptoms, including aggression, agitation, anger, anxiety, apathy, depersonalization, depression, emotional lability, hallucinations, hostility, irritability, and suicidal tendencies, have occurred with antiepileptic agents.

Major/overdose: Arrhythmias (e.g., bradycardia, cardiac arrest, heart block, tachycardia, ventricular fibrillation), coma, hyperreflexia, hypotension, lethargy, nausea, respiratory arrest, slurred speech, syncope, tonic seizures, tremor, and vomiting. Deaths have been reported.

ANTIDOTE

Notify physician of any side effects. Obtain serum plasma levels at first signs of toxicity; reduce dose. If symptoms persist or major side effects appear, discontinue fosphenytoin and notify physician. Treat symptomatically, maintain a patent airway, and resuscitate as necessary. Symptoms of bradycardia or heart block may be reversed with IV atropine. Epinephrine may also be useful. One source says hemodialysis may be helpful in overdose. Another source says hemodialysis, peritoneal dialysis, forced fluid diuresis, exchange transfusions, and plasmapheresis are ineffective. In overdose, measure ionized free calcium levels to guide treatment in phosphate toxicity.

FOSPROPOFOL DISODIUM
(**FOS**-proh-poh-fohl)

Sedative–hypnotic
Anesthetic
Anesthesia adjunct

Lusedra   pH 8.2 to 9

USUAL DOSE

Supplemental oxygen and continuous monitoring required; see Monitor. Dose must be individualized and titrated to desired level of sedation. Use the minimum dose required to facilitate the procedure. In clinical studies, fentanyl 50 mcg was administered as a premedication 5 minutes before the initial dose of fospropofol.

Standard dosing regimen for healthy adults under 65 years of age or those with mild systemic disease (ASA I or II): 6.5 mg/kg as an initial IV bolus. Follow with supplemental doses of 1.6 mg/kg (25% of initial dose) as an IV bolus as needed to achieve the desired level of sedation. Administer supplemental doses based on the patient's level of sedation. Give supplemental doses only when patients can demonstrate purposeful movement in response to verbal or light tactile stimulation and not more frequently than every 4 minutes. Dose is limited by the lower and upper weight limits of 60 kg and 90 kg. Patients who weigh over 90 kg should be dosed as if they weigh 90 kg. *No initial dose should exceed 16.5 mL; no supplemental dose should exceed 4 mL.* Patients who weigh less than 60 kg should be dosed as if they weigh 60 kg. However, doses lower than those specified for the lower weight limit may be used to achieve lesser levels of sedation. See the following table for the standard dosing regimen described earlier.

Fospropofol Standard Dosing Regimen for Adults Under 65 Years of Age Who Are Healthy or Have Mild Systemic Disease (ASA I or II)*				
	Initial Dose		Supplemental Dose (no more frequently than every 4 minutes)	
Weight (kg)	mg	mL	mg	mL
≤60	385	11	105	3
61 to 63	402.5	11.5	105	3
64 to 65	420	12	105	3
66 to 68	437.5	12.5	105	3
69 to 71	455	13	105	3
72 to 74	472.5	13.5	122.5	3.5
75 to 76	490	14	122.5	3.5
77 to 79	507.5	14.5	122.5	3.5
80 to 82	525	15	140	4
83 to 84	542.5	15.5	140	4
85 to 87	560	16	140	4
88 to 89	577.5	16.5	140	4
≥90	577.5	16.5	140	4

*Note: Doses in this table are rounded to the nearest half-milliliter volume to facilitate practical measurement; hence they may differ slightly from the dose recommended on the basis of mg/kg.

Continued

Modified dosing regimen for adults 65 years of age or older or those with severe systemic disease (ASA III or IV): Decrease initial and supplemental doses to 75% of the standard dosing regimen as listed in the following table.

Fospropofol Modified Dosing Regimen for Adults 65 Years of Age or Older or Those with Severe Systemic Disease (ASA III or IV)*				
	Initial Dose		Supplemental Dose (no more frequently than every 4 minutes)	
Weight (kg)	mg	mL	mg	mL
≤60	297.5	8.5	70	2
61 to 62	297.5	8.5	70	2
63 to 64	315	9	87.5	2.5
65 to 66	315	9	87.5	2.5
67 to 69	332.5	9.5	87.5	2.5
70 to 73	350	10	87.5	2.5
74 to 77	367.5	10.5	87.5	2.5
78 to 80	385	11	105	3
81 to 84	402.5	11.5	105	3
85 to 87	420	12	105	3
88 to 89	437.5	12.5	105	3
≥90	437.5	12.5	105	3

*Note: Doses in this table are rounded to the nearest half-milliliter volume to facilitate practical measurement; hence they may differ slightly from the dose recommended on the basis of mg/kg.

DOSE ADJUSTMENTS

See Usual Dose for specific reduced doses required for adults 65 years of age or older or ASA risk III or IV patients. ■ Reduced doses are required in the presence of other CNS depressants; see Drug/Lab Interactions. ■ Reduced doses are not required based on race, gender, age, alkaline phosphatase concentrations, or mild to moderate renal impairment. ■ Has not been adequately studied in patients with a CrCl less than 30 mL/min or in patients with hepatic impairment.

DILUTION

Supplied as a ready-to-use solution containing 35 mg/mL of fospropofol (1,050 mg/30 mL vial). Intended for single use. Strict aseptic technique is imperative. Draw solution into a sterile syringe immediately after vial is opened. Discard any unused portion at the end of the procedure.

Filter: Not required. Information not available.

Storage: Store at CRT. Draw up into syringe immediately after opening vial and discard any unused solution at the end of the procedure.

COMPATIBILITY

Manufacturer states, "Do not mix with other drugs or fluids prior to administration. Is **not physically compatible** with midazolam or meperidine, and **compatibility** with other agents has not been adequately evaluated. Flush the infusion line with NS before and after administration." Has been shown to be **compatible** with the following solutions: D5W, D5/¼NS, D5/½NS, NS, LR, D5LR, ½NS, D5/½NS, and 20 mEq KCl.

RATE OF ADMINISTRATION

Administer as a bolus injection.

ACTIONS

A sedative-hypnotic agent. A prodrug of propofol. Following injection, fospropofol is metabolized by alkaline phosphatases to propofol, which interacts with the GABA (gamma-aminobutyric acid) receptors of the CNS, resulting in sedation. In clinical studies, peak plasma levels of propofol released from fospropofol were noted within 12 minutes. In patients undergoing a colonoscopy, the median time to sedation was 8 minutes (range 2 to 28 minutes), and the median time to Fully Alert following the procedure was 5 minutes (range 0 to 47 minutes). In patients undergoing a bronchoscopy, the median time to sedation was 4 minutes (range 2 to 22 minutes), and the median time to Fully Alert following the procedure was 5.5 minutes (range 0 to 6 minutes). Both fospropofol and its active metabolite propofol are highly protein bound, primarily to albumin. Propofol is further metabolized in the liver. The half-lives of fospropofol and propofol are approximately 0.8 and 2 hours, respectively. Propofol is excreted as metabolites in the urine.

INDICATIONS AND USES

To initiate and maintain monitored anesthesia care (MAC) sedation in adult patients undergoing diagnostic or therapeutic procedures.

CONTRAINDICATIONS

Manufacturer states, "None." See Precautions.

PRECAUTIONS

Administered by persons trained in the administration of general anesthesia and not involved in the conduct of the diagnostic or therapeutic procedure. Patients should be continuously monitored, and facilities and supplies for responding to any medical emergency must be immediately available. ▪ Respiratory depression, including the loss of spontaneous respirations, may occur. Supplemental oxygen is recommended for all patients. Hypoxemia may occur and has been seen in patients who retained the ability to respond purposefully. The risk of hypoxemia is reduced by appropriate positioning of the patient and the administration of supplemental oxygen. ▪ Has not been studied for use in general anesthesia and is not recommended. Administration may inadvertently cause patients to become unresponsive or minimally responsive to vigorous tactile or painful stimulation. ▪ May cause hypotension. Patients with compromised myocardial function, reduced vascular tone (e.g., sepsis), or reduced intravascular volume may be at an increased risk for hypotension. ▪ Use with caution in patients with hepatic impairment or severe renal impairment (CrCl less than 30 mL/min). ▪ Safety for continuous sedation has not been established and is not recommended. ▪ See Drug/Lab Interactions. **Monitor:** Patients should be continuously monitored during sedation and through the recovery process with pulse oximetry, ECG, and frequent BP measurements for early signs of arrhythmia, hypotension, apnea, airway obstruction, and/or oxygen desaturation. Hypoxemia may be detected by pulse oximetry. ▪ Assess patients for the ability to demonstrate a purposeful response while sedated. Patients who are unable to demonstrate a purposeful response may lose protective reflexes. Airway assistance maneuvers may be required. ▪ Correct fluid volume deficiencies before administration.

Patient Education: Paresthesias and/or pruritus, usually manifested in the perineal region, are common side effects. Side effects are usually mild to moderate in intensity and of short duration. ▪ Avoid alcohol or other CNS depressants (e.g., antihistamines, benzodiazepines) for 24 hours following the procedure. ▪ Do not perform tasks that require mental alertness (e.g., driving, operating hazardous machinery, or signing legal documents) until the day after surgery or longer. All effects must have subsided.

Maternal/Child: Category B: use during pregnancy only if clearly needed. Use during labor and delivery, including cesarean section, is not recommended. It is not known if fospropofol crosses the placenta; however, propofol is known to cross the placenta, and as with other sedative-hypnotic agents, the administration of fospropofol may be associated with neonatal respiratory and cardiovascular depression. ▪ Use during breastfeeding not recommended. ▪ Safety and effectiveness for use in pediatric patients not established.

Elderly: Patients 65 years of age or older should receive the modified dosing regimen; see Usual Dose. Hypoxemia has been reported more frequently in the elderly.

DRUG/LAB INTERACTIONS

Potentiated by other medications that can depress cardiac or respiratory status (e.g., **narcotics** [e.g., morphine, meperidine (Demerol), fentanyl (Sublimaze)], **sedatives** [barbiturates, benzodiazepines (e.g., diazepam [Valium], midazolam [Versed])], chloral hydrate, droperidol [Inapsine]). ▪ Has been administered with fentanyl, meperidine, midazolam, and morphine.

SIDE EFFECTS

The most commonly reported side effects are paresthesia (burning, stinging, tingling) and/or pruritus, usually manifested in the perineal region. The most serious side effects reported include hypotension, hypoxemia, loss of purposeful responsiveness, and respiratory depression. The most commonly reported reasons for discontinuation of therapy are cough and paresthesia. Other reported side effects include headache, nausea, procedural pain, and vomiting.

Overdose: (Secondary to accumulation of formate and phosphate metabolites) Anion-gap metabolic acidosis, hypocalcemia with paresthesia, muscle spasms, and seizures.

ANTIDOTE

Notify physician of any side effects; most will be treated symptomatically. A short-acting drug, a patent airway, and continuous controlled ventilation with oxygen until normal function is ensured should be adequate. Treat hypotension with IV fluid replacement, Trendelenburg position, or vasopressors (e.g., dopamine) as indicated. Resuscitate as necessary.

660

FUROSEMIDE BBW
(fur-**OH**-seh-myd)

Diuretic (loop)
Antihypertensive
Antihypercalcemic

Lasix pH 8 to 9.3

USUAL DOSE
Adjust dose and dose schedule to individual patient needs.
Edema/congestive heart failure: 20 to 40 mg. May be repeated in 1 to 2 hours. If necessary, increase dosage by 20-mg increments (under close medical supervision and no sooner than 1 to 2 hours after previous dose) until desired diuresis is obtained. (Maximum recommended dose is 200 mg/dose.) Total of IV bolus doses should not exceed 1 Gm/day. If larger doses are required, give as an infusion. In severe refractory congestive heart failure, doses up to 4 Gm/24 hr have been given with extreme caution. After the initial diuresis the minimum effective dose may be given once or twice every 24 hours as required for maintenance.
New-onset pulmonary edema with hypovolemia: AHA guidelines recommend less than 0.5 mg/kg.
Hypertension: Up to 40 mg twice daily. If this dose does not reduce hypertension, the addition of other antihypertensive agents is recommended instead of larger doses of furosemide.
Hypertensive crisis: 40 to 80 mg concomitantly with other antihypertensive agents. AHA guidelines recommend 0.5 to 1 mg/kg over 1 to 2 minutes. If no response, increase dose to 2 mg/kg.
Hypertensive crisis with pulmonary edema or acute renal failure: 100 to 200 mg.
Acute pulmonary edema or post–cardiac arrest cerebral edema: 40 mg. If no response in 1 hour, increase to 80 mg. AHA guidelines recommend 0.5 to 1 mg/kg over 1 to 2 minutes. If no response, increase dose to 2 mg/kg.
Acute or chronic renal failure: Initial dose required can range from 100 mg to 2 Gm. Higher doses are well tolerated in these patients. Increase dose as needed to achieve desired effect. IV bolus dose should not exceed 1 Gm/day. If larger doses are required, give as an infusion. Has been doubled at 2- to 24-hour intervals in some studies. One protocol calls for an infusion of 250 mg over 1 hour. If urine output insufficient in 1 hour, increase to 500 mg infused over 2 hours. If urine output still insufficient after the first hour, increase to 1 Gm over 4 hours. For high-dose infusions, individualize dose and titrate to maximum therapeutic effect from the lowest dose. Highest total IV dose was 6 g.
Hypercalcemia: 80 to 100 mg at 1- to 2-hour intervals. Given concomitantly with NS. Total IV dose required has ranged from 160 mg to 3.2 g.
Diagnostic aid (renal imaging adjunct [unlabeled]): 0.3 to 0.5 mg/kg to maximum dose of 40 mg.
PEDIATRIC DOSE
See Maternal/Child.
Diuretic: 1 mg/kg of body weight. After 2 hours increase by 1-mg/kg increments to effect desired response. Effective dose may be given every 6 to 12 hours. Another source suggests 0.5 to 2 mg/kg/dose every 6 to 12 hours. Do not exceed 6 mg/kg/dose.

Hypercalcemia: 25 to 50 mg. Repeat every 4 hours to desired response. Do not exceed 6 mg/kg/dose.

NEONATAL DOSE

Diuretic: 0.5 to 1 mg/kg/dose every 8 to 24 hours. Maximum dose is 2 mg/kg/dose. See Maternal/Child.

DOSE ADJUSTMENTS

Higher doses may be required in renal insufficiency and acute or chronic renal failure. ■ Reduced dose or extended intervals may be appropriate in the elderly. ■ Extend dosing intervals in neonates because half-life is prolonged. ■ See Drug/Lab Interactions.

DILUTION

May be given undiluted. May be given through Y-tube or three-way stopcock of infusion set. Not usually added to IV solutions, but large doses may be added to NS, LR, D5W, D5NS and given as an infusion. pH of solution must be over 5.5. Some sources recommend protecting diluted solutions from light to prevent photodegradation (minimized at pH 7).

Filters: If obtaining large doses from ampules, use of a filter is recommended to eliminate possible pieces of glass.

Storage: If diluted for infusion, discard after 24 hours.

COMPATIBILITY (Underline Indicates Conflicting Compatibility Information)

Consider any drug NOT listed as compatible to be INCOMPATIBLE until consulting a pharmacist; specific conditions may apply.

One source suggests the following **compatibilities:**

Additive: Amikacin (Amikin), aminophylline, <u>amiodarone (Nexterone)</u>, ampicillin, atropine, bumetanide, calcium gluconate, cefuroxime (Zinacef), dexamethasone (Decadron), digoxin (Lanoxin), <u>epinephrine (Adrenalin)</u>, <u>gentamicin</u>, heparin, <u>hydrocortisone sodium succinate (Solu-Cortef)</u>, kanamycin (Kantrex), lidocaine, meropenem (Merrem IV), midazolam (Versed), morphine, nitroglycerin IV, penicillin G potassium, potassium chloride (KCl), ranitidine (Zantac), sodium bicarbonate, theophylline, tobramycin, <u>verapamil</u>.

Y-site: Allopurinol (Aloprim), amifostine (Ethyol), amikacin (Amikin), <u>amiodarone (Nexterone)</u>, amphotericin B cholesteryl (Amphotec), <u>anidulafungin (Eraxis)</u>, argatroban, aztreonam (Azactam), bivalirudin (Angiomax), bleomycin (Blenoxane), cefepime (Maxipime), ceftazidime (Fortaz), <u>cisatracurium (Nimbex)</u>, cisplatin (Platinol), cladribine (Leustatin), cyclophosphamide (Cytoxan), cytarabine (ARA-C), dexmedetomidine (Precedex), <u>dobutamine</u>, docetaxel (Taxotere), <u>dopamine</u>, doripenem (Doribax), <u>doxorubicin (Adriamycin)</u>, doxorubicin liposomal (Doxil), <u>drotrecogin alfa (Xigris)</u>, <u>epinephrine (Adrenalin)</u>, etoposide phosphate (Etopophos), <u>famotidine (Pepcid IV)</u>, fentanyl (Sublimaze), fludarabine (Fludara), fluorouracil (5-FU), foscarnet (Foscavir), gallium nitrate (Ganite), granisetron (Kytril), heparin, hetastarch in electrolytes (Hextend), hydrocortisone sodium succinate (Solu-Cortef), hydromorphone (Dilaudid), indomethacin (Indocin IV), kanamycin (Kantrex), leucovorin calcium, linezolid (Zyvox), lorazepam (Ativan), melphalan (Alkeran), <u>meperidine (Demerol)</u>, meropenem (Merrem IV), methotrexate, <u>micafungin (Mycamine)</u>, mitomycin (Mutamycin), <u>morphine</u>, <u>nitroglycerin IV</u>, nitroprusside sodium, norepinephrine (Levophed), oxaliplatin (Eloxatin), paclitaxel (Taxol), <u>pantoprazole (Protonix IV)</u>, piperacillin/tazobactam (Zosyn), potassium chloride (KCl), propofol (Diprivan), ranitidine (Zantac), remifentanil (Ultiva), sargramostim (Leukine), tacrolimus (Prograf), teniposide (Vumon), thiopental (Pentothal), thiotepa, tirofiban (Aggrastat), tobramycin.

RATE OF ADMINISTRATION

IV injection: Each 40 mg or fraction thereof should be given over 1 to 2 minutes. A 1-Gm bolus must be given over at least 30 minutes; up to 3 hours is preferred. In oliguric or anuric patients the total dose (undiluted) should be infused at a rate of 4 mg/min. Constant rate infusion pump required.

Infusion: *Adults:* 0.1 mg/kg/hr. ***Pediatric patients:*** 0.05 mg/kg/hr. Titrate to effect. High-dose therapy in an infusion should not exceed a rate of 4 mg/min. A 1-Gm dose should take at least 3 hours in an adult to prevent ototoxicity.

ACTIONS

A sulfonamide-type diuretic, related to the thiazides. Extremely potent and has a rapid onset of action. Effectiveness is noted within 5 minutes and may last for 2 hours. Apparently acts on the proximal and distal ends of the tubule and the ascending limb of the loop of Henle to excrete water, sodium, chlorides, and potassium. Will produce diuresis in alkalosis or acidosis. Highly protein bound. Metabolized and excreted in the urine. Crosses the placental barrier. Secreted in breast milk.

INDICATIONS AND USES

Edema associated with congestive heart failure, cirrhosis of the liver with ascites, and renal disease including the nephrotic syndrome. ▪ Acute pulmonary edema. ▪ Edema unresponsive to other diuretic agents. ▪ Hypercalcemia. ▪ Hypertension. ▪ Post–cardiac arrest cerebral edema. **Unlabeled uses:** Renal imaging radionuclide adjunct to increase urine flow and aid in differentiation of mechanical obstruction versus nonobstructive dilatation in patients with hydroureteronephrosis.

CONTRAINDICATIONS

Anuria, hypersensitivity to furosemide, severe progressive renal disease with increasing azotemia and oliguria; rarely used in pediatric patients, pregnancy, and breast-feeding.

PRECAUTIONS

May be used concurrently with aldosterone antagonists (e.g., spironolactone [Aldactone]) for more effective diuresis and to prevent excessive potassium loss. ▪ Use caution and improve basic condition first in hepatic coma, electrolyte depletion, and advanced cirrhosis of the liver. ▪ May precipitate excessive diuresis with water and electrolyte depletion. ▪ May increase risk of gastric hemorrhage during corticosteroid therapy. ▪ Use extreme caution in known sulfonamide sensitivity. ▪ Risk of ototoxicity increases with higher doses, rapid injection, decreased renal function, or concurrent use with other ototoxic drugs; see Drug/Lab Interactions. ▪ May activate or exacerbate systemic lupus erythematosus.

Monitor: Discontinue at least 2 days before elective surgery. ▪ Monitor BP frequently, especially during initial therapy. ▪ May precipitate excessive diuresis with water and electrolyte depletion. Routine checks on electrolyte panel, CO_2, and BUN are necessary during therapy. Replacement of KCl may be required. ▪ May increase blood glucose and has precipitated diabetes mellitus. ▪ May lower serum calcium level; may cause tetany. ▪ Hyperuricemia can occur. Rarely precipitates acute gout attack. ▪ See Drug/Lab Interactions.

Patient Education: Hypotension may cause dizziness; request assistance with ambulation. ▪ Report cramps, dizziness, muscle weakness, or nausea promptly. ▪ May cause a decrease in potassium levels and require a supplement. ▪ Skin may become photosensitive; avoid unprotected exposure to sun.

Maternal/Child: Category C: use during pregnancy only when clearly needed and benefits outweigh potential risks to fetus. ▪ Discontinue breastfeeding. ▪ Safety for use in pediatric patients not established. ▪ Prolonged use in premature infants may result in nephrocalcinosis. ▪ May increase risk of patent ductus arteriosus in pre-term infants with respiratory distress syndrome; use with caution before delivery. ▪ See Contraindications.

Elderly: Consider increased sensitivity to hypotensive and electrolyte effects. ▪ May be more susceptible to dehydration; observe carefully. ▪ Avoid rapid contraction of plasma volume and hemoconcentration. May cause thromboembolic episodes (e.g., CVA, pulmonary emboli).

DRUG/LAB INTERACTIONS
Causes excessive potassium depletion with **corticosteroids, thiazide diuretics** (e.g., hydrochlorothiazide [HydroDIURIL]), **amphotericin B** (all formulations). ▪ Potentiates **antihypertensive drugs** (e.g., nitroglycerin, nitroprusside sodium); reduced dose of the antihypertensive agent or both drugs may be indicated. ▪ May cause transient or permanent deafness with doses exceeding the usual or when given in conjunction with **other ototoxic drugs** (e.g., aminoglycosides [e.g., gentamicin], cisplatin). ▪ **Amphotericin B** (all formulations) may increase potential for ototoxicity and nephrotoxicity; avoid concurrent use. ▪ Nephrotoxicity increased by **other nephrotoxic agents** (e.g., acyclovir [Zovirax], aminoglycosides, ciprofloxacin [Cipro IV], cyclosporine [Sandimmune], vancomycin); avoid concurrent use. ▪ May increase activity of **anticoagulants** (e.g., warfarin [Coumadin], heparin, streptokinase); monitor PT. ▪ May increase serum levels of **beta-blockers** (e.g., propranolol) and of **lithium** (may cause toxicity). ▪ May cause cardiac arrhythmias with **amiodarone** (Nexterone) **or digoxin** (potassium depletion). ▪ Risk of cardiotoxicity increased with **pimozide** (Orap) **and sparfloxacin** (Zagam); concurrent use not recommended. ▪ May enhance or inhibit actions of **nondepolarizing muscle relaxants** (e.g., atracurium [Tracrium]) or **theophyllines.** ▪ May cause hyperglycemia with **insulin or sulfonylureas** (e.g., tolbutamide) by decreasing glucose tolerance. ▪ Effects may be inhibited by **ACE inhibitors** (e.g., captopril [Capoten]), **NSAIDs** (e.g., ibuprofen [Motrin]), **probenecid,** or in patients with **cirrhosis and ascites on salicylates.** ▪ May cause profound diuresis and serious electrolyte abnormalities with **thiazide diuretics** (e.g., chlorothiazide [Diuril]) because of synergistic effects. ▪ **Clofibrate** (Atromid-S) may cause increased diuresis. ▪ May be inhibited by **phenytoin** (Dilantin). ▪ Do not use concomitantly with **ethacrynic acid** (Edecrin); risk of ototoxicity markedly increased. ▪ **Smoking** may increase secretion of ADH-decreasing diuretic effects and cardiac output. ▪ See Precautions.

SIDE EFFECTS
Usually occur in prolonged therapy, seriously ill patients, or following large doses.

Anemia, anorexia, blurring of vision, deafness (reversible), diarrhea, dizziness, headache, hyperglycemia, hyperuricemia, hypokalemia, leg cramps, lethargy, leukopenia, mental confusion, nausea, paresthesia, postural hypotension, pruritus, rash, tinnitus, urinary frequency, urticaria, vomiting, weakness.

Major: Anaphylactic shock, blood volume reduction, circulatory collapse, dehydration, excessive diuresis, hypokalemia, metabolic acidosis, vascular thrombosis, and embolism.

ANTIDOTE

If minor side effects are noted, discontinue the drug and notify the physician, who may treat the side effects symptomatically and continue the drug. If side effects are progressive or any major side effect occurs, discontinue the drug immediately and notify the physician. Treatment of major side effects is symptomatic and aggressive. Resuscitate as necessary.

GALLIUM NITRATE BBW
(**GAL**-lee-yum **NIH**-trayt)

Ganite

Antihypercalcemic

pH 6 to 7

USUAL DOSE

Adequate hydration and specific testing required; see Monitor.

200 mg/M^2 daily for 5 consecutive days. Must be administered as an IV infusion. Discontinue treatment at any time the serum calcium levels are lowered into the normal range (8.5 to 10.5 mg/100 mL, corrected for serum albumin). Safety and effectiveness of retreatment not established. See Precautions.

DOSE ADJUSTMENTS

Consider reduction to 100 mg/M^2/day for 5 days in patients with mild hypercalcemia (12 mg/100 mL range corrected for serum albumin) and few symptoms. ▪ Reduced dose may be required in impaired renal function based on CrCl (2 to 2.5 mg/100 mL). See Contraindications.

DILUTION

A single daily dose must be diluted in 1,000 mL NS (preferred) or D5W. Less diluent may be used if absolutely necessary in patients with compromised cardiovascular status.

Filters: Use not required by manufacturer; however, use of a filter would not have an adverse effect.

Storage: Store at CRT before dilution. Stable after dilution for 48 hours at CRT and for 7 days if refrigerated.

COMPATIBILITY

Consider any drug NOT listed as compatible to be INCOMPATIBLE until consulting a pharmacist; specific conditions may apply.

One source suggests the following **compatibilities:**

Y-site: Acyclovir (Zovirax), allopurinol (Aloprim), amifostine (Ethyol), aminophylline, ampicillin/sulbactam (Unasyn), aztreonam (Azactam), cefazolin (Ancef), ceftazidime (Fortaz), ceftriaxone (Rocephin), ciprofloxacin (Cipro IV), cladribine (Leustatin), cyclophosphamide (Cytoxan), dexamethasone (Decadron), diphenhydramine (Benadryl), filgrastim (Neupogen), fluconazole (Diflucan), furosemide (Lasix), granisetron (Kytril), heparin, hydrocortisone sodium succinate (Solu-Cortef), ifosfamide (Ifex), magnesium sulfate, mannitol (Osmitrol), melphalan (Alkeran), meperidine (Demerol), mesna (Mesnex), methotrexate, metoclopramide (Reglan), ondansetron (Zofran), piperacillin, piperacillin/tazobactam (Zosyn), potassium chloride (KCl), ranitidine (Zantac), sodium bicarbonate, sulfamethoxazole/trimethoprim, teniposide (Vumon), thiotepa, ticarcillin/clavulanate (Timentin), vancomycin, vinorelbine (Navelbine).

RATE OF ADMINISTRATION
A single daily dose equally distributed over 24 hours as an IV infusion. Use of a microdrip (60 gtt/mL) or an infusion pump recommended for even distribution. Too-rapid injection may lead to overdose.

ACTIONS
A hypocalcemic agent that inhibits calcium resorption from bone. Thought to act by reducing increased bone turnover. Does not have cytotoxic effects on bone cells. Plasma levels achieve a steady state 24 to 48 hours after infusion initiated. In one study it normalized serum calcium in 75% of patients who began treatment with a serum calcium corrected for albumin greater than 12 mg/100 mL. Maintains duration of normocalcemia/hypocalcemia longer than calcitonin. Route of metabolism is unknown. Significant excretion occurs through the kidneys.

INDICATIONS AND USES
Treatment of clearly symptomatic cancer-related hypercalcemia that has not responded to adequate hydration. Serum calcium above 12 mg/100 mL corrected for serum albumin. Symptoms may include anorexia, cardiac arrest, coma, confusion, constipation, dehydration, depression, fatigue, muscle weakness, nausea and vomiting.
Unlabeled uses: Slow bone resorption and reduce calcium excretion in bone metastasis; treatment of malignant lymphoma.

CONTRAINDICATIONS
Severe renal impairment (SCr greater than 2.5 mg/100 mL).

PRECAUTIONS
In patients with cancer-related hypercalcemia, the risk of developing severe renal insufficiency is increased with concurrent use of other potentially nephrotoxic drugs (e.g., aminoglycosides [e.g., gentamicin], amphotericin B). If use of these drugs is necessary, discontinue gallium nitrate. Continue hydration for several days after administration of nephrotoxic drugs, and closely monitor serum creatinine and urine output during and after their administration. ▪ Calcium is bound to serum protein; concentration fluctuates with changes in blood volume. Changes in serum calcium (especially during rehydration) may not reflect true plasma levels. All calcium measurement should be corrected for albumin to establish a basis for treatment and evaluation of treatment. ▪ Mild or asymptomatic hypercalcemia will be treated with conservative measures (e.g., saline hydration, with or without diuretics). Consider patient's cardiovascular status.
Monitor: Baseline measurements of serum calcium corrected for serum albumin, serum phosphorus, electrolytes, plasma pH, SCr, and BUN are required. Monitor calcium daily, phosphorus twice weekly, and electrolytes, plasma pH, creatinine, and BUN closely as indicated by baseline results (may be daily). ▪ Patients with cancer-related hypercalcemia are frequently dehydrated. Must be adequately hydrated orally and/or intravenously before treatment is initiated. Hydration with saline is preferred to facilitate renal excretion of calcium and correct dehydration. A pretreat-

ment urine output of 2 L/day is recommended. ▪ Avoid overhydration in patients with compromised cardiovascular status. Observe frequently for signs of fluid overload. Correct hypovolemia before using diuretics. ▪ Maintain adequate hydration and urine output throughout treatment. ▪ See Precautions.

Patient Education: Regular visits and assessments of lab tests imperative. ▪ Restriction of dietary calcium and vitamin D may be required. ▪ Take only prescribed medications. ▪ Report abdominal cramps, chills, confusion, fever, muscle spasms, sore throat, and/or any new medical problem promptly.

Maternal/Child: Category C: use in pregnancy has not been studied; use only if clearly needed. ▪ Discontinue breast-feeding or do not use gallium nitrate. Consider importance of drug to mother. ▪ Safety for use in pediatric patients not established.

DRUG/LAB INTERACTIONS

Nephrotoxicity may be increased with **other nephrotoxic drugs** (e.g., aminoglycosides [gentamicin], amphotericin B [generic], Edecrin); see Precautions. ▪ Concomitant use with **oral cyclophosphamide and oral prednisone** may cause asthenia, dyspnea, and mouth soreness in a small number of patients with multiple myeloma.

SIDE EFFECTS

Acute renal failure, anemia, asymptomatic decrease in BP, confusion, constipation, diarrhea, dreams and hallucinations, dyspnea, edema of the lower extremities, fever, fluid overload, hearing loss, hypocalcemia, hypophosphatemia, hypothermia, lethargy, leukopenia, nausea and vomiting, optic neuritis (acute), paresthesia, pleural effusion, pulmonary infiltrates, rales and rhonchi, rash, respiratory alkalosis, tinnitus. Many other side effects, possibly from underlying disease, have occurred in less than 1% of patients.

Overdose: Acute renal failure, anemia, hypocalcemia, hypophosphatemia, nausea, vomiting.

ANTIDOTE

Discontinue drug if CrCl reaches 2.5 mg/100 mL at any time during treatment. Discontinue if concurrent use of nephrotoxic drugs is indicated, and continue hydration for several days after nephrotoxic drug regimen is complete. Discontinue drug for any symptoms of overdose. Monitor serum calcium; use vigorous IV hydration, with or without diuretics, for 2 to 3 days. Monitor intake and output to ensure adequacy and balance. For asymptomatic or mild to moderate hypocalcemia (6.5 to 8 mg/100 mL corrected for serum albumin), short-term calcium therapy may be indicated. Oral phosphorus may be required for hypophosphatemia. RBC transfusions may be required in anemia. Keep physician informed. Some side effects may respond to symptomatic treatment. Treat anaphylaxis and resuscitate as indicated.

GANCICLOVIR SODIUM BBW   Antiviral
(gan-**SYE**-kloh-veer **SO**-dee-um)
Cytovene IV   pH 9 to 11

USUAL DOSE
Adequate hydration and specific testing required; see Monitor.
CMV retinitis: 5 mg/kg of body weight every 12 hours for 14 to 21 days. Begin a maintenance dose the next day (Day 15 to 22) of 5 mg/kg daily for 7 days each week or 6 mg/kg daily for 5 days each week. See Precautions/Monitor. After IV induction and when retinitis is stable, Cytovene capsules may be used for maintenance therapy; see Precautions. If retinitis progresses during the maintenance regimen, initiate the twice-daily program again. Do not exceed recommended dose or infusion rate. Larger doses or increased rates of infusion have resulted in increased toxicity. For patients who have relapsed after induction and reinduction monotherapy with either ganciclovir or foscarnet, practitioners may consider an unlabeled combination therapy, which adds the alternate drug to the regimen. Information on this combination regimen is available from Roche and in the Clinical Trials section of the foscarnet sodium prescribing information.
Prevention of CMV disease in transplant recipients: 5 mg/kg every 12 hours for 7 to 14 days. Follow with maintenance regimen as outlined in CMV retinitis. Length of treatment based on immunosuppression degree and duration; 3 to 4 months or longer is common. CMV disease may occur if treatment stopped prematurely.
Prevention of CMV disease in HIV-infected adolescents and adults (unlabeled): 5 to 6 mg/kg/dose for 5 to 7 days each week. Cytovene capsules may be used.

PEDIATRIC DOSE
Safety for use in pediatric patients under 12 years of age not established. ■ Use extreme caution; long-term carcinogenicity and reproductive toxicity are probable. Benefit must outweigh risks. See Indications and Maternal/Child.
CMV retinitis in pediatric patients over 3 months of age (unlabeled): 2.5 mg/kg every 8 hours for 14 to 21 days followed by a maintenance dose of 6 to 6.5 mg/kg/day was used during clinical trials. When retinitis progressed, the adult dosing regimen for induction and maintenance was followed. Another source suggests the adult dose regimen listed in Usual Dose.
Prevention of CMV disease in transplant recipients (unlabeled): Same as adults; see Usual Dose.
Prevention of CMV disease in HIV-infected individuals (unlabeled): 5 mg/kg/dose IV daily.

DOSE ADJUSTMENTS
Dose selection should be cautious in the elderly. Reduced doses may be indicated based on the potential for decreased organ function and concomitant disease or drug therapy. Assess renal function before adminis-
Continued

tration to elderly patients and adjust dose appropriately; see Elderly. ■ Withhold dose if absolute neutrophil count (ANC) less than 500 cells/mm^3 or platelets less than 25,000 cells/mm^3. ■ See Drug/Lab Interactions. ■ With impaired renal function, reduce dose according to the following chart.

Ganciclovir Induction and Maintenance Dose Guidelines in Impaired Renal Function				
Creatinine Clearance (mL/min)	Ganciclovir IV Induction Dose (mg/kg)	Dosing Interval (hours)	Ganciclovir Maintenance Dose (mg/kg)	Dosing Interval (hours)
≥70	5 mg/kg	12 hours	5 mg/kg	24 hours
50-69	2.5 mg/kg	12 hours	2.5 mg/kg	24 hours
25-49	2.5 mg/kg	24 hours	1.25 mg/kg	24 hours
10-24	1.25 mg/kg	24 hours	0.625 mg/kg	24 hours
<10	1.25 mg/kg	3 times per week following hemodialysis	0.625 mg/kg	3 times per week following hemodialysis

DILUTION
Specific techniques required; see Precautions. Initially dissolve the 500-mg vial with 10 mL SW (50 mg/mL). Do not use bacteriostatic water containing parabens; will cause precipitation. Shake well to dissolve completely. Discard if particulate matter or discoloration observed. Withdraw desired dose and further dilute with NS, D5W, Ringer's, or LR to provide a concentration less than 10 mg/mL (70-kg adult at 5 mg/kg equals 350 mg; dissolved in 100 mL of solution equals 3.5 mg/mL).
Filters: Use not required by manufacturer; however, use of a filter would not have an adverse effect.
Storage: Store unopened vials below 40° C (104° F). Reconstituted solution in vial stable at CRT for 12 hours. Do not refrigerate. Solution fully diluted for administration must be refrigerated and used within 24 hours to reduce incidence of bacterial contamination. Stable for 14 days refrigerated at 5° C (41° F) if prepared in PVC bags and reconstituted with SW and further diluted with NS.

COMPATIBILITY   (Underline Indicates Conflicting Compatibility Information)
Consider any drug NOT listed as compatible to be INCOMPATIBLE until consulting a pharmacist; specific conditions may apply.
Because of physical **incompatibilities,** ganciclovir sodium and *foscarnet sodium* must never be mixed.
  One source suggests the following **compatibilities:**
Y-site: Allopurinol (Aloprim), amphotericin B cholesteryl (Amphotec), anidulafungin (Eraxis), caspofungin (Cancidas), cisatracurium (Nimbex), cisplatin (Platinol), cyclophosphamide (Cytoxan), docetaxel (Taxotere), doxorubicin liposomal (Doxil), enalaprilat (Vasotec IV), etoposide phosphate (Etopophos), filgrastim (Neupogen), fluconazole (Diflucan), granisetron (Kytril), linezolid (Zyvox), melphalan (Alkeran), methotrexate, paclitaxel (Taxol), pemetrexed (Alimta), propofol (Diprivan), remifentanil (Ultiva), teniposide (Vumon), thiotepa.

RATE OF ADMINISTRATION

A single dose must be administered at a constant rate over 1 hour as an infusion. Use of an infusion pump or microdrip (60 gtt/mL) recommended. *Do not give by rapid or bolus IV injection.* Excessive plasma levels and toxicity will occur with too-rapid rate of injection. Advisable to clear tubing with NS before and after administration through Y-tube or three-way stopcock.

ACTIONS

An antiviral agent that inhibits DNA synthesis and stops cytomegalovirus (CMV) from multiplying. Does not destroy existing viruses but stops them from reproducing and invading healthy cells. May allow a weakened immune system to defend the body against the CMV infection. May also be inhibitory against herpes simplex virus 1 and 2, Epstein-Barr virus, and varicella zoster virus, but clinical studies have not been done. Onset of action is prompt, and therapeutic levels are maintained for 3 to 6 hours with some drug remaining 11 hours after infusion. Widely distributed in tissues and body fluids. Half-life is 2.6 to 4.4 hours. Crosses the placental barrier. Suspected to be secreted in breast milk. Approximately 90% excreted unchanged in urine in patients with normal renal function.

INDICATIONS AND USES

Treatment of CMV retinitis in immunocompromised individuals, including patients with AIDS. ■ CMV disease prevention in at-risk transplant patients. ■ Safety and effectiveness for use in congenital or neonatal CMV disease, treatment of established CMV disease other than retinitis, or non-immunocompromised individuals not established. Use should be limited to treatment of conditions listed above. ■ Now available as an ophthalmic surgical aid (intravitreal implant) to treat CMV retinitis. ■ Ganciclovir (Cytovene) capsules are used for prevention of CMV retinitis in at-risk patients with advanced HIV infection and in the prevention of CMV disease in solid-organ transplant recipients; see Precautions. Valganciclovir (Valcyte) is an oral drug recently approved for the treatment of CMV retinitis, and it is also being used for maintenance.

Unlabeled uses: Treatment of other CMV infections (e.g., gastroenteritis, hepatitis, pneumonitis) in immunocompromised patients. ■ Treatment of polyradiculopathy caused by CMV infections. ■ Combination therapy (ganciclovir and foscarnet) to treat progressive retinitis refractory to single therapy.

CONTRAINDICATIONS

Hypersensitivity to ganciclovir or acyclovir; patients with a neutrophil count less than 500 cells/mm^3 or a platelet count less than 25,000 cells/mm^3; patients receiving zidovudine (AZT, Retrovir), since both drugs cause granulocytopenia.

PRECAUTIONS

A nucleoside analog; follow guidelines for handling and disposal of cytotoxic agents. See Appendix A, p. 1429. ■ For IV use only; IM or SC administration will cause severe tissue irritation. ■ Hematologic toxicity (anemia, granulocytopenia, thrombocytopenia) common; see Monitor. ■ Use with caution in patients with pre-existing cytopenias or a history of cytopenic reactions to other drugs, chemicals, or irradiation. ■ Ganciclovir is not a cure for CMV infections. Maintenance therapy is almost always necessary to prevent relapse in patients with AIDS. ■ Resistance has been reported to develop. May be higher in patients treated for a prolonged period. ■ Cidofovir is also an agent for treatment of CMV retinitis. ■ Risk

of a more rapid rate of disease progression is increased with oral ganciclovir. Use in maintenance recommended only if benefits of avoiding daily
IV infusions outweigh risk.
Monitor: Confirm diagnosis of CMV retinitis by indirect ophthalmoscopy.
Diagnosis may be supported by cultures of CMV (e.g., urine, blood,
throat); negative culture does not rule out CMV retinitis. ▪ Continue
ophthalmologic exams during induction and maintenance treatment to
monitor CMV status. ▪ CBC with differential and platelet counts, SCr, and
CrCl are required before treatment initiated. Monitor CBC and platelet
counts frequently, especially in patients with previous leukopenia from
ganciclovir or other nucleoside analogs or those with neutrophils less than
1,000 cells/mm³ at beginning of treatment and in patients undergoing
hemodialysis. Withhold dose if absolute neutrophil count (ANC) less than
500 cells/mm³ or platelets less than 25,000 cells/mm³. Monitor SCr or
CrCl every 2 weeks. ▪ Maintain adequate hydration and urine flow before
and during infusion. ▪ Phlebitis or pain may occur at site of infusion;
confirm patency of vein and use small needles and large veins to ensure
adequate blood flow for rapid dilution and distribution. ▪ Granulocytopenia usually occurs within 14 days but may occur at any time; recovery
should begin within 3 to 7 days of discontinuing ganciclovir. ▪ Consider
the possibility of viral resistance if retinitis does not show significant
improvement with treatment. ▪ See Drug/Lab Interactions.
Patient Education: Must use effective birth control throughout treatment.
Men should continue barrier contraception for at least 90 days. ▪ Not a
cure; retinitis may still progress. Frequent ophthalmoscopic examinations
important. ▪ Cooperation for close monitoring of blood cell counts is
imperative to control side effects (e.g., anemia, neutropenia, thrombocytopenia). ▪ Report any unexpected side effects promptly (e.g., chills,
fever, unusual bleeding or bruising). ▪ Patients with AIDS receiving zidovudine (AZT, Retrovir) may not tolerate ganciclovir. ▪ High frequency of
impaired renal function increased with concomitant use of nephrotoxic
agents (e.g., cyclosporine, amphotericin); high risk for transplant recipients.
Maternal/Child: Category C: avoid pregnancy. A potential carcinogen. Teratogenic and embryotoxic; has caused aspermatogenesis and will cause birth
defects. Do not use during pregnancy unless risk is justified. May cause
temporary or permanent infertility in men and women. ▪ Discontinue
nursing during treatment; minimum interval required before resuming
breast-feeding is unknown. ▪ Use extreme caution in pediatric patients
under 12 years of age. Long-term carcinogenicity and reproductive toxicity are probable. Benefit must outweigh risks.
Elderly: Dose selection should be cautious; see Dose Adjustments. Monitor
renal function during therapy and adjust dose as indicated.
DRUG/LAB INTERACTIONS
Because of physical **incompatibilities,** ganciclovir and **foscarnet** must
never be mixed. ▪ Additive toxicity may occur with concomitant use
of **other drugs that inhibit replication of rapidly dividing cell populations** (e.g.,
dapsone, pentamidine, flucytosine [Ancobon], vincristine, vinblastine,
doxorubicin [Adriamycin], amphotericin B [generic], sulfamethoxazole/
trimethoprim [Bactrim]). ▪ May cause severe anemia and neutropenia with
zidovudine (AZT, Retrovir). Combination used in patients with AIDS is
rarely tolerated. ▪ Concurrent treatment with **didanosine** (Videx) may

cause increased didanosine levels. ▪ May cause seizures with **imipenem-cilastatin** (Primaxin). ▪ Potentiated by **probenecid and other drugs that may reduce renal clearance;** will increase toxicity. ▪ Impaired renal function may be markedly increased with other **nephrotoxic agents** (e.g., cyclosporine, amphotericin B). ▪ Concurrent or consecutive use with **other bone marrow suppressants** (e.g., antineoplastics, amphotericin B, zidovudine and/or radiation therapy) may produce additive bone marrow suppression. ▪ Drug interaction studies with drugs commonly used in transplant recipients have not been conducted. ▪ See Contraindications.

SIDE EFFECTS

Anemia, leukopenia, and thrombocytopenia are most common and are generally reversible if treatment discontinued. Abdominal pain; anorexia; chills; diarrhea; fever; infection; nausea; neuropathy; pain, infection, and sepsis at injection site; phlebitis; pruritus; rash; retinal detachment; sepsis; sweating; and vomiting occur in some patients. Abnormal kidney function and/or failure, abnormal vision, alopecia, anxiety, arthralgia, asthenia, chest pain, confusion, constipation, cough, decreased CrCl, depression, dizziness, dry mouth, dry skin, dyspepsia, dyspnea, edema, eructation, headache, hypertension, increased ALT and AST, increased creatinine, insomnia, leg cramps, malaise, myalgia, myasthenia, pancytopenia, seizures, somnolence, stomatitis, taste perversion, tinnitus, tremor, and weight loss have occurred. Gastrointestinal perforation, multiple organ failure, pancreatitis, and sepsis have occurred and may be fatal. Numerous additional side effects may occur.

Overdose: Acute renal failure, hematuria, hepatitis, irreversible pancytopenia, persistent bone marrow suppression, and seizures have occurred.

ANTIDOTE

Notify physician of all side effects; most will be treated symptomatically. Filgrastim (Neupogen) 1 to 10 mcg/kg/day has been used to maintain the neutrophil count. Discontinue drug if neutrophils fall below 500 cells/mm^3 or platelets fall below 25,000 cells/mm^3. Hydration and hemodialysis (up to 50% removal) are useful in overdose. Treat anaphylaxis and resuscitate as necessary.

GEMCITABINE HYDROCHLORIDE
(jem-**SIGHT**-ah-been hy-droh-**KLOR**-eyed)
Gemzar

**Antineoplastic
(miscellaneous)**

pH 2.7 to 3.3

USUAL DOSE

Pancreatic cancer: 1,000 mg/M^2 once each week for up to 7 weeks (or until toxicity necessitates reducing or holding a dose). Follow with a week of rest. In subsequent cycles, 1,000 mg/M^2 or appropriate reduced or increased dose once each week for 3 consecutive weeks. Follow with a week of rest.

Non–small-cell lung cancer (NSCLC): 1,000 mg/M^2 as an infusion on Days 1, 8, and 15 of each 28-day cycle. Given in combination with cisplatin (Platinol). Administer cisplatin 100 mg/M^2 IV on Day 1 after the infusion of gemcitabine. An alternate schedule is gemcitabine 1,250 mg/M^2 on Days 1 and 8 of each 21-day cycle. Administer cisplatin 100 mg/M^2 IV on Day 1 after the infusion of gemcitabine. See cisplatin monograph for administration and hydration guidelines.

Breast cancer: 1,250 mg/M^2 as an infusion on Days 1 and 8 of each 21-day cycle. Given in combination with paclitaxel (Taxol). On Day 1, administer paclitaxel 175 mg/M^2 as a 3-hour infusion before the gemcitabine infusion. Premedication required; see paclitaxel monograph.

Ovarian cancer: 1,000 mg/M^2 as an infusion on Days 1 and 8 of a 21-day cycle. Given in combination with carboplatin (Paraplatin). On Day 1, administer carboplatin at AUC 4 after gemcitabine administration.

Bladder cancer (unlabeled): 1,000 to 1,200 mg/M^2 once each week for 3 weeks. Follow with a week of rest.

Hodgkin's or non-Hodgkin's lymphoma (unlabeled): 1,000 to 1,250 mg/M^2 on Days 1, 8, and 15 of a 28-day cycle. Doses up to 1,500 mg/M^2 have been used.

DOSE ADJUSTMENTS

Clearance decreased in women and the elderly. May be less likely to progress to subsequent cycles; see Precautions and Elderly. ■ For pancreatic cancer, NSCLC and unlabeled uses reduce dose based on the degree of hematologic toxicity according to the following chart.

Gemcitabine Dose Reduction Guidelines Indicated for Dose Reduction in Pancreatic Cancer, NSCLC, and Unlabeled Uses		
Absolute Granulocyte Count (cells/mm^3)	Platelet Count (cells/mm^3)	% of Full Dose to Be Administered
≥1,000 and	≥100,000	100%
500-999 or	50,000-99,999	75%
<500 or	<50,000	Hold

Treatment of pancreatic cancer: Dose may be increased by 25% (to 1,250 mg/M^2) in patients who complete an entire 7-week initial cycle or a subsequent 3-week cycle at a dose of 1,000 mg/M^2. Absolute granulocyte count nadir must exceed 1,500/mm^3 and platelet nadir must exceed

$100,000/mm^3$. Nonhematologic toxicity should not be greater than WHO Grade 1 (some examples are: able to eat, reasonable intake, no more than one emesis in 24 hours, asymptomatic heart and lungs, mild paresthesia). If this cycle is tolerated, dose for the next cycle may be increased to 1,500 mg/M^2 providing the same criteria have been met (e.g., granulocyte nadir, platelet nadir, nonhematologic toxicity).

Treatment of NSCLC: Treatment with gemcitabine and cisplatin should be held or decreased by 50% when Grade 3 or 4 nonhematologic toxicity occurs (except alopecia and nausea and vomiting). See cisplatin monograph for additional dose adjustment guidelines.

Treatment of breast cancer (combination with paclitaxel): Reduce dose based on degree of hematologic toxicity seen on Day 8 according to the following chart.

Dose Reduction Guidelines for Gemcitabine in Combination with Paclitaxel Indicated for Dose Reduction in Breast Cancer			
Absolute Granulocyte Count (cells/mm³)		Platelet Count (cells/mm³)	% of Full Dose to Be Administered
≥1,200	and	>75,000	100%
1,000-1,199	or	50,000-75,000	75%
700 to 999	and	≥50,000	50%
<700	or	<50,000	Hold

Treatment with gemcitabine and paclitaxel should be held or decreased by 50% when Grade 3 or 4 nonhematologic toxicity occurs. See paclitaxel monograph for additional dose adjustment guidelines.

Treatment of ovarian cancer in combination with carboplatin: Reduce dose based on the degree of hematologic toxicity that is seen on Day 8 according to the following chart.

Day 8 Dose Reduction Guidelines for Gemcitabine in Combination with Carboplatin Indicated for Dose Reduction in Ovarian Cancer			
Absolute Granulocyte Count (cells/mm³)		Platelet Count (cells/mm³)	% of Full Dose to Be Administered
≥1,500	and	≥100,000	100%
1,000-1,499	and/or	75,000-99,999	50%
<1,000	and/or	<75,000	Hold

Treatment with gemcitabine and carboplatin should be held or decreased by 50% when severe (Grade 3 or 4) nonhematologic toxicity (except nausea and vomiting) occurs. See carboplatin monograph for additional dose adjustment guidelines.

Dose adjustment for gemcitabine in combination with carboplatin for subsequent cycles is based on observed toxicity. In subsequent cycles,

Continued

reduce the dose of gemcitabine to 800 mg/M^2 on Days 1 and 8 in case of any of the following hematologic toxicities:

- Absolute granulocyte count <500 cells/mm^3 for more than 5 days
- Absolute granulocyte count <100 cells/mm^3 for more than 3 days
- Febrile neutropenia
- Platelets <25,000 cells/mm^3
- Cycle delay of more than 1 week due to toxicity

If any of the previous toxicities recur after the initial dose reduction, administer gemcitabine 800 mg/M^2 only on Day 1 of subsequent cycles.

DILUTION
Specific techniques required; see Precautions. Each 200 mg must be reconstituted with 5 mL NS without preservatives (25 mL NS for 1 Gm). Yields 38 mg/mL. Shake to dissolve. Do not use less solution to reconstitute; dissolution will be incomplete. The appropriate dose *must* be further diluted with NS to concentrations as low as 0.1 mg/mL. 1,500 mg diluted in 250 mL yields 6 mg/mL. 750 mg in 100 mL yields 7.5 mg/mL.
Filters: Reconstituted solution may be filtered through a 0.22- or 0.45-micron pre-filter.
Storage: Store unopened vials at CRT. Reconstituted or diluted solutions are stable at CRT for 24 hours. Do not refrigerate in any form; may crystallize. Discard unused portion.

COMPATIBILITY   (Underline Indicates Conflicting Compatibility Information)
Consider any drug NOT listed as compatible to be INCOMPATIBLE until consulting a pharmacist; specific conditions may apply.
Manufacturer states, "**Compatibilities** with other drugs have not been studied. No **incompatibilities** observed with IV bottles or PVC bags and administration sets."

One source suggests the following **compatibilities:**
Y-site: Amifostine (Ethyol), amikacin (Amikin), aminophylline, ampicillin, ampicillin/sulbactam (Unasyn), anidulafungin (Eraxis), aztreonam (Azactam), bleomycin (Blenoxane), bumetanide, buprenorphine (Buprenex), butorphanol (Stadol), calcium gluconate, carboplatin (Paraplatin), carmustine (BiCNU), cefazolin (Ancef), cefotetan (Cefotan), cefoxitin (Mefoxin), ceftazidime (Fortaz), ceftriaxone (Rocephin), cefuroxime (Zinacef), chlorpromazine (Thorazine), ciprofloxacin (Cipro IV), cisplatin (Platinol), clindamycin (Cleocin), cyclophosphamide (Cytoxan), cytarabine (ARA-C), dactinomycin (Cosmegen), daunorubicin (Cerubidine), dexamethasone (Decadron), dexrazoxane (Zinecard), diphenhydramine (Benadryl), dobutamine, docetaxel (Taxotere), dopamine, doripenem (Doribax), doxorubicin (Adriamycin), doxycycline, droperidol (Inapsine), enalaprilat (Vasotec IV), etoposide (VePesid), etoposide phosphate (Etopophos), famotidine (Pepcid IV), fluconazole (Diflucan), fludarabine (Fludara), fluorouracil (5-FU), gentamicin, granisetron (Kytril), haloperidol (Haldol), heparin, hydrocortisone sodium succinate (Solu-Cortef), hydromorphone (Dilaudid), idarubicin (Idamycin), ifosfamide (Ifex), leucovorin calcium, linezolid (Zyvox), lorazepam (Ativan), mannitol, meperidine (Demerol), mesna (Mesnex), metoclopramide (Reglan), metronidazole (Flagyl IV), mitoxantrone (Novantrone), morphine, nalbuphine, ondansetron (Zofran), oxaliplatin (Eloxatin), paclitaxel (Taxol), palonosetron (Aloxi), potassium chloride (KCl), promethazine (Phenergan), ranitidine (Zantac), sodium bicarbonate, streptozocin (Zanosar), sulfamethoxazole/trimethoprim, teni-

poside (Vumon), thiotepa, ticarcillin/clavulanate (Timentin), tobramycin, topotecan (Hycamtin), vancomycin, vinblastine, vincristine, vinorelbine (Navelbine), zidovudine (AZT, Retrovir).

RATE OF ADMINISTRATION

A single dose as an infusion equally distributed over 30 minutes. Do not extend infusion time beyond 60 minutes; will increase toxicity.

ACTIONS

A nucleoside analog with antineoplastic activity. Metabolized intracellularly to two active nucleosides. Cell phase specific, these nucleosides induce internucleosomal DNA fragmentation, primarily killing cells undergoing DNA synthesis (S-phase) and also blocking the progression of cells through the G_1/S-phase boundary. Very little is bound to plasma protein. Volume of distribution is increased by infusion length. Half-life is shorter (32 to 94 minutes) with a short infusion (less than 70 minutes), and longer (245 to 638 minutes) with a long infusion (more than 70 minutes). Half-life is slightly longer and rate of clearance is lower in women and in the elderly, resulting in higher concentrations for any given dose. Primarily excreted in urine.

INDICATIONS AND USES

First-line treatment for patients with nonresectable or metastatic cancer of the pancreas and for patients previously treated for cancer of the pancreas with fluorouracil. ■ First-line treatment in combination with cisplatin for the palliative treatment of locally advanced or metastatic non–small-cell lung cancer. ■ First-line treatment in combination with paclitaxil for treatment of metastatic breast cancer after failure of previous anthracycline chemotherapy unless anthracyclines (e.g., doxorubicin [Adriamycin], idarubicin [Idamycin]) were clinically contraindicated. ■ Treatment in combination with carboplatin for patients with advanced ovarian cancer that has relapsed at least 6 months after completion of platinum-based therapy. **Unlabeled uses:** Treatment of metastatic bladder cancer. ■ Treatment of relapsed or refractory testicular cancer. ■ Treatment of squamous cell cancer of the head and neck.

CONTRAINDICATIONS

Hypersensitivity to gemcitabine or any of its components.

PRECAUTIONS

Follow guidelines for handling cytotoxic agents. See Appendix A, p. 1429. ■ Administered by or under the direction of the physician specialist. ■ Adequate diagnostic and treatment facilities must be available. ■ For IV use only. May be administered on an outpatient basis. ■ Prolongation of the infusion time beyond 60 minutes and more frequent than weekly dosing have been shown to increase toxicity. ■ Clearance in women and the elderly is reduced; women, especially older women, were more likely not to proceed to a subsequent cycle and to experience Grade 3 or 4 neutropenia and thrombocytopenia. No age or gender dose adjustments recommended. ■ Use with caution in impaired renal or hepatic function. Clear dose recommendations are not available; data from clinical studies insufficient. ■ Hepatotoxicity, including liver failure and death, has been reported. Use in patients with concurrent liver metastases or a history of alcoholism, hepatitis, or liver cirrhosis may lead to exacerbation of the underlying hepatic insufficiency. ■ Hemolytic uremic syndrome (HUS) and/or renal toxicity, including renal failure leading to death or requiring dialysis, has been reported. ■ Gemcitabine is a potent radiosensitizer.

Depending on the site being radiated, concurrent use with gemcitabine may cause severe, life-threatening esophagitis and pneumonitis. Data suggest that gemcitabine can be started after the acute effects of radiation have resolved or at least 1 week after radiation is completed. ▪ Pulmonary toxicity has been reported. If gemcitabine-induced pneumonitis is confirmed or suspected, discontinue permanently. Dyspnea unrelated to underlying disease has been reported with gemcitabine therapy and has been occasionally accompanied by bronchospasm. ▪ Use caution in patients who have had previous cytotoxic chemotherapy or radiation therapy.

Monitor: Monitor for bone marrow suppression; myelosuppression (e.g., anemia, leukopenia, and thrombocytopenia) is the dose-limiting toxicity. See Dose Adjustments. ▪ Obtain a CBC, including differential and platelet count, before each dose. ▪ Obtain baseline renal function (e.g., SCr) and liver function tests (e.g., AST, ALT) and repeat periodically. ▪ Monitor serum calcium, magnesium, potassium, and SCr during combination therapy with cisplatin. ▪ Monitor vital signs. ▪ Maintain adequate hydration. ▪ Nausea and vomiting are frequent and were severe in 15% of patients; prophylactic administration of antiemetics will increase patient comfort. ▪ Observe closely for S/S of infection. May cause fever in the absence of infection or prophylactic antibiotics may be indicated pending results of C/S in a febrile or nonfebrile patient. ▪ Monitor for thrombocytopenia (platelet count less than 50,000/mm^3). Initiate precautions to prevent excessive bleeding (e.g., inspect IV sites, skin, and mucous membranes; use extreme care during invasive procedures; test urine, emesis, stool, and secretions for occult blood). ▪ Consider a diagnosis of HUS if anemia with evidence of microangiopathic hemolysis, elevation of bilirubin or LDH, reticulocytosis, severe thrombocytopenia, and/or evidence of renal failure (elevation of SCr or BUN) develops; discontinue gemcitabine. ▪ Not a vesicant, but monitor injection site for inflammation and/or extravasation.

Patient Education: Nonhormonal birth control recommended. ▪ See Appendix D, p. 1434. ▪ Report any unusual or unexpected symptoms or side effects (e.g., shortness of breath, blood in stool or urine, S/S of infection, unusual bruising or bleeding) as soon as possible.

Maternal/Child: Category D: avoid pregnancy. May cause fetal harm. ▪ Discontinue breast-feeding. ▪ Safety and effectiveness for use in pediatric patients not established. Small clinical studies have been performed with questionable results; see prescribing information.

Elderly: Clearance reduced in the elderly; hematologic toxicity requiring reduction, delay, or omission of subsequent doses is higher than in younger adults; however, incidence of nonhematologic toxicity is similar. Elderly men and women are more likely to experience grade 3 or 4 thrombocytopenia. Elderly women are also more likely to experience Grade 3 or 4 neutropenia. Usual dose adjustments based on toxicity are considered appropriate. Age-related impaired renal function may further reduce clearance and increase toxicity.

DRUG/LAB INTERACTIONS

Interaction of gemcitabine with other drugs has not been adequately studied. ▪ Additive bone marrow suppression may occur with **radiation therapy, other bone marrow–suppressing agents** (e.g., amphotericin B [traditional and lipid], azathioprine [Imuran], chloramphenicol, melphelan [Alkeran]), and/or **immunosuppressants** (e.g., chlorambucil [Leukeran], cyclophosphamide [Cytoxan], cyclosporine [Sandimmune], glucocorticoid corticosteroids [e.g., dexamethasone], muromonab-CD3 [Orthoclone], tacrolimus [Prograf]); dose reduction may be required. ▪ Do not administer **live virus vaccines** to patients receiving antineoplastic agents.

SIDE EFFECTS

Alopecia, anorexia, arrhythmias, arthralgia, bone marrow toxicity (e.g., anemia, leukopenia, neutropenia, thrombocytopenia), bone pain, bronchospasm, cerebrovascular accident, CHF, constipation, diarrhea, dyspnea, edema, elevated lab tests (e.g., BUN, creatinine, hematuria, proteinuria), fatigue, febrile neutropenia, fever, flu syndrome (e.g., anorexia, chills, cough, headache, myalgia, weakness), hemorrhage, hepatotoxicity, hypertension, increased liver function tests (e.g., ALT, AST, GGT, alkaline phosphatase, and bilirubin), infection, injection site reaction, myalgia, myocardial infarction, nausea and vomiting, neuropathy (motor and sensory), pain, paresthesias, peripheral vasculitis and gangrene, pruritus, pulmonary effects (including pulmonary edema, pulmonary fibrosis, interstitial pneumonitis, ARDS, respiratory failure), radiation recall reactions, rash, severe skin reactions (e.g., desquamation and bullous skin eruptions), somnolence, stomatitis. Anaphylaxis and hemolytic uremic syndrome have been reported.

ANTIDOTE

Keep physician informed of all side effects. Symptomatic and supportive treatment is indicated. Reduce dose or withhold gemcitabine until myelosuppression improves to specific criteria; see Dose Adjustments. If gemcitabine-induced pneumonitis or esophagitis is confirmed or suspected, discontinue permanently (in one study severe stomatitis and pharyngeal damage required patients to be fed by feeding tube for up to 12 months after receiving doses of 300 mg/M^2 [25% of the usual dose]). Anemia may require RBC transfusions. Other whole blood products (e.g., platelets, leukocytes) and/or blood modifiers (e.g., darbepoetin alfa [Aranesp], epoetin alfa [Epogen], filgrastim [Neupogen], oprelvekin [Neumega], pegfilgrastim [Neulasta], sargramostim [Leukine]) may be indicated to treat bone marrow toxicity. Most side effects are reversible with dose reduction or temporary withholding of gemcitabine. No known antidote for overdose. If hemolytic uremic syndrome occurs, discontinue gemcitabine; renal failure may not be reversible even with discontinuation of therapy and dialysis may be required. Treat hypersensitivity reactions as indicated; may require epinephrine, airway management, oxygen, IV fluids, antihistamines (e.g., diphenhydramine [Benadryl]), corticosteroids (e.g., hydrocortisone sodium succinate [Solu-Cortef]), and pressor amines (e.g., dopamine).

GENTAMICIN SULFATE BBW
(jen-tah-**MY**-sin **SUL**-fayt)

**Antibacterial
(aminoglycoside)**

pH 3 to 5.5

USUAL DOSE
3 mg/kg of body weight/24 hr equally divided into 3 doses (1 mg/kg every 8 hours). Up to 5 mg/kg/24 hr may be given if indicated. Reduce to usual dose as soon as feasible. Another source suggests 1 to 2.5 mg/kg/dose every 8 to 12 hours. A loading dose of 2 mg/kg is commonly used. **Dosage based on ideal body weight.** Studies suggest that a single daily dose of 4 to 7 mg/kg (instead of divided into 2 to 3 doses) may provide higher peak levels and enhance drug effectiveness while actually reducing or having no adverse effects on risk of toxicity. Various procedures for monitoring blood levels are in use. Some health facilities are monitoring with trough levels; others may draw levels at predetermined times and plot the concentration on nomograms. Depending on the protocol in place, doses or intervals may be adjusted. See Precautions/Monitor.

Prevention of bacterial endocarditis in dental, respiratory tract, GI or GU tract surgery or instrumentation: 1.5 mg/kg 30 minutes before procedure. Do not exceed 80 mg. Repeat in 8 hours. Given concurrently with ampicillin, vancomycin, or amoxicillin.

Pelvic inflammatory disease: 2 mg/kg as an initial dose. Follow with 1.5 mg/kg every 8 hours for 4 days or 48 hours after patient improves. Given concurrently with clindamycin.

PEDIATRIC DOSE
See Maternal/Child.

6 to 7.5 mg/kg of body weight/24 hr (2 to 2.5 mg/kg every 8 hours). A single daily dose is also being used in pediatric patients. See comments under Usual Dose. 10 mg/mL product available for pediatric use.

Prevention of bacterial endocarditis in dental, respiratory tract, GI or GU tract surgery or instrumentation: 2 mg/kg. See Adult Dose for instructions.

NEONATAL DOSE
See Maternal/Child.

2.5 mg/kg. Intervals adjusted based on age as follows:

0 to 7 days of age; less than 28 weeks' gestation: Every 24 hours.
28 to 34 weeks' gestation: Every 18 hours.
Over 34 weeks' gestation: Every 12 hours.
Over 7 days of age; less than 28 weeks' gestation: Every 18 hours.
28 to 34 weeks' gestation: Every 12 hours.
Over 34 weeks' gestation: Every 8 hours.

Another source suggests that higher doses (4 to 5 mg/kg/dose) at extended intervals (24 to 48 hours) may be used.

DOSE ADJUSTMENTS
Reduce daily dose commensurate with amount of renal impairment according to the following chart. Other protocols are in use; see literature. ■ Reduced dose or extended intervals may be indicated in elderly adults. ■ See Monitor and Drug/Lab Interactions.

Gentamicin Dosing Guidelines for Impaired Renal Function (Dose at 8-Hour Intervals After the Initial Dose)		
Serum Creatinine (mg%)	Approximate Creatinine Clearance Rate (mL/min/1.73 M^2)	Percent of Usual Dose to Be Administered q 8 hr
<1	>100	100%
1.1-1.3	71-100	80%
1.4-1.6	56-70	65%
1.7-1.9	46-55	55%
2-2.2	41-45	50%
2.3-2.5	36-40	40%
2.6-3	31-35	35%
3.1-3.5	26-30	30%
3.6-4	21-25	25%
4.1-5.1	16-20	20%
5.2-6.6	11-15	15%
6.7-8	≤10	10%

The recommended dose at the end of each dialysis period is 1 to 1.7 mg/kg depending on the severity of the infection. 2 mg/kg may be administered to pediatric patients. The amount of gentamicin removed by dialysis may vary; however, an 8-hour dialysis session may reduce serum concentrations by 50%. Another source suggests the following dose guidelines for impaired renal function.

Conventional Gentamicin Dosing Guidelines for Impaired Renal Function	
Approximate Creatinine Clearance Rate (mL/min/1.73 M^2)	Administer Conventional Dose at the Following Intervals
>60 mL/min	Every 8 hours
40 to 60 mL/min	Every 12 hours
20 to 40 mL/min	Every 24 hours
<20 mL/min	Loading dose, then monitor levels

High-dose therapy: Interval may be extended (e.g., every 48 hours) in patients with moderate renal impairment (CrCl 30 to 59 mL/min) and/or adjusted based on serum level determinations.
DILUTION
Available premixed in several concentrations. Vials equal 10 or 40 mg/mL. Further dilute each single dose in 50 to 200 mL of IV NS or D5W. Decrease volume of diluent for pediatric patients. Commercially diluted solutions available.

COMPATIBILITY (Underline Indicates Conflicting Compatibility Information)
Consider any drug NOT listed as compatible to be INCOMPATIBLE until consulting a pharmacist; specific conditions may apply.
Manufactuer states, "Do not physically premix with other drugs; administer separately." Inactivated in solution with beta-lactam antibiotics (e.g., cephalosporins, penicillins) and vancomycin. Do not mix in the same solution. Appropriate spacing required because of physical **incompatibilities.** See Drug/Lab Interactions.
One source suggests the following **compatibilities:**
Additive: *Not recommended by manufacturer.* Atracurium (Tracrium), aztreonam (Azactam), bleomycin (Blenoxane), ciprofloxacin (Cipro IV), clindamycin (Cleocin), cytarabine (ARA-C), dopamine, fluconazole (Diflucan), furosemide (Lasix), linezolid (Zyvox), metronidazole (Flagyl IV), midazolam (Versed), ranitidine (Zantac), verapamil.
Y-site: Acyclovir (Zovirax), alprostadil, amifostine (Ethyol), amiodarone (Nexterone), anidulafungin (Eraxis), atracurium (Tracrium), aztreonam (Azactam), bivalirudin (Angiomax), caspofungin (Cancidas), cefepime (Maxipime), ceftazidime (Fortaz), ciprofloxacin (Cipro IV), cisatracurium (Nimbex), cyclophosphamide (Cytoxan), cytarabine (ARA-C), daptomycin (Cubicin), dexmedetomidine (Precedex), diltiazem (Cardizem), docetaxel (Taxotere), doripenem (Doribax), doxapram (Dopram), doxorubicin liposomal (Doxil), enalaprilat (Vasotec IV), esmolol (Brevibloc), etoposide phosphate (Etopophos), famotidine (Pepcid IV), fenoldopam (Corlopam), filgrastim (Neupogen), fluconazole (Diflucan), fludarabine (Fludara), foscarnet (Foscavir), gemcitabine (Gemzar), granisetron (Kytril), hetastarch in electrolytes (Hextend), hydromorphone (Dilaudid), insulin (regular), labetalol (Trandate), levofloxacin (Levaquin), linezolid (Zyvox), lorazepam (Ativan), magnesium sulfate, melphalan (Alkeran), meperidine (Demerol), meropenem (Merrem IV), midazolam (Versed), milrinone (Primacor), morphine, multivitamins (M.V.I.), nicardipine (Cardene IV), ondansetron (Zofran), paclitaxel (Taxol), palonosetron (Aloxi), pancuronium, remifentanil (Ultiva), sargramostim (Leukine), tacrolimus (Prograf), teniposide (Vumon), theophylline, thiotepa, tigecycline (Tygacil), vasopressin, vecuronium, vinorelbine (Navelbine), zidovudine (AZT, Retrovir).
RATE OF ADMINISTRATION
Each single dose, properly diluted, over 30 to 60 minutes, up to 2 hours in pediatric patients. Studies suggest bolus dosing (versus infusion over 30 minutes) may produce an earlier bactericidal effect, which is sustained. No dose, dilution, or rate recommendations are available at this time.
ACTIONS
Aminoglycoside antibiotic with neuromuscular blocking action. Bactericidal against specific gram-negative bacilli, including *Escherichia coli, Klebsiella, Proteus,* and *Pseudomonas.* Not effective for fungi or viral infections. Well distributed throughout all body fluids; serum and urine levels remain adequate for 6 to 12 hours. Usual half-life is 2 hours. Half-life prolonged in infants, postpartum females, fever, liver disease and ascites, spinal cord injury, cystic fibrosis, and the elderly; shorter in severe burns. Crosses placental barrier. Excreted through kidneys.

INDICATIONS AND USES

Treatment of serious infections of the GI (peritonitis), respiratory, and urinary tracts; CNS (meningitis); skin; bone; soft tissue (burns); septicemia; and bacterial neonatal sepsis. ■ Primarily used when penicillin and other less toxic antibiotics are ineffective or contraindicated. ■ Prevention of bacterial endocarditis in dental, respiratory tract, GI, or GU surgery or instrumentation. ■ Used concurrently with clindamycin to treat pelvic inflammatory disease. ■ Considered initial therapy after culture and sensitivity is drawn in suspected or confirmed gram-negative infections or other serious infections. ■ Treat suspected infection in the immunosuppressed patient. ■ May be used synergistically in gram-positive infections.
■ Used concurrently with penicillin for endocarditis and neonatal sepsis.

CONTRAINDICATIONS

Known gentamicin or aminoglycoside sensitivity, renal failure. Sulfite sensitivity may be a contraindication.

PRECAUTIONS

Sensitivity studies indicated to determine susceptibility of the causative organism to gentamicin. ■ Use extreme caution if therapy is required over 7 to 10 days. ■ Superinfection may occur from overgrowth of nonsusceptible organisms. ■ Use caution in infants, children, and the elderly. ■ Advanced age and dehydration may increase risk of toxicity. ■ May contain sulfites; use caution in patients with asthma. ■ Aminoglycosides are nephrotoxic; risk for nephrotoxicity is increased in patients with impaired renal function and in patients who receive high doses or prolonged therapy. ■ Use extreme caution in patients with end-stage renal disease. ■ Single daily dosing has been used effectively in abdominal, pelvic inflammatory, and GU infections in patients with normal renal function. Not recommended in bacteremia caused by *Pseudomonas aeruginosa,* endocarditis, meningitis, during pregnancy, or in patients less than 6 weeks postpartum. Limited data available for use in all other situations (e.g., burns, cystic fibrosis, elderly, pediatrics, renal impairment). ■ Risk of neurotoxicity (e.g., auditory and vestibular ototoxicity) is increased in patients with pre-existing renal damage or in normal renal function with prolonged use. Partial or total irreversible deafness may continue to develop after gentamicin discontinued. ■ *Clostridium difficile*–associated diarrhea (CDAD) has been reported. May range from mild diarrhea to fatal colitis. Consider in patients who present with diarrhea during or after treatment with gentamicin.

Monitor: Narrow range between toxic and therapeutic levels. Periodically monitor peak and trough concentrations. Therapeutic level is between 4 and 8 mcg/mL. Avoid trough levels above 2 mcg/mL and prolonged peak levels above 12 mcg/mL; adjust dose as indicated. Risk of renal and eighth cranial nerve toxicity increased. Monitor frequently in patients with impaired renal function. ■ Watch for decrease in urine output and rising BUN and SCr. May require decreased dose. ■ Routine gentamicin serum levels and evaluation of hearing are recommended. ■ Closely monitor renal and eighth cranial nerve function, especially in patients with known or suspected reduced renal function at onset of therapy and in patients who develop signs of renal dysfunction during therapy. Monitor urine for decreased specific gravity, increased protein, and the presence of cells or casts. Serial audiograms are recommended, particularly in high-risk patients. ■ Maintain good hydration. ■ Monitor serum calcium, magnesium, sodium, and potassium; levels may decline. Depressed levels have caused mental confusion, paresthesia, positive Chvostek and Trousseau signs (provoked spasm of facial muscles and other muscles; occurs in tetany), and tetany in adults; muscle weakness and tetany in infants. ▪ Closely monitor patients with impaired renal function for nephrotoxicity and neurotoxicity (e.g., auditory and vestibular ototoxicity, convulsions, muscle twitching, numbness, tingling); nephrotoxicity may be reversible. ▪ In extended treatment, monitoring of serum levels, electrolytes, renal, auditory, and vestibular functions is recommended daily. ▪ See Drug/Lab Interactions.

Patient Education: Report promptly: dizziness, hearing loss, weakness, or any changes in balance. ▪ Promptly report diarrhea or bloody stools that occur during treatment or up to several months after an antibiotic has been discontinued; may indicate CDAD and require treatment. ▪ Consider birth control options.

Maternal/Child: Category D: avoid pregnancy. Potential hazard to fetus. ▪ Safety for use during breast-feeding not established; use extreme caution. ▪ Peak concentrations are generally lower in infants and young children.

Elderly: Consider less toxic alternatives. Half-life prolonged. Longer intervals between doses may be more important than reduced doses. ▪ Advanced age and dehydration may increase risk for toxicity. ▪ Monitor renal function and drug levels carefully. Measurement of CrCl more useful than BUN or SCr to assess renal function. ▪ See Precautions.

DRUG/LAB INTERACTIONS
Inactivated in solution with **penicillins** but is synergistic when used in combination with **beta-lactam antibiotics** (e.g., sulbactam sodium, clavulanate potassium, cephalosporins, penicillins) and **vancomycin.** Do not mix in the same solution. Dose adjustment and appropriate spacing required because of physical **incompatibilities** and interactions. Synergism may be inconsistent; measure aminoglycoside levels. ▪ Concurrent and/or sequential use topically or systemically with any other **neurotoxic or nephrotoxic agent** should be avoided (e.g., amikacin [Amikin], cephaloridine, cisplatin [Platinol], colistin [Coly-Mycin S, kanamycin [Kantrex], neomycin, polymyxin B, paromomycin [Humatin], streptomycin, tobramycin, vancomycin). ▪ May have dangerous additive effects with **anesthetics** (e.g., enflurane), **other neuromuscular blocking antibiotics** (e.g., kanamycin, streptomycin), **beta-lactam antibiotics** (e.g., cephalosporins), **diuretics** (e.g., furosemide [Lasix]), **vancomycin, and many others.** ▪ Neuromuscular blocking muscle relaxants (e.g., atracurium [Tracrium], succinylcholine) are potentiated by aminoglycosides. **Apnea can occur.** ▪ Aminoglycosides are also potentiated by **anticholinesterases** (e.g., edrophonium), **antineoplastics** (e.g., nitrogen mustard, cisplatin). ▪ May be antagonized by **bacteriostatic antibiotics** (e.g., chloramphenicol, erythromycin, tetracyclines); bactericidal action may be impacted.

SIDE EFFECTS
Occur more frequently with impaired renal function, higher doses, or prolonged administration, in dehydrated or elderly patients, and in patients receiving other ototoxic or nephrotoxic drugs.

Anorexia, burning, dizziness, fever, headache, hypertension, hypotension, itching, lethargy, muscle twitching, nausea, numbness, rash, roaring in ears, seizures, tingling sensation, tinnitus, urticaria, vomiting, weight loss.

Major: Acute organic brain syndrome; blood dyscrasias; CDAD; convulsions; elevated bilirubin, BUN, SCr, AST, and ALT; hearing loss; laryngeal edema; neuromuscular blockade; oliguria; respiratory depression or arrest.

ANTIDOTE

Notify the physician of all side effects. If minor side effects persist or any major symptom appears, notify the physician; may require dose adjustment or discontinuation of gentamicin. Treatment is symptomatic. In overdose or toxic reactions, hemodialysis may be indicated. Rate of gentamicin removal is lower with peritoneal dialysis. Monitor fluid balance, CrCl, and plasma levels carefully. Complexation with ticarcillin may be as effective as hemodialysis. Consider exchange transfusion in the newborn. Calcium salts or neostigmine may reverse neuromuscular blockade. Treat CDAD with fluids, electrolytes, protein supplements, and oral vancomycin (Vancocin) or metronidazole (Flagyl) as indicated. In severe cases, surgical evaluation may be indicated. Resuscitate as necessary.

GLUCAGON (rDNA ORIGIN)
(**GLOO**-kah-gon)

GlucaGen, Glucagon for Injection

Antihypoglycemic
Diagnostic agent
Antidote

pH 2.5 to 3.5

USUAL DOSE

Hypoglycemia in adults and pediatric patients weighing more than 20 kg (Glucagon [44 lbs]) to 25 kg (GlucaGen [55 lbs]): 1 mg. May be given IV, IM, or SC. Usually awakens an unconscious patient within 15 minutes. May be repeated in 20 minutes. For severe hypoglycemia or when patient fails to respond to glucagon, IV dextrose should be administered. Up to 2 mg of glucagon has been given as initial dose.

Diagnostic aid: stomach, duodenal bulb, duodenum, and small bowel: 0.2 to 0.5 mg IV or 1 mg IM before procedure begins. One source suggests 0.5 to 2 mg IV or 1 to 2 mg IM depending on the onset of action and duration of effect required for the specific examination. Upper range doses may be indicated during prolonged scan times (e.g., during an MRI [duration of action of glucagon is longer if given IM]). When diagnostic procedure is over, administer oral carbohydrates; see Monitor.

Diagnostic aid: colon: 0.5 to 0.75 mg IV or 1 to 2 mg IM before procedure begins. When diagnostic procedure is over, administer oral carbohydrates; see Monitor.

Management of cardiac effects of beta-blocker or calcium channel blocker overdose (unlabeled): 50 mcg/kg over 1 to 2 minutes. Doses up to 10 mg may be needed if the initial dose is ineffective. May be followed by an infusion of 2 to 5 mg/hr (up to a maximum of 10 mg/hr) diluted in D5W. Titrate to patient response. AHA guidelines recommend 3 to 10 mg slowly over 3 to 5 minutes, followed by an infusion of 3 to 5 mg/hr.

Treatment of foreign body obstruction in the esophagus (unlabeled): 0.5 to 2 mg IV. Repeat in 10 minutes if necessary.

PEDIATRIC DOSE

Hypoglycemia in infants and children weighing less than 20 kg (Glucagon [44 lbs]) to 25 kg (GlucaGen [55 lbs]): 20 to 30 mcg/kg or 0.5 mg. See comments under Usual Dose. If the weight is unknown, use 0.5 mg for pediatric patients younger than 6 years of age and 1 mg for those 6 years of age and older.

DOSE ADJUSTMENTS

For uses other than hypoglycemia, lower-end doses may be indicated in the elderly; consider impaired organ function and concurrent disease or other drug therapy.

DILUTION

Dilute 1 unit (1 mg) with 1 mL SW (may be supplied). Shake vial gently until completely dissolved. Concentrations greater than 1 mg/mL are not recommended. Do not add to IV solutions. May be given through Y-tube or three-way stopcock of infusion set if a dextrose solution is infusing. A 2-mg dose may be diluted with an equal amount of SW for injection.

Reverse effects of beta blockade: Reconstitute each 1 unit (1 mg) with 1 mL SW. For *continuous infusion* this reconstituted solution may be further diluted in D5W to deliver 1 to 5 mg/hr.

Storage: Use immediately after reconstitution. Discard any unused portion. Store *Glucagon for injection* at CRT before reconstitution. Before reconstitution, *GlucaGen* may be stored at CRT for up to 24 months in original package to protect from light. Do not freeze.

COMPATIBILITY

May form a precipitate with saline solutions and solutions with a pH of 3 to 9.5. Consider specific use; consult pharmacist.

RATE OF ADMINISTRATION

Too-rapid rate of injection or doses over 1 mg may increase incidence of side effects (e.g., nausea and vomiting).

1 unit (1 mg) or fraction thereof over 1 minute.

ACTIONS

An antihypoglycemic agent and a gastrointestinal motility inhibitor. A polypeptide hormone identical to naturally occurring human glucagon produced by recombinant DNA technology. Induces liver glycogen breakdown, releasing glucose from the liver. Blood glucose is raised within 10 minutes. Glucagon acts only on liver glycogen; hepatic stores of glycogen are necessary for glucagon to produce an antihypoglycemic effect. Extrahepatic effect produces relaxation of the smooth muscle of the stomach, duodenum, small bowel, and colon, inhibiting GI motility. Maximal glucose concentrations are seen about ½ hour after administration. Onset of smooth muscle relaxation is less than 1 minute. Duration of antihypoglycemic effect is 60 to 90 minutes. Duration of smooth muscle relaxation is dose-dependent and ranges from 9 to 25 minutes. Has a half-life of 8 to 18 minutes. Degraded in the liver, kidney, and plasma. Does not cross the placental barrier.

INDICATIONS AND USES

Treatment of severe hypoglycemia (e.g., during insulin therapy in the management of diabetes mellitus). ▪ As a diagnostic aid in the radiologic examination of the stomach, duodenum, small bowel, and colon when diminished intestinal motility would be advantageous.

Unlabeled uses: May be helpful in reversing adverse beta-blockade of beta-adrenergic blocking agents (e.g., propranolol) in overdose situations. ▪ If conventional therapy is ineffective, may be helpful in reversing myocardial depression of calcium channel blockers (e.g., diltiazem [Cardizem]). ▪ To decrease motility and aid in removing foreign bodies in the lower esophagus, including food boluses.

CONTRAINDICATIONS

Glucagon for injection: Known hypersensitivity to glucagon or its components, patients with known pheochromocytoma. **GlucaGen:** Known hypersensitivity to GlucaGen, lactose, or any of its components, patients with pheochromocytoma or insulinoma.

PRECAUTIONS

Easily absorbed IM or SC. ▪ If glucagon and glucose do not awaken patient, coma is probably caused by a condition other than hypoglycemia. ▪ Use caution in patients with a history suggestive of insulinoma, glucagonoma, and/or pheochromocytoma; secondary hypoglycemia may occur. Treat with adequate carbohydrate intake. ▪ May cause the release of catecholamines in patients with pheochromocytoma. ▪ Evaluation by a physician is recommended for all patients who experience severe hypoglycemia. ■ Use caution in patients with conditions that result in low levels of releasable glucose (e.g., adrenal insufficiency, chronic hypoglycemia, prolonged fasting, starvation). Will result in inadequate reversal of hypoglycemia. Treatment with dextrose is recommended. ■ Use caution; hypersensitivity reactions have occurred, usually in association with endoscopic examination during which other agents are administered (e.g., contrast media, local anesthetics). ■ As a smooth muscle relaxant, it is as effective as anticholinergic drugs and has fewer side effects. ■ When used to inhibit gastrointestinal motility, use caution in patients with known cardiac disease. ■ Hypotension has been reported for up to 2 hours after use as premedication for upper GI endoscopy procedures. ■ See Drug/Lab Interactions.

Monitor: Should awaken patient in 5 to 20 minutes. Prolonged hypoglycemic reactions may result in severe cortical damage. ■ Repeat dose if necessary. Supplement with IV dextrose (50%) to precipitate awakening and avoid complications of cerebral hypoglycemia. ■ Use blood glucose measurements to monitor patient response. ■ Emesis on awakening is common. Prevent aspiration by turning patient face down. ■ Depletes glycogen stores, especially in children and adolescents; supplement with oral carbohydrates on awakening to prevent secondary hypoglycemia. ■ In the treatment of beta-adrenergic blocker toxicity, may be used with isoproterenol (Isuprel) or dobutamine if indicated. Glucagon may decrease serum potassium levels; supplemental potassium may be indicated. ■ Monitor for S/S of hypersensitivity (e.g., dizziness, dyspnea, fever, flushing, hypotension, nausea, pruritus, rash, rigors, urticaria).

Patient Education: Eat some form of sugar if hypoglycemia recurs. ■ Report episodes of hypoglycemia and glucagon use at home. ■ Teach patient and family proper storage and preparation of glucagon from kits. Include signs of hypoglycemia and procedures to be followed after administration to an unconscious patient.

Maternal/Child: Category B: use during pregnancy only if clearly needed. Use caution during breast-feeding. Not absorbed through the GI tract; it would be unlikely to have any effect on the infant. ■ Does not cross the placental barrier. ■ Safety and effectiveness for treatment of hypoglycemia in pediatric patients has been demonstrated; however, safety and effectiveness for use in pediatric patients as a diagnostic aid has not been established.

Elderly: Cautious dosing may be indicated in the elderly; see Dose Adjustments. ■ Differences in response compared to younger adults not identified. ■ If used to inhibit gastrointestinal motility, use caution in elderly patients with known cardiac disease.

DRUG/LAB INTERACTIONS

Beta-blockers (e.g., metoprolol [Lopressor], sotalol) may cause a temporary increase in BP and pulse; treatment may be required in patients with cardiac disease or pheochromocytoma. ■ Concurrent use with **indomethacin** (Indocin) may cause glucagon to lose its ability to raise blood glucose and may produce hypoglycemia. ■ Coadministration with **anticholinergic** agents (e.g., atropine) is not recommended due to increased GI side effects. ■ May increase the anticoagulant effects of **warfarin** (Coumadin). ■ **Insulin** reacts antagonistically toward glucagon; use caution when used as a diagnostic aid in patients with diabetes.

SIDE EFFECTS

Rare in recommended doses: hyperglycemia (excessive dosage), hypersensitivity reactions (e.g., anaphylaxis, dyspnea, hypotension, rash), hypotension, increased BP, increased HR, nausea, vomiting. Increases in BP and HR may be greater in patients taking beta-blockers.

Overdose: Nausea and vomiting, increase in BP and HR, inhibition of GI tract motility, hypokalemia.

ANTIDOTE

Nausea and vomiting are tolerable and do occur in hypoglycemia. Antiemetics are indicated when larger doses are given. Increased BP and HR may require treatment in patients with coronary heart disease or pheochromocytoma. Treat sudden increases in BP with phentolamine 5 to 10 mg IV. For any other side effects, discontinue the drug and notify the physician. Treat hypersensitivity reactions and resuscitate as necessary. Insulin administration may be indicated in acute overdose. Effects of dialysis unknown; unlikely to provide benefit because of the short half-life of glucagon and the nature of the symptoms of overdose.

GLYCOPYRROLATE
(**GLYE**-koh-**pye**-roh-layt)

Anticholinergic
Antidote

pH 2 to 3

USUAL DOSE
Dose equivalents in mL are based on the 0.2 mg/mL concentration. Check vial for correct concentration.
Preanesthetic medication: 0.004 mg/kg (0.02 mL/kg) of body weight IM 30 to 60 minutes before anesthesia induction. Usually given at the same time as the preanesthetic narcotic and/or sedative.
Intraoperative medication: 0.1 mg (0.5 mL) IV. Repeat as needed at 2- to 3-minute intervals to counteract drug-induced or vagal traction reflexes and associated arrhythmias (e.g., bradycardia). Attempt to determine the etiology of arrhythmia and the procedures required to correct parasympathetic imbalance.
Reversal of neuromuscular blockade: 0.2 mg (1 mL) IV for each 1 mg of neostigmine or 5 mg of pyridostigmine (Regonol); to minimize the bradycardia and excessive secretions caused by these agents used to reverse the neuromuscular blockade of nondepolarizing muscle relaxants. May be administered simultaneously and may be mixed in the same syringe.
Peptic ulcer: 0.1 mg (0.5 mL) at 4-hour intervals 3 to 4 times/day. May be given IV or IM. Adjust frequency of administration based on patient response. Some may require only a single dose. If a more profound effect is required, dose may be increased to 0.2 mg (1 mL).
Respiratory antisecretory: 0.1 to 0.2 mg/dose (0.5 to 1 mL/dose) every 4 to 8 hours. Maximum dose suggested is 0.2 mg/dose or 0.8 mg/24 hr.

PEDIATRIC DOSE
See Maternal/Child.
Preanesthetic medication: Same as Usual Dose. *Infants 1 month to 2 years of age:* May require up to 0.009 mg/kg (0.045 mL/kg) of body weight.
Intraoperative medication: Rarely needed in pediatric patients because of the long duration of action from the preanesthetic dose. If required, administer 0.004 mg/kg (0.02 mL/kg) of body weight IV. Do not exceed 0.1 mg (0.5 mL) in a single dose. Repeat as needed at 2- to 3-minute intervals to counteract drug-induced or vagal traction reflexes and associated arrhythmias (e.g., bradycardia). Attempt to determine the etiology of arrhythmia and the procedures required to correct parasympathetic imbalance.
Reversal of neuromuscular blockade: Same as Usual Dose.
Peptic ulcer: Not recommended for treatment of peptic ulcer in pediatric patients; see Maternal/Child.
Respiratory antisecretory: 0.004 to 0.01 mg/kg/dose (0.02 to 0.05 mL/kg/dose) every 4 to 8 hours. Maximum dose suggested is 0.2 mg/dose or 0.8 mg/24 hr.

DOSE ADJUSTMENTS
Caution and lower-end dosing suggested for elderly patients based on potential for decreased organ function and concomitant disease or drug therapy. ▪ Elimination prolonged in patients with renal failure. Dose adjustment not provided; see Precautions. ▪ See Drug/Lab Interactions.

DILUTION

May be given undiluted. Administer through Y-tube or three-way stopcock of infusion tubing containing D5 or D10 in water or saline, D5/½NS, NS, or Ringer's. May be further diluted with D5 or D10 in water or saline.

Filters: No data available from manufacturer.

Storage: Store at CRT.

COMPATIBILITY   (Underline Indicates Conflicting Compatibility Information)

Consider any drug NOT listed as compatible to be INCOMPATIBLE until consulting a pharmacist; specific conditions may apply.

Manufacturer lists as **incompatible** with lactated Ringer's and states, "Stability is questionable above a pH of 6. May form a precipitate or a gas with chloramphenicol (Chloromycetin), diazepam (Valium), dimenhydrinate, methohexitol (Brevital), pentazocine (Talwin), pentobarbital (Nembutal), sodium bicarbonate, thiopental (Pentothal); do not combine in the same syringe." Dexamethasone (Decadron) will result in a pH above 6.

One source suggests the following **compatibilities:**

Y-site: <u>Palonosetron (Aloxi)</u>, propofol (Diprivan).

RATE OF ADMINISTRATION

0.2 mg or fraction thereof over 1 to 2 minutes.

ACTIONS

A synthetic anticholinergic agent. It inhibits the action of acetylcholine. It reduces the volume and free acidity of gastric secretions and controls excessive pharyngeal, tracheal, and bronchial secretions. Antagonizes muscarinic symptoms (e.g., bronchorrhea, bronchospasm, bradycardia, and intestinal hypermotility) induced by cholinergic drugs. Onset of action is within 1 minute. Vagal blocking effects last 2 to 3 hours, and antisialagogic (inhibited saliva flow) effects last up to 7 hours. Metabolism has not been studied. Half-life is 0.7 to 0.96 hours. Excreted primarily in urine and to a small extent in bile. Does not effectively cross the blood-brain barrier. Crosses the placental barrier in very small amounts.

INDICATIONS AND USES

Adjunctive therapy in peptic ulcer. ■ Protection against the peripheral muscarinic effects (e.g., bradycardia and excessive secretions) of cholinergic agents such as neostigmine and pyridostigmine (Regonol) given to reverse the neuromuscular blockade due to nondepolarizing muscle relaxants (e.g., atracurium [Tracrium]). ■ Reduction of salivary, tracheobronchial, and pharyngeal secretions preoperatively. ■ Reduction of volume and free acidity of gastric secretions. ■ Other intraoperative uses controlled by the anesthesiologist (counteract drug-induced or vagal traction reflexes and associated arrhythmias, prevent aspiration pneumonitis).

CONTRAINDICATIONS

Known hypersensitivity to glycopyrrolate. May be contraindicated in patients with glaucoma, obstructive uropathy, obstructive disease of the GI tract, paralytic ileus, intestinal atony of the elderly or debilitated, unstable cardiovascular status in acute hemorrhage, severe ulcerative colitis, toxic megacolon, and myasthenia gravis, when used for treatment of peptic ulcer disease because of long duration of therapy. ■ Do not use in neonates.

PRECAUTIONS

Use IV only when immediate drug effect is essential. ■ Use extreme caution in autonomic neuropathy, asthma, glaucoma, pregnancy, breastfeeding, cardiac arrhythmias, congestive heart failure, coronary artery disease, hepatic or renal disease, hiatal hernia, hypertension, hyperthyroidism, incomplete intestinal obstruction (diarrhea may be an early symptom), ulcerative colitis, and prostatic hypertrophy. Anticholinergic drugs may aggravate these conditions. ▪ Obtain cardiac history before administration of glycopyrrolate; may exacerbate pre-existing tachycardia. ▪ Heat prostration can occur with the use of anticholinergic agents in the presence of fever or high environmental temperatures. Pediatric patients and the elderly are at increased risk.

Monitor: Urinary retention can be avoided if the patient voids just before each dose. ▪ See Drug/Lab Interactions.

Patient Education: Use caution if a task requires alertness; may cause blurred vision, dizziness, or drowsiness. ▪ Report constipation, difficulty urinating, dry mouth, flushing, increased light sensitivity, or skin rash promptly. ▪ Use caution during exercise or hot weather. Increased heat sensitivity may result in heatstroke.

Maternal/Child: Category B: safety for use in pregnancy not established. ▪ It is not known whether this drug is secreted in breast milk; may suppress lactation; use caution. ▪ Safety and effectiveness for use in pediatric patients under 16 years of age not established for management of peptic ulcer. ▪ Dysrhythmias have been observed in pediatric patients. ▪ Pediatric patients may have an increased response to anticholinergics and be at increased risk for side effects (e.g., paradoxical hyperexcitability). Infants and young children, patients with Down syndrome, and pediatric patients with spastic paralysis or brain damage are especially susceptible to this increased response. ▪ *Contains benzyl alcohol; do not use in neonates;* see Contraindications.

Elderly: Differences in response compared to younger adults not observed. ▪ Dosing should be cautious; see Dose Adjustments. ▪ May produce excitement, agitation, confusion, or drowsiness in the elderly. ▪ May precipitate undiagnosed glaucoma. ▪ Risk of urinary retention and constipation increased. ▪ May increase memory impairment.

DRUG/LAB INTERACTIONS

Potentiated by other drugs with **anticholinergic activity** (e.g., amantadine [Symmetrel], **antiparkinson drugs** [e.g., levodopa (Larodopa, Dopar)], **atropine, phenothiazines** [e.g., prochlorperazine (Compazine)], **tricyclic antidepressants** [e.g., amitriptyline (Elavil), imipramine (Tofranil)]). Reduced dose of either or both drugs may be indicated. ▪ Concomitant administration with **KCl** in a wax matrix may increase the risk and severity of KCl-induced GI lesions (due to slower GI transit time). ▪ May decrease antipsychotic effects of **phenothiazines.** Dose adjustment may be required. ▪ Risk of ventricular arrhythmias increased when given in presence of **cyclopropane.** Risk is less than with atropine and when given in doses of 0.1 mg or less. ▪ Potentiates **atenolol** (Tenormin) and **digoxin.**

SIDE EFFECTS

Anaphylaxis, anticholinergic psychosis, arrhythmias, blurred vision, cardiac arrest, confusion, constipation, decreased sweating, dizziness, drowsiness, dry mouth, headache, heat prostration, hypertension, hypotension, impotence, increased ocular tension, injection site reactions, insomnia, loss of taste, malignant hyperthermia, muscular weakness, nausea and vomiting, nervousness, palpitation, paralysis, photophobia, pruritus, respiratory arrest, seizures, suppression of lactation, tachycardia, urinary hesitancy and retention, urticaria, weakness.

Overdose: A curare-like action may occur (i.e., neuromuscular blockade leading to muscular weakness and possible paralysis).

ANTIDOTE

Notify physician of all side effects. May be treated symptomatically or drug may be discontinued. Treat hypotension with IV fluids and/or pressor agents (e.g., dopamine). Initiate artificial respiration if overdose with paralysis of respiratory muscles occurs. Neostigmine, in 0.25-mg increments, may be used to counteract peripheral anticholinergic effects. May repeat every 5 to 10 minutes to a maximum dose of 2.5 mg. Need for repetitive doses of neostigmine should be based on close monitoring of the decrease in HR and the return of bowel sounds. Physostigmine, in increments of 0.5 to 2 mg, may be used to counteract CNS effects. May repeat as needed to a maximum dose of 5 mg. Proportionately smaller doses should be used in pediatric patients. Resuscitate as necessary.

GRANISETRON HYDROCHLORIDE

(gran-**ISS**-eh-tron hy-droh-**KLOR**-eyed)

Kytril

Antiemetic
(5-HT$_3$ receptor antagonist)

pH 4 to 6

USUAL DOSE

Chemotherapy-induced nausea and vomiting (prophylaxis): A single dose of 10 mcg/kg of body weight as an injection or as an infusion. Begin within 30 minutes before giving emetogenic cancer chemotherapy (e.g., cisplatin, carboplatin) and only on the day(s) chemotherapy is given. Clinical trials used doses up to 40 mcg/kg with effects similar to the recommended 10-mcg/kg dose. Some studies question the effectiveness of a 10-mcg/kg dose. Repeat doses are frequently required to prevent nausea with chemotherapy. Oral granisetron is available.

Prevention and treatment of postoperative nausea and vomiting: 1 mg before induction of anesthesia, immediately before reversal of anesthesia, or postoperatively.

PEDIATRIC DOSE

Chemotherapy-induced nausea and vomiting (prophylaxis) in pediatric patients 2 to 16 years of age: Identical to adult dose. See Maternal/Child.

DOSE ADJUSTMENTS

No dose adjustment required for the elderly or in renal failure or impaired hepatic function.

DILUTION

Read label carefully. Available in two concentrations (0.1 mg/mL and 1 mg/mL). The 0.1-mg/mL vial contains no preservatives. The 1-mg/mL single-dose and multidose vials contain benzyl alcohol. Sterile technique imperative when withdrawing a single dose from the multidose vial; see Storage.

A single dose may be given undiluted by IV injection or further diluted to a total volume of 20 to 50 mL with NS or D5W and given as an infusion.

Storage: Store vials at CRT or below. Do not freeze; protect from light. Should be administered after dilution (preservative free) but is stable up to

24 hours at room temperature. Discard multidose vial within 30 days of initial penetration.

COMPATIBILITY
Consider any drug NOT listed as compatible to be INCOMPATIBLE until consulting a pharmacist; specific conditions may apply. Manufacturer recommends not mixing in solution with other drugs as a general precaution.

One source suggests the following **compatibilities:**
Additive: *Not recommended by manufacturer.* Dexamethasone (Decadron), methylprednisolone (Solu-Medrol).

Y-site: Acyclovir (Zovirax), allopurinol (Aloprim), amifostine (Ethyol), amikacin (Amikin), aminophylline, amphotericin B cholesteryl (Amphotec), ampicillin, ampicillin/sulbactam (Unasyn), aztreonam (Azactam), bleomycin (Blenoxane), bumetanide, buprenorphine (Buprenex), butorphanol (Stadol), calcium gluconate, carboplatin (Paraplatin), carmustine (BiCNU), cefazolin (Ancef), cefepime (Maxipime), cefotaxime (Claforan), cefotetan (Cefotan), cefoxitin (Mefoxin), ceftazidime (Fortaz), ceftriaxone (Rocephin), cefuroxime (Zinacef), chlorpromazine (Thorazine), ciprofloxacin (Cipro IV), cisplatin (Platinol), cladribine (Leustatin), clindamycin (Cleocin), cyclophosphamide (Cytoxan), cytarabine (ARA-C), dacarbazine (DTIC), dactinomycin (Cosmegen), daunorubicin (Cerubidine), dexamethasone (Decadron), dexmedetomidine (Precedex), diphenhydramine (Benadryl), dobutamine, docetaxel (Taxotere), dopamine, doripenem (Doribax), doxorubicin (Adriamycin), doxorubicin liposomal (Doxil), doxycycline, droperidol (Inapsine), enalaprilat (Vasotec IV), etoposide (VePesid), etoposide phosphate (Etopophos), famotidine (Pepcid IV), fenoldopam (Corlopam), filgrastim (Neupogen), fluconazole (Diflucan), fludarabine (Fludara), fluorouracil (5-FU), furosemide (Lasix), gallium nitrate (Ganite), ganciclovir (Cytovene), gemcitabine (Gemzar), gentamicin, haloperidol (Haldol), heparin, hetastarch in electrolytes (Hextend), hydrocortisone sodium succinate (Solu-Cortef), hydromorphone (Dilaudid), idarubicin (Idamycin), ifosfamide (Ifex), imipenem-cilastatin (Primaxin), leucovorin calcium, levoleucovorin (Fusilev), linezolid (Zyvox), lorazepam (Ativan), magnesium sulfate, mechlorethamine (nitrogen mustard), melphalan (Alkeran), meperidine (Demerol), mesna (Mesnex), methotrexate, methylprednisolone (Solu-Medrol), metoclopramide (Reglan), metronidazole (Flagyl IV), mitomycin (Mutamycin), mitoxantrone (Novantrone), morphine, nalbuphine, oxaliplatin (Eloxatin), paclitaxel (Taxol), pemetrexed (Alimta), piperacillin, piperacillin/tazobactam (Zosyn), potassium chloride (KCl), prochlorperazine (Compazine), promethazine (Phenergan), propofol (Diprivan), ranitidine (Zantac), sargramostim (Leukine), sodium bicarbonate, streptozocin (Zanosar), sulfamethoxazole/trimethoprim, teniposide (Vumon), thiotepa, ticarcillin/clavulanate (Timentin), tobramycin, topotecan (Hycamtin), vancomycin, vinblastine, vincristine, vinorelbine (Navelbine), zidovudine (AZT, Retrovir).

RATE OF ADMINISTRATION
IV injection: A single dose over 30 seconds.
Intermittent infusion: A single dose equally distributed over 5 minutes.

ACTIONS
An antinauseant and antiemetic agent. A selective antagonist of specific serotonin ($5\text{-}HT_3$) receptors. Chemotherapeutic agents such as cisplatin

increase the release of serotonin from specific cells in the GI tract, causing emesis. By antagonizing these receptors, chemotherapy-induced nausea and vomiting are prevented. Has little effect on BP, HR, ECG, plasma prolactin, or aldosterone concentrations. Moderately bound to protein (65%). Distributes freely between plasma and RBCs. Metabolized in the liver by hepatic cytochrome P_{450} enzymes. Mean half-life is approximately 9 hours. Excreted in urine and feces.

INDICATIONS AND USES

Prevention of nausea and vomiting associated with initial and repeat courses of emetogenic cancer therapy, including high-dose cisplatin. Has been shown to be effective with most emetogenic antineoplastic agents. ▪ Prevention and treatment of postoperative nausea and vomiting in adults. **Unlabeled uses:** Prevention of nausea and vomiting associated with total body radiation or fractional abdominal radiation.

CONTRAINDICATIONS

Known hypersensitivity to granisetron.

PRECAUTIONS

Stool softeners or laxatives may be required to prevent constipation. ▪ See Drug/Lab Interactions. ▪ Hypersensitivity reactions have been reported. Use caution in patients who have exhibited hypersensitivity to other selective 5-HT$_3$ receptor antagonists. Cross-sensitivity has been reported between dolasetron (Anzemet) and other agents in this class (e.g., granisetron, ondansetron). ▪ The use in patients following abdominal surgery or in patients with chemotherapy-induced nausea and vomiting may mask a progressive ileus and/or gastric distention. ▪ Does not stimulate GI motility and should not be used instead of NG suction. ▪ QT prolongation has been reported. Use with caution in patients with pre-existing arrhythmias, cardiac conduction disorders, or electrolyte abnormalities or in patients who are taking other medications that can prolong the QT interval; see Drug/Lab Interactions. ▪ Not recommended if nausea and vomiting are not expected postoperatively unless nausea and vomiting must be avoided during the postoperative period.

Monitor: Ambulate slowly to avoid orthostatic hypotension. ▪ Monitor for S/S of hypersensitivity (e.g., anaphylaxis, hypotension, shortness of breath, urticaria).

Patient Education: Request assistance for ambulation. ▪ Report promptly if nausea persists for more than 10 minutes. ▪ Maintain adequate hydration. ▪ Stool softeners may be required to avoid constipation.

Maternal/Child: Category B: no evidence of impaired fertility or harm to fetus. Benzyl alcohol may cross the placenta; see Dilution. Use during pregnancy only if benefits justify risks. ▪ Use caution if required during breast-feeding. ▪ Safety and effectiveness for use in the treatment of chemotherapy-induced nausea and vomiting in pediatric patients under 2 years of age have not been established. ▪ Not recommended for prevention and treatment of postoperative nausea and vomiting in pediatric patients due to a lack of efficacy and QT prolongation observed in a clinical trial.

Elderly: Response similar to other age-groups. ▪ Clearance lower and half-life prolonged but has no clinical significance.

DRUG/LAB INTERACTIONS

Metabolism may be inhibited by **ketoconazole** (Nizoral). Clinical significance unknown. ▪ Does not induce or inhibit the cytochrome P_{450} drug metabolizing system, but definitive interaction studies have not been done.

Its clearance and half-life may be affected by **inducers of these enzymes** such as anticonvulsants (e.g., carbamazepine [Tegretol], phenobarbital [Luminal], phenytoin [Dilantin]) or rifampin (Rifadin) or by **inhibitors of these enzymes** (e.g., cimetidine [Tagamet], calcium channel blockers [e.g., diltiazem (Cardizem), verapamil], antiviral agents [e.g., indinavir (Crixivan), ritonavir [Norvir], saquinavir [Invirase]). ▪ Has been safely administered with **benzodiazepines** (e.g., lorazepam [Ativan], midazolam [Versed]), **neuroleptics** (e.g., chlordiazepoxide [Librium]), and **antiulcer drugs** (e.g., ranitidine [Zantac]) commonly prescribed with antiemetic treatment. ▪ Does not appear to interact with emetogenic cancer chemotherapies. ▪ Concurrent use with **drugs known to prolong the QT interval** (e.g., amiodarone [Nexterone], antihistamines, azole antifungals [e.g., itraconazole (Sporanox)], disopyramide [Norpace], fluoroquinolones [e.g., levofloxacin (Levaquin)], ibutilide [Corvert], mexiletine, phenothiazines [e.g., thioridazine (Mellaril)], procainamide [Pronestyl], quinidine, and tricyclic antidepressants [e.g., amitriptyline (Elavil), imipramine (Tofranil)]) may result in clinical consequences.

SIDE EFFECTS
Asthenia (5%), constipation (3%), diarrhea (4%), headache (14%), somnolence (4%), and weakness (5%) occur most frequently. Hypersensitivity reactions, including anaphylaxis (rare), have occurred. Transient elevation of AST or ALT may occur. Other side effects include abdominal pain, anemia, anxiety, bradycardia, coughing, dizziness, dyspepsia, fever, hypertension, hypotension, infection, insomnia, leukocytosis, oliguria, pain. Other side effects have occurred in fewer than 2% of patients but could not be clearly associated with granisetron.
Post-Marketing: QT prolongation.

ANTIDOTE
Most side effects will be treated symptomatically. Keep physician informed as indicated. There is no specific antidote. Treat anaphylaxis and resuscitate as necessary.

HEMIN BBW
(**HEE**-men)
Panhematin

Porphyrin inhibitor

USUAL DOSE
A single dose of 1 to 4 mg/kg of body weight/24 hr of hematin for 3 to 14 days. This dose could be repeated in 12 hours for severe cases. Never exceed a total dose of 6 mg/kg/24 hr. Length of treatment dependent on severity of symptoms and clinical response. See Precautions.

DILUTION
Each vial containing 313 mg of hemin must be diluted with 43 mL of SW for injection (provides 301 mg of hematin). Shake well for 2 to 3 minutes to ensure dissolution. Each 1 mL contains 7 mg hematin. Each 0.14 mL contains 1 mg hematin. May be given directly from vial as an infusion or through Y-tube or three-way stopcock of infusion set.

Filters: Use of a 0.45-micron or smaller in-line filter recommended.
Storage: Store in refrigerator at 2° to 8° C. Contains no preservative, decomposes rapidly; discard unused solution.

COMPATIBILITY

Undergoes rapid chemical decomposition in solution. Manufacturer states, "No drug or chemical agent should be added unless its effect on the chemical and physical stability has been determined." Specific information not available; consult pharmacist.

RATE OF ADMINISTRATION

A single dose evenly distributed over 10 to 15 minutes.

ACTIONS

An iron-containing metalloporphyrin enzyme inhibitor extracted from RBCs. Inhibits rate of porphyria/heme biosynthesis in the liver and bone marrow by an unknown mechanism. Induces remission of symptoms only; not curative. Some excretion occurs in urine and feces.

INDICATIONS AND USES

To control symptoms of recurrent attacks of acute intermittent porphyria in selected patients (often related to the menstrual cycle in susceptible women).

CONTRAINDICATIONS

Hypersensitivity to hemin; porphyria cutanea tarda.

PRECAUTIONS

Confirm diagnosis of acute porphyria before use (positive Watson-Schwartz or Hoechst test). Administered by or under the supervision of a physician experienced in the treatment of porphyrias and in facilities equipped to monitor the patient and respond to any medical emergency. ■ Alternate therapy of 400 Gm glucose/24 hr for 1 to 2 days should be tried before use of hemin is initiated. ■ Give as early as possible with onset of attack to achieve the most benefit. ■ Must be given before irreversible neuronal damage of porphyria has begun. ■ See Drug/Lab Interactions.
Monitor: Use of a large arm vein or central venous catheter recommended to avoid phlebitis. ■ Effectiveness monitored by decrease in urine concentration of S-aminolevulinic acid (ALA), uroporphyrinogen (UPG), or porphobilinogen (PBG).
Maternal/Child: Category C: safety for use during pregnancy, breast-feeding, and in pediatric patients not established.

DRUG/LAB INTERACTIONS

Action inhibited by **estrogens, barbiturates, and steroid metabolites.** Avoid concurrent use. ■ Has mild anticoagulant effects. Avoid concurrent use with **anticoagulants** (e.g., heparin, warfarin [Coumadin]).

SIDE EFFECTS

Almost nonexistent with usual dosage and appropriate technique; fever, phlebitis. Reversible renal shutdown has been reported with excessive doses.

ANTIDOTE

Discontinue temporarily if known or questionable side effect appears and notify physician. Renal shutdown of overdose has responded to ethacrynic acid (Edecrin) and mannitol. Treat anaphylaxis (antihistamines, epinephrine, corticosteroids) and resuscitate as necessary.

HEPARIN SODIUM

Anticoagulant

(**HEP**-ah-rin **SO**-dee-um)

❦Hepalean, Heparin Lock-Flush, Heparin Sodium PF, Hep-Flush 10, Hep-Lock, Hep-Lock U/P

pH 5 to 7.5

USUAL DOSE

As of 2009 USP heparin has a new reference standard and a new test method for manufacturers to use in determining accurate potency. The adjustment in reference standard results in approximately a 10% reduction in the potency of heparin and makes it commensurate with the World Health Organization International Standard unit dose. In most situations this new reference standard will not require a dose adjustment; however, dose adjustments and more frequent monitoring may be indicated in selected clinical situations.

Intermittent injection: 10,000 units initially. Dosage is repeated every 4 to 6 hours and adjusted according to coagulation test results. Usually 5,000 to 10,000 units.

IV infusion: 20,000 to 40,000 units/24 hr in NS or other **compatible** infusion solution. An initial bolus dose of 5,000 units is required. Adjust dose according to coagulation test results.

Adjuvant therapy in treatment of AMI: AHA guidelines recommend an initial bolus dose of 60 units/kg of body weight (maximum dose 4,000 units). Follow with an infusion of 12 units/kg/hr. The initial maximum recommended infusion rate is 1,000 units/hr. Adjust to maintain aPTT at 1.5 to 2 times control. Other protocols are in use.

Adjuvant therapy during treatment with thrombolytic agents (e.g., alteplase, reteplase, streptokinase) and glycoprotein GPIIb/IIIa receptor antagonists (e.g., abciximab, eptifibitide, tirofiban): See individual monographs for suggested doses.

Open heart surgery: 150 to 400 units/kg of body weight during surgical procedure.

Disseminated intravascular coagulation: Use and dose of heparin is based on severity of DIC and underlying cause and extent of thrombosis. Several dosing regimens have been used; see literature.

Maintain patency of indwelling venipuncture devices used with a continuous infusion: 500 to 1,000 units to each 1,000 mL IV fluid.

Maintain patency of indwelling venipuncture devices (e.g., central venous line, heparin plugs) intended for intermittent use: 10 to 100 units. Dilute in a sufficient quantity of NS to fill the entire device (e.g., needle, catheter, or implanted port) and inject via injection hub. Use after each medication injection or every 8 to 24 hours. From 100 units up to 500 units may be required in central venous lines. Confirm patency by aspirating before each injection. Flush with SW or NS before and after any medication **incompatible** with heparin. Re-instill heparin after second flush. If additional medications are not needed, each single dose of heparin will prevent clotting within the lumen of indwelling venipuncture devices for up to 24 hours. Consult device manufacturers instructions for specific requirements regarding its use.

Blood transfusion: 400 to 600 units/100 mL whole blood.

PEDIATRIC DOSE

Read label carefully. Comes in many strengths. Confirm use of the correct strength. Fatal hemorrhages have occurred in pediatric patients, including neonates, as a result of medication errors in which heparin sodium injection vials have been confused with heparin-lock flush vials.

Do not use products containing benzyl alcohol in neonates or infants. Preservative-free solution is required for neonates and infants. See Maternal/Child.

Full-dose continuous IV infusion: A *loading dose* of 50 units/kg followed by a *maintenance dose* of 25 units/kg/hr or up to 20,000 units/M^2 equally distributed over 24 hours. Another source suggests a *loading dose* of 75 to 100 units/kg and a *maintenance dose* (to maintain an aPTT of approximately 60 to 85 seconds or to a range corresponding to an anti-Factor Xa level of 0.35 to 0.7 units/mL [for 5 to 10 days]) based on age as follows: *Less than 1 year of age:* 28 units/kg/hr.

Over 1 year of age: 20 units/kg/hr.

Older pediatric patients: Dose similar to the weight-adjusted dose in adults (18 units/kg/hr) or a *loading dose* of 100 units/kg followed by 50 to 100 units/kg every 4 hours (12.5 to 25 units/kg every hour). Alternately, an initial dose of 50 units/kg of body weight may be followed by a maintenance dose of 10 to 25 units/kg/hr as a continuous infusion, an intermittent infusion of 50 to 100 units/kg every 4 hours, or 20,000 units/M^2/24 hr. All doses should be adjusted to coagulation tests.

Disseminated intravascular coagulation: Use and dose of heparin is based on severity of DIC and underlying cause and extent of thrombosis. Several dosing regimens have been used; see literature.

Patency of indwelling venipuncture devices: See Maternal/Child. Safety and effectiveness of the 100-USP units/mL heparin lock flush solution for pediatric patients not established. Patency for peripheral devices (e.g., single- and double-lumen central catheters) is usually accomplished with 10 units/mL heparin solution in younger infants (e.g., less than 10 kg) and with 100 units/mL for older infants, children, and adults. Avoid approaching therapeutic unit/kg dose. Follow catheter manufacturer's guidelines. See all comments under similar section in Usual Dose.

DOSE ADJUSTMENTS

Reduction of initial dose indicated in low-birth-weight infants and may be indicated in patients 60 years of age and older (especially women). Dose is based on coagulation tests; see Monitor. ■ Increased dose may be required in smokers (half-life shortened and elimination rate increased).

DILUTION

May be given undiluted or diluted in any given amount of NS, dextrose, or Ringer's solution for infusion and given by IV injection, as an intermittent IV, or continuous IV infusion. *In all situations,* invert container a minimum of 6 times to ensure adequate mixing of heparin with solution. Available in several strengths for administration or dilution as well as in several premixed concentrations and volumes and in ADD-Vantage vials for use with ADD-Vantage infusion containers. Unit-dose heparin flush syringes are not for multiple use; discard unused portions.

Intermittent infusion: Usually diluted in 50 to 100 mL of NS.

Continuous infusion: Usually diluted in 1,000 mL of NS/24-hour dose.

Blood transfusion: Add 7,500 units heparin to 100 mL NS. Add 6 to 8 mL of this sterile solution to each 100 mL of whole blood.

Filters: No significant reduction in potency when 10,000 units diluted in D5W or NS was filtered through a 0.22-micron cellulose ester membrane filter.

Storage: Store at CRT. Do not freeze. Do not use if solution is discolored or contains a precipitate.

COMPATIBILITY   (Underline Indicates Conflicting Compatibility Information)
Consider any drug NOT listed as compatible to be INCOMPATIBLE until consulting a pharmacist; specific conditions may apply.

Several sources recommend not mixing or administering through the same IV line with other drugs until **compatibility** confirmed. To avoid precipitation with heparin, they also caution to flush with SW or NS before and after any acidic or **incompatible** medication or solution.

One source suggests the following **compatibilities:**

Additive: Aminophylline, amphotericin B (generic), ampicillin, ascorbic acid, bleomycin (Blenoxane), calcium gluconate, cefepime (Maxipime), chloramphenicol (Chloromycetin), clindamycin (Cleocin), colistimethate (Coly-Mycin M), dimenhydrinate, dobutamine, dopamine, enalaprilat (Vasotec IV), esmolol (Brevibloc), fluconazole (Diflucan), flumazenil (Romazicon), furosemide (Lasix), hydrocortisone sodium succinate (Solu-Cortef), hydromorphone (Dilaudid), isoproterenol (Isuprel), lidocaine, lincomycin (Lincocin), magnesium sulfate, meropenem (Merrem IV), methyldopa, methylprednisolone (Solu-Medrol), mitomycin (Mutamycin), nafcillin (Nallpen), norepinephrine (Levophed), octreotide (Sandostatin), penicillin G potassium and sodium, potassium chloride, ranitidine (Zantac), sodium bicarbonate, teicoplanin (Targocid), vancomycin, verapamil.

Y-site: Acyclovir (Zovirax), aldesleukin (Proleukin), allopurinol (Aloprim), amifostine (Ethyol), aminophylline, ampicillin, ampicillin/sulbactam (Unasyn), anidulafungin (Eraxis), anti-thymocyte globulin (rabbit), atracurium (Tracrium), atropine, aztreonam (Azactam), bivalirudin (Angiomax), bleomycin (Blenoxane), calcium gluconate, cefazolin (Ancef), cefotetan (Cefotan), ceftazidime (Fortaz), ceftriaxone (Rocephin), chlorpromazine (Thorazine), cisatracurium (Nimbex), cisplatin (Platinol), cladribine (Leustatin), clindamycin (Cleocin), cyclophosphamide (Cytoxan), cytarabine (ARA-C), dacarbazine (DTIC), daptomycin (Cubicin), dexamethasone (Decadron), dexmedetomidine (Precedex), digoxin (Lanoxin), diltiazem (Cardizem), diphenhydramine (Benadryl), dobutamine, docetaxel (Taxotere), dopamine, doripenem (Doribax), doxapram (Dopram), doxorubicin (Adriamycin), doxorubicin liposomal (Doxil), droperidol (Inapsine), drotrecogin alfa (Xigris), edrophonium (Enlon), enalaprilat (Vasotec IV), epinephrine (Adrenalin), ertapenem (Invanz), erythromycin (Erythrocin), esmolol (Brevibloc), estrogens, conjugated (Premarin), ethacrynic acid (Edecrin), etoposide phosphate (Etopophos), famotidine (Pepcid IV), fenoldopam (Corlopam), fentanyl (Sublimaze), fluconazole (Diflucan), fludarabine (Fludara), fluorouracil (5-FU), foscarnet (Foscavir), furosemide (Lasix), gallium nitrate (Ganite), gemcitabine (Gemzar), granisetron (Kytril), hetastarch in electrolytes (Hextend), hydralazine, hydrocortisone sodium succinate (Solu-Cortef), hydromorphone (Dilaudid), insulin (regular), isoproterenol (Isuprel), kanamycin (Kantrex), labetalol (Trandate), leucovorin calcium, lidocaine, linezolid (Zyvox), lorazepam (Ativan), magnesium sulfate, melphalan (Alkeran), meperidine (Demerol), meropenem (Merrem IV), methotrexate, methyldopa, methylergonovine (Methergine), <u>methylprednisolone (Solu-Medrol)</u>, metoclopramide (Reglan), metronidazole (Flagyl IV), <u>micafungin (Mycamine)</u>, midazolam (Versed), milrinone (Primacor), mitomycin (Mutamycin), morphine, nafcillin (Nallpen), neostigmine, <u>nicardipine (Cardene IV)</u>, nitroglycerin IV, nitroprusside sodium, norepinephrine (Levophed), ondansetron (Zofran), oxacillin (Bactocill), oxaliplatin (Eloxatin), oxytocin (Pitocin), paclitaxel (Taxol), <u>palonosetron (Aloxi)</u>, pancuronium, pemetrexed (Alimta), penicillin G potassium, pentazocine (Talwin), phytonadione (vitamin K_1), piperacillin, piperacillin/tazobactam (Zosyn), potassium chloride (KCl), procainamide (Pronestyl), prochlorperazine (Compazine), <u>promethazine (Phenergan)</u>, propofol (Diprivan), propranolol, pyridostigmine (Regonol), <u>quinidine gluconate</u>, ranitidine (Zantac), remifentanil (Ultiva), sargramostim (Leukine), sodium bicarbonate, succinylcholine, tacrolimus (Prograf), theophylline, thiopental (Pentothal), thiotepa, ticarcillin/clavulanate (Timentin), tigecycline (Tygacil), tirofiban (Aggrastat), <u>vancomycin</u>, vasopressin, vecuronium, vinblastine, vincristine, <u>vinorelbine (Navelbine)</u>, warfarin (Coumadin), zidovudine (AZT, Retrovir).

RATE OF ADMINISTRATION

First 1,000 units or fraction thereof over 1 minute. After this test dose, any single injection (5,000 units or fraction thereof) may be given over 1 minute. A continuous IV infusion may be given over 4 to 24 hours, depending on specific dosage of heparin required, amount of heparin added, and amount of infusion fluid used as a diluent. Continuous IV infusion is the preferred method of administration. Use an infusion pump for accuracy.

ACTIONS

An anticoagulant with immediate and predictable effects on the blood. Inhibits reactions that lead to clotting of blood and the formation of fibrin clots. Heparin combines with other factors in the blood to inhibit the conversion of prothrombin to thrombin and fibrinogen to fibrin. Adhesiveness of platelets is reduced. Well-established clots are not dissolved, but growth is prevented and newer clots may be dissolved. Duration of action is short, about 4 to 6 hours. Average half-life is 30 to 180 minutes. The half-life of the anticoagulant effect of heparin is approximately 1.5 hours and does not increase with dose. The plasma half-life is prolonged by higher doses and in liver or kidney disease and shortened in patients with pulmonary embolism. Does not cross the placental barrier. Metabolized in the liver and excreted by the kidneys.

INDICATIONS AND USES

Prevention and/or treatment of all types of thromboses and emboli including deep vein thrombosis (DVT), pulmonary emboli (PE), and embolization associated with atrial fibrillation (AF). ▪ Diagnosis and treatment of disseminated intravascular coagulation (DIC). ▪ Prevention of clotting in surgery of the heart or blood vessels, during blood transfusion, and hemodialysis. ▪ Adjunct in treatment of coronary occlusion with acute myocardial infarction (MI). ▪ Prevention of rethrombosis or reocclusion during MI after thrombolytic therapy (e.g., alteplase, reteplase, streptokinase). ▪ Adjunct to use of glycoprotein GP IIb/IIIa receptor antagonists in percutaneous coronary intervention (PCI). ▪ Maintain patency of indwelling venipuncture devices (e.g., heparin-lock, needle, catheter, or implanted port) during prolonged IV infusion or for intermittent medication injection or vein access.

Unlabeled uses: Prevention of left ventricular thrombi and cerebrovascular accidents after MI. ■ Continuous infusion for treatment of myocardial ischemia in unstable angina refractory to conventional treatment. ■ Prevention of cerebral thrombosis in the evolving stroke.

CONTRAINDICATIONS

Severe thrombocytopenia. ■ Patients receiving full-dose heparin unless blood coagulation tests can be performed at appropriate intervals. ■ Hypersensitivity to heparin unless required in a clearly life-threatening situation. ■ Uncontrolled bleeding except in DIC. ■ Do not administer heparin preparations preserved with benzyl alcohol to neonates, infants, pregnant women, or breast-feeding mothers.

PRECAUTIONS

Read label carefully. Comes in many strengths. Confirm use of the correct strength. Fatal hemorrhages have occurred in pediatric patients, including neonates, as a result of medication errors in which heparin sodium injection vials have been confused with heparin-lock flush vials. ■ Unit-to-milligram conversions are not consistent. ■ For IV or SC use only; avoid IM administration (may cause hematomas). ■ Selected products are derived from animal protein. ■ Use extreme caution in any disease state or clinical condition where risk of hemorrhage may be increased such as subacute bacterial endocarditis; severe hypertension; during or following spinal tap, spinal anesthesia, or major surgery (especially major surgery involving the brain, spinal cord, or eye); hemophilia; thrombocytopenia; gastrointestinal ulcerative lesions; vascular purpuras; continuous tube drainage of the stomach or small intestine; menstruation; and severe liver disease with impaired hemostasis. ■ Resistance to heparin increased in cancer, fever, infections with thrombosing tendencies, MI, postsurgical patients, thrombophlebitis, and thrombosis. ■ Use caution if administering ACD-converted blood (variable). ■ May cause thrombocytopenia; monitor closely. ■ May develop heparin-induced thrombocytopenia (HIT, with or without thrombosis), an antibody-mediated reaction resulting from irreversible aggregation of platelets. HIT may progress to heparin-induced thrombocytopenia and thrombosis (HITT), which involves the development of venous and arterial thromboses. HIT and HITT may occur during heparin treatment or may be delayed for up to several weeks after heparin treatment is discontinued; see Monitor. ■ See Elderly for additional precautions. ■ Repeated flushing of an indwelling venipuncture device with heparin may result in a systemic anticoagulant effect. ■ Heparin-lock flush solution is intended for maintenance of patency of intravenous injection devices only and is not to be used for anticoagulant therapy. ■ See Maternal/Child.

Monitor: Whole blood clotting time (WBCT), activated coagulation time (ACT), or aPTT must be done before initial injection. Obtain a baseline platelet count. ■ During the early stages of treatment, coagulation tests are often done before each intermittent injection or every 4 hours with a continuous infusion. Usually repeated daily thereafter during IV therapy and more often if indicated (some sources recommend an aPTT every 6 hours). Depending on the test chosen the desired therapeutic level is approximately 1½ to 3 times greater than the control level (e.g., aPTT [1.5 to 2 times therapeutic level], WBCT [2.5 to 3 times control level]). Confirm desired control level with physician. Obtain test just before next dose due in intermittent injection. Notify the physician if aPTT, ACT, or

WBCT is above therapeutic level. ▪ Monitor platelet count periodically. Discontinue heparin if it falls below 100,000 or a thrombosis forms. May develop HIT (with or without thrombosis) or HITT (irreversible aggregation of platelets induced by heparin that may lead to severe thromboembolic complications [e.g., DVT; cerebral vein thrombosis, limb ischemia, mesenteric thrombosis, or renal artery thrombosis; skin necrosis; gangrene of the extremities that may lead to amputation; MI; pulmonary embolism; stroke; or death]). HIT and HITT may occur during heparin therapy or may be delayed. Evaluate patients for HIT and HITT if they present with thrombocytopenia or thrombosis after heparin is discontinued. Can occur up to several weeks after heparin is discontinued. ▪ Also monitor hematocrit and occult blood in stool. ▪ Hemorrhage can occur at any site and is the primary complication. Monitor closely. Consider the possibility of a hemorrhagic event with an unexplained fall in hematocrit, a fall in BP, or any other unexplained symptom. GI or urinary tract bleeding may indicate an underlying lesion. Certain hemorrhagic complications may be difficult to detect and can be very serious (e.g., adrenal [with resultant adrenal insufficiency], ovarian [corpus luteum], and retroperitoneal hemorrhage). ▪ Use extensive precautionary methods to prevent bleeding if patient requires IM injection, arterial puncture, or venipuncture.

Patency of indwelling venipuncture devices: Obtain a baseline aPTT prior to insertion of an indwelling venipuncture device. Repeated heparin injections can alter aPTT. ▪ To avoid precipitation, irrigate indwelling venipuncture devices with NS before and after injecting acidic or **incompatible** solutions. ▪ Heparin and/or NS may interfere with blood samples drawn from these devices, especially if drawn on a frequent basis. Clear the heparin flush solution by aspirating and discarding a volume of solution equal to that of the indwelling venipuncture device before the desired blood sample is drawn.

Patient Education: Report all episodes of bleeding and apply local pressure if indicated. ▪ Report tarry stools. ▪ Compliance with all measures to minimize bleeding is very important (e.g., avoid use of razors, toothbrushes, other sharp items). ▪ Use caution while moving to avoid excess bumping.

Maternal/Child: Category C: preferred anticoagulant in pregnancy but must be used with caution. Hemorrhage most likely to occur during the last trimester or postpartum. Has caused stillbirths and prematurity. ▪ Not secreted in breast milk. ▪ Some preparations may contain benzyl alcohol; do not use in neonates, infants, pregnant women, or breast-feeding mothers; see Contraindications. ▪ Use to maintain patency of umbilical artery catheters has been associated with an increased risk of intraventricular hemorrhage in low-birth-weight infants. ▪ Use heparin-lock flush with caution in infants with diseases with an increased risk of hemorrhage. The 100 units/mL concentration should not be used in neonates or infants who weigh less than 10 kg because of the risk of systemic anticoagulation. Use caution when using the 10 units/mL concentration in premature infants who weigh less than 1 kg and are receiving frequent flushes, because a therapeutic heparin dose may be given in a 24-hour period. Use minimal doses and preservative-free preparations, and monitor carefully. ▪ See Dose Adjustments and Precautions.

Elderly: Higher plasma levels of heparin and longer aPTTs may occur in patients over 60 years of age. Higher incidence of bleeding in patients

60 years of age and older (especially women). Lower doses of heparin may be indicated; see Dose Adjustments.

DRUG/LAB INTERACTIONS

Nitroglycerin IV may cause a decrease in PTT with a subsequent rebound effect when nitroglycerin is discontinued. Monitor PTT carefully and adjust heparin dose as needed. ▪ Increased risk of bleeding with **ACD-converted blood, adrenal cortical steroids** (especially chronic therapeutic use), **some cephalosporins** (e.g., cefotetan, moxalactam [Moxam]), **dextran, penicillins, platelet aggregation inhibitors** (e.g., dipyridamole [Persantine], glycoprotein GPIIb/IIIa receptor antagonists [e.g., abciximab (ReoPro), eptifibatide (Integrilin), tirofiban (Aggrastat)], ticlopidine [Ticlid]), **hydroxychloroquine** (Chloroquine), **NSAIDs** (e.g., ibuprofen [Motrin], indomethacin [Indocin], ketorolac [Toradol]), **plicamycin** (Mithracin), **salicylates** (e.g., aspirin), **other thrombolytic agents** (e.g., alteplase, streptokinase), **thyroid agents** (e.g., methimazole [Tapazole], propylthiouracil), **valproic acid** (Depakote), **or any drug that may cause hypothrombinemia, thrombocytopenia, GI ulceration, or hemorrhage.** ▪ Resistance to heparin anticoagulation may occur following administration of **streptokinase** as a systemic thrombolytic agent; adjust dose of heparin based on more frequent aPTTs. ▪ Inhibited by **antihistamines, digoxin, nicotine, tetracyclines, and others;** may counteract anticoagulant action of heparin. ▪ Potentiates **oral anticoagulants.** ▪ See Precautions/Monitor. ▪ Use caution when administered after **other anticoagulants.** Lab data may not provide an accurate baseline. ▪ **Blood gas sample errors** may occur with the therapeutic use of heparin. ▪ Numerous **lab values** (e.g., imaging studies, thyroid, AST, ALT, free fatty acid, triglycerides, cholesterol) may be altered. Notify lab of heparin use. Diagnostic results may not be attainable. See Monitor.

SIDE EFFECTS

Bruising, epistaxis, hematuria, hemorrhage, prolonged coagulation time (in excess of two to three times the control level), tarry stools or any other signs of bleeding, thrombocytopenia, HIT or HITT (platelet aggregation, clotting). Hypersensitivity reactions, including anaphylaxis, do occur. Vasospastic reactions resulting in a painful, ischemic, cyanotic limb may develop. Alopecia, arthralgias, chest pain, cutaneous necrosis, headache, hypertension, itching on the plantar surface of the feet, osteoporosis, priapism (painful penile erection), rebound hyperlipidemia, and suppressed aldosterone synthesis have been reported. Several studies have shown that moderately high doses of heparin can cause excessive internal bleeding that may lead to paralyzing or lethal strokes. Fewer side effects occur with controlled continuous IV infusion as compared to intermittent.

ANTIDOTE

Discontinue drug and notify physician of any side effects. Protamine sulfate is a heparin antagonist and specifically indicated in overdose or desired heparin reversal. Each milligram of protamine neutralizes approximately 100 units heparin. No more than 50 mg should be administered, very slowly, in any 10-minute period. Administration of protamine can cause severe hypotension and anaphylactoid reactions. Use with caution and have emergency equipment and mediations readily available. Whole blood transfusion may be indicated. If heparin-induced thrombocytopenia or white clot syndrome occurs, lepirudin (Refludan), which is an anticoagulant and a direct inhibitor of thrombin, may be indicated. Follow up with oral anticoagulation (e.g., warfarin [Coumadin]) may also be indicated.

HEPATITIS B IMMUNE GLOBULIN INTRAVENOUS (HUMAN)
(hep-ah-**TY**-tiss ih-**MUNE GLAW**-byoo-lin IV)

Immunizing agent (passive)

HepaGam B

pH 5.6

USUAL DOSE
(International units [IU])

Prevention of hepatitis B recurrence following liver transplantation: Administered by a set dosing regimen designed to attain serum levels of antibodies to hepatitis B surface antigen (anti-HBs) greater than 500 IU/L. Each dose should contain 20,000 IU calculated from the measured potency as stamped on the vial label. Administer the first dose of 20,000 IU concurrently with grafting of the transplanted liver (the anhepatic phase). Administer each subsequent dose of 20,000 IU as recommended in the following table.

Hepatitis B IGIV Dosing Regimen			
Anhepatic Phase	Week 1 Postoperative	Weeks 2-12 Postoperative	Month 4 Onwards
First dose of 20,000 IU	20,000 IU daily from Day 1 through Day 7; see Dose Adjustments	20,000 IU every 2 weeks from Day 14 (Week 2) through Week 12	20,000 IU monthly

DOSE ADJUSTMENTS
(International units [IU])

Increased doses may be required in patients who fail to reach anti-HBs levels of 500 IU/L within the first week after liver transplantation. Particularly susceptible to an extensive decrease of circulated anti-HBs are patients who have surgical bleeding or abdominal fluid drainage (greater than 500 mL) or those who undergo plasmapheresis. If the desired anti-HBs levels are not reached, increase the dosing regimen to a half-dose (10,000 IU [calculated from the measured potency as stamped on the vial label]) and administer IV every 6 hours until the target anti-HBs level is reached.

DILUTION

A ready-to-use liquid preparation; should be clear to opalescent. Multiple vials will be required. ***Do not shake vials; avoid foaming.*** Bring to room temperature before administration. Administer through a separate IV line using an IV administration set and an infusion pump.

Filters: No data available from manufacturer.

Storage: Store between 2° and 8° C (35.6° and 46.4° F). Do not freeze. Do not use after expiration date. Use within 6 hours of opening the vial, and discard partially used vials.

COMPATIBILITY

Manufacturer states, "Administer through a separate IV line using an IV administration set via infusion pump."

RATE OF ADMINISTRATION

Set infusion pump rate at 2 mL/min. Decrease to 1 mL/min or slower for patient discomfort, infusion-related adverse events, or concern about the speed of infusion.

ACTIONS

A solvent/detergent-treated sterile solution of purified gamma globulin containing anti-HBs. Prepared from plasma donated by healthy, screened donors with high titers of anti-HBs. Purified by an anion-exchange column chromatography manufacturing method. It provides passive immunization for individuals exposed to the hepatitis B virus by binding to the surface antigen and reducing the rate of hepatitis B infection. Following liver transplantation, hepatitis B virus re-infection can occur immediately at the time of liver reperfusion due to a circulating virus or later from a virus retained in extrahepatic sites. Provides an immediate immune response to the hepatitis B virus. Mechanism of action is not known but may occur through several pathways (e.g., through blockage of a putative HBV receptor, neutralization of circulating virions through immune precipitation and immune complex formation, triggering of an antibody-dependent cell-mediated cytotoxicity response that results in target cell lysis, or binding to hepatocytes and interaction with HBsAg within cells). Clinical effectiveness is dependent on dose, length of administration, and viral replication status of the patient at the time of transplant. Bioavailability is complete and immediate and is distributed quickly between plasma and extravascular fluid. Immune globulins are metabolized by being broken down in the reticuloendothelial system. IM injection results in mean peak concentrations within 4 to 5 days of administration and an elimination half-life of 22 to 25 days. A slightly decreased half-life is expected following IV administration.

INDICATIONS AND USES

Prevention of hepatitis B recurrence following liver transplantation in HBsAg-positive liver transplant patients. Recommended for use in patients who have no or low levels of viral replication at the time of liver transplantation. ■ Used IM for post-exposure prophylaxis in the following settings: acute exposure to blood containing HBsAg, perinatal exposure of infants born to HBsAg-positive mothers, sexual exposure to HBsAg-positive persons, and household exposure to persons with acute HBV infection.

CONTRAINDICATIONS

History of anaphylactic or severe systemic reactions to human globulins. ■ Weigh benefits versus risk of hypersensitivity reactions in IgA-deficient individuals; see Precautions.

PRECAUTIONS

Administer in a facility with adequate equipment and supplies to monitor the patient and respond to any medical emergency. ■ Hypersensitivity and/or infusion reactions may occur. ■ Individuals deficient in IgA may have the potential to develop IgA antibodies and have an anaphylactoid reaction. ■ Contains maltose, which can interfere with select blood glucose monitoring systems (those based on the glucose dehydrogenase pyrroloquinequinone [GDH-PQQ] method). May cause falsely elevated glucose readings, result in inappropriate insulin administration, and cause life-threatening hypoglycemia. In contrast, cases of true hypoglycemia may go untreated if the hypoglycemic state is masked by falsely elevated results. ■ Derived from human plasma. Despite screening and purification processes, may have the potential risk of transmitting infectious agents (e.g., viruses [e.g., HIV, hepatitis]) or the Creutzfeldt-Jacob disease agent. ■ Has not been evaluated in combination with antiviral therapy post-transplantation. ■ See Patient Education and Drug/Lab Interactions.

Monitor: Hepatitis B IGIV is most effective in patients with no or low levels of HBV replication at the time of transplantation. Monitor serum HBsAg and levels of anti-HBs antibody regularly and pre-infusion to track treatment response and adjust dose when indicated. ■ Infusion reactions may occur; usually related to rate of infusion. Monitor closely during and following an infusion. ■ Use caution and observe diabetic patients closely; see Precautions. Only glucose-specific testing systems can be used in patients receiving hepatitis IGIV. Review product information of the blood glucose testing system to confirm that it can be used with maltose-containing parenteral products. ■ Monitor for S/S of a hypersensitivity reaction.

Patient Education: Regular monitoring of serum HBsAg and anti-HBs antibody levels imperative. ■ Vaccination with live virus vaccines should be deferred until approximately 3 months after administration of hepatitis B IGIV. Revaccination may be required if the previous vaccination occurred within 2 weeks of the initial hepatitis IGIV dose.

Maternal/Child: Category C: use during pregnancy only if clearly indicated. ■ Use caution during breast-feeding. ■ Safety and effectiveness for use in pediatric patients under 18 years of age not established.

Elderly: Safety and effectiveness not established.

DRUG/LAB INTERACTIONS

May reduce the effectiveness of **live virus vaccines** (e.g., measles, mumps, rubella, varicella). Vaccination with live virus vaccines should be deferred until approximately 3 months after administration of hepatitis B IGIV. ■ Contains **maltose,** which can interfere with select blood glucose monitoring systems (those based on the glucose dehydrogenase pyrroloquinequinone [GDH-PQQ] method). May cause falsely elevated glucose readings. Use only glucose-specific testing systems in patients receiving hepatitis B IGIV. ■ Passively transferred antibodies may cause a misleading positive result in **serologic testing** (e.g., Coombs' test). ■ No data available on drug interactions with other medications.

SIDE EFFECTS

Arthralgia, chills, fever, headaches, hypersensitivity reactions, moderate or low back pain, nausea, and vomiting are the most common. Other reported side effects include agitation, amnesia, aphthous stomatitis, diarrhea, dyspepsia, edema, fatigue, gingival hyperplasia, hepatobiliary disease, hyperglycemia, hypertension, hypotension, infectious diarrhea, liver transplant rejection, nocturia, pleural effusion, pneumonia, presbyopia, pruritus, rash, sepsis, splenomegaly, tremors.

ANTIDOTE

Reduce rate of infusion for patient discomfort, infusion-related side effects, or other concerns. Discontinue the drug immediately for any signs of a hypersensitivity reaction. Notify the physician. Antihistamines (e.g., diphenhydramine [Benadryl]) or analgesic agents may be indicated for symptoms related to immune complex formation. Resume infusion at a slower rate if symptoms subside. Treat anaphylaxis immediately. Epinephrine, diphenhydramine (Benadryl), corticosteroids, and ventilation equipment must always be available.

HETASTARCH
(**HET**-ah-starch)

Hespan, Hextend

Plasma volume expander

pH 5.5 to 5.9

USUAL DOSE
HESPAN, HEXTEND
Shock: Variable, depending on amount of fluid loss and resultant hemo-concentration. Age, weight, and clinical condition of the patient are also considered. Usually 500 to 1,000 mL. Total dose usually does not exceed 1,500 mL/24 hr or 20 mL/kg of body weight. Higher doses, usually in conjunction with blood and/or blood products, have been used in postoperative and trauma patients who have had severe blood loss.

HESPAN
Leukapheresis: 250 to 700 mL in continuous flow centrifugation procedures. Do not use Hextend for leukapheresis.

DOSE ADJUSTMENTS
In patients with a CrCl less than 10 mL/min, the initial dose remains as in Usual Dose; however, subsequent doses should be reduced by 20% to 50%.

DILUTION
HESPAN: Available as a 6% solution in 500-mL containers properly diluted in NS and ready for use. Calculated osmolarity is approximately 310 mOsm/L.

HEXTEND: Available as a 6% solution in 500 mL and 1,000 mL containers properly diluted in lactated electrolyte solution and ready for use. Lactated electrolyte solution contains dextrose, normal physiologic levels of calcium and sodium, and slightly lower than normal physiologic levels of potassium and magnesium.

Storage: Store at CRT. Avoid excessive heat. Do not freeze. Do not use if color is a turbid deep brown or a crystalline precipitate is visible. Discard unused portions.

COMPATIBILITY   (Underline Indicates Conflicting Compatibility Information)
Consider any drug NOT listed as compatible to be INCOMPATIBLE until consulting a pharmacist; specific conditions may apply.

HESPAN
One source suggests the following **compatibilities:**

Additive: Fosphenytoin (Cerebyx).

Y-site: <u>Ampicillin</u>, <u>cefazolin (Ancef)</u>, diltiazem (Cardizem), <u>doxycycline</u>, enalaprilat (Vasotec IV), ertapenem (Invanz), nicardipine (Cardene IV).

HEXTEND
Safety and **compatibility** of other additives not established. Contains calcium; do not administer simultaneously through the same administration set as blood; coagulation likely.

One source suggests the following **compatibilities:**

Y-site: Alfentanil (Alfenta), amikacin (Amikin), aminophylline, amiodarone (Nexterone), ampicillin, ampicillin/sulbactam (Unasyn), atracurium (Tracrium), azithromycin (Zithromax), aztreonam (Azactam), bumetanide, butorphanol (Stadol), calcium gluconate, cefazolin (Ancef), cefepime (Maxipime), cefotaxime (Claforan), cefotetan (Cefotan), cefoxitin (Mefoxin), ceftazidime (Fortaz), cefuroxime (Zinacef), chlorpromazine (Thorazine), ciprofloxacin (Cipro IV), cisatracurium (Nimbex), clindamycin (Cleocin), dexamethasone (Decadron), digoxin (Lanoxin), diltiazem (Cardizem), diphenhydramine (Benadryl), dobutamine, dolasetron (Anzemet), dopamine, doxycycline, droperidol (Inapsine), enalaprilat (Vasotec IV), ephedrine, epinephrine (Adrenalin), erythromycin (Erythrocin), esmolol (Brevibloc), famotidine (Pepcid IV), fenoldopam (Corlopam), fentanyl (Sublimaze), fluconazole (Diflucan), furosemide (Lasix), gentamicin, granisetron (Kytril), haloperidol (Haldol), heparin, hydrocortisone sodium succinate (Solu-Cortef), hydromorphone (Dilaudid), inamrinone (Amrinone), isoproterenol (Isuprel), ketorolac (Toradol), labetalol (Trandate), levofloxacin (Levaquin), lidocaine, lorazepam (Ativan), magnesium sulfate, mannitol, meperidine (Demerol), methylprednisolone (Solu-Medrol), metoclopramide (Reglan), metronidazole (Flagyl IV), midazolam (Versed), milrinone (Primacor), morphine, nalbuphine, nitroglycerin IV, nitroprusside sodium, norepinephrine (Levophed), ondansetron (Zofran), palonosetron (Aloxi), pancuronium, phenylephrine (Neo-Synephrine), piperacillin, piperacillin/tazobactam (Zosyn), potassium chloride (KCl), procainamide (Pronestyl), prochlorperazine (Compazine), promethazine (Phenergan), ranitidine (Zantac), rocuronium (Zemuron), succinylcholine, sufentanil (Sufenta), sulfamethoxazole/trimethoprim, theophylline, thiopental (Pentothal), ticarcillin/clavulanate (Timentin), tobramycin, vancomycin, vecuronium, verapamil.

RATE OF ADMINISTRATION

Variable, depending on indication, present blood volume, and patient response. Initial 500 mL may be given at rates approaching 20 mL/kg of body weight per hour. Reduce rate in burns or septic shock. If additional hydroxyethyl starch is required, reduce flow to lowest rate possible to maintain hemodynamic status. If pressure infusion is used (flexible containers), withdraw all air through medication port before infusing. If a pumping device is used for administration, discontinue pumping action before the container runs dry or air embolism may result.

Leukapheresis: Usually infused at a constant ratio to venous whole blood (i.e., 1:8).

ACTIONS

A synthetic polymer with properties similar to dextran. Approximates colloidal properties of human albumin. Provides hemodynamically significant plasma volume expansion in excess of the amount infused for about 24 hours. Permits retention of intravascular fluid until hetastarch is replaced by blood proteins. **Hextend** supports oncotic pressure and provides electrolytes. Its electrolyte content resembles that of normal plasma. **Hespan** increases erythrocyte sedimentation rate. Granulocyte collection by centrifuging becomes more efficient. Both are enzymatically degraded to molecules small enough to be excreted through the kidneys attached to glucose units.

INDICATIONS AND USES

HESPAN AND HEXTEND: Treatment of hypovolemia when plasma volume expansion is desired. An adjunct in treatment of shock due to burns, hemorrhage, sepsis, surgery, or trauma. ■ Used when whole blood or blood products are not available or when cross-matching of blood products cannot be accomplished quickly enough.

HESPAN: Adjunct in leukapheresis to improve harvesting and increase yield of granulocytes.

CONTRAINDICATIONS

Severe bleeding disorders, severe congestive heart failure, hypersensitivity to hetastarch, renal disease with oliguria or anuria not related to hypovolemia. **Hextend** contains lactate; not for use in leukapheresis or in the treatment of lactic acidosis.

PRECAUTIONS

HESPAN AND HEXTEND: For IV use only. ■ Not a substitute for whole blood or plasma proteins. ■ Use caution in heart disease, renal shutdown, congestive heart failure, pulmonary edema, and liver disease. ■ Does not interfere with blood typing or cross-matching. ■ Anaphylactic reactions have occurred, even after solutions containing hetastarch have been discontinued. Patients allergic to corn may also be allergic to hetastarch. ■ Use extreme caution in shock not accompanied by hypovolemia; volume overload may result. ■ Contains dextrose; use caution in patients with overt diabetes. ■ Administration of large volumes may transiently alter the coagulation mechanism due to hemodilution and a mild direct inhibitory action on Factor VIII. Volumes greater than 25% of blood volume within 24 hours may cause significant hemodilution (decreased hematocrit and plasma proteins). Administration of packed RBCs, platelets, or fresh frozen plasma may be indicated. ■ When used over a period of days, hetastarch has been associated with coagulation abnormalities in conjunction with an acquired reversible von Willebrand's–like syndrome and/or Factor VIII deficiency. If a severe Factor VIII deficiency is identified, replacement therapy may be indicated. If coagulopathy develops, it may take days to resolve. ■ Not recommended for use as a cardiac bypass pump prime, while the patient is undergoing cardiopulmonary bypass, or in the immediate period after the pump has been discontinued. Risk of coagulopathies and bleeding increased.

HEXTEND: Use extreme caution in patients with metabolic or respiratory alkalosis; contains lactate ions. Excessive lactate may result in metabolic alkalosis. ■ Contains electrolytes; sodium or potassium retention may occur. Use caution in patients receiving corticosteroids, and in renal or cardiac disease particularly in digitalized patients.

Monitor: Monitor HR, BP, central venous pressure, and urine output every 5 to 15 minutes for the first hour and hourly thereafter while indicated. ■ Maintain adequate hydration of patient with additional IV fluids. ■ Change IV tubing or flush with NS before imposing blood. ■ May reduce coagulability of the circulating blood. Observe patient for increased bleeding and/or circulatory overload. Risk increased with higher doses. ■ Hemoglobin, hematocrit, platelet count, acid-base balance, electrolyte, and serum protein evaluation are necessary during therapy. During leukapheresis also monitor leukocyte and platelet count, leukocyte differential, PT, and PTT. ■ Observe frequent donors carefully; may have a marked decline in platelet count and hemoglobin levels resulting from hemodilution by hetastarch and saline. Temporary declines in total protein, albumin, calcium, and fibrinogen may also be present.

Maternal/Child: Category C: not recommended for use in pregnancy, especially early pregnancy; benefit must justify the potential risk to the fetus. Embryocidal to rabbits. ■ Use caution during breast-feeding. ■ Safety and effectiveness for use in pediatric patients not established, but has been used. Increased prothrombin time noted in pediatric patients who received more than 20 mL/kg/24 hr.

Elderly: Differences in response between elderly and younger patients not identified. Risk of toxic reactions may be greater in patients with impaired renal function. Monitoring of renal function suggested in the elderly.

DRUG/LAB INTERACTIONS

Use with caution in patients receiving other drugs that affect coagulation (e.g., **anticoagulants** [e.g., heparin, lepirudin (Refludan), warfarin (Coumadin)], **platelet aggregation inhibitors** [e.g., clopidogrel (Plavix), dipyridamole (Persantine), ticlopidine (Ticlid)], **glycoprotein GPIIb/IIIa receptor antagonists** [e.g., abciximab (ReoPro), eptifibatide (Integrilin), tirofiban (Aggrastat)], **plicamycin** [Mithracin], **valproic acid** [Depacon]). Close monitoring of aPTT and PT indicated. ▪ May increase **indirect bilirubin** levels. Total bilirubin remained normal.

SIDE EFFECTS

Anemia and/or bleeding due to hemodilution and/or Factor VIII deficiency, acquired von Willebrand's–like syndrome, and other coagulopathies, including DIC; chills; circulatory overload; congestive heart failure; elevated serum amylase; fever; headache; hypersensitivity reactions including anaphylaxis; increased urine specific gravity; intracranial bleeding; itching; metabolic acidosis; muscle pains; peripheral edema; pulmonary edema; submaxillary and parotid glandular enlargement; urticaria; and vomiting.

ANTIDOTE

Notify the physician of any side effect. Discontinue the drug immediately at the first sign of a hypersensitivity reaction, provided other means of sustaining the circulation are available. Antihistamines such as diphenhydramine (Benadryl) are helpful. Epinephrine (Adrenalin) may also be indicated. Not eliminated by dialysis. Many side effects can result in medical emergencies. Deaths from severe hypersensitivity reactions have occurred. Treat as indicated and resuscitate as necessary.

HYDRALAZINE HYDROCHLORIDE
(hy-**DRAL**-ah-zeen hy-droh-**KLOR**-eyed)

Antihypertensive
Vasodilator

pH 3.4 to 4

USUAL DOSE

10 to 40 mg. Begin with a low dose. Increase gradually as indicated. Repeat every 3 to 6 hours as necessary. Maximum dose is 300 to 400 mg/24 hr.

Eclampsia: 5 to 10 mg every 20 minutes. If no effect after a total dose of 20 mg, use another agent.

PEDIATRIC DOSE

See Maternal/Child (unlabeled).

0.1 to 0.5 mg/kg/dose every 4 to 6 hours. Initial dose should not exceed 20 mg. Maximum IV dose is 0.2 to 0.8 mg/kg/dose up to 40 mg. Another source suggests 0.1 to 0.2 mg/kg/dose (not to exceed 20 mg) every 4 to 6 hours as needed. Up to 1.7 to 3.5 mg/kg/day divided in 4 to 6 doses.

DOSE ADJUSTMENTS

Reduced dose may be required with advanced renal disease and in the elderly. ▪ See Drug/Lab Interactions.

DILUTION

May be given undiluted. Do not add to IV solutions. May be given through Y-tube or three-way stopcock of infusion set. Color changes occur in most 10% dextrose solutions and after drawing through a metal filter. Use immediately after drawing up solution.

Filters: See Dilution.

COMPATIBILITY   (Underline Indicates Conflicting Compatibility Information)

Consider any drug NOT listed as compatible to be INCOMPATIBLE until consulting a pharmacist; specific conditions may apply.

One source suggests the following **compatibilities:**

Additive: Dobutamine.

Y-site: <u>Caspofungin (Cancidas)</u>, heparin, hydrocortisone sodium succinate (Solu-Cortef), <u>nitroglycerin IV</u>, potassium chloride, verapamil.

RATE OF ADMINISTRATION

Adults: A single dose over 1 minute.

Pediatric patients: A single dose over 3 to 5 minutes.

ACTIONS

A potent antihypertensive drug. It lowers BP by direct relaxation of smooth muscle of arteries and arterioles. Peripheral vasodilation and decreased peripheral vascular resistance result. HR, cardiac output, and stroke volume are all increased. Renal blood flow increased in some cases, while cerebral blood flow maintained. Onset of action is 5 to 20 minutes. Average duration of action is 2 to 6 hours. Metabolized by the liver and excreted in urine. Crosses placental barrier. Secreted in breast milk.

INDICATIONS AND USES

Severe essential hypertension. ▪ Vasodilation in cardiogenic shock. ▪ Drug of choice for pregnancy-induced hypertension (eclampsia).

CONTRAINDICATIONS

Hypersensitivity to hydralazine, coronary artery disease, mitral valvular rheumatic heart disease.

PRECAUTIONS

IV use recommended only when the oral route is not feasible. ■ Rarely the drug of choice for hypertension unless used in combination (effectiveness increased and side effects decreased) with spironolactone (Aldactone), reserpine (Serpasil), guanethidine (Ismelin), and thiazide diuretics. ■ Tolerance is easily developed but subsides about 7 days after the drug is discontinued. ■ Use caution in advanced renal disease, cerebrovascular accidents, congestive heart failure, coronary insufficiency, headache, increased intracranial pressure, and tachycardia. ■ Use in pregnancy should be limited to treatment of eclampsia.

Monitor: Check BP every 5 minutes until stabilized at the desired level. Check every 15 minutes thereafter throughout crisis. Average maximum decrease occurs in 10 to 80 minutes. ■ Withdraw drug gradually to avoid rebound hypertension.

Patient Education: Report chest pain, fatigue, fever, joint or muscle pain promptly.

Maternal/Child: Category C: can cause fetal abnormalities; see Indications and Precautions. ■ Safety for use in pediatric patients not established. ■ May be used in breast-feeding women.

Elderly: Increased risk of hypotension. ■ Consider age-related renal impairment.

DRUG/LAB INTERACTIONS

Sometimes used with a **beta-adrenergic blocking drug** (e.g., propranolol) **or diuretics** (e.g., hydrochlorothiazide [Aldactazide]); use caution; may potentiate effects. ■ Potentiated by **anesthetics, MAO inhibitors** (e.g., selegiline [Eldepryl]), **and other antihypertensive agents.** ■ Inhibits **epinephrine, levarterenol** (Levophed). ■ Use with **diazoxide** can cause profound hypotension. ■ **NSAIDs** (e.g., ibuprofen [Motrin]) may decrease antihypotensive effect.

SIDE EFFECTS

May often be minimized by initiating therapy with a small dose and increasing the dose gradually.

Anxiety, depression, dry mouth, flushing, headache, nausea, numbness, palpitations, paresthesia, postural hypotension, tachycardia, tingling, unpleasant taste, vomiting.

Major: Angina, blood dyscrasias, chills, coronary insufficiency, delirium, dependent edema, fever, ileus, lupus erythematosus (simulated), myocardial ischemia and infarction, rheumatoid syndrome (simulated), toxic psychosis.

ANTIDOTE

If minor side effects occur, notify the physician, who will probably treat them symptomatically. Beta-adrenergic blocking agents (e.g., propranolol) will control tachycardia. Pyridoxine will relieve numbness, tingling, and paresthesia. Antihistamines, barbiturates, and salicylates may be required. Treat hypotension with a vasopressor that is least likely to precipitate cardiac arrhythmias. If side effects are progressive or any major side effects occur, discontinue the drug immediately and notify the physician. Treatment is symptomatic. Resuscitate as necessary. Occasionally methyldopa (Aldomet) will be used as a substitute, since it is effective for the same indications but has fewer side effects.

HYDROCORTISONE SODIUM SUCCINATE
(hy-droh-**KOR**-tih-zohn **SO**-dee-um **SUK**-sih-nayt)

**Hormone
(adrenocorticoid
glucocorticoid)
Anti-inflammatory
Antiemetic**

A-Hydrocort, Solu-Cortef

pH 7 to 8

USUAL DOSE

The IV route is usually used in an emergency situation or when oral dosing is not feasible. The lowest possible dose should be used to control condition. When reduction in dosage is possible, reduction should be gradual. Larger doses may be justified by patient condition. Repeat until adequate response, then decrease dose as indicated. Doses must be individualized and are not always reduced for pediatric patients. High dose treatment is utilized until patient condition stabilizes, usually no longer than 48 to 72 hours. Complications secondary to treatment with corticosteroids are dependent on the size of dose and duration of therapy.

Average dose range is 100 to 500 mg repeated as necessary every 2, 4, or 6 hours. For severe shock, doses up to 2 Gm or more every 2 to 10 hours have been given. Maximum dose is 8 Gm/24 hr. A minimum dose of no less than 25 mg/24 hr is recommended. Increased doses are indicated in patients undergoing corticosteroid therapy who are subjected to any unusual stressful situation (e.g., illness, surgery).

Other sources recommend:

Acute asthma: 1 to 2 mg/kg/dose every 6 hours for 24 hours. Follow with 0.5 to 1 mg/kg every 6 hours.

Anti-inflammatory or immunosuppressive: 15 to 240 mg every 12 hours.

Life-threatening shock: 50 mg/kg initially. Repeat in 4 hours and/or every 24 hours as needed *or*
0.5 to 2 Gm initially. Repeat every 2 to 6 hours as needed.

Adrenal insufficiency (acute): 100 mg as an IV bolus. Follow with 300 mg/day in divided doses every 8 hours or as a continuous infusion for 48 hours. Change to oral dosing when patient is stable.

Physiologic replacement: 20 to 30 mg/day (usually given PO).

PEDIATRIC DOSE

See Maternal/Child.

Average dose range in pediatric patients is 0.56 to 8 mg/kg/day in 3 to 4 divided doses (0.19 to 2.67 mg/kg every 8 hours or 0.14 to 2 mg/kg every 8 hours).

Other sources recommend:

Acute asthma: 1 to 2 mg/kg/dose every 6 hours for 24 hours; then 2 to 4 mg/kg/24 hr in equally divided doses every 6 hours (0.5 to 1 mg/kg every 6 hours). For status asthmaticus, another source suggests a *loading dose (optional)* of 4 to 8 mg/kg up to a maximum dose of 250 mg. *Maintenance dose:* 8 mg/kg/24 hr in equally divided doses every 6 hours (2 mg/kg every 6 hours).

Anti-inflammatory: 1 to 5 mg/kg/24 hr, or 0.5 to 2.5 mg/kg every 12 hours, or 30 to 150 mg/M^2/24 hr, or 15 to 75 mg/M^2 every 12 hours.

Adrenal insufficiency (acute): 1 to 2 mg/kg/dose bolus, then 25 to 150 mg/day in divided doses every 6 to 8 hours (8.33 to 50 mg every 8 hours or 6.25 to 37.5 mg every 6 hours) in infants and young children. In older children the bolus dose is the same, followed by 150 to 250 mg/day in divided doses every 6 to 8 hours (50 to 83.33 mg every 8 hours or 37.5 to 62.5 mg every 6 hours).

Physiologic replacement: 0.5 to 0.75 mg/kg/day given every 8 hours (usually given PO).

DOSE ADJUSTMENTS
Reduced dose may be required in the elderly. ▪ See Drug/Lab Interactions.

DILUTION
Available in Act-O-Vials and Univials, which are reconstituted by removing the protective cap, turning the rubber stopper a quarter turn, and pressing down, allowing the diluent into the lower chamber. Agitate gently. Using sterile techniques, a needle can be easily inserted through the center of the rubber stopper to withdraw the solution. Also available in flip-top vials. For these other preparations, reconstitute each 250 mg or fraction thereof with 2 mL bacteriostatic water for injection. Agitate gently to mix solution. May be given by IV injection, or each 100 mg (250 mg, 500 mg, or more) may be further diluted in at least 100 mL (250 mL, 500 mL, or more) but not more than 1,000 mL of D5W, NS, or D5NS.

Storage: Store vials and solutions at RT (20° to 25° C [68° to 77° F]). Protect solution from light. Discard unused solutions after 3 days. If fluid restriction is necessary, 100 to 3,000 mg may be added in 50 mL of compatible solution. Resultant solution is stable for 4 hours.

COMPATIBILITY   (Underline Indicates Conflicting Compatibility Information)
Consider any drug NOT listed as compatible to be INCOMPATIBLE until consulting a pharmacist; specific conditions may apply.
Manufacturer states, "Should not be diluted or mixed with other solutions."

One source suggests the following **compatibilities:**
Solution: Most commonly used IV solutions, fat emulsion 10% IV.
Additive: Amikacin (Amikin), aminophylline, amobarbital, amphotericin B (generic), ampicillin, calcium chloride, calcium gluconate, chloramphenicol (Chloromycetin), clindamycin (Cleocin), cytarabine (ARA-C), daunorubicin (Cerubidine), dimenhydrinate, diphenhydramine (Benadryl), dopamine, erythromycin (Erythrocin), furosemide (Lasix), heparin, kanamycin (Kantrex), lidocaine, magnesium sulfate, metronidazole (Flagyl IV), mitomycin (Mutamycin), mitoxantrone (Novantrone), norepinephrine (Levophed), penicillin G potassium and sodium, piperacillin, potassium chloride (KCl), thiopental (Pentothal), vancomycin, verapamil.
Y-site: Acyclovir (Zovirax), allopurinol (Aloprim), amifostine (Ethyol), aminophylline, amphotericin B cholesteryl (Amphotec), ampicillin, anidulafungin (Eraxis), anti-thymocyte globulin (rabbit), argatroban, atracurium (Tracrium), atropine, aztreonam (Azactam), bivalirudin (Angiomax), calcium gluconate, caspofungin (Cancidas), cefepime (Maxipime), chlorpromazine (Thorazine), cisatracurium (Nimbex), cladribine (Leustatin), cytarabine (ARA-C), dexamethasone (Decadron), digoxin (Lanoxin), diltiazem (Cardizem), diphenhydramine (Benadryl), docetaxel (Taxotere), dopamine, doripenem (Doribax), doxorubicin liposomal (Doxil), droperi-

dol (Inapsine), edrophonium (Enlon), enalaprilat (Vasotec IV), epinephrine (Adrenalin), esmolol (Brevibloc), estrogens, conjugated (Premarin), ethacrynic acid (Edecrin), etoposide phosphate (Etopophos), famotidine (Pepcid IV), fenoldopam (Corlopam), fentanyl (Sublimaze), filgrastim (Neupogen), fludarabine (Fludara), fluorouracil (5-FU), foscarnet (Foscavir), furosemide (Lasix), gallium nitrate (Ganite), gemcitabine (Gemzar), granisetron (Kytril), heparin, hetastarch in electrolytes (Hextend), hydralazine, inamrinone (Amrinone), insulin (regular), isoproterenol (Isuprel), kanamycin (Kantrex), lidocaine, linezolid (Zyvox), lorazepam (Ativan), magnesium sulfate, melphalan (Alkeran), meperidine (Demerol), methylergonovine (Methergine), methylprednisolone (Solu-Medrol), morphine, neostigmine, nicardipine (Cardene IV), norepinephrine (Levophed), ondansetron (Zofran), oxacillin (Bactocill), oxaliplatin (Eloxatin), oxytocin (Pitocin), paclitaxel (Taxol), pancuronium, penicillin G potassium, pentazocine (Talwin), phytonadione (vitamin K_1), piperacillin/tazobactam (Zosyn), procainamide (Pronestyl), prochlorperazine (Compazine), promethazine (Phenergan), propofol (Diprivan), propranolol, pyridostigmine (Regonol), remifentanil (Ultiva), sodium bicarbonate, succinylcholine, tacrolimus (Prograf), teniposide (Vumon), theophylline, thiotepa, vecuronium, vinorelbine (Navelbine).

RATE OF ADMINISTRATION
Each 100 mg or fraction thereof over 30 seconds to 1 minute. Extend to 10 minutes for larger doses (500 mg or more). IV injection is usually the route of choice and eliminates the possibility of overloading the patient with IV fluids. At the discretion of the physician, a continuous infusion may be given, properly diluted over the specified time desired.

ACTIONS
Contains the principal hormone secreted by the adrenal cortex and has both glucocorticoid and mineralocorticoid properties. Has potent metabolic, anti-inflammatory, and innumerable other effects. Peak plasma levels achieved promptly. Metabolized in the liver and excreted as inactive metabolites in the urine. Elimination half-life is 1 to 2 hours. Crosses placental barrier. Secreted in breast milk.

INDICATIONS AND USES
Agents of choice for adrenocortical insufficiency; total, relative, and operative. ■ Agents of choice for acute exacerbation of disease for patients on steroid therapy. ■ Occasionally used for asthma or shock, but non-mineralocorticoid steroids are preferred (e.g., dexamethasone, methylprednisolone).

CONTRAINDICATIONS
Absolute contraindications except in life-threatening situations: Hypersensitivity to any product component, including sulfites; systemic fungal infections. ■ Administration of live or live-attenuated vaccines in patients receiving an immunosuppressive dose of corticosteroids.
Relative contraindications: Active or latent peptic ulcer, active or latent tuberculosis, chickenpox, diverticulitis, fresh intestinal anastomoses, measles, myasthenia gravis, ocular herpes simplex, pregnancy, thromboembolic tendencies, vaccinia.

PRECAUTIONS
To avoid relative adrenocortical insufficiency, do not stop therapy abruptly. Taper off. Patient is observed carefully, especially under stress, for up to 2 years. The exception is very short-term therapy. ■ Anaphylactoid reac-

tions have occurred (incidence is rare). ■ Increased doses are indicated in patients undergoing corticosteroid therapy who are subjected to any unusual stressful situation (e.g., illness, surgery). ■ Should not be used for treatment of traumatic brain injury. May increase mortality. ■ Use with caution in patients who have had a recent MI. May be associated with left ventricular free wall rupture. ■ Kaposi's sarcoma has been reported in patients receiving corticosteroid therapy, most often for chronic conditions. Clinical improvement may occur if therapy is discontinued. ■ Use with caution in patients with CHF, hypertension, or renal insufficiency; see Monitor. ■ Use with caution in patients with active or latent peptic ulcer disease, diverticulitis, fresh intestinal anastomoses, and nonspecific ulcerative colitis; may increase risk of perforation. Prophylactic antacids may prevent peptic ulcer complications. ■ May induce psychological side effects (e.g., euphoria, insomnia, mood swings, depression, psychosis) or may aggravate existing emotional instability or psychotic tendencies.

Monitor: Monitor electrolytes. May cause sodium retention and potassium and calcium excretion. Dietary salt restriction and potassium supplementation may be necessary. May cause hypertension secondary to fluid and electrolyte disturbances. ■ May increase susceptibility to infection, reactivate latent infectious diseases, or mask signs of infection. ■ Monitor blood glucose. May increase insulin needs in diabetes. ■ Administer before 9 AM to reduce suppression of individual's own adrenocortical activity. ■ Periodic ophthalmic exams may be necessary with prolonged treatment. ■ See Drug/Lab Interactions.

Patient Education: Do not discontinue abruptly. ■ Advise all medical personnel of current or past corticosteroid use. ■ Report edema, tarry stools, or weight gain promptly. Anorexia, diarrhea, dizziness, fatigue, low blood sugar, nausea, weakness, weight loss, and vomiting may indicate adrenal insufficiency after dose reduction or discontinuing therapy; report any of these symptoms. ■ May mask signs of infection and/or decrease resistance. ■ Diabetics may have an increased requirement for insulin or oral hypoglycemics. ■ Avoid immunization with live virus vaccines. ■ Carry ID stating steroid dependent if receiving prolonged therapy.

Maternal/Child: Category C: could produce fetal abnormalities. ■ Discontinue breast-feeding. ■ Observe newborn for hypoadrenalism if mother has received large doses. ■ Observe growth and development in long-term use in pediatric patients.

Elderly: Reduced muscle mass and plasma volume may require a reduced dose. ■ Monitor BP, blood glucose, and electrolytes carefully; increased risk of hypertension. ■ Higher risk of glucocorticoid-induced osteoporosis.

DRUG/LAB INTERACTIONS

Aminoglutethimide (Cytadren) may increase the metabolism of hydrocortisone, thereby decreasing therapeutic effects. Monitor carefully if concurrent use is necessary. ■ Metabolism increased and effects reduced by **hepatic enzyme–inducing agents** (e.g., alcohol, barbiturates [e.g., phenobarbital], hydantoins [e.g., phenytoin (Dilantin)], and rifampin [Rifadin]); dose adjustment may be required when adding or deleting from drug profile. ■ Risk of hypokalemia increased with **amphotericin B or potassium-depleting diuretics** (e.g., thiazides, furosemide, ethacrynic acid). Monitor potassium levels and cardiac function. Increased risk of **digoxin** toxicity secondary to hypokalemia. ■ May also decrease effectiveness of **potassium supplements;** monitor serum potassium. ■ **Diuretics** decrease sodium and fluid retention effects of corticosteroids; corticosteroids decrease sodium excretion and diuretic effects of diuretics. ■ May antagonize effects of **anticholinesterases** (e.g., neostigmine), **isoniazid, salicylates, and somatrem;** dose adjustments may be required. ■ Clearance decreased and effects increased with **estrogens, oral contraceptives, macrolide antibiotics** (e.g., azithromycin [Zithromax]), **and ketoconazole** (Nizoral). ■ May interact with **anticoagulants, nondepolarizing muscle relaxants** (e.g., atracurium [Tracrium]), **or theophyllines;** may inhibit or potentiate action. ■ Monitor patients receiving **insulin or thyroid hormones** carefully; dose adjustments of either or both agents may be required. ■ Increased activity of both **hydrocortisone and cyclosporine** may occur with concurrent use. Therapeutic use is beneficial for organ transplants; however, toxicity may also be increased, and convulsions have been reported. ■ Concurrent use with **aspirin or NSAIDs** (e.g., ibuprofen [Motrin], naproxen [Aleve, Naprosyn]) may increase the risk of GI side effects. ■ Administration of **live or live-attenuated vaccines** is contraindicated in patients receiving immunosuppressive dose of corticosteroids. Inactivated vaccines may be administered; however, the response to these vaccines cannot be predicted. ■ Altered **protein-binding capacity** will impact effectiveness of this drug. ■ **Corticosteroids** may suppress reactions to skin tests. ■ See Dose Adjustments.

SIDE EFFECTS
Do occur but are usually reversible: alteration of glucose metabolism including hyperglycemia and glycosuria; Cushing's syndrome (e.g., moon face, fat pads); electrolyte and calcium imbalance; euphoria or other psychic disturbances; hypersensitivity reactions including anaphylaxis; increased BP; increased intracranial pressure; masking of infection; menstrual irregularities; perforation and hemorrhage from aggravation of peptic ulcer; protein catabolism with negative nitrogen balance; spontaneous fractures; sweating, headache, or weakness; thromboembolism; transitory burning or tingling; and many others.

ANTIDOTE
Notify the physician of any side effect. Will probably treat the side effect if necessary. Resuscitate as necessary for anaphylaxis and notify physician. Keep epinephrine immediately available.

HYDROMORPHONE
HYDROCHLORIDE BBW
(hy-droh-**MOR**-fohn hy-droh-**KLOR**-eyed)

Dilaudid, Dilaudid HP

Opioid analgesic
(agonist)

pH 4 to 5.5

USUAL DOSE

IV injection: Usual starting dose is 1 to 2 mg every 4 to 6 hours. Shorter intervals (3 to 4 hours) have been used. Use lower initial doses in opiate-naïve patients; one source suggests 0.2 to 0.6 mg.

Infusion: Used postoperatively with a patient-controlled analgesic device (PCA) and in selected terminally ill cancer patients; hydromorphone may be administered in doses as high as 2 to 9 mg/hr. Must be administered through a controlled infusion device that may be patient activated. The initial loading dose, the continuous background infusion to provide a level of pain relief and maintain patency of the vein, additional patient-activated doses with specific time interval, additional health care professional–provided boluses with specific time interval, and the total dose allowed per hour must be determined by the physician specialist and individualized for each patient. When seeking the required dose to achieve pain relief for an individual patient, increases in increments of at least 25% of the previous dose are suggested. May lower slightly if pain is controlled but patient is too drowsy or, alternately, lower dose and increase frequency.

PEDIATRIC DOSE

Individualized on the basis of age and weight. One source suggests 0.015 mg/kg/dose every 4 to 6 hours as needed in pediatric patients; see Contraindications and Maternal/Child.

DOSE ADJUSTMENTS

Dose selection should be cautious in the elderly. Reduced initial doses may be indicated based on the potential for increased sensitivity, decreased organ function, and concomitant disease or drug therapy. ▪ Reduced dose or extended intervals may be required in impaired renal or hepatic function and in elderly or debilitated patients. ▪ Doses appropriate for the general population may cause serious respiratory depression in vulnerable patients. ▪ Increase doses as required if analgesia is inadequate, tolerance develops, or pain severity increases. The first sign of tolerance is usually a reduced duration of effect. ▪ See Drug/Lab Interactions.

DILUTION

Available in more than one concentration, including a high-potency (10 mg/mL) formulation that carries a black box warning BBW because of its concentration and is usually reserved for compounding in the pharmacy or use in opioid-tolerant patients. Verify concentration to avoid overdose.

IV injection: May be given undiluted; further dilution with 5 mL SW or NS to facilitate titration is appropriate. May give through Y-tube or three-way stopcock of infusion set.

Infusion: Each 0.1 to 1 mg is usually diluted in 1 mL NS to provide 0.1 to 1 mg/mL for use in a narcotic syringe infusor system. Available in 1-, 2-, 4-, or 10-mg/mL ampules. Use concentrated preparations for larger doses. May be diluted in larger amounts of D5W, D5NS, D5/½NS, or NS (concentration is usually 1 mg/mL) for infusion and given through a standard infusion pump (requires very close titration).

Storage: Store at CRT and protect from light and freezing.

COMPATIBILITY   (Underline Indicates Conflicting Compatibility Information)
Consider any drug NOT listed as compatible to be INCOMPATIBLE until consulting a pharmacist; specific conditions may apply.

One source suggests the following **compatibilities:**

Additive: Fluorouracil (5-FU), heparin, midazolam (Versed), ondansetron (Zofran), potassium chloride (KCl), promethazine (Phenergan), verapamil.

Y-site: Acyclovir (Zovirax), allopurinol (Aloprim), amifostine (Ethyol), amikacin (Amikin), ampicillin, atropine, aztreonam (Azactam), bivalirudin (Angiomax), caspofungin (Cancidas), cefazolin (Ancef), cefepime (Maxipime), cefotaxime (Claforan), cefoxitin (Mefoxin), ceftazidime (Fortaz), cefuroxime (Zinacef), chloramphenicol (Chloromycetin), cisatracurium (Nimbex), cisplatin (Platinol), cladribine (Leustatin), clindamycin (Cleocin), cyclophosphamide (Cytoxan), cytarabine (ARA-C), dexamethasone (Decadron), dexmedetomidine (Precedex), diazepam (Valium), diltiazem (Cardizem), diphenhydramine (Benadryl), dobutamine, docetaxel (Taxotere), dopamine, doripenem (Doribax), doxorubicin (Adriamycin), doxorubicin liposomal (Doxil), doxycycline, epinephrine (Adrenalin), erythromycin (Erythrocin), etoposide phosphate (Etopophos), famotidine (Pepcid IV), fenoldopam (Corlopam), fentanyl (Sublimaze), filgrastim (Neupogen), fludarabine (Fludara), foscarnet (Foscavir), furosemide (Lasix), gemcitabine (Gemzar), gentamicin, granisetron (Kytril), haloperidol (Haldol), heparin, hetastarch in electrolytes (Hextend), kanamycin (Kantrex), ketorolac (Toradol), labetalol (Trandate), linezolid (Zyvox), lorazepam (Ativan), magnesium sulfate, melphalan (Alkeran), methotrexate, metoclopramide (Reglan), metronidazole (Flagyl IV), micafungin (Mycamine), midazolam (Versed), milrinone (Primacor), morphine, nafcillin (Nallpen), nicardipine (Cardene IV), nitroglycerin IV, norepinephrine (Levophed), ondansetron (Zofran), oxacillin (Bactocill), oxaliplatin (Eloxatin), paclitaxel (Taxol), palonosetron (Aloxi), pemetrexed (Alimta), penicillin G potassium, phenobarbital (Luminal), piperacillin, piperacillin/tazobactam (Zosyn), propofol (Diprivan), ranitidine (Zantac), remifentanil (Ultiva), sulfamethoxazole/trimethoprim, tacrolimus (Prograf), teniposide (Vumon), thiotepa, tobramycin, vancomycin, vecuronium, vinorelbine (Navelbine).

RATE OF ADMINISTRATION
Rapid IV administration increases the possibility of hypotension and respiratory depression.

IV injection: 2 mg or fraction thereof over a minimum of 2 to 3 minutes. Frequently titrated according to symptom relief and respiratory rate.

Infusion: All parameters (outlined in Usual Dose) should be ordered by the physician. Any dose requiring a controlled infusion device requires accurate titration and close monitoring.

ACTIONS
A pure opioid agonist closely related to morphine. Provides potent analgesia without significant hypnotic effects. Six times more potent than morphine milligram for milligram. Onset of action is 10 to 15 minutes and lasts 4 to 5 hours. Hydromorphone is metabolized in the liver and excreted in the urine. Crosses placental barrier. Secreted in breast milk.

INDICATIONS AND USES

Management of pain in patients for whom an opioid analgesic is appropriate. Reserve high-potency hydromorphone (10 mg/mL) for opioid-tolerant patients who require larger than usual doses of opioids to provide adequate pain relief.

CONTRAINDICATIONS

Hypersensitivity to hydromorphone, status asthmaticus, respiratory depression in the absence of resuscitation equipment, and obstetric analgesia. Dilaudid HP is contraindicated in patients who are not opioid tolerant.

PRECAUTIONS

Schedule II opioid agonists, including hydromorphone, morphine, oxymorphone, oxycodone, fentanyl, and methadone, have the highest potential for abuse and risk of producing respiratory depression. Alcohol, CNS depressants, and other opioids potentiate the respiratory depressant effects of hydromorphone, increasing the risk for respiratory depression that might result in death; see Drug/Lab Interactions. ■ Use caution in the elderly or debilitated and in patients with impaired hepatic or renal function, pulmonary disease, cor pulmonale, decreased respiratory reserve, hypoxia, hypercapnia, or pre-existing respiratory depression. ■ Use caution in patients with myxedema or hypothyroidism, adrenocortical insufficiency (e.g., Addison's disease), CNS depression or coma, toxic psychoses, prostatic hypertrophy or urethral stricture, acute alcoholism, delirium tremens, or kyphoscoliosis. ■ Use extreme caution in craniotomy, head injury, and increased intracranial pressure. Respiratory depression may cause an increased PCO_2, cerebral vasodilation, and increased intracranial pressure. Clinical course of head injury may be obscured. ■ Avoid administration in patients with GI obstruction, especially paralytic ileus. Diminishes peristalsis and may prolong obstruction. ■ Symptoms of acute abdominal conditions may be masked. Use with caution in patients with biliary tract disease, including acute pancreatitis; may diminish biliary and pancreatic secretions. ■ Cough reflex may be suppressed. ■ May cause apnea in the asthmatic. ■ Seizures and myoclonus have been reported in patients administered high doses for cancer and severe pain. May also aggravate pre-existing seizures in patients with a convulsive disorder. ■ Tolerance to hydromorphone gradually increases. A marked increase in dose may precipitate seizures. ■ Use with caution in patients in circulatory shock. Vasodilation caused by the drug may further reduce cardiac output and BP. ■ Physical dependence can develop but is not a factor in the presence of chronic cancer and non-cancer pain. ■ Some products may use a latex stopper and some may contain sulfites; may cause a hypersensitivity reaction in susceptible patients.

Monitor: Oxygen, controlled respiratory equipment, and naloxone (Narcan) must be available. ■ Assess baseline pain, then assess pain when vital signs are taken and/or more frequently if needed. Reassess after administration of hydromorphone and adjust dose or interval as required. ■ Monitor vital signs and observe patient frequently to continuously based on amount of dose. Keep patient supine; orthostatic hypotension and fainting may occur; less likely with continuous low doses, but observe closely during ambulation. ■ Uncontrolled pain causes sleep deprivation, decreases pain threshold, and increases pain. When pain is finally controlled, expect the patient to sleep more until recovery from sleep deprivation. ■ Laxatives with or without stool softeners will be required to

avoid constipation and fecal impaction, especially with increased doses and extended use. Maintain adequate hydration. ▪ May increase ventricular response rate in presence of supraventricular tachycardias.
Patient Education: Avoid alcohol or other CNS depressants (e.g., barbiturates, benzodiazepines [e.g., diazepam (Valium)]). ▪ May cause blurred vision, drowsiness, or dizziness; use caution in tasks that require alertness. ▪ Request assistance with ambulation. ▪ May be habit forming. ▪ Take only as directed. ▪ Report unrelieved pain or unacceptable side effects promptly.
Maternal/Child: Category C: safety for use during pregnancy or breastfeeding not established. Benefits must outweigh risks. Some sources list as Category D when used for a prolonged period if the mother is receiving a high dose at term. ▪ May cause respiratory compromise in newborns when administered during labor and delivery. ▪ See Contraindications. ▪ Infants born to mothers physically dependent on opioids will also be physically dependent and may exhibit respiratory difficulties and withdrawal symptoms. ▪ Pediatric patients may be more sensitive to effects (e.g., respiratory depression). ▪ Safety and effectiveness for use in pediatric patients not established. ▪ May cause paradoxical excitation.
Elderly: See Dose Adjustments and Precautions. ▪ May be more susceptible to effects (e.g., respiratory depression, urinary retention, constipation). ▪ Lower doses may provide effective analgesia.

DRUG/LAB INTERACTIONS

Potentiated by **phenothiazines and other CNS depressants** such as opioid analgesics, alcohol, anticholinergics, antihistamines, barbiturates, hypnotics, sedatives, MAO inhibitors (e.g., selegiline [Eldepryl]), neuromuscular blocking agents (e.g., atracurium [Tracrium]), psychotropic agents (e.g., antidepressants, antianxiety agents), and skeletal muscle relaxants (e.g., cyclobenzaprine [Flexeril]). Side effects (e.g., CNS or respiratory depression, constipation, hypotension) may be additive. Reduced dosages of both drugs may be indicated. ▪ Administration of **agonist/antagonist analgesics** (e.g., butorphanol [Stadol], buprenorphine [Buprenex]) to an opiate-dependent patient receiving a pure opiate may precipitate withdrawal symptoms. ▪ Plasma **amylase and lipase determinations** may be unreliable for 24 hours following opioid administration.

SIDE EFFECTS

Most frequently occurring side effects include constipation, dizziness, dry mouth, dysphoria, euphoria, flushing, light-headedness, nausea, pruritus, sweating, and vomiting. Other side effects may include alteration of moods, anorexia, bronchospasm, disorientation and hallucination, headache, hypotension, increased biliary tract pressure, increased intracranial pressure, miosis, tremor, urinary retention or hesitancy.
Major: Anaphylaxis, apnea, cardiac arrest, circulatory depression, hypotension, respiratory depression or arrest, and seizures.

ANTIDOTE

Notify the physician of any side effect. If minor side effects progress or any major side effect occurs, discontinue the drug and notify the physician. Treat anaphylaxis as indicated or resuscitate as necessary. Naloxone (Narcan) will reverse serious reactions. Naloxone use should be reserved for situations in which clinically significant respiratory or circulatory depression is present. Titrate naloxone dose carefully to avoid precipitating an acute abstinence syndrome or uncontrolled pain.

HYDROXOCOBALAMIN

(hy-**DROX**-oh-koh-**BAL**-ah-min)

Cyanokit

USUAL DOSE

Manufacturer provides a quick-use reference guide in carton to facilitate immediate administration. It covers reconstitution, mixing, infusion rate, common S/S of cyanide poisoning with or without smoke inhalation, **incompatibilities,** and alternate diluents.

Initial dose: 5 Gm administered by IV infusion over 15 minutes. Based on severity of poisoning and clinical response, a second 5-Gm dose may be administered for a total dose of 10 Gm.

PEDIATRIC DOSE

Safety and effectiveness for use in pediatric patients not established but has been used outside of the United States.

Initial dose (unlabeled): 70 mg/kg.

DOSE ADJUSTMENTS

No dose adjustments required in the elderly. ▪ Potential need for dose adjustment in patients with impaired hepatic or renal function has not been studied.

DILUTION

Each kit contains one 250-mL glass vial of lyophilized hydroxocobalamin, a sterile transfer spike, a sterile vented infusion tubing, a quick-use reference guide, and a package insert. The glass vial is marked with a fill line for diluent. Using a sterile spike, transfer 200 mL of NS diluent into the glass vial (to the fill line [25 mg/mL]). If NS is not available, LR or D5W may be used. *Do Not Shake!* Invert or rock vial for at least 60 seconds to mix. Solution should be clear and dark red. Attach infusion tubing and begin infusion of the first vial; see Rate of Administration.

Filters: Specific information not available.

Storage: Store kit at CRT. See package insert for allowable storage temperatures for kit transport in extreme weather conditions. Reconstituted product may be held at a temperature not to exceed 40° C (104° F) for up to 6 hours. Do not freeze. Discard any unused portion after 6 hours.

COMPATIBILITY

Manufacturer lists as **incompatible** with ascorbic acid, blood products (whole blood, packed red cells, platelet concentrate, and/or fresh frozen plasma), diazepam (Valium), dobutamine, dopamine, fentanyl (Sublimaze), nitroglycerin IV, pentobarbital (Nembutal), propofol (Diprivan), sodium nitrite, sodium thiosulfate, thiopental (Pentothal). Do not administer simultaneously through the same IV line. Use of a separate line on the opposing extremity is recommended.

RATE OF ADMINISTRATION

Each 5-Gm dose properly diluted and evenly distributed over 15 minutes. The rate of infusion for the second 5-Gm dose may range from 15 minutes (for a patient in extremis) to 2 hours based on patient condition.

ACTIONS

A high dose of cyanide can result in death within minutes by inhibiting the cells' ability to use oxygen (inhibition of cytochrome oxidase results in arrest of cellular respiration). Specifically, cyanide binds with a component of cytochrome oxidase (cytochrome a3), prevents the cell from using oxygen, and forces anaerobic metabolism; this results in lactate production, cellular hypoxia, and metabolic acidosis. Each molecule of hydroxocobalamin can bind one cyanide ion to form cyanocobalamin (vitamin B_{12}) and reverse the toxic process. Cyanocobalamin is then excreted in urine.

INDICATIONS AND USES

Treatment of known or suspected cyanide poisoning. Administer without delay if clinical suspicion of cyanide poisoning is high. Symptoms of cyanide poisoning include chest tightness, confusion, dyspnea, headache, nausea. Signs of cyanide poisoning include altered mental status (e.g., confusion, disorientation), seizures or coma, mydriasis (excessive dilation of the pupil of the eye), abnormally rapid or deep breathing (early), abnormally slow breathing or apnea (late), hypertension (early), hypotension (late), cardiovascular collapse, vomiting, plasma lactate concentration equal to or greater than 8 mmol/L. Smoke inhalation victims with cyanide poisoning have usually been exposed to fire and smoke in an enclosed area and may present with soot around mouth, nose, and/or oropharynx; or an altered mental status. They may have a plasma lactate concentration equal to or greater than 10 mmol/L.

CONTRAINDICATIONS

Manufacturer states, "None"; see Precautions.

PRECAUTIONS

For IV use only. ▪ In addition to treatment with hydroxocobalamin, immediate confirmation of airway patency, adequacy of oxygenation and hydration, cardiovascular support (may be hypotensive or hypertensive), and management of seizure activity is required. Decontamination measures may also be indicated. ▪ Use caution in patients with known hypersensitivity to hydroxocobalamin or cyanocobalamin (vitamin B_{12}). Consider alternative treatments if available (e.g., sodium nitrite and sodium thiosulfate). ▪ Collection of a pretreatment blood sample would be useful in confirming a diagnosis of cyanide poisoning but should not delay treatment. ▪ May cause photosensitivity. ▪ Use in patients with impaired hepatic or renal function has not been studied. ▪ See Drug/Lab Interactions.

Monitor: Immediately confirm airway patency, adequacy of oxygenation, and adequate hydration. ▪ If feasible, draw a pretreatment blood sample; see Precautions. ▪ Monitor BP (may be hypotensive or hypertensive [BP equal to or greater than 180 mm Hg systolic or equal to or greater than 110 mm Hg diastolic has been reported with this treatment]). Hypertension may occur at the beginning of the infusion, is usually at a maximum by the end of the infusion, and should return to baseline within 4 hours. Note Compatibility if treatment is required. ▪ Monitor for seizures. Note Compatibility if treatment is required. ▪ Monitor for S/S of hypersensitivity reactions (e.g., anaphylaxis, angioneurotic edema, chest tightness, dyspnea, edema, pruritus, rash, urticaria).

Patient Education: Skin redness may last up to 2 weeks. Avoid sun exposure while skin is red. ▪ Urine redness may last up to 5 weeks. ▪ An acne-like rash may appear 7 to 28 days after treatment. Has usually resolved without treatment. ▪ Discontinue breast-feeding; talk with your physician to see when and if you can resume. ▪ Report any side effect that is troublesome or doesn't go away.

Maternal/Child: Category C: has caused skeletal and visceral abnormalities in animal studies. Because cyanide readily crosses the placenta, maternal cyanide poisoning results in fetal cyanide poisoning that can be life threatening to the mother and fetus. Consider benefit versus risk before use in pregnancy and labor and delivery. ▪ Discontinue breast-feeding until cleared with physician. ▪ Safety and effectiveness for use in pediatric patients not established but has been used outside of the United States.

Elderly: Safety and effectiveness similar to that seen in younger adults.

DRUG/LAB INTERACTIONS

Formal drug interaction studies have not been conducted. ▪ **Sodium nitrite and sodium thiosulfate** are also used to treat cyanide poisoning. They are **incompatible** with hydroxocobalamin and must be administered in a separate IV line if used concurrently. Safety of coadministration has not been established. ▪ Because of its deep red color, hydroxocobalamin **interferes with numerous clinical laboratory tests.** Effects persist for varying lengths of time depending on test. See package insert for specifics. ▪ Deep red color may cause hemodialysis machines to shut down (an erroneous detection of a "blood leak"). Consider before hemodialysis is initiated in patients treated with hydroxocobalamin.

SIDE EFFECTS

Most common side effects include chromaturia, decreased lymphocytes, erythema, headache, hypertension, injection site reactions, nausea, and rash. Hypersensitivity reactions and hypertension are the most serious side effects associated with hydroxocobalamin. Other reactions that may occur include abdominal discomfort, chest discomfort, diarrhea, dizziness, dry throat, dyspepsia, dysphagia, dyspnea, hematochezia (blood in stool), hot flashes, impaired memory, irritation, peripheral edema, pruritus, redness and swelling of the eyes, restlessness, throat tightness, urticaria, and vomiting.

ANTIDOTE

Keep physician informed of all side effects; will be treated symptomatically. Note Compatibility before treating hypertension or seizures; use an alternate IV line if indicated. Severe hypersensitivity reactions may require epinephrine (Adrenalin), antihistamines (e.g., diphenhydramine [Benadryl]), corticosteroids (e.g., hydrocortisone), or bronchodilators (e.g., albuterol [Ventolin], theophylline). Data on overdose not available; manage symptomatically. Hemodialysis may be effective and is indicated for significant hydroxocobalamin toxicity. Cardiac and/or respiratory arrest may occur before treatment has an effect; resuscitate as indicated.

IBANDRONATE SODIUM
(i-**BAN**-dro-nate **SO**-dee-um)
Boniva

Bone resorption inhibitor
Bisphosphonate

USUAL DOSE
3 mg as an IV injection over 15 to 30 seconds every 3 months. Supplemental calcium and vitamin D are required. See Precautions. Do not administer more frequently than every 3 months; if a dose is missed, administer it as soon as it can be rescheduled, and schedule the next injection for 3 months from that date.

DOSE ADJUSTMENTS
No dose adjustment is indicated based on age, gender, or impaired hepatic function. ▪ No dose adjustment is indicated for impaired kidney function in patients with a CrCl equal to or greater than 30 mL/min; see Contraindications.

DILUTION
May be given undiluted. Available in a prefilled syringe with a 23-gauge needle and a needle-stick protection device.

Storage: Store at CRT. Syringes are for single use only; discard unused drug.

COMPATIBILITY
Manufacturer states, "Must not be mixed with calcium-containing solutions or other intravenously administered drugs."

RATE OF ADMINISTRATION
A single dose as an IV injection over 15 to 30 seconds.

ACTIONS
A nitrogen-containing bisphosphonate. Action is based on its affinity for hydroxyapatite, which is part of the mineral matrix of bone. Ibandronate inhibits osteoclast activity and reduces bone resorption and turnover. In postmenopausal women, it reduces the elevated rate of bone turnover and usually results in a net gain in bone mass. Either rapidly binds to bone (40% to 50% of a dose) or is excreted unchanged in urine (50% to 60%). No evidence that it is metabolized in humans. Terminal half-life ranges from 4.6 to 25.5 hours. Renal clearance is related to CrCl. Patients with a CrCl less than 30 mL/min have a more than twofold increase in exposure (AUC) than do patients with a CrCl greater than 90 mL/min.

INDICATIONS AND USES
Treatment of osteoporosis in postmenopausal women. Osteoporosis may be confirmed by the presence or history of osteoporotic fracture or by a finding of low bone mass (bone mass density [BMD] more than 2 standard deviations below the premenopausal mean [i.e., T-score]).

CONTRAINDICATIONS
Hypersensitivity to ibandronate or its excipients, uncorrected hypocalcemia, severe impaired renal function (CrCl less than 30 mL/min or SCr greater than 2.3 mg/dL).

PRECAUTIONS
For IV injection only. Confirm patency of vein. Intra-arterial or paravenous administration could lead to tissue damage. ▪ Disturbances of bone and

mineral metabolism (e.g., hypocalcemia, hypovitaminosis D) must be treated before administration of ibandronate. ▪ In one study, IV injection was demonstrated to be statistically superior to daily oral tablets. ▪ Bisphosphonates have been associated with a deterioration in renal function (e.g., increased SCr, acute renal failure [rare]). Use caution in patients who have concomitant diseases or are taking concomitant medications that may have adverse effects on the kidney. Risk of serious renal toxicity with other bisphosphonates appears to be inversely related to the rate of administration. ▪ Osteonecrosis of the jaw (ONJ) has been reported in patients receiving bisphosphonates. The majority of cases have been in cancer patients undergoing dental procedures. Risk factors include cancer, concomitant therapy (e.g., chemotherapy, radiotherapy, corticosteroids), and co-morbid conditions (e.g., anemia, coagulopathies, infection, pre-existing oral disease). Consider dental exam and appropriate preventive dentistry before beginning therapy with bisphosphonates. Avoid invasive dental procedures during bisphosphonate therapy. Dental surgery may exacerbate ONJ in patients who develop ONJ while on bisphosphonate therapy. ▪ Severe and occasionally incapacitating bone, joint, and muscle pain has been reported rarely. Symptoms may occur from one day to several months after initiation of treatment. In most cases, pain resolves when ibandronate is discontinued; in some patients, however, symptoms resolved slowly or persisted. ▪ Optimum duration of use has not been determined. Re-evaluate need for continued therapy on a periodic basis. ▪ Atypical, low-energy, or low-trauma fractures of the femoral shaft have been reported in bisphosphonate-treated patients. May be bilateral. Many patients report prodromal pain in the affected area, which usually presents as dull, aching thigh pain weeks to months before a complete fracture occurs. Patients presenting with thigh or groin pain should be evaluated to rule out an incomplete femur fracture. Patients presenting with an atypical fracture should also be assessed for S/S of fracture in the contralateral limb.

Monitor: Obtain baseline measurements of serum calcium, magnesium, phosphate, and serum creatinine; see Precautions. ▪ May cause a transient decrease in serum calcium values. ▪ Daily supplements of calcium and vitamin D are required during therapy with ibandronate. ▪ Monitor SCr before each dose. Nephropathy has been reported; see Precautions. Withhold treatment for renal deterioration. ▪ Influenza-like side effects (e.g., bone, muscle, or joint pains; chills; fever; fatigue) are consistent with an acute phase reaction. Incidence is higher with IV administration. Usually occurs within 3 to 7 days of injection. Symptoms generally subside within 24 to 48 hours, and treatment other than acetaminophen has not been required.

Patient Education: Read manufacturer's patient information sheet before each infusion. ▪ Daily supplements of calcium and vitamin D are required during therapy with ibandronate. ▪ Avoid pregnancy; report a suspected pregnancy immediately. ▪ Discuss your health history (e.g., kidney problems, diabetes, high blood pressure, heart disease, planned tooth extraction), and prescription and non-prescription medications with health care providers, including your dentist. ▪ Promptly report jaw problems following dental procedures. ▪ Report development of bone, joint, or muscle pain promptly. Onset of pain is variable. ▪ Promptly report thigh or groin pain. ▪ Do not administer more frequently than every 3 months; if a dose is

missed, administer it as soon as it can be rescheduled, and schedule the next injection for 3 months from that date.
Maternal/Child: Category C: use during pregnancy only if benefits justify risks to the mother and fetus. Bisphosphonates do cause fetal harm in animals. ▪ Found in milk of lactating animals; safety for use during breast-feeding not established. ▪ Safety and effectiveness for use in pediatric patients not established.
Elderly: Response similar to that seen in younger patients; however, greater sensitivity cannot be ruled out. ▪ Monitor renal function. Consider impaired renal function and concomitant disease or drug therapy.

DRUG/LAB INTERACTIONS

Does not inhibit cytochrome P_{450} isoenzymes. ▪ Secretory pathway does not appear to include known acidic or basic transport systems involved in the excretion of other drugs. ▪ Limited studies show no interaction between ibandronate and melphalan (Alkeran), oral prednisolone, or tamoxifen (Nolvadex). ▪ Bisphosphonates are known to interfere with the use of **bone-imaging agents;** ibandronate has not been studied.

SIDE EFFECTS

Common side effects are headache, increased SCr, influenza-like illness (bone, muscle, or joint pains; chills; fever; fatigue), and injection site reactions (redness or swelling). Other side effects include abdominal pain, arthralgia, back pain, bronchitis, constipation, cystitis, diarrhea, dizziness, dyspepsia, extremity pain, gastritis, gastroenteritis, hypercholesterolemia, hypertension, insomnia, localized osteoarthritis, myalgia, nasopharyngitis, nausea, rash, upper respiratory infection, urinary tract infection. Bisphosphonates may be associated with atypical, low-energy, or low-trauma fractures of the femoral shaft; ocular inflammation (e.g., uveitis, scleritis); and osteonecrosis of the jaw.
Overdose: Hypocalcemia, hypomagnesemia, and hypophosphatemia.

ANTIDOTE

Keep physician informed of side effects. Most will respond to symptomatic treatment. Withhold treatment for renal deterioration. Treat clinically relevant reductions in serum levels of calcium, magnesium, and phosphorus with IV administration of calcium gluconate, magnesium sulfate, and/or potassium or sodium phosphate as indicated. Discontinue ibandronate if severe bone, joint, or muscle pain develops. To be beneficial, dialysis must be administered within 2 hours of overdose. Treat anaphylaxis and/or resuscitate as indicated.

IBRITUMOMAB TIUXETAN BBW

(ib-rih-**TOO**-moh-mab ty-**UKS**-e-tan)

Radiopharmaceutical
Monoclonal antibody
Antineoplastic

Zevalin

pH 7.1 (Buffer Vial)

USUAL DOSE

A combination therapeutic regimen consisting of rituximab and two radiolabeled agents (Indium-111 [In-111] ibritumomab tiuxetan and Yttrium-90 [Y-90] ibritumomab tiuxetan). Specific timing of the course of treatment based on the availability of the radioactive components is necessary; see Dilution. These two radiolabeled agents should not be used without the rituximab pre-dose. *It is imperative that the rituximab monograph be consulted; all information in that monograph must be considered.* (Deaths from infusion reactions have occurred within 24 hours of rituximab infusion.) The rituximab dose in this combination regimen is reduced to 250 mg/M^2 versus 375 mg/M^2 when it is used as a single agent.

DAY 1

Premedication: Acetaminophen (Tylenol) 650 mg PO and diphenhydramine (Benadryl) 50 mg PO before rituximab to prevent or attenuate severe hypersensitivity reactions.

Rituximab: 250 mg/M^2 as an IV infusion.

In-111 ibritumomab tiuxetan (Zevalin): Within 4 hours following completion of the rituximab infusion, give 5 mCi (1.6 mg total antibody dose) In-111 ibritumomab as an IV injection over 10 minutes.

Assess biodistribution: *1st image:* 48 to 72 hours after In-111 ibritumomab injection. *2nd image:* Optional, other time points.

If biodistribution is not acceptable, stop therapy immediately. Do not administer Y-90 ibritumomab tiuxetan to patients with altered biodistribution as determined by imaging with In-111 ibritumomab tiuxetan. If biodistribution is acceptable, therapy can proceed on either Day 7, Day 8, or Day 9. Date is selected based on the availability of the radioactive component of Y-90 ibritumomab tiuxetan (may also be adjusted within these 3 days for patient convenience after the availability of the radioactive component is considered).

DAY 7, 8, OR 9 (SELECT ONE DATE)

Premedication: Acetaminophen (Tylenol) 650 mg PO and diphenhydramine (Benadryl) 50 mg PO before rituximab to prevent or attenuate severe hypersensitivity reactions.

Rituximab: 250 mg/M^2 as an IV infusion.

Y-90 ibritumomab tiuxetan (Zevalin): Within 4 hours following completion of rituximab infusion, give Y-90 ibritumomab tiuxetan as an IV injection through a free-flowing IV line over 10 minutes based on platelet count:

0.4 mCi/kg (14.8 MBq/kg) for patients with a normal platelet count *or*

0.3 mCi/kg (11.1 MBq/kg) in relapsed or refractory patients with a platelet count of 100,000-149,000 cells/mm^3

Do not treat patients with a platelet count less than 100,000/mm^3.

Do not exceed the maximum allowable dose of Y-90 ibritumomab tiuxetan (32 mCi [1184 MBq]), regardless of the patient's weight.

DOSE ADJUSTMENTS

See Usual Dose.

DILUTION

Specific timing of the course of treatment based on the availability of the radioactive components is necessary. The In-111 chloride sterile solution (the radioactive component of In-111 ibritumomab tiuxetan) is available from several sources. The Y-90 chloride sterile solution (the radioactive component of Y-90 ibritumomab tiuxetan) is available from only one source and can be delivered on only 2 or 3 days of the week. Specific timing of the course of treatment moves backwards from the day of availability of the Y-90 ibritumomab tiuxetan radioactive component. The radioactive component of In-111 ibritumomab tiuxetan is ordered for 7, 8, or 9 days before that availability.

Changing the ratio of any of the reactants in the radiolabeling process may adversely impact therapeutic results.

Rituximab: See rituximab monograph.

In-111 ibritumomab tiuxetan: A specific kit provides the vials required to produce a single dose. The In-111 chloride sterile solution (the radioactive component) must be ordered separately at the same time the kit is ordered. Other supplies (listed in the package insert) are required for preparation of ibritumomab tiuxetan with In-111 and radiolabeling.

Y-90 ibritumomab tiuxetan: A specific kit provides the vials required to produce a single dose. The Y-90 chloride sterile solution (the radioactive component) will be shipped with the kit when ordered. Other supplies (listed in package insert) are required for the preparation of ibritumomab tiuxetan with Y-90 and radiolabeling.

All preparation, calibration, confirmation of radiochemical purity, and administration of these kits will be by personnel authorized to handle radiopharmaceuticals. Each requires a specific order and specific timing of preparation.

Filters: Administration through a 0.22-micron, low–protein binding filter is required for both radiopharmaceuticals.

Storage:

In-111 ibritumomab tiuxetan: Store at 2° to 8° C (36° to 46° F) until use and administer within 12 hours of radiolabeling.

Y-90 ibritumomab tiuxetan: Store at 2° to 8° C (36° to 46° F) until use and administer within 8 hours of radiolabeling.

COMPATIBILITY

A radiopharmaceutical; use only the supplies provided in each specific kit. All components, including the rituximab, should not be mixed or diluted with other drugs.

RATE OF ADMINISTRATION

Rituximab: See rituximab monograph.

Both radiopharmaceuticals require the use of a 0.22-micron, low–protein binding filter and a vial and syringe shield. After injection of each radiopharmaceutical, the line should be flushed with at least 10 mL of NS.

In-111 ibritumomab tiuxetan: A single dose as an IV injection over 10 minutes.

Y-90 ibritumomab tiuxetan: A single dose as an IV injection through a free-flowing IV line over 10 minutes; see Monitor.

ACTIONS

A combination therapeutic regimen consisting of rituximab and two radiolabeled agents (Indium-111 [In-111] ibritumomab tiuxetan and Yttrium-90 [Y-90] ibritumomab tiuxetan). Ibritumomab tiuxetan is the immunoconjugate resulting from a stable thiourea covalent bond between the monoclonal antibody ibritumomab and the linker-chelator tiuxetan. This linker-chelator provides a high affinity, specific chelation site for In-111 or Y-90. The antibody (ibritumomab) is a murine IgG, kappa monoclonal antibody directed against the CD20 antigen found on the surface of normal and malignant B lymphocytes. The CD20 antigen is expressed on pre-B and mature B lymphocytes and on more than 90% of B-cell non-Hodgkin's lymphomas (NHL). Like rituximab, ibritumomab induces apoptosis (fragmentation of the cell). The In-111 component improves detection of the known disease sites. The beta emission from Y-90 induces cellular damage by the formation of free radicals in the target and neighboring cells. After calibration, In-111 decays by electron capture, with a physical half-life of 67.3 hours. After calibration, Y-90 decays by the emission of beta particles, with a physical half-life of 64.1 hours. A small amount of all components is excreted in urine. Administration of the prescribed regimen results in sustained depletion of circulating B-cells (median was zero at 4 weeks [range 0 to 1,084 cells/mm^3]). B-cell recovery begins approximately 12 weeks post-treatment and usually progresses to normal range (32 to 341 cells/mm^3) by 9 months post-treatment.

INDICATIONS AND USES

Treatment of relapsed or refractory low-grade or follicular B-cell non-Hodgkin's lymphoma (NHL). ▪ Treatment of previously untreated follicular NHL in patients who achieve a partial or complete response to first-line chemotherapy. Used in combination with rituximab.

CONTRAINDICATIONS

Manufacturer states, "None." Known hypersensitivity or anaphylactic reactions to murine proteins or any component of this regimen. ▪ Do not administer Y-90 ibritumomab tiuxetan to patients with 25% or greater lymphoma marrow involvement and/or impaired bone marrow reserve (e.g., prior myeloablative therapies, platelet count less than 100,000/mm^3, neutrophil count less than 1,500/mm^3, hypocellular bone marrow [equal to or greater than 15% cellularity or marked reduction in bone marrow precursors] or to patients with a history of failed stem cell collection). ▪ Do not administer Y-90 ibritumomab tiuxetan to patients with altered biodistribution as determined by imaging with In-111 ibritumomab tiuxetan. ▪ Do not treat patients with a platelet count less than 100,000/mm^3.

PRECAUTIONS

Radiopharmaceuticals are administered by or under the direction of the physician specialist whose experience and training in the safe use and handling of radionuclides have been approved by the appropriate government agency. ▪ Contents of the kits are not radioactive; however, during and after radiolabeling, care should be taken to minimize radiation exposure to patients and to medical personnel consistent with institutional good radiation safety practices and patient management procedures. Contact the radiation safety officer. ▪ If a splash occurs, flush eyes for at least 15 minutes. For skin contact, wash affected areas thoroughly with soap and water and blot dry; do not abrade skin. In both situations, notify the radiation safety officer and continue the process until no more radiation can be detected. ▪ Notify the radiation safety officer immediately if any ingestion occurs. ▪ Administer in a facility with adequate personnel, equipment, and supplies to monitor the patient and respond to any medical emergency. ■ Y-90 ibritumomab tiuxetan results in severe and prolonged cytopenias; see Contraindications, Monitor, and Antidote. ■ See prescribing information for descriptions of expected biodistribution and altered biodistribution. Regimen discontinued if biodistribution altered. ■ May cause severe, and potentially fatal, infusion reactions; see Monitor, Side Effects, and rituximab monograph. Deaths have occurred within 24 hours of rituximab infusion and were associated with hypoxia, pulmonary infiltrates, ARDS, MI, VF, or cardiogenic shock. ■ Use caution; hypersensitivity reactions and/or anaphylaxis can occur. As with all proteins, there is a potential for immunogenicity; patients who have received murine proteins should be screened for human anti-mouse antibodies (HAMA); may be at increased risk of hypersensitivity reactions. ■ Severe cutaneous and mucocutaneous reactions, some fatal, have been reported. Onset of these reactions is variable and may be acute (occurring within days) or delayed (occurring after 3 to 4 months); see Monitor and Side Effects. ■ Safety of ibritumomab tiuxetan for more than a single course of treatment or for use with other therapeutic regimens has not been established. ■ Contains albumin and carries a theoretical risk for transmission of viral diseases or Creutzfeldt-Jakob disease. Effective donor screening and product manufacturing processes make this risk extremely remote. ■ Secondary malignancies (e.g., myelodysplastic syndrome and/or acute myelogenous leukemia [AML]) have been reported. ■ Ability to generate a primary or anamnestic humoral response to any vaccine has not been studied.

Monitor: Obtain a baseline CBC, including differential and platelet count. Monitor weekly or more frequently if indicated (e.g., cytopenias, concurrent drugs). Continue until levels recover. Cytopenias (e.g., thrombocytopenia and neutropenia) can be severe; see Precautions, Contraindications, and Antidote. Median time to nadir was 7 to 9 weeks, and the median duration of cytopenias was 22 to 35 days. Some cytopenias extended beyond 12 weeks, and some patients died without recovering. ■ Monitor for infusion reactions. Typically occur within 30 to 120 minutes of the first rituximab infusion and may cause interruption of rituximab, In-111 ibritumomab tiuxetan, or Y-90 ibritumomab tiuxetan. S/S may include angioedema, bronchospasm, hypotension, and hypoxia; see Side Effects for additional symptoms. ■ Monitor for serious cutaneous or mucocutaneous reactions (e.g., bullous dermatitis, erythema multiforme, exfoliative dermatitis, Stevens-Johnson syndrome, toxic epidermal necrolysis). ■ To reduce unnecessary radiation exposure to vital organs (e.g., thyroid, kidneys, bladder), patients should be well hydrated before, during, and for at least 1 day after administration. Encourage fluid intake and frequent voiding. ■ Establish a free-flowing IV line before administration of Y-90 ibritumomab tiuxetan; avoid extravasation. Monitor closely; if any signs of extravasation occur, discontinue immediately and restart in another vein. ■ Hemorrhage, including fatal cerebral hemorrhage, has occurred. Monitor for thrombocytopenia (platelet count less than 50,000/mm^3) for up to 3 months. Initiate precautions to prevent excessive bleeding (e.g., inspect IV sites, skin, and mucous membranes; use extreme care during invasive procedures; test urine, emesis, stool, and secretions for occult blood). ■ Observe closely for signs of infection for up to 3 months. Prophylactic antibiotics may be indicated pending results of C/S in a febrile neutropenic patient. ■ See rituximab monograph; additional monitoring may be required. ■ See Precautions, Drug/Lab Interactions, and Antidote.

Patient Education: Avoid pregnancy; effective birth control recommended for males and females during treatment and for up to 12 months following therapy. Women should report a suspected pregnancy immediately. ■ Explain importance of increased fluid intake and frequent voiding. ■ Promptly report S/S of infection (e.g., fever, sore throat) or S/S of bleeding (e.g., bruising, nose bleed, dark stools).
Maternal/Child: Category D: avoid pregnancy; can cause fetal harm. Women of childbearing potential should avoid becoming pregnant. ■ Could cause toxic effects on testes and ovaries. Effective contraceptive methods recommended for men and women during treatment and for up to 12 months following therapy. ■ Discontinue breast-feeding. ■ Safety and effectiveness for use in pediatric patients not established.
Elderly: Response similar to that found in younger patients; however, the elderly may have a greater sensitivity to its effects.

DRUG/LAB INTERACTIONS
Formal drug interaction studies have not been performed. ■ Risk of bleeding may be increased by **any medicine that affects blood clotting,** including **anticoagulants** (e.g., heparin, lepirudin [Refludan], warfarin [Coumadin]); **glycoprotein GPIIb/IIIa receptor antagonists** (e.g., abciximab [ReoPro], eptifibatide [Integrilin], tirofiban [Aggrastat]); **any medication that may cause hypoprothrombinemia, thrombocytopenia, or GI ulceration or bleeding** (e.g., selected antibiotics [e.g., cefotetan], aspirin, NSAIDs [e.g., ibuprofen (Advil, Motrin), naproxen (Aleve, Naprosyn)]; **and/or any other medication that inhibits platelet aggregation** (e.g., clopidogrel [Plavix], dipyridamole [Persantine], plicamycin [Mithracin], sulfinpyrazone [Anturane], ticlopidine [Ticlid], valproate [Depacon, Depakene]). ■ Safety of immunization with **live virus vaccines** has not been studied. ■ Potential for additive effects with previously administered **bone marrow–suppressing agents and/or radiation therapy** has not been studied.

SIDE EFFECTS
The most common side effects are asthenia, cough, cytopenias (e.g., anemia, neutropenia, and thrombocytopenia), fatigue, fever, GI symptoms (e.g., abdominal pain, diarrhea, nausea, and vomiting), and sore throat. The most serious side effects are prolonged and severe cytopenias and secondary malignancies. Other side effects include anorexia, anxiety, arthralgias, dizziness, dyspnea, ecchymosis. Abdominal enlargement, asthenia, back pain, chills, constipation, flushing, headache, hypotension, immunogenicity (development of HAMA or HACA), insomnia, myalgia, peripheral edema, rhinitis, throat irritation, and many other side effects have been reported. Nonhematologic toxicities were considered mild in severity.
Major: Other major side effects include hemorrhage while thrombocytopenic (resulting in death), hypersensitivity reactions (e.g., anaphylaxis, angioedema, bronchospasm, hypotension, pruritus, rash), severe or fatal infusion reactions (e.g., ARDS, cardiogenic shock, hypoxia, MI, pulmonary infiltrates, VF), infections (predominantly bacterial in origin), and severe cutaneous or mucocutaneous reactions (e.g., bullous dermatitis, erythema multiforme, exfoliative dermatitis, Stevens-Johnson syndrome, toxic epidermal necrolysis).
Post-Marketing: Cutaneous and mucocutaneous reactions (e.g., erythema multiforme, Stevens-Johnson syndrome, toxic epidermal necrolysis, bullous dermatitis, and exfoliative dermatitis). Infusion site erythema and ulceration following extravasation, radiation injury, and complications that

occur within a month of administration in or near areas of lymphomatous involvement.

ANTIDOTE

Keep physician informed of all side effects. May constitute a medical emergency or will be treated symptomatically as indicated. Hypersensitivity or infusion-related side effects to any component of the regimen may resolve with slowing or interruption of the infusion and with supportive care (IV saline, diphenhydramine, bronchodilators such as albuterol [Ventolin] or aminophylline, and acetaminophen). Discontinue entire regimen (rituximab, In-111 ibritumomab tiuxetan, and Y-90 ibritumomab tiuxetan) in patients who develop severe infusion reactions (usually to rituximab). Treat anaphylaxis with oxygen, antihistamines (diphenhydramine), epinephrine, and corticosteroids. Maintain a patent airway. Autologous stem cell support, administration of whole blood products (e.g., packed RBCs, platelets, leukocytes), and/or blood modifiers (e.g., darbepoetin alfa [Aranesp], epoetin alfa [Epogen], filgrastim [Neupogen], pegfilgrastim [Neulasta], sargramostim [Leukine], oprelvekin [Neumega]) may be indicated to treat bone marrow toxicity or to treat moderate to severe bleeding. However, in clinical studies, patients were prohibited from receiving growth factor therapy for 2 weeks before the ibritumomab therapeutic regimen, as well as 2 weeks following completion of the regimen. Control minor bleeding by local pressure. For severe bleeding, discontinue therapy and obtain PT, aPTT, platelet count, and fibrinogen. Draw blood for type and cross-match. Antibiotic therapy is indicated for infections and may be indicated prophylactically. Patients who experience severe cutaneous or mucocutaneous reactions should not receive any further component of the therapeutic regimen and should seek prompt medical attention. Death may occur from the progression of some side effects. Resuscitate as indicated.

IBUPROFEN BBW

(**EYE**-bue-**PROE**-fen)

Caldolor

Analgesic
Antipyretic

pH 7.4

USUAL DOSE

Use the lowest effective dose for the shortest duration of time based on individual needs and response. Reevaluate after the initial dose. Adjust dose and frequency as indicated. Total daily dose should not exceed 3200 mg. Adequate hydration required before administration to reduce the risk of adverse renal reactions.

Analgesia: 400 to 800 mg every 6 hours as necessary.

Antipyretic: 400 mg every 4 to 6 hours or 100 to 200 mg every 4 hours as necessary.

DOSE ADJUSTMENTS

Lower-end initial and reduced doses may be indicated in the elderly and/or debilitated. Consider potential for decreased organ function and concomitant disease or drug therapy.

DILUTION

Must be diluted to a final concentration of 4 mg/mL or less. Infusion without dilution can cause hemolysis. Further dilute in NS, D5W, or LR. An 800-mg dose requires dilution with no less than 200 mL of infusion fluid; a 400-mg dose, 100 mL; a 200-mg dose, 50 mL; and a 100-mg dose, no less than 25 mL of infusion fluid.

Filters: Specific information not available; consult pharmacist.

Storage: Store vials at CRT. Diluted solutions stable for up to 24 hours at 20° to 25° C (68° to 77° F) and with ambient room lighting.

COMPATIBILITY

Specific information not available; consult pharmacist.

RATE OF ADMINISTRATION

A single dose as an infusion over no less than 30 minutes.

ACTIONS

A nonsteroidal anti-inflammatory drug (NSAID) that has anti-inflammatory, analgesic, and antipyretic activity. Mechanism of action may be related to prostaglandin synthetase inhibition. Ibuprofen is a mixture of two isomers: [-]R- and [+]S-. The [+]S- isomer is responsible for the activity of ibuprofen. The [-]R- isomer slowly converts to the active [+]S- isomer to maintain levels of the active drug in the circulation. Highly protein bound; the mean half-life of a 400-mg dose is 2.2 hours, and the mean half-life of an 800-mg dose is 2.44 hours.

INDICATIONS AND USES

Management of mild to moderate pain. ■ Management of moderate to severe pain as an adjunct to opioid analgesics. ■ Reduction of fever in adults.

CONTRAINDICATIONS

Known hypersensitivity (anaphylactoid reactions, serious skin reactions) to ibuprofen or other NSAIDs. ■ Known history of asthma, urticaria, or allergic-type reactions after taking aspirin or other NSAIDs. ■ Treatment of perioperative pain in patients undergoing coronary artery bypass graft (CABG) surgery. ■ See Maternal/Child.

PRECAUTIONS

For IV infusion only. ■ NSAIDs (especially with longer-term use) have been shown to increase the risk of numerous and serious events, which may occur with short-term use in patients with or without a history of the event. ■ May increase risk for serious cardiovascular (CV) thrombotic events (e.g., MI, stroke), which can be fatal. Patients with risk factors for CV disease or known CV disease may be at greater risk. ■ May increase the risk of serious GI ulceration, bleeding, and/or perforation with or without warning signs (can be fatal). Use extreme caution in patients with a prior history of ulcer disease or GI bleeding. Risk is also increased in elderly or debilitated patients and with concomitant use of aspirin, oral corticosteroids, anticoagulants, alcohol, or smoking. ■ May cause elevations of liver function tests (e.g., ALT, AST). Rare cases of serious hepatic reactions (jaundice, liver necrosis, hepatic failure) have occurred, and some have been fatal. ■ May cause fluid retention and edema; use caution in patients with CHF or edema. ■ May precipitate hypertension or worsen pre-existing hypertension; see Drug/Lab Interactions. ■ In addition to the usual caution in patients with reduced hepatic or renal function, NSAIDs may cause a dose-dependent reduction in renal prostaglandin formation and, secondarily, in renal blood flow, which can precipitate renal failure. Patients with impaired renal function, heart failure, or liver dysfunction; elderly patients; and patients receiving ACE inhibitors (e.g., enalaprilat [Vasotec], lisinopril [Zestril]) or diuretics are at greatest risk. ■ Use caution in dehydrated patients. ■ Anaphylactic reactions have occurred in patients without previous known exposure to ibuprofen; see Contraindications. Use caution in patients with pre-existing asthma. ■ May cause serious skin reactions (e.g., exfoliative dermatitis, Stevens-Johnson syndrome, toxic epidermal necrolysis) without warning; some have been fatal. ■ Anti-inflammatory and antipyretic effects may reduce the utility of these diagnostic signs in detecting other illnesses. ■ May cause anemia. ■ NSAIDs inhibit platelet aggregation and may cause a prolonged bleeding time. ■ Aseptic meningitis and ophthalmologic effects (e.g., blurred or diminished vision, changes in color vision) have been reported with oral ibuprofen. ■ See Maternal/Child.

Monitor: Correct hypovolemia before administration and maintain adequate hydration. ■ Obtain baseline vital signs and monitor frequently during therapy. CBC, liver function tests, and SCr or CrCl may be indicated for a baseline or as needed as symptoms develop. ■ Monitor patients with or without a previous history of CV disease for S/S of CV events (e.g., chest pain, dyspnea, edema, hypertension, limb or facial paralysis). ■ Observe for S/S of GI ulceration or bleeding and/or liver dysfunction. ■ Monitor renal function, especially in patients with impaired renal function. ■ Monitor for S/S of hypersensitivity reactions (e.g., anaphylaxis, pruritus, rash, urticaria, or wheezing). ■ Monitor patients who may be adversely affected by alterations in platelet function (e.g., patients with coagulation disorders or patients receiving anticoagulants).

Patient Education: Side effects have resulted in extended hospitalization and could be fatal. ■ Promptly report any unusual S/S (e.g., abdominal pain, bloody emesis, changes in vision, chest pain, dark stools, dizziness, numbness of face or limbs, rash, shortness of breath, unexplained weight gain or edema).

Maternal/Child: Category C before 30 weeks' gestation; Category D starting at 30 weeks' gestation. Avoid use starting at 30 weeks' gestation; premature closure of the ductus arteriosus in the fetus may occur. Use during pregnancy only if the potential benefit justifies the potential risk to the fetus. ■ Effects during labor and delivery unknown. ■ Discontinue breast-feeding. ■ Safety and effectiveness for use in pediatric patients not established.

Elderly: Response compared with younger patients unknown. ■ Increased risk for serious GI adverse events. ■ Dosing should be cautious; see Dose Adjustments.

DRUG/LAB INTERACTIONS

Concurrent use with **aspirin** not recommended; may increase risk of serious GI events. Aspirin also reduces the protein binding of ibuprofen; clinical significance not known. ■ Synergistic with **anticoagulants** (e.g., heparin, warfarin [Coumadin]); risk of GI bleeding increased. ■ NSAIDs may decrease the effectiveness of **ACE inhibitors** (e.g., enalaprilat [Vasotec], lisinopril [Zestril]). ■ Ibuprofen can reduce the natriuretic effects of **furosemide** (Lasix) and **thiazide diuretics** (e.g., hydrochlorothiazide [HydroDI-URIL]); observe for signs of renal failure and ensure diuretic effectiveness. ■ Concurrent use of **lithium** with NSAIDs may decrease lithium clearance, increasing plasma levels of lithium; observe for signs of lithium toxicity. ■ Concurrent use of NSAIDs with **methotrexate** may enhance methotrexate toxicity. ■ Coadministration of cimetidine (Tagamet) or ranitidine (Zantac) did not affect ibuprofen serum concentrations.

SIDE EFFECTS

The most common side effects are dizziness, flatulence, headache, hemorrhage, and nausea and vomiting. Other side effects include abdominal discomfort, anemia, bacteremia, bacterial pneumonia, cough, diarrhea, dyspepsia, eosinophilia, hypernatremia, hypertension, hypoalbuminemia, hypokalemia, hypoproteinemia, hypotension, increased blood urea, increased lactic dehydrogenase (LDH), neutropenia, peripheral edema, thrombocytosis, urinary retention, wound hemorrhage. See Precautions for potential major side effects.

ANTIDOTE

Keep the physician informed of significant side effects. With increasing severity or onset of symptoms of any major side effect (e.g., CHF; edema; hypersensitivity reactions; GI bleeding, ulceration, or perforation; hepatic or renal effects; hypertension; skin reactions; thrombotic events), discontinue the drug and notify the physician. A patent airway, artificial ventilation, oxygen therapy, and other symptomatic treatment must be instituted promptly if indicated. Treat anaphylaxis with epinephrine (Adrenalin), diphenhydramine (Benadryl), and corticosteroids as indicated. No known antidote.

IBUPROFEN LYSINE
(eye-byou-**PROH**-fen **LIE**-seen)

NeoProfen

NSAID
(patent ductus arteriosus adjunct)

pH 7

NEONATAL DOSE

All doses are based on birth weight. A course of therapy is three doses given at 24-hour intervals.

Initial dose: 10 mg/kg. Follow with a dose of 5 mg/kg in 24 hours and repeat at 48 hours; see Dose Adjustments.

After completion of the first course, no further doses are indicated if the ductus arteriosus closes or is significantly reduced in size. If the ductus arteriosus fails to close or reopens, a second course, alternative pharmacologic therapy, or surgery may be necessary.

DOSE ADJUSTMENTS

If urine output is less than 0.6 mL/kg/hr at any time a dose is to be given, withhold dose until lab studies confirm a return to normal renal function.

DILUTION

Each single dose must be diluted to an appropriate volume for administration as an infusion over 15 minutes with dextrose or saline. Prepare for infusion and begin administration within 30 minutes of preparation. A fresh solution should be prepared just before each administration. Contains no preservatives; discard any unused portion.

Filters: Specific information not available.

Storage: Store vials in cartons at CRT and protect from light until use. Use reconstituted solution within 30 minutes of preparation.

COMPATIBILITY

Manufacturer states, "Should not be simultaneously administered in the same IV line with Total Parenteral Nutrition" (TPN). If required, interrupt TPN for 15 minutes before and after ibuprofen administration. Maintain IV line patency with dextrose or saline infusion.

RATE OF ADMINISTRATION

Administer via the IV port nearest the insertion site.

A single dose, properly diluted, and infused continuously over 15 minutes.

ACTIONS

A nonsteroidal anti-inflammatory drug (NSAID). Mechanism of action by which it causes closure of a patent ductus arteriosus (PDA) is unknown; however, in adults it is an inhibitor of prostaglandin synthesis. By closing the patent ductus arteriosus, the need for surgical intervention is eliminated. Half-life varies inversely with postnatal age, but in general the half-life in infants is more than 10 times longer than in adults. In lower birth weight premature infants, half-life may range from 20 to 51 hours. Metabolism and excretion have not been studied. In adults, it is metabolized in the liver and excreted in the urine and feces.

INDICATIONS AND USES

Closure of a clinically significant patent ductus arteriosus in premature infants weighing between 500 and 1,500 Gm who are no more that 32 weeks' gestational age when usual medical management (e.g., fluid restriction, diuretics, respiratory support) is not effective. Consequences beyond 8 weeks after treatment have not been evaluated.

CONTRAINDICATIONS

Bleeding (especially active intracranial hemorrhage or GI bleeding), coagulation defects, suspected necrotizing enterocolitis, infants with congenital heart disease (e.g., pulmonary atresia, severe coarctation of the aorta, severe tetralogy of Fallot) who require patency of the ductus arteriosus for satisfactory pulmonary or systemic blood flow, proven or suspected untreated infection, significant renal impairment, thrombocytopenia.

PRECAUTIONS

For IV use only; see Monitor. ▪ Reserve for infants with clear evidence of a clinically significant PDA (three of the following five criteria: bounding pulse, hyperdynamic precordium, pulmonary edema, increased cardiac silhouette, systolic murmur) or as diagnosed by a neonatologist. ▪ For use only in a highly supervised setting such as an intensive care nursery. ▪ No long-term evaluations available. Effects of ibuprofen on neurodevelopmental outcome and growth and on disease processes associated with prematurity (e.g., retinopathy of prematurity, chronic lung disease) have not been assessed. ▪ May alter the usual signs of infection. Use with extreme caution in the presence of an existing controlled infection and in infants at risk for infection. ▪ Can inhibit platelet aggregation; observe for signs of bleeding. ▪ Can prolong bleeding time in adults; use caution in infants with underlying hemostatic defects; see Contraindications. ▪ Can displace bilirubin from albumin-binding sites; use with caution in infants with elevated total bilirubin. ▪ Surgery indicated if condition is not responsive to two courses of therapy.

Monitor: Confirm absolute patency of vein. Avoid extravasation; will irritate tissue. Administration via an umbilical arterial line has not been studied. ▪ Obtain baseline and monitor vital signs, oxygenation, acid-base status, fluid and electrolyte balance, and kidney function (SCr, BUN, urine output). ▪ Can cause a reduction in urine output, increased BUN and SCr, and a decreased CrCl; may progress to oliguria or renal failure. Monitor all infants closely, especially those with some degree of renal impairment. ▪ May inhibit platelet aggregation; monitor for signs of bleeding.

DRUG/LAB INTERACTIONS

Drug interactions have not been studied.

SIDE EFFECTS

Most commonly reported side effects include adrenal insufficiency, anemia, apnea, atelectasis, decreased urine output, edema, GI disorders (including non-necrotizing enterocolitis), hematuria, hypernatremia, hypocalcemia, hypoglycemia, increased BUN and SCr, intraventricular hemorrhage and other bleeding, renal failure, renal insufficiency, respiratory failure, respiratory infection, sepsis, skin lesion or irritation, and urinary tract infection. Other side effects of unknown association include abdominal distention, cardiac failure, cholestasis, convulsions, feeding problems, gastritis, gastroesophageal reflux, hypotension, ileus, infections, inguinal hernia, injection site reactions, jaundice, lab abnormalities (e.g., hyperglycemia, neutropenia, thrombocytopenia), and tachycardia.

Post-Marketing: GI perforation, necrotizing enterocolitis.

Overdose: Breathing difficulties, coma, drowsiness, hypotension, irregular heartbeat, kidney failure, seizures, and vomiting have occurred in individuals (not necessarily in premature infants) following overdose of oral ibuprofen.

ANTIDOTE

Discontinue the drug and notify the physician of all side effects. Based on severity, side effects may be treated symptomatically or drug will be completely discontinued in favor of surgical intervention. In case of overdose, there is no specific antidote. Treat symptomatically and follow for several days after apparent recovery; GI ulceration and hemorrhage may occur. Resuscitate as necessary.

IBUTILIDE FUMARATE   BBW   Antiarrhythmic
(ih-**BYOU**-tih-lyd   **FU**-mar-ayt)
Corvert   pH 4.6

USUAL DOSE

Guidelines for Ibutilide Dosing		
Patient Weight	Initial Infusion (over 10 minutes)	Second Infusion
60 kg (132 lb) or more	1 mg ibutilide fumarate (one vial [10 mL])	If the arrhythmia does not terminate within 10 minutes after the end of the initial infusion, a second 10-minute infusion of equal strength may be administered 10 minutes after completion of the first infusion.
Less than 60 kg (132 lb)	0.01 mg/kg ibutilide fumarate (0.1 mL/kg)	

Discontinue infusion promptly when the presenting arrhythmia is terminated (desired effect). Must also be discontinued immediately if sustained or nonsustained ventricular tachycardia or marked prolongation of QT or QTc occur (adverse effects). Postconversion treatment with appropriate antiarrhythmics (e.g., digoxin, verapamil, or propranolol) is usually required.

DOSE ADJUSTMENTS

Dose selection should be cautious in the elderly. Reduced doses may be indicated based on the potential for decreased organ function and concomitant disease or drug therapy. ▪ No adjustments required in patients with impaired hepatic or renal function; see Monitor. Lower doses may be indicated in post–cardiac surgery patients. In recent studies one or two infusions of 0.5 mg in patients weighing 60 kg or more or 0.005 mg/kg/dose for patients under 60 kg was effective in terminating atrial fibrillation and/or flutter.

DILUTION

May be given undiluted or may be diluted in 50 mL of NS or D5W and given as an infusion. 1 mg (10 mL of a 0.1-mg/mL solution) of ibutilide in 50 mL diluent yields 0.017 mg/mL.

Storage: Store at CRT in carton until use. Stable after dilution for 24 hours at room temperature, 48 hours if refrigerated.

COMPATIBILITY

Manufacturer lists as **compatible** with NS and D5W packaged in glass, polyvinyl chloride, or polyolefin infusion containers. Additional information not available; consult pharmacist.

RATE OF ADMINISTRATION

A single dose by injection or infusion over 10 minutes.

ACTIONS

A class III antiarrhythmic agent that produces mild slowing of the sinus rate and atrioventricular conduction. Delays repolarization by activation of a slow inward current (sodium) rather than blocking outward potassium currents. Prolonged atrial and ventricular action potential duration and refractoriness result. Produces dose-related prolongation of the QT interval (may result from dose of ibutilide or rate of injection). Conversion of atrial flutter/fibrillation usually occurs within 30 minutes but may take up to 90 minutes after the start of the infusion. Most patients remain in normal sinus rhythm (NSR) for 24 hours. At recommended doses, ibutilide has no clinically significant effects on cardiac output, mean pulmonary arterial pressure, or pulmonary capillary wedge pressure. Rapidly distributed and metabolized. Elimination half-life is 6 hours (range 2 to 12 hours). Primarily excreted in urine (7% as unchanged drug). Excreted in small amounts in feces.

INDICATIONS AND USES

Rapid conversion of recent onset atrial fibrillation or atrial flutter to sinus rhythm. Patients with more recent onset of arrhythmia have a higher rate of conversion. Effectiveness was less in those with a longer-duration arrhythmia.

CONTRAINDICATIONS

Known hypersensitivity to ibutilide or any of its components. ■ Not recommended in patients who have had a previous polymorphic ventricular tachycardia (e.g., torsades de pointes). ■ See Drug/Lab Interactions.

PRECAUTIONS

For IV infusion only. ■ Usually administered by or under the direction of the physician specialist. ■ Skilled personnel and proper equipment (e.g., cardiac monitors, intracardiac pacing facilities, cardioverter/defibrillator, emergency drugs) must be immediately available. ■ May cause life-threatening arrhythmias (e.g., torsades de pointes) with or without documented QT prolongation. ■ Correct hypokalemia and hypomagnesemia before use; may exaggerate a prolonged QT and cause arrhythmias. ■ Adequate anticoagulation (usually at least 2 weeks) is required for any patient with atrial fibrillation of more than 2 to 3 days' duration. ■ Select patients carefully; benefits (potential for maintaining sinus rhythm) must outweigh risks. Patients with chronic atrial fibrillation are more likely to revert back to atrial fibrillation after conversion to sinus rhythm. Patients with a QTc interval greater than 440 msec or a serum potassium less than 4.0 mEq/L are at very high risk to develop life-threatening arrhythmias. ■ Patients with a history of CHF may be more susceptible to sustained polymorphic VT. ■ Slightly more effective in atrial flutter than atrial fibrillation. ■ See Drug/Lab Interactions.

Monitor: Obtain weight, baseline vital signs, and ECG before administration. Continuous ECG monitoring during and after infusion indicated to observe for arrhythmias. Watch for QT or QTc prolongation; may cause arrhythmia (torsades de pointes) with or without QT prolongation. ■ Monitor BP and

HR. Bradycardia, a varying HR, and/or hypokalemia may increase risk of arrhythmia. ▪ Arrhythmia occurs most frequently within 40 minutes of completion of infusion but may occur for up to 3 hours after infusion. Monitor ECG for a minimum of 4 hours or until QTc has returned to baseline. Monitor longer if there are any episodes of arrhythmias or if the patient has impaired liver function.

Patient Education: Report promptly any feeling of faintness, difficulty breathing, or pain or stinging along injection site.

Maternal/Child: Category C: benefits must outweigh risks. Caused birth defects and was embryocidal in rats. ▪ Temporarily discontinue breastfeeding. ▪ Safety and effectiveness for use in pediatric patients under 18 years of age not established.

Elderly: No age-related differences observed. Median age in clinical trials was 65 years. ▪ Lower-end initial doses may be indicated; see Dose Adjustments.

DRUG/LAB INTERACTIONS

Should not be given concurrently with **Class Ia antiarrhythmics** (e.g., disopyramide [Norpace], procainamide [Pronestyl], quinidine) **or other Class III antiarrhythmics** (e.g., amiodarone [Nexterone], sotalol [Betapace]). Withhold any of these agents for at least 5 half-lives before ibutilide infusion and for 4 hours after. ▪ Incidence of arrhythmia may be increased with **other drugs that prolong the QT interval** (e.g., phenothiazines [e.g., promethazine (Phenergan)], tricyclic antidepressants [e.g., amitriptyline (Elavil)], tetracyclic antidepressants [e.g., maprotiline (Ludiomil)]). ▪ Monitor **serum digoxin levels** to avoid digoxin toxicity. ▪ Use with **digoxin, beta-blockers, or calcium channel blockers** does not alter safety or effectiveness of ibutilide. However, **sotalol** is a beta-blocker, and its use with ibutilide is restricted because it has Class III antiarrhythmic activity; see first sentence above.

SIDE EFFECTS

Sustained polymorphic VT (1.7%) and nonsustained polymorphic VT (2.7%) can deteriorate into ventricular fibrillation and be fatal. May cause many other arrhythmias (e.g., first-, second-, or third-degree AV block [1.5%], bradycardia [1.2%], bundle branch block [1.9%], nonsustained monomorphic VT [4.9%], prolonged QT segment [1.2%], PVCs [5.1%], tachycardia [2.7%]), CHF (0.5%), headache (3.6%), hypertension (1.2%), hypotension (2%), nausea (1.9%), palpitation (1%).

Overdose: Side effects exaggerated with overdose in humans. Acute overdose in animals resulted in CNS depression, rapid gasping breathing, convulsions.

ANTIDOTE

If proarrhythmias occur, discontinue ibutilide; correct electrolyte abnormalities (e.g., potassium and magnesium). Overdrive cardiac pacing, electrical cardioversion, or defibrillation may be required. Infusions of magnesium sulfate may be helpful. Avoid treatment with antiarrhythmic agents. VT that deteriorates to VF will require immediate defibrillation.

IDARUBICIN HYDROCHLORIDE BBW

(eye-dah-**ROOB**-ih-sin hy-droh-**KLOR**-eyed)

Idamycin PFS, Idarubicin PFS, IDR

Antineoplastic
(anthracycline antibiotic)

pH 5 to 7

USUAL DOSE

Adult acute myeloid leukemia (AML) induction therapy:
Induction: Idarubicin 12 mg/M^2/day for 3 days. Used in combination with cytarabine (Ara-C). Cytarabine 100 mg/M^2/day may be given as a continuous infusion on Days 1 to 7 (daily for 7 days), or alternately the cytarabine may be given as an IV injection of 25 mg/M^2 followed immediately by a continuous infusion of cytarabine 200 mg/M^2/day on Days 1 to 5 (daily for 5 days). See Precautions/Monitor. If unequivocal evidence of leukemia remains after the first course, a second course may be given; see Dose Adjustments. The benefit of an aggressive consolidation and maintenance program in prolonging the duration of remissions and survival has not been proven. See prescribing information for regimens used in clinical trials.

DOSE ADJUSTMENTS

Delay second course until full recovery if severe mucositis has occurred and reduce dose by 25%. ■ Consider dose reductions in impaired liver and kidney function based on bilirubin and/or creatinine levels above the normal range. Do not administer if bilirubin is above 5 mg/dL. In one Phase III clinical trial, patients with bilirubin levels between 2.6 and 5 mg/dL received a 50% reduction in dose.

DILUTION

Specific techniques required (see Precautions). Idamycin PFS is a liquid formulation; each 5 mg of powdered idamycin must be reconstituted with 5 mL of nonbacteriostatic NS for injection (1 mg/mL). Use extreme caution inserting the needle; vial contents are under negative pressure. Avoid any possibility of inhalation from aerosol or any skin contamination.
Filters: No data available from manufacturer.
Storage: PFS product must be refrigerated. Reconstituted idamycin is stable for 7 days under refrigeration (2° to 8° C [36° to 46° F]) or 3 days (72 hours) at room temperature (15° to 30° C [59° to 86° F]). Discard unused solution appropriately.

COMPATIBILITY

Consider any drug NOT listed as compatible to be INCOMPATIBLE until consulting a pharmacist; specific conditions may apply.
Manufacturer states, "Should not be mixed with other drugs unless specific **compatibility** data are available," and lists as **incompatible** with heparin. Prolonged contact with solutions of an alkaline pH (e.g., sodium lactate, sodium bicarbonate) will result in degradation of idarubicin.
One source suggests the following **compatibilities:**
Y-site: Amifostine (Ethyol), amikacin (Amikin), aztreonam (Azactam), cladribine (Leustatin), cyclophosphamide (Cytoxan), cytarabine (ARA-C), diphenhydramine (Benadryl), droperidol (Inapsine), erythromycin (Erythrocin), etoposide phosphate (Etopophos), filgrastim (Neupogen), gemcitabine (Gemzar), granisetron (Kytril), imipenem-cilastatin (Primaxin), magnesium sulfate, mannitol, melphalan (Alkeran), metoclopramide

(Reglan), potassium chloride (KCl), ranitidine (Zantac), sargramostim (Leukine), thiotepa, vinorelbine (Navelbine).

RATE OF ADMINISTRATION
A single dose of properly diluted medication over 10 to 15 minutes through Y-tube or three-way stopcock of a free-flowing infusion of D5W or NS.

ACTIONS
A highly toxic, synthetic, antibiotic, antineoplastic agent. An analog of daunorubicin. Rapidly distributed; has an increased rate of cellular uptake compared to other anthracyclines. It inhibits synthesis of DNA and interacts with the enzyme topoisomerase II. Results in a greater number of remissions and longer survival than previous protocols (daunorubicin and cytarabine). It is severely immunosuppressive. Extensive extrahepatic metabolism. Half-life averages 20 to 22 hours. Slowly excreted in bile and urine.

INDICATIONS AND USES
Treatment of acute myeloid leukemia (AML) in adults in combination with other approved antileukemic drugs.
Unlabeled uses: Treatment of acute lymphoblastic leukemia in pediatric patients; see Maternal/Child.

CONTRAINDICATIONS
Not absolute; pre-existing bone marrow suppression, impaired cardiac function, pre-existing infection; see Precautions/Monitor. ▪ Do not administer if bilirubin above 5 mg/dL.

PRECAUTIONS
Follow guidelines for handling cytotoxic agents. See Appendix A, p. 1429. ▪ Administered by or under the direction of the physician specialist, with facilities for monitoring the patient and responding to any medical emergency. ▪ For IV use only. Do not give IM or SC. ▪ Use extreme caution in pre-existing drug-induced bone marrow suppression, existing heart disease, previous treatment with other anthracyclines (e.g., daunorubicin), other cardiotoxic agents (e.g., bleomycin), or radiation therapy encompassing the heart. ▪ Myocardial toxicity may cause potentially fatal acute congestive heart failure, acute life-threatening arrhythmias, or other cardiomyopathies. Cardiac toxicity is more common in patients who have received prior anthracyclines (e.g., doxorubicin) or who have pre-existing cardiac disease. ▪ May cause severe myelosuppression. ▪ Use with caution in patients with hepatic or renal dysfunction. Metabolism and excretion of idarubicin may be impaired; see Dose Adjustments.
Monitor: Determine absolute patency of vein. A stinging or burning sensation indicates extravasation, but extravasation may occur without stinging or burning; severe cellulitis and tissue necrosis can occur with extravasation. Discontinue injection; use another vein. ▪ Monitoring of WBCs, RBCs, platelet count, liver function, kidney function, ECG, chest x-ray, echocardiography, and systolic ejection fraction indicated before and during therapy. ▪ Severe myelosuppression occurs with effective therapeutic doses. Observe closely for all signs of infection or bleeding. ▪ Monitor for thrombocytopenia (platelet count less than 50,000/mm^3). Initiate precautions to prevent excessive bleeding (e.g., inspect IV sites, skin, and mucous membranes; use extreme care during invasive procedures; test urine, emesis, stool, and secretions for occult blood). ▪ Prophylactic antibiotics may be indicated pending results of C/S in a febrile neutropenic patient. ▪ Prophylactic antiemetics may reduce nausea and vomiting and increase

patient comfort. ▪ Monitor uric acid levels; maintain hydration; allopurinol and urine alkalinization may be indicated. ▪ See Precautions.

Patient Education: Nonhormonal birth control recommended. ▪ Report IV site burning or stinging promptly. ▪ See Appendix D, p. 1434.

Maternal/Child: Category D: avoid pregnancy. May produce teratogenic effects on the fetus. Contraceptive measures indicated during childbearing years. ▪ Discontinue breast-feeding before taking idarubicin. ▪ Safety and efficacy for use in pediatric patients not established but has been used; consult literature.

Elderly: Cardiotoxicity or myelotoxicity may be more severe. Patients over 60 years of age who were undergoing induction experienced CHF, serious arrhythmias, chest pain, myocardial infarction, and asymptomatic declines in left ventricular ejection fraction more frequently than younger patients. ▪ Monitor renal, hepatic, and hematologic functions closely.

DRUG/LAB INTERACTIONS

Bone marrow toxicity is additive with **other chemotherapeutic agents.** ▪ Risk of cardiotoxicity increased in patients previously treated with maximum cumulative doses of **other anthracyclines** (e.g., doxorubicin [Adriamycin], mitoxantrone [Novantrone]) **and/or radiation encompassing the heart.** ▪ Leukopenic and/or thrombocytopenic effects may be increased with **drugs that cause blood dyscrasias** (e.g., anticonvulsants [e.g., carbamazepine (Tegretol), phenytoin (Dilantin)], NSAIDs [e.g., ibuprofen (Advil, Motrin), naproxen (Aleve, Naprosyn)]). Adjust dose based on differential and platelet count. ▪ Do not administer **live virus vaccines** to patients receiving antineoplastic drugs. ▪ See Precautions/Monitor.

SIDE EFFECTS

Acute congestive heart failure, alopecia (reversible), arrhythmias, bone marrow suppression (marked with average doses), cramping, decrease in systolic ejection fraction, depressed QRS voltage, diarrhea, erythema and tissue necrosis (if extravasation occurs), fever, headache, hemorrhage (severe), hepatic function changes, infection, mucositis, myocarditis, nausea, pericarditis, renal function changes, seizures, skin rash, urticaria (local), vomiting.

ANTIDOTE

Most side effects will be tolerated or treated symptomatically. Keep physician informed. Close monitoring of bone marrow, ECG, chest x-ray, echocardiography, and systolic ejection fraction may prevent most serious and potentially fatal side effects. There is no specific antidote, but adequate supportive care including platelet transfusions, antibiotics, and symptomatic treatment of mucositis is required. For extravasation, elevate the extremity and apply intermittent ice packs over the area immediately and 4 times a day for ½ hour. Continue for 3 days. Consider aspiration of as much infiltrated drug as possible, flooding of the site with NS, and injection of hydrocortisone sodium succinate (Solu-Cortef) throughout extravasated tissue. Use a 27- or 25-gauge needle. Site should be observed promptly by a reconstructive surgeon. If ulceration begins or there is severe persistent pain at the site, early wide excision of the involved area will be considered. Hemodialysis or peritoneal dialysis probably not effective in overdose.

IFOSFAMIDE BBW

(eye-**FOS**-fah-myd)

Ifex/Mesnex Kit, Ifosfamide/Mesna Kit

Antineoplastic
(alkylating agent/nitrogen mustard)

pH 6

USUAL DOSE

Specific testing recommended before each dose; see Monitor.
1.2 Gm/M^2/day for 5 consecutive days. Repeat every 3 weeks as hematologic recovery permits. To initiate this protocol, platelets must be above 100,000/mm^3 and WBCs must be above 4,000/mm^3. To prevent hemorrhagic cystitis, a protector such as mesna should be administered with every dose. Ifosfamide dose has been mixed with the initial mesna dose each day in the same solution. Appears to be **compatible.**

DOSE ADJUSTMENTS

Reduced dose may be required for adrenalectomized patients and in renal or hepatic impairment. Adequate data not available. ■ Severe myelosuppression is frequent, especially when ifosfamide is given with other chemotherapeutic agents. Dose adjustments of all agents may be required.

DILUTION

Specific techniques required; see Precautions. Each 1 Gm must be diluted with 20 mL SW or bacteriostatic water for injection (parabens or benzyl alcohol preserved only). Shake solution to dissolve. May be further diluted with D5W, NS, LR, or SW for injection. 1 Gm in 20 mL equals 50 mg/mL; 1 Gm in 50 mL equals 20 mg/mL; 1 Gm in 200 mL equals 5 mg/mL (additional diluent recommended by some researchers to reduce side effects). Available in a kit containing ifosfamide and mesna.

Filters: Studies measured potency of ifosfamide in combination with mesna through a 5-micron filter. No significant drug loss for ifosfamide; mesna was not measured.

Storage: Store dry powder at room temperature, never above 40° C (104° F). Diluted solution may be stored at room temperature up to 1 week except for solutions prepared with SW for injection without preservatives. These must be refrigerated and used within 6 hours.

COMPATIBILITY

(Underline Indicates Conflicting Compatibility Information)

Consider any drug NOT listed as compatible to be INCOMPATIBLE until consulting a pharmacist; specific conditions may apply.

One source suggests the following **compatibilities:**

Additive: Carboplatin (Paraplatin), cisplatin (Platinol), epirubicin (Ellence), etoposide (VePesid), fluorouracil (5-FU), mesna (Mesnex).

Y-site: Allopurinol (Aloprim), amifostine (Ethyol), amphotericin B cholesteryl (Amphotec), anidulafungin (Eraxis), aztreonam (Azactam), caspofungin (Cancidas), doripenem (Doribax), doxorubicin liposomal (Doxil), etoposide phosphate (Etopophos), filgrastim (Neupogen), fludarabine (Fludara), gallium nitrate (Ganite), gemcitabine (Gemzar), granisetron (Kytril), linezolid (Zyvox), melphalan (Alkeran), ondansetron (Zofran), oxaliplatin (Eloxatin), paclitaxel (Taxol), palonosetron (Aloxi), pemetrexed (Alimta), piperacillin/tazobactam (Zosyn), propofol (Diprivan), sargramostim (Leukine), sodium bicarbonate, teniposide (Vumon), thiotepa, topotecan (Hycamtin), vinorelbine (Navelbine).

RATE OF ADMINISTRATION

A single dose over a minimum of 30 minutes as an infusion. Extend administration time based on amount of diluent and patient condition.

ACTIONS

An alkylating agent. A synthetic analog of cyclophosphamide chemically related to the nitrogen mustard group. An inert compound; metabolic activation by microsomal liver enzymes is required to produce biologically active metabolites. These alkylated metabolites interact with DNA to effect regression in the size of malignant tumors. Elimination half-life for a usual dose is 7 to 15 hours. Larger doses extend half-life. Extensively metabolized (considerable individual variation); this drug or its metabolites are excreted in urine. Secreted in breast milk.

INDICATIONS AND USES

In combination with other specific antineoplastic agents to suppress or retard neoplastic growth in germ cell testicular cancer. Usually used after other chemotherapy protocols have failed.

Unlabeled uses: Lung, breast, ovarian, pancreatic, and gastric cancer; sarcomas; acute leukemias (except acute myelogenous); malignant lymphomas.

CONTRAINDICATIONS

Hypersensitivity to ifosfamide; patients with severely depressed bone marrow function.

PRECAUTIONS

Follow guidelines for handling cytotoxic agents. See Appendix A, p. 1429. ▪ Usually administered by or under the direction of the physician specialist. ▪ Use caution in impaired renal function; may increase CNS toxicity. Use caution in patients with compromised bone marrow reserve (e.g., leukopenia, granulocytopenia, extensive bone marrow metastases, prior radiation therapy, treatment with other cytotoxic agents) and patients with severe hepatic or renal disease. ▪ Severe myelosuppression has been reported. ▪ Urotoxic side effects (hemorrhagic cystitis) and CNS toxicities (e.g., confusion, coma) have also been reported. ▪ May interfere with normal wound healing. Consider waiting 5 to 7 days or more after a major surgical procedure before beginning treatment.

Monitor: Urinalysis before each dose recommended. Withhold drug if RBCs in urine exceed 10 per high-powered field. Reinstitute after complete resolution. Mesna given concurrently should prevent hemorrhagic cystitis. ▪ Differential WBC, platelet count, and hemoglobin are recommended before each daily dose and as clinically indicated. WBC count must be above $2,000/mm^3$ and platelet count above $50,000/mm^3$. ▪ Observe constantly for signs of infection (e.g., fever, sore throat, tiredness) or unusual bleeding or bruising. ▪ Monitor for thrombocytopenia (platelet count less than $50,000/mm^3$). Initiate precautions to prevent excessive bleeding (e.g., inspect IV sites, skin, and mucous membranes; use extreme care during invasive procedures; test urine, emesis, stool, and secretions for occult blood). ▪ Prophylactic antibiotics may be indicated pending results of C/S in a febrile neutropenic patient. ▪ Adequate hydration required; encourage fluid intake (minimum of 2 L/day) and frequent voiding to prevent cystitis. Bladder irrigation with acetylcysteine (2,000 mL/day) has also been used to prevent hematuria. ▪ Prophylactic administration of antiemetics recommended.

Patient Education: Nonhormonal birth control recommended. ▪ See Appendix D, p. 1434.

Maternal/Child: Category D: avoid pregnancy. Embryotoxic and teratogenic to the fetus. ▪ Discontinue breast-feeding. ▪ Safety and effectiveness for use in pediatric patients not established.

Elderly: Monitor renal, hepatic, and hematologic functions closely.

DRUG/LAB INTERACTIONS
See Dose Adjustments. ▪ Because it is a synthetic analog of cyclophosphamide, ifosfamide may share similar interactions with numerous drugs, including **allopurinol, antidiabetics, barbiturates, chloramphenicol, corticosteroids, succinylcholine, thiazide diuretics, and other alkylating agents** to produce potentially serious reactions. ▪ Do not administer **live virus vaccine** to patients receiving antineoplastic drugs.

SIDE EFFECTS
Hematuria, hemorrhagic cystitis, and bone marrow suppression are dose-limiting side effects. Alopecia, anorexia, confusion, constipation, diarrhea, depressive psychosis with hallucinations, nausea, somnolence, and vomiting occur frequently. Cardiotoxicity, coagulopathy, coma, cranial nerve dysfunction, dermatitis, dizziness, disorientation, fatigue, fever of unknown origin, hematuria, hemorrhagic cystitis, hypersensitivity reactions, hypertension, hypotension, infection, liver dysfunction, leukopenia, malaise, neutropenia, phlebitis, polyneuropathy, pulmonary symptoms, thrombocytopenia, or seizures may occur.

ANTIDOTE
Minor side effects will be treated symptomatically if necessary. Discontinue ifosfamide and notify physician immediately if hematuria, hemorrhagic cystitis, confusion, coma, WBC below 2,000/mm^3, or platelets below 50,000/mm^3 occur. Administration of whole blood products (e.g., packed RBCs, platelets, leukocytes) and/or blood modifiers (e.g., darbepoetin alfa [Aranesp], epoetin alfa [Epogen], filgrastim [Neupogen], pegfilgrastim [Neulasta], sargramostim [Leukine], oprelvekin [Neumega]) may be indicated to treat bone marrow suppression. There is no specific antidote. Supportive therapy as indicated will help sustain the patient in toxicity. May respond to hemodialysis.

IMIGLUCERASE ▪ VELAGLUCERASE ALFA

(em-ee-**GLUE**-sir-ace) ▪
(vel-a-**GLOO**-ser-ase **AL**-fa)

**Enzyme replenisher
(glucocerebrosidase)**

Cerezyme ▪ **VPRIV**

Imiglucerase pH 6.1

USUAL DOSE

Imiglucerase: *Adults and pediatric patients over 2 years of age:* Individualized to each patient based on the severity of illness and patient response. Initial doses range from 2.5 units/kg 3 times a week to 60 units/kg every 2 weeks. Imiglucerase should be given at least every 4 weeks. Patients with very severe Gaucher disease may require higher-range initial doses and/or increased frequency because they have accumulated more lipid throughout their bodies, requiring more enzyme to remove the excess stored lipid and bring their disease under control. See Maternal/Child.

Velaglucerase alfa: *Adult and pediatric patients over 4 years of age:* 60 units/kg every other week. Patients currently being treated with a stable dose of imiglucerase may be switched to velaglucerase alfa at that same dose.

DOSE ADJUSTMENTS

Both preparations: Dose may increase or decrease based on achievement of each patient's therapeutic goals. Optimal goal is to establish the lowest dose that is effective in maintaining control of the disease and preventing recurrence of symptoms for each patient. ▪ Consider potential co-morbid conditions and dose the elderly cautiously.

Imiglucerase: To utilize each bottle fully and reduce waste, a single dose may be increased or decreased slightly as long as the total monthly dose remains unaltered.

Velaglucerase alfa: Clinical studies have evaluated doses ranging from 15 units/kg to 60 units/kg every other week.

DILUTION

Both preparations: Available in 200-unit and 400-unit vials.

Weight in kg × dose/kg desired ÷ 200 or 400 (units/vial) = # of vials required

A 60-kg man requiring 60 units/kg would require 3,600 units. Number of vials required would be 18 vials at 200 units/vial or 9 vials at 400 units/vial. After patient is weighed and appropriate dose is calculated, remove sufficient vials from refrigerator.

Imiglucerase: Adjust number of vials up or down within monthly dose requirement to fully utilize each vial. Each 200-unit vial must be reconstituted with 5.1 mL of SW. Each 400-unit vial must be reconstituted with 10.2 mL of SW. Both equal 40 units/mL. Gently swirl to mix the solution. *Do not shake.* Let stand for several minutes to allow product to dissolve and bubbles to dissipate. Withdraw exactly 5 mL from the 200-unit vial or 10 mL from the 400-unit vial. A total dose must be further diluted with NS to a volume of 100 to 200 mL. Do not use if discolored or opaque or if particulate matter is present. After dilution, slight flocculation (thin translucent fibers) may occur.

Velaglucerase alfa: Reconstitute each 200-unit vial with 2.2 mL SW and each 400-unit vial with 4.3 mL SW. Both equal 100 unit/mL. Mix gently. *Do not shake.* Should be clear to slightly opalescent. Do not use if discolored or opaque or if particulate matter is present. Withdraw the calculated volume of drug from vials. A total dose must be further diluted in 100 mL of NS. Mix gently. *Do not shake.*

Filters: *Both preparations:* Administration through a low–protein binding, 0.2-micron in-line filter is recommended.

Storage: *Imiglucerase:* Refrigerate before use. Do not use after expiration date on bottle. Return of unsuitable vials (reconstituted, before reconstitution, or expired) may be authorized; contact manufacturer. Contains no preservative; do not store opened vials for future use. Should be promptly diluted after reconstitution but has been shown to be stable after reconstitution for up to 12 hours at RT or under refrigeration. Diluted solutions stable for up to 24 hours under refrigeration.

Velaglucerase alfa: Refrigerate at 2° to 8° C (36° to 46° F) in carton before use. Do not use after expiration date on vial. Protect from light; do not freeze. Immediate use is preferred, but reconstituted and fully diluted solutions are stable for up to 24 hours if refrigerated and protected from light. Do not freeze. Complete infusion within 24 hours of reconstitution. For single use only; discard unused solution.

COMPATIBILITY

Imiglucerase: Specific information not available. Consider specific use; consult pharmacist.

Velaglucerase alfa: Manufacturer states, "Should not be infused with other products in the same infusion tubing." **Compatibility** studies have not been done.

RATE OF ADMINISTRATION

Both preparations: Use of an in-line, low–protein binding, 0.2-micron filter is recommended. Use of an infusion pump is helpful. Flush the IV line with NS at the end of the infusion to ensure the total dose is received.

Imiglucerase: A single dose equally distributed over 1 to 2 hours.

Velaglucerase alfa: A single dose equally distributed over 60 minutes.

ACTIONS

Imiglucerase is an analog of the human enzyme beta-glucocerebrosidase produced by recombinant DNA technology. **Velaglucerase alfa** is produced by gene activation technology in a human fibroblast cell line. Both have the same amino acid sequence as the naturally occurring human enzyme glucocerebrosidase. Gaucher disease is characterized by a functional deficiency in beta-glucocerebrosidase enzymatic activity and the resultant accumulation of lipid glucocerebroside in tissue macrophages (Gaucher cells). These cells are found in the liver, spleen, bone marrow, and occasionally in the lung, kidney, and intestine. These agents act like glucocerebrosidase, catalyzing the hydrolysis of glucocerebroside to glucose and ceramide. Effective in controlling and actually reversing disease symptoms. Increase in appetite and energy level and improvement in hemoglobin are often the first observable effects and may occur in 2 to 4 months. Cachexia and wasting in pediatric patients are reduced. Within 6 months splenomegaly and hepatomegaly are significantly reduced, and hemoglobin, hematocrit, erythrocyte, and platelet counts improved. Replenishment of bone marrow and improving mineralization of bone may take several years.

INDICATIONS AND USES

Imiglucerase: Long-term enzyme replacement therapy for pediatric and adult patients with confirmed diagnosis of Type I Gaucher disease, which results in one or more of the following conditions: anemia, thrombocytopenia, bone disease, hepatomegaly, or splenomegaly.

Velaglucerase alfa: Long-term enzyme replacement therapy for pediatric and adult patients with Type 1 Gaucher disease.

CONTRAINDICATIONS

Imiglucerase: None known. Reevaluate if there is significant clinical evidence of hypersensitivity to imiglucerase.

Velaglucerase alfa: Manufacturer states, "None."

PRECAUTIONS

Both preparations: Hypersensitivity and infusion reactions have been reported. Administer further enzyme replacement therapy treatment with caution in patients who have exhibited symptoms of hypersensitivity to other enzyme replacement therapy; see Antidote. ▪ Effective only via IV route. ▪ Should be used under the direction of a physician knowledgeable in the management of Gaucher disease. Administer in a facility with adequate diagnostic and treatment facilities to monitor the patient and respond to any medical emergency.

Imiglucerase: A recombinant product; risk of transmission of any bacterial, mycoplasmal, fungal, or viral agent is remote. ▪ Approximately 15% of patients have developed IgG antibodies. Most patients who develop antibodies to imiglucerase do so within 12 months of treatment. Patients with antibodies to imiglucerase are at increased risk for developing hypersensitivity reactions. Monitor periodically for IgG antibody formation during the first year of therapy. Patients who develop hypersensitivity reactions to imiglucerase may be premedicated (see Antidote) or consideration may be given to treatment with velaglucerase alfa (VPRIV). Most patients who previously received alglucerase (Ceredase) have been transferred to imiglucerase and will remain on imiglucerase or velaglucerase alfa unless a severe hypersensitivity reaction develops. Alglucerase availability is restricted to patients with severe hypersensitivity reactions who are not responsive to premedication. ▪ Pulmonary hypertension and pneumonia have been reported. They are known complications of Gaucher disease and have been observed in these patients whether or not they are receiving imiglucerase. Evaluate patients with respiratory symptoms in the absence of fever for the presence of pulmonary hypertension.

Velaglucerase alfa: Infusion reactions have occurred usually during the first 6 months of treatment and occurred less frequently with time. Generally mild (e.g., asthenia, dizziness, fatigue, fever, headache, hypertension, hypotension, nausea). Development of IgG antibodies has been rare but is possible.

Monitor: Evaluate hemoglobin, hematocrit, platelets, WBC, acid phosphatase (AP), plasma glucocerebroside, liver and/or spleen size, and bone changes before and during therapy. Frequency determined by patient response; more frequent when determining response to initial dose and when dose is being adjusted. Blood tests will be done more frequently because anemia is the first symptom to improve. ▪ Monitor weight before each dose (used to calculate dose) and monitor vital signs. ▪ Observe for S/S of a hypersensitivity reaction; see Antidote. ▪ MRI may be used to evaluate liver and spleen. ▪ Standard x-rays provide adequate evaluation of bone changes. ▪ Observe patient closely for signs of improvement (e.g., increased energy, reduced bleeding tendency, reduction in size of liver and/or spleen, reduced joint swelling, reduced bone pain). ▪ Continue to monitor for antibodies in patients who have developed an immune response to either alglucerase or imiglucerase and are transferred to velaglucerase alfa. ▪ See Precautions.

Patient Education: Treatment required for life. ▪ Promptly report S/S of a hypersensitivity or infusion reaction (e.g., chills, dizziness, fatigue, fever, headache, itching, nausea, rash, shortness of breath, wheezing).

Maternal/Child: *Imiglucerase:* Category C: use in pregnancy only if potential benefit justifies the risk. ▪ Has been used in pediatric patients under 2 years of age, but safety and effectiveness have not been established.

Velaglucerase alfa: Category B: use in pregnancy only if clearly needed.

Both preparations: Safety for use during breast-feeding not established. Not known if imiglucerase or velaglucerase are secreted in breast milk.

Elderly: *Imiglucerase:* Specific information not available in product information.

Velaglucerase alfa: Numbers in clinical studies insufficient to determine if the elderly respond differently from younger subjects; see Dose Adjustments.

DRUG/LAB INTERACTIONS
None indicated. Specific information not available.

SIDE EFFECTS

Imiglucerase: Headache, pruritus, and rash were most commonly reported. In addition, abdominal discomfort; backache; burning, discomfort, and pruritus at injection site; chills; diarrhea; dizziness; fatigue; fever; hypotension (mild); nausea; peripheral edema (transient); swelling or sterile abscess at venipuncture site; and tachycardia were reported.

Pediatric patients 2 to 12 years: Coughing, dyspnea, fever, flushing, nausea, and vomiting were most commonly reported in this age-group.

Velaglucerase alfa: Adults: Infusion-related reactions were the most common, and hypersensitivity reactions were the most serious. Other reported side effects include abdominal pain, asthenia, back pain, dizziness, fatigue, fever, headache, joint pain, nausea, prolonged aPTT, and upper respiratory infections.

Pediatric patients: Adverse reactions similar to adults; however, fever, prolonged aPTT, rash, and upper respiratory infections were seen more commonly in pediatric patients.

Both preparations: A protein immune reaction may develop. Side effects may improve with continued therapy because antibody levels decrease. Hypersensitivity reactions (e.g., anaphylaxis, angioedema, chest discomfort, cyanosis, flushing, hypotension, pruritus, rash, respiratory symptoms, urticaria) have occurred.

ANTIDOTE

Keep physician informed of side effects; may be treated symptomatically if indicated. Based on the severity of the reaction, temporarily interrupt or discontinue infusion for clinical evidence of hypersensitivity or an infusion reaction. Patients have successfully continued therapy after mild hypersensitivity or infusion reactions with pretreatment with antipyretics, antihistamines (e.g., diphenhydramine [Benadryl]), and/or corticosteroids (e.g., dexamethasone [Decadron]) and/or a reduction in rate of administration. Treat anaphylaxis as necessary.

IMIPENEM-CILASTATIN
(em-ee-**PEN**-em sigh-lah-**STAT**-in)

Primaxin

**Antibacterial
(carbapenem)**

pH 6.5 to 8.5

USUAL DOSE

Range is from 250 mg to 1 Gm every 6 to 8 hours. Dose based on severity of disease, susceptibility of pathogens, condition of the patient, age, weight, and CrCl. Adult doses in the following chart are limited to patients with a CrCl equal to or greater than 71 mL/min/1.73 M^2 and a body weight equal to or greater than 70 kg; see Dose Adjustments. Because of high antimicrobial activity, do not exceed the lower of 50 mg/kg/24 hr or 4 Gm/24 hr in adult or pediatric patients. Continue for at least 2 days after all symptoms of infection subside.

Imipenem-Cilastatin Dosing Guidelines				
Type or Severity of Infection	Fully Susceptible Organisms	Total Daily Dose	Moderately Susceptible Organisms	Total Daily Dose
Mild	250 mg q 6 hr	1 Gm	500 mg q 6 hr	2 Gm
Moderate	500 mg q 8 hr or 500 mg q 6 hr	1.5 Gm 2 Gm	500 mg q 6 hr or 1 Gm q 8 hr	2 Gm 3 Gm
Severe/life-threatening	500 mg q 6 hr	2 Gm	1 Gm q 8 hr or 1 Gm q 6 hr	3 Gm 4 Gm
Uncomplicated UTI	250 mg q 6 hr	1 Gm	250 mg q 6 hr	1 Gm
Complicated UTI	500 mg q 6 hr	2 Gm	500 mg q 6 hr	2 Gm

Adult and pediatric patients over 12 years of age with cystic fibrosis and normal renal function: Higher doses up to 90 mg/kg/day have been used. Do not exceed 4 Gm/24 hr.

PEDIATRIC DOSE

Not recommended for use in pediatric patients with CNS infections because of the risk of seizures, or in pediatric patients weighing less than 30 kg with impaired renal function (no data available). Because of high antimicrobial activity, do not exceed the lower of 50 mg/kg/24 hr or 4 Gm/24 hr in adult or pediatric patients.

Infants 3 months of age or less, weighing 1,500 Gm or more: For non-CNS infections:

Less than 1 week of age: 25 mg/kg every 12 hours.

1 to 4 weeks of age: 25 mg/kg every 8 hours.

4 weeks to 3 months of age: 25 mg/kg every 6 hours.

Premature infants weighing from 670 to 1,890 Gm in the first week of life were given 20 mg/kg every 12 hours in one study (see package insert).

Infants and other pediatric patients over 3 months of age: For non-CNS infections: 15 to 25 mg/kg/dose every 6 hours. See statements in Usual

Dose. Maximum dose is 2 Gm/day for treatment of infections caused by fully susceptible organisms and 4 Gm/day for moderately susceptible organisms.

DOSE ADJUSTMENTS
Dose adjustments are extensive and required for all patients weighing less than 70 kg, as well as all patients with a CrCl less than 71 mL/min/ 1.73 M^2. Dose adjustments also vary based on total daily dose required (e.g., 1, 1.5, 2, 3, or 4 Gm). See charts in package insert. ▪ Reduced doses may be required in the elderly based on weight and/or decreased renal function. ▪ Cleared by hemodialysis; administer after hemodialysis and at 12-hour intervals thereafter. ▪ See Precautions/Monitor and Drug/Lab Interactions.

DILUTION
Reconstitute each single dose with 10 mL of **compatible** infusion solutions (e.g., D5W, D10W, NS [see chart on inside back cover or literature]); also **compatible** in D5W with 0.15% KCl and mannitol 5% and 10%. Shake well and transfer the resulting suspension to 100 mL of the same infusion solution. Rinse vial with an additional 10 mL of infusion solution to ensure complete transfer of vial contents to the infusion solution. Agitate until clear. Also available in ADD-Vantage vials for use with ADD-Vantage infusion containers.

Neonatal dilution: Use preservative-free solutions for reconstitution of neonatal doses.

Filters: Manufacturer's data limited; indicates that use of a filter system when withdrawing the suspension from the vial would probably result in filter clogging and decrease the available antibiotic. An in-house study documented **compatibility** of the final diluted solution with a 0.22-micron in-line filter.

Storage: Store dry powder below 25° C (77° F). Diluted solutions are stable at room temperature for 4 hours after preparation or 24 hours if refrigerated. Do not freeze.

COMPATIBILITY   (Underline Indicates Conflicting Compatibility Information)
Consider any drug NOT listed as compatible to be INCOMPATIBLE until consulting a pharmacist; specific conditions may apply.
Manufacturer states, "Should not be mixed with or physically added to other antibiotics." See Drug/Lab Interactions.

One source suggests the following **compatibilities:**
Y-site: Acyclovir (Zovirax), amifostine (Ethyol), <u>anidulafungin (Eraxis)</u>, aztreonam (Azactam), <u>caspofungin (Cancidas)</u>, <u>cefepime (Maxipime)</u>, cisatracurium (Nimbex), diltiazem (Cardizem), docetaxel (Taxotere), famotidine (Pepcid IV), <u>filgrastim (Neupogen)</u>, fludarabine (Fludara), foscarnet (Foscavir), granisetron (Kytril), idarubicin (Idamycin), insulin (regular), linezolid (Zyvox), melphalan (Alkeran), methotrexate, ondansetron (Zofran), propofol (Diprivan), remifentanil (Ultiva), tacrolimus (Prograf), teniposide (Vumon), thiotepa, tigecycline (Tygacil), vasopressin, vinorelbine (Navelbine), zidovudine (AZT, Retrovir).

RATE OF ADMINISTRATION
Intermittent IV: Each 500 mg or fraction thereof over 20 to 30 minutes. Doses greater than 500 mg should be infused over 40 to 60 minutes. Slow infusion rate if patient develops nausea and vomiting, dizziness, hypotension, or sweating. May be given through Y-tube or three-way stopcock of infusion set.

ACTIONS

A potent broad-spectrum antibacterial agent. Imipenem is a carbapenem antibiotic; cilastatin inhibits the kidney enzyme responsible for the metabolism of imipenem. Both components are present in equal amounts. Bactericidal to many gram-negative, gram-positive, and anaerobic organisms. Bactericidal activity results from the inhibition of bacterial wall synthesis. Effective against many otherwise resistant organisms. Has a high degree of stability in the presence of beta-lactamases produced by gram-negative and gram-positive bacteria. Rapidly and widely distributed into many body fluids and tissues. Metabolized in the kidneys. Half-life is approximately 1 hour. Excreted in the urine. May cross the placental barrier.

INDICATIONS AND USES

Treatment of serious lower respiratory tract, urinary tract, skin and skin structure, bone and joint, gynecologic, intra-abdominal, and polymicrobic infections; bacterial septicemia, and endocarditis. Most effective against specific organisms (see literature).

Unlabeled uses: Treatment of febrile neutropenia and melioidosis (a rare infection in humans and animals).

CONTRAINDICATIONS

Known sensitivity to any component of this product. ▪ See Maternal/Child and Precautions.

PRECAUTIONS

Specific sensitivity studies are indicated to determine susceptibility of the causative organism to imipenem-cilastatin. ▪ To reduce the development of drug-resistant bacteria and maintain its effectiveness, imipenem-cilastatin should be used to treat or prevent only those infections proven or strongly suspected to be caused by bacteria. ▪ Serious and occasionally fatal hypersensitivity reactions have been reported in patients receiving therapy with beta-lactams (e.g., carbapenems, cephalosporins, penicillins). More likely in patients with a history of sensitivity to multiple allergens; obtain a careful history. Cross-sensitivity is possible. ▪ Avoid prolonged use of drug; superinfection caused by overgrowth of nonsusceptible organisms may result. ▪ CNS adverse effects, including confusional states, myoclonic activity, and seizures, have been reported. Incidence increases with higher doses, compromised renal function, or pre-existing CNS disorders. ▪ Not recommended in patients with a CrCl less than 5 mL/min/1.73 M^2 unless hemodialysis is instituted within 48 hours. ▪ For patients on hemodialysis, benefits of use must outweigh risk of seizures. ▪ *Clostridium difficile*–associated diarrhea (CDAD) has been reported. May range from mild diarrhea to fatal colitis. Consider in patients who present with diarrhea during or after treatment with imipenem-cilastatin. ▪ Safety and effectiveness for use in meningitis not established. ▪ Clinical improvement has been observed in patients with cystic fibrosis, COPD, and lower respiratory tract infections caused by *Pseudomonas aeruginosa;* however, effective bacterial eradication may not occur. ▪ See Maternal/Child and Drug/Lab Interactions.

Monitor: May cause thrombophlebitis. Use small needles and large veins, and rotate infusion sites. ▪ Electrolyte imbalance and cardiac irregularities resulting from sodium content are possible. Contains 3.2 mEq of sodium/Gm. ▪ Monitor renal, hepatic, and hemopoietic systems in prolonged therapy. ▪ Some strains of *Pseudomonas aeruginosa* may develop resistance fairly rapidly during treatment. Periodic susceptibility testing should be done when clinically indicated. ▪ See Drug/Lab Interactions. **Patient Education:** Promptly report diarrhea or bloody stools that occur during treatment or up to several months after an antibiotic has been discontinued; may indicate CDAD and require treatment. ▪ Patients with a history of seizures should review medication profile with physician before taking imipenem; see Drug/Lab Interactions.

Maternal/Child: Category C: use only if potential benefit outweighs potential risk during pregnancy and breast-feeding.

Elderly: Consider weight and age-related renal impairment. See Dose Adjustments. ▪ Response similar to that seen in younger patients; however, greater sensitivity in the elderly cannot be ruled out.

DRUG/LAB INTERACTIONS

Carbapenems may reduce serum **valproic acid** concentrations to subtherapeutic levels, resulting in loss of seizure control. Monitor valproic acid levels. Consider alternative antibacterial therapy. If administration of imipenem is necessary, supplemental anticonvulsant therapy should be considered. ▪ May be used concomitantly with **aminoglycosides and other antibiotics,** but these drugs must never be mixed in the same infusion or given concurrently. ▪ Use with **ganciclovir** (Cytovene) may cause generalized seizures. Use only if benefit outweighs risk. ▪ Half-life and plasma levels slightly increased by **probenecid.** Avoid concurrent use. ▪ Concurrent use with **cyclosporine** (Sandimmune) may decrease cyclosporine metabolism. Elevated cyclosporine levels and neurotoxicity (e.g., agitation, confusion, tremor) have been reported.

SIDE EFFECTS

Full scope of hypersensitivity reactions including anaphylaxis, pruritus, rash, and urticaria. Abdominal pain; abnormal clotting time; altered CBC and electrolytes; anuria; burning, discomfort, and pain at injection site; CDAD; confusion; diarrhea; dizziness; dyspnea; elevated alkaline phosphotase, AST, ALT, bilirubin, creatinine, BUN, LDH; fever; gastroenteritis; glossitis; headache; heartburn; hemorrhagic colitis; hepatic failure; hepatitis (including fulminant hepatitis); hyperventilation; hypotension; increased salivation; myoclonus; nausea and vomiting; paresthesia; pharyngeal pain; polyarthralgia; polyuria; positive direct Coombs' test; presence of WBCs or RBCs, protein casts, bilirubin, or urobilinogen in urine; seizures; somnolence; thrombophlebitis; tinnitus; tongue papillar hypertrophy; transient hearing loss in the hearing impaired; vertigo; and many others.

ANTIDOTE

Notify physician of any side effects. Discontinue the drug if indicated. Treat hypersensitivity reactions as indicated; may require epinephrine, airway management, oxygen, IV fluids, antihistamines (e.g., diphenhydramine [Benadryl]), corticosteroids (e.g., hydrocortisone sodium succinate [Solu-Cortef]), and pressor amines (e.g., dopamine). Resuscitate as necessary. Begin anticonvulsants if focal tremors, myoclonus, or seizures occur. If symptoms continue, decrease dose or discontinue the drug. Infusion rate reactions (e.g., dizziness, hypotension, N/V, and sweating) may respond to a decrease in rate of infusion. Mild cases of CDAD may respond to discontinuation of the drug. Treat CDAD with fluids, electrolytes, protein supplements, and oral vancomycin (Vancocin) or metronidazole (Flagyl) as indicated. In severe cases, surgical evaluation may be indicated. Hemodialysis may be useful in overdose.

IMMUNE GLOBULIN INTRAVENOUS BBW
(im-**MUNE GLAW**-byoo-lin IV)

Carimune NF, Flebogamma, Gamimune S/D, Gammagard Liquid, Gammagard S/D, Gammar P-IV, Gamunex-C, IGIV, Iveegam EN, Privigen

Immunizing agent
(passive)
Platelet count stimulator
Antibacterial
Antiviral
Antipolyneuropathy agent

pH 4 to 7.2

USUAL DOSE

PRIMARY IMMUNODEFICIENCY (PID) DISEASES

Carimune NF: 200 mg/kg as a single-dose IV infusion. May be repeated monthly if indicated. If adequate IgG levels in the circulation or clinical response not achieved, may be increased to 300 mg/kg, or the 200 mg/kg dose may be given more frequently.

Gammagard S/D: 300 to 600 mg/kg as a single-dose IV infusion every 3 to 4 weeks.

Gammar P-IV: 200 to 400 mg/kg as a single-dose IV infusion every 3 to 4 weeks. Up to 600 mg/kg may be required. High-end doses may be given initially and for several doses at more frequent intervals based on individual patient response and adequate IgG levels. Reduce dose 100 to 200 mg/kg and/or increase interval when therapeutic IgG levels are achieved.

Flebogamma, Gamunex-C: 300 to 600 mg/kg as a single-dose IV infusion every 3 to 4 weeks. Individualize dose and interval based on clinical response. A target serum IgG trough level before the next infusion of at least 5 Gm/L is suggested. Gamunex-C may be given SC for PID at an initial dose 1.37 times the current IV dose in mg/kg. Do not administer SC for ITP patients. Must be given by IV infusion in ITP patients. See prescribing information for individualizing the SC dose, converting from monthly to weekly injections, and increasing the SC dose based on target serum IgG trough level.

Gammagard Liquid: 300 to 600 mg/kg as a single-dose IV infusion every 3 to 4 weeks. Individualize dose and interval based on clinical response.

Iveegam EN: 200 mg/kg/month as a single-dose IV infusion. If adequate IgG levels in the circulation or clinical response are not achieved, may be increased up to 800 mg/kg or intervals shortened. Do not exceed 800 mg/kg/month.

Privigen: 200 to 800 mg/kg as a single-dose IV infusion every 3 to 4 weeks. Adjust dose to achieve desired serum trough levels and clinical response.

IDIOPATHIC THROMBOCYTOPENIC PURPURA (ITP)

Carimune NF: 400 mg/kg for 2 to 5 consecutive days based on platelet count and clinical response. May be discontinued in acute ITP of childhood if an initial platelet count response to the first two doses is adequate (30,000 to 50,000/mm^3). If clinically significant bleeding occurs or the platelet count falls below 30,000/mm^3, a maintenance dose of 400 mg/kg may be given as a single infusion. If response inadequate, increase to 800 to 1,000 mg/kg. May be given intermittently to maintain platelet count.

Gammagard S/D: 1 Gm/kg. Up to 3 doses can be given on alternate days based on clinical response and platelet count.

Gamunex-C: Do not administer SC for ITP patients due to a potential risk of hematoma formation. 1 Gm/kg/day (10 mL/kg/day) for 2 consecutive days or 0.4 Gm/kg/day (4 mL/kg/day) for 5 consecutive days. With either regimen the total dose is 2 Gm/kg. Dose is based on platelet count and clinical response. The second 1 Gm/kg dose may be withheld if an adequate increase in platelet count is observed at 24 hours. The high-dose regimen (1 Gm/kg/day for 1 to 2 days) is not recommended for individuals with expanded fluid volumes or where fluid volume may be a concern.

Privigen: *Chronic ITP:* 1 Gm/kg IV daily for 2 consecutive days for a total dose of 2 Gm/kg.

B-CELL CHRONIC LYMPHOCYTIC LEUKEMIA (CLL)

Gammagard S/D: 400 mg/kg every 3 to 4 weeks.

CHRONIC INFLAMMATORY DEMYELINATING POLYNEUROPATHY (CIDP)

Gamunex-C: The initial total loading dose of 2 Gm/kg should be given in divided doses (1 Gm/kg/day [10 mL/kg/day] for 2 consecutive days or 500 mg/kg/day [5 mL/kg/day] for 4 consecutive days). Follow with maintenance infusions of 1 Gm/kg every 3 weeks. The maintenance dose may be given as a total dose of 1 Gm/kg (10 mL/kg) on Day 1 or divided into 2 doses of 500 mg/kg given over 2 consecutive days.

PREVENTION OF INFECTION IN BONE MARROW TRANSPLANT PATIENTS

Gamimune N, which is no longer available, was the only IGIV preparation approved for this indication. Other IGIV preparations may be considered as an unlabeled use; consult literature for recommendations. Gamimune N was indicated only in transplant patients over 20 years of age and was given in a 500 mg/kg dose on Day 7 and Day 2 pre-transplant (or at time that conditioning therapy for transplant began). The same dose was given each week through day 90 post-transplant.

PREVENTION OF BACTERIAL INFECTIONS IN HIV-INFECTED CHILDREN AND ADULTS

Gamimune N, which is no longer available, was the only IGIV preparation approved for this indication. Other IGIV preparations may be considered as an unlabeled use; consult literature for recommendations. Gamimune N was given in a 400 mg/kg dose every 28 days.

KAWASAKI SYNDROME

Iveegam EN: 2 Gm/kg as a single dose over 10 to 12 hours. If symptoms persist an additional 2 Gm/kg dose may be given over 10 to 12 hours. Alternately, *Iveegam EN* may be given at 400 mg/kg/day for 4 days. Initiate within 10 days of onset of disease. Concomitantly give aspirin 80 to 100 mg/kg/day equally divided into 4 doses through 14th day after onset of symptoms or until fever subsides, then 3 to 10 mg/kg/day for 5 weeks or 3 to 5 mg/kg/day for 6 to 8 weeks or longer. Repeat regimen if symptoms persist or recur due to active Kawasaki disease.

PEDIATRIC DOSE

See mg/kg or Gm/kg dose recommendations under Usual Dose. Begin with the lowest recommended dose. With most brands, clinical studies suggested that no difference in dosing is necessary and no special precautions are indicated. According to the manufacturers, infants and neonates were not included in clinical studies for primary immunodeficiency diseases or Kawasaki disease. All age-groups were represented in clinical studies for idiopathic thrombocytopenic purpura. See Maternal/Child.

Continued

Another source recommends the following doses, some of which may be unlabeled in the pediatric population:

Primary immunodeficiency disease: 300 to 400 mg/kg monthly. Optimum dose and frequency are determined by monitoring clinical response and IgG trough levels (increases of 300 to 400 mg/dL over initial pretreatment level are considered ideal).

Idiopathic thrombocytopenic purpura (ITP): *Initial therapy for acute ITP:* 0.8 to 1 Gm/kg given in 1 or 2 doses. *Maintenance therapy:* Individualized.

Kawasaki disease: 2 Gm/kg as a single dose over 10 to 12 hours or 400 mg/kg daily on four consecutive days. Start within 10 days of illness. Treatment should include aspirin (see Usual Dose).

Pediatric HIV infection: 400 mg/kg every 28 days.

Bone marrow transplantation: 500 mg/kg on Day 7 and Day 2 pretransplant. Repeat 500 mg/kg once each week through Day 90 posttransplant. May reduce incidence of infection and death; does not decrease graft-versus-host disease.

Low-birth-weight infants (less than 1,500 Gm): Variable. 500 mg/kg has been used each week or three times in the first week of life and then weekly (target IgG around 700 mg/dL). Not recommended for routine use in preterm infants to prevent late-onset infection.

Parvovirus B19 infection: 400 mg/kg/day for 5 consecutive days or 1 Gm/kg/day for 2 consecutive days.

DILUTION

All formulations: Do not mix with IGIV products from other manufacturers.

Flebogamma, Gamunex-C, Gammagard Liquid, and *Privigen* are liquid preparations and are ready to use; see complete information in the following sections.

For all other formulations, absolute sterile technique is required at all steps of the reconstitution process. Gently rotate to dissolve completely. Complete dilution may take 20 minutes or more. Check label for sucrose content; see Precautions. For most preparations, filtration is required as drawn into a syringe for administration or as administered through IV tubing. Check each brand for specific equipment. If prepared in a sterile laminar air flow hood, may be pooled into plastic IV infusion bags and refrigerated for up to 24 hours. Mark with date and time of reconstitution and pooling.

Carimune NF: Contains sucrose; see Precautions. Reconstitute with diluent provided. Makes a 3% solution. Invert quickly so that the vacuum allows diluent to flow into the IV bottle. May also be reconstituted with desired amounts of NS, D5W, or SW. Available as 1 (3, 6, or 12) Gm with 33 (100 or 200) mL diluent. For a 6% solution, use one half the diluent provided. Remove diluent bottle and swirl vigorously; *do not shake;* should dissolve within a few minutes. Package insert has a chart with dilution requirements for 9% and 12% concentrations. Immediate use is recommended unless reconstituted under a sterile laminar flow hood; then it may be refrigerated and administration must begin within 24 hours. Must be warmed to room temperature before dilution if it has been refrigerated. pH 6.4 to 6.8.

Flebogamma: Contains sorbitol; does not contain sucrose. A ready-to-use 5% sterile solution; available as 0.5 Gm in 10 mL, 2.5 Gm in 50 mL, 5 Gm in 100 mL, and 10 Gm in 200 mL. Further dilution with other solutions not recommended. See Filters. pH 5 to 6.

Gammagard Liquid: Contains no added sugars. A ready-to-use 10% solution available as 1 Gm in 10 mL, 2.5 Gm in 25 mL, 5 Gm in 50 mL, 10 Gm in 100 mL, and 20 Gm in 200 mL. Warm to room temperature before use. May be further diluted only with D5W. See Filters. pH 4.6 to 5.1.

Gammagard S/D: Must be warmed to room temperature before dilution. Diluent (SW for injection), transfer device, administration set with integral airway, and filter provided with each single-use vial. Available in 2.5-, 5-, and 10-Gm single-dose vials with diluent. Use full amount of diluent (50, 96, 192 mL) to prepare a 5% solution (50 mg/mL) or one half the amount of diluent (25, 48, 96 mL) to prepare a 10% solution (100 mg/mL). Must be used within 2 hours of dilution. pH 6.4 to 7.2.

Gammar P-IV: Contains sucrose; see Precautions. Must be warmed to room temperature before dilution. Diluent (SW for injection) is provided. May provide a transfer device (plastic piercing pin to diluent vial; metal needle to product vial), administration set with integral airway. Available in 1-, 2.5-, 5-, and 10-Gm single-dose vials with diluent (50 mg/mL) and a bulk pack without diluent. *Do not shake* to dissolve; rotate or agitate vial. Must be used within 3 hours of dilution. pH 6.4 to 7.2. (Supplies limited.)

Gamunex-C: Does not contain sucrose. A ready-to-use 10% sterile solution. Available in 1-, 2.5-, 5-, 10-, and 20-Gm single-dose vials. Bring to room temperature before administration. Use an 18-gauge needle to penetrate the stopper of the 1-Gm size. Use a 16-gauge needle to penetrate the stopper of the 2.5- to 20-Gm sizes. Penetration of the stopper in the center of the raised ring and perpendicular to it is recommended. May be further diluted with D5W if required. Do not use any other diluent. Filtration during administration is not required. Content of vials may be pooled under aseptic conditions into sterile infusion bags but must be infused within 8 hours of pooling. pH 4 to 4.5.

Iveegam EN: Diluent (SW for injection), transfer device, administration set with integral airway, and filter provided with each vial. Available in 0.5-, 1-, 2.5-, and 5-Gm vials with 10, 20, 50, or 100 mL diluent providing 50 mg/mL. *Do not shake* to dissolve; rotate or agitate vial. Use immediately after dilution. May be further diluted with a given amount of D5W or NS.

Privigen: Does not contain sucrose. A ready-to-use 10% sterile solution. Available in 5-, 10-, and 20-Gm single-dose vials. *Do not shake.* May be further diluted with D5W if required. Do not use any other diluent. Filtration during administration is not required. Content of vials may be pooled under aseptic conditions into sterile infusion bags but should be infused as soon as possible; contains no preservatives.

Filters: Filter or filter needle is provided by most manufacturers. *Carimune NF, Flebogamma,* and *Gammar P-IV* may be filtered with a larger pore filter size but is not required by manufacturers (filters greater than or equal to 15 microns will be less likely to slow infusion [0.2-micron antibacterial filters may be used with *Carimune NF and Flebogamma*]). *Carimune NF* is nano-filtered. Filtration of *Gamunex-C* during administration is not required; however, use of a non–protein binding, 0.22-micron filter is permissible. Use of an in-line filter is optional with *Gammagard Liquid.*

Storage: Storage requirements are brand specific and vary considerably; see manufacturer's package insert. Do not use after expiration date. Discard partially used vials. Do not use if solution is turbid or has been frozen.

COMPATIBILITY

Consider any drug NOT listed as compatible to be INCOMPATIBLE until consulting a pharmacist; specific conditions may apply.

Manufacturers recommend administration through a separate IV line without admixture with other drugs and state, "Do not combine one IGIV product with an IGIV product from another manufacturer." *Gammagard Liquid* and *Gamunex-C* are **incompatible** with NS. *Flebogamma* should not be further diluted with any solution.

Most preparations may be infused sequentially into a primary IV of D5W or NS, or the tubing may be flushed with D5W or NS before and after administration. No **compatibility** studies available for *Gamunex-C* or *Gammagard Liquid*. Both are **compatible** only with D5W.

One source suggests the following **compatibilities:**

Y-site: Fluconazole (Diflucan), sargramostim (Leukine).

RATE OF ADMINISTRATION

Too-rapid infusion may cause a precipitous hypotensive reaction. Decrease rate in patients at risk for thrombotic events and/or neuromuscular disorders. In patients at risk for developing renal dysfunction, administer at the minimum concentration available and the minimum rate of infusion that is practicable. *Another source suggests decreasing the rate of infusion by one half (5% solution) to one quarter (10% solution). For specific rates recommended by various manufacturers, see prescribing information.* See Precautions and the following specific recommendations for each product. Decrease rate of infusion at onset of patient discomfort or any adverse reactions; see Antidote. Administer via separate IV tubing with filter or filter needle (provided by most manufacturers if required). Do not mix with IGIV products from other manufacturers or with other drugs or IV solutions. An infusion pump will facilitate an accurate rate of administration.

Carimune NF: Contains sucrose; see Precautions. 0.5 to 1 mL/min for 15 to 30 minutes. May then be increased to 1.5 to 2.5 mL/min. After the first infusion, the rate may be initiated at 2 to 2.5 mL/min. The first dose must be a 3% solution. After the first dose, a 6% solution may be used to facilitate the administration of larger doses. Begin at 1 to 1.5 mL/min and increase in 15 to 30 minutes to 2 to 2.5 mL/min. To keep the amount of sucrose infused at less than 3 mg/kg/min in patients at risk for developing renal dysfunction, the concentration and infusion rate should be the minimum practicable.

Flebogamma: 0.01 mL/kg/min (0.5 mg/kg/min) for the first 30 minutes. If no discomfort or adverse effects, may be gradually increased to a maximum rate of 0.10 mL/kg/min (5 mg/kg/min). In patients at risk for developing renal dysfunction, the infusion rate should be the minimum practicable.

Gammagard Liquid: 0.5 mL/kg/hr for the first 30 minutes. If no discomfort or adverse effects, may be gradually increased every 30 minutes to a maximum rate of 5 mL/kg/hr. In patients at risk for developing renal dysfunction or thrombotic episodes, the maximum infusion rate should be less than 2 mL/kg/hr.

Gammagard S/D: 5% solution 0.5 mL/kg/hr. May be gradually increased to 4 mL/kg/hr if no discomfort or adverse effects. If 5% solution well tolerated at 4 mL/kg/hr, a 10% solution can be used. Begin with 0.5 mL/kg/hr. If no adverse effects, gradually increase up to a maximum of 8 mL/kg/hr. In patients at risk for developing renal dysfunction, the concentration and infusion rate should be the minimum practicable.

Gammar P-IV: Contains sucrose; see Precautions. 0.01 mL/kg/min. May be increased to 0.02 mL/kg/min after 15 to 30 minutes. May be gradually increased to 0.03 to 0.06 mL/kg/min if no discomfort or adverse effects. To keep the amount of sucrose infused at less than 3 mg/kg/min in patients at risk for developing renal dysfunction, the concentration and infusion rate should be the minimum practicable.

Gamunex-C: 0.01 mL/kg/min (1 mg/kg/min) for the first 30 minutes. If no discomfort or adverse effects, may be gradually increased to a maximum rate of 0.08 mL/kg/min (8 mg/kg/min). In patients at risk for developing renal dysfunction, the infusion rate should be the minimum practicable. The initial infusion rate in CIDP may begin at 0.02 mL/kg/min (2 mg/kg/min).

Iveegam EN: 1 mL/min. May be increased to a maximum of 2 mL/min in the standard 5% solution. Rate may be adjusted proportionately with further dilution. Note rate for single-dose regimen in Kawasaki disease. In patients at risk for developing renal dysfunction, the concentration and infusion rate should be the minimum practicable.

Privigen: IV line may be flushed with D5W or NS.

Primary immunodeficiency: 0.005 mL/kg/min (0.5 mg/kg/min) initially. If no discomfort or adverse effects, may be gradually increased to a maximum rate of 0.08 mL/kg/min (8 mg/kg/min). In patients at risk for developing renal dysfunction or thrombotic events, the infusion rate should be the minimum practicable.

Chronic immune thrombocytopenic purpura: 0.005 mL/kg/min (0.5 mg/kg/min) initially. If no discomfort or adverse effects, may be gradually increased to a maximum rate of 0.04 mL/kg/min (4 mg/kg/min). In patients at risk for developing renal dysfunction or thrombotic events, the infusion rate should be the minimum practicable.

Pediatric rate of administration: Begin at 0.01 mL/kg/min. Double rate every 15 to 30 minutes up to a maximum of 0.08 mL/kg/min. If side effects occur, discontinue infusion until they subside. Restart at previously tolerated rate.

ACTIONS

An immune serum containing immune globulin. Obtained, purified, and standardized from human serum or plasma. Specific methods (e.g., cold ethanol fractionation, detergents, solvents) inactivate blood-borne viruses (e.g., hepatitis, HIV). Provides antibodies that bind and neutralize pathogenic autoantibodies with immediate antibody levels against bacterial, viral, parasitic, and mycoplasmic antigens. Half-life variable; approximately 3 to 6 weeks but may be decreased by fever or infection (increased catabolism or consumption). Distribution into extravascular fluid, tissue, and cells causes a rapid fall in serum IgG in the first week after infusion. Crosses placental barrier.

INDICATIONS AND USES

Selected products are approved for different uses; see Usual Dose. All provide rapid onset, short-term passive immunization. Labeled uses include: *Primary immunodeficiency diseases:* Maintenance and treatment of adults, adolescents, and other pediatric patients unable to produce adequate amounts of IgG antibodies, especially in the following situations: need for immediate increase in intravascular immunoglobulin levels, small muscle mass or bleeding tendencies that contraindicate IM injection, and selected disease states (e.g., congenital agammaglobulinemia, common variable hypogammaglobulinemia, combined immunodeficiency, Wiskott-Aldrich syndrome). ▪ *Treatment of acute and chronic idiopathic thrombocytopenic purpura:* Temporary increase in platelet counts in patients with idiopathic thrombocytopenic purpura and with thrombocytopenia associated with bone marrow transplant. ▪ *Treatment of chronic inflammatory demyelinating polyneuropathy (CIDP):* Improvement of neuromuscular disability and impairment and maintenance therapy to prevent relapse. ▪ *Adjunct in chronic lymphocytic leukemia:* Prevention of bacterial infections in patients with hypogammaglobulinemia or recurrent bacterial infection associated with B-cell CLL. ▪ *Kawasaki syndrome:* Prevention of coronary artery aneurysms associated with Kawasaki syndrome. ▪ Gamunex-C is approved for SC humoral administration for primary immunodeficiency disease (PID). **Unlabeled uses:** *Infection prophylaxis or control* and to improve immunologic parameters in select patients with symptomatic AIDS or ARC and pediatric patients with HIV. ▪ *Bone marrow transplant:* Reduce risk of serious infections and graft-versus-host disease in bone marrow transplant patients. ▪ Infection prophylaxis and control in low-birth-weight neonates, patients with iatrogenically induced or disease-associated immunosuppression (major surgery [e.g., bone marrow or cardiac transplants], hematologic malignancies, extensive burns, or collagen-vascular diseases). ▪ Treatment of post-transfusion purpura. ▪ Treatment of chronic Parvovirus B19 infection in immunodeficient patients. ▪ Prevention of recurrent bacterial infections in patients with IgG subclass deficiencies (e.g., allergies, HIV). ▪ Treatment or adjunct in the treatment of dermatomyositis, intractable epilepsy, multiple sclerosis, myasthenia gravis, polymyositis, polyneuropathies, rheumatoid arthritis, and other autoimmune disease (e.g., autoimmune neutropenia, pediatric patients with type 1 diabetes, chronic fatigue syndrome, Guillain-Barré syndrome, hyperimmunoglobulinemia E syndrome, multifocal motor neuropathy, and many others).

CONTRAINDICATIONS

Individuals known to have anaphylactic or severe hypersensitivity responses to gamma globulin or its components (e.g., thimerosal); patients with isolated or selective IgA deficiency, IgA deficiency when the patient has IgE-mediated antibodies to IgA, or pre-existing anti-IgA antibodies and/or a history of hypersensitivity. Manufacturer of *Flebogamma* adds anaphylactic or severe reactions to blood or blood-derived products. Manufacturer of *Gamunex-C* suggests IgA-deficient patients with antibodies against IgA are at greater risk for developing severe hypersensitivity reactions. Manufacturer of *Gammagard S/D* states, "None known." *Privigen* is contraindicated in patients with selective IgA deficiency; it contains L-proline as a stabilizer and is contraindicated in patients with hyperprolinemia.

PRECAUTIONS

Check label; must state, "For IV use." ▪ Do not use IM or SC. Do not skin test. Will cause a localized chemical skin reaction. ▪ Hypersensitivity reactions have occurred; administer in a facility with adequate equipment and supplies to monitor the patient and respond to any medical emergency. ▪ Use extreme caution in individuals with a history of prior systemic hypersensitivity reactions. Incidence of anaphylaxis may be increased, especially with repeated injections. ▪ Some packaging of these products may contain latex; use caution in sensitive individuals. ▪ IGIV products have been associated with renal dysfunction, acute renal failure, osmotic nephrosis, and death. Use extreme caution in patients with any degree of renal insufficiency; in patients age 65 years and older; in patients with diabetes mellitus, paraproteinemia, sepsis, volume depletion; and/or in patients receiving known nephrotoxic drugs. If used, should be administered at the minimum concentration available and at the minimum rate of infusion practicable. **Products containing sucrose as a stabilizer (Carimune NF and Gammar P-IV) have demonstrated an increased risk of renal dysfunction.** Consider benefit versus risk before use. ▪ Increases in SCr and/or BUN may progress to oliguria and anuria requiring dialysis; however, some patients improve spontaneously with discontinuation of IGIV. ▪ May cause aseptic meningitis syndrome (AMS), especially with 2-Gm/kg doses. May begin from 2 hours to 2 days after treatment. Symptoms are drowsiness, fever, headache (severe), nausea and vomiting, nuchal rigidity, painful eye movements, and photophobia. Cerebrospinal fluid (CSF) studies are often positive with pleocytosis, predominantly from the granulocyte series and elevated protein levels. ▪ Hyperproteinemia, increased serum viscosity, and hyponatremia may occur. Distinguish true hyponatremia from pseudohyponatremia to determine correct treatment. Volume depletion with a further increase in serum viscosity may predispose to thromboembolic events. ▪ IGIV products have been associated with thrombotic events; use caution in patients with advanced age, impaired cardiac output, a history of cardiovascular disease, thrombotic episodes, and thrombotic risk factors (e.g., cerebrovascular disease, coronary artery disease, diabetes, hypertension, prolonged periods of immobilization). Octagam has been voluntarily withdrawn from the market until the root cause of reported thromboembolic events with this formulation can be determined. ▪ Baseline assessment of blood viscosity should be made in patients at risk for hyperviscosity, including chylomicronemia, markedly high triglycerides, or monoclonal gammopathies. ▪ May rarely cause hemolysis, which can result in hemolytic anemia. ▪ Noncarcinogenic pulmonary edema (transfusion-related acute lung injury [TRALI]) has been reported; see Monitor. ▪ Derived from human blood. Despite purification processes, may carry risk of transmitting infectious agents (e.g., viruses [e.g., HIV, hepatitis] or Creutzfeldt-Jakob disease [CJD] agent).

Monitor: Use of larger veins recommended to reduce infusion-site discomfort, especially with 10% solutions. ▪ Correct volume depletion before administration in all patients, especially patients with pre-existing renal insufficiency. ▪ Recording of lot number on vials is recommended. ▪ Monitor vital signs and observe patient continuously during infusion. A precipitous drop in BP or anaphylaxis can occur at any time. Emergency equipment and supplies must be at bedside. ▪ Monitor renal function (e.g., BUN, SCr) and urine output in patients at increased risk for renal failure. Obtain baseline studies, monitor at intervals, and discontinue IGIV if renal function deteriorates. See Precautions. ▪ Monitor for hyperproteinemia with resultant changes in serum viscosity and electrolyte imbalances. ▪ Monitor for S/S of hemolysis (e.g., lysis of red blood cells, liberation of hemoglobin) and hemolytic anemia. ▪ Monitor for S/S of TRALI (e.g., fever, hypoxemia, normal left ventricular function, pulmonary edema, severe respiratory distress). Usually occurs within 1 to 6 hours after completion of the transfusion. Manage with oxygen and adequate ventilatory support. If TRALI is suspected, both the product and the patient serum should be tested for the presence of antineutrophil antibodies. ▪ Monitor for volume overload. ▪ Minimum serum level of IgG after infusion should exceed 300 mg/dL.

Patient Education: Report a burning sensation in the head, chills, cyanosis, diaphoresis, dyspnea, faintness or light-headedness, fatigue, fever, hives, itching or rash, neck pain or difficulty moving neck, tachycardia, wheezing. ▪ Report chest pain or tightness, difficulty passing urine, decreased urine output, fluid retention, edema, shortness of breath, or sudden weight gain. ▪ Remote risk of viral or CJD infection; consider risk versus benefit of therapy. See Drug/Lab Interactions.

Maternal/Child: Category C: use with caution in pregnancy; no adverse effects documented, but adequate studies are not available. ▪ Safety for use in breast-feeding not established. ▪ Response in pediatric patients usually exceeds response in adults. ▪ Gamimune-N contains maltose and may cause osmotic diuresis. ▪ Use of *Privigen* to treat primary immunodeficiency in pediatric patients under 3 years of age or to treat chronic immune thrombocytopenic purpura in pediatric patients under 15 years of age not established.

Elderly: Use with extreme caution. Incidence of renal insufficiency and other side effects increased due to age, potential for decreased organ function, and pre-existing medical conditions; see Precautions.

DRUG/LAB INTERACTIONS

Do not administer **live virus vaccines** from 2 weeks before to at least 3 months after immune globulin IV. Passive transfer of antibodies may transiently interfere with the response to live virus vaccines, such as measles, mumps, and rubella; see prescribing information if there is a risk of measles exposure or if accidental exposure has occurred. ▪ Provides immediate antibody levels that last for about 3 weeks. In selected patients, may have an immune-modulating effect that may alter their response to **corticosteroids or antineoplastic agents.** ▪ Concurrent use with **nephrotoxic drugs** (e.g., aminoglycosides [e.g., gentamicin], amphotericin B [Amphotec, generic], cidofovir [Vistide], rifampin [Rifadin]) may increase risk of renal insufficiency. ▪ Products that contain **maltose** may interfere with blood and urine glucose tests. ▪ Various antibody titers may be raised temporarily, resulting in **false-positive serologic testing.**

SIDE EFFECTS

Arthralgia, asthenia, back pain, chills, fatigue, fever, headache, hypertension, infusion site reactions, nausea and vomiting, and rash were reported most commonly. Full range of hypersensitivity symptoms, including anaphylaxis, is possible. Angioedema, erythema, fever, and urticaria are most frequently observed. Anxiety, chest tightness, cough, difficulty breathing, elevated ALT and AST (temporary), flushing, hemolytic anemia (reversible), increased BUN and SCr (may occur as soon as 1 to 2 days following infusion), leg cramps, light-headedness, malaise, pharyngitis, tachycardia, and urticaria have been reported. Severe reactions (e.g., circulatory collapse, fever, loss of consciousness, nausea and vomiting, sudden onset of dyspnea) have occurred and are more common in patients with antibody deficiencies. Noncarcinogenic pulmonary edema (transfusion-related acute lung injury [TRALI]) has been reported. Acute renal failure, acute tubular necrosis, osmotic nephrosis, and proximal tubular nephropathy have been reported; may result in death. Is made from human plasma;

process attempts to eliminate risk of hepatitis or HIV infection. A precipitous hypotensive reaction can occur and is most frequently associated with too-rapid rate of injection. Aseptic meningitis syndrome and hemolysis occur infrequently. See Precautions.

ANTIDOTE

Reduce rate for patient discomfort, any sign of adverse reaction, and in patients at risk for renal insufficiency. If symptoms subside promptly, the infusion may be resumed at a lower rate. Decreasing the volume of subsequent infusions may also prevent or decrease the incidence of adverse reactions. Loop diuretics (e.g., furosemide [Lasix]) may be helpful in the management of fluid overload. Patients who continue to experience adverse reactions, after rate and/or volume have been reduced, may be premedicated with hydrocortisone 1 to 2 mg/kg 30 minutes prior to the immune globulin infusion. Pretreatment with acetaminophen (Tylenol) and diphenhydramine (Benadryl) or trying a different brand of immune globulin may also be useful. Discontinue the drug immediately for any signs of a hypersensitivity reaction or renal insufficiency. Notify the physician. May be treated symptomatically, and infusion resumed at slower rate if symptoms subside. Treat anaphylaxis immediately. Epinephrine (Adrenalin), diphenhydramine (Benadryl), oxygen, vasopressors (e.g., dopamine), corticosteroids, and ventilation equipment must always be available. Manage TRALI with oxygen and ventilatory support. Resuscitate as necessary.

INDOMETHACIN SODIUM
(in-doh-**METH**-ah-sin **SO**-dee-um)

**Prostaglandin inhibitor
(patent ductus
arteriosus adjunct)**

Indocin IV

pH 6 to 7.5

USUAL DOSE

Neonates: Three IV doses, specific to age at first dose, given at 12- to 24-hour intervals constitute a course of therapy.

Less than 48 hours of age: First dose (0.2 mg/kg of body weight), second dose (0.1 mg/kg), third dose (0.1 mg/kg).

2 to 7 days of age: 0.2 mg/kg for each of 3 doses.

Over 7 days of age: First dose (0.2 mg/kg), then 0.25 mg/kg for the next 2 doses.

If ductus arteriosus reopens, a second course of 1 to 3 doses as described for each neonate age may be repeated one time given at 12- to 24-hour intervals. If neonate remains unresponsive to indomethacin therapy after 2 courses, surgery may be required for closure of the ductus arteriosus.

DOSE ADJUSTMENTS

If urine output is less than 0.6 mL/kg/hr at any time a dose is to be given, withhold dose until lab studies confirm normal renal function.

DILUTION

Each 1 mg must be diluted with at least 1 mL NS or SW for injection without preservatives (0.1 mg/0.1 mL); may be diluted with 2 mL diluent (0.05 mg/0.1 mL). The preservative benzyl alcohol is toxic in neonates. A fresh solution should be prepared just before each administration. Discard any unused portion.

Filters: No data available from manufacturer.

Storage: Store unopened vials in carton at CRT. Protect from light. Use reconstituted solution immediately.

COMPATIBILITY   (Underline Indicates Conflicting Compatibility Information)
Consider any drug NOT listed as compatible to be INCOMPATIBLE until consulting a pharmacist; specific conditions may apply.
Manufacturer states, "Prepare only with preservative-free NS or SW"; further dilution with IV solutions is not recommended and may precipitate with solutions with a pH below 6.

One source suggests the following **compatibilities:**
Y-site: <u>Dextrose</u>, furosemide (Lasix), insulin (regular), potassium chloride (KCl), sodium bicarbonate, nitroprusside sodium.

RATE OF ADMINISTRATION
A single dose, properly diluted, by IV injection over 20 to 30 minutes.

ACTIONS
A potent inhibitor of prostaglandin synthesis. Through an unconfirmed method of action (thought to be inhibition of prostaglandin synthesis), it causes closure of a patent ductus arteriosus 75% to 80% of the time, eliminating the need for surgical intervention. Plasma half-life varies inversely with postnatal age and weight and ranges from 12 to 20 hours. Metabolized in the liver and eventually excreted in urine and bile.

INDICATIONS AND USES
Closure of a hemodynamically significant patent ductus arteriosus in premature infants weighing between 500 and 1,750 Gm if usual medical management (e.g., fluid restriction, diuretics, digoxin, respiratory support) has not been effective after 48 hours.

CONTRAINDICATIONS
Bleeding, especially active intracranial hemorrhage or GI bleeding; coagulation defects; necrotizing enterocolitis; infants with congenital heart disease (e.g., pulmonary atresia, severe coarctation of the aorta, severe tetralogy of Fallot) who require patency of the ductus arteriosus for satisfactory pulmonary or systemic blood flow; proven or suspected untreated infection; significant renal impairment; thrombocytopenia.

PRECAUTIONS
Clinical evidence of a hemodynamically significant patent ductus arteriosus (respiratory distress, a continuous murmur, a hyperactive precordium, cardiomegaly and pulmonary plethora on chest x-ray) should be present before use is considered. ■ For use only in a highly supervised setting such as an intensive care nursery. ■ May increase potential for GI or intraventricular bleeding. ■ Use caution in presence of existing controlled infection; may mask signs and symptoms of exacerbation. ■ May suppress water excretion to a greater extent than sodium excretion. Hyponatremia may result. ■ For IV use only. ■ Surgery indicated if condition is not responsive to two courses of therapy.

Monitor: Vital signs, oxygenation, acid-base status, fluid and electrolyte balance, and kidney function (SCr, BUN, urine output) must be monitored and maintained. ■ Can cause marked reduction in urine output (over 50%), increase BUN and SCr, and reduce glomerular filtration rate and CrCl. These symptoms usually disappear when therapy completed but may cause acute renal failure, especially in infants with impaired renal function from other causes. ■ May inhibit platelet aggregation; monitor for signs of bleeding. ■ Discontinue drug if signs of impaired liver function appear. ■ Confirm absolute patency of vein. Avoid extravasation; will irritate tissue. ■ See Drug/Lab Interactions.

DRUG/LAB INTERACTIONS

May reduce elimination and increase serum concentrations of **drugs that are renally excreted** (e.g., aminoglycosides [e.g., gentamicin], digoxin [Lanoxin]). Monitor drug levels and adjust doses as needed to avoid toxicity. ■ Observe neonate closely for signs of **digoxin toxicity;** frequent monitoring of ECG and digoxin serum levels is indicated. ■ Use with **furosemide** (Lasix) may help to maintain renal function. ■ Concomitant use with **anticoagulants** may increase risk of bleeding; monitoring of PT suggested. ■ Coadministration with **ACE inhibitors** (e.g., enalaprilat [Vasotec IV]) may result in deterioration of renal function, including renal failure.

SIDE EFFECTS

Abdominal distention; acidosis; alkalosis; apnea; bleeding into the GI tract (gross or microscopic); bradycardia; DIC; elevated BUN or creatinine; exacerbation of pre-existing pulmonary infection; fluid retention; gastric perforation; hyperkalemia; hypoglycemia; hyponatremia; intracranial bleeding; necrotizing enterocolitis; oliguria; oozing from needle puncture sites; pulmonary hemorrhage; pulmonary hypertension; reduced urine sodium, chloride, potassium, urine osmolality, free water clearance, or glomerular filtration rate; renal failure, retrolental fibroplasia; thrombocytopenia; transient ileus; uremia; vomiting.

ANTIDOTE

Discontinue the drug and notify the physician of all side effects. Based on severity, side effects may be treated symptomatically or drug will be completely discontinued in favor of surgical intervention. Resuscitate as necessary.

INFLIXIMAB BBW

(in-**FLIX**-ih-mab)

Monoclonal antibody
Inflammatory bowel disease agent
Antirheumatic agent

Remicade

pH 7.2

USUAL DOSE

Preliminary patient evaluation required; see Monitor.

Premedication: Administer at the physician's discretion. May include antihistamines (e.g., diphenhydramine [Benadryl]), H_2 blockers (e.g., famotidine [Pepcid IV]), acetaminophen, and/or corticosteroids (e.g., hydrocortisone).

Crohn's disease and fistulizing Crohn's disease: Begin with an initial dose of 5 mg/kg as an infusion. Repeat at 2 and 6 weeks and every 8 weeks thereafter. For patients who respond and then lose their response, a 10 mg/kg dose may be given on Day 1, repeated at 2- and 6-week intervals, and then repeated in 8 weeks (a total of 14 weeks elapsed). If

Continued

there is no response by Week 14, response with continued dosing is unlikely; consider discontinuing infliximab. See Precautions.

Rheumatoid arthritis: 3 mg/kg as an infusion. Repeat dose at 2 and 6 weeks, then every 8 weeks thereafter. Given in combination with methotrexate at a minimum dose of 12.5 mg/week (median dose of 15 mg/week). See methotrexate monograph. If response to infliximab is incomplete, dose may be adjusted up to 10 mg/kg or interval decreased to every 4 weeks. Risk of infection may be increased at higher doses.

Ankylosing spondylitis: 5 mg/kg as an infusion. Repeat at 2 and 6 weeks, then every 6 weeks thereafter.

Psoriatic arthritis: 5 mg/kg as an infusion. Repeat dose at 2 and 6 weeks, then every 8 weeks thereafter. May be used with or without methotrexate.

Ulcerative colitis and plaque psoriasis: 5 mg/kg as an infusion. Repeat dose at 2 and 6 weeks, then every 8 weeks thereafter.

PEDIATRIC DOSE

Preliminary patient evaluation required; see Monitor. See Maternal/Child.

Crohn's disease: 5 mg/kg as an infusion. Repeat dose at 2 and 6 weeks. Follow with a maintenance regimen of 5 mg/kg every 8 weeks.

DOSE ADJUSTMENTS

Dose adjustment not required based on gender, age, weight, or hepatic or renal function. ■ Do not exceed a dose of 5 mg/kg in patients with moderate to severe CHF (NYHA class III/IV); see Contraindications.

DILUTION

Each vial contains 100 mg of infliximab. When reconstituted as directed below, each milliliter of solution contains 10 mg of infliximab. Calculate the dose and the number of vials required and the total volume of reconstituted infliximab solution required. Reconstitute each 100-mg vial with 10 mL of SW, using a syringe equipped with a 21-gauge or smaller needle. Direct the stream of SW to side of vial. Do not use vial if vacuum is absent. Swirl gently; do not shake. Allow reconstituted solution to stand for 5 minutes. Solution should be colorless to light yellow and opalescent and may develop a few translucent particles as infliximab is a protein. Do not use if opaque particles, discoloration, or other foreign particles are present. The total dose of reconstituted solution must be further diluted with NS to a final volume of 250 mL. (May withdraw a volume of NS equal to the calculated volume of reconstituted infliximab from a 250-mL bottle or bag of NS and slowly add reconstituted solution.) Mix gently. Infusion concentration should range between 0.4 mg/mL and 4 mg/mL.

Filters: Must be administered through an infusion set with an in-line, sterile, non-pyrogenic, low–protein binding filter (pore size equal to or less than 1.2 micron). Flush and prime tubing/filter system with NS before administration of infusion.

Storage: Refrigerate unopened vials at 2° to 8° C (36° to 46° F). Do not freeze. Discard any unused portion.

COMPATIBILITY

Manufacturer recommends not infusing concomitantly in the same IV line with other agents until specific **compatibility** data are available.

RATE OF ADMINISTRATION

Flush and prime tubing/filter system with NS before administration. A single dose should be given over a period of not less than 2 hours. Upon completion of infusion, IV line should be flushed thoroughly with 15 to 20 mL of NS to ensure all active drug is delivered to the patient. A slower rate of infusion may reduce the occurrence or severity of infusion reactions; see Antidote.

ACTIONS

A chimeric IgG1 monoclonal antibody that binds specifically to human tumor necrosis factor alpha (TNFα). Is composed of human constant and murine variable regions. Neutralizes the biologic activity of TNFα by binding with high affinity to the soluble and transmembrane forms of TNFα and inhibiting binding of TNFα with its receptors. Infliximab does not neutralize TNFβ. Biologic activities attributed to TNFα include induction of pro-inflammatory cytokines such as IL-1 and IL-6, enhancement of leukocyte migration by increasing endothelial layer permeability and expression of adhesion molecules by endothelial cells and leukocytes, activation of neutrophil and eosinophil functional activity, and induction of acute phase and other liver proteins. Elevated concentrations of TNFα have been found in involved tissues and fluids of patients with Crohn's disease, rheumatoid arthritis, ankylosing spondylitis, ulcerative colitis, psoriatic arthritis, and plaque psoriasis. These elevated concentrations correlate with elevated disease activity. Treatment with infliximab reduces infiltration of inflammatory cells and TNFα production in inflamed areas of the joint and of the intestine and reduces the proportion of mononuclear cells from the lamina propria able to express TNFα and interferon γ. After treatment, patients have decreased levels of serum IL-6 and C-reactive protein compared to baseline. Infliximab is distributed predominantly within the vascular space. Has a prolonged terminal half-life of 7.7 to 9.5 days. Studies suggest median onset of response to be 2 to 4 weeks and median duration of response to be 12 weeks. Produced by a recombinant cell line cultured by continuous perfusion and is purified by a series of steps that include measures to inactivate and remove viruses.

INDICATIONS AND USES

Adult and pediatric patients: Reduce the S/S and induce and maintain clinical remission in patients with moderately to severely active Crohn's disease who have had an inadequate response to conventional therapy. **Adult patients:** Reduce the number of draining enterocutaneous and rectovaginal fistula(s) and maintain fistula closure in fistulizing Crohn's disease. ■ Given in combination with methotrexate to improve physical function, inhibit progression of structural damage, and reduce S/S in patients with rheumatoid arthritis who have had an inadequate response to methotrexate. ■ Reduce S/S in active ankylosing spondylitis. ■ Reduce the S/S of active arthritis, inhibit progression of structural damage, and improve physical function in psoriatic arthritis. ■ Reduce the S/S, induce and maintain clinical remission and mucosal healing, and eliminate corticosteroid use in patients with moderately to severely active ulcerative colitis who have had inadequate response to conventional therapy. ■ Used for treatment of patients with chronic severe (i.e., extensive and/or disabling) plaque psoriasis who are candidates for systemic treatment and when other systemic treatments are less appropriate.

CONTRAINDICATIONS

Known hypersensitivity to infliximab, murine proteins, or other components of the product. ■ Administration of doses exceeding 5 mg/kg in patients with moderate to severe (NYHA class III/IV) CHF.

PRECAUTIONS

TNFα mediates inflammation and modulates cellular immune response. Anti-TNF therapies, including infliximab, may affect normal immune responses. Serious infections, including sepsis and pneumonia, have been reported. Fatalities have occurred. Many of the serious infections have occurred in patients undergoing concomitant immunosuppressive therapy that, in addition to their underlying disease, may predispose them to infections; see Drug/Lab Interactions. Not recommended for patients with a clinically important active infection. Use caution in patients with a chronic infection or a history of recurrent infection. ▪ Tuberculosis (often disseminated or extrapulmonary at clinical presentation), invasive fungal infections, or opportunistic infections (e.g., aspergillosis, blastomycosis, candidiasis, coccidioidomycosis, histoplasmosis, listeriosis, and pneumocystosis) have been observed in patients receiving infliximab. Some of these infections have been fatal. Antituberculosis treatment of patients with a reactive TB skin test reduces the risk of TB reactivation in patients receiving infliximab. However, active TB has developed in patients receiving infliximab who had a negative skin test before initiating infliximab therapy. Consider risk versus benefit in patients who have resided or traveled in areas of endemic tuberculosis or endemic mycoses, such as histoplasmosis, coccidiodomycosis, or blastomycosis. ▪ A higher incidence of worsening CHF and increased mortality have been seen in patients with moderate to severe CHF. Occurs more frequently in patients receiving a 10 mg/kg dose. Do not use doses greater than 5 mg/kg in patients with CHF. Discontinue for new-onset CHF or for worsening CHF, and consider discontinuing in patients with CHF who have not had a significant response to infliximab. Use with caution in patients with mild CHF (NYHA Class I/II); monitor closely. ▪ Hypersensitivity reactions characterized by urticaria, dyspnea, and/or hypotension have occurred in association with infliximab infusion. Most occur during or within 2 hours of the infusion. Discontinue infusion if severe reaction occurs. Medications for management of hypersensitivity reaction (e.g., acetaminophen [Tylenol], diphenhydramine [Benadryl], corticosteroids [e.g., hydrocortisone] and/or epinephrine) should be readily available. ▪ Serum sickness–like reactions (dyspnea, fever, hand and facial edema, headache, myalgias, polyarthralgias, sore throat) have been reported and have occurred as early as after the second dose and when infliximab was interrupted and then reinitiated after an extended period. These reactions are associated with a marked increase in antibodies to infliximab, a loss of detectable serum concentrations of infliximab, and a possible loss of drug efficacy. ▪ Readministration of infliximab after a period of no treatment resulted in a higher incidence of infusion reactions relative to regular maintenance treatment in clinical trials. Evaluate risk versus benefit of re-administration after a period of no treatment, especially if considering a re-induction regimen given at 0, 2, and 6 weeks. For cases in which maintenance therapy for psoriasis has been interrupted, infliximab should be reinitiated with a single dose followed by maintenance therapy. ▪ Anti-TNF therapy may result in formation of autoimmune antibodies and, rarely, in the development of a lupus-like syndrome. Discontinue therapy if this occurs. In clinical studies, symptoms resolved with discontinuation of therapy. ▪ Lymphoma and other malignancies, some fatal, have been reported in children and adolescent patients treated with TNF blockers, including infliximab. Most of the affected patients were receiving concomitant immunosuppressants. ▪ Cases of hepatosplenic T-cell lymphoma have been reported. They have primarily occurred in adolescents and young adult males being treated with infliximab for Crohn's disease or ulcerative colitis. This type of lymphoma has a very aggressive disease course and is usually fatal. All affected patients received concomitant treatment with azathioprine (Imuran) or 6-mercaptopurine (Purinethol) at or before diagnosis. When treating patients with inflammatory bowel disease, particularly adolescents and young adults, the decision whether to use infliximab alone or in combination with other immunosuppressants should consider the possibility that there is a higher risk of hepatosplenic T-cell lymphoma (HSTCL) with combination therapy versus an observed increased risk of immunogenicity and hypersensitivity reactions with infliximab monotherapy. ▪ The potential role of TNF-blocking therapy in the development of malignancies is not known. Patients with Crohn's disease, ulcerative colitis, rheumatoid arthritis, or plaque psoriasis, particularly with highly active disease and/or exposure to immunosuppressant therapies, may be at higher risk (up to several-fold) than the general population for the development of lymphoma, leukemia, and other malignancies, even in the absence of TNF-blocking therapy. ▪ Use caution in patients with moderate to severe COPD; may have an increased risk of malignancy, especially of the lungs and head or neck. ▪ In studies of extended treatment, systemic accumulation of infliximab did not occur, clinical benefit was maintained, and retreatment was well tolerated. ▪ Rare cases with CNS manifestations of systemic vasculitis, seizures, and new-onset or exacerbation of clinical symptoms and/or radiographic evidence of CNS demyelinating disorders (e.g., multiple sclerosis, optic neuritis) and peripheral demyelinating disorders (e.g., Guillain-Barré syndrome) have been reported. Use with caution in patients with any of these existing neurologic disorders. Consider discontinuing therapy if any of these disorders develop. ▪ Patients with invasive fungal infections (e.g., aspergillosis, blastomycosis, candidiasis, coccidioidomycosis, histoplasmosis, pneumocystosis) may present with disseminated, rather than localized, disease. Antigen and antibody testing may be negative. Empiric antifungal therapy should be considered in patients at risk for invasive fungal infections who develop severe systemic illness. ▪ Bacterial, viral, and other infections due to opportunistic pathogens have also been reported. ▪ Severe hepatic reactions, including liver failure, jaundice, hepatitis, cholestasis, and autoimmune hepatitis, have been reported. Reactions have occurred anywhere from 2 weeks to more than a year after initiation of treatment and have resulted in death or the need for a liver transplant. ▪ Reactivation of hepatitis B has occurred in chronic carriers of the virus who are being treated with infliximab. ▪ Leukopenia, neutropenia, thrombocytopenia, and pancytopenia have been reported. ▪ Use caution when switching between Biological Disease-Modifying Antirheumatic Drugs (DMARDS [e.g., methotrexate, leflunomide, sulfasalazine]); overlapping biological activity may further increase the risk of infection.

Monitor: Evaluate patients for latent tuberculosis (TB) with a TB skin test. Initiate treatment of latent TB before therapy with infliximab. Monitor patients for S/S of active TB (chest x-ray, cough [progressively more productive], dyspnea), including patients who had a negative skin test. ▪ Monitor cardiac status closely for new-onset or worsening CHF; see Precautions. ▪ Patients receiving infliximab may develop human antichimeric antibody (HACA). Patients who are HACA-positive may be more likely to experience an infusion reaction. The incidence of positive HACA is lower among patients receiving immunosuppressant therapies (e.g., 6-mercaptopurine, azathioprine, corticosteroids). ■ Monitor for S/S of hepatotoxicity (e.g., jaundice and/or marked liver enzyme elevations [equal to or greater than 5 times the upper limit of normal]). ■ Evaluation and monitoring of patients who are chronic carriers of hepatitis B is required before, during, and for several months after treatment with infliximab. ■ Monitor CBC with differential and platelet count periodically. ■ Monitor BP and pulse every 30 minutes during infusion. If patient experiences a significant change in vital signs (e.g., drop in diastolic BP of 15 to 20 mm Hg) or exhibits any symptoms that may indicate hypersensitivity, stop infusion. Evaluate symptoms and treat appropriately. Continue to monitor patient for at least 30 minutes after completion of the infusion. ■ Monitor for S/S of infection; discontinue if a serious infection occurs and initiate appropriate antimicrobial treatment; see Precautions. ■ Monitor psoriasis patients, particularly those who have had prolonged phototherapy treatment; may be at increased risk for nonmelanoma skin cancers. ■ Monitor for S/S of malignancies such as HSTCL (e.g., abdominal pain, hepatomegaly, night sweats, persistent fever, weight loss).

Patient Education: Read manufacturer's supplied information sheet before each treatment with infliximab. ■ Tell health care professionals of heart conditions, previous or current infections, and recent or past exposure to TB or histoplasmosis. ■ Review all medicines and disease history with pharmacist or physician before initiating treatment. ■ Promptly report abdominal pain, fever, S/S of heart failure (e.g., shortness of breath, swelling feet), infection, numbness, tingling, or visual disturbances. ■ Report S/S of hypersensitivity reactions (e.g., itching, rash, swelling in the throat). Usually occur during or immediately following the infusion but may occur from 3 to 12 days later.

Maternal/Child: Category B: use during pregnancy only if clearly needed. ■ Has potential for harm to the nursing infant; discontinue breastfeeding. ■ Safety and effectiveness for use in pediatric patients with ulcerative colitis, plaque psoriasis, and/or Crohn's disease who are less than 6 years of age not established. ■ Safety and effectiveness for use in pediatric patients with juvenile rheumatoid arthritis was evaluated in a multi-center trial. The study failed to establish effectiveness; see prescribing information for details. ■ Before initiating infliximab therapy in pediatric patients with Crohn's disease, all vaccinations should be brought up-to-date. ■ Long-term (greater than 1 year) safety and effectiveness in pediatric patients with Crohn's disease not established.

Elderly: Specific differences in safety and effectiveness not noted; the incidence of serious side effects may be increased. Because the impact of infliximab on the incidence of infection is unknown and there is a higher incidence of infections in the elderly population in general, caution should be used in treating the elderly. See Precautions.

DRUG/LAB INTERACTIONS

Specific interaction studies have not been performed. ■ Concurrent administration with **anakinra** (Kineret), an interleukin-1 antagonist, **or abatacept** (Orencia), an anti-rheumatic agent, may be associated with an increased risk of serious infections. The added benefit of combination therapy has not been documented. Anakinra is also associated with an increased risk of neutropenia. Concurrent administration of TNF α-blocking agents (e.g., infliximab) with anakinra or abatacept is not recommended. ■ May cause increased immunosuppression and increased risk of infection with **tocilizumab** (Actemra); concurrent use should be avoided. ■ The majority of patients with Crohn's disease, rheumatoid arthritis, or psoriatic arthritis received one or more of the following concomitant medications without evidence of any type of negative drug interaction: aminosalicylates, antibiotics, antivirals, corticosteroids, 6-mercaptopurine (Purinethol), azathioprine (Imuran), folic acid, methotrexate, narcotics, NSAIDs (e.g., ibuprofen [Motrin, Advil], naproxen [Aleve, Naprosyn]), and sulfasalazine. ■ Patients receiving **immunosuppressants** (e.g., 6-mercaptopurine, azathioprine, corticosteroids) tended to experience fewer infusion reactions as compared to patients on no immunosuppressants. ■ Concomitant **methotrexate** use may decrease incidence of anti-infliximab antibody production and increase infliximab concentrations. ■ **Corticosteroid** use increases the volume of distribution of infliximab. May be due to corticosteroid-mediated changes in fluid and electrolyte balance. ■ Concurrent administration of **live virus vaccines** is not recommended.

SIDE EFFECTS

Most common reasons for discontinuation of therapy were infusion-related reactions (e.g., chest pain, chills, dyspnea, fever, hypertension, hypotension, pruritus, or urticaria) occurring during or within 2 hours of infusion or infections (bacterial, fungal, protozoal, and viral). See Precautions. Most commonly reported side effects include abdominal pain, coughing, fatigue, headache, nausea, pharyngitis, upper respiratory tract infections, and vomiting. Other less common side effects include abscess, anaphylactic-like reactions (including laryngeal/pharyngeal edema and severe bronchospasm), anemia, anxiety, arthralgia, autoantibodies/lupus-like syndrome, back pain, conjunctivitis, constipation, depression, diarrhea, dizziness, dyspepsia, dysuria, flushing, hot flashes, HACA development, hepatitis B virus reactivation, hepatotoxicity (autoimmune hepatitis, increased liver function tests, jaundice, liver failure), insomnia, intestinal obstruction, lymphoproliferative disorders, malignancies including lymphoma, moniliasis, myalgia, pain, paresthesia, peripheral edema, rash, seizures, serum sickness–like reactions, stomatitis, tachycardia, vertigo, and visual disturbances. See Precautions. Infections (bacterial, fungal, protozoal, and viral) including TB, invasive opportunistic infections (e.g., histoplasmosis, listeriosis, and pneumocystosis), new-onset or worsening CHF, CNS demyelinating disorders, and deaths have been reported.

Post-Marketing: Cholestasis, erythema multiforme, hepatitis, hepatosplenic T-cell lymphomas, idiopathic and/or thrombotic thrombocytopenic purpura, interstitial lung disease (including pulmonary fibrosis/interstitial pneumonitis and, very rarely, rapidly progressive disease), jaundice, liver failure, myocardial ischemia/infarction, neuropathies, neutropenia, pericardial effusion, peripheral demyelinating disorders (e.g., Guillain-Barré syndrome, chronic inflammatory demyelinating polyneuropathy, and multifocal motor neuropathy), psoriasis (including new-onset and pustular, primarily palmar/plantar), Stevens-Johnson syndrome, systemic and cutaneous vasculitis, toxic epidermal necrolysis, and transverse myelitis have been reported; fatalities have occurred.

Pediatric patients with Crohn's disease: Anemia, bacterial infection, blood in stool, bone fracture, flushing, leukopenia, neutropenia, respiratory tract allergic reactions, and viral infections were reported more commonly in pediatric patients than in adult patients receiving similar treatment regimens. Serious side effects were infections (some fatal), including opportunistic infections and tuberculosis, infusion reactions, and hypersensitivity reactions. Malignancies (including hepatosplenic T-cell lymphomas), transient hepatic enzyme abnormalities, lupus-like syndromes, and the development of autoantibodies were less common, yet serious, reactions.

ANTIDOTE

Notify physician of any side effects; most will be treated symptomatically. Discontinue infliximab if patient experiences a serious infection, significant changes in vital signs, new or worsening S/S of heart failure, a hypersensitivity reaction, or a lupus-like syndrome (fever, pleuritic pain, pleural effusion). Treat with acetaminophen (Tylenol), antihistamines (diphenhydramine [Benadryl]), corticosteroids, dopamine, and epinephrine as indicated. If infusion is stopped but reaction is not severe and does not require treatment with drugs such as epinephrine or corticosteroids, infusion may be restarted with caution. Restart at lower rate and/or premedicate patient; see Usual Dose. A physician should be present during initiation of any subsequent infusion for a patient who has had a previous reaction. Lupus-like syndrome usually subsides within 10 days of discontinuing infliximab.

INSULIN INJECTION (REGULAR) ▪
INSULIN ASPART rDNA origin ▪
INSULIN GLULISINE rDNA origin

Hormone
Antidiabetic agent

(**IN**-sue-lin in-**JEK**-shun ▪ **IN**-sue-lin **AS**-part)

Humulin R, ✿ Novolin ge Toronto,
Novolin R ▪ NovoLog ▪ Apidra   pH 7 to 7.8 ▪ pH 7.2 to 7.6 ▪ pH 7.3

USUAL DOSE

Only regular insulin, insulin aspart, and insulin glulisine may be given IV. Confirm by label or package insert that a particular insulin product is for IV use; see Precautions.

Dose varies greatly. Will be dependent on patient's condition and response. It is imperative that dosing is individualized and adjusted based on blood glucose determinations because of the marked loss of insulin from adsorption to glass and plastic infusion containers and tubing; see Precautions.

Low-dose treatment in ketoacidosis: The American Diabetes Association recommends 0.15 units/kg as a loading dose (10.5 units for a 70-kg patient), followed by a continuous infusion of 0.1 units/kg/hr (7 units/hr for a 70-kg patient). Plasma glucose should decrease at a rate of 50 to 75 mg/dL/hr. If plasma glucose concentrations do not fall by 50 mg/dL within the first hour of insulin therapy, the insulin infusion rate may be doubled every hour, provided the patient is adequately hydrated. Decrease the rate of infusion when plasma glucose reaches 300 to 250 mg/dL. Start a separate IV of D5/½NS when plasma glucose reaches 300 mg/dL. Administer insulin to maintain serum glucose concentrations between 150 and 200 mg/dL in patients with diabetic ketoacidosis. Continue until metabolic acidosis is corrected. Administer an appropriate dose of insulin SC 30 minutes before discontinuing the insulin infusion (intermediate-acting insulin recommended).

Diabetes mellitus with hyperosmolar coma, nonketotic: An initial bolus dose of 0.1 unit/kg followed by a continuous infusion of 0.1 unit/kg/hr until the blood glucose falls to 250 mg/dL.

Hyperkalemia (unlabeled): Insulin may be used in patients with or without diabetes mellitus to treat hyperkalemia. Must be administered with a dextrose solution in nondiabetic patients. Begin with an initial dose of 5 to 10 units of regular insulin and 50 mL of dextrose 50% as an IV bolus. Follow with a continuous infusion of 10% dextrose with regular insulin 20 units/L. Administer at 50 mL/hr to prevent fasting hyperkalemia.

Diagnosis of growth hormone deficiency (regular insulin [unlabeled use]): 0.05 to 0.15 units/kg of body weight as a rapid, one-time injection.

Myocardial infarction (glucose, insulin, potassium therapy [GIK therapy]; regular insulin [unlabeled use]): Insulin 20 or 50 units/liter in combination with potassium chloride 40 or 80 mEq/liter respectively and a liter of 10% or 25% IV dextrose solution (20 units insulin with 40 mEq KCl in 1 liter of D10W or 50 units insulin with 80 mEq KCl in 1 liter of D25W). Low-dose regimen is infused at 1 mL/kg/hr for 24 hours, high-dose regimen at 1.5 mL/kg/hr for 24 hours. High-dose regimen may be more effective.

PEDIATRIC DOSE

Ketoacidosis: *Regular insulin and insulin aspart:* 0.1 unit/kg as an IV bolus. Follow with a continuous infusion of 0.1 unit/kg/hr. Rate of glucose fall should not exceed 80 to 100 mg/dL/hr. Increase insulin to 0.14 to 0.2 unit/kg/hr if glucose falls less than 50 mg/dL/hr. If glucose falls faster than 100 mg/dL/hr, continue insulin infusion (0.1 unit/kg/hr) and add 5% dextrose to IV fluids. As glucose approaches 250 to 300 mg/dL, add 5% dextrose to IV fluids.

DOSE ADJUSTMENTS

A reduced dose of insulin may be indicated when infusions are discontinued and SC administration is indicated. As in Usual Dose, base on blood glucose determinations and patient's response to therapy. ▪ Dose requirements may be reduced in patients with renal or hepatic impairment.

DILUTION

Regular insulin and insulin aspart: Use only if clear. May be given undiluted either directly into the vein or through a Y-tube or three-way stopcock. Fifty units of insulin added to 500 mL of infusion solution given at a rate of 1 mL/min will deliver 6 units/hr. Another regimen adds 100 units of insulin (1 mL) to 100 mL of NS. This solution yields 1 unit/mL and is usually given at a rate of 0.1 unit/kg of body weight/hr (70-kg adult would receive 7 units/hr). May be diluted in NS, D5W, or D10W with 40 mmol/L of KCl to a final concentration of 0.05 to 1 unit/mL. Use a polypropylene infusion bag. See Precautions.

Humulin R U-100: Must be diluted with NS to achieve a final concentration of 0.1 to 1 unit/mL (100 units of insulin [1 mL] to 100 mL of NS yields 1 unit/mL). Use polyvinyl chloride (PVC) infusion bags.

Insulin glulisine: May be diluted with NS to achieve a final concentration of 0.05 unit/mL to 1 unit/mL (e.g., dilute 100 units in 100 mL NS). Polyvinyl chloride (PVC) Viaflex infusion bags and PVC tubing must be used. Use of other bags and tubings has not been studied.

Storage: *Regular insulin and insulin aspart:* Infusion bags prepared as indicated in Dilution are stable at RT for 24 hours. A certain amount of insulin will be initially absorbed into the infusion bag and tubing. *Insulin glulisine:* Infusion bags prepared as indicated in dilution are stable at RT for 48 hours. *Regular insulin:* Store unopened vials in refrigerator; vial that is in use may be stored in a cool, dark room. Protect from sunlight and freezing. Discard any open vial not used for several weeks. *Insulin aspart and insulin glulisine:* Store unopened vials in refrigerator. Vial that is in use may be stored at RT (below 30° C) for up to 28 days. Do not expose to excessive heat or sunlight.

COMPATIBILITY   (Underline Indicates Conflicting Compatibility Information)
Consider any drug NOT listed as compatible to be INCOMPATIBLE until consulting a pharmacist; specific conditions may apply.
Manufacturer lists **insulin glulisine** as **incompatible** with dextrose solution and Ringer's solutions and therefore cannot be mixed with these solutions. The use of **insulin glulisine (Apidra)** with other solutions has not been studied and is not recommended.

One source suggests the following **compatibilities:**
These compatibilities refer to regular insulin only; information on specific compatibilities for insulin aspart and insulin glulisine are not available.
Additive: Lidocaine, meropenem (Merrem IV), ranitidine (Zantac), verapamil.
Y-site: Amiodarone (Nexterone), ampicillin, ampicillin/sulbactam (Unasyn), aztreonam (Azactam), caspofungin (Cancidas), cefazolin (Ancef), cefepime (Maxipime), cefotetan, ceftazidime (Fortaz), digoxin (Lanoxin), diltiazem (Cardizem), dobutamine, doripenem (Doribax), doxapram (Dopram), esmolol (Brevibloc), famotidine (Pepcid IV), gentamicin, heparin, imipenem-cilastatin (Primaxin), indomethacin (Indocin IV), levofloxacin (Levaquin), magnesium sulfate, meperidine (Demerol), meropenem (Merrem IV), midazolam (Versed), milrinone (Primacor), morphine, nitroglycerin IV, nitroprusside sodium, oxytocin (Pitocin), pantoprazole (Protonix IV), pentobarbital (Nembutal), potassium chloride (KCl), propofol (Diprivan), sodium bicarbonate, tacrolimus (Prograf), ticarcillin/clavulanate (Timentin), tobramycin, vancomycin, vasopressin.

RATE OF ADMINISTRATION
Each 50 units or fraction thereof over 1 minute. When given in an IV infusion, the rate should be ordered by the physician and will depend on insulin and fluid needs; see Dilution for example. Decrease rate when plasma glucose reaches 300 mg/dL.

ACTIONS
A hormone produced by the pancreas that controls the storage and metabolism of carbohydrates, proteins, and fat. Responsible for regulation of glucose metabolism. Binds to insulin receptors on muscle and fat cells and lowers blood glucose by facilitating cellular uptake of glucose and inhibiting output of glucose from the liver. Also inhibits lipolysis and proteolysis and enhances protein synthesis. Rapidly and widely distributed. Half-life with IV administration varies with each product. The glucose-lowering activities of regular insulin, insulin aspart, and insulin glulisine are equipotent when administered by the IV route. The average elimination half-life is 81 minutes for insulin aspart, 98 minutes for insulin glulisine,

and 141 to 161 minutes for regular human insulin. Eliminated to some extent renally. Does not cross the placenta.

INDICATIONS AND USES

Regular insulin: Treatment of diabetes mellitus (Type I, Type II, and gestational). ▪ Treatment of complications associated with diabetes (e.g., diabetic coma, hyperosmolar hyperglycemia with or without coma [hyperglycemia and dehydration], ketoacidosis with or without coma [plasma glucose exceeding 250 mg/dL with arterial pH of 7 to 7.24 or less and serum bicarbonate of 10 to 15 mEq/L or less]). ▪ In combination with glucose to treat hyperkalemia. ▪ Add to total parenteral nutrition to control hyperglycemia.

Humulin R U-100, insulin aspart, and insulin glulisine: Treatment of patients with diabetes mellitus for control of hyperglycemia. Usually used as part of a SC injection regimen or as a SC infusion administered via an external insulin pump. May be given IV under proper medical supervision to prevent hypoglycemia and hypokalemia.

Unlabeled uses: Diagnosis of growth hormone deficiency. ▪ Continuous intravenous infusions administered via a special pump have been used to treat severe brittle diabetics who have failed more conventional therapy. ▪ GIK therapy for metabolic modulation post MI. May have potential beneficial effects on morbidity and mortality. Has been used in combination with thrombolytics or percutaneous coronary intervention (PCI).

CONTRAINDICATIONS

Contraindicated during episodes of hypoglycemia and in patients hypersensitive to regular human insulin, insulin aspart, insulin glulisine, or one of the excipients of any of these products.

PRECAUTIONS

Only regular insulin, insulin aspart, and insulin glulisine may be given IV. All insulin formulations are standardized at 100 units/mL.

Regular insulin, insulin aspart, and insulin glulisine: Circulating levels of insulin may be increased in patients with renal or hepatic failure; see Dose Adjustments. ▪ Hypoglycemia and hypokalemia are potential side effects of insulin therapy. Use caution in patients in whom these side effects may be clinically relevant (e.g., patients who are fasting, have autonomic neuropathy, are using potassium-lowering drugs [e.g., diuretics], or are taking drugs sensitive to serum potassium levels [e.g., digoxin]). ▪ Insulin requirements may be altered during illness or stress. ▪ Anti-insulin antibodies have been reported. Clinical significance of anti-insulin antibodies is unknown. ▪ Systemic hypersensitivity reactions have been reported. May include hypotension, pruritus, rash, shortness of breath, sweating, tachycardia, and/or wheezing. Anaphylaxis has occurred.

Regular insulin: Insulin potency may be reduced by at least 20% and possibly up to 80% via the glass or plastic infusion container and plastic IV tubing before it actually reaches the venous system in an infusion. The percentage adsorbed is inversely proportional to the concentration of insulin (the larger the dose, the less adsorption) and takes place within 30 to 60 minutes. Albumin is sometimes added to reduce this adsorption. Other additives (e.g., electrolytes, other drugs, vitamins) may also reduce adsorption. Other methods of compensation for insulin loss include the addition of added insulin to saturate binding sites or the use of a syringe pump (instead of infusion containers) to reduce surface area for adsorption.

Monitor: Response to insulin measured by blood glucose, blood pH, acetone, BUN, sodium, potassium, chloride, and CO_2 levels. Monitor patient carefully in all situations. Glucose and potassium levels must be monitored closely during IV administration of insulin to avoid potentially fatal hypoglycemia and hypokalemia. Glycosylated hemoglobin (HgbA1c) may be measured to assess long-term glycemic control. ▪ Hypovolemia is a common complication of diabetic acidosis. ▪ See Drug/Lab Interactions. ▪ Insulin is inactivated at pH above 7.5.

Patient Education: Monitor blood glucose as directed. ▪ Adhere to consistent diet and exercise programs. ▪ Avoid alcohol. ▪ Review medications or changes in medication regimen with a health care professional. ▪ Review S/S of hypoglycemia and hyperglycemia with a health care professional. Be familiar with the treatment for each. ▪ Insulin requirements may change with onset of illness. Monitor glucose carefully and adjust insulin therapy as required.

Maternal/Child: *Regular insulin:* Category B: human insulin is drug of choice for control of diabetes in pregnancy. Additional insulin may be required to control serum glucose and avoid ketoacidosis. Monitor carefully; insulin requirements may drop immediately postpartum. Normal prepregnancy dose should be achieved within 6 weeks. Patients with gestational diabetes usually do not require insulin therapy following childbirth. ▪ Use caution in breast-feeding. ▪ Breast-feeding may decrease insulin requirements. ▪ Inadequately controlled maternal blood glucose late in pregnancy may cause increased insulin production in the fetus. Monitor and treat neonatal hypoglycemia postpartum.

Insulin aspart: Category B: careful monitoring of glucose control is essential; see comments under regular insulin. ▪ Use caution during breast-feeding.

Insulin glulisine: Category C: use caution and assess risk versus benefit. Careful monitoring of glucose control is essential; see comments under regular insulin. ▪ Safety and effectiveness of IV administration for use in pediatric patients not established.

DRUG/LAB INTERACTIONS

Hypoglycemic effect is potentiated by **ACE inhibitors** (e.g., enalaprilat [Vasotec], lisinopril [Prinivil]), **anabolic steroids** (e.g., nandrolone [Durabolin]), **disopyramide** (Norpace), **fluoxetine** (Prozac), **fibrates** (e.g., fenofibrate [Tricor]), **guanethidine, MAO inhibitors** (e.g., selegiline [Eldepryl]), **oral antidiabetic agents** (e.g., glyburide [DiaBeta]), **pentoxifylline** (Trental), **propoxyphene** (Darvon-N), **salicylates, sulfonamides, tetracyclines, and many others.** ▪ Inhibited by **atypical antipsychotic medications** (e.g., olanzapine [Zyprexa], clozapine [Clozaril]), **corticosteroids, danazol** (Cyclomen), **diazoxide, diuretics** (e.g., furosemide [Lasix]), **dobutamine, glucagon, isoniazid** (INH), **niacin, oral contraceptives, phenothiazine derivatives** (e.g., chlorpromazine [Thorazine]), **protease inhibitors** (e.g., indinavir [Crixivan]), **somatropin** (Humatrope), **sympathomimetic agents** (e.g., epinephrine [Adrenalin], albuterol [Ventolin]), **thyroid preparations, and others.** ▪ **Alcohol, beta-adrenergic blockers including ophthalmics** (e.g., propranolol, metoprolol [Lopressor]), **clonidine** (Catapres), **and lithium** may either potentiate or inhibit the blood glucose–lowering effect of insulin. ▪ Hypoglycemic effects may be decreased in **smokers;** dose adjustment may be required. ▪ Will affect serum potassium levels; use caution in patients taking **digoxin.** ▪ **Octreotide** (Sandostatin) may alter insulin, glucagon, and growth hormone secretion, resulting in hypoglycemia or hyperglycemia. Monitor serum glucose and adjust insulin dose as indicated. Octreotide also markedly increases adsorption of insulin to glass and plastic and reduces availability. ▪ **Pentamidine** is toxic to the beta cells of the pancreas. Patients may develop hypoglycemia initially as insulin is released. This may be followed by hypoinsulinemia and hyperglycemia with continued pentamidine therapy. ▪ S/S of hypoglycemia may be masked in the presence of **beta-blockers, clonidine** (Catapres), **guanethidine** (Ismelin), **and reserpine.**

SIDE EFFECTS

Hypoglycemia with overdose. *Early:* Ashen color, clammy skin, drowsiness, faintness, fatigue, headache, hunger, nausea, nervousness, sweating, tremors, weakness. *Advanced:* Coma, convulsions, disorientation, hypokalemia (with ECG changes), psychic disturbances, unconsciousness. Hypersensitivity reactions including anaphylaxis may occur; death is rare.

ANTIDOTE

Discontinue the drug immediately and notify physician. *Glucagon* 1 to 2 mg IM or SC is the specific antidote for insulin overdose. It may be supplemented by glucose 50% IV and/or oral carbohydrates such as glucose gel or orange juice. Oral carbohydrates may be sufficient to combat early symptoms of hypoglycemia. Correct hypokalemia as indicated. Hypersensitivity reactions usually respond to symptomatic treatment.

INTERFERON ALFA-2b, RECOMBINANT BBW

(in-ter-**FEER**-on **AL**-fah)

Intron A

Biologic response modifier
Antineoplastic

pH 6.9 to 7.5

USUAL DOSE

(International units [IU])

Pretreatment with acetaminophen may lessen flu-like side effects.

Malignant melanoma: *Induction:* 20,000,000 IU/M^2 as an infusion each day for 5 consecutive days per week for 4 weeks. Begin therapy within 56 days of surgical resection.

Maintenance: Follow with 10,000,000 IU/M^2 as a SC injection three times each week for 48 weeks.

Total treatment regimen lasts for 1 year and should be completed unless there is progression of disease or the drug is discontinued because of specific side effects.

DOSE ADJUSTMENTS

Temporarily discontinued for serious adverse reactions, if granulocytes decrease to less than 500/mm^3, or ALT/AST increases to more than 5 times upper limit of normal. When adverse reactions subside or improvement of granulocytes or liver function tests occur, treatment can be restarted at 50% of the previous dose. Discontinue permanently if serious adverse reactions persist, if granulocytes decrease to less than 250/mm^3, or if ALT/AST increases to more than 10 times the upper limit of normal. ▪ See Elderly.

DILUTION (International units [IU])

Prepare immediately before use. Only the sterile powder is suitable for dilution for IV use. Do not use different brands of interferon in any single treatment regimen; variations exist and may adversely affect dosage and response to treatment. Available in 10, 18, and 50 million IU vials; select one most appropriate for desired dose. Reconstitute with the diluent provided. Gently swirl to dissolve. Withdraw desired dose and inject into 100 mL of NS. Final concentration should be at least 10 million IU/100 mL.

Storage: Unopened vials of powder for injection should be refrigerated. After reconstitution, solution should be used immediately but can be refrigerated at 2° to 8° C (36° to 46° F) for 24 hours.

COMPATIBILITY

Specific information not available. Consider specific use; consult pharmacist. One source indicates **compatibility** with NS, LR, and R solutions and **incompatibility** with dextrose solutions.

RATE OF ADMINISTRATION

A single dose equally distributed over 20 minutes. Administration at bedtime and the use of acetaminophen may prevent or partially reduce common side effects (e.g., fever, headache, "flu-like" symptoms).

ACTIONS

A naturally occurring small protein and glycoprotein of the interferon family produced by recombinant DNA techniques. It binds to specific membrane receptors on the cell surface and initiates a complex sequence of intracellular events (e.g., induction of specific enzymes, suppression of cell proliferation, immunomodulating activities [e.g., enhancement of phagocytic activity of macrophages, augmentation of the specific cytotoxicity of lymphocytes for target cells, inhibition of virus replication in virus-infected cells]). Peak concentration achieved within 30 minutes. Half-life about 2 hours; undetectable 4 hours after infusion. Has produced a significant increase in relapse-free and overall survival in patients with malignant melanoma. The kidney may be the site of interferon catabolism.

INDICATIONS AND USES

Adjuvant to surgical treatment in patients with malignant melanoma who are free of disease but at high risk for systemic recurrence within 56 days of surgery. ■ Used IM or SC to treat hairy cell leukemia, follicular non-Hodgkin's lymphoma, AIDS-related Kaposi's sarcoma, chronic hepatitis B, chronic hepatitis C in patients unresponsive to previous therapy, in combination with recombinant ribavirin to treat chronic hepatitis C in patients with compensated liver disease who have relapsed following interferon alfa therapy, and intralesionally to treat condylomata acuminata.

CONTRAINDICATIONS

Hypersensitivity to interferon alfa or any of its components (benzyl alcohol, glycine, human albumin, and sodium phosphate dibasic and monobasic). ■ Not recommended for patients with a pre-existing psychiatric condition, especially depression or a history of severe psychiatric disorder. ■ Not recommended for patients with pre-existing thyroid abnormalities if thyroid function cannot be maintained within the normal range with medication. ■ Not recommended for patients with decompensated liver disease, autoimmune hepatitis, or a history of autoimmune disease or for patients who are immunosuppressed transplant recipients.

PRECAUTIONS

Use cautiously in patients with a history of pulmonary disease (e.g., COPD), diabetes mellitus prone to ketoacidosis, coagulation disorders (e.g., thrombophlebitis, pulmonary embolism) or severe myelosuppression. ■ Use cautiously in patients with a history of cardiovascular disease (e.g., unstable angina, uncontrolled CHF, recent MI, and previous or current arrhythmic disorder). ■ May cause or aggravate depression and suicidal behavior; see Maternal/Child. ■ May cause or aggravate life-threatening or fatal neuropsychiatric (e.g., depression, aggressive and/or suicidal behavior), autoimmune, ischemic, or infectious disorders. Close monitoring with periodic clinical and laboratory evaluations required. Discontinue therapy if S/S of any of the previous conditions worsen. Symptoms may resolve. ■ Severe cytopenias, including rare cases of aplastic anemia, have been reported; see Monitor. ■ Ophthalmologic disorders (e.g., decreased vision or loss of vision; retinopathy including macular edema, retinal artery or vein thrombosis, retinal hemorrhages, and cotton wool spots; optic neuritis; papilledema) may be induced or aggravated by treatment with interferons; see Monitor. ■ Use caution in patients with psoriasis and sarcoidosis; may exacerbate disease. ■ Rare cases of autoimmune diseases (e.g., lupus erythematosus, Raynaud's phenomenon, rhabdomyolysis, rheumatoid arthritis, thrombocytopenia, and vasculitis) have been reported; may require discontinuation of therapy. ■ Use caution as combination therapy with ribavirin (Rebetol). Hemolytic anemia (less than 10 Gm/dL) can occur within 1 to 2 weeks. Combination should not be used in patients with creatinine clearance less than 50 mL/min. ■ Serum neutralizing antibodies have been detected in some patients; clinical significance unknown. ■ Ischemic and hemorrhagic cerebrovascular events have been reported. A causal relationship between interferon therapy and these side effects is difficult to establish.

Monitor: Obtain baseline CBC including differential and platelet count, blood chemistries (electrolytes, liver function tests, and TSH), chest x-ray. Obtain baseline eye exam for all patients and periodically for patients with pre-existing ophthalmologic disorders (e.g., diabetic or hypertensive retinopathy). Obtain baseline ECG if there is a history of cardiovascular disease and/or patient is in advanced stages of cancer. Monitor all tests periodically during therapy. ■ Monitor CBC with differential and platelet count and liver function tests weekly during the induction phase and monthly during maintenance. Dose adjustments will be determined by results. Discontinue therapy if neutrophil count drops below 500 cells/mm^3. ■ Monitor for thrombocytopenia (platelet count less than 50,000/mm^3). Discontinue therapy if platelet count drops below 25,000/mm^3. Initiate precautions to prevent excessive bleeding (e.g., inspect IV sites, skin, and mucous membranes; use extreme care during invasive procedures; test urine, emesis, stool, and secretions for occult blood). ■ Closely monitor any patient with a history of cardiovascular disease (see Precautions); arrhythmias including tachycardia, hypotension, and transient reversible cardiomyopathy have occurred. ■ Monitor for S/S of a hypersensitivity reaction (e.g., anaphylaxis, angioedema, bronchoconstriction, urticaria). ■ Hypotension may occur during administration or up to 2 days posttherapy; monitor frequently. May require fluid replacement. ■ Maintain adequate hydration, particularly during initial states of treatment. ■ Monitor for signs of depression and/or aggressive or suicidal behavior. If psychiatric problems develop, patients should be carefully monitored during treatment and in the 6-month follow-up period. ▪ Use of narcotics, hypnotics, or sedatives may be required to manage adverse effects; use with caution and monitor carefully. ▪ Monitor thyroid function, liver function tests, blood glucose, and triglyceride levels; abnormalities not normalized by medication may require discontinuing interferon. ▪ Determine cause of persistent fever. ▪ Repeat chest x-ray if cough, dyspnea, fever, or other respiratory symptoms occur. Monitor closely if pulmonary infiltrates or evidence of pulmonary function impairment is present; may require discontinuing interferon. ▪ Obtain an eye exam for any patient who complains of changes in visual acuity, visual fields, or other ophthalmologic symptoms. ▪ See Precautions.

Patient Education: Must use effective birth control throughout treatment; nonhormonal birth control preferred. ▪ Cooperation for close monitoring and reporting of side effects is imperative. Side effects may include depression, cardiovascular toxicity (e.g., chest pain), ophthalmologic toxicity (e.g., loss of or change in vision), pancreatitis, cytopenias. ▪ Manufacturer provides a patient information sheet. ▪ Home use may require extensive patient education. ▪ See Appendix D, p. 1434. ▪ Do not change brands of interferon without medical consultation. ▪ Do not drive or operate machinery; mental alertness may be impaired. ▪ Administration at bedtime and/or use of acetaminophen may be helpful to prevent the most common "flu-like" side effects. Remain well hydrated. ▪ Side effects may decrease in severity as treatment continues. Avoid excessive sunlight or artificial ultraviolet light. Potential for photosensitivity; wear protective clothing, sunscreens, and sunglasses. ▪ Dental and periodontal disorders have been reported in patients receiving combination therapy with interferon and ribavirin (Rebetol). Proper dental hygiene and regular dental exams recommended.

Maternal/Child: Category C: has abortifacient effects. Should be used only if benefits justify risks. ▪ Discontinue breast-feeding. ▪ Safety for use in pediatric patients under 18 years of age for indications other than chronic hepatitis B or C has not been established. ▪ Suicidal ideation or attempts have occurred more often among pediatric patients (primarily adolescents) compared to adult patients. ▪ For use in pediatric patients for indications other than SC administration in chronic hepatitis B and chronic hepatitis C; see prescribing literature.

Elderly: Incidence of encephalopathy, obtundation, and coma has occurred, especially at higher doses. ▪ Cardiovascular adverse events and confusion have been reported more frequently in the elderly. ▪ Consider age-related decreases in organ function and concomitant disease and drug therapy. Careful monitoring required. Make dose adjustments based on symptoms and/or lab abnormalities.

DRUG/LAB INTERACTIONS
Specific information not available. Use caution with any **other potentially myelosuppressive agent** (e.g., cisplatin [Platinol], zidovudine [AZT, Retrovir]). ▪ May increase serum levels of **theophylline;** monitoring of theophylline levels recommended. ▪ May have synergistic additive effects with **zidovudine** (AZT, Retrovir) and increase incidence of neutropenia; monitor WBC closely. ▪ See Precautions.

SIDE EFFECTS

Occur in high percentages of patients; may be serious enough to require a decreased dose or discontinuation of drug. Usually rapidly reversible after therapy discontinued, but may require up to 3 weeks to resolve. Alopecia, anemia, anorexia, arrhythmias, autoimmune disorders, bleeding, coughing, depression, diarrhea, dizziness, dyspnea, elevated triglycerides, "flu-like" symptoms (e.g., chills, fatigue, fever, headache, myalgia), granulocytopenia, hyperglycemia, increased AST and/or ALT, leukopenia, nausea, ophthalmologic disorders, pain (variable), paresthesia, psychiatric disorders (e.g., depression, aggressive or suicidal behavior), pulmonary disorders, rash, taste alteration, thrombocytopenia, vomiting. Many other side effects may occur. Acute serious hypersensitivity reactions (e.g., anaphylaxis, angioedema, bronchoconstriction, urticaria) are rare but have occurred. **Post-Marketing:** Stevens-Johnson syndrome, toxic epidermal necrolysis, erythema multiforme, injection site necrosis, myositis, hearing loss, and a wide variety of autoimmune and immune-mediated disorders (e.g., idiopathic thrombocytopenic purpura and thrombotic thrombocytopenic purpura) have been identified in post-marketing reports.

ANTIDOTE

Keep physician informed of all side effects. Some will be tolerated or treated symptomatically. Discontinue interferon immediately for any acute serious hypersensitivity reactions and treat as appropriate; may require epinephrine, airway management, oxygen, IV fluids, antihistamines (e.g., diphenhydramine [Benadryl]), corticosteroids (e.g., hydrocortisone sodium succinate [Solu-Cortef]), and pressor amines (e.g., dopamine). Discontinue drug for any patient who develops severe depression or other psychiatric disorder. Close patient monitoring and psychiatric intervention may be indicated. Discontinue for myelosuppression that persists after dose reduction, endocrine thyroid abnormalities not normalized by medication, serious liver function abnormalities, new or worsening ophthalmologic disorders, serious pulmonary function impairment, or pulmonary infiltrates. Treatment of overdose with hemodialysis or peritoneal dialysis is not considered effective. Resuscitate as necessary.

IRINOTECAN HYDROCHLORIDE BBW

(**eye**-rih-noh-**TEE**-kan hy-droh-**KLOR**-eyed)

Camptosar, CPT-11

Antineoplastic
(topoisomerase 1 inhibitor)

pH 3 to 3.8

USUAL DOSE

Premedication with antiemetics recommended. Dexamethasone 10 mg and a 5-HT$_3$ blocker (e.g., ondansetron or granisetron) should be given on the day of treatment. Begin at least 30 minutes before giving irinotecan. See Monitor.

First-line treatment of colorectal cancer: The Saltz regimen or Regimen 1 is a combination therapy. It is administered once each week for 4 weeks (Days 1, 8, 15, and 22) followed by a 2-week rest period. Premedication

Continued

as described above is recommended. In addition prophylactic or therapeutic atropine may be indicated in patients experiencing cholinergic symptoms. Initiate regimen with the dose of irinotecan over 90 minutes. Follow immediately with the dose of leucovorin calcium (see leucovorin calcium monograph). Follow the leucovorin immediately with the dose of fluorouracil (see fluorouracil monograph). Doses and modified dosing recommendations are based on the chart Combination-Agent Dosage Regimens and Dose Modifications. Doses of irinotecan and fluorouracil may require modification based on toxicity. See Dose Adjustments, combination therapy and/or package insert.

Regimen 2, called the Douillard or European regimen, is another regimen. Used primarily in Europe, doses are considerably higher, intervals are different, and side effects more pronounced. See the following chart, Combination-Agent Dosage Regimens and Dose Modifications, and see Dose Adjustments, combination therapy and/or package insert.

Combination-Agent Dosage Regimens and Dose Modifications* (Irinotecan/Fluorouracil [5-FU]/Leucovorin Calcium [LV])				
Regimen 1 6-wk course with bolus 5-FU/LV (next course begins on Day 43)	irinotecan leucovorin 5-FU	125 mg/M^2 IV over 90 min, Day 1,8,15,22 20 mg/M^2 IV bolus, Day 1,8,15,22 500 mg/M^2 IV bolus, Day 1,8,15,22		
		Starting Dose and Modified Dose Levels (mg/M^2)		
		Starting Dose	Dose Level −1	Dose Level −2
	irinotecan	125 mg/M^2	100 mg/M^2	75 mg/M^2
	leucovorin	20 mg/M^2	20 mg/M^2	20 mg/M^2
	5-FU	500 mg/M^2	400 mg/M^2	300 mg/M^2
Regimen 2 6-wk course with infusional 5-FU/LV (next course begins on Day 43)	irinotecan leucovorin 5-FU Bolus 5-FU Infusion†	180 mg/M^2 IV over 90 min, Day 1,15,29 200 mg/M^2 IV over 2 hr, Day 1,2,15,16,29,30 400 mg/M^2 IV bolus, Day 1,2,15,16,29,30 600 mg/M^2 IV over 22 hr, Day 1,2,15,16,29,30		
		Starting Dose and Modified Dose Levels (mg/M^2)		
		Starting Dose	Dose Level −1	Dose Level −2
	irinotecan	180 mg/M^2	150 mg/M^2	120 mg/M^2
	leucovorin	200 mg/M^2	200 mg/M^2	200 mg/M^2
	5-FU Bolus	400 mg/M^2	320 mg/M^2	240 mg/M^2
	5-FU Infusion†	600 mg/M^2	480 mg/M^2	360 mg/M^2

*Dose reductions beyond dose level −2 by decrements of ~20% may be warranted for patients continuing to experience toxicity. Provided intolerable toxicity does not develop, treatment with additional courses may be continued indefinitely as long as patients continue to experience clinical benefit.
†Infusion follows bolus administration.

Treatment of colorectal cancer after failure of treatment with fluorouracil: Irinotecan: Administer as an infusion based on the following chart, Irinotecan Single-Agent Regimens and Dose Modifications. See Premedication. After adequate recovery, additional doses may be repeated in a similar cycle and continued indefinitely in patients who attain a response or in those whose disease remains stable.

Irinotecan Single-Agent Regimens and Dose Modifications		
Weekly Regimen*	125 mg/M² IV over 90 min, Day 1, 8, 15, 22 then 2-wk rest	
	Starting Dose and Modified Dose Levels‡ (mg/M²)	
	Starting Dose	Dose Level −1	Dose Level −2
	125 mg/M²	100 mg/M²	75 mg/M²
Once-Every-3-Week Regimen†	350 mg/M² IV over 90 min, once every 3 wks‡	
	Starting Dose and Modified Dose Levels (mg/M²)	
	Starting Dose	Dose Level −1	Dose Level −2
	350 mg/M²	300 mg/M²	250 mg/M²

*Subsequent doses may be adjusted as high as 150 mg/M² or to as low as 50 mg/M² in 25 to 50 mg/M² decrements depending upon individual patient tolerance.

†Subsequent doses may be adjusted as low as 200 mg/M² in 50 mg/M² decrements depending upon individual patient tolerance.

‡Provided intolerable toxicity does not develop, treatment with additional courses may be continued indefinitely as long as patients continue to experience clinical benefit.

DOSE ADJUSTMENTS

Consider decreasing the **starting dose** by at least one level of irinotecan when administered in combination with other agents or as a single agent to a patient known to be homozygous for the UGT1A1*28 allele (an allele is an alternative form of a gene). The precise dose reduction for this patient population is not known. Subsequent dose modification should be based on individual patient tolerance as outlined in the following tables. Heterozygous patients (patients who carry one variant allele) appear to tolerate normal starting doses. ▪ See Precautions.

Combination therapy: Decrease dose based on toxicity as described in the following chart, Guidelines for Dose Adjustments in Combination Schedules.

Guidelines for Dose Adjustments in Combination Schedules (Irinotecan Fluorouracil [5-FU]/Leucovorin Calcium [LV])		
Patients should return to pretreatment bowel function without requiring antidiarrhea medications for at least 24 hours before the next chemotherapy administration. A new course of therapy should also not begin until the granulocyte count has recovered to ≥1,500/mm³, and the platelet count has recovered to ≥100,000/mm³. Treatment should be delayed 1 to 2 weeks to allow for recovery from treatment-related toxicities. If the patient has not recovered after a 2-week delay, consideration should be given to discontinuing therapy.		
Toxicity CTCAE Grade* (Value)	During a Course of Therapy	At the Start of Subsequent Courses of Therapy†
No toxicity	Maintain dose level	Maintain dose level
Neutropenia 1 (1,500 to 1,999/mm³) 2 (1,000 to 1,499/mm³) 3 (500 to 999/mm³) 4 (<500/mm³)	Maintain dose level ↓1 dose level Omit dose until resolved to ≤Grade 2, then ↓1 dose level Omit dose until resolved to ≤Grade 2, then ↓2 dose levels	Maintain dose level Maintain dose level ↓1 dose level ↓2 dose levels
Neutropenic fever	Omit dose, then ↓2 dose levels when resolved	

Continued

Guidelines for Dose Adjustments in Combination Schedules
(Irinotecan Fluorouracil [5-FU]/Leucovorin Calcium [LV])—cont'd

Patients should return to pretreatment bowel function without requiring antidiarrhea medications for at least 24 hours before the next chemotherapy administration. A new course of therapy should also not begin until the granulocyte count has recovered to ≥1,500/mm³, and the platelet count has recovered to ≥100,000/mm³. Treatment should be delayed 1 to 2 weeks to allow for recovery from treatment-related toxicities. If the patient has not recovered after a 2-week delay, consideration should be given to discontinuing therapy.

Toxicity CTCAE Grade* (Value)	During a Course of Therapy	At the Start of Subsequent Courses of Therapy†
Other hematologic toxicities	Dose modifications for leukopenia or thrombocytopenia during a course of therapy and at the start of subsequent courses of therapy are also based on Common Terminology Criteria for Adverse Events and are the same as previously recommended for neutropenia.	
Diarrhea		
1 (2-3 stools/day >pretx‡)	Delay dose until resolved to baseline, then give same dose	Maintain dose level
2 (4-6 stools/day >pretx)	Omit dose until resolved to baseline, then ↓1 dose level	Maintain dose level
3 (7-9 stools/day >pretx)	Omit dose until resolved to baseline, then ↓1 dose level	↓1 dose level
4 (≥10 stools/day >pretx)	Omit dose until resolved to baseline, then ↓2 dose levels	↓2 dose levels
Other nonhematologic toxicities		
Grade 1	Maintain dose level	Maintain dose level
Grade 2	Omit dose until resolved to ≤Grade 1, then ↓1 dose level	Maintain dose level
Grade 3	Omit dose until resolved to ≤Grade 2, then ↓1 dose level	↓1 dose level
Grade 4	Omit dose until resolved to ≤Grade 2, then ↓2 dose levels *For mucositis/stomatitis decrease only 5-FU, not irinotecan*	↓2 dose levels *For mucositis/stomatitis decrease only 5-FU, not irinotecan*

*Common Terminology Criteria for Adverse Events.
†All dose modifications should be based on the worst preceding toxicity.
‡Pretreatment.

Single agent therapy: Reduce dose based on toxicity levels in the following chart, Irinotecan Guidelines for Dose Adjustments in Single-Agent Schedules. Most common reasons for dose reduction are late diarrhea, neutropenia, and leukopenia. ■ A reduction in the starting dose by one dose level may be required in patients with a performance status of 2, in patients who have previously received pelvic/abdominal irradiation, or in patients with increased bilirubin levels; see Elderly.

Guidelines for Irinotecan Dose Adjustments in Single-Agent Schedules*

A new course of therapy should not begin until the granulocyte count has recovered to ≥1,500/mm³, and the platelet count has recovered to ≥100,000/mm³, and treatment-related diarrhea is fully resolved. Treatment should be delayed 1 to 2 weeks to allow for recovery from treatment-related toxicities. If the patient has not recovered after a 2-week delay, consideration should be given to discontinuing irinotecan.

Worst Toxicity CTCAE Grade† (Value)	During a Course of Therapy	At the Start of the Next Courses of Therapy (After Adequate Recovery). Compared with the Starting Dose in the Previous Course*	
	Weekly	Weekly	Once Every 3 Weeks
No toxicity	Maintain dose level	↑25 mg/M² up to a maximum dose of 150 mg/M²	Maintain dose level
Neutropenia			
1 (1,500 to 1,999/mm³)	Maintain dose level	Maintain dose level	Maintain dose level
2 (1,000 to 1,499/mm³)	↓25 mg/M²	Maintain dose level	Maintain dose level
3 (500 to 999/mm³)	Omit dose until resolved to ≤Grade 2, then ↓25 mg/M²	↓25 mg/M²	↓50 mg/M²
4 (<500/mm³)	Omit dose until resolved to ≤Grade 2, then ↓50 mg/M²	↓50 mg/M² dose levels	↓50 mg/M²
Neutropenic fever	Omit dose until resolved, then ↓50 mg/M²	↓50 mg/M²	↓50 mg/M²
Other hematologic toxicities	Dose modifications for leukopenia, thrombocytopenia, and anemia during a course of therapy and at the start of subsequent courses of therapy are also based on Common Terminology Criteria for Adverse Events and are the same as recommended for neutropenia above.		
Diarrhea			
1 (2-3 stools/day >pretx‡)	Maintain dose level	Maintain dose level	Maintain dose level
2 (4-6 stools/day >pretx)	↓25 mg/M²	Maintain dose level	Maintain dose level
3 (7-9 stools/day >pretx)	Omit dose until resolved to ≤Grade 2, then ↓25 mg/M²	↓25 mg/M²	↓50 mg/M²
4 (≥10 stools/day >pretx)	Omit dose until resolved to ≤Grade 2, then ↓50 mg/M²	↓50 mg/M²	↓50 mg/M²
Other nonhematologic toxicities			
Grade 1	Maintain dose level	Maintain dose level	Maintain dose level
Grade 2	↓25 mg/M²	↓25 mg/M²	↓50 mg/M²
Grade 3	Omit dose until resolved to ≤Grade 2, then ↓25 mg/M²	↓25 mg/M²	↓50 mg/M²
Grade 4	Omit dose until resolved to ≤Grade 2, then ↓50 mg/M²	↓50 mg/M²	↓50 mg/M²

*All dose modifications should be based on the worst preceding toxicity.
†Common Terminology Criteria for Adverse Events.
‡Pretreatment.

DILUTION
Specific techniques required; see Precautions. Must be diluted for infusion with D5W (preferred) or NS to concentrations between 0.12 to 2.8 mg/mL. Usually diluted in 250 to 500 mL D5W.

Storage: Packaged in a blister pack to protect against accidental breakage and leakage. Store in carton protected from light at CRT. Do not freeze. If damaged, incinerate the unopened package. Recommended that diluted solution be used within 24 hours if refrigerated, within 6 hours if kept at CRT. However, when mixed with D5W, is stable for 48 hours if refrigerated and protected from light and 24 hours at CRT. Do not refrigerate if mixed with NS; a precipitate may form. Stable for 24 hours at CRT when mixed in NS. Avoid freezing.

COMPATIBILITY   (Underline Indicates Conflicting Compatibility Information)
Consider any drug NOT listed as compatible to be INCOMPATIBLE until consulting a pharmacist; specific conditions may apply.

Manufacturer states, "Other drugs should not be added to the infusion solution." Consider specific use and toxicity.

One source suggests the following **compatibilities:**
Y-site: Oxaliplatin (Eloxatin) and palonosetron (Aloxi).

RATE OF ADMINISTRATION
A single dose as an infusion equally distributed over 90 minutes.

ACTIONS
A semi-synthetic derivative of camptothecin. An alkaloid extract from plants such as *Camptotheca acuminata.* A class of antineoplastic agent that inhibits the enzyme topoisomerase I required for DNA replication. Together with its active metabolite SN-38 it causes cell death by damaging DNA produced during the S-phase of cell synthesis. Maximum plasma SN-38 levels are reached within 1 hour of infusion end. Extensively distributed to body tissues. Terminal half-life of irinotecan is about 6 to 12 hours; SN-38 is 10 to 20 hours. Irinotecan is moderately bound to plasma proteins (35%), but SN-38 is highly bound (95%). Metabolic conversion of irinotecan to SN-38 primarily occurs in the liver. SN-38 is conjugated to a glucuronide metabolite by the enzyme UDP-glucuronosyltransferase 1A1 (UGT1A1). Approximately 25% to 50% excreted through bile and urine.

INDICATIONS AND USES
First-line therapy for the treatment of metastatic colorectal cancer in combination with fluorouracil and leucovorin calcium. ■ As a single agent in the treatment of metastatic carcinoma of the colon or rectum that has recurred or progressed following treatment with fluorouracil.

CONTRAINDICATIONS
Hypersensitivity to irinotecan or any of its components. ■ Concomitant administration of St. John's wort and ketoconazole (Nizoral) is contraindicated; see Drug/Lab Interactions.

PRECAUTIONS
Follow guidelines for handling cytotoxic agents. See Appendix A, p. 1429.
■ Administered by or under the direction of the physician specialist. ■ Adequate diagnostic and treatment facilities must be available. ■ Can induce both early and late forms of diarrhea that appear to be mediated by different mechanisms. Both forms may be severe. ■ Hepatic dysfunction may impair the metabolism of both irinotecan and SN-38. Patients with a bilirubin of 1 to 2 mg/dL are at increased risk for developing Grade 3 or 4 neutropenia. The

manufacturer does not recommend a dose for patients with a bilirubin greater than 2 mg/dL and states that insufficient information is available. However, some clinicians recommend administering 75% of the recommended dose to patients who have a bilirubin of 1.5 to 3 mg/dL. ▪ May cause severe myelosuppression. Deaths due to sepsis following severe neutropenia have been reported. ▪ Use with caution in patients with renal impairment. Has not been studied. Not recommended for use in patients on dialysis. ▪ Patients who are homozygous for the UGT1A1*28 allele have decreased UGT1A1 enzyme activity. This leads to a higher exposure to SN-38 and an increased risk for neutropenia; see Dose Adjustments. A laboratory test is available to determine the UGT1A1 status of patients. ▪ Use caution in the elderly (may have an increased incidence and severity of diarrhea) and in patients who have had previous cytotoxic therapy or previous pelvic/abdominal irradiation (likely to have an increased incidence and severity of myelosuppression). Monitor closely. ▪ Use caution in patients with poor performance status. Patients with a baseline performance status of 2 had higher rates of hospitalization, neutropenic fever, thromboembolism, first-cycle treatment discontinuation, and early deaths than patients with a performance status of 0 or 1. ▪ Use caution in patients with a history of allergies. Severe hypersensitivity reactions, including anaphylaxis, have been reported. ▪ Use caution in patients with pleural effusions and/or with impaired pulmonary function. Interstitial pulmonary disease has been reported rarely. Can be fatal. Risk factors may include pre-existing lung disease, use of pneumotoxic agents (e.g., amiodarone [Nexterone]), radiation therapy, or colony-stimulating factors; see Antidote. ▪ Colitis complicated by ulceration, ileus, and what was described as toxic megacolon has been reported. Any bowel obstruction must be resolved before treatment with irinotecan is initiated. ▪ Contains sorbital. Do not use in patients with hereditary fructose intolerance. ▪ The Mayo Clinic regimen of 5-FU/LV (administered for 4 to 5 days every 28 days) should not be used in combination with irinotecan outside of a carefully controlled, well-designed clinical study. Regimen has caused increased toxicity and death. ▪ Thromboembolic events have been observed; a specific cause has not been determined. ▪ See Monitor.

Monitor: Obtain a WBC with differential, hemoglobin, and platelet count before each dose. Expected nadir for platelets is 14 days, and 21 days for hemoglobin, neutrophils, and leukocytes. ▪ Prophylactic antiemetics are recommended; see Usual Dose. To reduce nausea and vomiting and increase patient comfort after initial dosing, additional antiemetics should be available (e.g., ondansetron, granisetron). ▪ Obtain baseline electrolytes and liver function tests. ▪ Not a vesicant, but monitor injection site for inflammation and/or extravasation. ▪ Monitor vital signs. ▪ Obtain an accurate bowel history to evaluate changes in bowel habits after administration of irinotecan. ▪ Monitor for "early" diarrhea. Occurs during or within 24 hours of irinotecan administration and is cholinergic in nature. Usually transient and only infrequently is severe. May be accompanied by other cholinergic symptoms (e.g., abdominal cramping, diaphoresis, flushing, increased salivation, lacrimation, miosis, rhinitis). Patients who have a cholinergic reaction to irinotecan will probably have similar reactions to subsequent doses. Atropine 0.25 to 1 mg IV or SC may be considered for treatment or for prophylactic use unless clinically contraindicated. ▪ Monitor for "late" diarrhea (more than 24 hours after irinotecan administration), which probably results from cytotoxic effects on GI epithelium. May be prolonged; cause dehydration, electrolyte imbalances, or sepsis; and can be life threatening. At first onset give loperamide (Imodium) 4 mg; give 2 mg every 2 hours (4 mg every 4 hours during the night) until diarrhea-free for a minimum of 12 hours. An alternate regimen suggests loperamide 4 mg every 3 hours in combination with diphenhydramine (Benadryl) 25 mg every 6 hours. Monitor carefully; replace fluids and electrolytes as needed; see Patient Education. ■ Premedication or prophylaxis with loperamide is not recommended. If Grade 3 or 4 late diarrhea develops, hold irinotecan therapy until patient recovers, then decrease subsequent doses; see Dose Adjustments. ■ Use of laxatives is not recommended; however, they may be used in patients requiring them for constipation caused by narcotics. Close supervision is required. ■ Initiate antibiotic therapy in patients who develop ileus, fever, or severe neutropenia. After the first treatment, subsequent weekly chemotherapy treatments should be delayed until the return of pretreatment bowel function for at least 24 hours without the need for antidiarrheal medication. ■ Closely monitor patients with pulmonary risk factors for adverse respiratory symptoms; see Precautions and Antidote. ■ Maintain adequate hydration. Orthostatic hypotension or dizziness may indicate dehydration. Rare cases of renal impairment or acute renal failure have been reported, usually in patients who became dehydrated from vomiting and/or diarrhea. ■ Be alert for signs of bone marrow suppression or infection. Prophylactic antibiotics may be indicated pending results of C/S in a febrile or nonfebrile neutropenic patient. ■ Monitor for thrombocytopenia (platelet count less than 50,000/mm^3). Initiate precautions to prevent excessive bleeding (e.g., inspect IV sites, skin, and mucous membranes; use extreme care during invasive procedures; test urine, emesis, stool, and secretions for occult blood). ■ See Dose Adjustments.

Patient Education: Manufacturer provides a patient education brochure, "Important Facts About Your Chemotherapy." ■ Report any unusual or unexpected symptoms or side effects as soon as possible. ■ Report black or bloody stools, diarrhea not under control within 24 hours, dry mouth, fever or chills, inability to retain oral fluids due to nausea and vomiting, infections, symptoms of dehydration (e.g., light-headedness, dizziness, fainting), urine changes, or vomiting immediately; each must be treated promptly. Have loperamide (Imodium) available. Dose of loperamide prescribed for late diarrhea is higher than the usual dose recommendation. Limit use at this dose to 48 hours to avoid risk of paralytic ileus. ■ May cause dizziness or visual disturbances (usually within 24 hours of administration); use caution in tasks that require alertness. ■ Compliance with regimen imperative (e.g., taking temperature, obtaining lab work, adequate rest, nourishment, and fluids). ■ Avoid caffeine and alcohol. May worsen dehydration. ■ Avoid raw fruits and vegetables, bran, fatty foods, or any other food that may aggravate diarrhea. ■ Nonhormonal birth control recommended. ■ Inform health care professionals of any problems with previous treatments. ■ See Appendix D, p. 1434.

Maternal/Child: Category D: avoid pregnancy. May cause fetal harm. ■ Discontinue breast-feeding. ■ Safety and effectiveness for use in pediatric patients not established. Results from a few open-label studies have been evaluated. Significant Grade 3 and 4 toxicities were noted. See package insert.

Elderly: Half-life slightly extended. ▪ Reduce starting dose by one dose level to 300 mg/M² in patients 70 years and older in the single agent once every 3-week regimen. No change in the starting dose is recommended for elderly patients receiving the weekly dose schedule of irinotecan. See Usual Dose and Dose Adjustments. ▪ Risk of early and late diarrhea increased in the elderly. ▪ Monitor carefully; may dehydrate more quickly from diarrhea. Begin loperamide therapy promptly. Avoid laxatives.

DRUG/LAB INTERACTIONS
Interaction of irinotecan with other drugs has not been adequately studied. ▪ Additive bone marrow suppression may occur with **radiation therapy and/or other bone marrow–suppressing agents** (e.g., azathioprine [Imuran], chloramphenicol, melphalan [Alkeran]). Dose reduction may be required. ▪ Concurrent administration with **irradiation** is not recommended. ▪ **Dexamethasone** for antiemetic prophylaxis may increase lymphocytopenia and may contribute to hyperglycemia in patients with diabetes. ▪ Administration of **prochlorperazine** (Compazine) and irinotecan on the same day may increase the risk of akathisia (inability to sit still, urge to move about constantly). ▪ Use caution or withhold **diuretics** (e.g., furosemide [Lasix]) **and laxatives** during treatment; may increase risk of dehydration secondary to vomiting and/or diarrhea. ▪ Concomitant use with **phenytoin** (Dilantin), **phenobarbital, or carbamazepine** (Tegretol) may increase the metabolism of irinotecan, which decreases concentrations and effectiveness. Discontinue treatment with these agents at least 2 weeks before starting irinotecan. Consider alternate anticonvulsant therapy. ▪ **Rifampin** (Rifadin) **and rifabutin** (Mycobutin) may also increase metabolism and decrease the serum concentrations and effectiveness of irinotecan. ▪ **Ketoconazole** (Nizoral) **and atazanavir** (Reyataz) may decrease metabolism, which increases serum concentrations and the risk of toxicity. Discontinue ketoconazole at least 1 week before starting irinotecan. ▪ **St. John's wort** may decrease serum levels and effectiveness. Discontinue St. John's wort at least 2 weeks before starting irinotecan. ▪ May prolong neuromuscular blockade of **depolarizing neuromuscular blocking agents** (e.g., succinylcholine) and antagonize neuromuscular blockade of **nondepolarizing neuromuscular blocking agents** (e.g., cisatracurium [Nimbex], vecuronium). ▪ Do not administer **live virus vaccines** to patients receiving antineoplastic drugs.

SIDE EFFECTS
Myelosuppression (anemia, leukopenia, neutropenia) and diarrhea ("early" [e.g., abdominal cramping or pain, diaphoresis] or "late") occur in patients and are the most common dose-limiting toxicities. Nausea and vomiting occur in most patients and can be severe, may occur early (within 24 hours of administration) or late (more than 24 hours after administration). Abdominal bloating, alopecia, anorexia, asthenia, back pain, chills, confusion, constipation, coughing, dehydration, dizziness, dyspepsia, dyspnea, edema, exfoliative dermatitis, fever, flatulence, flushing, headache, hypersensitivity reactions (including anaphylaxis), hyponatremia, hypotension, increased alkaline phosphatase and AST, increased bilirubin, infection, insomnia, interstitial pulmonary disease, mucositis, muscular contractions or cramps, myocardial infarction, neutropenic fever, neutropenic infection, paresthesia, pneumonia, pulmonary embolism, rash, rhinitis, somnolence, stomatitis, thrombocytopenia, thrombophlebitis, and weight loss may occur. Death was preceded by cyanosis, tremors, respiratory distress, and convulsions. In addition, ileus without preceding colitis

has occurred. Renal impairment or failure has occurred usually in patients who became volume depleted from severe vomiting and/or diarrhea. **Post-Marketing:** Asymptomatic elevated pancreatic enzymes (e.g., amylase, lipase), dysarthria (transient), ischemic or ulcerative colitis, megacolon, myocardial ischemic events, pancreatitis.

ANTIDOTE

Keep physician informed of all side effects and monitor carefully. Adjust or omit dose as indicated for toxicity; see Dose Adjustments. Treat diarrhea immediately; see Monitor. In the event of an acute onset of new or progressive, unexplained pulmonary symptoms (e.g., cough, dyspnea, fever), interrupt irinotecan and other co-prescribed chemotherapeutic agents pending diagnostic evaluation. If interstitial pulmonary disease is diagnosed, discontinue irinotecan and other chemotherapy and initiate appropriate treatment as needed. Administration of whole blood products (e.g., packed RBCs, platelets, leukocytes) and/or blood modifiers (e.g., darbepoetin alfa [Aranesp], epoetin alfa [Epogen], filgrastim [Neupogen], pegfilgrastim [Neulasta], sargramostim [Leukine], oprelvekin [Neumega]) may be indicated to treat bone marrow toxicity. Death may occur from the progression of many side effects. No known antidote for overdose. Maximum supportive care (e.g., to prevent dehydration due to diarrhea and to treat any infectious complications) will help sustain patient in toxicity. If extravasation occurs, flush site with SW, elevate the extremity, and apply ice.

IRON DEXTRAN INJECTION BBW

(EYE-ern DEKS-tran in-JEK-shun)

DexFerrum, ♣DexIron, InFeD, ♣Infufer, Proferdex

Hematinic
Antianemic
Iron supplement

pH 4.5 to 7

USUAL DOSE

Iron-deficiency anemia: *Test dose:* 0.5 mL (25 mg) on the first day as a test dose. Wait 1 hour. If no adverse reactions, administer a total dose of 2 mL (100 mg)/24 hr and repeat daily until results achieved or maximum calculated dosage reached (see dosage tables in literature or formula below). A total calculated dose has been given as an infusion. Though not FDA approved, this method is preferred by some to multiple small-dose infusions or injections. To calculate the total amount of iron dextran (mL) required to restore hemoglobin and to replenish iron stores in adults and pediatric patients weighing over 15 kg (lean body weight [LBW]):

Dose (mL) = 0.0442 (Desired Hb − Observed Hb) ×
$$\text{LBW in kg} + (0.26 \times \text{LBW in kg})$$

If actual weight is less than LBW or in pediatric patients between 5 and 15 kg, use actual weight in kg. Calculated dose is in **mL**.

Iron replacement for blood loss: Dose should represent the equivalent amount of iron represented in blood loss. Begin with a test dose of 0.5 mL (25 mg). Wait 1 hour. If no adverse reactions, calculate the desired dose with the following formula and administer the balance of the replacement dose over 2 to 3 daily doses:

$$\text{Amount of replacement iron } (\text{mg}) = \text{Blood loss } (\text{mL}) \times \text{Hematocrit}$$

Calculated dose is in **mg**; convert to **mL** before administration.

Formula is based on the approximation that 1 mL of normocytic, normochromic red cells contains 1 mg of elemental iron.

PEDIATRIC DOSE

Injectable iron not normally used in infants less than 4 months of age. See Maternal/Child.

Iron-deficiency anemia: *Test dose:* 0.5 mL (25 mg) for pediatric patients or 0.25 mL (12.5 mg) for infants over at least 5 minutes on the first day. Wait 1 hour. If no adverse reactions, may give remainder of daily dose. Direct IV push is not recommended; diluting with NS for infusion may lower the incidence of phlebitis. If actual weight is less than LBW or for pediatric patients between 5 and 15 kg, use actual weight in kg. The following daily doses have been recommended for IM injection by one source: ***less than 5 kg,*** 25 mg; ***5 to 10 kg,*** 50 mg; ***more than 10 kg,*** 100 mg. Repeat daily until results achieved or maximum calculated dosage reached (see dosage tables in literature or the formula listed earlier).

Iron replacement for blood loss: Calculate dose by formula used for adult dose. Dose should represent the equivalent amount of iron represented in blood loss. Begin with a test dose of 0.5 mL (25 mg) for pediatric patients or 0.25 mL (12.5 mg) for infants over at least 5 minutes on the first day. Wait 1 hour. If no adverse reactions, administer the balance of the replacement dose over 2 to 3 daily doses.

DILUTION

Given undiluted, or up to the total desired dose may be further diluted in 50 to 1,000 mL NS for infusion. D5W may cause additional local pain and phlebitis.

Filters: No data available from manufacturer.

Storage: Store unopened vials at CRT, protect from freezing.

COMPATIBILITY

Manufacturer states, "Do not mix with other medications or add to parenteral nutrition solutions."

RATE OF ADMINISTRATION

Test dose: 25 mg over 5 minutes (DexFerrum) or over 30 seconds (InFeD). Specific rates of test dose infusions not available for other manufacturers.

IV injection: If no adverse reactions to the test dose, administer 1 mL (50 mg) or a fraction thereof over 1 minute or more. Extend injection time in pediatric patients.

Infusion: If no adverse reactions to the test dose, infuse remaining dose over 1 to 8 hours (based on amount of dose, amount of diluent, and patient comfort).

ACTIONS

Iron dextran is removed from the plasma by cells of the reticuloendothelial system, which split the complex into its components of iron and dextran. Iron is immediately bound to protein moieties to form hemosiderin or ferritin, the physiologic forms of iron, or to a lesser extent to transferrin. This iron replenishes hemoglobin and depleted iron stores. Serum ferritin peaks approximately 7 to 9 days after iron dextran administration and slowly returns to baseline after about 3 weeks. Dextran is metabolized or excreted. Negligible amounts of iron are lost via the urinary or alimentary pathways after administration of iron dextran. Some placental transfer of iron dextran may occur. Trace amounts of unmetabolized iron dextran are excreted in breast milk.

INDICATIONS AND USES
Iron deficiency anemia in patients for whom oral administration is unsatisfactory or impossible; identify and treat the cause of the anemia.
Unlabeled uses: Iron supplementation for patients taking epoetin alfa (Epogen).

CONTRAINDICATIONS
Manifestation of hypersensitivity reactions; any anemia other than iron deficiency.

PRECAUTIONS
Anaphylactic-type reactions, including fatalities, have been reported. Fatal reactions have occurred both after the test dose and in situations in which the test dose was tolerated. Administer in facilities equipped to monitor the patient and respond to any medical emergency. Patients with a history of drug allergy or multiple drug allergies may be at increased risk for anaphylactic-type reactions. Concomitant use of angiotensin-converting enzyme inhibitors (e.g., enalaprilat [Vasotec], lisinopril [Zestril]) may also increase the risk of reactions. Facilities for monitoring the patient and responding to any medical emergency must be readily available. ▪ Iron dextran products are not clinically interchangeable. They differ in chemical characteristics and may differ in clinical and adverse effects. ▪ Large IV doses have been associated with an increased incidence of side effects, including arthralgia, backache, chills, dizziness, fever, headache, malaise, myalgia, nausea, and vomiting. The onset of these side effects is often delayed (1 to 2 days) and symptoms generally subside within 3 to 4 days. Maximum daily recommended dose is 100 mg (2 mL) of undiluted iron dextran. ▪ Use with caution in patients with severe liver impairment, cardiovascular disease, or a history of significant allergies and/or asthma. ▪ Do not administer during the acute phase of infectious kidney disease. ▪ Patients with rheumatoid arthritis may experience increased joint pain and swelling after administration of iron dextran. ▪ Administration of parenteral iron therapy should be limited to patients in whom clinical and laboratory investigations have established an iron-deficient state. Unwarranted therapy may cause excess storage of iron and possible exogenous hemosiderosis.
Monitor: Keep patient lying down after injection to prevent postural hypotension. ▪ Observe continuously for a hypersensitivity reaction during an infusion. Monitor vital signs. ▪ Monitor hemoglobin, hematocrit, reticulocyte count, total iron-binding capacity (TIBC), and percent of saturation of transferrin as indicated to monitor therapy and iron status. May take up to 3 weeks to see response. ▪ Monitor serum ferritin assays in prolonged therapy. Consider possibility of false results for months after injection caused by delayed utilization. ▪ In patients undergoing chronic renal dialysis who are receiving iron dextran complex, the correlation of body iron stores and serum ferritin may not be valid.
Patient Education: Promptly report S/S of hypersensitivity (e.g., rash, itching, SOB). ▪ Promptly report any other side effects, immediate or delayed.
Maternal/Child: Category C: use only if absolutely necessary in pregnancy, breast-feeding, or childbearing years. ▪ Injectable iron not normally used in infants younger than 4 months of age.

DRUG/LAB INTERACTIONS

Inhibited by **chloramphenicol**. ▪ Concurrent administration of medicinal iron with **dimercaprol** (BAL in Oil) will result in the formation of a toxic complex. Either postpone iron therapy or treat severe iron deficiency with transfusions. ▪ Effectiveness negated by **deferoxamine** (Desferal), an iron chelating agent. May be affected by **other chelating agents** (e.g., edetate disodium). Give iron dextran at least 2 hours after a chelating agent. ▪ May cause **false serum iron values** within 1 to 2 weeks of large doses of iron dextran. ▪ May cause a **false elevated bilirubin, false decreased calcium, or affect numerous other tests or scans.** ▪ See Monitor.

SIDE EFFECTS

Backache, dizziness, headache, itching, local phlebitis at injection site, malaise, nausea, rash, shivering, transitory paresthesias.

Major: Anaphylaxis (fatalities have occurred); arthritic reactivation; dyspnea; febrile episodes; hypotension; leukocytosis; local phlebitis; lymphadenopathy; peripheral vascular flushing, especially with too-rapid injection; urticaria; tachycardia; shock (severe iron toxicity increases vasodilation and venous pooling and decreases circulating blood volume. Results in decreased cardiac output, hypotension, increased peripheral vascular resistance, and shock).

Overdose: Serum iron levels greater than 300 mcg/dL may indicate iron poisoning. Overdose with iron dextran is unlikely. May result in hemosiderosis, and excess iron may increase susceptibility to infection. If acute toxicity is seen, it may present as:

Early: Abdominal pain, diarrhea, vomiting.

Late: Bluish-colored lips, fingernails, and palms of hands; acidosis, drowsiness, shallow and rapid breathing, clammy skin, weak and fast heartbeat, hypotension, hypoglycemia, cardiovascular collapse.

ANTIDOTE

Discontinue the drug and notify the physician of early symptoms. For severe symptoms, discontinue drug, treat hypersensitivity reactions, or resuscitate as necessary, and notify physician. Epinephrine (Adrenalin) and diphenhydramine (Benadryl) should always be available. In overdose, monitor CBC, iron studies, vital signs, blood gases, and glucose and electrolytes. Maintain fluid and electrolyte balance. Correct acidosis with sodium bicarbonate. Deferoxamine is an iron chelating agent and may be useful in iron toxicity or overdose. Dialysis will not remove iron alone but will remove the iron deferoxamine complex and is indicated if oliguria or anuria is present.

IRON SUCROSE
(EYE-ern SOO-kros)

Venofer

Hematinic
Iron supplement
Antianemic

pH 10.5 to 11.1

USUAL DOSE

Dose is expressed in terms of mg of elemental iron.

Test dose (optional): 50 mg. Test dose is not required but was administered in some of the clinical trials. May be given at the physician's discretion.

Non–dialysis dependent chronic kidney disease patients (NDD-CKD): 200 mg as a slow IV injection. Administer on 5 different days within a 14-day period to a total cumulative dose of 1,000 mg. Alternately, there is limited experience with administering a 500-mg dose on Day 1 and Day 14 as a 3.5- to 4-hour infusion in a maximum of 250 mL of NS.

Hemodialysis-dependent chronic kidney disease patients (HDD-CKD): 100 mg as a slow IV injection one to three times a week to a total dose of 1,000 mg in 10 doses. Administered during the dialysis session. Repeat as needed to maintain target levels of hemoglobin, hematocrit, and laboratory parameters of iron stores within acceptable limits. Frequency of dosing should be no more than three times weekly.

Peritoneal dialysis–dependent chronic kidney disease patients (PDD-CKD): 300 mg as an infusion on Day 1 and Day 14. Follow with 400 mg as an infusion on Day 28. A total cumulative dose of 1,000 mg given in 3 doses over 28 days. Each infusion is diluted in a maximum of 250 mL NS and administered over 1.5 to 2.5 hours; see Rate of Administration.

DOSE ADJUSTMENTS

Begin at the low end of the dosing range in elderly patients. Consider the potential for decreased organ function and concomitant disease or drug therapy. ■ Withhold in patients with evidence of tissue iron overload; see Monitor.

DILUTION

Available in several sizes of single-dose vials. Check vial carefully and select the size that is closest to the desired dose. All contain 20 mg/mL of elemental iron.

Test dose (optional): 50 mg should be diluted in 50 mL of NS.

Non–dialysis dependent chronic kidney disease patients (NDD-CKD): 200-mg dose may be given undiluted. The 500-mg dose may be further diluted in a maximum of 250 mL of NS and given as an infusion.

Hemodialysis-dependent chronic kidney disease patients (HDD-CKD): 100-mg dose may be given undiluted or may be further diluted in a maximum of 100 mL of NS and given as an infusion.

Peritoneal dialysis–dependent chronic kidney disease patients (PDD-CKD): Each 300- or 400-mg dose must be diluted in a maximum of 250 mL NS and given as an infusion.

Filters: No data available from manufacturer.

Storage: Store unopened vials in original carton at CRT. Do not freeze. Diluted iron infusions should be used immediately after preparation. Discard any unused portion.

COMPATIBILITY

Manufacturer states, "Do not mix with other medications or add to parenteral nutrition solutions."

RATE OF ADMINISTRATION

Too-rapid administration may cause hypotension or symptoms of overdose; see Side Effects.

Test dose (optional): A single dose over 3 to 10 minutes.

Slow IV injection: A single undiluted dose over 2 to 5 minutes. In dialysis patients, administer into the dialysis line during the dialysis session.

Infusion: This method of administration may reduce the risk of hypotensive episodes.

Non–dialysis dependent chronic kidney disease patients (NDD-CKD): A single 200-mg dose as a slow IV injection over 2 to 5 minutes. Has also been administered as an infusion in a 500-mg dose equally distributed over 3.5 to 4 hours.

Hemodialysis-dependent chronic kidney disease patients (HDD-CKD): A single 100-mg dose given as a slow IV injection over 2 to 5 minutes. Alternately may be given as an infusion equally distributed over at least 15 minutes.

Peritoneal dialysis–dependent chronic kidney disease patients (PDD-CKD): A single 300-mg dose equally distributed over 1.5 hours or a single 400-mg dose equally distributed over 2.5 hours.

ACTIONS

An aqueous, complex of polynuclear iron (III)-hydroxide in sucrose. Used to replenish the total body iron stores in patients with iron deficiency. Iron is critical for normal hemoglobin synthesis to maintain oxygen transport and necessary for metabolism and synthesis of DNA and various other processes. Following intravenous administration, iron sucrose is dissociated by the reticuloendothelial system into iron and sucrose. Iron distributes into liver, spleen, and bone marrow. Since iron disappearance from serum depends on the need for iron in the iron stores and iron-utilizing tissues of the body, serum clearance of iron is expected to be more rapid in iron deficient patients as compared to healthy individuals. Half-life of the iron component is 6 hours. The sucrose component is eliminated mainly by urinary excretion. Most iron is stored in the body in hemoglobin, bone marrow, spleen, liver, and ferritin. Small amounts are eliminated in the urine. Significant increases in serum iron and ferritin and significant decreases in total iron-binding capacity occur within 4 weeks of beginning iron sucrose treatment.

INDICATIONS AND USES

Treatment of iron deficiency anemia in hemodialysis-dependent chronic kidney disease (HDD-CKD) patients receiving an erythropoietin. ▪ Treatment of iron deficiency anemia in non–dialysis dependent chronic kidney disease (NDD-CKD) patients who may or may not be receiving an erythropoietin. ▪ Treatment of iron deficiency anemia in peritoneal dialysis–dependent chronic kidney disease (PDD-CKD) patients who are receiving an erythropoietin.

CONTRAINDICATIONS

Patients with evidence of iron overload. Anemia not caused by iron deficiency. Known hypersensitivity to iron sucrose or any of its inactive components.

PRECAUTIONS
Use only when truly indicated to avoid excess storage of iron. Not recommended for use in patients with iron overload. ▪ Potentially fatal hypersensitivity reactions characterized by anaphylactic shock, loss of consciousness, collapse, hypotension, dyspnea, or convulsions have been reported. Medications and equipment for resuscitation must be readily available. ▪ Hypotension has been reported frequently and may be related to rate of administration and/or total dose administered. Follow guidelines for dosing and administration. See Usual Dose and Rate of Administration.
Monitor: Monitor vital signs during and immediately following administration. Recumbent position during and after administration may help to prevent postural hypotension. Hypotensive effects may be additive to transient hypotension during dialysis and/or from too-rapid rate of administration. ▪ Monitor for S/S of hypersensitivity reactions; see Precautions. ▪ Periodic monitoring of hematologic and hematinic parameters (hemoglobin, hematocrit, serum ferritin and transferrin saturation) is indicated during parenteral iron replacement therapy. Takes about 4 weeks of treatment to see increased serum iron and ferritin and decreased TIBC (total iron-binding capacity). Transferrin saturation values increase rapidly after IV adminstration of iron sucrose; thus serum iron values may be reliably obtained 48 hours after the last IV dose.
Patient Education: Report S/S of a hypersensitivity reaction promptly.
Maternal/Child: Category B: use in pregnancy only if clearly needed. ▪ Safety for use during breast-feeding and in pediatric patients not established. ▪ Necrotizing enterocolitis in 5 premature infants (weight less than 1,250 Gm) with 2 deaths has been reported in one country in which iron sucrose is approved for use in pediatric patients. No causal relationship to drugs could be established; it may be a complication of prematurity in very-low-birth-weight infants.
Elderly: Differences in response between elderly and younger patients have not been identified. Lower-end initial doses may be appropriate in the elderly; see Dose Adjustments.

DRUG/LAB INTERACTIONS
Drug interactions involving iron sucrose have not been studied. May reduce the absorption of concomitantly administered **oral iron preparations,** concurrent use not recommended. ▪ Concurrent administration of medicinal iron with **dimercaprol** (BAL in Oil) will result in the formation of a toxic complex. Either postpone iron therapy or treat severe iron deficiency with transfusions.

SIDE EFFECTS
Frequent: Cramps/leg cramps, diarrhea, headache, hypotension, nausea, and vomiting.
Less frequent: Varied according to the type of chronic kidney disease patient who is receiving iron sucrose (e.g., hemodialysis dependent, peritoneal dialysis–dependent, non–dialysis dependent): Abdominal pain, altered taste, arthritis, asthenia, back pain, catheter site infection, chest pain, conjunctivitis, constipation, cough, dizziness, dyspnea, ear pain, fecal occult blood positive, fever, gout, graft complications, hyperglycemia, hypersensitivity reactions, hypertension, hypervolemia, hypoesthesia, hypoglycemia, injection site burning or pain, malaise, musculoskeletal pain, nasopharyngitis, peripheral edema, peritoneal infection, pharyngitis, sinusitis, upper respiratory infection.

Overdose: Serum iron levels greater than 300 mcg/dL may indicate iron poisoning. May result in hemosiderosis. Excess iron may increase susceptibility to infection. If acute toxicity is seen, it may present as abdominal and muscle pain, cardiovascular collapse, diarrhea, dizziness, edema, headache, hemosiderosis, hypotension, joint aches, nausea, pale eyes, paresthesia, sedation, vomiting.

Post-Marketing: Life-threatening hypersensitivity reactions (e.g., anaphylactic shock, bronchospasm, collapse, convulsions, dyspnea, hypotension, loss of consciousness, pruritus, rash, wheezing).

ANTIDOTE

Reduce rate of infusion for hypotension or other symptoms. Most symptoms are successfully treated with IV fluids, hydrocortisone sodium succinate (Solu-Cortef), and/or antihistamines (e.g., diphenhydramine [Benadryl]). Volume expanders (e.g., albumin, dextran, hetastarch [Hespan]) may be indicated. Keep physician informed of all side effects. Discontinue drug if severe hypersensitivity reactions occur. Treat hypersensitivity reactions as indicated; may require epinephrine, airway management, oxygen, IV fluids, antihistamines (e.g., diphenhydramine [Benadryl]), corticosteroids (e.g., hydrocortisone sodium succinate [Solu-Cortef]), and pressor amines (e.g., dopamine). Resuscitate as needed. Not removed by dialysis.

ISOPROTERENOL HYDROCHLORIDE
(eye-so-**PROH**-ter-ih-nohl hy-droh-**KLOR**-eyed)

Isuprel

**Cardiac stimulant
(inotropic/chronotropic)
Bronchodilator
Antiarrhythmic**

pH 3.5 to 4.5

USUAL DOSE
In all situations, adjust the rate of infusion based on HR, CVP, BP, respiratory rate, and urine output.

Recommended Isoproterenol Dose for Adults with Atropine-Resistant Hemodynamically Significant Bradycardia, Heart Block, Adams-Stokes Attacks, and Cardiac Arrest			
Route of Administration	Preparation of Dilution	Initial Dose	Subsequent Dose Range*
Bolus intravenous injection	Dilute 1 mL (0.2 mg) to 10 mL with NS or D5W	0.02 to 0.06 mg (1 to 3 mL of diluted solution)	0.01 to 0.2 mg (0.5 to 10 mL of diluted solution)
Intravenous infusion	Dilute 10 mL (2 mg) in 500 mL D5W	5 mcg/min (1.25 mL of diluted solution per minute)	
Intracardiac	Use solution 1:5,000 undiluted	0.02 mg (0.1 mL)	

*Subsequent dose depends on the ventricular rate and the rapidity with which the cardiac pacemaker can take over when the drug is gradually withdrawn.
AHA recommendation is 2 to 10 mcg/min if an external pacemaker is not available.

Recommended Isoproterenol Dose for Adults with Shock (Cardiogenic, CHF, Hypoperfusion [Low Cardiac Output], Hypovolemic, Septic)		
Route of Administration	Preparation of Dilution*	Infusion Rate†
Intravenous infusion	Dilute 5 mL (1 mg) in 500 mL of D5W	0.5 to 5 mcg per minute (0.25 to 2.5 mL of diluted solution)

*Concentrations up to 10 times greater have been used when limitation of volume is essential.
†Rates over 30 mcg/min have been used in advanced stages of shock. Adjust infusion rate based on HR, CVP, BP, and urine flow. If HR exceeds 110 beats/min, consider decreasing rate or temporarily discontinue the infusion.

Recommended Isoproterenol Dose for Adults with Bronchospasm Occurring During Anesthesia			
Route of Administration	Preparation of Dilution	Initial Dose	Subsequent Dose
Bolus intravenous injection	Dilute 1 mL (0.2 mg) to 10 mL with NS or D5W	0.01 to 0.02 mg (0.5 to 1 mL of diluted solution)	Repeat initial dose as necessary

Complete heart block following closure of ventricular septal defects: 0.04 to 0.06 mg (2 to 3 mL of a 1:50,000 dilution) as a bolus injection. May maintain a sinus rhythm with a HR above 90 to 100 beats/min or may relapse into complete heart block again.

Diagnosis of mitral regurgitation (unlabeled): 4 mcg/min as an infusion (1 mL/min of a 1:250,000 dilution).

Diagnosis of coronary artery disease or lesions (unlabeled): 1 to 3 mcg/min as an infusion (0.25 to 0.75 mL/min of a 1:250,000 dilution).

Refractory torsades de pointes, bradycardia in heart transplant patients, beta-adrenergic blocker poisoning: AHA recommends 2 to 10 mcg/min (0.5 to 2.5 mL/min of a 1:250,000 dilution [4 mcg/mL]). Titrate to adequate heart rate. In torsades de pointes titrate to increase heart rate until VT is suppressed.

PEDIATRIC DOSE
See Dilution and Maternal/Child.
0.05 to 2 mcg/kg/min. Begin with 0.1 mcg/kg/min as an infusion. Increase by 0.1 mcg/kg/min until desired effect. Titrate to patient response and monitor cardiac status carefully. Maximum dose is 2 mcg/kg/min. Another source suggests a maximum dose of 1 mcg/kg/min.

Complete heart block after closure of ventricular septal defects in infants: 0.01 to 0.03 mg (0.5 to 1.5 mL of a 1:50,000 dilution) as a bolus injection. See comments in Usual Dose.

DOSE ADJUSTMENTS
Lower-end initial doses may be appropriate in the elderly; consider the potential for decreased organ function and concomitant disease or drug therapy.

DILUTION
IV injection: Available in a 1:50,000 solution or dilute 0.2 mg (1 mL) of a 1:5,000 solution with 10 mL NS or D5W to provide a concentration of 0.02 mg/mL (1:50,000 solution).

Infusion: Dilute 10 mL (2 mg) in 500 mL D5W (4 mcg/mL). **Shock:** Dilute 5 mL (1 mg) in 500 mL D5W (2 mcg/mL). Use an infusion pump or microdrip (60 gtt equals 1 mL) to administer. Less diluent may be used to reduce fluid intake.

Pediatric infusion: 0.6 mg/kg isoproterenol in 100 mL D5W. 1 mL/hr equals 0.1 mcg/kg/min.

Filters: No data available from manufacturer. Another source sites no significant loss in drug potency in several studies using various types and sizes of filters from 0.22 to 5 microns in size.

Storage: Store between 8° and 15° C (46° to 59° F) unless otherwise specified by manufacturer. Do not use if pink or brown in color or contains a precipitate.

COMPATIBILITY
Consider any drug NOT listed as compatible to be INCOMPATIBLE until consulting a pharmacist; specific conditions may apply.
One source suggests the following **compatibilities:**
Additive: Atracurium (Tracrium), calcium chloride, dobutamine, heparin, magnesium sulfate, multivitamins (M.V.I.), potassium chloride (KCl), ranitidine (Zantac), succinylcholine, verapamil.
Y-site: Amiodarone (Nexterone), atracurium (Tracrium), bivalirudin (Angiomax), cisatracurium (Nimbex), dexmedetomidine (Precedex), fa-

motidine (Pepcid IV), fenoldopam (Corlopam), heparin, hetastarch in electrolytes (Hextend), hydrocortisone sodium succinate (Solu-Cortef), inamrinone (Amrinone), levofloxacin (Levaquin), milrinone (Primacor), nitroprusside sodium, pancuronium, potassium chloride (KCl), propofol (Diprivan), remifentanil (Ultiva), tacrolimus (Prograf), vecuronium.

RATE OF ADMINISTRATION

IV injection: Each 1 mL of a 1:50,000 (0.02 mg) solution or fraction thereof over 1 minute. Follow with a 20 mL flush of NS if indicated to ensure distribution to circulation.

Infusion: Titrate to desired dose, HR, and rhythm; see the following infusion rate chart. Decrease rate of infusion as necessary. Ventricular rate generally should not exceed 110 beats/min.

	Isoproterenol (Isuprel) Infusion Rates*						
Desired Dose	1 mg in 500 mL D5W (2 mcg/mL)			1 mg in 250 mL D5W 2 mg in 500 mL D5W (4 mcg/mL)			
mcg/min	mcg/hr	mL/min	mL/hr	mcg/hr	mL/min	mL/hr	
2	120	1	60	120	0.5	30	
5	300	2.5	150	300	1.25	75	
10	600	5	300	600	2.5	150	
15	900	7.5	450	900	3.75	225	
20	1,200	10	600	1,200	5	300	
25	1,500	12.5	750	1,500	6.25	375	
30	1,800	15	900	1,800	7.5	450	

*Pediatric infusion: 0.6 mg/kg in 100 mL D5W 1 mL/hr = 0.1 mcg/kg/min.

ACTIONS

A non-selective synthetic cardiac beta receptor stimulant (sympathomimetic amine) similar to epinephrine and norepinephrine. Has positive inotropic and chronotropic actions more potent than those of epinephrine. It increases cardiac output, cardiac work, coronary flow, and venous return. Improves atrioventricular conduction. Stimulates only the higher ventricular foci, allowing a more normal cardiac pacemaker to take over, thus suppressing ectopic pacemaker activity. Decreases peripheral vascular resistance by relaxing arterial smooth muscle and is a most effective bronchial smooth muscle relaxant. Onset of action is immediate and lasts 1 to 2 hours. Metabolized by the liver and inactivated by various enzyme systems. Excreted in the urine.

INDICATIONS AND USES

Treatment of mild or transient episodes of heart block that do not require cardioversion or pacemaker therapy. ■ Treatment of serious episodes of heart block and Adams-Stokes attacks (except when caused by VT or VF). ■ May be used in cardiac arrest until defibrillation or pacemaker (the treatments of choice) are available. ■ Treatment of refractory torsades de pointes until pacemaker implanted. ■ Temporary control of symptomatic bradycardia in denervated hearts of heart transplant patients until pacemaker implanted. ▪ Bronchospasm during anesthesia. ▪ Management of shock (cardiogenic, CHF, hypoperfusion [low cardiac output], hypovolemic, septic). Adequate fluid and electrolyte replacement required. ▪ Pulmonary embolism, to increase pulmonary blood volume and decrease pulmonary arterial pressure and vascular resistance. ▪ AHA recommends cautious use in symptomatic bradycardia if a pacemaker is not available, and use in the treatment of refractory torsades de pointes unresponsive to magnesium sulfate, and poisoning from beta-adrenergic blockers (e.g., metoprolol [Lopressor]).

Unlabeled uses: Aid in diagnosis of the etiology of mitral regurgitation. ▪ Aid in diagnosis of coronary artery disease or lesions.

CONTRAINDICATIONS

Tachyarrhythmias, patients with tachycardia or heart block caused by digoxin intoxication, angina pectoris, ventricular arrhythmias that require inotropic therapy.

PRECAUTIONS

IV injection in cardiac standstill must be accompanied by cardiac massage to perfuse drug into the myocardium. Current JAMA recommendations do not include isoproterenol in the treatment of cardiac arrest or hypotension. ▪ Fourth-line agent for bradycardia; considered possibly helpful but may be harmful. ▪ Can cause a severe drop in BP and can be very harmful in bradycardia. ▪ Use extreme caution when inhalant anesthetics (e.g., cyclopropane) are being administered and supplementary to digoxin administration. ▪ Use caution in coronary insufficiency, diabetes, hyperthyroidism, known sensitivity to sympathomimetic amines, history of seizures, hypertension, and pre-existing cardiac arrhythmias with tachycardia. ▪ Increased cardiac output and work can increase ischemia and worsen arrhythmias. ▪ Contains sulfites; use caution in allergic patients.

Monitor: Decrease rate of infusion as necessary. Ventricular rate generally should not exceed 110 beats/min. Maintain adequate blood volume and correct acidosis. ▪ Continuous cardiac monitoring, central venous pressure readings, BP, respiratory rate, and urine flow measurements are advisable during therapy with isoproterenol. ▪ Monitoring of serum glucose, magnesium, and potassium may be indicated. ▪ See Drug/Lab Interactions and Maternal/Child.

Maternal/Child: Category C: safety for use in pregnancy or breast-feeding not established. Benefits must outweigh risks. ▪ Safety and effectiveness in pediatric patients not established. ▪ In asthmatic pediatric patients, IV infusion of isoproterenol has caused clinical deterioration, myocardial necrosis, CHF, and death. Risks of cardiac toxicity may be increased by other factors such as acidosis, hypoxemia, coadministration of corticosteroids or methylxanthines (e.g., aminophylline). Continuous assessment of VS, frequent ECGs, and daily measurement of cardiac enzymes (e.g., CPK, MB) is suggested if isoproterenol infusion is required.

Elderly: Difference in response from younger adults not known. May be more sensitive to the effects of beta-adrenergic agents (e.g., hypertension, hypokalemia, tachycardia, tremor). Patients with cardiac disease may be at increased risk for cardiac effects. ▪ Lower-end initial doses may be appropriate; see Dose Adjustments.

DRUG/LAB INTERACTIONS

May be used alternately with epinephrine (Adrenalin), but they may not be used together. Both are direct cardiac stimulants; serious arrhythmias and death may result. An adequate interval between doses must be maintained. ▪ Do not use concomitantly with other **sympathomimetic agents** (e.g., ephedrine, dopamine). Additive effects may cause toxicity. May be used after effects of previous drug have subsided. ▪ Simultaneous use with **oxytoxics** may cause hypertensive crisis. ▪ May cause hypertension with **guanethidine** (Ismelin). ▪ **Digoxin, quinidine, and halogenated hydrocarbon anesthetics** (e.g., halothane) may sensitize myocardium and cause serious arrhythmias. ▪ Antagonized by **propranolol.** May be used to treat tachycardia caused by isoproterenol, but tachycardia and hypotension secondary to peripheral vasodilation may occur. ▪ Potentiated by **tricyclic antidepressants** (e.g., imipramine [Tofranil]). ▪ Concomitant use with **theophylline** increases the risk of cardiotoxicity. ▪ See Contraindications.

SIDE EFFECTS
Anginal pain, cardiac arrhythmias, flushing, headache, hyperglycemia, hypokalemia, nausea, nervousness, palpitations, sweating, tachycardia, vomiting. Cardiac dilation, marked hypotension, pulmonary edema, and death may occur with prolonged use or overdose. Adams-Stokes attacks have been reported.

ANTIDOTE
Notify the physician of any side effect. Treatment will probably be symptomatic. For ventricular rate over 110 beats/min, PVCs, or ECG changes, decrease rate of infusion or discontinue drug. Vasodilators (e.g., nitrates) may be useful for treatment of hypertension. For accidental overdose, discontinue drug immediately, resuscitate and sustain patient, and notify physician.

IXABEPILONE BBW
(ix-ab-**EP**-i-lone)

Ixempra Kit

Antineoplastic
(microtubule inhibitor)

USUAL DOSE
Premedication: An H_1 antagonist (e.g., diphenhydramine [Benadryl]) and an H_2 antagonist (e.g., ranitidine [Zantac], famotidine [Pepcid]) should be administered 60 minutes prior to ixabepilone to minimize the chance of a hypersensitivity reaction. Patients who experience a hypersensitivity reaction require premedication with a corticosteroid (e.g., dexamethasone 20 mg IV 30 minutes before infusion or orally 60 minutes before infusion) in addition to pretreatment with the H_1 and H_2 antagonists.

Ixabepilone: 40 mg/M^2 as an infusion over 3 hours every 3 weeks. Doses for patients with a body surface area (BSA) greater than 2.2 M^2 should be calculated based on 2.2 M^2. Administered alone or in combination with capecitabine (Xeloda) 1,000 mg/M^2 twice daily for 2 weeks followed by 1 week of rest.

DOSE ADJUSTMENTS

If toxicities are present, therapy should be delayed to allow recovery. ■ Dosing adjustment guidelines for monotherapy and combination therapy are listed in the following table. *If toxicities recur, an additional 20% dose reduction should be made.*

Dose Adjustments Guidelines	
Ixabepilone (Monotherapy or Combination Therapy)	**Ixabepilone Dose Modification**
NONHEMATOLOGIC	
Grade 2 neuropathy (moderate) lasting ≥7 days	Decrease the dose by 20%
Grade 3 neuropathy (severe) lasting <7 days	Decrease the dose by 20%
Grade 3 neuropathy (severe) lasting ≥7 days or disabling neuropathy	Discontinue treatment
Any Grade 3 toxicity (severe) other than neuropathy	Decrease the dose by 20%
Transient Grade 3 arthralgia/myalgia or fatigue	No change in dose required
Grade 3 hand-foot syndrome (palmar-plantar erythrodysesthesia)	No change in dose required
Any Grade 4 toxicity (disabling)	Discontinue treatment
HEMATOLOGIC	
Neutrophils <500 cells/mm^3 for ≥7 days	Decrease the dose by 20%
Febrile neutropenia	Decrease the dose by 20%
Platelets <25,000/mm^3 or platelets <50,000/mm^3 with bleeding	Decrease the dose by 20%
Capecitabine (When Used in Combination with Ixabepilone)	**Capecitabine Dose Modification**
NONHEMATOLOGIC	Follow capecitabine prescribing information
HEMATOLOGIC	
Platelets <25,000/mm^3 or platelets <50,000/mm^3 with bleeding	Hold for concurrent diarrhea or stomatitis until platelet count >50,000/mm^3, then continue at same dose
Neutrophils <500 cells/mm^3 for ≥7 days or febrile neutropenia	Hold for concurrent diarrhea or stomatitis until neutrophil count >1,000/mm^3, then continue at same dose

Dose adjustments at the start of a cycle should be based on nonhematologic toxicity or blood counts from the preceding cycle following the previous guidelines. Patients should not begin a new cycle unless the neutrophil count is at least 1,500 cells/mm^3, the platelet count is at least 100,000 cells/mm^3, and nonhematologic toxicities have improved to Grade 1 (mild) or have resolved. ■ Combined use with capecitabine is

Continued

contraindicated in patients who have AST or ALT >2.5 times the ULN or bilirubin >1 times the ULN; see Contraindications and Precautions. ▪ Patients with hepatic impairment who are receiving monotherapy should be dosed according to the guidelines listed in the following table.

Dose Adjustments for Ixabepilone as Monotherapy in Patients with Hepatic Impairment			
	Transaminase Levels	Bilirubin Levels*	Ixabepilone Dose† (mg/M²)
Mild	AST and ALT ≤2.5 × ULN	and ≤1 × ULN	40
	AST or ALT ≤10 × ULN	and ≤1.5 × ULN	32
Moderate	AST and ALT ≤10 × ULN	and >1.5 × ULN to ≤3 × ULN	20-30
Severe	AST or ALT >10 × ULN	or >3 × ULN	Not recommended

*Excluding patients whose total bilirubin is elevated due to Gilbert's disease.
†Dosage recommendations are for the first course of therapy; further decreases in subsequent courses should be based on individual tolerance.

Patients with moderate hepatic impairment should start with 20 mg/M². The dose in subsequent cycles may be increased up to, but should not exceed, 30 mg/M² if tolerated. ▪ Reduce dose to 20 mg/M² when coadministered with a strong CYP3A4 inhibitor; see Drug Interactions. If the strong inhibitor is discontinued, wait for at least 1 week before adjusting the ixabepilone dose upward to the indicated dose. ▪ If coadministration of a strong CYP3A4 inducer is required and alternatives are not feasible (e.g., the patient has been maintained on a strong CYP3A4 inducer), the dose may be gradually increased from 40 mg/M² to 60 mg/M² if tolerated; see Drug Interactions. Increase infusion duration of 60 mg/M² dose to 4 hours and monitor patient closely for toxicity. If CYP3A4 inducer is discontinued, return to original dose. ▪ No dose adjustment indicated based on age, race, and gender. ▪ Minimally excreted by the kidney; no studies conducted in patients with renal impairment.

DILUTION

Specific techniques required; see Precautions. Available as a 15-mg or 45-mg IXEMPRA Kit that contains two vials; one vial contains the indicated amount of ixabepilone, and the other contains a manufacturer-supplied diluent. Only the manufacturer-supplied diluent may be used for reconstitution. Calculate dose and remove required number of kits from refrigerator. Let stand at RT for approximately 30 minutes. A white precipitate may appear in the diluent vial. This will dissolve as the vial warms to RT. Withdraw diluent and slowly inject it into the ixabepilone vial. (The 15-mg vial is reconstituted with 8 mL of diluent, and the 45-mg vial is reconstituted with 23.5 mL.) Gently swirl and invert until completely dissolved. Concentration of reconstituted solution is 2 mg/mL. Must be further diluted to a final concentration of 0.2 to 0.6 mg/mL with LR, Plasma-Lyte A Injection pH 7.4, or NS 250 to 500 mL (the pH of the NS must be adjusted to between 6 and 9 by adding 2 mEq [i.e., 2 mL of an 8.4% w/v solution or 4 mL of a 4.2% w/v solution] of sodium bicarbonate injection before adding the ixabepilone). A 250-mL bag will be sufficient for most doses. Withdraw the calculated dose from the ixabepilone vials and transfer to a DEHP-free IV bag containing an appropriate volume of infusion solution to achieve the final desired concentration. Thoroughly mix by manual rotation. Should be administered through a DEHP-free, polyethylene-lined administration set.

Filter: Must be administered through an in-line filter with a microporous membrane of 0.2 to 1.2 microns.

Storage: Store unopened vials at 2° to 8° C (36° to 46° F) in original carton. Protect from light. Reconstituted solution may be stored in vial for 1 hour at RT and room light. Once diluted, solution is stable for a maximum of 6 hours at RT. Administration must be completed within this 6-hour period.

COMPATIBILITY

Manufacturer states, "DEHP-free infusion containers and administration sets must be used." Must be reconstituted with manufacturer-supplied diluent only and further diluted with the infusion solutions noted in Dilution. Indicated solutions have a pH between 6 to 9, which is required for ixabepilone stability.

RATE OF ADMINISTRATION

A single dose as an infusion equally distributed over 3 hours. In patients who experience a hypersensitivity reaction, increase duration of infusion and premedicate with corticosteroids and H_1 and H_2 antagonists; see Usual Dose. Increase duration of infusion to 4 hours in patients receiving 60 mg/M^2 dose; see Dose Adjustments.

ACTIONS

A microtubule inhibitor belonging to a class of antineoplastic agents, the epothilones. A semi-synthetic analog of epothilone B. Binds directly to β-tubulin subunits on microtubules, leading to suppression of microtubule dynamics. Blocks cells in the mitotic phase of the cell division cycle, leading to cell death. Has antitumor activity against multiple human tumor xenografts and is active in xenografts that are resistant to multiple agents, including taxanes, anthracyclines, and vinca alkaloids. Has demonstrated synergistic antitumor activity in combination with capecitabine. In addition to direct antitumor activity, ixabepilone has antiangiogenic activity. 67% to 77% bound to plasma proteins. Extensively metabolized in the liver, primarily by CYP3A4. Eliminated primarily as metabolized drug in feces and urine. Half-life is approximately 52 hours.

INDICATIONS AND USES

In combination with capecitabine (Xeloda) for the treatment of patients with metastatic or locally advanced breast cancer resistant to treatment with an anthracycline and a taxane or for patients whose cancer is taxane resistant and for whom further anthracycline therapy is contraindicated. Anthracycline resistance is defined as progression while on therapy or within 6 months in the adjuvant setting or 3 months in the metastatic setting. Taxane resistance is defined as progression while on therapy or within 12 months in the adjuvant setting or 4 months in the metastatic setting. ■ As monotherapy for the treatment of metastatic or locally advanced breast cancer in patients whose tumors are resistant or refractory to anthracyclines, taxanes, and capecitabine.

CONTRAINDICATIONS

History of severe (CTCAE Grade 3 or 4) hypersensitivity reaction to agents containing Cremophor® EL or its derivatives. ■ Neutrophil count less than 1,500 cells/mm^3 or platelet count less than 100,000 cells/mm^3. ▪ In combination with capecitabine in patients with AST or ALT greater than 2.5 times the ULN or bilirubin greater than 1 times the ULN.

PRECAUTIONS
Follow guidelines for handling cytotoxic agents. See Appendix A, p. 1429. ▪ Should be administered by or under the direction of the physician specialist in facilities equipped to monitor the patient and respond to any medical emergency. ▪ Ixabepilone in combination with capecitabine is contraindicated in patients with significant hepatic insufficiency due to increased risk of toxicity and neutropenia-related death; see Contraindications. ▪ Use caution in patients with hepatic insufficiency receiving monotherapy. Risk of toxicity is increased and data are limited; see Dose Adjustments. ▪ Premedication is required to minimize the chance of a hypersensitivity reaction; see Usual Dose. ▪ Peripheral neuropathy is a common side effect and was the most common cause of treatment discontinuation in clinical studies. It is cumulative and generally reversible. May require dose reduction or delay in therapy; see Dose Adjustments. Use caution in patients with diabetes mellitus or pre-existing peripheral neuropathy. Risk of severe neuropathy may be increased. ▪ Myelosuppression is dose dependent and primarily manifested as neutropenia. Hold therapy in patients with a neutrophil count less than 1,500 cells/mm^3; see Dose Adjustments and Contraindications. ▪ Use caution in patients with a history of cardiac disease. Adverse cardiac events (e.g., myocardial ischemia, ventricular dysfunction, and supraventricular arrhythmias) have been reported. ▪ Not studied in patients with renal impairment.

Monitor: Obtain baseline and periodic CBC with differential and platelet count. ▪ Obtain baseline and periodic bilirubin, AST, and ALT. ▪ Monitor for S/S of a hypersensitivity reaction (e.g., bronchospasm, dyspnea, flushing, rash). ▪ Monitor for S/S of peripheral neuropathy (primarily sensory [e.g., burning sensation, discomfort, hyperesthesia, hypoesthesia, neuropathic pain or paresthesia]). Most cases of new onset or worsening neuropathy occurred during the first 3 cycles. ▪ Monitor for thrombocytopenia (platelet count less than 50,000/mm^3); see Dose Adjustments and Contraindications. Initiate precautions to prevent excessive bleeding (e.g., inspect IV sites, skin, and mucous membranes; use extreme care during invasive procedures; test urine, emesis, stool, and secretions for occult blood).

Patient Education: Promptly report any numbness or tingling of feet, S/S of infection (fever, chills cough), or S/S of a hypersensitivity reaction (chest tightness, dyspnea, flushing, pruritus, rash, urticaria). ▪ Avoid pregnancy. Use of nonhormonal birth control is required. ▪ Promptly report chest pain, difficulty breathing, palpitations, or unusual weight gain; these may be signs of adverse cardiac events.

Maternal/Child: Category D: avoid pregnancy; may cause fetal harm. ▪ Discontinue breast-feeding. ▪ Safety and effectiveness for use in pediatric patients not established.

Elderly: The incidence of Grade 3 and 4 adverse reactions was higher when used in combination with capecitabine in clinical studies. As monotherapy, no overall difference in safety was seen in the elderly compared with younger adults.

DRUG/LAB INTERACTIONS

Use of concomitant strong **CYP3A4 inhibitors** (e.g., amprenavir [Agenerase], atazanavir [Reyataz], clarithromycin [Biaxin], delavirdine [Rescriptor], indinavir [Crixivan], itraconazole [Sporanox], ketoconazole [Nizoral], nefazodone, nelfinavir [Viracept], ritonavir [Norvir], saquinavir [Invirase], telithromycin [Ketek], or voriconazole [VFEND]) may increase plasma concentrations of ixabepilone. Avoid concomitant use if possible. If required, decrease dose of ixabepilone to 20 mg/M^2 and monitor closely for acute toxicity. If strong inhibitor is discontinued, wait for at least 1 week before adjusting ixabepilone dose upward to indicated dose. ▪ **Grapefruit juice** may increase plasma concentrations of ixabepilone and should be avoided. ▪ **Rifampin** (Rifadin), a potent CYP3A4 inducer, decreases ixabepilone plasma concentrations. Other strong **CYP3A4 inducers** (e.g., carbamazepine [Tegretol], dexamethasone [Decadron], phenobarbital [Luminal], phenytoin [Dilantin], rifabutin [Mycobutin]) may also decrease ixabepilone plasma concentrations, decreasing effectiveness. Avoid use if possible; see Dose Adjustments. ▪ **St. John's wort** may decrease ixabepilone plasma concentrations, decreasing effectiveness. Avoid use. ▪ Ixabepilone does not inhibit CYP enzymes and is not expected to alter plasma concentrations of other drugs.

SIDE EFFECTS

The most common side effects in patients receiving monotherapy included alopecia, anemia, arthralgia, asthenia, diarrhea, fatigue, leukopenia, mucositis, musculoskeletal pain, myalgia, nausea, neutropenia, peripheral sensory neuropathy, stomatitis, thrombocytopenia, and vomiting. In combination therapy, the following additional side effects were commonly reported: abdominal pain, anorexia, constipation, nail disorder, and handfoot syndrome (palmar-plantar erythrodysesthesia). Other less commonly reported side effects included chest pain, cough, dehydration, dizziness, dyspnea, edema, febrile neutropenia, fever, gastroesophageal reflux disease, headache, hot flush, hypersensitivity reactions (including anaphylaxis), increased lacrimation, infection, insomnia, pain, pruritus, rash, skin exfoliation, skin hyperpigmentation, taste disorder.

Overdose: Fatigue, GI symptoms (e.g., abdominal pain, anorexia, diarrhea, nausea, stomatitis), musculoskeletal pain/myalgia, and peripheral neuropathy.

Post-Marketing: Radiation recall has been reported.

ANTIDOTE

Keep physician informed of all side effects. Most minor side effects will be treated symptomatically. Monitor patient closely. Discontinuation should be considered in patients who develop cardiac ischemia or impaired cardiac function. Discontinue ixabepilone at the first sign of a severe hypersensitivity reaction. Treat hypersensitivity reactions as indicated; may require epinephrine, airway management, oxygen, IV fluids, antihistamines (e.g., diphenhydramine [Benadryl]), corticosteroids, (e.g., hydrocortisone sodium succinate [Solu-Cortef]), and pressor amines (e.g., dopamine). Patients who experience a hypersensitivity reaction may be able to continue therapy. Rate reduction and additional pretreatment with corticosteroids may be attempted in subsequent cycles; see Usual Dose.

KETOROLAC TROMETHAMINE BBW

(kee-toh-**ROH**-lack tro-**METH**-ah-meen)

Toradol

Analgesic
(NSAID)

pH 6.9 to 7.9

USUAL DOSE

Adults less than 65 years: 30 mg. May repeat every 6 hours. Maximum dose is 120 mg/24 hr. Do not increase the dose or frequency for breakthrough pain. Consider alternating with low doses of opioids (e.g., morphine or meperidine). Ketorolac oral may be used only as continuation therapy to parenteral dosing. Maximum oral dose is 40 mg/24 hr. Do not administer for longer than 5 days (IV/IM alone or combined use with oral).

Adults over 65 years, patients with impaired renal function, and/or patients under 50 kg (110 lb): 15 mg. May repeat every 6 hours. Maximum dose is 60 mg in 24 hours. Note all restrictions for adults less than 65 years outlined above.

PEDIATRIC DOSE

See Maternal/Child.

Pediatric patients 2 to 16 years of age: One dose of 0.5 mg/kg up to a maximum dose of 15 mg. 0.5 mg/kg IV every 6 hours has been administered in a limited number of patients (unlabeled).

Short-term postoperative pain management (unlabeled): 1 mg/kg alone or as an adjunct.

DOSE ADJUSTMENTS

Required for patients under 50 kg (110 lb), patients over 65 years of age, and patients with reduced renal function (moderately elevated SCr); see Usual Dose. Further dose reductions may be required with high-dose salicylates; see Drug/Lab Interactions.

DILUTION

Confirm IV use. Some 2 mL tubex syringes are for IM use only. May be given undiluted through Y-tube or three-way stopcock of infusion set. Administration through a free-flowing IV is preferred.

Storage: Store at CRT; protect from light.

COMPATIBILITY

Consider any drug NOT listed as compatible to be INCOMPATIBLE until consulting a pharmacist; specific conditions may apply.

May form a precipitate if admixed with drugs with a low pH (e.g., meperidine [Demerol], morphine, promethazine [Phenergan]).

One source suggests the following **compatibilities:**

Solution: D5W, NS, D5NS, LR, R.

Y-site: Cisatracurium (Nimbex), dexmedetomidine (Precedex), fentanyl (Sublimaze), hetastarch in electrolytes (Hextend), hydromorphone (Dilaudid), methadone (Dolophine), morphine, remifentanil (Ultiva), sufentanil (Sufenta).

RATE OF ADMINISTRATION

A single dose over a minimum of 15 seconds; evenly distributed over 1 to 2 minutes is preferred.

ACTIONS

A nonsteroidal anti-inflammatory drug (NSAID) with peripheral analgesic, anti-inflammatory, and antipyretic actions. Inhibits prostaglandin synthesis. 30 to 60 mg produces analgesia similar to morphine 12 mg or Demerol 100 mg. Studies reflect less drowsiness, nausea, and vomiting. Not a narcotic agonist or antagonist. Cardiac and hemodynamic parameters are not altered. Onset of action is 30 to 60 minutes. Half-life varies from 3.8 to 8.6 hours based on age and clinical status. Relief in some patients may last 6 to 8 hours. Excreted primarily in urine. Secreted in breast milk.

INDICATIONS AND USES

Short-term management of moderately severe, acute pain (no longer than 5 days). ▪ NOT indicated for minor or chronic painful conditions.

Unlabeled uses: Postoperative short-term pain management in pediatric patients.

CONTRAINDICATIONS

Hypersensitivity to ketorolac, its components, or ASA or other NSAIDs; labor and delivery; breast-feeding; preoperative or intraoperative medication when hemostasis is critical due to increased risk of bleeding; patients currently receiving ASA or NSAIDs (e.g., ibuprofen [Advil, Motrin], naproxen [Aleve, Naprosyn]); active peptic ulcer disease; recent GI bleeding or perforation; patients with a history of peptic ulcer disease or GI bleeding; suspected or confirmed cerebrovascular bleeding; hemorrhagic diathesis; incomplete hemostasis; high risk of bleeding; advanced renal impairment; or patients at risk for renal failure because of volume depletion. Do not use for epidural or intrathecal administration; contains alcohol. See Drug/Lab Interactions.

PRECAUTIONS

Use only recommended doses; increased doses will not be more effective and will increase the risk of serious adverse events. ▪ Hypersensitivity reactions, including anaphylaxis, have been reported. Administer in a facility with adequate diagnostic and treatment facilities to monitor the patient and respond to any medical emergency. ▪ Inhibits platelet aggregation and may prolong bleeding time. ▪ May cause serious GI ulceration and bleeding without warning. ▪ In addition to the usual caution in patients with reduced hepatic or renal function, ketorolac may also cause a dose-dependent reduction in renal prostaglandin formation. Can precipitate renal failure in patients with impaired renal function, heart failure, or liver dysfunction; in the elderly or in patients receiving diuretics. ▪ Use caution in patients with cardiac decompensation, hypertension, or similar conditions; may cause fluid retention and edema. ▪ Use caution in patients with pre-existing asthma, especially aspirin-sensitive asthma. Severe bronchospasm has been reported.

Monitor: Correct hypovolemia before giving ketorolac and maintain adequate hydration. ▪ Observe patient frequently, especially for heartburn or signs and symptoms of GI upset or bleeding, and monitor vital signs. ▪ Monitor BUN, SCr, liver enzymes, occult blood loss, urinalysis, urine output, and signs of pain relief (e.g., increased appetite and activity). ▪ Observe closely during ambulation. ▪ Low doses of narcotics may be required to treat breakthrough pain.

Patient Education: Side effects have resulted in extended hospitalization and could be fatal. ▪ Discard any remaining oral ketorolac at end of 5-day total cumulative maximum time for use.

Maternal/Child: See Contraindications. ▪ Category C: safety for use not established. Use only if other alternatives are not available. ▪ Discontinue breast-feeding. ▪ Multiple dose treatment in pediatric patients has not been studied; limited data available.

Elderly: See Dose Adjustments and Precautions. ■ More sensitive to side effects. ■ Incidence of GI bleeding and acute renal failure increases with age.

DRUG/LAB INTERACTIONS

Probenecid inhibits clearance and may triple plasma levels of ketorolac. Concomitant use is contraindicated. ■ Potentiated by **salicylates** (especially high-dose regimens). May double plasma levels of ketorolac. Reduce dose of ketorolac by half. ■ May decrease clearance and increase toxicity of **methotrexate.** ■ Additive if used with other **NSAIDs** (see Contraindications); side effects may increase markedly. ■ May potentiate **lithium** levels. ■ May increase risk of bleeding, especially from the GI tract, when given concomitantly with **anticoagulants** (e.g., warfarin [Coumadin], heparin) or **thrombolytic agents** (e.g., alteplase [tPA]). ■ May increase risk of bleeding when given with agents that may cause **hypoprothrombinema or inhibit platelet aggregation** (e.g., cefaperazone [Cefobid], valproic acid [Depacon]). ■ Can precipitate renal failure concomitantly with **diuretics** (e.g., furosemide [Lasix]); see Precautions. ■ Can reduce response to **furosemide** (Lasix) in normovolemic healthy individuals. ■ May increase risk of renal impairment with **ACE inhibitors** (e.g., enalapril [Vasotec]). ■ Nephrotoxicity of both agents may be increased with **other nephrotoxic agents** (e.g., aminoglycosides [e.g., gentamicin], cyclosporine [Sandimmune]). ■ May potentiate **nondepolarizing muscle relaxants** (e.g., atracurium [Tracrium]). ■ Has caused seizures in a few patients taking **antiepileptics** (e.g., phenytoin [Dilantin], carbamazepine [Tegretol]). ■ May cause hallucinations with **antipsychotics** (e.g., thiothixene [Navane]), **antidepressants** (e.g., fluoxetine [Prozac]). ■ May cause **elevations of liver function tests** AST and ALT.

SIDE EFFECTS

Average dose: Diarrhea, dizziness, dyspepsia, drowsiness, edema, GI bleeding, GI pain, headache, injection site pain, nausea, and sweating are most common. Capable of all side effects of other NSAIDs, especially with extended use: abnormal taste, abnormal vision, asthenia, asthma, confusion, constipation, depression, dry mouth, dypsnea, euphoria, excessive thirst, flatulence, inability to concentrate, insomnia, liver function abnormalities, melena, myalgia, nervousness, oliguria, pallor, paresthesia, peptic ulcer, rectal bleeding, stimulation, stomatitis, pruritus, purpura, urinary frequency, urticaria, vasodilation, vertigo, vomiting.

Overdose: Abdominal pain, diarrhea, labored breathing, metabolic acidosis, pallor, peptic ulcer, rales, vomiting.

ANTIDOTE

With increasing severity of any side effect or onset of symptoms of overdose, discontinue the drug and notify the physician. A patent airway, artificial ventilation, oxygen therapy, and other symptomatic treatment must be instituted promptly if indicated. Treat anaphylaxis with epinephrine (Adrenalin), diphenhydramine (Benadryl), and corticosteroids as indicated. Not significantly cleared by dialysis.

LABETALOL HYDROCHLORIDE
(lah-**BET**-ah-lohl hy-droh-**KLOR**-eyed)

Trandate

Alpha/beta-adrenergic
blocking agent
Antihypertensive

pH 3 to 4

USUAL DOSE
Dose must be individualized based on degree of hypertension and patient response.

20 mg as an initial dose by IV injection. May repeat with injections of 40 to 80 mg at 10-minute intervals until desired BP is achieved, or may be diluted and given as a continuous infusion. Usually effective with 50 to 200 mg. Do not exceed a total dose of 300 mg. Initiate oral labetalol after desired BP has been achieved and the supine diastolic pressure starts to rise. See literature for dose regimen. AHA recommends 10 mg IV over 1 to 2 minutes. May repeat or double dose every 10 minutes to a maximum dose of 150 mg. Or initial dose may be given by IV injection followed by an infusion of 2 to 8 mg/min. Titrate slowly to achieve desired results without exceeding maximum dose.

DOSE ADJUSTMENTS
See Precautions and Drug/Lab Interactions.

DILUTION
IV injection: May be given undiluted in a 5 mg/mL concentration.

Continuous infusion: May be diluted in most commonly used IV solutions (see chart on inside back cover). Addition of 200 mg (40 mL) to 160-mL solution yields 1 mg/mL, 300 mg (60 mL) to 240 mL yields 1 mg/mL, or 200 mg (40 mL) to 250 mL yields 2 mg/3 mL. Amount of solution may be decreased if required by fluid restrictions of the patient.

Storage: Store unopened vial between 2° and 30° C (36° and 86° F). Do not freeze. Protect from light. Stable after dilution for 24 hours at room temperature or refrigerated.

COMPATIBILITY (Underline Indicates Conflicting Compatibility Information)
Consider any drug NOT listed as compatible to be INCOMPATIBLE until consulting a pharmacist; specific conditions may apply.

Manufacturer lists 5% sodium bicarbonate as **incompatible** and indicates to use care when administering alkaline drugs, including furosemide (Lasix).

One source suggests the following **compatibilities:**

Y-site: Amikacin (Amikin), aminophylline, amiodarone (Nexterone), ampicillin, bivalirudin (Angiomax), butorphanol (Stadol), calcium gluconate, cefazolin (Ancef), ceftazidime (Fortaz), chloramphenicol (Chloromycetin), clindamycin (Cleocin), dexmedetomidine (Precedex), diltiazem (Cardizem), dobutamine, dopamine, doripenem (Doribax), enalaprilat (Vasotec IV), epinephrine (Adrenalin), erythromycin (Erythrocin), esmolol (Brevibloc), famotidine (Pepcid IV), fenoldopam (Corlopam), fentanyl (Sublimaze), gentamicin, <u>heparin</u>, hetastarch in electrolytes (Hextend), hydromorphone (Dilaudid), <u>insulin (regular)</u>, lidocaine, linezolid (Zyvox), lorazepam (Ativan), magnesium sulfate, meperidine (Demerol), metronidazole (Flagyl IV), midazolam (Versed), milrinone (Primacor), morphine, nicardipine (Cardene IV), nitroglycerin IV, nitroprusside sodium, norepinephrine (Levophed), oxacillin (Bactocill), penicillin G potassium, piperacillin, potassium chloride (KCl), potassium phosphates, propofol (Diprivan), ranitidine (Zantac), sodium acetate, sulfamethoxazole/trimethoprim, tobramycin, vancomycin, vecuronium.

RATE OF ADMINISTRATION

IV injection: Each 20 mg or fraction thereof over at least 2 minutes.
Continuous infusion: Begin at 2 mg/min. Adjust according to orders of physician and BP response. Another source suggests 0.5 to 2 mg/min. Use of a microdrip (60 gtt/mL) or an infusion pump may be helpful.

ACTIONS

An adrenergic receptor blocking agent with both selective alpha 1-adrenergic and nonselective beta-adrenergic receptor blocking activity. Causes dose-related falls in BP without reflex tachycardia or significant reduction in HR. Maximum effect of each dose is reached in 5 minutes. Half-life is 5.5 hours, but some effects last up to 16 hours. Metabolized and excreted as metabolites in urine and through bile to feces. Crosses the placental barrier. Present in small amounts in breast milk.

INDICATIONS AND USES

Control of BP in severe hypertension.
Unlabeled uses: Treatment of clonidine withdrawal hypertension. ■ Decrease BP and relieve symptoms in patients with pheochromocytoma.

CONTRAINDICATIONS

Obstructive airway disease including asthma, cardiogenic shock, greater than first-degree heart block, overt cardiac failure, severe bradycardia, other conditions associated with severe and prolonged hypotension, and hypersensitivity to labetalol or its components.

PRECAUTIONS

Use caution in impaired liver function. ■ Hepatic injury has been reported. Has occurred after both short-term and long-term treatment. Usually reversible, but hepatic necrosis and death have been reported. ■ Use extreme caution in patients with any degree of cardiac failure; may further depress myocardial contractility. Does not alter effectiveness of digoxin on heart muscle. ■ Effective in lowering BP in pheochromocytoma but has caused a paradoxical hypertensive response in some patients. ■ Use with extreme caution in diabetics or patients with a history of hypoglycemia. May mask the symptoms of hypoglycemia and reduce the release of insulin in response to hyperglycemia. ■ Routine withdrawal of chronic beta-blocker therapy before surgery is not recommended. However, the effect of the alpha-adrenergic activity of labetalol has not been evaluated in the surgical setting. Deaths have occurred when labetalol has been used during surgery. ■ Intraoperative floppy iris syndrome has been observed during cataract surgery in some patients treated with alpha-1 blockers. Characterized by a combination of a flaccid iris, progressive miosis despite preoperative dilation with standard mydriatic drugs, and potential prolapse of the iris. Modification of the surgical technique may be required. ■ See Drug/Lab Interactions.

Monitor: Keep patient supine. Postural hypotension can occur for up to 3 hours after administration. Ambulate with care and assistance. ■ Monitor BP before and 5 and 10 minutes after each direct IV injection. Monitor at least every 5 minutes during infusion. Avoid rapid or excessive falls in either systolic or diastolic BP. When severely elevated BP drops too rapidly, catastrophic reactions can occur (e.g., cerebral infarction, optic nerve infarction, angina, ischemic ECG changes). ▪ Monitor for S/S of CHF. ▪ Although rebound angina, myocardial infarction, or ventricular arrhythmias have not been a problem with labetalol, it is recommended that the dose of beta-adrenergic blockers be reduced gradually to avoid these conditions. ▪ See Drug/Lab Interactions.

Patient Education: Report cough, dizziness, irregular pulse, or shortness of breath promptly. ▪ May cause dizziness or fainting; request assistance with ambulation.

Maternal/Child: Category C: use in pregnancy only when clearly indicated and benefit outweighs risk. Hypotension, bradycardia, hypoglycemia, and respiratory depression have been reported in infants of mothers who were treated with labetalol for hypertension during pregnancy. Has been used during labor and delivery. ▪ Use caution during breast-feeding. ▪ Safety and effectiveness for use in pediatric patients not established.

Elderly: Use with caution in age-related peripheral vascular disease; risk of hypothermia increased. ▪ May exacerbate mental impairment.

DRUG/LAB INTERACTIONS
Inhibits **beta-agonist bronchodilators** (e.g., albuterol [Ventolin]); increased doses may be required, especially in asthmatics. ▪ Synergistic with **halothane anesthesia.** High concentrations of halothane (3% or above) should not be used. The degree of hypotension will be increased, and the possibility of a large reduction in cardiac output and an increase in central venous pressure exists. Notify anesthesiologist that patient is receiving labetalol. ▪ Potentiated by **cimetidine** (Tagamet). May blunt the reflex tachycardia produced by **nitroglycerin.** May cause further hypotension with **nitroglycerin.** ▪ The use of labetalol with **calcium channel blockers** (e.g., diltiazem [Cardizem], verapamil) may potentiate both drugs and result in severe depression of myocardium, AV conduction, and severe hypotension. ▪ May mask the hypoglycemic effects of **insulin and other antidiabetic agents.** May inhibit the mobilization of glucose from hepatic stores. Monitor glucose carefully in diabetic patients. ▪ Patients receiving betablockers who have a history of severe anaphylactic reaction to a variety of allergens may be unresponsive to the usual doses of **epinephrine** used to treat an allergic reaction. ▪ May interfere with lab tests in the **diagnosis of pheochromocytoma.** ▪ May cause a **false-positive urine test** for amphetamine use.

SIDE EFFECTS
Diaphoresis, dizziness, flushing, moderate hypotension, numbness, severe postural hypotension, nausea, somnolence, tingling of scalp, and ventricular dysrhythmias (e.g., intensified atrioventricular block) occur most frequently.

ANTIDOTE
Notify the physician of all side effects. Decrease rate or discontinue drug if hypotension occurs. Notify physician immediately. Trendelenburg position may be appropriate. May require treatment with IV fluids or vasopressors (e.g., norepinephrine [levarterenol], dopamine). Use atropine or epinephrine for severe bradycardia; digoxin, diuretics, dopamine, or dobutamine for cardiac failure; norepinephrine (Levophed) for hypotension;

epinephrine (Adrenalin) and/or albuterol (Ventolin) for bronchospasm; and diazepam (Valium) for seizures. Unresponsive hypotension and bradycardia may be reversed by glucagon 5 to 10 mg over 30 seconds followed by a continuous infusion of 5 mg/hr. Reduce rate as condition improves. Treat other side effects symptomatically and resuscitate as necessary. Hemodialysis is not effective.

LACOSAMIDE
(la-**KOE**-sa-mide)

Vimpat

Anticonvulsant

pH 3.5 to 5

USUAL DOSE

Serum levels similar by oral or IV route; no dose or frequency adjustment is necessary. Transfer to oral therapy as soon as practical.

Initiate treatment: Begin with a daily dose of 100 mg/day equally divided into 2 doses (50 mg twice daily). May be increased at weekly intervals by 100 mg/day given as 2 divided doses up to the recommended maintenance dose of 200 to 400 mg/day based on individual patient response and tolerability. Titrate dose with caution in patients with renal or hepatic impairment and in the elderly. Twice-daily IV infusions have been used for up to 5 days. There is no evidence that doses greater than 400 mg/day offer additional benefit, and they have been associated with a higher incidence of side effects.

Transfer from an IV dose to an oral dose: Transfer at the equivalent daily dose and frequency of the IV dose.

DOSE ADJUSTMENTS

No dose adjustment is indicated for patients with mild to moderate renal impairment. ▪ 300 mg is the maximum recommended dose for patients with severe renal impairment (a CrCl equal to or less than 30 mL/min) and for patients with end-stage renal disease. A supplemental dose of up to 50% should be considered after a 4-hour hemodialysis treatment. ▪ A maximum dose of 300 mg/day is recommended for patients with mild or moderate hepatic impairment. ▪ Not recommended for patients with severe hepatic impairment. ▪ Dose adjustment not required based on gender or race or in the elderly; see Elderly.

DILUTION

May be given undiluted or may be further diluted with NS, D5W, or LR. See Rate of Administration.

Filters: Specific information not available.

Storage: Store unopened vials at CRT. Diluted solutions are stable at ambient RT for 24 hours in glass or PVC bags. Discard unused portions of vial.

COMPATIBILITY

Solutions: Compatible with NS, D5W, and LR. Additional information not available.

RATE OF ADMINISTRATION

A single dose as an infusion over 30 to 60 minutes.

ACTIONS

An antiepileptic (anticonvulsant) drug. The precise mechanism of action is unknown. *In vitro* studies have shown that it selectively enhances the slow inactivation of voltage-gated sodium channels, resulting in stabilization of hyperexcitable neuronal membranes and inhibition of repetitive neuronal firing. Some effects are reached at the end of infusion. Steady-state plasma concentrations are achieved after 3 days of administration. Doses above 400 mg/day do not appear to have additional benefit. Less than 15% bound to plasma proteins. Partially metabolized. Half-life is approximately 13 hours. Excreted as metabolites and as unchanged drug in urine.

INDICATIONS AND USES

Adjunctive therapy in the treatment of partial-onset seizures in adult patients (17 years of age and older) with epilepsy. IV injection is used as a temporary alternative to oral therapy. Usually given in combination with other antiepileptic drugs.

CONTRAINDICATIONS

Manufacturer indicates none; see Precautions.

PRECAUTIONS

For IV use only. ▪ Psychotic symptoms and other behavioral changes have been reported with AEDs (antiepileptic drugs) and may include aggression, agitation, anger, anxiety, apathy, depersonalization, depression, emotional lability, hallucinations, hostility, irritability, and suicidal tendencies. In an analysis of AED clinical trials, symptoms occurred as early as 1 week after starting AEDs and persisted for the duration of treatment. May require a dose reduction or discontinuation of lacosamide. Many illnesses for which AEDs are prescribed, including epilepsy, are associated with morbidity and mortality and an increased risk of suicidal thoughts and behavior. Consider that these symptoms may also be related to the illness being treated. ▪ Associated with CNS side effects in addition to behavioral problems and psychotic tendencies (e.g., ataxia, dizziness, somnolence). ▪ Dose-dependent prolongations in PR intervals have been observed. Use caution in patients with known conduction problems (e.g., marked first-degree AV block, second-degree or higher AV block, and sick sinus syndrome without a pacemaker) or severe cardiac disease such as myocardial ischemia or heart failure. ▪ May cause atrial arrhythmias (atrial fibrillation or atrial flutter), especially in patients with diabetic neuropathy or cardiovascular disease. ▪ Dizziness and loss of consciousness also occurred in patients with diabetic neuropathy. ▪ A delayed multiorgan hypersensitivity reaction (also known as Drug Reaction with Eosinophilia and Systemic Symptoms, or DRESS) occurred in one patient and manifested as symptomatic hepatitis and nephritis, which resolved over time. DRESS has been reported with other AEDs and typically presents with a fever and rash associated with other organ involvement, such as eosinophilia, hepatitis, nephritis, lymphadenopathy, and/or myocarditis. ▪ Not recommended for patients with severe hepatic impairment. ▪ To minimize the potential for increased seizure frequency, withdraw AEDs (including lacosamide) gradually (over a minimum of 1 week).

Monitor: Baseline CBC and CrCl indicated; monitor as needed. ▪ Monitor vital signs. ▪ Monitor for seizure activity. ▪ Monitor for the emergence or worsening of depression, suicidal thoughts or behavior, and/or any unusual changes in mood or behavior. ▪ Observe patient closely for signs of CNS side effects, prolonged PR interval, and/or symptoms of DRESS; see

Precautions. ▪ Obtain a baseline ECG in patients with known conduction problems and/or severe cardiac disease. Repeat after lacosamide is titrated to steady-state concentrations.

Patient Education: May cause dizziness, fainting, and somnolence; use caution performing tasks that require alertness (e.g., operating machinery, driving). ▪ Inform your health care professional if you are pregnant or breast-feeding. ▪ May cause alterations in mood (e.g., aggression, agitation, anger, anxiety, apathy, decreased ability to cope, depression, hostility, irritability, thoughts of suicide); report these changes promptly. ▪ Has caused atrial arrhythmias. Promptly report palpitations, rapid pulse, and/or shortness of breath. ▪ Promptly report S/S of hypersensitivity (e.g., fever, rash) or liver toxicity (e.g., fatigue, jaundice, dark urine). ▪ Women who are pregnant or who become pregnant should be encouraged to enroll in the North American Antiepileptic Drug (NAAED) Pregnancy Registry.

Maternal/Child: Category C: animal studies demonstrated developmental toxicity (increased embryofetal and perinatal mortality, growth deficit). Use during pregnancy only if the potential benefit justifies the potential risk to the fetus. Manufacturer has established a pregnancy registry to evaluate safety and outcomes; see manufacturer's literature and Patient Education. ▪ Effects during labor and delivery unknown. ▪ Discontinue breast-feeding. ▪ Safety and effectiveness for use in pediatric patients under 17 years of age not established.

Elderly: Higher plasma concentrations seen in the elderly may be due to differences in total body water and age-associated impaired renal function.

DRUG/LAB INTERACTIONS

Coadministration with **other drugs that can affect cardiac conduction** may lead to conduction abnormalities (e.g., drugs that increase QT interval prolongation such as **antiarrhythmics** [e.g., amiodarone (Nexterone), disopyramide (Norpace), ibutilide (Corvert), mexiletine, procainamide (Pronestyl), quinidine], **antihistamines, azole antifungals** [e.g., itraconazole (Sporanox)], **fluoroquinolones** [e.g., levofloxacin (Levaquin)], **phenothiazines** [e.g., thioridazine (Mellaril)], and **tricyclic antidepressants** [e.g., amitriptyline (Elavil), imipramine (Tofranil)]). ▪ No evidence of any relevant drug/drug interaction with **other antiepileptic drugs** (AEDs) such as carbamazepine (Tegretol), clonazepam (Klonopin), gabapentin (Neurontin), lamotrigine (Lamictal), levetiracetam (Keppra), oxcarbazepine (Trileptal), phenobarbital (Luminal), phenytoin (Dilantin), topiramate (Topamax), valproic acid (e.g., Depacon, Depakote), and zonisamide (Zonegran). ▪ Concurrent administration with **carbamazepine, phenobarbital, or phenytoin** has resulted in small reductions in lacosamide plasma concentrations. ▪ Minimal protein binding; unlikely to have interactions with drugs requiring protein-binding sites. ▪ Has been administered with oral contraceptives (containing ethinyl estradiol and levonorgestrel), digoxin (Lanoxin), metformin (Glucophage), and omeprazole (Prilosec) with no interference on the pharmacokinetics of either drug. ▪ Does not induce or inhibit the enzyme activity of many drugs metabolized by selected cytochrome P_{450} isoforms; see prescribing information.

SIDE EFFECTS

The most common side effects are diplopia, dizziness, headache, and nausea. Ataxia, blurred vision, diplopia, dizziness, nausea, vertigo, and vomiting led to discontinuation of lacosamide. Incidence of side effects increased with doses above 400 mg/day. Most side effects at recommended doses were considered mild or moderate and included asthenia; balance disorder; confusion; depression; diarrhea; elevated liver function tests (e.g., ALT, AST); fatigue; gait disturbance; injection site pain, discomfort, irritation, or erythema; nystagmus; pruritus; skin laceration; somnolence; and tremor. Psychiatric disorders, including aggression, agitation, anger, anxiety, apathy, depersonalization, depression, emotional lability, hallucinations, hostility, irritability, and suicidal tendencies, have been reported. May produce euphoria-type reactions. One patient experienced profound bradycardia; another developed symptoms of DRESS, including hepatitis and nephritis. Both improved with discontinuation of lacosamide.

ANTIDOTE
Keep physician informed of all side effects. Some may not require intervention, and others may improve with a reduced dose or discontinuation of lacosamide; see Precautions and Side Effects. Discontinue lacosamide for symptoms of DRESS; use of an alternate treatment is recommended. Support patient as required in treatment of overdose. No specific antidote in overdose; however, hemodialysis will remove approximately 50% of a dose in 4 hours.

LANSOPRAZOLE
(lan-**SAHP**-rah-zohl)

Prevacid IV

Proton pump inhibitor (Gastric acid inhibitor)

pH 9.5 to 11

USUAL DOSE
30 mg as an infusion once daily for up to 7 days.

Given as an alternative to continued oral therapy. Resume oral therapy as soon as practical. Dose and serum levels similar by IV or oral route. See Rate of Administration.

DOSE ADJUSTMENTS
No dose adjustment is required based on age, race, or gender; in the elderly; or in patients with renal insufficiency. ■ Consider dose adjustment in patients with impaired hepatic function; half-life is increased and mean AUC is increased up to 500%.

DILUTION
Reconstitution in vial: Each 30-mg dose must be reconstituted with 5 mL of SW (6 mg/mL). The use of other solutions for reconstitution may result in precipitation. Mix gently until powder is dissolved. Must be further diluted for infusion in 50 mL of NS, LR, or D5W.

Reconstitution with Baxter MINI-BAG Plus Container: May be reconstituted directly into 50 mL of NS or D5W in a Baxter MINI-BAG Plus Container. Refer to specific instructions included with the MINI-BAG Plus Container.

Filters: Must be administered through the provided 1.2-micron in-line filter to remove precipitate that may form when the reconstituted drug is further diluted with IV solutions.

Storage: Store vials in carton at CRT to protect from light.

Vials: Reconstituted solution is stable for 1 hour at 25° C (77° F) before further dilution (pH 11). Fully diluted solutions are stable at 25° C (77° F) and should be administered within 24 hours when diluted in NS (pH 10.2) or LR (pH 10) and within 12 hours when diluted in D5W (pH 9.5). **MINI-BAG:** Store admixture at 25° C (77° F). Administer within 24 hours in NS (pH 10.2) and within 8 hours in D5W (pH 9.5).

COMPATIBILITY

Consider any drug NOT listed as compatible to be INCOMPATIBLE until consulting a pharmacist; specific conditions may apply.

Manufacturer states, "Do not mix with other drugs or diluents." A dedicated line is not required; however, the IV line should be flushed with a **compatible** IV solution (NS, LR, or D5W) before and after administration of lansoprazole.

One source suggests the following **compatibilities:**

Y-site: Acyclovir (Zovirax), amikacin (Amikin), ceftriaxone (Rocephin), cyclosporine (Sandimmune), dexamethasone (Decadron), fentanyl (Sublimaze), fluconazole (Diflucan), ganciclovir (Cytovene), gentamicin, heparin, ifosfamide (Ifex), mannitol (Osmitrol), methotrexate, nalbuphine, paclitaxel (Taxol), piperacillin, piperacillin/tazobactam (Zosyn), sulfamethoxazole/trimethoprim, sufentanil (Sufenta).

RATE OF ADMINISTRATION

Flush the IV line with at least 5 mL of a **compatible** IV solution (NS, LR, or D5W) before and after administration of lansoprazole. Must be administered through the provided in-line filter. Refer to package insert for manufacturer's specific instructions for priming this filter and specific precautions required with the use of this filter.

A single 30-mg dose properly diluted as an infusion evenly distributed over 30 minutes. Remove and discard the administration set and filter after lansoprazole infusion is complete. Flush the IV port with at least 5 mL of a **compatible** solution. If the port is not flushed and the set is not removed, a brown/black particulate produced from lansoprazole degradation may appear in the tubing or filter.

ACTIONS

A proton pump inhibitor. A compound that does not exhibit anticholinergic or histamine H_2-receptor antagonist properties. It suppresses gastric acid secretion by specific inhibition of the (H^+, K^+)-ATPase enzyme system at the secretory surface of the gastric parietal cell. Blocks the final step of acid production. Effects are dose related, and both basal and stimulated gastric acid secretions are inhibited for at least 24 hours. Does not accumulate, and pharmacokinetics are not altered with multiple daily dosing (with the exception of patients with impaired hepatic function). Distributed in extracellular fluid and highly bound to serum protein. Extensively metabolized in the liver by the cytochrome P_{450} isoenzyme system (CYP3A and CYP2C19 isozymes). Half-life is 1.3 hours (range is 0.8 to 1.8 hours) and does not reflect the duration of suppression of gastric acid secretion. Primarily excreted in bile and feces, with some excretion in urine.

INDICATIONS AND USES

Short-term treatment (up to 7 days) of all grades of erosive esophagitis as an alternative to oral therapy in patients who are unable to continue taking lansoprazole oral formulations. Safety and effectiveness for use in the initial treatment of erosive esophagitis not demonstrated.

CONTRAINDICATIONS

Known hypersensitivity to lansoprazole or its components.

PRECAUTIONS

For IV use only; do not give IM or SC. ▪ Gastric malignancy may be present even though patient's symptoms improve. ▪ May be associated with an increased risk for osteoporosis-related fractures of the hip, wrist, or spine. Risk is increased in patients receiving high-dose (multiple daily doses) and long-term therapy (a year or longer). Use lowest dose and shortest duration of therapy appropriate for the condition being treated. ▪ Discontinue as soon as the patient is able to resume oral therapy.

Monitor: Observe for S/S of allergic reaction; anaphylaxis has been reported in post-marketing reports. ▪ Monitor vital signs, pain levels, and injection site.

Patient Education: Review prescription and non-prescription drugs with physician. ▪ Oral route preferred.

Maternal/Child: Category B: use during pregnancy only if clearly needed. Animal studies did not show harm to the fetus. ▪ If the drug is indicated for the mother, breast-feeding should be discontinued. May have serious reactions in the infant and has a potential for tumorigenicity. ▪ Safety and effectiveness for use in pediatric patients not established.

Elderly: Safety and effectiveness similar to that seen in younger adults. ▪ Consider potential for impaired liver function; see Dose Adjustments.

DRUG/LAB INTERACTIONS

Because of profound and long-lasting inhibition of gastric acid secretion, lansoprazole may **interfere with the absorption of drugs** in which gastric pH is an important determinant of their bioavailability (e.g., ampicillin esters [Omnipen], digoxin [Lanoxin], iron salts [ferrous sulfate], ketoconazole [Nizoral]). ▪ Increases in INR and PT have been reported when administered concurrently with **warfarin;** monitoring of INR and PT indicated. ▪ Studies suggest that the metabolism and serum concentrations of lansoprazole are not significantly altered when used concurrently with other drugs metabolized by the cytochrome P_{450} system (e.g., clarithromycin [Biaxin], diazepam [Valium], indomethacin [Indocin], ibuprofen [Advil, Motrin], phenytoin [Dilantin], propranolol, prednisone). ▪ May cause a minor increase in the clearance of **theophylline;** certain patients may require some dose titration when lansoprazole is started or discontinued. ▪ Concomitant administration with **tacrolimus** (Prograf) may increase whole blood levels of tacrolimus, especially in patients who are intermediate or poor metabolizers of CYP2C19.

SIDE EFFECTS

Most common side effects are headache, injection site pain or reaction, and nausea. Other side effects include abdominal pain, constipation, diarrhea, dizziness, dyspepsia, paresthesia, rash, taste perversion, vasodilation, and vomiting. Numerous other side effects may occur in fewer than 1% of patients. Other side effects reported with oral lansoprazole include abnormal albumin-to-globulin (A/G) ratio, abnormal or increased liver function tests (e.g., AST and ALT, alkaline phosphatase, bilirubinemia, LDH), abnormal RBC count, eosinophilia, hyperlipidemia, increased/decreased cholesterol, increased creatinine, increased/decreased electrolytes, increased/decreased/abnormal platelets, increased/decreased/abnormal WBC count, increased gastrin levels, increased GGTP (gamma-glutamyl transpeptidase), increased globulins, increased glucocorticoids, and urine abnormalities (e.g., albuminuria, glycosuria, hematuria).

Overdose: Ataxia, decreased locomotor response, ptosis, and tonic convulsions were symptoms of acute toxicity in heavily overdosed mice and rats.

Post-Marketing: Agranulocytosis, anaphylaxis, aplastic anemia, bone fracture, hemolytic anemia, hepatotoxicity, hypomagnesemia, leukopenia, pancreatitis, pancytopenia, serious dermatologic reactions (including erythema multiforme, Stevens-Johnson syndrome, and toxic epidermal necrolysis [some fatal]), speech disorder, thrombocytopenia, thrombotic thrombocytopenic purpura, urinary retention.

ANTIDOTE

Keep physician informed of significant side effects. May be treated symptomatically. Discontinue and initiate appropriate treatment if S/S associated with post-marketing reports or overdose occur; see Side Effects. Not removed by hemodialysis.

LEPIRUDIN
(leh-**PEER**-you-din)

Refludan

Anticoagulant

pH 7

USUAL DOSE

A baseline aPTT should be determined before initiation of therapy with lepirudin. To avoid a potential overdose, therapy should not be started in patients with a baseline aPTT ratio of 2.5 or more. The aPTT ratio is the aPTT in a given patient at a given time over an aPTT reference value; usually median of the laboratory normal range for aPTT.

Anticoagulation in adult patients with heparin-induced thrombocytopenia (HIT) and associated thromboembolic disease. *Bolus dose:* 0.4 mg/kg body weight (up to 110 kg).

Lepirudin Standard Bolus Injection Volumes According to Body Weight for a 5 mg/mL Concentration		
	Injection Volume	
Body Weight (kg)	Dosage 0.4 mg/kg	Dosage 0.2 mg/kg*
50 kg	4 mL	2 mL
60 kg	4.8 mL	2.4 mL
70 kg	5.6 mL	2.8 mL
80 kg	6.4 mL	3.2 mL
90 kg	7.2 mL	3.6 mL
100 kg	8 mL	4 mL
≥110 kg	8.8 mL	4.4 mL

*Dosage recommended for all patients with renal insufficiency.

Maintenance infusion: 0.15 mg/kg body weight (up to 110 kg)/hr for 2 to 10 days or longer as clinically indicated. Adjust rate to maintain an aPTT ratio of 1.5 to 2.5. See Dose Adjustments and Precautions/Monitor. In general, an infusion rate of 0.21 mg/kg/hr should not be exceeded without checking for coagulation abnormalities, which might prevent an appropriate aPTT response.

Alternate-dosing regimen (unlabeled): 0.2 mg/kg as a bolus dose (used only if life- or limb-threatening thrombosis is present) followed by a continuous infusion of 0.05 to 0.1 mg/kg/hr has been recommended due to higher rates of bleeding associated with the FDA-approved dosing regimen. Further dose reduction may be required in patients with renal dysfunction.

DOSE ADJUSTMENTS

Normally the initial dose depends on body weight. This is valid up to a body weight of 110 kg. In patients weighing more than 110 kg, the initial dose should not be increased beyond the 110-kg body weight dose (i.e., the initial bolus dose should not exceed 44 mg and the initial infusion rate should not exceed 16.5 mg/hr). ▪ If possible, an aPTT ratio outside of the target range (aPTT 1.5 to 2.5) should be confirmed before any dose adjustment. If the confirmed aPTT ratio is above the target range, the infusion should be stopped for 2 hours and then restarted at half the previous infusion rate. If the confirmed aPTT ratio is below the target range, the infusion rate should be increased in 20% increments. ▪ Dose reduction is required in patients with renal impairment as measured by a CrCl of less than 60 mL/min or a SCr of greater than 1.5 mg/dL. Reduce bolus dose to 0.2 mg/kg body weight. Adjust infusion rate as indicated in the following chart.

Reduction of Lepirudin Infusion Ratio in Patients with Renal Impairment			
		Adjusted Infusion Rate	
Creatinine Clearance (mL/min)	Serum Creatinine (mg/dL)	(% of Standard Initial Infusion Rate)	(mg/kg/hr)
45-60 mL/min	1.6-2 mg/dL	50%	0.075 mg/kg/hr
30-44 mL/min	2.1-3 mg/dL	30%	0.045 mg/kg/hr
15-29 mL/min	3.1-6 mg/dL	15%	0.0225 mg/kg/hr
Below 15 mL/min*	Above 6 mg/dL*	Avoid or STOP infusion*	

*In hemodialysis patients or in case of acute renal failure (CrCl <15 mL/min or SCr >6 mg/dL). Infusion of lepirudin is to be avoided or stopped. Additional intravenous bolus doses of 0.1 mg/kg body weight should be considered every other day only if the aPTT ratio falls below the lower therapeutic limit of 1.5.

▪ There are limited data regarding concomitant use of lepirudin with thrombolytic therapy (e.g., alteplase [tPA, Activase], streptokinase [Streptase]). A dose reduction of 0.2 mg/kg of body weight for the bolus dose and 0.1 mg/kg of body weight/hr for the continuous infusion has been recommended. ▪ In patients scheduled to receive a coumarin derivative for oral anticoagulation after lepirudin therapy, the rate should be decreased gradually until an aPTT ratio just above 1.5 is reached. Initiate oral

Continued

anticoagulant therapy at this point. Coumarin derivatives should be initiated only when platelet counts are normalizing. Do not use a loading dose; administer the intended maintenance dose. Discontinue lepirudin when target INR is reached. May take 4 to 5 days. See package insert. ▪ Clearance of lepirudin is lower in women and in the elderly. Dose adjustments may be necessary.

DILUTION

Warm preparation to room temperature before administration.

Bolus: Reconstitute 50-mg vial with 1 mL of SW or NS and shake gently. Transfer the contents of the vial to a sterile syringe and further dilute with NS, SW, or D5W to a total volume of 10 mL. This provides a final concentration of 5 mg/mL, which is suitable for bolus injection. Calculate volume of dilution to be administered. See Usual Dose. Discard any unused solution.

Infusion: Reconstitute 2 vials with 1 mL each of SW or NS. Add the contents of both vials (100 mg) to 250 mL or 500 mL of NS or D5W to obtain a final concentration of 0.4 mg/mL or 0.2 mg/mL, respectively.

Filters: Use not required by manufacturer; however, no loss of drug potency expected with use of any size low-flex membrane, in-line filter.

Storage: Store unopened vials at 2° to 25° C (36° to 77° F). Once reconstituted, lepirudin should be used immediately. Stable for 24 hours at room temperature (e.g., during infusion).

COMPATIBILITY

Manufacturer states, "Should not be mixed with other drugs except for SW, NS, or D5W." One source suggests **compatibility** at the **Y-site** with amiodarone (Nexterone); consult pharmacist.

RATE OF ADMINISTRATION

Bolus: A single dose over 15 to 20 seconds.

Infusion: Administer at the determined rate according to body weight. See Usual Dose, Dose Adjustments, and the following chart. An infusion rate of 0.21 mg/kg/hr should not be exceeded without checking for coagulation abnormalities, which might prevent an appropriate aPTT response.

Lepirudin Standard Infusion Rates According to Body Weight		
	Infusion Rate at 0.15 mg/kg/hr	
Body Weight (kg)	500-mL Infusion Bag (0.2 mg/mL)	250-mL Infusion Bag (0.4 mg/mL)
50 kg	38 mL/hr	19 mL/hr
60 kg	45 mL/hr	23 mL/hr
70 kg	53 mL/hr	26 mL/hr
80 kg	60 mL/hr	30 mL/hr
90 kg	68 mL/hr	34 mL/hr
100 kg	75 mL/hr	38 mL/hr
≥110 kg	83 mL/hr	41 mL/hr

ACTIONS

An anticoagulant that is a highly specific direct inhibitor of thrombin. A recombinant hirudin that is derived from yeast cells. One molecule of lepirudin binds to one molecule of thrombin, thereby blocking the thrombogenic activity of thrombin. Inhibits both free and clot-bound thrombin without requiring endogenous cofactors (i.e., mode of action is independent of antithrombin III and heparin cofactor II and is not inhibited by platelet factor 4). Produces a dose-dependent increase in aPTT and PT/INR. Distribution is restricted primarily to the extracellular space. Thought to be partially metabolized by hydrolysis. Excreted almost exclusively by the kidneys as metabolites and unchanged drug. Terminal half-life approximately 1.3 hours.

INDICATIONS AND USES

Anticoagulation in patients with heparin-induced thrombocytopenia (HIT) and associated thromboembolic disease to prevent further thromboembolic complications.

CONTRAINDICATIONS

Known hypersensitivity to hirudins or to any of the components of lepirudin.

PRECAUTIONS

Hemorrhage can occur at any site. Consider a hemorrhagic event if there is an unexplained fall in hemoglobin or BP or any other unexplained symptom. ■ Intracranial bleeding in the absence of concomitant thrombolytic therapy has been reported. Concomitant therapy with thrombolytic agents (e.g., alteplase [tPA, Activase], streptokinase [Streptase]) may increase the risk of bleeding, including life-threatening intracranial bleeding. See Dose Adjustments and Drug/Lab Interactions. ■ Use with extreme caution and weigh risk versus benefit in all patients with an increased risk of bleeding. Conditions of concern include recent significant surgery, anomaly of vessels or organs, bacterial endocarditis, severe uncontrolled hypertension, advanced renal impairment, hemorrhagic diathesis, recent puncture of large vessels, recent CVA, stroke, intracerebral surgery or other neuraxial procedures, recent organ biopsy, and recent major bleeding (e.g., intracranial, gastrointestinal, intraocular, or pulmonary bleeding or recent active peptic ulcer). ■ Hepatic impairment may enhance the anticoagulant effect of lepirudin due to coagulation defects secondary to reduced generation of vitamin K–dependent coagulation factors. ■ There are limited data regarding re-exposure to lepirudin. Allergic reactions ranging from a mild allergic skin reaction to anaphylaxis resulting in shock or death have been reported and have occurred during initial administration and on re-exposure. ■ Antihirudin antibody formation has been reported in about 40% of patients receiving lepirudin. This may increase the drug's anticoagulant effect. To date, there is no evidence that antibody formation may lead to neutralization of lepirudin or development of hypersensitivity reactions.

Monitor: Monitor renal function. CrCl is preferred method of monitoring. May use SCr if CrCl is not available. See Dose Adjustments. ■ Determine a baseline aPTT ratio. Infusion rate should be adjusted according to the aPTT ratio. See Dose Adjustments. An aPTT ratio should be determined 4 hours after the start of the infusion and 4 hours after any change in infusion rate. Follow-up aPTT ratios should be determined at least once daily. More frequent monitoring is recommended in patients with renal or hepatic impairment. ▪ Obtain baseline and monitor platelet count, hemoglobin, hematocrit, and occult blood in stool. ▪ Strict monitoring of aPTT indicated in prolonged therapy to monitor for antihirudin antibodies. ▪ See Precautions.

Patient Education: Report all episodes of bleeding. ▪ Report tarry stools. ▪ Compliance with all measures to minimize bleeding is very important (e.g., avoid use of razors, toothbrushes, other sharp items). ▪ Use caution while moving to avoid excess bumping.

Maternal/Child: Category B: safety for use in pregnancy not established. Benefits must outweigh risks. ▪ In lactating women, the decision should be made to discontinue breast-feeding or to discontinue the drug, taking into account the importance of the drug to the mother. ▪ Safety and efficacy have not been established for pediatric patients. Was used during trials in two older children without adverse events.

Elderly: Clearance is reduced in the elderly, possibly due to age-related renal impairment. See Dose Adjustments.

DRUG/LAB INTERACTIONS

Concomitant treatment with **thrombolytics** (e.g., alteplase [tPA, Activase], reteplase [Retavase], streptokinase [Streptase]) may increase the risk of bleeding complications and enhance the effect of lepirudin on aPTT prolongation. See Dose Adjustments. ▪ Concomitant treatment with **coumarin derivatives** (warfarin [Coumadin]) **and drugs that affect platelet function** such as dipyridamole (Persantine), glycoprotein GPIIb/IIIa receptor antagonists (e.g., abciximab [ReoPro], eptifibatide [Integrilin], tirofiban [Aggrastat]), NSAIDs (e.g., ibuprofen [Advil, Motrin], naproxen [Aleve, Naprosyn]) may also increase the risk of bleeding. ▪ Other **thrombin-dependent coagulation assays** will be changed by lepirudin.

SIDE EFFECTS

Bleeding is the most frequent adverse event. May occur as bleeding from a puncture site, anemia, epistaxis, hematoma, hematuria, hemothorax, GI bleeding, or intracranial bleeding.

Abnormal kidney or liver function, allergic reactions (including anaphylaxis), fever, heart failure, infection, intracranial bleeding, multi-organ failure, pericardial effusion, pneumonia, ventricular fibrillation.

ANTIDOTE

No specific antidote is available. If life-threatening bleeding develops and excessive plasma levels of lepirudin are suspected, immediately stop lepirudin infusion. Determine aPTT and hemoglobin and prepare for blood transfusion as appropriate. Follow current guidelines for treatment of shock as indicated (fluid, vasopressors [e.g., dopamine], Trendelenburg position, plasma expanders [e.g., albumin, hetastarch]). Hemodialysis or hemofiltration may be useful in overdose situation; see package insert for specifics.

LEUCOVORIN CALCIUM
(loo-koh-**VOR**-in **KAL**-see-um)

**Citrovorum Factor, Folinic Acid,
Leucovorin Calcium PF**

Antidote
Antineoplastic adjunct

pH 6 to 8.1

USUAL DOSE
May be given IV/IM or PO. If GI toxicity is present, should be administered parenterally.

Delayed excretion or overdose of methotrexate (MTX): 10 mg/M^2 every 6 hours until the serum MTX level is less than 0.05 micromolar. Milligram for milligram or greater than the dose of MTX is common. Administer within the first hour (or as soon as possible) in overdose or within 24 hours of MTX dose if there is delayed excretion. At least every 24 hours, obtain a SCr and MTX level. If SCr is more than 50% above pretreatment level, increase the leucovorin dose to 100 mg/M^2 every 3 hours until the serum MTX level is less than 0.05 micromolar.

Leucovorin rescue after high-dose MTX therapy: With high-dose methotrexate (12 to 15 Gm/M^2 as an infusion over 4 hours); begin leucovorin 15 mg (approximately 10 mg/M^2) 24 hours after MTX infusion started. Repeat every 6 hours for 10 doses. If MTX elimination is delayed, extend every-6-hour dosing until MTX level is less than 0.05 micromolar. If there is evidence of acute renal injury, increase leucovorin to 150 mg every 3 hours until MTX level is less than 1 micromolar, then 15 mg every 3 hours until MTX level is less than 0.05 micromolar. In both situations obtain SCr and MTX level at least every 24 hours. Other protocols are in use. Amount of leucovorin is dependent on MTX dose, MTX serum levels, and SCr.

Megaloblastic anemia: Up to 1 mg daily.

Advanced colorectal cancer: 200 mg/M^2 followed by fluorouracil (5-FU) 370 mg/M^2 or leucovorin 20 mg/M^2 followed by 5-FU 425 mg/M^2 daily for 5 days. Repeat at 4-week intervals twice, then repeat every 28 to 35 days based on complete recovery from toxic effects. Reduce 5-FU dose based on tolerance to previous course, 20% for moderate hematologic or GI toxicity, 30% for severe. Leucovorin doses remain the same. Increase 5-FU dose 10% if no toxicity. Other protocols are in use. Also approved for use with irinotecan and 5-FU.

Pemetrexed toxicity (unlabeled): A single dose of 100 mg/M^2. Follow with 50 mg/M^2 every 6 hours for 8 days.

DOSE ADJUSTMENTS
See adjustments in Usual Dose; larger reductions may be required in the elderly based on the potential for decreased renal function, especially in combination with fluorouracil. ■ See Precautions/Monitor.

DILUTION
Each 50-mg, 100-mg, or 350-mg vial should be diluted to a 10 mg/mL to 20 mg/mL solution. For total doses less than 10 mg/M^2, dilute with bacteriostatic water for injection (contains benzyl alcohol as a preservative). Use SW for injection without a preservative for any dose 10 mg/M^2 or greater. May be further diluted in 100 to 500 mL of D5W, D10W, NS, R, or LR. 1-mL (3-mg) ampules may be given undiluted (contain benzyl alcohol).

Storage: If prepared without a preservative, use immediately; stable up to 7 days with a preservative.

COMPATIBILITY (Underline Indicates Conflicting Compatibility Information)
Consider any drug NOT listed as compatible to be INCOMPATIBLE until consulting a pharmacist; specific conditions may apply.
Several sources, including the manufacturer, cite **incompatibility** with fluorouracil (5-FU) as an additive; may form a precipitate.
One source suggests the following **compatibilities:**
Additive: Cisplatin (Platinol).
Y-site: Amifostine (Ethyol), <u>anidulafungin (Eraxis)</u>, aztreonam (Azactam), bleomycin (Blenoxane), cefepime (Maxipime), cisplatin (Platinol), cladribine (Leustatin), cyclophosphamide (Cytoxan), docetaxel (Taxotere), doxorubicin (Adriamycin), doxorubicin liposomal (Doxil), etoposide phosphate (Etopophos), filgrastim (Neupogen), fluconazole (Diflucan), <u>fluorouracil (5-FU)</u>, furosemide (Lasix), gemcitabine (Gemzar), granisetron (Kytril), heparin, linezolid (Zyvox), methotrexate, metoclopramide (Reglan), mitomycin (Mutamycin), oxaliplatin (Eloxatin), pemetrexed (Alimta), piperacillin/tazobactam (Zosyn), tacrolimus (Prograf), teniposide (Vumon), thiotepa, vinblastine, vincristine.

RATE OF ADMINISTRATION
Because of calcium content, do not exceed a rate of 160 mg/min (16 mL of a 10-mg/mL or 8 mL of a 20-mg/mL solution). May be given more slowly. Large doses may be infused equally distributed over 1 to 6 hours. Never exceed above limits.

ACTIONS
Potent agent for neutralizing immediate toxic effects of methotrexate (and other folic acid antagonists) on the hematopoietic system. Preferentially rescues normal cells without reversing the oncolytic effect of methotrexate. Also enhances the therapeutic and toxic effects of fluoropyrimidines (e.g., fluorouracil [5-FU]).

INDICATIONS AND USES
Treatment of accidental folic acid antagonist (e.g., methotrexate) overdose or delayed excretion of MTX. ▪ Folinic acid rescue to prevent or decrease the toxicity of massive MTX doses used to treat resistant neoplasms. ▪ Treatment of megaloblastic anemia due to folic acid deficiency when oral therapy not appropriate. ▪ In combination with fluorouracil or fluorouracil and irinotecan (Camptosar) to treat colorectal cancer.
Unlabeled uses: Adjunct in the treatment of Ewing's sarcoma, head and neck cancer, non-Hodgkin's lymphomas, and trophoblastic tumors. ▪ Treatment of pemetrexed toxicity.

CONTRAINDICATIONS
Pernicious anemia and other megaloblastic anemias secondary to lack of vitamin B_{12}. None when used as indicated for other specific uses.

PRECAUTIONS
Usually administered in the hospital by or under the direction of the physician specialist. ▪ Permits use of massive doses of methotrexate. ▪ Do not discontinue leucovorin calcium until methotrexate serum levels fall below toxic levels. ▪ Much less effective in accidental overdose after a 1-hour delay. ▪ Delayed MTX excretion may occur from third-space fluid accumulation (ascites, pleural effusion), renal insufficiency, or inadequate hydration. ▪ All doses over 25 mg should be given IM or IV (no more than 25 mg can be absorbed orally). ▪ IM or IV dosing required in presence of

GI toxicity, nausea, or vomiting. ▪ Benzyl alcohol associated with gasping syndrome in premature infants.

Monitor: Monitor serum blood levels of MTX and SCr levels at least daily until level is less than 0.05 micromolar. Death can occur in 5 to 10 days if MTX remains at toxic levels longer than 48 hours. ▪ Minimum fluid intake of 3 L/24 hr and alkalinization of urine to a pH of 7 or more with oral sodium bicarbonate recommended. Begin 12 hours before MTX dose and continue for 48 hours after final dose in each sequence. Does not reduce nephrotoxicity of MTX from drug or metabolite precipitation in the kidney. ▪ See methotrexate or fluorouracil monograph.

Maternal/Child: Category C: safety for use in pregnancy and breast-feeding not established. Benefits must outweigh risks. ▪ Contains benzyl alcohol; do not use in neonates or dilute with SW if indicated; see Dilution.

Elderly: Response similar to that seen in younger patients; however, use caution, may have greater sensitivity to its toxic effects (e.g., greater risk for GI toxicity and severe diarrhea in combination with fluorouracil). Monitoring of renal function suggested. ▪ See Dose Adjustments.

DRUG/LAB INTERACTIONS

May inhibit **phenytoins** (e.g., Dilantin), **phenobarbital, and primidone;** may cause increased frequency of seizures. ▪ Is used in combination with **fluorouracil;** use caution; leucovorin calcium may increase toxic as well as therapeutic effects of fluorouracil. ▪ When given with **MTX,** avoid any drug that may interfere with MTX elimination or binding to serum albumin (e.g., **NSAIDs** [e.g., ibuprofen (Advil, Motrin), indomethacin, ketoprofen, naproxen (Aleve, Naprosyn)], **probenecid, procarbazine** [Matulane], **salicylates, sulfonamides**). Consider as a possible cause of toxicity. ▪ High doses of leucovorin may reduce the effectiveness of intrathecally administered **methotrexate.** ▪ Leucovorin may enhance the toxic effects of **capecitabine** (Xeloda); monitor closely. ▪ Concurrent use with **sulfamethoxazole and trimethoprim** may cause treatment failure and increased morbidity in HIV patients being treated for *Pneumocystis jiroveci* pneumonia.

SIDE EFFECTS

Allergic reactions including anaphylaxis have occurred rarely. Methotrexate or fluorouracil may cause many serious and dose-limiting side effects; see individual monographs.

ANTIDOTE

Keep physician informed of patient's condition. Symptomatic treatment indicated.

LEVETIRACETAM INJECTION

(lee-ve-tye-**RA**-se-tam in-**JEK**-shun)

Anticonvulsant

Keppra

pH 5.5

USUAL DOSE

Serum levels similar by oral or IV route; no dose or frequency adjustment is necessary. Transfer to oral therapy as soon as practical.

Transfer to an IV dose from an oral dose: The IV dose should be equivalent to the total daily dose and frequency of the oral dose prescribed for the individual patient (e.g., 500, 1,000, or 1,500 mg every 12 hours to achieve a total daily dose of 1,000, 2,000, or 3,000 mg).

Initiate treatment: Begin with a daily dose of 1,000 mg/day equally divided into 2 doses (500 mg every 12 hours). Monitor for 2 weeks. If needed, dose may be increased by a 1,000 mg/day increment (total dose of 2,000 mg/day equally divided into 2 doses [1,000 mg every 12 hours]). Monitor for another 2 weeks. If needed, increase dose by another 1,000 mg/day increment (total dose of 3,000 mg/day equally divided into 2 doses [1,500 mg every 12 hours]).

Patients with partial-onset seizures: There is no evidence that doses ***greater*** than 3,000 mg/day offer additional benefit.

Patients with primary generalized tonic-clonic seizures or those with myoclonic seizures in juvenile myoclonic epilepsy: The effectiveness of doses ***lower*** than 3,000 mg/day has not been adequately studied.

DOSE ADJUSTMENTS

No dose adjustment is required for gender, race, or impaired hepatic function. ■ Dose adjustment may be required in the elderly based on impaired renal function. ■ Dose adjustment in impaired renal function is calculated based on CrCl and is adjusted according to the following chart.

Levetiracetam Dose Adjustment in Adults with Impaired Renal Function		
Creatinine Clearance	Dose in mg	Frequency
>80 mL/min	500 to 1,500 mg	Every 12 hours
50 to 80 mL/min	500 to 1,000 mg	Every 12 hours
30 to 49 mL/min	250 to 750 mg	Every 12 hours
<30 mL/min	250 to 500 mg	Every 12 hours
ESRD patients on dialysis	500 to 1,000 mg	Every 24 hours*

*Administration of a 250- to 500-mg supplemental dose following dialysis is recommended.

DILUTION

A single dose (500, 1,000, or 1,500 mg [1, 2, or 3 vials]) must be diluted in 100 mL of NS, LR, or D5W for infusion.

Filters: Specific information not available.

Storage: Store at CRT. Diluted solution stable for at least 24 hours at CRT stored in polyvinyl chloride (PVC) bags. Discard any unused portion of vial.

COMPATIBILITY

Consider any drug NOT listed as compatible to be INCOMPATIBLE until consulting a pharmacist; specific conditions may apply.

Manufacturer lists solutions NS, LR, and D5W and other antiepileptic drugs lorazepam (Ativan), diazepam (Valium), and valproate sodium (Depacon) as **compatible** for at least 24 hours stored in polyvinyl chloride (PVC) bags at CRT.

RATE OF ADMINISTRATION

A single dose (500, 1,000, or 1,500 mg) properly diluted as an infusion over 15 minutes.

ACTIONS

An antiepileptic (anticonvulsant) drug. The precise mechanism of action is unknown. In animal studies it inhibited burst firing without affecting normal neuronal excitability, which suggests that it may selectively prevent hypersynchronization of epileptiform burst firing and propagation of seizure activity in human complex partial seizures. Less than 10% bound to plasma proteins. Not extensively metabolized in humans and not liver (cytochrome P_{450}) dependent. Half-life is 6 to 8 hours. Undergoes enzymatic hydrolysis. Primarily excreted in urine as unchanged drug and metabolites. Crossed the placental barrier in animal studies. Secreted in breast milk.

INDICATIONS AND USES

IV injection is used as a temporary alternative to oral therapy in adult patients (16 years and older). ▪ Adjunctive therapy in the treatment of the following seizure types: partial-onset seizures in adults with epilepsy, myoclonic seizures in adults with juvenile myoclonic epilepsy (JME), and primary generalized tonic-clonic seizures in adults with idiopathic generalized epilepsy.

CONTRAINDICATIONS

Known hypersensitivity to levetiracetam or its active ingredients (sodium chloride, glacial acetic acid, sodium acetate trihydrate).

PRECAUTIONS

For IV use only. ▪ Associated with CNS side effects (somnolence and fatigue, coordination difficulties [abnormal gait, ataxia, incoordination], and behavioral abnormalities [depression, hallucinations, psychotic symptoms, including psychosis and suicidal tendencies]). Somnolence and fatigue and coordination difficulties occurred most frequently within the first 4 weeks of treatment and resolved or improved with dose reduction or discontinuation of levetiracetam. ▪ Psychotic symptoms and other behavioral changes have been reported and may include aggression, agitation, anger, anxiety, apathy, depersonalization, depression, emotional lability, hallucinations, hostility, irritability, and suicidal tendencies. Some resolved without intervention. Others required dose reduction or discontinuation of levetiracetam. ▪ To minimize the potential of increased seizure frequency, withdraw antiepileptic drugs (including levetiracetam) gradually.

Monitor: Baseline CBC and CrCl indicated; monitor as needed. ▪ Monitor for seizure activity. ▪ Observe patient closely for signs of CNS side effects; see Precautions. ▪ Monitor vital signs.

Patient Education: May cause dizziness and somnolence; use caution performing tasks that require alertness (e.g., operating machinery, driving). ▪ Inform your health care professional if you are pregnant or breast-feeding. ▪ May cause alterations in mood (e.g., aggression, agitation, anger, anxi-

ety, apathy, decreased ability to cope, depression, hostility, irritability, thoughts of suicide); report these changes promptly. ■ Women who are pregnant or who become pregnant should be encouraged to enroll in the North American Antiepileptic Drug (NAAED) Pregnancy Registry.
Maternal/Child: Category C: animal studies demonstrated fetal skeletal abnormalities and delayed offspring growth. Use during pregnancy only if potential benefit justifies the potential risk to the fetus. Manufacturer has established a pregnancy registry to evaluate safety and outcomes; see manufacturer's literature and Patient Education. ■ Physiologic changes during pregnancy may decrease levetiracetam concentration. ■ Effects during labor and delivery unknown. ■ Discontinue breast-feeding. ■ Safety and effectiveness for use in pediatric patients younger than 16 years of age not established.
Elderly: Safety similar to that seen in younger adults; however, total body clearance is decreased and half-life is increased. ■ Reduced doses may be indicated; see Dose Adjustments. Monitoring of renal function suggested.
DRUG/LAB INTERACTIONS
Manufacturer states that levetiracetam "is unlikely to produce, or be subject to, pharmacokinetic interactions." ■ Other antiepileptic drugs (AEDs) such as carbamazepine (Tegretol), gabapentin (Neurontin), lamotrigine (Lamictal), phenobarbital (Luminal), phenytoin (Dilantin), primidone (Mysoline), and valproate (Depacon) do not influence the pharmacokinetics of levetiracetam, and it does not influence their pharmacokinetics. ■ Not an inhibitor or a substrate of cytochrome P_{450} isoforms; unlikely to have interactions with drugs metabolized by these isoenzymes in the liver. ■ Minimal protein binding; unlikely to have interactions with drugs requiring protein-binding sites. ■ Has been administered with oral contraceptives, digoxin (Lanoxin), and warfarin (Coumadin) with no interference on the pharmacokinetics of either drug. ■ **Probenecid** (Benemid) decreases renal clearance and increases serum concentrations of one of the metabolites of levetiracetam.
SIDE EFFECTS
Asthenia, dizziness, infection, and somnolence occurred most frequently during the first 4 weeks of treatment. Other side effects presented anywhere from 1 to 4 weeks and include amnesia; anger; anorexia; anxiety; apathy; ataxia; cough; decreased RBC, WBC, Hct, and Hgb; depersonalization; depression; diplopia; emotional lability; headache; hostility; hypersomnia; influenza; insomnia; irritability; neck pain; nervousness; pain; paresthesia; pharyngitis; rhinitis; seizures; sinusitis; and vertigo.
Post-Marketing: Abnormal liver function tests, alopecia, hepatic failure, hepatitis, leukopenia, neutropenia, pancreatitis, pancytopenia (with bone marrow suppression), suicidal behavior, thrombocytopenia, and weight loss.
Overdose: Aggression, agitation, coma, depressed level of consciousness, respiratory depression, and somnolence.
ANTIDOTE
Keep physician informed of all side effects. Some may not require intervention, and others may improve with a reduced dose or discontinuation of levetiracetam; see Precautions and Side Effects. Support patient as required in treatment of overdose. No specific antidote in overdose; however, hemodialysis will remove approximately 50% of a dose in 4 hours.

LEVOFLOXACIN BBW

(**lee**-voh-**FLOX**-ah-sin)

Antibacterial
(fluoroquinolone)

Levaquin

pH 3.8 to 5.8

USUAL DOSE

250 to 750 mg once every 24 hours. Dose and duration of treatment are based on degree of infection and specific diagnosis. CrCl equal to or greater than 50 mL/min is required. Dose and serum levels similar by oral or IV route. Transfer to oral dose as soon as practical.

Levofloxacin Dosing Guidelines		
Type of Infection[a]	Dose Every 24 Hours	Duration (Days)
Acute Bacterial Exacerbation of Chronic Bronchitis	500 mg	7 days
Nosocomial Pneumonia	750 mg	7-14 days
Comm. Acquired Pneumonia	500 mg or 750 mg	7-14 days 5 days
Acute Bacterial Sinusitis	500 mg or 750 mg	10-14 days 5 days
Chronic Bacterial Prostatitis	500 mg	28 days
Complicated SSSI[b]	750 mg	7-14 days
Uncomplicated SSSI[b]	500 mg	7-10 days
Complicated UTI[c] or Acute Pyelonephritis	750 mg	5 days
Complicated UTI[c] or Acute Pyelonephritis	250 mg	10 days
Uncomplicated UTI[c]	250 mg	3 days
Inhalation Anthrax (post-exposure) in adults[d]	500 mg	60 days
Inhalation Anthrax (post-exposure) in pediatric patients >50 kg and ≥6 months of age[d]	500 mg	60 days[e]
Inhalation Anthrax (post-exposure) in pediatric patients <50 kg and ≥6 months of age[d]	8 mg/kg q 12 hr (not to exceed 250 mg/dose)	60 days[e]

[a]DUE TO THE DESIGNATED PATHOGENS (See Indications and Usage.)
[b]Skin and Skin Structure Infections.
[c]Urinary Tract Infections.
[d]Begin drug administration as soon as possible after suspected or confirmed exposure to aerosolized *Bacillus anthracis*.
[e]See Precautions and Maternal/Child.

Continued

DOSE ADJUSTMENTS

Clearance is reduced and half-life is prolonged in patients with a CrCl equal to or less than 80 mL/min. See the following chart for dosing guidelines. See Important IV Therapy Facts on p. xxvii for formula to convert SCr to CrCl. ▪ Supplemental doses are not required after hemodialysis or peritoneal dialysis. ▪ No dose adjustment is required specifically for age, gender, race, or in impaired hepatic function.

Levofloxacin Dosing Guidelines in Impaired Renal Function			
Dosage in Normal Renal Function Every 24 hours	Creatinine Clearance 20 to 49 mL/min	Creatinine Clearance 10 to 19 mL/min	Hemodialysis or Chronic Ambulatory Peritoneal Dialysis (CAPD)
750 mg	750 mg q 48 hr	750 mg initial dose, then 500 mg q 48 hr	750 mg initial dose, then 500 mg q 48 hr
500 mg	500 mg initial dose, then 250 mg q 24 hr	500 mg initial dose, then 250 mg q 48 hr	500 mg initial dose, then 250 mg q 48 hr
250 mg	No dose adjustment required	250 mg q 48 hr; no dose adjustment required if treating uncomplicated UTI	No information on dose adjustment available

DILUTION

Available in single-use vials and as prediluted, ready-to-use infusions.

Single-use vials: Withdraw desired dose from single-use vial (10 mL for 250 mg, 20 mL for 500 mg, 30 mL for 750 mg). Each 10 mL (250 mg) must be further diluted with a minimum of 40 mL NS, D5W, D5NS, D5LR, D5/plasma-Lyte 56, D5/½NS with 0.15% KCl, or ⅙ M sodium lactate. Desired concentration is 5 mg/mL. No preservatives; enter vial only once. When 500-mg (20-mL) vial is used to prepare two 250-mg doses, withdraw entire contents of vial at once into separate syringes, prepare and store second dose for subsequent use.

Premix flexible containers: No further dilution necessary. Available as 250 mg in 50 mL, 500 mg in 100 mL, or 750 mg in 150 mL D5W. Instructions for access to and use of premix flexible containers are on its storage carton. Do not use flexible containers in series connections.

Filters: Not required; however, contents of both vials and premixed solutions were filtered during manufacturing with polyvinyl mixed ester cellulose filters. Size not specified by manufacturer. No significant loss of potency expected.

Storage: Store vials at CRT; protect from light. Store premix at or below 25° C (77° F); protect from freezing, light, and excessive heat. Both are stable to expiration date. Solutions diluted from vials are stable at CRT for 3 days, up to 14 days if refrigerated. May be frozen for up to 6 months. Do not force thaw (e.g., microwave or water bath) and do not refreeze. Discard any unused portion of premixed solutions and/or opened vials. Premixed flexible containers must be used within 6 days (250 mg) or 7 days (500 and 750 mg) after foil over-wrap is removed.

COMPATIBILITY (Underline Indicates Conflicting Compatibility Information)
Consider any drug NOT listed as compatible to be INCOMPATIBLE until consulting a pharmacist; specific conditions may apply.
Manufacturer states, "Limited compatibility information available; other intravenous substances, additives, or other medications should not be added to levofloxacin or infused simultaneously through the same intravenous line." Never administer in the same IV or through the same tubing with any solution containing multivalent cations (e.g., calcium, magnesium). Flush line with a **compatible** solution before and after administration of levofloxacin and/or any other drug through the same IV line.

One source suggests the following **compatibilities:**
Y-site: Amikacin (Amikin), aminophylline, ampicillin, anidulafungin (Eraxis), bivalirudin (Angiomax), caffeine citrate (Cafcit), caspofungin (Cancidas), cefotaxime (Claforan), clindamycin (Cleocin), daptomycin (Cubicin), dexamethasone (Decadron), dexmedetomidine (Precedex), dobutamine, dopamine, doripenem (Doribax), epinephrine (Adrenalin), fenoldopam (Corlopam), fentanyl (Sublimaze), gentamicin, hetastarch in electrolytes (Hextend), insulin (regular), isoproterenol (Isuprel), lidocaine, linezolid (Zyvox), lorazepam (Ativan), metoclopramide (Reglan), morphine, oxacillin (Bactocill), pancuronium, penicillin G sodium, phenobarbital (Luminal), phenylephrine (Neo-Synephrine), sodium bicarbonate, vancomycin.

RATE OF ADMINISTRATION
Each 250- or 500-mg dose must be equally distributed over 60 minutes as an infusion. A 750-mg dose must be equally distributed over 90 minutes as an infusion. Too-rapid administration may cause hypotension. May be given through a Y-tube or three-way stopcock of infusion set. Temporarily discontinue other solutions infusing at the same site and flush tubing with **compatible** solutions before and after levofloxacin.

ACTIONS
A synthetic, broad-spectrum, fluoroquinolone antibacterial agent. Bactericidal to a wide range of aerobic gram-negative and gram-positive organisms, as well as some anaerobic organisms through interference with an enzyme (topoisomerase II) needed for synthesis of bacterial DNA. May be active against bacteria resistant to aminoglycosides, beta-lactam antibiotics, and macrolides. Onset of action is prompt, and serum levels are dose related. Mean terminal half-life is 6 to 8 hours. Steady state is achieved within 48 hours. Widely distributed into body tissues, including blister fluid and lung tissues. Moderately bound to serum protein (24% to 38%). Metabolism is minimal; primarily excreted as unchanged drug in urine. Very small amounts found in bile and feces. May cross placental barrier. May be secreted in breast milk.

INDICATIONS AND USES
Treatment of adults with mild, moderate, and severe infections caused by susceptible strains of microorganisms in conditions including acute bacterial sinusitis, acute bacterial exacerbation of chronic bronchitis, and nosocomial pneumonia. ■ Treatment of community-acquired pneumonia due to many organisms, including *Streptococcus pneumoniae* (including multidrug-resistant strains (MDRSP). MDRSP strains are resistant to two or more of the following antibiotics: penicillin, second-generation cephalosporins (e.g., cefuroxime [Zinacef]), macrolides, tetracyclines, and sulfamethoxazole/trimethoprim. ■ Treatment of complicated skin and skin

structure infections, mild to moderate uncomplicated skin and skin structure infections, complicated and uncomplicated urinary tract infections, and acute pyelonephritis. ▪ To reduce the incidence and progression of inhalational anthrax following exposure to *Bacillus anthracis.* Begin administration as soon as possible after suspected or confirmed exposure. Transfer to oral therapy when practical. ▪ Treatment of chronic bacterial prostatitis (usually oral therapy).

CONTRAINDICATIONS

History of hypersensitivity to levofloxacin, its components, or any other quinolone antimicrobial agents (e.g., ciprofloxacin [Cipro], norfloxacin [Noroxin]).

PRECAUTIONS

For IV use only. ▪ Culture and sensitivity studies indicated to determine susceptibility of the causative organism to levofloxacin. ▪ *Pseudomonas aeruginosa* may develop resistance during treatment. Ongoing culture and sensitivity studies indicated. ▪ The emergence of bacterial resistance to fluoroquinolones and the occurrence of cross-resistance with other fluoroquinolones have been observed and are of concern. Proper use of fluoroquinolones and other classes of antibiotics is encouraged to avoid the emergence of resistant bacteria from overuse. ▪ Prolonged use may cause superinfection because of overgrowth of nonsusceptible organisms. ▪ Use with caution in patients with known CNS disorders that predispose to seizures or alter seizure threshold (e.g., epilepsy, severe cerebral arteriosclerosis, concomitant drug therapy). Convulsions, toxic psychosis, increased intracranial pressure, and CNS stimulation have been reported. ▪ Use caution in patients with impaired renal function; see Dose Adjustments. ▪ May be used by patients who are allergic to penicillin or intolerant of macrolides (e.g., erythromycin). ▪ Cross-resistance may occur with other fluoroquinolones, but some microorganisms resistant to other fluoroquinolones may be susceptible to levofloxacin. ▪ Severe, sometimes fatal hepatotoxicity has been reported. Symptoms appeared within 6 to 14 days of initiating therapy, and most cases were not associated with hypersensitivity and occurred in patients 65 years of age or older; see Patient Education and Antidote. ▪ Tendinitis and tendon rupture that required surgical repair or resulted in prolonged disability have been reported in patients of all ages receiving quinolones. Most frequently involves the Achilles tendon but has also been reported with the shoulder, hand, biceps, thumb, and other tendon sites. ▪ Tendon rupture or tendinitis may occur during or after fluoroquinolone therapy. Risk may be increased in patients over 60 years of age; in patients taking corticosteroids; in patients with heart, kidney, or lung transplants; with strenuous physical activity; and in patients with renal failure or previous tendon disorders such as rheumatoid arthritis. ▪ Prolongation of the QT interval on ECG and infrequent cases of arrhythmia (including torsades de pointes) have been reported. The risk of arrhythmia may be reduced by avoiding use of levofloxacin in the presence of hypokalemia, significant bradycardia, cardiomyopathy, or concurrent treatment with class IA antiarrhythmic agents (e.g., quinidine [Quinidex], procainamide [Procanbid, Procan SR]) or Class III antiarrhythmic agents (e.g., amiodarone [Nexterone], sotalol [Betapace]) and any other drug that can prolong the QT interval; avoid coadministration; see Drug/Lab Interactions. ▪ Fluoroquinolones have neuromuscular blocking activity. Serious adverse events, including ventilatory support and deaths, have been reported in patients with myasthenia gravis. Avoid use in patients with a known history of myasthenia gravis; may exacerbate muscle weakness. ▪ Rare cases of peripheral neuropathy (e.g., paresthesias, hypoesthesias, dysesthesias [impairment of sensitivity or touch], or weakness) have been reported. ▪ *Clostridium difficile*–associated diarrhea (CDAD) has been reported. May range from mild diarrhea to fatal colitis. Consider in patients who present with diarrhea during or after treatment with levofloxacin. ▪ Other serious events (sometimes fatal) due to hypersensitivity or uncertain etiology have been reported with fluoroquinolones; see Side Effects, Post-Marketing. Discontinue levofloxacin at the first appearance of a skin rash, jaundice, or other signs of hepatotoxicity or hypersensitivity. ▪ Moderate to severe photosensitivity/phototoxicity reactions have been reported in patients receiving quinolones; see Patient Education. ▪ Not tested in humans for post-exposure prevention of inhalation anthrax; however, plasma concentrations are considered to be in a range to produce effective results. ▪ Safety for use in adults beyond 28 days or in pediatric patients beyond 14 days not studied; use only for prescribed indication; benefits must outweigh risks. An increased incidence of musculoskeletal adverse events has been observed in pediatric patients.

Monitor: Hypersensitivity reactions, including anaphylaxis with the first or succeeding doses, has been reported in patients receiving quinolones, even in those without known hypersensitivity. Emergency equipment must always be available; see Precautions. ▪ Obtain baseline CBC with differential, CrCl, and blood glucose. Periodic monitoring of organ systems, including hematopoietic, hepatic, and renal, is recommended. ▪ Monitor for S/S of peripheral neuropathy. Discontinue levofloxacin at the first symptoms of neuropathy (e.g., pain, burning, tingling, numbness and/or weakness) or if patient is found to have deficits in light touch, pain, temperature, position sense, vibratory sensation, and/or motor strength. ▪ Maintain adequate hydration to prevent concentrated urine throughout treatment. Other quinolones have formed crystals. ▪ Monitor infusion site for inflammation and/or extravasation. ▪ Symptomatic hyperglycemia or hypoglycemia may occur, usually in diabetic patients receiving oral hypoglycemic agents (e.g., glyburide) or insulin. Monitor blood glucose closely. ▪ See Precautions, Drug/Lab Interactions, and Antidote.

Patient Education: A patient medication guide is available from the manufacturer. ▪ Review all medicines and disease history with pharmacist or physician before initiating treatment. ▪ Inform physician of any history of myasthenia gravis. ▪ Patients with a history of myasthenia gravis should promptly report breathing problems or worsening muscle weakness. ▪ Drink fluids liberally. ▪ Promptly report skin rash or any other hypersensitivity reaction. ▪ Promptly report pain, burning, tingling, numbness and/or weakness. ▪ Photosensitivity has occurred in a minimal number of patients, but it is best to avoid excessive sunlight or artificial ultraviolet light. May cause severe sunburn; wear protective clothing, use sunscreen, and wear dark glasses outdoors. Report a sunburn-like reaction or skin eruption promptly. ▪ Dizziness or light-headedness may interfere with ambulation and motor coordination. Use caution in tasks that require alertness. ▪ Effects of caffeine, theophylline preparations, and/or warfarin

(Coumadin) may be increased; notify your physician if you take any of these agents. If diabetic and on medication, monitor your blood glucose carefully. If a hypoglycemia reaction occurs, discontinue levofloxacin and consult physician. ▪ Promptly report S/S of liver injury (e.g., dark-colored urine, fever, itching, jaundice [yellowing of skin or whites of eyes], light-colored bowel movements, loss of appetite, nausea, right upper quadrant tenderness, tiredness, vomiting, weakness). ▪ Promptly report tendon pain or inflammation; rest and refrain from exercise. ▪ Promptly report diarrhea or bloody stools that occur during treatment or up to several months after an antibiotic has been discontinued; may indicate CDAD and require treatment. ▪ See Precautions, Monitor, Drug/Lab Interactions, and Antidote.

Maternal/Child: Category C: safety for use in pregnancy not established; benefits must outweigh risks. ▪ Discontinue breast-feeding. ▪ Safety for use in pediatric patients under 18 years of age not established. Indicated in pediatric patients 6 months of age or older only for prevention of inhalation anthrax (post-exposure). An increased incidence of musculoskeletal disorders (arthralgia, arthritis, tendinopathy, and gait abnormality) compared with controls has been observed in pediatric patients receiving levofloxacin.

Elderly: Half-life may be slightly extended due to age-related renal impairment. Dose reduction required only in the elderly with a CrCl of 50 mL/min or less. ▪ Safety and effectiveness similar to that in younger adults; however, they may experience an increased risk of side effects (e.g., CNS effects, hepatotoxicity, tendinitis, tendon rupture, risk of QT prolongation). Monitoring of renal function may be useful. ▪ See Dose Adjustments and Precautions.

DRUG/LAB INTERACTIONS

May cause ventricular arrhythmias or torsades de pointes with **drugs that prolong the QT interval,** such as class IA antiarrhythmic agents (e.g., quinidine [Quinidex], procainamide [Procanbid, Procan SR]), class III antiarrhythmic agents (e.g., amiodarone [Nexterone], sotalol [Betapace]), anticonvulsants (e.g., fosphenytoin [Cerebyx]), antihistamines (e.g., diphenhydramine [Benedryl]), astemizole (has been removed from market), antineoplastics (e.g., doxorubicin [Adriamycin]), phenothiazines (e.g., chlorpromazine [Thorazine]), serotonin reuptake inhibitors (e.g., fluoxetine [Prozac], paroxetine [Paxil]), tricyclic antidepressants (e.g., imipramine [Tofranil], amitryptyline [Elavil]). Avoid coadministration. ▪ Risk of CNS stimulation and convulsive seizures may be increased with **NSAIDs** (e.g., ibuprofen [Advil, Motrin], naproxen [Aleve, Naprosyn]). ▪ May cause hyperglycemia and hypoglycemia with concurrent administration of **antidiabetic agents** (e.g., metformin [Glucophage], insulin); monitoring of blood glucose recommended. ▪ Concomitant administration with **cimetidine or probenecid** reduces levofloxacin renal clearance by 24% and 35% respectively, but dose adjustment is not required. ▪ Interactions with **theophylline** that occur with other quinolones have not been noted, but monitoring of theophylline levels is recommended with concomitant use. ▪ May enhance effects of **warfarin** (Coumadin); monitoring of PT or INR is recommended with concomitant use. ▪ No dose adjustment required for either drug when levofloxacin is administered concomitantly with **cyclosporine or digoxin.** ▪ See Precautions. ▪ May cause **false-positive when testing urine for opiates;** more specific testing methods may be indicated.

SIDE EFFECTS

Abdominal pain, anorexia, anxiety, cerebrovascular disorders, constipation, decreased glucose, decreased lymphocytes, diarrhea, dizziness, dry mouth, dyspepsia, dysphonia, ear disorders, edema, fatigue, flatulence, genital moniliasis, headache, increased INR/PT, infection, injection site reaction, insomnia, leukorrhea, malaise, nausea, photosensitivity/phototoxicity (sun sensitivity), pruritus, rash, sweating, taste disturbances, tremor, urticaria, vaginitis, vomiting. Capable of numerous other reactions in fewer than 1% of patients.

Major: Allergic pneumonitis; cardiovascular effects (e.g., cardiac arrest, palpitations, QT interval prolongation, tachycardia, torsades de pointes, vasodilation, ventricular tachyarrhythmias); CDAD; CNS stimulation (e.g., anxiety, confusion, depression, encephalopathy, hallucinations, nightmares, paranoia and, rarely, suicidal thoughts or acts); convulsions, increased intracranial pressure, and toxic psychoses; eosinophilia; fever, rash, and severe dermatologic reactions (e.g., toxic epidermal necrolysis, Stevens-Johnson syndrome); hemolytic anemia; hypersensitivity reactions (e.g., anaphylaxis, cardiovascular collapse, death, dyspnea, edema [facial, laryngeal, or pharyngeal]); hypoglycemic reactions; multisystem organ failure; pain, inflammation, and ruptures of the shoulder, hand, and Achilles tendons; peripheral neuropathy (e.g., pain, burning, tingling, numbness and/or weakness [see Precautions, Monitor]); and rhabdomyolysis have all been reported in patients receiving quinolones.

Post-Marketing: Allergic pneumonitis; arthralgia; hematologic abnormalities (agranulocytosis, anemia [hemolytic and aplastic], leukopenia, pancytopenia, thrombocytopenia, thrombotic thrombocytopenic purpura); interstitial nephritis; hepatotoxicity (sometimes fatal), including acute hepatic necrosis or failure, acute hepatitis, jaundice; myalgia; rash; serum sickness; severe dermatologic reactions (e.g., toxic epidermal necrolysis [Lyell's syndrome], Stevens-Johnson syndrome); vasculitis.

ANTIDOTE

Keep physician informed of all side effects. Most minor side effects will be treated symptomatically; monitor closely. Discontinue levofloxacin at the first sign of any major side effect (CDAD, CNS symptoms, dermatologic reactions, hepatotoxicity, hypersensitivity, hypoglycemic reactions, phototoxicity, or tendon rupture). Treat hypersensitivity reactions as indicated with epinephrine, airway management, oxygen, IV fluids, antihistamines (e.g., diphenhydramine [Benadryl]), corticosteroids (e.g., Solu-Cortef), and pressor amines (e.g., dopamine). Treat CNS symptoms as indicated; may require diazepam (Valium) for seizures. Mild cases of CDAD may respond to discontinuation of levofloxacin. Treat CDAD with fluids, electrolytes, protein supplements, and oral vancomycin (Vancocin) or metronidazole (Flagyl) as indicated. In severe cases, surgical evaluation may be indicated. Complete rest is indicated for an affected tendon until treatment is available. Maintain hydration in overdose. No specific antidote; not removed by hemodialysis or peritoneal dialysis. Maintain patient until drug is excreted and symptoms subside.

LEVOLEUCOVORIN
(lee-voh-loo-koh-**VOR**-in)
Fusilev

USUAL DOSE

Dosed at one-half the usual dose of the racemic form (leucovorin calcium). **Levoleucovorin rescue after high-dose methotrexate therapy:** Dose is based on a methotrexate dose of 12 Gm/M^2 infused over 4 hours; see methotrexate monograph. Obtain serum creatinine and methotrexate levels at least once daily. Additional hydration and urinary alkalinization (pH 7 or greater) is indicated and should be continued until the methotrexate level is less than 0.05 micromolar. Administer and/or adjust the levoleucovorin dose or extend rescue based on the following guidelines. See Dose Adjustments, Precautions, and Monitor.

Guidelines for Levoleucovorin Administration, Adjustment, or Extension of Rescue		
Clinical Situation	Laboratory Findings	Levoleucovorin Dose and Duration
Normal methotrexate elimination	Serum methotrexate level approximately 10 micromolar at 24 hours, 1 micromolar at 48 hours, and less than 0.2 micromolar at 72 hours after methotrexate administration.	7.5 mg IV every 6 hours for 60 hours (10 doses starting at 24 hours after start of methotrexate infusion).
Delayed late methotrexate elimination	Serum methotrexate level remains above 0.2 micromolar at 72 hours and more than 0.05 micromolar at 96 hours after methotrexate administration.	Continue 7.5 mg IV every 6 hours until methotrexate level is less than 0.05 micromolar.
Delayed early methotrexate elimination and/or evidence of acute renal injury	Serum methotrexate level of 50 micromolar or more at 24 hours or 5 micromolar or more at 48 hours after methotrexate administration. **OR** 100% or greater increase in serum creatinine level at 24 hours after methotrexate administration (e.g., an increase from 0.5 mg/dL to a level of 1 mg/dL or more).	75 mg IV every 3 hours until methotrexate level is less than 1 micromolar; then 7.5 mg IV every 3 hours until methotrexate level is less than 0.05 micromolar.

Inadvertent methotrexate overdose: 7.5 mg IV every 6 hours (approximately 5 mg/M^2) until the serum methotrexate level is less than 5×10^{-8} M (0.05 micromolar). Begin levoleucovorin rescue as soon as possible after an inadvertent methotrexate overdose and within 24 hours of methotrexate administration when there is delayed excretion. The effectiveness of levoleucovorin in counteracting toxicity may decrease as the time interval between methotrexate administration and levoleucovorin rescue increases. See Dose Adjustments and Monitor.

Colorectal cancer: Several regimens are in use. See fluorouracil (5-FU) monograph for 5-FU specific information. Administer 5-FU and levoleucovorin separately to avoid the formation of a precipitate. Consider flushing the IV line with NS between drugs.

Levoleucovorin 100 mg/M^2 by IV injection over a minimum of 3 minutes (see Rate of Administration) followed by *5-FU* 370 mg/M^2 by IV injection *or levoleucovorin* 10 mg/M^2 by IV injection followed by *5-FU* at 425 mg/M^2 by IV injection. Repeat either regimen daily for 5 days. This 5-day course is repeated at 4-week intervals for 2 courses and then at 4- to 5-week intervals provided that complete recovery from the toxic effects of the previous course has occurred. See Dose Adjustments.

PEDIATRIC DOSE
See Usual Dose.

DOSE ADJUSTMENTS

Levoleucovorin rescue after high-dose methotrexate therapy: Some patients may have significant but less severe abnormalities in methotrexate elimination or renal function following methotrexate administration than the abnormalities described in the preceding table. These abnormalities may or may not be associated with significant clinical toxicity. If significant clinical toxicity is observed, levoleucovorin rescue should be extended for an additional 24 hours (a total of 14 doses over 84 hours) in subsequent courses of therapy. If lab abnormalities or clinical toxicities are observed, consider the possibility that the patient is taking other medications that interact with methotrexate (e.g., medications that may interfere with methotrexate elimination or binding to serum albumin [see methotrexate monograph]). ■ Delayed methotrexate excretion may also be caused by accumulation in a third space fluid collection (i.e., ascites, pleural effusion), inadequate hydration, or renal insufficiency. Higher doses of levoleucovorin or prolonged administration may be indicated.

Inadvertent methotrexate overdose: If the 24-hour serum creatinine has increased 50% over baseline or if the 24-hour methotrexate level is greater than 5×10^{-6} M (5 micromolar) or the 48-hour level is greater than 9×10^{-7} M (0.9 micromolar), increase the dose of levoleucovorin to 50 mg/M^2 IV every 3 hours until the methotrexate level is less than 0.05 micromolar. Hydrate with a minimum of 3 liters/day and use sodium bicarbonate for urinary alkalinization (adjust to maintain a urine pH of 7 or greater).

Colorectal cancer: In subsequent courses, adjust the dose of 5-FU based on patient tolerance of the previous treatment course. Reduce 5-FU dose by 20% for patients who experienced moderate hematologic or GI toxicity in the previous course and 30% for patients who experienced severe toxicity. 5-FU dose may be increased by 10% if no toxicity was experienced in the previous course. Levoleucovorin doses are not adjusted for toxicity.

DILUTION

Levoleucovorin for injection: Reconstitute each 50-mg vial of lyophilized powder with 5.3 mL of preservative-free NS (concentration equals 10 mg/mL). Do not use other diluents. A single dose may be further diluted immediately in NS or D5W to a concentration of 0.5 mg/mL to 5 mg/mL. Do not use if solution is cloudy or a precipitate is observed.

Levoleucovorin injection: Available in ready-to-use single-use vials containing 175 mg (17.5 mL) or 250 mg (25 mL). Concentration equals

10 mg/mL. A single dose of these solutions may be further diluted to a concentration of 0.5 mg/mL in NS or D5W.

Filters: Specific information not available.

Storage: *Levoleucovorin for injection (reconstituted lyophilized powder):* Store unopened vials in carton at CRT. Protect from light. Solutions reconstituted or further diluted in NS are stable for not more than 12 hours at RT. Reconstituted solutions further diluted in D5W are stable for not more than 4 hours at RT. *Levoleucovorin injection (ready-to-use solution):* Refrigerate unopened vials in carton at 2° to 8° C (36° to 46° F). Protect from light. Solutions diluted to 0.5 mg/mL in NS or D5W are stable for not more than 4 hours at RT.

COMPATIBILITY

Manufacturer states, "Due to the risk of precipitation, do not coadminister levoleucovorin with other agents in the same admixture." Dilute only with preservative-free NS; do not use other diluents or NS with preservatives.

RATE OF ADMINISTRATION

Because of the calcium content of the solution, do not exceed a rate of injection of 16 mL/min of reconstituted solution (160 mg of levoleucovorin). When given in combination with 5-FU, consider flushing the IV line with NS between drugs.

ACTIONS

A folate analog. An active isomer of 5-formyl tetrahydrofolic acid, the pharmacologically active isomer of leucovorin calcium. A replacement for leucovorin calcium, which also contains the pharmacologically inactive dextro isomer. Does not require reduction by the enzyme dihydrofolate reductase. Actively and passively transported across cell membranes. Converted *in vivo* to the primary circulating form of active reduced folate. Levoleucovorin can counteract the therapeutic and toxic effects of folic acid antagonists such as methotrexate, which act by inhibiting dihydrofolate reductase. Terminal half-life is from 5.1 to 6.8 hours.

INDICATIONS AND USES

Levoleucovorin rescue is indicated after high-dose methotrexate therapy in patients with osteosarcoma. ■ Also indicated to diminish the toxicity and counteract the effects of impaired methotrexate elimination and of inadvertent overdose of folic acid antagonists (e.g., methotrexate, pemetrexed [Alimta]). ■ Indicated for use in combination chemotherapy with 5-fluorouracil (5-FU) in the palliative treatment of advanced metastatic colorectal cancer. ■ Not indicated for the treatment of pernicious anemia and megaloblastic anemias secondary to vitamin B_{12} deficiency; improper use may cause a hematologic remission while neurologic manifestations continue to progress.

CONTRAINDICATIONS

Contraindicated in patients who have had previous hypersensitivity reactions to folic acid or folinic acid.

PRECAUTIONS

For IV use only; do not administer by any other route. ■ Contains calcium; limit rate of administration to no more than 16 mL/min (160 mg of levoleucovorin per minute). ■ Toxicities during combination use with 5-fluorouracil (5-FU) are similar to those observed with 5-FU alone; however, GI toxicities (particularly stomatitis and diarrhea) are observed more commonly and may be more severe or of prolonged duration. ■ Concomitant use with sulfamethoxazole/trimethoprim for the acute treatment of *Pneumocystis jiroveci* pneumonia in patients with HIV infection may cause treatment failure and morbidity.

Monitor: *All situations with methotrexate:* Obtain baseline serum methotrexate, serum creatinine, electrolytes, and urine pH. Monitor at least daily. ▪ Adequate hydration and maintenance of a urinary pH of 7 or greater with sodium bicarbonate is indicated.

Levoleucovorin rescue after high-dose methotrexate therapy: Patients who experience delayed early methotrexate elimination are likely to develop reversible renal failure. Continuing hydration and urinary alkalinization and close monitoring of fluid and electrolyte status is required until the serum methotrexate level has fallen to below 0.05 micromolar and the renal failure has resolved.

Inadvertent methotrexate overdose: See Dose Adjustments; hydration with a minimum of 3 liters/day and the use of sodium bicarbonate for urinary alkalinization (adjust to maintain a urine pH of 7 or greater) may be indicated.

Combination with 5-FU: Monitor for S/S of GI toxicity. See the 5-fluorouracil monograph for hematologic monitoring requirements.

Maternal/Child: Category C: use during pregnancy only if clearly needed. ▪ Not known if levoleucovorin is excreted in human milk; has potential for harmful effects; discontinue breast-feeding.

Elderly: Studies of levoleucovorin in the treatment of osteosarcoma did not include adults age 65 or older. ▪ Dehydration, diarrhea, and severe enterocolitis have been reported in elderly patients receiving weekly levoleucovorin and 5-fluorouracil (5-FU).

DRUG/LAB INTERACTIONS

May ameliorate the hematologic toxicity associated with **high-dose methotrexate,** but levoleucovorin has no effect on other established toxicities of methotrexate, such as nephrotoxicity resulting from drug and/or metabolite precipitation in the kidney. ▪ Folic acid in large amounts may counteract the antiepileptic effects of **phenobarbital** (Luminal), **phenytoin** (Dilantin), **and primidone** (Mysoline). Seizure activity may be increased in susceptible patients. Levoleucovorin may or may not have the same effect due to shared metabolic pathways; use caution when administering concurrently with anticonvulsant drugs. ▪ Small amounts of systemically administered levoleucovorin may enter the cerebrospinal fluid (CSF). *Do not give levoleucovorin intrathecally;* see Precautions. ▪ Increases the toxicity of **5-fluorouracil** (5-FU); dehydration, diarrhea, and severe enterocolitis have been reported in elderly patients receiving weekly levoleucovorin and 5-fluorouracil. ▪ Concomitant use with **sulfamethoxazole/trimethoprim** for the acute treatment of *Pneumocystis jiroveci* pneumonia in patients with HIV infection may cause treatment failure and morbidity. ▪ High doses of levoleucovorin may reduce the effectiveness of intrathecally administered **methotrexate.** ▪ Levoleucovorin may enhance the toxic effects of **capecitabine** (Xeloda); monitor closely.

SIDE EFFECTS

Nausea and vomiting and stomatitis were reported most commonly. Abnormal renal function, confusion, dermatitis, diarrhea, dyspepsia, dyspnea, hypersensitivity reactions, leukopenia, neuropathy, thrombocytopenia, typhlitis (inflammation of the cecum), and taste perversion have been reported.

Combination therapy with 5-fluorouracil (5-FU): Abdominal pain, alopecia, anorexia, dermatitis, diarrhea, fatigue, nausea, stomatitis, vomiting. Hypersensitivity reactions have been reported.

Post-Marketing: Dyspnea, pruritus, rash, rigors, temperature change.

ANTIDOTE

Keep physician informed of patient's condition. Symptomatic treatment indicated.

LEVOTHYROXINE SODIUM [BBW]
(lee-voh-thigh-**ROX**-een **SO**-dee-um)

Hormone (thyroid)

T_4, L-Thyroxine

USUAL DOSE

When oral ingestion is not practical, IV dose should be ½ of any previously established oral dose. Adjust in small increments as indicated. Initiate oral treatment as soon as possible. 0.05 to 0.06 mg (50 to 60 mcg) equals approximately 60 mg (gr 1) thyroid hormone.

Hypothyroidism: Usual IV starting dose would be 6.25 to 12.5 mcg/day. Increase in increments of 12.5 mcg every 2 to 4 weeks. Base dosing on clinical response and serum thyroid and TSH levels. Average maintenance dose is 50 to 100 mcg/day PO.

Myxedema coma: 400 mcg as initial dose. Range is 200 to 500 mcg. 100 to 300 mcg may be repeated the next day unless considerable improvement has occurred, as indicated by patient response or serum protein-bound iodine levels. Maintenance dose ranges from 50 to 200 mcg. See Precautions. Liothyronine (Triostat) is the drug of choice for myxedema coma.

Thyroid suppression therapy: Usually given PO. 1.3 mcg/kg/day for 7 to 10 days; usually yields normal serum T_4 and T_3 levels and lack of response to TSH. Doses greater than 2 mcg/kg/day may be required.

PEDIATRIC DOSE

Given orally (may be crushed in food or liquid). See Precautions. Any IV dose should be 75% of oral dose. Size of *oral* dose is inversely proportional to age from 8 to 10 mcg/kg/24 hr at 0 to 6 months to 2 to 3 mcg/kg/24 hr for over 12 years.

DOSE ADJUSTMENTS

See Drug/Lab Interactions. Reduce dose in elderly, functional or ECG evidence of cardiovascular disease including angina, long-standing thyroid disease, other endocrinopathies, and severe hypothyroidism.

DILUTION

Available in different strengths; read label carefully. Each vial of lyophilized powder is diluted with 5 mL of NS for injection (without preservatives). Shake well to dissolve completely. Reconstituted concentrations will be 40 mcg/mL for the 200-mcg vial and 100 mcg/mL for the 500-mcg vial. Do not add to IV solutions. May be given through Y-tube or three-way stopcock of infusion set. Must be used immediately after dilution; any remaining solution is discarded.

COMPATIBILITY

Specific information not available. Consider specific use; consult pharmacist.

RATE OF ADMINISTRATION

100 mcg or fraction thereof over 1 minute.

ACTIONS

A synthetic thyroid hormone. Effective replacement for decreased or absent thyroid function. Requires peripheral metabolic conversion to active hormone T_3 to be effective. Process inhibited by illness or stress. Onset of action is slow. Up to 5 or 6 hours is required before any noticeable improvements occur, and 24 hours may be required to note full benefits. Thyroid hormone is essential to many body functions, including rate of metabolism.

INDICATIONS AND USES

Specific replacement therapy for reduced or absent thyroid function due to any cause. ■ An emergency measure in myxedema coma. ■ Thyroid suppression therapy.

CONTRAINDICATIONS

Relative contraindications include myocardial infarction, thyrotoxicosis, and uncorrected adrenal insufficiency. ■ Not indicated for use in treatment of obesity. Risk can outweigh benefit.

PRECAUTIONS

Correct adrenocortical insufficiency before administration or acute adrenal crisis and death may result. ■ Corticosteroid therapy is also required concomitantly to prevent acute adrenal insufficiency in myxedema coma or any pre-existing manifestation of adrenal insufficiency. ■ Use caution in diabetes and cardiovascular disease. ■ Larger doses (e.g., 0.3 to 0.4 mg) may cause cardiovascular side effects; use with extreme caution.

Monitor: Observe patient closely and monitor vital signs. ■ Monitor thyroid function tests (e.g., free T_4 index, TSH). ■ Monitor TSH every 6 to 9 weeks until normalized, every 8 to 12 weeks after dose changes, and every 6 to 12 months throughout therapy.

Maternal/Child: Category A: may be used during pregnancy. ■ Presumed safe in breast-feeding; use caution and observe infant. ■ Avoid excessive dose in pediatric patients; can cause brain damage in thyrotoxicosis during infancy. Can also accelerate bone age and cause craniosynotosis (premature closing of sutures in the skull).

Elderly: See Dose Adjustments; more sensitive to effects.

DRUG/LAB INTERACTIONS

Increases rate of metabolism and requires dose adjustment for **anticoagulants, antidepressants, oral antidiabetics, barbiturates, digoxin, catecholamines** (e.g., epinephrine), **beta-adrenergic blockers** (e.g., propranolol), **insulin, estrogens, theophylline, and others.** Cardiac arrhythmias, hypoglycemia, and bleeding can occur with unadjusted dose of some of these drugs.

SIDE EFFECTS

Arrhythmias, chest pain, diarrhea, heart palpitations, heat intolerance, muscle cramps, nervousness, perspiration, tachycardia, vomiting.

ANTIDOTE

Notify the physician of any side effect. A reduction in dose will usually decrease symptoms. In massive overdose control fever, hypoglycemia, and fluid loss. Digitalis may be indicated for CHF; propranolol has been used to treat increased sympathetic activity (1 to 3 mg IV over 10 minutes). Adrenal insufficiency may be unrecognized.

LIDOCAINE HYDROCHLORIDE

Antiarrhythmic

(**LYE**-doh-kayn hy-droh-**KLOR**-eyed)

Lidocaine PF, Xylocaine PF, ✤Xylocard

pH 5 to 7

USUAL DOSE

Ventricular arrhythmia: 50 to 100 mg as a *loading dose* (0.7 to 1.4 mg/kg). Repeat after 5 minutes if desired clinical response is not produced. Follow with an infusion of 1 to 4 mg/min (0.014 to 0.057 mg/kg/min). Should not exceed 200 to 300 mg/hr.

Refractory ventricular fibrillation or pulseless ventricular tachycardia: 1 to 1.5 mg/kg of body weight (50 to 100 mg) as a *loading dose.* May repeat 0.5 to 1.5 mg/kg every 5 to 10 minutes to desired effect, up to a total of 3 mg/kg. Should not exceed 200 to 300 mg/hr. AHA recommends 0.5 to 0.75 mg/kg up to 1 to 1.5 mg/kg. A dose of 0.5 to 0.75 mg/kg may be repeated every 5 to 10 minutes to a maximum total dose of 3 mg/kg.

Maintenance dose: With return of perfusion, initiate an infusion of 20 to 50 mcg/kg/min (1 to 4 mg/min in an average 70-kg adult). *Do not exceed 4 mg/min rate.* If arrhythmias occur during an infusion, give a small bolus of 0.5 mg/kg to increase plasma concentration.

Seizures unresponsive to other therapy (unlabeled): 1 mg/kg as a loading dose. If seizure does not terminate in 2 minutes, give an additional 0.5 mg/kg to prevent recurrences; a maintenance infusion of 30 mcg/kg/ min has been used. Another source suggests a loading dose of 100 mg. Give an additional 50 mg in 20 minutes. Follow with a maintenance infusion of 1 to 3 mg/min. Reduce infusion rate gradually based on patient response; complete withdrawal may take several days.

Cardiac arrest: AHA guidelines recommend a single dose of 1 to 1.5 mg/kg. An additional dose of 0.5 to 0.75 mg/kg may be given in 5 to 10 minutes to a maximum of 3 doses or a total dose of 3 mg/kg.

PEDIATRIC DOSE

See Maternal/Child (unlabeled).

Antiarrhythmic: AHA recommends 1 mg/kg as an IV injection followed immediately by an infusion of 20 to 50 mcg/kg/min (average of 30 mcg/kg/min). If 15 minutes have elapsed since the initial bolus dose before the infusion is started, administration of an additional bolus (1 mg/ kg/min) is recommended when the infusion is initiated. Another source recommends 1 mg/kg IV. May repeat in 10 to 15 minutes × 2 if indicated. Maximum total dose is 3 to 4.5 mg/kg/hr. Follow with an infusion of 20 to 50 mcg/kg/min. Intratracheal dose suggested should be 2 to 2.5 times the IV dose.

DOSE ADJUSTMENTS

Reduce loading dose in digoxin toxicity with AV block. ▪ Consider loading dose reduction (not universally recommended) in congestive heart failure, reduced cardiac output and liver disease. ▪ Lower-end initial doses may be indicated in the elderly based on potential for decreased organ function and concomitant disease or drug therapy. ▪ Reduce maintenance dose by one half in presence of decreased cardiac output (e.g., acute MI, congestive heart failure, or shock from any cause), impaired liver function, the elderly (over 65), and in patients receiving drugs that may decrease clearance of lidocaine or decrease liver blood flow (e.g., beta-blockers [propranolol, cimetidine (Tagamet)]). ■ Reduce maintenance dose after 24 hours or monitor blood levels; half-life of lidocaine increases with prolonged administration.

DILUTION
Label must state, "for IV use" and be preservative free. Bolus dose may be given undiluted.

Infusion: Add 1 Gm of lidocaine to 500 or 250 mL of D5W (preferred), D5/½NS, D5NS, LR, or other **compatible** solutions; see chart on inside back cover. Solution gives 2 or 4 mg/mL of lidocaine. Available prediluted (2, 4, or 8 mg/mL). Titrate to desired response.

Pediatric infusion: Add 120 mg of lidocaine to 100 mL of diluent (1,200 mcg/mL). 1 to 2.5 mL/kg/hr will deliver 20 to 50 mcg/kg/min or add 6 mg/kg to 100 mL diluent. 1 mL/hr equals 1 mcg/kg/min.

Storage: Store at CRT. Discard diluted solution after 24 hours.

COMPATIBILITY   (Underline Indicates Conflicting Compatibility Information)
Consider any drug NOT listed as compatible to be INCOMPATIBLE until consulting a pharmacist; specific conditions may apply.
Additives should not be introduced into premixed solutions of lidocaine.
    One source suggests the following **compatibilities:**
Additive: *Physically* **compatible** *with numerous drugs. Combination may not be practical because of extensive individualized rate adjustments of lidocaine to achieve desired effects; consult pharmacist.* Alteplase (Activase, tPA), aminophylline, amiodarone (Nexterone), atracurium (Tracrium), calcium chloride, calcium gluconate, chloramphenicol (Chloromycetin), chlorothiazide (Diuril), ciprofloxacin (Cipro IV), dexamethasone (Decadron), digoxin (Lanoxin), diphenhydramine (Benadryl), dobutamine, dopamine, ephedrine sulfate, erythromycin (Erythrocin), fentanyl (Sublimaze), flumazenil (Romazicon), furosemide (Lasix), heparin, hydrocortisone sodium succinate (Solu-Cortef), insulin (regular), nafcillin (Nallpen), nitroglycerin IV, penicillin G potassium, pentobarbital (Nembutal), phenylephrine (Neo-Synephrine), potassium chloride (KCl), procainamide (Pronestyl), prochlorperazine (Compazine), ranitidine (Zantac), sodium bicarbonate, sodium lactate, theophylline, verapamil.
Y-site: Alteplase (Activase, tPA), amiodarone (Nexterone), argatroban, bivalirudin (Angiomax), cefazolin (Ancef), ciprofloxacin (Cipro IV), cisatracurium (Nimbex), daptomycin (Cubicin), dexmedetomidine (Precedex), diltiazem (Cardizem), dobutamine, dopamine, enalaprilat (Vasotec IV), eptifibatide (Integrilin), etomidate (Amidate), famotidine (Pepcid IV), fenoldopam (Corlopam), haloperidol (Haldol), heparin, hetastarch in electrolytes (Hextend), inamrinone (Amrinone), labetalol (Trandate), levofloxacin (Levaquin), linezolid (Zyvox), meperidine (Demerol), micafungin (Mycamine), morphine, nicardipine (Cardene IV), nitroglycerin IV, nitroprusside sodium, palonosetron (Aloxi), potassium chloride (KCl), propofol (Diprivan), remifentanil (Ultiva), streptokinase, theophylline, tigecycline (Tygacil), tirofiban (Aggrastat), vasopressin, warfarin (Coumadin).

RATE OF ADMINISTRATION
Bolus dose: 25 to 50 mg or fraction thereof over 1 minute. Too-rapid injection may cause seizures.
Infusion: Using a microdrip (60 gtt/mL) or an infusion pump delivers lidocaine in recommended doses. Adjust as indicated by progress in patient's condition. See Dose Adjustments and the Infusion Rate chart.

Lidocaine Infusion Rates						
Desired Dose	1 Gm in 500 mL Diluent (2 mg/mL)			1 Gm in 250 mL Diluent (4 mg/mL)		
mg/min	mg/hr	mL/min	mL/hr	mg/hr	mL/min	mL/hr
1	60 mg/hr	0.5 mL/min	30 mL/hr	60 mg/hr	0.25 mL/min	15 mL/hr
2	120 mg/hr	1 mL/min	60 mL/hr	120 mg/hr	0.5 mL/min	30 mL/hr
3	180 mg/hr	1.5 mL/min	90 mL/hr	180 mg/hr	0.75 mL/min	45 mL/hr
4	240 mg/hr	2 mL/min	120 mL/hr	240 mg/hr	1 mL/min	60 mL/hr

Pediatric infusion: 120 mg to 100 mL diluent = 1,200 mcg/mL
1 to 2.5 mL/kg/hr = 20 to 50 mcg/kg/min or
6 mg/kg to 100 mL diluent 1 mL/hr = 1 mcg/kg/min

ACTIONS

A local anesthetic agent. Exerts an antiarrhythmic effect similar to procainamide but is more potent. Decreases ventricular excitability. In usual therapeutic doses, produces no change in myocardial contractility, systemic arterial pressure, or absolute refractory period by increasing the stimulation threshold of the ventricle during diastole. Decreases cell membrane permeability and prevents loss of sodium and potassium ions. Onset of action should occur within 2 minutes and last approximately 10 to 20 minutes. Crosses placental barrier. Metabolized in the liver and excreted in the urine.

INDICATIONS AND USES

Treatment of ventricular arrhythmias (e.g., PVCs, ventricular tachycardia [VT], ventricular fibrillation [VF]) occurring during acute myocardial infarction or during cardiac manipulations, such as cardiac surgery. ■ Wide-complex tachycardia of uncertain origin. ■ Wide-complex PSVT.

Unlabeled uses: Pediatric cardiac arrest, seizures unresponsive to other therapy.

CONTRAINDICATIONS

Known sensitivity to lidocaine or any other local anesthetic of the amide type; Wolff-Parkinson-White syndrome, Stokes-Adams syndrome or any other severe first-, second-, or third-degree heart block without an artificial pacemaker in place. ■ Solutions containing dextrose may be contraindicated in patients with known allergies to corn or corn products.

PRECAUTIONS

Oral antiarrhythmic drugs are preferred for maintenance. ■ Use caution in severe liver or renal disease, hypovolemia, shock, all forms of heart block, and untreated bradycardia. ■ Systemic toxicity may result in CNS depression (sedation) or irritability (twitching). May progress to frank convulsions with respiratory depression and/or arrest. ■ Vasopressors (e.g., dopamine) may be used if circulatory depression occurs. ■ Has been associated with malignant hyperthermia.

Monitor: Monitor IV flow rate and the patient's ECG continuously. Therapeutic serum levels range from 1.5 to 5 mcg/mL; above 6 mcg/mL is usually toxic. ■ Monitor electrolytes, fluid balance, and acid-base balance. ■ Half-life increases over time. Reduce dose of continuous infusion after 24 hours and monitor blood levels. ■ Keep patient lying down to reduce hypotensive effects. ▪ Discontinue lidocaine when patient's cardiac condition is stable or any signs of toxicity become apparent. ▪ Keep a bolus dose, 100 mg (5 mL), available at all times for emergency use in myocardial infarction.

Patient Education: May cause dizziness; remain at bed rest; request assistance if ambulation permitted.

Maternal/Child: Category B: use during pregnancy only if clearly needed. ▪ Safety for use in breast-feeding and pediatric patients not established.

Elderly: Lower-end initial dosing and/or mg/kg dose may be appropriate. See Dose Adjustments. ▪ Decreased lidocaine clearance and increased sensitivity to adverse effects. ▪ Consider age-related renal and hepatic impairment.

DRUG/LAB INTERACTIONS

Cross-sensitivity and/or potentiation may occur with **other antiarrhythmics** (e.g., procainamide or quinidine); may cause conduction abnormalities. ▪ **Amiodarone** (Nexterone), **beta-blocking agents** (e.g., propranolol), **and cimetidine** (Tagamet) may decrease lidocaine clearance and increase lidocaine toxicity. ▪ Monitor cardiac function. ▪ May produce excessive cardiac depression with **phenytoin** (Dilantin). ▪ Potentiates neuromuscular blockade of **muscle relaxants** (e.g., succinylcholine) **and aminoglycoside antibiotics** (e.g., gentamicin). ▪ Use caution in patients with **digitalis toxicity** and AV block. ▪ Effects may be altered by **smoking;** monitor carefully.

SIDE EFFECTS

Transient because of short duration of action of lidocaine.

Apprehension, blurred vision, confusion, dizziness, "doom" anxiety, drowsiness, edema, euphoria, hallucinations, light-headedness, mood changes, nervousness, sensations of heat, cold, and numbness, slurred speech, tinnitus, urticaria, vomiting.

Major: Anaphylaxis, bradycardia, cardiac arrest, cardiovascular collapse, convulsions, hypotension, malignant hyperthermia (tachycardia, tachypnea, metabolic acidosis, fever), PR interval prolonged, QRS complex widening, respiratory depression, tremors, twitching, unconsciousness.

ANTIDOTE

Notify the physician of any side effects. For major side effects, discontinue the drug immediately and institute appropriate measures. Ensure patency of airway and adequacy of ventilation. Treat anaphylaxis immediately with oxygen, epinephrine (Adrenalin), antihistamines (e.g., diphenhydramine [Benadryl]), vasopressors (e.g., dopamine), corticosteroids, albuterol (Ventolin), IV fluids, and ventilation equipment as indicated. To correct CNS stimulation use diazepam (Valium), rapid ultra-short-acting barbiturates (e.g., thiopental [Pentothal]), or if under anesthesia, muscle relaxants (e.g., succinylcholine). Use vasopresssors (e.g., dopamine) and IV fluids to correct hypotension. Maintain and support patient; resuscitate as necessary.

LINEZOLID
(lih-**NAY**-zoh-lid)

Zyvox

**Antibacterial
(oxazolidinone)**

USUAL DOSE

Dose and duration of therapy are based on diagnosis and designated pathogens. May be transferred to oral dosing when appropriate; no dose adjustment is necessary. See Precautions.

Recommended Linezolid Doses in Pediatric and Adult Patients			
Infection*	Dosage and Route of Administration		Recommended Duration of Treatment (Consecutive Days)
	Pediatric Patients† (Birth Through 11 Years of Age)	Adults and Adolescents (12 Years of Age and Older)	
Complicated skin and skin structure infections	10 mg/kg IV or PO‡ q 8 hr	600 mg IV or PO‡ q 12 hr	10 to 14
Community-acquired pneumonia, including concurrent bacteremia			
Nosocomial pneumonia			
Vancomycin-resistant *Enterococcus faecium* infections, including concurrent bacteremia	10 mg/kg IV or PO‡ q 8 hr	600 mg IV or PO‡ q 12 hr	14 to 28
Uncomplicated skin and skin structure infections	Less than 5 years: 10 mg/kg PO‡ q 8 hr 5-11 years: 10 mg/kg PO‡ q 12 hr	Adults: 400 mg PO‡ q 12 hr Adolescents: 600 mg PO‡ q 12 hr	10 to 14

*Due to the designated pathogens (see Indications and Uses and package insert).
†Neonates less than 7 days of age: Most preterm neonates less than 7 days of age (gestational age less than 34 weeks) have lower systemic linezolid clearance values and larger AUC values than many full-term neonates and older infants. These neonates should be initiated with a dosing regimen of 10 mg/kg q 12 hr. Consideration may be given to the use of 10 mg/kg q 8 hr regimen in neonates with a suboptimal clinical response. All neonatal patients should receive 10 mg/kg q 8 hr by 7 days of life.
‡Oral dosing using either linezolid tablets or linezolid for oral suspension.

PEDIATRIC DOSE

See Usual Dose and Maternal/Child.

DOSE ADJUSTMENTS

Dose adjustment based on age, gender, renal insufficiency, or hepatic insufficiency is not required. ■ 30% of a dose is removed during a 3-hour dialysis session. Administer linezolid after hemodialysis.

DILUTION

Available in ready-to-use flexible plastic infusion bags in a foil laminate overwrap. Available as a 2 mg/mL solution in 200-, 400-, and 600-mg infusion bags. Prior to use, remove overwrap and check for leaks by squeezing the bag. Do not use flexible containers in series connections. **Storage:** Store at CRT. Protect from light and freezing. Keep in overwrap until ready to use. Solution may exhibit a yellow color that can intensify with time. Will not adversely affect potency.

COMPATIBILITY   (Underline Indicates Conflicting Compatibility Information)

Consider any drug NOT listed as compatible to be INCOMPATIBLE until consulting a pharmacist; specific conditions may apply.

Manufacturer states, "Additives should not be added to the infusion bag." If administered through the same tubing as other medications, flush line before and after infusion of linezolid with a solution that is **compatible** with linezolid (e.g., D5W, NS, LR) and with any medications administered through the common line. Manufacturer lists as **incompatible** at the **Y-site** with amphotericin B (generic), ceftriaxone (Rocephin), chlorpromazine (Thorazine), diazepam (Valium), erythromycin (Erythrocin), pentamidine, phenytoin (Dilantin), and sulfamethoxazole/trimethoprim.

One source suggests the following **compatibilities:**

Solutions: D5W, NS, LR.

Additive: *Not recommended by manufacturer.* Aztreonam (Azactam), cefazolin (Ancef), ceftazidime (Fortaz), ciprofloxacin (Cipro IV), gentamicin, levofloxacin (Levaquin), piperacillin, tobramycin.

Y-site: Acyclovir (Zovirax), alfentanil (Alfenta), amikacin (Amikin), aminophylline, ampicillin, ampicillin/sulbactam (Unasyn), anidulafungin (Eraxis), aztreonam (Azactam), buprenorphine (Buprenex), butorphanol (Stadol), calcium gluconate, carboplatin (Paraplatin), caspofungin (Cancidas), cefazolin (Ancef), cefotetan, cefoxitin (Mefoxin), ceftazidime (Fortaz), ceftriaxone (Rocephin), cefuroxime (Zinacef), ciprofloxacin (Cipro IV), cisatracurium (Nimbex), cisplatin (Platinol), clindamycin (Cleocin), cyclophosphamide (Cytoxan), cyclosporine (Sandimmune), cytarabine (ARA-C), dexamethasone (Decadron), dexmedetomidine (Precedex), D5/½NS, D5NS, digoxin (Lanoxin), diphenhydramine (Benadryl), dobutamine, dopamine, doripenem (Doribax), doxorubicin (Adriamycin), doxycycline, droperidol (Inapsine), enalaprilat (Vasotec IV), esmolol (Brevibloc), etoposide phosphate (Etopophos), famotidine (Pepcid IV), fenoldopam (Corlopam), fentanyl (Sublimaze), fluconazole (Diflucan), fluorouracil (5-FU), furosemide (Lasix), ganciclovir (Cytovene), gemcitabine (Gemzar), gentamicin, granisetron (Kytril), haloperidol (Haldol), heparin, hydrocortisone sodium succinate (Solu-Cortef), hydromorphone (Dilaudid), ifosfamide (Ifex), imipenem-cilastatin (Primaxin), labetalol (Trandate), leucovorin calcium, levofloxacin (Levaquin), lidocaine, lorazepam (Ativan), magnesium sulfate, mannitol, meperidine (Demerol), meropenem (Merrem IV), mesna (Mesnex), methotrexate, methylprednisolone (Solu-Medrol), metoclopramide (Reglan), metronidazole (Flagyl IV), midazolam (Versed), mitoxantrone (Novantrone), morphine, nalbuphine (Nubain), naloxone (Narcan), nicardipine (Cardene IV), nitroglycerin IV, ondansetron (Zofran), paclitaxel (Taxol), pentobarbital (Nembutal), phenobarbital (Luminal), piperacillin, piperacillin/tazobactam (Zosyn), potassium chloride (KCl), prochlorperazine (Compazine), promethazine (Phenergan), propranolol, ranitidine (Zantac), remifentanil (Ultiva), Ringer's solution, sodium bicarbonate, sufentanil (Sufenta), theophylline, tigecycline (Tygacil), tobramycin, vancomycin, vasopressin, vecuronium, verapamil, vincristine, zidovudine (AZT, Retrovir).

RATE OF ADMINISTRATION

Administer as an infusion over 30 to 120 minutes. Flush line before and after administration if indicated; see Compatibility.

ACTIONS

A synthetic antibacterial agent. The first agent of a new class of antibiotics, the oxazolidinones. Clinically useful in the treatment of infections caused by aerobic gram-positive bacteria. See Indications and Uses and manufacturer's literature. Inhibits bacterial protein synthesis through a mechanism of action different from that of other antibacterial agents; therefore, cross-resistance between linezolid and other classes of antibiotics is unlikely. Bacteriostatic against enterococci and staphylococci. Bactericidal against most strains of streptococci. Readily distributes into well-perfused tissues. Metabolized to two inactive metabolites. Metabolic pathway is not fully understood. Half-life is 4.8 hours. Approximately 30% of a dose is excreted in the urine as linezolid and 50% is excreted as metabolites.

INDICATIONS AND USES

Treatment of adults, adolescents, and other pediatric patients with the following infections caused by susceptible strains of the designated microorganisms: vancomycin-resistant *Enterococcus faecium* infections, including cases with concurrent bacteremia; nosocomial pneumonia caused by *Staphylococcus aureus* (methicillin-susceptible and methicillin-resistant strains) or *Streptococcus pneumoniae* (including multidrug-resistant strains [MDRSP]); complicated skin and skin-structure infections (including diabetic foot infections without concomitant osteomyelitis) caused by *Staphylococcus aureus* (methicillin-susceptible and methicillin-resistant strains), *Streptococcus pyogenes,* or *Streptococcus agalactiae;* uncomplicated skin and skin-structure infections caused by *Staphylococcus aureus* (methicillin-susceptible strains only) or *Streptococcus pyogenes;* and community-acquired pneumonia caused by *Streptococcus pneumoniae* (including multidrug-resistant strains [MDRSP] and cases with concurrent bacteremia) or *Staphylococcus aureus* (methicillin-susceptible strains only). ▪ Treatment of decubitus ulcers has not been studied. ▪ Given orally to treat uncomplicated skin and skin-structure infections. ▪ Not indicated for treatment of gram-negative infections. Critical that specific gram-negative therapy be initiated immediately if a concomitant gram-negative pathogen is documented or suspected. ▪ Not approved for and should not be used for treatment of patients with catheter-related bloodstream infections or catheter-site infections.

CONTRAINDICATIONS

History of hypersensitivity to linezolid or any of its components. ▪ Avoid use in patients taking any medicinal products that inhibit monoamine oxidase A or B (e.g., isocarboxazid [Marplan], phenelzine [Nardil]) or within 2 weeks of taking any such product. ▪ Unless closely monitored for potential increases in BP, avoid use in patients with uncontrolled hypertension, pheochromocytoma, or thyrotoxicosis and/or in patients taking any of the following types of medications: directly and indirectly acting sympathomimetic agents (e.g., pseudoephedrine [Sudafed]), vasopressive agents (e.g., epinephrine [Adrenalin], norepinephrine [Levophed]), dopaminergic agents (e.g., dobutamine, dopamine); see Precautions and Drug/Lab Interactions. ▪ Unless closely monitored for S/S of serotonin syndrome, avoid use in patients with carcinoid syndrome and/or in patients taking any of the following medications: serotonin reuptake inhibitors (e.g., fluoxetine [Prozac], sertraline [Zoloft]), tricyclic antidepressants (e.g., amitriptyline [Elavil]), serotonin 5-HT$_1$ receptor agonists (e.g., triptans [e.g., sumatriptan (Imitrex)]), meperidine (Demerol), or buspirone (BuSpar); see Precautions and Drug/Lab Interactions.

PRECAUTIONS
Culture and sensitivity studies are indicated to determine susceptibility of the causative organism to linezolid. ▪ To reduce the development of drug-resistant bacteria and maintain its effectiveness, linezolid should be used to treat or prevent only those infections proven or strongly suspected to be caused by bacteria. ▪ Reports of vancomycin-resistant *Enterococcus faecium* (VRE) becoming resistant to linezolid during its clinical use have been published. ▪ There has been a report of methicillin-resistant *Staphylococcus aureus* (MRSA) developing resistance to linezolid during its clinical use. ▪ Combination therapy may be clinically indicated in treatment of nosocomial pneumonia or complicated skin and skin-structure infections if the documented or presumptive pathogens include gram-negative organisms. ▪ Should not be used for treatment of patients with catheter-related bloodstream infections or catheter site infections. ▪ Use with caution in patients with renal failure. Although dose adjustments are not recommended in this patient population, the metabolites may accumulate. The clinical significance of this accumulation is unknown. Dose should be given after hemodialysis. ▪ Use with caution in patients with uncontrolled hypertension, severe hepatic insufficiency, pheochromocytoma, carcinoid syndrome, or untreated hyperthyroidism; see Contraindications. Use has not been studied in these patient populations. ▪ Safety and efficacy of linezolid given for longer than 28 days have not been evaluated. ▪ Neuropathy (peripheral and optic) has been reported, primarily in patients treated for longer than the maximum recommended duration of 28 days. May occur in patients treated with linezolid for shorter periods, as well as in patients treated for more than 28 days. ▪ Superinfection, caused by the overgrowth of nonsusceptible organisms, may occur with antibiotic use. Treat as indicated. ▪ *Clostridium difficile*–associated diarrhea (CDAD) has been reported. May range from mild diarrhea to fatal colitis. Consider in patients who present with diarrhea during or after treatment with linezolid. ▪ Lactic acidosis has been reported. In most cases, patients experienced repeated episodes of N/V. ▪ Serotonin syndrome (e.g., cognitive dysfunction, hyperpyrexia, hyperreflexia, incoordination) has been reported in patients receiving linezolid and concomitant serotonergic agents; see Drug/Lab Interactions. ▪ Convulsions have been reported; however, a history of seizures was reported in some of the cases. ▪ See Monitor, Patient Education, and Drug/Lab Interactions.

Monitor: Myelosuppression (including anemia, leukopenia, pancytopenia, and thrombocytopenia) has been reported. CBC with differential and platelet count should be monitored weekly, especially in patients who receive linezolid for longer than 2 weeks; those with pre-existing myelosuppression; those receiving concomitant drugs that produce bone marrow suppression (e.g., antineoplastics [cisplatin (Platinol), gemcitabine

(Gemzar)], chloramphenicol, immunosuppressants [e.g., azathioprine (Imuran)]) or affect platelet function (e.g., aspirin, epoprostenol [Flolan], NSAIDs [e.g., ibuprofen (Advil, Motrin), naproxen (Aleve, Naprosyn)], platelet aggregation inhibitors [e.g., abciximab (ReoPro), clopidogrel (Plavix), dipyridamole (Persantine), eptifibatide (Integrilin)], selected antibiotics [e.g., piperacillin], valproic acid [Depacon, Depakene]); or those with a chronic infection who have received previous or concomitant antibiotics. Consider discontinuing therapy in patients who develop or have worsening myelosuppression. Myelosuppression appears to be reversible following discontinuation of linezolid. ■ Prompt ophthalmic evaluation is recommended in patients taking linezolid for extended periods (3 months or more) or if symptoms of visual impairment appear (e.g., blurred vision, changes in visual acuity or color vision, or visual field defect). ■ Monitor for S/S of lactic acidosis (e.g., recurrent N/V, unexplained acidosis, or a low bicarbonate level); immediate medical evaluation is indicated. ■ Monitor for S/S of serotonin syndrome (cognitive dysfunction, hyperpyrexia, hyperreflexia, incoordination) when administered concurrently with serotonergic agents; see Drug/Lab Interactions. ■ Monitor dietary intake of tyramine; see Patient Education. Hypertension may result from excessive tyramine intake (less than 100 mg/day). ■ See Precautions and Drug/Lab Interactions.

Patient Education: Avoid foods or beverages high in tyramine (e.g., aged cheeses, fermented or air-dried meats, sauerkraut, soy sauce, tap beers, red wines). ■ Inform physician of any history of hypertension or seizures. See Precautions. ■ Inform physician if taking any medications containing pseudoephedrine or phenylpropanolamine (found in many cold or allergy preparations or diet aids), or if taking serotonin re-uptake inhibitors (e.g., fluoxetine [Prozac], sertraline [Zoloft], paroxetine [Paxil]) or other antidepressants. ■ Promptly report diarrhea or bloody stools that occur during treatment or up to several months after an antibiotic has been discontinued; may indicate CDAD and require treatment. ■ Report any vision changes promptly. See Drug Interactions.

Maternal/Child: Category C: safety for use in pregnancy and breast-feeding not established; benefits must outweigh risks. ■ Volume of distribution is similar regardless of age in pediatric patients; however, clearance varies as a function of age. Clearance is most rapid in the youngest age-groups (ranging from less than 1 week old to 11 years of age), resulting in lower single-dose systemic exposure (AUC) and shorter half-life. ■ AUC values in patients from birth to 11 years of age dosed every 8 hours are similar to adolescents and adults dosed every 12 hours. ■ Therapeutic concentrations are not consistent in CSF; not indicated for empiric treatment of CNS infections in pediatric patients.

Elderly: No overall difference in safety or effectiveness has been observed between these patients and younger patients. Pharmacokinetics are not significantly altered in the elderly. See Dose Adjustments.

DRUG/LAB INTERACTIONS

Linezolid is a reversible, nonselective inhibitor of monoamine oxidase and therefore has the potential to interact with **adrenergic and serotonergic agents and with tyramine-containing foods.** ■ A reversible enhancement of the pressor response to **indirect-acting sympathomimetic agents or vasopressor or dopaminergic agents** (e.g., pseudoephedrine [Sudafed], phenylpropanolamine, epinephrine [Adrenalin], dopamine) may be seen with concomitant use. Initial doses of adrenergic agents, such as epinephrine or dopamine, should be reduced and titrated to achieve the desired response; see Contraindications. ▪ In clinical trials, coadministration of linezolid and **serotonergic agents** (e.g., dextromethorphan [Benylin DM], fluoxetine [Prozac], paroxetine [Paxil], sertraline [Zoloft]) was not associated with serotonin syndrome (e.g., blushing, cognitive dysfunction, confusion, diaphoresis, delirium, hyperpyrexia, restlessness, and tremors). However, post-marketing cases have been reported. Patients receiving both therapies should be monitored for the development of serotonin syndrome. If S/S of serotonin syndrome develop, consider discontinuing either the linezolid or the serotonergic agent. If the serotonergic agent is discontinued, specific symptoms due to the discontinuation may be observed; see prescribing information for the specific agent; see Contraindications. ▪ Does not appear to induce, inhibit, or be induced by the cytochrome P_{450} system and should therefore not affect drugs metabolized by this system (e.g., warfarin [Coumadin], phenytoin [Dilantin]); however, coadministration with **rifampin** (Rifadin) led to an observed reduction in linezolid plasma concentrations. The mechanism is unclear. **Other strong inducers of hepatic enzymes** (e.g., carbamazepime [Tegretol], phenytoin [Dilantin], phenobarbital [Luminal]) may also cause a decrease in linezolid concentration. ▪ Has been coadministered with aztreonam (Azactam) and gentamicin. When linezolid was coadministered with either one of these agents, no alteration of pharmacokinetics occurred in either drug. ▪ Severe myelosuppression may occur with **bone marrow suppressants and other drugs that affect platelet function;** see Monitor.

SIDE EFFECTS

Most common side effects are diarrhea, headache, and nausea. Other reported side effects include abdominal pain; CDAD; constipation; dizziness; dysgeusia (change in sense of taste); dyspepsia; fever; hypertension; increased AST, BUN, SCr, total bilirubin; insomnia; lactic acidosis; myelosuppression (anemia, leukopenia, neutropenia, pancytopenia, thrombocytopenia); neuropathy (peripheral and optic [optic neuropathy may progress to vision loss]); oral moniliasis; pruritus; rash; seizures; serotonin syndrome (cognitive dysfunction, hyperpyrexia, hyperreflexia, lack of coordination); tongue discoloration; vaginal moniliasis; and vomiting.

Post-Marketing: Anaphylaxis, angioedema, bullous skin disorders such as Stevens-Johnson syndrome, and superficial tooth and tongue discoloration.

ANTIDOTE

Keep physician informed of all side effects. Discontinue drug if indicated. If S/S of serotonin syndrome develop, consider discontinuing linezolid or the serotonergic agent. Consider discontinuing linezolid in patients who develop or have worsening myelosuppression. Mild cases of CDAD may respond to discontinuation of linezolid. Treat CDAD with fluids, electrolytes, protein supplements, and oral vancomycin (Vancocin) or metronidazole (Flagyl) as indicated. In severe cases, surgical evaluation may be indicated. In the event of an overdose, initiate supportive care and maintain glomerular filtration. Both linezolid and its metabolites are partially removed by hemodialysis.

LIOTHYRONINE SODIUM BBW

(lye-oh-**THIGH**-roh-neen **SO**-dee-um)

T₃, Triostat

Hormone
(thyroid)

pH 9.5 to 11.5

USUAL DOSE

Preadministration testing and adjunctive therapy with corticosteroids required (see Precautions/Monitor).

Initial and subsequent doses must be determined on the basis of continuous monitoring of clinical condition and response to liothyronine therapy. An adequate dose is important in determining clinical outcome.

Myxedema coma: 25 to 50 mcg as an initial dose. At least 4 hours but no more than 12 hours should elapse between doses; allows sufficient time to evaluate response and avoids fluctuation in hormone levels. Myxedematous patients have an increased sensitivity to thyroid hormones. Begin with lower doses and increase gradually. Use caution in adjusting dose to avoid large changes that may precipitate adverse cardiovascular events. A total daily dose of 65 mcg/day in the initial days of treatment has decreased mortality. Experience with doses above 100 mcg/day is limited.

Transfer to oral therapy: Initiate oral therapy as soon as condition is stabilized and patient is able to take oral medications. With oral liothyronine, discontinue IV liothyronine and begin with low doses. Increase gradually based on response. If levothyroxine (L-thyroxine, T₄) is used, discontinue IV therapy gradually to compensate for several-day delay in effectiveness of oral levothyroxine.

DOSE ADJUSTMENTS

Reduce initial dose to 10 to 20 mcg in known or suspected cardiovascular disease. ■ Begin with lower doses in the elderly based on the potential for decreased organ function and concomitant disease or drug therapy. ■ See Drug/Lab Interactions.

DILUTION

May be given undiluted. Available as 10 mcg/mL in 1-mL vials.

Storage: Must be refrigerated until administration. Discard unused portion.

COMPATIBILITY

Specific references not available. Consider specific use; consult pharmacist.

RATE OF ADMINISTRATION

Each 10 mcg or fraction thereof over 1 minute.

ACTIONS

A synthetic form of the natural thyroid hormone triiodothyronine (T₃). Enters peripheral tissues readily and binds to specific nuclear receptor(s) to initiate hormonal, metabolic effects. Affinity for these receptors is 10-fold higher than prohormone T₄ (levothyroxine) and no additional conversion (T₄ to T₃) is required. Increases metabolic rate and reverses the loss of consciousness, hypothermia, lactic acidosis, and other symptoms of myxedema coma. Thyroid hormones have many beneficial effects on general metabolism and the cardiovascular system. Liothyronine produces a detectable metabolic response in 2 to 4 hours. Achieves maximum therapeutic response within 48 hours. Has a rapid cutoff of activity, permitting quick dose adjustments and/or control of overdose. Metabolized in the liver to an inactive metabolite. Does not readily cross the placental barrier. Minimal secretion in breast milk.

INDICATIONS AND USES

Treatment of myxedema coma and precoma (patient not completely unconscious). ▪ May be used in patients allergic to desiccated thyroid or thyroid extract derived from pork or beef.

CONTRAINDICATIONS

Concomitant use with artificial patient rewarming; generally contraindicated in diagnosed but uncorrected adrenal cortical insufficiency or untreated thyroxicosis; hypersensitivity to any components (no documented evidence of true hypersensitivity idiosyncratic reactions). Not indicated for use in treatment of obesity or male or female infertility without hypothyroidism. Risk can outweigh benefit.

PRECAUTIONS

For IV use only. ▪ Myxedema coma is a medical emergency usually precipitated in a hypothyroid patient by illness, sedatives, or anesthetics. Has a 50% to 70% mortality rate even with aggressive therapy. ▪ Use with caution in presence of any compromised cardiac function or cardiac disease, particularly of the coronary arteries. ▪ May precipitate a hyperthyroid state or may aggravate existing hyperthyroidism. ▪ Due to the rarity of myxedema coma and precoma, no systematic studies have been performed with IV liothyronine.

Monitor: Confirm diagnosis with serum TSH (greater than 60 mcU/mL), serum total T_4 and free T_4 (low), and serum total T_3 and free T_3 (normal or low). Repeat as indicated to evaluate response to treatment. ▪ ECG, chest x-ray, CBC, AST, CPK, LDH, lipids, serum electrolytes, serum cortisol, cerebrospinal fluid examination, and EEG are helpful before dose administration. Monitor progress by repeat evaluations at selected intervals. ▪ Correct adrenocortical insufficiency before administration or acute adrenal crisis and death may result. Corticosteroids (e.g., dexamethasone [Decadron], methylprednisolone [Solu-Medrol]) should be administered routinely in the initial emergency treatment of all myxedema coma patients; required before starting liothyronine or simultaneously with administration in pituitary myxedema; recommended in primary myxedema. During therapy metabolism increases at a greater rate than adrenocortical activity; can precipitate adrenocortical insufficiency and shock; corticosteroids may be needed throughout therapy. ▪ In any patient with compromised cardiac function, monitoring of cardiac function is required. ▪ Assisted or artificial ventilation may be required. ▪ Treatment should correct electrolyte disturbances, possible infection, or other illness. ▪ IV fluids will be required, but use caution to prevent cardiac decompensation and be alert for water intoxication from inappropriate secretion of ADH. ▪ Do not rewarm patient artificially; may further decrease circulation to vital internal organs and increase shock. Normal body temperature can be restored in 24 to 48 hours by preventing heat loss. Keep patient covered with blankets in a warm room. ▪ See Drug/Lab Interactions.

Maternal/Child: Category A: clinical experience does not indicate adverse effect on fetus. ▪ Observe infant carefully for any adverse symptoms if breast-feeding; minimal amounts secreted in breast milk. ▪ Experience with pediatric patients under 18 years of age is limited; safety and effectiveness not established.

Elderly: Response similar to other age-groups; however, may be more sensitive to effects. Evaluate carefully for any occult cardiac disease; see Precautions/Monitor. ▪ Reduced dose may be indicated; see Dose Adjustments.

DRUG/LAB INTERACTIONS

Metabolic requirements are markedly reduced in hypothyroid patients. Concomitant use with **vasopressors** (e.g., epinephrine, dopamine) may increase risk of coronary insufficiency, arrhythmias, or circulatory collapse. Use lower doses and extreme caution. ▪ Observe any patient previously stabilized on **anticoagulants** carefully; dose reduction may be required. Monitor PT. ▪ Increased doses of **insulin or oral hypoglycemics** may be required. ▪ Higher doses of levothyroxine may be required with **estrogens or estrogen-containing oral contraceptives** in the patient with a nonfunctioning thyroid. ▪ May cause transient cardiac arrhythmias with **tricylic antidepressants** (e.g., imipramine [Tofranil]). ▪ May potentiate toxic effects of **digoxin,** whereas increased metabolism may require a higher digoxin dose. ▪ Hypertension and tachycardia are probable with **ketamine anesthesia.** Be prepared to treat promptly. ▪ Pregnancy, as well as many drugs (e.g., androgens, corticosteroids, estrogens, estrogen oral contraceptives, iodine preparations, salicylates) in combination with thyroid preparations, **interfere with accurate interpretation of lab tests.** Consult with lab personnel.

SIDE EFFECTS

Average dose: Arrhythmia (6%), cardiopulmonary arrest (2%), hypotension (2%), myocardial infarction (2%), tachycardia (3%). Angina, congestive heart failure, fever, hypertension, phlebitis, and twitching occurred in 1% or less.

Overdose: Acute myocardial infarction, angina pectoris, arrhythmia, congestive heart failure, headache, increased bowel motility, irritability, menstrual irregularities, nervousness, shock, sweating, tachycardia, thyroid storm, tremor.

ANTIDOTE

Keep physician informed of all side effects. If side effects progress or overdose occurs, reduce or temporarily discontinue liothyronine. Restart at lower doses when feasible. Treatment is symptomatic and supportive. Oxygen and artificial ventilation may be required. Treat increased sympathetic activity with beta-adrenergic antagonists (e.g., esmolol [Brevibloc]). Monitor fever, hypoglycemia, and fluid loss and treat as needed. Digoxin (Lanoxin) may be required in congestive heart failure.

LORAZEPAM
(lor-**AYZ**-eh-pam)

Benzodiazepine
Sedative-hypnotic
Antianxiety agent
Anticonvulsant
Amnestic
Skeletal muscle relaxant
Antiemetic

Ativan, Lorazepam PF

USUAL DOSE

Dose must be individualized, especially when used in conjunction with other medications that may cause CNS depression. See Dose Adjustments, Precautions, and Drug/Lab Interactions.

Antianxiety/amnestic: 2 mg or 0.044 mg/kg of body weight, whichever is smaller, 15 to 20 minutes before procedure. For greater lack of recall 0.05 mg/kg up to 4 mg may be given. 2 mg is usually the maximum dose for patients over 50 years of age.

Sedation: 2 mg as the initial dose (may not be necessary if patient is receiving intermittent benzodiazepines [e.g., diazepam, midazolam]). Follow with an infusion of 0.5 to 1 mg/hr (0.25 to 0.5 mg/hr if less agitated or has cardiorespiratory problems). Titrate to achieve adequate sedation. Increase in 1 mg/hr increments. Up to 5 to 10 mg/hr has been used. When sedation is adequate, reduce to lowest amount needed.

Status epilepticus: 4 mg as the initial dose. May repeat once in 10 to 15 minutes if seizures continue. Experience with further doses is very limited. Additional intervention (e.g., concomitant administration of phenytoin) may be required. Another source suggests 0.05 mg/kg of body weight to a total dose of 4 mg. May repeat once in 10 to 15 min. If still not effective, use another anticonvulsant agent (e.g., phenytoin). Do not exceed a total dose of 8 mg in 12 hours.

High-dose therapy for refractory status epilepticus (unlabeled): With continuous EEG monitoring, begin a continuous infusion of lorazepam at 1 mg/hr. Increase by 1 mg/hr at 15-minute intervals until patient is seizure free. Maintain seizure-free state with lorazepam for 24 hours. Use therapeutic doses of phenytoin and phenobarbital in addition to lorazepam. At the end of 24 hours, begin to reduce the lorazepam by 1 mg/hr at hourly intervals. Observe closely and monitor EEG for signs of recurrent seizures. Repeat process if seizures recur.

Management of emetic-inducing chemotherapy (unlabeled): 0.025 mg/kg to 0.05 mg/kg (maximum dose is 4 mg) 30 minutes before chemotherapy is begun. Supplement with oral lorazepam 1 to 2 mg/hr as needed. Another source suggests 1.5 mg/M^2 (up to a maximum of 3 mg/M^2) over 5 minutes. Administer 30 to 45 minutes before administration of antineoplastic agent. May be given in combination with other antiemetics (e.g., ondansetron [Zofran], dexamethasone). Repeat every 4 hours as needed.

Continued

PEDIATRIC DOSE

Safety for use in pediatric patients under 12 years of age has not been fully studied, but it has been used for status epilepticus in neonates, infants, and children; see Maternal/Child.

Sedation: 0.05 mg/kg up to a maximum of 2 mg/dose every 4 to 8 hours.

Status epilepticus (unlabeled): *Neonates, infants, and children:* 0.05 to 0.1 mg/kg up to a maximum of 4 mg/dose. May repeat 0.05 mg/kg once in 5 to 10 minutes if needed.

Antiemetic, adjunct therapy (unlabeled): 0.02 to 0.05 mg/kg/dose up to a maximum of 2 mg/dose. May repeat every 6 hours as needed.

DOSE ADJUSTMENTS

Start with a small dose in the elderly and increase gradually based on response. Consider the potential for decreased organ function and concomitant disease or drug therapy. ■ Dose adjustments are not required with impaired liver function. ■ Dose adjustments are not required with impaired renal function unless frequent doses are given over a short period of time. ■ Reduced dose may be indicated in the presence of other CNS depressants. ■ Reduce dose by 50% when given concurrently with probenicid (Benemid) or valproate (Depacon). ■ See Drug/Lab Interactions.

DILUTION

IV injection: Dilute immediately before use with an equal volume of SW, D5W, or NS. Do not shake vigorously, will result in air entrapment. Gently invert repeatedly until completely in solution. May be given by IV injection or through Y-tube or three-way stopcock of infusion tubing.

Infusion (unlabeled): Has been further diluted in D5W or NS and given as an infusion. Best solubility is in concentrations of 0.1 mg/mL or 0.2 mg/mL.

Lorazepam Guidelines for Dilution and Infusion				
Base Concentration	2 mg/mL		4 mg/mL	
Desired Concentration	0.1 mg/mL	0.2 mg/mL	0.1 mg/mL	0.2 mg/mL
Volume of diluent required for each 1 mL lorazepam	19 mL	9 mL	39 mL	19 mL

Very viscous; mix well and observe for crystallization. Crystallization does occur and is thought to be due to propylene glycol preservative. May occur more frequently in NS than in D5W and with 4-mg/mL vials of lorazepam base than with 2-mg/mL vials. Prepare only enough to last for 12 hours. If necessary for fluid restriction, a 2-mg/mL vial has been stable for 24 hours when diluted in a 1 mg (lorazepam base) to 1 mL diluent (D5W preferred). Monitor carefully.

Storage: Refrigerate before dilution; protect from light. Use only freshly prepared solutions; discard if discolored or precipitate forms. Infusions stable at room temperature for 12 hours in plastic, 24 hours in glass.

COMPATIBILITY   (Underline Indicates Conflicting Compatibility Information)

Consider any drug NOT listed as compatible to be INCOMPATIBLE until consulting a pharmacist; specific conditions may apply.

One source suggests the following **compatibilities:**

Y-site: Acyclovir (Zovirax), albumin (Albuminar), allopurinol (Aloprim), amifostine (Ethyol), amikacin (Amikin), amiodarone (Nexterone), amphotericin B cholesteryl (Amphotec), atracurium (Tracrium), bivalirudin (Angiomax), bumetanide, caspofungin (Cancidas), cefepime (Maxipime), cefotaxime (Claforan), ciprofloxacin (Cipro IV), cisatracurium (Nimbex), cisplatin (Platinol), cladribine (Leustatin), cyclophosphamide (Cytoxan), cytarabine (ARA-C), dexamethasone (Decadron), dexmedetomidine (Precedex), diltiazem (Cardizem), dobutamine, docetaxel (Taxotere), dopamine, doripenem (Doribax), doxorubicin (Adriamycin), doxorubicin liposomal (Doxil), epinephrine (Adrenalin), erythromycin (Erythrocin), etomidate (Amidate), etoposide phosphate (Etopophos), famotidine (Pepcid IV), fenoldopam (Corlopam), fentanyl (Sublimaze), filgrastim (Neupogen), fluconazole (Diflucan), fludarabine (Fludara), foscarnet (Foscavir), fosphenytoin (Cerebyx), furosemide (Lasix), gemcitabine (Gemzar), gentamicin, granisetron (Kytril), haloperidol (Haldol), heparin, hetastarch in electrolytes (Hextend), hydrocortisone sodium succinate (Solu-Cortef), hydromorphone (Dilaudid), labetalol (Trandate), levofloxacin (Levaquin), linezolid (Zyvox), melphalan (Alkeran), methadone (Dolophine), methotrexate, metronidazole (Flagyl IV), micafungin (Mycamine), midazolam (Versed), milrinone (Primacor), morphine, nicardipine (Cardene IV), nitroglycerin IV, norepinephrine (Levophed), oxaliplatin (Eloxatin), paclitaxel (Taxol), palonosetron (Aloxi), pancuronium, pemetrexed (Alimta), piperacillin, piperacillin/tazobactam (Zosyn), potassium chloride (KCl), propofol (Diprivan), ranitidine (Zantac), remifentanil (Ultiva), sulfamethoxazole/trimethoprim, tacrolimus (Prograf), teniposide (Vumon), thiopental (Pentothal), thiotepa, vancomycin, vecuronium, vinorelbine (Navelbine), zidovudine (AZT, Retrovir).

RATE OF ADMINISTRATION
IV injection: Each 2 mg or fraction thereof over 1 to 5 minutes.
Infusion: Use a microdrip or infusion pump for accuracy to deliver desired dose and/or titrate to desired level of sedation.
Pediatric rate: 1 mg or fraction thereof over 2 to 5 minutes.

ACTIONS
A benzodiazepine with antianxiety, sedative, and anticonvulsant effects. Inhibits ability to recall events. Interacts with the GABA-benzodiazepine receptor complex in the brain. Effective in 15 to 30 minutes. Effects last an average of 6 to 8 hours, but may last as long as 12 to 24 hours. Half-life is 9.5 to 19.5 hours. Distributed in body fluids. Metabolized by the liver to inactive metabolites; some is slowly excreted in urine. Crosses the placental barrier. Excreted in breast milk.

INDICATIONS AND USES
Preanesthetic medication for adult patients. ■ Produce sedation, relieve anxiety, and provide anterograde amnesia. ■ Management of status epilepticus.
Unlabeled uses: High-dose therapy for status epilepticus clinically or EEG diagnosed as refractory to high doses of phenytoin and phenobarbital. ■ Management of emetic-inducing chemotherapy. ■ Antipanic agent. ■ Treatment of alcohol withdrawal. ■ Amnestic during endoscopic procedures. ■ Skeletal muscle relaxant adjunct. ■ Treatment of tension headaches.

CONTRAINDICATIONS
Hypersensitivity to benzodiazepines (diazepam [Valium]) or the components (e.g., polyethylene glycol, propylene glycol, or benzyl alcohol). Patients with acute narrow angle glaucoma, sleep apnea syndrome, or

severe respiratory insufficiency (except patients requiring relief of anxiety and/or diminished recall of events while being mechanically ventilated). Intra-arterial injection.

PRECAUTIONS
Rapidly and completely absorbed IM. ▪ When given as a sedative, patient is able to respond to simple instructions. ▪ Increased risk of respiratory depression; airway support, emergency drugs, and equipment must be immediately available. ▪ Dependence is possible with prolonged use or high dose. ▪ Use with extreme caution in the elderly, the very ill, or patients with limited pulmonary reserve; risk of hypoventilation and/or hypoxic cardiac arrest is increased. ▪ Use as a premedicant before local or regional anesthesia may cause excessive drowsiness and interfere with assessment of levels of anesthesia. More likely to occur with doses greater than 0.05 mg/kg or when narcotic agents are used concomitantly. ▪ Use with caution in patients with mild to moderate renal or hepatic disease. ▪ There have been reports of possible propylene and polyethylene glycol toxicity (e.g., lactic acidosis, hyperosmolality, hypotension, acute tubular necrosis) when lorazepam has been administered at higher than recommended doses. Patients with renal impairment may be at increased risk of developing toxicity. Paradoxical reactions may occur. ▪ See Antidote (e.g., risk of seizure with flumazenil).

Monitor: To reduce incidence of thrombophlebitis, avoid smaller veins. Extravasation is hazardous; arterial administration may cause arteriospasms and gangrene and/or require amputation. ▪ Bed rest required for a minimum of 3 hours after IV injection and assistance required for up to 8 hours. ▪ Monitor and maintain patent airway. Respiratory assistance and flumazenil (Romazicon) must be available. ▪ Establish an IV and monitor vital signs. **Status epilepticus:** In addition to the above, observe for and correct any other possible cause of seizure (e.g., hypoglycemia, hyponatremia, other metabolic disorders). ▪ Sedative effects may add to the impairment of consciousness seen in the post-ictal state (e.g., after a seizure). ▪ Neurologic consult is suggested for any patient who fails to regain consciousness.

Patient Education: May produce drowsiness or dizziness; request assistance with ambulation and use caution performing tasks that require alertness for 24 to 48 hours or until the effects of the drug have subsided. ▪ Avoid use of alcohol or other CNS depressants (e.g., antihistamines, barbiturates) for 24 to 48 hours or until the effects of the drug have subsided. ▪ May be habit-forming with long-term use or high-dose therapy. ▪ Has amnestic potential; may impair memory. ▪ Consider birth control options.

Maternal/Child: Category D: avoid pregnancy. May cause fetal damage. Not recommended during pregnancy, labor and delivery, breast-feeding, or in pediatric patients under 12 years of age. ▪ Has FDA approval for treatment of status epilepticus in adults over 18 years of age. Safety for use in pediatric patients has not been fully studied, but has been used for status epilepticus in neonates, infants, and children. ▪ May cause paradoxical excitement in pediatric patients. ▪ Seizure activity and myoclonus have been reported in low-birth-weight neonates. ▪ Contains benzyl alcohol, which has been associated with a fatal "gasping syndrome" in neonates. ▪ Half-life prolonged in pediatric patients.

Elderly: Dosing should be cautious in the elderly; see Dose Adjustments. ▪ More sensitive to therapeutic and adverse effects (e.g., ataxia, dizziness, oversedation). ▪ IV injection may be more likely to cause apnea, brady-cardia, CNS depression, hypotension, respiratory depression, and cardiac arrest. ▪ See Precautions and Drug/Lab Interactions.

DRUG/LAB INTERACTIONS
Concurrent use with **other CNS depressants** such as alcohol, antihistamines, barbiturates, MAO inhibitors (e.g., selegiline [Eldepryl]), narcotics (e.g., morphine, meperidine [Demerol], fentanyl), phenothiazines (e.g., prochlor-perazine [Compazine]), and tricyclic antidepressants (e.g., imipramine [Tofanil-PM]) may result in additive effects for up to 48 hours. Reduced dose may be indicated. ▪ Concurrent administration with **valproate** (Depa-con) **or probenicid** (Benemid) will decrease clearance of lorazepam. Re-duce dose of lorazepam by one half in patients receiving concurrent valproate or probenicid. ▪ Apnea, arrhythmia, bradycardia, cardiac arrest, coma, and death have been reported when used concurrently with **halo-peridol** (Haldol). ▪ Significant hypotension, respiratory depression, and stupor have been reported (rare) with concomitant use of **loxapine** (Loxapac). ▪ May increase serum concentrations of **digoxin and phenytoin** (Dilantin); monitor digoxin and phenytoin serum levels. ▪ Use with **rifam-pin** (Rifadin) increases clearance and reduces effects of benzodiazepines. ▪ **Theophyllines** (Aminophylline) antagonize the sedative effects of benzo-diazepines. ▪ Marked sedation, salivation, ataxia and, rarely, death have been reported with concomitant use of **clozapine** (Clozaril) and lorazepam. ▪ Estrogen-containing **oral contraceptives** increase clearance and decrease effects. ▪ Inhibits antiparkinson effectiveness of **levodopa.** ▪ Incidence of hallucinations and irrational behavior and an increased incidence of seda-tion have been observed with concurrent use of scopolamine.

SIDE EFFECTS
Airway obstruction, apnea, blurred vision, confusion, crying, delirium, depression, excessive drowsiness, hallucinations, hypotension, injection site reaction, respiratory depression, restlessness, somnolence.
Overdose: Ataxia, coma, hypotension, hypotonia, hypnosis, and very rarely death.

ANTIDOTE
Notify physician of all symptoms. Reduction of dose may be required. Treat hypotension with dopamine or norepinephrine (Levophed). In over-dose, flumazenil (Romazicon) will reverse all sedative effects of benzo-diazepines. See flumazenil monograph (risk of seizures). A patent airway, artificial ventilation, oxygen therapy, and other symptomatic and support-ive treatment must be instituted promptly. Monitor vital signs and fluid status carefully. Forced diuresis and osmotic diuretics (e.g., mannitol) may increase rate of lorazepam elimination. The value of dialysis has not been adequately determined.

LYMPHOCYTE IMMUNE GLOBULIN BBW
(**LIM**-foh-sight ih-**MUNE GLAW**-byoo-lin)

Anti-Thymocyte Globulin [Equine], Atgam

Immunosuppressant

pH 6.8

USUAL DOSE

Intradermal skin test required before administration. Use 0.1 mL of a 1:1,000 dilution in NS and a saline control. If a systemic reaction (rash, dyspnea) occurs, do not administer. If a limited reaction (10 mm wheal or erythema) occurs, proceed with extreme caution. Anaphylaxis can occur even if skin test is negative.

Range is 10 to 30 mg/kg of body weight/24 hr. Actual potency and activity may vary from lot to lot. Given concomitantly with other immunosuppressive therapy (antimetabolites such as azathioprine [Imuran] and corticosteroids).

Delay onset of renal allograft rejection: 15 mg/kg/24 hr for 14 days, then every other day for 7 more doses. Initial dose should be given 24 hours before or after the transplant.

Treat allograft rejection: 10 to 15 mg/kg/24 hr for 14 days, then every other day for 7 more doses (optional). Initial dose should be given when first rejection episode is diagnosed.

Aplastic anemia: 10 to 20 mg/kg/24 hr for 8 to 14 days. Additional alternate-day therapy up to a total of 21 doses may be given.

PEDIATRIC DOSE

Experience with pediatric patients is limited and unlabeled. Intradermal skin test required; see Usual Dose. Has been administered to treat aplastic anemia, to manage renal allograft rejection, and to delay onset of renal allograft rejection using mg/kg doses recommended for adults.

DILUTION

Total daily dose must be further diluted with NS, D5/¼NS, or D5/½NS for infusion. Invert solution while injecting drug so contact is not made with air in infusion bottle. Gently rotate diluted solution. Do not shake. Concentration should not exceed 4 mg/mL. May be infused into a vascular shunt, AV fistula, or high-flow central vein.

Filters: Use of a 0.2- to 1-micron filter recommended.

Storage: Keep refrigerated before and after dilution. Discard diluted solution after 24 hours.

COMPATIBILITY

Manufacturer states lymphocyte immune globulin may precipitate in dextrose solutions and may be unstable with highly acidic solutions.

RATE OF ADMINISTRATION

A total daily dose equally distributed over a minimum of 4 hours.

ACTIONS

A lymphocyte-selective immunosuppressant. Reduces the number of thymus-dependent lymphocytes and contains low concentrations of antibodies against other formed elements in blood. Effective without causing severe lymphopenia. Supports an increase in the frequency of resolution of an acute rejection episode. Has a serum half-life of 5 to 8 days.

INDICATIONS AND USES

Management of allograft rejection in renal transplant patients. ■ Adjunctive to other immunosuppressive therapy to delay onset of initial rejection episode. ■ Treatment of moderate to severe aplastic anemia in patients who are not candidates for bone marrow transplant.

CONTRAINDICATIONS

Systemic hypersensitivity reaction to previous injection of lymphocyte immune globulin or any other equine gamma-globulin preparation.

PRECAUTIONS

Administered only under the direction of a physician experienced in immunosuppressive therapy and management of renal transplant patients in a facility with adequate laboratory and supportive medical resources. ■ Use caution in repeated courses of therapy; observe for signs of hypersensitivity reactions.

Monitor: Will cause chemical phlebitis in peripheral veins. ■ Monitor carefully for signs of infection, leukopenia, or thrombocytopenia. Thrombocytopenia is usually transient in renal transplant patients. Platelet transfusions may be necessary in patients with aplastic anemia. Notify physician immediately so prompt treatment can be instituted and/or drug discontinued. ■ Prophylactic antibiotics may be indicated pending results of C/S. ■ Masked reactions may occur as dose of corticosteroids and antimetabolites is decreased. Observe carefully. ■ Antihistamines (e.g., diphenhydramine [Benadryl]) may be required to control itching. ■ Anaphylaxis can occur at any time. Monitor closely for S/S of a hypersensitivity reaction. Emergency equipment and supplies must be at bedside.

Patient Education: See Appendix D, p. 1434.

Maternal/Child: Category C: no studies conducted in pregnant patients. Use caution. ■ Safety for use in breast-feeding not established. ■ Limited experience on use in pediatric patients; see Pediatric Dose.

DRUG/LAB INTERACTIONS

See Monitor.

SIDE EFFECTS

Full range of hypersensitivity reactions, including anaphylaxis, is possible. Arthralgia, back pain, chest pain, chills, clotted AV fistula, diarrhea, dyspnea, fever, headache, hypotension, infusion site pain, leukopenia, nausea, night sweats, pruritus, rash, stomatitis, thrombocytopenia, thrombophlebitis, urticaria, vomiting, wheal and flare. Other reactions occur in fewer than 1% of patients.

ANTIDOTE

Notify physician of all side effects. Discontinue if anaphylaxis, severe and unremitting thrombocytopenia, and/or severe and unremitting leukopenia occur; see Monitor. May be discontinued if infection or hemolysis present even if appropriately treated. Clinically significant hemolysis may require erythrocyte transfusion, IV mannitol, furosemide, sodium bicarbonate, and fluids. Prophylactic or therapeutic antihistamines (e.g., diphenhydramine [Benadryl]) or corticosteroids should control chills caused by release of endogenous leukocyte pyrogens. Treat anaphylaxis immediately. Epinephrine (Adrenalin), diphenhydramine (Benadryl), oxygen, vasopressors (e.g., dopamine), corticosteroids, and ventilation equipment must always be available. Resuscitate as necessary.

MAGNESIUM SULFATE
(mag-**NEE**-see-um **SUL**-fayt)

Electrolyte replenisher
Anticonvulsant
Antiarrhythmic
Uterine relaxant

pH 5.5 to 7

USUAL DOSE

Individualize dose based on patient requirement and response. Discontinue as soon as desired response is obtained.

Eclampsia: 4 Gm (32 mEq [40 mL of a 10% solution]) over 3 to 4 minutes. Subsequent doses may be given IM every 4 hours as needed, or a continuous infusion of 1 to 2 Gm/hr may be initiated. Do not exceed 30 to 40 Gm/24 hr. Frequent monitoring required; see Dose Adjustments, Precautions, and Monitor.

Seizures associated with epilepsy, glomerulonephritis, or hypothyroidism: 1 Gm.

Hypomagnesemia (mild): 1 Gm every 6 hours for 4 doses.

Hypomagnesemia (severe): 5 Gm (40 mEq) in 1,000 mL D5W or NS as an infusion evenly distributed over 3 hours.

Hyperalimentation in adults: 8 to 24 mEq/24 hr (1 to 3 Gm).

Paroxysmal atrial tachycardia (unlabeled): 3 to 4 Gm (30 to 40 mL of a 10% solution) over 30 seconds with extreme caution. Reserve for patients in whom simpler measures have failed and in whom there is no evidence of myocardial damage.

Reduction of cerebral edema (unlabeled): 2.5 Gm (25 mL of a 10% solution).

Cardiac arrest (hypomagnesemia or torsades de pointes): AHA recommends 1 to 2 Gm (2 to 4 mL of a 50% solution) diluted in 10 mL D5W.

Torsades de pointes (with pulses) or AMI with hypomagnesemia: AHA recommends a loading dose of 1 to 2 Gm in 50 to 100 mL D5W as an infusion over 5 to 60 minutes. Follow with an infusion of 0.5 to 1 Gm/hr and titrate to control the torsades.

Refractory ventricular tachycardia/ventricular fibrillation (unlabeled): A loading dose of 1 to 2 Gm (8 to 16 mEq) in 50 to 100 mL D5W as an infusion over 5 to 60 minutes. Follow with an infusion of 0.5 to 1 Gm/hr.

Myocardial infarction (unlabeled): To reduce cardiovascular morbidity and mortality, administer 2 Gm as an IV injection over 5 to 15 minutes. Follow with an infusion of 18 Gm equally distributed over 24 hours (approximately 12.5 mg/min). Begin administration as soon as possible after onset of symptoms, preferably no later than 6 hours after symptom onset.

Barium poisoning: 1 to 2 Gm.

Alleviate bronchospasm in acute asthma (unlabeled): 2 Gm given IV over 20 minutes. Usually given concurrently with inhaled albuterol (Proventil) and IV corticosteroids.

PEDIATRIC DOSE

Hypomagnesemia or hypocalcemia: 25 to 50 mg/kg of body weight. May repeat at 4- to 6-hour intervals for 3 or 4 doses. Maximum recommended single dose is 2 Gm. Maintain with 30 to 60 mg/kg/24 hr (approximately 0.25 to 0.5 mEq/kg/24 hr). Maximum dose is 1 Gm/24 hr.

Pulseless VT with torsades de pointes: AHA recommends 25 to 50 mg/kg IV push. A 50% solution equals 500 mg/mL. Maximum recommended dose is 2 Gm.

Torsades de pointes (with pulses) or hypomagnesemia: 25 to 50 mg/kg as an infusion over 10 to 20 minutes. A 50% solution equals 500 mg/mL. Maximum recommended dose is 2 Gm.

Status asthmaticus: 25 to 50 mg/kg as an infusion over 15 to 30 minutes. A 50% solution equals 500 mg/mL. Another source recommends 25 to 75 mg/kg as an infusion over 20 minutes. Maximum recommended dose is 2 Gm.

Acute nephritis in pediatric patients (unlabeled): 100 to 200 mg/kg as a 1% to 3% solution (1 Gm in 100 mL = 1% solution, 3 Gm in 100 mL = 3%). One-half dose should be given slowly over 15 to 20 minutes. Complete balance of dose within 1 hour. Monitor BP closely.

Alleviate bronchospasm in acute asthma (unlabeled): 25 to 50 mg/kg. Given IV over 20 minutes. Do not exceed 2 Gm. Usually given concurrently with inhaled albuterol (Proventil) and IV corticosteroids. Monitor BP and HR closely.

Hyperalimentation: *Infants:* 2 to 10 mEq (0.25 to 1.25 Gm daily). *Other pediatric patients:* 0.25 to 0.5 mEq/24 hr or 30 to 60 mg/kg/24 hr.

DOSE ADJUSTMENTS

Reduce dose of other CNS depressants (e.g., narcotics, barbiturates) when given in conjunction with magnesium sulfate. ■ Reduce dose in impaired renal function and in the elderly. ■ Decrease maximum daily dose to 10 Gm/24 hr in patients with severe renal insufficiency. Frequent serum magnesium concentrations must be obtained.

DILUTION

Must be diluted to a concentration of 20% (200 mg/mL) or less for IV administration. D5W or NS are the most common diluents. Available in vials or syringes as 10% (100 mg/mL), 12.5% (125 mg/mL), 20% (200 mg/mL), and 50% (500 mg/mL); premixed in SW as a 4% solution (40 mg/mL) in 100, 500, or 1,000 mL containers; premixed as an 8% solution (80 mg/mL) in 50 mL; and premixed as a 1% solution (10 mg/mL) in 100 or 1,000 mL D5W or a 2% solution (20 mg/mL) in 500 or 1,000 mL D5W. See Usual Dose for specific dilutions. May be given through Y-tube or three-way stopcock of infusion set.

Storage: Store at CRT.

COMPATIBILITY   (Underline Indicates Conflicting Compatibility Information)

Consider any drug NOT listed as compatible to be INCOMPATIBLE until consulting a pharmacist; specific conditions may apply.

Will form various precipitates with alkali carbonates and bicarbonates, alkali hydroxides, arsenates, barium, calcium, clindamycin (Cleocin), hydrocortisone sodium succinate (Solu-Cortef), lead, phosphates, salicylates, strontium, and tartrates. Use caution; consult pharmacist.

One source suggests the following **compatibilities:**

Additive: Calcium gluconate, chloramphenicol (Chloromycetin), cisplatin (Platinol), heparin, hydrocortisone sodium succinate (Solu-Cortef), isoproterenol (Isuprel), linezolid (Zyvox), meropenem (Merrem IV), methyldopate, norepinephrine (Levophed), penicillin G potassium, potassium chloride (KCl), potassium phosphate, verapamil.

Y-site: Acyclovir (Zovirax), aldesleukin (Proleukin), amifostine (Ethyol), amikacin (Amikin), amiodarone (Nexterone), ampicillin, aztreonam

(Azactam), bivalirudin (Angiomax), caspofungin (Cancidas), cefazolin (Ancef), cefotaxime (Claforan), cefoxitin (Mefoxin), chloramphenicol (Chloromycetin), ciprofloxacin (Cipro IV), cisatracurium (Nimbex), clindamycin (Cleocin), dexmedetomidine (Precedex), dobutamine, docetaxel (Taxotere), doripenem (Doribax), doxorubicin liposomal (Doxil), doxycycline, enalaprilat (Vasotec IV), erythromycin (Erythrocin), esmolol (Brevibloc), etoposide phosphate (Etopophos), famotidine (Pepcid IV), fenoldopam (Corlopam), fludarabine (Fludara), gallium nitrate (Ganite), gentamicin, granisetron (Kytril), heparin, hetastarch in electrolytes (Hextend), hydrocortisone sodium succinate (Solu-Cortef), hydromorphone (Dilaudid), idarubicin (Idamycin), insulin (regular), kanamycin (Kantrex), labetalol (Trandate), linezolid (Zyvox), meperidine (Demerol), metronidazole (Flagyl IV), micafungin (Mycamine), milrinone (Primacor), morphine, nafcillin (Nallpen), nicardipine (Cardene IV), nitroprusside sodium, ondansetron (Zofran), oxacillin (Bactocill), oxaliplatin (Eloxatin), paclitaxel (Taxol), penicillin G potassium, piperacillin, piperacillin/tazobactam (Zosyn), potassium chloride (KCl), propofol (Diprivan), remifentanil (Ultiva), sargramostim (Leukine), sulfamethoxazole/trimethoprim, thiotepa, tobramycin, vancomycin.

RATE OF ADMINISTRATION

IV injection: 150 mg/min (1.5 mL of a 10% solution or its equivalent) over at least 1 minute or as directed in Usual Dose. Too-rapid administration may cause hypotension and asystole.

IV infusion: As directed in Usual Dose.

ACTIONS

An important cofactor for enzymatic reactions and plays an important role in neurochemical transmission and muscular excitability. A CNS depressant and a depressant of smooth, skeletal, and cardiac muscle. It also possesses a mild diuretic effect and vasodilating effect. It prevents or controls seizures by blocking neuromuscular transmission and decreasing the amount of acetylcholine release. Can reverse refractory VF caused by hypomagnesemia and help replenishment of intracellular potassium. Onset of action is immediate and effective for about 30 minutes. Excreted in the urine. Secreted in breast milk. Crosses the placental barrier.

INDICATIONS AND USES

Replacement therapy in magnesium deficiency (e.g., acute hypomagnesemia accompanied by signs of tetany similar to those seen in hypocalcemia); also used in magnesium deficiency associated with acute pancreatitis, alcoholism, cirrhosis of the liver, malabsorption syndromes, and prolonged IV therapy with magnesium-free fluids. ■ Correct or prevent hypomagnesemia in patients receiving TPN. ■ Prevention and control of seizures in toxemia of pregnancy (eclampsia and/or preeclampsia).

Unlabeled uses: Prevention and control of convulsive states (epilepsy, glomerulonephritis, hypoparathyroidism). ■ Cerebral edema. ■ Inhibit uterine contractions in premature labor. ■ Acute nephritis in pediatric patients to control hypertension, encephalopathy, and convulsions. ■ Treatment of torsades de pointes, recurrent and refractory ventricular tachycardia, and ventricular fibrillation (VT/VF). ■ Reduce the incidence of post-infarction arrhythmias by counteracting post-infarction hypomagnesemia (given on admission to CCU of a patient with suspected myocardial infarction). ■ Counteract muscle-stimulating effects of barium poisoning. ▪ Treatment of paroxysmal atrial tachycardia. ▪ Treatment of acute asthma in patients who do not respond to conventional therapy.

CONTRAINDICATIONS

Presence of heart block or myocardial damage, within 2 hours of delivery; see Maternal/Child.

PRECAUTIONS

IV use in eclampsia should be reserved for immediate control of life-threatening conditions. ▪ Each 1 Gm contains 8.12 mEq of magnesium. A normal adult body contains 20 to 30 Gm of magnesium. ▪ Use caution in impaired renal function and in patients receiving digoxin. Even in normal renal function, use caution to prevent exceeding renal excretory capacity. ▪ Some solutions may contain aluminum. In impaired kidney function, aluminum may reach toxic levels. Premature neonates are particularly at risk because of their immature kidneys and requirement for calcium and phosphate, which also contain aluminum. Research indicates that patients with impaired renal function who receive greater than 4 to 5 mcg/kg/day of parenteral aluminum are at risk for developing CNS or bone toxicity associated with aluminum accumulation. ▪ Hypomagnesemia can precipitate refractory VF and hinder potassium replacement.

Monitor: Discontinue IV administration when the desired therapeutic effect is obtained. ▪ Monitor magnesium levels. Deep tendon reflexes decrease at plasma magnesium levels above 4 mEq/L and disappear as levels approach 10 mEq/L. Respiratory paralysis will occur at this level. Heart block may occur at or below this level. Levels above 12 mEq/L may be fatal. ▪ Test knee jerks and observe respirations before each additional dose. If the knee jerk is absent or respirations are less than 16/min, do not give additional magnesium sulfate. ▪ Equipment to maintain artificial ventilation must be available at all times. Patient must be continuously observed. Maintain minimum of 100 mL of urine output every 4 hours. ▪ Closely monitor patients with suspected or probable MI for hypotension or asystole and measure magnesium levels.

Maternal/Child: See Precautions. ▪ Category A: appears to be safe for use during pregnancy. May cause magnesium toxicity in the newborn if given IV to the mother within 2 hours of delivery. Risk may be decreased with IV administration. ▪ A continuous infusion given to control convulsions in toxemic mothers before delivery (especially in the 24 hours preceding) may cause signs of magnesium toxicity in the newborn (e.g., respiratory depression); see Drug/Lab Interactions. ▪ Some literature indicates possible harm to the fetus during pregnancy if mother is not toxic. ▪ Use caution during breast-feeding. ▪ Safety for use in pediatric patients not established.

Elderly: See Dose Adjustments.

DRUG/LAB INTERACTIONS

Additive CNS depressant effects when used concomitantly with **barbiturates, hypnotics, narcotics, or systemic anesthetics.** See Dose Adjustments and Monitor. ▪ Potentiates **neuromuscular blocking agents** (e.g., vecuronium, succinylcholine). ▪ If **calcium** is used to treat magnesium toxicity, use in digitalized patients may cause serious changes in cardiac conduction, resulting in heart block. Use with extreme caution.

SIDE EFFECTS

Usually the result of magnesium intoxication. Absence of knee-jerk reflex; cardiac arrest; circulatory collapse; CNS depression; complete heart block; flaccid paralysis; flushing; hypocalcemia with signs of tetany; hypotension; hypothermia; increased PR interval; increased QRS complex; prolonged QT interval; respiratory depression, paralysis, and failure; stupor; sweating.

ANTIDOTE
Discontinue the drug and notify the physician of the occurrence of any side effect. Calcium gluconate and calcium gluceptate are specific antidotes; 5 to 10 mEq should reverse respiratory depression and heart block; see Drug/Lab Interactions. Physostigmine 0.5 to 1 mg SC may be helpful. Treat hypotension with dopamine. Employ artificial ventilation as necessary and resuscitate as necessary. Peritoneal dialysis or hemodialysis are effective in overdose.
Newborn resuscitation: Will require endotracheal intubation, assisted ventilation, and calcium 1 mEq as an antidote.

MANNITOL
(**MAN**-nih-tol)
Osmitrol

Diuretic
(osmotic)

pH 4.5 to 7

USUAL DOSE
Total dose, concentration, and rate of administration should be based on the nature and severity of the condition being treated, fluid requirements, and urine output. The usual adult dose may range from 20 to 100 Gm/24 hr. In most instances, an adequate response is achieved with doses of 50 to 100 Gm/24 hr. The rate of administration is usually adjusted to maintain a urine output of at least 30 to 50 mL/hr. See Precautions and Monitor.
A test dose may be required (e.g., patients with marked oliguria or inadequate renal function).
Test dose: Give 200 mg/kg of body weight over 3 to 5 minutes. 30 to 50 mL of urine should be produced in 1 hour. If adequate urine not produced, repeat once. If still ineffective, reevaluate patient.
1 Gm equal to approximately 5.5 mOsm.
Available as:
5% solution (50 Gm/L)
10% solution (50 Gm/500 mL, 100 Gm/L)
15% solution (75 Gm/500 mL)
20% solution (50 Gm/250 mL, 100 Gm/500 mL)
25% solution (12.5 Gm/50 mL)
Prevention of oliguric phase of acute renal failure: 50 to 100 Gm as a 5% to 25% solution. A concentrated solution may be used initially followed by a 5% to 10% solution.
Treatment of oliguria: 50 to 100 Gm of a 15% to 25% solution.
Management of intracranial pressure in neurologic emergencies: Manufacturer recommends 0.25 Gm/kg every 6 to 8 hours. AHA recommends 0.5 to 1 Gm/kg over 5 to 10 minutes through an in-line filter. Repeat 0.25 to 2 Gm/kg every 4 to 6 hours as needed. A third source suggests 1.5 to 2 Gm/kg of body weight as a 15% to 25% solution. An osmotic

gradient between the blood and cerebrospinal fluid of approximately 10 mOsm should yield a satisfactory reduction in intracranial pressure.

Reduction of intraocular pressure: 1.5 to 2 Gm/kg of body weight as a 15% or 20% solution. To obtain maximal effect, this dose may be administered over a period as short as 30 minutes. May be used 60 to 90 minutes before surgery.

Promotion of urinary excretion of toxic substances: 50 to 200 Gm. Manufacturer recommends a 5% or 25% solution as indicated if urine output remains adequate. Numerous regimens are in use. Urine output of 100 to 500 mL/hr and a positive fluid balance of 1 to 2 L should be maintained. One regimen suggests an initial loading dose of 25 Gm followed by an infusion at a rate to maintain urine output at 100 mL/hr. Discontinue if no benefit derived from 200 Gm.

Diuretic for adjunctive treatment of ascites or edema: 100 Gm of a 10% to 20% solution over 2 to 6 hours.

PEDIATRIC DOSE

See Maternal/Child. *Test dose may be required (e.g., oliguria or anuria).*

Test dose: Give 200 mg/kg of body weight or 6 Gm/M^2 over 3 to 5 minutes. 30 to 50 mL of urine should be produced in 1 hour. If adequate urine not produced, repeat once. If still ineffective, reevaluate patient. Maximum test dose is 12.5 Gm.

Cerebral or ocular edema: 2 Gm/kg of body weight or 60 Gm/M^2 of body surface as a 15% to 20% solution over 30 to 60 minutes.

Promotion of urinary excretion of toxic substances: 2 Gm/kg or 60 Gm/M^2 as a 5% or 10% solution as needed if urine output remains adequate. Concentration depends on fluid requirement and urine output.

Anuria/oliguria: 0.5 to 1 Gm/kg as an initial dose. Maintain with 0.25 to 0.5 Gm/kg every 4 to 6 hours. Another source suggests 2 Gm/kg or 60 Gm/M^2 over 90 minutes to several hours.

Edema and ascites: 2 Gm/kg or 60 Gm/M^2 as a 15% to 20% solution over 2 to 6 hours.

DOSE ADJUSTMENTS

Reduce dose by one half for small or debilitated patients. ■ Dose selection in the elderly should be cautious (usually starting at the low end of the dosing range), reflecting the greater frequency of decreased organ function and of concomitant disease or drug therapy. ■ Reduced dose may be required in oliguria or impaired renal function; see Monitor.

DILUTION

No further dilution is necessary; however, if there are any crystals present in the solution, they must be completely dissolved before administration. Warm ampule or bottle in hot water (to 50° C [122° F]) and shake vigorously at intervals. Cool to at least body temperature before administration.

Glomerular filtration rate: See Usual Dose.

Filters: Use an in-line filter for 15%, 20%, and 25% solutions.

Storage: Store below 40° C. Discard unused portions.

COMPATIBILITY   (Underline Indicates Conflicting Compatibility Information)

Consider any drug NOT listed as compatible to be INCOMPATIBLE until consulting a pharmacist; specific conditions may apply.

Sources list as **incompatible** with strongly acidic or alkaline solutions. 20% or 25% solutions of mannitol may precipitate with potassium chloride (KCl) or sodium chloride. Concomitant administration of electrolyte-free mannitol solutions with whole blood may cause pseudoagglutination. If blood must be given simultaneously, at least 20 mEq of NaCl should be added to each liter of mannitol solution; consult pharmacist. Do not use PVC infusion bags with 25% mannitol; may form a precipitate.

One source suggests the following **compatibilities:**

Additive: Amikacin (Amikin), cefoxitin (Mefoxin), cisplatin (Platinol), dopamine, fosphenytoin (Cerebyx), furosemide (Lasix), gentamicin, levofloxacin (Levaquin), metoclopramide (Reglan), ondansetron (Zofran), sodium bicarbonate, tobramycin, verapamil.

Y-site: Allopurinol (Aloprim), amifostine (Ethyol), amphotericin B cholesteryl (Amphotec), aztreonam (Azactam), bivalirudin (Angiomax), cisatracurium (Nimbex), cladribine (Leustatin), docetaxel (Taxotere), doripenem (Doribax), etoposide phosphate (Etopophos), fenoldopam (Corlopam), fludarabine (Fludara), fluorouracil (5-FU), gallium nitrate (Ganite), gemcitabine (Gemzar), hetastarch in electrolytes (Hextend), idarubicin (Idamycin), linezolid (Zyvox), melphalan (Alkeran), ondansetron (Zofran), oxaliplatin (Eloxatin), paclitaxel (Taxol), palonosetron (Aloxi), pemetrexed (Alimta), piperacillin/tazobactam (Zosyn), propofol (Diprivan), remifentanil (Ultiva), sargramostim (Leukine), teniposide (Vumon), thiotepa, vinorelbine (Navelbine).

RATE OF ADMINISTRATION

Variable; may be adjusted to obtain a urine output of at least 30 to 50 mL/hr. A single dose should be given over 30 to 90 minutes. Up to 3 Gm/kg have been given over this time span. A test dose (see Monitor) or loading doses may be given over 3 to 5 minutes.

Oliguria: A single dose over 90 minutes to several hours.

Reduction of intracranial pressure and brain mass: A single dose over 30 to 60 minutes.

Treatment of edema or ascites: A single dose over 2 to 6 hours.

ACTIONS

A sugar alcohol and most effective osmotic diuretic. It is a stable, inert, nontoxic solution. Distribution in the body is limited to extracellular compartments. Increases osmolarity of glomerular filtrate and the extracellular space. An increase in extracellular osmolarity causes the movement of water to the extracellular and vascular spaces. This action is responsible for the ability of mannitol to decrease intracranial pressure and edema and to reduce elevated intraocular pressure. Mannitol is not reabsorbed or secreted by the tubules of the kidneys. It is excreted almost completely in the urine along with water, sodium, and chloride. Onset of diuresis is 1 to 3 hours. Reduction in cerebrospinal and intraocular fluid occurs within 15 minutes and lasts 4 to 8 hours. Rebound may occur within 12 hours.

INDICATIONS AND USES

Promotion of diuresis in the prevention and/or treatment of the oliguric phase of acute renal failure before irreversible renal failure becomes established. ■ Reduction of intracranial pressure and treatment of cerebral edema by reducing brain mass. ■ Reduction of extremely high intraocular pressure. ■ Promotion of excretion of toxic substances. ■ Reduction of generalized edema and ascites.

CONTRAINDICATIONS

Anuria, hypersensitivity to mannitol, intracranial bleeding except during craniotomy, progressive heart failure or pulmonary congestion after initiation of mannitol therapy, severe dehydration, severe pulmonary congestion or frank pulmonary edema, severe renal impairment or progressive renal dysfunction after initiation of mannitol therapy, including increasing azotemia or oliguria.

PRECAUTIONS

For IV use only. ▪ Evaluate cardiac status to avoid fulminating congestive heart failure. Use caution in renal failure; fluid overload may result. ▪ Loss of water in excess of electrolytes can cause hypernatremia. ▪ May cause osmotic nephrosis, which may progress to severe irreversible nephrosis. ▪ Use with caution in neurosurgical patients. May increase cerebral blood flow and increase risk of postoperative bleeding. ▪ Increased cerebral blood flow may worsen intracranial hypertension in pediatric patients who develop a generalized cerebral hyperemia within 48 hours of injury.

Monitor: Test dose should be used in patients with marked oliguria or impaired renal functions; see Usual Dose. ▪ Observe urine output continuously; should exceed 30 to 50 mL/hr. Insert Foley catheter if necessary. ▪ Monitor fluid status and osmolality (not to exceed 310 mOsm/kg). ▪ May obscure signs of inadequate hydration or hypovolemia. Electrolyte depletion (especially sodium and potassium) may occur. Administration of water and electrolytes is required to maintain fluid balance due to losses of these substances from urine, sweat, and expired air. Check with laboratory studies and replace as necessary. Monitor renal, cardiac, and pulmonary function. ▪ Before attempting to reduce intracranial pressure and brain mass, evaluate circulatory and renal reserve, fluid and electrolyte balance, body weight, and total input and output before and after mannitol infusion. Support with adequate ventilation and oxygenation. Reduced cerebrospinal fluid pressure must be observed within 15 minutes after starting infusion. ▪ Observe infusion site to prevent infiltration.

Maternal/Child: Category C: safety for use in pregnancy, labor, or delivery not established. Benefits must outweigh risks. ▪ Use caution in breast-feeding. ▪ Safety and effectiveness for use in pediatric patients under 12 years of age not established; however, doses are used clinically.

Elderly: Response similar to that seen in younger patients. Lower-end initial doses may be appropriate; see Dose Adjustments.

DRUG/LAB INTERACTIONS

May increase **lithium** excretion, thereby decreasing its effectiveness. ▪ Mannitol-induced hypokalemia may increase the potential for **digoxin** toxicity.

SIDE EFFECTS

Rare when used as directed but may include acidosis, backache, blurred vision, chest pain, chills, convulsions, decreased chloride levels, decreased sodium levels, dehydration, diuresis, dizziness, dryness of mouth, edema, fever, fulminating congestive heart failure, headache, hyperosmolality, hypertension, hypotension, nausea, polyuria then oliguria, pulmonary edema, rhinitis, tachycardia, thirst, thrombophlebitis, and urinary retention.

ANTIDOTE

If minor side effects persist, notify the physician. For all major side effects or if urine output is under 30 to 50 mL/hr, discontinue the drug and notify the physician. Treatment will be supportive to correct fluid and electrolyte imbalances. Hemodialysis may be used to clear mannitol and reduce serum osmolality.

MELPHALAN HYDROCHLORIDE BBW Antineoplastic

(**MEL**-fah-lan hy-droh-**KLOR**-eyed)   (alkylating agent/nitrogen mustard)

**Alkeran, L-PAM, Phenylalanine
Mustard, L-Sarcolysin**

pH 6.5 to 7

USUAL DOSE

Multiple myeloma: 16 mg/M^2 every 2 weeks for 4 doses. After recovery from toxicity, repeat a dose every 4 weeks. Prednisone is administered concurrently. No exact dosage conversion from oral to parenteral or parenteral to oral.

High-dose therapy as part of a bone marrow transplant protocol (unlabeled): 140 to 240 mg/M^2 as a single dose or divided into 2 to 5 daily doses. Infuse over 20 to 60 minutes.

PEDIATRIC DOSE

See Maternal/Child.

Pediatric rhabdomyosarcoma (unlabeled): 10 to 35 mg/M^2/dose every 21 to 28 days.

High-dose melphalan with bone marrow transplantation for neuroblastoma (unlabeled): 70 to 100 mg/M^2/day on Days 7 and 6 before BMT or

140 to 220 mg/M^2 as a single dose before BMT or

50 mg/M^2/day for 4 days before BMT or

70 mg/M^2/day for 3 days before BMT.

DOSE ADJUSTMENTS

Manufacturer recommends reducing dose by 50% if BUN greater than 30 mg/dL. Other recommendations have been suggested in the literature. ■ Dose reduction based on myelotoxicity should be considered. In one clinical study, the following reductions based on cell count were followed: reduce dose by 25% if WBC between 3,000 and 4,000/mm^3 and platelets between 75,000 and 100,000/mm^3; by 50% if WBC between 2,000 and 3,000/mm^3 and platelets between 50,000 and 75,000/mm^3. Withhold dose for WBC below 2,000/mm^3 and platelets below 50,000/mm^3. ■ Lower-end initial doses may be indicated in the elderly. Consider impaired organ function and concomitant disease or drug therapy. ■ Somewhat reduced dose may be appropriate for patients undergoing hemodialysis.

DILUTION

Specific techniques required; see Precautions. Reconstitution to completion of administration must take place within 60 minutes due to instability of melphalan (rapid hydrolysis). Rapidly inject 10 mL of supplied diluent into vial. Shake vigorously until a clear solution results (5 mg/mL). Use only clear solutions. Further dilute in NS to a concentration of 0.1 to 0.45 mg/mL (45 mg in 100 mL equals 0.45 mg/mL). Keep the time from reconstitution to dilution to administration to a minimum. Drug is very unstable and may begin to deteriorate within 30 minutes.

Filters: No data available from manufacturer. Another source indicates minimal adsorption with several types of filters from 0.2 to 0.45 microns in size.

Storage: Protect from light and store at room temperature before reconstitution. Reconstituted solution is stable for up to 2 hours maximum.

Stable at a concentration of 0.1 to 0.45 mg/mL for only 60 minutes or less. Will precipitate if refrigerated.

COMPATIBILITY   (Underline Indicates Conflicting Compatibility Information)
Consider any drug NOT listed as compatible to be INCOMPATIBLE until consulting a pharmacist; specific conditions may apply.
One source suggests the following **compatibilities:**
Y-site: Acyclovir (Zovirax), amikacin (Amikin), aminophylline, ampicillin, aztreonam (Azactam), bleomycin (Blenoxane), bumetanide, buprenorphine (Buprenex), butorphanol (Stadol), calcium gluconate, carboplatin (Paraplatin), carmustine (BiCNU), caspofungin (Cancidas), cefazolin (Ancef), cefepime (Maxipime), cefotaxime (Claforan), cefotetan, ceftazidime (Fortaz), ceftriaxone (Rocephin), cefuroxime (Zinacef), cisplatin (Platinol), clindamycin (Cleocin), cyclophosphamide (Cytoxan), cytarabine (ARA-C), dacarbazine (DTIC), dactinomycin (Cosmegen), daunorubicin (Cerubidine), dexamethasone (Decadron), diphenhydramine (Benadryl), doxorubicin (Adriamycin), doxycycline, droperidol (Inapsine), enalaprilat (Vasotec IV), etoposide (VePesid), famotidine (Pepcid IV), filgrastim (Neupogen), fluconazole (Diflucan), fludarabine (Fludara), fluorouracil (5-FU), furosemide (Lasix), gallium nitrate (Ganite), ganciclovir (Cytovene), gentamicin, granisetron (Kytril), haloperidol (Haldol), heparin, hydrocortisone sodium succinate (Solu-Cortef), hydromorphone (Dilaudid), idarubicin (Idamycin), ifosfamide (Ifex), imipenem-cilastatin (Primaxin), lorazepam (Ativan), mannitol, mechlorethamine (nitrogen mustard), meperidine (Demerol), mesna (Mesnex), methotrexate, methylprednisolone (Solu-Medrol), metoclopramide (Reglan), metronidazole (Flagyl IV), mitomycin (Mutamycin), mitoxantrone (Novantrone), morphine, nalbuphine, ondansetron (Zofran), pentostatin (Nipent), piperacillin, potassium chloride (KCl), prochlorperazine (Compazine), promethazine (Phenergan), ranitidine (Zantac), sodium bicarbonate, streptozocin (Zanosar), sulfamethoxazole/trimethoprim, teniposide (Vumon), thiotepa, ticarcillin/clavulanate (Timentin), tobramycin, vancomycin, vinblastine, vincristine, vinorelbine (Navelbine), zidovudine (AZT, Retrovir).

RATE OF ADMINISTRATION
Keep the time from reconstitution to dilution to administration to a minimum. Drug is very unstable and may begin to deteriorate within 30 minutes. Do not administer directly into a peripheral vein. Administration by injecting slowly into a fast-running IV solution via an injection port or via a central venous line is recommended.
Intravenous infusion: A single dose over 15 to 20 minutes. Unlabeled high-dose regimens have been infused over 20 to 60 minutes.

ACTIONS
A phenylalanine derivative of nitrogen mustard that is a bifunctional alkylating antineoplastic agent. Cytotoxicity is related to the extent of its interstrand cross-linking with DNA. Not dependent on cell cycle phase. Active against both resting and dividing tumor cells. Binding to plasma proteins ranges from 60% to 90%. Approximately 30% is irreversibly bound to proteins. Eliminated from plasma primarily by chemical hydrolysis rather than metabolism. Half-life is approximately 75 minutes. About 10% excreted as unchanged drug in urine.

INDICATIONS AND USES

Palliative treatment of patients with multiple myeloma when oral therapy is not appropriate.

Unlabeled uses: Treatment of multiple myeloma in combination with other cytotoxic agents. ■ Treatment of cancers of the breast, thyroid, and testes when oral therapy is not appropriate. ■ Treatment of chronic myelocytic leukemia. ■ Component of an induction regimen before bone marrow transplantation. ■ Component of combination therapy to treat relapsed, resistant Hodgkin's lymphomas. ■ Pediatric rhabdomyosarcoma. ■ High-dose melphalan with BMT for pediatric neuroblastoma. ■ Intra-arterial injection (hyperthermic isolated limb perfusion) is used with surgery for extremity melanoma and as a palliative treatment with locally advanced, unresectable malignant melanoma of the extremity.

CONTRAINDICATIONS

Prior resistance to or hypersensitivity to melphalan.

PRECAUTIONS

Follow guidelines for handling cytotoxic agents. See Appendix A, p. 1429. ■ Administered by or under the direction of the physician specialist, with facilities for monitoring the patient and responding to any medical emergency. ■ Use extreme caution in patients whose bone marrow is compromised by or recovering from previous radiation or chemotherapy. ■ Severe myelotoxicity (WBC below 1,000/mm^3 and platelets below 25,000/mm^3) with resulting infection or bleeding is more common with IV dosing. ■ Do not abandon treatment prematurely. Improvement may continue slowly over many months with repeated courses. ■ Patients with an elevated BUN had a greater incidence of severe bone marrow suppression. ■ Secondary malignancies, including acute nonlymphocytic leukemia, myeloproliferation syndrome, and carcinoma have been reported in patients treated with alkylating agents, including melphalan. ■ See Drug/Lab Interactions.

Monitor: Determine absolute patency of vein. A stinging or burning sensation indicates extravasation; cellulitis and tissue necrosis may result. Discontinue injection; use another vein. ■ Monitor platelet count, hemoglobin, white blood cell count, and differential frequently. Indicated before each dose as well as between doses to determine optimal dose and avoid toxicity. Nadirs occur 2 to 3 weeks after treatment, recovery should occur in 4 to 5 weeks. ■ Severe myelosuppression can occur with effective doses. Withhold further doses until blood cell counts have recovered if thrombocytopenia and/or leukopenia occur. ■ Monitor kidney function before and during therapy. ■ Hypersensitivity reactions may occur with initial treatment but often are delayed and occur after multiple courses. Observe closely; anaphylaxis and death have occurred. ■ Observe closely for all signs of infection or bleeding. Prophylactic antibiotics may be indicated pending results of C/S in a febrile neutropenic patient. ■ Prophylactic antiemetics may reduce nausea and vomiting and increase patient comfort. ■ Some facilities are using ice pops to help prevent stomatitis. ■ Monitor for thrombocytopenia (platelet count less than 50,000/mm^3). Initiate precautions to prevent excessive bleeding (e.g., inspect IV sites, skin, and mucous membranes; use extreme care during invasive procedures; test urine, emesis, stool, and secretions for occult blood). ■ See Drug/Lab Interactions.

Patient Education: Avoid pregnancy; nonhormonal birth control recommended. ■ Promptly report IV site burning or stinging, S/S of a hypersensitivity reaction, or any potential side effects (e.g., bleeding, cough, fever, rash). ▪ See Appendix D, p. 1434.

Maternal/Child: Category D: avoid pregnancy. Can cause chromosomal damage and severe birth defects in the fetus and impairment of fertility in men and women. ▪ Discontinue breast-feeding. ▪ Safety and effectiveness for use in pediatric patients not established; see Unlabeled Uses.

Elderly: Response similar to that seen in younger adults. ▪ See Dose Adjustments.

DRUG/LAB INTERACTIONS

Coadministration with **cyclosporine** (Sandimmune) may result in acute renal failure. May occur after the first dose of each drug. ▪ Renal dysfunction and increased toxicity may occur with concurrent **cisplatin.** ▪ Threshold for lung toxicity associated with **carmustine** (BiCNU) may be reduced with concurrent use. ▪ **Interferon alfa** may decrease serum concentrations of melphalan. ▪ Use with **nalidixic acid** (NegGram) may cause severe hemorrhagic necrotic enterocolitis in pediatric patients. ▪ Do not administer **live virus vaccines** to immunocompromised patients receiving antineoplastic agents.

SIDE EFFECTS

Reversible bone marrow suppression is dose-limiting. Irreversible bone marrow failure has been reported. Alopecia, diarrhea, hemolytic anemia, hepatic toxicity (including veno-occlusive disease), hypersensitivity reactions (2% [e.g., anaphylaxis, bronchospasm, dyspnea, edema, hypotension, pruritus, urticaria, tachycardia]), interstitial pneumonitis, nausea and vomiting, oral ulceration, pulmonary fibrosis, secondary malignancies (longterm use), skin ulceration at injection site, vasculitis.

Overdose: Severe bone marrow suppression, cholinomimetic effects (e.g., bradycardia, increased peristalsis and salivation, incontinence), convulsions, decreased consciousness, hyponatremia (inappropriate secretion of ADH), muscular paralysis, severe nausea and vomiting.

ANTIDOTE

Keep physician informed of all side effects. Close monitoring of bone marrow may prevent most serious and potentially fatal side effects. WBC and platelet count nadirs occur 2 to 3 weeks after treatment with recovery in 4 to 5 weeks. Withhold further doses until blood cell counts have recovered if leukopenia or thrombocytopenia occur. There is no specific antidote, but adequate supportive care including administration of whole blood products (e.g., packed RBCs, platelets, leukocytes) and/or blood modifiers (e.g., darbepoetin alfa [Aranesp], epoetin alfa [Epogen], filgrastim [Neupogen], oprelvekin [Neumega], pegfilgrastim [Neulasta], sargramostim [Leukine]) may be indicated to treat bone marrow toxicity. Appropriate antibiotics may be indicated. Monitor closely until recovery (6 weeks or more). Discontinue the infusion and treat hypersensitivity reactions with antihistamines, corticosteroids, pressor agents, or volume expanders; do not readminister melphalan (IV or oral). Hemodialysis probably not effective in overdose. For extravasation, elevate the extremity and apply intermittent ice packs over the area immediately and 4 times daily for ½ hour. Continue for several days.

MEPERIDINE HYDROCHLORIDE
(meh-**PER**-ih-deen hy-droh-**KLOR**-eyed)

Demerol, Demerol HCl, Meperidine HCl PF

Opioid analgesic
(agonist)
Anesthesia adjunct

pH 3.5 to 6

USUAL DOSE
IV injection: 5 to 10 mg every 5 minutes as needed. Do not exceed 600 mg/24 hr. IV dosing in acute pain should be limited to 48 hours or less; see Precautions.
Infusion: Must be administered through a controlled infusion device. May be patient activated. *Based on a 10 mg/mL dilution,* an initial loading dose of 10 to 25 mg (1 to 2.5 mL) is average. The continuous background infusion to provide a level of pain relief and maintain patency of the vein may range from 10 to 35 mg/hr (1 to 3.5 mL/hr). One source suggests a rate of 0.5 to 1 mg/min. Additional doses of 5 to 10 mg (0.5 to 1 mL) may be activated by the patient at selected intervals every 3 to 60 minutes (averaging 10 to 15 minutes). Additional boluses (averaging 5 to 10 mg [0.5 to 1 mL]) may be given by health care professionals (e.g., every 30 min prn).
Supplement anesthesia: 1 to 10 mg/mL dilution is usually used. Titrate under the direct observation and control of the anesthesiologist. Dose dependent on premedication, type of anesthesia, type and duration of procedure and patient's condition.
Treatment or prevention of shaking chills (unlabeled): 0.5 mg/kg 20 minutes before shaking chills are expected to begin or 50 mg after onset of chills. Up to 150 mg has been required within 30 minutes if administered after onset.

PEDIATRIC DOSE
1 to 1.5 mg/kg/dose. May repeat every 3 to 4 hours. Maximum dose 100 mg; see Maternal/Child.

DOSE ADJUSTMENTS
Reduced dose may be required in the elderly or debilitated, in hepatic or renal disease, or in numerous other disease entities; see Precautions. ■ Doses appropriate for the general population may cause serious respiratory depression in vulnerable patients. ■ Increase doses as required if analgesia is inadequate, tolerance develops, or pain severity increases. The first sign of tolerance is usually a reduced duration of effect. ■ See Drug/Lab Interactions.

DILUTION
IV injection: May be given undiluted; however, further dilution with 5 mL of SW, NS, or other IV solutions to facilitate titration is appropriate; see chart on inside back cover.
Infusion: Available as 10, 25, 50, 75, or 100 mg/mL for infusion. Each 10 mg must be diluted in at least 1 mL of NS, D5W, D5NS, or other **compatible** infusion solution. Usually diluted in NS for use in narcotic syringe infusor systems.
Filters: No data available from manufacturer.
Storage: Before use, store at CRT protected from light. Do not freeze.

COMPATIBILITY (Underline Indicates Conflicting Compatibility Information)
Consider any drug NOT listed as compatible to be INCOMPATIBLE until consulting a pharmacist; specific conditions may apply.
One source suggests the following **compatibilities:**

Additive: Cefazolin (Ancef), dobutamine, metoclopramide (Reglan), ondansetron (Zofran), sodium bicarbonate, succinylcholine, verapamil.

Y-site: Acyclovir (Zovirax), amifostine (Ethyol), amikacin (Amikin), ampicillin, ampicillin/sulbactam (Unasyn), anidulafungin (Eraxis), aztreonam (Azactam), bivalirudin (Angiomax), bumetanide, caspofungin (Cancidas), cefazolin (Ancef), cefotaxime (Claforan), cefotetan, cefoxitin (Mefoxin), ceftazidime (Fortaz), ceftriaxone (Rocephin), cefuroxime (Zinacef), chloramphenicol (Chloromycetin), cisatracurium (Nimbex), cladribine (Leustatin), clindamycin (Cleocin), dexamethasone (Decadron), dexmedetomidine (Precedex), digoxin (Lanoxin), diltiazem (Cardizem), diphenhydramine (Benadryl), dobutamine, docetaxel (Taxotere), dopamine, doripenem (Doribax), doxycycline, droperidol (Inapsine), erythromycin (Erythrocin), etoposide phosphate (Etopophos), famotidine (Pepcid IV), fenoldopam (Corlopam), filgrastim (Neupogen), fluconazole (Diflucan), fludarabine (Fludara), furosemide (Lasix), gallium nitrate (Ganite), gemcitabine (Gemzar), gentamicin, granisetron (Kytril), heparin, hetastarch in electrolytes (Hextend), hydrocortisone sodium succinate (Solu-Cortef), insulin (regular), kanamycin (Kantrex), labetalol (Trandate), lidocaine, linezolid (Zyvox), magnesium sulfate, melphalan (Alkeran), methyldopate, methylprednisolone (Solu-Medrol), metoclopramide (Reglan), metoprolol (Lopressor), metronidazole (Flagyl IV), nafcillin (Nallpen), ondansetron (Zofran), oxacillin (Bactocill), oxaliplatin (Eloxatin), oxytocin (Pitocin), paclitaxel (Taxol), palonosetron (Aloxi), pemetrexed (Alimta), penicillin G potassium, piperacillin, piperacillin/tazobactam (Zosyn), potassium chloride (KCl), propofol (Diprivan), propranolol, ranitidine (Zantac), remifentanil (Ultiva), sargramostim (Leukine), sulfamethoxazole/trimethoprim, teniposide (Vumon), thiotepa, ticarcillin/clavulanate (Timentin), tobramycin, vancomycin, verapamil, vinorelbine (Navelbine).

RATE OF ADMINISTRATION
IV injection: A single dose over 4 to 5 minutes. Frequently titrated according to symptom relief and respiratory rate. Rapid IV administration increases the possibility of hypotension and respiratory depression.

Infusion: Must be administered through a controlled infusion device. May be patient activated. Initial loading dose, basal rate (continuous rate of infusion), patient self-administered dose and interval, additional boluses permitted, and total dose for 1 hour should be ordered by physician. Do not exceed direct IV rate. For continuous infusion note range of mg/hr under Usual Dose; distribute evenly via infusion device.

ACTIONS
A synthetic narcotic analgesic and descending CNS depressant, similar to but slightly less potent than morphine. Onset of action occurs in about 5 minutes and lasts for about 2 to 4 hours. Crosses the placental barrier. Readily absorbed and distributed throughout the body. Metabolized to an active, toxic metabolite (normeperidine) in the liver, its extended half-life (15 to 30 hours) may lead to cumulative effects. Excreted in the urine. Crosses placental barrier. Secreted in breast milk.

INDICATIONS AND USES
Short-term relief of moderate to severe pain. ▪ Preoperative medication. ▪ Support of anesthesia.
Unlabeled uses: Treatment or prevention of shaking chills (rigors) caused by some medications (e.g., amphotericin B [all formulations], aldesleukin [Proleukin]).

CONTRAINDICATIONS
Acute bronchial asthma, hypersensitivity to meperidine, patients who have received MAO inhibitors (e.g., selegiline [Eldepryl]) in the previous 2 to 3 weeks, diarrhea resulting from poisoning until toxic material eliminated, pregnancy before labor, premature infants or labor and delivery of premature infants, pulmonary edema caused by chemical respiratory irritant, upper airway obstruction.

PRECAUTIONS
Use of meperidine as a first-line analgesic for pain is discouraged due to its short duration of action and the risk of accumulation of its toxic metabolite, normeperidine. Accumulation of normeperidine may increase the risk of toxicity (e.g., seizures). If its use in acute pain (in patients without renal or CNS disease) cannot be avoided, the American Pain Society and ISMP recommend limiting treatment to 48 hours or less and not exceeding 600 mg/24 hr. ▪ Use with caution in glaucoma, head injuries, increased intracranial pressure (elevates spinal fluid pressure), asthma, chronic obstructive pulmonary disease, decreased respiratory reserve or respiratory depression, supraventricular tachycardia, convulsions, acute abdominal conditions before diagnosis, the elderly and debilitated, and hepatic or renal insufficiency. ▪ Use with caution and in reduced doses in patients receiving concurrent therapy with other narcotic analgesics, general anesthetics, phenothiazines (e.g., promethazine [Phenergan], prochlorperazine [Compazine]), sedative-hypnotics (including barbiturates [e.g., phenobarbital]), tricyclic antidepressants (e.g., imipramine [Tofranil]), and other CNS depressants, including alcohol. Use may result in respiratory depression, hypotension, and profound sedation or coma. See Drug/Lab Interactions. ▪ Use with caution in patients with renal dysfunction; normeperidine may accumulate resulting in increased CNS toxicity. ▪ Use with caution in patients with sickle cell anemia, hypothyroidism, Addison's disease, pheochromocytoma, and prostatic hypertrophy or urethral stricture; may cause hypertension. Reduced doses may be indicated; see Dose Adjustments. ▪ Cough reflex is suppressed. ▪ Morphine is usually preferred for pain during cardiac arrhythmias. ▪ IM route frequently used. Frequent IM injections may lead to severe fibrosis of muscle tissue. ▪ Do not use in patients for any long-term pain relief (e.g., cancer).
Monitor: Oxygen, controlled respiratory equipment, and naloxone (Narcan) must always be available. ▪ Observe patient frequently to continuously based on amount of dose and monitor vital signs. ▪ Assess baseline pain, then assess pain with vital signs and/or more frequently if needed. Reassess after administration of meperidine and adjust dose or interval as required. ▪ Keep patient supine; orthostatic hypotension and fainting may occur; less likely with continuous low doses, but observe closely during ambulation. ▪ Uncontrolled pain causes sleep deprivation, decreases pain threshold, and increases pain. When pain is finally controlled, expect the patient to sleep more until recovery from sleep deprivation. ▪ With use the

active metabolite normeperidine accumulates to toxic levels; will lower seizure threshold. Monitor for twitching, jerking, shaky hands, tremors; may lead to grand mal seizure. ▪ Laxatives with or without stool softeners may be required to avoid constipation and fecal impaction. Maintain adequate hydration.

Patient Education: Avoid alcohol or other CNS depressants (e.g., barbiturates, benzodiazepines [e.g., diazepam (Valium)]). ▪ May cause blurred vision, dizziness, or drowsiness; use caution in tasks that require alertness. ▪ Request assistance with ambulation. ▪ May be habit forming.

Maternal/Child: Category C: see Contraindications. ▪ Use during delivery may cause depression of respiration and psychophysiologic functions in the newborn requiring resuscitation. ▪ May cause serious adverse reactions in nursing infants; discontinue breast-feeding or discontinue meperidine. ▪ Not recommended for IV use in pediatric patients but is used. Consider risk versus benefit before use in neonates or young infants. Rate of elimination is slower in neonates and young infants compared to older children or adults. May be more sensitive to effects (e.g., respiratory depression) and may cause paradoxical excitation.

Elderly: See Dose Adjustments and Precautions. ▪ Elimination rate is slower than in younger adults. ▪ May be more sensitive to effects (e.g., respiratory depression, constipation, urinary retention). ▪ Lower doses may provide effective analgesia. ▪ Consider age-related organ impairment.

DRUG/LAB INTERACTIONS

Potentiated by **acyclovir** (Zovirax), **antacids, anticholinergics, cimetidine** (Tagamet), **tricyclic antidepressants** (e.g., imipramine [Tofranil]), **isoniazid** (Nydrazid), **neostigmine, neuromuscular blocking agents** (e.g., atracurium [Tracrium]), **oral contraceptives, phenothiazines, general anesthetics, other narcotic analgesics, and CNS depressants including alcohol.** Side effects (e.g., CNS depression, constipation, hypotension) may be additive. Reduced dosage of both drugs may be indicated. ▪ Do not use with **MAO inhibitors** (e.g., selegiline [Eldepryl]); may cause cardiovascular collapse. ▪ Concurrent use with **protease inhibitors** (e.g., saquinavir [Invirase], ritonavir [Norvir]) not recommended. May increase meperidine serum concentrations and increase the risk of side effects, including seizures and cardiac arrhythmias. ▪ May increase clearance and decrease serum levels and effectiveness of **hydantoins** (e.g., phenytoin [Dilantin]). ▪ Metabolism increased and analgesic effects may be decreased or delayed in **smokers.** ▪ May aggravate adverse effects of **isoniazid** with concomitant use.

SIDE EFFECTS

Dizziness, flushing, light-headedness, nausea, postural hypotension, rash, restlessness, sedation, sweating, syncope, vomiting. Side effects associated with histamine release, convulsions, and constipation may be more common with meperidine than with most other narcotic analgesics.

Major: Apnea, cardiac arrest, cardiovascular collapse, cold and clammy skin, convulsions, dilated pupils, hypersensitivity reactions (e.g., anaphylaxis, pruritus), normeperidine toxicity (jerking, tremor, twitching, shaky hands, grand mal seizure), respiratory depression, shock, tremor.

ANTIDOTE

With increasing severity of minor side effects or onset of any major side effect, discontinue the drug and notify the physician. A patent airway, artificial respiration, oxygen therapy, and other symptomatic treatment must be instituted promptly. Naloxone hydrochloride (Narcan) will reverse serious reactions. In patients who are physically dependent on narcotics, either avoid the use of a narcotic antagonist or use extreme caution and doses as small as one-fifth to one-tenth of the usual initial dose to avoid precipitating an acute withdrawal syndrome. In all patients, adjust and titrate the dose of a narcotic antagonist to reverse side effects without reversing pain control. Avoid total reversal of pain control. Resuscitate as necessary.

MEROPENEM
(**mer**-oh-**PEN**-em)

Merrem I.V.

Antibacterial (carbapenem)

pH 7.3 to 8.3

USUAL DOSE

Dose ranges from 500 mg to 2 Gm and depends on type and severity of infection.

Skin and skin structure infections (complicated) in adults and pediatric patients weighing 50 kg or more: 500 mg every 8 hours. Increase to 1 Gm every 8 hours in diabetic foot infections.

Intra-abdominal infections in adults and pediatric patients weighing 50 kg or more: 1 Gm every 8 hours.

Febrile neutropenia in adults and pediatric patients weighing 50 kg or more (unlabeled): 1 Gm every 8 hours.

Meningitis (unlabeled): 40 mg/kg every 8 hours (up to 6 Gm daily). Other clinicians recommend the use of a total dose of 6 Gm daily (2 Gm every 8 hours). Has been given concurrently with ceftriaxone (Rocephin) or cefotaxime (Claforan).

Burkholderia infections (melioidosis [unlabeled]): 25 mg/kg every 8 hours (up to 6 Gm daily) with concomitant administration of sulfamethoxazole/trimethoprim (8 mg/kg of oral trimethoprim daily in four divided doses). Other clinicians recommend meropenem 0.5 to 1 Gm every 8 hours with or without sulfamethoxazole/trimethoprim. Continue treatment for at least 14 days or until clinical improvement.

Liver abscess (unlabeled): 1 Gm every 8 hours for 2 to 3 weeks. Transfer to oral therapy and continue for 2 to 3 additional weeks.

Mild to moderate infection, other severe infections (unlabeled): 500 mg to 1 Gm every 8 hours.

Complicated urinary tract infections (unlabeled): 500 mg to 1 Gm every 8 hours.

PEDIATRIC DOSE

Skin and skin structure infections in pediatric patients over 3 months of age and less than 50 kg: 10 mg/kg every 8 hours. Maximum single dose every 8 hours is 500 mg.

Intra-abdominal infections in pediatric patients over 3 months of age and less than 50 kg: 20 mg/kg every 8 hours. Maximum single dose every 8 hours is 1 Gm.

Meningitis in pediatric patients over 3 months of age and less than 50 kg: 40 mg/kg every 8 hours. Maximum single dose every 8 hours is 2 Gm.

Meningitis in pediatric patients weighing 50 kg or more: 2 Gm every 8 hours.
Febrile neutropenia in pediatric patients 3 months of age and older and less than 50 kg (unlabeled): 20 mg/kg every 8 hours.
Burkholderia infections in pediatric patients over 3 months of age and less than 40 kg (unlabeled): 10 to 20 mg/kg every 8 hours for **melioidosis or glanders.** Concomitant administration of sulfamethoxazole/trimethoprim may be indicated in severely ill patients.
Burkholderia infections in pediatric patients weighing 40 kg or more (unlabeled): Same as adult dose.

DOSE ADJUSTMENTS
Reduce dose required if CrCl is less than 51 mL/min based on the following chart.

Meropenem Recommended IV Dosage Schedule for Adults with Impaired Renal Function		
Creatinine Clearance (mL/min)	Dose (dependent on type of infection)	Dosing Interval
26-50 mL/min	Recommended dose	Every 12 hours
10-25 mL/min	One half recommended dose	Every 12 hours
<10 mL/min	One half recommended dose	Every 24 hours

Consult package insert or front matter of this text for formula to convert SCr to CrCl. ▪ No dose adjustment necessary in impaired hepatic function. ▪ Reduced dose may be required in the elderly based on decreased renal function. ▪ Information is inadequate for use in patients on hemodialysis, and there is no experience with peritoneal dialysis. ▪ No experience in pediatric patients with renal impairment.

DILUTION
Injection: Reconstitute each 500 mg with 10 mL SW (1 Gm with 20 mL). Yields 50 mg/mL. Shake to dissolve and let stand until clear. May be given as an IV injection or further diluted with 50 to 250 mL of **compatible** infusion solutions (see Infusion and Compatibility).
Infusion: Available as infusion vials that may be directly reconstituted with a **compatible** solution and then infused. Concentration may range from 2.5 to 50 mg/mL. Alternately, withdraw 10 or 20 mL of a **compatible** solution (see Compatibility) from an infusion bag for the reconstitution. Inject the reconstituted solution into the same infusion bag for administration.
Storage: Store unopened vials (dry powder) at RT (20° to 25° C [68° to 77° F]). Use of freshly prepared solutions preferred. Vials for injection stable at room temperature for 2 hours after reconstitution and for 12 hours refrigerated. Infusion vials reconstituted with NS having a final concentration of 2.5 to 50 mg/mL are stable for up to 2 hours at CRT and up to 18 hours at 4° C (39° F). Stability of all other dilutions (syringe for injection or solutions for infusion) is dependent on diluent and room temperature or refrigeration. Range is from 1 hour to 4 hours at 15° to 25° C (59° to 77° F) and 4 to 24 hours at 4° C (39° F); see package insert or consult pharmacist. Do not freeze.

COMPATIBILITY   (Underline Indicates Conflicting Compatibility Information)
Consider any drug NOT listed as compatible to be INCOMPATIBLE until consulting a pharmacist; specific conditions may apply.
Manufacturer states, "Meropenem should not be mixed or physically added to solutions containing other drugs; **compatibility** not established."
  One source suggests the following **compatibilities:**
Solution: Compatible under specific conditions (see Storage) with NS, D5W, D10W, D5NS, D5/¼NS, KCl 0.15% in D5W, Na Bicarbonate 0.02% in D5W, D5 in Normosol-M, D5LR, D2½ in ½NS, Mannitol 2.5%, R, LR, Na Lactate ⅙ M, Na Bicarbonate 5%.
Additive: *Not recommended by manufacturer.* Acyclovir (Zovirax), aminophylline, atropine, dexamethasone (Decadron), dobutamine, dopamine, doxycycline, enalaprilat (Vasotec IV), fluconazole (Diflucan), furosemide (Lasix), gentamicin, heparin, insulin (regular), magnesium sulfate, metoclopramide (Reglan), morphine, norepinephrine (Levophed), ondansetron (Zofran), phenobarbital (Luminal), ranitidine (Zantac), vancomycin, zidovudine (AZT, Retrovir).
Y-site: Acyclovir (Zovirax), aminophylline, anidulafungin (Eraxis), atropine, calcium gluconate, caspofungin (Cancidas), dexamethasone (Decadron), digoxin (Lanoxin), diphenhydramine (Benadryl), docetaxel (Taxotere), doxycycline, enalaprilat (Vasotec IV), fluconazole (Diflucan), furosemide (Lasix), gentamicin, heparin, insulin (regular), linezolid (Zyvox), metoclopramide (Reglan), milrinone (Primacor), morphine, norepinephrine (Levophed), ondansetron (Zofran), phenobarbital (Luminal), potassium chloride (KCl), vancomycin, vasopressin, zidovudine (AZT, Retrovir).

RATE OF ADMINISTRATION
Same rate is used for adults and pediatric patients over 3 months of age.
IV injection: A single dose (up to 1 Gm [20 mL] after dilution) over 3 to 5 minutes.
Intermittent infusion: A single dose over 15 to 30 minutes.

ACTIONS
A synthetic, broad-spectrum, carbapenem antibiotic. Bactericidal to selected gram-negative, gram-positive, and anaerobic organisms. Bactericidal activity results from the inhibition of cell wall synthesis. Readily penetrates the cell wall of susceptible organisms to reach penicillin-binding protein targets. Has significant stability to hydrolysis by penicillinases and cephalosporinases produced by gram-positive and gram-negative bacteria. Peak plasma concentrations reached by the end of an infusion. Penetrates well into most body fluids and tissues, including cerebrospinal fluid. Peak fluid and tissue concentrations reached in 0.5 to 1.5 hours. Minimal protein binding. Elimination half-life averages 1 hour in adults, 1.5 hours in pediatric patients age 3 months to 2 years. 70% recovered as unchanged drug in urine within 12 hours. Not yet known if it crosses the placental barrier or is secreted in breast milk.

INDICATIONS AND USES
Treatment of intra-abdominal infections (e.g., complicated appendicitis, peritonitis) caused by specific susceptible organisms. ■ Treatment of complicated skin and skin structure infections, including diabetic foot infections, caused by specific susceptible organisms. ■ Treatment of bacterial meningitis in pediatric patients 3 months of age and older caused by specific susceptible organisms.

Unlabeled uses: Treatment of febrile neutropenia. ▪ Treatment of meningitis in adults. ▪ Treatment of Burkholderia infections. ▪ Treatment of acute pulmonary exacerbations in cystic fibrosis patients with chronic lower respiratory tract infections with susceptible organisms (orphan drug status). ▪ Treatment of liver abscess, complicated urinary tract infections, and other mild, moderate, or severe infections.

CONTRAINDICATIONS

History of hypersensitivity to meropenem, its components, any other carbapenem antibiotic (e.g., imipenem-cilastatin [Primaxin]), or patients with hypersensitivity to beta-lactams; see Precautions.

PRECAUTIONS

Specific sensitivity studies are indicated to determine susceptibility of the causative organism to meropenem. ▪ To reduce the development of drug-resistant bacteria and maintain its effectiveness, meropenem should be used to treat or prevent only those infections proven or strongly suspected to be caused by bacteria. ▪ Serious and occasionally fatal hypersensitivity reactions have been reported in patients receiving therapy with beta-lactams (e.g., penicillins, cephalosporins, carbapenems). More likely in patients with a history of sensitivity to multiple allergens; obtain a careful history. Cross-sensitivity is possible. ▪ May cause seizures in patients with a history of CNS disorders (e.g., brain lesions, history of seizures) or with bacterial meningitis and/or compromised renal function. Use extreme caution; continue administration of anticonvulsants in patients with known seizure disorders. ▪ Use with caution in patients with moderately severe impaired renal function (CrCl 10 to 26 mL/min); thrombocytopenia may occur and incidence of heart failure, kidney failure, and shock may be increased; see Dose Adjustments. ▪ Staphylococci resistant to methicillin/oxacillin must be considered resistant to meropenem. ▪ May have cross-resistance with strains resistant to other carbapenems (e.g., imipenem-cilastatin [Primaxin]). ▪ Has been found to eliminate concurrent bacteremia associated with bacterial meningitis. ▪ Avoid prolonged use of drug; superinfection caused by overgrowth of nonsusceptible organisms may result. ▪ *Clostridium difficile*–associated diarrhea (CDAD) has been reported. May range from mild diarrhea to fatal colitis. Consider in patients who present with diarrhea during or after treatment with meropenem. ▪ See Drug/Lab Interactions.

Monitor: Anaphylaxis has been reported. Emergency equipment must always be available. ▪ Monitor infusion site for inflammation and/or extravasation. May cause thrombophlebitis. ▪ Monitor for S/S of CNS reactions (e.g., focal tremors, myoclonus, seizures). ▪ Monitor renal, hepatic, and hemopoietic systems in prolonged therapy. ▪ Each 1 Gm contains 3.92 mEq of sodium; monitoring of electrolytes may be indicated. ▪ See Drug/Lab Interactions and Side Effects.

Patient Education: Report any itching, rash, shortness of breath, or twitching sensation immediately. ▪ Report any burning, pain, or stinging at injection site. ▪ Promptly report diarrhea or bloody stools that occur during treatment or up to several months after an antibiotic has been discontinued; may indicate CDAD and require treatment. ▪ Patients with a history of seizures should review medication profile with physician before taking meropenem; see Drug/Lab Interactions.

Maternal/Child: Category B: safety for use in pregnancy not established; use only if clearly needed. ▪ Use caution during breast-feeding. Not known if meropenem is secreted in breast milk; safety not established. ■ Approved only for use in infants and other pediatric patients over 3 months of age. **Elderly:** Consider age-related renal impairment; plasma clearance is decreased with decreased renal function; see Dose Adjustments. Monitoring of renal function is suggested. Response is similar to that seen in younger patients; however, greater sensitivity in the elderly cannot be ruled out. See Precautions.

DRUG/LAB INTERACTIONS

Carbapenems may reduce serum **valproic acid** concentrations to subtherapeutic levels, resulting in a loss of seizure control. Monitor valproic acid levels. Consider alternative antibacterial therapy. If administration of meropenem is necessary, supplemental anticonvulsant therapy should be considered. ■ **Probenecid** inhibits renal excretion and increases serum levels of meropenem, extending its half-life and increasing systemic exposure; coadministration is not recommended. ■ May be synergistic with **aminoglycosides** against some isolates of *Pseudomonas aeruginosa*.

SIDE EFFECTS

Toxicity rate is usually low. *Pediatric patients:* Diarrhea, diaper area moniliasis, glossitis, oral moniliasis, rash, vomiting. *Adults:* Anemia, constipation, diarrhea, headache, nausea and vomiting, rash. Injection site reactions (e.g., edema, inflammation, pain, phlebitis, pruritus) are most common. Apnea, pruritus, sepsis, and shock also occurred in more than 1% of patients. Many other side effects including increases or decreases in hematologic, hepatic, and renal lab tests may occur in fewer than 1% of patients. *Adults and pediatric patients:* Full scope of hypersensitivity reactions, including anaphylaxis, have occurred in a few patients. **Post-Marketing:** Agranulocytosis, angioedema, bleeding events (e.g., GI bleeding, epistaxis), CDAD, erythema multiforme, hemolytic anemia, leukopenia, neutropenia, positive direct or indirect Coombs' test, Stevens-Johnson syndrome, seizures, shock, sepsis, thrombocytopenia, and toxic epidermal necrolysis can occur.

ANTIDOTE

Notify physician of all side effects. Most treated symptomatically. Discontinue immediately if a hypersensitivity reaction occurs. Treat hypersensitivity reactions as indicated; may require epinephrine, airway management, oxygen, IV fluids, antihistamines (e.g., diphenhydramine [Benadryl]), corticosteroids (e.g., hydrocortisone sodium succinate [Solu-Cortef]), and pressor amines (e.g., dopamine). If focal tremors, myoclonus, or seizures occur, evaluate neurologically, initiate anticonvulsant therapy, and decide whether to decrease or discontinue meropenem. Mild cases of CDAD may respond to discontinuation of meropenem. Treat CDAD with fluids, electrolytes, protein supplements, and oral vancomycin (Vancocin) or metronidazole (Flagyl) as indicated. In severe cases, surgical evaluation may be indicated. Readily removed by hemodialysis.

MESNA
(**MEZ**-nah)

Ifex/Mesnex Kit, Ifosfamide/Mesna Kit, Mesnex, ✚Uromitexan

Antidote
Antineoplastic adjunct
Prophylactic for hemorrhagic cystitis

pH 6.5 to 8.5

USUAL DOSE
Specific testing recommended before each dose of ifosfamide; see Monitor.

Intravenous dose: Total daily dose is 60% of the ifosfamide dose equally divided into 3 doses. A single dose of mesna equal to 20% of the ifosfamide dose is given at the time of the ifosfamide injection and repeated 4 hours and 8 hours later (e.g., ifosfamide 1.2 Gm/M^2 would require mesna 240 mg/M^2 with the ifosfamide, 240 mg/M^2 in 4 hours, and again at 8 hours). The initial mesna dose each day may be mixed with the ifosfamide. Appears to be **compatible.** Available combined in solution with ifosfamide and as a single agent in tablet form.

Combination of intravenous and oral doses: At the time of the ifosfamide injection, give a single IV dose of mesna equal to 20% of the ifosfamide dose. At 2 hours and at 6 hours after each dose of ifosfamide, administer mesna tablets PO in a dose equal to 40% of the ifosfamide dose. The total daily dose of mesna (IV [20%] and PO [80%] combined) is 100% of the ifosfamide dose.

DOSE ADJUSTMENTS
Dose of mesna must be repeated each day ifosfamide is administered and adjusted with each increase or decrease of the ifosfamide dose.

DILUTION
Each 100 mg (1 mL) must be diluted in a minimum of 4 mL D5W, D5NS, D5/¼NS, D5/⅓NS, D5/½NS, NS, or LR. Desired concentration is 20 mg/mL.

Filters: Manufacturer's studies measured the potency of ifosfamide in combination with mesna through a 5-micron filter. No significant drug loss for ifosfamide; mesna was not measured.

Storage: Store at CRT before use. Opened multidose vials may be stored at CRT and used for up to 8 days. Diluted solutions are stable for 24 hours at 25° C (77° F). Mesna oxidizes to disulfide dimesna when exposed to oxygen.

COMPATIBILITY (Underline Indicates Conflicting Compatibility Information)
Consider any drug NOT listed as compatible to be INCOMPATIBLE until consulting a pharmacist; specific conditions may apply.
One source suggests the following **compatibilities:**

Additive: <u>Cyclophosphamide (Cytoxan)</u>, ifosfamide (Ifex).

Y-site: Allopurinol (Aloprim), amifostine (Ethyol), aztreonam (Azactam), cefepime (Maxipime), cladribine (Leustatin), docetaxel (Taxotere), doxorubicin liposomal (Doxil), etoposide phosphate (Etopophos), filgrastim (Neupogen), fludarabine (Fludara), gallium nitrate (Ganite), gemcitabine (Gemzar), granisetron (Kytril), linezolid (Zyvox), melphalan (Alkeran), methotrexate, <u>micafungin (Mycamine)</u>, ondansetron (Zofran), oxaliplatin (Eloxatin), paclitaxel (Taxol), pemetrexed (Alimta), piperacillin/tazobactam (Zosyn), sargramostim (Leukine), sodium bicarbonate, teniposide (Vumon), thiotepa, vinorelbine (Navelbine).

RATE OF ADMINISTRATION

A single dose over a minimum of 1 minute given as a single agent. Administer at rate for ifosfamide if given together. Another source recommends administering as an infusion over 15 to 30 minutes or as a continuous infusion maintained for 12 to 24 hours after completion of the ifosfamide infusion.

ACTIONS

A detoxifying agent. Reacts chemically in the kidney with urotoxic ifosfamide metabolites to detoxify them and inhibit hemorrhagic cystitis. Remains in the intravascular compartment and much of a single dose is excreted within 4 hours in urine. Does not appear to interfere with the antitumor efficacy of ifosfamide.

INDICATIONS AND USES

A prophylactic agent used to reduce the incidence of hemorrhagic cystitis caused by ifosfamide.

Unlabeled uses: May reduce the incidence of hemorrhagic cystitis caused by cyclophosphamide.

CONTRAINDICATIONS

Hypersensitivity to mesna or other thiol compounds.

PRECAUTIONS

Repeated doses are required to maintain adequate levels of mesna in the kidneys and bladder to detoxify urotoxic ifosfamide metabolites. ■ Hemorrhagic cystitis caused by ifosfamide is dose dependent. Mesna is most effective when ifosfamide dose is less than 1.2 $Gm/M^2/24$ hr. Somewhat less effective when ifosfamide dose is 2 to 4 $Gm/M^2/24$ hr. If hematuria develops with appropriate doses of mesna, ifosfamide dose may need to be reduced or discontinued. ■ Does not inhibit any other side effects or toxicities caused by ifosfamide therapy. ■ Not effective in preventing hematuria caused by other conditions (e.g., thrombocytopenia). ■ Hypersensitivity reactions ranging from mild to anaphylaxis have been reported. Patients with autoimmune disorders who are treated with cyclophosphamide and mesna may have a higher incidence of hypersensitivity reactions.

Monitor: Before administering each dose of ifosfamide, obtain a morning specimen of urine and test for hematuria. Depending on the severity of the hematuria, dose reduction or discontinuation of ifosfamide may be required. ■ If emesis occurs within 2 hours of taking PO mesna, either repeat the PO dose or administer an IV dose.

Patient Education: Drink at least one quart of liquid daily. ▪ Report pink or red urine immediately. ▪ Report emesis within 2 hours of taking PO mesna.

Maternal/Child: Category B: use during pregnancy only if benefits clearly outweigh risks. ▪ Discontinue breast-feeding. ▪ Multidose vial contains benzyl alcohol. Do not use in neonates or infants.

Elderly: Dosing should be cautious; however, the ratio of ifosfamide to mesna should remain the same.

DRUG/LAB INTERACTIONS

May cause a false-positive reaction for **urinary ketones.** If a red-violet color develops, glacial acetic acid returns the coloring to violet.

SIDE EFFECTS

Average dose: Anorexia, bad taste in the mouth, coughing, decreased platelets associated with hypersensitivity reactions, diarrhea, dizziness, fever, flushing, headache, hyperesthesia, hypersensitivity reactions, hypertension, hypotension, increased liver enzymes, influenza-like symptoms, injection site reactions, malaise, myalgia, nausea, pharyngitis, soft stool, somnolence, ST-segment elevation, tachycardia, tachypnea, vomiting.

Overdose: Convulsions, cyanosis, diarrhea, dyspnea, fatigue, headache, hematuria, hypersensitivity reactions, hypotension, limb pain, nausea, tremor.

ANTIDOTE

No specific antidote. Keep physician informed of all side effects. Notify promptly if signs of overdose occur. Resuscitate as necessary.

METHADONE HYDROCHLORIDE BBW

(**METH**-ah-dohn hy-droh-**KLOR**-eyed)

Opioid analgesic
(agonist)
Narcotic abstinence
syndrome suppressant

Dolophine

pH 4.5 to 6.5

USUAL DOSE

Parenteral administration permitted only under specific conditions; see Indications and Precautions.

Dosing is complex and requires extensive individualization. Extended half-life, potential for prolonged respiratory depressant effects, retention in the liver (prolonging the potential duration of action), and high interpatient variability in absorption, metabolism, and relative analgesic potency must be considered.

Treatment of pain: Consider the following factors for each patient before determining an initial dose:

- Total daily dose, potency, and specific characteristics of any previously administered opioid.
- Will it be used for acute or chronic methadone dosing?
- Patient's degree of opioid tolerance.
- Patient's age, general condition, and medical status.
- Concurrent medications; see Drug/Lab Interactions.
- Type, severity, and expected duration of patient's pain.
- Acceptable balance between pain control and adverse effects.

Initial analgesic in patients who are not being treated with other opioids and are not tolerant to other opioids: 2.5 to 10 mg every 8 to 12 hours. Titrate slowly to effect. More frequent dosing may be required to maintain adequate analgesia; use extreme caution, consider extended half-life, and avoid overdose.

Conversion from oral to parenteral methadone: Begin with a 2:1 ratio (e.g., 10 mg oral methadone to 5 mg parenteral methadone); see Precautions.

Switching from other chronic opioids to parenteral methadone: Dose conversion ratios and cross-tolerance are uncertain; deaths have occurred in opioid-tolerant patients during conversion to methadone. Individualize dose based on patient's prior opioid exposure, general medical condition, concomitant medication, and anticipated breakthrough medication use. Titrate to achieve adequate pain relief balanced against tolerability of side effects. Adjust dose and/or dosing interval as necessary. The following charts are examples of conversions.

Conversion from Oral Morphine to IV Methadone for Chronic Administration		
Total Daily Baseline Oral Morphine Dose	Estimated Total Daily Oral Methadone Dose as a Percentage of Total Daily Morphine Dose*	Estimated Daily IV Methadone Dose as a Percentage of Total Daily Oral Morphine Dose*
<100 mg	20% to 30%	10% to 15%
100 mg to 300 mg	10% to 20%	5% to 10%
300 mg to 600 mg	8% to 12%	4% to 6%
600 mg to 1,000 mg	5% to 10%	3% to 5%
>1,000 mg	Less than 5%	Less than 3%

*Divide total daily methadone dose as necessary to achieve desired dosing schedule (e.g., divide by 3 for administration every 8 hours).

Conversion from Parenteral Morphine to IV Methadone for Chronic Administration	
Total Daily Baseline Parenteral Morphine Dose	Estimated Daily IV Methadone Dose as a Percentage of Total Daily Morphine Dose*
10 mg to 30 mg	40% to 66%
30 mg to 50 mg	27% to 66%
50 mg to 100 mg	22% to 50%
100 mg to 200 mg	15% to 34%
200 mg to 500 mg	10% to 20%

*Divide total daily methadone dose as necessary to achieve desired dosing schedule (e.g., divide by 3 for administration every 8 hours).

DOSE ADJUSTMENTS
Lower-end initial doses are indicated in the elderly; consider impaired organ function and concomitant disease or drug therapy. ▪ Reduced initial doses are indicated in debilitated patients and in those with severe impaired hepatic or renal function. ▪ Clearance may be increased and half-life decreased during pregnancy. Increased doses or shorter intervals between doses may be indicated; see Maternal/Child.

DILUTION
May be given undiluted; however, to facilitate titration, further dilution of each mL with 1 to 5 mL of NS is appropriate. May be given through Y-tube or three-way stopcock of infusion set.

Storage: A multidose vial; store in carton at CRT protected from light until contents have been used.

COMPATIBILITY   (Underline Indicates Conflicting Compatibility Information)
Consider any drug NOT listed as compatible to be INCOMPATIBLE until consulting a pharmacist; specific conditions may apply.
One source suggests the following **compatibilities**:
Y-site: Atropine, dexamethasone (Decadron), diazepam (Valium), diphenhydramine (Benadryl), haloperidol (Haldol), ketorolac (Toradol), lorazepam (Ativan), metoclopramide (Reglan), midazolam (Versed), phenobarbital (Luminal).

RATE OF ADMINISTRATION

A single dose as an injection over a minimum of several minutes. Titrate according to symptom relief and respiratory rate; side effects may be increased if rate of injection is too rapid.

ACTIONS

A synthetic opioid analgesic with actions similar to those of morphine. Duration of analgesic action is from 4 to 8 hours. Respiratory depressant effects occur later and persist longer than its peak analgesic effects. With repeated dosing, methadone may be retained in the liver and then slowly released, thereby prolonging the duration of action while plasma concentrations are low. Highly protein bound (85% to 90%). Metabolized in the liver by various enzymes (including cytochrome P_{450} enzymes) to inactive metabolites. Half-life is prolonged (ranges from 8 to 59 hours). Eliminated by extensive biotransformation followed by renal and fecal elimination. Secreted in saliva, breast milk, amniotic fluid, and umbilical cord plasma.

INDICATIONS AND USES

Treatment of moderate to severe pain not responsive to non-narcotic analgesics. ▪ Temporary treatment in opioid-dependent patients unable to take oral medication. ▪ Used PO for detoxification or maintenance in opioid addiction. ▪ Parenteral products are not approved for outpatient use.

CONTRAINDICATIONS

Known hypersensitivity to methadone or any of its components. ▪ Any situation in which opioids are contraindicated (e.g., patients with respiratory depression [where resuscitative equipment is not readily available or in unmonitored settings], patients with acute bronchial asthma or hypercarbia). ▪ Other sources add paralytic ileus and concurrent use of selegiline (Zelapar, Eldepryl).

PRECAUTIONS

If the parenteral route is indicated, the IV route is preferred; absorption by the IM or SC routes is unpredictable and may cause local tissue reaction. ▪ Schedule II opioid agonists, including hydromorphone, morphine, oxymorphone, oxycodone, fentanyl, and methadone, have the highest potential for abuse and risk of producing respiratory depression. Alcohol, CNS depressants, and other opioids potentiate the respiratory depressant effects of hydromorphone, increasing the risk of respiratory depression that might result in death; see Drug/Lab Interactions. ▪ Deaths, cardiac and respiratory, have been reported during initiation and conversion of pain patients to methadone treatment from treatment with other opioid agonists. Close monitoring is required during these times as well as during dose titration. ▪ The peak respiratory depressant effects of methadone usually occur later and last longer than the peak analgesic effects. Iatrogenic overdose may occur with short-term use, particularly during treatment initiation and dose titration. ▪ Patients tolerant to other opioids may still be sensitive to methadone. This incomplete cross-tolerance makes dose selection difficult when converting to methadone. Deaths have been reported. A high degree of "opioid tolerance" does not eliminate the possibility of methadone toxicity. ▪ Prolongation of the QT interval and infrequent cases of arrhythmia (including torsades de pointes) have been reported. May occur with any dose but appears to be more common with higher dose treatment (greater than 200 mg/day). ▪ Use with caution in patients at risk for development of prolonged QT interval (e.g., cardiac conduction abnormalities, cardiac hypertrophy, hypokalemia, hypomagnesemia) and in patients receiving

concurrent treatment with other drugs that may induce electrolyte disturbances (e.g., diuretics, laxatives and, rarely, mineralocorticoid hormones)
or other drugs that may prolong the QT interval; see Drug/Lab
Interactions. ■ Initiate treatment for analgesic therapy in patients with
acute or chronic pain only if benefits outweigh the increased risk of QT
prolongation with high doses. ■ Use extreme caution in patients with
potential respiratory insufficiency (e.g., elderly or debilitated patients,
conditions accompanied by hypoxia or hypercapnia or decreased respiratory reserve [e.g., asthma, COPD, pulmonary disease or cor pulmonale,
severe obesity, sleep apnea syndrome, myxedema, kyphoscoliosis, CNS
depression, or coma]). Usual doses may decrease respiratory drive and
simultaneously increase airway resistance, resulting in apnea. Consider use
of non-opioid analgesics. If methadone is required, administer at lowest
effective dose under close medical supervision. ■ Use caution in elderly or
debilitated patients, severe impaired hepatic or renal function, Addison's
disease, hypothyroidism, prostatic hypertrophy, or urethral stricture; see
Dose Adjustments. ■ Use with caution in patients with head injury, other
intracranial lesions, or pre-existing increased intracranial pressure. Cerebrospinal fluid pressure may be markedly exaggerated, and the clinical
course of head injuries may be obscured. ■ May mask symptoms and
make diagnosis of acute abdominal conditions difficult. ■ May cause
severe hypotension in patients whose ability to maintain normal blood
pressure is compromised (e.g., severe volume depletion). ■ Patients with
impaired hepatic function may be at increased risk of accumulating
methadone after multiple dosing. ■ Because of their opioid tolerance,
patients receiving maintenance doses may require increased or more
frequent doses of opioids to treat physical trauma, postoperative pain, or
other acute pain. ■ Do not increase methadone dose for symptoms of
anxiety. ■ Abrupt discontinuation of methadone is not recommended; may
result in withdrawal symptoms (e.g., chills, lacrimation, myalgia, mydriasis, perspiration, restlessness, rhinorrhea, yawning), and may lead to
relapse of illicit drug use.

Monitor: Oxygen, controlled ventilation equipment, and naloxone (Narcan)
must always be available. ■ Observe patient frequently to continuously
based on amount of dose, and monitor VS. ■ Assess baseline pain, then
assess pain with vital signs or more frequently if needed. Reassess after
administration of methadone and adjust dose or interval as required. Keep
patient supine; orthostatic hypotension and fainting may occur; monitor
closely during ambulation. ■ Uncontrolled pain causes sleep deprivation,
decreases pain threshold, and increases pain. When pain is finally controlled, expect the patient to sleep more until recovered from sleep
deprivation. ■ Monitor ECG in patients who develop QT prolongation and
assess for modifiable risk factors (e.g., drugs with cardiac effects, drugs
that may cause electrolyte abnormalities, or drugs that may inhibit the
metabolism of methadone); see Drug/Lab Interactions. Consider alternate
therapies for pain management. ■ Laxatives with or without stool softeners
will be required to avoid constipation and fecal impaction, especially with
increased doses and extended use. Maintain adequate hydration. ■ See
Precautions and Drug/Lab Interactions.

Patient Education: Promptly report dizziness, light-headedness, palpitations, or syncope; may indicate a need for ECG monitoring. ■ Avoid
alcohol or other CNS depressants (e.g., barbiturates, benzodiazepines [e.g.,

diazepam (Valium)]). ▪ May cause blurred vision, dizziness, or drowsiness; use caution in tasks that require alertness. ▪ Request assistance with ambulation. ▪ May be habit forming.
Maternal/Child: Category C: potential benefit should justify potential risk to fetus. Compare the benefit of methadone to the risk of untreated addiction to illicit drugs. ▪ Total body clearance is increased during pregnancy and half-life is decreased (during 2nd and 3rd trimesters). May lead to withdrawal symptoms. Increases in dose or dosing at more frequent intervals may be indicated. ▪ Data is insufficient; however, women treated with methadone during pregnancy had improved prenatal care and did not appear to have an increased risk of miscarriage or premature delivery. Methadone in amniotic fluid and cord plasma has similar concentrations to maternal plasma. Newborn urine concentrations are less than maternal. ▪ Infants born to women treated with methadone during pregnancy may experience respiratory depression (consider methadone's long duration of action), and may be born physically dependent. Onset of withdrawal may occur in days or be delayed for 2 to 4 weeks. Withdrawal signs include fever, hyperactive reflexes, increased respiratory rate, increased stools, irritability and excessive crying, sneezing, tremors, vomiting, and yawning. May have reduced birth weight, length, and/or head circumference and some deficits in psychometric and behavioral tests. ▪ Discontinue or do not start breast-feeding. Women who are breast-feeding should wean gradually to prevent withdrawal symptoms in their infants. ▪ Safety and effectiveness for use in pediatric patients under 18 years of age not established. ▪ See Drug/Lab Interactions.
Elderly: Dosing should be cautious; see Dose Adjustments. ▪ Differences in response compared to younger adults not identified. ▪ See Precautions.
DRUG/LAB INTERACTIONS
May have additive effects with **other CNS depressants** (e.g., alcohol, general anesthetics, hypnotics or sedatives [e.g., benzodiazepines (e.g., diazepam [Valium], midazolam [Versed]), barbiturates [e.g., phenobarbital (Luminal)], other opioid analgesics, phenothiazines [e.g., prochlorperazine (Compazine)]). Concurrent use may result in hypotension, profound sedation, respiratory depression, coma, or death. ▪ Not recommended for concurrent administration with **opioid antagonists** (e.g., naloxone [Narcan], naltrexone [ReVia]), **mixed agonist/antagonists, or partial agonists** (e.g., buprenorphine [Buprenex], butorphanol [Stadol], nalbuphine, pentazocine [Talwin]); may precipitate withdrawal symptoms and/or reduce analgesic effect in patients maintained on methadone. ▪ Metabolism increased and serum concentrations decreased by **cytochrome P$_{450}$ inducers** (e.g., carbamazepine [Tegretol], phenobarbital [Luminal], phenytoin [Dilantin], rifampin [Rifadin], St. John's wort), efavirenz (Sustiva), nevirapine (Viramune), ritonavir (Norvir), and ritonavir/lopinavir combination (Kaletra). With concurrent administration, the effects of methadone are decreased; monitor for S/S of withdrawal, and adjust methadone dose as indicated. ▪ Metabolism decreased and serum concentrations increased by **cytochrome P$_{450}$ inhibitors** (e.g., azole antifungal agents [e.g., itraconazole (Sporanox), ketoconazole (Nizoral)], macrolide antibiotics [e.g., erythromycin], selective serotonin reuptake inhibitors (SSRIs) [e.g., fluvoxamine (Luvox), sertraline (Zoloft)]). With concurrent administration, monitor methadone serum concentrations to prevent methadone toxicity. ▪ May increase serum levels of **desipramine** (Norpramin). ▪ May increase AUC of

zidovudine and result in zidovudine toxicity. ▪ May decrease AUC and peak levels of **didanosine** (Videx) **and stavudine** (Zerit). ▪ Use caution with **MAO inhibitors** (e.g., selegiline [Eldepryl]) administered within 14 days and test for sensitivity. MAO inhibitors have caused cardiovascular collapse with other opioids (e.g., meperidine [Demerol]), not reported with methadone; see Contraindications. ▪ Use extreme caution with other **drugs that prolong the QT interval** (e.g., class IA antiarrhythmic agents [e.g., quinidine, procainamide (Pronestyl)], class III antiarrhythmic agents [e.g., amiodarone (Nexterone), sotalol (Betapace)], calcium channel blockers [e.g., diltiazem (Cardizem), verapamil], some neuroleptics [e.g., phenothiazines (e.g., chlorpromazine [Thorazine])], and tricyclic antidepressants [e.g., amitriptyline (Elavil), imipramine (Tofranil)]).

SIDE EFFECTS

Hypotension and respiratory depression are dose limiting. Respiratory arrest, shock, cardiac arrest, and death have occurred.

Dizziness, light-headedness, nausea and vomiting, sedation, and sweating occur most frequently. Other reported side effects include abdominal pain, agitation, anorexia, antidiuretic effect, arrhythmias, asthenia, biliary tract spasm, cardiomyopathy, confusion, constipation, chronic hepatitis, dry mouth, edema, euphoria, flushing, glossitis, headache, heart failure, hypokalemia, hypomagnesemia, hypotension, palpitations, phlebitis, prolonged QT interval, pulmonary edema, pruritus, seizures, skin rashes, syncope, thrombocytopenia (reversible), torsades de pointes, urticaria, urinary retention or hesitancy, visual disturbances.

Overdose: Bradycardia, cold and clammy skin, constricted pupils, hypotension, respiratory depression (decrease in respiratory rate and/or tidal volume, Cheyne-Stokes respiration, cyanosis), skeletal muscle flaccidity, somnolence progressing to stupor or coma. Apnea, circulatory collapse, cardiac arrest, and death may occur.

ANTIDOTE

Keep physician informed of all side effects; may be treated symptomatically. During prolonged administration (patients on maintenance), side effects usually decrease with time. Lower doses of methadone may be indicated for dizziness, light-headedness, nausea and vomiting, sedation, and sweating. Management of major side effects or overdose requires establishing a patent airway, instituting assisted or controlled ventilation, IV fluids, vasopressors, and other supportive measures as indicated. Nontolerant patients may be treated with naloxone (Narcan). These opioid antagonists have a much shorter duration of action than methadone and may need repeating for up to 48 hours. Continuous monitoring is required. Do not administer opioid antagonists to physically dependent patients unless clinically significant respiratory or cardiovascular depression occurs. May precipitate an acute withdrawal syndrome. Forced diuresis, peritoneal dialysis, hemodialysis, or charcoal hemoperfusion may not be useful to increase methadone or metabolite elimination; however, urine acidification has been shown to increase renal elimination of methadone.

METHOTREXATE SODIUM BBW

(meth-oh-**TREKS**-ayt **SO**-dee-um)

Methotrexate PF, MTX

Antineoplastic (antimetabolite)
Antipsoriatic
Antirheumatic

pH 8.5

USUAL DOSE

Many dose limitations based on patient condition, renal and hepatic function, and concomitant drugs or therapies; see Precautions/Monitor. Doses between 100 and 500 mg/M^2 *may require* leucovorin calcium rescue. Doses over 500 mg/M^2 *require* leucovorin calcium rescue; see leucovorin calcium or levoleucovorin (Fusilev) monograph. Part of numerous protocols that change as new advances in antileukemic therapy are developed for all diagnoses. Selections from those protocols are included in the following text.

Acute lymphoblastic leukemia: *Induction:* 3.3 mg/M^2 in combination with prednisone 60 mg/M^2. Give daily if tolerated, and continue for up to 8 weeks or until satisfactory response (usually 4 to 6 weeks). Usually given PO.

Maintenance: Dose individualized; 15 mg/M^2/dose administered 2 times weekly IM or PO (a total dose of 30 mg/M^2) or 2.5 mg/kg IV every 14 days has been used.

Gastric cancers (unlabeled): One regimen administers methotrexate 1.5 Gm/M^2 on Day 1 followed by 1.5 Gm/M^2 of fluorouracil on Day 1 (administer 1 hour after methotrexate infusion is complete), leucovorin calcium 15 mg/M^2 PO every 6 hours for 48 hours starting 24 hours after methotrexate, and doxorubicin 30 mg/M^2 IV on Day 15. Repeated every 4 weeks.

Mycosis fungoides: 5 to 50 mg once weekly in the early stages of disease. Adjust dose or discontinue as indicated by patient response and hematologic monitoring. 15 to 37.5 mg twice weekly may be used in patients who respond poorly to weekly therapy. Usually given PO or IM, but combination chemotherapy regimens, including higher doses of IV methotrexate with leucovorin calcium rescue, have been used in advanced stages of the disease.

Breast cancer (unlabeled): 40 mg/M^2 on Days 1 and 8 of each cycle. Given in combination with PO cyclophosphamide 100 mg/M^2 on Days 1 through 14 of each cycle and fluorouracil 600 mg/M^2 on Days 1 and 8 of each cycle. In patients over 60 years of age, reduce the initial methotrexate dose to 30 mg/M^2 and the initial fluorouracil dose to 400 mg/M^2. Repeat monthly (allows a 2-week rest period between cycles) for 6 to 12 cycles. Another source suggests methotrexate 30 to 60 mg/M^2 on Days 1 and 8 every 3 to 4 weeks.

Psoriasis and rheumatoid arthritis: 10 to 25 mg once a week. Some references suggest an initial test dose of 10 mg followed by gradually increased doses until adequate response. Sources suggest 30 mg/week as a maximum dose. Use smallest effective dose. Usually given PO or IM. May be used in combination with infliximab; see infliximab monograph.

Osteosarcoma: One regimen recommends 12 Gm/M^2 as a single dose given as an infusion over 4 hours. Begin the fourth week after surgery and repeat weekly at Weeks 5, 6, 7, 11, 12, 15, 16, 29, 30, 44, and 45. A peak serum concentration of 1,000 micromolars/L at the end of the infusion is desired. Dose may be increased to 15 Gm/M^2 if required. Must be accompanied by leucovorin calcium rescue; see leucovorin calcium or levoleucovorin (Fusilev) monograph. Leucovorin calcium may be given IV or PO; levoleucovorin is IV only. *Osteosarcoma also requires combination chemotherapy.* Protocols vary but may include methotrexate in combination with doxorubicin, with cisplatin, and with the combination of bleomycin, cyclophosphamide, and dactinomycin (BCD regimen). These massive doses are highly individualized and require exacting calculations and constant patient monitoring; see Precautions/Monitor.

PEDIATRIC DOSE

Safety for use in pediatric patients is limited to chemotherapy and in polyarticular-course juvenile rheumatoid arthritis. May contain benzyl alcohol; not recommended for use in neonates. See Maternal/Child.

DOSE ADJUSTMENTS

Administer 75% of dose if bilirubin is between 3.1 and 5 or if transaminases are greater than 3 times the ULN; if bilirubin above 5, omit dose. ▪ Reduced doses may be required in patients with impaired renal function. Suggested guidelines are to administer 75% of a dose with a CrCl of 61 to 80 mL/min, 70% of a dose with a CrCl of 51 to 60 mL/min, 30% to 50% of a dose with a CrCl of 10 to 50 mL/min, and avoid use with a CrCl of less than 10 mL/min. Supplemental doses are not necessary in hemodialysis or peritoneal dialysis patients; methotrexate is not dialyzable. ▪ Reduced dose may be required in patients with ascites or pleural effusions, in the very young or very elderly, in the debilitated, and in other diseases; see Precautions. ▪ Often used with other antineoplastic drugs to achieve tumor remission. ▪ See Drug/Lab Interactions.

DILUTION

Specific techniques required; see Precautions. 25 mg/mL is the maximum concentration that can be given IV. Reconstitution of each 5 mg with 2 mL of preservative-free D5W or NS is preferred. Each milliliter equals 2.5 mg of methotrexate. Available in preservative-free solution. Do not use formulations or diluents with preservatives (e.g., bacteriostatic) for high-dose therapy or intrathecal injection. 1-Gm vial available for high-dose use with appropriate dilution. Not usually added to IV solutions when given in smaller doses (less than 100 mg). Discard solution if a precipitate forms. May be given through Y-tube or three-way stopcock of a free-flowing IV.

A single dose may be further diluted with D5W or NS immediately before use as an infusion with higher (100 mg or more) methotrexate doses.

Filters: No data available from manufacturer. Another source indicates no significant drug loss filtered through a nylon 0.2-micron filter.

Storage: Store in unopened container at CRT; protect from light. If prepared without a preservative, use immediately. May be stable up to 24 hours with a preservative.

COMPATIBILITY   (Underline Indicates Conflicting Compatibility Information)
Consider any drug NOT listed as compatible to be INCOMPATIBLE until consulting a pharmacist; specific conditions may apply.
One source suggests the following **compatibilities:**
Additive: Cyclophosphamide (Cytoxan), cytarabine (ARA-C), fluorouracil (5-FU), ondansetron (Zofran), sodium bicarbonate, vincristine. Other sources add dacarbazine (DTIC), furosemide (Lasix), hydrocortisone sodium succinate (Solu-Cortef), leucovorin calcium.
Y-site: Allopurinol (Aloprim), amifostine (Ethyol), amphotericin B cholesteryl (Amphotec), asparaginase (Elspar), aztreonam (Azactam), bleomycin (Blenoxane), cefepime (Maxipime), ceftriaxone (Rocephin), cisplatin (Platinol), cyclophosphamide (Cytoxan), cytarabine (ARA-C), daunorubicin (Cerubidine), dexamethasone (Decadron), diphenhydramine (Benadryl), doripenem (Doribax), doxorubicin (Adriamycin), doxorubicin liposomal (Doxil), droperidol (Inapsine), etoposide (VePesid), etoposide phosphate (Etopophos), famotidine (Pepcid IV), filgrastim (Neupogen), fludarabine (Fludara), fluorouracil (5-FU), furosemide (Lasix), gallium nitrate (Ganite), ganciclovir (Cytovene), granisetron (Kytril), heparin, hydromorphone (Dilaudid), imipenem-cilastatin (Primaxin), leucovorin calcium, linezolid (Zyvox), lorazepam (Ativan), melphalan (Alkeran), mesna (Mesnex), methylprednisolone (Solu-Medrol), metoclopramide (Reglan), mitomycin (Mutamycin), morphine, ondansetron (Zofran), oxacillin (Bactocill), oxaliplatin (Eloxatin), paclitaxel (Taxol), piperacillin/tazobactam (Zosyn), prochlorperazine (Compazine), ranitidine (Zantac), sargramostim (Leukine), teniposide (Vumon), thiotepa, vancomycin, vinblastine, vincristine, vinorelbine (Navelbine).
RATE OF ADMINISTRATION
IV injection: Each 10 mg or fraction thereof over 1 minute.
Infusion: A single dose equally distributed over 30 minutes to 4 hours or as prescribed by protocol.
ACTIONS
An antimetabolite and folic acid antagonist. Cell cycle–specific for the S phase, it interrupts the mitotic process during nucleic acid synthesis. Rapidly proliferating malignant cells are inhibited by a cytostatic effect. Widely distributed, average doses of methotrexate are excreted unchanged in the urine within 24 hours. Clearance rates decrease with higher doses. Does not cross blood-brain barrier. Secreted in breast milk.
INDICATIONS AND USES
Used for life-threatening neoplastic disease alone or in combination with other anti-cancer agents in the treatment of acute lymphocytic leukemia, breast cancer, epidermal tumors of the head and neck, small-cell and non–small-cell lung cancer, non-Hodgkin's lymphoma, advanced mycosis fungoides (cutaneous T-cell lymphoma). ■ Severe disabling psoriasis or rheumatoid arthritis unresponsive to other treatment. ■ High-dose regimen for treatment of osteosarcoma. ■ Given PO or IM for early-stage mycosis fungoides, trophoblastic disease, polyarticular-course juvenile rheumatoid arthritis, and other diagnoses and intrathecally for meningeal leukemia.
Unlabeled uses: Treatment of cancers of the cervix, ovaries, bladder, colon, rectum, esophagus, stomach, pancreas, and penis. Treatment of acute nonlymphocytic leukemia, Crohn's disease, ectopic pregnancy, Hodgkin's lymphomas, soft tissue sarcomas, and CNS lymphomas. High-dose regi-

mens for neoplastic diseases other than osteosarcoma are investigational, and therapeutic effects are not established.

CONTRAINDICATIONS

Hypersensitivity to methotrexate; breast-feeding mothers. Not absolute, but methotrexate is not recommended during pregnancy or with hepatic, renal, or bone marrow damage. Contraindicated in psoriasis or rheumatoid arthritis patients with immunodeficiency syndromes, pre-existing blood dyscrasias, or chronic liver disease.

PRECAUTIONS

Follow guidelines for handling cytotoxic agents. See Appendix A, p. 1429. ▪ Administered by or under the direction of the physician specialist. ▪ Deaths have been reported with methotrexate use in the treatment of malignancy, psoriasis, and rheumatoid arthritis. ▪ Methotrexate elimination is reduced in patients with ascites or pleural effusions. Careful monitoring of dose reduction and, in some cases, discontinuation of therapy is required; consider evacuating excess fluid from ascites and pleural effusions before treatment if possible. ▪ Serious and sometimes fatal bone marrow suppression, aplastic anemia, and GI toxicity have been reported with concomitant use of methotrexate (usually high doses) and some NSAIDs; see Drug/Lab Interactions. ▪ Leukoencephalopathy has been reported in patients who have received both IV methotrexate and craniospinal irradiation. ▪ A transient stroke-like encephalopathy has been reported with high-dose methotrexate therapy. Symptoms may include confusion, hemiparesis, transient blindness, seizures, and coma. ▪ Methotrexate-induced lung disease, including acute or chronic interstitial pneumonitis, may occur at any time, may occur even with low doses, and has been fatal. Patients may present with fever, dry cough, dyspnea, hypoxemia, and an infiltrate on chest x-ray. May require interruption of therapy. ▪ Severe skin reactions can occur at any time and have been fatal. ▪ Elevated liver enzymes may occur early during treatment, but hepatotoxicity (may be fatal) occurs more frequently with prolonged use. ▪ Use with extreme caution in patients with ascites, bone marrow suppression, folate deficiency, GI obstruction, infection, impaired renal or liver function, peptic ulcer, pleural effusion, or ulcerative colitis; in debilitated patients; and in the very young or very elderly. ▪ Diarrhea and ulcerative stomatitis will require interrupting therapy; otherwise hemorrhagic enteritis and death from intestinal perforation may occur. ▪ *Clostridium difficile*–associated diarrhea (CDAD) has been reported. May range from mild to life threatening. Consider in patients who present with diarrhea during or after treatment with methotrexate. ▪ Tumor lysis syndrome may occur, and S/S include hyperkalemia, hyperphosphatemia, hyperuricemia, hypocalcemia, metabolic acidosis, urate crystalluria, and renal failure. Prevent or alleviate tumor lysis syndrome with appropriate supportive and pharmacologic measures; see Monitor. ▪ Potentially fatal opportunistic infections, especially *Pneumocystis jiroveci* pneumonia, may occur. ▪ Risk of soft tissue necrosis and osteonecrosis may be increased with concomitant use of methotrexate and radiotherapy. ▪ Painful plaque erosions have been reported (rare) with use of methotrexate for treatment of psoriasis. ▪ May cause renal damage that may lead to acute renal failure. Nonreversible oliguric renal failure is likely to develop in patients who experience delayed early methotrexate elimination. ▪ Malignant lymphomas have been reported. May occur in patients receiving low-dose methotrexate and may not require cytotoxic treatment;

discontinue methotrexate first and initiate appropriate treatment if the lymphoma does not regress.

Monitor: Close patient observation is mandatory. Course of therapy is not repeated until all signs of toxicity from the previous course subside. ■ CBC with platelets, chest x-ray, and renal and liver function tests before, during, and after therapy are essential to comprehensive treatment. ■ Monitor closely for bone marrow, liver, lung, kidney, and skin toxicities. ■ Nadir of leukocyte and platelet count usually occurs after 7 to 10 days, with recovery 7 days later. Liver biopsy, pulmonary studies, and bone marrow studies may be indicated in high-dose or long-term therapy. ■ Monitor renal function closely; verify by CrCl levels; see Precautions. Maintain continuing adequate hydration and urine alkalinization. ■ Prevention and treatment of hyperuricemia due to tumor lysis syndrome may be accomplished with adequate hydration and, if necessary, allopurinol and alkalinization of urine. ■ Monitor serum methotrexate levels. ■ Use prophylactic antiemetics to reduce nausea and vomiting and increase patient comfort. ■ Observe closely for signs of infection. Prophylactic antibiotics may be indicated pending results of C/S in a febrile neutropenic patient. ■ Monitor for thrombocytopenia (platelet count less than 50,000/mm^3). Initiate precautions to prevent excessive bleeding (e.g., inspect IV sites, skin, and mucous membranes; use extreme care during invasive procedures; test urine, emesis, stool, and secretions for occult blood). ■ *Administration of high-dose methotrexate* requires a WBC count greater than 1,500 mm^3; neutrophil count greater than 200/mm^3; platelet count greater than 75,000 mm^3; serum bilirubin less than 1.2 mg/dL; alanine aminotransferase (ALT) level less than 450 units; any mucositis must be healing; ascites or pleural effusion must be drained dry; SCr must be normal; CrCl greater than 60 mL/min; 1 L/M^2 of IV fluid over 6 hours before dosing and 3 L/M^2/day on day of infusion and for 2 days after; alkalinization of urine with sodium bicarbonate; and repeat serum methotrexate and SCr levels at least daily until methotrexate level is below 0.05 micromolar. ■ See Drug/Lab Interactions.

Patient Education: Avoid pregnancy. Nonhormonal birth control recommended for both females and males. Continue for at least 3 months after treatment is complete in male patients and for at least one ovulatory cycle after therapy is complete for female patients. ■ Avoid alcohol and take only prescribed medications. Reactions can be lethal. ■ Close follow-up with physician is imperative. ■ See Appendix D, p. 1434.

Maternal/Child: Category X: avoid pregnancy. Has caused fetal death and congenital anomalies. ■ Discontinue breast-feeding. ■ Safety for use in pediatric patients established for cancer chemotherapy and polyarticular-course juvenile rheumatoid arthritis. Not a labeled use but has been used in pediatric patients 2 to 16 years of age to treat rheumatoid arthritis.

Elderly: See Dose Adjustments. Dose selection should be cautious and based on the potential for decreased organ function, decreased folate stores, and concomitant disease or drug therapy. ■ Consider monitoring CrCl and methotrexate levels. ■ Monitor for early signs of hepatic, renal, or bone marrow toxicity. ■ In chronic administration, certain toxicities may be decreased by folate supplementation. ■ Post-marketing experience suggests that the occurrence of bone marrow suppression, thrombocytopenia, and pneumonitis may increase with age.

DRUG/LAB INTERACTIONS

The following drugs may enhance methotrexate toxicity when administered concomitantly: **alcohol, amiodarone** (Nexterone), **antibacterials** (e.g., tetracycline, chloramphenicol), **cyclosporine** (Sandimmune), **any hepatotoxic drug** (e.g., azathioprine [Imuran], retinoids [vitamin A, sulfasalazine]), **etretinate** (Tegison), **acetylated salicylates** (e.g., aspirin), **NSAIDs** (e.g., ibuprofen [Advil, Motrin], ketoprofen, naproxen [Aleve, Naprosyn]), **penicillins** (e.g., amoxicillin, mezlocillin), **probenecid, salicylates, sulfonamides, para-aminobenzoic acid** (PABA), **phenytoin** (Dilantin), **pyrimethamine, trimethoprim** (component of sulfamethoxazole/trimethoprim), **and vancomycin** (given up to 10 days prior to methotrexate); interactions may be life threatening. Monitoring serum levels and/or reduced doses of methotrexate may be indicated or a longer duration of leucovorin calcium rescue may be required. One source suggests delaying administration of aspirin, NSAIDs, and probenecid for 48 hours after larger doses of methotrexate; see Precautions. ▪ **NSAIDs** are used in the treatment of rheumatoid arthritis in combination with low doses of methotrexate (e.g., 7.5 to 15 mg/week). Do not administer NSAIDs before or concomitantly with high doses of methotrexate (e.g., treatment of osteosarcoma); deaths have been reported. ▪ Use caution if high-dose methotrexate is administered in combination with **nephrotoxic chemotherapy agents** (e.g., cisplatin [Platinol]). ▪ **Omeprazole** (Prilosec) increases serum levels of methotrexate. Discontinue several days before methotrexate administration. Consider an H_2 antagonist (e.g., ranitidine [Zantac]). ▪ **Asparaginase** antagonizes methotrexate; separate administration by 24 hours. ▪ **Doxycycline** may increase toxicity of methotrexate in high-dose regimens. ▪ **Vitamins with folic acid** may inhibit the antifolate effects of methotrexate. ▪ Methotrexate interacts with many drugs such as **anticoagulants, antidiabetics, charcoal, corticosteroids, other antineoplastics** (e.g., procarbazine), **and others** to produce potentially serious reactions. ▪ May increase serum levels of **mercaptopurine** (Purinethol); dose adjustment may be required. ▪ Do not administer **live virus vaccines** to patients receiving antineoplastic drugs. ▪ May decrease **phenytoin** (Dilantin) serum levels. ▪ **Procarbazine** (Matulane) may increase nephrotoxicity of methotrexate. Allow 72 hours between last dose of procarbazine and first dose of methotrexate. ▪ Monitor for signs of increased bone marrow suppression with **sulfonamides** (e.g., sulfisoxazole [Gantrisin], SMZ-TMP [Bactrim]), **bone marrow–suppressing agents** (e.g., antineoplastics), **and radiation therapy.** May also cause SMZ-TMP (Bactrim)-induced megaloblastic anemia. ▪ May decrease **theophylline** clearance and increase serum levels; monitor theophylline serum levels with concurrent use. ▪ **Urinary alkalinizers** increase renal excretion and may reduce effectiveness.

SIDE EFFECTS

Toxicity usually dose related. Death can occur from average doses, high doses, drug interactions (e.g., NSAIDs), bone marrow toxicity, GI toxicity, hepatic toxicity, pulmonary toxicity, and/or severe skin reactions. Abdominal distress, chills, decreased resistance to infection, dizziness, fatigue, fever, leukopenia, malaise, nausea, and ulcerative stomatitis occur most frequently. Other side effects reported include abortion (spontaneous), acne, acute hepatitis, agranulocytosis, alopecia, alveolitis, anaphylaxis, anemia, anorexia, aplastic anemia, azotemia, blurred vision, chronic fibrosis and cirrhosis, convulsions, COPD, cystitis, decreased serum albumin, defective oogenesis or spermatogenesis, diabetes, diarrhea, drowsiness, enteritis, eosinophilia, erythema multiforme, erythematous rashes, exfoliative dermatitis, fetal defects or death, furunculosis, gingivitis, GI ulceration and bleeding, gynecomastia, headache, hematemesis, hematuria, hemiparesis, hepatic failure, hepatotoxicity, hypotension, infertility, interstitial pneumonitis, liver enzyme elevations, lymphadenopathy and lymphoproliferative disorders, melena (passage of dark tarry stools), menstrual dysfunction, nephropathy (severe), neutropenia, oligospermia (transient), opportunistic infections (e.g., cytomegalovirus infection, herpes zoster, histoplasmosis, *Pneumocystis jiroveci* pneumonia), pancreatitis, pancytopenia, paresis, pericardial effusion, pericarditis, pharyngitis, photosensitivity, pigmentary changes, proteinuria, pruritus, pseudomembranous colitis, renal failure, respiratory failure, respiratory fibrosis, skin necrosis, skin ulceration, speech impairment (aphasia, dysarthria), Stevens-Johnson syndrome, stomatitis, suppressed hematopoiesis (blood cell formation), telangiectasia, thrombocytopenia, thromboembolic events (e.g., arterial thrombosis, cerebral thrombosis, deep vein thrombosis, pulmonary embolus, retinal vein thrombosis, thrombophlebitis), toxic epidermal necrolysis, transient blindness, tumor lysis syndrome, urticaria, vaginal discharge, vomiting.

ANTIDOTE

Discontinue methotrexate and notify the physician of any side effects. **Leucovorin calcium (citrovorum factor, folinic acid)** may be given PO, IM, or IV promptly to counteract inadvertent overdose. Leucovorin calcium is also indicated as a planned rescue mechanism for large doses of methotrexate required to treat some malignancies. Doses equal to dose of methotrexate are frequently required. Should be given within 1 hour in overdose, 24 hours in rescue. See specific process for overdose and for rescue for high-dose MTX; in leucovorin calcium monograph. Doses up to 150 mg or 100 mg/M^2 every 3 hours may be required if SCr is 50% or greater than baseline measurement before methotrexate administration. Serum methotrexate must come down to below 0.05 micromolar. Continuing hydration and urinary alkalinization are mandatory to prevent precipitation in renal tubules. Monitor fluid and electrolyte status until serum methotrexate has fallen to less than 0.05 micromolar and renal failure has resolved. Administration of whole blood products (e.g., packed RBCs, platelets, leukocytes) and/or blood modifiers (e.g., darbepoetin alfa [Aranesp], epoetin alfa [Epogen], filgrastim [Neupogen], oprelvekin [Neumega], pegfilgrastim [Neulasta], sargramostim [Leukine]) may be indicated to treat bone marrow toxicity. Death may occur from the progression of most of these side effects. Symptomatic and supportive therapy is indicated. Charcoal hemoperfusion may be helpful, and/or acute intermittent hemodialysis with a high-flux dialyzer may be used to counteract toxicity or inadvertent overdose.

METHYLERGONOVINE MALEATE
(meth-ill-er-**GON**-oh-veen **MAL**-ee-ayt)

Methergine

Uterine stimulant
(oxytocic)

pH 2.7 to 3.5

USUAL DOSE
1 mL (0.2 mg); may be repeated every 2 to 4 hours as necessary. A maximum of 5 doses is usually not exceeded.

DILUTION
Check expiration date on vial; methylergonovine deteriorates with age. May be given undiluted. Some clinicians recommend dilution with 5 mL of NS. Do not add to IV solutions. May be given through Y-tube or three-way stopcock of infusion set.

Filters: No data available from manufacturer; suggests following hospital protocol for filtering from ampules.

Storage: Store in refrigerator (2° to 8° C [36° to 46° F]); protect from light.

COMPATIBILITY
Consider any drug NOT listed as compatible to be INCOMPATIBLE until consulting a pharmacist; specific conditions may apply.

One source suggests the following **compatibilities:**

Y-site: Heparin, hydrocortisone sodium succinate (Solu-Cortef).

RATE OF ADMINISTRATION
0.2 mg or fraction thereof over 1 minute. Too-rapid injection may cause severe nausea and vomiting. See Precautions.

ACTIONS
A semi-synthetic ergot alkaloid used for prevention and control of post-partum hemorrhage. An oxytocic. It exerts a direct stimulation on the smooth muscle of the uterus. Increases tone, rate, and amplitude of rhythmic contractions. Shortens third-stage labor and reduces blood loss. In therapeutic doses the prolonged initial contraction of the uterus is followed by periods of relaxation and contraction. Preferred because it is less likely to cause hypertension. Also produces vasoconstriction, increases CVP, elevates BP, and may rarely produce peripheral ischemia. Effective within minutes. Half-life approximately 3.4 hours. It is probably metabolized in the liver and excreted in feces. Secreted in breast milk.

INDICATIONS AND USES
Routine management after delivery of the placenta. ▪ Postpartum atony and hemorrhage. ▪ Subinvolution. ▪ Under full obstetric supervision (the obstetrician directs and is present), may be given in the second stage of labor following delivery of the anterior shoulder.

CONTRAINDICATIONS
Hypersensitivity, hypertension, pregnancy before third stage of labor (delivery of the placenta) except as stated in Indications, toxemia. ▪ Contraindicated for concomitant use with potent CYP3A4 inhibitors (e.g., protease inhibitors [ritonavir (Norvir)], macrolide antibiotics [erythromycin], and azole antifungals [ketoconazole (Nizoral)]); see Drug/Lab Interactions.

PRECAUTIONS
IV administration is for emergency use only. IM or oral routes are preferred and should be used after the initial IV dose. ▪ IV use may induce

hypertension and/or CVA. Give slowly and monitor BP. ▪ Use caution in presence of sepsis, obliterative vascular disease, and cardiac, hepatic, or renal disease. ▪ Use with caution during the second stage of labor. The necessity for manual removal of a retained placenta should occur rarely with proper technique and adequate allowance of time for a spontaneous separation. ▪ Avoid intra-arterial or peri-arterial injection. ▪ See Contraindications.

Monitor: Monitor BP. ▪ Uterine response may be poor in calcium-deficient patients; calcium replacement may be required for effective response. Avoid or use extreme caution if calcium replacement is needed in patients taking digoxin. ▪ See Drug/Lab Interactions.

Maternal/Child: Category C: see Contraindications and Precautions. Administration before delivery of the placenta may cause hypoxia and intracranial hemorrhage in the infant, captivation of the placenta, or missed diagnosis of a second infant. ▪ May be given orally with caution during breast-feeding for up to 1 week after delivery. ▪ Safety and effectiveness for use in pediatric patients not established.

Elderly: Difference in safety and effectiveness compared to younger adults not observed. ▪ If used in the elderly, dose selection should be cautious.

DRUG/LAB INTERACTIONS

Severe hypertension and cerebrovascular accidents can result with **ephedrine and other vasopressors.** Chlorpromazine (Thorazine) or hydralazine IV will reduce this hypertension. ▪ *Do not administer with potent CYP3A4 inhibitors,* such as **macrolide antibiotics** (e.g., erythromycin [Erythrocin], troleandomycin [TAO], clarithromycin [Biaxin]), **HIV protease inhibitors** (e.g., indinavir [Crixivan], nelfinavir [Viracept], ritonavir [Norvir]), **reverse transcriptase inhibitors** (e.g., delavirdine [Rescriptor]), **or azole antifungals** (e.g., ketoconazole [Nizoral], voriconazole [VFEND]). Serum levels increased. Elevated levels of ergot alkaloids can cause ergotism (i.e., risk for vasospasm potentially leading to cerebral ischemia and/or ischemia of the extremities). ▪ May be used cautiously with **less potent CYP3A4 inhibitors** (e.g., saquinavir [Invirase], nefazodone, fluconazole [Diflucan], grapefruit juice, fluoxetine [Prozac], fluvoxamine [Luvox], zileuton [Zyflo], and clotrimazole [Gyne-Lotrimin, Mycelex]).

SIDE EFFECTS

Rare in therapeutic doses but may include the following:
Arterial spasm (coronary and peripheral), bradycardia, chest pain (temporary), diaphoresis, diarrhea, dilated pupils, dizziness, dyspnea, hallucinations, headache, hematuria, hypertension (transient), hypersensitivity reactions, hypotension, leg cramps, MI, nausea, palpitations, rash, seizures, tachycardia, thrombophlebitis, tinnitus, vomiting, water intoxication, weakness.

Overdose: Abortion, blindness, cerebrovascular accident, coma, convulsions, excitement, gangrene, hypercoagulability, hypertension (followed by hypotension in severe cases), hypothermia, palpitations, respiratory depression, severe nausea and vomiting, shock, tachycardia, thirst, tingling of the extremities, tremor, uterine bleeding.

ANTIDOTE

Discontinue the drug immediately at the onset of any side effect and notify the physician. Most side effects are transient unless there is severe toxicity and will be treated symptomatically. Use antiemetics (e.g., prochlorperazine [Compazine], ondansetron [Zofran] for nausea and vomiting.

Treat seizures with anticonvulsants (e.g., diazepam [Valium], phenytoin [Dilantin]). Treat peripheral ischemia with vasodilators (e.g., nitroprusside sodium, papaverine, phentolamine [Regitine]). Hypertension has been treated with chlorpromazine (Thorazine). Severe poisoning is treated with vasodilator drugs, sedatives, calcium gluconate to relieve muscular pain, and other supportive treatment. Heparin is used to control hypercoagulability.

METHYLPREDNISOLONE SODIUM SUCCINATE

(meth-ill-pred-**NISS**-oh-lohn **SO**-dee-um **SUK**-sih-nayt)

A-Methapred, Solu-Medrol

**Hormone
(adrenocorticoid/glucocorticoid)
Anti-inflammatory**

pH 7 to 8

USUAL DOSE

Average dose range is 10 to 40 mg initially. May be repeated every 4 to 6 hours as necessary. IV methylprednisolone is usually given in an emergency situation or when oral dosing is not feasible. Larger doses may be justified by patient condition. Repeat until adequate response, then decrease dose as indicated. Total dose usually does not exceed 1.5 Gm/24 hr, but higher doses have been used in life-threatening shock. Dose is individualized according to the severity of the disease and the response of the patient and is not necessarily reduced for pediatric patients. High-dose treatment is utilized until patient condition stabilizes, usually no longer than 48 to 72 hours.

Anti-inflammatory: 10 to 40 mg. May be repeated every 4 to 6 hours as necessary.

Acute spinal cord injury high-dose therapy (unlabeled): Spinal cord injury must be less than 8 hours old and above L-2. The earlier methylprednisolone therapy begins, the better the results. *Loading dose:* 30 mg/kg of a specifically diluted solution (see Dilution) evenly distributed over 15 minutes. Maintain IV line with standard IV fluids for 45 minutes, then begin a *maintenance dose* of 5.4 mg/kg/hr for 23 hours. Discontinue 24 hours after loading dose initiated.

Status asthmaticus: Newer asthma guidelines recommend 40 to 80 mg/day in 1 to 2 divided doses until peak expiratory flow is 70% of predicted or personal best. Another source recommends a *loading dose* of 2 mg/kg followed by 0.5 to 1 mg/kg/dose every 6 hours for up to 5 days.

Acute exacerbation of multiple sclerosis: 160 mg as a single dose each day for 7 days. Follow with 64 mg every other day for 1 month.

***Pneumocystis jiroveci* pneumonia (unlabeled):** Initiate within 24 to 72 hours of initial antibiotic PCP therapy. 30 mg twice daily for 5 days. Follow with 30 mg once daily for 5 days (Days 6 to 10). Then reduce to 15 mg once daily for 11 days (Days 11 to 21) or until antibiotic regimen is complete.

Severe lupus nephritis (unlabeled): 1 Gm as an infusion over 1 hour for 3 days. Follow with long-term prednisolone oral therapy.

Continued

PEDIATRIC DOSE

See Maternal/Child.

Anti-inflammatory/immunosuppressive: The range of initial doses is 0.11 to 1.6 mg/kg/day (3.2 to 48 mg/M^2/day) in 3 to 4 divided doses (0.275 to 0.4 mg/kg every 6 hours or 0.036 to 0.53 mg/kg every 8 hours, or 0.8 to 12 mg/M^2 every 6 hours or 1.06 to 16 mg/M^2 every 8 hours). Another source recommends 0.5 to 1.7 mg/kg/day or 5 to 25 mg/M^2/day in divided doses every 6 to 12 hours (0.125 to 0.425 mg/kg or 1.25 to 6.25 mg/M^2 every 6 hours, or 0.25 to 0.85 mg/kg or 2.5 to 12.5 mg/M^2 every 12 hours).

Status asthmaticus: Newer asthma guidelines recommend 0.5 to 1 mg/kg every 12 hours (maximum 60 mg/day) until peak expiratory flow is 70% of predicted or personal best. Another source recommends 2 mg/kg as a *loading* dose. *Maintain* with 0.5 to 1 mg/kg every 6 hours for up to 5 days.

Severe lupus nephritis (unlabeled): 30 mg/kg every other day for 6 doses. Follow with long-term prednisolone oral therapy.

DOSE ADJUSTMENTS

Reduced dose may be required; see Precautions and Drug/Lab Interactions. ■ Clearance of corticosteroids is decreased in patients with hypothyroidism and increased in patients with hyperthyroidism. Dose adjustment may be required.

DILUTION

Available in Act-O-Vials containing 40 mg, 125 mg, 500 mg, 1,000 mg, and 2,000 mg. Each vial has an appropriate amount of diluent. Reconstitute by removing the protective cap, turning the rubber stopper a quarter turn, and pressing down, allowing the diluent into the lower chamber. Agitate gently. Using sterile technique, insert a needle through the center of the rubber stopper to withdraw diluted solution. To be diluted only with diluent supplied in Act-O-Vial. Also available in vials. Should be diluted with accompanying diluent or BWFI with benzyl alcohol. May be given direct IV, as an infusion, or further diluted in desired amounts of D5W, D5NS, or NS.

Acute spinal cord injury loading and maintenance doses: Each 1-Gm vial must be diluted to 16 mL with bacteriostatic water to maintain potency and avoid precipitation (62.5 mg/mL). Further dilute in D5W, D5NS, or NS with an amount to facilitate dose of 5.4 mg/kg/hr. (Example for a patient weighing 50 kg: [50 kg × 5.4 mg/hr = 270 mg/hr. 270 mg/hr × 23 hours = 6,210 mg total dose]. With a total dose of 6,210 mg at 62.5 mg/mL, you will have 99.36 [100] mL of reconstituted methylprednisolone. Add an additional 100 mL diluent to achieve 31.25 mg/mL. 270 mg/hr is the desired dose for this patient. 270 mg/hr divided by 31.25 mg/mL [strength of solution] equals 8.6. Administer at 8.6 mL/hr to achieve desired dose over 23 hours.)

Storage: Protect from light. Store both unreconstituted product and solution at RT (20° to 25° C [68° to 77° F]). Use solution within 48 hours of mixing. Heat sensitive; do not autoclave.

COMPATIBILITY   (Underline Indicates Conflicting Compatibility Information)

Consider any drug NOT listed as compatible to be INCOMPATIBLE until consulting a pharmacist; specific conditions may apply.

Manufacturer states, "Because of possible physical incompatibilities, should not be diluted or mixed with other solutions."

One source suggests the following **compatibilities:**

Additive: Aminophylline, chloramphenicol (Chloromycetin), clindamycin (Cleocin), cytarabine (ARA-C), dopamine, granisetron (Kytril), heparin, norepinephrine (Levophed), penicillin G potassium, ranitidine (Zantac), theophylline, verapamil.

Y-site: Acyclovir (Zovirax), alprostadil, amifostine (Ethyol), amiodarone (Nexterone), amphotericin B cholesteryl (Amphotec), anidulafungin (Eraxis), aztreonam (Azactam), bivalirudin (Angiomax), cefepime (Maxipime), ceftazidime (Fortaz), cisatracurium (Nimbex), cisplatin (Platinol), cladribine (Leustatin), cyclophosphamide (Cytoxan), cytarabine (ARA-C), dexmedetomidine (Precedex), diltiazem (Cardizem), dopamine, doripenem (Doribax), doxorubicin (Adriamycin), doxorubicin liposomal (Doxil), enalaprilat (Vasotec IV), famotidine (Pepcid IV), fludarabine (Fludara), granisetron (Kytril), heparin, hetastarch in electrolytes (Hextend), inamrinone (Amrinone), linezolid (Zyvox), melphalan (Alkeran), meperidine (Demerol), methotrexate, metronidazole (Flagyl IV), midazolam (Versed), milrinone (Primacor), morphine, nicardipine (Cardene IV), oxaliplatin (Eloxatin), pemetrexed (Alimta), piperacillin/tazobactam (Zosyn), potassium chloride (KCl), remifentanil (Ultiva), sodium bicarbonate, tacrolimus (Prograf), teniposide (Vumon), theophylline, thiotepa, topotecan (Hycamtin).

RATE OF ADMINISTRATION

IV injection: A single dose of 10 to 40 mg over several minutes. When higher doses are needed, administer up to 30 mg/kg over 30 minutes or more. Too-rapid administration of high doses (greater than 500 mg administered over a period of less than 10 minutes) may precipitate hypotension, cardiac arrhythmia, and sudden death. Direct IV administration of lower doses (10 to 40 mg) is usually the route of choice and eliminates the possibility of overloading the patient with IV fluids. May be given as an *infusion* in its own diluent. At the discretion of the physician, a continuous infusion may be given, properly diluted, over a specified time. Another source suggests the following:

A single dose of up to 1.8 mg/kg or 125 mg may be given *IV push* over 3 to 15 minutes.

A single dose of 2 mg/kg or 250 mg or more may be given as an *infusion* over 15 to 30 minutes.

A single dose of 15 mg/kg or greater than 500 mg may be given as an *infusion* over 30 minutes or more.

Acute spinal cord injury: See Usual Dose and Dilution.

ACTIONS

An adrenocortical steroid with potent metabolic, anti-inflammatory actions and innumerable other effects. Has a greater anti-inflammatory potency than prednisolone and less tendency to cause excessive potassium and calcium excretion and sodium and water retention. Has five times the potency of hydrocortisone sodium succinate. Has minimal mineralocorticoid activity. Primarily used for anti-inflammatory and immunosuppressive effects. May be used in conjunction with other forms of therapy, such as epinephrine for acute hypersensitivity reactions. Demonstrable effects seen within 1 hour of administration. Primarily metabolized in the liver and excreted in the urine and feces. Dose almost completely excreted after 12 hours, which allows the use of very large doses with reasonable safety. Crosses the placental barrier. Secreted in breast milk.

INDICATIONS AND USES

Includes treatment of allergic states, dermatologic diseases, endocrine disorders, gastrointestinal diseases, hematologic disorders, neoplastic diseases, nervous system disorders, ophthalmic diseases, renal diseases, respiratory diseases, and rheumatic disorders. See prescribing information for a complete list. Used primarily as an anti-inflammatory or immunosuppressant agent. Oral therapy should be used when appropriate.

Unlabeled uses: High-dose therapy as an adjunct to traditional spinal cord injury management; to improve neurologic recovery in an acute (less than 8 hours old) spinal cord injury above L-2. ■ Treatment of *Pneumocystis jiroveci* pneumonia as an adjunct to antibiotics.

CONTRAINDICATIONS

Absolute contraindications in long-term therapy, except in life-threatening situations: Hypersensitivity to any product component, including sulfites; systemic fungal infections. ■ Formulations containing benzyl alcohol are contraindicated in neonates and for intrathecal administration.

Relative contraindications: Active or healed tuberculosis, amebiasis (latent or active), cerebral malaria, chickenpox, ocular herpes simplex, pregnancy.

PRECAUTIONS

Not the drug of choice to treat acute adrenocortical insufficiency. ■ May produce hypothalamic-pituitary-adrenal (HPA) axis suppression with resulting glucocorticosteroid insufficiency in patients undergoing chronic or prolonged therapy. To avoid relative adrenocortical insufficiency, do not stop therapy abruptly; taper off. Patient is observed carefully, especially under stress, for up to 2 years; exception is very short-term therapy. ■ Formulation may contain benzyl alcohol; see Contraindications and Maternal/Child. ■ Rare instances of anaphylactoid reactions have been reported in patients receiving corticosteroid therapy. ■ In one study, an increase in mortality was seen in patients with cranial trauma who had no other clear indication for corticosteroid treatment. Should not be used for treatment of traumatic brain injury. ■ Use with caution in patients who have had a recent MI. Ventricular free wall rupture has been reported. ■ Patients taking corticosteroids may be more susceptible to infections. Latent disease may be activated. Intercurrent infections may be exacerbated; see Contraindications. ■ Use with caution in patients with CHF, hypertension, or renal insufficiency. May affect fluid and electrolyte balance. ■ Use with caution in patients with thyroid dysfunction; see Dose Adjustments. ■ Use with caution in patients with active or latent peptic ulcers, diverticulitis, fresh intestinal anastomoses, and nonspecific ulcerative colitis. May be at increased risk for perforation. ■ Metabolism of corticosteroids is decreased in patients with cirrhosis; effects may be enhanced. ■ Use with caution in patients at risk for osteoporosis. Corticosteroids decrease bone formation, increase bone resorption, and decrease protein matrix of the bone. May lead to inhibition of bone growth in pediatric patients and the development of osteoporosis at any age. ■ An acute myopathy has been reported with the use of high doses of corticosteroids. Most often seen in patients with disorders of neuromuscular transmission (e.g., myasthenia gravis) or in patients receiving concomitant therapy with neuromuscular blocking drugs. Myopathy is generalized, may involve ocular and respiratory muscles, and may result in quadriparesis. Clinical improvement following discontinuation of corticosteroids may take weeks to years. ▪ May induce psychological changes (e.g., depression, euphoria, insomnia, mood swings, personality changes, psychosis). May aggravate existing emotional instability or psychotic tendencies. ▪ Prophylactic antacids may prevent peptic ulcer complications.

Monitor: Monitor electrolytes. May cause sodium retention and potassium and calcium excretion. May cause hypertension secondary to fluid and electrolyte disturbances. ▪ May mask signs of infection. ▪ May increase insulin needs in diabetics. ▪ Administer single dose before 9 AM to reduce suppression of adrenocortical activity. ▪ May increase intraocular pressure. Periodic ophthalmic exams may be necessary with prolonged treatment. ▪ See Drug/Lab Interactions.

Patient Education: Report edema, tarry stools, or weight gain promptly. Report anorexia, diarrhea, dizziness, fatigue, low blood sugar, nausea, weakness, weight loss, or vomiting; may indicate adrenal insufficiency after dose reduction or discontinuing therapy. ▪ May mask signs of infection and/or decrease resistance. ▪ Diabetics may have increased requirement for insulin or oral hypoglycemics. ▪ Avoid immunizations with live virus vaccines. ▪ Avoid exposure to measles or chickenpox. Seek immediate medical advice if exposure occurs. ▪ Carry ID stating steroid dependent if receiving prolonged therapy.

Maternal/Child: Category C: corticosteroids have been shown to be teratogenic in many species. ▪ Discontinue breast-feeding. ▪ Infants born to mothers who received corticosteroids during pregnancy should be carefully monitored for signs of hypoadrenalism. ▪ May contain benzyl alcohol, which has been associated with a fatal "gasping syndrome" in neonates. ▪ Monitor growth and development of pediatric patients receiving prolonged treatment.

Elderly: Differences in response between the elderly and younger patients have not been identified. Dose selection should be cautious based on the possibility of age-related organ impairment (e.g., bone marrow reserve, renal, hepatic). May be more sensitive to effects.

DRUG/LAB INTERACTIONS

Aminoglutethimide (Cytadren) **and mitotane** (Lysodren) decrease serum concentration of corticosteroids; monitor carefully if concurrent use is necessary. ▪ Metabolism increased and effects reduced by **hepatic enzyme–inducing agents** (e.g., alcohol, barbiturates [e.g., phenobarbital], hydantoins [e.g., phenytoin (Dilantin)], rifampin [Rifadin]); dose adjustments may be required when adding or deleting from drug profile. ▪ Risk of hypokalemia increased with **amphotericin B, or potassium-depleting diuretics** (e.g., thiazides, furosemide, ethacrynic acid). Monitor potassium levels and cardiac function. Increased risk of **digoxin** toxicity secondary to hypokalemia. ▪ May decrease effectiveness of **potassium supplements;** monitor serum potassium. ▪ **Diuretics** decrease sodium and fluid retention effects of corticosteroids; corticosteroids decrease sodium excretion and diuretic effects of diuretics. ▪ Use with **cyclosporine** in organ transplants is therapeutic but may increase cyclosporine toxicity; seizures have been reported; use caution. ▪ Clearance decreased and effects increased with **estrogens, oral contraceptives, triazole antifungals** (e.g., itraconazole [Sporanox]), **and macrolide antibiotics** (e.g., azithromycin [Zithromax], erythromycin, troleandomycin [TAO]). ▪ Coadmistration of **aprepitant** (fosaprepitant [Emend]) may increase methylprednisolone levels. Dose reduction of methylprednisolone may be indicated. ▪ May interact with **anticoagulants, nondepolarizing muscle relaxants** (e.g., atracurium [Tracrium]), **or theophyllines;** may inhibit or potentiate action; monitor carefully. ▪ Monitor patients receiving **antidiabetic agents** (e.g., insulin, glyburide) **or thyroid hormones** carefully; dose adjustments of either or both agents may be required. ▪ May antagonize effects of **isoniazid and salicylates;** dose adjustments may be required. ▪ Administration of live or live-attenuated vaccines is contraindicated in patients receiving immunosuppressive doses of corticosteroids. Inactivated vaccines may be administered, but the response to such vaccines cannot be predicted. ▪ Concomitant use with **NSAIDs** (e.g., ibuprofen [Advil, Motrin], naproxen [Aleve, Naprosyn]), may increase the risk of adverse GI effects. ▪ Concomitant use with **anticholinesterase agents** (e.g., neostigmine) may produce severe weakness in patients with myasthenia gravis. If possible, anticholinesterase agents should be withdrawn at least 24 hours before initiating corticosteroid therapy. ▪ Altered **protein-binding capacity** will impact effectiveness of this drug. ▪ Corticosteroids may **suppress reactions to skin tests.** ▪ See Dose Adjustments.

SIDE EFFECTS
Do occur but are usually reversible: Cushing's syndrome; electrolyte and calcium imbalance; euphoria; glycosuria; hyperglycemia; hypersensitivity reactions, including anaphylaxis; hypertension; increased appetite; increased intracranial pressure; menstrual irregularities; peptic ulcer perforation and hemorrhage; protein catabolism; spontaneous fractures; transitory burning or tingling; sweating, headache, or weakness; thromboembolism and many others.

ANTIDOTE
Notify the physician of any side effect. Will probably treat the side effect if necessary. Resuscitate as necessary for anaphylaxis and notify physician. Keep epinephrine immediately available.

METOCLOPRAMIDE
HYDROCHLORIDE BBW
(**meh**-toe-kloh-**PRAH**-myd hy-droh-**KLOR**-eyed)

Reglan

GI stimulant
Antiemetic

pH 4.5 to 6.5

USUAL DOSE
Small bowel intubation and/or radiologic examination of the small bowel: 10 mg (2 mL) as a single dose.
Antiemetic: High-dose regimen for highly emetogenic chemotherapy is rarely used; 5HT$_3$ receptor antagonists (e.g., granisetron [Kytril], ondansetron [Zofran]) preferred. 2 mg/kg of body weight 30 minutes before giving emetogenic cancer chemotherapy (e.g., cisplatin, dacarbazine). Repeat every 2 hours for 2 doses, then every 3 hours for 3 doses; see Dose Adjustments. For less emetogenic regimens, 1 mg/kg/dose may be adequate.

Diabetic gastroparesis: 10 mg immediately before each meal and at bedtime. Use IV for up to 10 days if symptoms are severe. Continue treatment PO for 2 to 8 weeks.

Prevention of postoperative nausea and vomiting: 10 mg, usually given IM toward the end of surgery. Up to 20 mg may be used.

PEDIATRIC DOSE

Small bowel intubation and/or radiologic examination of the small bowel: *6 to 14 years:* 2.5 to 5 mg. *Under 6 years:* 0.1 mg/kg of body weight.

Gastroesophageal reflux or GI dysmotility (unlabeled): 0.1 to 0.2 mg/kg/dose. May be given every 6 hours if required. Maximum dose 0.8 mg/kg/24 hr (0.2 mg/kg/dose every 6 hours).

Antiemetic (unlabeled): Rarely used. $5HT_3$-receptor antagonists preferred. A high-dose regimen for highly emetogenic chemotherapy of 1 to 2 mg/kg/dose every 2 to 6 hours has been administered but is rarely used. Premedicate with diphenhydramine (Benadryl) to reduce extrapyramidal symptoms.

DOSE ADJUSTMENTS

Antiemetic dose may be reduced to 1 mg/kg if initial doses suppress vomiting. Initial doses may be reduced to 1 mg/kg for less emetogenic regimens. ▪ Reduce initial dose by half in any patient with a CrCl less than 40 mL/min. Adjust subsequent doses as indicated. ▪ Caution and lower-end dosing suggested in elderly patients. Consider potential for decreased organ function and concomitant disease or drug therapy. ▪ See Drug/Lab Interactions.

DILUTION

May be given undiluted if dose does not exceed 10 mg. For doses exceeding 10 mg dilute in at least 50 mL of D5W, NS, D5/½NS, R, or LR, and give as an infusion.

Storage: Light sensitive; store in carton before use. Diluted solutions stable for 24 hours in normal light, 48 hours if protected from light. Do not freeze unless diluted in NS. Discard if color or particulate matter is observed.

COMPATIBILITY   (Underline Indicates Conflicting Compatibility Information)

Consider any drug NOT listed as compatible to be INCOMPATIBLE until consulting a pharmacist; specific conditions may apply.

Manufacturer lists as **incompatible** with chloramphenicol (Chloromycetin) and sodium bicarbonate.

Sources suggest the following **compatibilities:**

Additive: Manufacturer lists <u>ampicillin</u>, ascorbic acid, benztropine (Cogentin), <u>cisplatin (Platinol)</u>, <u>clindamycin (Cleocin)</u>, <u>cyclophosphamide (Cytoxan)</u>, cytarabine (ARA-C), dexamethasone (Decadron), diphenhydramine (Benadryl), doxorubicin (Adriamycin), <u>erythromycin (Erythrocin)</u>, heparin, <u>insulin (regular)</u>, lidocaine, mannitol, <u>methotrexate</u>, <u>multivitamins (M.V.I.)</u>, <u>penicillin G potassium</u>, potassium acetate, and potassium phosphate. Other sources add meperidine (Demerol), meropenem (Merrem IV), morphine, potassium chloride (KCl), verapamil.

Y-site: All drugs listed by the manufacturer as **compatible** under *Additive.* Other sources add acyclovir (Zovirax), aldesleukin (Proleukin), amifostine (Ethyol), aztreonam (Azactam), bivalirudin (Angiomax), bleomycin (Blenoxane), ciprofloxacin (Cipro IV), cisatracurium (Nimbex), cisplatin (Platinol), cladribine (Leustatin), cyclophosphamide (Cytoxan), cytarabine (ARA-C), dexmedetomidine (Precedex), diltiazem (Cardizem), docetaxel (Taxotere), doripenem (Doribax), doxapram (Dopram), doxorubicin

(Adriamycin), droperidol (Inapsine), etoposide phosphate (Etopophos), famotidine (Pepcid IV), fenoldopam (Corlopam), fentanyl (Sublimaze), filgrastim (Neupogen), fluconazole (Diflucan), fludarabine (Fludara), fluorouracil (5-FU), foscarnet (Foscavir), gallium nitrate (Ganite), gemcitabine (Gemzar), granisetron (Kytril), heparin, hetastarch in electrolytes (Hextend), hydromorphone (Dilaudid), idarubicin (Idamycin), leucovorin calcium, levofloxacin (Levaquin), linezolid (Zyvox), melphalan (Alkeran), meperidine (Demerol), meropenem (Merrem IV), methadone (Dolophine), methotrexate, mitomycin (Mutamycin), morphine, ondansetron (Zofran), oxaliplatin (Eloxatin), paclitaxel (Taxol), palonosetron (Aloxi), pemetrexed (Alimta), piperacillin/tazobactam (Zosyn), quinupristin/dalfopristin (Synercid), remifentanil (Ultiva), sargramostim (Leukine), sufentanil (Sufenta), tacrolimus (Prograf), teniposide (Vumon), thiotepa, tigecycline (Tygacil), topotecan (Hycamtin), vinblastine, vincristine, vinorelbine (Navelbine), zidovudine (AZT, Retrovir).

RATE OF ADMINISTRATION
Too-rapid IV injection will cause intense anxiety, restlessness, and then drowsiness.

IV injection: 10 mg or fraction thereof over 2 minutes. Reduce rate of injection in pediatric patients.

Infusion: Administer over a minimum of 15 minutes.

ACTIONS
A dopamine antagonist. Antiemetic properties appear to be the result of antagonism of central and peripheral dopamine receptors. Blocks the stimulation of medullary chemoreceptor trigger zones by dopamine. Inhibits nausea and vomiting. Increases tone and amplitude of gastric contractions, relaxes the lower pyloric sphincter and duodenal bulb, and increases peristalsis of the duodenum and jejunum, resulting in accelerated gastric emptying. Does not stimulate gastric, biliary, or pancreatic secretions. Acts even if vagal innervation not present. Action negated by anticholinergic drugs. Distributes extensively into tissues. Onset of action occurs in 1 to 3 minutes and lasts 1 to 2 hours. Average half-life is 5 to 6 hours. Excreted in urine. Secreted in breast milk.

INDICATIONS AND USES
Facilitate small bowel intubation. ▪ Stimulate gastric and intestinal emptying of barium to permit radiologic examination of the stomach and small intestine. ▪ Prevention of nausea and vomiting associated with emetogenic cancer chemotherapy. ▪ Prophylaxis of postoperative nausea and vomiting when nasogastric suction is not indicated. ▪ Diabetic gastroparesis.

CONTRAINDICATIONS
Situations in which gastric motility is contraindicated, i.e., gastric hemorrhage, obstruction, or perforation; known hypersensitivity to metoclopramide; patients with epilepsy or patients taking drugs that may also cause extrapyramidal reactions; pheochromocytoma.

PRECAUTIONS
May produce sedation, extrapyramidal symptoms, or Parkinson-like symptoms, similar to those seen with phenothiazines. Use caution in patients with pre-existing disease. ▪ Acute dystonic reactions (a type of extrapyramidal symptom [EPS]) are usually seen during the first 24 to 48 hours of treatment and are more common in pediatric patients, in adults under 30 years of age, and at higher doses used for prophylaxis of N/V due to

chemotherapy. ▪ Tardive dyskinesia may develop and is usually related to duration of treatment and total cumulative dose. Avoid use for longer than 12 weeks unless benefit outweighs risk of tardive dyskinesia. ▪ Neuroleptic malignant syndrome (NMS) has been reported rarely. Potentially fatal. Discontinue metoclopramide immediately; see Monitor. ▪ Produces a transient increase in plasma aldosterone, patients with cirrhosis or CHF may develop fluid retention and volume overload. If S/S occur, discontinue metoclopramide. ▪ Use with caution in patients with hypertension. May cause release of catecholamines, exacerbating the condition. ▪ A prolactin-elevating compound; may be carcinogenic. Risk with a single dose almost nonexistent. ▪ May cause serious depression and suicidal tendencies; use extreme caution in any patient with a history of depression. ▪ Patients with NADH-cytochrome b_5 reductase deficiency are at increased risk for developing methemoglobinemia and/or sulfhemoglobinemia. In patients with G6PD deficiency who develop methemoglobinemia, methylene blue treatment is not recommended. Can cause hemolytic anemia. ▪ See Maternal/Child.

Monitor: Monitor vital signs. ▪ Pretreatment with diphenhydramine may reduce incidence of extrapyramidal symptoms with larger doses (e.g., antiemetic). ▪ Monitor for S/S of NMS (e.g., hyperthermia, muscle rigidity, altered consciousness, and evidence of autonomic instability [irregular pulse or BP, tachycardia, diaphoresis, and arrhythmias]). ▪ Discontinue therapy in patients who develop S/S of tardive dyskinesia (syndrome of potentially irreversible involuntary movements of the tongue, face, mouth, jaw, trunk, or extremities). ▪ See Precautions and Drug/Lab Interactions.

Patient Education: Use caution performing any task that requires alertness, coordination, or physical dexterity; may produce dizziness and drowsiness. ▪ If any involuntary movement of eyes, face, or limbs occurs, notify physician promptly. ▪ Avoid alcohol or other CNS depressants (e.g., barbiturates, benzodiazepines [e.g., diazepam (Valium)]).

Maternal/Child: Category B: use caution in pregnancy and breast-feeding. ▪ May increase milk production (elevates prolactin). ▪ Pharmacokinetics highly variable in children and neonates. ▪ Safety and effectiveness for use in pediatric patients not established except when administered to facilitate small bowel intubation. ▪ Dystonic reactions are more common in pediatric patients. ▪ Prolonged clearance in neonates may produce excessive serum concentrations. ▪ May cause methemoglobinemia in premature and full-term neonates at doses exceeding 0.5 mg/kg/24 hr. ▪ See Precautions and Side Effects.

Elderly: May be more sensitive to therapeutic or adverse effects. ▪ Long-term use increases risk of extrapyramidal effects (e.g., parkinsonism, tardive dyskinesia). ▪ See Dose Adjustments and Precautions.

DRUG/LAB INTERACTIONS

Antagonized by **anticholinergic drugs** (e.g., atropine) **and narcotic analgesics** (e.g., morphine). ▪ May potentiate **alcohol and cyclosporine.** ▪ Drugs ingested orally may be absorbed more slowly or more rapidly depending on the absorption site (e.g., inhibits **cimetidine, digoxin**). ▪ Potentiates **MAO inhibitors** (e.g., selegiline [Eldepryl]); use extreme caution or do not use. ▪ **Insulin** reactions may result from gastric stasis, making diabetic control difficult. Dose or timing of insulin may need adjustment. ▪ Extrapyramidal effects may be potentiated with concomitant use of **phenothiazines, butyrophenones, and thioxanthines** (antipsychotic drugs). ▪ Used concurrently, metoclopramide and **levodopa** have opposite effects on dopamine receptors; metoclopramide is inhibited and levodopa is potentiated.

SIDE EFFECTS
Usually mild, transient, and reversible after metoclopramide discontinued. Hypersensitivity reactions can occur. Acute CHF, anxiety, arrhythmias, bowel disturbances, confusion, convulsions, depression (severe, may have suicidal tendencies), dizziness, drowsiness, extrapyramidal reactions, fatigue, fluid retention, hallucinations, headache, hypertension, hypotension, insomnia, methemoglobinemia in neonates, nausea, NMS (hyperthermia, muscle rigidity, altered consciousness, and evidence of autonomic instability [irregular pulse or BP, tachycardia, diaphoresis, and arrhythmias]), restlessness, sulfhemoglobinemia in adults, tardive dyskinesia. Numerous other side effects may occur.
Overdose: Disorientation, drowsiness, and extrapyramidal reactions.

ANTIDOTE
Notify physician of all side effects. Most will respond to a reduced dose or discontinuation of metoclopramide. Treat overdose or extrapyramidal reactions with diphenhydramine (Benadryl) or benztropine (Cogentin). Symptoms should disappear within 24 hours. To manage NMS, immediately discontinue metoclopramide. Intensive symptomatic treatment and monitoring is required. Bromocriptine (Parlodel) and dantrolene (Dantrium) have been used to treat NMS, but effectiveness not established. Discontinue therapy in patients who develop S/S of tardive dyskinesia; symptoms may resolve. Treat methemoglobinemia with IV methylene blue. Hemodialysis is not likely to be useful in an overdose. Resuscitate as necessary.

METOPROLOL TARTRATE BBW
(me-toe-**PROH**-lohl **TAHR**-trayt)

Lopressor

Beta-adrenergic
blocking agent
Antiarrhythmic (post MI)

pH 7.5

USUAL DOSE
Treatment of myocardial infarction: 2.5 to 5 mg as an IV bolus dose. Initiate as soon as the patient's hemodynamic condition has stabilized. Repeat at 2-minute intervals for 2 more doses; a total dose of 15 mg (AHA recommends 5 mg at 5-minute intervals to a total dose of 15 mg). If IV doses are well tolerated, give 50 mg PO every 6 hours for 48 hours beginning 15 minutes after the last bolus. Follow with an oral maintenance dose of 100 mg twice daily. In patients who do not tolerate the full IV dose start 25 to 50 mg PO within 15 minutes of the last IV dose. Dosage based on degree of intolerance. May have to discontinue metoprolol.
Treatment of atrial fibrillation (unlabeled): 2.5 to 5 mg as an IV injection over 2 to 5 minutes as necessary to control rate up to a total dose of 15 mg in a 10- to 15-minute period if indicated.

Treatment of ventricular rate control/hypertension (unlabeled): 1.25 to 5 mg every 6 to 12 hours. Begin with a lower initial dose and titrate to response. Up to 15 mg every 3 to 6 hours has been used.

DOSE ADJUSTMENTS

See Drug/Lab Interactions. ▪ Not required in impaired renal function.

DILUTION

May be given undiluted.

Storage: Store at CRT. Protect from light.

COMPATIBILITY

Consider any drug NOT listed as compatible to be INCOMPATIBLE until consulting a pharmacist; specific conditions may apply.

One source suggests the following **compatibilities:**

Y-site: Abciximab (ReoPro), alteplase (tPA), argatroban, bivalirudin (Angiomax), meperidine (Demerol), morphine, nesiritide (Natrecor).

RATE OF ADMINISTRATION

A single dose over 1 minute. Monitor ECG, HR, and BP and discontinue metoprolol if adverse symptoms occur (bradycardia less than 45 beats/min, heart block greater than first degree, systolic BP less than 100 mm Hg, or moderate to severe cardiac failure).

ACTIONS

Metoprolol is a cardioselective (B_1) adrenergic blocking agent. Its mechanism of action in patients with suspected or definite myocardial infarction is not known. It reduces the incidence of recurrent myocardial infarctions and reduces the size of the infarct and the incidence of fatal arrhythmias. Reduces HR, systolic BP, and cardiac output. Well distributed throughout the body, it acts within 1 to 2 minutes and lasts about 3 to 4 hours. Maximum beta blockade is achieved in approximately 20 minutes. Metabolized in the liver by the cytochrome P_{450} enzyme system, primarily CYP2D6. Excreted as metabolites in the urine. Secreted in breast milk.

INDICATIONS AND USES

To reduce cardiac mortality in hemodynamically stable individuals with suspected or definite myocardial infarction. ▪ Treatment of hypertension, angina pectoris, and CHF in oral dosage form.

Unlabeled uses: Treatment of atrial fibrillation and unstable angina. ▪ Has been used in the perioperative period to reduce cardiac morbidity and mortality in patients at risk. ▪ Treatment of ventricular rate control and hypertension in patients who cannot take PO medications.

CONTRAINDICATIONS

HR below 45 beats/min, second- or third-degree heart block, significant first-degree heart block (PR interval equal to or greater than 0.24 second), systolic BP below 100 mm Hg, or moderate to severe cardiac failure. ▪ Hypersensitivity to metoprolol. Use caution in patients with hypersensitivity to other beta-blockers (e.g., atenolol [Tenormin], esmolol [Brevibloc], propranolol). Cross-sensitivity between beta-blockers can occur. ▪ Pheochromocytoma, severe peripheral arterial circulatory disorders, sick sinus syndrome.

PRECAUTIONS

Use caution in CHF. Beta blockade may depress myocardial contractility and precipitate or exacerbate heart failure. ▪ Use caution in presence of heart failure controlled by digoxin. Both drugs slow AV conduction. ▪ May produce significant first- (PR interval equal to or greater than 0.26 second),

second-, or third-degree heart block. Acute MI can also cause heart block. ▪ Metoprolol decreases sinus heart rate. MI may also produce significant lowering of HR; see Antidote. ▪ May mask tachycardia occurring with hypoglycemia in diabetes and tachycardia of hyperthyroidism. ▪ In general, patients with bronchospastic disease should not receive beta-blockers, including metoprolol. Because of its relative beta selectivity, metoprolol may be used with extreme caution in these patients. Monitor pulmonary function closely; see Antidote. ▪ Use with caution in patients with impaired hepatic function. ▪ May cause arrhythmia, angina, MI, or death if stopped abruptly (more of an issue with chronic oral therapy). ▪ May cause severe bradycardia in patients with Wolff-Parkinson-White syndrome. ▪ Contraindicated in patients known to have or suspected of having a pheochromocytoma. If metoprolol is required, it should be given in combination with an alpha-blocker (e.g., phenoxybenzamine [Dibenzyline]) and only after the alpha-blocker has been initiated. ▪ See Drug/Lab Interactions.

Monitor: Continuous ECG, HR, and BP monitoring is mandatory with use of IV metoprolol. ▪ Hemodynamic status must be closely monitored. If heart failure or hypotension occurs or persists despite appropriate treatment, metoprolol should be discontinued. Assess extent of myocardial damage. Invasive monitoring of central venous, pulmonary capillary wedge, and arterial pressure may be required. ▪ See Drug/Lab Interactions.

Patient Education: Report any breathing difficulty promptly.

Maternal/Child: Category C: safety for use in pregnancy and breast-feeding and in pediatric patients not established.

Elderly: Age-related differences in safety and effectiveness not identified; however, greater sensitivity of some elderly cannot be ruled out. Dose with caution. ▪ May exacerbate mental impairment.

DRUG/LAB INTERACTIONS

Concurrent use with **calcium channel blockers** (e.g., diltiazem, verapamil) may potentiate both drugs and result in severe depression of myocardium and AV conduction and severe hypotension. ▪ Concurrent use with **antihypertensive agents** may result in excessive hypotension. Dose adjustment may be required. ▪ **Potent inhibitors of the CYP2D6 enzyme** may increase plasma concentrations of metoprolol. These inhibitors include antidepressants (e.g., fluoxetine [Prozac], paroxetine [Paxil], and bupropion [Wellbutrin]), antipsychotics (e.g., thioridazine [Mellaril]), antiarrhythmics (e.g., quinidine, propafenone [Rythmol]), antiretrovirals (e.g., ritonavir [Norvir]), antihistamines (e.g., diphenhydramine [Benadryl]), antimalarials (e.g., hydroxychloroquine [Plaquenil], quinidine), allylamine antifungals (e.g., terbinafine [Lamisil]) and medications for stomach ulcers (e.g., cimetidine [Tagamet]). ▪ Concurrent use within 14 days of **MAO inhibitors** (selegiline [Eldepryl]) may cause severe hypertension. ▪ Use with **sympathomimetic agents** (e.g., epinephrine, norepinephrine, phenylephrine) **or xanthines** (e.g., aminophylline) may negate therapeutic effects of both drugs. ▪ Effects of beta-adrenergic blocking agents may be decreased by **ampicillin, anti-inflammatory drugs** (e.g., NSAIDs), **barbiturates, calcium salts, rifampin, salicylates, and others.** ▪ **Inhalation anesthetics, phenytoin** (Dilantin), **and quinolone antibiotics** (e.g., ciprofloxacin) may increase myocardial depressant effects and hypotension. ▪ Beta-adrenergic blocking agents may be continued during the perioperative period in most patients; however, use caution with **selected anesthetic agents** that may depress the myocardium. ■ Potentiates effects of **oral antidiabetics, catecholamine-depleting drugs** (e.g., reserpine), insulin, lidocaine, narcotics, and skeletal muscle relaxants; monitor carefully. Dose adjustment may be required. ■ Concurrent use with **clonidine** may precipitate acute hypertension if one or both agents are stopped abruptly. Withdraw metoprolol first. ■ Effects decreased when hypothyroid patient is **converted to a euthyroid state;** adjust dose as indicated. ■ Used concurrently with **digoxin or alpha-adrenergic blockers** (e.g., phentolamine [Regitine]) as indicated. ■ Use caution; both **digoxin** and beta-blockers (e.g., atenolol, esmolol, metoprolol, propranolol) slow AV conduction. May increase risk of bradycardia. ■ Patients taking beta-blockers who are exposed to a potential allergen may be unresponsive to the usual dose of **epinephrine** used to treat a hypersensitivity reaction.

SIDE EFFECTS

Abdominal pain, bradyarrhythmias, bronchospasm, cardiac failure, claudication, confusion, dizziness, dyspnea, elevated liver function tests, first-degree heart block, hallucinations, headache, hepatitis, hypotension, jaundice, nausea, nightmares, pruritus, rash, reduced libido, respiratory distress, second- or third-degree heart block, sleep disturbances, syncopal attacks, tiredness, unstable diabetes, vertigo, visual disturbances.

ANTIDOTE

For any side effect, discontinue drug and notify physician immediately. Patients with myocardial infarction may be more hemodynamically unstable; treat with caution. Use atropine (0.25 to 0.5 mg) for bradycardia or heart block; use isoproterenol with caution if atropine is not effective. Glucagon 5 to 10 mg IV may be effective if atropine and isoproterenol are not (investigational use). Transvenous cardiac pacing may be needed. Treat hypotension with IV fluids if indicated or vasopressors (dopamine or norepinephrine [Levarterenol]); treat cause of hypotension (e.g., bradycardia). Use all vasopressors with extreme caution; severe hypotension can result. Use digoxin and diuretics at first sign of cardiac failure; dobutamine, isoproterenol, or glucagon may be required. Use aminophylline or isoproterenol (with extreme care) for bronchospasm, and glucagon or IV glucose for hypoglycemia. Treat other side effects symptomatically; resuscitate as necessary.

METRONIDAZOLE
HYDROCHLORIDE BBW
(meh-troh-**NYE**-dah-zohl hy-droh-**KLOR**-eyed)

Flagyl IV, Flagyl IV RTU, Metronidazole RTU

Antibacterial
Antiprotozoal

pH 4.5 to 7

USUAL DOSE

May transfer to oral therapy when condition warrants (usual PO dose is 7.5 mg/kg every 6 hours).

Anaerobic infections: Begin with an initial loading dose of 15 mg/kg of body weight. Follow with 7.5 mg/kg (up to 1 Gm/dose) in 6 hours and every 6 hours thereafter for 7 to 10 days or longer if indicated. Do not exceed 4 Gm in 24 hours.

Complicated intra-abdominal infections: 500 mg every 6 hours given in combination with ciprofloxacin 400 mg every 12 hours or cefepime 2 Gm every 12 hours.

Prevent postoperative infection in contaminated or potentially contaminated colorectal surgery: 15 mg/kg infused over 30 to 60 minutes and completed 1 hour before surgery. Follow with 7.5 mg/kg over 30 to 60 minutes in 6 hours and in 12 hours. If *Bacteroides fragilis* is the suspected or confirmed organism, an alternate regimen is to give a 1,500-mg dose at the beginning of surgery to ensure adequate metronidazole levels.

PEDIATRIC DOSE

Safety for use in infants and other pediatric patients not established, but is used for anaerobic infections; see Maternal/Child.

Anaerobic infections: *Pediatric patients more than 7 days of age:* An initial loading dose of 15 mg/kg. Follow with 7.5 mg/kg every 6 hours. Another source recommends 7.5 mg/kg every 6 hours with a maximum dose of 4 Gm/24 hr.

Preterm infants: An initial loading dose of 15 mg/kg. 48 hours after loading dose, begin 7.5 mg/kg every 12 hours.

Term infants: Same as preterm except begin maintenance dose (7.5 mg/kg) 24 hours after loading dose.

Another source recommends age- and weight-specific doses as follows:
Less than 7 days of age weighing less than 1.2 kg: 7.5 mg/kg every 48 hours.
Less than 7 days of age weighing 1.2 to 2 kg: 7.5 mg/kg every 24 hours.
Less than 7 days of age weighing 2 or more kg: 7.5 mg/kg every 12 hours.
7 days of age or older weighing less than 1.2 kg: 7.5 mg/kg every 24 hours.
7 days of age or older weighing 1.2 to 2 kg: 7.5 mg/kg every 12 hours.
7 days of age or older weighing 2 or more kg: 15 mg/kg every 12 hours.

DOSE ADJUSTMENTS

Reduce dose in severe hepatic disease and in the elderly. Increase intervals in neonates; see Pediatric Dose. ■ No dose adjustment is indicated in mild to moderate impaired renal function. Recommendations vary for patients with a CrCl of less than 10 mL/min who are not on dialysis; consider reducing dose by 50% or increasing the interval to every 12 hours. ■ Dose adjustment not indicated in anuric patients; accumulated metabolites readily removed by dialysis. ■ Continuous NG suction may remove sufficient metronidazole in gastric aspirate to reduce serum levels. No dose adjustment is recommended.

DILUTION

All solutions are prediluted and ready to use (5 mg/mL) except Flagyl IV. Do not use plastic containers in series connections. Risk of air embolism is present. Avoid all contact with aluminum in needles and syringes in all situations. Color change will occur. The powder form (Flagyl IV) is not readily available, but it requires a specific dilution process; initially add 4.4 mL SW or NS for injection (100 mg/mL). Solution must be clear. Will be yellow to yellow-green in color with a pH of 0.5 to 2. Must be further diluted to at least 8 mg/mL with NS, D5W, or LR and be neutralized before infusion with 5 mEq of sodium bicarbonate per 500 mg metronidazole. Mix thoroughly. CO_2 gas will be generated and may require venting.

Storage: Store at room temperature before and after dilution. Discard diluted and neutralized solutions in 24 hours. Do not refrigerate; a precipitate will result. Protect from light when storing.

COMPATIBILITY   (Underline Indicates Conflicting Compatibility Information)

Consider any drug NOT listed as compatible to be INCOMPATIBLE until consulting a pharmacist; specific conditions may apply.

Manufacturer recommends, "Administer separately, discontinue the primary IV during administration, and do not introduce additives into the solution." Do not use equipment containing aluminum.

One source suggests the following **compatibilities:**

Additive: *Not recommended by manufacturer.* Ampicillin, cefazolin (Ancef), cefepime (Maxipime), cefotaxime (Claforan), cefoxitin (Mefoxin), ceftazidime (Fortaz), ceftriaxone (Rocephin), cefuroxime (Zinacef), ciprofloxacin (Cipro IV), fluconazole (Diflucan), gentamicin, hydrocortisone sodium succinate (Solu-Cortef), midazolam (Versed), penicillin G potassium, tobramycin.

Y-site: Acyclovir (Zovirax), allopurinol (Aloprim), amifostine (Ethyol), anidulafungin (Eraxis), bivalirudin (Angiomax), caspofungin (Cancidas), cefepime (Maxipime), cisatracurium (Nimbex), cyclophosphamide (Cytoxan), dexmedetomidine (Precedex), diltiazem (Cardizem), dimenhydrinate, docetaxel (Taxotere), dopamine, doripenem (Doribax), doxapram (Dopram), doxorubicin liposomal (Doxil), enalaprilat (Vasotec IV), esmolol (Brevibloc), etoposide phosphate (Etopophos), fenoldopam (Corlopam), fluconazole (Diflucan), foscarnet (Foscavir), gemcitabine (Gemzar), granisetron (Kytril), heparin, hetastarch in electrolytes (Hextend), hydromorphone (Dilaudid), labetalol (Trandate), linezolid (Zyvox), lorazepam (Ativan), magnesium sulfate, melphalan (Alkeran), meperidine (Demerol), methylprednisolone (Solu-Medrol), midazolam (Versed), milrinone (Primacor), morphine, nicardipine (Cardene IV), palonosetron (Aloxi), piperacillin/tazobactam (Zosyn), remifentanil (Ultiva), sargramostim (Leukine), tacrolimus (Prograf), teniposide (Vumon), theophylline, thiotepa, vasopressin, vinorelbine (Navelbine).

RATE OF ADMINISTRATION

Must be given as a slow intermittent or continuous IV infusion, each single dose evenly distributed over 1 hour. Discontinue primary IV during administration. Rate should be ordered by physician.

Surgical prophylaxis: Administer each single dose over 30 to 60 minutes.

ACTIONS

A bactericidal agent with cytotoxic effects, active against specific anaerobic bacteria and protozoa. Widely distributed in therapeutic levels to all body fluids (including abscesses). Levels are directly proportional to dose given. Onset of action is prompt. Metabolized in the liver. Half-life is 8 hours. Crosses placental and blood-brain barriers. Excreted in urine, some in feces. Secreted in breast milk.

INDICATIONS AND USES

Treatment of serious intra-abdominal, skin and skin structure, gynecologic, bone and joint, CNS, and lower respiratory tract infections; bacterial septicemia; and endocarditis caused by susceptible anaerobic bacteria. ■ Perioperative prophylaxis to reduce infection rates in contaminated or potentially contaminated colorectal surgery. ■ Given orally for antibiotic-related CDAD, amebiasis, and other indications.

CONTRAINDICATIONS

Hypersensitivity to metronidazole or nitroimidazole derivatives; first trimester of pregnancy.

PRECAUTIONS

A mixed (anaerobic/aerobic) infection will require use of additional appropriate antibiotics. ■ Sensitivity studies indicated to determine susceptibility of the causative organism to metronidazole. ■ To reduce the development of drug-resistant bacteria and maintain its effectiveness, metronidazole should be used to treat or prevent only those infections proven or strongly suspected to be caused by bacteria. ■ Avoid prolonged use of the drug; superinfection caused by overgrowth of nonsusceptible organisms may result. ■ Symptoms of candidiasis may be exacerbated and require treatment. ■ Encephalopathy has been reported in association with cerebellar toxicity characterized by ataxia, dizziness, and dysarthria. CNS lesions have been seen on MRI. Generally reversible within days to weeks after metronidazole is discontinued. ■ Optic neuropathy and peripheral neuropathy (mainly sensory with S/S of numbness or paresthesia of extremities) have been reported. ■ May cause seizures. ■ Aseptic meningitis has been reported. Symptoms may occur within hours of dose administration and generally resolve after metronidazole is discontinued. ■ Use caution in patients predisposed to edema and/or taking corticosteroids, in patients with impaired cardiac function (contains 27 to 28 mEq sodium/Gm), CNS disease, hepatic disease or impairment, or a history of blood dyscrasias. ■ *Clostridium difficile*–associated diarrhea (CDAD) has been reported. May range from mild diarrhea to fatal colitis. Consider in patients who present with diarrhea during or after treatment with metronidazole. ■ Carcinogenic in rodents; use only when necessary.

Monitor: Rotate IV site frequently to avoid thrombophlebitis. Avoid extravasation. ■ Mild leukopenia has been reported. Obtain total and differential leukocyte counts before and after therapy. ■ Monitor serum levels (suggested) and observe for toxicity in patients with hepatic disease receiving reduced doses and in the elderly. ■ Monitor for neurologic S/S (e.g., ataxia, dizziness, dysarthrias, numbness, paresthesia, and seizures). Prompt evaluation of risk versus benefit of continuing metronidazole required. ■ Transfer to oral dosing as soon as practical. ■ See Drug/Lab Interactions.

Patient Education: Avoid alcohol, alcohol-containing preparations, and disulfiram; toxic reactions will occur. ■ Promptly report diarrhea or bloody stools that occur during treatment or up to several months after an antibiotic has been discontinued; may indicate CDAD and require treatment. **Maternal/Child:** Category B: use during pregnancy only if clearly needed. ▪ Discontinue breast-feeding. ▪ Safety for use in pediatric patients and neonates not established. Half-life markedly extended in newborns; adjust intervals; see Pediatric Dose. ▪ See Contraindications. **Elderly:** Pharmacokinetics altered in the elderly; monitor serum levels if possible and adjust dose accordingly.

DRUG/LAB INTERACTIONS

Avoid **alcohol and alcohol-containing preparations** for at least 3 days after taking any dose of metronidazole; avoid for 2 weeks after disulfiram. Toxic reactions will occur. ▪ Concurrent use with **drugs that induce microsomal enzyme activity** (e.g., phenobarbital, phenytoin [Dilantin]) may increase metabolism of metronidazole and decrease plasma levels. ▪ May be antagonized by **bacteriostatic antibiotics** (e.g., chloramphenicol, erythromycin, and tetracyclines); bactericidal action may be negated. ▪ Administration with **drugs that inhibit microsomal liver enzyme activity** (e.g., cimetidine [Tagamet]) may prolong the half-life of metronidazole and increase metronidazole plasma levels. ▪ Potentiates **hydantoins** (e.g., phenytoin [Dilantin]). ▪ May decrease metabolism and increase anticoagulant effects of **warfarin** (Coumadin). Monitor PT/INR periodically. ▪ May increase **lithium** levels and cause toxicity. ▪ May interfere with **selected chemical studies** (e.g., AST, ALT, LDH, triglycerides, hexokinase glucose).

SIDE EFFECTS

The most serious side effects include aseptic meningitis, encephalopathy, and optic and peripheral neuropathy. Abdominal cramping; anorexia; ataxia; CDAD; constipation; cystitis; darkened deep red urine; decreased libido; diarrhea; dizziness; dryness of the mouth, vagina, or vulva; dysuria; epigastric distress; fever; fleeting joint pain; flushing; furry tongue; glossitis; headache; incontinence; metallic taste (expected); nasal congestion; nausea; neutropenia (reversible); numbness; painful coitus; paresthesia; pelvic pressure; polyuria; proctitis; pruritus; rash; seizures; Stevens-Johnson syndrome; stomatitis; syncope; thrombocytopenia (reversible); thrombophlebitis; T-wave flattening; urticaria; and vomiting have occurred.

ANTIDOTE

Notify physician of all side effects. Treatment will be symptomatic and supportive. Discontinue metronidazole with onset of seizures or signs of peripheral neuropathy (e.g., numbness or paresthesia of an extremity); benefit/risk of therapy must be reconsidered with onset of convulsions or peripheral neuropathy. Treat CDAD with fluids, electrolytes, protein supplements, and oral vancomycin (Vancocin) or metronidazole (Flagyl) as indicated. In severe cases, surgical evaluation may be indicated. Rapidly removed by hemodialysis. Treat anaphylaxis and resuscitate as necessary.

MICAFUNGIN SODIUM
(my-kah-**FUN**-gin **SO**-dee-um)
Mycamine

Antifungal

pH 5 to 7

USUAL DOSE
Treatment of candidemia, acute disseminated candidiasis, *Candida* peritonitis and abscesses: 100 mg/day as an infusion. Mean duration of treatment during clinical studies was 15 days (range 10 to 47 days).
Treatment of esophageal candidiasis: 150 mg/day as an infusion. Mean duration of treatment during clinical studies was 15 days (range 10 to 30 days).
Prophylaxis of *Candida* infections in hematopoietic stem cell transplant (HSCT) recipients: 50 mg/day as an infusion. Mean duration of treatment in patients who responded successfully during clinical studies was 19 days (range 6 to 51 days).

DOSE ADJUSTMENTS
No dose adjustment indicated based on gender or race, in the elderly, or in patients with severe renal dysfunction or mild to moderate hepatic insufficiency (Child-Pugh score 7 to 9). ▪ Has not been studied in patients with severe hepatic insufficiency. ▪ Not dialyzable; a supplementary dose following hemodialysis should not be required. ▪ See Drug/Lab Interactions.

DILUTION
Each 50- or 100-mg vial must be reconstituted with 5 mL of NS without a bacteriostatic agent (preferred). Alternately, 5 mL of D5W may be used. The use of strict aseptic technique is required. Swirl vial(s) gently to dissolve. **Do not shake.** Do not use if precipitation or foreign matter is observed. Each single dose (50, 100, or 150 mg) must be further diluted in 100 mL NS (preferred) or D5W for infusion.
Filters: No study data available; if filtering is necessary, contact manufacturer.
Storage: Store unopened vials at CRT. Reconstituted solution in original vial or diluted solution is stable up to 24 hours at 25° C (77° F). Protect diluted solution from light. Discard partially used vials.

COMPATIBILITY
(Underline Indicates Conflicting Compatibility Information)
Consider any drug NOT listed as compatible to be INCOMPATIBLE until consulting a pharmacist; specific conditions may apply.
Manufacturer states, "Do not mix or co-infuse micafungin with other medications. Has been shown to precipitate when mixed directly with a number of other commonly used medications." Flush IV line with NS before and after infusion.
  One source suggests the following **compatibilities:**
Y-site: Aminophylline, bumetanide, calcium chloride, calcium gluconate, carboplatin (Paraplatin), cyclosporine (Sandimmune), dopamine, doripenem (Doribax), eptifibatide (Integrilin), esmolol (Brevibloc), etoposide (VePesid), fenoldopam (Corlopam), furosemide (Lasix), heparin, hydromorphone (Dilaudid), lidocaine, lorazepam (Ativan), magnesium sulfate, mesna (Mesnex), milrinone (Primacor), nitroglycerin IV, nitroprusside (Nitropress), norepinephrine (Levophed), phenylephrine (Neo-

Synephrine), potassium chloride, potassium phosphate, sodium phosphate, tacrolimus (Prograf), theophylline, vasopressin.

RATE OF ADMINISTRATION

Flush IV line with NS before and after infusion.

A single dose as an infusion equally distributed over 1 hour. Rapid infusion may result in more frequent histamine-mediated reactions (e.g., facial swelling, pruritus, rash, vasodilation).

ACTIONS

A semisynthetic lipopeptide and the first of a new class of antifungal agents, the echinocandins. Acts by inhibiting the synthesis of 1,3-beta-D-glucan, an integral component of the fungal cell wall not present in mammalian cells. The AUC increases as doses are increased (e.g., from 50 to 150 mg or from 3 to 8 mg/kg). Highly protein bound primarily to albumin but does not competitively displace bilirubin binding to albumin. 85% of steady-state concentration achieved after three daily doses. Metabolized in the liver. A substrate and weak inhibitor of CYP3A, but CYP3A is not a major pathway for metabolism. Half-life ranges from 11 to 21.3 hours. Primarily excreted in feces, with some excretion in urine.

INDICATIONS AND USES

Treatment of patients with candidemia, acute disseminated candidiasis, and *Candida* peritonitis and abscesses. ■ Treatment of esophageal candidiasis. ■ Prophylaxis of *Candida* infections in patients undergoing hematopoietic stem cell transplantation. ■ Efficacy against infections caused by fungi other than *Candida* not established.

CONTRAINDICATIONS

Hypersensitivity to micafungin, any of its components, or other echinocandins (e.g., anidulafungin [Eraxis]), caspofungin (Cancidas).

PRECAUTIONS

Do not give as an IV bolus; for IV infusion only. ■ Isolated anaphylactoid reactions (including shock) and anaphylaxis have been reported. ■ Abnormal liver function tests have been reported. Isolated cases of significant hepatic dysfunction, hepatitis, or worsening hepatic failure have occurred. Incidence may be increased in patients with serious underlying conditions who are receiving additional concomitant medications. Evaluate risk versus benefit of continued micafungin therapy. ■ Elevations in BUN and creatinine have been reported. Isolated cases of significant renal dysfunction or acute renal failure have occurred. ■ Intravascular hemolysis and hemoglobinuria have been reported. Isolated cases of significant hemolysis and hemolytic anemia have occurred. Evaluate risk versus benefit of continued micafungin therapy. ■ Potential for development of drug resistance not known. Mutants of *Candida* with reduced susceptibility to micafungin have been identified, suggesting a potential for development of drug resistance. ■ See Monitor and Antidote.

Monitor: Specimens for fungal culture, serologic testing, and histopathologic testing should be obtained before therapy to isolate and identify causative organisms. Therapy may begin as soon as all specimens are obtained and before results are known. Reassess after test results are known. ■ Baseline CBC with differential and platelet count, BUN, SCr, and liver function tests (e.g., ALT, AST) may be indicated. ■ Monitor for S/S of a hypersensitivity reaction (e.g., bronchospasm, dyspnea, hives, hypotension, rash, pruritus, swelling of eyelids, lips, or face); discontinue infusion if a hypersensitivity reaction occurs. ■ Monitor for evidence of worsening hepatic function (e.g., increased ALT, AST, serum alkaline phosphatase). ▪ Monitor for evidence of worsening renal function (e.g., increased BUN, SCr). ▪ Monitor for S/S of hemolytic anemia, hemolysis, and hemoglobinuria as indicated (lysis of RBCs, liberation of hemoglobin, blood in the urine). ▪ Hematologic, hepatic, and renal effects may require discontinuation of micafungin.

Patient Education: Promptly report shortness of breath, dizziness or fainting, itching, rash, or swelling of extremities. ▪ Report S/S of liver dysfunction (anorexia, fatigue, jaundice, nausea and vomiting, dark urine, or pale stools). ▪ Report any S/S of hemoglobinuria (blood in the urine). ▪ Report S/S of renal dysfunction (decrease in urine output). ▪ Review list of current medications with physician. Drug interactions are possible; see Drug/Lab Interactions.

Maternal/Child: Pregnancy category C: use during pregnancy only if benefits justify risk to fetus. Some abnormalities, including abortion, occurred in animal studies. ▪ Use caution if required during breastfeeding. Secreted in milk of drug-treated rats; not known if micafungin is secreted in human milk. ▪ Safety and effectiveness for use in pediatric patients not established.

Elderly: Differences in response compared to younger adults not identified; however, greater sensitivity in the elderly cannot be ruled out.

DRUG/LAB INTERACTIONS

No alteration of micafungin pharmacokinetics observed with concurrent administration of amphotericin B, cyclosporine (Sandimmune), fluconazole (Diflucan), itraconazole (Sporanox), mycophenolate (CellCept), nifedipine (ProCardia XL), prednisolone, rifampin (Rifadin), ritonavir (Norvir), sirolimus (Rapamune), tacrolimus (Prograf), or voriconazole (VFEND). ▪ Concurrent doses of micafungin did not appear to alter the pharmacokinetics of cyclosporine, mycophenolate, fluconazole, prednisolone, tacrolimus, or voriconazole. ▪ The effects of **itraconazole, nifedipine, and sirolimus** are increased with concurrent administration of micafungin. Monitor for itraconazole, nifedipine, or sirolimus toxicity and reduce their dose as indicated. ▪ Effects of micafungin on the pharmacokinetics of **rifampin and ritonavir** not available. ▪ Not expected to alter effects of drugs metabolized by the CYP3A system.

SIDE EFFECTS

Abdominal pain, anemia, chills, delirium, dizziness, fever, headache, increased liver function tests (e.g., alkaline phosphatase, ALT, AST, BUN, transaminases), injection site reactions (including inflammation, phlebitis, and thrombophlebitis), leukopenia, lymphopenia, nausea, neutropenia, somnolence, thrombocytopenia, vomiting occurred in patients treated for esophageal candidiasis. In addition, constipation, decreased appetite, diarrhea, dysgeusia (altered sense of taste), dyspepsia, fatigue, febrile neutropenia, flushing, hiccups, hyperbilirubinemia, hypertension, hypocalcemia, hypokalemia, hypomagnesemia, hypophosphatemia, hypotension, increased drug levels, increased SCr, and mucosal inflammation occurred in patients undergoing prophylactic use during HSCT. Most serious side effects that may occur regardless of indication include acute intravascular hemolysis, decreased WBC, hemoglobinuria, hemolytic anemia, histamine-mediated reactions (e.g., facial swelling, pruritus, rash, vasodilation), hypersensitivity reactions (e.g., anaphylaxis and anaphylactoid reactions [including shock]), significant hepatic dysfunction (e.g., hepatitis, hepatocellular damage, hyperbilirubinemia, or worsening hepatic failure), significant renal dysfunction and/or acute renal failure.

Other side effects varied with each indication, but all three indications reported abdominal pain, anemia, diarrhea, fever, headache, insomnia, nausea, and vomiting.

Patients with esophageal candidiasis: Also reported rash and phlebitis.

Patients with candidemia and other *Candida* infections and prophylaxis of *Candida* infection in HSCT: Both reported bacteremia, hypertension, hypokalemia, hypomagnesemia, hypotension, peripheral edema, tachycardia, and thrombocytopenia.

Patients with candidemia and other *Candida* infections: Also reported aggravated anemia, atrial fibrillation, bradycardia, decubitus ulcer, hyperkalemia, hypernatremia, hypoglycemia, increased blood alkaline phosphatase, pneumonia, sepsis, septic shock, vascular disorders.

Prophylaxis of *Candida* infection in HSCT: Also reported anorexia, anxiety, constipation, cough, dizziness, dyspepsia, dyspnea, epistaxis, erythema, fatigue, febrile neutropenia, fluid overload, fluid retention, flushing, hypocalcemia, mucosal inflammation, neutropenia, pruritus, rash, and rigors.

ANTIDOTE

Notify physician of all side effects; most will be treated symptomatically. If a hypersensitivity reaction occurs, discontinue micafungin and treat as indicated. Appropriate treatment may include oxygen, epinephrine, antihistamines (e.g., diphenhydramine [Benadryl]), vasopressors (e.g., dopamine), corticosteroids, IV fluids, and ventilation equipment. S/S indicative of hepatic, renal, or hematologic side effects may require evaluation of benefits versus risk of continuing micafungin therapy. Not removed by hemodialysis. Resuscitate as indicated.

MIDAZOLAM HYDROCHLORIDE `BBW`
(my-**DAYZ**-oh-lam hy-droh-**KLOR**-eyed)

Benzodiazepine
Sedative-hypnotic
Anesthetic adjunct
Amnestic

Midazolam HCl PF, Versed   pH 3

USUAL DOSE

Dose requirements for each patient may vary and will depend on the type and amount of premedication used. Doses given below are general guidelines. Individualize dose and titrate slowly to effect. Allow 3 to 5 minutes between each small injection to evaluate the full effect before administering additional doses.

SEDATION, ANXIOLYSIS (ANTI-ANXIETY), AND/OR AMNESIA FOR SHORT DIAGNOSTIC, ENDOSCOPIC, AND THERAPEUTIC PROCEDURES

The desired endpoint for conscious sedation can usually be achieved in 3 to 6 minutes. Time will depend on total dose and type or dose of narcotic premedication used concomitantly.

Healthy adults less than 60 years of age: 1 to 2.5 mg immediately before the procedure. Begin with 1 mg and titrate slowly up to slurred speech or 2.5 mg. Some patients respond adequately to 1 mg. If additional medication is needed, wait a full 2 minutes, then titrate additional dosage slowly in small increments (usually no more than 1 mg). Wait a full 2 minutes between each increment. A total dose exceeding 5 mg is rarely necessary. Reduce dose by 30% in the presence of narcotic premedication or other CNS depressants. 25% of the sedating dose can be used for maintenance only when clearly indicated by clinical evaluation.

Patients over 60 years of age or debilitated or chronically ill patients: 1 to 1.5 mg. Begin with 1 mg and titrate slowly up to slurred speech or 1.5 mg. May respond adequately to 1 mg. If additional medication is needed, wait a full 2 minutes, then titrate additional dosage in small increments (no more than 1 mg). Wait a full 2 minutes between each increment. A total dose exceeding 3.5 mg is rarely necessary. Reduce dose by 50% in the presence of narcotic premedication or other CNS depressants. 25% of the sedating dose can be used for maintenance only when clearly indicated by clinical evaluation.

INDUCTION OF ANESTHESIA BEFORE ADMINISTRATION OF OTHER ANESTHETIC AGENTS AND/OR MAINTENANCE OF ANESTHESIA AS A COMPONENT OF BALANCED ANESTHESIA DURING SURGICAL PROCEDURES

In all patients (unpremedicated and premedicated), allow 2 minutes from initial dose to reach peak effect. If necessary, complete induction with 25% of initial dose or use inhalational anesthesia (e.g., halothane). Doses of any agents used after induction of anesthesia with midazolam may need to be reduced to as little as 25% of the usual initial dose. 25% of the induction dose can be repeated when indicated by lightening of anesthesia.

Unpremedicated patients under 55 years of age: 0.3 to 0.35 mg/kg as an initial dose. A total dose of up to 0.6 mg/kg has been required; recovery may be prolonged.

Unpremedicated patients over 55 years of age (ASA I or II): 0.15 to 0.3 mg/kg as an initial dose.

Unpremedicated debilitated patients or those with severe systemic disease (ASA III or IV): 0.15 to 0.25 mg/kg as an initial dose. As little as 0.15 mg/kg may be adequate.

Patients premedicated with sedatives or narcotics under 55 years of age: 0.25 mg/kg as an initial dose may be adequate. Range is 0.15 to 0.35 mg/kg of body weight.

Patients premedicated with sedatives or narcotics over 55 years of age (Good risk [ASA I & II]): 0.2 mg/kg as an initial dose may be adequate.

Patients premedicated with sedatives or narcotics who are debilitated or those with severe systemic disease (ASA III or IV): 0.15 mg/kg as an initial dose may be adequate.

Premedication usually includes narcotics (e.g., fentanyl 1.5 to 2 mcg/kg IV 5 minutes before induction, or morphine [up to 0.15 mg/kg IM] or meperidine [up to 1 mg/kg IM]) 1 hour before induction with midazolam. Sedative premedication usually includes hydroxyzine (Vistaril) 100 mg PO or a barbiturate PO 1 hour before induction.

SEDATION FOR ANESTHESIA OR TREATMENT IN A CRITICAL CARE SETTING FOR INTUBATED AND MECHANICALLY VENTILATED PATIENTS

Continuous infusion (concentration 0.5 mg/mL): Begin with a *loading dose* of 0.01 to 0.05 mg/kg (0.5 to 4 mg for a typical adult) to rapidly initiate sedation. Infuse over several minutes. May be repeated at 10- to 15-minute intervals until adequate sedation achieved.

For maintenance of sedation: An initial infusion rate of 0.02 to 0.1 mg/kg/hr (1 to 7 mg/hr) may be used. Upper-end doses may be required, but use the lowest recommended doses in patients with residual effects from anesthetic drugs or in those concurrently receiving other sedatives or opioids. Initial infusion rate may be titrated up or down by 25% to 50% to maintain desired level of sedation. Decrease by 10% to 25% every few hours to find the minimum effective infusion rate. The lowest rate that produces the desired level of sedation is recommended. Agitation, hypertension, or tachycardia in response to stimulation in adequately sedated patients may indicate need for an opioid analgesic. Reduced rate of midazolam infusion may be indicated with the addition of an opioid analgesic. Taper dose gradually if midazolam has been used for more than a few days. Abrupt discontinuation may result in withdrawal symptoms.

REFRACTORY STATUS EPILEPTICUS (UNLABELED)

0.15 to 0.3 mg/kg (usual dose 5 to 15 mg); may repeat every 10 to 15 minutes or has been given as a continuous infusion at a rate of 0.05 to 0.6 mg/kg/hr.

PEDIATRIC DOSE

In all situations dose is based on lean body weight in obese pediatric patients. See Precautions and Maternal/Child.

SEDATION, ANXIOLYSIS (ANTIANXIETY), AND/OR AMNESIA BEFORE AND DURING PROCEDURES OR BEFORE ANESTHESIA

All increments of midazolam are on a mg/kg basis. Initial dose is age, procedure, and route dependent. Total dose will depend on patient response, type and duration of the procedure, and type and dose of concomitant medications. Titrate dose of midazolam and other concomitant medications slowly to the desired clinical effect. With concomitant medications, dose of midazolam

Continued

should be reduced (usually by 25% to 30%). Before beginning a procedure or repeating a dose, wait a full 2 to 3 minutes to fully evaluate the sedative effect. If further sedation is necessary, continue to titrate with small increments at 2- to 3-minute intervals until desired level of sedation achieved. Prolonged sedation and risk of hypoventilation may be associated with higher-end doses.

Nonintubated infants less than 6 months of age: Uncertain when patient transfers from neonatal physiology to pediatric physiology; manufacturer has no specific dosing recommendations. Titrate with very small increments to clinical effect and monitor very carefully for airway obstruction and hypoventilation.

Pediatric patients 6 months to 5 years of age: Begin with an initial dose of 0.05 to 0.1 mg/kg. Up to 0.6 mg/kg may be required, but a total dose of 6 mg is usually not exceeded.

Pediatric patients 6 to 12 years of age: Begin with an initial dose of 0.025 to 0.05 mg/kg. Up to 0.4 mg/kg may be required, but a total dose of 10 mg is usually not exceeded.

Pediatric patients 12 to 16 years of age: See Usual Dose. May require higher-than-recommended adult doses, but total dose usually does not exceed 10 mg.

SEDATION, ANXIOLYSIS, AMNESIA

Intubated pediatric patients in critical care settings: Begin with a loading dose of 0.05 to 0.2 mg/kg. May be allowed to breathe on own through intubation tube but assisted ventilation recommended in pediatric patients receiving other CNS depressants. In hemodynamically compromised pediatric patients, titrate the loading dose in small increments and monitor for hypotension, respiratory rate, and oxygen saturation. May be followed by a continuous IV infusion at 0.06 to 0.12 mg/kg/hr (1 to 2 mcg/kg/min). Increase or decrease infusion in 25% increments or use supplemental IV injection to maintain desired effect.

SEDATION OF INTUBATED NEONATES IN CRITICAL CARE SETTINGS

Neonates less than 32 weeks: A continuous infusion at a rate of 0.03 mg/kg/hr (0.5 mcg/kg/min).

Neonates 32 weeks or older: A continuous infusion at a rate of 0.06 mg/kg/hr (1 mcg/kg/min).

Do not use loading doses in neonates. Infusion may be run more rapidly for the first several hours to establish therapeutic plasma levels. Reassess rate carefully and frequently to use the lowest possible effective dose and reduce the potential for drug accumulation. Midazolam contains benzyl alcohol and must be used with extreme caution in neonates.

REFRACTORY STATUS EPILEPTICUS (UNLABELED)

Pediatric patients 2 months of age or older: *Loading dose:* 0.15 mg/kg followed by a continuous infusion of 1 mcg/kg/min. Titrate dose upward every 5 minutes to effect. Mean dose is 2.3 mcg/kg/min (range is 1 to 18 mcg/kg/min).

DOSE ADJUSTMENTS

Reduce dose by 30% to 50%, depending on age, in the presence of narcotic premedication or other CNS depressants; see Usual Dose. ■ Reduce dose in congestive heart failure, chronic obstructive pulmonary disease, impaired hepatic or renal function, debilitated patients, and patients over 55 years of age. Half-life is extended and depressant effects will be potentiated; see Usual Dose. ▪ Dose based on lean body weight in obese pediatric patients. ▪ See Drug/Lab Interactions.

DILUTION

Read Label Carefully and Confirm mg Dose. Available in Two Strengths, 1 mg/mL and 5 mg/mL.

IV injection: May be diluted with D5W or NS. Dilute in a sufficient amount to permit slow titration (i.e., 1 mg in 4 mL or 5 mg in 20 mL [0.25 mg/m]). Maximum concentration after dilution should not exceed 0.5 mg/mL.

Infusion: Dilute in either of the previously listed solutions to a maximum concentration of 0.5 mg/mL. 5 mL of a 1 mg/mL (5 mg) in 5 mL of diluent yields 0.5 mg/mL. 5 mL of a 5 mg/mL (25 mg) in 45 mL diluent is usually a 24-hour supply and also yields 0.5 mg/mL. Use a controlled infusion device or at the very least a metriset (60 gtt/mL) to facilitate titration and control flow to prevent overdose.

COMPATIBILITY   (Underline Indicates Conflicting Compatibility Information)

Consider any drug NOT listed as compatible to be INCOMPATIBLE until consulting a pharmacist; specific conditions may apply.

One source suggests the following **compatibilities:**

Additive: Cefuroxime (Zinacef), ciprofloxacin (Cipro IV), furosemide (Lasix), gentamicin, hydromorphone (Dilaudid), metronidazole (Flagyl IV), ranitidine (Zantac).

Y-site: Abciximab (ReoPro), amikacin (Amikin), amiodarone (Nexterone), anidulafungin (Eraxis), argatroban, atracurium (Tracrium), bivalirudin (Angiomax), calcium gluconate, caspofungin (Cancidas), cefazolin (Ancef), cefotaxime (Claforan), ciprofloxacin (Cipro IV), cisatracurium (Nimbex), clindamycin (Cleocin), digoxin (Lanoxin), diltiazem (Cardizem), dobutamine, dopamine, doripenem (Doribax), epinephrine (Adrenalin), erythromycin (Erythrocin), esmolol (Brevibloc), etomidate (Amidate), famotidine (Pepcid IV), fenoldopam (Corlopam), fentanyl (Sublimaze), fluconazole (Diflucan), gentamicin, haloperidol (Haldol), heparin, hetastarch in electrolytes (Hextend), hydromorphone (Dilaudid), insulin (regular), labetalol (Trandate), linezolid (Zyvox), lorazepam (Ativan), methadone (Dolophine), methylprednisolone (Solu-Medrol), metronidazole (Flagyl IV), milrinone (Primacor), morphine, nicardipine (Cardene IV), nitroglycerin IV, nitroprusside sodium, norepinephrine (Levophed), palonosetron (Aloxi), pancuronium, piperacillin, potassium chloride (KCl), propofol (Diprivan), ranitidine (Zantac), remifentanil (Ultiva), sufentanil (Sufenta), theophylline, tirofiban (Aggrastat), tobramycin, vancomycin, vecuronium.

RATE OF ADMINISTRATION

IV injection: *Sedation:* Any single increment of a total dose titrated slowly over at least 2 minutes. Stop at any point that the speech becomes slurred.

Induction of anesthesia: Any single increment of a total dose over 20 to 30 seconds. Rapid injection in any situation may cause respiratory depression or apnea.

Infusion: See Usual Dose. The American Academy of Critical Care recommends limiting the use of midazolam in the critical care setting to 24 hours because its metabolites accumulate in peripheral tissue, especially with long-term infusion.

Pediatric rate: Any single increment of a total dose over a minimum of 2 to 3 minutes. Rapid injection or infusion may cause severe hypotension or seizures in infants and neonates; incidence increased with concomitant fentanyl. See comments under Infusion.

ACTIONS

A short-acting benzodiazepine CNS depressant 3 to 4 times as potent as diazepam. Has anxiolytic, hypnotic, anticonvulsant, muscle relaxant, and anterograde amnestic effects. Depressant effects are dependent on dose, route of administration, and the presence or absence of other premedications. Can depress the ventilatory response to CO_2 stimulation. Mechanics of respiration are not adversely affected with usual doses. Mean arterial pressure, cardiac output, stroke volume, and systemic vascular resistance may be slightly decreased. May cause HRs of less than 65/min to rise and more than 85/min to fall. Produces sleepiness and relief of apprehension, and diminishes patient recall very effectively. Widely distributed. Onset of action occurs within 1.5 to 5 minutes. Half-life is approximately 2.5 hours (range is 1 to 5 hours), shorter than that of diazepam (Valium). Time to recovery is usually within 2 hours but may take as long as 6 hours. Metabolized in the liver by cytochrome P_{450} mediation and excreted as metabolites in urine. Crosses the placental barrier. Secreted in breast milk.

INDICATIONS AND USES

To produce sedation, relieve anxiety, and impair memory of perioperative events. ■ May be used with or without narcotic sedation for conscious sedation before short diagnostic, endoscopic, or therapeutic procedures (e.g., bronchoscopy, gastroscopy, cystoscopy, coronary angiography, cardiac catheterization). ■ Induction of anesthesia before administration of other anesthetic agents. ■ As a component in the induction and maintenance of balanced anesthesia in short surgical procedures. ■ Continuous infusions may be used in intubated and mechanically ventilated patients for sedation as a component of anesthesia or during treatment in a critical care setting.

Unlabeled use: Treatment of refractory status epilepticus.

CONTRAINDICATIONS

Acute narrow-angle glaucoma, known hypersensitivity to midazolam, open-angle glaucoma unless receiving appropriate treatment. Not recommended in pregnancy, childbirth, breast-feeding, shock, coma, acute alcohol intoxication with depression of vital signs. Contraindicated with ritonavir (Norvir).

PRECAUTIONS

Respiratory depression and/or respiratory arrest may occur. Should be used only in a hospital or ambulatory care setting with continuous monitoring of respiratory and cardiac function (e.g., pulse oximetry). Resuscitative drugs (including flumazenil [Romazicon]) and age- and size-appropriate equipment for bag/valve/mask ventilation and intubation must be immediately available. Personnel must be skilled in airway management. ■ A dedicated individual with no other responsibilities should monitor deeply sedated patients throughout any procedure. ■ A topical anesthetic agent should be used with midazolam during perioral endoscopy, and premedication with a narcotic is recommended in bronchoscopy since increased cough reflex and laryngospasm frequently occur. Premedication with a narcotic is also recommended with balanced anesthesia. ■ For IV/IM use only. Contains benzyl alcohol. Do not use for intrathecal or epidural administration. ■ Use caution in neonates. At recommended doses benzyl alcohol is not expected to be toxic, but excessive benzyl alcohol may result in hypotension, metabolic acidosis, and increased incidence of kernicterus, especially in small preterm infants. ▪ Use extreme caution in the elderly, in patients with chronic disease states, decreased pulmonary reserve, hepatic or renal impairment, neuromuscular disorders, and in those with uncompensated acute illness (e.g., severe fluid or electrolyte disturbances); may have increased risks of hypoventilation, airway obstruction, or apnea. Peak effect may take longer. ▪ Use with caution in obese patients and patients with CHF. Half-life is prolonged. ▪ See Pediatric Dose and Maternal/Child for additional precautions with infants and other pediatric patients. ▪ Does not protect against increased intracranial pressure or circulatory changes noted with succinylcholine or pancuronium or associated with intubation under light general anesthesia. ▪ Some clinicians prefer midazolam over diazepam because of effectiveness, minimum pain if any on injection, and miscibility with many drugs and solutions.

Monitor: Obtain a careful presedation history (e.g., medical conditions, concomitant meds), and complete a physical exam. Check for airway abnormalities. ▪ Monitor respiratory and cardiac function (e.g., BP, HR, pulse oximetry) continuously. *Has caused apnea and cardiac arrest.* Monitoring of ECG desirable. Maintain a patent airway and support adequate ventilation. Record assessments using standard assessment charts for scoring, especially in pediatric patients. Monitor for both adequate and excessive sedation. ▪ Extravasation or arterial administration hazardous. ▪ Bed rest required for a minimum of 3 hours after IV injection. ▪ See Drug/Lab Interactions.

Patient Education: Do not drive or operate hazardous machinery until the day after surgery or longer. All effects must have subsided. Avoid use of alcohol or other CNS depressants (e.g., antihistamines, barbiturates) for 24 hours after last dose. ▪ May impair memory; request written postop instructions. ▪ Consider birth control options.

Maternal/Child: Category D: avoid pregnancy. ▪ Not recommended during pregnancy, labor and delivery, or breast-feeding. ▪ Elimination rate is faster in infants and children. ▪ Neonate has reduced or immature organ function. Clearance is decreased and half-life is increased in critically ill neonates. May be susceptible to profound and/or prolonged respiratory effects. ▪ See Precautions and Monitor.

Elderly: See Usual Dose and Dose Adjustments. Start with a small dose and increase gradually based on response. ▪ Clearance is reduced compared to younger adults, and time to recovery may be prolonged. ▪ All elderly are more sensitive to therapeutic and adverse effects (e.g., oversedation, ataxia, dizziness). Patients over 70 years of age may be particularly sensitive. IV injection may be more likely to cause apnea, bradycardia, hypotension, and cardiac arrest. ▪ See Precautions and Drug/Lab Interactions.

DRUG/LAB INTERACTIONS

Concurrent use with **other CNS depressants** (e.g., alcohol, antihistamines, barbiturates, inhalation anesthetics [e.g., halothane], MAO inhibitors [e.g., selegiline (Eldepryl)], narcotics [e.g., morphine, meperidine (Demerol), fentanyl], phenothiazines [e.g., prochlorperazine (Compazine)], thiopental, and tricyclic antidepressants [e.g., imipramine (Tofranil)]) may result in additive effects for up to 48 hours. May produce apnea or prolonged effect, depress ventilatory response to CO_2, or cause hypotension. Reduce doses of midazolam. ▪ **Agents that inhibit cytochrome P_{450} activity** (e.g., triazole antifungals [e.g., itraconazole (Sporanox), ketoconazole (Nizoral), miconazole (Monistat)], cimetidine [Tagamet], diltiazem [Cardizem], verapamil, macrolide antibiotics [e.g., erythromycin], omeprazole [Prilosec], and ranitidine [Zantac]) decrease clearance and increase effects of midazolam resulting in prolonged sedation. ▪ Reduce doses of **inhalation anesthetics** (e.g., halothane) **and/or thiopental** when used with midazolam. ▪ **Protease inhibitors** (e.g., indinavir [Crixivan], nelfinavir [Viracept], and saquinavir [Invirase]) may increase risk of prolonged sedation and respiratory depression. Concurrent use not recommended. Half-life may double with saquinavir. *Contraindicated with ritonavir (Norvir);* may cause life-threatening increased sedation and respiratory depression. Benzodiazepines metabolized by alternate routes may be safer (e.g., lorazepam [Ativan], oxazepam [Serax], temazepam [Restoril]). ▪ May increase serum concentrations of **digoxin;** monitor digoxin serum levels. ▪ Hypotensive effects of benzodiazepines may be increased by any **agent that induces hypotension** (e.g., antihypertensives, CNS depressants, diuretics, lidocaine, paclitaxel). Monitor BP during and after use. ▪ Use with **rifampin** (Rifadin) increases clearance and reduces effects of benzodiazepines. ▪ **Theophyllines** (Aminophylline) antagonize sedative effects of benzodiazepines. ▪ **Smoking** increases metabolism and clearance of midazolam, decreasing plasma levels and sedative effects.

SIDE EFFECTS
The incidence of cardiorespiratory events is higher in patients undergoing procedures involving the upper airway (e.g., upper endoscopy or dental procedures). Serious cardiorespiratory events may include airway obstruction, apnea, hypotension (especially with narcotic premedication), oxygen desaturation, respiratory arrest, and/or cardiac arrhythmias or arrest. Inadequate or excessive dosing may cause agitation, combativeness, involuntary movements (e.g., clonic, tonic, muscle tremor), and hyperactivity; may be caused by cerebral hypoxia or be true paradoxical reactions. Other common reactions are coughing, drowsiness, fluctuation in vital signs, headache, hiccups, nausea and vomiting, nystagmus (especially in pediatric patients), induration, redness, or phlebitis at injection site. Capable of numerous other side effects. Has caused death and hypoxic encephalopathy. Withdrawal may be seen in patients receiving an infusion for extended periods of time.
Overdose: Sedation, somnolence, confusion, impaired coordination, diminished reflexes, coma, and untoward effect on vital signs.

ANTIDOTE
Notify the physician of all side effects. Reduction of dosage may be required or will be treated symptomatically. Discontinue the drug for major side effects or paradoxical reactions. Flumazenil (Romazicon) will reverse all sedative effects of benzodiazepines. A patent airway, artificial ventilation, oxygen therapy and other symptomatic treatment must be instituted promptly. Treat hypotension with IV fluids, Trendelenburg position, or vasopressors (e.g., dopamine) as indicated. May cause emesis; observe closely. Treat hypersensitivity reactions and resuscitate as necessary.

MILRINONE LACTATE
(**MILL**-rih-nohn **LAK**-tayt)

Primacor

USUAL DOSE
50 mcg/kg (0.05 mg/kg) of body weight as the initial loading dose.
Follow with a maintenance infusion according to the following chart.

Milrinone Maintenance Dose Guidelines			
	Infusion Rate (mcg/kg/min)	Total Daily Dose (24 Hours)	
Minimum	0.375 mcg/kg/min	0.59 mg/kg	Administer as a continuous IV infusion.
Standard	0.50 mcg/kg/min	0.77 mg/kg	
Maximum	0.75 mcg/kg/min	1.13 mg/kg	

Titrate the infusion dose between 0.375 mcg/kg/min to 0.75 mcg/kg/min
(26 mcg/min to 52 mcg/min for a 70-kg person) based on hemodynamic
and clinical response. Do not exceed a total dose of 1.13 mg/kg/24 hr.
Duration of infusion usually does not exceed 48 hours.

DOSE ADJUSTMENTS
Reduced dose required in impaired renal function based on CrCl according
to the following chart.

Milrinone Dose Guidelines in Impaired Renal Function	
Creatinine Clearance (mL/min/1.73 M^2)	Infusion Rate (mcg/kg/min)
5 mL/min/1.73 M^2	0.2 mcg/kg/min
10 mL/min/1.73 M^2	0.23 mcg/kg/min
20 mL/min/1.73 M^2	0.28 mcg/kg/min
30 mL/min/1.73 M^2	0.33 mcg/kg/min
40 mL/min/1.73 M^2	0.38 mcg/kg/min
50 mL/min/1.73 M^2	0.43 mcg/kg/min

DILUTION
Loading dose: May be given undiluted, or each 1 mg (1 mL) may be diluted
in 1 mL NS or ½NS for injection. Alternately, the loading dose may be
diluted with NS, ½NS, or D5W to a total volume of 10 or 20 mL for
injection.
Infusion: Dilute with NS, ½NS, or D5W. Available prediluted as
200 mcg/mL in D5W. Amount of diluent may be increased or decreased
based on patient fluid requirements. Another source suggests dilution
with LR.

Guidelines for Dilution of Milrinone for Infusion			
Desired Infusion Concentration (mcg/mL)	Milrinone 1 mg/mL (mL)	Diluent (mL)	Total Volume (mL)
200 mcg/mL	10 mL	40 mL	50 mL
200 mcg/mL	20 mL	80 mL	100 mL

May be given through Y-tube or three-way stopcock of IV infusion set but should never come in contact with furosemide (Lasix). Use only freshly prepared solutions.

Filters: No data available from manufacturer.

Storage: Store at room temperature before dilution; avoid freezing.

COMPATIBILITY (Underline Indicates Conflicting Compatibility Information)
Consider any drug NOT listed as compatible to be INCOMPATIBLE until consulting a pharmacist; specific conditions may apply.

Manufacturer states, "Do not add supplementary medications." Forms an immediate precipitate with furosemide (Lasix).

One source suggests the following **compatibilities:**

Additive: *Not recommended by manufacturer.* Quinidine gluconate.

Y-site: Acyclovir (Zovirax), amikacin (Amikin), amiodarone (Nexterone), ampicillin, argatroban, atracurium (Tracrium), bivalirudin (Angiomax), bumetanide, calcium chloride, calcium gluconate, caspofungin (Cancidas), cefazolin (Ancef), cefepime (Maxipime), cefotaxime (Claforan), ceftazidime (Fortaz), cefuroxime (Zinacef), ciprofloxacin (Cipro IV), clindamycin (Cleocin), dexamethasone (Decadron), dexmedetomidine (Precedex), digoxin (Lanoxin), diltiazem (Cardizem), dobutamine, dopamine, doripenem (Doribax), epinephrine (Adrenalin), fenoldopam (Corlopam), fentanyl (Sublimaze), gentamicin, heparin, hetastarch in electrolytes (Hextend), hydromorphone (Dilaudid), insulin (regular), isoproterenol (Isuprel), labetalol (Trandate), lorazepam (Ativan), magnesium sulfate, meropenem (Merrem IV), methylprednisolone (Solu-Medrol), metronidazole (Flagyl IV), micafungin (Mycamine), midazolam (Versed), morphine, nesiritide (Natrecor), nicardipine (Cardene IV), nitroglycerin IV, nitroprusside sodium, norepinephrine (Levophed), oxacillin (Bactocill), pancuronium, piperacillin, piperacillin/tazobactam (Zosyn), potassium chloride (KCl), propofol (Diprivan), propranolol, quinidine gluconate, ranitidine (Zantac), rocuronium (Zemuron), sodium bicarbonate, theophylline, thiopental (Pentothal), ticarcillin/clavulanate (Timentin), tobramycin, torsemide (Demadex), vancomycin, vasopressin, vecuronium, verapamil.

RATE OF ADMINISTRATION

Loading dose: A single dose evenly distributed over 10 minutes.

Infusion: Use an infusion pump to deliver milrinone in recommended doses. The following manufacturer's dose chart defines selected dose in mcg/kg/min in infusion rate of mL/hr. Adjust as indicated by physician's orders and progress in patient's condition. Reduce rate or stop infusion for excessive drop in BP.

Milrinone Infusion Rate (mL/hr) Using 200 mcg/mL Concentration									
Maintenance Dose (mcg/kg/min)	Patient Body Weight (kg)								
	30	40	50	60	70	80	90	100	110	120
0.375	3.4	4.5	5.6	6.8	7.9	9	10.1	11.3	12.4	13.5
0.4	3.6	4.8	6	7.2	8.4	9.6	10.8	12	13.2	14.4
0.5	4.5	6	7.5	9	10.5	12	13.5	15	16.5	18
0.6	5.4	7.2	9	10.8	12.6	14.4	16.2	18	19.8	21.6
0.7	6.3	8.4	10.5	12.6	14.7	16.8	18.9	21	23.1	25.2
0.75	6.8	9	11.3	13.5	15.8	18	20.3	22.5	24.8	27

ACTIONS
A class of cardiac inotropic agent different in chemical structure and mode of action from digitalis glycosides and catecholamines. Similar to inamrinone (Amrinone), with fewer side effects. With a loading dose, peak effect occurs within 10 minutes. Continuous administration is required to maintain serum levels. It has positive inotropic action with vasodilator activity. Reduces afterload and preload by direct relaxant effect on vascular smooth muscle. Produces slight enhancement of AV node conduction. Cardiac output is improved without significant increases in HR or myocardial oxygen consumption or changes in arteriovenous oxygen difference. Pulmonary capillary wedge pressure, total peripheral resistance, diastolic BP, and mean arterial pressure are decreased. HR generally remains the same. Mean half-life is 2.4 hours. Primary route of excretion is in urine.

INDICATIONS AND USES
Short-term management of patients with acute decompensated heart failure.

CONTRAINDICATIONS
Hypersensitivity to milrinone or inamrinone (Amrinone).

PRECAUTIONS
Not shown to be safe or effective for use longer than 48 hours. No improvement in symptoms and an increased risk of death have been reported. ■ Use caution in impaired renal function; serum levels may increase considerably. ■ May be given to digitalized patients without causing signs of digoxin toxicity; correct hypokalemia with potassium supplements. ■ May increase ventricular response in atrial flutter/fibrillation. Consider pretreatment with digoxin. ■ Additional fluids and electrolytes may be required to facilitate appropriate response in patients who have been vigorously diuresed and may have insufficient cardiac filling pressure. Use caution. ■ Safety for use in the acute phase of myocardial infarction not established. ■ Should not be used in patients with severe obstructive aortic or pulmonary valvular disease in lieu of surgical relief of the obstruction. May aggravate outflow tract obstruction in hypertrophic subaortic stenosis.

Monitor: Observe closely. Continuous ECG monitoring required to allow for prompt detection and management of cardiac events, including life-threatening ventricular arrhythmias. Emergency equipment must be readily available. ■ Monitoring of BP, urine output, renal function, fluid and electrolyte changes (especially potassium), liver function tests, and body weight are recommended. ■ Monitoring of cardiac index, pulmonary capillary wedge pressure, central venous pressure, and plasma concentration is very useful. ■ Observe for orthopnea, dyspnea, and fatigue. ■ Reduce rate or stop infusion for excessive drop in BP. ■ As cardiac output and diuresis improves, a reduction in diuretic dose may be indicated. ■ Possible risk of arrhythmias. Risk further increased with excessive diuresis and/or hypokalemia. Replace potassium as indicated. ■ Infusion site reactions may occur. Monitor site carefully.

Maternal/Child: Category C: safety for use during pregnancy, breastfeeding, and in pediatric patients not established. Use during pregnancy only if potential benefit justifies potential risk.

Elderly: Consider impaired renal function; may require a reduced dose.

DRUG/LAB INTERACTIONS

Theoretical potential for interaction with **calcium channel blockers** (e.g., verapamil); no clinical evidence to date. ■ May cause additive hypotensive effects with **any drug that produces hypotension** (e.g., alcohol, benzodiazepines [e.g., diazepam, midazolam], lidocaine, paclitaxel). ■ No untoward drug interactions observed when used in a limited number of patients concurrently with captopril (Capoten), chlorthalidone (Hygroton), diazepam (Valium), digoxin (Lanoxin), furosemide (Lasix), heparin, hydralazine, hydrochlorothiazide, insulin, isosorbide dinitrate (Sorbitrate), lidocaine, nitroglycerin, prazosin (Minipress), quinidine, spironolactone (Aldactone), warfarin (Coumadin), and potassium supplements. ■ See Monitor.

SIDE EFFECTS

Supraventricular and ventricular arrhythmias including nonsustained ventricular tachycardia do occur; rare cases of torsades de pointes have been reported. Abnormal liver function tests, anaphylactic shock (rare), angina, bronchospasm, chest pain, headaches, hypokalemia, hypotension, infusion site reactions, rash, and tremor have been reported.

ANTIDOTE

Notify the physician of any side effect. Based on degree of severity and condition of the patient, may be treated symptomatically, and dose may remain the same, be decreased, or the milrinone may be discontinued. Reduce rate or discontinue the drug at the first sign of marked hypotension and notify the physician. May be resolved by these measures alone or vasopressors (e.g., dopamine) may be required. Treat dysrhythmias with the appropriate drug. Resuscitate as necessary.

MITOMYCIN BBW

(my-toe-**MY**-sin)

MTC, Mutamycin

Antineoplastic
(antibiotic)

pH 6 to 8

USUAL DOSE

10 to 20 mg/M^2 as a single dose. May be repeated in 6 to 8 weeks after adequate bone marrow recovery; see Dose Adjustments. Discontinue drug if no response after two courses of treatment.

DOSE ADJUSTMENTS

Subsequent doses based on post-treatment leukocyte and platelet counts. Withhold dose for leukocytes below 4,000/mm^3 or platelet count below 100,000/mm^3. Adjust subsequent doses based on nadir after the prior dose according to the following chart. ■ Lower usual dose range is indicated when used with other antineoplastic drugs and radiation.

Guide to Mitomycin Dose Adjustment		
Nadir After Prior Dose		
Leukocytes/mm^3	Platelets/mm^3	Percentage of Prior Dose to Be Given
≥4,000	≥100,000	100%
3,000 to 3,999	75,000 to 99,999	100%
2,000 to 2,999	25,000 to 74,999	70%
<2,000	<25,000	50%

DILUTION

Specific techniques required; see Precautions. Each 5 mg must be diluted with 10 mL SW for injection. Allow to stand at room temperature until completely in solution. May be given through Y-tube or three-way stopcock of a free-flowing infusion of NS or D5W or further diluted in either of the same solutions or sodium lactate ⅙ M and given as an infusion.

Storage: Store unopened vial at CRT. Stable after initial reconstitution at room temperature for 7 days, up to 14 days if refrigerated. When further diluted to a concentration of 20 to 40 mcg/mL, it is stable at room temperature for 3 hours in D5W, 12 hours in NS, and 24 hours in sodium lactate ⅙ M.

COMPATIBILITY   (Underline Indicates Conflicting Compatibility Information)

Consider any drug NOT listed as compatible to be INCOMPATIBLE until consulting a pharmacist; specific conditions may apply.

Sources suggest the following **compatibilities**:

Additive: Manufacturer states that mitomycin (5 to 15 mg) and heparin (1,000 to 10,000 units) in 30 mL NS is stable at CRT for 48 hours. Other sources list dexamethasone (Decadron), <u>heparin</u>, hydrocortisone sodium succinate (Solu-Cortef).

Y-site: Amifostine (Ethyol), bleomycin (Blenoxane), <u>caspofungin (Cancidas)</u>, cisplatin (Platinol), cyclophosphamide (Cytoxan), doxorubicin

(Adriamycin), droperidol (Inapsine), fluorouracil (5-FU), furosemide (Lasix), granisetron (Kytril), heparin, leucovorin calcium, melphalan (Alkeran), methotrexate, metoclopramide (Reglan), ondansetron (Zofran), teniposide (Vumon), thiotepa, vinblastine, vincristine.

RATE OF ADMINISTRATION
IV injection: A single dose over 5 to 10 minutes.
Infusion: Rate determined by amount and type of solution, typically 15 to 30 minutes.

ACTIONS
A highly toxic antibiotic, antineoplastic agent. Cell cycle phase–nonspecific, it is most useful in G and S phases. Interferes with cell division by binding with DNA to slow production of RNA. Rapidly distributed to body tissues and ascitic fluid. Does not cross blood-brain barrier. Metabolized primarily in the liver, but some metabolism occurs in other tissues as well. Some excreted in urine.

INDICATIONS AND USES
Treatment of disseminated adenocarcinoma of the stomach or pancreas. Used in combination with other drugs. Used intravesically in bladder cancer.
Unlabeled uses: Combination chemotherapy in anal, cervical, head and neck, metastatic breast, non–small cell lung cancers, and malignant mesothelioma.

CONTRAINDICATIONS
Not recommended as single-agent primary therapy. Known hypersensitivity to mitomycin, thrombocytopenia, coagulation disorders, increased bleeding from other causes, potentially serious infections, SCr greater than 1.7 mg/100 mL.

PRECAUTIONS
Follow guidelines for handling cytotoxic agents. See Appendix A, p. 1429. ■ Administered by or under the direction of the physician specialist in a facility with adequate diagnostic and treatment facilities for monitoring the patient and responding to any medical emergency. ■ Use extreme caution in impaired renal function; see Contraindications. ■ Acute shortness of breath and bronchospasm have occurred within minutes to hours following administration of vinca alkaloids (e.g., vincristine) in patients who have received mitomycin previously or are receiving mitomycin simultaneously. Bronchodilators, steroids and/or oxygen may be used to treat respiratory distress. ■ Bone marrow suppression (leukopenia and thrombocytopenia) may be severe and contribute to overwhelming infections in an already compromised patient. ■ Hemolytic uremic syndrome (hemolytic anemia, thrombocytopenia, and irreversible renal failure) has occurred in patients receiving mitomycin as a single agent or in combination with other agents. It can occur at any time during treatment, but most cases have occurred with a cumulative dose greater than 60 mg. Administration of blood products may exacerbate the symptoms.
Monitor: Monitor WBC, RBC, platelet count, PT, bleeding time, differential, and hemoglobin before, during, and 7 to 10 weeks after therapy. ■ Monitor all patients, especially those nearing a cumulative dose of 60 mg, for unexplained anemia with fragmented cells on peripheral blood smear, thrombocytopenia, and decreased renal function; see Precautions. ■ Determine absolute patency of vein; use of an IV catheter is preferred because severe cellulitis and tissue necrosis will result from extravasation.

If extravasation occurs, discontinue injection and use another vein. Elevate extremity and apply cold compresses to extravasated area. Delayed erythema with or without ulceration has occurred at or distant to the injection site. May occur weeks to months after mitomycin administration, even when no obvious evidence of extravasation was observed during administration. ■ May precipitate acute respiratory distress syndrome. Oxygen can be toxic to the lungs; monitor intake carefully and use only enough to provide adequate arterial saturation. ■ Monitor fluid balance; avoid overhydration. ■ Be alert for signs of bone marrow suppression or infection. ■ Monitor for thrombocytopenia (platelet count less than 50,000/mm^3). Initiate precautions to prevent excessive bleeding (e.g., inspect IV sites, skin, and mucous membranes; use extreme care during invasive procedures; test urine, emesis, stool, and secretions for occult blood). ■ Prophylactic antibiotics may be indicated pending results of C/S in a febrile neutropenic patient. ■ Prophylactic antiemetics may reduce nausea and vomiting and increase patient comfort. ■ See Precautions and Drug/Lab Interactions.

Patient Education: Nonhormonal birth control recommended. ■ Report shortness of breath and IV site burning and stinging promptly. ■ See Appendix D, p. 1434.

Maternal/Child: Avoid pregnancy; may produce teratogenic effects on the fetus. ■ Information on safety in breast-feeding or in pediatric patients not available; discontinue breast-feeding.

Elderly: Consider diminished hepatic function; monitor for early signs of toxicity.

DRUG/LAB INTERACTIONS

Do not administer **live virus vaccines** to patients receiving antineoplastic drugs. ■ May cause shortness of breath, severe bronchospasm, and acute pneumonitis with **vinca alkaloids** (e.g., vinblastine).

SIDE EFFECTS

Alopecia, anaphylaxis, anorexia, bleeding, blurring of vision, cellulitis at injection site, confusion, CHF (patient has usually received doxorubicin [Adriamycin, Doxil]), coughing, diarrhea, drowsiness, dyspnea with nonproductive cough, edema, elevated BUN or SCr, fatigue, fever, headache, hematemesis, hemolytic uremic syndrome (microangiopathic hemolytic anemia [hematocrit less than 25%], irreversible renal failure [SCr greater than 1.6 mg/dL], and thrombocytopenia [less than 100,000/mm^3]), hemoptysis, hypertension, leukopenia, mouth ulcers, nausea, paresthesias, pneumonia, pruritus, pulmonary edema, purple discoloration of vein, radiographic evidence of pulmonary infiltrates, rash, renal failure, respiratory distress syndrome (acute), skin toxicity, stomatitis, syncope, thrombocytopenia, thrombophlebitis, vomiting.

ANTIDOTE

Most side effects will be treated symptomatically. Keep the physician informed. All are potentially serious and many can be life threatening. Hematopoietic depression requires cessation of therapy until recovery occurs. Discontinue drug if dyspnea, nonproductive cough, or radiographic evidence of pulmonary infiltrates is present. Discontinue drug for any symptoms of hemolytic uremic syndrome. There is no specific antidote. Supportive therapy as indicated will help sustain the patient in toxicity. Administration of whole blood products (e.g., packed RBCs, platelets, leukocytes) and/or blood modifiers (e.g., darbepoetin alfa (Aranesp], epo-etin alfa [Epogen], filgrastim [Neupogen], oprelvekin [Neumega], peg-filgrastrim [Neulasta], sargramostim [Leukine]) may be indicated to treat bone marrow toxicity; see Precautions. If extravasation has occurred, L.A. dexamethasone injected into the indurated area with a fine hypodermic needle may be helpful; elevate extremity.

MITOXANTRONE HYDROCHLORIDE BBW
(my-toe-**ZAN**-trohn hy-droh-**KLOR**-eyed)

Novantrone

Antineoplastic
(antibiotic)

pH 3 to 4.5

USUAL DOSE
Preliminary evaluations and testing required; see Monitor.

Combination initial therapy for acute nonlymphocytic leukemia (ANLL) in adults:
Induction: 12 mg/M^2/day of mitoxantrone on Days 1 through 3 and cytarabine 100 mg/M^2/day as a continuous 24-hour infusion on Days 1 through 7. Should a complete remission not be achieved, repeat mitox-antrone, 12 mg/M^2/day for only 2 days, and cytarabine 100 mg/M^2/day for 5 days after all signs or symptoms of severe or life-threatening nonhema-tologic toxicity have cleared.

Consolidation: After full hematologic recovery (usually 6 weeks after induction therapy), administer mitoxantrone 12 mg/M^2/day by IV infusion on Days 1 and 2 and cytarabine 100 mg/M^2/day as a continuous 24-hour infusion on Days 1 to 5. May repeat in 4 weeks. Severe myelosuppression occurred in these subsequent courses. See Monitor.

Prostate cancer: 12 to 14 mg/M^2 as a short IV infusion once every 21 days. Used concurrently with steroids.

Multiple sclerosis (MS): 12 mg/M^2 as an infusion over 5 to 15 minutes. Repeat every 3 months. May be given for up to 2 years or until a cumulative dose of 140 mg/M^2 has been administered.

DOSE ADJUSTMENTS
Adjust dose based on clinical response and development and severity of toxicity. ▪ Clearance is reduced by impaired hepatic function. Treat pa-tients with impaired hepatic function with caution, dose adjustment may be indicated. Specific recommendations not available; see Precautions.

DILUTION
Specific techniques required; see Precautions. A single dose must be diluted with at least 50 mL of NS or D5W. May be further diluted in NS, D5W, or D5NS. Must be given through Y-tube or three-way stopcock of a free-flowing infusion of D5W or NS, or may be diluted in larger amounts of the same solutions and given as a continuous infusion.

Filters: No data available from manufacturer.

Storage: Store unopened vial at RT (15° to 25° C [59° to 77° F]). Do not freeze. Diluted solution should be used immediately. After penetration of the stopper on a multidose vial, the undiluted mitoxantrone may be stored at RT for 7 days or refrigerated for up to 14 days. Do not freeze.

COMPATIBILITY

Consider any drug NOT listed as compatible to be INCOMPATIBLE until consulting a pharmacist; specific conditions may apply.

Manufacturer recommends not mixing in the same infusion with other drugs until **compatibility** data available, and states that it may form a precipitate if mixed in the same infusion with heparin.

One source suggests the following **compatibilities:**

Additive: *Not recommended by manufacturer.* Cyclophosphamide (Cytoxan), cytarabine (ARA-C), etoposide (VePesid), fluorouracil (5-FU), hydrocortisone sodium succinate (Solu-Cortef), potassium chloride (KCl).

Y-site: Allopurinol (Aloprim), amifostine (Ethyol), cladribine (Leustatin), etoposide (VePesid), etoposide phosphate (Etopophos), filgrastim (Neupogen), fludarabine (Fludara), gemcitabine (Gemzar), granisetron (Kytril), linezolid (Zyvox), melphalan (Alkeran), ondansetron (Zofran), oxaliplatin (Eloxatin), sargramostim (Leukine), teniposide (Vumon), thiotepa, vinorelbine (Navelbine).

RATE OF ADMINISTRATION

IV injection: A single dose of properly diluted medication over at least 3 to 5 minutes. Must be given through Y-tube or three-way stopcock of a free-flowing infusion of D5W or NS.

Intermittent infusion: A single dose over 15 to 30 minutes.

Infusion: Sometimes a single dose is given as a continuous infusion over 24 hours. Is combined with cytarabine.

ACTIONS

An anthracenedione, a synthetic antibiotic antineoplastic agent. Has achieved complete remissions with a single course of combination therapy. Has a cytocidal effect on proliferating and nonproliferating cells. Probably not cell-cycle specific. Inhibits DNA and RNA synthesis. Thought to reduce the number of relapses and slow down progression of MS through its ability to suppress the activity of T-cells, B-cells, and macrophages. These cells attack the myelin sheath around nerve cells, causing the symptoms of MS. Improves the presentation of brain lesions on MRI studies. Extensive distribution to tissue occurs rapidly. Partially metabolized. Exact pathways unknown. Half-life varies from 23 to 213 hours (median 75 hours). Slowly excreted in bile, urine, and feces as either unchanged drug or as inactive metabolites.

INDICATIONS AND USES

Treatment of acute nonlymphocytic leukemia in adults; includes erythroid, monocytic, myelogenous, and promyelocytic acute leukemias. Given in combination with other approved drugs. ■ Treatment of bone pain in patients with advanced prostate cancer resistant to hormones. Used concurrently with steroids. ■ To reduce neurologic disability and/or the frequency of clinical relapses in patients with secondary (chronic) progressive, progressive relapsing, or worsening relapsing-remitting multiple sclerosis (i.e., patients whose neurologic status is significantly abnormal between relapses). Not indicated in the treatment of patients with primary progressive MS.

Unlabeled uses: Treatment of acute lymphocytic leukemia (ALL), breast cancer, Hodgkin's lymphoma, non-Hodgkin's lymphomas, myelodysplastic syndrome, pediatric acute leukemias, pediatric sarcoma, and part of a conditioning regimen for autologous hematopoietic stem cell transplantation (HSCT).

CONTRAINDICATIONS

Hypersensitivity to mitoxantrone or other anthracyclines. ■ Not for intrathecal use; severe injury with permanent sequelae can result.

PRECAUTIONS

For IV use only. Do not administer SC, IM, intra-arterially, or intrathecally. ■ Follow guidelines for handling cytotoxic agents. See Appendix A, p. 1429. ■ Use of goggles, gloves, and protective gown recommended. Flush skin copiously with warm water should any contact occur. Irrigate eyes immediately in case of contact. Clean spills with 5.5 parts calcium hypochlorite to 13 parts by weight of water for each 1 part of mitoxantrone. ■ Usually administered by or under the direction of the physician specialist with facilities for monitoring the patient and responding to any medical emergency. ■ Will cause severe myelosuppression; use extreme caution in pre-existing drug-induced bone marrow suppression. ■ Should not be given to patients with baseline neutrophil counts of less than 1,500 cells/mm^3 (except for the treatment of acute nonlymphocytic leukemia). ■ MS patients with a baseline left ventricular ejection fraction (LVEF) below the lower limit of normal or patients who have received a cumulative dose equal to or greater than 140 mg/M^2 should not be treated with mitoxantrone. ■ May cause severe cardiac toxicity (e.g., acute congestive heart failure) in all patients, even if cardiac risk factors are not present. May occur early during therapy or months to years after completion. Risk increased with cumulative doses (equal to or greater than 140 mg/M^2), in patients with pre-existing heart disease, and in patients previously treated with anthracyclines (see Drug/Lab Interactions), other cardiotoxic drugs, or radiation therapy encompassing the heart. ■ Use caution in impaired liver function. Clearance is decreased; see Dose Adjustments. Patients with MS who have hepatic impairment should ordinarily not be treated with mitoxantrone. ■ Use caution if renal function is impaired; has not been studied. ■ Urine and sclera may turn bluish in color. ■ Therapy with mitoxantrone increases the risk of developing secondary leukemia in patients with multiple sclerosis and in patients with cancer. Most commonly reported types are acute promyelocytic leukemia and acute myelocytic leukemia. The occurrence is more common when mitoxantrone is given in combination with other cytotoxic agents and/or radiotherapy or when doses of anthracyclines (e.g., doxorubicin [Adriamycin], idarubicin [Idamycin]) have been escalated. ■ Rapid lysis of cancer cells may cause tumor lysis syndrome. ■ See Monitor.

Monitor: Obtain baseline CBC with differential and platelet count; repeat before each dose and if S/S of infection occur. ■ Complete a physical exam and ECG and obtain a complete history to assess for S/S of pre-existing cardiac disease. ■ In all patients, obtain an evaluation of left ventricular ejection fraction (LVEF) by echocardiogram or MUGA (multiple-gated acquisition) before therapy begins. ■ Evaluation of LVEF and assessment of cardiotoxicity by history, physical exam, and ECG should be repeated before each dose in MS patients. ■ Obtain repeat LVEF as indicated in all patients. ■ Mitoxantrone should not ordinarily be administered to MS patients who have received a cumulative dose equal to or greater than 140 mg/M^2 or to patients who experience a drop in LVEF to below the lower limit of normal or a clinically significant reduction in LVEF. MS patients should have an annual quantitative evaluation of LVEF after discontinuing mitoxantrone therapy to monitor for late-occurring cardiotoxicity. ■ Monitoring of liver function is indicated before and during therapy. ■ Because of rapid lysis of cancer cells, initiate hypouricemic therapy with allopurinol or similar agents before beginning treatment. Monitor uric acid levels, maintain hydration, and alkalinize urine if necessary. ▪ Observe closely and frequently for all signs of bleeding or infection. ▪ Prophylactic antibiotics may be indicated pending results of C/S in a febrile neutropenic patient. ▪ Determine absolute patency of vein. Severe local tissue damage may occur with extravasation. Phlebitis at the infusion site has also been reported. Should extravasation or phlebitis occur, discontinue injection and use another vein. ▪ Prophylactic antiemetics may reduce nausea and vomiting and increase patient comfort. ▪ Monitor for thrombocytopenia (platelet count less than 50,000/mm³). Initiate precautions to prevent excessive bleeding (e.g., inspect IV sites, skin, and mucous membranes; use extreme care during invasive procedures; test urine, emesis, stool, and secretions for occult blood). ▪ Monitor for S/S of acute leukemia (secondary leukemia); may include excessive bruising, bleeding, and recurrent infections. ▪ See Precautions and Drug/Lab Interactions.

Patient Education: Nonhormonal birth control recommended; see Maternal/Child. ▪ Blood and cardiac tests are imperative; keep all appointments. ▪ Report IV site burning or stinging promptly. ▪ Urine may turn blue-green for 24 hours following administration. Bluish discoloration of sclera may also occur. ▪ See Appendix D, p. 1434.

Maternal/Child: Category D: avoid pregnancy. May produce teratogenic effects on the fetus. Women with MS who are biologically capable of becoming pregnant should have a pregnancy test before each dose of mitoxantrone regardless of other methods of birth control used, including birth control pills. ▪ Secreted in breast milk. Discontinue breast-feeding. ▪ Safety for use in pediatric patients not established.

Elderly: Specific age-related differences have not been identified; consider age-related organ impairment (e.g., bone marrow reserve, renal, hepatic) and possibility of increased sensitivity.

DRUG/LAB INTERACTIONS

Additive bone marrow suppression may occur with **radiation therapy and/or other bone marrow–suppressing agents** (e.g., azathioprine [Imuran], chloramphenicol, melphalan [Alkeran]). Dose reduction may be required. ▪ Risk of cardiotoxicity increased in patients previously treated with maximum cumulative doses of **other anthracyclines** (e.g., doxorubicin [Adriamycin], epirubicin [Ellence], idarubicin [Idamycin]) **and/or radiation encompassing the heart.** ▪ Do not administer **live virus vaccines** to patients receiving antineoplastic drugs.

SIDE EFFECTS

Alopecia (reversible), bladder infections, menstrual disorders, mucositis, and nausea occur frequently. Other side effects include abdominal pain, acute congestive heart failure, altered electrolytes, altered liver function tests (e.g., increased ALT, AST, BUN), arrhythmias, arthralgias, bleeding, bone marrow suppression (severe with standard doses), cardiotoxicity, conjunctivitis, cough, decrease in LVEF, diarrhea, dyspnea, erythema, fever, GI bleeding, headache, hematuria, hypersensitivity reactions (e.g., dyspnea, hypotension, rash, urticaria), infections, injection site burning, jaundice, leukemia (including secondary AML), mucositis, myalgias, nail bed changes, phlebitis, renal failure, seizures, skin discoloration, stomatitis, swelling, vomiting. Interstitial pneumonitis has been reported. Anaphylaxis has been reported rarely.

Post-Marketing: Secondary acute myelogenous leukemia (AML).

ANTIDOTE

There is no specific antidote. Notify physician of all side effects. Most will be treated symptomatically. Blood and blood products, antibiotics and other adjunctive therapies must be available. Blood modifiers (e.g., darbepoetin alfa [Aranesp], epoetin alfa [Epogen], filgrastim [Neupogen], oprelvekin [Neumega], pegfilgrastim [Neulasta], sargramostim [Leukine]) may be indicated to treat bone marrow toxicity. Nadir of leukocyte count occurs within 10 days. Recovery is within 21 days. For extravasation, elevate extremity and apply ice. Monitor closely and obtain surgical consult if necessary. Overdose has resulted in death. Peritoneal dialysis or hemodialysis not effective. Supportive therapy as indicated will help sustain the patient in toxicity.

MORPHINE SULFATE `BBW`
(**MOR**-feen **SUL**-fayt)

Opioid analgesic (agonist)
Adjunct, pulmonary edema
Anesthesia adjunct

Astramorph PF, Duramorph PF

pH 2.5 to 7

USUAL DOSE

IV injection: Manufacturer recommends an initial dose of 2 to 10 mg/70 kg of body weight. Repeat every 3 to 4 hours as necessary. Doses may range from 2 to 20 mg based on patient requirements and response. Titrate to achieve pain relief with lowest dose. Frequent, repeated doses (e.g., up to every 5 minutes if needed) in small-dose increments (e.g., 1 to 4 mg) may be associated with fewer side effects than the administration of larger, less frequent doses.

Cancer patients suffering with severe chronic pain often require higher doses because of increased tolerance (up to 150 mg/hr has been given). Very high doses (275 to 440 mg/hr) are occasionally used for short periods of time (hours to days) for extreme exacerbations of pain in these drug-tolerant individuals. 1 to 3 mg/kg over 15 to 20 minutes will induce unconsciousness.

Acute MI: 2 to 4 mg initially. May give additional doses of 2 to 8 mg at 5- to 15-minute intervals as needed (AHA guidelines).

Infusion: 1 mg/mL (range is 0.1 to 1 mg/mL) in NS or D5W per controlled infusion device (may be patient activated). *Based on a 1 mg/mL dilution,* an initial loading dose may be as high as 15 mg (15 mL). The continuous background infusion to provide a level of pain relief and maintain patency of the vein may range from 1 to 2.5 mg/hr (1 to 2.5 mL). Additional doses averaging 0.5 to 1.5 mg (0.5 to 1.5 mL) may be activated by the patient at selected intervals every 3 to 60 minutes (averaging 10 to 15 min). Additional boluses averaging 1 to 2 mg (1 to 2 mL) may be given by health care professionals (e.g., every 30 min prn). In selected cancer patients all of these doses may be considerably higher.

Open heart surgery: 0.5 to 3 mg/kg as the sole anesthetic or with an anesthetic agent. Cardiovascular function not depressed if oxygen is used and adequate ventilation maintained.

Dyspnea during end-of-life care (unlabeled): 2 to 5 mg IV every 5 to 10 minutes until relief. Patient-controlled anesthesia (PCA) is recommended in the inpatient setting. Higher doses may be needed for patients taking chronic opioids.

PEDIATRIC DOSE
Analgesic: Usual range is 0.05 to 0.1 mg/kg. Administer very slowly.
Postoperative analgesia: 0.01 to 0.04 mg/kg/hr (10 to 40 mcg/kg/hr).
Selected pediatric patients with severe chronic cancer pain: 0.025 to 2.6 mg/kg/hr (average 0.04 to 0.07 mg/kg/hr).
Selected pediatric patients with severe pain during sickle cell crisis: 0.025 to 2.6 mg/kg/hr (average 0.04 to 0.07 mg/kg/hr).

NEONATAL DOSE
Elimination is reduced in neonates, and they have an increased susceptibility to CNS side effects.
Analgesia/tetralogy (cyanotic) spells (unlabeled): 0.05 to 0.2 mg/kg/dose every 4 hours. Titrate to individual response. Another source suggests an *IV injection* of 0.05 to 0.1 mg/kg/dose every 4 to 8 hours or an *IV infusion* of 0.01 to 0.02 mg/kg/hr. Titrate to individual response.
Mechanical ventilation of neonates (unlabeled): 50 mcg/kg as an initial loading dose. Administer over 30 to 60 minutes. Follow with a continuous infusion of 10 to 30 mcg/kg/hr. Titrate to individual response.
Postoperative analgesia (unlabeled): 50 mcg/kg as an initial loading dose. Administer over 30 to 60 minutes. Follow with a continuous infusion of 15 mcg/kg/hr. Titrate to individual response.

DOSE ADJUSTMENTS
Reduced dose and/or extended intervals may be required in impaired renal or hepatic function and in the elderly. ■ Doses appropriate for the general population may cause serious respiratory depression in vulnerable patients. ■ Increase doses as required if analgesia is inadequate, tolerance develops, or pain severity increases. The first sign of tolerance is usually a reduced duration of effect. ■ See Drug/Lab Interactions.

DILUTION
IV injection: May be given undiluted; however, further dilution with 5 mL of SW or NS for injection or other IV solutions to facilitate titration is appropriate. May be given through Y-tube or three-way stopcock of infusion set.
Infusion: Each 0.1 to 1 mg is usually diluted in 1 mL NS or D5W and administered via a controlled infusion device that may be patient activated (e.g., a narcotic syringe infuser system). Available in 60-mL ampules containing 1 to 2 mg/mL for direct transfer to syringe infuser systems. (*Astramorph PF and Duramorph* are preservative free and expensive; can be used IV, but are the only choice for epidural or intrathecal injection; see drug literature. *Duramorph* is **NOT** for use in continuous microinfusion devices. *Infumorph* is **NOT** for IV use.) Fluid restriction or high doses may require more concentrated solutions. Concentrations above 5 mg/mL are rarely exceeded. Available in vials containing 25 mg/mL, which must be further diluted before infusion. Also available in ADD-Vantage vials for

use with ADD-Vantage infusion containers. Is sometimes added to larger amounts (500 mL to 1 L) of IV solution in selected situations and infused via a large volume controlled infusion pump (requires close titration). **Storage:** Store at CRT. Protect from light and freezing.

COMPATIBILITY   (Underline Indicates Conflicting Compatibility Information)
Consider any drug NOT listed as compatible to be INCOMPATIBLE until consulting a pharmacist; specific conditions may apply.

One source suggests the following **compatibilities:**
Additive: Alteplase (tPA, Activase), atracurium (Tracrium), dobutamine, fluconazole (Diflucan), furosemide (Lasix), ketamine (Ketalar), meropenem (Merrem IV), metoclopramide (Reglan), ondansetron (Zofran), succinylcholine, verapamil.

Y-site: Acyclovir (Zovirax), allopurinol (Aloprim), amifostine (Ethyol), amikacin (Amikin), aminophylline, amiodarone (Nexterone), ampicillin, ampicillin/sulbactam (Unasyn), anidulafungin (Eraxis), argatroban, atracurium (Tracrium), atropine, aztreonam (Azactam), bivalirudin (Angiomax), bumetanide, calcium chloride, caspofungin (Cancidas), cefazolin (Ancef), cefepime (Maxipime), cefotaxime (Claforan), cefotetan, cefoxitin (Mefoxin), ceftazidime (Fortaz), ceftriaxone (Rocephin), cefuroxime (Zinacef), chloramphenicol (Chloromycetin), cisatracurium (Nimbex), cisplatin (Platinol), cladribine (Leustatin), clindamycin (Cleocin), cyclophosphamide (Cytoxan), cytarabine (ARA-C), dexamethasone (Decadron), diazepam (Valium), digoxin (Lanoxin), diltiazem (Cardizem), diphenhydramine (Benadryl), dobutamine, docetaxel (Taxotere), dopamine, doripenem (Doribax), doxorubicin (Adriamycin), doxycycline, enalaprilat (Vasotec IV), epinephrine (Adrenalin), erythromycin (Erythrocin), esmolol (Brevibloc), etomidate (Amidate), etoposide phosphate (Etopophos), famotidine (Pepcid IV), fenoldopam (Corlopam), fentanyl (Sublimaze), filgrastim (Neupogen), fluconazole (Diflucan), fludarabine (Fludara), foscarnet (Foscavir), furosemide (Lasix), gemcitabine (Gemzar), gentamicin, granisetron (Kytril), haloperidol (Haldol), heparin, hetastarch in electrolytes (Hextend), hydrocortisone sodium succinate (Solu-Cortef), hydromorphone (Dilaudid), insulin (regular), kanamycin (Kantrex), ketorolac (Toradol), labetalol (Trandate), levofloxacin (Levaquin), lidocaine, linezolid (Zyvox), lorazepam (Ativan), magnesium sulfate, melphalan (Alkeran), meropenem (Merrem IV), methotrexate, methyldopate, methylprednisolone (Solu-Medrol), metoclopramide (Reglan), metoprolol (Lopressor), metronidazole (Flagyl IV), midazolam (Versed), milrinone (Primacor), nafcillin (Nallpen), nicardipine (Cardene IV), nitroglycerin IV, nitroprusside sodium, norepinephrine (Levophed), ondansetron (Zofran), oxacillin (Bactocill), oxaliplatin (Eloxatin), oxytocin (Pitocin), paclitaxel (Taxol), palonosetron (Aloxi), pancuronium, pantoprazole (Protonix IV), pemetrexed (Alimta), penicillin G potassium, phenobarbital (Luminal), piperacillin, piperacillin/tazobactam (Zosyn), potassium chloride (KCl), propofol (Diprivan), propranolol, ranitidine (Zantac), remifentanil (Ultiva), sodium bicarbonate, sulfamethoxazole/trimethoprim, tacrolimus (Prograf), teniposide (Vumon), thiopental (Pentothal), thiotepa, ticarcillin/clavulanate (Timentin), tirofiban (Aggrastat), tobramycin, vancomycin, vecuronium, vinorelbine (Navelbine), warfarin (Coumadin), zidovudine (AZT, Retrovir).

RATE OF ADMINISTRATION

Frequently titrated according to symptom relief and respiratory rate. Side effects markedly increased if rate of injection too rapid. Rapid IV administration may result in chest wall rigidity.

IV injection: 15 mg or fraction thereof over 4 to 5 minutes.

Infusion: Initial loading dose, basal rate (continuous rate of infusion), patient self-administered dose and interval, additional boluses permitted, and total dose for 1 hour should be ordered by physician. Administer initial dose and boluses at rate for IV injection. For continuous infusion and self-administered dose and interval, note range of mL/hr under Usual Dose.

ACTIONS

An opium-derivative, opioid analgesic, which is a descending CNS depressant. Produces a wide spectrum of pharmacologic effects, including analgesia, diminished GI mobility, dysphoria, euphoria, physical dependence, respiratory depression, and somnolence. Pain relief is effected almost immediately and lasts up to 4 to 5 hours (mean is 2 hours). Morphine induces sleep and inhibits perception of pain by binding to opiate receptors, decreasing sodium permeability, and inhibiting transmission of pain impulses. Depresses many other senses or reflexes. Relieves pulmonary congestion, lowers myocardial oxygen requirements, and reduces anxiety. Metabolized in the liver and primarily excreted in the urine and feces. Crosses the blood-brain barrier, but plasma concentration of morphine is higher than CSF concentration. Crosses the placental barrier. Secreted in breast milk.

INDICATIONS AND USES

Relief of moderate to severe acute and chronic pain (e.g., postop or cancer pain). ▪ Analgesic of choice in pain associated with myocardial infarction. ▪ Treatment of acute pulmonary edema associated with left ventricular failure. ▪ Used before surgery to sedate, decrease anxiety, and facilitate induction of anesthesia. ▪ Management of neonatal opiate withdrawal.

Unlabeled uses: Treatment of dyspnea in end-of-life care. ▪ Control of pain during mechanical ventilation in neonates. ▪ Control of postoperative pain in neonates.

CONTRAINDICATIONS

Hypersensitivity to morphine sulfate or any component of the formulation, bronchial asthma (acute or severe), and upper airway obstruction. Other sources include paralytic ileus, premature infants, or labor and delivery of premature infants. Specific formulations may have additional contraindications; see prescribing information. ▪ *Duramorph* is **NOT** for use in continuous microinfusion devices.

PRECAUTIONS

Schedule II opioid agonists, including hydromorphone, morphine, oxymorphone, oxycodone, fentanyl, and methadone, have the highest potential for abuse and risk of producing respiratory depression. Alcohol, CNS depressants, and other opioids potentiate the respiratory depressant effects of hydromorphone, increasing the risk of respiratory depression that might result in death; see Drug/Lab Interactions. ▪ Use caution in the elderly, in patients with impaired hepatic or renal function, and in pulmonary disease. ▪ May cause severe hypotension in an individual whose ability to maintain BP has been compromised by a depleted blood volume or a concurrent administration of drugs such as phenothiazines or general anesthetics; see

Drug/Lab Interactions. ▪ Use extreme caution in craniotomy, head injury, and increased intracranial pressure; respiratory depression and intracranial pressure may be further increased. ▪ May cause sedation and pupillary changes (miosis) that may obscure the existence, extent, and course of intracranial pathology. ▪ May cause apnea in asthmatic patients. ▪ Symptoms of acute abdominal conditions may be masked. ▪ May increase ventricular response rate in presence of supraventricular tachycardias. ▪ Cough reflex is suppressed. ▪ Tolerance as well as psychological and physical dependence can develop. Tolerance for the drug gradually increases, but abstinence for 1 to 2 weeks will restore effectiveness. Risk of using a narcotic antagonist in patients chronically receiving narcotic therapy should be considered. ▪ A marked increase in dose may precipitate seizures. Use with caution in patients with known seizure disorders.

Monitor: Oxygen, controlled respiratory equipment, and naloxone (Narcan) must always be available. ▪ Observe patient frequently to continuously based on amount of dose and monitor vital signs. ▪ Assess baseline pain, then assess pain with vital signs and/or more frequently if needed. Reassess after administration of morphine and adjust dose or interval as required. ▪ Keep patient supine; orthostatic hypotension and fainting may occur; less likely with continuous low doses, but observe closely during ambulation. ▪ Uncontrolled pain causes sleep deprivation, decreases pain threshold, and increases pain. When pain is finally controlled, expect the patient to sleep more until recovery from sleep deprivation. ▪ Adhere to prescribed bowel care regimen to avoid constipation and/or impaction. Maintain adequate hydration. ▪ See Drug/Lab Interactions.

Patient Education: Avoid alcohol or other CNS depressants (e.g., barbiturates, benzodiazepines [e.g., diazepam (Valium)]). ▪ May cause blurred vision, dizziness, or drowsiness; use caution in tasks that require alertness. ▪ Request assistance with ambulation. ▪ May be habit forming.

Maternal/Child: Category C: safety for use in pregnancy or breast-feeding not established. Benefits must outweigh risks. ▪ May reduce strength, duration, and frequency of uterine contractions during labor and delivery. ▪ See Contraindications. ▪ Pediatric patients may be more sensitive to effects, especially respiratory depressant effects. ▪ May cause paradoxical excitation. ▪ May cause respiratory depression in the neonate when given during labor and delivery. Have naloxone and resuscitative equipment available. ▪ Infants born to mothers who have been taking morphine chronically may exhibit withdrawal symptoms.

Elderly: See Dose Adjustments and Precautions. ▪ May be more sensitive to effects (e.g., respiratory depression, constipation, urinary retention). ▪ Lower doses may provide effective analgesia. ▪ Consider age-related organ impairment.

DRUG/LAB INTERACTIONS

Alcohol, other CNS depressants (e.g., narcotic analgesics, general anesthetics, antidepressants [e.g., amitriptyline (Elavil), imipramine (Tofranil), nortriptyline (Aventyl)], barbiturates, hypnotics, sedatives), H_2 antagonists (e.g., cimetidine [Tagamet]), and some phenothiazines (e.g., chlorpromazine [Thorazine]) may increase CNS depression, respiratory depression, and hypotension; reduced dose of one or both agents indicated. ▪ **Anticholinergics** (e.g., atropine) **and antidiarrheals** may increase risk of constipation or paralytic ileus. ▪ Hypotensive effects will be increased with **diuretics** (e.g., furosemide [Lasix]), **antihypertensive agents** (especially ganglionic blockers [e.g., guanethidine (Ismelin)]), **or hypotension-producing agents** (e.g., antidepressants, benzodiazepines [e.g., diazepam], adrenergic blocking agents [e.g., propranolol], calcium channel blocking agents [e.g., diltiazem], calcium, nitroprusside sodium, nitroglycerin). ■ Concurrent use with **rifampin** (Rifadin) may decrease analgesic effects of morphine; an alternate analgesic may be required. ■ Markedly reduced doses of **MAO inhibitors** (e.g., selegiline [Eldepryl]) required with opiates. ■ Administration of **agonist/antagonist analgesics** (e.g., butorphanol [Stadol] or buprenorphine [Buprenex]) to an opiate-dependent patient receiving a pure opiate may precipitate withdrawal symptoms. ■ May potentiate anticoagulant effect of oral **warfarin.**

SIDE EFFECTS

Average dose: Anxiety, bradycardia, confusion, constipation, depression of cough reflex, decreased libido in men and women, delayed absorption of oral medications, dizziness, drowsiness/sedation, euphoria, histamine-related reactions (e.g., local tissue irritation, pruritus, urticaria, wheals), hypersensitivity reactions, hypothermia, increased intracranial pressure, interference with thermal regulation, menstrual irregularities (including amenorrhea), nausea, neonatal apnea, oliguria, orthostatic hypotension, physical or psychological dependence, reduced male potency, respiratory depression (slight), skeletal muscle rigidity, tremors, urinary retention, vomiting. Side effects associated with histamine and constipation may be more common with morphine than with most other narcotic analgesics. **Higher doses:** CNS excitation (convulsions), respiratory depression (severe).

Overdose: Anaphylaxis, cardiac arrest, Cheyne-Stokes respiration, circulatory collapse, coma, excitation, hypotension (severe), inverted T-wave on ECG, myocardial depression (severe), pinpoint pupils, respiratory depression or arrest, tachycardia, death.

ANTIDOTE

With increasing severity of any side effect or onset of symptoms of overdose, discontinue the drug and notify the physician. Naloxone (Narcan) will reverse serious reactions. Question the diagnosis of narcotic-induced toxicity if no response is observed after administration of 10 mg of naloxone. A patent airway, artificial ventilation, oxygen therapy, and other symptomatic treatment must be instituted promptly. Resuscitate as necessary.

MOXIFLOXACIN HYDROCHLORIDE BBW Antibacterial
(mox-ee-**FLOX**-ah-sin hy-droh-**KLOR**-eyed) (fluoroquinolone)

Avelox   pH 4.1 to 4.6

USUAL DOSE
400 mg once every 24 hours. Duration of therapy is based on diagnosis as listed in the following chart. Serum levels similar by oral or IV route. Transfer to oral therapy as soon as practical; no dose adjustment necessary. The magnitude of QT prolongation may increase with increasing serum concentrations. Do not exceed recommended dose.

Moxifloxacin Dosing Guidelines		
Infection*	Daily Dose (mg)	Duration (days)
Acute bacterial sinusitis	400 mg	10 days
Acute bacterial exacerbation of chronic bronchitis	400 mg	5 days
Community-acquired pneumonia	400 mg	7-14 days
Uncomplicated skin and skin structure infections	400 mg	7 days
Complicated skin and skin structure infections	400 mg	7-21 days
Complicated intra-abdominal infections†	400 mg	5-14 days

*Due to the designated pathogens.
†Therapy should usually be started with the IV formulation.

DOSE ADJUSTMENTS
Dose adjustment is not indicated based on age, gender, or race; in impaired renal function (including patients on hemodialysis or CAPD); or in mild, moderate, or severe impaired hepatic function (Child Pugh Classes A, B, and C). See Precautions.

DILUTION
Available in ready-to-use latex-free plexibags containing 400 mg moxifloxacin in 0.8% saline. No further dilution is necessary. Refer to directions provided with administration set.

Filters: No data available from manufacturer.

Storage: Store at CRT. Do not refrigerate; a precipitate will form. Discard unused portions.

COMPATIBILITY
Consider any drug NOT listed as compatible to be INCOMPATIBLE until consulting a pharmacist; specific conditions may apply.

Limited **compatibility** data available. Manufacturer states, "Other IV substances, additives, or other medications should not be added to moxifloxacin or infused simultaneously through the same IV line." Flush line with a solution **compatible** to both drugs before and after administration of moxifloxacin and/or any other drug through the same IV line. May be administered through a Y-tube or three-way stopcock. Temporarily discontinue other solutions infusing at the same site.

Y-site: Manufacturer lists as **compatible** with NS, D5W, D10W, SW, LR at ratios from 1:10 to 10:1.

One source suggests the following **compatibilities:**

Y-site: Doripenem (Doribax), vasopressin.

RATE OF ADMINISTRATION
Single dose equally distributed over 60 minutes as an infusion. Avoid rapid or bolus IV infusion. Incidence and magnitude of QT prolongation may increase with increasing concentrations or increasing rates of infusion. Flush tubing before and after moxifloxacin with a **compatible** solution.

ACTIONS
A synthetic broad-spectrum methoxy fluoroquinolone antibacterial agent. Effective against a wide range of gram-negative and gram-positive organisms, including common respiratory pathogens such as *Streptococcus pneumoniae, Haemophilus influenzae,* and *Moraxella catarrhalis,* and atypicals such as *Chlamydophila pneumoniae* and *Mycoplasma pneumoniae.* Bactericidal action results from inhibition of topoisomerase II and IV, which are required for bacterial DNA replication, transcription, repair, and recombination. Mode of action helps minimize selection of resistant mutants of gram-positive bacteria, which cause many respiratory tract infections. Mechanism of fluoroquinolones differs from that of aminoglycosides, cephalosporins, macrolides, penicillins, and tetracyclines, and fluoroquinolones may be active against pathogens resistant to these antibiotics. There is no cross-resistance between fluoroquinolones and these other antibiotics. Widely distributed throughout the body. Concentrations in most target tissues are higher than those found in serum. Mean half-life is approximately 10.7 to 13.3 hours. Partially metabolized in the liver by glucuronide and sulfate conjugation. Excreted as unchanged drug and metabolites in feces and urine. May be secreted in breast milk.

INDICATIONS AND USES
Treatment of adults with infections caused by susceptible strains of microorganisms in conditions, including acute bacterial sinusitis, acute bacterial exacerbation of chronic bronchitis, complicated and uncomplicated skin and skin structure infections, and complicated intra-abdominal infections. ■ Treatment of community-acquired pneumonia caused by many organisms, including *Streptococcus pneumoniae* (including multidrug-resistant strains [MDRSP]). MDRSP strains are resistant to two or more of the following antibiotics: penicillin, second-generation cephalosporins (e.g., cefuroxime [Zinacef]), macrolides, tetracyclines, and sulfamethoxazole/trimethoprim.

CONTRAINDICATIONS
History of hypersensitivity to moxifloxacin or other quinolone antibiotics (e.g., ciprofloxacin [Cipro], levofloxacin [Levaquin], norfloxacin [Noroxin]).

PRECAUTIONS
For IV use only. ■ Culture and sensitivity studies indicated to determine susceptibility of the causative organism to moxifloxacin. ■ Prolonged use may cause superinfection because of overgrowth of nonsusceptible organisms. ■ Cross-resistance has been observed between moxifloxacin and other fluoroquinolones against gram-negative bacteria. However, gram-positive bacteria resistant to other fluoroquinolones may still be

susceptible to moxifloxacin. The emergence of bacterial resistance to fluoroquinolones and the occurrence of cross-resistance with other fluoroquinolones have been observed and are of concern. Proper use of fluoroquinolones and other classes of antibiotics is encouraged to avoid the emergence of resistant bacteria from overuse. ■ Prolongation of the QTc interval on ECG has been reported with moxifloxacin. Infrequent cases of arrhythmia (including torsades de pointes) have been reported with the use of other fluoroquinolones. The risk of arrhythmia may be reduced by avoiding quinolone use in patients with known prolongation of the QTc interval and in the presence of hypokalemia, significant bradycardia, acute myocardial ischemia, or concurrent treatment with class IA antiarrhythmic agents (e.g., quinidine [Quinidex], procainamide [Procanbid, Procan SR]) or class III antiarrhythmic agents (e.g., amiodarone [Nexterone], sotalol [Betapace]); see Rate of Administration. ■ Use with caution in patients receiving drugs that prolong the QTc interval (e.g., antipsychotics, cisapride [Propulsid], erythromycin, and tricyclic antidepressants). ■ Use caution in patients with mild, moderate, or severe hepatic insufficiency; associated metabolic disturbances may lead to QT prolongation. ■ Use with caution in patients with known or suspected CNS disorders, such as severe cerebral atherosclerosis, epilepsy, or other factors that may predispose to seizures. Convulsions, increased intracranial pressure, psychosis, and CNS stimulation have been reported; see Side Effects. ■ Tendinitis and tendon rupture that required surgical repair or resulted in prolonged disability have been reported in patients of all ages receiving quinolones. Most frequently involves the Achilles tendon but has also been reported with the shoulder, hand, biceps, thumb, and other tendon sites. ■ Tendinitis or tendon rupture may occur during or after fluoroquinolone therapy. Risk may be increased in patients over 60 years of age; in patients taking corticosteroids; in patients with heart, kidney, or lung transplants; with strenuous physical activity; and in patients with renal failure or previous tendon disorders such as rheumatoid arthritis. ■ Fluoroquinolones have neuromuscular blocking activity. Serious adverse events, including ventilatory support and deaths, have been reported. Avoid use in patients with a known history of myasthenia gravis; may exacerbate muscle weakness. ■ Rare cases of peripheral neuropathy (e.g., paresthesias, hypoesthesias, dysesthesias [impairment of sensitivity or touch], or weakness) have been reported. ■ *Clostridium difficile*–associated diarrhea (CDAD) has been reported. May range from mild diarrhea to fatal colitis. Consider in patients who present with diarrhea during or after treatment with moxifloxacin. ■ Other serious events (sometimes fatal) due to hypersensitivity or uncertain etiology have been reported with fluoroquinolones; see Side Effects, Post-Marketing. Discontinue moxifloxacin at the first appearance of a skin rash, other signs of hypersensitivity, or jaundice. ■ Moderate to severe photosensitivity/phototoxicity reactions have been reported in patients receiving quinolones; see Patient Education. ■ See Monitor.

Monitor: Serious and occasionally fatal hypersensitivity reactions have been reported in patients receiving quinolone therapy. May be seen with first or subsequent doses. Emergency equipment must be readily available; see Side Effects. Watch for early symptoms of a hypersensitivity reaction. ■ Monitor for S/S of peripheral neuropathy. Discontinue moxifloxacin at first symptoms of neuropathy (e.g., pain, burning, tingling, numbness and/or weakness) or if patient is found to have deficits in light touch, pain, temperature, position sense, vibratory sensation, and/or motor strength. ■ Obtain baseline and periodic CBC with differential. ■ ECG monitoring for QT prolongation may be indicated in select patients. ■ Maintain adequate hydration to prevent concentrated urine throughout treatment. Other quinolones have formed crystals. ■ See Precautions, Drug/Lab Interactions, and Antidote.

Patient Education: A patient medication guide is available from the manufacturer. ■ Drink fluids liberally. ■ Inform physician of any history of myasthenia gravis. ■ Patients with a history of myasthenia gravis should promptly report breathing problems or worsening muscle weakness. ■ Report skin rash or any other hypersensitivity reaction promptly. ■ Dizziness or light-headedness may interfere with ambulation or motor coordination. Use caution in tasks that require alertness. ■ Discontinue moxifloxacin and promptly report CNS side effects such as confusion, depression, dizziness, hallucinations, seizures, suicidal thoughts, or tremors. ■ Report tendon pain or inflammation promptly; rest and refrain from exercise. ■ May produce changes in ECG. Report fainting spells or palpitations promptly. ■ Review medicines and disease states with physician or pharmacist before initiating therapy. ■ Photosensitivity has occurred in patients receiving other quinolones and, infrequently, moxifloxacin. It is best to avoid excessive sunlight or artificial ultraviolet light. May cause severe sunburn; wear protective clothing, use sunscreen, and wear dark glasses outdoors. Report a sunburn-like reaction or skin eruption promptly. ■ Promptly report diarrhea or bloody stools that occur during treatment or up to several months after an antibiotic has been discontinued; may indicate CDAD and require treatment. ■ See Precautions, Monitor, Drug/Lab Interactions, and Antidote.

Maternal/Child: Category C: safety for use in pregnancy not established. Benefit must outweigh risk to fetus. ■ Has potential for harmful effects on breast-feeding infants; either discontinue breast-feeding or choose an alternate drug. ■ Safety and effectiveness for use in pediatric patients under 18 years of age not established. ■ Quinolones have caused erosion of cartilage in weight-bearing joints and other signs of arthropathy in juvenile animals; however, they have been used in infants and children to treat serious infections unresponsive to other antibiotic regimens.

Elderly: Safety and effectiveness similar to that of younger adults; however, they may experience an increased risk of side effects (e.g., CNS effects, tendinitis, tendon rupture, risk of QT prolongation). ■ See Precautions.

DRUG/LAB INTERACTIONS

May cause ventricular arrhythmias or torsades de pointes with **drugs that prolong the QT interval;** avoid concurrent administration with Class IA and Class III antiarrhythmics; see Precautions. ■ Risk of CNS stimulation and seizures may be increased with concurrent use of **NSAIDs** (e.g., ibuprofen [Advil, Motrin], naproxen [Aleve, Naprosyn]). ■ Not metabolized by the cytochrome P_{450} isoenzyme system. Drug-drug interactions with atenolol (Tenormin), digoxin, glyburide (DiaBeta), itraconazole (Sporanox), oral contraceptives, theophylline, and warfarin have not been observed. ■ Does not inhibit the P_{450} isoenzyme system. Drugs metabolized by this system (e.g., cyclosporine [Sandimmune], midazolam [Versed], theophylline, or warfarin [Coumadin]) are not affected by coadministration of moxifloxacin. ■ Digoxin, itraconazole, morphine, probenecid, ranitidine (Zan-

tac), theophylline, and warfarin (Coumadin) have been shown not to alter the pharmacokinetics of moxifloxacin; dose adjustments are not indicated.
- Some quinolones may enhance the effects of **warfarin** (Coumadin); monitoring of PT or INR is recommended with concomitant use. ■ See literature for additional drug/drug interactions on transfer to oral moxifloxacin. ■ May cause a false-positive when **testing urine for opiates;** more specific testing methods may be indicated.

SIDE EFFECTS
Diarrhea, dizziness, headache, and nausea were most common and described as mild to moderate in severity. Capable of numerous other reactions in less than 1% of patients.

Major: Cardiovascular effects (e.g., cardiac arrest, palpitations, QT interval prolongation, tachycardia, torsades de pointes, vasodilation, ventricular tachyarrhythmias); CDAD; CNS stimulation (e.g., anxiety, confusion, depression, hallucinations, insomnia, nightmares, paranoia, restlessness, seizures, tremor); hepatic failure; hepatitis and jaundice (predominantly cholestatic); hyperglycemia; hypersensitivity reactions (e.g., anaphylaxis, cardiovascular collapse, death, dyspnea, edema [facial, laryngeal, or pharyngeal], hypotension, itching, rash, shock, urticaria); hypotension; increased bilirubin; increased intracranial pressure; pain, inflammation, and ruptures of the shoulder, hand, and Achilles tendon; peripheral neuropathy (e.g., pain, burning, tingling, numbness and/or weakness [see Precautions, Monitor]); photosensitivity/phototoxicity; prolonged PT and INR; Stevens-Johnson syndrome; syncope; and toxic psychoses; see Precautions.

Post-Marketing: Allergic pneumonitis, arthralgia, exacerbation of myasthenia gravis, hematologic abnormalities (agranulocytosis, anemia [hemolytic and aplastic], leukopenia, pancytopenia, thrombocytopenia, thrombotic thrombocytopenic purpura), interstitial nephritis, jaundice, liver abnormalities (e.g., acute hepatic necrosis or failure, hepatitis, jaundice), myalgia, rash, serum sickness, severe dermatologic reactions (e.g., toxic epidermal necrolysis [Lyell's syndrome], Stevens-Johnson syndrome), vasculitis.

ANTIDOTE
Keep physician informed of all side effects. Most minor side effects will be treated symptomatically or will resolve with continued dosing (e.g., dizziness, light-headedness); monitor closely. Discontinue moxifloxacin at the first sign of hypersensitivity (e.g., skin rash), CDAD, CNS symptoms, dermatologic reactions, hypoglycemic reactions, phototoxicity, or tendon rupture. Treat allergic reactions as indicated with epinephrine, airway management, oxygen, IV fluids, antihistamines (e.g., diphenhydramine [Benadryl]), corticosteroids (e.g., Solu-Cortef), and pressor amines (e.g., dopamine). Treat CNS symptoms as indicated; may require anticonvulsants (e.g., phenytoin [Dilantin], diazepam [Valium]) for seizures and discontinuation of moxifloxacin. Mild cases of CDAD may respond to discontinuation of drug. Treat CDAD with fluids, electrolytes, protein supplements, and oral vancomycin (Vancocin) or metronidazole (Flagyl) as indicated. In severe cases, surgical evaluation may be indicated. Complete rest is indicated for an affected tendon until treatment is available. Discontinue if photosensitivity occurs. Monitoring of the ECG and adequate hydration are indicated in overdose. No specific antidote. Less than 10% of moxifloxacin and its glucuronide metabolite are removed by CAPD or hemodialysis.

MULTIVITAMIN INFUSION

Nutritional supplement (vitamin)

(mul-ti-**VI**-tah-min in-**FU**-zhun)

Infuvite Adult, Infuvite Pediatric, M.V.I.-12, M.V.I. Adult, M.V.I. Pediatric

USUAL DOSE

Multiples of the daily dose may be given for 2 or more days in patients (adult and pediatric patients) with multiple vitamin deficiencies or markedly increased requirements. Individual components may be indicated in specific or long-standing deficiencies. Monitor blood vitamin concentrations to ensure maintenance of adequate levels. Formulations differ in the amount of each vitamin supplied and in their content (some contain vitamin K [e.g., *M.V.I. Adult and Pediatric, Infuvite (Adult and Pediatric)*], and others do not [e.g., *M.V.I.-12*]); see Drug/Lab Interactions.

All adult formulations: One 5- to 10-mL dose every 24 hours.

PEDIATRIC DOSE

See Maternal/Child.

INFUVITE PEDIATRIC

Supplemental vitamin A may be required for low-birth-weight infants.

Less than 1 kg: 30% of the contents of vial 1 and vial 2 (1.2 mL of vial 1 and 0.3 mL of vial 2).

1 to 3 kg: 65% of the contents of vial 1 and vial 2 (2.6 mL of vial 1 and 0.65 mL of vial 2).

Over 3 kg to 11 years of age: Entire contents of vial 1 (4 mL) and entire contents of vial 2 (1 mL).

M.V.I. PEDIATRIC

Less than 1 kg: 1.5 mL/24 hr.

1 to 3 kg: 3.25 mL/24 hr.

Over 3 kg to 11 years of age: 5 mL/24 hr.

DILUTION

Various preparations. Most may be reconstituted with 5 mL of SW or supplied diluent. All preparations must be further diluted in at least 500 mL but preferably 1,000 mL of IV fluids. Soluble in commonly used infusion fluids, including dextrose, saline, electrolyte replacement fluids, plasma, and selected protein amino acid products. Do not use if any crystals have formed. When reconstituted as directed, *Infuvite Adult* contains no more than 70 mcg/L of aluminum.

Pediatric dilution: *Infuvite Pediatric and M.V.I. Pediatric:* Each dose should be added to at least 100 mL of dextrose, saline, or other **compatible** infusion solution. When reconstituted as directed, *M.V.I. Pediatric* contains no more than 42 mcg/L of aluminum, and *Infuvite Pediatric* contains no more than 30 mcg/L of aluminum; see Precautions. See Maternal/Child.

Storage: Before use, refrigerate at 2° to 8° C (36° to 46° F) protected from light. Manufacturers recommend immediate use of fully diluted Infuvite Pediatric and M.V.I. Adult and Pediatric. Fully diluted Infuvite Adult should be refrigerated and used within 24 hours.

COMPATIBILITY

Consider any drug NOT listed as compatible to be INCOMPATIBLE until consulting a pharmacist; specific conditions may apply.

Compatibility may vary with preparation; consult prescribing information for specifics of a preparation. Direct addition to IV fat emulsions is not recommended. Some manufacturers suggest that admixture or **Y-site** administration with vitamin solutions should be avoided. Alkaline or moderately alkaline solutions (e.g., acetazolamide [Diamox], aminophylline, chlorothiazide [Diuril], sodium bicarbonate), as well as ampicillin and tetracycline, are listed as **incompatible** by one manufacturer. Folic acid may be unstable with calcium salts. *All formulations must be diluted in infusion solutions.*

One source suggests the following **compatibilities:**

Additive: Cefoxitin (Mefoxin), isoproterenol (Isuprel), methyldopa, metoclopramide (Reglan), norepinephrine (Levophed), sodium bicarbonate, verapamil.

Y-site: *All formulations must be diluted in infusion solutions before administration at the Y-site.* Acyclovir (Zovirax), ampicillin, cefazolin (Ancef), clindamycin (Cleocin), diltiazem (Cardizem), erythromycin (Erythrocin), fludarabine (Fludara), gentamicin, tacrolimus (Prograf).

RATE OF ADMINISTRATION

A single dose given as an infusion at prescribed rate of infusion fluids.

ACTIONS

A multiple vitamin solution containing fat-soluble and water-soluble vitamins in an aqueous solution. Provides B complex and vitamins A, D, and E. Some multivitamin preparations presently available do not contain vitamin K. *Infuvite Adult, M.V.I. Adult, Infuvite Pediatric, and M.V.I. Pediatric* do contain vitamin K. Provides daily requirements or corrects an existing deficiency.

INDICATIONS AND USES

A daily multivitamin maintenance supplement for patients receiving parenteral nutrition. Provides the necessary vitamins required to maintain the body's normal resistance and repair processes. Used in situations such as surgery, trauma, burns, severe infectious disease, and comatose states which may provoke a stress response and alteration in the body's metabolic demands. Used when oral administration is contraindicated, not possible, or insufficient.

CONTRAINDICATIONS

Known hypersensitivity to thiamine hydrochloride or other product components; pre-existing hypervitaminosis. ▪ Contraindicated prior to blood sampling for detection of megaloblastic anemia. Folic acid and cyanocobalamin in formulation may mask serum deficits.

PRECAUTIONS

Do not wait for the development of clinical signs of vitamin deficiency before initiating vitamin therapy. ▪ Hypersensitivity reactions have occurred following IV administration of multivitamin solutions containing vitamin B_1 (thiamine) and vitamin K. ▪ Use caution in patients receiving vitamin A from other sources. Use vitamin A in patients with renal failure with caution. ▪ Vitamin A may adhere to plastic, resulting in inadequate vitamin A administration in the doses recommended; see Maternal/Child. ▪ Elevated blood levels of vitamin E may result if doses larger than recommended or oral or parenteral vitamin E are administered. ▪ Solutions containing multivitamins may contain aluminum. In impaired kidney function, aluminum may reach toxic levels. Premature neonates are particularly at risk because of their immature kidneys and requirement for calcium and phosphate, which also contain aluminum. Research indicates that patients with impaired renal function who receive more than 4 to 5 mcg/kg/day of parenteral aluminum are at risk for developing CNS or bone toxicity associated with aluminum accumulation. ▪ See Drug/Lab Interactions.

Monitor: Monitor VS. ▪ Monitor for any symptoms of a hypersensitivity reaction. ▪ Moderate increase in ALT may occur in patients with active inflammatory enterocolitis. Usually reversible following discontinuation of vitamin infusion. Monitoring of ALT levels suggested. ▪ Monitor lipid-soluble vitamin levels in patients with impaired renal function. ▪ Measure blood vitamin concentrations periodically in patients receiving parenteral nutrition to determine if vitamin deficiencies or excesses are developing. Blood levels of A, C, D, and folic acid may decline in patients receiving parenteral multivitamins as their sole source of vitamins for 4 to 6 months. ▪ See Precautions and Maternal/Child.

Maternal/Child: Recommendations for use during pregnancy vary by product. Range is from vitamin needs may exceed those of nonpregnant women to Category C: safety for use in pregnancy not established; use only if clearly needed. ▪ Recommendations for use during breast-feeding vary by product. Range is from vitamin needs may exceed those of nonpregnant women to not known if secreted in breast milk; use caution if required during breast-feeding. ▪ Vitamin A may adhere to plastic resulting in inadequate vitamin A administration in the doses recommended. Additional vitamin A supplementation may be necessary, especially in low-birth-weight infants. ▪ Polysorbates (a component of some multivitamins) have been associated with E-Ferol syndrome (ascites, cholestasis, hepatomegaly, hypotension, metabolic acidosis, renal dysfunction, and thrombocytopenia) in low-birth-weight infants; however, this has not been reported with the use of pediatric multivitamins. ▪ See Precautions.

Elderly: Consider age-related decreased organ function and/or medical problems.

DRUG/LAB INTERACTIONS

Folic acid may lower serum concentration of **phenytoin,** resulting in increased seizure frequency; monitor serum levels of both drugs. ▪ **Phenytoin** may decrease serum folic acid concentrations; avoid during pregnancy. ▪ Folic acid may obscure pernicious anemia and may decrease the patient's response to **methotrexate** therapy. ▪ Pyridoxine may reduce effectiveness of **levodopa.** ▪ Concomitant administration of **hydralazine or isoniazid** (INH) may increase pyridoxine requirements. ▪ Vitamin K may antagonize the anticoagulant effects of **warfarin** (Coumadin) and reduce its effectiveness; monitor INR/PT. ▪ The hematologic response to vitamin B_{12} therapy in patients with pernicious anemia may be inhibited by concomitant administration of **chloramphenicol.** ▪ Thiamine, riboflavin, pyridoxine, niacinamide, and ascorbic acid may decrease the antibiotic activity of **erythromycin, kanamycin, streptomycin, doxycycline, and lincomycin.** ▪ **Bleomycin** is inactivated in vitro by ascorbic acid and riboflavin. ▪ Ascorbic acid in the urine may cause **false-negative urine glucose** determinations.

SIDE EFFECTS

Rare when administered as recommended: Agitation; allergic reactions including anaphylaxis, angioedema, shortness of breath, urticaria, and wheezing; anxiety; diplopia; dizziness; erythema; fainting; headache; pruritus; rash. Vitamin A and vitamin D hypervitaminosis (symptomatology related to hypercalcemia) may occur with prolonged use of significant doses.

ANTIDOTE

With onset of any side effect, discontinue administration immediately and notify physician. Treat anaphylaxis or resuscitate as necessary.

MUROMONAB-CD3   BBW

(myour-oh-**MON**-ab)

Orthoclone OKT3

Monoclonal antibody
Immunosuppressant

pH 6.5 to 7.5

USUAL DOSE

Do not give initial or subsequent doses unless patient temperature is less than 37.8° C (100° F). Administration of IV methylprednisolone sodium succinate 8 mg/kg of body weight 1 to 4 hours before muromonab-CD3 is recommended to reduce the side effects of cytokine release syndrome (CRS) associated with the first two to three doses. Acetaminophen and antihistamines may also be used concomitantly. See Monitor.

Renal allograft rejection: 5 mg/24 hr for 10 to 14 days. Initiate on diagnosis of acute renal rejection.

Cardiac/hepatic allograph rejections: 5 mg/24 hr for 10 to 14 days if rejection has not been reversed by corticosteroid therapy.

PEDIATRIC DOSE

Initiate on diagnosis of acute renal rejection. Initiate in cardiac/hepatic allograft rejections if rejection has not been reversed by corticosteroid therapy. See comments under Usual Dose for patient temperature and premedication requirements. See Dose Adjustments and Maternal/Child.

Pediatric patients 1 month to 16 years of age:

Weight 30 kg or less: 2.5 mg/day for 10 to 14 days.

Weight more than 30 kg: 5 mg/day for 10 to 14 days.

Another source recommends:

Less than 12 years of age: 0.1 mg/kg/day.

12 years of age or older: See adult dose.

DOSE ADJUSTMENTS

Adults and pediatric patients: Doses of concomitant immunosuppressive therapy must be reduced to the lowest level compatible with a therapeutic response during muromonab-CD3 therapy. Resume maintenance doses 3 days before completion of muromonab-CD3 therapy.

Pediatric patients: Pediatric patients have higher CD3 lymphocyte counts than adults. Daily increases in 2.5-mg increments may be required to achieve depletion of CD3-positive cells (less than 25 cells/mm^3) and to ensure therapeutic serum concentrations (greater than 800 ng/mL).

DILUTION

May be given undiluted. Must be withdrawn from vial through a low–protein binding 0.2- or 0.22-micron filter. Discard filter and attach needle for direct IV administration. Do not shake.

Filters: Use of a low–protein binding, 0.2- or 0.22-micron filter is recommended to withdraw from vial; see Dilution.

Storage: Keep unopened ampules under refrigeration. May have some fine translucent particles. Will not affect potency, and use of filter will clear. Do not freeze or shake.

COMPATIBILITY

Until specific data are available, the manufacturer states, "Other IV medications/substances should not be added or infused simultaneously through the same IV line," and recommends flushing line with NS before and after administration of muromonab-CD3 and/or any other drug through the same IV line. Also states, "Do not give by IV infusion or in conjunction with other drug solutions."

RATE OF ADMINISTRATION

A single dose as an IV bolus in less than 1 minute.

ACTIONS

A murine monoclonal antibody to the T3 (CD3) antigen of human T cells. An immunosuppressive agent that reverses graft rejection by blocking all known T-cell functions. Binds to and blocks the function of CD3 in the membrane of the T-cells. Results in early activation of T-cells, which leads to cytokine release and, later, to blocking of T-cell functions. The released cytokines/lymphokines are believed to be responsible for many of the acute clinical manifestations seen following muromonab-CD3 administration. Reacts with most peripheral blood T-cells and T-cells in some body tissues but has not been found to react with other hematopoietic elements or other tissues of the body. Onset of action is within minutes. CD3-positive cells reappear within several days and reach pretreatment levels in 1 week after daily injections are stopped.

INDICATIONS AND USES

Treatment of acute allograft rejection in renal transplant patients. ▪ Treatment of acute rejection in heart and liver transplant patients resistant to standard steroid therapy.

Unlabeled uses: Prophylaxis of cardiac and renal transplant rejection. ▪ Treatment of rejection of lung or pancreas transplant.

CONTRAINDICATIONS

Hypersensitivity to muromonab-CD3 or any product of murine origin; anti-mouse antibody titer equal to or greater than 1:1,000; patients in uncompensated heart failure or fluid overload as evidenced by chest x-ray or greater than 3% weight gain within the week before treatment; history of seizures or patients who may be predisposed to seizures; uncontrolled hypertension; pregnancy and breast-feeding.

PRECAUTIONS

Usually administered in the hospital by or under the direction of a physician experienced in immunosuppressive therapy and management of organ transplant patients. Adequate laboratory and supportive medical resources, including airway management, emergency drugs, and equipment, must be available. ▪ Serious and occasionally fatal immediate (usually within 10 minutes) hypersensitivity (anaphylactic) reactions have been reported. S/S may include airway obstruction, angioedema (including facial, laryngeal, or pharyngeal edema), bronchospasm, cardiorespiratory arrest, cardiovascular collapse, dyspnea, hypotension/shock, loss of consciousness, tachycardia, tingling, urticaria, and pruritus. ■ Serious, occasionally life-threatening or lethal, systemic, cardiovascular, and CNS reactions have been reported, including blindness, cardiac or respiratory arrest, cardiac collapse, coma, cerebral edema, cerebral herniation, coma, paralysis, pulmonary edema (especially in patients with volume overload), seizures, and shock. ■ A protein substance that induces antibodies; use extreme caution if a second course of therapy is needed. Serious hypersensitivity events, including anaphylactic reactions, have been reported in patients re-exposed to muromonab-CD3 subsequent to their initial course of therapy. In this setting, pretreatment with steroids and/or antihistamines may not be effective in preventing anaphylaxis. Weigh benefits versus risk. ■ Most patients develop an acute clinical syndrome called cytokine release syndrome (CRS), which is temporarily associated with the first few doses of muromonab-CD3. CRS typically begins 30 to 60 minutes after administration and may persist for several hours. May range from a mild, flu-like illness to a severe, life-threatening, shock-like reaction that may include serious cardiovascular and CNS manifestations. Common clinical manifestations may include abdominal pain, arthralgia/myalgia, chills/rigors, fever (high), headache, malaise, and tremor. Cardiorespiratory findings may include adult respiratory distress syndrome, angina, apnea, arrhythmias, bronchospasm, cardiac arrest, cardiovascular collapse, dyspnea, heart failure, hemodynamic instability, hypertension, hypotension, hypoxemia, MI, pulmonary edema, respiratory distress/arrest/failure, SOB, tachycardia, and tachypnea. ■ Patients with pre-existing cardiovascular disease, cerebrovascular disease, a history of seizures, pulmonary disease, or intravascular volume overload or depletion of any etiology are at risk for more serious complications of CRS. Correct or stabilize background conditions before initiating therapy. ■ Acute and transient declines in GFR and diminished urine output have occurred. ■ Immunosuppression may increase the risk of lymphomas, skin cancers, or lymphoproliferative disorders. ■ Also increases the risk of serious infections, including bacterial, viral (CMV, HSV, EBV), and other opportunistic infections. ■ Neuropsychiatric events, including seizures, encephalopathy, cerebral edema, aseptic meningitis, and headache have been reported. Patients at increased risk for CNS adverse events include those with known or suspected CNS disorders (e.g., seizures), cardiovascular disease (small or large vessel), conditions with associated neurologic problems (e.g., head trauma), or underlying vascular disease, or patients who are receiving a medication that may affect the CNS. ■ Arterial, venous, and capillary thromboses of allografts and other vascular beds (e.g., heart, lungs, brain, bowel) have been reported. Patients with a history of thrombosis or vascular disease may be at increased risk; consider benefits versus risk.

Monitor: To reduce the incidence of serious side effects, evaluate patients for fluid overload. Monitor fluid status carefully during administration. Must have a clear chest x-ray within 24 hours and have gained no more than 3% above minimal weight present 7 days before injection. ■ Monitor WBC count and differential, circulating T cells as CD3 antigen, and 24-hour trough values of muromonab-CD3 (rise rapidly for the first 3 days of treatment and then average 0.9 mcg/mL thereafter during treatment). ■ Monitor renal and hepatic function. ■ Testing for human-mouse antibody titers is strongly recommended; see Contraindications. ■ Monitor for S/S of anaphylaxis/hypersensitivity and CRS; see Precautions. ■ Anaphylaxis may occur immediately. ■ May be difficult to distinguish between CRS and anaphylaxis. If hypersensitivity is suspected, do not reexpose patient to muromonab-CD3. ■ Monitor for S/S of CNS side effects such as aseptic meningitis, manifestations of encephalopathy, or seizures. ■ Increased susceptibility to infection; observe closely. Prophylactic antibiotics may be indicated pending results of C/S in a febrile neutropenic patient. ■ Treat any fever over 37.8° C (100° F) with antipyretics to lower before giving any single dose. ■ See Dose Adjustments.

Patient Education: Side effects from first few doses are expected. Incidence lessens with subsequent doses. ■ Avoid pregnancy; consider birth control options. ■ See Appendix D, p. 1434. ■ Review potentially serious symptoms of CRS. ■ Report difficulty in breathing, swallowing, rapid heartbeat, rash, or itching immediately. ■ Use caution performing tasks that require mental alertness.

Maternal/Child: Category C: safety for use in pregnancy and men and women capable of conception not established. Use only when absolutely necessary. ■ Discontinue breast-feeding. ■ Response in pediatric patients with renal or hepatic transplants is similar to adults. Data insufficient to compare results in cardiac transplants. ■ Pediatric patients may be at increased risk for cerebral edema with or without herniation and thrombosis.

DRUG/LAB INTERACTIONS

Do not administer **live virus vaccines** to patients receiving immunosuppressive drugs. ■ **Immunosuppressive agents** (e.g., azathioprine, cyclophosphamide, corticosteroids, cyclosporine) increase the risk of infection and development of lymphoproliferative disorders. Use reduced doses with caution.

SIDE EFFECTS

Cytokine release syndrome (chills, dyspnea, fever, and malaise) is very common with early doses and can progress to shock; incidence lessens with subsequent doses. Abnormal chest sounds, anaphylaxis, arthralgia, asthenia, chest pain, diarrhea, dyspnea, edema, fever (high), headache, hypertension, hypotension, infections (e.g., cytomegalovirus, Epstein Barr, herpes simplex, *Staphylococcus epidermidis, Pneumocystis jiroveci, Legionella, Cryptococcus, Serratia*), lymphoproliferative disorders (including lymphomas), nausea, rash, rigors, serum sickness, severe pulmonary edema, tachycardia, tremors, vomiting, wheezing, and many others have occurred; see Precautions.

ANTIDOTE

Notify the physician of all side effects. Most can be treated symptomatically. Pretreat as indicated in Usual Dose to reduce side effects with early doses. Use antipyretics and antihistamines as indicated. Proper patient screening should reduce the incidence of pulmonary edema, anaphylaxis, or shock. Shock from CRS may require epinephrine, O_2, IV fluids, corticosteroids, pressor amines (e.g., dopamime [Intropin]), antihistamines (e.g., diphenhydramine [Benadryl]), and intubation. Drug may be decreased or discontinued or other immunosuppressive agents utilized. Resuscitate as necessary.

MYCOPHENOLATE MOFETIL HYDROCHLORIDE BBW

(**my**-koh-**FEN**-oh-layt **MAH**-fuh-teel hy-droh-**KLOR**-eyed)

Immunosuppressant

CellCept Intravenous

pH 2.4 to 4.1

USUAL DOSE

Used in combination with cyclosporine (Sandimmune) and corticosteroids. IV and oral doses are therapeutically equivalent. Oral form should be used as soon as tolerated by the patient. Initial dose should be given within 24 hours of transplantation. The IV preparation may be used for up to 14 days.

Kidney or liver transplant: 1 Gm as an infusion twice daily (total daily dose of 2 Gm).

Heart transplant: 1.5 Gm as an infusion twice daily (total daily dose of 3 Gm).

PEDIATRIC DOSE

Limited data available; see Indications and product insert. Safety and efficacy of IV formulation not established. Usually given orally.

DOSE ADJUSTMENTS

No dose adjustments are indicated in renal transplant patients who experience delayed graft function postoperatively. ▪ Avoid doses greater than 1 Gm twice a day in renal transplant patients with severe chronic renal impairments (GFR less than 25 mL/min/1.73 M^2) outside the immediate posttransplant period. ▪ Data not available for cardiac or hepatic transplant patients with severe chronic renal impairment; potential benefits must outweigh risks. ▪ Reduce dose or interrupt the dosing cycle if neutropenia (ANC less than 1.3×10^3 [1,300 cells/mm³]) occurs. ▪ Dose adjustment not indicated in impaired liver function. ▪ See Precautions/Monitor.

DILUTION

Specific techniques required; see Precautions. Use caution in handling and preparation. Avoid skin contact with the solution. If skin contact occurs, wash thoroughly with soap and water; rinse eyes with plain water.

Reconstitute each 500-mg vial with 14 mL of D5W (500 mg/15 mL). Shake gently to dissolve. Discard if particulate matter or discoloration is observed or if a lack of vacuum in vial is noted when diluent is added. To achieve a final concentration of 6 mg/mL, each 500 mg must be further diluted with 70 mL of D5W (1 Gm with 140 mL; 1.5 Gm with 210 mL).

Filters: Not required by manufacturer; however, no significant loss of potency is expected with the use of a filter.

Storage: Store powder and reconstituted or diluted solutions at 15° to 30° C (59° to 86° F). Most desired storage temperature is 25° C (77° F). Reconstituted or diluted solutions are best used immediately after preparation. Keep reconstituted or diluted solutions at CRT; the infusion must begin within 4 hours of reconstitution/dilution.

COMPATIBILITY   (Underline Indicates Conflicting Compatibility Information)
Consider any drug NOT listed as compatible to be INCOMPATIBLE until consulting a pharmacist; specific conditions may apply.

Manufacturer states, "Mycophenolate is **incompatible** with other IV solutions and should not be mixed or administered concurrently via the same infusion catheter with other intravenous drugs or infusion admixtures."
One source lists the following **compatibilities:**
Y-site: Anidulafungin (Eraxis), caspofungin (Cancidas), cefepime (Maxipime), dopamine, norepinephrine (Levophed), tacrolimus (Prograf), vancomycin.

RATE OF ADMINISTRATION
A single dose must be given as an infusion over a minimum of 2 hours. **Do Not** administer by rapid or bolus IV injection.

ACTIONS
A hydrochloride salt of mycophenolate mofetil. A potent immunosuppressive agent, inhibiting proliferation of both B- and T-lymphocytes. Has been shown to prolong the survival of allogeneic transplants (kidney, heart, liver, intestine, limb, small bowel, pancreatic islets, and bone marrow) and to reverse ongoing acute rejection episodes in animal models. Rapidly and completely metabolized to MPA, its active metabolite. MPA is then metabolized predominantly to its inactive metabolite, MPAG. Secondary peak in plasma MPA concentration is usually noted 6 to 12 hours postdose. Enterohepatic recirculation is thought to contribute to MPA concentrations. Both MPA and MPAG are highly bound to albumin. In patients with renal impairment or delayed graft function, levels of MPAG may be elevated. Binding of MPA may then be reduced as a result of competition between MPAG and MPA. Plasma concentrations of metabolites are increased in patients with renal impairment. Half-life is 11.4 to 24.4 hours. Excreted primarily as MPAG in urine. Small amount excreted in feces. May cross the placental barrier. May be secreted in breast milk.

INDICATIONS AND USES
Used as part of an immunosuppressive regimen that includes cyclosporine and corticosteroids. ■ Prophylaxis of acute organ rejection in patients receiving allogeneic kidney, heart or liver transplants. ■ Capsules, tablets, and oral solution approved for prevention of rejection in pediatric renal transplant patients.

CONTRAINDICATIONS
Hypersensitivity to mycophenolate mofetil, mycophenolic acid, any component of the drug product, or polysorbate 80 (TWEEN).

PRECAUTIONS
For IV use only. ■ Use caution in handling and preparation. Avoid skin contact of the solution. If contact occurs, wash thoroughly with soap and water; rinse eyes with plain water. Follow guidelines for handling cytotoxic agents. See Appendix A, p. 1429. ■ Usually administered by or under the direction of a physician experienced in immunosuppressive therapy and the management of organ transplant patients. Adequate laboratory and supportive medical resources must be available. ■ Use caution; hypersensitivity reactions have been observed; emergency equipment and drugs for treatment of severe hypersensitivity reactions must be immediately available. ■ Risk of developing lymphoproliferative diseases, lymphomas, and other malignancies, particularly of the skin, is increased. Appears to be related to the intensity and duration of immunosuppression rather than to any specific

agent. ▪ Oversuppression of the immune system can also increase susceptibility to infection, including opportunistic infections, sepsis, fatal infections, and activation of latent viral infections (e.g., PML and BKVAN). ▪ Progressive multifocal leukoencephalopathy (PML) has been reported. PML is a serious progressive neurologic disorder caused by infection of the CNS by JC virus, a member of the papovavirus family. It typically occurs in immunocompromised patients. PML is rare but may result in irreversible neurologic deterioration and death, and there is no known effective treatment. Hemiparesis, apathy, confusion, cognitive deficiencies, and ataxia are the most commonly observed clinical signs. ▪ BK virus–associated nephropathy (BKVAN) has been reported. May lead to deterioration in renal function and renal graft loss. Reduction in immunosuppression may be indicated. ▪ Pure red cell aplasia (PRCA) has been reported in patients receiving mycophenolate in combination with other immunosuppressive agents. May be reversible with dose reduction or discontinuation of mycophenolate. In transplant patients, reduced immunosuppression may place the graft at risk. ▪ Has been associated with an increased incidence of GI adverse effects (e.g., GI tract ulceration, hemorrhage, and/or perforation). Use caution in patients with active serious digestive system disease. ▪ Use with caution in patients with hepatic insufficiency. Metabolism of MPA may be affected by certain types of hepatic disease. ▪ Use caution in patients with severe chronic renal impairment; see Dose Adjustments. ▪ Avoid use in patients with selected rare hereditary deficiency diseases (e.g., Lesch-Nyhan, Kelley-Seegmiller syndrome). ▪ See Monitor, Patient Education, and Maternal/Child.

Monitor: Obtain baseline CBC with differential before treatment. Repeat weekly during the first month, twice monthly for the second and third months, then monthly thereafter. ▪ Monitor for neutropenia. Has been observed most frequently in the period from 31 to 180 days posttransplant. May be due to mycophenolate, concomitant medications, viral infections, or some combination of these causes. If neutropenia develops (ANC less than 1,300 cells/mm^3), mycophenolate should be interrupted or the dose reduced. Appropriate diagnostic tests and treatment should be instituted. ▪ Assess neurologic status frequently. ▪ Monitor patients with severe chronic renal impairment and patients with delayed graft function closely. See Dose Adjustments and Actions.

Patient Education: In women of childbearing age, a negative pregnancy test is indicated within 1 week of starting mycophenolate; effective contraception must be used for 4 weeks before beginning mycophenolate, during therapy, and for 6 weeks following cessation of therapy. Either total abstinence is required or two reliable forms of contraception must be used simultaneously even in patients with a history of infertility unless due to hysterectomy. Birth control pills may be ineffective. If a pregnancy occurs, do not stop mycophenolate; call your health care provider. ▪ Promptly report any S/S of infection or bone marrow suppression (e.g., unexpected bruising, bleeding). May cause serious infections. ▪ Routine laboratory monitoring is required. ▪ May increase risk of lymphoproliferative disease and some other malignancies. ▪ Although most vaccinations may be less effective, the manufacturer suggests that flu vaccinations may be of value. ▪ Risk of skin cancer may be increased. Reduce exposure to sunlight and UV light. Wear protective clothing and use a sunscreen with a high protection factor. ▪ Cooperation with repeated laboratory tests imperative. ▪ Review medications with the physician responsible for mycophenolate therapy. ■ Manufacturer provides a patient information Medication Guide. ■ See Appendix D, p. 1434.

Maternal/Child: Category D: avoid pregnancy. Increased risk of first-trimester pregnancy loss and increased risk of congenital malformations, including cleft lip and palate and microtia. See manufacturer's literature for details. A negative serum or urine pregnancy test with a sensitivity of at least 25 mIU/mL within 1 week of beginning therapy is indicated in all women of childbearing age. Contraception required before, during, and after use. See Patient Education. Use during pregnancy only if benefit justifies risk; should pregnancy occur during treatment, discuss the desirability of continuing the pregnancy. Women using mycophenolate at any time during pregnancy are encouraged to enroll in the National Transplantation Pregnancy Registry. ■ Discontinue breast-feeding. ■ Safety and effectiveness for use in pediatric patients not established; see Indications.

Elderly: No specific recommendations. Consider age-related decreased organ function and/or additional medical problems and medications. May be at increased risk of adverse reactions. Observe carefully.

DRUG/LAB INTERACTIONS

Cyclosporine (Sandimmune) may decrease serum levels of MPA (mycophenolate). Monitor levels closely when cyclosporine is added or removed from a drug regimen containing mycophenolate. ■ **Tacrolimus** may increase serum levels of mycophenolate. Monitor serum levels and adjust dose as indicated. ■ Has been administered in combination with **antithymocyte globulin** (ATGAM), **cyclosporine, corticosteroids, and muromonab-CD3** (Orthoclone). Safety for use with other agents has not been determined. ■ Manufacturer recommends not administering concomitantly with **azathioprine.** Both agents may cause bone marrow suppression and concomitant administration has not been studied. ■ Use caution with **drugs that interfere with enterohepatic recirculation or alter the intestinal flora** (e.g., cholestyramine [Questran]). ■ In impaired renal function, **acyclovir** (Zovirax) **and/or ganciclovir** (Cytovene) and mycophenolate may compete for tubular secretion, further increasing the serum levels of each drug; monitor patients closely. ■ Coadministration with **probenicid** (Benemid) results in an increase in the AUC of MPAG and MPA. **Other agents that undergo renal tubular secretion** (e.g., acyclovir, ganciclovir) may also result in increased serum levels of mycophenolate. ■ Salicylates (e.g., aspirin) increase the free fraction of MPA. Cyclosporine, digoxin, naproxen (Naprosyn), prednisone, propranolol, tacrolimus (Prograf), theophylline (Aminophylline), tolbutamide, and warfarin (Coumadin) did not increase the free fraction of MPA. ■ MPA may slightly decrease protein binding of **phenytoin** (Dilantin) **and theophylline,** increasing the free fraction of these drugs. ■ **Oral contraceptives** may be ineffective; use additional birth control measures. ■ Not recommended for concurrent administration with a combination of **metronidazole** (Flagyl) **and norfloxacin** (Noroxin); may decrease mycophenolate levels. Interaction not observed when mycophenolate is administered with either antibiotic separately. ■ Not recommended for concurrent use with **rifampin** (Rifadin); may decrease mycophenolate levels. ■ Coadministration with **ciprofloxacin** (Cipro) or **amoxicillin/clavulanic acid** (Augmentin) may cause a reduction in median MPA trough concentrations. Clinical significance unknown. ■ Do not use **live virus vaccines** in patients receiving mycophenolate; other types of vaccinations may be less effective. See Patient Education.

SIDE EFFECTS

Principal side effects include diarrhea, infection, leukopenia, phlebitis, thrombosis, and vomiting occur most frequently. Abdominal pain, acne, asthenia, back pain, bone marrow suppression (e.g., anemia, hypochromic anemia, leukocytosis, leukopenia, neutropenia, thrombocytopenia), chest pain, colitis, constipation, cough, dizziness, dyspepsia, dyspnea, edema, fever, GI hemorrhage (3%), headache, hematuria, hypercholesterolemia, hyperglycemia, hyperkalemia, hypertension, hypokalemia, hypomagnesemia, hypophosphatemia, infection (a higher frequency of opportunistic infections including TB and atypical mycobacterial infections [fatal infections occurred in less than 2% of patients]), insomnia, kidney tubular necrosis, nausea, oral moniliasis, pain, pancreatitis, peripheral edema, pharyngitis, progressive multifocal leukoencephalopathy, rash, severe neutropenia (2% to 3% of patients), tremor, and UTI may occur. In renal transplant patients, those receiving 2 Gm/day demonstrated an overall better safety profile than those receiving 3 Gm/day. In addition, arrhythmias, abnormal kidney function, accidental injury, bradycardia, ecchymosis, heart failure, hypotension, increased kidney and liver function tests, oliguria, pericardial effusion, tachycardia, and other side effects occurred in cardiac transplant patients.

Post-marketing: BK virus–associated nephropathy and pure red cell aplasia.

ANTIDOTE

Notify the physician of all side effects. Most can be treated symptomatically. Drug may be decreased or discontinued or other immunosuppressive agents utilized. Some side effects (e.g., neutropenia) may require temporary reduction of dosage or withholding of treatment. Consider reducing the amount of immunosuppression in patients who develop PML, taking into account the risk this may represent to the graft. At clinically encountered concentrations, MPA and MPAG are not usually removed by hemodialysis. However, at high concentrations (greater than 100 mcg/mL) small amounts of MPAG are removed. MPA may be removed by bile and acid sequestrants such as cholestyramine (Questran).

NAFCILLIN SODIUM
(naf-**SILL**-in **SO**-dee-um)

Nallpen

Antibacterial
(penicillinase-resistant penicillin)

pH 6 to 8.5

USUAL DOSE

500 mg to 1 Gm every 4 hours. Up to 12 Gm in 24 hours has been used in severe infections. Continue therapy for at least 48 hours after patient is afebrile and asymptomatic and cultures are negative. Usual duration of therapy is at least 14 days for severe staphylococcal infections and longer (4 to 6 weeks) for endocarditis and osteomyelitis.

Endocarditis, meningitis, osteomyelitis, or pericarditis: 1.5 to 2 Gm every 4 to 6 hours.

PEDIATRIC DOSE

Safety and effectiveness for use in pediatric patients not established. All pediatric doses are unlabeled; see Maternal/Child. Limited clinical experience with IV route in neonates and infants. Maximum dose is 12 Gm/24 hr.

Pediatric patients less than 40 kg and over 1 month of age: *Moderate infections:* 50 to 100 mg/kg/24 hr in equally divided doses every 6 hours (12.5 to 25 mg/kg every 6 hours).

Serious infections (e.g., osteomyelitis, pericarditis, endocarditis): 100 to 200 mg/kg/24 hr in equally divided doses every 4 to 6 hours (16.6 to 33.3 mg/kg every 4 hours or 25 to 50 mg/kg every 6 hours).

NEONATAL DOSE

Safety and effectiveness for use in neonates not established. All pediatric doses are unlabeled; see Maternal/Child. Limited clinical experience with IV route in neonates and infants.

10 to 20 mg/kg every 8 to 12 hours, or 25 mg/kg with the interval adjusted based on age and weight as follows:

0 to 7 days of age and under 2,000 Gm: Every 12 hours.

Over 7 days of age and under 1,200 Gm: Every 12 hours.

Over 7 days of age and 1,200 to 2,000 Gm: Every 8 hours.

0 to 7 days of age and over 2,000 Gm: Every 8 hours.

Over 7 days of age and over 2,000 Gm: Every 6 hours.

Increase dose to 50 mg/kg every 6, 8, or 12 hours in meningitis.

DOSE ADJUSTMENTS

Dose adjustment not required for patients with renal dysfunction, including those receiving hemodialysis. ■ Measure nafcillin serum levels and adjust dose accordingly in patients with hepatic insufficiency and renal failure.

DILUTION

Each 500-mg vial is diluted with 1.7 mL of SW for injection (1-Gm vial with 3.4 mL, 2-Gm vial with 6.8 mL). Each 1 mL equals 250 mg. Further dilute each dose with a minimum of 15 to 30 mL of SW, NS, or ½NS, or other **compatible** IV solutions (see chart on inside back cover or literature). Concentration should be 2 to 40 mg/mL. Available prediluted and in ADD-Vantage vials for use with ADD-Vantage infusion containers. May be given through Y-tube, three-way stopcock, or with additive tubing, or may be added to larger volume of **compatible** solutions.

Filters: Not required by manufacturer. Premixed and frozen solutions are filtered during manufacturing.

Storage: Store unopened vials at CRT. Refrigerate unused medication after initial dilution and discard after 7 days. Stable in specific solutions at concentrations of 2 to 40 mg/mL for 24 hours at room temperature and 96 hours if refrigerated. Frozen, premixed solutions should be stored at −20° C (−4° F). Thaw at room temperature or under refrigeration. Thawed solutions are stable for 72 hours at RT or 21 days refrigerated. Do not refreeze.

COMPATIBILITY   (Underline Indicates Conflicting Compatibility Information)
Consider any drug NOT listed as compatible to be INCOMPATIBLE until consulting a pharmacist; specific conditions may apply.
Inactivated in solution with aminoglycosides (e.g., amikacin [Amikin], gentamicin). Do not mix in the same solution. Appropriate spacing and/or separate sites required. See Drug/Lab Interactions.

One source suggests the following **compatibilities:**
Additive: Aminophylline, chloramphenicol (Chloromycetin), chlorothiazide (Diuril), dexamethasone (Decadron), diphenhydramine (Benadryl), ephedrine sulfate, heparin, lidocaine, potassium chloride (KCl), prochlorperazine (Compazine), sodium bicarbonate, sodium lactate, verapamil.
Y-site: Acyclovir (Zovirax), atropine, cyclophosphamide (Cytoxan), diazepam (Valium), diltiazem (Cardizem), enalaprilat (Vasotec IV), esmolol (Brevibloc), famotidine (Pepcid IV), fentanyl (Sublimaze), fluconazole (Diflucan), foscarnet (Foscavir), heparin, hydromorphone (Dilaudid), magnesium sulfate, meperidine (Demerol), morphine, nicardipine (Cardene IV), propofol (Diprivan), theophylline, vancomycin, zidovudine (AZT, Retrovir).

RATE OF ADMINISTRATION
IV injection: Each 500 mg or fraction thereof properly diluted over 5 to 10 minutes.
Intermittent IV: Administration over 30 to 60 minutes may decrease incidence of thrombophlebitis.
Infusion: When diluted in large volumes of infusion fluids, give at rate prescribed.

ACTIONS
A semisynthetic penicillinase-resistant penicillin, used for its bactericidal activity against gram-positive organisms, primarily penicillinase-producing staphylococci. Mode of action involves inhibition of bacterial cell wall biosynthesis. Highly resistant to inactivation by staphylococcal penicillinase. Readily distributes into most body fluids and tissues except spinal fluid. Binds to serum proteins, primarily albumin. Mainly eliminated by hepatic inactivation and excretion in bile; a small amount is excreted in urine. Half-life is 30 to 60 minutes. Crosses the placental barrier. Secreted in breast milk.

INDICATIONS AND USES
Treatment of infections caused by penicillinase-producing staphylococci.

CONTRAINDICATIONS
Known hypersensitivity to any penicillin or cephalosporin (not absolute); see Precautions. Prediluted solutions containing dextrose may be contraindicated with known allergies to corn products.

PRECAUTIONS

Sensitivity studies necessary to determine susceptibility of the causative organism to nafcillin. Nafcillin should not be used in infections caused by an organism susceptible to penicillin G or due to an organism other than a resistant staphylococcus. Modify antimicrobial treatment as indicated by C/S. ▪ To reduce the development of drug-resistant bacteria and maintain its effectiveness, nafcillin should be used to treat or prevent only those infections proven or strongly suspected to be caused by bacteria. ▪ Use with caution in patients with both impaired hepatic and renal function; elevated serum concentrations may cause neurotoxic reactions. See Dose Adjustments. ▪ Hypersensitivity reactions, including fatalities, have been reported in patients undergoing penicillin therapy; most likely to occur in patients with a history of penicillin hypersensitivity or sensitivity to multiple allergens. There have been reports of individuals with a history of penicillin hypersensitivity experiencing severe reactions when treated with cephalosporins. Check history of previous hypersensitivity reactions to penicillins, cephalosporins, or other allergens. Actual incidence of cross-allergenicity not established but may be more common with first-generation cephalosporins. ▪ Avoid prolonged use of the drug; superinfection caused by overgrowth of nonsusceptible organisms may result. ▪ *Clostridium difficile*–associated diarrhea (CDAD) has been reported. May range from mild diarrhea to fatal colitis. Consider in patients who present with diarrhea during or after treatment with nafcillin. ▪ Manufacturer's premixed solutions contain dextrose; may be contraindicated in patients with an allergy to corn or corn products.

Monitor: Obtain baseline CBC with differential and monitor during treatment. Monitor urinalysis, SCr, BUN, ALT, and AST periodically, especially with prolonged treatment. ▪ Watch for early symptoms of a hypersensitivity reaction, especially in individuals with a history of allergic problems. ▪ Test patients with syphilis for HIV. ▪ May cause thrombophlebitis, especially in the elderly or with too-rapid injection. Limit IV treatment to 24 to 48 hours when possible. Change to oral therapy as soon as practical. ▪ Electrolyte imbalance and cardiac irregularities from sodium content are possible. Contains up to 3.3 mEq sodium/Gm. May aggravate CHF. Observe for hypokalemia. ▪ See Drug/Lab Interactions.

Patient Education: May require alternate birth control. ▪ Promptly report diarrhea or bloody stools that occur during treatment or up to several months after an antibiotic has been discontinued; may indicate CDAD and require treatment.

Maternal/Child: Category B: use only if clearly needed. ▪ Safety and effectiveness for use in pediatric patients not established, but it is used; see Pediatric Dose. ▪ May cause diarrhea, candidiasis, or allergic response in nursing infants. ▪ Elimination rate markedly reduced in neonates and infants due to immature hepatic and renal function.

Elderly: Response similar to that seen in younger adults. Consider age-related organ impairment and concomitant disease or drug therapy. ▪ May be at increased risk for thrombophlebitis. ▪ See Precautions/Monitor and Dose Adjustments.

DRUG/LAB INTERACTIONS

May be antagonized by **bacteriostatic antibiotics** (e.g., chloramphenicol, erythromycin, tetracyclines), may interfere with bactericidal action. ▪ Potentiated by **probenecid** (Benemid); toxicity may result. ▪ Synergistic when used in combination with **aminoglycosides** (e.g., amikacin [Amikin], gentamicin). Synergism may be inconsistent; see Compatibility. ▪ Concomitant use with **beta-adrenergic blockers** (e.g., propranolol) may increase risk of anaphylaxis and inhibit treatment. ▪ Risk of bleeding with **anticoagulants** (e.g., heparin) is increased. ▪ May decrease serum levels and effectiveness of **cyclosporine** (Sandimmune). ▪ Inhibits effectiveness of **oral contraceptives;** breakthrough bleeding or pregnancy could result. ▪ High doses (9 to 12 Gm daily) may decrease serum half-life of **warfarin** (Coumadin); monitor PT up to 30 days after nafcillin completed. ▪ May reduce effectiveness of **nifedipine** (Procardia XL) by reducing its serum plasma levels. ▪ May cause **false values in common lab tests;** see literature.

SIDE EFFECTS

Bleeding abnormalities, bone marrow suppression (e.g., agranulocytosis, neutropenia), diarrhea, hypersensitivity reactions (e.g., anaphylaxis, bronchospasm, pruritus, rash, serum sickness–like symptoms, urticaria [may be immediate or delayed]), local reactions (e.g., pain, phlebitis, thrombophlebitis, and occasionally skin sloughing with extravasation), nausea and vomiting, renal tubular damage, and interstitial nephritis have been reported. CDAD and hypersensitivity myocarditis (fever, eosinophilia, rash, sinus tachycardia, ST-T changes, and cardiomegaly) can occur. Higher-than-normal doses may cause neurologic adverse reactions, including convulsions, especially with concomitant impaired hepatic insufficiency and renal dysfunction.

ANTIDOTE

Notify physician immediately of any adverse symptoms. For severe symptoms discontinue the drug, treat hypersensitivity reaction (antihistamines, epinephrine, corticosteroids), and resuscitate as necessary. Hemodialysis or peritoneal dialysis is minimally effective in overdose. Treat CDAD with fluids, electrolytes, protein supplements, and oral vancomycin (Vancocin) or metronidazole (Flagyl) as indicated. In severe cases, surgical evaluation may be indicated. Mild cases may respond to drug discontinuation alone.

NALBUPHINE HYDROCHLORIDE
(**NAL**-byoo-feen hy-droh-**KLOR**-eyed)

Narcotic analgesic
(agonist-antagonist)
Anesthesia adjunct

pH 3.5 to 3.7

USUAL DOSE
Pain control: 10 mg/70 kg. May repeat every 3 to 6 hours. In nontolerant patients, the recommended single maximum dose is 20 mg. Maximum total daily dose is 160 mg. Adjust dose and interval according to severity of pain, physical status of patient, and other medications administered concomitantly; see Dose Adjustments.

Adjunct to balanced anesthesia: A loading dose of 300 mcg (0.3 mg) to 3 mg/kg over 10 to 15 minutes. Maintain desired level of balanced anesthesia with 250 to 500 mcg (0.25 to 0.5 mg)/kg as required. Administered only under the direction of the anesthesiologist.

DOSE ADJUSTMENTS
In patients dependent on opioids, initiate a dose of nalbuphine at one-fourth the usual dose if their previous medication was a narcotic. Observe for symptoms of withdrawal. Increase to effective dose gradually. ▪ Reduced dose may be required in the elderly or debilitated; in impaired liver or renal function; in patients with limited pulmonary reserve; and in the presence of other CNS depressants. ▪ See Drug/Lab Interactions.

DILUTION
May be given undiluted.

Filters: No data available from manufacturer.

Storage: Store at CRT. Avoid freezing and/or prolonged exposure to light.

COMPATIBILITY
Consider any drug NOT listed as compatible to be INCOMPATIBLE until consulting a pharmacist; specific conditions may apply.

Manufacturer lists as **incompatible** with nafcillin (Nallpen) and ketorolac (Toradol).

One source suggests the following **compatibilities:**

Solution: D5NS, D10W, LR, NS.

Y-site: Amifostine (Ethyol), aztreonam (Azactam), bivalirudin (Angiomax), cisatracurium (Nimbex), cladribine (Leustatin), dexmedetomidine (Precedex), etoposide phosphate (Etopophos), fenoldopam (Corlopam), filgrastim (Neupogen), fludarabine (Fludara), gemcitabine (Gemzar), granisetron (Kytril), hetastarch in electrolytes (Hextend), linezolid (Zyvox), melphalan (Alkeran), oxaliplatin (Eloxatin), paclitaxel (Taxol), propofol (Diprivan), remifentanil (Ultiva), teniposide (Vumon), thiotepa, vinorelbine (Navelbine).

RATE OF ADMINISTRATION
Pain control: Each 10 mg or fraction thereof over 3 to 5 minutes. Frequently titrated according to symptom relief and respiratory rate.

Anesthesia adjunct: See Usual Dose.

ACTIONS
A synthetic narcotic agonist-antagonist analgesic. Binds to kappa, mu, and delta receptors. Acts as an agonist at kappa receptors and as a partial

antagonist at mu receptors. It equals morphine in analgesic effect. Does produce respiratory depression, but this does not increase markedly with increased doses. Onset of pain relief occurs within 2 to 3 minutes and lasts about 3 to 6 hours. Metabolized in the liver. Some excretion in urine. Crosses the placental barrier. Secreted in breast milk.

INDICATIONS AND USES
Relief of moderate to severe pain. ▪ Preoperative and postoperative analgesia. ▪ Surgical anesthesia supplement. ▪ Obstetric analgesia during labor and delivery.

Unlabeled uses: 10 mg SC to reduce pruritus from epidural morphine.

CONTRAINDICATIONS
Hypersensitivity to nalbuphine or its components.

PRECAUTIONS
May precipitate withdrawal symptoms if stopped too quickly after prolonged use or if patient has been on opiates. ▪ Use caution in patients with impaired respiration (e.g., from other medications, uremia, asthma, severe infection, cyanosis, or respiratory obstruction); see Dose Adjustments. ▪ Use caution in patients with myocardial infarction who have nausea and vomiting or compromised cardiac function; effect on heart not fully evaluated. ▪ Use caution in ambulatory patients; see Patient Education. ▪ Use caution in patients with head injuries, intracranial lesions, or pre-existing increases in intracranial pressure. Nalbuphine may elevate CSF pressure and may produce effects that can obscure the clinical course of patients with head injuries (e.g., pupillary changes, sedation). ▪ Use caution in patients with a history of drug abuse or emotional instability; close monitoring is required. ▪ Use caution in the elderly and debilitated and in patients with renal or hepatic impairment; see Dose Adjustments. ▪ Use caution in patients about to undergo surgery of the biliary tract. Can cause spasm of the sphincter of Oddi. ▪ Administration during labor has caused severe fetal bradycardia; naloxone (Narcan) may reverse effects; see Maternal/Child. ▪ Should be administered as a supplement to general anesthesia only by persons specifically trained in the use of IV anesthetics and in the management of the respiratory effects of potent opioids. ▪ When used with anesthesia, a high incidence of bradycardia has been reported in patients who did not receive atropine preoperatively.

Monitor: Naloxone (Narcan), oxygen, and controlled respiratory equipment must be available. ▪ Observe frequently; monitor vital signs. ▪ Keep patient supine to minimize side effects; orthostatic hypotension and fainting may occur. Observe closely during ambulation. ▪ Pain control usually more effective with routinely administered doses. Determine appropriate interval through clinical assessment ▪ See Drug/Lab Interactions.

Patient Education: Avoid use of alcohol or other CNS depressants (e.g., antihistamines, diazepam [Valium]). ▪ Request assistance for ambulation. ▪ Use caution performing any task that requires alertness; may cause dizziness, euphoria, and sedation. ▪ May be habit forming. Can cause withdrawal if stopped too quickly after prolonged use or if other opioids are used.

Maternal/Child: Category B: use during pregnancy (other than labor and delivery) only if benefits justify risks. Take appropriate measures (e.g., fetal monitoring) to detect and manage potential adverse effects to the fetus. ▪ Safety for use during breast-feeding not established. ▪ Fetal and neonatal bradycardia, respiratory depression at birth, apnea, cyanosis, and

hypotonia have been reported. Maternal or neonatal administration of naloxone (Narcan) may reverse these effects. Fetal death has been reported when mothers received nalbuphine during labor and delivery. Use during labor and delivery only if clearly indicated and if benefit outweighs risk. Newborns should be monitored for respiratory depression, apnea, bradycardia, and arrhythmias if nalbuphine has been used. ▪ Not recommended for pediatric patients under 18 years of age.
Elderly: May be more sensitive to effects (e.g., respiratory depression, constipation, dizziness, urinary retention). ▪ Analgesia should be effective with lower doses. ▪ Consider age-related organ impairment.

DRUG/LAB INTERACTIONS
Potentiated by **cimetidine** (Tagamet), **phenothiazines** (e.g., chlorpromazine [Thorazine]), by **other CNS depressants** such as narcotic analgesics, general anesthetics, alcohol, anticholinergics, antihistamines, barbiturates, hypnotics, neuromuscular blocking agents (e.g., atracurium [Tracrium]), psychotropic agents, and sedatives. Reduced doses of both drugs may be indicated. ▪ May decrease analgesic effects of **other narcotics;** avoid concurrent use. ▪ Plasma **amylase and lipase** determinations may be unreliable for 24 hours following narcotic administration. ▪ Depending on the test used, nalbuphine may interfere with enzymatic methods for the detection of **opiates.** Consult test manufacturer's literature.

SIDE EFFECTS
Abdominal pain, agitation, anaphylaxis, anxiety, blurred vision, bradycardia, clammy skin, dizziness, dry mouth, fever, headache, hypertension, hypotension, injection site reaction, nausea, psychotomimetic effect (symptoms resembling a psychosis), pulmonary edema, respiratory depression, sedation, seizures, symptoms associated with histamine release, tachycardia, tremor, urinary urgency, vertigo, vomiting.

ANTIDOTE
With increasing severity of any side effect or onset of symptoms of overdose, discontinue the drug and notify the physician. Naloxone hydrochloride (Narcan) will reverse severe reactions. A patent airway, artificial ventilation, oxygen therapy, and other symptomatic treatment (e.g., fluids, vasopressors) must be instituted promptly.

NALOXONE HYDROCHLORIDE
(nal-**OX**-ohn hy-droh-**KLOR**-eyed)

Antidote
Narcotic antagonist

pH 3 to 4

USUAL DOSE

Narcotic overdose: 0.4 to 2 mg. Repeat in 2 to 3 minutes if indicated. The diagnosis of narcotic overdose should be questioned if no response is observed after 10 mg of naloxone. If effective, dosage may be repeated as necessary for recurrence of symptoms.

Postoperative narcotic depression: 0.1 to 0.2 mg at 2- to 3-minute intervals to desired response. Titrate to avoid excessive reduction of narcotic analgesic action.

Challenge test for suspected opioid dependence: 0.2 mg. Observe for 30 seconds for S/S of withdrawal (e.g., abdominal cramps, diaphoresis, dysphoria, nausea and vomiting, rhinorrhea). If no evidence of withdrawal, inject 0.6 mg of naloxone and observe for an additional 20 minutes. Monitor VS and observe patient again for S/S of opiate withdrawal.

PEDIATRIC DOSE

Ampules containing 0.02 mg/mL are available, but larger doses are frequently required. Adult strength is often used to reduce amount of injection and to effect desired response, which may require increased or repeat doses. One source states, "Up to 10 times a dose has been required."

Narcotic overdose: *Less than 20 kg:* 0.01 to 0.1 mg/kg of body weight initially. Based on estimated degree of overdose and respiratory depression. May repeat every 2 to 3 minutes. May dilute with SW. American Academy of Pediatrics recommends 0.1 mg/kg. Manufacturer recommends 0.01 mg/kg.

Over 20 kg or over 5 years of age: 2 mg. Repeat every 2 to 3 minutes as needed. A continuous infusion may be used after initial effective dose. Add 75% to 100% of effective dose to a specific amount of IV fluid and infuse evenly distributed over 1 hour. For some overdoses (e.g., methadone), weaning in 50% increments may take up to 48 hours. For others, 6 to 12 hours is adequate. If symptoms recur, rebolus and go back to 100%.

Postoperative narcotic depression: 0.005 to 0.01 mg IV at 2- to 3-minute intervals to desired response.

NEONATAL DOSE

Neonatal opiate depression: Administration into umbilical vein is preferred. 0.01 to 0.1 mg/kg of body weight initially. Based on estimated degree of overdose and respiratory depression. May repeat every 2 to 3 minutes to achieve a satisfactory response. May dilute with SW. American Academy of Pediatrics recommends 0.1 mg/kg repeated every 2 to 3 minutes. Manufacturer recommends 0.01 mg/kg repeated every 2 to 3 minutes. Another source suggests an initial dose of 0.01 mg/kg. If response is not satisfactory, increase subsequent doses to 0.1 mg/kg.

DILUTION

May be given undiluted, diluted with SW for injection, or further diluted in NS or D5W and given as an infusion (2 mg in 500 mL equals a concentration of 0.004 mg/mL). Discard infusions after 24 hours.

Storage: Store below 40° C. Protect from light.

COMPATIBILITY

Consider any drug NOT listed as compatible to be INCOMPATIBLE until consulting a pharmacist; specific conditions may apply.

Manufacturer lists as **incompatible** with bisulfites, sulfites, long-chain or high-molecular-weight anions, solutions with an alkaline pH.

One source suggests the following **compatibilities:**

Additive: Verapamil.

Y-site: Fenoldopam (Corlopam), linezolid (Zyvox), propofol (Diprivan).

RATE OF ADMINISTRATION

Each 0.4 mg or fraction thereof over 15 seconds. Titrate infusion to patient response.

ACTIONS

A potent narcotic antagonist. Overcomes effects of narcotic overdose including respiratory depression, sedation, and hypotension. Unlike other narcotic antagonists, it does not have any narcotic effect itself. Onset of action is within 2 minutes. Duration of action is dependent on dose and route of naloxone administration. Requirement for repeat doses is dependent on amount, type, and route of narcotic administration. Metabolized in the liver and excreted in urine.

INDICATIONS AND USES

Reversal of narcotic depression. ▪ Antidote for natural (e.g., morphine) and synthetic narcotics (e.g., butorphanol, methadone, nalbuphine, pentazocine, and propoxyphene). ▪ Diagnosis of suspected opioid tolerance or acute opiate overdose.

Unlabeled uses: Reversal of alcoholic coma and improvement of circulation in refractory shock.

CONTRAINDICATIONS

Known hypersensitivity to naloxone. ▪ The naloxone challenge test should not be performed in patients showing S/S of withdrawal or whose urine contains opioids.

PRECAUTIONS

Does not produce respiratory depression with non-narcotic drug overdose, a beneficial action. ▪ It is ineffective against respiratory depression caused by barbiturates, anesthetics, other non-narcotic agents, or pathologic conditions. ▪ Will precipitate acute withdrawal symptoms in narcotic addicts; use caution, especially in newborns of narcotic-dependent mothers. ▪ Use caution in cardiac disease patients or those receiving cardiotoxic drugs.

Monitor: Symptomatic treatment with oxygen and artificial ventilation as necessary should be continued until naloxone is effective. Observe patient continuously. Duration of narcotic action may exceed that of naloxone.

Maternal/Child: Category B: use in pregnancy and breast-feeding only when clearly needed. Safety for use not established. ▪ See Precautions.

DRUG/LAB INTERACTIONS

Specific information not available.

SIDE EFFECTS

Hypertension, irritability and increased crying in the newborn, nausea and vomiting, sweating, tachycardia, tremulousness. Overdose postoperatively may result in excitement, hypertension, hypotension, reversal of analgesia, pulmonary edema, ventricular tachycardia and fibrillation.

ANTIDOTE

Notify the physician of any side effect. Treatment will probably be symptomatic. Resuscitate as necessary.

NATALIZUMAB BBW
(nah-tah-**LIZZ**-u-mab)

Tysabri

Monoclonal antibody
Immunomodulator

pH 6.1

USUAL DOSE
Multiple sclerosis (MS): 300 mg as an infusion every 4 weeks.
Crohn's disease (CD): 300 mg as an infusion every 4 weeks. Discontinue if no benefit is seen after 12 weeks of therapy. For patients with CD who initiate natalizumab therapy while on chronic corticosteroids, begin steroid tapering as soon as therapeutic benefit of natalizumab has occurred. Discontinue natalizumab if the patient cannot be tapered off of steroids within 6 months. Consider discontinuing therapy in patients who require more than 3 months of steroid use (excluding the original 6-month taper) in a calendar year to control their CD. Aminosalicylates may be continued during therapy with natalizumab.

DOSE ADJUSTMENTS
None indicated. Pharmacokinetics have not been studied in patients with renal or hepatic insufficiency.

DILUTION
Available in 300 mg/15 mL single-use vials. Withdraw 15 mL of concentrate (300 mg) from the vial and inject into 100 mL of NS. Gently invert to mix completely. Do not shake. No other IV diluents may be used to prepare the solution. Solution is a colorless, clear to slightly opalescent concentrate. Do not use if particulates are present or if solution is discolored.
Filters: Use of filtration devices during administration not evaluated.
Storage: Refrigerate vials at 2° to 8° C (36° to 46° F). Do not use beyond the expiration date on the vial. Do not shake or freeze. Protect from light. Following dilution, solution should be infused immediately. However, it may be refrigerated and used within 8 hours of preparation. If refrigerated, allow to warm to room temperature before infusion.

COMPATIBILITY
Manufacturer states, "Other medications should not be injected into infusion set side ports or mixed with natalizumab." Flush line with NS before and after infusion.

RATE OF ADMINISTRATION
Do not administer as an IV push or bolus injection. Infuse over approximately 1 hour. Flush line with NS before and after infusion.

ACTIONS
A recombinant humanized IgG4κ monoclonal antibody produced in murine myeloma cells. Natalizumab is thought to bind to a subunit on the surface of all leukocytes except neutrophils and inhibit the adhesion of leukocytes to their counterreceptors. The receptors for the α4 family of integrins include vascular cell adhesion molecule-1 (VCAM-1), which is expressed on activated vascular endothelium, and mucosal addressin cell adhesion molecule-1 (MAdCAM-1), which is present on vascular endothelial cells of the GI tract. Disruption of these molecular interactions prevents transmigration of leukocytes across the endothelium into inflamed parenchymal tissue. Specific mechanisms of how natalizumab exerts its effects in MS and CD have not been fully defined. In multiple

sclerosis (MS), lesions are believed to occur when activated inflammatory cells, including T-lymphocytes, cross the blood-brain barrier (BBB). Leukocyte migration across the BBB involves the interaction between adhesion molecules on inflammatory cells and their counterreceptors on the endothelial cells of the vessel wall, thereby preventing immune cells from migrating from the bloodstream into the brain, where they can cause inflammation and potentially damage nerve fibers and their insulation. This action may be secondary to blockade of the molecular interaction of α4β1 integrins expressed by inflammatory cells with VCAM-1 on vascular endothelial cells and with CS-1 and/or osteopontin expressed by parenchymal cells in the brain. In clinical trials, natalizumab reduced the rate of clinical relapse and the appearance of new or newly enlarging T2 hyperintense lesions on MRI studies. The number of gadolinium-enhancing lesions on the 1-year MRI scan follow-up was also reduced. In Crohn's disease (CD), the α4β7 integrin with the endothelial receptor MAdCAM-1 expression has been found to be increased at active sites of inflammation in the mucosa and to contribute to the inflammatory response characteristic of CD. It is mainly expressed on gut endothelial cells. The action of natalizumab may be secondary to blockade of MAdCAM-1 and reduce this inflammatory response in the GI tract. Distribution is limited primarily to vascular space (plasma volume). Half-life is 3 to 17 days.

INDICATIONS AND USES

Monotherapy for the treatment of patients with relapsing forms of multiple sclerosis (MS) to delay the accumulation of physical disability and to reduce the frequency of clinical exacerbations. Should be reserved for patients who have had an inadequate response to or are unable to tolerate alternate MS therapies. ■ Safety and efficacy in patients with chronic progressive MS not established. ■ Induction and maintenance of clinical response and remission in adults with moderately to severely active Crohn's disease with evidence of inflammation who have had an inadequate response to or are unable to tolerate conventional therapy and inhibitors of TNFα (e.g., infliximab [Remicade]). Should not be used in combination with immunosuppressants (e.g., 6-mercaptopurine, azathioprine [Imuran], cyclosporine [Sandimmune], or methotrexate) or inhibitors of TNFα; see Precautions.

CONTRAINDICATIONS

Hypersensitivity to natalizumab or any of its components, patients who have or have had progressive multifocal leukoencephalopathy (PML).

PRECAUTIONS

Has been associated with hypersensitivity reactions, including anaphylaxis. Reactions usually occur within 2 hours of the start of the infusion. Generally associated with antibodies to natalizumab. ■ Anti-natalizumab antibodies have been detected in some patients. Persistently positive antibodies were associated with a substantial decrease in effectiveness and an increase in infusion-related reactions. 90% of patients who became persistently antibody-positive developed detectable antibodies by 12 weeks. Patients who receive therapeutic monoclonal antibodies, including natalizumab, after an extended period without treatment may be at increased risk of hypersensitivity reactions with re-exposure. Consider testing for the presence of antibodies in patients who want to resume therapy after a dose interruption. ■ Effects on immune system may increase the risk of infection, including opportunistic infection. ■ **Progressive multifocal** leukoencephalopathy (PML) has been reported. PML is a serious progressive neurologic disorder caused by infection of the CNS by JC virus, a member of the papovavirus family. It typically occurs in immunocompromised patients. PML is rare but may result in irreversible neurologic deterioration and death, and there is no known effective treatment. Most cases of PML have occurred in patients with recent or concomitant exposure to immunomodulators (e.g., interferon beta-1a [Avonex]) or immunosuppressants (e.g., azathioprine [Imuran]). However, there have been reports of PML in patients receiving natalizumab monotherapy. Because of the risk of PML, natalizumab is available only through a special restricted distribution program called the TOUCH™ Prescribing Program. See prescribing information or contact manufacturer for specific details and requirements. ■ Use of a gadolinium-enhanced MRI scan of the brain is recommended for diagnosis and, when indicated, CSF analysis for JC viral DNA.

■ The risk for developing PML increases with longer treatment durations. ■ The risk for PML is also increased in patients who have been treated with an immunosuppressant (excluding short courses of corticosteroids) before natalizumab treatment. ■ Patients who develop PML and have discontinued natalizumab have developed immune reconstitution inflammatory syndrome (IRIS). In most cases IRIS occurred after plasma exchange was used to eliminate circulating natalizumab. This syndrome has not been seen in patients discontinuing treatment for reasons unrelated to PML. ■ Liver injury has been reported; it has occurred as early as 6 days after the first dose and after multiple doses. The combination of ALT, AST, and bilirubin elevations without evidence of obstruction is generally recognized as an important predictor of severe liver injury that may lead to death or the need for liver transplantation. ■ No data available on secondary transmission of infections by live virus vaccines.

Monitor: Obtain baseline CBC and differential. Monitor periodically during treatment. ■ Obtain a baseline MRI before initiating treatment and periodically throughout treatment. In MS patients it may be helpful in differentiating subsequent MS symptoms from PML and assessing disease progression. In CD patients it may be helpful in distinguishing pre-existing lesions from newly developed lesions. ■ Observe patients during the infusion and for 1 hour after the infusion is complete. Discontinue infusion at the first sign of any hypersensitivity reaction (e.g., chest pain, dizziness, dyspnea, fever, flushing, hypotension, nausea, pruritus, rash, rigors, urticaria). ■ Antibodies detected within the first 6 months of therapy may be transient and disappear. Repeat testing in 3 months. If antibodies are persistent, consider risk versus benefit of continued therapy; see Precautions. ■ Monitor for S/S of infection. ■ Monitor for signs of clinical relapse. ■ Assess neurologic status frequently. S/S associated with PML are diverse and occur over days to weeks. May include progressive weakness on one side of the body, clumsiness of limbs, disturbances of vision, or changes in thinking, memory, and orientation leading to confusion and personality changes. Progression of deficits usually leads to severe disability or death over weeks to months. Withhold natalizumab if PML is suspected. If clinical suspicion of PML remains after initial evaluations are negative, continue to withhold natalizumab and repeat evaluations. ■ Monitor for S/S of IRIS; may occur within days to weeks after plasma exchange. IRIS presents as a clinical decline in condition (may occur after clinical improvement); decline may be rapid and cause serious neurologic complications or death. Associated with characteristic changes in the MRI. ▪ Monitor for S/S of liver injury (e.g., elevated bilirubin or liver function tests, jaundice).

Patient Education: Read medication guide carefully. ▪ Review medical conditions and medications with health care provider. ▪ Promptly report any new medical problems (e.g., new or sudden change in thinking, eyesight, balance, or strength). ▪ Report infections. ▪ Report jaundice and any symptoms of infusion or hypersensitivity reactions immediately (e.g., difficulty breathing, dizziness, feeling faint, itching, nausea). ▪ Discuss potential risks and benefits of treatment (e.g., risk of PML). ▪ Scheduled follow-up visits are required as part of the TOUCH™ Program.

Maternal/Child: Category C: if a woman becomes pregnant while taking natalizumab, consider discontinuing natalizumab. If continued, encourage enrollment in TYSARBI Pregnancy Exposure Registry. ▪ Has been detected in breast milk. Discontinue nursing or natalizumab, taking into account the importance of therapy to the mother. ▪ Safety and effectiveness in pediatric patients with MS or CD under 18 years of age has not been studied.

Elderly: Studies did not include sufficient numbers of patients 65 years of age and older to determine whether they respond differently than younger patients.

DRUG/LAB INTERACTIONS

Formal studies not completed. Concurrent use with **antineoplastic, immunosuppressant, or immunomodulating agents** may further increase the risk of infection, including PML and other opportunistic infections, over the risk observed with the use of natalizumab alone. Safety and efficacy of natalizumab in combination with any of these agents not established. ▪ Concurrent use of short courses of **corticosteroids** was associated with an increase in infections in clinical trials. However, the increase in infections in both the natalizumab-treated and placebo-treated patients who received steroids was similar. Corticosteroids should be tapered in patients with CD who are initiating natalizumab therapy; see Usual Dose. ▪ No data are available on the effects of **vaccination** in patients receiving natalizumab. ▪ Increases circulating **lymphocytes, monocytes, eosinophils, basophils, and nucleated red blood cells.** A return to baseline usually occurs within 16 weeks after the last dose. Elevations of **neutrophils** are not observed. ▪ May induce mild decreases in **hemoglobin,** frequently transient.

SIDE EFFECTS

Most commonly reported serious adverse reactions were infections (including influenza, pneumonia, and UTIs), hypersensitivity reactions (including anaphylaxis), depression (including suicidal ideation), and cholelithiasis. The most commonly reported adverse reactions resulting in clinical intervention (i.e., discontinuation of natalizumab) were urticaria and other hypersensitivity reactions. Infusion-related reactions (defined as any adverse event occurring within 2 hours of the start of an infusion) included headache, dizziness, fatigue, hypersensitivity reactions, nausea, pruritus, rigors, urticaria, and vomiting. Other reported adverse reactions included abdominal discomfort, abnormal liver function tests, amenorrhea, antibody formation, arthralgia, chest discomfort, dermatitis, diarrhea, fatigue, gastroenteritis, irregular menstruation/dysmenorrhea, local bleeding, muscle cramps, night sweats, pain in extremities, pruritus, rash, somnolence, syncope, tonsillitis, tremor, urinary urgency and frequency, vaginitis, and vertigo. Adverse reactions reported in persistently antibody-positive patients included anxiety, dyspnea, hypertension, myalgia, and tachycardia. **Post-Marketing:** Herpes encephalitis (1 MS patient), herpes meningitis (1 MS patient), PML in patients treated with natalizumab monotherapy.

ANTIDOTE

Keep physician informed of all side effects. Most will be treated symptomatically. Discontinue natalizumab at the first sign of liver injury, S/S suggestive of PML, or with any change in neurologic status. Discontinue infusion if any S/S of a hypersensitivity or infusion reaction occur. Treat with epinephrine, corticosteroids, diphenhydramine, bronchodilators, and oxygen as indicated. Patients who experience a hypersensitivity reaction should not be retreated with natalizumab.

NELARABINE BBW
(nell-ah-**RA**-ben)
Arranon

Antineoplastic

pH 5 to 7

USUAL DOSE

1,500 mg/M^2 administered as an infusion over 2 hours on Days 1, 3, and 5. Repeat every 21 days. The recommended duration of treatment has not been clearly established. In clinical trials, treatment was generally continued until there was evidence of disease progression or until the patient experienced unacceptable toxicity, became a candidate for bone marrow transplant, or no longer continued to benefit from treatment.

PEDIATRIC DOSE

650 mg/M^2 administered as an infusion over 1 hour daily for 5 consecutive days. Repeat every 21 days; see Usual Dose.

DOSE ADJUSTMENTS

Discontinue therapy for neurologic events of Common Terminology Criteria for Adverse Events (CTCAE) Grade 2 or greater. Dosage may be delayed for other toxicity, including hematologic toxicity. ■ Has not been studied in patients with hepatic or renal impairment. Because nelarabine and ara-G are partially eliminated by the kidneys, clearance may be reduced in patients with renal insufficiency. Dose recommendations are not available; see Precautions. ■ Use caution in dose selection for the elderly.

DILUTION

Specific techniques required; see Precautions. Nelarabine is not diluted prior to administration. Available in a 250 mg/50 mL (5 mg/mL) vial. Transfer the appropriate dose into a polyvinylchloride (PVC) infusion bag or glass container and administer as an infusion. Example: An adult patient with a body surface area of 2 M^2 would require a dose of 3,000 mg (1,500 mg/M^2 × 2 M^2 = 3,000 mg). 3,000 mg ÷ 250 mg/vial = 12 vials. **Filters:** Specific information not available. **Storage:** Store unopened vials at CRT. Stable in PVC infusion bags or glass containers for up to 8 hours at up to 30° C (86° F).

COMPATIBILITY

Specific information not available. Consider specific use; consult pharmacist.

RATE OF ADMINISTRATION
Adult dose: A single dose evenly distributed over 2 hours.
Pediatric dose: A single dose evenly distributed over 1 hour.

ACTIONS
A prodrug of ara-G, a T-cell selective nucleoside analog. Nelarabine is demethylated to ara-G and then converted through various metabolic processes to the active 5′-triphosphate, ara-GTP. Ara-GTP is incorporated into DNA, leading to inhibition of DNA synthesis and cell death. Nelarabine and ara-G are extensively distributed throughout the body and are rapidly eliminated from the plasma, with a mean half-life of 18 minutes and 3.2 hours, respectively. They are partially eliminated by the kidneys.

INDICATIONS AND USES
Treatment of patients with T-cell acute lymphoblastic leukemia and T-cell lymphoblastic lymphoma whose disease has not responded to treatment or has relapsed following treatment with at least two chemotherapy regimens. This use is based on the induction of complete responses. Randomized trials demonstrating increased survival or other clinical benefit have not been conducted.

CONTRAINDICATIONS
Hypersensitivity to nelarabine or any of its components.

PRECAUTIONS
Follow guidelines for handling cytotoxic agents. See Appendix A, p. 1429. ▪ For IV use only. ▪ Administered by or under the direction of a physician specialist in a facility with adequate diagnostic and treatment facilities to monitor the patient and respond to any medical emergency. ▪ Neurotoxicity is the dose-limiting toxicity. Severe neurologic events have been reported and may include altered mental states (e.g., coma, confusion, severe somnolence), central nervous system effects (e.g., ataxia, convulsions), and peripheral neuropathy ranging from numbness and paresthesias to motor weakness and paralysis. Events associated with demyelination and ascending peripheral neuropathies similar in appearance to Guillain-Barré syndrome have also been reported. Full recovery from these events has not always occurred with cessation of therapy. ▪ Patients treated previously or concurrently with intrathecal chemotherapy or previously with craniospinal irradiation may be at increased risk for neurologic adverse events. ▪ Hematologic toxicity (e.g., anemia, leukopenia, neutropenia [including febrile neutropenia], thrombocytopenia) is common. ▪ Use caution in patients with renal or hepatic impairment. Use has not been studied. Patients with a CrCl less than 50 mL/min or a bilirubin greater than 3 times the ULN may be at increased risk for toxicity. Monitor closely. ▪ May develop tumor lysis syndrome. ▪ See Drug/Lab Interactions.

Monitor: Close monitoring for neurologic events is strongly recommended; see Precautions and Antidote. ▪ Obtain a baseline CBC with platelets and monitor regularly. ▪ Monitor renal and hepatic function (BUN, SCr, bilirubin). ▪ Monitor for S/S of tumor lysis syndrome (e.g., hyperkalemia, hyperphosphatemia, hyperuricemia, hypocalcemia, metabolic acidosis, urate crystalluria, and renal failure). ▪ Adequate hydration, alkalinization of urine, and allopurinol are indicated to prevent and/or treat hyperuricemia due to tumor lysis syndrome. ▪ Monitor for S/S of infection. Prophylactic antibiotics may be indicated pending results of C/S in a febrile neutropenic patient. ▪ Monitor for thrombocytopenia (platelet count less than $50,000/mm^3$). Initiate precautions to prevent excessive bleeding (e.g., inspect IV sites, skin, and mucous membranes; use extreme care during invasive procedures; test urine, emesis, stool, and secretions for occult blood). ▪ Avoid administration of live virus vaccines to immunocompromised patients.

Patient Education: Avoid pregnancy; nonhormonal birth control is recommended. ▪ Use caution in tasks that require alertness. ▪ Notify physician at first sign of infection or of new or worsening neurotoxicity (e.g., numbness, tingling, difficulty with fine motor coordination, unsteadiness, weakness, seizures).

Maternal/Child: Category D: avoid pregnancy; may cause fetal harm. ▪ Discontinue breast-feeding. ▪ The mean clearance of nelarabine is about 30% higher in pediatric patients than in adult patients. Half-lives of nelarabine and ara-G are shorter than those seen in adults—13 minutes and 2 hours, respectively.

Elderly: May be at increased risk of neurologic adverse events. Clearance may be reduced in the elderly due to age-related renal impairment; see Dose Adjustments and Precautions.

DRUG/LAB INTERACTIONS

Formal drug interaction studies have not been completed. ▪ Concurrent administration with **adenosine deaminase inhibitors** (e.g., pentostatin [Nipent]) is not recommended; may decrease conversion of nelarabine to its active form and decrease its effectiveness. ▪ Nelarabine and ara-G do not appear to inhibit the activities of human hepatic cytochrome P_{450} isoenzymes. ▪ Fludarabine does not appear to affect the pharmacokinetics of nelarabine, ara-G, or ara-GTP. ▪ Do not administer **live virus vaccines** to immunocompromised patients receiving antineoplastic agents.

SIDE EFFECTS

Adults: Side effects most frequently reported were anemia, constipation, cough, diarrhea, dizziness, dyspnea, fatigue, fever, headache, hyperuricemia, hypoesthesia, nausea, neutropenia, paresthesia, peripheral neurologic disorders, somnolence, thrombocytopenia, and vomiting. Other reported side effects included abdominal distention, abdominal pain, abnormal gait, anorexia, arthralgia, asthenia, back pain, blurred vision, chest pain, chills, confusion, dehydration, depression, edema, epistaxis, exertional dyspnea, extremity pain, febrile neutropenia, hyperglycemia, hypotension, increased AST, infection, insomnia, pain, muscular weakness, myalgia, peripheral edema, petechiae, pleural effusion, pneumonia, sinusitis, sinus tachycardia, stomatitis, and wheezing. *Neurologic* side effects in adults were mostly Grade 1 or 2 and included amnesia, ataxia, balance disorder, depressed level of consciousness, headache, hypoesthesia, neuropathy (peripheral, peripheral motor, and peripheral sensory), paresthesia, sensory loss, taste alteration, and tremor. Grade 3 events included aphasia, convulsion, hemiparesis, and loss of consciousness. Cerebral hemorrhage, coma, intracranial hemorrhage, leukoencephalopathy, and metabolic encephalopathy also were reported. One patient had a cerebral hemorrhage (fatal), coma, and leukoencephalopathy.

Pediatric patients: Side effects most frequently reported were anemia, decreased blood albumin and potassium levels, headache, increased transaminase levels, leukopenia, neutropenia, peripheral neurologic disorders, thrombocytopenia, and vomiting. Other reported side effects included asthenia; decreased calcium, glucose, and magnesium levels; increased bilirubin and SCr; and infection. *Neurologic* side effects that were greater than Grade 2 included ataxia, headache, hypertonia, hypoesthesia, motor dysfunction, neuropathy (peripheral, peripheral motor, and peripheral sensory), paralysis of the third and sixth nerves, paresthesia, seizures (convulsions, grand mal convulsions, status epilepticus), somnolence, tremor. **Overdose:** Myelosuppression, severe neurotoxicity (coma, paralysis), and potentially death.

Post-Marketing: Demyelination and ascending peripheral neuropathies similar in appearance to Guillain-Barré syndrome, opportunistic infections (fatal), tumor lysis syndrome.

ANTIDOTE

Notify physician of any side effects. Most will be treated symptomatically. Discontinue therapy for neurologic events of Common Terminology Criteria for Adverse Events (CTCAE) Grade 2 or greater. Dosage may be delayed for other toxicity, including hematologic toxicity. Blood and blood products, antibiotics, and other adjunctive therapies must be available. Blood modifiers (e.g., darbepoetin alfa [Aranesp], epoetin alfa [Epogen], filgrastim [Neupogen], oprelvekin [Neumega], pegfilgrastim [Neulasta], sargramostim [Leukine]) may be indicated to treat bone marrow toxicity. No known antidote; provide supportive care in overdose. Resuscitate as necessary.

NEOSTIGMINE METHYLSULFATE
(nee-oh-**STIG**-meen **METH**-ill-**SUL**-fayt)

Cholinergic
Cholinesterase inhibitor
Antidote
Antimyasthenic

pH 5.9

USUAL DOSE

Muscle relaxant antagonist: *Atropine:* Administer atropine sulfate 0.6 to 1.2 mg for each 0.5 to 2 mg of neostigmine. Administer in a separate syringe a few minutes before neostigmine.

Neostigmine: 0.5 to 2 mg. Administer neostigmine when patient is being hyperventilated and carbon dioxide level of blood is low. Repeat as required to restore voluntary respiration. 5 mg is the normal maximum total dose. Use caution and monitor pulse rate. Pulse rate must be at least 80 beats/min. Alternately, glycopyrrolate 0.2 mg for each 1 mg of neostigmine can be used and can be mixed in the same syringe as neostigmine.

Treatment of myasthenia gravis: 0.5 mg; titrate carefully; usually given IM.

PEDIATRIC DOSE

Muscle relaxant antagonist: 40 mcg (0.04 mg)/kg of body weight with 20 mcg (0.02 mg)/kg of atropine. An alternate dose regimen is:

Infants: 0.025 to 0.1 mg/kg with atropine 0.0125 to 0.05 mg/kg.

Other pediatric patients: 0.025 to 0.08 mg/kg with atropine 0.0125 to 0.04 mg/kg. Maximum dose is 2.5 mg. Glycopyrrolate 0.2 mg for each 1 mg of neostigmine can be used instead of atropine. See all comments under Usual Dose.

Treatment of myasthenia gravis: 0.01 to 0.04 mg/kg. May repeat every 2 to 3 hours. Usually given IM. See Maternal/Child.

Continued

DOSE ADJUSTMENTS

Use extreme caution and minimum effective dose in small children, cardiac disease, asthma, epilepsy, hypothyroidism, vagotonia, peptic ulcer, and severely ill patients. Titrate exact dose; evaluate response with a peripheral nerve stimulator device.

DILUTION

Confirm ampule or vial is for IV use. May be given undiluted through Y-tube or three-way stopcock of infusion set. Do not add to IV solutions.

Storage: Store below 40° C. Protect from light.

COMPATIBILITY (Underline Indicates Conflicting Compatibility Information)

Consider any drug NOT listed as compatible to be INCOMPATIBLE until consulting a pharmacist; specific conditions may apply.

Consider specific use and potential toxicity.

One source suggests the following **compatibilities:**

Y-site: Heparin, hydrocortisone sodium succinate (Solu-Cortef), palonosetron (Aloxi), potassium chloride (KCl).

RATE OF ADMINISTRATION

0.5 mg or fraction thereof over 1 minute.

ACTIONS

An anticholinesterase and antagonist of nondepolarizing neuromuscular blocking agents. Inhibits the enzyme cholinesterase, allowing acetylcholine to accumulate at the myoneural junction. Restores normal transmission of nerve impulses and makes muscle contraction stronger and more prolonged. Onset of action is 4 to 8 minutes. Duration of action is 2 to 4 hours. Hydrolyzed by cholinesterases and metabolized by microsomal enzymes in the liver. Excreted primarily in urine.

INDICATIONS AND USES

Antidote for nondepolarizing muscle relaxants (e.g., atracurium [Tracrium]), atropine, hyoscine. ▪ Treatment of myasthenia gravis.

CONTRAINDICATIONS

High concentrations of inhalant anesthesia (e.g., halothane, cyclopropane); known sensitivity to bromides and neostigmine, mechanical intestinal or urinary obstruction, peritonitis.

PRECAUTIONS

A physician should be present when this drug is used IV. ▪ Has many additional uses given IM or orally. ▪ Edrophonium (Tensilon) can differentiate between myasthenic and cholinergic crisis. ▪ See Dose Adjustments. **Monitor:** A peripheral nerve stimulator device should be used to monitor effectiveness. ▪ *Caution:* Atropine may mask symptoms of neostigmine overdose. ▪ Epinephrine should always be available. ▪ Maintain airway and ensure adequate ventilation until complete recovery of normal respiration; see Antidote. ▪ Hyperventilate the patient before administration; carbon dioxide level of blood should be low. ▪ See Dose Adjustments and Drug/Lab Interactions.

Maternal/Child: Category C: may induce premature labor in pregnancy near term. ▪ Transient muscular weakness in swallowing, sucking, and breathing has been observed in neonates of myasthenic mothers. Confirm distinction between cholinergic or myasthenic crisis in neonate with edrophonium test. Treat neonate with IM pyridostigmine 0.05 to 0.15 mg/kg of body weight if indicated. ▪ Discontinue breast-feeding.

Elderly: Duration of antagonism of neuromuscular blockade prolonged.

DRUG/LAB INTERACTIONS

Potentiates **narcotic analgesics** (e.g., morphine, codeine, meperidine) **and succinylcholine.** ▪ Antagonized by **ganglionic blocking agents** (e.g., trimethaphan [Arfonad], guanethidine [Ismelin], mecamylamine [Inversine]) **and aminoglycoside antibiotics** (e.g., gentamicin). ▪ May be inhibited by **corticosteroids and magnesium.**

SIDE EFFECTS

Usually caused by overdose: abdominal cramps, anorexia, anxiety, bradycardia, cardiac arrhythmias and arrest, cholinergic crises, cold moist skin, convulsion, diaphoresis, diarrhea, hypotension, increased bronchial secretions, increased lacrimation, increased salivation, miosis, muscle cramps, muscle weakness, nausea, pulmonary edema, vomiting.

ANTIDOTE

Atropine sulfate. If side effects occur, discontinue drug and notify the physician. Atropine sulfate in doses of 0.6 mg IV will counteract most side effects and may be repeated every 3 to 10 minutes. Endotracheal intubation or tracheostomy is considered prophylactic in anesthesia or crises. Artificial ventilation, oxygen therapy, cardiac monitoring, adequate suctioning, and treatment of shock or convulsions must be instituted and maintained as necessary. Treat hypersensitivity reactions with epinephrine. Pralidoxime chloride (PAM) 2 Gm IV followed by 250 mg every 5 minutes may be required to reactivate cholinesterase and reverse paralysis.

NESIRITIDE
(nih-**SIR**-ih-tide)

Natrecor

Cardiotonic
Vasodilator

USUAL DOSE

Prime the IV tubing with the diluted nesiritide solution before connecting to the patient and before giving the bolus dose and infusion. *Bolus must be drawn from the prepared infusion bag.*

An initial dose of 2 mcg/kg of diluted solution is given as an IV bolus over 60 seconds. Follow immediately with the diluted solution as an infusion of 0.01 mcg/kg/min (0.1 mL/kg/hr); see Dilution and Rate of Administration. Experience is limited in the use of the infusion for more than 48 hours. *Use only the recommended dose;* see Dose Adjustments and Precautions.

DOSE ADJUSTMENTS

Reduced doses are not required in impaired renal function or based on age, gender, race, baseline endogenous human B-type natriuretic peptide (hBNP) concentration, severity of CHF, or concomitant administration of an ACE inhibitor (e.g., enalapril [Vasotec, Lexxel]). ▪ During clinical studies, if indicated and after 3 hours had passed, a bolus of 1 mcg/kg was given and infusion was increased by 0.005 mcg/kg/min in select patients (with central hemodynamic monitoring, a pulmonary capillary wedge pressure [PCWP] equal to or greater than 20 mm Hg, and a systolic blood pressure [SBP] equal to or greater than 100 mm Hg). Bolus and infusion increase of 0.005 mcg/kg/min may be repeated only once every 3 hours to a maximum dose of 0.03 mcg/kg/min; see Precautions. ▪ See Antidote.

DILUTION

Each 1.5-mg vial must be reconstituted with 5 mL of diluent withdrawn from a pre-filled, preservative-free, 250 mL plastic IV bag of D5W, NS, D5/½NS, or D5/¼NS. Do not shake. Ensure complete dilution by rotating the vial gently so all surfaces, including the stopper, are in contact with the diluent. Withdraw the entire contents of the vial and add to the 250-mL plastic IV bag used for the initial reconstitution. Invert several times to ensure complete mixing. Yields a concentration of 6 mcg/mL. *Prime the tubing and withdraw the bolus dose from this final dilution.* The IV tubing should be primed with 5 mL of the infusion solution before connecting to the IV access port and before withdrawing the bolus. Use the remaining solution for the infusion.

Filters: Manufacturer did two studies. Data indicate no loss of drug potency through a 5-micron needle filter in a 500 mcg/mL concentration. With the use of an in-line, 0.22-micron filter and concentrations of 2 and 50 mcg/mL at a rate of 9 mL/hr, drug potency was initially lower but recovered to 90% in 1 hour and 100% at 2 hours.

Storage: Vials should be stored in the carton at CRT or refrigerated (2° to 8° C [36° to 46° F]). Reconstituted vials may be stored at CRT or refrigerated for up to 24 hours.

COMPATIBILITY

Consider any drug NOT listed as compatible to be INCOMPATIBLE until consulting a pharmacist; specific conditions may apply.

Manufacturer lists as **incompatible** with bumetanide, enalaprilat (Vasotec IV), ethacrynic acid (Edecrin), furosemide (Lasix), heparin, hydralazine, insulin (regular), and any injectable drug that contains the preservative sodium metabisulfite. Manufacturer states, "Do not coadminister as infusions with nesiritide through the same IV catheter." If an **incompatible** drug has been administered, the IV catheter must be flushed with a **compatible** solution (see Dilution) before and after the administration of nesiritide. Do not administer through a heparin-coated catheter (central or peripheral). Binds to heparin and could bind to the lining of a heparin-coated catheter and decrease the amount of nesiritide delivered to the patient.

One source suggests the following **compatibilities:**

Y-site: Amiodarone (Nexterone), argatroban, digoxin (Lanoxin), diltiazem (Cardizem), fentanyl (Sublimaze), metoprolol (Lopressor), milrinone (Primacor), nicardipine (Cardene IV), nitroglycerin IV, nitroprusside (Nitropress), propranolol, quinidine gluconate, torsemide (Demadex), verapamil.

RATE OF ADMINISTRATION

If the IV line has been used to administer other drugs, flush it with a solution **compatible** to nesiritide before administration and then prime it with nesiritide solution. The IV tubing should be primed with 5 mL of the infusion solution before connecting to the IV access port and before withdrawing the bolus.

IV bolus: A single dose over 60 seconds through an IV port in the tubing.

IV infusion: Use a volume-controlled infusion pump and administer at a flow rate of 0.1 mL/kg/hr to deliver the desired dose of 0.01 mcg/kg/min.

Adjust bolus volumes and rates of infusion by weight according to the following chart.

Nesiritide Weight-Adjusted Bolus Volume and Infusion Flow Rate (2 mcg/kg Bolus Followed by a 0.01 mcg/kg/min Infusion)		
Patient Weight (kg)	Volume of Bolus (mL)	Rate of Infusion (mL/hr)
60 kg	20 mL	6 mL/hr
70 kg	23.3 mL	7 mL/hr
80 kg	26.7 mL	8 mL/hr
90 kg	30 mL	9 mL/hr
100 kg	33.3 mL	10 mL/hr
110 kg	36.7 mL	11 mL/hr

Alternately, the following formulas can be used to calculate the correct bolus volume and infusion rate:

$$\text{Bolus volume (mL)} = \text{Patient weight (kg)} \div 3$$

$$\text{Infusion flow rate (mL/hr)} = 0.1 \times \text{Patient weight (kg)}$$

ACTIONS

A recombinant form of human B-type natriuretic peptide (hBNP). Has the same 32–amino acid sequence as the endogenous peptide produced by the ventricular myocardium. Binds to specific receptors of vascular smooth muscle and endothelial cells, resulting in increased intracellular concentrations of cGMP and smooth muscle cell relaxation. Dilates veins and arteries. Produces dose-dependent reductions in PCWP and systemic arterial pressure in patients with heart failure. Has no effect on cardiac contractility or measures of cardiac electrophysiology (e.g., atrial and ventricular refractory times or atrioventricular node conduction) in animals. 60% of the 3-hour effect on PCWP reduction and 70% of the 3-hour effect on SBP reduction is achieved within 15 minutes. Half-life is approximately 18 minutes. Duration of action may be longer than predicted based on half-life and may be dose dependent. At steady state, plasma hBNP levels increase from baseline levels by 3-fold to 6-fold, with infusion doses ranging from 0.01 to 0.03 mcg/kg/min. Cleared from circulation through three independent mechanisms: cellular internalization and lysosomal proteolysis after binding to cell surface receptors, proteolytic cleavage by endopeptidases, and renal filtration.

INDICATIONS AND USES

Treatment of acutely decompensated CHF in patients who have dyspnea at rest or with minimal activity. Has been shown to reduce PCWP and improve dyspnea.

CONTRAINDICATIONS

Hypersensitivity to nesiritide or its components (a recombinant protein manufactured using *Escherichia coli*). ■ Not recommended as primary therapy for patients with cardiogenic shock or patients with a systolic BP less than 90 mm Hg. ■ Not recommended in patients for whom vasodilating agents are not appropriate (e.g., restrictive or obstructive cardiomyopathy, constrictive pericarditis, pericardial tamponade, significant valvular stenosis), for other conditions in which cardiac output is dependent on venous return, or for patients who may have or are known to have low cardiac filling pressures.

PRECAUTIONS

Safety and effectiveness for use longer than 48 hours not established. ■ Administered by or under the supervision of a physician experienced in its use and in a facility equipped to monitor the patient and respond to any medical emergency. ■ An *E. coli*–derived protein product; hypersensitivity reactions have been reported. ■ May cause azotemia in patients with severe CHF whose renal function may depend on the activity of the renin-angiotensin-aldosterone system. Some patients have required first-time dialysis. ■ Use with caution in patients with a baseline SBP of less than 100 mm Hg; risk of hypotension may be increased. ■ Increased risk of hypotensive episodes of greater intensity and duration with bolus doses larger than 2 mcg/kg and infusion doses ranging from 0.015 to 0.03 mcg/kg/min. ■ Recently published reports question whether nesiritide may have adverse effects on survival and kidney function compared to control agents (e.g., nitroglycerin and diuretics). Outcome studies are currently underway. In addition, an expert panel of cardiology and heart failure clinicians has provided a consensus statement on each issue and has provided recommendations regarding the appropriate use of nesiritide; see literature.

Monitor: Incidence of hypotension is similar to nitroglycerin, but duration of hypotension is longer. Monitor BP closely. Reduce rate or stop infusion for excessive drop in BP; see Antidote. ■ Observe patient continuously; monitor ECG, urine output, renal function, fluid and electrolyte changes, and body weight. Monitoring of cardiac index and PCWP useful. ■ Observe for orthopnea, dyspnea, and fatigue. ■ As cardiac output and diuresis improves, a reduction in diuretic dose may be indicated. ■ Possible risk of arrhythmias. Risk increased with excessive diuresis and/or hypokalemia. Replace potassium as indicated. ■ See Precautions and Drug/Lab Interactions.

Patient Education: Report dizziness or faintness; request assistance for ambulation.

Maternal/Child: Pregnancy Category C: use only if potential benefit justifies possible risk to the fetus. ■ Not known if nesiritide is secreted in breast milk; use caution in women who are breast-feeding. ■ Safety and effectiveness for use in pediatric patients not established.

Elderly: Response similar to that found in younger patients; however, use with caution in the elderly; may have a greater sensitivity to its effects.

DRUG/LAB INTERACTIONS

May cause additive hypotension with oral **ACE inhibitors** (e.g., enalapril [Vasotec, Lexxel]) **and other drugs that may cause hypotension** (e.g., antidepressants [e.g., amitriptyline (Elavil)], antihypertensives, benzodiazepines [e.g., diazepam (Valium), lorazepam (Ativan)], magnesium sulfate). ■ Has been administered with angiotensin II receptor antagonists, anticoagulants, beta-blockers (e.g., atenolol [Tenormin]), calcium channel blockers (e.g., diltiazem [Cardizem], verapamil), class III antiarrhythmic agents (e.g., amiodarone [Nexterone], sotalol [Betapace]), digoxin, diuretics, dobutamine, dopamine, oral ACE inhibitors, oral nitrates, and statins (e.g., simvastatin [Zocor]). No specific effect on the action of nesiritide was noted, but hypotensive effects are additive. ■ Effects of concurrent use with **other IV vasodilators** (e.g., IV ACE inhibitors, milrinone, nitroglycerin, or nitroprusside sodium) have not been studied, but hypotensive effects would be additive.

SIDE EFFECTS

Hypotension is the primary side effect; may be symptomatic and can be dose limiting; see Antidote. Other reported side effects include abdominal pain, amblyopia (vision impairment), anemia, angina, anxiety, apnea, arrythmias (e.g., atrial fibrillation, AV node conduction abnormalities, bradycardia, PVCs, tachycardia, VT), back pain, catheter pain, confusion, dizziness, fever, headache, hemoptysis, increased cough, increased serum creatinine, injection site reaction, insomnia, leg cramps, nausea, paresthesia, pruritus, rash, somnolence, sweating, tremor, and vomiting. Hypersensitivity reactions and anaphylaxis may occur.

ANTIDOTE

Notify the physician of any side effects. Based on degree of severity and condition of the patient; may be treated symptomatically; dose may remain the same, be decreased, or be discontinued. Reduce rate or discontinue nesiritide at the first sign of marked hypotension and notify the physician. Hypotension may respond to a Trendelenburg position and IV fluids (avoid fluid overload). Hypotension may last for hours; observation for a prolonged period may be indicated before restarting nesiritide. After hypotension is stabilized, nesiritide may be restarted; do not administer a bolus dose and reduce the rate of infusion by 30%. Treat hypersensitivity reactions as indicated. Treat arrhythmias with the appropriate drug.

NICARDIPINE HYDROCHLORIDE
(nye-**KAR**-dih-peen hy-droh-**KLOR**-eyed)

Cardene IV

Calcium channel blocker
Antihypertensive

pH 3.7 to 4.7

USUAL DOSE

Must be individualized based on the severity of hypertension and the response of each patient. Blood pressure decrease is dependent on the rate of infusion and frequency of dose adjustments. Gradual reduction based on clinical situation is best. Avoid too-rapid or excessive drop in BP. See Precautions. Transfer to oral medication as soon as clinical condition permits.

To substitute for oral nicardipine therapy: 0.5 mg/hr will achieve similar plasma concentration to an oral dose of 20 mg every 8 hours; 1.2 mg/hr to an oral dose of 30 mg every 8 hours; 2.2 mg/hr to an oral dose of 40 mg every 8 hours.

Gradual reduction of BP in a drug-free patient: Initiate therapy at 5 mg/hr. May be increased by 2.5 mg/hr every 15 minutes until desired BP reduction is achieved. Do not exceed 15 mg/hr.

Rapid reduction of BP in a drug-free patient: Initiate a 5-mg/hr dose as above, but increases of 2.5 mg/hr may be given every 5 minutes until desired BP reduction is achieved (AHA guidelines recommend 5 to 15 minutes). Do not exceed 15 mg/hr.

Maintenance: When desired BP is achieved, reduce rate to 3 mg/hr. This is the average maintenance rate. Adjust as needed to maintain desired response.

Transfer to an oral antihypertensive agent: The first dose of oral nicardipine should be given 1 hour before discontinuing infusion. Initiate any other oral antihypertensive agent on discontinuation of infusion.

DOSE ADJUSTMENTS

Lower doses and slower titration suggested in heart failure and impaired hepatic or renal function; see Precautions. ▪ Lower-end initial doses may be indicated in the elderly. Consider potential for decreased organ function and concomitant disease or drug therapy.

DILUTION

Available as a premixed solution containing 0.1 mg/mL in D5W or NS or in a vial that requires further dilution. Each vial (25 mg in 10 mL) must be diluted with 240 mL of **compatible** infusion solution to equal a concentration of 0.1 mg/mL; in this 0.1 mg/mL concentration, 2.5 mg/hr equals 25 mL/hr, 3 mg/hr equals 30 mL/hr, 5 mg/hr equals 50 mL/hr, and 15 mL/hr equals 150 mL/hr. **Compatible** in ½NS, NS, D5W, D5/½NS, D5NS. Also **compatible** in D5W with 40 mEq of potassium added.

Fluid-restricted or pediatric patients: One source recommends mixing up to 50 mg in 100 mL (0.5 mg/mL). To avoid superficial phlebitis, administration via a central line is recommended for this concentration.

Filters: No data available from manufacturer.

Storage: Store vials in carton, protected from light at CRT. Has a light yellow color. Diluted solution is stable at room temperature for 24 hours. Store prediluted solutions at CRT; protect from light and excessive heat and avoid freezing.

COMPATIBILITY (Underline Indicates Conflicting Compatibility Information)
Consider any drug NOT listed as compatible to be INCOMPATIBLE until consulting a pharmacist; specific conditions may apply.
Manufacturer states, "Do not combine with any product in the same IV line or premixed container. Do not add supplementary medication to the bag." Manufacturer lists as **incompatible** with sodium bicarbonate 5% and LR.

One source suggests the following **compatibilities:**
Additive: *Not recommended by manufacturer.* Potassium chloride (KCl).
Y-site: *Not recommended by manufacturer.* Amikacin (Amikin), aminophylline, aztreonam (Azactam), butorphanol (Stadol), calcium gluconate, cefazolin (Ancef), ceftazidime (Fortaz), chloramphenicol (Chloromycetin), clindamycin (Cleocin), dextran 40 in 5% dextrose, diltiazem (Cardizem), dobutamine, dopamine, enalaprilat (Vasotec IV), epinephrine (Adrenalin), erythromycin (Erythrocin), esmolol (Brevibloc), famotidine (Pepcid IV), fenoldopam (Corlopam), fentanyl (Sublimaze), gentamicin, heparin, hetastarch in NS (Hespan), hydrocortisone sodium succinate (Solu-Cortef), hydromorphone (Dilaudid), labetalol (Trandate), lidocaine, linezolid (Zyvox), lorazepam (Ativan), magnesium sulfate, methylprednisolone (Solu-Medrol), metronidazole (Flagyl IV), midazolam (Versed), milrinone (Primacor), morphine, nafcillin (Nallpen), nesiritide (Natrecor), nitroglycerin IV, nitroprusside sodium, norepinephrine (Levophed), penicillin G potassium, piperacillin, potassium chloride (KCl), potassium phosphate, ranitidine (Zantac), sodium acetate, sulfamethoxazole/trimethoprim, tobramycin, vancomycin, vecuronium.

RATE OF ADMINISTRATION
Must be administered as a slow continuous infusion. Adjust as indicated in Usual Dose and Dose Adjustments.

ACTIONS
The first dihydropyridine calcium channel blocker for IV use. Inhibits influx of calcium ions into cardiac muscle and smooth muscle without altering serum calcium. Contractile processes are dependent on calcium movement through specific channels. Effects seen are more selective to vascular smooth muscle than cardiac muscle. Causes coronary and peripheral blood vessels to dilate and relax, reducing systemic vascular resistance. Increases cardiac output, coronary blood flow, and myocardial oxygen supply without increasing cardiac oxygen demand. Reduces BP without significantly affecting cardiac conduction and usually does not depress cardiac function. Produces dose-dependent decreases in BP. Begins to reduce BP in minutes; achieves 50% of ultimate decrease in 45 minutes. When discontinued, can lose 50% of effect within 30 minutes, but gradually decreasing effects persist for up to 50 hours. Effects more prominent in hypertensive than in normotensive volunteers. Highly protein bound. Extensively metabolized in the liver. Half-life is 14.4 hours. Excreted in urine and feces. Crosses placental barrier. Minimally secreted in breast milk.

INDICATIONS AND USES
Short-term treatment of hypertension when oral therapy is not feasible or not desirable.

CONTRAINDICATIONS

Advanced aortic stenosis (reduced diastolic pressure may worsen rather than improve myocardial oxygen balance). ▪ Known hypersensitivity to nicardipine.

PRECAUTIONS

Use caution in patients with coronary artery disease. May cause increase in frequency, duration, or severity of angina. ▪ Has improved left ventricle function after beta-blockade. ▪ Use caution and titrate slowly in patients with heart failure or significant left ventricular dysfunction, particularly when used in combination with a beta-blocker; possible negative inotropic effects may occur. ▪ Use caution with impaired hepatic or renal function; lower doses, slower titration, and close monitoring indicated. ▪ May produce symptomatic hypotension or tachycardia. Avoid systemic hypotension (systolic BP less than 90 mm Hg), and use with caution in patients with acute cerebral infarction or hemorrhage.

Monitor: To reduce the possibility of venous thrombosis, phlebitis, local irritation, swelling, extravasation, and/or vascular impairment, administer through a central vein or large peripheral vein rather than a small peripheral vein. Avoid intra-arterial administration. If administered via a peripheral vein, change the infusion site every 12 hours. ▪ Avoid tachycardia or too-rapid or excessive reduction in either systolic or diastolic BP. Monitor BP and HR continually during infusion and frequently after infusion. Additional monitoring of BP and HR is indicated when used in combination with a beta-blocker in patients with HF or significant left ventricular dysfunction ▪ Transfer to oral therapy as soon as clinical condition permits. ▪ See Precautions and Drug/Lab Interactions.

Patient Education: Request assistance to change position or ambulate.

Maternal/Child: Category C: use during pregnancy only if benefit justifies potential risk to the fetus. ▪ Dizziness, flushing, headache, hypotension, nausea, postpartum hemorrhage, reflex tachycardia, and tocolysis have occurred in pregnant women treated for hypertension during pregnancy. Produced hypotension in some neonates. ▪ During use in preterm labor, dyspnea, headache, hypotension, hypoxia, phlebitis at the injection site, and pulmonary edema have been reported. Neonatal side effects included acidosis (pH less than 7.25). ▪ Use caution during breast-feeding; infant exposure may occur. ▪ Safety and effectiveness for use in pediatric patients under 18 years of age not established.

Elderly: Response similar to that seen in younger adults; however, greater sensitivity in the elderly cannot be ruled out. ▪ Half-life may be prolonged. ▪ See Dose Adjustments.

DRUG/LAB INTERACTIONS

May cause possible negative inotropic effects with concurrent administration of a **beta-blocker** (e.g., atenolol [Tenormin], metoprolol [Lopressor]); see Precautions. ▪ **Cimetidine** (Tagamet) increases oral nicardipine plasma concentrations; monitor patients receiving IV nicardipine carefully. ▪ Oral nicardipine does not appear to alter **digoxin** levels. However, as a precaution, evaluate digoxin levels with concomitant use. ▪ Will increase plasma levels of **cyclosporine** (Sandimmune); monitor and decrease cyclosporine dose if indicated. ▪ May potentiate the effects of **other antihypertensives.** Monitor BP closely and adjust doses as indicated. ▪ Metabolism may be increased and serum concentrations decreased by **rifampin** (Rifadin). Adjust dose as needed. ▪ Plasma protein binding of nicardipine not altered with therapeutic concentrations of furosemide (Lasix), propranolol, dipyridamole (Persantine), warfarin (Coumadin), quinidine, or naproxen (Naprosyn).

SIDE EFFECTS

Average dose: Most common side effects include headache, hypotension, nausea and vomiting, and tachycardia. Many other side effects, including ECG abnormality (e.g., angina pectoris, atrioventricular block, ST-segment depression, inverted T wave), confusion, conjunctivitis, deep vein thrombophlebitis, dyspepsia, ear disorder, fever, hypertonia, hypophosphatemia, neck pain, peripheral edema, respiratory difficulties, thrombocytopenia, tinnitus, and urinary frequency, occurred in fewer than 3% of patients. Hypersensitivity reactions (e.g., angioedema, rash, wheezing) have been reported.

Overdose: Bradycardia (following initial tachycardia), confusion, drowsiness, flushing, hypotension (marked), palpitations, slurred speech. Progressive AV block may occur with lethal overdose.

ANTIDOTE

Keep physician informed of all side effects. Headache, hypotension, and tachycardia have required a reduction in dose or discontinuation of nicardipine. When symptoms subside, nicardipine may be restarted at low doses (e.g., 3 to 5 mg/hr [30 to 50 mL/hr of a 0.1 mg/mL solution or 15 to 25 mL/hr of a 0.2 mg/mL solution]) and adjusted to maintain desired BP. In overdose, monitor BP, cardiac and respiratory functions; put patients in Trendelenburg position; use vasopressors (e.g., dopamine) for excessive hypotension. IV calcium gluconate may reverse effects of calcium entry blockade. Not removed by hemodialysis.

NITROGLYCERIN IV
(**NYE**-troe-**GLIS**-er-in)

Antianginal
Antihypertensive
Vasodilator

pH 3 to 6.5

USUAL DOSE

See Compatibility; these doses are recommended for use with non-PVC administration sets. Increased doses are required if using PVC administration sets. Effectiveness is short term; see Actions. Initiate concurrent therapy before tolerance develops (e.g., doses exceeding 200 mcg/min or administration over 12 to 24 hours).

Unstable angina, persistent ischemia, and/or congestive heart failure associated with MI: An IV bolus of 12.5 to 25 mcg followed by a continuous infusion of 10 to 20 mcg/min; increase by 5 to 10 mcg/min every 5 to 10 minutes until desired hemodynamic response. AHA recommends an IV bolus of 12.5 to 25 mcg followed by an infusion at 10 mcg/min. Increase rate by 10 mcg/min every 3 to 5 minutes until desired effect. 200 mcg/min is the usual maximum dose.

Treatment of angina in patients unresponsive to therapeutic doses of nitrates or beta-blockers: 5 mcg/min initially. Increase by 5 mcg/min increments every 3 to 5 minutes until some BP response is noted. Reduce increments and/or increase time to fine-tune to desired hemodynamic response. If no response at 20 mcg/min, 10 mcg/min increases may be used. Incremental increases of up to 20 mcg/min may be needed to achieve desired effect. No fixed optimum dose. Tolerance may develop if administered over 12 to 24 hours.

Severe hypertension or hypertensive emergency: Doses up to 100 mcg/min may be required (range is 5 to 100 mcg/min). Doses that will reduce mean arterial BP by no more than 25% over several minutes to 1 hour are suggested to prevent overaggressive therapy. If stable, follow with further reductions toward 160/100 to 110 mm Hg within the next 2 to 6 hours. When an initial response is achieved, increases in dosage increments should be reduced and/or the intervals between dose increases lengthened.

PEDIATRIC DOSE

0.25 to 0.5 mcg/kg/min initially. May increase by 0.5 to 1 mcg/kg/min increments every 3 to 5 minutes until desired response. See Maternal/Child. AHA guidelines recommend titrating by 1 mcg/kg/min every 15 to 20 minutes and states the typical dose range is 1 to 5 mcg/kg/min.

DOSE ADJUSTMENTS

Reduced dose may be required with persistent headache unrelieved by analgesics. Reduce dose gradually when weaning to prevent rebound symptoms. ■ Lower-end initial doses may be appropriate in the elderly based on potential for decreased organ function, concomitant disease, or other drug therapy.

DILUTION

Available premixed in D5W with various concentrations of nitroglycerin. All other preparations must be diluted and administered as an infusion. Use only non-PVC plastic or glass infusion bottles and specific (nonpolyvinyl chloride) infusion tubing (provided by manufacturer). Do not use filters.

Dilute in a given amount of D5W or NS for infusion. Concentration dependent on initial preparation (0.5 mg/mL or 5 mg/mL) and patient fluid tolerances. 10 mL of 0.5 mg/mL in 250 mL diluent equals 20 mcg/mL (in 1,000 mL, 5 mcg/mL). 10 mL of 5 mg/mL in 250 mL diluent equals 200 mcg/mL (in 1,000 mL, 50 mcg/mL). See the following dilution chart.

Guidelines for Dilution of Nitroglycerin IV for Infusion		
Diluent Volume (mL)	Quantity of Nitroglycerin (5 mg/mL)	Approximate Final Concentration (mcg/mL)
100 mL	10 mg (2 mL)	100 mcg/mL
100 mL	20 mg (4 mL)	200 mcg/mL
100 mL	40 mg (8 mL)	400 mcg/mL
250 mL	25 mg (5 mL)	100 mcg/mL
250 mL	50 mg (10 mL)	200 mcg/mL
250 mL	100 mg (20 mL)	400 mcg/mL
500 mL	50 mg (10 mL)	100 mcg/mL
500 mL	100 mg (20 mL)	200 mcg/mL
500 mL	200 mg (40 mL)	400 mcg/mL

May be used in dilutions from 25 to 400 mcg/mL.
Pediatric dilution: 6 mg/kg nitroglycerin IV in 100 mL D5W at an infusion rate of 1 mL/hr equals 1 mcg/kg/min.
Filters: Do not use filters; see Dilution.
Storage: Protect vials from light. Solution stable for up to 24 hours.
COMPATIBILITY   (Underline Indicates Conflicting Compatibility Information)
Consider any drug NOT listed as compatible to be INCOMPATIBLE until consulting a pharmacist; specific conditions may apply.
Manufacturer states, "Do not admix with any other drug." See Dilution. Non-PVC plastic or glass infusion bottles and nonpolyvinyl chloride infusion tubing is required to deliver accurate dosing with minimal adsorption. Calculated dose will not be correct if other infusion containers or tubing are used because of excess adsorption.
   One source suggests the following **compatibilities:**
Additive: *Not recommended by manufacturer.* Alteplase (tPA, Activase), aminophylline, dobutamine, dopamine, enalaprilat (Vasotec IV), furosemide (Lasix), lidocaine, verapamil.
Y-site: Amiodarone (Nexterone), amphotericin B cholesteryl (Amphotec), argatroban, atracurium (Tracrium), bivalirudin (Angiomax), cisatracurium (Nimbex), dexmedetomidine (Precedex), diltiazem (Cardizem), dobutamine, dopamine, drotrecogin alfa (Xigris), epinephrine (Adrenalin), esmolol (Brevibloc), famotidine (Pepcid IV), fenoldopam (Corlopam), fentanyl (Sublimaze), fluconazole (Diflucan), furosemide (Lasix), haloperidol (Haldol), heparin, hetastarch in electrolytes (Hextend), hydralazine, hydromorphone (Dilaudid), inamrinone (Amrinone), insulin (regular), labetalol (Trandate), lidocaine, linezolid (Zyvox), lorazepam (Ativan), micafungin (Mycamine), midazolam (Versed), milrinone (Primacor), morphine, nesiritide (Natrecor), nicardipine (Cardene IV), nitroprusside sodium, norepinephrine (Levophed), pancuronium, pantoprazole (Pro-

tonix IV), propofol (Diprivan), ranitidine (Zantac), remifentanil (Ultiva), tacrolimus (Prograf), theophylline, thiopental (Pentothal), tirofiban (Aggrastat), vasopressin, vecuronium, warfarin (Coumadin).

RATE OF ADMINISTRATION

Dependent on patient response and effective dose. Specific adjustments required; see Usual Dose. Use extreme caution in patients responsive to initial 5 mcg/min dose. Decrease adjustments and increase time between doses as patient begins to respond. Use of an infusion pump or microdrip (60 gtt/mL) required. Exact and constant delivery mandatory. See the following chart.

Nitroglycerin IV Guidelines for Infusion				
Concentration (mcg/mL)	50	100	200	400
Desired Dose (mcg/min)	60 Microdrops = 1 mL Flow Rate (microdrops/min = mL/hr)			
5 mcg/min	6	3	—	—
10 mcg/min	12	6	3	—
15 mcg/min	18	9	—	—
20 mcg/min	24	12	6	3
30 mcg/min	36	18	9	—
40 mcg/min	48	24	12	6
60 mcg/min	72	36	18	9
80 mcg/min	96	48	24	12
120 mcg/min	—	72	36	18
160 mcg/min	—	96	48	24
240 mcg/min	—	—	72	36
320 mcg/min	—	—	96	48
480 mcg/min	—	—	—	72
640 mcg/min	—	—	—	96

ACTIONS

A vascular smooth-muscle relaxant and vasodilator. Affects arterial and venous beds. Reduces myocardial oxygen consumption, preload, and afterload by reducing systolic, diastolic, and mean arterial blood pressure; central venous and pulmonary capillary wedge pressures; and pulmonary and systemic vascular resistance. Effective coronary perfusion is usually maintained. Low doses (30 to 40 mcg/min) produce venodilation; high doses (150 to 500 mcg/min) produce arteriolar dilation. Widely distributed throughout the body. Onset of action occurs in 1 to 2 minutes and lasts 3 to 5 minutes. Metabolized in the liver and excreted in urine.

INDICATIONS AND USES

Control of BP in perioperative hypertension (especially cardiovascular procedures). ■ Drug of choice in unstable angina or congestive heart failure associated with acute myocardial infarction. May be used in combination with dobutamine 2 to 20 mcg/kg/min to produce hemodynamic improvement while reducing risk of ischemic damage. ▪ Treatment of angina pectoris if patient unresponsive to therapeutic doses of organic nitrates and/or a beta-blocker. ▪ Controlled hypotension during surgical procedures.

CONTRAINDICATIONS

Anemia (severe), hypersensitivity to nitrates, hypotension or uncorrected hypovolemia, cerebral hemorrhage, closed-angle glaucoma, head trauma, increased intracranial pressure, patients taking sildenafil (Viagra), pericardial tamponade, constrictive pericarditis.

PRECAUTIONS

Special tubing causes problems with infusion pump control. Patient may still be receiving nitroglycerin IV even though pump is off or tubing clamped. Low flow rates may actually be higher and not deliver accurate dosage. ▪ Plastic (polyvinyl chloride) tubing or containers will absorb up to 80% of diluted nitroglycerin IV. Use extreme caution and adjust dose if changing infusion equipment (e.g., IV tubing, extension tubing). Absorption greatest with slowest rate. ▪ If changing preparations from 0.8 mg/mL to 5 mg/mL, use new tubing or clear tubing with a minimum of 15 mL, adjust dose carefully, and observe effects. ▪ Use caution in patients with low left ventricular filling pressure or low pulmonary capillary wedge pressure. May have exaggerated response to low dosage. ▪ Use caution in hepatic or renal disease, pericarditis, or postural hypotension.

Monitor: Maintain adequate systemic BP and coronary perfusion pressure. HR and BP measurements mandatory; pulmonary wedge pressure recommended. ▪ Observe for tachycardia, which can decrease diastolic filling time. ▪ Observe for fall in pulmonary wedge pressure. Precedes arterial hypotension and impending shock. Reduce or discontinue drug temporarily. ▪ Headache may improve with analgesics or slightly lower dose; usually improves with time. ▪ See Drug/Lab Interactions.

Maternal/Child: Category C: safety for use in pregnancy, breast-feeding, and in pediatric patients not established.

Elderly: Hypotensive effects may be increased. ▪ Differences in response compared to younger patients not identified. ▪ Lower-end initial doses may be indicated; see Dose Adjustments.

DRUG/LAB INTERACTIONS

May cause irreversible hypotension if given within 24 to 48 hours of **impotence agents** (e.g., sildenafil citrate [Viagra, Revatio], tadalafil [Cialis], vardenafil [Levitra]). ▪ Potentiated by **alcohol** (may cause hypotension and cardiovascular collapse), **antihypertensives, aspirin, beta-adrenergic blockers** (e.g., propranolol), **other vasodilators, phenothiazines** (e.g., prochlorperazine [Compazine]), **and tricyclic antidepressants.** ▪ Inhibited by **dihydroergotamine and sympathomimetics** (e.g., vasopressors [phenylephrine], bronchodilators, decongestants, glaucoma agents, mydriatics). ▪ Inhibits **acetylcholine, histamine, norepinephrine.** ▪ Potentiates **nondepolarizing muscle relaxants** (e.g., atracurium [Tracrium]); may cause apnea. ▪ May cause marked orthostatic hypotension with **calcium channel blockers** (e.g., verapamil). ▪ May antagonize anticoagulant effects of **heparin;** monitor. ▪ Concurrent use with **alteplase** (tPA); reduces the thrombolytic effects of alteplase.

SIDE EFFECTS

Abdominal pain, angina, apprehension, dizziness, headache, hypersensitivity reactions (e.g., itching, tracheobronchitis, wheezing), hypotension, methemoglobinemia, muscle twitching, nausea, palpitations, postural hypotension, restlessness, retrosternal discomfort, tachycardia, vomiting.
Overdose: Bloody diarrhea, colic, confusion, diaphoresis, dyspnea, flushing, heart block, paralysis, tachycardia, visual disturbances. Severe hypotension may result in shock, reflex paradoxical bradycardia, inadequate cerebral circulation, constrictive pericarditis, pericardial tamponade, decreased organ perfusion, and death.

ANTIDOTE

Notify physician of all side effects. Discontinue if blurred vision or dry mouth occur. For accidental overdose with severe hypotension and reflex tachycardia and/or fall in pulmonary wedge pressure, reduce rate or temporarily discontinue until condition stabilizes. Lower head of bed (Trendelenburg position). Administer IV fluids. Use O_2 and assisted ventilation if indicated. An alpha-adrenergic agonist (e.g., phenylephrine [Neo-Synephrine]) is rarely required. Epinephrine and related compounds (dopamine) are contraindicated. Monitor levels and treat methemoglobinemia if indicated with methylene blue 0.2 mL/kg of body weight (1 to 2 mg/kg) IV and high-flow oxygen. Treat anaphylaxis and resuscitate as necessary.

NITROPRUSSIDE SODIUM BBW
(nye-troh-**PRUS**-eyed **SO**-dee-um)
Nitropress

Antihypertensive
Vasodilator
pH 3.5 to 6

USUAL DOSE
Begin with 0.25 to 0.3 mcg/kg of body weight/min. Under continuous BP monitoring, titrate upward very gradually (small increments every 2 to 3 minutes). 3 mcg/kg/min is the average effective dose; range is 0.1 to 10 mcg/kg/min. AHA guidelines recommend beginning with 0.1 mcg/kg/min. Titrate upward every 3 to 5 minutes to desired effect (up to 5 mcg/kg/min). Small adjustments can lead to major fluctuations in BP. Never exceed 10 mcg/kg/min. If 10 mcg/kg/min does not promote adequate BP reduction in 10 minutes, discontinue administration and use another antihypertensive agent. Cyanide toxicity can occur with as little as 2 mcg/kg/min and could begin to occur after 10 minutes at the maximum dose.

Acute CHF: Titrate as described previously until one of the following occurs: cardiac output is no longer increasing, perfusion of vital organs would be compromised by further reduction of BP, or maximum infusion rate (10 mcg/kg/min) is reached.

PEDIATRIC DOSE
Begin with 0.3 mcg/kg/min. Adjust slowly to individual response as in Usual Dose. AHA guidelines recommend 0.3 to 1 mcg/kg/min initially; titrate up to 8 mcg/kg/min as needed.

DOSE ADJUSTMENTS
Average effective dose may be as little as 0.5 mcg/kg/min in patients who are receiving other antihypertensive agents by any route. ▪ Reduced dose may be required in the elderly.

DILUTION
Available in a liquid formulation (25 mg/mL), or each 50 mg must be reconstituted with 2 to 3 mL of D5W or SW for injection without a preservative. Must be further diluted in a minimum of 250 mL of D5W (manufacturer's recommendation). JAMA suggests NS may be used. Must be administered as an infusion. Larger amounts of solution may be used. 50 mg in 250 mL equals 200 mcg/mL. 50 mg in 500 mL equals 100 mcg/mL. Immediately after mixing, wrap infusion bottle in opaque material (e.g., aluminum foil) to protect from light. Use only freshly prepared solutions; usually discard infusion within 4 hours of mixing. (Literature now states, "Stable for 24 hours if properly protected.") ▪ Solution has a faint brownish tint; discard immediately if highly colored, blue, green, or dark red.

Pediatric dilution: Add 0.6 mg/kg to 100 mL diluent. 1 mL/hr equals 0.1 mcg/kg/min.

COMPATIBILITY   (Underline Indicates Conflicting Compatibility Information)
Consider any drug NOT listed as compatible to be INCOMPATIBLE until consulting a pharmacist; specific conditions may apply.
One source suggests the following **compatibilities:**
Additive: Enalaprilat (Vasotec IV), ranitidine (Zantac), verapamil.

Y-site: Alprostadil, amiodarone (Nexterone), argatroban, atracurium (Tracrium), bivalirudin (Angiomax), calcium chloride, cisatracurium (Nimbex), dexmedetomidine (Precedex), diltiazem (Cardizem), dobutamine, dopamine, enalaprilat (Vasotec IV), epinephrine (Adrenalin), esmolol (Brevibloc), famotidine (Pepcid IV), furosemide (Lasix), haloperidol (Haldol), heparin, hetastarch in electrolytes (Hextend), inamrinone (Amrinone), indomethacin (Indocin IV), insulin (regular), isoproterenol (Isuprel), labetalol (Trandate), lidocaine, magnesium sulfate, micafungin (Mycamine), midazolam (Versed), milrinone (Primacor), morphine, nesiritide (Natrecor), nicardipine (Cardene IV), nitroglycerin IV, norepinephrine (Levophed), pancuronium, potassium chloride (KCl), potassium phosphate, procainamide (Pronestyl), propofol (Diprivan), tacrolimus (Prograf), theophylline, vecuronium.

RATE OF ADMINISTRATION

Use of an infusion pump (volumetric preferred) required to regulate dose accurately. Increase mcg/kg/min rate as outlined in Usual Dose to reduce BP gradually to preset or desired levels. Do not exceed maximum dose. Response should be noted almost immediately. Manufacturer provides the following infusion rate chart in mL/hr to achieve initial (0.3 mcg/kg/min) and maximal (10 mcg/kg/min) for 50-, 100-, and 200-mcg/mL dilutions.

Nitroprusside Sodium Guidelines for Infusion						
Volume		250 mL		500 mL		1,000 mL
Nitroprusside Sodium		50 mg		50 mg		50 mg
Injection Concentration		200 mcg/mL		100 mcg/mL		50 mcg/mL
Patient Weight		Infusion Rate (mL/hr)				
kg	lbs	Initial	Maximum	Initial	Maximum	Initial	Maximum
10	22	1	30	2	60	4	120
20	44	2	60	4	120	7	240
30	66	3	90	5	180	11	360
40	88	4	120	7	240	14	480
50	110	5	150	9	300	18	600
60	132	5	180	11	360	22	720
70	154	6	210	13	420	25	840
80	176	7	240	14	480	29	960
90	198	8	270	16	540	32	1,080
100	220	9	300	18	600	36	1,200

ACTIONS

A potent, rapid-acting antihypertensive agent. Produces peripheral vasodilation through direct action on smooth muscle of the blood vessels. Effective almost immediately. Will lower diastolic BP 30% to 40% or more below pretreatment levels. May increase HR and/or cardiac output slightly. Effectiveness ends when IV infusion is stopped. BP will return to pretreatment levels in 1 to 10 minutes. Rapidly converted to thiocyanate and eventually excreted in the urine.

INDICATIONS AND USES

Drug of choice for hypertensive emergencies. ▪ Cardiogenic shock. ▪ Controlled hypotension during surgery. ▪ Acute congestive heart failure. **Unlabeled uses:** In combination with dopamine to reduce afterload in hypertensive patient with myocardial infarction. ▪ Treatment of left ventricular failure in combination with oxygen, morphine, and a loop diuretic.

CONTRAINDICATIONS

Compensatory hypertension, e.g., arteriovenous shunt or coarctation of the aorta; known inadequate cerebral circulation; emergency surgery on moribund patients.

PRECAUTIONS

Use only when adequate personnel and appropriate equipment are available for continuous monitoring. ▪ Precipitous decreases in BP can occur quickly. Can lead to irreversible ischemic injuries or death. ▪ Cyanide toxicity can occur with doses less than the average effective dose and will begin to occur as the maximum dose of 10 mcg/kg/min is approached. May be rapid, serious, and lethal. ▪ Methemoglobinemia may begin to occur within 16 hours if larger doses are required. ▪ Use caution in hypothyroidism, increased intracranial pressure, liver or renal impairment, and the elderly. ▪ May increase ischemia in myocardial infarction.

Monitor: Determine patency of vein; avoid extravasation. ▪ Continuous automatic BP monitoring is mandatory (intra-arterial pressure sensor preferred). Never allow systolic BP to fall below 60 mm Hg. ▪ Monitor pulmonary wedge pressure in patients with myocardial infarction or severe congestive heart failure. ▪ Monitor acid/base balance and venous oxygen concentration; may indicate cyanide toxicity. ▪ Oral antihypertensive agents may be given concomitantly to maintain ongoing BP regulation. Reduced nitroprusside sodium dose may be indicated; see Dose Adjustments. ▪ Measure blood thiocyanate levels daily if dose is 3 mcg/kg/min (1 mcg/kg/min in the anuric patient). Desired level of steady-state thiocyanate is less than 1 mmol/L. Coadministration of sodium thiosulfate in doses 5 to 10 times that of nitroprusside sodium has been used to avoid toxicity with larger doses or necessary long-term therapy. May potentiate hypotensive action; use with extreme caution. ▪ In controlled hypotension, monitor blood loss and correct hypovolemia before and during surgery. ▪ Persistent hypotension (lasting more than 1 to 10 minutes) after nitroprusside sodium is discontinued is due to another source. Monitor for sodium retention.

Patient Education: Report IV site burning or stinging promptly. ▪ Request assistance to ambulate.

Maternal/Child: Category C: safety for use in pregnancy and in pediatric patients not yet established. Has caused cyanide toxicity in fetuses of ewes, but not in humans. ▪ Discontinue breast-feeding.

Elderly: See Dose Adjustments and Precautions. ▪ Hypotensive effects may be increased. ▪ Consider age-related renal impairment.

DRUG/LAB INTERACTIONS

Potentiated by **ganglionic blocking agents** (e.g., trimethaphan [Arfonad]), **volatile liquid anesthesia** (e.g., halothane), **and circulatory depressants.** ▪ Will cause profound hypotension with **diazoxide.**

SIDE EFFECTS

Usually occur with too-rapid rate of infusion and are reversible: abdominal pain, apprehension, bradycardia, coma, decreased platelet aggregation, diaphoresis, dizziness, ECG changes, flushing, headache, hypotension (profound), ileus, increased intracranial pressure, muscle twitching, nausea, palpitations, rash, restlessness, retching, retrosternal discomfort, venous streaking. With prolonged therapy or overdose, cyanide intoxication (air hunger, bright red venous blood, confusion, elevated cyanide levels, marked clinical deterioration, metabolic acidosis, and death), hypothyroidism, or methemoglobinemia (chocolate brown blood, impaired oxygen delivery even though cardiac output and arterial PO_2 are adequate) can occur.

ANTIDOTE

At first sign of side effects, decrease rate of administration. Never allow systolic BP to fall below 60 mm Hg. If BP begins to rise or side effects persist, notify the physician. Hemodialysis or peritoneal dialysis may be indicated for thiocyanate levels over 10 mg/dL. For massive overdose with signs of cyanide toxicity or tachyphylaxis, discontinue nitroprusside sodium. Cyanide antidote kits contain all needed medications (see sodium nitrite/sodium thiosulfate monograph for complete information). Administer amyl nitrite inhalations for 15 to 30 seconds each minute until 3% sodium nitrite solution can be initiated as an IV infusion or immediately start the infusion (4 to 6 mg/kg) over 2 to 4 minutes. Monitor BP carefully; may cause hypotension that will also require treatment. Next, inject sodium thiosulfate 150 to 200 mg/kg (usually about 12.5 Gm or 50 mL of the 25% solution) in 50 mL of 5% dextrose in water IV over 10 minutes. Observe patient. If signs of overdose reappear, may repeat the previously described process after 2 hours; but use one half the original dosage. Sodium nitrite provides a buffer for cyanide by converting HgB into methemoglobin; sodium thiosulfate converts cyanide into thiocyanate, which is then excreted in urine. For hypotension, slow or discontinue the IV and put the patient in Trendelenburg position. Should improve in 1 to 10 minutes. Correct hypotension with vasopressors (e.g., dopamine). Treat methemoglobinemia with methylene blue 1 to 2 mg/kg. Use with caution if considerable amounts of cyanide are bound to methemoglobin.

NOREPINEPHRINE BITARTRATE BBW

Vasopressor

(nor-ep-ih-NEF-rin by-TAR-trayt)

Levarterenol Bitartrate, Levophed

pH 3 to 4.5

USUAL DOSE

8 to 12 mcg/min initially. Other clinicians suggest an initial dose of 0.5 to 1 mcg/min titrated to maintain the desired BP range. Usual maintenance dose is 2 to 4 mcg/min (AHA recommendation is 0.1 to 0.5 mcg/kg/min; titrate to response). Larger doses may be given safely as long as the patient remains hypotensive and blood volume depletion is corrected. Up to 30 mcg/min may be required in patients with refractory shock. 2 mg bitartrate equals 1 mg of norepinephrine. All doses are expressed in terms of norepinephrine.

PEDIATRIC DOSE

Safety and effectiveness for use in pediatric patients not established. Begin with an initial dose of 0.05 to 0.1 mcg/kg/min. Titrate up to a maximum dose of 2 mcg/kg/min to maintain desired BP. AHA recommends 0.1 to 2 mcg/kg/min in advanced life support. Another source suggests 0.05 to 0.3 mcg/min. Initiate the infusion at 0.1 mcg/kg/min and titrate to desired BP. A third source suggests 2 mcg/M^2/min. Titrate to maintain desired BP, but do not exceed 6 mcg/min.

DOSE ADJUSTMENTS

Lower-end initial doses may be indicated in the elderly based on potential for decreased organ function and concomitant disease or drug therapy.

DILUTION

Must be diluted in 250 to 1,000 mL of D5W or D5NS and given as an infusion. 4 mg (4 mL) in 1 L of diluent equals 4 mcg/mL. Final concentration based on fluid volume requirements of the patient. Administration in a dextrose solution reduces loss of potency resulting from oxidation. NS without dextrose is not recommended. Phentolamine (Regitine) 5 to 10 mg and/or heparin sodium to provide 100 to 200 units/hr may be added to the diluent to prevent any sloughing, necrosis, and/or thrombosis from slight leakage along the vein pathway.

Storage: Before dilution, store at CRT; protect from light.

COMPATIBILITY

(Underline Indicates Conflicting Compatibility Information)

Consider any drug NOT listed as compatible to be INCOMPATIBLE until consulting a pharmacist; specific conditions may apply.

Consult pharmacist; may be inactivated by solutions with a pH above 6. **Incompatible** with whole blood; administer through **Y-site** or a separate IV line. Avoid contact with iron salts, alkalis, or oxidizing agents.

One source suggests the following **compatibilities:**

Additive: Amikacin (Amikin), calcium chloride, calcium gluconate, ciprofloxacin (Cipro IV), dimenhydrinate, dobutamine, heparin, hydrocortisone sodium succinate (Solu-Cortef), magnesium sulfate, meropenem (Merrem IV), methylprednisolone (Solu-Medrol), multivitamins (M.V.I.), potassium chloride (KCl), ranitidine (Zantac), succinylcholine, verapamil.

Y-site: Amiodarone (Nexterone), anidulafungin (Eraxis), argatroban, bivalirudin (Angiomax), caspofungin (Cancidas), cisatracurium (Nimbex), dexmedetomidine (Precedex), diltiazem (Cardizem), dobutamine, dopamine, doripenem (Doribax), epinephrine (Adrenalin), esmolol (Brevibloc), famotidine (Pepcid IV), fenoldopam (Corlopam), fentanyl (Sublimaze), furosemide (Lasix), haloperidol (Haldol), heparin, hetastarch in electrolytes (Hextend), hydrocortisone sodium succinate (Solu-Cortef), hydromorphone (Dilaudid), inamrinone (Amrinone), labetalol (Trandate), lorazepam (Ativan), meropenem (Merrem IV), micafungin (Mycamine), midazolam (Versed), milrinone (Primacor), morphine, mycophenolate mofetil (CellCept IV), nicardipine (Cardene IV), nitroglycerin IV, nitroprusside sodium, pantoprazole (Protonix IV), potassium chloride (KCl), propofol (Diprivan), ranitidine (Zantac), remifentanil (Ultiva), vasopressin, vecuronium.

RATE OF ADMINISTRATION

See Usual Dose. Use the slowest possible flow rate to correct hypotension gradually and maintain adequate or preset BP. Some response should be noted within 1 to 2 minutes of IV administration. Use of an infusion pump or microdrip (60 gtt/mL) is an aid to correct evaluation of dose. Reduce infusion rate gradually. Avoid sudden discontinuation.

	Norepinephrine (Levophed) Infusion Rate					
Desired Dose	4 mg in 1,000 mL D5W or D5NS 2 mg in 500 mL D5W or D5NS 4 mcg/mL			8 mg in 1,000 mL D5W or D5NS 4 mg in 500 mL D5W or D5NS 8 mcg/mL		
mcg/min	mcg/hr	mL/min	mL/hr	mcg/hr	mL/min	mL/hr
2 mcg/min	120	0.5	30	120	0.25	15
3 mcg/min	180	0.75	45	180	0.375	22.5
4 mcg/min	240	1	60	240	0.5	30
6 mcg/min	360	1.5	90	360	0.75	45
8 mcg/min	480	2	120	480	1	60
9 mcg/min	540	2.25	135	540	1.125	67.5
10 mcg/min	600	2.5	150	600	1.25	75
11 mcg/min	660	2.75	165	660	1.375	82.5
12 mcg/min	720	3	180	720	1.5	90

ACTIONS

Levarterenol is the levo-isomer of norepinephrine. It is a sympathomimetic drug that functions as a peripheral vasoconstrictor (alpha-adrenergic action) and inotropic stimulator of the heart and dilator of coronary arteries (beta-adrenergic action). Dilates the coronary arteries more than twice as much as epinephrine can. It is rapidly inactivated in the body by various enzymes and excreted in changed form in the urine.

INDICATIONS AND USES

All hypotensive states, including those associated with spinal anesthesia, blood reactions, drug reactions, hemorrhage, myocardial infarction, pheochromocytomectomy, septicemia, surgery, sympathectomy, and trauma. ■ Adjunct in treatment of cardiac arrest and profound hypotension.

CONTRAINDICATIONS
Do not use in hypotension from blood loss unless an emergency, in mesenteric or peripheral vascular thrombosis, or with cyclopropane or halothane (inhalant) anesthesia.

PRECAUTIONS
Whole blood or plasma should be given in a separate IV site. May be given through Y-tube connection. ■ Use caution in the elderly and in those with peripheral vascular disease or ischemic heart disease. ■ Use caution in previously hypertensive patients. Raise BP no more than 40 mm Hg below pre-existing systolic pressure. ■ Use caution in patients with allergies; some formulations contain sulfites. ■ Therapy may be continued until the patient can maintain own BP. Decrease dosage gradually.

Monitor: Check BP every 2 minutes until stabilized at the desired level. Check every 5 minutes thereafter during therapy. Avoid hypertension. One source suggests limiting rise in BP in previously hypertensive patients to no more than 40 mm Hg below previously systolic normal. ■ Observe for hypovolemia and replace fluids immediately. In an emergency, norepinephrine can be effective in a hypovolemic state before fluid replacement has been accomplished. ■ Check flow rate and injection site constantly. ■ Infusion should be through a large vein, preferably the antecubital vein, to prevent complications of prolonged peripheral vasoconstriction. Avoid veins in the hands, ankles, and legs. Use of the femoral vein may be considered. ■ Causes severe tissue necrosis, sloughing, and gangrene. Insert a plastic IV catheter or similar intravascular device at least 6 inches long well into the large vein chosen to prevent extravasation into any surrounding tissue; see Dilution. ■ Blanching along the vein pathway is a preliminary sign of extravasation. Change the injection site. ■ See Drug/Lab Interactions.

Patient Education: Report IV site burning or stinging promptly. ■ Request assistance to ambulate.

Maternal/Child: Category C: use only if clearly needed; benefits must outweigh risks. ■ Use caution in breast-feeding.

Elderly: See Precautions. ■ Lower-end initial doses may be indicated; see Dose Adjustments. ■ Differences in response versus younger patients not documented.

DRUG/LAB INTERACTIONS
Pressor effects may be potentiated by **amphetamines, anesthetics, antihistamines, tricyclic antidepressants** (e.g., desipramine [Norpramin]), **rauwolfia alkaloids** (e.g., reserpine), **thyroid preparations, and methylphenidate** (Ritalin). ■ May cause severe hypertension with **ergot alkaloids and guanethidine** (Ismelin), and severe prolonged hypertension with **MAO inhibitors** (e.g., selegiline [Eldepryl]). ■ May cause hypotension and bradycardia with **hydantoins** (e.g., phenytoin [Dilantin]). ■ **Halogenated hydrocarbon anesthetics** (e.g., halothane) may cause serious arrhythmias. ■ Interacts in numerous and sometimes contradictory ways with many drugs.

SIDE EFFECTS
Rare when used as directed; anxiety, arrhythmias (e.g., bradycardia and VT), chest pain, decreased cardiac output, dyspnea, headache, ischemia, necrosis caused by extravasation, pallor, photophobia, seizures, vomiting. Persistent headache may indicate overdose and severe hypertension. Gangrene has been reported.

ANTIDOTE

To prevent sloughing and necrosis in areas where extravasation has occurred, use a fine hypodermic needle to inject 5 to 10 mg of phentolamine (Regitine) diluted in 10 to 15 mL of NS liberally throughout the tissue in the extravasated area. Phentolamine causes immediate and conspicuous local hyperemic changes if the area is infiltrated within 12 hours. Treatment should be started as soon as extravasation is recognized. Atropine may be used to counteract the bradycardia. Notify physician of any side effect. Should a sudden or uncontrolled hypertensive state occur, discontinue levarterenol, notify the physician, and if necessary, treat with an adrenergic blocking agent (e.g., phentolamine [Regitine] or phenoxybenzamine [Dibenzyline]).

OCTREOTIDE ACETATE
(ok-**TREE**-oh-tide **AS**-ah-tayt)

Octreotide Acetate PF, Sandostatin

Antidiarrheal
Growth hormone suppressant

pH 3.9 to 4.5

USUAL DOSE

Usually given SC. Check label, confirm for IV use; Sandostatin LAR Depot is for IM use only; see Precautions. In most situations begin with a lower dose to allow gradual tolerance to GI side effects. Increase gradually based on patient response and tolerance. Begin SC or IM (LAR Depot) dosing as soon as practical.

Antidiarrheal (GI tumor): 50 mcg once or twice daily. Increase gradually if indicated.

Antidiarrheal (unlabeled for AIDS): 100 mcg as an IV bolus over 10 minutes. Follow with a continuous infusion, intermittent infusion, or bolus dose of 10 mcg/hr. Increase gradually to 100 mcg/hr. When adequate control is achieved, decrease to 75 mcg/hr. SC dose range is from 100 mcg up to 3,000 mcg/24 hr.

Carcinoid tumors: 100 to 600 mcg/24 hr in equally divided doses 2 to 4 times daily during first 2 weeks of therapy (50 to 300 mcg every 12 hours or 25 to 150 mcg every 6 hours). Average total daily dose ranges from 300 to 450 mcg, but therapeutic response is obtained with ranges from 50 to 750 mcg. Up to 1,500 mcg/day has been used in selected patients.

Carcinoid crisis (unlabeled): 100 mcg as an IV bolus. May be given to treat carcinoid crisis during anesthesia or given before induction of anesthesia as a prophylactic measure.

Vasoactive intestinal peptide tumors: Average dose range is 200 to 300 mcg/24 hr in equally divided doses 2 to 4 times daily during first 2 weeks of therapy (100 to 150 mcg every 12 hours or 50 to 75 mcg every 6 hours). Average total daily dose ranges from 150 to 750 mcg but therapeutic response usually achieved with doses under 450 mcg/24 hr.

Treatment of GI bleeding (unlabeled): Begin with a loading dose of 50 to 100 mcg. Follow with a continuous infusion of 25 to 50 mcg/hr for 1 to 5 days. Intermittent infusion or bolus doses may be substituted for the continuous infusion.

Growth hormone suppression (acromegaly): 50 mcg every 8 hours is the initial dose. Increase dose gradually as indicated by IGF-1 levels; see Monitor. Acromegaly has been suppressed at doses of 300 to 500 mcg/24 hr. May be maintained at home with infusions through an implantable IV or SC pump or SC dosing of 50 to 100 mcg every 8 hours.

Antihypoglycemic: Life-threatening hypoglycemia secondary to insulinoma (unlabeled): 100 mcg as an IV bolus.

Reduce output from GI or pancreatic fistulas (unlabeled): 50 to 200 mcg every 8 hours. In one study, 250 mcg/hr was given as a continuous infusion for 48 hours, followed with SC dosing. Fistula became dry within 72 hours and eventually closed.

PEDIATRIC DOSE

Experience is limited, and doses are **unlabeled.** See Maternal/Child.

Intractable diarrhea: 1 to 10 mcg/kg of body weight/24 hr. May be given as a single daily dose or divided and given every 12 hours. Dose may be increased within the recommended range by 0.3 mcg/kg/dose every 3 days as needed. Maximum dose is 1,500 mcg/24 hr.

Diarrhea associated with graft versus host: 1 mcg/kg/dose bolus followed by 1 mcg/kg/hr as a continuous infusion has been used.

DOSE ADJUSTMENTS

In all situations dose adjustment may be required on a daily basis to maintain symptomatic control. After initial 2 weeks of therapy, gradually decrease dose to achieve therapeutically effective maintenance dose. ■ Reduce dose in the elderly; half-life extended and clearance decreased. Start at the lower end of the dosing range. Consider the greater frequency of decreased organ function and of concomitant disease or drug therapy. ■ Half-life markedly extended in severe renal failure requiring dialysis. Reduction of maintenance dose indicated. ■ See Drug/Lab Interactions.

DILUTION

Available in several different concentrations and formulations; read label carefully. May be given undiluted or may be diluted with 50 to 200 mL of NS or D5W and given as an intermittent infusion or further diluted and given as a continuous infusion.

Storage: Before use store in refrigerator (2° to 8° C [36° to 46° F]) or at CRT for 14 days; protect from light. May store at room temperature on day of use. Diluted solution stable for 24 hours. Multi-dose vial must be dated on opening and discarded after 14 days.

COMPATIBILITY   (Underline Indicates Conflicting Compatibility Information)

Consider any drug NOT listed as compatible to be INCOMPATIBLE until consulting a pharmacist; specific conditions may apply.

Manufacturer lists TPN as **incompatible** (forms a conjugate that decreases effectiveness). If used as an additive with insulin, octreotide markedly increases adsorption of insulin and reduces insulin availability.

One source suggests the following **compatibilities:**

Additive: Heparin.

Y-site: Pantoprazole (Protonix IV).

RATE OF ADMINISTRATION

IV injection: A single dose over 3 minutes.

Intermittent infusion: A single dose over 15 to 30 minutes.

Continuous infusion: Give at a rate consistent with the required hourly dose in an amount of fluid appropriate for the specific patient.

ACTIONS

A long-acting octapeptide. Mimics the actions of the natural hormone somatostatin, suppressing secretion of serotonin, gastroenteropancreatic peptides (e.g., gastrin, vasoactive intestinal peptide, insulin, glucagon, secretin, motilin, pancreatic polypeptide), and growth hormone. Decreases splanchnic blood flow. Stimulates fluid and electrolyte absorption from GI tract and prolongs GI transit time. These pharmacologic actions provide a means of treating the symptoms associated with metastatic carcinoid tumors (flushing and diarrhea) and vasoactive intestinal peptide (VIP)–secreting tumors (watery diarrhea). Other actions include inhibition of gallbladder contractility and bile secretion and suppression of thyroid-stimulating hormone (TSH) secretion. Distribution from plasma is rapid. About 65% bound to plasma protein. Half-life longer than the natural hormone (1.7 to 1.9 hours compared to 1 to 3 minutes). Action may extend to 12 hours. Some excreted unchanged in urine.

INDICATIONS AND USES

To suppress or inhibit the severe diarrhea and flushing episodes associated with carcinoid tumor. ▪ Treatment of profuse watery diarrhea associated with vasoactive intestinal peptide tumors (VIPomas). ▪ Treatment of acromegaly to suppress growth hormone and achieve normalization of growth hormone and IGF-1 levels.

Unlabeled uses: Treatment of severe diarrhea in patients with AIDS; treatment of chemotherapy-induced diarrhea. Carcinoid crisis during anesthesia, adjunct to treatment of life-threatening hypoglycemia, treatment of GI bleeding. Adjunct to pancreatectomy and treatment of GI or pancreatic fistulas.

CONTRAINDICATIONS

Sensitivity to octreotide acetate or any of its components.

PRECAUTIONS

IV use is limited to emergency situations. SC injection with rotation of injection sites is preferred route of administration. ▪ Sandostatin LAR Depot must be administered intragluteally but has the advantage of extending the interval between injections to every 4 weeks. ▪ May decrease size of tumors and slow rate of growth and metastases. Data not definitive. ▪ May inhibit gallbladder contractility and decrease bile secretion. ▪ Use caution in patients with diabetes. In patients with type I diabetes, octreotide is likely to affect glucose regulation, and insulin requirements may be decreased. Severe, symptomatic hypoglycemia has been reported. In nondiabetics and type II diabetics with partially intact insulin reserves, octreotide may result in decreased insulin levels and hyperglycemia. Glucose tolerance and antidiabetic treatment should be closely monitored. ▪ Cardiac abnormalities (e.g., arrhythmias, bradycardia, conduction abnormalities, QT prolongation) have been reported. More common in patients with acromegaly; see Side Effects. ▪ Suppresses thyroid-stimulating hormone. May cause hypothyroidism.

Monitor: Observe for transient hyperglycemia or hypoglycemia during induction and dose changes because of changes in balance of hormones (e.g., insulin, glucagon, and growth hormone). ▪ Monitor fluids and electrolytes carefully. ▪ 5-HIAA, plasma serotonin, and plasma substance P may be useful lab studies to evaluate patient response with carcinoid tumor. Measurement of plasma vasoactive intestinal peptide will be helpful in VIPoma. ▪ In acromegaly, initial response may be monitored with growth hormone levels at 1- to 4-hour intervals for 8 to 12 hours after a dose. IGF-1 levels every 2 weeks and/or multiple growth hormone levels taken 0 to 8 hours after administration may be used to make dose adjustments. Goal is to achieve growth hormone levels less than 5 ng/mL or IGF-1 (somatomedin C) levels less than 1.9 units/mL in males and less than 2.2 units/mL in females. After stabilization, IGF-1 or growth hormone levels should be re-evaluated at 6-month intervals. ■ In patients with acromegaly who have received irradiation, octreotide should be withdrawn yearly for 4 weeks to assess disease activity. If growth hormone or IGF-1 levels increase and S/S recur, octreotide therapy should be resumed. ■ Can alter fat absorption and decrease gallbladder motility; observe for gall-bladder disease. Baseline and periodic ultrasound of gallbladder and bile ducts indicated in long-term SC therapy. Periodic fecal fat and carotene studies also indicated. ■ Pancreatitis has been reported. Monitor pancreatic enzymes as indicated. ■ Depressed B_{12} levels have been observed. Monitor in prolonged therapy. ■ Monitor baseline and periodic thyroid function tests (TSH, total, and/or free T_4), especially in long-term SC therapy. ■ See Dose Adjustments and Drug/Lab Interactions.

Patient Education: Instruct patient and/or family in appropriate skills if self-administration indicated. To avoid or lessen incidence of GI side effects, schedule injections between meals and at bedtime. ■ In women with acromegaly being treated with octreotide, normalization of GH and IGF-1 may restore fertility. Adequate contraception is recommended.

Maternal/Child: Category B: although studies do not indicate harm to the fetus or infants, use in pregnancy and breast-feeding only if clearly needed. ■ Safety and effectiveness for use in pediatric patients not established; see Literature. In post-marketing reports, hypoxia, necrotizing enterocolitis, and death have been reported, most notably in pediatric patients under 2 years of age, many of which had serious underlying co-morbid conditions. Relationship to octreotide not established.

Elderly: See Dose Adjustments. ■ Response similar to that seen in younger patients; however, may be more sensitive to side effects; observe carefully.

DRUG/LAB INTERACTIONS

Use caution in patients receiving concomitant **beta-blockers** (e.g., atenolol [Tenormin], propranolol), **calcium channel blockers** (e.g., diltiazem [Cardizem], verapamil), **or any agents used for fluid and electrolyte balance.** Will require adjustment in these therapies as symptoms are controlled by octreotide. ■ May affect absorption of **orally administered medications.** ■ May inhibit effectiveness of **cyclosporine** and may result in transplant rejection. ■ Markedly increases adsorption of **insulin** and reduces availability. ■ Concurrent use with **oral antidiabetic agents, glucagon, growth hormone, or insulin** may cause hypoglycemia or hyperglycemia. Monitor patient carefully and give adjunct dose of these agents as indicated. ■ May increase availability of **bromocriptine** (Parlodel). ■ Suppression of growth hormones may cause a decreased clearance of drugs metabolized by selected cytochrome P_{450} enzymes. Use caution with concurrent use of **drugs metabolized by CYP3A4** (e.g., cisapride [Propulsid], erythromycin, HMG-CoA reductase inhibitors [lovastatin (Mevacor) and simvastatin (Zocor)], itraconazole [Sporanox], oral midazolam [Versed], quinidine, terfenadine).

SIDE EFFECTS

Most side effects are of mild to moderate severity and of short duration. Abdominal pain/discomfort, abnormal stools, anorexia, anxiety, biliary sludge, cholelithiasis, constipation, convulsions, depression, diarrhea, dizziness, drowsiness, fatigue, fat malabsorption, flatulence, fluttering sensation, GI bleeding, headache, heartburn, hepatitis, hyperesthesia, hyperglycemia, hypoglycemia, increase in liver enzymes, insomnia, irritability, jaundice, nausea, pancreatitis, pounding in the head, rectal spasm, swollen stomach, vomiting. In rare cases, GI side effects may resemble intestinal obstruction with progressive abdominal distention, severe epigastric pain, abdominal tenderness, and guarding. Many other side effects occur in fewer than 1% of patients. Side effects that occur more often in patients with acromegaly include cardiac abnormalities (e.g., sinus bradycardia, ECG changes [including QT prolongation], conduction abnormalities, and arrhythmias) and hypothyroidism.

ANTIDOTE

Keep physician informed of all side effects. A dose adjustment of either octreotide or other concomitant therapies may be required. Symptomatic and supportive treatment may be indicated. Overdose will cause hyperglycemia or hypoglycemia depending on tumor involved and endocrine status of patient. Discontinue octreotide temporarily, notify the physician, and monitor the patient carefully. Symptomatic treatment should be sufficient.

OFATUMUMAB
(oh-**FAT**-oo-moo-mab)

Arzerra

Monoclonal antibody
Antineoplastic

pH 6.5

USUAL DOSE

Premedication: 30 minutes to 2 hours before ofatumumab administration, premedicate with oral acetaminophen 1,000 mg (or equivalent), an oral antihistamine (cetirizine [Zyrtec] 10 mg [or equivalent]), or an IV antihistamine (diphenhydramine [Benadryl] 50 mg), and an IV corticosteroid (prednisolone 100 mg or equivalent [e.g., methylprednisolone (Solu-Medrol) 80 mg]).

Ofatumumab: 300 mg as the initial dose (Dose 1). Follow 1 week later with 2,000 mg weekly for 7 doses (Doses 2 through 8), followed 4 weeks later with 2,000 mg every 4 weeks for 4 doses (Doses 9 through 12).

DOSE ADJUSTMENTS

Ofatumumab: Interrupt infusion for an infusion reaction of any severity. ■ Do not resume the infusion for a Grade 4 infusion reaction. ■ If a Grade 1, 2, or 3 infusion reaction resolves with interruption or remains less than or equal to Grade 2, resume infusion with the following modifications based on the initial grade of the infusion reaction: *Grade 1 or 2:* infuse at one-half of the previous infusion rate. *Grade 3:* infuse at 12 mL/hr. After resuming the infusion, the rate may be increased according to the chart in Rate of Administration. ■ No dose adjustment is indicated for age, body weight, gender, or renal impairment.

Premedication: Do not reduce the corticosteroid dose for Doses 1, 2, and 9.
■ Doses 3 through 8: If a Grade 3 or greater infusion reaction did not occur with the preceding dose, gradually reduce the corticosteroid dose with successive infusions. ■ Doses 10 through 12: If a Grade 3 or greater infusion reaction did not occur with Dose 9, administer prednisolone 50 to 100 mg or equivalent (e.g., methylprednisolone [Solu-Medrol] 40 to 80 mg).

DILUTION

Do not shake ofatumumab in vial or solution. Should be a colorless solution and may have some visible translucent-to-white particles. Prepare all doses in 1,000 mL polyolefin bags of NS.

300-mg dose: Withdraw and discard 15 mL from a 1,000 mL bag of NS. Withdraw 5 mL from each of 3 vials of ofatumumab and add to the bag of NS.

2,000 mg dose: Withdraw and discard 100 mL from a 1,000 mL bag of NS. Withdraw 5 mL from each of 20 vials of ofatumumab and add to the bag of NS.

Mix diluted solution by gentle inversion. Administer using an infusion pump, the provided in-line filter, and PVC administration sets.

Filters: Must be administered with the in-line filter provided by the manufacturer.

Storage: Refrigerate vials and prepared solutions between 2° to 8° C (36° to 46° F). Protect vials from light and do not freeze. Start infusion within 12 hours of preparation and discard the prepared solution after 24 hours.

COMPATIBILITY

Manufacturer states, "Do not mix ofatumumab with, or administer as an infusion with, other medicinal products." Flush the IV line with NS before and after each dose.

RATE OF ADMINISTRATION

Use of an in-line filter (provided by manufacturer), an infusion pump, and PVC administration set is required. Flush the IV line with NS before and after each dose.

Dose 1: Initiate infusion at a rate of 3.6 mg/hr (12 mL/hr).
Dose 2: Initiate infusion at a rate of 24 mg/hr (12 mL/hr).
Doses 3 through 12: Initiate infusion at a rate of 50 mg/hr (25 mL/hr).

If there is no infusion reaction, the rate may be increased every 30 minutes as described in the following table. Do not exceed these infusion rates.

Ofatumumab Infusion Rates			
Interval After Start of Infusion	Dose 1*	Dose 2†	Doses 3 to 12†
0 to 30 minutes	12 mL/hr	12 mL/hr	25 mL/hr
31 to 60 minutes	25 mL/hr	25 mL/hr	50 mL/hr
61 to 90 minutes	50 mL/hr	50 mL/hr	100 mL/hr
91 to 120 minutes	100 mL/hr	100 mL/hr	200 mL/hr
>120 minutes	200 mL/hr	200 mL/hr	400 mL/hr

*Dose 1 = 300 mg (0.3 mg/mL).
†Doses 2 and 3 through 12 = 2,000 mg (2 mg/mL).

ACTIONS

A CD20-directed cytolytic monoclonal antibody (also known as an IgGlk human monoclonal antibody). The CD20 molecule is expressed on normal B lymphocytes and on B-cell CLL. Ofatumumab binds specifically to both the small and large extracellular loops of the CD20 molecule, resulting in B-cell lysis. Possible mechanisms of cell lysis include complement-dependent cytotoxicity and antibody-dependent, cell-mediated cytotoxicity. Decreases circulating CD19-positive B-cells. With depletion of B-cells, the clearance of ofatumumab decreases substantially after subsequent infusions compared with the first infusion.

INDICATIONS AND USES

Treatment of patients with chronic lymphocytic leukemia (CLL) refractory to fludarabine (Fludara) and alemtuzumab (Campath).

CONTRAINDICATIONS

Manufacturer states, "None."

PRECAUTIONS

Do not administer as an IV push or bolus. For IV infusion only. ▪ Administered under the supervision of a physician experienced in the use of antineoplastic therapy in a facility equipped to monitor the patient and respond to any medical emergency. ▪ Serious infusion reactions have occurred and seem to occur more frequently with the first 2 infusions; see Monitor. ▪ Prolonged (1 week or longer) severe neutropenia and thrombocytopenia can occur. ▪ Progressive multifocal leukoencephalopathy (PML) can occur. ▪ Screen patients at high risk for hepatitis B virus (HBV) before initiating therapy. Hepatitis B reactivation, including fulminant hepatitis and death, may occur. Insufficient data exist regarding the safety of ofatumumab administration in patients with active hepatitis. ▪ Obstruction of the small intestine can occur. ▪ A protein substance, it has the potential for producing immunogenicity. ▪ No studies of ofatumumab use in impaired hepatic or renal function have been conducted; use with caution. ▪ Not approved for use in patients with moderate to severe COPD. ▪ See Monitor.

Monitor: Obtain baseline CBC and platelet counts and monitor at regular intervals during therapy. Increase the frequency of monitoring in patients who develop Grade 3 or 4 cytopenias. ▪ Monitor for S/S of infusion reactions. S/S have included abdominal pain, angioedema, back pain, bronchospasm, cardiac ischemia/infarction, dyspnea, fever, flushing, hypertension, hypotension, laryngeal edema, pulmonary edema, rash, syncope, and urticaria. ▪ Monitor for new onset of or changes in pre-existing neurologic signs or symptoms. Evaluation for PML includes consultation with a neurologist, brain MRI, and lumbar puncture. ▪ Monitor carriers of hepatitis B closely for clinical and laboratory signs of active HBV infection during treatment and for 6 to 12 months after the last infusion. ▪ Monitor for S/S of bowel obstruction. ▪ Monitor for thrombocytopenia (platelet count less than 50,000/mm^3). Initiate precautions to prevent excessive bleeding (e.g., inspect IV sites, skin, and mucous membranes; use extreme care during invasive procedures; test urine, emesis, stool, and secretions for occult blood). ▪ Use of prophylactic antiemetics may be indicated to reduce nausea and/or vomiting and to increase patient comfort. ▪ Observe closely for signs of infection. Prophylactic antibiotics may be indicated.

Patient Education: Blood counts will be required at regular intervals. ▪ Avoid vaccination with live virus vaccines. ▪ Promptly report symptoms of the following potential side effects: bleeding, easy bruising or petechiae, fatigue, infection (e.g., cough, fever), infusion reactions (e.g., breathing problems, chills, fever, rash that occurs within 24 hours of infusion), pallor or worsening weakness, new or worsening abdominal pain or nausea, new or worsening neurologic S/S, worsening fatigue or yellow discoloration of skin or eyes. ▪ See Appendix D, p. 1434.

Maternal/Child: Category C: use during pregnancy only if the potential benefit justifies the potential risk to the fetus. ▪ Use caution if breastfeeding. The effects of local gastrointestinal and limited systemic exposure to ofatumumab are unknown. ▪ Safety and effectiveness for use in pediatric patients not established.

Elderly: Numbers of patients over 65 years of age in studies were not sufficient to determine a response that might differ from younger patients.

DRUG/LAB INTERACTIONS

Formal drug-drug interaction studies have not been conducted. ▪ Do not administer **live virus vaccines** to patients who have recently received ofatumumab.

SIDE EFFECTS

Most common side effects are anemia, bronchitis, cough, diarrhea, dyspnea, fatigue, fever, nausea, neutropenia, pneumonia, rash and upper respiratory infections. Fever, infections (some fatal) including pneumonia and sepsis, infusion reactions, and neutropenia were the most common serious side effects. Other side effects reported include back pain, chills, headache, hepatitis B reactivation, herpes zoster, hypertension, hypotension, insomnia, intestinal obstruction, muscle spasms, nasopharyngitis, peripheral edema, PML, sinusitis, tachycardia, thrombocytopenia, and urticaria.

ANTIDOTE

Notify physician of significant side effects. Temporarily discontinue the infusion for an infusion reaction, angina, or S/S of myocardial ischemia. Delay therapy for serious infection or serious hematologic toxicity until the infection or adverse event resolves. Treatment of most reactions will be supportive. Discontinue medication permanently for severe reactions, including Grade 4 infusion reactions or S/S of PML or in patients who develop viral hepatitis or reactivation of viral hepatitis. Infusion reactions may be treated with acetaminophen, antiemetics (e.g., ondansetron [Zofran]), antihistamines (e.g., diphenhydramine [Benadryl]), or corticosteroids (e.g., hydrocortisone) as indicated. Discontinue ofatumumab and provide supportive therapy in overdose. Treat hypersensitivity reactions with epinephrine, antihistamines, and corticosteroids as needed. Resuscitate as indicated.

ONDANSETRON HYDROCHLORIDE

(on-**DAN**-sih-tron hy-droh-**KLOR**-eyed)

Antiemetic

5HT$_3$ receptor antagonist

Ondansetron HCl PF, Zofran, Zofran PF

pH 3 to 4

USUAL DOSE

Nausea associated with emetogenic agents: A single 32-mg dose once daily or 0.15 mg/kg of body weight (first in a sequence of three doses) 30 minutes before giving emetogenic cancer chemotherapy (e.g., cisplatin, methotrexate). Given as an intermittent infusion. Repeat 0.15 mg/kg dose at 4 and 8 hours after the first dose. Do not repeat the 32-mg dose. Concurrent use with dexamethasone may improve the effectiveness of ondansetron in controlling cisplatin-induced nausea and vomiting.

Postoperative nausea in adults and pediatric patients weighing 40 kg or more: 4 mg before anesthesia induction or postoperatively if the patient experiences nausea or vomiting. Although repeat doses are not recommended by the manufacturer, they have been given.

PEDIATRIC DOSE

See Maternal/Child.

Nausea associated with emetogenic agents in pediatric patients 6 months to 18 years of age: 0.15 mg/kg of body weight as an intermittent infusion 30 minutes before giving emetogenic cancer chemotherapy. Repeat 0.15 mg/kg/dose at 4 and 8 hours after the first dose. For highly emetogenic cancer chemotherapy, one source suggests a single dose of 0.45 mg/kg/day 30 minutes before administration. Maximum dose is 32 mg.

Postoperative nausea in pediatric patients 1 month to 12 years of age: Given immediately before or following anesthesia induction or postoperatively if the patient experiences nausea or vomiting. See comments under Usual Dose.

Weight 40 kg or less: 0.1 mg/kg.

Weight more than 40 kg: See Adult dose.

DOSE ADJUSTMENTS

No dose adjustment required for the elderly or in renal disease. ▪ Before emetogenic chemotherapy, a single maximum daily dose of 8 mg is suggested for patients with severe hepatic disease (Child-Pugh score of 10 or greater).

DILUTION

IV injection: 4 mg dose may be given undiluted.

Intermittent infusion: A single dose should be diluted in 50 mL of NS or D5W. Also available as 32 mg in 50 mL D5W.

Continuous infusion: Available prediluted and ready to use or may be further diluted in larger amounts of the above solutions. Also **compatible** in D5/½NS, D5NS, 3% NaCl injection, 10% mannitol, and Ringer's injection. A precipitate will form in alkaline solutions.

Storage: Store unopened vials at CRT or refrigerate. Protect from light. Stable at CRT for 48 hours after dilution with NS, D5W, D5/½NS, D5NS, and 3% NaCl injection. However, manufacturer recommends that the dilution not be used beyond 24 hours. Shake vigorously to resolubilize if a precipitate forms at the stopper/vial interface.

COMPATIBILITY (Underline Indicates Conflicting Compatibility Information)
Consider any drug NOT listed as compatible to be INCOMPATIBLE until consulting a pharmacist; specific conditions may apply.

One source suggests the following **compatibilities**:

Additive: Cisplatin (Platinol), cyclophosphamide (Cytoxan), cytarabine (ARA-C), dacarbazine (DTIC), dexamethasone (Decadron), doxorubicin (Adriamycin), etoposide (VePesid), hydromorphone (Dilaudid), meperidine (Demerol), meropenem (Merrem IV), methotrexate, morphine.

Y-site: Aldesleukin (Proleukin), amifostine (Ethyol), amikacin (Amikin), azithromycin (Zithromax), aztreonam (Azactam), bleomycin (Blenoxane), carboplatin (Paraplatin), carmustine (BiCNU), caspofungin (Cancidas), cefazolin (Ancef), cefotaxime (Claforan), cefoxitin (Mefoxin), ceftazidime (Fortaz), cefuroxime (Zinacef), chlorpromazine (Thorazine), cisatracurium (Nimbex), cisplatin (Platinol), cladribine (Leustatin), clindamycin (Cleocin), cyclophosphamide (Cytoxan), cytarabine (ARA-C), dacarbazine (DTIC), dactinomycin (Cosmegen), daunorubicin (Cerubidine), dexamethasone (Decadron), dexmedetomidine (Precedex), diphenhydramine (Benadryl), docetaxel (Taxotere), dopamine, doripenem (Doribax), doxorubicin (Adriamycin), doxorubicin liposomal (Doxil), doxycycline, droperidol (Inapsine), etoposide (VePesid), etoposide phosphate (Etopophos), famotidine (Pepcid IV), fenoldopam (Corlopam), filgrastim (Neupogen), fluconazole (Diflucan), fludarabine (Fludara), fluorouracil (5-FU), gallium nitrate (Ganite), gemcitabine (Gemzar), gentamicin, haloperidol (Haldol), heparin, hetastarch in electrolytes (Hextend), hydrocortisone sodium succinate (Solu-Cortef), hydromorphone (Dilaudid), ifosfamide (Ifex), imipenem-cilastatin (Primaxin), linezolid (Zyvox), magnesium sulfate, mannitol, mechlorethamine (nitrogen mustard), melphalan (Alkeran), meperidine (Demerol), meropenem (Merrem IV), mesna (Mesnex), methotrexate, metoclopramide (Reglan), mitomycin (Mutamycin), mitoxantrone (Novantrone), morphine, oxaliplatin (Eloxatin), paclitaxel (Taxol), pentostatin (Nipent), piperacillin/tazobactam (Zosyn), potassium chloride (KCl), prochlorperazine (Compazine), promethazine (Phenergan), ranitidine (Zantac), remifentanil (Ultiva), sodium acetate, streptozocin (Zanosar), teniposide (Vumon), thiotepa, ticarcillin/clavulanate (Timentin), topotecan (Hycamtin), vancomycin, vinblastine, vincristine, vinorelbine (Navelbine), zidovudine (AZT, Retrovir).

RATE OF ADMINISTRATION
IV injection: (Postop N/V): A single 4-mg dose over at least 30 seconds; 2 to 5 minutes preferred.

Intermittent infusion adults and pediatric patients: A single dose equally distributed over 15 minutes.

Continuous infusion: Evenly distributed over 12 to 24 hours.

ACTIONS
A selective antagonist of serotonin ($5HT_3$) receptors. $5\text{-}HT_3$ receptors are found both peripherally on vagal nerve terminals and centrally in the chemoreceptor trigger zone. It is unclear whether antiemetic action in chemotherapy-induced nausea and vomiting is mediated centrally, peripherally, or at both sites. Chemotherapeutic agents such as cisplatin increase the release of serotonin from specific cells in the GI tract, causing emesis. By antagonizing these receptors, chemotherapy-induced nausea and vomiting are prevented. Lacks the activity at dopamine receptors of metoclopramide (Reglan), so it does not cause the same level of sedation. No

correlation between plasma levels and antiemetic activity. Metabolized by specific hepatic enzymes of the cytochrome P_{450} isoenzyme system; onset of action is prompt. Half-life is 3.5 to 5.5 hours. Excreted in feces and urine.

INDICATIONS AND USES

Prevention of nausea and vomiting associated with initial and repeat courses of emetogenic cancer chemotherapy, including high-dose cisplatin. ▪ Prevention or treatment of postoperative nausea. ▪ Used orally (available as liquid, tablets, and orally disintegrating tablets) for prevention of nausea and vomiting, including postoperative N/V, and N/V associated with chemotherapy and radiotherapy (including total body irradiation). Approved for IM injection as an alternative to IV in the prevention of postoperative nausea and vomiting.

CONTRAINDICATIONS

Hypersensitivity to ondansetron. ▪ Concomitant use of apomorphine.

PRECAUTIONS

Sterile technique imperative in withdrawing a single dose from the multidose vial. Available as a single-dose vial and in 4- and 8-mg tablets. ▪ Cross-sensitivity has been reported between ondansetron and other $5HT_3$ receptor agonists (e.g., dolasetron [Anzemet] or granisetron [Kytril]). ▪ Use with caution in patients with hepatic impairment. Clearance is decreased; see Dose Adjustments. ▪ Not indicated instead of gastric suction. Use in abdominal surgery or in patients with chemotherapy-induced nausea and vomiting may mask a progressive ileus or gastric distension. ▪ May cause transient ECG changes, including QT-interval prolongation. **Monitor:** Observe closely. Ambulate slowly to avoid orthostatic hypotension. ▪ Stool softeners or laxatives may be required to prevent constipation.

Patient Education: May cause dizziness or fainting; request assistance to ambulate. ▪ Promptly report difficulty breathing, tightness in the chest, or wheezing.

Maternal/Child: Category B: no evidence of impaired fertility or harm to fetus. Use in pregnancy only if potential benefit justifies potential risk. ▪ Use caution if required during breast-feeding. ▪ Information limited in pediatric cancer patients under 6 months of age and in pediatric surgical patients under 1 month of age. ▪ In general, surgical and cancer pediatric patients younger than 18 years tend to have a higher clearance compared with adults, leading to a shorter half-life (2.9 hours). Infants 1 to 4 months of age have a lower clearance, resulting in a longer half-life (6.7 hours).

Elderly: See Dose Adjustments.

DRUG/LAB INTERACTIONS

Does not appear to induce or inhibit the **cytochrome P_{450} isoenzyme system.** However, it is metabolized by this system, and medications that induce or inhibit this system may affect its clearance and half-life. ▪ **Phenytoin** (Dilantin), **carbamazepine** (Tegretol), and **rifampin** (Rifadin) increase clearance and decrease levels of ondansetron. Dose adjustment not recommended. ▪ Concomitant use of **apomorphine** may result in profound hypotension and loss of consciousness; see Contraindications. ▪ Carmustine (BiCNU), etoposide (VePesid), etoposide phosphate (Etopophos), and cisplatin (Platinol) do not affect the pharmacokinetics of ondansetron. ▪ Ondansetron does not increase the concentrations of high-dose methotrexate. ▪ Has been used with cyclophosphamide (Cytoxan), doxorubicin (Adriamycin), etoposide (VePesid), fluorouracil (5-FU), ifosfamide (Ifex), methotrexate, mitoxantrone (Novantrone), and vincristine.

SIDE EFFECTS

Adults: Agitation, arrhythmias (including ventricular and superventricular tachycardia, PVCs, atrial fibrillation, and bradycardia), chest pain, cold sensation, constipation, cramps, diarrhea, dizziness, drowsiness, ECG alterations (including second-degree heart block, QT-interval prolongation, and ST segment depression), faintness, fatigue, fever, flushing, headache, hypersensitivity reactions (e.g., anaphylaxis, angioedema, bronchospasm, cardiopulmonary arrest, hypotension, laryngospasm, shock, shortness of breath, stridor, urticaria), hiccups, hypokalemia, injection site reactions, oculogyric crisis, pain (abdominal, joint, musculoskeletal, rib cage, shoulder), palpitations, paresthesia, pruritus, shivering, transient blurred vision or blindness, transient elevation of AST or ALT, urinary retention. Other side effects have occurred (e.g., extrapyramidal reaction, rash) in fewer than 1% of patients. Overdose caused sudden blindness in one patient.

Infants 1 to 24 months: Bronchospasm, diarrhea, fever, post-procedural pain.

Pediatric patients 2 to 12 years of age: Anxiety/agitation, drowsiness/sedation, fever, headache, wound problems.

Post-Marketing: Arthralgia; dyspnea; erythema; hepatitis, hepatic necrosis, hepatic failure, and death (in patients receiving potentially hepatotoxic cytotoxic chemotherapy and antibiotics; etiology unclear); hyperhidrosis; increased alkaline phosphatase (ALP), gamma-glutamyl transferase (GGT), and bilirubin; jaundice; laryngeal edema; lethargy; torsades de pointes; ventricular fibrillation.

ANTIDOTE

Most side effects will be treated symptomatically. Keep physician informed as indicated. Overdose of 10 times the usual dose has not caused significant problems. Treat anaphylaxis and resuscitate as necessary.

OXACILLIN SODIUM
(ox-ah-**SILL**-in **SO**-dee-um)

Bactocill

Antibacterial
(penicillinase-resistant penicillin)

pH 6 to 8.5

USUAL DOSE
Mild to moderate infections: 250 to 500 mg every 4 to 6 hours.
Severe infections: Increase to 1 Gm every 4 to 6 hours. Up to 1.5 to 2 Gm every 4 to 6 hours has been used to treat *acute or chronic osteomyelitis.* Continue therapy for at least 48 hours after patient becomes afebrile and asymptomatic and cultures are negative. Usual duration of therapy is at least 14 days for severe staphylococcal infections and longer (4 to 6 weeks) for endocarditis and osteomyelitis.

PEDIATRIC DOSE
Infants and pediatric patients under 40 kg: *Mild to moderate infections:* 50 mg/kg of body weight/24 hr in equally divided doses every 6 hours (12.5 mg/kg of body weight every 6 hours).
Severe infections: Increase to 100 to 200 mg/kg/24 hr in equally divided doses every 4 to 6 hours (16.7 mg/kg to 33.3 mg/kg every 4 hours or 25 mg/kg to 50 mg/kg every 6 hours). Maximum dose is 12 Gm/24 hr.

NEONATAL DOSE
Under 1,200 Gm; less than 7 days of age: 25 mg/kg every 12 hours.
Under 2,000 Gm; less than 7 days of age: 25 to 50 mg/kg every 12 hours.
Under 2,000 Gm; 1 to 4 weeks of age: 25 to 50 mg/kg every 8 hours.
Under 1,200 Gm; 1 to 4 weeks of age: 25 mg/kg every 12 hours.
2,000 Gm or more; less than 7 days of age: 25 to 50 mg/kg every 8 hours.
2,000 Gm or more; 1 to 4 weeks of age: 25 to 50 mg/kg every 6 hours.
    Another source suggests 6.25 mg/kg every 6 hours for premature infants and neonates.

DOSE ADJUSTMENTS
Decreased dose may be required in severe renal impairment.

DILUTION
Each 500 mg or fraction thereof should be diluted in 5 mL of SW or NS for injection. May be further diluted for intermittent or continuous infusion in 50 to 1,000 mL of D5W, D5NS, NS, LR, or other **compatible** IV solutions to a final concentration of 0.5 to 40 mg/mL (see literature or chart on inside back cover). Available prediluted and in ADD-Vantage vials for use with ADD-Vantage infusion containers.
Storage: Diluted solution stable for at least 6 hours. See literature.

COMPATIBILITY
(Underline Indicates Conflicting Compatibility Information)
Consider any drug NOT listed as compatible to be INCOMPATIBLE until consulting a pharmacist; specific conditions may apply.
Manufacturer states, "Do not physically mix with other agents." May degrade in infusion solutions containing acidic agents. Inactivated in solution with aminoglycosides (e.g., amikacin [Amikin], gentamicin). Do not mix in the same solution. Appropriate spacing and/or separate sites required. See Drug/Lab Interactions.
    One source suggests the following **compatibilities:**
Additive: *Not recommended by manufacturer.* Chloramphenicol (Chloromycetin), dopamine, potassium chloride (KCl), verapamil.

Y-site: Acyclovir (Zovirax), cyclophosphamide (Cytoxan), diltiazem (Cardizem), doxapram (Dopram), famotidine (Pepcid IV), fluconazole (Diflucan), foscarnet (Foscavir), heparin, hydrocortisone sodium succinate (Solu-Cortef), hydromorphone (Dilaudid), labetalol (Trandate), levofloxacin (Levaquin), magnesium sulfate, meperidine (Demerol), methotrexate, milrinone (Primacor), morphine, potassium chloride (KCl), tacrolimus (Prograf), zidovudine (AZT, Retrovir).

RATE OF ADMINISTRATION

Too-rapid rate may cause seizures.

IV injection: 1 Gm (10 mL) or fraction thereof slowly over 10 minutes.

Intermittent IV: A single dose over 10 to 30 minutes.

Infusion: May be administered in specific IV solutions (check literature) over up to a 6-hour period.

ACTIONS

A semi-synthetic penicillinase-resistant penicillin used for its bactericidal activity against gram-positive organisms, primarily penicillinase-producing staphylococci. Mode of action involves inhibition of bacterial cell wall biosynthesis. Highly resistant to inactivation by staphylococcal penicillinase. Readily distributes into most body fluids and tissues except spinal fluid. Binds to serum proteins, primarily albumin. Excreted primarily as unchanged drug in urine. Nonrenal elimination includes hepatic inactivation and excretion in bile. Half-life is 30 minutes. Crosses the placental barrier. Secreted in breast milk.

INDICATIONS AND USES

Infection caused by penicillinase-producing staphylococci.

CONTRAINDICATIONS

Known sensitivity to any penicillin or cephalosporin (not absolute; see Precautions).

PRECAUTIONS

Hypersensitivity reactions, including fatalities, have been reported in patients undergoing penicillin therapy; most likely to occur in patients with a history of penicillin hypersensitivity or sensitivity to multiple allergens. ▪ There have been reports of individuals with a history of penicillin hypersensitivity experiencing severe reactions when treated with cephalosporins. Check history of previous hypersensitivity reactions to penicillins, cephalosporins, or other allergens. Actual incidence of cross-allergenicity not established but may be more common with first-generation cephalosporins. ▪ Sensitivity studies necessary to determine susceptibility of the causative organism to oxacillin. ▪ To reduce the development of drug-resistant bacteria and maintain its effectiveness, oxacillin should be used to treat or prevent only those infections proven or strongly suspected to be caused by bacteria. ▪ Superinfection caused by overgrowth of nonsusceptible organisms is a possibility. ▪ *Clostridium difficile*–associated diarrhea (CDAD) has been reported. May range from mild diarrhea to fatal colitis. Consider in patients who present with diarrhea during or after treatment with oxacillin. ▪ Change to oral therapy as soon as practical.

Monitor: Periodic liver, kidney, and hematopoietic studies are advised. ▪ Test patients with syphilis for HIV. ▪ Electrolyte imbalance and cardiac irregularities from sodium content are possible. Contains up to 4.02 mEq sodium/Gm. May aggravate CHF. Observe for hypokalemia. ▪ May cause thrombophlebitis; observe carefully and rotate infusion sites. ▪ See Drug/ Lab Interactions.

Patient Education: May require alternate birth control. ▪ Promptly report diarrhea or bloody stools that occur during treatment or up to several months after an antibiotic has been discontinued; may indicate CDAD and require treatment.

Maternal/Child: Category B: use only if clearly needed. ▪ May cause diarrhea, candidiasis, or allergic response in nursing infants. ▪ Limited experience in use on premature infants and neonates. Use with caution. Elimination rate markedly reduced in neonates.

Elderly: Response similar to that seen in younger patients. Consider age-related organ impairment and concomitant disease or drug therapy. ▪ See Precautions/Monitor and Dose Adjustments.

DRUG/LAB INTERACTIONS

Synergistic when used in combination with **aminoglycosides** (e.g., amikacin [Amikin], gentamicin). Synergism may be inconsistent; see Compatibility. ▪ May be antagonized by **bacteriostatic antibiotics** (e.g., chloramphenicol, erythromycin, tetracyclines); may interfere with bactericidal action. ▪ Potentiated by **probenecid** (Benemid); toxicity may result. ▪ May potentiate **heparin.** ▪ Concomitant use with **beta-adrenergic blockers** (e.g., propranolol) may increase risk of anaphylaxis and inhibit treatment. ▪ May decrease clearance and increase toxicity of **methotrexate.** ▪ May inhibit effectiveness of **oral contraceptives;** breakthrough bleeding or pregnancy could result. ▪ May cause false values in **common lab tests;** see literature.

SIDE EFFECTS

Relatively infrequent: diarrhea, elevated AST, hepatic dysfunction, hypersensitivity with anaphylaxis, nausea, pruritus, skin rash, thrombophlebitis, transient hematuria in newborns, urticaria, vomiting. Hypersensitivity myocarditis (fever, eosinophilia, rash, sinus tachycardia, ST-T changes, and cardiomegaly) and CDAD can occur. Higher-than-normal doses may cause neurologic adverse reactions including convulsions, especially with impaired renal function.

ANTIDOTE

Notify the physician of any adverse symptoms. For severe symptoms, discontinue the drug, treat hypersensitivity reactions (antihistamines, epinephrine, corticosteroids), and resuscitate as necessary. Treat CDAD with fluids, electrolytes, protein supplements, and oral vancomycin (Vancocin) or metronidazole (Flagyl) as indicated. In severe cases, surgical evaluation may be indicated. Hemodialysis or peritoneal dialysis are minimally effective in overdose.

OXALIPLATIN BBW

(**OX**-al-ee-**plah**-tin)

Eloxatin

Antineoplastic

USUAL DOSE

Both indications: Given in combination with 5-FU and leucovorin calcium in a dose schedule that repeats every 2 weeks. When used as adjuvant therapy in patients with stage III colon cancer, a treatment period repeated every 2 weeks for 6 months is recommended (a total of 12 cycles). For advanced disease, treatment is recommended until disease progression or unacceptable toxicity. For information on 5-FU and leucovorin calcium, see respective monographs. Prehydration is not required. Premedication with antiemetics recommended; see Monitor. Some clinicians are administering magnesium and calcium before and after oxaliplatin to decrease neurotoxicity.

Day 1: Oxaliplatin 85 mg/M^2 and leucovorin calcium 200 mg/M^2, both given as an IV infusion over 120 minutes at the same time in separate bags using a Y-line. Follow with 5-FU 400 mg/M^2 IV bolus given over 2 to 4 minutes, followed by 5-FU 600 mg/M^2 in 500 mL D5W (recommended) as a 22-hour continuous infusion.

Day 2: Leucovorin calcium 200 mg/M^2 IV infusion over 120 minutes. Follow with 5-FU 400 mg/M^2 IV bolus given over 2 to 4 minutes, followed by 5-FU 600 mg/M^2 in 500 mL D5W (recommended) as a 22-hour continuous infusion.

DOSE ADJUSTMENTS

Advanced colorectal cancer: Dose adjustments are based on clinical toxicities. Reduce dose of oxaliplatin to 65 mg/M^2 in patients who experience persistent Grade 2 neurosensory events that do not resolve. (See Monitor for study-specific neurotoxicity scale.) The infusional 5-FU/leucovorin calcium regimen need not be altered. ▪ Reduce dose of oxaliplatin to 65 mg/M^2 and 5-FU by 20% (300 mg/M^2 bolus and 500 mg/M^2 as a 22-hour infusion) in patients who develop Grade 3 or 4 gastrointestinal toxicity (despite prophylactic treatment), Grade 4 neutropenia, or Grade 3 or 4 thrombocytopenia. Delay next dose until neutrophils are greater than or equal to 1.5×10^9/L [1,500 cells/mm^3] and platelets are greater than or equal to 75×10^9/L [75,000 cells/mm^3]).

Adjuvant therapy in stage III colon cancer (postoperative): Reduce dose of oxaliplatin to 75 mg/M^2 in patients who experience persistent Grade 2 neurosensory events that do not resolve (NCICTC scale version 1 used). The infusional 5-FU/leucovorin calcium regimen need not be altered. ▪ Reduce dose of oxaliplatin to 75 mg/M^2 and 5-FU by 20% (300 mg/M^2 bolus and 500 mg/M^2 as a 22-hour infusion) in patients who develop Grade 3 or 4 gastrointestinal toxicity (despite prophylactic treatment), Grade 4 neutropenia, or Grade 3 or 4 thrombocytopenia. Delay next dose until neutrophils are greater than or equal to 1.5×10^9/L (1,500 cells/mm^3) and platelets are greater than or equal to 75×10^9/L (75,000 cells/mm^3).

Both indications: Consider discontinuing therapy in patients with persistent Grade 3 neurosensory events.

DILUTION

Specific techniques required; see Precautions.
Do not reconstitute or dilute with a sodium chloride solution (e.g., NS, ½NS, ¼NS) or other chloride-containing solutions. Available as a powder for solution and as a concentrate for solution. To reconstitute powder for solution, add 10 mL (for the 50-mg vial) or 20 mL (for the 100-mg vial) of SW or D5W. Both the reconstituted powder for solution and the concentrate for solution must be further diluted with 250 to 500 mL of D5W. *Do not use NS or any chloride-containing solutions; see Compatibility.* Do not use needles or administration sets with aluminum parts; a precipitate may form, and potency may decrease.

Storage: Store unopened vials containing powder for solution under normal lighting conditions at CRT. Store vials with concentrate in the original carton at CRT. Protect vials with concentrate from light and do not freeze. The reconstituted solution may be stored up to 24 hours under refrigeration. After final dilution with 250 to 500 mL of D5W, the solution may be stored for up to 6 hours at CRT or up to 24 hours under refrigeration.

COMPATIBILITY   (Underline Indicates Conflicting Compatibility Information)

Consider any drug NOT listed as compatible to be INCOMPATIBLE until consulting a pharmacist; specific conditions may apply.

Manufacturer states oxaliplatin "is **incompatible** in solution with alkaline medications or media (such as basic solutions of 5-FU) and must not be mixed with these or administered simultaneously through the same infusion line. *The infusion line should be flushed with D5W prior to administration of any concomitant medication.*" Reconstitution or final dilution must not be performed with a sodium chloride solution or other chloride-containing solutions. Do not use needles or administration sets with aluminum parts; a precipitate may form, and potency may decrease.

Sources suggest the following **compatibilities:**

Y-site: Manufacturer lists leucovorin calcium. Another source lists bumetanide, buprenorphine (Buprenex), butorphanol (Stadol), calcium gluconate, carboplatin (Paraplatin), chlorpromazine (Thorazine), cyclophosphamide (Cytoxan), dexamethasone (Decadron), diphenhydramine (Benadryl), dobutamine, docetaxel (Taxotere), dolasetron (Anzemet), dopamine, doxorubicin (Adriamycin), droperidol (Inapsine), enalaprilat (Vasotec IV), epirubicin (Ellence), etoposide phosphate (Etopophos), famotidine (Pepcid IV), fentanyl (Sublimaze), furosemide (Lasix), gemcitabine (Gemzar), granisetron (Kytril), haloperidol (Haldol), heparin, hydrocortisone sodium succinate (Solu-Cortef), hydromorphone (Dilaudid), ifosfamide (Ifex), irinotecan (Camptosar), leucovorin calcium, lorazepam (Ativan), magnesium sulfate, mannitol (Osmitrol), meperidine (Demerol), mesna (Mesnex), methotrexate, methylprednisolone (Solu-Medrol), metoclopramide (Reglan), mitoxantrone (Novantrone), morphine, nalbuphine, ondansetron (Zofran), paclitaxel (Taxol), palonosetron (Aloxi), potassium chloride (KCl), prochlorperazine (Compazine), promethazine (Phenergan), ranitidine (Zantac), theophylline, topotecan (Hycamtin), verapamil, vincristine, vinorelbine (Navelbine).

RATE OF ADMINISTRATION

The infusion line should be flushed with D5W prior to administration of any concomitant medication.

Day 1: Oxaliplatin and leucovorin calcium are given as infusions and equally distributed over 120 minutes. Given at the same time in separate bags using a Y-line. When complete, flush the IV line with D5W. Follow with a **5-FU bolus** administered over 2 to 4 minutes, followed by a **5-FU continuous infusion** equally distributed over 22 hours. ▪ Increasing the infusion time of oxaliplatin from 2 to 6 hours may mitigate acute toxicities. The infusion times for 5-FU and leucovorin calcium need not be altered.

Day 2: Leucovorin calcium is given as an infusion equally distributed over 120 minutes. Follow with a **5-FU bolus** administered over 2 to 4 minutes, followed by a **5-FU continuous infusion** equally distributed over 22 hours.

ACTIONS

A platinum-based antineoplastic agent. Undergoes nonenzymatic conversion to active derivatives that inhibit DNA replication and transcription. Cytotoxicity is cell-cycle nonspecific. Rapidly distributed into tissues or eliminated in the urine. Highly protein bound. Undergoes rapid and extensive nonenzymatic biotransformation. No evidence of cytochrome P_{450}-mediated metabolism. Major route of elimination is renal excretion.

INDICATIONS AND USES

Used in combination with infusional 5-FU and leucovorin calcium for the treatment of patients with advanced colorectal cancer and for adjuvant therapy of stage III colon cancer patients who have undergone complete resection of the primary tumor.

CONTRAINDICATIONS

Hypersensitivity to oxaliplatin or other platinum-containing compounds (e.g., carboplatin [Paraplatin], cisplatin [Platinol]).

PRECAUTIONS

Follow guidelines for handling cytotoxic agents. See Appendix A, p. 1429. ▪ Administered by or under the direction of the physician specialist. ▪ Adequate diagnostic and treatment facilities and emergency resuscitation equipment and supplies must always be available. ▪ Hypersensitivity and anaphylactic-like reactions, some fatal, have been reported and may occur within minutes of administration and during any cycle. See Side Effects and Antidote. ▪ Use with caution in patients with renal impairment. Safety and effectiveness have not been evaluated. ▪ Associated with two types of neuropathy. *The first type is an acute, reversible, primarily peripheral sensory neuropathy that is of early onset, occurs within hours or 1 to 2 days of dosing, resolves within 14 days, and frequently recurs with further dosing.* Symptoms may be precipitated or exacerbated by exposure to cold temperature or cold objects. Usually presents as transient paresthesia (abnormal sensation [e.g., burning, prickling]), dysesthesia (decreased sensitivity to stimulation), and hypoesthesia (impairment of any sense, especially touch) in the hands, feet, perioral area, or throat. *The second type is a persistent (lasting more than 14 days), primarily peripheral, sensory neuropathy that is usually characterized by paresthesias, dysesthesias, and hypoesthesias but may also include deficits in proprioception (stimulus of the sensory end organs [e.g., muscles, tendons]), which can interfere with daily activities (e.g., writing, buttoning, swallowing, and walking).* May occur without any prior acute neuropathy event. Symptoms may or may not improve with discontinuation of oxaliplatin. ▪ Has been associated with pulmonary fibrosis, which may be fatal; see Monitor. ▪ Hepatotoxicity has been reported; see Monitor. ▪ See Drug/Lab Interactions.

Monitor: CBC with differential, platelet count, and blood chemistries (including ALT, AST, bilirubin, and creatinine) are recommended before each cycle. See Dose Adjustments and Precautions. ▪ Monitor for S/S of a hypersensitivity reaction (e.g., chest pain, dizziness, dyspnea, fever, flushing, hypotension, nausea, pruritus, rash, rigors, urticaria). ▪ Monitor for unexplained respiratory symptoms such as nonproductive cough, dyspnea, crackles, or radiologic pulmonary infiltrates. Discontinue oxaliplatin until pulmonary investigation rules out interstitial lung disease or pulmonary fibrosis. ▪ Monitor for S/S of neuropathy (e.g., transient paresthesia [abnormal sensation (e.g., burning, prickling)], dysesthesia [decreased sensitivity to stimulation], and hypoesthesia [impairment of any sense, especially touch] in the hands, feet, perioral area, or throat). Neurotoxicity scale used during advanced colorectal cancer studies differed from National Cancer Institute toxicity grading. Grading scale for paresthesias/dysesthesias was as follows: Grade 1, resolved and did not interfere with functioning; Grade 2, interfered with function but not daily activities; Grade 3, pain or functional impairment that interfered with daily activities; Grade 4, persistent impairment that is disabling or life threatening. ▪ Nausea and vomiting may be severe. Prophylactic administration of antiemetics, including $5HT_3$ blockers (e.g., ondansetron [Zofran]), with or without dexamethasone (Decadron), is recommended. ▪ Observe closely for signs of infection. Prophylactic antibiotics may be indicated pending results of C/S in a febrile neutropenic patient.

Patient Education: Avoid pregnancy. Nonhormonal birth control recommended. ▪ Report any neurologic toxicities. Acute neurosensory toxicity may be precipitated or exacerbated by exposure to cold. Avoid cold drinks and use of ice. Cover exposed skin prior to exposure to cold temperature. ▪ Promptly report persistent vomiting, diarrhea, breathing difficulty, cough, or any sign or infection, allergic reaction, or dehydration. ▪ Use caution while driving or using machines; neurologic symptoms (e.g., dizziness), nausea and vomiting, and vision abnormalities (e.g., transient vision loss) may interfere with abilities. ▪ Manufacturer supplies a patient information leaflet. ▪ See Appendix D, p. 1434.

Maternal/Child: Category D: avoid pregnancy; may cause fetal harm. ▪ Discontinue breast-feeding. ▪ Safety and effectiveness for use in pediatric patients not established. Has been studied in a small number of solid tumors in pediatric patients. No significant response was observed. See manufacturer's literature.

Elderly: The overall rates of adverse events, including Grade 3 and 4 events, were similar for all age-groups. However, the incidence of dehydration, diarrhea, fatigue, Grade 3 to 4 granulocytopenia, hypokalemia, leukopenia, and syncope were higher in patients 65 years of age or older. Adjustment of starting dose is not required.

DRUG/LAB INTERACTIONS
Formal studies have not been performed. ▪ Do not administer **live virus vaccines** to patients receiving antineoplastic agents. ▪ Platinum-containing species are eliminated primarily through the kidney; clearance of these products may be decreased by coadministration of potentially **nephrotoxic compounds** (e.g., aminoglycosides [e.g., gentamicin], amphotericin B [all formulations], NSAIDs [e.g., ibuprofen (Advil, Motrin), naproxen (Aleve, Naprosyn)], pamidronate [Aredia], tacrolimus [Prograf]). ▪ Oxaliplatin is not metabolized by, nor does it inhibit, cytochrome P_{450} isoenzymes. P_{450}-mediated interactions are not anticipated. ▪ A prolonged PT and INR

(occasionally associated with hemorrhage) has been reported when oxaliplatin is used concomitantly with **anticoagulants** (e.g., warfarin [Coumadin]); close monitoring of PT and INR recommended.

SIDE EFFECTS

Are frequent and numerous. Most common adverse reactions are anemia, diarrhea, fatigue, increased liver function tests (e.g., alkaline phosphatase, total bilirubin, and transaminases), nausea, neutropenia, peripheral sensory neuropathies, stomatitis, thrombocytopenia, and vomiting; see Precautions. Other reported reactions include abdominal pain, alopecia, angioedema, anorexia, arthralgia, back pain, chest pain, colitis (including *Clostridium difficile* diarrhea), conjunctivitis, constipation, coughing, deafness, dehydration, dizziness, dyspepsia, dyspnea, dysuria, edema, elevated serum creatinine, epistaxis, fever, flushing, gastroesophageal reflux, hand-foot syndrome, headache, hematuria, hemolytic uremic syndrome, hypersensitivity reactions (e.g., anaphylaxis, angioedema, bronchospasm, erythema, hypotension, pruritis, rash, urticaria), hypokalemia, immunoallergic hemolytic anemia, injection site reaction, insomnia, intestinal obstruction, lacrimation abnormalities, metabolic acidosis, mucositis, pain, pancreatitis, persistent vomiting, pharyngitis, pulmonary fibrosis, rhinitis, rigors, secondary malignancies, stomatitis, taste perversion, thromboembolism, veno-occlusive disease of the liver, visual disorders (e.g., decrease of visual acuity, visual field disturbance, optic neuritis), weight gain. Many other side effects have been reported and may occur.

Overdose: Chest pain, dehydration, diarrhea, dyspnea, enlarged abdomen and Grade 4 intestinal obstruction, hypersensitivity reactions, myelosuppression, nausea and vomiting, neurotoxicity, paresthesia, respiratory failure, severe bradycardia, stomatitis, wheezing, and death.

Post-Marketing: Acute interstitial nephritis, acute tubular necrosis, acute renal failure, colitis (including *Clostridium difficile* diarrhea), convulsions, cranial nerve palsies, dysarthria, fasciculations, hemolytic uremic syndrome, ileus, immunoallergic thrombocytopenia, Lhermitte's sign, metabolic acidosis, perisinusoidal fibrosis, pulmonary fibrosis and other interstitial lung diseases (sometimes fatal), severe diarrhea/vomiting resulting in hypokalemia, transient vision loss (reversible after oxaliplatin is discontinued).

ANTIDOTE

Notify physician of all side effects. Oxaliplatin may need to be discontinued permanently or until recovery. Slowing of infusion rate may help mitigate acute toxicities. Symptomatic and supportive treatment is indicated. Administration of whole blood products (e.g., packed RBCs, platelets, leukocytes) and/or blood modifiers (e.g., darbepoetin alfa [Aranesp], epoetin alfa [Epogen], filgrastim [Neupogen], oprelvekin [Neumega], pegfilgrastim [Neulasta], sargramostim [Leukine]) may be indicated to treat bone marrow toxicity. Treat anaphylaxis with epinephrine, corticosteroids, oxygen, and antihistamines (diphenhydramine). There is no specific antidote. Resuscitate as indicated.

1026

OXYMORPHONE HYDROCHLORIDE
(ox-ee-**MOR**-fohn hy-droh-**KLOR**-eyed)

Opana

Opioid analgesic
(agonist)

pH 2.7 to 4.5

USUAL DOSE
Individualize dose. Consider age, general condition, and medical status of the patient as well as type and severity of pain and prior analgesic treatment experience.

0.5 mg initially. May repeat every 2 to 4 hours. Up to 1.5 mg may be required.

When seeking the required dose to achieve pain relief for an individual patient, increases in increments of at least 25% of the previous dose are suggested. Lower slightly if pain controlled but patient is too drowsy, or lower dose and increase frequency.

DOSE ADJUSTMENTS
Reduced dose or extended intervals may be required in the elderly, in hepatic or renal disease, and in emphysema. ■ Doses appropriate for the general population may cause serious respiratory depression in vulnerable patients. ■ Reduce dose by one third to one half in patients who are concurrently receiving other CNS depressants; see Drug/Lab Interactions. ■ Increase doses as required if analgesia is inadequate, tolerance develops, or pain severity increases. The first sign of tolerance is usually a reduced duration of effect.

DILUTION
May be given undiluted; however, further dilution with 5 mL of SW or NS to facilitate titration is appropriate. May give through Y-tube or three-way stopcock of infusion set.

Storage: Store at CRT. Protect from light.

COMPATIBILITY
Specific information not available.

RATE OF ADMINISTRATION
Rapid IV administration increases the possibility of hypotension and respiratory depression.

A single dose over 2 to 5 minutes. Usually titrated according to symptom relief and respiratory rate.

ACTIONS
A semi-synthetic opioid analgesic closely related to morphine. Ten times more potent than morphine milligram for milligram. Produces a wide range of pharmacologic effects, including analgesia, anxiolysis, cough suppression, diminished GI motility, dysphoria, euphoria, physical dependence, respiratory depression, and somnolence. Onset of action is 5 to 10 minutes. Duration of action is 3 to 6 hours. Metabolized in the liver and excreted in urine and feces. Crosses placental barrier. Secreted in breast milk.

INDICATIONS AND USES
Relief of moderate to severe pain. ■ Support of anesthesia. ■ Obstetric analgesia. ■ Relief of anxiety in patients with dyspnea associated with pulmonary edema secondary to acute left ventricular dysfunction.

CONTRAINDICATIONS

Acute bronchial asthma, pediatric patients under 12 years of age, diarrhea caused by poisoning until toxic material eliminated, hypercarbia, known hypersensitivity to oxymorphone or other morphine analogs (e.g., codeine), moderate to severe hepatic impairment, paralytic ileus, premature infants and labor and delivery of premature infants, pulmonary edema caused by chemical respiratory irritant, upper airway obstruction.

PRECAUTIONS

Schedule II opioid agonists, including hydromorphone, morphine, oxymorphone, oxycodone, fentanyl, and methadone, have the highest potential for abuse and risk of producing respiratory depression. Alcohol, CNS depressants, and other opioids potentiate the respiratory depressant effects of hydromorphone, increasing the risk of respiratory depression that might result in death; see Drug/Lab Interactions. ■ Use extreme caution in patients with conditions accompanied by hypoxia, hypercapnia, or decreased respiratory reserve such as asthma, COPD, cor pulmonale, severe obesity, sleep apnea syndrome, myxedema, kyphoscoliosis, CNS depression, or coma. May decrease respiratory drive and increase airway resistance to the point of apnea. ■ Use with caution in the elderly or debilitated and in patients known to be sensitive to CNS depressants, such as those with cardiovascular, pulmonary, renal, or hepatic disease. ■ Use extreme caution in craniotomy, head injury, and increased intracranial pressure; respiratory depression and intracranial pressure may be further increased. ■ Can also produce effects on pupillary response and consciousness, which may obscure neurologic signs of further increases in intracranial pressure. ■ Use with caution in patients in circulatory shock. May further reduce cardiac output or BP. ■ Use with caution in acute alcoholism, adrenocortical insufficiency (e.g., Addison's disease), CNS depression, delirium tremens, prostatic hypertrophy, or urethral stricture. ■ Symptoms of acute abdominal conditions may be masked. Can cause spasm of the sphincter of Oddi. Use with caution in patients with biliary tract disease, including acute pancreatitis. ■ May increase ventricular response rate in presence of supraventricular tachycardias. ■ Cough reflex is suppressed. ■ Tolerance to oxymorphone gradually increases. A marked increase in dose may precipitate seizures. ■ Concerns about abuse, addiction, and diversion should not prevent proper management of pain.

Monitor: Oxygen, controlled respiratory equipment, and naloxone (Narcan) must be available. ■ Assess baseline pain, then assess pain with vital signs and/or more frequently if needed. Reassess after administration of oxymorphone and adjust dose or interval as required. ■ Keep patient supine; orthostatic hypotension and fainting may occur. Uncontrolled pain causes sleep deprivation, decreases pain threshold, and increases pain; when pain is finally controlled, expect the patient to sleep more until recovery from sleep deprivation. ■ Adhere to prescribed bowel care regimen to avoid constipation and/or impaction. Maintain adequate hydration.

Patient Education: Avoid alcohol or other CNS depressants (e.g., barbiturates, benzodiazepines [e.g., diazepam (Valium)]). ■ May cause blurred vision, dizziness, or drowsiness; use caution in tasks that require alertness. ■ Request assistance with ambulation. ■ May be habit forming.

Maternal/Child: Category C: safety for use in pregnancy or breast-feeding not established; see Contraindications. ■ Use with caution during labor.

May cause respiratory depression in the newborn. ▪ Safety for use in pediatric patients under 18 years of age not established.
Elderly: See Dose Adjustments and Precautions. ▪ May be more sensitive to effects (e.g., respiratory depression, constipation, urinary retention). Adverse effects more commonly observed in the elderly include confusion, dizziness, nausea, and somnolence. ▪ Lower doses may provide effective analgesia. ▪ Consider age-related organ impairment.

DRUG/LAB INTERACTIONS

Potentiated by **phenothiazines and other CNS depressants** such as narcotic analgesics, alcohol, antihistamines, barbiturates, cimetidine (Tagamet), hypnotics, sedatives, MAO inhibitors (e.g., selegiline [Eldepryl]), neuromuscular blocking agents (e.g., atracurium [Tracrium]), and psychotropic agents. Interactive effects resulting in respiratory depression, hypotension, profound sedation, or coma may result with concomitant use. Reduced dosages of both drugs may be indicated. ▪ Administration of **agonist/ antagonist analgesics** (e.g., butorphanol [Stadol], buprenorphine [Buprenex]) to an opiate-dependent patient receiving a pure opiate may reduce the analgesic effect of the pure opiate and/or precipitate withdrawal symptoms. ▪ Concomitant use with **anticholinergics or medications with anticholinergic activity** (e.g., diphenhydramine [Benadryl]) may result in an increased risk of urinary retention and/or severe constipation, which may lead to paralytic ileus. ▪ Concomitant use with **propofol** (Diprivan) for the induction of anesthesia may increase the incidence of bradycardia. ▪ Plasma **amylase and lipase determinations** may be unreliable for 24 hours following opioid administration.

SIDE EFFECTS

At equianalgesic doses, may cause more nausea, vomiting, and euphoria than morphine.

Abdominal pain, anorexia, biliary colic, blurred vision, bradycardia, bronchospasm, confusion, constipation, diplopia, dizziness, dry mouth, flushing, hallucinations, miosis, paralytic ileus, pruritus, skin rash, urinary retention, urticaria.

Major: Anaphylaxis, hypotension, respiratory depression, somnolence.

ANTIDOTE

Notify the physician of any side effect. If minor side effects progress or any major side effect occurs, discontinue the drug and notify the physician. Treat anaphylaxis as indicated or resuscitate as necessary. Naloxone hydrochloride (Narcan) will reverse serious reactions.

OXYTOCIN INJECTION BBW
(ox-eh-**TOE**-sin in-**JEK**-shun)
Pitocin

Oxytocic
Antihemorrhagic
pH 2.5 to 4.5

USUAL DOSE

Determined by uterine response and intended use, dilution, and rate of administration. Oxytocins must be administered by only one route at a time. For instance, do not combine oral and IV routes. Piggyback oxytocin into a physiologic electrolyte IV solution (e.g., NS) without oxytocins; see Precautions.

Induction of labor: 0.5 to 1 milliunit/min (mU/min) will deliver 3 to 6 mL/hr of properly diluted solution. See Dilution and Rate of Administration.

Control of postpartum bleeding: A total dose of 10 units delivered at 10 to 40 mU/min, following delivery of the infant(s) and preferably the placenta(s). See Dilution and Rate of Administration.

Incomplete or inevitable abortion: A total of 10 units delivered at 10 to 20 mU/min; a second source says 10 to 40 mU/min. See Dilution and Rate of Administration.

Postabortion hemorrhage (unlabeled): A total of 10 units delivered at 20 to 100 mU/min. See Dilution and Rate of Administration.

Oxytocin challenge test (unlabeled): Infuse properly diluted oxytocin (10 mU/mL) at an initial rate of 0.5 mU/min. Rate may be gradually increased at 15- to 30-minute intervals to a maximum of 20 mU/min. Discontinue infusion when 3 moderate contractions occur in a 10-minute interval and compare baseline and oxytocin-induced fetal HR. Monitor fetal HR concurrently. Observe signs of fetal distress with contractions. Distress indicates inadequate fetal respiratory capabilities and placental reserve. Stop infusion.

DILUTION

In all situations rotate gently to distribute medication through solution.

Induction of labor: Dilute 1 mL (10 units) in 1 liter of NS, D5W, LR, or D5NS for infusion (10 mU/mL). This dilution is also used for the *oxytocin challenge test.*

Control of postpartum bleeding: Dilute 1 to 4 mL (10 to 40 units) in 1 liter of above infusion fluids (10 to 40 mU/mL).

Incomplete or inevitable abortion/postabortion hemorrhage: Dilute 1 mL (10 units) in 500 mL of above infusion fluids (20 mU/mL).

Storage: Check package insert. Some preparations may require refrigeration; others can be stored at RT.

COMPATIBILITY

Consider any drug NOT listed as compatible to be INCOMPATIBLE until consulting a pharmacist; specific conditions may apply.

Rapidly decomposes in the presence of sodium bisulfate.

One source suggests the following **compatibilities:**

Additive: Chloramphenicol (Chloromycetin), sodium bicarbonate, thiopental (Pentothal), verapamil.

Y-site: Heparin, hydrocortisone sodium succinate (Solu-Cortef), insulin (regular), meperidine (Demerol), morphine, potassium chloride (KCl), warfarin (Coumadin), zidovudine (AZT, Retrovir).

RATE OF ADMINISTRATION

Given only as an IV infusion. Use of an infusion pump or other accurate control device is required. In all situations, use the minimum effective rate and monitor strength, frequency, and duration of contractions; resting uterine tone, fetal HR (in induction of labor), and maternal BP at least every 15 minutes or more often if indicated.

Induction of labor: Begin with 0.5 to 1 mU/min (0.05 to 0.1 mL), increase in increments of 1 to 2 mU/min at 30- to 60-minute intervals until contractions simulate normal labor. Maximum dose rarely exceeds 9 to 10 mU/min at term, average is 2 to 5 mU/min. Reduce by similar increments when desired frequency of contractions is reached and labor has progressed to 5 to 6 cm. 6 mU/min provides oxytocin levels similar to spontaneous labor. Preterm inductions may require somewhat higher doses (one source suggests a maximum of 20 mU/min); use caution.

Control of postpartum bleeding: Adjust rate of infusion to sustain contractions and control uterine atony. Begin with 10 to 40 mU/min. Increase or decrease rate as indicated. Proceed quickly but with caution because of strength of solution.

Incomplete or inevitable abortion: 10 to 40 mU/min.

Postabortion hemorrhage: 20 to 100 mU/min.

ACTIONS

A synthetic posterior pituitary hormone that will produce rhythmic contraction of uterine smooth muscle. Its effectiveness depends on the level of uterine excitability, which usually increases as a pregnancy progresses. Very rapid acting, it has a shorter duration of action than ergot derivatives (half-life of 1 to 6 minutes). Duration of action is approximately 1 hour. Is the drug of choice for induction of delivery. Probably detoxified in the liver and through enzymatic processes and excreted in the urine. May exhibit antidiuretic and pressor effects at higher doses. Probably crosses the placental barrier in small amounts.

INDICATIONS AND USES

After selective patient evaluation by the physician, it is used to induce or stimulate labor at term or before. ■ Control of postpartum bleeding. ■ Adjunctive therapy in the management of incomplete or inevitable abortion. ■ Treatment of post-abortion hemorrhage. ■ Not indicated for elective induction of labor (i.e., no medical indication for induction).

Unlabeled uses: Oxytocin challenge test.

CONTRAINDICATIONS

Cephalopelvic disproportion, fetal malpresentation, hypersensitivity, hypertonic uterine contractions, lack of satisfactory progress with adequate uterine activity, obstetrical emergencies (e.g., abruptio placentae), prolonged use in uterine inertia, serious medical or obstetric conditions (past or present), toxemia (severe), vaginal delivery contraindicated (e.g., active herpes genitalis, cord presentation or prolapse, invasive cervical carcinoma, total placenta previa and vasa previa). See Precautions.

PRECAUTIONS

A NS IV without oxytocins must be hung, connected by Y-tube or three-way stopcock, and ready for use in adverse reactions. ■ Should be administered only in the hospital; the physician must be immediately available. ■ The use of oxytocin for fetal distress, hydramnios, partial placenta previa, prematurity, borderline cephalopelvic disproportion, or any condition that may cause uterine rupture (e.g., cesarean section [previous], uterine surgery, uterine overdistention, past history of uterine sepsis) is not recommended except in unusual circumstances. ▪ Maternal deaths due to hypertensive episodes, subarachnoid hemorrhage, and uterine rupture, as well as fetal deaths due to various causes, have been reported. ▪ When used for induction or reinforcement of already existing labor, patients should be carefully selected. Evaluate pelvic adequacy and maternal and fetal conditions before use. ▪ Oxytocin challenge test is an antepartum test of uteroplacental insufficiency in high-risk pregnancy. Test done only by a qualified physician.

Monitor: When properly administered, oxytocin should stimulate uterine contractions comparable to normal labor. Monitor BP, fetal heart tones, strength and timing of contractions, and resting uterine tone at least every 15 minutes or more often if indicated. Continuous observation of patient required. ▪ Electronic fetal monitoring provides the best means of early detection of overdose. A fetal scalp electrode provides a more accurate recording of fetal HR than external monitoring. ▪ Monitor oral fluid intake and observe for signs of fluid retention. Water intoxication has caused maternal death. ▪ See Precautions and Drug/Lab Interactions.

Maternal/Child: Has no use before induction of labor; see Contraindications.

DRUG/LAB INTERACTIONS

Severe hypertension can result in the presence of **local anesthesia, regional anesthesia** (caudal or spinal), **and with dopamine, ephedrine, epinephrine, and other vasopressors. Chlorpromazine** (Thorazine) IV will reduce this hypertension. ▪ Concurrent use with **cyclopropane anesthesia** may cause hypotension and/or sinus bradycardia with abnormal atrioventricular rhythms.

SIDE EFFECTS

Maternal: Anaphylaxis, cardiac arrhythmias, fatal afibrinogenemia, fluid retention leading to water intoxication and coma, convulsion, and death; hypertension, increased blood loss, nausea, pelvic hematoma, PVCs, postpartum hemorrhage, severe uterine hypertonicity, spasm or contraction; subarachnoid hemorrhage, uterine rupture, vomiting.

Fetal: Bradycardia, brain damage, CNS damage, death, low Apgar scores, neonatal jaundice, retinal hemorrhage, seizures.

ANTIDOTE

Nausea and vomiting are tolerable and can be treated symptomatically. Immediately call the physician's attention to any side effect noted or suspected; many can be fatal. Discontinue the drug immediately for any signs of fetal distress, uterine hyperactivity, tetanic contractions, uterine resting tone exceeding 15 to 20 mm H_2O, or water intoxication. Use of a Y-connection or three-way stopcock, allowing the oxytocin drip to be discontinued while the vein is kept open, is required. Turn mother on side (to prevent fetal anoxia) and administer oxygen. Restriction of fluids, diuresis, hypertonic saline solutions IV, correction of electrolyte imbalance, control of convulsions with cautious use of barbiturates, or the use of magnesium sulfate may be required. These side effects can occur during labor and delivery and into the postpartum period. Careful evaluation and selection of patients eliminate many hazards, but be prepared for an emergency.

PACLITAXEL ▪ PACLITAXEL PROTEIN-BOUND PARTICLES FOR INJECTABLE SUSPENSION (ALBUMIN-BOUND) BBW

(PACK-lih-tax-el)

Onxol, Taxol ▪ Abraxane

Antineoplastic
(taxane)

pH 4.4 to 5.6 ▪ not available

USUAL DOSE

Assessment required before dosing: see Precautions, Monitor, and Dose Adjustments.

CONVENTIONAL PACLITAXEL

Several regimens of paclitaxel, alone or in combination with other antineoplastics, are in use. Doses vary, depending on the regimen used. Consult literature. ▪ For all uses, premedication, specific parameters, and specific equipment are required before or during administration; see Premedication, Dose Adjustments, and Precautions/Monitor.

Premedication: Must be premedicated before each dose to prevent severe hypersensitivity reactions. Usual regimen includes IV or oral dexamethasone (Decadron) 20 mg 12 and 6 hours before; IV diphenhydramine (Benadryl) 50 mg 30 to 60 minutes before; and an H_2 antagonist (e.g., ranitidine [Zantac] 50 mg or famotidine [Pepcid IV] 20 mg) 30 to 60 minutes before dosing with paclitaxel. When premedicating patients with AIDS-related Kaposi's sarcoma, reduce the dose of dexamethasone to 10 mg at 12 and 6 hours before paclitaxel. The doses of IV diphenhydramine and IV H_2 antagonists remain as above.

Ovarian cancer in previously untreated patients: 135 mg/M^2 as an infusion over 24 hours. Follow with cisplatin 75 mg/M^2 as an infusion over 6 to 8 hours. Repeat every 3 weeks. An alternative regimen is paclitaxel 175 mg/M^2 as an infusion over 3 hours. Follow with cisplatin 75 mg/M^2 (one source suggests an infusion over 24 hours; another suggests 6 to 8 hours, which would allow for outpatient therapy). Repeat every 3 weeks. See comments under Usual Dose.

Ovarian cancer in patients previously treated with chemotherapy: 135 or 175 mg/M^2 as an infusion over 3 hours. An alternate regimen suggests the same dose given as a 24-hour infusion. Repeat every 3 weeks. Larger doses, with or without filgrastim (G-CSF, Neupogen), have produced similar responses. See comments under Usual Dose.

Adjuvant treatment of node-positive breast cancer: 175 mg/M^2 as an infusion over 3 hours. Repeat every 3 weeks for four courses. Administered sequentially to doxorubicin-containing combination therapy. Clinical trials used four courses of doxorubicin and cyclophosphamide. Administer filgrastim (G-CSF) 5 mcg/kg/dose on days 3 through 10. See comments under Usual Dose.

Breast cancer in patients previously treated with chemotherapy: 175 mg/M^2 as an infusion over 3 hours. Repeat every 3 weeks. An alternate regimen suggests 175 to 250 mg/M^2 over 3 hours every 3 weeks. See comments under Usual Dose.

First-line treatment of non–small-cell lung cancer: 135 mg/M^2 as an infusion over 24 hours. Follow with cisplatin 75 mg/M^2 over 6 to 8 hours. Repeat every 3 weeks. See comments under Usual Dose. A Canadian source recommends 175 mg/M^2 as an infusion over 3 hours followed with cisplatin 75 mg/M^2 over 6 to 8 hours and repeated every 3 weeks.

AIDS-related Kaposi's sarcoma: 135 mg/M^2 as an infusion over 3 hours. An alternate regimen suggests the same dose given as a 24-hour infusion. Repeat every 3 weeks. Another regimen is 100 mg/M^2 as an infusion over 3 hours repeated every 2 weeks. Toxicity somewhat increased with 135 mg/M^2 dose in clinical studies. See comments under Usual Dose.

Fallopian tube and peritoneal cancers of ovarian origin (unlabeled): 135 to 175 mg/M^2 as a 3-hour infusion in combination with carboplatin AUC 5 to 6, every 3 weeks. Repeat for 5 to 9 cycles. Extend infusion time of paclitaxel if appropriate (e.g., patient comfort, level of toxicity).

ABRAXANE

Premedication: Not required.

Breast cancer in patients previously treated with chemotherapy: 260 mg/M^2 as an infusion over 30 minutes every 3 weeks.

DOSE ADJUSTMENTS

CONVENTIONAL PACLITAXEL

Reduce dose by 20% for subsequent courses in patients who experience severe peripheral neuropathy or severe neutropenia (neutrophils less than 500 cells/mm^3) for 1 week or longer. ▪ Withhold therapy if neutrophils below 1,500/mm^3 or platelets below 100,000/mm^3. ▪ Dose reduction not required in impaired renal function. ▪ In AIDS-related Kaposi's sarcoma the parameters are slightly different. Initiate or repeat paclitaxel only if neutrophil count is equal to or greater than 1,000/mm^3; reduce dose of dexamethasone to 10 mg/dose; reduce dose of paclitaxel by 20% in patients who experience severe neutropenia (neutrophils less than 500/mm^3 for a week or longer); use concomitant filgrastim (G-CSF) as clinically indicated. ▪ Recommendations for dose adjustment of the initial course of therapy in patients with impaired hepatic function are listed in the following chart.

Guidelines for Dose Adjustment of Paclitaxel in Impaired Hepatic Function*		
Degree of Hepatic Impairment		
Transaminase Levels	Bilirubin Levels†	Recommended TAXOL Dose‡
24-Hour Infusion		
<2 × ULN and	≤1.5 mg/dL	135 mg/M^2
2 to <10 × ULN and	≤1.5 mg/dL	100 mg/M^2
<10 × ULN and	1.6-7.5 mg/dL	50 mg/M^2
≥10 × ULN or	>7.5 mg/dL	Not recommended

Continued

Guidelines for Dose Adjustment of Paclitaxel in Impaired Hepatic Function*—cont'd			
Degree of Hepatic Impairment			
Transaminase Levels		Bilirubin Levels†	Recommended TAXOL Dose‡
3-Hour Infusion			
<10 × ULN	and	≤1.25 × ULN	175 mg/M^2
<10 × ULN	and	1.26-2 × ULN	135 mg/M^2
<10 × ULN	and	2.01-5 × ULN	90 mg/M^2
≥10 × ULN	or	>5 × ULN	Not recommended

*These recommendations are based on clinical trials of dosages for patients without hepatic impairment of 135 mg/M^2 over 24 hours or 175 mg/M^2 over 3 hours; data are not available to make dose adjustment recommendations for other regimens (e.g., for AIDS-related Kaposi's sarcoma).

†Differences in criteria for bilirubin levels between the 3- and 24-hour infusion are due to differences in clinical trial design.

‡Dosage recommendations are for the first course of therapy; further dose reduction in subsequent courses should be based on individual tolerance.

ABRAXANE

Withhold therapy if neutrophils below 1,500/mm^3 or platelets below 100,000/mm^3. Reduce dose to 220 mg/M^2 in patients who experience severe neutropenia (neutrophils less than 500 cells/mm^3) or severe sensory neuropathy. ▪ Further reduce dose to 180 mg/M^2 for subsequent courses if severe neutropenia (less than 500 cells/mm^3 for 7 days or more) or severe sensory neuropathy recur. ▪ If Grade 3 sensory neuropathy occurs, withhold treatment until resolution to Grade 1 or 2, followed by a dose reduction for all subsequent courses. ▪ No dose adjustment is necessary for patients with mild hepatic impairment. Recommendations for a starting dose in patients with hepatic impairment are shown in the following table. Doses for subsequent cycles should be based on patient tolerance.

Starting Dose Recommendations for Patients with Hepatic Impairment			
Degree of Hepatic Impairment	SGOT (AST) Levels	Bilirubin Levels	Abraxane
Mild	<10 × ULN	>ULN to ≤1.25 × ULN	260 mg/M^2
Moderate	<10 × ULN and	1.26 to 2 × ULN	200 mg/M^2
Severe	<10 × ULN	2.01 to 5 × ULN	130 mg/M^2*
Severe	>10 × ULN or	>5 × ULN	Not eligible

*Dose increase to 200 mg/M^2 in subsequent courses should be considered based on individual tolerance.

DILUTION

Specific techniques required; see Precautions.

CONVENTIONAL PACLITAXEL

Must be diluted and given as an infusion. May leach the toxic plasticizer DEHP from PVC infusion bags or sets; prepare and store in bottles (glass, polypropylene) or plastic bags (polypropylene, polyolefin) and administer through polyethylene-lined administration sets. **Compatible** with NS, D5W, D5NS, or D5R. Final concentration of 0.3 to 1.2 mg/mL required. For a 135 mg/M^2 dose, a large adult (body surface about 2 M^2) will receive 270 mg (45 mL of paclitaxel at 6 mg/mL). Will require dilution in an additional 180 mL to make a 1.2 mg/mL concentration or 855 mL to make a 0.3 mg/mL concentration. Solution may appear hazy. Do not use a chemo-dispensing pin; can cause the stopper to collapse and result in loss of sterility.

ABRAXANE
Available in single-use vials, each containing 100 mg (5 mg/mL after reconstitution with 20 mL of NS). Calculate the exact number of vials needed to achieve the total dosing volume of suspension required.

Total # of vials required = Total dose (mg) ÷ 100 mg
Dosing volume (mL) = Total dose (mg) ÷ 5 (mg/mL)

For example, a patient with a body surface area (BSA) of 1.73 M^2 would need a dose of 449.8 mg of Abraxane. 449.8 mg divided by 100 mg equals 4.498 vials, so 5 vials of Abraxane would be needed. 449.8 mg divided by 5 (mg/mL) equals a dosing volume of 90 mL of reconstituted solution.

Reconstitute each 100-mg vial with 20 mL of NS. A specific process is required to avoid foaming or clumping. Over a minimum of 1 minute, slowly inject the NS, directing it to the inside wall of the vial. Do not allow the NS to flow directly onto the lyophilized cake (will cause foaming). Allow each vial to sit for a minimum of 5 minutes while the NS wets the cake. Gently swirl and/or invert each vial slowly for at least 2 minutes until complete dissolution. Avoid generation of foam. If foaming or clumping occurs, allow solution to stand for at least 15 minutes until foam subsides. Solution should be milky and homogenous without visible particulates. If particulates are visible, gently invert to ensure complete resuspension before use.

Inject the calculated volume from each vial into an empty and sterile polyvinyl chloride (PVC) container or a PVC or non–PVC-type infusion bag (a total dosing volume of 90 mL in the previous example).
Filters: *Conventional paclitaxel:* Use of an in-line filter not greater than 0.22 microns required for administration. ***Abraxane:*** Use of an in-line filter not required or recommended.
Storage: *Conventional paclitaxel:* May be stored at CRT or refrigerated before dilution (may appear precipitated under refrigeration; will redissolve at room temperature). Diluted for infusion, it is stable at room temperature for up to 27 hours. ***Abraxane:*** Store vials in original package at 20° to 25° C (68° to 77° F). Protect from light. Refrigeration or freezing does not affect stability of the product. Immediate use of reconstituted solution is preferred, but reconstituted vial may be refrigerated for a maximum of 8 hours if necessary. If refrigeration required, return to original carton to protect from light. Ensure complete resuspension after removing from refrigerator by gently inverting. Reconstituted solution in an infusion bag should be used immediately; however, it is stable at 25° C with ambient lighting conditions for up to 8 hours. Discard unused portions of the vial.

COMPATIBILITY (Underline Indicates Conflicting Compatibility Information)
Consider any drug NOT listed as compatible to be INCOMPATIBLE until consulting a pharmacist; specific conditions may apply.
CONVENTIONAL PACLITAXEL
Leaches out plasticizers; see Dilution.

One source suggests the following **compatibilities:**
CONVENTIONAL PACLITAXEL
Additive: Carboplatin (Paraplatin), cisplatin (Platinol), doxorubicin (Adriamycin); see Drug/Lab Interactions.

Y-site: Acyclovir (Zovirax), amikacin (Amikin), aminophylline, ampicillin/ sulbactam (Unasyn), anidulafungin (Eraxis), bleomycin (Blenoxane), butorphanol (Stadol), calcium chloride, carboplatin (Paraplatin), cefepime (Maxipime), cefotetan, ceftazidime (Fortaz), ceftriaxone (Rocephin), cisplatin (Platinol), cladribine (Leustatin), cyclophosphamide (Cytoxan), cytarabine (ARA-C), dacarbazine (DTIC), dexamethasone (Decadron), diphenhydramine (Benadryl), doripenem (Doribax), doxorubicin (Adriamycin), droperidol (Inapsine), etoposide (VePesid), etoposide phosphate (Etopophos), famotidine (Pepcid IV), fluconazole (Diflucan), fluorouracil (5-FU), furosemide (Lasix), ganciclovir (Cytovene), gemcitabine (Gemzar), gentamicin, granisetron (Kytril), haloperidol (Haldol), heparin, hydrocortisone sodium succinate (Solu-Cortef), hydromorphone (Dilaudid), ifosfamide (Ifex), linezolid (Zyvox), lorazepam (Ativan), magnesium sulfate, mannitol, meperidine (Demerol), mesna (Mesnex), methotrexate, metoclopramide (Reglan), morphine, nalbuphine, ondansetron (Zofran), oxaliplatin (Eloxatin), palonosetron (Aloxi), pemetrexed (Alimta), pentostatin (Nipent), potassium chloride (KCl), prochlorperazine (Compazine), propofol (Diprivan), ranitidine (Zantac), sodium bicarbonate, thiotepa, topotecan (Hycamtin), vancomycin, vinblastine, vincristine, zidovudine (AZT, Retrovir).

ABRAXANE
Manufacturer states, "Use of specialized DEHP-free solution containers or administration sets is not necessary." Additional specific information not available.

RATE OF ADMINISTRATION
CONVENTIONAL PACLITAXEL
A single dose properly diluted must be equally distributed over 3 hours or as indicated in Usual Dose. Use of an in-line filter not greater than 0.22 microns required. Use of a metriset (60 gtt/mL) or an infusion pump appropriate to control flow. Rate extended to 24 hours in some regimens.

ABRAXANE
A single dose properly reconstituted and equally distributed over 30 minutes. Volume is small; use of an infusion pump or syringe pump is indicated. Use of an in-line filter is not recommended.

ACTIONS
ALL FORMULATIONS
An antineoplastic. A novel antimicrotubule agent. Paclitaxel derived from the bark of pacific yew has now been replaced by paclitaxel produced semisynthetically from a renewable source (needles and twigs of the Himalayan yew). Both are chemically identical. Through specific processes it stabilizes microtubules by preventing depolymerization. This action inhibits the normal dynamic reorganization of the microtubule network essential for vital interphase and mitotic cellular functions. Also

induces abnormal bundles of microtubules throughout the cell cycle and multiple asters of microtubules during mitosis. More active in patients who have not received previous chemotherapy. Distribution and/or tissue binding is extensive. Evidence suggests metabolism in the liver via the cytochrome P_{450} isoenzyme system (CYP2C8 and CYP3A4). Terminal half-life ranges from 13.1 to 52.7 hours (average is 27 hours). High concentrations occur and are probably excreted through bile and feces. Minimal excretion of unchanged drug occurs in urine.

ABRAXANE

A new class of "protein-bound particle" drugs manufactured by a new nanoparticle albumin-bound technology. Consists of albumin-bound paclitaxel nanoparticles. Free of toxic solvents and has demonstrated a response rate almost double that of solvent-based Taxol in clinical trials of patients with metastatic breast cancer. Clearance may be larger and distribution may be higher than with conventional paclitaxel.

INDICATIONS AND USES

CONVENTIONAL PACLITAXEL

Treatment of metastatic carcinoma of the ovary after failure of first-line or subsequent chemotherapy. ▪ First-line treatment for ovarian cancer in combination with cisplatin. ▪ Adjuvant treatment of node-positive breast cancer administered sequentially to standard doxorubicin-containing combination chemotherapy. Most effective in estrogen- and progesterone–receptor–negative tumors. ▪ Metastatic breast cancer refractory to initial chemotherapy or for a relapse within 6 months. ▪ First-line treatment, in combination with cisplatin, for non–small-cell lung cancer in patients who are not candidates for potentially curative surgery or radiation therapy. ▪ Second-line treatment of AIDS-related Kaposi's sarcoma.

ABRAXANE

Treatment of breast cancer after failure of combination chemotherapy for metastatic disease or relapse within 6 months of adjuvant chemotherapy. Prior therapy should have included an anthracycline unless clinically contraindicated.

Unlabeled uses: *Conventional paclitaxel:* Advanced head and neck cancer. ▪ Cancers of the bladder, cervix, endometrium, esophagus, and upper GI tract. ▪ Hormone-refractory prostate cancer. ▪ Previously untreated extensive-stage small-cell lung cancer. ▪ Non-Hodgkin's lymphomas. ▪ Treatment of fallopian tube and peritoneal cancer of ovarian origin. ▪ First-line therapy alone and in combination with other agents for treatment of metastatic breast cancer. ▪ Treatment of testicular germ cell tumors in patients refractory to cisplatin-based therapy.

CONTRAINDICATIONS

CONVENTIONAL PACLITAXEL

Baseline neutropenia less than 1,500 cells/mm^3 in patients with solid tumors or baseline neutropenia less than 1,000 cells/mm^3 in patients with AIDS-related Kaposi's sarcoma. History of prior severe hypersensitivity reactions to paclitaxel or other drugs formulated in polyoxyethylated castor oil (Cremophor EL [e.g., cyclosporine, teniposide]).

ABRAXANE

Baseline neutrophil count less than 1,500 cells/mm^3.

PRECAUTIONS

ALL FORMULATIONS

Follow guidelines for handling cytotoxic agents. See Appendix A, p. 1429. ▪ Usually administered by or under the direction of the physician specialist in a facility with adequate diagnostic and treatment facilities to monitor the patient and respond to any medical emergency.

CONVENTIONAL PACLITAXEL

Use caution in patients with cardiac conduction abnormalities, CHF, and MI within previous 6 months. ▪ Myelosuppression may be more frequent and more severe in patients who have received prior radiation therapy. ▪ Pre-existing neuropathies resulting from prior therapies are not a contra-indication for paclitaxel therapy. ▪ Various studies show that incidence and severity of neurotoxicity and hematologic toxicity increase with dose, especially above 190 mg/M^2. ▪ Use with caution in patients with a total bilirubin greater than 2 times the ULN. May be at increased risk of toxicity, especially profound myelosuppression; see Dose Adjustments.

ABRAXANE

Do not substitute for or with other paclitaxel formulations. ▪ Use of gloves recommended. Wash skin immediately if contact occurs. Flush mucous membranes thoroughly with water if contact occurs. Topical exposure may result in tingling, burning, and redness. ▪ Premedication to prevent hyper-sensitivity reactions is not required; rare reports of severe hypersensitivity reactions have occurred. ▪ Neutropenia is dose dependent and is a dose-limiting toxicity. Subsequent cycles of Abraxane should not be adminis-tered until neutrophils recover to a level greater than 1,500 cells/mm^3 and platelets recover to a level greater than 100,000 cells/mm^3. ▪ Sensory neuropathy occurs frequently; see Dose Adjustments. ▪ Has not been studied in patients with renal dysfunction (patients with a baseline SCr greater than 2 mg/dL were excluded from trials). ▪ Use with caution in patients with hepatic impairment. Patients with AST greater than 10 times the ULN and bilirubin greater than 5 times the ULN have not been studied; see Dose Adjustments. ▪ A protein substance; may carry a risk of viral disease or Creutzfeldt-Jakob disease; risk considered ex-tremely remote. ▪ Use with concurrent radiotherapy has not been studied. ▪ Has not been studied in patients who have had a hypersensitivity reaction to conventional paclitaxel.

Monitor: ALL FORMULATIONS: Neutropenia is dose dependent and is the dose-limiting toxicity. Obtain baseline CBC with differential and platelet count. Mon-itor frequently during therapy and before each dose. ▪ Monitor injection site carefully; avoid extravasation. ▪ Observe closely for signs of infection. Prophylactic antibiotics may be indicated pending results of C/S in a febrile neutropenic patient. ▪ Use prophylactic antiemetics to reduce nau-sea and vomiting and increase patient comfort. ▪ Monitor for thrombocy-topenia (platelet count less than 50,000/mm^3). Initiate precautions to prevent excessive bleeding (e.g., inspect IV sites, skin, and mucous membranes; use extreme care during invasive procedures; test urine, emesis, stool, and secretions for occult blood).

CONVENTIONAL PACLITAXEL: Neutrophil nadir occurs around day 11; see Dose Adjustments. ▪ Obtain baseline ECG; arrhythmias occur frequently. Con-tinuous cardiac monitoring required for all patients with an abnormal baseline ECG or those who experienced conduction arrhythmias during administration of a previous dose. ▪ Monitoring of cardiac function is

recommended when paclitaxel is used in combination with doxorubicin; see doxorubicin monograph. ▪ Anaphylaxis and severe hypersensitivity reactions have been reported. Fatal reactions have occurred despite premedication.
▪ Most severe hypersensitivity reactions occur in the first hour; chest pain, dyspnea, flushing, and tachycardia were the most frequent initial symptoms; abdominal pain, diaphoresis, extremity pain, and hypertension also occurred. Monitor all vital signs, including BP continuously for the first 30 minutes of the infusion and at frequent intervals after that. Incidence seems to decrease with subsequent doses. ▪ Treatment can often be continued in patients with mild hypersensitivity reactions if proper premedication is given. ▪ Monitor injection site carefully; avoid extravasation. Incidence of inflammation increased with 24-hour infusions. Injection site reactions may occur during administration or be delayed by 7 to 10 days. Recurrence of skin reactions at a site of previous extravasation following administration of paclitaxel ("recall") has been reported.

ABRAXANE: Limited infusion time (30 minutes) reduces the likelihood of infusion-related reactions; however, they have been reported; monitor for S/S; see Precautions. ▪ Based on patient history, a baseline ECG may be indicated.

Patient Education: ALL FORMULATIONS: Males and females should avoid conception; nonhormonal birth control recommended. ▪ Review of monitoring requirements and adverse events before therapy imperative. ▪ Report any unusual or unexpected symptoms, side effects, pain or burning at injection site, signs of infection (e.g., chills, fever, night sweats), signs of sensory neuropathy (e.g., numbness, tingling, or burning in hands and/or feet), or signs of bleeding (e.g., bruising, tarry stools, blood in urine, pinpoint red spots on skin) as soon as possible. ▪ Avoid tasks that require mental alertness (e.g., driving, operating machinery) until the effect of the medication is known. Side effects such as fatigue, lethargy, and malaise may affect the ability to perform these tasks. ▪ See Appendix D, p. 1434. ▪ Obtain name and telephone number of a contact person for emergencies, questions, or problems. ▪ Seek resources for counseling or supportive therapy. ▪ Manufacturer provides a patient information booklet.

Maternal/Child: ALL FORMULATIONS: Category D: males and females should avoid pregnancy. May cause fetal harm. ▪ Discontinue breast-feeding. ▪ Safety and effectiveness for use in pediatric patients not established.

CONVENTIONAL PACLITAXEL: CNS toxicity (rarely associated with death) was reported in one pediatric trial using high-dose paclitaxel. Use of antihistamines and the ethanol contained in the paclitaxel may have contributed to toxicity noted.

Elderly: ALL FORMULATIONS: Studies suggest response is similar to that seen in younger patients.

CONVENTIONAL PACLITAXEL: Incidence of side effects, including myelosuppression, neuropathy, and cardiovascular events, may be increased in the elderly.

DRUG/LAB INTERACTIONS

ALL FORMULATIONS

Do not administer **chloroquine or live virus vaccines** to patients receiving antineoplastic agents.

CONVENTIONAL PACLITAXEL

Formal drug interaction studies have not been conducted.
To reduce potential for profound myelosuppression when using paclitaxel

and **cisplatin** concurrently, give paclitaxel first, then cisplatin. ▪ Neurotoxicity and symptomatic motor dysfunction occurring with higher doses (greater than 250 mg/M²) may be potentiated by **cisplatin and filgrastim (G-CSF)**. ▪ May cause additive effects with **bone marrow–suppressing agents, radiation therapy, or agents that cause blood dyscrasias** (e.g., amphotericin B, antithyroid agents [methimazole (Tapazole)], azathioprine [Imuran], chloramphenicol, ganciclovir [Cytovene], interferon, plicamycin [Mithracin], zidovudine [AZT, Retrovir]). Reduced doses may be required. ▪ May increase levels of **doxorubicin** and its active metabolite when drugs are used in combination. ▪ Metabolized by **cytochrome P₄₅₀ isoenzymes CYP3A4 and CYP2C8.** Use caution when administered concomitantly with known **substrates** (e.g., buspirone [BuSpar], eletriptan [Relpax], felodipine [Plendil], midazolam [Versed], sildenafil [Viagra, Revatio], simvastatin [Zocor], and triazolam [Halcion]), **inhibitors** (e.g., atazanavir [Reyataz], clarithromycin [Biaxin], indinavir [Crixivan], itraconazole [Sporanox], ketoconazole [Nizoral], nefazodone, nelfinavir [Viracept], ritonavir [Norvir], saquinavir [Invirase], and telithromycin [Ketek]), and **inducers** (e.g., rifampin [Rifadin] and carbamazepine [Tegretol]) of **CYP3A4.** ▪ **Other medications that are substrates and/or inducers of CYP3A4** (e.g., ritonavir [Norvir], saquinavir [Invirase], indinavir [Crixivan], and nelfinavir [Viracept]) may alter the metabolism of paclitaxel but have not been evaluated in clinical trials. ▪ Dexamethasone (Decadron), diphenhydramine (Benadryl), cimetidine (Tagamet), and ranitidine (Zantac) do not affect the protein binding of paclitaxel.

ABRAXANE
Drug interaction studies have not been conducted. See All Formulations above. ▪ Use caution when administering with medicines **known to inhibit or induce CYP2C8 or CYP3A4.** Drugs that may inhibit these enzymes include ketoconazole (Nizoral) and other imidazole antifungals, erythromycin, fluoxetine (Prozac), gemfibrozil (Lopid), cimetidine (Tagamet), ritonavir (Norvir), saquinavir (Invirase), indinavir (Crixivan), and nelfinavir (Viracept). Drugs that may induce these enzymes include rifampin (Rifadin), carbamazepine (Tegretol), phenytoin (Dilantin), efavirenz (Sustiva), nevirapine (Viramune).

SIDE EFFECTS
CONVENTIONAL PACLITAXEL
Dose dependent and generally reversible, but may be fatal. All patients were premedicated to prevent hypersensitivity reactions. Abnormal ECG, alopecia, arthralgia/myalgia, asthenia, autonomic neuropathy resulting in paralytic ileus, bleeding, bone marrow suppression (anemia, leukopenia, neutropenia, thrombocytopenia), bradycardia, CHF (including cardiac dysfunction and reduction in left ventricular ejection fraction or ventricular failure [more common in patients receiving combination therapy with anthracyclines]), diarrhea, elevated bilirubin, elevated alkaline phosphatase, elevated AST, febrile neutropenia, fever, fluid retention and edema, hypersensitivity reactions (moderate, [e.g., dyspnea, flushing, hypotension, rash, tachycardia]; severe [e.g., chest pain, dyspnea requiring bronchodilators, hypotension requiring treatment, generalized urticaria]), hypertension, hypotension, infections including opportunistic infections (chills, fever, night-sweats), injection site reactions (cellulitis, fibrosis, induration, necrosis, phlebitis, skin exfoliation), mucositis, nausea and vomiting, numbness, peripheral neuropathy, optic nerve and/or visual disturbances,

respiratory reactions (interstitial pneumonia, lung fibrosis, pleural effusions, pulmonary embolism, respiratory failure), Stevens-Johnson syndrome, toxic epidermal necrolysis, and visual disturbances. A grand mal seizure occurred in one patient. Other side effects (e.g., cardiac arrest, cardiac ischemia/infarction, CVA, hepatic necrosis, and hepatic encephalopathy leading to death, intestinal obstruction, intestinal perforation, ischemic colitis, pancreatitis, thrombosis/embolism) and many others have been reported rarely. A higher incidence of elevated liver function tests and renal toxicity is seen in Kaposi's sarcoma patients.

Post-Marketing: Diffuse edema, thickening, and sclerosing of the skin; exacerbation of S/S of scleroderma; ototoxicity.

ABRAXANE

Most of the same side effects can occur with Abraxane as occur with Onxol or Taxol. Hypersensitivity reactions have occurred but are not usually severe; premedication is not indicated. Frequency of sensory neuropathy may increase with cumulative dose. Diarrhea and nausea and vomiting occur with moderately more frequency.

Post-Marketing: Cranial nerve palsies and skin reactions, including erythema, generalized or maculopapular rash, photosensitivity, radiation recall phenomenon, and palmar-plantar erythrodysaesthesia (in patients previously exposed to capecitabine [Xeloda]). Rare reports of severe hypersensitivity reactions have occurred with Abraxane.

ANTIDOTE

Keep physician informed of all side effects. Most will be treated symptomatically as indicated. Most hypersensitivity reactions will subside with temporary discontinuation of paclitaxel, and incidence seems to decrease with subsequent doses. Moderate reactions such as dyspnea, flushing, hypotension, skin reactions, or tachycardia do not usually require interruption of treatment. Severe reactions may require epinephrine (Adrenalin), antihistamines (e.g., diphenhydramine [Benadryl]), corticosteroids (e.g., dexamethasone [Decadron]), or bronchodilators (e.g., albuterol [Ventolin], theophylline [aminophylline]). Most severe reactions should not be rechallenged, but some patients tolerated subsequent doses of **conventional paclitaxel;** see Contraindications. Neutropenia can be profound, and the nadir usually occurs about day 11 with **conventional paclitaxel.** Recovery is generally rapid and spontaneous but may be treated with filgrastim (G-CSF, Neupogen, pegfilgrastim [Neulasta]). Severe thrombocytopenia (nadir day 8 or 9 with **conventional paclitaxel**) may require platelet transfusions; has been treated with oprelvekin (Neumega). Severe anemia (less than 8 Gm/dL) may require packed cell transfusions, moderate anemia (less than 11 Gm/dL) may be treated with darbepoetin alfa (Aranesp) or epoetin alfa (Epogen). Hypotension and bradycardia do not usually occur at the same time except in hypersensitivity. Treat only if symptomatic. Some arrhythmias (e.g., nonspecific repolarization abnormalities, sinus tachycardia, and PVCs) are common and may not require intervention. Treat any serious or symptomatic arrhythmia (e.g., conduction abnormalities, ventricular tachycardia) promptly and monitor continuously during subsequent doses. Neurologic symptoms tend to worsen with each course; see Dose Adjustments. Usually improve within several months. Severe peripheral neuropathies or seizure may necessitate discontinuation of paclitaxel. There is no specific antidote for overdose. Supportive therapy will help sustain the patient in toxicity. Resuscitate if indicated.

PALIFERMIN
(**PAL**-lih-fur-min)
Kepivance, KGF

Growth factor

pH 6.5

USUAL DOSE

Administered as an IV bolus injection for 3 consecutive days before and 3 consecutive days after myelotoxic therapy (a total of 6 doses). Do not administer within 24 hours before, during infusion of, or within 24 hours after administration of myelotoxic chemotherapy. Has resulted in increased severity and duration of oral mucositis. Myelotoxic therapy is high-dose chemotherapy, with or without radiation, that is destructive to bone marrow or any of its components. Followed by bone marrow transplant/hematopoietic stem cell support.

Pre-myelotoxic therapy (first 3 doses): Administer 60 mcg/kg/day for 3 consecutive days before myelotoxic therapy, with the third dose 24 to 48 hours before myelotoxic therapy.

Post-myelotoxic therapy (last 3 doses): Administer 60 mcg/kg/day for 3 consecutive days post-myelotoxic therapy; the first of these doses should be administered after, but on the same day of, hematopoietic stem cell infusion and at least 4 days after the most recent administration of palifermin. See Precautions.

DOSE ADJUSTMENTS

None indicated. Gender-related differences were not observed. ▪ No dose adjustment is recommended in impaired renal function. ▪ Pharmacokinetic studies have not been performed for pediatric patients or for patients with hepatic insufficiency.

DILUTION

Available as a lyophilized powder in a 6.25-mg single vial. Reconstitute by slowly injecting 1.2 mL SW into vial. Final concentration is 5 mg/mL. Swirl contents gently. **Do not shake.** Dissolution should take less than 3 minutes. Solution is clear and colorless. Do not use if particulates are present or if solution is discolored.

Filters: Manufacturer states, "Do not filter the reconstituted solution during preparation or administration."

Storage: Keep vials in carton until use. Store at 2° to 8° C (36° to 46° F). Protect from light. Do not use beyond expiration date on vial. Reconstituted product should be used immediately but can be stored up to 24 hours if refrigerated and stored in its carton. Do not freeze. Solution may be warmed to RT before injection but should not be left at RT for more than 1 hour and must be protected from light.

COMPATIBILITY

Specific information not available; however, manufacturer states, "If heparin is used to maintain an IV line, saline should be used to flush the line before and after administration since palifermin has been shown to bind to heparin in vitro."

RATE OF ADMINISTRATION

A single dose administered as an IV bolus injection. If heparin is used to maintain an IV line, flush the line with NS before and after administration.

ACTIONS

Human keratinocyte growth factor (KGF) produced by recombinant DNA technology. Binding of KGF to its receptor results in proliferation, differentiation, and migration of epithelial cells. KGF receptors are present on the epithelial cells in many tissues, including the tongue, buccal mucosa, esophagus, stomach, intestine, salivary gland, lung, liver, pancreas, kidney, bladder, mammary gland, skin (hair follicles and sebaceous gland), and the lens of the eye. KGF stimulates the growth of cells in tissues such as the skin and the epithelial layer of the mouth, stomach, and colon. Protects the epithelial cells that line the mouth and GI tract from the damage caused by chemotherapy and radiation and stimulates the growth and development of new epithelial cells. Average half-life is 4.5 hours (range: 3.3 to 5.7 hours).

INDICATIONS AND USES

To decrease the incidence and duration of severe oral mucositis in patients with hematologic malignancies who are receiving myelotoxic therapy (high-dose chemotherapy), with or without radiation therapy, and who require hematopoietic stem cell support. ▪ Safety and efficacy for use in patients with nonhematologic malignancies not established; see Precautions.

Investigational uses: Studies to determine whether palifermin can be used safely in other types of cancer are in progress.

CONTRAINDICATIONS

Hypersensitivity to palifermin, *E. coli*-derived proteins, or any other component of the product (e.g., L-histidine, mannitol, polysorbate 20, sucrose).

PRECAUTIONS

Safety and efficacy has not been established in patients with nonhematologic malignancies. Effect of palifermin on stimulation of KGF receptor–expressing, non-hematopoietic tumors in patients is not known. There is some evidence of tumor growth and stimulation in cell cultures and in animal models of non-hematopoietic human tumors.

Monitor: Monitor improvement in symptoms of oral mucositis. ▪ Monitor for the appearance of mucocutaneous adverse effects (e.g., edema, erythema, oral/perioral dysesthesia [impairment of sensitivity to touch], rash, taste alteration, tongue discoloration, tongue thickening).

Patient Education: Review possible side effects. ▪ Promptly report side effects (e.g., edema, impairment of sensitivity to touch [especially around the mouth], rash, taste alteration, tongue discoloration, tongue thickening). ▪ Inform patient of the evidence of tumor growth and stimulation in cell cultures and animal models of non-hematopoietic human tumors.

Maternal/Child: Category C: potential benefit to mother must justify potential risk to fetus. ▪ Use caution in breast-feeding; risk to infant unknown. ▪ Safety and effectiveness for use in pediatric patients not established.

Elderly: Age-related differences have not been observed.

DRUG/LAB INTERACTIONS

Formal studies have not been conducted. ▪ Binds to **heparin** in vitro. If heparin is used to maintain an IV line, NS should be used to flush the line before and after palifermin administration. ▪ Do not administer within 24 hours before, during infusion of, or within 24 hours after administration of **myelotoxic chemotherapy.** Has resulted in increased severity and duration of oral mucositis.

SIDE EFFECTS

The most common serious side effects are fever, GI events, respiratory events, and skin rash. Other commonly reported reactions include arthralgia, edema, elevated serum amylase and lipase, hypertension, oral toxicities (alteration of taste, oral/perioral dysesthesia, tongue discoloration, tongue thickening), pain, paresthesia, proteinuria, and skin toxicities (erythema, pruritus, rash). Has the potential for immunogenicity, but the clinical significance is unknown.

Post-Marketing: Anaphylaxis, edema of the face and mouth, palmar-plantar erythrodysesthesia syndrome (dysesthesia, edema on the palms and soles, erythema), tongue disorders (e.g., bumps, edema, redness), transient hyperpigmentation of the skin, vaginal edema and erythema.

ANTIDOTE

Notify physician of all side effects. Most will be treated symptomatically.

PALONOSETRON
(**pal**-oh-**NOH**-seh-tron)
Aloxi

Antiemetic
(5HT$_3$ receptor antagonist)

pH 4.5 to 5.5

USUAL DOSE

Chemotherapy-induced nausea and vomiting: A single dose of 0.25 mg approximately 30 minutes before the start of chemotherapy. Safety and effectiveness of consecutive or alternate-day dosing has not been evaluated. Has been coadministered with corticosteroids (e.g., dexamethasone [Decadron]) and metoclopramide (Reglan); see Drug/Lab Interactions.

Postoperative nausea and vomiting: A single dose of 0.075 mg immediately before induction of anesthesia.

DOSE ADJUSTMENTS

No dose adjustment required based on age or race or in patients with any degree of renal or hepatic impairment.

DILUTION

Available in 0.25 mg/5 mL and 0.075 mg/1.5 mL single-use vials. May be given undiluted.

Filters: No data available from manufacturer.

Storage: Before use, store at CRT. Protect from freezing and light.

COMPATIBILITY   (Underline Indicates Conflicting Compatibility Information)

Consider any drug NOT listed as compatible to be INCOMPATIBLE until consulting a pharmacist; specific conditions may apply.

Manufacturer states, "Should not be mixed with other drugs. Flush the infusion line with NS before and after administration."

One source suggests the following **compatibilities:**

Additive: *Not recommended by manufacturer.* Dexamethasone (Decadron).

Y-site: Ampicillin/sulbactam (Unasyn), atropine, carboplatin (Paraplatin), cefazolin (Ancef), cefotetan, cisatracurium (Nimbex), cisplatin (Platinol), cyclophosphamide (Cytoxan), dacarbazine (DTIC), docetaxel (Taxotere), famotidine (Pepcid IV), fentanyl (Sublimaze), fluorouracil (5-FU), gemcitabine (Gemzar), gentamicin, glycopyrrolate (Robinul), heparin, hetastarch in lactated electrolyte (Hextend), hydromorphone (Dilaudid), ifosfamide (Ifex), irinotecan (Camptosar), lidocaine, lorazepam (Ativan), mannitol (Osmitrol), meperidine (Demerol), metoclopramide (Reglan), metronidazole (Flagyl IV), midazolam (Versed), neostigmine, morphine, oxaliplatin (Eloxatin), paclitaxel (Taxol), potassium chloride, prometha-zine (Phenergan), rocuronium (Zemuron), succinylcholine (Anectine), sufentanil (Sufenta), topotecan (Hycamtin), vancomycin, vecuronium (Norcuron).

RATE OF ADMINISTRATION
Flush the infusion line with NS before and after administration.

Chemotherapy-induced nausea and vomiting: A single dose as an IV injection equally distributed over 30 seconds.

Postoperative nausea and vomiting: A single dose as an IV injection equally distributed over 10 seconds.

ACTIONS
A long-acting (up to 120 hours [5 days]) antinauseant and antiemetic agent. A selective antagonist of specific serotonin ($5HT_3$) receptors. Has a strong binding affinity for this receptor and little or no affinity for other receptors. Chemotherapeutic agents such as cisplatin increase the release of serotonin from specific cells in the GI tract, causing emesis. By antagonizing these receptors, the incidence and severity of chemotherapy-induced nausea and vomiting are decreased. 62% bound to plasma protein. Partially metabo-lized to selected metabolites. These metabolic pathways are mediated by multiple CYP enzymes; however, it is not an inhibitor or an inducer of CYP enzyme activity. Eliminated slowly from the body through both metabolic pathways and renal excretion. Has a prolonged half-life of approximately 40 hours. 80% of a single dose was recovered in urine within 144 hours.

INDICATIONS AND USES
Prevention of acute nausea and vomiting associated with initial and repeat courses of *moderately and highly emetogenic* cancer chemotherapy. ▪ Prevention of delayed nausea and vomiting associated with initial and repeat courses of *moderately emetogenic* cancer chemotherapy. Studies identified cisplatin (Platinol) in doses equal to or greater than 70 mg/M^2 and cyclophosphamide (Cytoxan) in doses equal to or greater than 1,100 mg/M^2 as *highly emetogenic*. Studies identified cisplatin in doses equal to or less than 50 mg/M^2, cyclophosphamide in doses less than 1,100 mg/M^2, doxorubicin (Adriamycin) in doses greater than 25 mg/M^2, methotrexate in doses greater than 250 mg/M^2, and carboplatin (Parapla-tin), epirubicin (Ellence), and irinotecan (Camptosar) in standard doses as *moderately emetogenic*. ▪ Prevention of postoperative nausea and vomit-ing (PONV) for up to 24 hours following surgery. Efficacy beyond 24 hours has not been demonstrated.

CONTRAINDICATIONS
Known hypersensitivity to palonosetron or any of its components. ▪ See Precautions.

PRECAUTIONS
Cross-sensitivity may occur with other selective $5HT_3$ receptor antagonists (e.g., dolasetron [Anzemet], granisetron [Kytril], ondansetron [Zofran]). ▪ Routine prophylaxis is not recommended for patients in whom there is little expectation of PONV. However, for patients in whom nausea and vomiting must be avoided during the postoperative period, prophylaxis is

recommended even when the incidence of PONV is low. ▪ Palonosetron does not appear to have any effect on ECG intervals, including QT$_C$ duration.

Monitor: Observe closely. Monitor VS. ▪ Ambulate slowly to avoid orthostatic hypotension. ▪ Stool softeners or laxatives may be required to prevent constipation.

Patient Education: Request assistance with ambulation. ▪ Used to prevent and/or treat both early and late N/V caused by chemotherapy. Report persistent N/V promptly. ▪ Maintain adequate hydration. ▪ Review prescription and nonprescription medications with health care provider. Drug interactions are possible, especially with diuretics or antiarrhythmics. ▪ Review other medical conditions with health care provider.

Maternal/Child: Category B: use during pregnancy only if clearly needed. Animal studies did not identify evidence of impaired fertility or harm to rat or rabbit fetuses. ▪ Safety for use during breast-feeding not established; effects unknown, but potential for tumorigenicity is a concern. Discontinue breast-feeding. ▪ Safety and effectiveness for use in pediatric patients under 18 years of age not established.

Elderly: Safety and effectiveness similar to younger adults; however, greater sensitivity in some elderly cannot be ruled out. No dose adjustment or special monitoring required.

DRUG/LAB INTERACTIONS

Eliminated through both renal excretion and metabolic pathways; potential for clinically significant drug interactions is considered to be low. ▪ Does not induce or inhibit the cytochrome P$_{450}$ drug metabolizing system. ▪ Has been safely administered with analgesics, antiemetics/antinauseants, antispasmodics, anticholinergic agents, and corticosteroids. ▪ Has been safely administered with PO metoclopramide (10 mg 4 times daily). ▪ Has been administered with oral aprepitant (Emend). ▪ Does not appear to inhibit the antitumor activity of emetogenic cancer chemotherapies. ▪ See Precautions.

SIDE EFFECTS

Abdominal pain, constipation, diarrhea, dizziness, fatigue, headache, and insomnia occur in 2% or more patients. Among other reported side effects in 1% or more patients were anxiety, hyperkalemia, and nonsustained tachycardia, bradycardia, or hypotension.

Overdose: Doses more than 20 times the recommended dose did not cause significant problems. Collapse, convulsions, cyanosis, gasping, and pallor occurred in animal studies with rats and mice.

Post-Marketing: Hypersensitivity reactions, including anaphylaxis and injection site reactions (burning, induration, pain) (rare).

ANTIDOTE

Most side effects will be treated symptomatically. Keep physician informed. There is no specific antidote. Has a large volume of distribution; dialysis not likely to be effective in overdose. Treat hypersensitivity reactions and resuscitate as indicated.

PAMIDRONATE DISODIUM
(pah-**MIH**-droh-nayt **DYE**-so-dee-um)

APD, Aredia

Bone resorption inhibitor
Antihypercalcemic
(bisphosphonate)

pH 6 to 7.4

USUAL DOSE

Prehydration required. Do not exceed a single dose of 90 mg. See Precautions and Monitor.

Moderate hypercalcemia (corrected serum calcium of 12 to 13.5 mg/dL): One dose of 60 to 90 mg as an infusion.

Severe hypercalcemia (corrected serum calcium greater than 13.5 mg/dL): One dose of 90 mg as an infusion. Serum calcium levels should fall into the normal range (8.5 to 10.5 mg/100 mL [1 dL], corrected for serum albumin).

Experience is limited, but retreatment with the same dose may be considered if hypercalcemia recurs; wait at least 7 days from completion of first infusion to allow full response. Always used in conjunction with adequate hydration and appropriate testing. See Precautions/Monitor.

Paget's disease: 30 mg/day as an infusion for 3 consecutive days. Selected patients have been retreated with the same dose when indicated. Experience limited. Prehydration required; see Precautions and Monitor.

Osteolytic bone lesions of multiple myeloma: 90 mg as an infusion once every 30 days. Optimal duration of therapy not known. Withhold dose if renal function has deteriorated; see Dose Adjustments, Precautions, and Monitor.

Osteolytic bone metastases of breast cancer: 90 mg as an infusion every 3 to 4 weeks. Optimum duration of therapy not known. Withhold dose if renal function has deteriorated; see Dose Adjustments, Precautions, and Monitor.

DOSE ADJUSTMENTS

Lower-dose regimen may be appropriate in impaired renal or hepatic function and in the elderly. No experience with creatinine above 5 mg/100 mL (1 dL). ▪ See Precautions and Elderly.

Osteolytic bone lesions of multiple myeloma and osteolytic bone metastases of breast cancer: Withhold dose if renal function has deteriorated. Renal deterioration is defined as an increase of 0.5 mg/dL in patients with a *normal* baseline creatinine or an increase of 1 mg/dL in patients with *abnormal* baseline creatinine. One study suggests that treatment should not be resumed until SCr has returned to within 10% of baseline value.

DILUTION

Reconstitute each 30- or 90-mg vial with 10 mL SW for injection. Dissolve completely (3 or 9 mg/mL).

Hypercalcemia of malignancy: Further dilute a single dose in 1,000 mL NS, ½NS, or D5W. A minimum of 500 mL diluent may be used if absolutely necessary in patients with compromised cardiovascular status.

Paget's disease: Further dilute a single daily dose in 500 mL NS, ½NS, or D5W.

Osteolytic bone lesions of multiple myeloma: Further dilute each 90-mg dose in 500 mL NS, ½NS, or D5W.

Osteolytic bone metastases of breast cancer: Further dilute each 90-mg dose in 250 mL NS, ½NS, or D5W.

Storage: Before reconstitution, store at CRT. After reconstitution, may be refrigerated for up to 24 hours. Stable after dilution for 24 hours at room temperature.

COMPATIBILITY

Manufacturer states, "Should be given in a single intravenous solution and line separate from all other drugs, and do not mix with calcium-containing solutions (e.g., Ringer's solutions)."

RATE OF ADMINISTRATION

Use of a microdrip (60 gtt/mL) or an infusion pump recommended for even distribution. Do not exceed recommended rate of infusion. Duration should be no less than 2 hours. Too-rapid infusion rate may lead to overdose, elevated BUN and creatinine levels, and renal tubular necrosis. Rate recommendations vary considerably. They are based on specific clinical trials for each diagnosis. In some trials a rate of up to 1 mg/min has been used with caution.

Hypercalcemia of malignancy: A 60-mg dose or 90-mg dose equally distributed over 2 to 24 hours. Longer infusion times (i.e., greater than 2 hours) may reduce the risk of renal toxicity, particularly in patients with pre-existing renal insufficiency.

Paget's disease: A single dose over 4 hours.

Osteolytic bone lesions of multiple myeloma: A single dose over 4 hours.

Osteolytic bone metastases of breast cancer: A single dose over 2 hours.

ACTIONS

A bisphosphonate hypocalcemic agent. Reduces serum calcium concentrations by inhibiting accelerated bone resorption. Binds to preformed bone surfaces and may block bone mineral dissolution. Effectively inhibits accelerated bone resorption resulting from osteoclast hyperactivity induced by various tumors. Does not inhibit bone formation and mineralization. Plasma levels achieve some reduction in calcium levels in 24 to 48 hours, and maximal response in 4 to 7 days. Rapidly adsorbed by bone. Is not metabolized. Half-life is approximately 21 to 35 hours. Slowly excreted in urine.

INDICATIONS AND USES

Treatment of moderate to severe hypercalcemia of malignancy in patients with or without bone metastasis, in conjunction with adequate hydration. Symptoms of hypercalcemia may include anorexia, bone pain, confusion, constipation, dehydration, depression, fatigue, lethargy, muscle weakness, nausea and vomiting, and polyuria. Severe dehydration may lead to renal insufficiency. With high levels of serum calcium, cardiac manifestations (e.g., bradycardia, cardiac arrest, ventricular arrhythmias), and neurologic symptoms (e.g., coma, seizures, and death) may occur. ■ Treatment of Paget's disease. ■ Adjunct in treatment of osteolytic lesions of multiple myeloma and osteolytic bone metastases of breast cancer.

Unlabeled uses: Prevent or decrease bone loss in women undergoing chemotherapy.

CONTRAINDICATIONS

Hypersensitivity to pamidronate or other bisphosphonates (e.g., alendronate [Fosamax], risedronate [Actonel], zoledronic acid [Reclast, Zometa]).

PRECAUTIONS

Calcium is bound to albumin. Total serum calcium levels in patients who have hypercalcemia of malignancy may not reflect the severity of the hypocalcemia because concomitant hypoalbuminemia is commonly present. Measurement with ionized calcium levels is preferred. If unavailable, all calcium measurement should be corrected for albumin to establish a basis for treatment and evaluation of treatment. ■ Mild or asymptomatic hypercalcemia will be treated with conservative measures (e.g., saline hydration, with or without diuretics [after correcting hypovolemia]). Consider patient's cardiovascular status. Corticosteroids may be indicated if the underlying cancer is sensitive (e.g., hematologic cancers). ■ May be used adjunctively with chemotherapy, radiation, or surgery. ■ May cause renal toxicity. Deterioration in renal function progressing to renal failure has been reported and has occurred after the initial or a single dose of pamidronate. Patients with pre-existing renal impairment may be at increased risk for developing toxicity. Do not exceed dose of 90 mg. ■ Osteonecrosis of the jaw (ONJ) has been reported in patients receiving bisphosphonates. The majority of cases have been in cancer patients. Risk factors include cancer, concomitant therapy (e.g., chemotherapy, radiotherapy, corticosteroids), and co-morbid conditions (e.g., anemia, coagulopathies, infection, pre-existing oral disease). Literature and case reports suggest a higher frequency of ONJ in advanced breast cancer or multiple myeloma based on tumor type (breast cancer, multiple myeloma) and dental status (dental extraction, periodontal disease, local trauma including poorly fitting dentures). Cancer patients should maintain good oral hygiene. Consider dental exam and appropriate preventive dentistry before beginning therapy with bisphosphonates. Avoid invasive dental procedures during bisphosphonate therapy. Dental surgery may exacerbate ONJ in patients who develop ONJ while on bisphosphonate therapy. ■ Severe and occasionally incapacitating bone, joint, and/or muscle pain has been reported rarely. Onset of symptoms varied from one day to several months after beginning treatment with pamidronate. In most cases, pain resolves when pamidronate is discontinued; however, in some patients symptoms resolved slowly or persisted. ■ Patients with a history of thyroid surgery may have relative hypoparathyroidism that may predispose them to hypocalcemia with pamidronate. *Osteolytic bone lesions of multiple myeloma and osteolytic bone metastases of breast cancer:* Patients being treated for multiple myeloma and bone metastases should have the dose withheld if renal function has deteriorated; see Dose Adjustments. Use is not recommended in patients with severe renal impairment being treated for bone metastases. See Monitor and Dose Adjustments. Limited information available on use in multiple myeloma patients with a CrCl less than 30 mL/min. In clinical trials, patients with a SCr above 3 mg/dL were excluded. ■ In the absence of hypercalcemia, patients with *multiple myeloma* or *Paget's disease of the bone* or patients with *predominantly lytic bone metastases* who are at risk for calcium and vitamin D deficiency should be given oral calcium and vitamin D to reduce the risk of hypocalcemia.

Monitor: Obtain baseline measurements of serum calcium (corrected for serum albumin), electrolytes, phosphate, magnesium, and creatinine and CBC with differential and hematocrit/hemoglobin. Monitor all closely as indicated by baseline results (may be daily). Serum phosphate levels will decrease and usually require treatment. ■ Monitor renal function before each treatment; nephropathy has been reported; see Precautions. ▪ Monitor serum alkaline phosphatase during therapy for Paget's disease. ▪ Patients with cancer-related hypercalcemia are frequently dehydrated. Must be adequately hydrated orally and/or IV before treatment is initiated. Hydration with saline is preferred to facilitate renal excretion of calcium and correct dehydration. A pretreatment urine output of 2 L/day is recommended. Maintain adequate hydration and urine output throughout treatment. ▪ Avoid overhydration in patients with compromised cardiovascular status. Observe frequently for signs of fluid overload. Correct hypovolemia before using diuretics. ▪ Monitor patients with pre-existing anemia, leukopenia, or thrombocytopenia very carefully during treatment and the first 2 weeks following treatment. *Osteolytic bone lesions of multiple myeloma:* Adequately hydrate patients with marked Bence-Jones proteinuria and dehydration before pamidronate infusion.

Patient Education: Regular visits and assessment of lab tests imperative. ▪ Dietary restriction of calcium and vitamin D may be required. ▪ Take only prescribed meds. ▪ Report abdominal cramps, chills, confusion, fever, muscle spasms, sore throat, and/or any new medical problems promptly. ▪ Report development of bone, joint, or muscle pain promptly. Onset of pain is variable. ▪ Avoid pregnancy; use of nonhormonal birth control suggested.

Maternal/Child: Category D: should not be used during pregnancy. May cause fetal harm. Avoid pregnancy; use of birth control necessary during treatment and for an undetermined time after treatment; see prescribing information. ▪ Safety for use during breast-feeding not established. ▪ Safety for use in pediatric patients not established.

Elderly: Response similar to that seen in younger patients. ▪ Use with caution based on age-related impaired organ function and concomitant disease or drug therapy; monitor renal function closely. See Dose Adjustments. ▪ Monitor fluid and electrolyte status carefully to avoid overhydration or electrolyte imbalance. Use of lower fluid volume may be required; see Dilution.

DRUG/LAB INTERACTIONS

Use caution when administered with other **potentially nephrotoxic drugs** (e.g., aminoglycosides [tobramycin, gentamicin], cisplatin [Platinol]). ▪ Concurrent administration with **furosemide** (Lasix) does not affect calcium-lowering action of pamidronate. ▪ Does not interfere with any known primary cancer therapy. ▪ Effects may be antagonized by **calcium-containing preparations or vitamin D**; avoid use. ▪ Concurrent use with **thalidomide** (Thalomid) may increase risk of renal toxicity in patients with multiple myeloma.

SIDE EFFECTS

Average dose: Abdominal pain, anemia, anorexia, bone pain, confusion and visual hallucinations (sometimes in conjunction with electrolyte imbalance), constipation, fever (mild and transient), generalized pain, hypertension, hypocalcemia (abdominal cramps, confusion, muscle spasms), infusion site reaction (e.g., induration and pain on palpation, redness, swelling), musculoskeletal pain (bone, joint, and/or muscle pain), pruritus, rash, renal toxicity, seizures, urinary tract infections, vomiting. Fluid overload, hypokalemia, hypomagnesemia, and hypophosphatemia occur frequently with use of concurrent fluid and diuretics. Rare instances of hypersensitivity reactions, including anaphylaxis, angioedema, dyspnea, and hypotension, have occurred. Osteonecrosis (primarily of the jaw) has been reported (see Precautions).

Overdose: Occurs less frequently with lower dose range (30 to 60 mg). Fever (high), hypocalcemia, hypotension, leukopenia or lymphopenia (fever, chills, sore throat), transient taste perversion. Elevated BUN and CrCl levels and renal tubular necrosis may occur with excessive dose or rate of administration.

Post-Marketing: Conjunctivitis, focal segmental glomerulosclerosis (including the collapsing variant), hematuria, hypernatremia, influenza-like symptoms, nephrotic syndrome, orbital inflammation, reactivation of herpes simplex and herpes zoster.

ANTIDOTE

Keep physician informed of side effects. Some may respond to symptomatic treatment. Magnesium, phosphorus, and potassium may require replacement if depletion too severe. If mild, all will probably return toward normal in 7 to 10 days. For asymptomatic or mild to moderate hypocalcemia (6.5 to 8 mg/100 mL [1 dL] corrected for serum albumin), short-term calcium therapy (e.g., calcium gluconate) may be indicated. Discontinue drug for any symptoms of overdose. Monitor serum calcium and use vigorous IV hydration, with or without diuretics, for 2 to 3 days. Monitor intake and output to ensure adequacy and balance. Use short-term IV calcium therapy if indicated. High fever may respond to steroids. RBC transfusions may be required in anemia. Treat anaphylaxis and resuscitate as indicated.

PANCURONIUM BROMIDE BBW
(pan-kyou-**ROH**-nee-um **BRO**-myd)

Neuromuscular
blocking agent
(nondepolarizing)
Anesthesia adjunct

pH 4

USUAL DOSE
Adjunct to general anesthesia for adults and pediatric patients: Must be individualized, depending on previous drugs administered and degree and length of muscle relaxation required. Must be used with adequate anesthesia and/or sedation and after unconsciousness induced. Succinylcholine must show signs of wearing off before pancuronium is given. 0.04 to 0.1 mg/kg of body weight initially. 0.01 mg/kg in increments as required to maintain muscle relaxation; usually 25- to 60-minute intervals.
Endotracheal intubation: 0.06 to 0.1 mg/kg.
Support of intubated mechanically ventilated or respiratory-controlled adult ICU patients (unlabeled): *IV bolus injection:* 0.1 to 0.2 mg/kg every 1 to 3 hours. *Continuous infusion:* begin with a *loading dose* of 0.03 to 0.1 mg/kg followed by a *maintenance dose* of 0.06 to 0.1 mg/kg/hr. A lower-end or reduced dose may be indicated if administered more than 5 minutes after the start of an inhalation agent, when steady-state has been achieved, or in patients with organ dysfunction (e.g., impaired renal function). Adjust dose according to clinical assessment of the patient's response. Use of a peripheral nerve stimulator is recommended.

NEONATAL DOSE
Adjunct to general anesthesia: Extreme sensitivity to pancuronium exists during the first month of life. Begin with a test dose of 0.02 mg/kg and assess responsiveness. See Maternal/Child.

DOSE ADJUSTMENTS
See Drug/Lab Interactions; marked reduction of pancuronium dose may be required. ■ A higher total dose may be required in biliary or hepatic disease, but onset is slower and neuromuscular block is prolonged.

DILUTION
May be given undiluted or diluted in D5W, D5/½NS, D5NS, NS, or LR for use as an infusion.
Storage: Best if stored in refrigerator. Will maintain potency at room temperature for up to 6 months.

COMPATIBILITY
(Underline Indicates Conflicting Compatibility Information)
Consider any drug NOT listed as compatible to be INCOMPATIBLE until consulting a pharmacist; specific conditions may apply.
One source suggests the following **compatibilities:**
Additive: Ciprofloxacin (Cipro IV), verapamil.
Y-site: Aminophylline, cefazolin (Ancef), cefuroxime (Zinacef), dobutamine, dopamine, epinephrine (Adrenalin), esmolol (Brevibloc), etomidate (Amidate), fenoldopam (Corlopam), fentanyl (Sublimaze), fluconazole (Diflucan), gentamicin, heparin, hetastarch in electrolytes (Hextend), hydrocortisone sodium succinate (Solu-Cortef), isoproterenol (Isuprel), levofloxacin (Levaquin), lorazepam (Ativan), midazolam (Versed),

milrinone (Primacor), morphine, nitroglycerin IV, nitroprusside sodium, propofol (Diprivan), ranitidine (Zantac), sulfamethoxazole/trimethoprim, vancomycin.

RATE OF ADMINISTRATION
Adjunct to general anesthesia: A single dose over 60 to 90 seconds.
Mechanical ventilation support in ICU: See Usual Dose for specific rates and criteria.

ACTIONS
A skeletal muscle relaxant. Causes paralysis by interfering with neural transmission at the myoneural junction. Onset of action is dose dependent. Peak effect occurs in 3 to 4 minutes and lasts 30 to 45 minutes. It may take another 30 minutes or up to several hours before complete recovery occurs. Excreted in the urine.

INDICATIONS AND USES
Adjunctive to general anesthesia to facilitate endotracheal intubation and to relax skeletal muscles during surgery or mechanical ventilation.
Unlabeled uses: Support of intubated, mechanically ventilated, or respiratory-controlled patients in ICU.

CONTRAINDICATIONS
Known hypersensitivity to pancuronium or bromides; first trimester of pregnancy.

PRECAUTIONS
Usually administered by or under the direct observation of the anesthesiologist. Appropriate emergency drugs and equipment for monitoring the patient and responding to any medical emergency must be readily available. ▪ Severe anaphylactic reactions have been reported with neuromuscular blocking agents; some have been fatal. Use caution in patients who have had an anaphylactic reaction to another neuromuscular blocking agent (depolarizing or nondepolarizing); cross-reactivity has occurred. ▪ Repeated doses may produce a cumulative effect. ▪ Impaired pulmonary function or respiratory deficiencies can cause critical reactions. ▪ Use caution in impaired liver or kidney function, in patients with tachycardia, and in any patient who might develop adverse effects from an increase in HR. ▪ Myasthenia gravis increases sensitivity to drug. ▪ Long-term use (i.e., intensive care) may result in prolonged paralysis or skeletal muscle weakness. ▪ Acid base and/or electrolyte imbalance, debilitation, hypoxic episodes, and/or the use of other drugs (e.g., broad-spectrum antibiotics, narcotics, steroids) may prolong the effects of pancuronium.
Monitor: *All uses:* This drug produces apnea. Controlled artificial ventilation with oxygen must be continuous and under direct observation at all times. Maintain a patent airway. ▪ Use a peripheral nerve stimulator to monitor response to pancuronium and avoid overdose. ▪ Patient may be conscious and completely unable to communicate by any means. Pancuronium has no analgesic or sedative properties. ▪ Action is altered by dehydration, electrolyte imbalance, body temperatures, and acid-base imbalance. ▪ Hyperkalemia may cause cardiac arrhythmias and increased paralysis. ▪ See Precautions and Drug/Lab Interactions.
Mechanical ventilation support in ICU: Physical therapy is recommended to prevent muscular weakness, atrophy, and joint contracture. Muscular weakness may first be noticed during attempts to wean patients from the ventilator.

Maternal/Child: Category C: unknown potential hazards to fetus. Benefits must outweigh risks. Not recommended in first trimester. ▪ Has caused rare severe skeletal muscle weakness in neonates undergoing mechanical ventilation.

Elderly: Delay in onset time may be caused by slower circulation time in cardiovascular disease, old age, or edematous states; allow more time for drug to achieve maximum effect.

DRUG/LAB INTERACTIONS

May cause severe arrhythmias with **inhalant anesthetics** (e.g., enflurane, halothane) and in patients on chronic **tricyclic antidepressant therapy** (e.g., amitriptyline [Elavil]). ▪ Potentiated by **hypokalemia, some carcinomas, many antibiotics** (e.g., aminoglycosides [kanamycin (Kantrex), gentamicin], bacitracin, colistin [Coly-Mycin S], colistimethate [Coly-Mycin M], polymixin-B [Aerosporin], tetracyclines, piperacillin), **calcium salts, CO_2, diuretics, diazepam** (Valium) **and other muscle relaxants, digoxin, magnesium sulfate, quinidine, morphine, lidocaine, meperidine, propranalol** (Inderal), **succinylcholine, and others.** May need to reduce dose of pancuronium; use with caution. ▪ Recurrent paralysis may occur with **quinidine.** ▪ Effects may be decreased by **acetylcholine, anticholinesterases, aminophylline, azathioprine, carbamazepine, and potassium.** ▪ **Succinylcholine** must show signs of wearing off before pancuronium is given. Use caution.

SIDE EFFECTS

Increased HR, decrease in mean arterial pressure, prolonged action resulting in respiratory insufficiency or apnea and tachycardia. Airway closure caused by relaxation of epiglottis, pharynx, and tongue muscles. Hypersensitivity reactions are possible. Anaphylaxis, histamine release (e.g., bronchospasm, vasodilation, hypotension, cutaneous flushing), and shock may occur. Muscular weakness and atrophy may occur with long-term use (1 to 3 weeks).

ANTIDOTE

All side effects are medical emergencies. Treat symptomatically. Controlled artificial ventilation must be continuous. Pyridostigmine (Regonol) or neostigmine given with atropine will probably reverse the muscle relaxation. Not effective in all situations; may aggravate severe overdose. Resuscitate as necessary.

PANITUMUMAB BBW
(pan-i-**TUE**-moo-mab)

Vectibix

Antineoplastic
Immunosuppressant
Monoclonal Antibody

pH 5.6 to 6

USUAL DOSE

6 mg/kg as an infusion once every 14 days.

DOSE ADJUSTMENTS

Hold panitumumab for dermatologic toxicities that are Grade 3 or higher or are considered intolerable. If toxicity does not improve to less than or equal to Grade 2 within a month, permanently discontinue therapy. If dermatologic toxicity improves to less than or equal to Grade 2 and the patient is symptomatically improved after withholding no more than 2 doses of panitumumab, treatment may be resumed at 50% of the original dose. If toxicity recurs, permanently discontinue therapy. If toxicity does not recur, subsequent doses may be increased by increments of 25% of the original dose until the recommended dose of 6 mg/kg is reached. ▪ No dose adjustment indicated based on age (21 to 88 years), gender, race, mild-to-moderate renal or hepatic dysfunction, and EGFR (epidermal growth factor receptor) membrane-staining intensity (1+, 2+, 3+).

DILUTION

Solution may contain a small amount of visible, translucent-to-white, amorphous, and proteinaceous panitumumab particulates (will be removed by in-line filter). Do not use if solution is discolored. **Do not shake.** Withdraw calculated dose from vial. Dilute to a total volume of 100 mL with NS. Doses higher than 1,000 mg should be diluted to a volume of 150 mL. (Withdraw a volume of NS equal to the volume of the calculated dose from the infusion bag.) Final concentration should not exceed 10 mg/mL. Mix diluted solution by gentle inversion. **Do not shake.**

Filters: Must be administered through a low–protein binding, 0.2- or 0.22-micron, in-line filter.

Storage: Store unopened vials in refrigerator (2° to 8° C [36° to 46° F]). Protect from direct sunlight. Do not freeze. Diluted solutions should be discarded within 6 hours of preparation if stored at RT and within 24 hours if stored in refrigerator. Do not freeze. Single-dose vial; discard any unused product after entry into vial.

COMPATIBILITY

Manufacturer states, "Should not be mixed with, or administered as an infusion, with other medicinal products. No other medications should be added to solutions containing panitumumab."

RATE OF ADMINISTRATION

Flush line before and after panitumumab administration with NS. **Do not administer as an IV push or bolus.** Administer with an IV infusion pump using a low–protein binding, 0.2- or 0.22-micron, in-line filter.

A single dose equally distributed over 60 minutes. Doses over 1,000 mg should be administered over 90 minutes. Reduce rate of infusion by 50% in patients experiencing a Grade 1 or 2 infusion reaction.

ACTIONS

A genetically engineered recombinant, human IgG2 kappa monoclonal antibody that binds specifically to the human epidermal growth factor receptor (EGFR). EGFR is a transmembrane glycoprotein that is expressed in many normal epithelial tissues, including skin and hair follicles. Over-expression of EGFR is detected in many human cancers, including those of the colon and rectum. Interaction of EGFR with its normal ligands leads to a series of reactions that regulate the transcription of molecules involved with cellular growth and survival, motility, proliferation, and transformation. Panitumumab binds to EGFR on both normal and tumor cells, inhibiting the binding of normal ligands to EGFR. This competitive binding results in inhibition of cell growth, induction of apoptosis, decreased proinflammatory cytokine and vascular growth factor production, and internalization of EGFR. The end result is inhibition of growth and survival of selected human tumor cells that express EGFR. Half-life is approximately 7.5 days (range 3.6 to 10.9 days).

INDICATIONS AND USES

As a single agent in the treatment of EGFR-expressing, metastatic colorectal carcinoma with disease progression on or following chemotherapy regimens that contain fluoropyrimidine (fluorouracil [5-FU]), oxaliplatin (Eloxatin), and irinotecan (Camptosar). ■ Not recommended for treatment of colorectal cancer in patients whose tumor has KRAS mutations in codon 12 or 13. The benefit in this patient population has not been shown. ■ Not indicated for use in combination with fluorouracil (5-FU), oxaliplatin (Eloxatin), irinotecan (Camptosar), or any other chemotherapy agent with or without bevacizumab (Avastin). Combination use resulted in decreased progression-free survival and increased incidence of CTCAE Grade 3 to 5 adverse reactions.

CONTRAINDICATIONS

None known. Use with IFL (irinotecan [Camptosar], bolus fluorouracil [5-FU], and leucovorin calcium) chemotherapy is not recommended; see Precautions.

PRECAUTIONS

Panitumumab should be used only in patients whose tumor shows EGFR expression. Immunohistochemical evidence of EGFR expression should be obtained using specific test kits. Assessment of EGFR expression should be performed by qualified laboratories with demonstrated proficiency in the technology required for testing. ■ Dermatologic toxicities were reported in 89% of patients and were severe (CTCAE Grade 3 or higher) in 12% of patients. Manifestations included dermatitis acneform, dry skin, erythema, paronychia, pruritus, rash, skin exfoliation, and skin fissures. Severe dermatologic toxicities were complicated by infection, including sepsis, septic death, and abscesses requiring incision and drainage; see Dose Adjustments and Antidote. ■ Sunlight may exacerbate dermatologic toxicity. Protection from sun is advised; see Patient Education. ■ Infusion reactions, some severe, have been reported. Fatal reactions have occurred with other monoclonal antibody products. Administer in a facility with adequate emergency medical equipment and medications for treating these reactions and for responding to any medical emergency; see Rate of Administration and Antidote. ■ Pulmonary fibrosis has been reported (rare); see Monitor. ■ A protein substance. Potential for immunogenicity exists. Anti-panitumumab antibodies have been detected in a small number of patients. Significance unknown.

Monitor: Monitor vital signs prior to, during (as needed), and at the completion of the infusion. ▪ Monitor for S/S of hypersensitivity or infusion-related reactions. Severe reactions may include anaphylaxis, bronchospasm, chills, fever, and hypotension; see Side Effects. Mild to moderate infusion reactions may respond to a reduction in the rate of infusion; see Rate of Administration. Utility of premedication to minimize or prevent infusion-related reactions has not been determined. ▪ Monitor skin integrity. ▪ Monitor lung function. Discontinue therapy in patients who develop interstitial lung disease, pneumonitis, or lung infiltrates. ▪ Obtain baseline and monitor electrolytes periodically during and for 8 weeks after completion of therapy. Hypomagnesemia and hypocalcemia have been reported. Oral or IV electrolyte replacement may be required.

Patient Education: Avoid pregnancy. Nonhormonal birth control recommended for both men and women during and for 6 months following completion of therapy. ▪ Review side effects, including dermatologic toxicity, infusion reactions, pulmonary fibrosis, and potential for fetal harm. ▪ Report skin or ocular changes, cough, dyspnea, or infusion-related reactions promptly. ▪ Limit sun exposure. Use of sunscreen and hats recommended. ▪ Compliance with periodic lab work required.

Maternal/Child: Category C: safety for use in pregnancy has not been established. EGFR has been implicated in the control of prenatal development and may be essential for normal organogenesis, proliferation, and differentiation in the developing embryo. Human IgG crosses the placental barrier. Therefore, it is possible that panitumumab may be transmitted from the mother to the developing fetus. Appropriate contraceptive measures must be used during treatment with panitumumab; see Patient Education. ▪ Women who become pregnant during panitumumab therapy are encouraged to enroll in Amgen's Pregnancy Surveillance Program. ▪ Discontinue breast-feeding during and for 2 months after the completion of therapy. ▪ Safety and effectiveness for use in pediatric patients not established.

Elderly: Specific differences in safety and effectiveness compared to younger adults not noted.

DRUG/LAB INTERACTIONS

Formal drug interaction studies have not been conducted. ▪ Incidence and severity of GI toxicity (diarrhea) increased with **concomitant use of IFL chemotherapy** and panitumumab. Combination use is not recommended; see Precautions.

SIDE EFFECTS

The most commonly reported side effects are abdominal pain, constipation, diarrhea (including diarrhea resulting in dehydration), fatigue, hypomagnesemia, paronychia, nausea, and skin toxicity (e.g., dermatitis acneiform, erythema, exfoliation fissures, pruritus, rash). The most serious side effects reported include abdominal pain, constipation, hypomagnesemia, infusion reactions (e.g., anaphylaxis, bronchospasm, chills, dyspnea, fever, hypotension), nausea, pulmonary embolism, pulmonary fibrosis, severe dermatologic toxicity complicated by infectious sequelae and septic death, and vomiting. Other reported side effects include cough, fatigue, mucosal inflammation, ocular toxicity (conjunctivitis, eyelid/eye irritation, increased lacrimation, ocular hyperemia), peripheral edema, and stomatitis. Reactions requiring discontinuation of therapy included infusion reactions, paronychia, pulmonary fibrosis, and severe dermatologic toxicity. **Post-Marketing:** Angioedema.

ANTIDOTE

Notify physician of any side effects; most will be treated symptomatically. Replace electrolytes parenterally or orally as indicated. Reduce infusion rate by 50% if a mild or moderate (Grade 1 or 2) infusion reaction occurs. Discontinue panitumumab for a serious infusion reaction (Grade 3 or 4). Depending on the severity and/or persistence of the reaction, discontinue permanently. Hold or discontinue panitumumab if dermatologic toxicities Grade 3 or higher occur or if they are considered intolerable. See Dose Adjustments for criteria to resume or permanently discontinue treatment. Discontinue at the first sign of pulmonary toxicity. Treat hypersensitivity or infusion reaction as indicated (e.g., oxygen, antihistamines [e.g., diphenhydramine (Benadryl)], epinephrine (Adrenalin), corticosteroids, vasopressors [e.g., dopamine], ventilation equipment, and/or fluids). Resuscitate as necessary.

PANTOPRAZOLE SODIUM
(pan-**TOH**-prah-zohl **SO**-dee-um)

Protonix IV

Proton pump inhibitor
(Gastric acid inhibitor)

pH 9 to 10.5

USUAL DOSE

Given as an alternative to continued oral therapy. Resume oral therapy as soon as practical.

Treatment of gastroesophageal reflux disease (GERD): 40 mg as an infusion once daily for 7 to 10 days.

Treatment of Zollinger-Ellison syndrome (ZES): 80 mg as an infusion every 12 hours. Adjust to patient needs based on acid output measurements. If an increased dose is required, 80 mg every 8 hours is expected to maintain gastric acid output at less than 10 mEq/hr. Daily doses in excess of 240 mg or for more than 6 days have not been studied.

Recurrent gastrointestinal bleeding, prophylaxis (unlabeled): 80 mg as an IV injection followed by a continuous infusion of 8 mg/hr for 72 hours.

DOSE ADJUSTMENTS

No dose adjustments are necessary based on race or gender, in the elderly, or in patients with mild, moderate, or severe renal insufficiency, on hemodialysis; or with mild to severe impaired hepatic function. Doses higher than 40 mg/day have not been studied in patients with hepatic impairment.

DILUTION

40-mg dose: Reconstitute each single dose with 10 mL NS. May be further diluted with 100 mL D5W, NS, or LR to achieve a final concentration of approximately 0.4 mg/mL for infusion.

80-mg dose: Combining of two 40-mg vials is required; reconstitute each 40-mg vial with 10 mL NS. This total 80-mg dose may be further diluted with 80 mL D5W, NS, or LR (a total volume of 100 mL) to achieve a final concentration of approximately 0.8 mg/mL for infusion.

Filters: No longer required. Filtration during preparation or administration not studied with this new formulation.

Storage: Store unopened vials at CRT. Protect from light. Do not freeze. Vials reconstituted for the 2-minute infusion may be stored for up to 24 hours at RT. Vials reconstituted for the 15-minute infusion may be stored for up to 6 hours at RT prior to further dilution. Fully diluted solution may then be stored at RT but must be used within 24 hours of initial reconstitution. Protection from light is not required for reconstituted or fully diluted solutions.

COMPATIBILITY   (Underline Indicates Conflicting Compatibility Information)

Consider any drug NOT listed as compatible to be INCOMPATIBLE until consulting a pharmacist; specific conditions may apply.

Manufacturer states, "Administer through a dedicated line, should not be simultaneously administered through the same line with other intravenous solutions." See Rate of Administration. Manufacturer lists as **incompatible** at the **Y-site** with midazolam (Versed) and states, "May not be **compatible** with products containing zinc." ***Discontinue if discoloration or precipitation occurs with any drug at the Y-site.***

One source suggests the following **compatibilities:**

Y-site: Ampicillin, anidulafungin (Eraxis), caspofungin (Cancidas), cefazolin (Ancef), ceftriaxone (Rocephin), dimenhydrinate, dopamine, doripenem (Doribax), epinephrine (Adrenalin), furosemide (Lasix), insulin (regular), morphine, nitroglycerin IV, norepinephrine (Levophed), octreotide (Sandostatin), potassium chloride (KCl), vasopressin.

RATE OF ADMINISTRATION

A dedicated line is preferred, but a **Y-site** may be used. In all situations the IV line must be flushed before and after administration of pantoprazole with **compatible** infusion solutions (D5W, NS, or LR).

Concentration determines the rate of administration.

40 mg/10 mL or 80 mg/20 mL: As an injection evenly distributed over at least 2 minutes.

40 mg/100 mL or 80 mg/100 mL: As an infusion evenly distributed over at least 15 minutes (approximately 7 mL/min).

ACTIONS

A proton pump inhibitor (PPI) that suppresses the final step in gastric acid production. Acts at the secretory surface of the gastric parietal cell. Inhibits both basal and stimulated gastric acid secretion irrespective of the stimulus. Does not accumulate and pharmacokinetics are not altered with multiple daily dosing. Half-life is approximately one hour. Duration of antisecretory effect persists longer than 24 hours. Distributed mainly in extracellular fluid. Highly bound by serum protein (primarily albumin). Extensively metabolized in the liver through the cytochrome P_{450} (CYP) system. Metabolism is independent of the route of administration (intravenous or oral). Primarily excreted in urine with some excretion in feces.

INDICATIONS AND USES

Short-term treatment (7 to 10 days) of gastroesophageal reflux disease (GERD) with a history of erosive esophagitis, as an alternative to oral therapy. ▪ Treatment of pathological hypersecretion associated with Zollinger-Ellison syndrome or other neoplastic conditions.

Unlabeled uses: Prophylaxis against recurrent GI bleed (peptic ulcer bleed).

CONTRAINDICATIONS

Known hypersensitivity to pantoprazole or its components.

PRECAUTIONS

For IV use only; do not give IM or SC. ▪ Gastric malignancy may be present even though patient's symptoms improve with pantoprazole therapy. ▪ May have carcinogenic potential. ▪ Formulation contains edetate disodium, which can chelate zinc; see Monitor. ▪ Should be discontinued as soon as the patient is able to resume treatment with pantoprazole delayed-release tablets. ▪ Data on safe and effective dosing for other conditions (including life-threatening upper GI bleeds) not available. 40 mg IV of pantoprazole daily does not raise gastric pH levels sufficiently to treat such life-threatening conditions. ▪ Hypersensitivity reactions, including anaphylaxis, have been reported. ▪ May be associated with an increased risk for osteoporosis-related fractures of the hip, wrist, or spine. Risk increased in patients receiving high-dose (multiple daily doses) and long-term therapy (a year or longer). Use lowest dose and shortest duration of therapy appropriate for the condition being treated.

Monitor: Observe for S/S of a hypersensitivity reaction. ▪ Monitor vital signs and pain levels. ▪ Concomitant use of antacids may be indicated. ▪ In hypersecretory states, acid output measurements may be indicated to guide dose adjustment. ▪ Monitor injection site. Thrombophlebitis has been reported. ▪ Zinc supplementation may be indicated in patients who are prone to zinc deficiency; see Precautions. ▪ Change to oral dosing when appropriate. ▪ See Drug/Lab Interactions.

Patient Education: Review prescription and non-prescription drugs with your physician. ▪ Oral route preferred.

Maternal/Child: Category B: use during pregnancy only when clearly needed. ▪ Has potential for serious harm to nursing infants; discontinue breast-feeding. ▪ Safety and effectiveness for pediatric patients under 18 years of age not established.

Elderly: Safety and effectiveness similar to that of younger patients.

DRUG/LAB INTERACTIONS

Because of profound and long lasting inhibition of gastric acid secretion, pantoprazole may interfere with **absorption of drugs where gastric pH is an important determinant of their bioavailability** (e.g., ampicillin, esters, iron salts [ferrous sulfate], ketoconazole [Nizoral]). ▪ Increases in INR and PT have been reported when administered concurrently with **warfarin** (Coumadin); monitoring of INR and PT indicated. ▪ Concurrent use with **atazanavir** (Reyataz) is not recommended. Coadministration of proton pump inhibitors (e.g., esomeprazole [Nexium], pantoprazole [Protonix]) results in a significant reduction in **atazanavir** plasma concentrations, thereby inhibiting atazanavir's therapeutic effect. ▪ Studies suggest that with concurrent use the metabolism and serum concentrations of pantoprazole are not significantly altered by other drugs metabolized by the Cytochrome P_{450} system (e.g., diazepam [Valium], diclofenac [Apo-Diclo], metoprolol [Lopressor], nifedipine [ProCardia XL], phenytoin [Dilantin], theophylline). ▪ Studies also suggest that concurrent use with pantoprazole has not been found to significantly alter the metabolism and serum concentrations of the above agents as well as other drugs metabolized by a similar process (e.g., carbamazepine [Tegretol], cisapride [Propulsid], oral contraceptives). Concurrent administration should not require dose adjustment of either drug. ▪ Antipyrine (Allergen), caffeine, digoxin (Lanoxin), and glyburide (DiaBeta) had no clinically relevant interactions during clinical studies. ▪ May cause false-positive **urine screening test for tetrahydrocannabinol** (THC).

SIDE EFFECTS

Abscess, abdominal pain, blurred vision, chest pain, confusion, diarrhea, dyspnea, gastroenteritis, headache, hemorrhage, hyperglycemia, hypokinesia, increased salivation, injection site reactions including thrombophlebitis, nausea, pruritus, rash, speech disorder, tinnitus, transient elevations of serum transaminase, urinary tract infection, and vertigo are reported. Numerous other side effects have been associated with oral pantoprazole. **Post-Marketing:** Anterior ischemic optic neuropathy, bone fracture, elevated creatine phosphokinase (CPK), hepatocellular damage leading to jaundice and hepatic failure, hypersensitivity reactions (e.g., anaphylaxis, angioedema), hypomagnesemia, interstitial nephritis, pancreatitis, pancytopenia, rhabdomyolysis, severe dermatologic reactions (e.g., erythema multiforme, Stevens-Johnson syndrome, toxic epidermal necrolysis [some fatal]).

ANTIDOTE

Keep physician informed of all side effects. May be treated symptomatically. Discontinue and initiate appropriate treatment if S/S associated with post-marketing reports occur; see Side Effects. Adverse effects from overdose (up to 240 mg/day in healthy subjects) did not occur during clinical trials. Not removed by hemodialysis.

PAPAVERINE HYDROCHLORIDE
(pah-**PAV**-er-een hy-droh-**KLOR**-eyed)

Vasodilator
(peripheral)

pH 3 to 4.5

USUAL DOSE

1 to 4 mL (30 to 120 mg) every 3 hours as indicated. Second dose may be given in 10 minutes only when treating extrasystoles.

PEDIATRIC DOSE

1.5 mg/kg of body weight every 6 hours; see Maternal/Child.

DOSE ADJUSTMENTS

See Drug/Lab Interactions.

DILUTION

May be given undiluted or may be diluted in an equal amount of SW for injection. Usually not added to IV solutions. May be given through Y-tube or three-way stopcock of infusion set.

COMPATIBILITY

Consider any drug NOT listed as compatible to be INCOMPATIBLE until consulting a pharmacist; specific conditions may apply.

Will form a precipitate with LR.

One source suggests the following **compatibilities:**
Additive: Theophylline.

RATE OF ADMINISTRATION
1 mL (30 mg) or fraction thereof over 2 minutes. Rapid IV injection may cause death.

ACTIONS
A non-narcotic opium alkaloid, it is a direct smooth muscle relaxant and antispasmodic. Relaxation is noted in vascular system and bronchial musculature and in GI, biliary, and urinary tracts. More effective on muscle in spasm, it has an affinity for the smooth muscle of blood vessels. Affects cardiac muscle to depress conduction and increase refractory period. Improved circulation and muscle relaxation decrease pain. Metabolized in the liver and excreted in the urine.

INDICATIONS AND USES
Vascular spasm associated with an acute myocardial infarction. ▪ Peripheral or pulmonary embolism. ▪ Peripheral vascular disease and cerebral angiospastic states. ▪ Visceral spasm of ureteral, biliary, or GI colic. ▪ Angina pectoris.

CONTRAINDICATIONS
Complete AV heart block.

PRECAUTIONS
Rarely used; active therapeutic value is questioned. ▪ Rapid IV injection may cause death. ▪ IM injection is preferred. ▪ Use with caution in glaucoma and impaired liver function. ▪ Large doses can depress AV and intraventricular conduction, resulting in arrhythmias.
Monitor: Observe patient continuously; monitor vital signs. ▪ See Drug/Lab Interactions.
Patient Education: Avoid alcohol and other CNS depressants. ▪ May cause dizziness and drowsiness; request assistance for ambulation. ▪ Use caution in any task requiring alertness.
Maternal/Child: Category C: safety for use in pregnancy and breast-feeding and in pediatric patients not established.
Elderly: Risk of hypothermia may be increased.

DRUG/LAB INTERACTIONS
May be used with **narcotics** if the relaxant effect is not adequate to relieve discomfort. Narcotic dosage should be reduced. ▪ Antagonizes effects of **levodopa.**

SIDE EFFECTS
Blurred or double vision, diaphoresis, discomfort (generalized), flushing, hypertension (slight), hypotension, respiratory depth increase, scleral jaundice, sedation, tachycardia.
Major: Respiratory depression, seizures, ventricular ectopic rhythms, sudden death.

ANTIDOTE
Notify the physician of any minor side effects. If minor symptoms progress or any major side effect appears, discontinue the drug immediately and notify the physician. Treatment of toxicity will be symptomatic and supportive. Consider diazepam (Valium) or phenytoin (Dilantin) for convulsions. Anesthesia with thiopental and paralysis with a neuromuscular blocking agent may be required. Use dopamine for hypotension. Calcium gluconate may reduce toxic cardiovascular effects. Monitor ECG. Resuscitate as necessary.

PARICALCITOL
(pair-ee-**KAL**-sih-tohl)
Zemplar

Vitamin D analog

USUAL DOSE

The currently accepted target range for intact parathyroid hormone (iPTH) in chronic kidney disease (CKD) Stage 5 patients is no more than 1.5 to 3 times the non-uremic upper limit of normal.

Recommended initial dose is 0.04 to 0.1 mcg/kg administered no more frequently than every other day at any time during dialysis. Doses as high as 0.24 mcg/kg have been safely administered.

Information supplied by the manufacturer suggests that the relative dosing of paricalcitol to calcitriol is 4:1. When converting a patient from calcitriol to paricalcitol, the initial dose of paricalcitol should be four times greater than the patient's dose of calcitriol.

PEDIATRIC DOSE

Dose recommendations are based on severity of disease in addition to body weight. A dose is administered at any time during dialysis.

Pediatric patients 5 to 19 years of age (unlabeled): Doses used in clinical trials were:

Baseline iPTH level less than 500 pg/mL: 0.04 mcg/kg 3 times a week.

Baseline iPTH level equal to or greater than 500 pg/mL: 0.08 mcg/kg 3 times a week.

See Dose Adjustments.

DOSE ADJUSTMENTS

Adults: Adjust dosing based on patient response. If a satisfactory response is not observed, dose may be increased by 2 to 4 mcg at 2- to 4-week intervals. Monitor serum calcium, phosphorus, and calcium × phosphorus product (Ca × P) frequently during any dose adjustment period. See Monitor.

Pediatric patients: Adjust dose in 0.04-mcg/kg increments based on the levels of serum iPTH, calcium, and Ca × P (from clinical trials).

Adults and pediatric patients: Reduce dose or interrupt therapy if elevated calcium level or a Ca × P product of greater than 75 is noted. Reinitiate therapy at a lower dose when parameters have normalized. ▪ Paricalcitol dose may need to be reduced as parathyroid hormone (PTH) levels decrease in response to therapy. The currently accepted target range for intact parathyroid hormone (iPTH) in patients with chronic kidney disease (CKD) is no more than 1.5 to 3 times the non-uremic upper limit of normal. Incremental dosing must be individualized and commensurate with PTH, serum calcium, and phosphorus levels. The following chart is a suggested approach to dose titration. *Continued*

Paricalcitol Suggested Dosing Guidelines	
PTH Level	Paricalcitol Dose
The same or increasing	Increase
Decreasing by <30%	Increase
Decreasing by >30%, <60%	Maintain
Decreasing by >60%	Decrease
One and one-half to three times upper limit of normal	Maintain

DILUTION
May be given undiluted. Available as a 2 mg/mL and a 5 mcg/mL solution in 1- and 2-mL vials.
Filters: Not required by manufacturer; no further data available.
Storage: Store single- and multi-dose vials at CRT before use. Discard unused portions of single-dose vials. Multi-dose vial is stable for up to 7 days at CRT after entry into vial.

COMPATIBILITY
Specific information not available. Consider specific use; consult pharmacist.

RATE OF ADMINISTRATION
Administer as a bolus dose at any time during dialysis.

ACTIONS
A synthetic analog of calcitriol, the metabolically active form of vitamin D indicated for the prevention and treatment of secondary hyperparathyroidism associated with chronic kidney disease (CKD) Stage 5. In the diseased kidney, activation of vitamin D is diminished, resulting in a rise in parathyroid hormone (PTH), subsequently leading to secondary hyperparathyroidism and disturbances in calcium and phosphorus homeostasis. Paricalcitol binds to vitamin D receptors present in the parathyroid gland, intestine, kidney, and bone to maintain parathyroid function and calcium and phosphorus homeostasis. Studies suggest that paricalcitol may cause less hypercalcemia and hyperphosphatemia than calcitriol. Serum paricalcitol levels decrease rapidly after a bolus injection. Extensively bound to plasma proteins. Extensively metabolized by multiple hepatic and nonhepatic enzymes. Mean half-life is approximately 15 hours. Eliminated primarily by hepatobiliary excretion in feces and, to a much smaller extent, by the kidneys.

INDICATIONS AND USES
Prevention and treatment of secondary hyperparathyroidism associated with chronic kidney disease (CKD) Stage 5.

CONTRAINDICATIONS
Patients with evidence of vitamin D toxicity, hypercalcemia, or hypersensitivity to any ingredient in this product; see Precautions.

PRECAUTIONS
Acute overdose may cause hypercalcemia and require emergency attention. If clinically significant hypercalcemia develops, dose should be reduced or held. Chronic administration may place patient at risk of hypercalcemia, elevated $Ca \times P$ product, and metastatic calcification. Chronic hypercalcemia can lead to generalized vascular calcification and

other soft tissue calcification. See Side Effects and Antidote. ▪ Phosphate or vitamin D–related compounds should not be taken concomitantly with paricalcitol. High intake of calcium and phosphate concomitant with vitamin D compounds (paricalcitol) may lead to serum abnormalities and require more frequent monitoring and individualized dose titration. ▪ Adynamic bone lesions may develop if PTH levels are suppressed to abnormal levels. ▪ Avoid chronic administration of aluminum-containing preparations (e.g., antacids, phosphate binders); may increase blood levels of aluminum and cause aluminum bone toxicity.

Monitor: During initiation of therapy, obtain baseline serum calcium and phosphorus levels and determine levels at least twice a week. Once dosage has been established, serum calcium and phosphorus should be monitored at least monthly. See Dose Adjustments. ▪ Calculate Ca × P (should be less than 75). ▪ Measurements of serum or plasma PTH are recommended every 3 months. ▪ Monitor for signs and symptoms of hypercalcemia. See Side Effects.

Patient Education: Report symptoms of hypercalcemia promptly (e.g., constipation, difficulty thinking clearly, fatigue, increased thirst, increased urination, loss of appetite, nausea or vomiting, weight loss). Dose adjustment or treatment may be required. Strict adherence to dietary supplementation of calcium and restriction of phosphorus is required to ensure optimal effectiveness of therapy. Phosphate-binding compounds (e.g., calcium acetate [Phos-lo], sevelamer [Renagel]) may be needed to control serum phosphorus levels in patients with CKD, but excessive use of aluminum-containing products (e.g., aluminum hydroxide gel [Alternagel]) should be avoided.

Maternal/Child: Category C: safety for use in pregnancy not established. Benefits must outweigh risks. ▪ Discontinue breast-feeding. ▪ Has not been studied in pediatric patients under 5 years of age.

Elderly: No overall differences in effectiveness or safety have been observed in the elderly.

DRUG/LAB INTERACTIONS

Specific interaction studies have not been performed. ▪ Paricalcitol is partially metabolized by the **cytochrome P$_{450}$ enzyme CYP3A.** Use with caution when administered concomitantly **with known inhibitors of this enzyme** (e.g., atazanavir [Reyataz], clarithromycin [Biaxin], indinavir [Crixivan], itraconazole [Sporanox], ketoconazole [Nizoral], nefazodone, nelfinavir [Viracept], ritonavir [Norvir], saquinavir [Invirase], telithromycin [Ketek], voriconazole [VFEND]). ▪ Digitalis toxicity is potentiated by hypercalcemia. Use caution when paricalcitol is prescribed concomitantly with **digoxin** compounds. ▪ **Phosphate or vitamin D–related compounds** should not be taken concomitantly with paricalcitol; see Precautions. ▪ May reduce **serum total alkaline phosphatase** levels.

SIDE EFFECTS

Most commonly reported side effects include arthralgia, chills, dry mouth, edema, fever, gastrointestinal hemorrhage, influenza, malaise, nausea, palpitations, pneumonia, sepsis, and vomiting. Many other side effects occurred in fewer than 2% of patients. Overdose or chronic administration may lead to hypercalcemia. Signs and symptoms of vitamin D intoxication associated with hypercalcemia include: **Early:** bone pain, constipation, dry mouth, headache, metallic taste, muscle pain, nausea, somnolence, vomiting, and weakness. **Late:** Anorexia, cardiac arrhythmias, conjunctivitis (calcific), death, decreased libido, ectopic calcification, elevated AST and ALT, elevated BUN, hypercholesterolemia, hypertension, hyperthermia, overt psychosis (rare), pancreatitis, photophobia, pruritus, rhinorrhea, somnolence, and weight loss.

Post-Marketing: Hypersensitivity reactions (e.g., angioedema [including laryngeal edema]), rash, urticaria.

ANTIDOTE
Notify physician of any side effects. Treatment should consist of general supportive measures and serial serum electrolyte determinations (especially calcium). Monitor rate of urinary calcium excretion. Treatment of patients with clinically significant hypercalcemia consists of immediate dose reduction or interruption of the therapy and includes a low-calcium diet, withdrawal of calcium supplements, patient mobilization, attention to fluid and electrolyte imbalances, assessment of electrocardiographic abnormalities (critical in patients receiving digoxin), and hemodialysis or peritoneal dialysis against a calcium-free dialysate, as warranted. Monitor serum calcium levels frequently until calcium levels return to within normal limits. Paricalcitol may be restarted at a lower dose when serum calcium levels return to within normal limits. Not significantly removed by dialysis.

PEGASPARGASE
(peg-**ASS**-pair-gays)

Oncaspar, PEG-L-Asparaginase

**Antineoplastic
(miscellaneous)**

pH 7.3

USUAL DOSE (International units [IU])
2,500 International units (IU)/M^2 every 14 days as an infusion. Most frequently used as a component of a multiple agent protocol.

PEDIATRIC DOSE (International units [IU])
Over 1 year of age with body surface area less than 0.6 M²: 82.5 IU/kg of body weight every 14 days.
Body surface area greater than 0.6 M²: Same as adult dose.

DOSE ADJUSTMENTS
Adjust dose based on patient response and toxicity.

DILUTION (International units [IU])
Available preservative free in 5-mL vials containing 750 IU/mL. Must be further diluted with 100 mL of NS or D5W and administered through the Y-tube or three-way stopcock of a free-flowing infusion of similar solutions. Do not shake; mix gently. Use only clear solutions.

Storage: Appearance the same but activity is destroyed if accidentally frozen. *Do not administer!* Refrigerate before dilution. For single-dose use only. Do not reenter vial; discard unused portions. Discard any time solution is cloudy or after 48 hours at room temperature.

COMPATIBILITY
Specific information not available. Consider specific use and toxicity; consult pharmacist.

RATE OF ADMINISTRATION

A single dose evenly distributed over 1 to 2 hours. Slow rate of infusion as indicated by side effects.

ACTIONS

An oncolytic agent. A modified version of L-asparaginase (native asparaginase derived from *Escherichia coli*) that rapidly depletes asparagine from cells. Some malignant cells have a metabolic defect that makes them unable to synthesize asparagine as normal cells do. They are dependent on exogenous asparagine for survival. Depletion of asparagine kills the leukemic cells without affecting normal cells that synthesize their own asparagine. Plasma half-life range is from 2.5 to 8.5 days and does not appear to be influenced by dose levels, nor does it correlate with age, sex, surface area, renal or hepatic function, diagnosis, or extent of disease. Measurable for up to 15 days. Cannot be detected in urine.

INDICATIONS AND USES

First-line treatment of patients with acute lymphoblastic leukemia (ALL). ■ Treatment of patients with ALL and hypersensitivity to native forms of L-asparaginase. Used as a component of a multi-agent regimen for both indications. Occasionally used as a single agent when multiagent chemotherapy is considered inappropriate. Safety and effectiveness have been established in patients between 1 and 21 years of age with known previous hypersensitivity to native L-asparaginase.

Unlabeled uses: Treatment of acute lymphocytic leukemia.

CONTRAINDICATIONS

Pancreatitis, history of pancreatitis, serious thrombosis, or significant hemorrhagic events associated with prior L-asparaginase therapy, and patients who have had previous serious hypersensitivity reactions (e.g., bronchospasm, generalized urticaria, hypotension, laryngeal edema, hypotension) or other unacceptable adverse reactions to pegaspargase (Oncaspar).

PRECAUTIONS

Must be administered by or under the direction of the physician specialist (e.g., medical oncologist). ■ Incidence of hypersensitivity reactions, hepatotoxicity, coagulopathy, and gastrointestinal and renal disorders are lower if given by intramuscular injection. ■ Serious hypersensitivity reactions can occur. Risk increased in patients with known hypersensitivity to other forms of L-asparaginase. ■ Serious thrombotic events have occurred. ■ Pancreatitis has been reported. Evaluate patients with abdominal pain for evidence of pancreatitis. ■ Glucose intolerance has occurred; may be irreversible. ■ Increased PT, PTT, or hypofibrinogenemia are possible. ■ See Monitor, Drug/Lab Interactions, and Antidote.

Monitor: Observe patient carefully during and for at least 1 hour after infusion. ■ Appropriate treatment for resuscitation and/or anaphylaxis must always be available. Risk may be increased if patient has had reactions to native asparaginase. ■ Frequent monitoring of blood cell counts, bone marrow evaluation, serum amylase, blood sugar, uric acid, and liver and kidney function are necessary. ■ Monitoring of fibrinogen, PT, and PTT may be indicated to determine effects on coagulation. ■ Allopurinol, increased fluid intake, and alkalinization of the urine may be required to reduce uric acid levels. ■ Nausea and vomiting can be severe.

Prophylactic administration of antiemetics recommended to increase patient comfort. ▪ Predisposition to infection probable. ▪ Prophylactic antibiotics may be indicated pending results of C/S in febrile neutropenic patient. ▪ Monitor for thrombocytopenia (platelet count less than 50,000/mm^3). Initiate precautions to prevent excessive bleeding (e.g., inspect IV sites, skin, and mucous membranes; use extreme care during invasive procedures; test urine, emesis, stool, and secretions for occult blood).

Patient Education: Report all side effects promptly, especially abdominal pain, allergic reactions, bleeding, increased thirst, or S/S of thrombosis (chest pain, headache, shortness of breath, swelling); incidence of hypersensitivity reactions is significant and risk of bleeding is increased. ▪ All meds including nonprescription drugs must be evaluated. Contact physician before changing any meds. ▪ Verbalize all questions. ▪ Assess birth control requirements. ▪ See Appendix D, p. 1434.

Maternal/Child: Category C: effect on fetus unknown. Evaluation of benefit versus risk is necessary for anyone who is pregnant or may become pregnant. ▪ Discontinue breast-feeding.

Elderly: Consider age-related organ toxicity.

DRUG/LAB INTERACTIONS

Manufacturer states that specific drug interaction studies have not been performed; other sources suggest that the combination regimen used may have the following effects:

Potential for increased risk of bleeding or thrombosis; may be exacerbated with concurrent administration of **drugs with anticoagulant effects** (e.g., heparin, coumadin, dipyridamole [Persantine], aspirin, or NSAIDs [e.g., ibuprofen (Advil, Motrin), naproxen (Aleve, Naprosyn)]). ▪ Use caution with **hepatotoxic agents** (e.g., other chemotherapeutic agents, alcohol, NSAIDs, phenytoin [Dilantin]), especially in the presence of liver dysfunction. May cause hepatic and CNS toxicity. ▪ May inhibit action of **drugs dependent on protein synthesis or cell replication** (e.g., methotrexate). One source suggests administering pegaspargase 24 hours after **methotrexate**. ▪ May **interfere with the enzymatic detoxification** of other drugs, particularly in the liver. ▪ **Depletes serum protein;** may increase the toxicity of protein-bound drugs.

SIDE EFFECTS

May be more toxic in adults than in pediatric patients. Hypersensitivity reactions, including anaphylaxis, occur more frequently in patients hypersensitive to native asparaginase (60% versus 12% in nonsensitized patients) and may be dose limiting. CNS thrombosis, coagulopathy, fever, hepatotoxicity, hyperbilirubinemia, hyperglycemia requiring insulin therapy (3%), hypersensitivity reactions (e.g., anaphylaxis, bronchospasm, chills, dyspnea, edema, erythema, fever, hypotension, laryngeal edema, pain, rash, urticaria), increased ALT, malaise, nausea and vomiting (over 5%), pancreatitis (clinical) (1%), thrombosis (4%). Has caused fatal fulminating pancreatitis. Capable of causing numerous other side effects in 1% to 5% of all patients.

ANTIDOTE

Notify physician of all side effects. Reduced rate of administration may be helpful. Pegaspargase may have to be discontinued until recovery or permanently discontinued. Discontinue pegaspargase in patients who experience severe hypersensitivity reactions, thrombosis, or coagulopathies. Symptomatic and supportive treatment is indicated. Treat hypersensitivity reactions as indicated; may require epinephrine, airway management, oxygen, IV fluids, antihistamines (e.g., diphenhydramine [Benadryl]), corticosteroids (e.g., hydrocortisone sodium succinate [Solu-Cortef]), and pressor amines (e.g., dopamine). Consider administration of fresh frozen plasma (FFP) to patients with severe or symptomatic coagulopathy. There is no specific antidote.

PEGLOTICASE BBW

(peg-LOE-ti-kase)

Krystexxa

Anti-gout agent

USUAL DOSE

Gout flare prophylaxis: Use of an NSAID or colchicine is recommended beginning at least 1 week before the start of pegloticase therapy and lasting at least 6 months unless medically contraindicated or not tolerated.

Premedication: Patients should be premedicated before each dose with antihistamines and corticosteroids to reduce the risk of infusion reactions, including anaphylaxis or other hypersensitivity reactions. An oral antihistamine and an IV corticosteroid and/or acetaminophen have been used.

Pegloticase: 8 mg as an IV infusion every 2 weeks. Optimum treatment duration not established.

DOSE ADJUSTMENTS

No dose adjustment is required based on age, gender, race, or renal impairment.

DILUTION

Withdraw 1 mL (8 mg) from the 2-mL vial. A clear, colorless solution that must be further diluted by injecting it into a 250-mL bag of NS or ½NS for infusion. Ensure thorough mixing by inverting the infusion bag a number of times. Do not shake. If diluted solution has been refrigerated, bring to RT before administration (do not subject to artificial heating [e.g., hot water, microwave]).

Filters: No study data available; if filtering is necessary, contact manufacturer.

Storage: Before use, refrigerate in carton at 2° to 8° C (36° to 46° F). Protect from light. Do not shake or freeze. Do not use beyond the expiration date stamped. Diluted infusion bags are stable for 4 hours refrigerated or at RT (20° to 25°C [68° to 77° F]). Manufacturer recommends storing under refrigeration, not frozen, protected from light, and used within 4 hours of dilution. Discard unused product remaining in the 2-mL vial.

COMPATIBILITY

Manufacturer states, "Do not mix or dilute with other drugs."

RATE OF ADMINISTRATION

A single dose properly diluted as an infusion over no less than 2 hours. Do not administer by IV push or as a bolus. Administer by gravity feed with a syringe-type pump or infusion pump.

ACTIONS

A uric acid–specific enzyme; a PEGylated product that consists of recombinant modified mammalian urate oxidase (uricase) produced by a genetically modified strain of *Escherichia coli*. Achieves its therapeutic effect by catalyzing the oxidation of uric acid to allantoin, thereby lowering serum uric acid. Duration of suppression of plasma uric acid appears to be dose related. Allantoin is an inert and water-soluble purine metabolite that is readily eliminated, primarily by renal excretion.

INDICATIONS AND USES

Treatment of chronic gout in adult patients refractory to conventional therapy. ■ Not recommended for the treatment of asymptomatic hyperuricemia.

CONTRAINDICATIONS

Patients with glucose-6-phosphate dehydrogenase (G6PD) deficiency due to risk of hemolysis and methemoglobinemia.

PRECAUTIONS

Administer under the direction of a physician knowledgeable in its use in a facility with adequate diagnostic and treatment facilities to monitor the patient and respond to any medical emergency. ■ Anaphylaxis and infusion reactions have been reported to occur during and after administration of pegloticase. ■ Anaphylaxis may occur with any infusion, including a first infusion, and generally manifests within 2 hours of the infusion. However, delayed-type hypersensitivity reactions have also been reported. ■ Infusion reactions, including anaphylaxis, occurred in patients premedicated with one or more doses of an oral antihistamine and an IV corticosteroid and/or acetaminophen. ■ Risk of infusion reaction, including anaphylaxis, is higher in patients who have lost therapeutic response (e.g., uric acid levels increase to above 6 mg/dL). ■ An increase in gout flares is often observed with the initiation of anti-hyperuricemic therapy because changing serum uric acid levels result in the mobilization of urate from tissue deposits. Gout flare prophylaxis with an NSAID (e.g., indomethacin [Indocin], ketoprofen, naproxen [Aleve, Naprosyn]) or colchicine is recommended. Pegloticase does not need to be discontinued because of a gout flare. ■ Exacerbation of CHF has occurred; use with caution in patients with CHF. ■ Data not available for safety and efficacy of retreatment with pegloticase after stopping treatment for longer than 4 weeks. May increase risk of infusion reactions, including anaphylaxis. ■ Anti-pegloticase antibodies developed in most patients treated. High titers were associated with a failure to maintain pegloticase-induced normalization of uric acid. These patients also had a higher incidence of infusion reactions. Anti-PEG antibodies were also detected; the impact on patients' responses to other PEG-containing therapeutics is unknown. ■ Effects of either renal or hepatic impairment on pegloticase pharmacokinetics were not studied.

Monitor: Before initiating treatment, screening for G6PD deficiency is recommended in patients at higher risk (e.g., African or Mediterranean ancestry); see Contraindications. ■ Monitor serum uric acid levels before each infusion. Consider discontinuing treatment if levels increase to above 6 mg/dL, particularly when two consecutive levels above 6 mg/dL are observed. ▪ Closely monitor for S/S of potential anaphylaxis for an appropriate period (e.g., during and for at least 2 or more hours after administration). Dyspnea, erythema, flushing, and urticaria were most commonly observed. Hemodynamic instability, perioral or lingual edema, and wheezing have been observed. Slow or stop the infusion (depending on the severity) if an infusion reaction occurs. ▪ Closely monitor patients with a history of CHF during and after infusion. ▪ Patients being restarted on therapy after a drug-free interval longer than 4 weeks should be monitored carefully.

Patient Education: Immediately report S/S of an infusion or hypersensitivity reaction (e.g., chest pain, dizziness, dyspnea, fever, flushing, hypotension, nausea, pruritus, rash, rigors, urticaria). ▪ Review prescription and nonprescription drugs with physician. ▪ Report side effects of pegloticase that are bothersome or do not go away (e.g., nausea, vomiting).

Maternal/Child: Category C: use during pregnancy only if clearly needed. ▪ Not recommended for use during breast-feeding. ▪ Safety and effectiveness for use in pediatric patients less than 18 years of age not established.

Elderly: Response similar to other age-groups; however, greater sensitivity in the elderly cannot be ruled out.

DRUG/LAB INTERACTIONS

Formal drug interaction studies have not been conducted. ▪ Antipegloticase antibodies appear to bind to the PEG portion of the drug; there may be the potential for binding with other PEGylated products (e.g., interferon alpha [Pegasys, Peg-Intron], L-asparaginase [Oncaspar], recombinant methionyl human granulocyte colony-stimulating factor [Neulasta], liposome-containing doxorubicin [Doxil, Caelyx]). Impact of anti-PEG antibodies on patients' responses to other PEG-containing therapeutics is unknown.

SIDE EFFECTS

Most common side effects include chest pain, contusion or ecchymosis, constipation, gout flares, nausea, nasopharyngitis, and vomiting. Most serious reactions are infusion reactions, including anaphylaxis or other hypersensitivity reactions.

ANTIDOTE

Keep physician informed of all side effects. Some will be tolerated or treated symptomatically. Discontinue immediately for any acute serious infusion or hypersensitivity reaction and treat as appropriate; may require epinephrine (Adrenalin), airway management, oxygen, antihistamines (e.g., diphenhydramine [Benadryl]), vasopressors (e.g., dopamine), corticosteroids, albuterol (Ventolin), IV fluids, and ventilation equipment as indicated. Resuscitate as necessary. Slow or stop the infusion (depending on the severity) if an infusion reaction occurs. May be restarted at a slower rate if symptoms subside. Pegloticase does not need to be discontinued because of a gout flare. No specific antidote; monitor and support as indicated in overdose. Resuscitate as necessary.

PEMETREXED
(peh-meh-**TREX**-ed)

Alimta

Antineoplastic
(Antifolate)

pH 6.6 to 7.8

USUAL DOSE

Premedication required. Regimen begins 1 week before the first infusion of pemetrexed.

Folic acid supplementation: Prophylaxis to reduce treatment-related hematologic and GI toxicity (pemetrexed is an antifolate; severe myelosuppression can occur); 350 to 1,000 mcg of folic acid *must* be taken for at least 5 days out of the 7 days *before* the first dose of pemetrexed. Must be continued daily throughout the treatment regimen and for 21 days after treatment is complete. May be taken as a folic acid preparation or as a multivitamin with folic acid. The most commonly used dose of oral folic acid in clinical trials was 400 mcg.

Vitamin B_{12} supplementation: Prophylaxis to reduce treatment-related hematologic and GI toxicity; 1,000 mcg of vitamin B_{12} *must* be given as an injection in the week *before* the first dose of pemetrexed. This dose will be repeated every 3 cycles (about every 9 weeks) during treatment, and these subsequent doses may be given on the same day as the pemetrexed infusion.

Corticosteroid: To reduce the incidence and severity of skin rashes, administer dexamethasone (Decadron) 4 mg PO (or equivalent) twice daily the day before, the day of, and the day after the pemetrexed infusion. Repeat with each planned dose of pemetrexed.

Prehydration: Required with cisplatin; see cisplatin monograph.

Pretesting required: See Monitor. Do not begin a new cycle of treatment unless the ANC (absolute neutrophil count) is equal to or greater than 1,500 cells/mm³, the platelet count is equal to or greater than 100,000 cells/mm³, and the CrCl is equal to or greater than 45 mL/min.

Nonsquamous non–small-cell lung cancer (NSCLC) and malignant pleural mesothelioma: *Pemetrexed:* 500 mg/M² as an infusion over 10 minutes on Day 1 of each 21-day cycle.

Cisplatin: Begin 30 minutes after the end of the pemetrexed infusion. 75 mg/M² as an infusion over 2 hours.

As a single agent in nonsquamous NSCLC: *Pemetrexed:* 500 mg/M² as an infusion over 10 minutes on Day 1 of each 21-day cycle.

DOSE ADJUSTMENTS

Other than those recommended for all patients, no dose adjustments are required based on age, gender, or race or in patients with a CrCl equal to or greater than 45 mL/min. ■ Dose adjustments in impaired hepatic function are the same as those for nonhematologic toxicities. ■ Dose Adjustments are based on the nadir ANC of the previous dose cycle for hematologic toxicities and the common toxicity criteria (CTC) for nonhematologic toxicities and neurotoxicity. Therapy may be delayed to allow sufficient time for recovery; when recovery occurs, reinitiate therapy according to the following charts:

Pemetrexed and Cisplatin Dose Reduction (Single Agent or in Combination): Hematologic Toxicities	
ANC and Platelet Count	Dose of Pemetrexed (mg/M^2) and Cisplatin (mg/M^2)
Nadir ANC <500/mm^3 and nadir platelets ≥50,000/mm^3	75% of previous dose (both drugs)
Nadir platelets <50,000/mm^3 without bleeding, regardless of nadir ANC	75% of previous dose (both drugs)
Nadir platelets <50,000/mm^3 with bleeding, regardless of nadir ANC	50% of previous dose (both drugs)

Pemetrexed and Cisplatin Dose Reduction (Single Agent or in Combination) in Neurotoxicity		
CTC Grade*	Dose of Pemetrexed (mg/M^2)	Dose of Cisplatin (mg/M^2)
0 or 1	100% of previous dose	100% of previous dose
2	100% of previous dose	50% of previous dose
3 or 4	Discontinue therapy	Discontinue therapy

*Common Terminology Criteria for Adverse Events (CTCAE).

Excluding neurotoxicity, if patients develop nonhematologic toxicities equal to or greater than Grade 3 (the exception is Grade 3 transaminase elevations), pemetrexed should be withheld until pretherapy values are achieved. Resume treatment according to the following chart.

Pemetrexed and Cisplatin Dose Reduction (Single Agent or in Combination): Nonhematologic Toxicities and Impaired Hepatic Function*		
CTC Grade†	Dose of Pemetrexed (mg/M^2)	Dose of Cisplatin (mg/M^2)
Any Grade 3‡ or 4 toxicities except mucositis	75% of previous dose	75% of previous dose
Any diarrhea requiring hospitalization or Grade 3 or 4 diarrhea	75% of previous dose	75% of previous dose
Grade 3 or 4 mucositis	50% of previous dose	100% of previous dose

*Excluding neurotoxicity.
†Common Terminology Criteria for Adverse Events (CTCAE).
‡Except Grade 3 transaminase elevation.

Discontinue therapy if hematologic or nonhematologic Grade 3 or 4 toxicity occurs after two dose reductions (the exception is Grade 3 transaminase elevations) or immediately if Grade 3 or 4 neurotoxicity is observed.
DILUTION
Specific techniques required; see Precautions. Calculate the dose and number of vials needed. Reconstitute each 100-mg vial with 4.2 mL of preservative-free NS and each 500-mg vial with 20 mL of preservative-free NS. Concentration equals 25 mg/mL. Gently swirl to completely

dissolve the powder. Solution ranges in color from colorless to yellow or green-yellow. Withdraw the required volume to provide the calculated dose of pemetrexed. *Must* be further diluted to a total volume of 100 mL with preservative-free NS.

Filters: No data available from manufacturer.

Storage: Store unopened vials at CRT. Reconstituted and diluted solutions are chemically and physically stable for 24 hours either refrigerated or at CRT. Contains no preservatives; discard unused portions.

COMPATIBILITY

Consider any drug NOT listed as compatible to be INCOMPATIBLE until consulting a pharmacist; specific conditions may apply.

Manufacturer states, "Is physically **incompatible** with diluents containing calcium, including lactated Ringer's and Ringer's injection. Co-administration with other diluents has not been studied." **Compatible** with standard PVC administration sets and bags.

One source suggests the following **compatibilities:**

Y-site: Acyclovir (Zovirax), amifostine (Ethyol), amikacin (Amikin), aminophylline, ampicillin, ampicillin/sulbactam (Unasyn), aztreonam (Azactam), bumetanide, buprenorphine (Buprenex), butorphanol (Stadol), carboplatin (Paraplatin), ceftriaxone (Rocephin), cefuroxime (Zinacef), cisplatin (Platinol), clindamycin (Cleocin), cyclophosphamide (Cytoxan), cytarabine (ARA-C), dexamethasone (Decadron), dexrazoxane (Zinecard), diphenhydramine (Benadryl), docetaxel (Taxotere), dopamine, enalaprilat (Vasotec IV), famotidine (Pepcid IV), fluconazole (Diflucan), fluorouracil (5-FU), ganciclovir (Cytovene), granisetron (Kytril), haloperidol (Haldol), heparin, hydromorphone (Dilaudid), ifosfamide (Ifex), leucovorin calcium, lorazepam (Ativan), mannitol (Osmitrol), meperidine (Demerol), mesna (Mesnex), methylprednisolone (Solu-Medrol), metoclopramide (Reglan), morphine, paclitaxel (Taxol), potassium chloride (KCl), promethazine (Phenergan), ranitidine (Zantac), sodium bicarbonate, sulfamethoxazole/trimethoprim, ticarcillin/clavulanate (Timentin), vancomycin, vinblastine, vincristine, zidovudine (AZT, Retrovir).

RATE OF ADMINISTRATION

A single dose as an infusion equally distributed over 10 minutes.

ACTIONS

An antifolate antineoplastic agent. It disrupts folate-dependent metabolic processes essential for cell replication. Transported into cells by both the reduced folate carrier and the membrane folate-binding protein transport systems. Converts to a polyglutamate form. Polyglutamation is a time- and concentration-dependent process that occurs in tumor cells and, to a lesser extent, in normal tissues. Polyglutamated metabolites have an increased intracellular half-life, resulting in prolonged drug action in malignant cells. Inhibited the in vitro growth of mesothelioma cell lines and showed synergistic effects when used concurrently with cisplatin. Folic acid and vitamin B_{12} supplementation is required during treatment. 81% bound to plasma protein. Not appreciably metabolized. Half-life is 3.5 hours. Primarily eliminated in urine as an unchanged drug. Clearance decreases and exposure (AUC) increases as renal function decreases.

INDICATIONS AND USES

Used in combination with cisplatin (Platinol) for the treatment of malignant pleural mesothelioma in patients whose disease is unresectable or who are not candidates for curative surgery. ■ As a single agent for treatment of patients with locally advanced or metastatic nonsquamous NSCLC after prior chemotherapy. ■ Used in combination with cisplatin for the initial treatment of patients with locally advanced or metastatic nonsquamous NSCLC. ■ Maintenance treatment of patients with locally advanced or metastatic NSCLC whose disease has not progressed after 4 cycles of platinum-based first-line chemotherapy. ■ Not indicated for treatment of squamous cell NSCLC.

CONTRAINDICATIONS

History of severe hypersensitivity reaction to pemetrexed or any of its components. ■ Should not be administered to patients with a CrCl less than 45 mL/min.

PRECAUTIONS

Follow guidelines for handling cytotoxic agents. See Appendix A, p. 1429. ■ Use of gloves recommended. If a solution of pemetrexed contacts the skin, wash the skin immediately and thoroughly with soap and water. If there is contact with mucous membrane, flush thoroughly with water. ■ Should be administered by or under the direction of a physician specialist in a facility equipped to monitor the patient and respond to any medical emergency. ■ Use caution in patients with a CrCl less than 80 mL/min if NSAIDs (e.g., ibuprofen [Advil, Motrin], naproxen [Aleve, Naprosyn]) are administered concurrently. ■ Bone marrow suppression (e.g., anemia, neutropenia, thrombocytopenia) is a dose-limiting toxicity; see Dose Adjustments. ■ Folic acid and vitamin B_{12} supplementation is required; a prophylactic measure to reduce treatment-related hematologic and GI toxicity. ■ In patients with pleural effusion and/or ascites, consider drainage of third-space fluid before administration; the effects of this fluid accumulation on pemetrexed are not known. ■ Coadministration with cisplatin has not been studied in patients with moderate renal impairment. ■ Cutaneous reactions (skin rash) occur more frequently in patients not pretreated with a corticosteroid. Men had a slightly increased incidence of rash compared to women. ■ See Contraindications and Drug/Lab Interactions.

Monitor: Pretreatment with folic acid, vitamin B_{12}, dexamethasone, and adequate hydration required; see Usual Dose. ■ Obtain baseline CBC, including platelet count, CrCl, and liver function tests. Repeat CBC and platelet count before each dose and on days 8 and 15 of each cycle. Do not begin a new cycle of treatment unless the ANC is equal to or greater than 1,500 cells/mm^3, the platelet count is equal to or greater than 100,000 cells/mm^3, and the CrCl is equal to or greater than 45 mL/min. ■ Monitor CBC and platelets for nadir and recovery. Time to ANC nadir ranged between 8 and 9.6 days. Return to baseline ANC occurred 4.2 to 7.5 days after the nadir. Has no cumulative effect on ANC nadir over multiple treatment cycles. ■ Repeat CrCl before each dose to evaluate renal function. Plasma clearance of pemetrexed given concurrently with cisplatin decreases as renal function decreases; see Dose Adjustments and Contraindications. ■ Repeat liver function tests periodically to evaluate hepatic function. Effects of AST, ALT, or total bilirubin are not known; see Dose Adjustments. ■ Monitor patients who have been or are taking NSAIDs carefully for signs of toxicity, especially myelosuppression and renal or GI toxicity; see Drug/Lab Interactions. ■ Monitor for thrombocytopenia (platelet count less than 50,000/mm^3). Initiate precautions to prevent excessive bleeding (e.g., inspect IV sites, skin, and mucous membranes;

use extreme care during invasive procedures; test urine, emesis, stool, and secretions for occult blood). ▪ See Precautions, Drug/Lab Interactions, and Antidote.

Patient Education: Avoid pregnancy; use of nonhormonal birth control recommended. See Maternal/Child. Women should report a suspected pregnancy immediately. ▪ Adherence to regimen (medication [folic acid, vitamin B_{12}, dexamethasone, avoidance or limiting of aspirin or NSAIDs], required lab work, follow-up visits with health care professional) is imperative. ▪ Promptly report S/S of anemia, bleeding, dehydration from diarrhea or vomiting, fatigue, infection (e.g., fever), rash, or other symptoms. ▪ See Appendix D, p. 1434.

Maternal/Child: Category D: avoid pregnancy; may cause fetal harm. Fetotoxic and teratogenic in mice. ▪ Reduced fertility, hypospermia, and testicular atrophy occurred in mice. ▪ Discontinue breast-feeding. ▪ Safety and effectiveness for use in pediatric patients not established.

Elderly: See Dose Adjustments; required only based on general patient criteria. ▪ Incidence of common toxicity criteria (CTC) Grade 3 and 4 for fatigue, hypertension, leukopenia, neutropenia, and thrombocytopenia were greater in patients 65 years of age or older even though they were fully supplemented with vitamins.

DRUG/LAB INTERACTIONS

Concomitant use with **nephrotoxic agents** (e.g., aminoglycosides [e.g., gentamicin], amphotericin B, cisplatin [Platinol], NSAIDs, vancomycin) and **agents that are tubularly secreted** (e.g., probenecid) may delay clearance of pemetrexed. ▪ **NSAIDs** (e.g., ibuprofen [Advil, Motrin], naproxen [Aleve, Naprosyn]) decrease clearance and increase AUC in patients with normal renal function. Ibuprofen 400 mg four times daily was administered to patients with normal renal function (CrCl equal to or greater than 80 mL/min) who were receiving pemetrexed. Effects of larger doses unknown; see Precautions. All patients taking NSAIDs should avoid taking them for from 2 days (short-acting NSAIDs) to 5 days (long-acting NSAIDs) before, the day of, and at least 2 days after a dose of pemetrexed. Monitoring for toxicity required. ▪ Pharmacokinetics of both drugs (pemetrexed and cisplatin) are not affected by each other. ▪ Coadministration of oral folic acid or IM vitamin B_{12} does not adversely affect pemetrexed. ▪ Is not a clinically significant inhibitor of drugs metabolized by cytochrome P_{450} enzymes. Used as recommended (every 21 days), it would not be expected to cause any significant enzyme induction. ▪ May be used concurrently with aspirin in low to moderate doses (325 mg every 6 hours). Effect of higher doses not known.

SIDE EFFECTS

The most common side effects with single-agent use are anorexia, fatigue, and nausea. When used in combination with cisplatin, additional common side effects include constipation, hematologic toxicity (anemia, leukopenia, neutropenia, thrombocytopenia), pharyngitis, stomatitis, and vomiting. Bone marrow suppression (anemia, leukopenia, neutropenia, thrombocytopenia), selected nonhematologic toxicities (e.g., Grade 3 or 4 toxicities, diarrhea requiring hospitalization, mucositis), and neurotoxicity are dose-limiting toxicities. Other frequently occurring side effects include fever, infection, and rash with desquamation. Infections and rash leading to bullous conditions (e.g., Stevens-Johnson syndrome and toxic epidermal necrolysis) have been fatal. Other side effects may include hypersensitivity reactions, alopecia, anorexia, arthralgia, chest pain, decreased CrCl, dehydration, depression, diarrhea, dysphagia, dyspnea, edema, elevated ALT, elevated AST, embolism or thrombosis, esophagitis, fatigue, febrile neutropenia, mood alteration, myalgia, neuropathy (sensory), odynophagia (pain produced by swallowing), renal failure.

Overdose: Bone marrow suppression (e.g., anemia, neutropenia, thrombocytopenia), diarrhea, infection with or without fever, mucositis, rash.

Post-Marketing: Colitis, edema, interstitial pneumonitis, radiation recall.

ANTIDOTE

Keep physician informed of dose parameters and other side effects. Pemetrexed may be delayed or discontinued based on the degree of side effects. Symptomatic and supportive therapy is indicated. Death may occur from the progression of some side effects. Begin leucovorin treatment immediately for Grade 4 thrombocytopenia, bleeding associated with Grade 3 thrombocytopenia, or Grade 3 or 4 mucositis. Leucovorin treatment is also indicated if Grade 4 neutropenia or Grade 4 leukopenia lasting 3 or more days occurs. Regimen recommended is leucovorin 100 mg/M^2 IV as an initial dose followed by 50 mg/M^2 IV every 6 hours for 8 days. Administration of whole blood products (e.g., packed RBCs, platelets, leukocytes) and/or blood modifiers (e.g., darbepoetin alfa [Aranesp], epoetin alfa [Epogen], filgrastim [Neupogen], oprelvekin [Neumega], pegfilgrastim [Neulasta], sargramostim [Leukine]) may be indicated to treat bone marrow toxicity. Effect of hemodialysis on pemetrexed is unknown.

PENICILLIN G AQUEOUS

(pen-ih-**SILL**-in **A**-kwe-us)

Penicillin G Potassium, Penicillin G Sodium, Pfizerpen

Antibacterial
(penicillin)

pH 5.5 to 8

USUAL DOSE

Adults and pediatric patients 12 years of age and older: 1 to 20 million units/24 hr equally distributed over 24 hours as a continuous infusion or equally divided in 4 to 6 intermittent infusions (250,000 to 5 million units every 6 hours or 166,000 to 3,333,333 units every 4 hours). Doses up to 80 million units/24 hr have been given in life-threatening infections. (400,000 units equals approximately 250 mg.) See package insert for specific indications.

PEDIATRIC DOSE

Administration by intermittent infusion over 15 to 30 minutes is preferred. Dose is based on age or weight and the severity of the infection.

Serious infections (e.g., pneumonia, endocarditis): 25,000 units/kg every 4 hours or 37,500 units/kg every 6 hours (150,000 units/kg/24 hr).

Meningitis: 41,666 units/kg every 4 hours (250,000 units/kg/24 hr). Continue treatment for 7 to 14 days. Maximum dose is 12 to 20 million units/24 hr.

Disseminated gonococcal infections (arthritis), weight less than 45 kg: 25,000 units/kg every 6 hours (100,000 units/kg/24 hr) for 7 to 10 days.

Disseminated gonococcal infections (meningitis), weight less than 45 kg: 41,666 units/kg every 4 hours (250,000 units/kg/24 hr) for 10 to 14 days.

Disseminated gonococcal infections (endocarditis), weight less than 45 kg: 41,666 units/kg every 4 hours (250,000 units/kg/24 hr) for 4 weeks.

Disseminated gonococcal infections (arthritis, meningitis, endocarditis), weight 45 kg or greater: 2,500,000 units every 6 hours (10,000,000 units/24 hr). Duration of therapy is dependent on diagnosis.

Syphilis (congenital or neurosyphilis) after the newborn period: 50,000 units/kg every 4 to 6 hours (200,000 to 300,000 units/kg/24 hr). Continue treatment for 10 to 14 days.

Diphtheria (adjunctive to antitoxin and prevention of carrier state): 37,500 to 62,500 units/kg every 6 hours (150,000 to 250,000 units/kg/24 hr) for 7 to 10 days.

Rat-bite fever, Haverhill fever (caused by a specific organism): 25,000 to 41,666 units/kg every 4 hours (150,000 to 250,000 units/kg/24 hr) for 4 weeks.

The American Association of Pediatrics (AAP) recommends:

Infants and other pediatric patients from 1 month to less than 12 years of age:
Mild to moderate bacterial infections: 6,250 to 12,500 units/kg every 6 hours (25,000 to 50,000 units/kg/24 hr).

Severe bacterial infections and Group B streptococcal meningitis: 62,500 to 100,000 units/kg every 6 hours or 41,666 to 66,666 units/kg every 4 hours (250,000 to 400,000 units/kg/24 hr).

Another source recommends:

Pediatric patients under 12 years of age: 100,000 to 400,000 units/kg/24 hr in equally divided doses every 4 to 6 hours as an intermittent infusion (25,000 to 100,000 units/kg every 6 hours or 16,666 to 66,666 units/kg every 4 hours). Dosage can vary greatly and must be adjusted according to the severity of the infection. Maximum dose is 24,000,000 units/24 hr.

Treatment of congenital syphilis over 4 weeks of age: 50,000 to 75,000 units/kg every 6 hours (200,000 to 300,000 units/kg/24 hr). Total course of treatment is 10 to 14 days.

NEONATAL DOSE

Administration by intermittent infusion over 15 to 30 minutes is preferred. Dose is based on weight and age and the severity of the infection. The AAP recommends 25,000 to 50,000 units/dose. Adjust interval based on weight and age as follows:

Moderate to severe bacterial infections:
Weight less than 1,200 Gm; 4 weeks of age or younger: Every 12 hours.
Weight 1,200 to 2,000 Gm; less than 7 days of age: Every 12 hours.
Weight 1,200 to 2,000 Gm; 1 to 4 weeks of age: Every 8 hours.
Weight over 2,000 Gm; less than 7 days of age: Every 8 hours.
Weight over 2,000 Gm; 1 to 4 weeks of age: Every 6 hours.
Meningitis caused by beta streptococci:
7 days of age or younger: 83,333 to 133,333 units/kg every 8 hours (250,000 to 400,000 units/kg/24 hr).
Older than 7 days of age: 112,500 units/kg every 6 hours (450,000 units/kg/24 hr).
Treatment of congenital syphilis less than 4 weeks of age: 50,000 units/kg every 12 hours (100,000 units/kg/24 hr) for the first week, then 50,000 units/kg every 8 hours (150,000 units/kg/24 hr) for an additional 3 to 7 days. Total course of treatment is 10 to 14 days.

DOSE ADJUSTMENTS

Reduce dose in severe impaired renal function; additional reductions may be indicated if liver function is also impaired. ■ If CrCl is greater than 10 mL/min in uremic patients, give a full loading dose followed by one-half loading dose every 4 to 5 hours. ■ If CrCl is less than 10 mL/min/1.73 M^2, administer a full loading dose followed by one half of the loading dose every 8 to 10 hours. Another source recommends giving 75% of a normal dose every 4 to 6 hours to patients with a CrCl of 10 to 50 mL/min and 20% to 50% of a normal dose every 4 to 6 hours to patients with a CrCl less than 10 mL/min. ■ See Drug/Lab Interactions.

DILUTION

Available premixed, or reconstitute each vial with SW for injection or NS. Direct flow of diluent against sides of the vial while gently rotating vial. Shake vigorously. Directions on vial should be followed to provide desired number of units per milliliter. Available with 1, 5, 10, and 20 million units per vial. May be added to NS or dextrose solutions for infusion. See chart on inside back cover.

Storage: Dry powder stored at CRT. Reconstituted solutions stable for 1 week if refrigerated. Infusion solutions stable at CRT for 24 hours.

COMPATIBILITY   (Underline Indicates Conflicting Compatibility Information)

Consider any drug NOT listed as compatible to be INCOMPATIBLE until consulting a pharmacist; specific conditions may apply.

Penicillins are rapidly inactivated in alkaline carbohydrate solutions, reducing agents, alcohols, and glycols; optimum pH range is 6 to 7. To preserve bactericidal action, consult pharmacist before mixing other agents with penicillin in the infusion solution. May form a precipitate with vancomycin. Inactivated in solution with aminoglycosides (e.g., amikacin

[Amikin], gentamicin). Do not mix in the same solution. Appropriate spacing and/or separate sites required. See Drug/Lab Interactions.

One source suggests the following **compatibilities:**

PENICILLIN G POTASSIUM

Additive: *See general comments under Compatibility.* Amikacin (Amikin), ascorbic acid, calcium chloride, calcium gluconate, chloramphenicol (Chloromycetin), colistimethate (Coly-Mycin M), dimenhydrinate, diphenhydramine (Benadryl), ephedrine, erythromycin (Erythrocin), heparin, hydrocortisone sodium succinate (Solu-Cortef), kanamycin (Kantrex), lidocaine, lincomycin (Lincocin), magnesium sulfate, methylprednisolone (Solu-Medrol), metronidazole (Flagyl IV), potassium chloride (KCl), prochlorperazine (Compazine), promethazine (Phenergan), ranitidine (Zantac), sodium bicarbonate, verapamil.

Y-site: Acyclovir (Zovirax), amiodarone (Nexterone), cyclophosphamide (Cytoxan), diltiazem (Cardizem), enalaprilat (Vasotec IV), esmolol (Brevibloc), fluconazole (Diflucan), foscarnet (Foscavir), heparin, hydromorphone (Dilaudid), labetalol (Trandate), magnesium sulfate, meperidine (Demerol), morphine, nicardipine (Cardene IV), potassium chloride (KCl), tacrolimus (Prograf), theophylline, verapamil.

PENICILLIN G SODIUM

Additive: *See general comments under Compatibility.* Calcium chloride, calcium gluconate, chloramphenicol (Chloromycetin), colistimethate (Coly-Mycin M), diphenhydramine (Benadryl), erythromycin (Erythrocin), gentamicin, heparin, hydrocortisone sodium succinate (Solu-Cortef), kanamycin (Kantrex), lincomycin (Lincocin), potassium chloride (KCl), ranitidine (Zantac), verapamil.

Y-site: Levofloxacin (Levaquin).

RATE OF ADMINISTRATION

Penicillin is not given by IV injection. Administer as ordered as continuous IV drip; for example, 5 million units in 1,000 mL of D5W over 12 hours. Is sometimes given by intermittent infusion (⅙ or ¼ of a daily dose in 100 mL over 1 to 2 hours every 4 to 6 hours). Because of its short half-life, frequent dosing is required to maintain serum concentration above the MIC (minimum inhibitory concentration) for most of the dosing interval. Too-rapid administration or excessive doses may cause electrolyte imbalance and/or seizures. Stable at room temperature for at least 24 hours. **Pediatric rate:** Administration by intermittent infusion over 15 to 30 minutes is preferred for infants and children.

ACTIONS

Bactericidal against penicillin-sensitive microorganisms during the stage of active multiplication. Inhibits bacterial cell wall synthesis. Distributed into most body fluids. Distribution into spinal fluid is minimal unless inflammation is present. Half-life is approximately 40 minutes. Crosses the placental barrier. Excreted in the urine via glomerular filtration and tubular secretion. Secreted in breast milk. Available in a potassium salt containing 1.02 mEq of potassium and 0.3 mEq sodium in 1 million units or a sodium salt containing 2 mEq sodium in 1 million units.

INDICATIONS AND USES

Severe infections caused by penicillin G–sensitive gram-positive, gram-negative, and anaerobic microorganisms (e.g., streptococcal, pneumococcal, Vincent's gingivitis, spirochetal infections, meningitis, endocarditis). **Unlabeled uses:** Arthritis, carditis.

CONTRAINDICATIONS

Known sensitivity to any penicillin or cephalosporin (not absolute; see Precautions).

PRECAUTIONS

Hypersensitivity reactions, including fatalities, have been reported in patients undergoing penicillin therapy; most likely to occur in patients with a history of penicillin allergy or sensitivity to multiple allergens. There have been reports of individuals with a history of penicillin hypersensitivity experiencing severe reactions when treated with cephalosporins. Check history of previous hypersensitivity reactions to penicillins, cephalosporins, or other allergens. Actual incidence of cross-allergenicity not established but may be more common with first-generation cephalosporins. ■ Sensitivity studies necessary to determine susceptibility of the causative organism to penicillin. ■ To reduce the development of drug-resistant bacteria and maintain its effectiveness, penicillin should be used to treat or prevent only those infections proven or strongly suspected to be caused by bacteria. ■ Continue treatment for 48 to 72 hours after symptoms subside. To reduce the risk of rheumatic fever, patients being treated for Group A beta-hemolytic streptococcal infections should be treated for at least 10 days. ■ Avoid prolonged use of drug; superinfection caused by overgrowth of nonsusceptible organisms may result. ■ *Clostridium difficile*–associated diarrhea (CDAD) has been reported. May range from mild diarrhea to fatal colitis. Consider in patients who present with diarrhea during or after treatment with penicillin. ■ Potassium penicillin most frequently used. Doses over 10,000,000 units may cause fatal hyperkalemia, especially in patients with renal insufficiency.

Monitor: Periodic evaluation of renal, hepatic, and hematopoietic systems is recommended in prolonged therapy. ■ Test patients with gonococcal infections and syphilis for HIV. Test patients with gonococcal infections for syphilis. ■ Electrolyte imbalance from potassium or sodium content is very possible. Monitor closely. Penicillin G potassium contains 1.02 mEq sodium/million units. May aggravate CHF. ■ May cause thrombophlebitis; observe carefully and rotate infusion sites. ■ See Drug/Lab Interactions.

Patient Education: May require alternate birth control. ■ Promptly report diarrhea or bloody stools that occur during treatment or up to several months after an antibiotic has been discontinued; may indicate CDAD and require treatment.

Maternal/Child: Category B: use only if clearly needed. ■ May cause diarrhea, candidiasis, or allergic response in nursing infants. ■ Elimination rate markedly reduced in neonates.

Elderly: Response similar to that seen in younger adults. ■ Consider age-related organ impairment and concomitant disease or drug therapy. Monitor renal function. ■ See Dose Adjustments.

DRUG/LAB INTERACTIONS

Synergistic when used in combination with **aminoglycosides** (e.g., amikacin [Amikin], gentamicin). Synergism may be inconsistent; see Compatibility. ▪ May be antagonized by **bacteriostatic antibiotics** (e.g., chloramphenicol, erythromycin, tetracyclines); may interfere with bactericidal action. ▪ **ASA, ethacrynic acid** (Edecrin), **furosemide** (Lasix), **indomethacin** (Indocin), **sulfonamides** (Bactrim), **and thiazide diuretics** (e.g., chlorothiazide [Diuril]) may interfere with tubular secretion of penicillin, increasing serum concentration and risk of toxicity. ▪ Risk of bleeding with **anticoagulants** (e.g., heparin) is increased. ▪ **Probenecid** decreases elimination of penicillin resulting in prolonged half-life and increased serum levels. May be desirable or may cause toxicity. ▪ May decrease effectiveness of **oral contraceptives;** breakthrough bleeding or pregnancy could result. ▪ Concomitant use with **potassium supplements, potassium-sparing diuretics** (e.g., spironolactone [Aldactone]), **or ACE inhibitors** (e.g., enalaprilat [Vasotec IV]) may increase risk of hyperkalemia. ▪ May decrease clearance and increase toxicity of **methotrexate.** ▪ May cause false values in common **lab tests;** see literature.

SIDE EFFECTS
Arthralgia, chills, edema, fever, pain at the injection site, prostration, skin rash, thrombophlebitis, urticaria.

Major: Acute interstitial nephritis, anaphylaxis, convulsions, hemolytic anemia, hyperreflexia, neurotoxicity, potassium poisoning with coma, sodium-induced congestive heart failure. Hypersensitivity myocarditis (fever, eosinophilia, rash, sinus tachycardia, ST-T changes and cardiomegaly) and CDAD can occur. Higher-than-normal doses may cause neurologic adverse effects including convulsions, especially with impaired renal function.

ANTIDOTE
For all side effects, discontinue the drug, treat hypersensitivity reactions or resuscitate as necessary, and notify the physician. Treat minor side effects symptomatically according to physician's order. Mild cases of CDAD may respond to discontinuation of the drug. Treat CDAD with fluids, electrolytes, protein supplements, and oral vancomycin (Vancocin) or metronidazole (Flagyl) as indicated. In severe cases, surgical evaluation may be indicated. Removed by hemodialysis.

PENTAMIDINE ISETHIONATE
(pen-**TAM**-ih-deen is-ah-**THIGH**-oh-nayt)

Antiprotozoal

pH 4.09 to 5.4

USUAL DOSE

Treatment of *Pneumocystis jiroveci*: 4 mg/kg of body weight once daily for 14 days. See Precautions/Monitor. Has been used up to 21 days; benefits not defined.

Pneumocystis prophylaxis: 4 mg/kg once each month. May be given every 2 weeks if indicated.

Leishmania, visceral (unlabeled): 2 to 4 mg/kg once daily for up to 15 days.

Leishmania, cutaneous (unlabeled): 2 to 4 mg/kg once or twice a week until lesions heal.

Trypanosoma gambiense (unlabeled): 4 mg/kg once daily for 10 days.

PEDIATRIC DOSE

***Pneumocystis jiroveci*:** 4 mg/kg once daily for 12 to 14 days.

Pneumocystis prophylaxis: See Usual Dose.

Leishmania donovani: 2 to 4 mg/kg once daily for 15 days. Up to 21 days have been suggested, but risks with therapy over 14 days may be increased.

Trypanosoma gambiense: See Usual Dose.

DOSE ADJUSTMENTS

Reduced dose in renal failure may be indicated. One source recommends 4 mg/kg every 24 hours with a CrCl of 10 to 50 mL/min or 4 mg/kg every 24 to 36 hours with a CrCl less than 10 mL/min.

DILUTION

Initially dilute each 300 mg or fraction thereof in 3 to 5 mL SW or D5W. A single dose must be further diluted in 50 to 250 mL of D5W and given as an infusion.

Storage: Stable at room temperature for 24 hours. Discard unused portion. Protect dry product and reconstituted solution from light.

COMPATIBILITY

Consider any drug NOT listed as compatible to be INCOMPATIBLE until consulting a pharmacist; specific conditions may apply.

Will form a precipitate with NS; do not use for dilution or infusion. Manufacturer states, "Do not mix pentamidine solutions with any other drugs."

One source suggests the following **compatibilities:**

Y-site: Diltiazem (Cardizem), zidovudine (AZT, Retrovir).

RATE OF ADMINISTRATION

A single dose should be evenly distributed over 60 minutes.

Leishmania, visceral and cutaneous: A single dose evenly distributed over 1 to 2 hours.

ACTIONS

An antiprotozoal agent. Specifically active against *Pneumocystis jiroveci*. It is thought to interfere with nuclear metabolism and inhibit the synthesis of DNA, RNA, phospholipids, and proteins. Route of metabolism is unknown. Excreted partially in urine. May accumulate in renal failure.

INDICATIONS AND USES
Treatment and prophylaxis of *Pneumocystis jiroveci* pneumonia (PCP). **Unlabeled uses:** Treatment of trypanosomiasis and visceral and cutaneous leishmaniasis. Aerosol used prophylactically to prevent PCP in high-risk patients.

CONTRAINDICATIONS
None if the diagnosis of *Pneumocystis jiroveci* pneumonia is confirmed.

PRECAUTIONS
Specific use only; establish correct diagnosis. ▪ Sulfamethoxazole/ trimethoprim is the drug of choice for treatment of *Pneumocystis* pneumonia. Pentamidine causes numerous and serious side effects and is indicated only if the patient does not respond to or tolerate SMX-TMP. ▪ Use extreme caution in patients with hypertension, hypotension, hypoglycemia, hyperglycemia, hypocalcemia, leukopenia, thrombocytopenia, anemia, hepatic or renal dysfunction, ventricular tachycardia, pancreatitis, and Stevens-Johnson syndrome.

Monitor: Before, during, and after therapy obtain a BUN and SCr (daily), CBC, platelet count, alkaline phosphatase, bilirubin, AST, ALT, serum calcium, and ECG. ▪ Has caused fatalities resulting from severe hypotension, hypoglycemia, and cardiac arrhythmias even with the administration of the first dose. Keep patient supine, observe continuously for any sign of adverse reaction, and monitor BP continuously during infusion and afterward until stable. ▪ Emergency equipment for resuscitation must be immediately available. ▪ Monitor blood glucose levels daily during therapy and several times after therapy is complete. Pancreatic necrosis and very high plasma insulin levels have occurred. May also cause hyperglycemia and diabetes mellitus.

Patient Education: May cause severe hypotension; remain lying down until BP is stable. ▪ Report any unusual bleeding or bruising.

Maternal/Child: Category C: use only when clearly needed during pregnancy and breast-feeding. Hazards to fetus or infant are unknown. ▪ Discontinue breast-feeding.

DRUG/LAB INTERACTIONS
Nephrotoxic effects may be additive with concomitant use with **other nephrotoxic drugs** (e.g., aminoglycosides [e.g., gentamicin], amphotericin B, cisplatin [Platinol], foscarnet [Foscavir], vancomycin). Monitoring of renal function, dose reductions, and/or dose interval adjustments may be required.

SIDE EFFECTS
Occur in over 50% of patients and may be life threatening. Some occur after course of treatment is completed. Acute renal failure, anemia, anorexia, bad taste in mouth, cardiac arrhythmias including ventricular tachycardia, confusion, dizziness, elevated SCr and liver function tests, fever, hallucinations, hyperglycemia, hyperkalemia, hypocalcemia, hypoglycemia, hypotension, leukopenia, nausea, neuralgia, phlebitis, rash, thrombocytopenia.

ANTIDOTE
Discontinue drug for any life-threatening side effects. Notify physician of all side effects. Symptomatic treatment indicated. Resuscitate as necessary.

PENTAZOCINE (LACTATE)
(pen-**TAZ**-oh-seen **LAK**-tayt)

Talwin

USUAL DOSE
30 mg. May repeat every 3 to 4 hours or decrease to 5 to 15 mg and repeat every 2 hours. 360 mg equals maximum dose in 24 hours. Use oral form of pentazocine when appropriate.

Patients in labor: 20 mg when contractions become regular. May repeat every 2 to 3 hours as needed for two or three additional doses.

DOSE ADJUSTMENTS
Reduced dose may be required in the elderly or debilitated, in impaired hepatic or renal function, in patients with limited pulmonary reserve, and in the presence of other CNS depressants; use caution. ■ Increased dose may be required in smokers. ■ See Precautions, Drug/Lab Interactions, and Elderly.

DILUTION
May be given undiluted. It is preferable to dilute each 5 mg with at least 1 mL of SW for injection.

Storage: Store at CRT. Avoid freezing.

COMPATIBILITY
Consider any drug NOT listed as compatible to be INCOMPATIBLE until consulting a pharmacist; specific conditions may apply.

Manufacturer states, "Do not mix in the same syringe with soluble barbiturates (e.g., phenobarbital [Luminal]); precipitation will occur."

One source suggests the following **compatibilities:**

Y-site: Heparin, hydrocortisone sodium succinate (Solu-Cortef), potassium chloride (KCl).

RATE OF ADMINISTRATION
Each 5 mg or fraction thereof over 1 minute.

ACTIONS
A synthetic narcotic agonist-antagonist with a potent analgesic action, pentazocine is somewhat less effective than morphine and meperidine in equivalent doses. May produce respiratory depression, but does not increase markedly with increased doses. Onset of action is prompt, 2 to 3 minutes, and lasts about 2 to 3 hours. Metabolized in the liver. Excreted in urine. Crosses the placental barrier. Secreted in breast milk.

INDICATIONS AND USES
Relief of moderate to severe pain. ■ Preoperative medication. ■ Support of anesthesia. ■ Obstetric analgesia.

CONTRAINDICATIONS
Hypersensitivity to pentazocine or its components (contains sulfites); pathologic brain conditions.

PRECAUTIONS
Use with caution in bronchial asthma, relief of biliary pain, history of drug abuse, decreased renal or hepatic function, respiratory depression from any cause, a history of seizures, and in patients with head injury or increased intracranial pressure. ■ Some formulations contain sulfites, use caution in

patients with allergies; see Contraindications. ■ Use with caution in patients with acute MI accompanied by hypertension or left ventricular failure. May increase systemic and pulmonary arterial pressure and systemic vascular resistance. ■ Mild narcotic antagonist. May precipitate withdrawal symptoms in patients accustomed to narcotics. ■ May provide less effective analgesia in heavy smokers.

Monitor: Naloxone (Narcan), oxygen, and controlled respiratory equipment must always be available. ■ Observe patient continuously during injection and frequently thereafter. Monitor vital signs. Keep patient supine to minimize side effects; orthostatic hypotension and fainting may occur. Observe closely during ambulation. ■ Pain control usually more effective with routinely administered doses. Determine appropriate interval through clinical assessment. ■ See Drug/Lab Interactions.

Patient Education: Avoid use of alcohol or other CNS depressants (e.g., antihistamines, diazepam [Valium]). ■ Request assistance for ambulation. ■ May be habit forming.

Maternal/Child: Category C: safety for use in pregnancy, (other than labor) and breast-feeding not established. ■ Respiratory depression, dyspnea, and transient apnea have been reported in a small number of newborn infants whose mothers received pentazocine during labor. ■ Use extreme caution if necessary during delivery of premature infants. ■ Safety and effectiveness for IV use in pediatric patients under 12 years of age not established.

Elderly: May be more sensitive to effects (e.g., respiratory depression, confusion, constipation, dizziness, oversedation, urinary retention). ■ Analgesia should be effective with lower doses. ■ Consider age-related organ impairment, monitoring of renal function may be indicated. ■ Half-life longer and clearance lower compared to younger patients. ■ See Dose Adjustments.

DRUG/LAB INTERACTIONS

Potentiated by **cimetidine** (Tagamet), **and other CNS depressants** such as narcotic analgesics, general anesthetics, alcohol, anticholinergics, antihistamines, barbiturates, hypnotics, sedatives, psychotropic agents, MAO inhibitors, and neuromuscular blocking agents (e.g., atracurium [Tracrium]). Reduced doses of both drugs may be indicated. ■ May decrease analgesic effects of **other narcotics;** avoid concurrent use. ■ Metabolism and clearance increased in **smokers;** analgesic effects may be decreased.

SIDE EFFECTS

Apprehension, blurred vision, circulatory depression, confusion, constipation, cramps, depression, diarrhea, disorientation, dizziness, double vision, dreams, drug dependence, dry mouth, dyspnea, euphoria, facial edema, floating feeling, flushing, hallucinations, headache, hypersensitivity reactions, hypertension, injection site reactions, insomnia, muscle tremor, nausea, neonatal apnea, nervousness, nystagmus, paresthesias, perspiration, pruritus, respiratory depression, sedation, seizures, shock, tachycardia, taste alteration, urinary retention, uterine contraction depression.

ANTIDOTE

For any side effect, discontinue the drug and notify the physician. Treat side effects symptomatically. For overdose or respiratory depression, naloxone hydrochloride (Narcan) is the antidote of choice. If naloxone is not available, methylphenidate (Ritalin) may be of value in respiratory depression (only available in oral form).

PENTETATE CALCIUM TRISODIUM INJECTION ▪ PENTETATE ZINC TRISODIUM INJECTION   Antidote

(**PEN**-teh-tayt **KAL**-see-um try-**SO**-dee-um in-**JEK**-shun ▪
PEN-teh-tayt **ZINK** try-**SO**-dee-um in-**JEK**-shun)

Ca-DTPA ▪ **Zn-DTPA**   pH 7.3 to 8.3 ▪ pH 6.5 to 7.5

USUAL DOSE

Chelation therapy with either pentetate calcium trisodium (Ca-DTPA) or pentetate zinc trisodium (Zn-DTPA) is most effective when administered within the first 24 hours after internal contamination; however, it should be started as soon as possible after suspected or known internal contamination, even if more than 24 hours have passed. *Initiation of therapy with a single dose of pentetate calcium trisodium (Ca-DTPA) is preferred because it is more effective than pentetate zinc trisodium (Zn-DTPA) in the first 24 hours.* After 24 hours, both drugs are equally effective. However, *if Ca-DTPA is not available, initiate therapy with pentetate zinc trisodium (Zn-DTPA).* Preliminary lab tests desired; see Monitor. See Maternal/Child.

Adults and pediatric patients 12 years of age or older: *Initial dose:* 1 Gm IV (dose is the same for either agent).

After the initial dose, *maintenance treatment is recommended with pentetate zinc trisodium (Zn-DTPA).* If Zn-DTPA is not available, therapy may be continued with Ca-DTPA. Ca-DTPA has more toxicity (e.g., depletion of more trace metals, higher rate of mortality, the presence of kidney and liver vacuolization [air or fluid in the tissues], and small bowel hemorrhagic lesions), and concomitant mineral supplements containing zinc are required. Zn-DTPA results in minimal depletion of manganese and magnesium.

Maintenance dose: 1 Gm IV daily (dose is the same for either agent; however, Zn-DTPA is preferred). If Ca-DTPA is used for maintenance doses, transfer to Zn-DTPA as soon as it is available. Zn-DTPA may be administered for days, months, or years depending on the extent of internal contamination and individual response to therapy. Usually continued until the excretion enhancement factor (EEF) approaches 1.

PEDIATRIC DOSE

Pediatric patients less than 12 years of age: *Initial dose:* 14 mg/kg IV (dose is the same for either agent). Do not exceed 1 Gm. See all comments under Usual Dose.

Maintenance dose: 14 mg/kg IV daily. See all comments under Usual Dose.

DOSE ADJUSTMENTS

No dose adjustment is required in patients with impaired renal function; however, renal impairment may reduce the rate at which the chelators remove radiocontaminants from the body. Hemodialysis may be used to increase the rate of elimination in heavily contaminated patients with renal impairment. The use of high flux dialysis is recommended. The dialysis fluid requires handling with radiation precautions.

DILUTION

Both agents: *IV:* A single dose may be given undiluted as an IV injection or diluted in 100 to 250 mL of D5W, NS, or LR and given as an infusion. To open the ampule, face the point upward and break off the neck with a downward movement.

Nebulized inhalation: Dilute in a 1:1 ratio with SW or NS (equal amounts of drug and diluent).

Filters: Manufacturer states product may be filtered.

Storage: Store between 15° to 30° C (59° to 86° F).

COMPATIBILITY

Specific information not available.

RATE OF ADMINISTRATION

Both agents: *IV injection:* A single dose evenly distributed over 3 to 4 minutes.

IV infusion: A single dose properly diluted and infused over 30 minutes.

ACTIONS

Both agents: Hyperosmolar solutions. Form stable chelates with radioactive contaminants (metal ions) found in the circulation, interstitial fluid, and tissues by exchanging calcium or zinc for a metal of greater binding capacity. Most effective with plutonium, americium, or curium. Chelating capacity is greatest immediately and up to approximately 24 hours after internal contamination, when the radiocontaminant is still circulating and readily available for chelation. The ability to chelate decreases with time as the radioactive contaminants incorporate into tissues and become sequestered in the liver and bone. Rapidly distributed throughout the extracellular fluid space. Significant amounts do not penetrate into erythrocytes or other cells. Accumulation in specific organs has not been observed. Metabolism is minimal. Cleared by glomerular filtration. Activity in plasma was not detectable 24 hours after injection. Excreted in urine.

Pentetate calcium trisodium (Ca-DTPA): More effective than pentetate zinc trisodium (Zn-DTPA) in the first 24 hours. After 24 hours, both drugs are equally effective.

INDICATIONS AND USES

Treatment of individuals with known or suspected internal contamination with radiocontaminants (e.g., plutonium, americium, or curium) to increase the rates of elimination. ▪ If Ca-DTPA is not available, initiate therapy with Zn-DTPA. ▪ May also be inhaled as treatment for inhalation contamination; it is absorbed, and inhalation results in comparable elimination of the radiocontaminants.

CONTRAINDICATIONS

None known when used for primary indication.

PRECAUTIONS

Both agents: For IV use, safety of IM injection not established. ▪ Begin chelation treatment as soon as possible after known or suspected internal contamination with radiocontaminants. The ability of both agents to chelate decreases with time as the radioactive contaminants incorporate into tissues. ▪ Radioactive iodine is not bound by DTPA. ▪ Not expected to be effective for uranium and neptunium because less stable chelates are formed, which results in the deposition of these elements in tissues (including the bone). ▪ Studies in patients with impaired renal or hepatic function have not been conducted. Impaired renal function is expected to increase the half-life of Ca-DTPA and Zn-DTPA and decrease the rate of elimination of the radiocontaminants; see Dose Adjustments. ▪ Nebulized chelation therapy may exacerbate asthma; use caution. ▪ Contamination with multiple or unknown radiocontaminants may require additional therapies (e.g., Prussian blue, potassium iodide). ▪ Manufacturer requests collection of patient treatment data; see prescribing information.

Pentetate calcium trisodium (Ca-DTPA): Loss of zinc, manganese, and magnesium from the small intestine, skeleton, pancreas, and testes is significant; see Monitor. The rate and amount of endogenous metal depletion has been shown to increase with split daily dosing, increased doses, and/or duration of treatment. Depletion of these endogenous metals can interfere with necessary mitotic cellular processes and has resulted in transient inhibition of a metalloenzyme-D-aminolevulinic acid dehydrase (ALAD) in the blood and suppressed hematopoiesis (formation of blood cells). Concomitant supplements containing zinc are required. ▪ Use with caution in patients with severe hemochromatosis (a disorder of iron metabolism); deaths have been reported.

Pentetate zinc trisodium (Zn-DTPA): Results in minimal depletion of manganese and magnesium.

Monitor: *Both agents:* If possible, obtain baseline CBC with differential, BUN, serum chemistries and electrolytes, urinalysis, and blood and urine radioassays before initiating treatment. Monitor regularly throughout treatment. ▪ When possible, establish an elimination curve. A quantitative baseline estimate of total internalized transuranium elements(s) and measures of elimination of radioactivity should be obtained by appropriate whole-body counting, bioassay (e.g., biodosimetry), or fecal/urine sample.
▪ Care should be taken to minimize radiation exposure to patients ·and to medical personnel from patients' contaminated excrement (e.g., blood, sputum, urine); this is consistent with institutional good radiation safety practices and patient management procedures. Contact the radiation safety officer. ▪ Encourage fluid intake and frequent voiding. Promotes dilution of the radiocontaminant in urine and minimizes radiation exposure to the bladder. ▪ Document adverse reactions. ▪ See Precautions, Maternal/Child, and Drug/Lab Interactions.

Pentetate calcium trisodium (Ca-DTPA): If more than one dose of Ca-DTPA is used, monitor lab tests more frequently (with specific attention to serum zinc), and initiate vitamin or mineral supplements containing zinc when appropriate.

Pentetate zinc trisodium (Zn-DTPA): Based on lab tests, initiate mineral or vitamin plus mineral supplements as appropriate.

Patient Education: *Both agents:* The following steps are required to minimize contamination of others by the radiocontaminants. Use a toilet instead of a urinal and flush several times after each voiding, because treatment increases excretion of radioactivity in the urine. Completely clean up spilled urine or feces, and wash hands thoroughly. Wash clothes that come in contact with blood or urine separately. Drink plenty of fluids; fluid intake is important to aid in flushing radiocontaminants from the system. Void frequently to limit the time that radiocontaminants remain in the bladder. Carefully dispose of expectorant from coughing; do not swallow expectorant. ▪ Parents and caregivers need to take extra precautions in handling the urine, feces, and expectorants of children to avoid additional exposure to the caregiver or child.

Maternal/Child: *Both agents:* Discontinue breast-feeding whether or not chelation therapy is received. Radiocontaminants are secreted in breast milk. Take precautions when disposing of breast milk. ▪ Safety and effectiveness of the nebulized route of administration in pediatric patients has not been established.

Pentetate calcium trisodium (Ca-DTPA): Category C: depletion of body stores of zinc is known to affect DNA and RNA synthesis in humans. Teratogenicity in humans cannot be ruled out. Birth defects in animals increased with dose, and incidences were higher in early and mid gestation. ▪ Treatment of pregnant women with pentetate zinc trisodium (if available) is preferred, except in cases of high internal radioactive contamination. The risk of immediate and delayed radiation-induced toxicity to both the mother and the fetus should be considered in comparison to the risk of pentetate calcium trisodium because it is more effective than pentetate zinc trisodium in the first 24 hours after internal contamination. The use of a single dose of Ca-DTPA with vitamin or mineral supplements containing zinc may be considered as the initial treatment.

Pentetate zinc trisodium (Zn-DTPA): Category B: treatment of pregnant women should begin and continue with Zn-DTPA. Use only if clearly needed; however, animal studies revealed no evidence of impaired fertility or harm to the fetus.

Elderly: Specific information not available.

DRUG/LAB INTERACTIONS

Specific drug interactions have not been studied. ▪ Contamination with **multiple or unknown radiocontaminants** may require the use of additional therapies (e.g., Prussian blue, potassium iodide).

SIDE EFFECTS

Pentetate calcium trisodium (Ca-DTPA): Allergic reactions, chest pain, dermatitis, diarrhea, headache, injection site reactions, light-headedness, metallic taste, and nausea have occurred. Prolonged treatment may result in depletion of manganese, magnesium, zinc and, possibly, metalloproteinases. Cough and/or wheezing occurred with nebulized Ca-DTPA.

Pentetate zinc trisodium (Zn-DTPA): Headache, light-headedness, and pelvic pain have been reported. Allergic reactions may occur.

ANTIDOTE

Keep physician informed of side effects; symptomatic treatment is indicated. Treat a hypersensitivity reaction as indicated (oxygen, antihistamines [e.g., diphenhydramine (Benadryl)], epinephrine [Adrenalin], and corticosteroids [e.g., methylprednisolone (Solu-Medrol)]). Maintain a patent airway. Resuscitate as necessary.

PENTOBARBITAL SODIUM

(**PEN**-toh-**bar**-bih-tal **SO**-dee-um)

Nembutal Sodium

Barbiturate
Sedative-hypnotic
Anticonvulsant

pH 9 to 10.5

USUAL DOSE

100 mg initially. Wait 1 full minute between each dose to determine drug effect. Additional doses in increments of 25 to 50 mg may be given as indicated. Maximum dosage ranges from 200 to 500 mg.
Barbiturate coma: *Loading dose:* 3 to 10 mg/kg over 30 minutes to 3 hours. *Maintenance dose:* 1.5 to 2 mg/kg every 1 to 2 hours or an infusion of 0.5 to 3 mg/kg/hr. Adjust to maintain pentobarbital blood level between 110 and 177 mm/L (25 to 40 mg/dL) or ICP below 25 Torr.

PEDIATRIC DOSE

See Maternal/Child.
1 to 3 mg/kg slowly until asleep. Maximum dose 100 mg/24 hr.
Barbiturate coma: See Usual Dose. An alternate source suggests *Loading dose:* 10 to 15 mg/kg over 1 to 2 hours. *Maintenance dose:* Begin with 1 mg/kg/hr; increase to 2 to 3 mg/kg/hr to maintain EEG burst suppression.

DOSE ADJUSTMENTS

Reduce dose in impaired renal or hepatic function; usually required in the debilitated or elderly. ▪ See Drug/Lab Interactions.

DILUTION

May be given undiluted or, preferably, may be further diluted in SW, NS, or Ringer's injection. Any desired amount of diluent may be used. 9 mL of diluent with 1 mL of pentobarbital (50 mg) equals 5 mg/mL. Use only absolutely clear solutions.

COMPATIBILITY

Consider any drug NOT listed as compatible to be INCOMPATIBLE until consulting a pharmacist; specific conditions may apply.
Manufacturer states, "Should not be admixed with any other medication or solution." Do not mix in a syringe with pentazocine (Talwin); precipitation will occur. May precipitate in acidic solutions.
One source suggests the following **compatibilities:**
Additive: *Not recommended by manufacturer.* Amikacin (Amikin), aminophylline, calcium chloride, chloramphenicol (Chloromycetin), dimenhydrinate, erythromycin (Erythrocin), lidocaine, thiopental (Pentothal), verapamil.
Y-site: Acyclovir (Zovirax), insulin (regular), linezolid (Zyvox), propofol (Diprivan).

RATE OF ADMINISTRATION

50 mg or fraction thereof over 1 minute. Titrate slowly to desired effect. Rapid injection rate may cause symptoms of overdose (e.g., serious respiratory depression).
Barbiturate coma: See specific dose recommendations.

ACTIONS

A sedative, hypnotic barbiturate of short duration with anticonvulsant effects. Pentobarbital is a CNS depressant. Onset of action is prompt by the IV route and lasts about 3 to 4 hours. Will effectively depress the motor cortex if adequate doses are administered. Pain perception is unimpaired. Reportedly reduces cerebral blood flow and thus reduces cerebral edema and intracranial pressure. Detoxified in the liver and excreted fairly quickly in the urine in changed form. Crosses the placental barrier. Secreted in breast milk.

INDICATIONS AND USES

Preanesthetic sedation. ■ Dental and minor surgical sedation. ■ Control of convulsions caused by disease and drug poisoning. ■ Short-term hypnotic. ■ Sedation in psychotic states.

Unlabeled uses: High doses have been used to induce coma in the management of cerebral ischemia and increased intracranial pressure. Has been most effective in patients under 35 years of age or in closed head injuries.

CONTRAINDICATIONS

Acute or chronic pain, delivery (when maximum drug effect would be at the time of delivery), history of porphyria, known hypersensitivity to barbiturates, severely impaired liver function especially with any signs of hepatic coma, severe respiratory disease or depression.

PRECAUTIONS

IV route usually reserved for critical situations. ■ Use caution in status asthmaticus, shock, severe renal or liver disease, depressive states after convulsions, shock, and in the elderly. ■ Use caution in acute or chronic pain. ■ Status epilepticus can occur from too-rapid withdrawal. ■ May be habit forming. Use caution in the presence of fever, diabetes, hyperthyroidism, or severe anemia; may increase side effects. ■ Benzodiazepines (diazepam [Valium], midazolam [Versed]) generally preferred for sedation.

Monitor: Record BP, pulse, and respirations every 3 to 5 minutes. Keep patient under constant observation. ■ Maintain a patent airway. ■ Treat the cause of a convulsion. ■ Highly alkaline; determine absolute patency of vein; use of large veins preferred to prevent thrombosis. Avoid extravasation. Intra-arterial injection will cause gangrene. ■ Monitor phenytoin and barbiturate levels when both drugs are used concurrently. ■ Monitor hematopoietic, renal, and hepatic systems in extended therapy. ■ See Drug/Lab Interactions.

Patient Education: Avoid alcohol and other CNS depressants (e.g., antihistamines, diazepam [Valium]). ■ May be habit forming. ■ May require alternate birth control.

Maternal/Child: Category D: avoid pregnancy; will cause birth defects. ■ May cause drowsiness in the nursing infant. ■ See Contraindications. ■ May cause paradoxical excitement in pediatric patients.

Elderly: Often have increased sensitivity to barbiturates; may cause marked excitement, depression, confusion, and increased risk of barbiturate-induced hypothermia. ■ See Dose Adjustments and Precautions. ■ Consider age-related hepatic or renal impairment and concomitant disease or drug therapy.

DRUG/LAB INTERACTIONS

Use extreme caution if any **other CNS depressants** have been given, such as alcohol, narcotic analgesics, anesthetics, antidepressants, antihistamines, hypnotics, MAO inhibitors, phenothiazines, sedatives, aminoglycoside antibiotics, or tranquilizers; potentiation with respiratory depression may occur. ■ Inhibits effectiveness of **propranolol, corticosteroids, doxycycline, oral anticoagulants, oral contraceptives, quinidine, and theophylline.** Capable of innumerable interactions with many drugs. ■ May increase orthostatic hypotension with **furosemide** (Lasix). ■ Monitor **phenytoin** and barbiturate levels when both drugs are used concurrently. ■ May inhibit **vitamin D** metabolism with extended use.

SIDE EFFECTS

Average dose: Depression, dermatitis, facial edema, fever, hypotension, neonatal apnea, pain at or below injection site, respiratory depression (hypoventilation), thrombocytopenic purpura.

Overdose: Apnea, coma, cough reflex depression, flat EEG (reversible unless hypoxic damage has occurred), hypotension, laryngospasm, lowered body temperature, pulmonary edema, renal shutdown, respiratory depression, sluggish or absent reflexes.

ANTIDOTE

Discontinue drug immediately for pain at or below injection site. Notify the physician of any side effects. Symptomatic and supportive treatment are most important in overdose. Maintain an adequate airway with artificial ventilation if indicated. Keep the patient warm. IV volume expanders (dextran) and IV fluids will help maintain adequate circulation. Diuretics or hemodialysis will promote the elimination of the drug. Vasopressors (dopamine) will maintain BP.

PENTOSTATIN `BBW`

(**PEN**-toh-**stah**-tin)

2-Deoxycoformycin, Nipent

Antineoplastic (antibiotic)

pH 7 to 8.5

USUAL DOSE

Evaluation and prehydration is required before administration; see Monitor.

4 mg/M^2 every other week. Do not exceed recommended dose; see Precautions. If there is no major toxicity and improvement is continuous, treat until a complete response is achieved, then administer two additional doses. Do not treat beyond 12 months.

DOSE ADJUSTMENTS

Reduced dose and benefit-versus-risk assessment may be required with impaired renal function (CrCl below 60 mL/min); insufficient data available. Two patients with impaired renal function (CrCl 50 to 60 mL/min) achieved complete response without unusual adverse events when treated with 2 mg/M^2. ▪ Withhold dose if SCr elevated; obtain CrCl. ▪ Withhold dose if the absolute neutrophil count falls from a baseline of greater than 500 cells/mm^3 before therapy to less than 200 cells/mm^3 during treatment. Resume treatment when count returns to predose levels.

DILUTION

Specific techniques required; see Precautions. Diluent (5 mL SW) provided; dissolve completely; will yield 2 mg/mL. May be given by IV injection or further diluted in 25 to 50 mL NS or D5W; 25 mL yields 0.33 mg/mL, 50 mL yields 0.18 mg/mL. Treat spills or waste with a 5% sodium hypochlorite solution before disposal.

Storage: Refrigerate before initial reconstitution. Store at room temperature and use within 8 hours after initial reconstitution or dilution for infusion.

COMPATIBILITY

Consider any drug NOT listed as compatible to be INCOMPATIBLE until consulting a pharmacist; specific conditions may apply.

Does not interact with PVC infusion containers or administration sets at concentrations specified for dilution.

One source suggests the following **compatibilities:**

Y-site: Melphalan (Alkeran), ondansetron (Zofran), paclitaxel (Taxol), sargramostim (Leukine). Physically **compatible** at the **Y-site** with fludarabine (Fludara); however, the two drugs are not recommended for concurrent use; see Drug/Lab Interactions.

RATE OF ADMINISTRATION

Follow each dose with an additional 500 mL of prehydration infusion fluids.

IV injection: A single dose over 1 minute.

Infusion: A single dose over 20 to 30 minutes.

ACTIONS

Mechanism of action is not known, but it is cytotoxic as a result of its potent inhibition of the enzyme adenosine deaminase (ADA). Blocks DNA and RNA synthesis and causes DNA damage. Average terminal half-life of 6 hours is extended to 18 hours in patients with impaired renal function (CrCl less than 50 mL/min). Inhibits ADA for up to 1 week; actual response may not occur for months. Primarily excreted in urine.

INDICATIONS AND USES
Single-agent treatment of both untreated patients and alpha-interferon–refractory hairy cell leukemia (HCL) patients with active disease as defined by clinically significant anemia, neutropenia, thrombocytopenia, or disease-related symptoms.

Unlabeled uses: Treatment of chronic lymphocytic leukemia, prolymphocytic leukemia, non-Hodgkin's lymphoma, cutaneous T-cell lymphoma, and peripheral T-cell lymphomas.

CONTRAINDICATIONS
Hypersensitivity to pentostatin; see Drug/Lab Interactions.

PRECAUTIONS
Follow guidelines for handling cytotoxic agents. See Appendix A, p. 1429.
■ Assess drug profile before administration. ■ Severe renal, liver, pulmonary, and CNS toxicities have occurred at higher doses; do not exceed recommended dose. ■ Usually administered by or under the supervision of a physician specialist. ■ Myelosuppression, especially neutropenia, is most severe during the first few courses of treatment. ■ Must consider risk/benefit in patients with some bone marrow suppression, the possibility of chickenpox or herpes zoster, a history of gout or urate renal stones, renal function impairment, or previous cytotoxic drug or radiation therapy. Use extreme caution. ■ After 6 months of treatment, assess for response; if partial or complete response is not evident, discontinue treatment. If partial response is evident, reevaluate as indicated but do not treat beyond 12 months.

Monitor: Monitor CBC (including differential and platelet count) and SCr before each dose and as indicated. Blood chemistries including serum uric acid, and a CrCl assay is required before and during treatment. ■ Prehydration with 500 to 1,000 mL D5/½NS or an equivalent is required. An additional 500 mL is required postadministration. ■ Treatment of patients with infection may exacerbate symptoms and cause death. Control infection before treatment initiated. Withhold treatment if an active infection occurs; resume when infection is controlled. ■ Prophylactic antiemetics recommended (e.g., prochlorperazine [Compazine], ondansetron [Zofran]); continue for 48 to 72 hours. ■ Observe closely for severe rashes, nervous system toxicity, and myelosuppression (especially after initial cycles); pentostatin may have to be withheld or discontinued. ■ For severe neutropenia beyond the initial cycles, evaluate for disease status, including a bone marrow examination. ■ Assess response to treatment with periodic monitoring of peripheral blood for hairy cells. Bone marrow aspirates and biopsies may be required at 2- to 3-month intervals. ■ Monitor for thrombocytopenia (platelet count less than 50,000/mm^3). Initiate precautions to prevent excessive bleeding (e.g., inspect IV sites, skin, and mucous membranes; use extreme care during invasive procedures; test urine, emesis, stool, and secretions for occult blood).

Patient Education: Consider birth control options; nonhormonal birth control recommended. ■ Report rashes, symptoms of infection, or bruising and bleeding immediately. ■ See Appendix D, p. 1434.

Maternal/Child: Category D: avoid pregnancy; can cause fetal harm. ■ Discontinue breast-feeding. ■ Safety for use in pediatric patients under 18 years of age not established.

Elderly: Consider decreased renal function.

DRUG/LAB INTERACTIONS

Assess drug profile before administration. ▪ Do not use with **fludarabine** (Fludara); may increase risk of fatal pulmonary toxicity. ▪ Combination therapy with **carmustine** (BiCNU), **etoposide** (VePesid), **and high-dose cyclophosphamide** as part of the ablative regimen for bone marrow transplant has caused acute pulmonary edema and hypotension. Deaths have occurred. ▪ Pentostatin enhances the effects of **vidarabine** (Ara-A). Combined use of these agents may result in an increase in adverse reactions associated with each drug. The therapeutic benefit of this drug combination has not been established. ▪ May cause skin rash with **allopurinol.** ▪ Elevates **liver function tests;** usually reversible. ▪ Do not administer **live virus vaccines** to patients receiving antineoplastic drugs. ▪ Uric acid levels may increase, increased dose of **gout agents** (e.g., colchicine, probenicid, sulfinpyrazone [Anturane]) may be indicated. ▪ Leukopenia and thrombocytopenia increased by **agents causing blood dyscrasias** (e.g., anticonvulsants [phenytoin (Dilantin)], penicillins, phenothiazines, and many others).

SIDE EFFECTS

Anemia, anorexia, chills, cough, diarrhea, fatigue, fever, GU disorders, headache, hepatic disorders/elevated liver function tests, hypersensitivity reactions, infection, leukopenia, lung disorders, myalgia, nausea, neurologic disorders/CNS, pain, rashes, skin disorders, thrombocytopenia, upper respiratory infections, and vomiting occur in 10% of patients and may require discontinuation of treatment. Abdominal pain, abnormal thinking, abnormal vision, abnormal ECG, anxiety, arthralgia, asthenia, back pain, bronchitis, cardiac arrhythmias, chest pain, confusion, conjunctivitis, constipation, depression, dizziness, dry skin, dyspnea, dysuria, ear pain, ecchymosis, eczema; elevated BUN, creatinine, and LDH; epistaxis, eye pain, flatulence, flu syndrome, hematuria, hemorrhage, herpes simplex, herpes zoster, insomnia, lung edema, lymphadenopathy, maculopapular rash, malaise, neoplasm, nervousness, paresthesia, peripheral edema, petechia, pharyngitis, pneumonia, pruritus, rhinitis, seborrhea, sinusitis, skin discoloration, somnolence, stomatitis, sweating, thrombophlebitis, vesiculobullous rash, weight loss, and death have occurred in 3% to 10% or more of patients.

ANTIDOTE

Keep physician informed of all side effects; most will be treated symptomatically if indicated. Withhold dose and notify physician for elevated SCr, absolute neutrophil count below 200 cells/mm^3, myelosuppression, infection, CNS toxicity, or severe rash. Administration of whole blood products (e.g., packed RBCs, platelets, leukocytes) and/or blood modifiers (e.g., darbepoetin alfa [Aranesp], epoetin alfa [Epogen], filgrastim [Neupogen], oprelvekin [Neumega], pegfilgrastim [Neulasta], sargramostim [Leukine]) may be indicated to treat bone marrow toxicity. Overdose may cause death due to severe renal, hepatic, pulmonary, or CNS toxicity. There is no specific antidote. Supportive therapy as indicated will help sustain the patient.

PHENOBARBITAL SODIUM
(fee-no-**BAR**-bih-tal **SO**-dee-um)

Luminal Sodium

Barbiturate
Sedative-hypnotic
Anticonvulsant

pH 8.5 to 10.5

USUAL DOSE

Use only enough medication to achieve the desired effect. May take up to 15 minutes to reach peak levels in the brain; guard against overdose and excessive respiratory depression.

Hypnotic: 100 to 325 mg.

Sedative: 30 to 120 mg/day in 2 or 3 divided doses (15 to 60 mg every 12 hours or 10 to 40 mg every 8 hours).

Anticonvulsant: 200 to 320 mg. May be repeated if necessary. Maximum dose usually does not exceed 600 mg.

Status epilepticus: *Loading dose:* 10 to 20 mg/kg in single or divided doses. May give an additional 5 mg/kg every 15 to 30 minutes up to a maximum dose of 30 mg/kg.

Maintenance dose: 1 to 3 mg/kg/24 hr or 0.5 to 1.5 mg/kg every 12 hours.

PEDIATRIC DOSE

See comments under Usual Dose.

Preoperative sedation: 1 to 3 mg/kg of body weight 60 to 90 minutes before procedure.

Status epilepticus: *Loading dose:* 15 to 18 mg/kg as a single dose or in divided doses. May give an additional 5 mg/kg every 15 to 30 minutes up to a maximum total dose of 30 mg/kg.

Maintenance dose: Infants: 2.5 to 3 mg/kg every 12 hours.

Ages 1 to 5: 3 to 4 mg/kg every 12 hours.

Ages 6 to 12: 2 to 3 mg/kg every 12 hours.

Over 12 years of age: 0.5 to 1.5 mg/kg every 12 hours. Up to 12 mg/kg/24 hours has been used in maintenance doses.

NEONATAL DOSE

See comments under Usual Dose.

Status epilepticus: *Loading dose:* 15 to 20 mg/kg as a single dose or in divided doses.

Maintenance dose: 1.5 to 2 mg/kg every 12 hours; may be increased to 2.5 mg/kg every 12 hours if needed. Therapeutic range is 15 to 40 mg/L. Because of its long half-life, it may take 2 to 3 weeks to reach steady-state levels.

DOSE ADJUSTMENTS

Reduce dose in impaired renal or hepatic function; usually required in the debilitated or elderly. ■ See Drug/Lab Interactions.

DILUTION

Sterile powder must be slowly diluted with SW for injection. Use a minimum of 3 mL of diluent. Also available in sterile vials and tubexes. Best if further diluted up to 10 mL with SW for injection. Solutions from powder form must be freshly prepared. Use only absolutely clear solutions. Discard powder or solution exposed to air for 30 minutes.

COMPATIBILITY   (Underline Indicates Conflicting Compatibility Information)
Consider any drug NOT listed as compatible to be INCOMPATIBLE until consulting a pharmacist; specific conditions may apply.

One source suggests the following **compatibilities:**

Additive: Amikacin (Amikin), aminophylline, calcium chloride, calcium gluconate, colistimethate (Coly-Mycin M), dimenhydrinate, meropenem (Merrem IV), thiopental (Pentothal), verapamil.

Y-site: Doripenem (Doribax), doxapram (Dopram), enalaprilat (Vasotec IV), fentanyl (Sublimaze), fosphenytoin (Cerebyx), <u>hydromorphone (Dilaudid)</u>, levofloxacin (Levaquin), linezolid (Zyvox), meropenem (Merrem IV), methadone (Dolophine), morphine, propofol (Diprivan), sufentanil (Sufenta).

RATE OF ADMINISTRATION
60 mg (gr 1) or fraction thereof over 1 minute. Titrate slowly to desired effect. Rapid injection rate may cause symptoms of overdose (e.g., serious respiratory depression).

Status epilepticus: A single loading dose over 10 to 15 minutes.

ACTIONS
A sedative, hypnotic barbiturate of long duration with potent anticonvulsant effects. Phenobarbital is a CNS depressant. Onset of action is prompt by the IV route and becomes rapidly more intense. Effects last from 6 to 10 hours. Will effectively depress the motor cortex with small doses. Pain perception is unimpaired. Rapidly absorbed by all body tissues and excreted in changed form in the urine. Excreted more readily in alkaline urine. Crosses the placental barrier. Secreted in breast milk.

INDICATIONS AND USES
Prolonged sedation (medical and psychiatric). ▪ Anticonvulsant.

CONTRAINDICATIONS
History of porphyria, impaired renal function, impaired hepatic function especially with any signs of hepatic coma, known hypersensitivity to barbiturates, previous addiction, severe respiratory depression including dyspnea, obstruction, or cor pulmonale.

PRECAUTIONS
IV route usually reserved for critical situations. ▪ Use caution in elderly and debilitated patients and those with asthma, pulmonary disease, shock, and impaired renal or hepatic function. ▪ Status epilepticus can occur from too-rapid withdrawal. ▪ May be habit forming. Use caution in acute or chronic pain. ▪ Benzodiazepines (diazepam [Valium], midazolam [Versed]) generally preferred for sedation.

Monitor: Keep patient under constant observation. Record vital signs every hour, or more often if indicated. ▪ Maintain a patent airway. ▪ Monitor hematopoietic, renal and hepatic systems in any extended therapy. ▪ Treat the cause of a convulsion. ▪ Keep equipment for artificial ventilation available. ▪ Highly alkaline. Determine absolute patency of vein; use of large veins preferred to prevent thrombosis. Avoid extravasation. Intra-arterial injection will cause gangrene. ▪ Monitor serum levels as indicated; the therapeutic range in adults is 20 to 40 mcg/mL (15 to 40 mcg/mL in pediatric patients). Because of its long half-life, it may take 2 to 3 weeks to reach steady-state levels. ▪ See Drug/Lab Interactions.

Patient Education: Avoid alcohol or other CNS depressants (e.g., antihistamines, diazepam [Valium]). May be habit forming. ▪ May require alternate birth control.

Maternal/Child: Category D: avoid pregnancy; will cause birth defects. ▪ May cause drowsiness in the nursing infant. ▪ See Precautions.

Elderly: See Dose Adjustments and Precautions. ▪ Often have increased sensitivity to barbiturates; may cause marked excitement, depression, confusion, and increased risk of barbiturate-induced hypothermia. ▪ Consider age-related hepatic or renal impairment and concomitant disease or drug therapy.

DRUG/LAB INTERACTIONS

Use extreme caution if any other **CNS depressants** have been given, such as alcohol, narcotic analgesics, anesthetics, antidepressants, antihistamines, hypnotics, MAO inhibitors, phenothiazines, sedatives, aminoglycoside antibiotics, tranquilizers. Potentiation with respiratory depression may occur. ▪ Inhibits effectiveness of **propranolol, corticosteroids, doxycycline, oral anticoagulants, oral contraceptives, quinidine, and theophylline.** Capable of innumerable interactions with many drugs. ▪ May increase orthostatic hypotension with **furosemide** (Lasix). ▪ Monitor **phenytoin** (Dilantin), **felbamate** (Felbatol), **carbamazepine** (Tegretol), **valproic acid and phenobarbital** levels when any combination of these drugs is used concurrently. ▪ May decrease the pharmacologic effect of **vitamin D.** ▪ May decrease plasma concentrations and effectiveness of **triazole antifungals** (e.g., itraconazole [Sporanox]).

SIDE EFFECTS

Rarely occur with slow injection of average doses.

Average dose: Depression, dermatitis, facial edema, fever, headache, hypotension, nausea, neonatal apnea, respiratory depression (hypoventilation), thrombocytopenic purpura, vertigo.

Overdose: Apnea, coma, cough reflex depression, delirium, flat EEG (reversible unless hypoxic damage has occurred), hypotension, laryngospasm, lowered body temperature, pulmonary edema, renal shutdown, respiratory depression, sluggish or absent reflexes, stupor.

ANTIDOTE

Notify the physician of any side effects. Symptomatic and supportive treatment is most important in overdose. Maintain an adequate airway with artificial ventilation if indicated. Keep the patient warm. IV volume expanders (dextran) and other IV fluids will help maintain adequate circulation. Diuretics may promote the elimination of the drug. Vasopressors (e.g., dopamine) will maintain BP.

PHENTOLAMINE MESYLATE
(fen-**TOLL**-ah-meen **MES**-ih-layt)

Alpha-adrenergic blocking agent
Antihypertensive
Vasodilator

Regitine

pH 4.5 to 6.5

USUAL DOSE
Preoperative: 5 mg 1 to 2 hours before surgery. May be repeated. During surgery the same doses are used as indicated to control epinephrine intoxication.

Prevent necrosis caused by norepinephrine (Levophed): Add 10 mg to each 1,000 mL of IV solution containing norepinephrine or dopamine.

Test dose for diagnosis of pheochromocytoma: 2.5 to 5 mg.

Treatment of congestive heart failure (unlabeled): 5 to 10 mg in 500 mL of D5W given at a rate of 0.17 to 0.4 mg/min.

PEDIATRIC DOSE
Preoperative: 1 mg, 0.1 mg/kg of body weight, or 3 mg/M^2 1 to 2 hours before surgery. Repeat as indicated; see Usual Dose.

Prevent necrosis caused by norepinephrine (Levophed): Add 0.1 to 0.2 mg/kg up to a maximum of 10 mg to each 1,000 mL of IV solution containing norepinephrine.

Test dose for diagnosis of pheochromocytoma: 1 mg.

DILUTION
Each 5 mg should be reconstituted with 1 mL of SW for injection. May be further diluted with 5 to 10 mL of SW or NS. Use only freshly prepared solutions.

Storage: Store below 40° C.

COMPATIBILITY
Consider any drug NOT listed as compatible to be INCOMPATIBLE until consulting a pharmacist; specific conditions may apply.

One source suggests the following **compatibilities:**

Additive: Dobutamine, verapamil.

Y-site: Amiodarone (Nexterone).

RATE OF ADMINISTRATION
Each 5 mg or fraction thereof over 1 minute.

Test dose: Inject rapidly after pressor response to venipuncture has subsided.

ACTIONS
An alpha-blocking agent that competitively antagonizes endogenous and exogenous alpha agents (e.g., epinephrine and norepinephrine). Has positive chronotropic and inotropic effects on cardiac muscle, as well as vasodilator effects on vascular smooth muscle. Onset of action is prompt. Half-life is approximately 19 minutes. Metabolic fate is undetermined.

INDICATIONS AND USES
Prevention and treatment of hypertensive episodes of pheochromocytoma preoperatively and during surgery. ■ Prevention and treatment of necrosis and sloughing occurring with dopamine and norepinephrine (Levophed). ■ Definitive diagnosis of pheochromocytoma.

Unlabeled uses: Treatment of congestive heart failure, hypertensive crisis due to MAO inhibitor/sympathomimetic amine interactions, and rebound hypertension after discontinuation of clonidine, propranolol, or other hypertensive agents.

CONTRAINDICATIONS

Coronary artery disease, coronary insufficiency, hypersensitivity to phentolamine, myocardial infarction (previous or present).

PRECAUTIONS

Use caution in gastritis or peptic ulcer disease. ■ Use care in the presence of any arrhythmia. It is preferable to have a normal sinus rhythm. ■ MI, cerebrovascular spasm, and cerebrovascular occlusion have occurred following administration, usually in association with marked hypotensive episodes. ■ For diagnosis of pheochromocytoma, urinary tests such as vanillylmandelic acid (VMA) are safer and more accurate. Phentolamine is used only when absolutely necessary. Specific procedure must be followed. Consult with physician and pharmacist.

Monitor: Monitor vital signs every 2 minutes.

Maternal/Child: Category C: safety for use during pregnancy and breast-feeding not established. Use with extreme caution and only when clearly indicated.

Elderly: Risk of phentolamine-induced hypothermia may be increased.

DRUG/LAB INTERACTIONS

Antagonizes effects of **epinephrine** and **ephedrine.**

SIDE EFFECTS

Abdominal pain, diarrhea, dizziness, hypotension, nasal stuffiness, nausea, tachycardia, tingling of skin, weakness, vomiting.

Major: Cardiac arrhythmias, cerebrovascular occlusion, cerebrovascular spasm, hypotension (severe), myocardial infarction, shock, tachycardia, vomiting under anesthesia.

ANTIDOTE

For minor side effects, notify the physician. If symptoms progress or any major side effect occurs, discontinue drug and notify the physician immediately. Elevation of legs, volume expanders (e.g., albumin, hetastarch), and administration of norepinephrine are recommended for treatment of hypotension. Do not use epinephrine. Maintain the patient as indicated. If tachycardia or cardiac arrhythmias occur, defer use of digoxin if possible until rhythm returns to normal.

PHENYLEPHRINE HYDROCHLORIDE BBW
(fen-ill-**EF**-rin hy-droh-**KLOR**-eyed)
Neo-Synephrine

Vasopressor

pH 3 to 6.5

USUAL DOSE
Mild to moderate hypotension or hypotensive emergencies during spinal anesthesia: 0.2 mg. From 0.1 to 0.5 mg may be used initially. May be repeated every 10 to 15 minutes. Never exceed 0.5 mg in a single dose. Highly individualized. Start with a small dose, giving only as much of the drug as required to alleviate undesirable symptoms.

Severe hypotension and shock- or drug-related hypotension: Begin infusion at 100 to 180 mcg/min (0.1 to 0.18 mg/min) until BP stabilized at a low normal for specific individual. Maintain with 40 to 60 mcg/min (0.04 to 0.06 mg/min). Titrate to desired effect.

Paroxysmal supraventricular tachycardia: 0.25 to 0.5 mg has been given as a rapid IV bolus. If additional doses are required to achieve adequate response, increase in increments of 0.1 to 0.2 mg and never exceed a total single dose of 1 mg. Adenosine may be the drug of choice. Monitor BP. Systolic BP should not be raised above 160 mm Hg.

PEDIATRIC DOSE
Mild to moderate hypotension: 5 to 20 mcg/kg of body weight per dose. May be repeated every 10 to 15 minutes. Do not exceed adult dose.

Severe hypotension and shock- or drug-related hypotension: Begin an infusion at 0.1 to 0.5 mcg/kg/min. Titrate to desired effect.

DOSE ADJUSTMENTS
Hypotension of powerful peripheral adrenergic blocking agents, chlorpromazine, or pheochromocytomectomy may require carefully calculated increased dose therapy.

DILUTION
IV injection: Dilute 1 mL of a 10 mg/mL solution with 9 mL of SW for injection to prepare a final concentration of 1 mg/mL.

Infusion: Dilute 10 mg in 500 mL of NS or D5W to provide a 1:50,000 solution (20 mcg/mL). May increase to 20 or 30 mg in 500 mL if necessary (40 to 60 mcg/mL).

Pediatric infusion: Add 0.6 mg/kg to 100 mL diluent. 1 mL/hr equals 0.1 mcg/kg/min.

Storage: Protect from light.

COMPATIBILITY
(Underline Indicates Conflicting Compatibility Information)

Consider any drug NOT listed as compatible to be INCOMPATIBLE until consulting a pharmacist; specific conditions may apply.

One source suggests the following **compatibilities:**

Additive: Chloramphenicol (Chloromycetin), dobutamine, lidocaine, potassium chloride (KCl), sodium bicarbonate.

Y-site: Amiodarone (Nexterone), anidulafungin (Eraxis), argatroban, bivalirudin (Angiomax), caspofungin (Cancidas), cisatracurium (Nimbex), dexmedetomidine (Precedex), doripenem (Doribax), etomidate (Amidate), famotidine (Pepcid IV), fenoldopam (Corlopam), haloperidol (Haldol), hetastarch in electrolytes (Hextend), inamrinone (Amrinone), levofloxacin (Levaquin), micafungin (Mycamine), propofol (Diprivan), remifentanil (Ultiva), vasopressin, zidovudine (AZT, Retrovir).

RATE OF ADMINISTRATION

IV injection: Single dose over 20 to 30 seconds to treat paroxysmal supraventricular tachycardia; over 1 minute in other situations.

Infusion: Regulate drip rate to provide and maintain individual's low normal BP. Use an infusion pump or microdrip (60 gtt/mL) to administer.

ACTIONS

Sympathomimetic, similar to epinephrine. Acts primarily on alpha-adrenergic receptors. Potent, long-lasting vasoconstrictor. Unique in that it slows HR, increases stroke volume, and does not induce any change in rhythm of the pulse. Renal vessel constriction will occur. Repeated injections produce comparable results. Effective within seconds and lasts about 15 minutes. Metabolic fate and route of excretion not determined. Uptake of drug into tissue and some metabolism by liver have been documented.

INDICATIONS AND USES

Maintain adequate BP in inhalation and spinal anesthesia, shocklike states, drug-induced hypotension, and hypersensitivity reactions. ▪ Treat paroxysmal supraventricular tachycardia. ▪ Prolong anesthesia.

Unlabeled uses: Specific antidote for hypotension produced by chlorpromazine hydrochloride (Thorazine).

CONTRAINDICATIONS

Hypertension, ventricular tachycardia, hypersensitivity to phenylephrine.

PRECAUTIONS

Usually administered by or under the supervision of a physician knowledgeable in its use. ▪ Blood volume depletion should be corrected. May be administered concurrently with blood volume replacement. ▪ Use extreme caution in the elderly, hyperthyroidism, bradycardia, partial heart block, myocardial disease, or severe arteriosclerosis. ▪ Contains bisulfites; use caution in allergic individuals.

Monitor: Check BP every 2 minutes until stabilized at desired level. ▪ Discontinue IV administration if vein infiltrates or is thrombosed; can cause tissue necrosis, sloughing. ▪ See Precautions, Drug/Lab Interactions.

Maternal/Child: Category C: safety for use in pregnancy or breast-feeding not established.

Elderly: See Precautions; may have increased sensitivity to effects.

DRUG/LAB INTERACTIONS

Potentiated by **tricyclic antidepressants** (e.g., desipramine [Norpramin]), **guanethidine, MAO inhibitors** (e.g., selegiline [Eldepryl]), **other vasopressors** (epinephrine [Adrenalin]); **ergot alkaloids or oxytocic agents** (e.g., methylergonovine, oxytocin); hypertensive crisis and death can result. ▪ Use caution with **digoxin or halogenated hydrocarbon anesthetics** (e.g., halothane, isoflurane); arrhythmias may occur.

SIDE EFFECTS

Bradycardia, fullness of head, headache, hypertension, tingling of extremities, tremulousness, ventricular extrasystoles, ventricular tachycardia (short paroxysms), vertigo.

ANTIDOTE

To prevent sloughing and necrosis in areas of extravasation, with a fine hypodermic needle inject 5 to 10 mg of phentolamine (Regitine) diluted in 10 to 15 mL of NS liberally throughout the tissue in the extravasated area. Treatment should be started as soon as extravasation is recognized. Notify the physician of all side effects. IM injection may be preferable. Treat hypertension with phentolamine (Regitine). Treat cardiac arrhythmias as indicated. Treat bradycardia with atropine. Resuscitate as necessary.

PHENYTOIN SODIUM BBW

(**FEN**-ih-toyn **SO**-dee-um)

Dilantin

Hydantoin
Anticonvulsant
Antiarrhythmic

pH 12

USUAL DOSE

In all situations, transfer to oral therapy 12 to 24 hours after a loading dose or as soon as practical. See Precautions.

Status epilepticus, anticonvulsant: A *loading dose* of 10 to 15 mg/kg. Do not exceed a total dose of 1.5 Gm. Lethal dose estimated at 2 to 5 Gm. Another source suggests that 15 to 20 mg/kg is generally recommended. Follow with **maintenance doses** of 100 mg every 6 to 8 hours. Adjust dose based on phenytoin levels; see Monitor. If seizure is not terminated, consider other anticonvulsants, barbiturates, or anesthesia. IV diazepam may be the drug of choice for initial treatment. Concurrent administration of phenytoin in the lesser doses is suggested by clinicians to maintain control.

Antiarrhythmic: 50 to 100 mg at 5- to 15-minute intervals until the arrhythmia is abolished or side effects occur. Do not exceed a total dose of 15 mg/kg or 1 Gm.

PEDIATRIC DOSE

Status epilepticus, anticonvulsant: 250 mg/M^2 as a *loading dose,* followed by **maintenance doses** of 4 to 8 mg/kg/24 hr in divided doses every 8 to 12 hours (2 to 4 mg/kg every 12 hours or 1.33 to 2.66 mg/kg every 8 hours). An alternate regimen for pediatric patients of all ages is a *loading dose* of 15 to 20 mg/kg. Follow with a *maintenance dose for age* (listed below): **Neonates:** Begin with 5 mg/kg/24 hr in equally divided doses every 8 to 12 hours. Range is 5 to 8 mg/kg/24 hr (2.5 to 4 mg/kg every 12 hours or 1.6 to 2.67 mg/kg every 8 hours).

Infants and other pediatric patients: Begin with 5 mg/kg/24 hr in equally divided doses every 8 to 12 hours (2.5 mg/kg every 12 hours or 1.67 mg/kg every 8 hours). Range varies according to age:

6 months to 3 years: 8 to 10 mg/kg/24 hr (4 to 5 mg/kg every 12 hours or 2.67 to 3.33 mg/kg every 8 hours).

4 to 6 years: 7.5 to 9 mg/kg/24 hr (3.75 to 4.5 mg/kg every 12 hours or 2.5 to 3 mg/kg every 8 hours).

7 to 9 years: 7 to 8 mg/kg/24 hr (3.5 to 4 mg/kg every 12 hours or 2.3 to 2.6 mg/kg every 8 hours).

10 to 16 years: 6 to 7 mg/kg/24 hr (3 to 3.5 mg/kg every 12 hours or 2 to 2.3 mg/kg every 8 hours).

Maintenance dose should not exceed 20 mg/kg/24 hr. Loading dose not included in this total. See comments in Usual Dose.

Antiarrhythmic: 1.25 mg/kg every 5 minutes until arrhythmia abolished or side effects occur. Do not exceed a total dose of 15 mg/kg. Maintenance dose is 2.5 to 5 mg/kg every 12 hours.

DOSE ADJUSTMENTS

Use caution, lower dose, and slower rate of administration in the seriously ill, elderly, cachetic patients, and in impaired liver or renal function. ▪ In obesity calculate dose on ideal body weight plus 1.33 of excess over ideal; phenytoin preferentially distributes into fat. ▪ Dose adjustment may be required based on serum albumin levels. ▪ See Drug/Lab Interactions.

DILUTION

Available as 100- or 250-mg ampules, syringes, or vials. Usually not added to IV solutions. May be injected through Y-tube or three-way stopcock of infusion set of a **compatible** solution. Use solution only when completely dissolved and clear; discard if hazy or if a precipitate forms. May be light yellow in color. Recent studies have utilized NS for infusion solutions that should be prepared immediately before use in suitable concentrations (less than 6.7 mg/mL) to facilitate required rate and fluid limitations or requirements. Method not recommended by manufacturer but is in common use; see Compatibility. Use within 1 to 2 hours is recommended.

Filters: According to most studies, a 0.22-micron in-line filter is required.

Storage: Store between 15° and 30° C.

COMPATIBILITY

Consider any drug NOT listed as compatible to be INCOMPATIBLE until consulting a pharmacist; specific conditions may apply.

Manufacturer recommends not adding to IV solutions or mixing with other medications. May precipitate if pH is altered. Always flush line with NS before and after administration of any other drug through the same IV line. See Dilution.

One source suggests the following **compatibilities:**

Additive: *Not recommended by manufacturer.* Verapamil.

Y-site: Esmolol (Brevibloc), famotidine (Pepcid IV), fluconazole (Diflucan), foscarnet (Foscavir), tacrolimus (Prograf).

RATE OF ADMINISTRATION

Very alkaline; administer slowly and follow each injection with sterile NS to reduce local venous irritation. Best to flush before and after with NS.

Anticonvulsant: *Adults:* 25 to 50 mg or fraction thereof over 1 minute. Do not exceed 50 mg/min.

Neonates and other pediatric patients: Do not exceed 1 to 3 mg/kg/min in neonates. Another source suggests 0.5 mg/kg/min in neonates or 1 mg/kg/min in infants and other pediatric patients not to exceed 50 mg/min.

Elderly: Limit rate to 25 mg/min.

Antiarrhythmic: 25 mg or fraction thereof over 2 to 3 minutes.

Infusion: Should be completed within 1 hour. Do not exceed 25 to 50 mg/min rate. Best if piggybacked to a **compatible** primary IV so phenytoin can be discontinued if side effects occur, but IV can be kept open.

ACTIONS

A synthetic anticonvulsant, chemically related to barbiturates. Selectively stabilizes seizure threshold and depresses seizure activity in the motor cortex. Effective control in emergency treatment of seizures may take 15 to 20 minutes because of rate of injection required. Also exerts a depressant effect on the myocardium by selectively elevating the excitability threshold of the cell, reducing the cell's response to stimuli. Readily absorbed, phenytoin is metabolized in the liver and excreted in changed form in the urine. Crosses placental barrier. Secreted in breast milk.

INDICATIONS AND USES

Control of grand mal and psychomotor seizures. ▪ Treatment of status epilepticus (grand mal seizures).

Unlabeled uses: Treatment of supraventricular and ventricular arrhythmias, including those caused by digoxin intoxication. Especially useful for patients who are unable to tolerate quinidine or procainamide.

CONTRAINDICATIONS

Bradycardia, sinoatrial, second- or third-degree heart block, Stokes-Adams syndrome; known sensitivity to hydantoin derivatives.

PRECAUTIONS

Because of benefits provided by fosphenytoin (Cerebyx)—e.g., solubility in IV solutions, improved infusion site tolerance, more rapid rate of administration, and well-tolerated IM option—Parke-Davis wants to discontinue injectable phenytoin (Dilantin). Generic products will still be available. ▪ Status epilepticus can occur from abrupt withdrawal of hydantoins. ▪ Not effective for petit mal seizures; combined therapy required if both conditions present. ▪ Use caution in hypotension and severe myocardial insufficiency. ▪ Use caution with low serum albumin level, and adjust dose as indicated. Phenytoin is 90% bound to serum protein, and a reduced albumin causes an increase in free drug availability. ▪ Lymphadenopathy has been reported. Monitoring and change in anticonvulsant therapy may be indicated. ▪ Discontinue phenytoin if skin rash appears. ▪ Hyperglycemia and blood dyscrasias have been reported. ▪ Psychotic symptoms and other behavioral changes have been reported with antiepileptic drugs and may include aggression, agitation, anger, anxiety, apathy, depersonalization, depression, emotional lability, hallucinations, hostility, irritability, and suicidal tendencies. Some resolved without intervention. Others required dose reduction or discontinuation of the antiepileptic agent. ▪ Selected patients of Asian ancestry (e.g., Han Chinese, Filipinos, Malaysians, South Asian Indians, and Thais) with a specific human leukocyte antigen allele may have an increased risk of serious skin reactions (e.g., Stevens-Johnson syndrome and toxic epidermal necrolysis) from phenytoin therapy

Monitor: Narrow margin of error between therapeutic and toxic dose. Plasma levels above 10 mcg/mL usually control seizure activity. The acceptable range is 5 to 20 mcg/mL. Consider monitoring free phenytoin levels in patients with hypoalbuminemia or renal insufficiency (therapeutic range is 1 to 2 mcg/mL). Toxicity begins with nystagmus and may be seen at levels less than 20 mcg/mL. ▪ Periodic monitoring of CBC, platelets, albumin, urinalysis, hepatic and renal function is recommended. ▪ Monitor ECG and BP continuously. ▪ Observation of patient symptoms and effectiveness of all medications is imperative. ▪ Determine absolute patency of vein. Avoid extravasation. Very alkaline; follow each injection with sterile NS to reduce local venous irritation. ▪ Patients maintained with phenytoin should be given a dose the morning of surgery to maintain adequate serum levels. ▪ Observe patient closely for signs of CNS side effects; see Precautions. ▪ See Drug/Lab Interactions.

Patient Education: May cause alterations in mood (e.g., aggression, agitation, anger, anxiety, apathy, decreased ability to cope, depression, hostility, irritability, thoughts of suicide); report these changes promptly. ▪ Women who are pregnant or who become pregnant should be encouraged to enroll in the North American Antiepileptic Drug (NAAED) Pregnancy Registry. **Maternal/Child:** Capable of numerous interactions in pregnant women. May cause birth defects (see literature). ▪ Alterations in phenytoin kinetics in pregnant women may necessitate periodic monitoring of serum levels. ▪ Discontinue nursing. ▪ May decrease folic acid serum concentrations; avoid during pregnancy.

Elderly: See Dose Adjustments and Rate of Administration. ▪ May have elevated serum concentrations because of slow metabolism. ▪ Low serum albumin causing a decrease in protein binding may result in increased sensitivity to phenytoin.

DRUG/LAB INTERACTIONS

Interactions are numerous and potentially life threatening. Review of drug profile by pharmacist imperative. ▪ Serum levels may be increased by **alcohol** (acute ingestion), **anticoagulants, antidepressants, antifungal agents** (e.g., fluconazole, miconazole, ketoconazole), **antihistamines, benzodiazepines** (e.g., diazepam [Valium]), **chloramphenicol, cimetidine** (Tagamet), **disulfiram** (Antabuse), **estrogens, fluorouracil, fluoxetine** (Prozac), **metronidazole, myocardial depressants, paroxetine** (Paxil), **phenothiazines, sulfonamides, tacrolimus** (Prograf), **valproic acid, and others.** Toxicity and fatality may result. ▪ Serum levels may be decreased by **chronic alcohol ingestion, antineoplastics, antituberculosis drugs, barbiturates, folic acid, leucovorin calcium, rifampin, theophylline, and others** resulting in reduced phenytoin effect. ▪ Phenytoin serum levels may be increased or decreased by **carbamazepine** (Tegretol). ▪ May increase serum levels of **CNS depressants, folic acid antagonists, and muscle relaxants.** ▪ May decrease effectiveness of **corticosteroids, digoxin, diuretics, itraconazole** (Sporanox), **levodopa, quetiapine** (Seroquel), **quinidine, ranitidine** (Zantac), **and others.** ▪ Severe hypotension and bradycardia result with concomitant administration with **dopamine and all other sympathomimetic antihypertensive drugs.** ▪ In one case report, a patient stabilized on phenytoin and valproic acid experienced seizures and a reduction in antiepileptic drug serum concentration when **acyclovir** was added to the regimen. ▪ Alters **some clinical laboratory tests.**

SIDE EFFECTS

Ataxia, confusion, dizziness, drowsiness, fever, hyperplasia of gums, nervousness, nystagmus, skin eruptions, tremors, visual disturbances. Psychotic symptoms, including aggression, agitation, anger, anxiety, apathy, depersonalization, depression, emotional lability, hallucinations, hostility, irritability, and suicidal tendencies, have occurred with antiepileptic agents.

Major: Bradycardia, cardiac arrest, heart block, hypotension, respiratory arrest, tonic seizures, ventricular fibrillation.

ANTIDOTE

Notify the physician of any side effects. If minor symptoms progress or any major side effect occurs, discontinue the drug and notify the physician. Maintain a patent airway and resuscitate as necessary. Symptoms of heart block or bradycardia may be reversed with IV atropine. Epinephrine may also be useful. Hemodialysis may be required in overdose.

PHOSPHATE
(**FOS**-fayt)

Potassium Phosphate, Sodium Phosphate

Electrolyte replenisher
Antihypophosphatemic

pH 5 to 7.8

USUAL DOSE

Dependent on individual needs of the patient.

TPN, adults and pediatric patients: 10 to 15 mM (310 to 465 mg) of phosphorus/liter of TPN solution should maintain normal serum phosphate. Larger amounts may be required. 1 mM equals 31 mg.

Acute hypophosphatemia: Adults and pediatric patients: 0.08 to 0.32 mM/kg of body weight as a *loading dose* equally distributed over 6 hours. *Maintain pediatric patients* with 0.5 to 1.5 mM/kg/24 hr. *Maintain adults* with 48.4 to 64.5 mM/24 hr.

INFANT DOSE

Infants receiving TPN: 1.5 to 2 mM/kg of body weight/day.

DOSE ADJUSTMENTS

Lower-end initial doses may be indicated in the elderly based on the potential for decreased organ function and concomitant disease or drug therapy.

DILUTION

Must be diluted in a larger volume of suitable IV solution and given as an infusion. Soluble in most commonly used IV solutions (see chart on inside back cover) except protein hydrolysate. Mix thoroughly. See Compatibility.

COMPATIBILITY

Consider any drug NOT listed as compatible to be INCOMPATIBLE until consulting a pharmacist; specific conditions may apply.

ALL FORMULATIONS

Mix thoroughly after each addition of supposedly **compatible** drugs or solutions. TPN solutions requiring the addition of phosphates and calcium salts must be mixed by the pharmacist to avoid a precipitate of calcium phosphate. Specific amounts, calculations, order and temperature (precipitate forms more readily at room temperature) are required. Deaths have been reported.

One source suggests the following **compatibilities:**

POTASSIUM PHOSPHATE

Additive: *See comments under All Formulations.* Mix thoroughly. Magnesium sulfate, metoclopramide (Reglan), verapamil.

Y-site: Diltiazem (Cardizem), enalaprilat (Vasotec IV), esmolol (Brevibloc), famotidine (Pepcid IV), labetalol (Trandate), micafungin (Mycamine), nicardipine (Cardene IV), nitroprusside sodium.

SODIUM PHOSPHATE

Y-site: Doripenem (Doribax), micafungin (Mycamine).

RATE OF ADMINISTRATION

A usual dose is usually equally distributed over 6 hours. Other sources suggest administering up to 15 mM over 2 hours, up to 30 mM over 4 hours, and up to 45 mM over 6 hours. Potassium phosphate will be further limited by the maximum rate for potassium. Consider sodium/potassium content. Infuse slowly. Rapid infusion may cause phosphate or potassium intoxication. Serum calcium may be reduced rapidly, causing hypocalcemic tetany.

ACTIONS

Involved in bone deposition. Helps to maintain calcium levels, has a buffering effect on acid-base equilibrium, and influences renal excretion of the hydrogen ion. Normal levels in adults, 3 to 4.5 mg/dL of serum; in pediatric patients, 4 to 7 mg/dL. Excreted in urine.

INDICATIONS AND USES

To prevent or correct hypophosphatemia in patients with restricted or no oral intake.

CONTRAINDICATIONS

Any disease with high phosphate or low calcium levels, hyperkalemia (potassium phosphate), hypernatremia (sodium phosphate).

PRECAUTIONS

Rapid infusion may cause phosphate, sodium, or potassium intoxication. Serum calcium may be reduced, rapidly causing hypocalcemic tetany. ▪ Use sodium phosphate with caution in renal impairment, cirrhosis, cardiac failure, or any edematous, sodium-retaining state. ▪ Use potassium phosphate with caution in cardiac disease, renal disease, and digitalized patients. ▪ See Compatibility.

Monitor: Monitor serum calcium, potassium, phosphate, chlorides, and sodium. Discontinue when serum phosphate exceeds 2 mg/dL. ▪ See Drug/Lab Interactions.

Maternal/Child: Category C: safety for use in pregnancy not established.

Elderly: Differences in response between elderly and younger patients have not been identified. Lower end initial doses may be appropriate in the elderly; see Dose Adjustments.

DRUG/LAB INTERACTIONS

May cause hyperkalemia with **potassium-sparing diuretics** (e.g., amiloride) **or angiotensin-converting enzyme inhibitors** (e.g., enalapril [Vasotec]).

SIDE EFFECTS

Elevated phosphates, reduced calcium levels and hypocalcemic tetany, elevated potassium levels causing cardiac arrhythmias, flaccid paralysis, heaviness of the legs, hypotension, listlessness, mental confusion, paresthesia of the extremities.

ANTIDOTE

For any side effect, discontinue the drug and notify the physician. Restore serum calcium with calcium gluconate or chloride. Shift potassium from serum to cells with 150 mL of ⅙ M sodium lactate or 10% to 20% dextrose with 10 units regular insulin for each 20 Gm dextrose at 300 to 500 mL/hr. Correct acidosis with sodium bicarbonate. Reduce sodium by restriction, diuretics, or hemodialysis. Resuscitate as necessary.

PHYSOSTIGMINE SALICYLATE
(fye-zoh-**STIG**-meen sah-**LIS**-ah-layt)

Cholinergic
Cholinesterase inhibitor
Antidote

pH 5.8

USUAL DOSE
Anticholinergic toxicity: 0.5 to 2 mg initially. 1 to 4 mg may be repeated as necessary as life-threatening signs recur (arrhythmias, convulsions, deep coma). Maximum dose is 4 mg in 30 minutes.

Postanesthesia: 0.5 to 1 mg initially. Repeat at 10- to 30-minute intervals until desired results obtained.

PEDIATRIC DOSE
To be used in life-threatening situations only. 0.02 mg/kg/dose. May be repeated at 5- to 10-minute intervals only if toxic effects persist and there is no sign of cholinergic effects. Maximum total dose is 2 mg. See Maternal/Child.

DILUTION
May be given undiluted. Do not add to IV solutions. May be given through Y-tube or three-way stopcock of infusion set.

COMPATIBILITY
Specific information not available. Consider specific use; consult pharmacist.

RATE OF ADMINISTRATION
Rapid IV administration may cause bradycardia, hypersalivation, respiratory distress, and convulsions.

1 mg or fraction thereof over 1 to 3 minutes.

Pediatric rate: 0.5 mg or fraction thereof over at least 1 minute.

ACTIONS
An extract of *Physostigma venenosum* seeds. It inhibits the destructive action of acetylcholinesterase and prolongs and exaggerates the effects of acetylcholine. Stimulates parasympathetic nerve stimulation (pupil contraction, increased intestinal musculature tonus, bronchial constriction, salivary and sweat gland stimulation). Does enter the CNS. Onset of action occurs in 5 minutes and lasts about 1 hour. Rapidly hydrolyzed by cholinesterases.

INDICATIONS AND USES
To reverse CNS toxic effects caused by drugs capable of producing anticholinergic poisoning (e.g., atropine), other anticholinergic/antispasmodic agents (e.g., phenothiazines, antihistamines), anticholinergic antiparkinson agents (e.g., benztropine [Cogentin], trihexyphenidyl [Artane]), and tricyclic antidepressants (e.g., imipramine [Tofranil]).

Unlabeled uses: Treatment of delirium tremens.

CONTRAINDICATIONS
Asthma, cardiovascular disease, diabetes, gangrene, mechanical obstruction of the intestines or urogenital tract, vagotonic states, patients receiving choline esters, depolarizing neuromuscular blocking agents (succinylcholine), or tricyclic antidepressants (e.g., amitriptyline [Elavil]).

PRECAUTIONS

Rapid IV administration may cause bradycardia, hypersalivation, respiratory distress, and convulsions. ▪ Contains bisulfites; use caution in allergic individuals.

Monitor: Atropine must always be available. ▪ Monitor vital signs. ▪ See Drug/Lab Interactions.

Maternal/Child: Safety for use in pregnancy and breast-feeding not established. ▪ Has caused muscular weakness in neonates of mothers treated with other cholinesterase inhibitors for myasthenia gravis. ▪ May contain benzyl alcohol; do not use in neonates.

DRUG/LAB INTERACTIONS

Potentiates **succinylcholine** and **other choline esters** (e.g., bethanecol). ▪ May antagonize CNS depressant effects of **diazepam** (Valium). ▪ May cause serious complications, including death, with **tricyclic antidepressants** (e.g., amitriptyline [Elavil]).

SIDE EFFECTS

Anxiety, bradycardia, cholinergic crisis (overdose), coma, convulsions, defecation, delirium, disorientation, emesis, hallucinations, hyperactivity, hypersalivation, hypersensitivity, nausea, respiratory distress, salivation, seizures, sweating, urination.

ANTIDOTE

Keep physician informed of side effects. For excessive nausea or sweating, reduce dose. Discontinue drug for bradycardia; convulsions; excessive defecation, emesis, salivation, or urination; or respiratory distress. Treat cholinergic side effects (e.g., arrhythmias, bronchoconstriction) or hypersensitivity with the specific antagonist atropine sulfate in doses of 0.6 mg IV. May be repeated every 3 to 10 minutes. Endotracheal intubation or tracheostomy are considered prophylactic in anesthesia or crisis. Artificial ventilation, oxygen therapy, cardiac monitoring, adequate suctioning, and treatment of shock or convulsions must be instituted and maintained as necessary.

PHYTONADIONE BBW
(fye-toe-nah-**DYE**-ohn)

Vitamin (prothrombinogenic)
Antidote
Antihemorrhagic

Vitamin K₁

pH 5 to 7

USUAL DOSE

Should be given by the SC or oral route whenever possible; parenteral route administration has caused death; see Precautions. A single dose is preferred, but it may be repeated if clinically indicated.

Vitamin K deficiency: Up to 10 mg may be added to TPN solutions as indicated.

Anticoagulant-induced (warfarin or dicumarol) hypoprothrombinemia: 2.5 to 10 mg. Doses up to 25 mg and, rarely, 50 mg may be needed. May repeat in 6 to 8 hours if initial response is not adequate. Doses as low as 1 to 2 mg may be effective. Use the smallest dose that achieves effective results to prevent clotting hazards.

Hypoprothrombinemia from other causes: 2 to 25 mg (rarely 50 mg), depending on the severity of the deficiency and the response obtained.

PEDIATRIC DOSE

See Usual Dose, Precautions, and Maternal/Child.

Vitamin K deficiency: 1 to 2 mg may be added to TPN solutions as indicated.

Anticoagulant-induced (warfarin or dicumarol) hypoprothrombinemia in infants and children: 1 to 2 mg/dose.

Hypoprothrombinemia from other causes in infants and children: A single dose of 1 to 2 mg.

NEWBORN DOSE

See Usual Dose, Precautions, and Maternal/Child. Rarely given IV in the newborn. SC injection preferred.

Prophylaxis of hemorrhagic disease of the newborn: 0.5 to 1 mg IM within 1 hour of birth.

Treatment of hemorrhagic disease of the newborn: 1 to 2 mg/24 hr SC or IM. Higher doses may be necessary if the mother has been receiving oral anticoagulants (e.g., warfarin [Coumadin]) or anticonvulsants (e.g., phenytoin [Dilantin]). Whole blood or blood components may be indicated for excessive bleeding. Give phytonadione concurrently to correct the underlying disorder.

DOSE ADJUSTMENTS

See Drug/Lab Interactions.

DILUTION

Use only preservative-free solutions. May be diluted only with NS, D5NS, or D5W. Dilution with at least 10 mL of diluent is recommended to facilitate prescribed rate of administration. Photosensitive; protect from light in all dilutions. Use immediately after preparation.

Filters: Not required by manufacturer; however, there should be no significant loss of potency with the use of a 0.22-micron filter.

Storage: Photosensitive; protect from light before use and in all dilutions. Store unopened ampules below 40° C (104° F), preferably between 15° C and 30° C (59° F and 86° F). Protect from light and freezing. Discard diluted solution and drug remaining in ampule after single use.

COMPATIBILITY

Consider any drug NOT listed as compatible to be INCOMPATIBLE until consulting a pharmacist; specific conditions may apply.

One source suggests the following **compatibilities:**

Additive: Amikacin (Amikin), chloramphenicol (Chloromycetin), sodium bicarbonate.

Y-site: Ampicillin, epinephrine (Adrenalin), famotidine (Pepcid IV), heparin, hydrocortisone sodium succinate (Solu-Cortef), potassium chloride (KCl).

RATE OF ADMINISTRATION

Each 1 mg or fraction thereof over 1 minute or longer. Too-rapid injection has caused severe reactions, including fatalities.

ACTIONS

Vitamin K, a fat-soluble vitamin, is essential for hepatic production of four blood coagulation factors including prothrombin. These are required for normal blood clotting. Onset of action is within 1 to 2 hours. Usually controls hemorrhage in 3 to 6 hours; normal prothrombin levels should be obtained in 12 to 14 hours. Metabolized by the liver and eliminated in urine and bile.

INDICATIONS AND USES

Coagulation disorders due to faulty formation of factors II, VII, IX, and X when caused by vitamin K deficiency or interference with vitamin K activity. Indicated in anticoagulant-induced prothrombin deficiency (warfarin or dicumarol). ▪ Prophylaxis and treatment of hemorrhagic disease of the newborn. ▪ Hypoprothrombinemia resulting from antibacterial therapy. ▪ Hypoprothrombinemia secondary to factors limiting the absorption or synthesis of vitamin K (e.g., obstructive jaundice, biliary fistula, sprue, ulcerative colitis, celiac disease, intestinal resection, cystic fibrosis of the pancreas, and regional enteritis). ▪ Other drug-induced hypoprothrombinemia where it is definitely shown that the result is due to interference with vitamin K metabolism (e.g., salicylates).

CONTRAINDICATIONS

Hypersensitivity to components.

PRECAUTIONS

IV and/or IM is not the route of choice; used only when SC or oral route cannot be used. Use extreme caution; has caused severe reactions, including death, with the first injection, even when the product has been diluted and infused slowly. ▪ As an alternative to administering phytonadione, discontinuation or reduction of the doses of drugs interfering with coagulation mechanisms (e.g., antibiotics, salicylates) should be considered. The severity of the coagulation disorder should determine if phytonadione is required in addition to discontinuing or reducing the doses of interfering drugs. To correct excess anticoagulation after the use of warfarin (Coumadin) (e.g., returning an increased INR to the desired range), consider the degree of elevation and the presence of clinically significant bleeding. ▪ Supplement with whole blood transfusion or blood components if indicated. ▪ Now the only vitamin K product for IV use. ▪ Do not use to counteract anticoagulant effects of heparin, not effective; protamine sulfate is indicated. ▪ Does not restore abnormal platelet function to normal. ▪ Does not correct hypoprothrombinemia due to hepatocellular damage. ▪ When phytonadione is used in a patient for whom anticoagulant therapy is indicated, the same clotting hazards that existed before beginning anticoagulant therapy will recur. Use the smallest dose of phytonadione possible and monitor PT. **Monitor:** See Neonatal Dose, Precautions, and Drug/Lab Interactions. ▪ Dose and effect determined by PT/INR. Repeat PT/INR 6 to 8 hours after a dose. Keep the physician informed. ▪ Pain and swelling at injection site can occur.

Maternal/Child: Category C: safety for use not established. ▪ Use caution during breast-feeding. ▪ Use extreme caution in premature infants and neonates. Hemolysis, jaundice, and hyperbilirubinemia in newborns may be related to the dose of phytonadione. The recommended dose should not be exceeded. Severe hemolytic anemia, hemoglobinuria, kernicterus, brain damage, and death may occur. ▪ Neonates with hemorrhagic disease of the newborn should respond to administration of phytonadione with a shortening of the PT within 2 to 4 hours. If shortening of the PT is not seen, consider other coagulation disorders. ▪ May contain benzyl alcohol. When used as recommended, there is no evidence to suggest that this small amount is associated with toxicity.

DRUG/LAB INTERACTIONS
Discontinue drugs **adversely affecting the coagulation mechanism** if possible (e.g., salicylates, antibiotics). ▪ May cause temporary resistance to **prothrombin-depressing oral anticoagulants** by increasing amount of phytonadione in the liver and blood. Anticoagulation will require larger doses of same or use of heparin sodium.

SIDE EFFECTS
Cyanosis, diaphoresis, dizziness, dyspnea, hyperbilirubinemia, hypotension, injection site reactions, peculiar taste sensations, rapid and weak pulse, tachycardia, transient flushing sensation. Anaphylaxis, cardiac and/or respiratory arrest, shock, and death have occurred with parenteral route.

ANTIDOTE
Should not be necessary if dosage is accurately calculated before administration. Action can be reversed by warfarin or heparin if indicated. Discontinue the drug and notify the physician of any side effects. For most side effects the physician will probably choose to continue the drug at a decreased rate of administration. Treat hypersensitivity reactions as necessary.

PIPERACILLIN SODIUM
(pie-**PER**-ah-sill-in **SO**-dee-um)

Antibacterial
(extended-spectrum penicillin)

pH 5.5 to 7.5

USUAL DOSE

3 to 4 Gm every 4 to 6 hours depending on severity of infection. Maximum dose usually 24 Gm/24 hr. Usual duration of therapy is 7 to 10 days (3 to 10 days for treatment of gynecologic infections). Continue at least 2 days after symptoms of infection disappear. Dosage recommendations for different types of infections are listed in the following chart.

Piperacillin Dose Guidelines	
Type of Infection	**Usual Total Daily Dose**
Serious infections such as septicemia, nosocomial pneumonia, intra-abdominal infections, aerobic and anaerobic gynecologic infections, and skin and soft tissue infections	12 to 18 Gm/day (200 to 300 mg/kg/day) in divided doses every 4 to 6 hours (2 to 3 Gm [33.3 to 50 mg/kg/dose] every 4 hours or 3 to 4.5 Gm [50 to 75 mg/kg/dose] every 6 hours)
Complicated urinary tract infections	8 to 16 Gm/day (125 to 200 mg/kg/day) in divided doses every 6 to 8 hours (2 to 4 Gm [31.25 to 50 mg/kg/dose] every 6 hours or 2.66 to 5.33 Gm [41.6 to 66.6 mg/kg/dose] every 8 hours)
Uncomplicated urinary tract infections and most community-acquired pneumonia	6 to 8 Gm/day (100 to 125 mg/kg/day) in divided doses every 6 to 12 hours (1.5 to 2 Gm [25 to 31.25 mg/kg/dose] every 6 hours or 3 to 4 Gm [50 to 62.5 mg/kg/dose] every 12 hours)
Empiric therapy in febrile neutropenic patients	50 mg/kg every 4 hours not to exceed 24 Gm/day or 300 mg/kg/day; given in combination with ciprofloxacin 400 mg every 8 hours
Perioperative prophylaxis	2 Gm administered as a 20- to 30-minute infusion just before starting anesthesia Repeat every 4 to 6 hours for up to 24 hours if indicated Specific doses for specific procedures; see literature

PEDIATRIC DOSE

Safety and effectiveness not established for pediatric patients less than 12 years of age. All IV doses are unlabeled; see Maternal/Child. Do not exceed adult dose.

200 to 300 mg/kg/24 hr in equally divided doses every 4 to 6 hours (33.3 to 50 mg/kg every 4 hours or 50 to 75 mg/kg every 6 hours).

Cystic fibrosis in pediatric patients under 12 years of age: 350 to 600 mg/kg/24 hr in equally divided doses every 4 to 6 hours (58.33 to 100 mg/kg every 4 hours or 87.5 to 150 mg/kg every 6 hours). *Continued*

NEONATAL DOSE

See comments under Pediatric Dose.

Premature infants (less than 36 weeks' gestation) less than 7 days of age: 75 mg/kg every 12 hours. **7 days of age or older:** 75 mg/kg every 8 hours. **Full-term infants less than 7 days of age:** 75 mg/kg every 8 hours. **7 days of age or older:** 75 mg/kg every 6 hours.

Another source suggests the following doses for bacterial meningitis:

7 days of age or younger and 2 kg or less: 50 mg every 12 hours; **over 2 kg:** 50 mg every 8 hours.

Over 7 days of age and 2 kg or less: 50 mg every 8 hours; **over 2 kg:** 50 mg every 6 hours.

DOSE ADJUSTMENTS

Reduced dose may be required in the elderly; see Elderly. ■ Reduce dose in patients with impaired renal function according to the following chart.

Pi_eracillin Dose Guidelines in Impaired Renal Function*			
Creatinine Clearance (mL/min)	Urinary Tract Infection (uncomplicated)	Urinary Tract Infection (complicated)	Serious Systemic Infection
>40 mL/min	No dose adjustment necessary		
20 to 40 mL/min	No dose adjustment necessary	9 Gm/day total; give 3 Gm q 8 hr	12 Gm/day total; give 4 Gm q 8 hr
<20 mL/min	6 Gm/day total; give 3 Gm q 12 hr	6 Gm/day total; give 3 Gm q 12 hr	8 Gm/day total; give 4 Gm q 12 hr
Hemodialysis†	6 Gm/day total; give 2 Gm q 8 hr	6 Gm/day total; give 2 Gm q 8 hr	6 Gm/day total; give 2 Gm q 8 hr

*Measure serum levels of piperacillin to guide dose adjustment in patients with renal failure and hepatic insufficiency.

†Hemodialysis removes 30% to 50% of piperacillin. Administer an additional 1-Gm dose following each dialysis session.

DILUTION

Each 1 Gm or fraction thereof should be reconstituted with at least 5 mL of SW, NS, D5W, or D5NS. Shake vigorously to dissolve. May be further diluted to desired volume (50 to 100 mL) with D5W, NS, D5NS, LR, or Dextran 6%/NS, and given as an intermittent infusion.

Storage: Store unopened vials at CRT. Stable at room temperature for 24 hours. Reconstituted vials are stable for 24 hours at RT and 48 hours if refrigerated. Diluted solutions stable for 24 hours at RT, up to 1 week refrigerated, and up to 1 month frozen. Use solutions diluted with LR within 2 hours. Do not refrigerate or freeze ADD-Vantage formulations.

COMPATIBILITY   (Underline Indicates Conflicting Compatibility Information)

Consider any drug NOT listed as compatible to be INCOMPATIBLE until consulting a pharmacist; specific conditions may apply.

Inactivated in solution with aminoglycosides (e.g., amikacin [Amikin], gentamicin). Do not mix in the same solution. Appropriate spacing and/or separate sites required. See Drug/Lab Interactions. Manufacturer states, "**Compatible** with KCl 40 mEq in D5W, NS, D5NS, LR, or Dextran 6%/NS."

One source suggests the following **compatibilities:**
Additive: *See general comments under Compatibility.* Clindamycin (Cleocin), fluconazole (Diflucan), hydrocortisone sodium succinate (Solu-Cortef), linezolid (Zyvox), potassium chloride (KCl), verapamil.

Y-site: Acyclovir (Zovirax), aldesleukin (Proleukin), allopurinol (Aloprim), amifostine (Ethyol), aztreonam (Azactam), bivalirudin (Angiomax), ciprofloxacin (Cipro IV), cisatracurium (Nimbex), cyclophosphamide (Cytoxan), dexmedetomidine (Precedex), diltiazem (Cardizem), docetaxel (Taxotere), doxorubicin liposomal (Doxil), enalaprilat (Vasotec IV), esmolol (Brevibloc), etoposide phosphate (Etopophos), famotidine (Pepcid IV), fenoldopam (Corlopam), fludarabine (Fludara), foscarnet (Foscavir), gallium nitrate (Ganite), granisetron (Kytril), heparin, hetastarch in electrolytes (Hextend), hydromorphone (Dilaudid), labetalol (Trandate), linezolid (Zyvox), lorazepam (Ativan), magnesium sulfate, melphalan (Alkeran), meperidine (Demerol), midazolam (Versed), milrinone (Primacor), morphine, nicardipine (Cardene IV), propofol (Diprivan), ranitidine (Zantac), remifentanil (Ultiva), tacrolimus (Prograf), teniposide (Vumon), theophylline, thiotepa, vancomycin, verapamil, zidovudine (AZT, Retrovir).

RATE OF ADMINISTRATION

Too-rapid injection may cause seizures.
IV injection: A single dose over 3 to 5 minutes.
Intermittent infusion: A single dose properly diluted over 20 to 30 minutes. Discontinue primary IV infusion during administration. Slow infusion rate for pain along venipuncture site.

ACTIONS

An extended-spectrum penicillin. Bactericidal against a variety of gram-negative and gram-positive bacteria, including aerobic and anaerobic strains. Especially effective against *Klebsiella* and *Pseudomonas*. Mode of action involves inhibition of both septum and cell wall synthesis. Widely distributed in tissues and body fluids, including bone, prostate, and heart. Reaches high concentrations in bile and penetrates into CSF through inflamed meninges. Onset of action is prompt. Eliminated primarily by glomerular filtration and tubular secretion. Excreted rapidly as unchanged drug in the urine and to a lesser extent in bile. Crosses the placental barrier. Secreted in breast milk.

INDICATIONS AND USES

Treatment of serious lower respiratory tract, intra-abdominal, urinary tract, gynecologic, hepatobiliary, skin and skin structure, bone and joint, and gonococcal infections and septicemia caused by susceptible organisms. May be used in either liver or renal impairment since excretion occurs in bile and urine. Frequently used to initiate therapy in serious infections because of broad spectrum. ▪ Perioperative prophylaxis.

CONTRAINDICATIONS

History of a hypersensitivity reaction to any penicillin or cephalosporin (not absolute; see Precautions).

PRECAUTIONS

Hypersensitivity reactions, including fatalities, have been reported in patients on penicillin therapy; most likely to occur in patients with a history of penicillin allergy or sensitivity to multiple allergens. There have been reports of individuals with a history of penicillin hypersensitivity experiencing severe reactions when treated with cephalosporins. Check history of previous hypersensitivity reactions to penicillins, cephalosporins, or other allergens. Actual incidence of cross-allergenicity not established but may be more common with first-generation cephalosporins. ▪ Sensitivity studies indicated to determine susceptibility of the causative organism to piperacillin. ▪ ▪ To reduce the development of drug-resistant bacteria and maintain its effectiveness, piperacillin should be used to treat or prevent only those infections proven or strongly suspected to be caused by bacteria. ▪ Avoid prolonged use of drug; superinfection caused by overgrowth of nonsusceptible organisms may result. ▪ Incidence of side effects (e.g., fever and rash) increased in patients with cystic fibrosis. ▪ *Clostridium difficile*–associated diarrhea (CDAD) has been reported. May range from mild diarrhea to fatal colitis. Consider in patients who present with diarrhea during or after treatment with piperacillin. ▪ Bleeding manifestations have been reported and may be associated with abnormal coagulation tests (e.g., clotting time, platelet aggregation, and PT). ▪ Patients with impaired renal function may be at increased risk for bleeding tendencies. ▪ Administration of higher than recommended doses has resulted in neuromuscular excitability and convulsions. ▪ Leukopenia and neutropenia have been reported. Usually reversible and is more likely to occur in patients receiving prolonged therapy at high doses or in association with drugs known to cause this reaction.

Monitor: Watch for early symptoms of a hypersensitivity reaction. ▪ Periodic evaluation of renal, hepatic, and hematopoietic systems and serum potassium is recommended in prolonged therapy. Observe for hypokalemia and increased bleeding tendencies. ▪ All patients with gonorrhea (IM indication) should be tested for syphilis at the time of diagnosis and have a follow-up test 3 months after treatment with piperacillin. ▪ Observe for electrolyte imbalance and cardiac irregularities. Contains 1.85 mEq sodium/Gm. May aggravate CHF. ▪ May cause thrombophlebitis; observe carefully and rotate infusion sites. ▪ See Drug/Lab Interactions.

Patient Education: May require alternate birth control. ▪ Promptly report diarrhea or bloody stools that occur during treatment or up to several months after an antibiotic has been discontinued; may indicate CDAD and require treatment.

Maternal/Child: Category B: use only if absolutely necessary in pregnancy and breast-feeding. ▪ May cause diarrhea, candidiasis, or allergic response in nursing infants. ▪ Safety for use in pediatric patients under 12 years not established but is used. ▪ Half-life in neonates is two- to four-fold longer than that seen in infants 1 month of age and above or in adults. Half-life is shorter in infants and other pediatric patients compared to adults.

Elderly: No problems documented. Caution and lower-end dosing suggested based on potential for decreased organ function and concomitant disease or drug therapy. Age-related decrease in renal function may require decreased dose.

DRUG/LAB INTERACTIONS

Synergistic when used in combination with **aminoglycosides** (e.g., amikacin [Amikin], gentamicin). Synergism may be inconsistent; see Compatibility. ▪ Concomitant use with **beta-adrenergic blockers** (e.g., propranolol) may increase risk of anaphylaxis and inhibit treatment. ▪ Risk of bleeding may be increased with **anticoagulants** (e.g., heparin); monitoring of coagulation tests may be indicated. Use caution. ▪ May be antagonized by

bacteriostatic antibiotics (e.g., chloramphenicol, erythromycin, tetracyclines); may interfere with bactericidal action. ▪ May inhibit effectiveness of **oral contraceptives;** could result in breakthrough bleeding or pregnancy. ▪ **Probenecid** decreases rate of piperacillin elimination resulting in higher and more prolonged blood levels. May be desirable or may cause toxicity. ▪ May prolong neuromuscular blockade with **vecuronium.** ▪ May decrease clearance and increase toxicity of **methotrexate.** If concurrent use is necessary, monitor for S/S of methotrexate toxicity and monitor methotrexate levels. ▪ May cause **false urine protein reactions** with various tests; see Side Effects and/or literature. ▪ **False-positive test** results using the Bio-Rad Laboratories Platelia Aspergillus EIA test in patients receiving piperacillin/tazobactam (Zosyn) have been reported.

SIDE EFFECTS

Agranulocytosis; anaphylaxis; CDAD; convulsions; diarrhea; dizziness; elevated SCr, BUN, alkaline phosphatase, LDH, serum bilirubin, AST, and ALT; erythema multiforme; fatigue; fever; headache; hemolytic anemia; hypokalemia; increased creatinine or BUN; injection site reactions; interstitial nephritis; leukopenia; muscle relaxation (prolonged); nausea; neutropenia; prolonged bleeding time; pruritus; renal failure; skin rash; Stevens-Johnson syndrome; thrombocytopenia; thrombophlebitis; toxic epidermal necrolysis; urticaria; vomiting. Hypersensitivity myocarditis can occur (cardiomegaly, fever, eosinophilia, rash, sinus tachycardia, and ST-T changes). Higher than normal doses may cause neurologic adverse reactions, including convulsions, especially with impaired renal function.

ANTIDOTE

Notify the physician immediately of any adverse symptoms. For severe symptoms, discontinue the drug, treat hypersensitivity reactions (antihistamines, epinephrine, corticosteroids, airway management, and oxygen), and resuscitate as necessary. Treat CDAD with fluids, electrolytes, protein supplements, and oral vancomycin (Vancocin) or metronidazole (Flagyl) as indicated. In severe cases, surgical evaluation may be indicated. Mild cases may respond to drug discontinuation alone. Hemodialysis is effective in overdose.

PIPERACILLIN SODIUM AND TAZOBACTAM SODIUM
(pie-**PER**-ah-sill-in **SO**-dee-um and tay-zoh-**BAC**-tam **SO**-dee-um)

Zosyn

Antibacterial
(extended-spectrum penicillin
and beta-lactamase inhibitor)

USUAL DOSE
Measurement of both drugs is included in the total dose; for every 1 Gm of piperacillin there is 0.125 Gm of tazobactam (8:1 ratio).

12 Gm piperacillin/1.5 Gm tazobactam/24 hours given as 3.375 (3 Gm piperacillin/0.375 Gm tazobactam) every 6 hours. Usual duration of therapy is 7 to 10 days, based on severity of infection and patient progress. **Nosocomial pneumonia:** 4.5 Gm every 6 hours. Also use an aminoglycoside. Continue aminoglycoside if *P. aeruginosa* is isolated; may be discontinued if it is not isolated. Usual duration of therapy is 7 to 14 days.

PEDIATRIC DOSE
2 months to 9 months of age: 80 mg piperacillin/10 mg tazobactam per kg of body weight every 8 hours.

Over 9 months of age weighing up to 40 kg: 100 mg piperacillin/12.5 mg tazobactam per kg of body weight every 8 hours.

Pediatric patients over 40 kg: See Usual Dose.

DOSE ADJUSTMENTS
No dose adjustment needed in impaired liver function. ▪ Dose reduction may be required in the elderly. ▪ Adjust dose in adult patients with impaired renal function based on the following chart. Dose recommendations for pediatric patients with impaired renal function are not available.

Piperacillin/Tazobactam Dose Guidelines in Adults with Impaired Renal Function		
Renal Function (Creatinine Clearance, mL/min)	All Indications (Except Nosocomial Pneumonia)	Nosocomial Pneumonia
>40 mL/min	3.375 Gm q 6 hr	4.5 Gm q 6 hr
20-40 mL/min*	2.25 Gm q 6 hr	3.375 Gm q 6 hr
<20 mL/min*	2.25 Gm q 8 hr	2.25 Gm q 6 hr
Hemodialysis†	2.25 Gm q 12 hr	2.25 Gm q 8 hr
CAPD	2.25 Gm q 12 hr	2.25 Gm q 8 hr

*Creatinine clearance for patients not receiving hemodialysis.
†Hemodialysis removes 30% to 40% of piperacillin/tazobactam. Give an additional dose of 0.75 Gm following each dialysis session. No additional dose is necessary for CAPD patients.

DILUTION
Available in two different formulations: one with EDTA (edetate disodium dihydrate) and one without. **Compatibility** information differs; consult pharmacist. See Compatibility.

Each 1 Gm of piperacillin content should be reconstituted with at least 5 mL of suitable diluent (e.g., SW or NS with or without preservatives,

D5W, Dextran 6% in Saline, LR [EDTA containing formulation only]). Swirl until dissolved. Should be further diluted to desired volume (50 to 150 mL) with the **compatible** infusion solutions above and given as an intermittent infusion. If further diluted with SW, maximum recommended volume of SW per dose is 50 mL. Also available premixed and in ADD-Vantage vials for use with ADD-Vantage infusion containers. May be used in ambulatory IV infusion pumps. Considered stable at RT for 12 hours when reconstituted and diluted to a final volume of 25 to 37.5 mL. See manufacturer's literature for additional information.

Storage: Store unopened vials at CRT. Use single-dose vials immediately after reconstitution; discard any unused portion after 24 hours at room temperature or 48 hours if refrigerated. Stable for 24 hours at CRT or for up to 7 days after dilution if refrigerated, 3 months if frozen. Do not refrigerate or freeze ADD-Vantage vials after reconstitution.

COMPATIBILITY (Underline Indicates Conflicting Compatibility Information)
Consider any drug NOT listed as compatible to be INCOMPATIBLE until consulting a pharmacist; specific conditions may apply.

Manufacturer states, "Should not be mixed with other drugs in a syringe or infusion bottle. Not chemically stable in solutions containing only sodium bicarbonate and/or solutions that significantly alter the pH. **Incompatible** with LR (EDTA-free formulation only) and should not be added to blood products or albumin hydrolysates." One source recommends temporarily discontinuing other solutions infusing at the same site to avoid compatibility problems. May be inactivated in solution with aminoglycosides (e.g., amikacin [Amikin], gentamicin). Do not mix in the same solution. Appropriate spacing and/or separate sites required. Formulation containing EDTA **may be compatible** at the **Y-site** with amikacin or gentamicin. Selected doses, specific diluents, and amounts of diluent are required. Consult pharmacist or manufacturer's literature. See Drug/Lab Interactions.

One source suggests the following **compatibilities:**
Y-site: *See general comments under Compatibility.* Aminophylline, anidulafungin (Eraxis), aztreonam (Azactam), bivalirudin (Angiomax), bleomycin (Blenoxane), bumetanide, buprenorphine (Buprenex), butorphanol (Stadol), calcium gluconate, carboplatin (Paraplatin), carmustine (BiCNU), cefepime (Maxipime), cisatracurium (Nimbex), clindamycin (Cleocin), cyclophosphamide (Cytoxan), cytarabine (ARA-C), dexamethasone (Decadron), dexmedetomidine (Precedex), diphenhydramine (Benadryl), docetaxel (Taxotere), dopamine, enalaprilat (Vasotec IV), etoposide (VePesid), etoposide phosphate (Etopophos), fenoldopam (Corlopam), fluconazole (Diflucan), fludarabine (Fludara), fluorouracil (5-FU), furosemide (Lasix), gallium nitrate (Ganite), granisetron (Kytril), heparin, hetastarch in electrolytes (Hextend), hydrocortisone sodium succinate (Solu-Cortef), hydromorphone (Dilaudid), ifosfamide (Ifex), leucovorin calcium, linezolid (Zyvox), lorazepam (Ativan), magnesium sulfate, mannitol, meperidine (Demerol), mesna (Mesnex), methotrexate, methylprednisolone (Solu-Medrol), metoclopramide (Reglan), metronidazole (Flagyl IV), milrinone (Primacor), morphine, ondansetron (Zofran), potassium chloride (KCl), ranitidine (Zantac), remifentanil (Ultiva), sargramostim (Leukine), sodium bicarbonate, sulfamethoxazole/trimethoprim, thiotepa, tigecycline (Tygacil), vasopressin, vinblastine, vincristine, zidovudine (AZT, Retrovir).

RATE OF ADMINISTRATION

A single dose over 30 minutes as an intermittent infusion. Discontinue primary IV infusion during administration. Slow infusion rate for pain along venipuncture site. See Compatibility.

ACTIONS

An antimicrobial agent that combines the extended-spectrum penicillin piperacillin with the potent beta-lactamase inhibitor tazobactam. May be used in suspected polymicrobial infections due to its broad spectrum of activity; spectrum is superior to many other agents. Acts by inhibiting septum formation and cell wall synthesis of susceptible bacteria. Bactericidal against all three classes of bacterial pathogens; gram-positive and gram-negative aerobes, and anaerobes that may be resistant to other antibiotics. Well distributed in all body fluids and tissues. Mean tissue concentrations are 50% to 100% of plasma concentrations. Peak levels are achieved immediately at the completion of an infusion. Plasma half-life ranges from 0.7 to 1.2 hours. Extended two-fold (piperacillin) to four-fold (tazobactam), if CrCl less than 20 mL/min. Metabolized and excreted in urine and, to a small extent, in bile. Crosses the placental barrier. Secreted in breast milk.

INDICATIONS AND USES

Treatment of infections caused by piperacillin-resistant, piperacillin/tazobactam–susceptible, beta-lactamase–producing strains of specific microorganisms in the following conditions: intra-abdominal (e.g., appendicitis complicated by rupture or abscess and peritonitis), gynecologic (e.g., postpartum endometritis and pelvic inflammatory disease), skin and skin structure (complicated and uncomplicated, e.g., cellulitis, cutaneous abscesses, and ischemic/diabetic foot infection), and pneumonia (moderately severe community-acquired and nosocomial). ▪ Used in combination with aminoglycosides for infections in neutropenic patients or nosocomial pneumonia caused by *Pseudomonas aeruginosa*.

Unlabeled uses: Treatment of septicemia.

CONTRAINDICATIONS

History of hypersensitivity reaction to any penicillin, cephalosporin, or beta-lactamase inhibitors (not absolute; see Precautions).

PRECAUTIONS

Hypersensitivity reactions, including fatalities, have been reported in patients on penicillin therapy; most likely to occur in patients with a history of penicillin allergy or sensitivity to multiple allergens. There have been reports of individuals with a history of penicillin hypersensitivity experiencing severe reactions when treated with cephalosporins. Check history of previous hypersensitivity reactions to penicillins, cephalosporins, or other allergens. Actual incidence of cross-allergenicity not established but may be more common with first-generation cephalosporins. ▪ Sensitivity studies indicated determine susceptibility of the causative organism to piperacillin. ▪ To reduce the development of drug-resistant bacteria and maintain its effectiveness, piperacillin/tazobactam should be used to treat or prevent only those infections proven or strongly suspected to be caused by bacteria. ▪ Avoid prolonged use of drug; superinfection caused by overgrowth of nonsusceptible organisms may result. ▪ Bleeding manifestations have been reported and may be associated with abnormal coagulation tests (e.g., clotting time, platelet aggregation, and PT). Patients with impaired renal function may be at increased risk for bleeding tendencies. ▪ Use caution in patients with CHF or those with a history of bleeding disorders or GI disease (e.g., colitis). ▪ *Clostridium difficile*–associated diarrhea (CDAD) has been reported. May range from mild diarrhea to fatal colitis. Consider in patients who present with diarrhea during or after treatment with piperacillin/tazobactam. ▪ Incidence of side effects (e.g., fever and rash) may be increased in patients with cystic fibrosis. ▪ Administration of higher than recommended doses has resulted in neuromuscular excitability and convulsions. Patients with renal impairment are at increased risk. ▪ Continue at least 2 days after symptoms of infection disappear.

Monitor: Watch for early symptoms of a hypersensitivity reaction. ▪ Periodic evaluation of renal, hepatic, and hematopoietic systems and serum potassium recommended in prolonged therapy. May cause hypokalemia; observe closely. ▪ Consider testing patients with gonorrhea for syphilis. ▪ Contains 2.79 mEq (64 mg) of sodium/Gm. At the usual recommended doses, patients would receive 33.5 to 44.6 mEq (768 to 1,024 mg) per day. ▪ Observe for electrolyte imbalance and cardiac irregularities. May aggravate CHF. ▪ May cause thrombophlebitis; observe carefully, rotate infusion sites. ▪ Observe for increased bleeding tendencies in all patients, especially those with impaired renal function. ▪ See Drug/Lab Interactions.

Patient Education: Report promptly: fever, rash, sore throat, unusual bleeding or bruising, severe stomach cramps, and/or diarrhea, seizures. ▪ May require alternate birth control. ▪ Promptly report diarrhea or bloody stools that occur during treatment or up to several months after an antibiotic has been discontinued; may indicate CDAD and require treatment.

Maternal/Child: Category B: use during pregnancy only if clearly needed. ▪ May cause diarrhea, candidiasis, or allergic response in nursing infants. ▪ Safety and effectiveness for use in pediatric patients under 2 months of age not established.

Elderly: No problems documented. Consider age-related organ function and concomitant disease or drug therapy.

DRUG/LAB INTERACTIONS

Synergistic when used in combination with **aminoglycosides** (e.g., amikacin [Amikin], gentamicin). Synergism may be inconsistent; see Compatibility. ▪ Does not affect pharmacokinetics of vancomycin; may be given without dose adjustment. ▪ Concomitant administration with **probenecid** decreases rate of elimination of piperacillin/tazobactam, resulting in higher and more prolonged blood levels. May be desirable or may cause toxicity. ▪ Use caution with **anticoagulants** (e.g., heparin, warfarin [Coumadin]), **platelet aggregation inhibitors** (e.g., aspirin, NSAIDs [e.g., ibuprofen (Advil, Motrin), naproxen (Aleve, Naprosyn)], dextran, dipyridamole, glycoprotein GPIIb/IIIa receptor antagonists [e.g., abciximab (ReoPro), eptifibatide (Integrilin), tirofiban (Aggrastat)], plicamycin). Risk of bleeding is increased. Monitoring of coagulation tests may be indicated. Concurrent use of piperacillin/tazobactam with **thrombolytic agents** (e.g., alteplase [tPA]) is not recommended; may increase risk of severe hemorrhage. ▪ May be antagonized by **bacteriostatic antibiotics** (e.g., chloramphenicol, erythromycin, and tetracyclines); may interfere with bactericidal action. ▪ May decrease clearance and increase toxicity of **methotrexate**; monitor methotrexate levels. ▪ May inhibit effectiveness of **oral contraceptives**; could result in breakthrough bleeding or pregnancy. ▪ May prolong neuromuscular blockade with **vecuronium** or other nondepolarizing muscle relaxants. ▪ May cause **false urine protein reactions** with various tests and **false-positive glucose** with Clinitest. ▪ **False-positive test results** using the Bio-Rad Laboratories Platelia Aspergillus EIA test in patients receiving piperacillin/tazobactam (Zosyn) have been reported. ▪ See Side Effects.

SIDE EFFECTS

Hypokalemia, prolonged PTT, prolonged PT, and increased bleeding time. Most other side effects are usually mild or moderate and transient. Abdominal pain; abscess; agitation; anxiety; CDAD; chest pain; cholestatic jaundice; constipation; diarrhea; dizziness; dyspnea; dyspepsia; edema; electrolyte abnormalities; fever; headache; hematuria; hematologic abnormalities (agranulocytosis, anemia, hemolytic anemia, pancytopenia, thrombocytopenia, thrombocytosis); hepatitis; hypertension; increased AST, BUN, and serum creatinine; insomnia; interstitial nephritis; local reactions; moniliasis; nausea; pain; pharyngitis; positive Coombs' test; pruritus; pseudomembranous colitis; rash (e.g., bullous, eczematoid, erythema multiforme, maculopapular, Stevens-Johnson syndrome, toxic epidermal necrolysis, urticarial); rhinitis; seizures; and vomiting have been reported. Anaphylaxis can occur. Transient leukopenia and eosinophilia can occur with prolonged therapy.

ANTIDOTE

Notify the physician immediately of any adverse symptoms. For severe symptoms, discontinue the drug, treat hypersensitivity reactions (antihistamines, epinephrine, corticosteroids, airway management, oxygen), and resuscitate as necessary. Use anticonvulsants (e.g., diazepam [Valium]) or barbiturates (e.g., phenobarbital) for seizures. Treat CDAD with fluids, electrolytes, protein supplements, and oral vancomycin (Vancocin) or metronidazole (Flagyl) as indicated. In severe cases, surgical evaluation may be indicated. Mild cases may respond to drug discontinuation alone. Hemodialysis is effective in overdose.

PLASMA PROTEIN FRACTION
Plasma volume expander
(**PLAZ**-ma **PRO**-teen **FRAK**-shun)
Plasmanate, Plasmatein, Protenate
pH 6.7 to 7.3

USUAL DOSE

Variable, depending on indication for use, condition of patient, and response to therapy. Range is from 250 to 1,500 mL/24 hr. Each 500-mL bottle yields 25 Gm of plasma protein. Suggested initial doses are as follows:

Shock: 250 to 500 mL.
Burns: 500 to 1,000 mL.
Hypoproteinemia: 1,000 to 1,500 mL/24 hr.

PEDIATRIC DOSE

Treatment of acute shock: 6.6 to 30 mL/kg of body weight.

DILUTION

Available as a 5% solution buffered with saline in 250- and 500-mL bottles with injection sets. Plasmanate also available in a 50-mL size. No further dilution is required. Do not use if solution is turbid or a sediment is visible. Use immediately after opening and discard any unused portion. Contains no preservatives.

Storage: Store at CRT.

COMPATIBILITY

Consider any drug NOT listed as compatible to be INCOMPATIBLE until consulting a pharmacist; specific conditions may apply.

Manufacturer lists as **incompatible** with solutions containing alcohol, protein hydrolysates, or amino acid products. Manufacturer states, "**Compatible** with the usual carbohydrate and electrolyte solutions."

RATE OF ADMINISTRATION

Variable, depending on indication, present blood volume, and patient response. Adjust or slow rate according to clinical response and rising BP. Averages are:

Normal blood volume: 1 mL/min.

Treatment of shock and burns in adult: 5 to 8 mL/min. Higher rates may be tolerated if necessary. Rapid infusion (over 10 mL/min) may cause hypotension. Decrease flow rate as patient improves.

Treatment of shock in infants and other pediatric patients: 5 to 10 mL/min. Do not exceed 10 mL/min in pediatric patients.

Treatment of hypoproteinemia: Single 500-mL dose over 1 hour. For larger amounts the maximum rate is 100 mL/hr.

ACTIONS

A sterile, natural, plasma protein substance containing at least 83% albumin, no more than 17% alpha and beta globulins, and no more than 1% gamma globulin. Contains 130 to 160 mEq sodium/liter. It expands intravascular volume, prevents marked hemoconcentration, and maintains appropriate electrolyte balance in burns.

INDICATIONS AND USES

Emergency treatment of hypovolemic shock caused by burns, infections, surgery, or trauma (may also be due to dehydration in infants and other pediatric patients). ■ Temporary treatment of hemorrhage when whole blood unavailable. ■ Hypoproteinemia until cause determined and corrected. ■ Prevention of hemoconcentration and maintenance of electrolyte balance in burn patients.

CONTRAINDICATIONS

Cardiac failure, cardiopulmonary bypass, history of hypersensitivity reactions to albumin, normal or increased intravascular volume, severe anemia.

PRECAUTIONS

May be given without regard to blood group or type. ■ Not effective for coagulation mechanism defects. ■ Added protein, fluid, and sodium load requires caution in hepatic or renal impairment. ■ If continuous protein loss occurs or edema is present, normal serum albumin (25%) may be the preferred product.

Monitor: Monitor vital signs (including central venous pressure if possible) and urine output every 5 to 15 minutes for 1 hour and hourly thereafter depending on condition. ■ For treatment of shock, observe carefully for bleeding points that may not have been evident at lower pressures. ■ Whole blood may be indicated for considerable RBC loss or anemia caused by administration of large amounts of plasma protein fraction. ▪ Additional fluids are required for dehydrated patients. Tissue dehydration caused by osmotic action of plasma proteins can be acute. ▪ May cause vascular overload; monitor for signs of pulmonary edema or heart failure (e.g., dyspnea, fluid in the lungs, abnormal increases in BP or CVP). ▪ Hemoglobin, hematocrit, electrolyte, and serum protein evaluations are necessary during therapy.

Maternal/Child: Category C: safety for use in pregnancy not established.

DRUG/LAB INTERACTIONS

May cause an **elevated alkaline phosphatase** level.

SIDE EFFECTS

Hypersensitivity and/or pyrogenic reactions can occur. Incidence of toxicity is low when administered with appropriate caution. Slight nausea can occur. Hypotension can be sudden if administered too rapidly.

ANTIDOTE

Notify the physician of all symptoms and side effects. Discontinue infusion for sudden hypotension. Decrease flow rate if indicated and treat symptomatically. Resuscitate as necessary.

PORFIMER SODIUM
(**POOR**-fih-mer **SO**-dee-um)

Photofrin

Photosensitizing agent
Antineoplastic

pH 7 to 8

USUAL DOSE

A course is a two-stage process requiring administration of both drug and light.

Stage one: Administration of porfimer: A single IV injection of 2 mg/kg. No further injection of porfimer sodium should be given in any one course of therapy.

Stage two: Illumination: Illumination with nonthermal laser light at 40 to 50 hours post-injection.

ESOPHAGEAL AND ENDOBRONCHIAL CANCER

2 mg/kg of porfimer sodium as an IV injection. Approximately 40 to 50 hours after the injection, standard endoscopic techniques are used for light administration and débridement. The laser system must be approved for delivery of a stable power output at a wavelength of 630 ± 3 nm. Light is delivered to the tumor by cylindrical OPTIGUIDE fiber-optic diffusers passed through the operating channel of an endoscope/bronchoscope. The choice of diffuser tip length depends on the length of the tumor. Diffuser length should be sized to avoid exposure of nonmalignant tissue to light and to prevent overlapping of previously treated malignant tissue. A second laser light application may be given 96 to 120 hours after injection. Before providing a second laser light treatment, the residual tumor should be gently débrided. Vigorous débridement may cause esophageal tumor bleeding; see Precautions.

Up to three courses may be given, but each must be separated by at least 30 days. Evaluate patients with esophageal cancer for the presence of a tracheoesophageal or bronchoesophageal fistula before each course. Evaluate all patients for possible erosion of the tumor into a major blood vessel. **Esophageal cancer:** 2 mg/kg of porfimer sodium as an IV injection. A light dose of 300 joules/cm of diffuser length should be delivered by the specific process outlined previously. Light exposure time is set to 12 minutes and 30 seconds. Débridement of tumor should be performed 2 to 3 days later; see Precautions.

Endobronchial non–small-cell lung cancer: 2 mg/kg of porfimer sodium as an IV injection. A light dose of 200 joules/cm of diffuser length should be delivered by the specific process outlined previously. Light exposure time is set to 8 minutes and 20 seconds. Débridement of tumor should be performed 2 to 3 days later; see Precautions.

HIGH-GRADE DYSPLASIA (HGD IN BARRETT'S ESOPHAGUS [BE])

2 mg/kg of porfimer sodium as an IV injection. Approximately 40 to 50 hours after the injection, administration of light should be delivered by an X-cell Photodynamic Therapy (PDT) balloon with a fiber optic diffuser. The choice of fiber optic/balloon diffuser combination will depend on the length of Barrett's mucosa to be treated (see manufacturer's information). The objective of therapy is to expose and treat all areas of HGD and the entire length of Barrett's esophagus. The light dose administered is 130 joules/cm of diffuser length. Acceptable light intensity for the balloon/diffuser combinations ranges from 200 to 270 mW/cm of diffuser. Treatment time is dependent on the fiber optic/balloon diffuser combination used (see manufacturer's information). A maximum of 7 cm of esophageal mucosa may be treated at the first light session. If possible, the area treated should include normal tissue margins of a few millimeters at both the proximal and distal ends. Nodules are pretreated at a light dose of 50 joules/cm of diffuser length with a short (2.5 cm) fiber optic diffuser placed directly against the nodule. A second laser light application may be given to a previously treated segment that shows a "skip" area using a 2.5-cm fiber optic diffuser at a light dose of 50 joules/cm of the diffuser length. Patients with Barrett's esophagus greater than 7 cm should have the remaining untreated length of Barrett's epithelium treated with a second PDT course at least 90 days later. See Precautions.

Up to 3 courses (each separated by 90 days) may be given to a previously treated segment that still shows high-grade dysplasia, low-grade dysplasia, or Barrett's metaplasia, or to a new segment if the initial Barrett's segment was greater than 7 cm in length.

DOSE ADJUSTMENTS

No adjustments required.

DILUTION

Specific techniques required; see Precautions. Prepare immediately before use. Each vial of porfimer sodium must be reconstituted with 31.8 mL of D5W or NS. Concentration will be 2.5 mg/mL. Shake well until dissolved. An opaque solution; detection of particulate matter by visual inspection is difficult. Withdraw desired dose. Must be protected from bright light and used immediately.

Storage: Store unopened vials at CRT in carton to protect from light.

COMPATIBILITY

Manufacturer states, "Do not mix porfimer sodium with other drugs in the same solution."

RATE OF ADMINISTRATION

A single dose equally distributed over 3 to 5 minutes.

ACTIONS

The first light-activated drug (photosensitizing agent) for use in photodynamic therapy (PDT) to be approved in the United States. Treatment consists of a two-step process involving administration of drug and light. Cytotoxic and anti-tumor actions are light and oxygen related. After IV infusion of drug, it is allowed to circulate. It accumulates and is retained in tumors, skin, and organs of the reticuloendothelial system (e.g., liver, spleen) while largely clearing from other tissues. Has no apparent effect on tumors until it is activated by selective delivery of light (usually 40 to 50 hours postinfusion). Light activation induces a photochemical, not a thermal, effect that produces an active form of oxygen and releases thromboxane A_2. This process causes vasoconstriction, activation and aggregation of platelets, and increased clotting that contribute to ischemic necrosis leading to tissue and tumor death. The necrotic reaction and associated inflammatory response may evolve over several days. In patients with esophageal cancer, ability to swallow is improved, as is quality of life. Elimination half-life is very prolonged, up to several weeks. Highly protein bound.

INDICATIONS AND USES

Palliative treatment of patients with completely obstructing esophageal cancer or partially obstructing esophageal cancers that are unsuitable for treatment with thermal laser therapy. ■ Treatment of microinvasive endobronchial non–small-cell lung cancer (NSCLC) in patients for whom surgery and radiotherapy are not indicated. ■ Reduction of obstruction and palliation of symptoms in patients with completely or partially obstructing endobronchial non–small-cell lung cancer. ■ Ablation of high-grade dysplasia (HGD) of Barrett's esophagus patients who do not undergo esophagectomy.

Unlabeled uses: Treatment of bladder cancer (approved for use in Canada). Studies are in progress on other tumors accessible by scope and fiberoptics to deliver light (e.g., various cutaneous carcinomas, head and neck carcinomas).

CONTRAINDICATIONS

Known allergies to porphyrins, an existing tracheoesophageal or bronchoesophageal fistula, porphyria, or tumors eroding into a major blood vessel. ■ Photodynamic therapy (PDT) is not suitable for emergency treatment of patients with severe acute respiratory distress caused by an obstructing endobronchial lesion because 40 to 50 hours are required between injection with porfimer sodium and laser light treatment. ■ PDT is not suitable for patients with esophageal varices or for patients with esophageal or gastric ulcers greater than 1 cm in diameter.

PRECAUTIONS

Use rubber gloves and eye protection during preparation and administration. Avoid any skin or eye contact since that area will become photosensitive. Wipe up spills with a damp cloth. Dispose of all contaminated materials in a polyethylene bag to avoid accidental contact by others. Protection from light will be necessary if accidental exposure or overexposure occurs. See process in Patient Education. ■ Administered by or under the direction of the physician specialist with appropriate knowledge of the selected laser system. Facilities for monitoring the patient and responding to any medical emergency must be available. ▪ Requires laser systems and a fiber-optic diffuser to activate. The FDA has approved several photodynamic lasers and the Optiguide fiber-optic diffuser for use with porfimer sodium. ▪ Avoid exposure of skin and eyes to direct sunlight or bright indoor light; see Patient Education. Porfimer elimination may be prolonged in patients with hepatic or renal impairment, and they may require longer precautionary measures for photosensitivity. ▪ In the original studies for esophageal tumors, some experienced investigators indicated that natural sloughing action in the esophagus might be sufficient and débridement could needlessly traumatize the area. However, débridement is now recommended after each light activation to minimize the potential for obstruction caused by necrotic debris. ▪ A minimum of 4 weeks after radiation therapy is complete is recommended before treatment with PDT. This allows the acute inflammation produced by radiotherapy to subside. ▪ 2 to 4 weeks should be allowed after PDT is complete before beginning any radiotherapy.

Esophageal tumors: Not recommended if the esophageal tumor is eroding into the trachea or bronchial tree; tracheoesophageal or bronchoesophageal fistula may result from treatment. ▪ Use extreme caution in patients with esophageal varices. Light should not be given directly to the variceal area because of the high risk of bleeding.

Endobronchial cancer: Interstitial fiber placement is preferred to intraluminal activation in noncircumferential endobronchial tumors that are soft enough to penetrate. Results in less exposure of the normal bronchial mucosa to light. ▪ Patients with obstructing lung cancer who have received prior radiation therapy or who have tumors that are large, centrally located, cavitating, or extensive and extrinsic to the bronchus have a higher incidence of fatal hemoptysis. ▪ An endobronchial tumor that invades deeply into the bronchial wall may create a fistula as the tumor resolves. ▪ Use with extreme caution in endobronchial tumors located where treatment-induced inflammation could obstruct the airway (e.g., long or circumferential tumors of the trachea, tumors of the carina that involve both mainstem bronchi circumferentially, or circumferential tumors in the mainstem bronchus in patients with prior pneumonectomy).

HGD in Barrett's esophagus: Before initiating treatment with porfimer PDT, a diagnosis of HGD in Barrett's esophagus should be confirmed by a GI pathologist. ▪ Long-term effect of PDT on HGD in Barrett's esophagus is unknown. There may be a risk of leaving cancerous cells behind or of leaving residual abnormal epithelium beneath the new squamous cell epithelium. ▪ Esophageal strictures are a common adverse effect seen in patients treated with PDT for HGD in Barrett's esophagus. Usually occur within 6 months following PDT. May be managed with esophageal dilation; several dilations may be required.

Monitor: Obtain baseline CBC and monitor for anemia due to tumor bleeding. ▪ Prevent extravasation at the injection site. Should extravasation occur, area must be protected from light. ▪ Opiates may be required to control pain. ▪ Observe patients carefully; most are critically ill, and many complications could occur. Monitor patients with ***endobronchial tumors*** closely between the laser light therapy and the mandatory débridement bronchoscopy for any evidence of respiratory distress, inflammation, mucositis, or necrotic debris that may cause obstruction of the airway. Immediate bronchoscopy may be required to remove secretions and debris to open the airway. ▪ Monitor for hemoptysis; may be a sign of progressive disease, or may result from resolution of a tumor that has eroded into a pulmonary artery. ▪ In patients who have received PDT for **HGD in Barrett's esophagus,** endoscopic biopsy surveillance should be conducted every 3 months until 4 consecutive negative evaluations for HGD have been recorded. Further follow-up should be performed every 6 to 12 months. ▪ Photosensitivity not transferable through skin to caregivers. ▪ See Precautions, Patient Education, and Drug/Lab Interactions.

Patient Education: Must observe precautions to avoid exposure of skin and eyes to direct sunlight or bright indoor light for at least 30 days. Some patients may remain photosensitive for up to 90 or more days. Photosensitivity is due to residual drug, which is present in all parts of the skin. Ambient indoor light is beneficial as it gradually inactivates the remaining drug through a photobleaching reaction. Do not remain in a darkened room. Do expose skin to ambient indoor light. Avoid bright indoor light from examination lamps, dental lamps, operating room lamps, and unshaded light bulbs. Limit time outdoors to necessary excursions and completely cover body with clothing and shade face before going out. Conventional ultraviolet sunscreens are of no value because photoactivation is caused by visible light, not UV rays. Eyes will be sensitive to sun, bright lights, and car headlights; wear dark sunglasses with an average white light transmittance of less than 4%. After several weeks and before exposing any area of skin to direct sunlight or bright indoor light, test a small area of skin (not the face) for residual photosensitivity. Expose the small area of skin for 10 minutes. If no photosensitivity reaction (redness, swelling, or blistering) occurs within 24 hours, gradually resume normal outdoor activities. Exercise caution and increase skin exposure gradually. If some photosensitivity reaction occurs, continue precautions for 2 more weeks and then retest. Retest level of photosensitivity if traveling to a different geographic area with greater sunshine. ▪ Report chest pain (caused by inflammatory response within the area of treatment); may require prescription pain medication. ▪ Effective contraception necessary for women of childbearing age.

Maternal/Child: Category C: use during pregnancy only if benefits justify potential risk to fetus. Effective contraception necessary for women of childbearing age. Has caused maternal and fetal toxicity in rats and rabbits (increased resorptions, decreased litter size, and reduced fetal body weight). ▪ Discontinue breast-feeding; not known if it is secreted in breast milk, but serious reactions could occur in the infant. ▪ Safety and effectiveness for use in pediatric patients not established.

Elderly: Dose modification based on age is not required.

DRUG/LAB INTERACTIONS
No specific studies have been completed, but the following interactions are likely to occur. ▪ Use with **other photosensitizing agents** (e.g., griseofulvin, fluoroquinolones [e.g., ciprofloxacin (Cipro IV)], phenothiazines [e.g., prochlorperazine (Compazine)], sulfonamides [sulfisoxazole (Gantrisin), ophthalmic solutions (AK-Sulf)], sulfonylurea hypoglycemic agents [tolbutamide], tetracyclines [doxycycline], thiazide diuretics [chlorothiazide (Diuril)]) could increase the photosensitivity reaction. ▪ Antitumor activity may be decreased by **dimethyl sulfoxide, beta-carotene, ethanol, formate, mannitol.** ▪ Anti-tumor activity may also be decreased by **allopurinol** (Aloprim), **calcium channel blockers** (e.g., diltiazem [Cardizem]),

prostaglandin synthesis inhibitors (NSAIDs [e.g., ibuprofen (Advil, Motrin), naproxen (Aleve, Naprosyn)]), **and tissue ischemia.** ▪ Effectiveness may be reduced by **drugs that decrease clotting** (e.g., heparin, alteplase [tPA]), **vasoconstriction** (e.g., nicardipine [Cardene]), **or platelet aggregation** (e.g., dipyridamole [Persantine], ticlopidine [Ticlid]). ▪ **Glucocorticoid hormones** (e.g., dexamethasone [Decadron]) given before or with PDT may reduce the effectiveness of porfimer by inhibiting the production of thromboxane A_2.

SIDE EFFECTS

All diagnoses: May cause constipation. Most toxicities are local effects in the region of illumination and occasionally in surrounding tissues. Usually an inflammatory response induced by the photodynamic effects. Photosensitivity reactions occurred in 20% of patients in clinical studies. Reactions were usually mild to moderate erythema, but also included blisters, burning sensation, itching, and swelling. Less common skin manifestations included increased hair growth, skin discoloration, skin nodules, increased wrinkles, and skin fragility. Cases of fluid imbalance have been reported. Cataracts have been reported in one man with a family history of cataracts. Relationship to porfimer sodium unknown.

Esophageal tumors: Bronchoesophageal or tracheoesophageal fistula can occur as a result of the disease or treatment, including débridement. Abdominal pain, anemia (more prevalent if tumor is located in the lower third of the esophagus), anorexia, arrhythmias (atrial fibrillation [more prevalent if tumor is located in the middle third of the esophagus], tachycardia), candidiasis, chest pain, coughing, dyspepsia, dysphagia, dyspnea, edema, eructation, esophageal edema (more prevalent if tumor is located in the upper third of the esophagus), esophageal tumor bleeding, esophageal stricture, esophagitis, fever, hematemesis, hypertension, hypotension, insomnia, nausea, pleural effusion, and vomiting may occur, as well as numerous others.

Endobronchial tumors: Coughing, dysphagia, dyspnea (may be life threatening), mucositis reaction (e.g., edema, exudate, and mucous plug obstruction), stricture, ulceration. Fatal hemoptysis has occurred (higher incidence in patients who have received radiation therapy).

High-grade dysplasia (HGD in Barrett's esophagus [BE]): Esophageal narrowing and esophageal stricture are common side effects and may require multiple dilations. Other side effects may include abdominal pain, anorexia, anxiety, arthralgia, back pain, chest discomfort or pain, dehydration, depression, diarrhea, dyspepsia, dysphagia, dyspnea, eructation, esophageal pain, fatigue, fever, headache, hiccups, hypertension, infections (bronchitis, sinusitis), insomnia, nausea and vomiting, odynophagia (pain on swallowing), pleural effusion.

ANTIDOTE

If an overdose of porfimer sodium is given, do not give the laser light treatment. Porfimer sodium is not dialyzable. Increased side effects and damage to normal tissue can be expected if an overdose of light is given. Keep physician informed of all side effects; most will be treated symptomatically. Some may be life threatening. Respiratory obstruction may require immediate bronchoscopy and removal of the obstruction with suction or forceps. Stent placement may be required in endobronchial stricture. Chest pain may require the use of opiates.

POTASSIUM ACETATE AND POTASSIUM CHLORIDE

(po-**TASS**-ee-um **AS**-ah-tayt,
po-**TASS**-ee-um **KLOR**-eyed)

Electrolyte replenisher
Antihypokalemic

pH 4 to 8

USUAL DOSE

Concentrated potassium solutions must be diluted before administration; direct injection of any concentrated solution can be instantly fatal.

Dose and rate of administration are dependent on specific patient condition.

Normal daily requirements: *Adults:* 40 to 80 mEq/24 hr.

Starting dose based on losses, desired replacement, or maintenance. 20 to 60 mEq/24 hr. 200 mEq/24 hr is usually not exceeded. Up to 400 mEq/24 hr has been given in selected situations (e.g., serum potassium less that 2 mEq/L) with extreme caution. Potassium acetate may contain up to 200 mcg/L of aluminum; see Precautions.

PEDIATRIC DOSE

Normal daily requirements: *Newborn:* 2 to 6 mEq/kg/24 hr. *Other pediatric patients:* 2 to 3 mEq/kg/24 hr.

1 to 4 mEq/kg of body weight/24 hr. Do not exceed 40 mEq/day. Potassium acetate may contain up to 200 mcg/L of aluminum; see Precautions and Maternal/Child.

DOSE ADJUSTMENTS

Reduce dose in impaired renal function. ■ Lower-end initial doses may be appropriate in the elderly based on potential for decreased organ function and concomitant disease or drug therapy.

DILUTION

Each individual dose must be diluted in a larger volume of suitable IV solution and given as an infusion. Check labels for aluminum content; see Precautions. Soluble in commonly used IV solutions; see chart on inside back cover. 40 mEq/L is the preferred dilution. 80 mEq/L is the usual maximum concentration and must be administered with caution. In replacement therapy more concentrated doses may be used and must be administered with extreme caution. 40 mEq/100 mL is commonly used and must be controlled by an infusion pump. *Up to 100 mEq/100 mL has been administered through a central line (to avoid phlebitis); must be controlled by an infusion pump.* **Direct injection of any concentrated solution can be instantly fatal.** Avoid layering of potassium by thoroughly agitating the prepared IV solution. Do not add potassium to an IV bottle in the hanging position; remove from hanger to guarantee dispersion throughout solution. In severe hypokalemia, solutions without dextrose are preferred (dextrose might decrease serum potassium level). Use only clear solutions.

COMPATIBILITY   (Underline Indicates Conflicting Compatibility Information)

Consider any drug NOT listed as compatible to be INCOMPATIBLE until consulting a pharmacist; specific conditions may apply.

One source suggests the following **compatibilities**:

POTASSIUM ACETATE

Additive: Metoclopramide (Reglan).

Y-site: Ciprofloxacin (Cipro IV).

POTASSIUM CHLORIDE

Additive: Amikacin (Amikin), aminophylline, amiodarone (Nexterone), atracurium (Tracrium), calcium gluconate, cefepime (Maxipime), chloramphenicol (Chloromycetin), ciprofloxacin (Cipro IV), clindamycin (Cleocin), cytarabine (ARA-C), dimenhydrinate, dobutamine, dopamine, enalaprilat (Vasotec IV), erythromycin (Erythrocin), fluconazole (Diflucan), foscarnet (Foscavir), fosphenytoin (Cerebyx), furosemide (Lasix), heparin, hydrocortisone sodium succinate (Solu-Cortef), hydromorphone (Dilaudid), isoproterenol (Isuprel), lidocaine, magnesium sulfate, methyldopate, metoclopramide (Reglan), mitoxantrone (Novantrone), nafcillin (Nallpen), norepinephrine (Levophed), oxacillin (Bactocill), penicillin G potassium, penicillin G sodium, phenylephrine (Neo-Synephrine), piperacillin, ranitidine (Zantac), sodium bicarbonate, thiopental (Pentothal), vancomycin, verapamil.

Y-site: Acyclovir (Zovirax), aldesleukin (Proleukin), allopurinol (Aloprim), amifostine (Ethyol), aminophylline, amiodarone (Nexterone), ampicillin, anidulafungin (Eraxis), atropine, aztreonam (Azactam), bivalirudin (Angiomax), calcium gluconate, caspofungin (Cancidas), ceftazidime (Fortaz), chlorpromazine (Thorazine), ciprofloxacin (Cipro IV), cisatracurium (Nimbex), cladribine (Leustatin), dexamethasone (Decadron), dexmedetomidine (Precedex), digoxin (Lanoxin), diltiazem (Cardizem), diphenhydramine (Benadryl), dobutamine, docetaxel (Taxotere), dopamine, doripenem (Doribax), doxorubicin liposomal (Doxil), droperidol (Inapsine), drotrecogin alfa (Xigris), edrophonium (Enlon), enalaprilat (Vasotec IV), epinephrine (Adrenalin), ertapenem (Invanz), esmolol (Brevibloc), estrogens, conjugated (Premarin), ethacrynic acid (Edecrin), etoposide phosphate (Etopophos), famotidine (Pepcid IV), fenoldopam (Corlopam), fentanyl (Sublimaze), filgrastim (Neupogen), fludarabine (Fludara), fluorouracil (5-FU), furosemide (Lasix), gallium nitrate (Ganite), gemcitabine (Gemzar), granisetron (Kytril), heparin, hetastarch in electrolytes (Hextend), hydralazine, idarubicin (Idamycin), inamrinone (Amrinone), indomethacin (Indocin IV), insulin (regular), isoproterenol (Isuprel), kanamycin (Kantrex), labetalol (Trandate), lidocaine, linezolid (Zyvox), lorazepam (Ativan), magnesium sulfate, melphalan (Alkeran), meperidine (Demerol), meropenem (Merrem IV), methylprednisolone (Solu-Medrol), micafungin (Mycamine), midazolam (Versed), milrinone (Primacor), morphine, neostigmine, nicardipine (Cardene IV), nitroprusside sodium, norepinephrine (Levophed), ondansetron (Zofran), oxacillin (Bactocill), oxaliplatin (Eloxatin), oxytocin (Pitocin), paclitaxel (Taxol), palonosetron (Aloxi), pantoprazole (Protonix IV), pemetrexed (Alimta), penicillin G potassium, pentazocine (Talwin), phytonadione (vitamin K_1), piperacillin/tazobactam (Zosyn), procainamide (Pronestyl), prochlorperazine (Compazine), promethazine (Phenergan), propofol (Diprivan), propranolol, pyridostigmine (Regonol), quinupristin/dalfopristin (Synercid in KCl 40 mEq/L), remifentanil (Ultiva), sargramostim (Leukine), sodium bicarbonate, succinylcholine, tacrolimus (Prograf), teniposide (Vumon), theophylline, thiotepa, tigecycline (Tygacil), tirofiban (Aggrastat), vinorelbine (Navelbine), warfarin (Coumadin), zidovudine (AZT, Retrovir).

RATE OF ADMINISTRATION

A maximum of 10 mEq/hr of potassium chloride in any given amount of infusion fluid should not be exceeded. With serious potassium depletion (under 2 mEq/L serum), 20 to 40 mEq/hr has been given with extreme

caution. Use of an infusion pump is recommended in all situations and required with any dose exceeding 60 mEq/24 hr. Too-rapid infusion of hypertonic solutions may cause local pain and, rarely, vein irritation. Adjust rate of administration according to patient tolerance.
Pediatric rate: 0.5 to 1 mEq/kg/hr. Do not exceed 10 mEq/hr.

ACTIONS
Potassium: Principal cation of intracellular fluid. Important for maintenance of body fluid composition and electrolyte balance. Participates in carbohydrate utilization and protein synthesis. Critical in the regulation of nerve conduction and muscle contraction, particularly in the heart. The normal serum potassium range is 3.5 to 5 mEq/L. The kidney normally regulates potassium balance but does not conserve potassium balance as well or as promptly as it conserves sodium. Excreted in urine.
Chloride: The major extracellular anion. Closely follows the metabolism of sodium. Changes in the acid-base balance of the body are reflected by the changes in chloride concentration.
Acetate: An alternate source of bicarbonate by metabolic conversion in the liver.

INDICATIONS AND USES
Prophylaxis or treatment of potassium deficiency (e.g., hypokalemia due to diuretic therapy, adjunct to treatment of digoxin toxicity, low dietary potassium intake, vomiting and diarrhea, diabetic acidosis, metabolic alkalosis, corticosteroid therapy, increased renal excretion resulting from acidosis, hemodialysis). ▪ Utilized when oral replacement therapy is not feasible.

CONTRAINDICATIONS
Any disease or condition in which high potassium levels may occur through potassium retention or other processes (e.g., acute dehydration, adrenocortical insufficiency [untreated Addison's disease]), adynamica episodica hereditaria [periodic loss of strength or weakness], anuria, azotemia, crush syndrome, heat cramps, hyperkalemia from any cause, oliguria, patients taking digoxin with severe or complete heart block, postoperative oliguria (early [except during GI drainage]), renal failure, severe hemolytic reactions.

PRECAUTIONS
Impaired renal function or adrenal insufficiency can cause potassium intoxication, which can develop rapidly and without symptoms. ▪ Loss of chloride usually accompanies potassium depletion and may cause hypochloremic alkalosis. Treat cause of potassium depletion in addition to giving potassium. ▪ Potassium phosphate is preferred for specific intracellular deficiency not caused by alkalosis, since phosphate is the usual ion attached to potassium in the body. Not used in the presence of kidney failure. ▪ Alkalyzing potassiums (e.g., acetate, citrate) are preferred for potassium-deficient patients with renal tubular acidosis. Metabolic acidosis and hyperchloremia are most likely present. ▪ Use potassium acetate with caution in patients with metabolic or respiratory alkalosis and in patients with severe hepatic insufficiency. ▪ Administration of IV solutions can cause fluid and/or solute overload, resulting in dilution of serum electrolyte concentrations, overhydration, congested states, or pulmonary edema. The risk of dilutional states is inversely proportional to the electrolyte concentration (increased fluids may dilute electrolyte concentration). The risk of solute overload causing congested states with peripheral

and pulmonary edema is directly proportional to the electrolyte concentration (higher electrolytes pull in fluid, leading to fluid overload). ▪ Use solutions containing potassium with caution in patients with cardiac disease, particularly in the presence of renal disease. Cardiac monitoring is recommended. ▪ Some solutions of potassium may contain aluminum. In impaired kidney function, aluminum may reach toxic levels. Premature neonates are particularly at risk because of their immature kidneys and requirement for calcium and phosphate, which also contain aluminum. Research indicates that patients with impaired renal function who receive more than 4 to 5 mcg/kg/day of parenteral aluminum are at risk for developing CNS or bone toxicity associated with aluminum accumulation.
Monitor: Monitor changes in fluid balance, electrolyte concentration, and acid-base balance (e.g., serum potassium, sodium, chloride, bicarbonate, urinary output, pH). Only extracellular potassium can be measured; intracellular potassium equals 98% of total body potassium. Entire clinical picture must be considered. ▪ Potassium replacement should be monitored whenever possible by continuous or serial ECG, especially in patients taking digoxin. Serum potassium levels are not necessarily dependable indicators of tissue potassium levels. ▪ Continuous cardiac monitoring is preferable for infusion of over 10 mEq of potassium in 1 hour. ▪ Confirm absolute patency of vein. Extravasation will cause necrosis. Local pain and phlebitis may occur with concentrations greater than 40 mEq/L. ▪ See Drug/Lab Interactions.
Patient Education: Report burning or stinging at IV site promptly.
Maternal/Child: Category C: effect unknown; use caution and only if clearly needed in pregnancy and breast-feeding. ▪ Safety and effectiveness for use of KCl in pediatric patients not established. However, use for treatment of potassium deficiency when oral therapy is not feasible is referenced in medical literature. Safety and effectiveness of potassium acetate for use in pediatric patients has been established.
Elderly: See Dose Adjustments. Monitoring of renal function suggested. ▪ Increased risk of hyperkalemia.

DRUG/LAB INTERACTIONS
Potentiated by **angiotensin-converting enzyme inhibitors** (e.g., captopril [Capoten], enalaprilat [Vasotec], lisinopril [Prinivil, Zestril]) and **angiotensin receptor blockers** (e.g., losartan [Cozaar], valsartan [Diovan]); risk of hyperkalemia increased. ▪ Digitalis intoxication may occur with hypokalemia. Use caution if discontinuing potassium after stabilization in patients taking **digoxin.** ▪ **Potassium-sparing diuretics** (e.g., spironolactone [Aldactone], triamterene [Dyrenium], amiloride [Midamor], and a component of Dyazide and Maxzide) may cause hyperkalemia.

SIDE EFFECTS
Abdominal pain, diarrhea, nausea, and vomiting are common side effects of potassium administration and may progress to potassium intoxication. Extravasation, fever, hyperkalemia, hypervolemia, infection or pain at the site of injection, phlebitis, or venous thrombosis may occur.
Potassium intoxication: Areflexia (absence of reflexes), cardiac arrest, cardiac arrhythmias (e.g., bradycardia, ventricular fibrillation), ECG abnormalities (including increased amplitude of T wave, decreased amplitude of R wave, below-baseline depression of S wave, disappearing P wave, PR prolongation), heart block, hypotension, mental confusion, muscular or

respiratory paralysis, paresthesias of the extremities, weakness. Progression of side effects may cause death.

Potassium deficit: Disruption of neuromuscular function, intestinal ileus, and dilatation.

ANTIDOTE

For any side effect, discontinue the drug and notify the physician. Death may result from potassium levels of 8 mEq/L. For severe hyperkalemia (over 6.5 mEq/L plasma), use IV sodium bicarbonate 40 to 160 mEq over 5 minutes to correct acidosis. Repeat in 10 to 15 minutes if ECG still abnormal. Initially, one ampule of 50% dextrose may be given into a large vein. Follow with IV dextrose, 10% to 25%, containing 10 units of regular insulin per 20 Gm of dextrose and infuse at 300 to 500 mL over 1 hour. 150 mL of ⅙ M sodium lactate is rarely used as a substitute. Eliminate potassium-containing foods and medicines. Monitor ECG continuously. If P waves are absent, give calcium gluconate or chloride 0.5 to 1 Gm over 2 minutes (exceeds usual rate of administration). Do not use if patient receiving digoxin. All of these measures cause a shift of potassium into the cells and may be used simultaneously. Sodium polystyrene sulfonate (Kayexalate) orally or as retention enemas is used to actually remove potassium from the body. Hemodialysis or peritoneal dialysis may be useful. Use caution in the digitalized patient; too-rapid removal of potassium may cause digoxin toxicity. Resuscitate as necessary. For extravasation, apply warm, moist compresses.

PRALATREXATE
(pral-a-**TREX**-ate)

Folotyn

Antineoplastic
(Antifolate)

pH 7.5 to 8.5

USUAL DOSE

Premedication: Begin folic acid 1 to 1.25 mg PO daily within the 10 days before starting pralatrexate. Continue daily throughout the full course of therapy and for 30 days after the last dose of pralatrexate. Administer vitamin B_{12} (1 mg) IM within the 10 weeks before starting pralatrexate and every 8 to 10 weeks thereafter. Subsequent vitamin B_{12} injections may be given the same day as pralatrexate.

Pralatrexate: 30 mg/M^2 by IV push over 3 to 5 minutes via the side port of a free-flowing infusion of NS. Administer once weekly for 6 weeks in 7-week cycles until progressive disease or unacceptable toxicity occurs. Management of severe or intolerable side effects may require dose omission or reduction or interruption of therapy; see Dose Adjustments.

DOSE ADJUSTMENTS

Before administering any dose of pralatrexate, mucositis should be equal to or less than Grade 1, platelet count should be equal to or more than 100,000 cells/mm^3 for the first dose and equal to or greater than 50,000 cells/mm^3 for all subsequent doses, and the absolute neutrophil count (ANC) should be equal to or greater than 1,000 cells/mm^3. Doses may be omitted or reduced based on patient tolerance. Do not make up omitted doses at the end of the cycle, and do not re-escalate once a dose reduction occurs for toxicity. See the following charts for dose modifications based on patient symptoms.

Guidelines for Pralatrexate Dose Modifications for Mucositis		
Mucositis Grade* on Day of Treatment	Action	Dose on Recovery to ≤ Grade 1
Grade 2	Omit dose	Continue prior dose
Grade 2 recurrence	Omit dose	20 mg/M^2
Grade 3	Omit dose	20 mg/M^2
Grade 4	Stop therapy	

*Per National Cancer Institute Common Terminology Criteria for Adverse Events (NCI CTCAE), Version 3.

Guidelines for Pralatrexate Dose Modifications for Hematologic Toxicities			
Blood Count on Day of Treatment	Duration of Toxicity	Action	Dose on Restart
Platelets <50,000/mm^3	1 week	Omit dose	Continue prior dose
	2 weeks	Omit dose	20 mg/M^2
	3 weeks	Stop therapy	
ANC 500 to 1,000/mm^3 and no fever	1 week	Omit dose	Continue prior dose
ANC 500 to 1,000/mm^3 with fever or ANC <500/mm^3	1 week	Omit dose, give G-CSF or GM-CSF support	Continue prior dose with G-CSF or GM-CSF support
	2 weeks or recurrence	Omit dose, give G-CSF or GM-CSF support	20 mg/M^2 with G-CSF or GM-CSF support
	3 weeks or 2nd recurrence	Stop therapy	

Guidelines for Pralatrexate Dose Modifications for All Other Treatment-Related Toxicities		
Toxicity Grade* on Day of Treatment	Action	Dose Upon Recovery to ≤ Grade 2
Grade 3	Omit dose	20 mg/M^2
Grade 4	Stop therapy	

*Per National Cancer Institute Common Terminology Criteria for Adverse Events (NCI CTCAE), Version 3.

DILUTION

Specific techniques for handling required; see Precautions. A clear yellow solution. ***Do Not Dilute.*** Aseptically withdraw the calculated dose directly into a syringe for immediate use. Available in vials containing 20 mg or 40 mg. Concentration of both is 20 mg/mL.

Filters: Specific information not available.

Storage: Refrigerate vials at 2° to 8° C (36° to 46° F) in original carton to protect from light until use. Unopened vial(s) are stable in original carton at RT for up to 72 hours. Discard if left at RT for more than 72 hours.

COMPATIBILITY
Manufacturer recommends administration via the side port of a free-flowing infusion of NS.

RATE OF ADMINISTRATION
A single dose by IV push over 3 to 5 minutes via the side port of a free-flowing infusion of NS.

ACTIONS
A folate analog metabolic inhibitor. It interferes with the growth of and leads to the destruction of cancer cells. It competitively inhibits dihydrofolate reductase and folylpolyglutamyl synthetase. This inhibition results in the depletion of thymidine and other biologic molecules. May also affect healthy cells. Approximately 67% bound to plasma proteins. Half-life is 12 to 18 hours. Some drug excreted unchanged in urine (approximately 31%).

INDICATIONS AND USES
Treatment of patients with relapsed or refractory peripheral T-cell lymphoma (PTCL).

CONTRAINDICATIONS
Manufacturer states, "None."

PRECAUTIONS
Follow guidelines for handling cytotoxic agents; see Appendix A, p. 1429. ■ Administered under the direction of a physician knowledgeable in its use and in a facility with adequate diagnostic and treatment facilities to monitor the patients and respond to any medical emergency. ■ Bone marrow suppression can occur (e.g., anemia, neutropenia, and thrombocytopenia). Dose modification based on ANC and platelet count is required before each dose; see Dose Adjustments. ■ May cause mucositis; see Dose Adjustments. ■ To potentially reduce treatment-related hematologic toxicity and mucositis, folic acid and vitamin B_{12} supplementation is required. ■ Severe dermatologic reactions, including skin exfoliation, toxic epidermal necrolysis, and ulceration, have been reported. May increase in severity with continued treatment, may involve skin and subcutaneous sites of known lymphoma, and may result in death. ■ Tumor lysis syndrome has been reported. ■ Has not been studied in patients with moderate to severe renal impairment; administer with caution. ■ Elevated liver enzymes have been observed. Persistent liver function test abnormalities may be indicators of liver toxicity. Patients with selected liver test elevations were excluded from clinical trials.

Monitor: Obtain baseline CBC and platelets and serum chemistry tests, including renal and hepatic function. Monitor CBC and platelets and severity of mucositis weekly. Repeat serum chemistry tests, including renal and hepatic function, before the start of the first and fourth dose of a given cycle. ■ Monitor patients with moderate to severe renal function closely; may have systemic toxicity due to increased pralatrexate exposure. ■ Monitor patients with elevated liver enzymes closely (e.g., AST, ALT, transaminases). If liver functions test abnormalities are greater than or equal to Grade 3, omit or modify dose; see Dose Adjustments. ■ Observe for S/S of skin reactions (e.g., blisters, peeling and loss of skin, rash, sores); see Antidote. ■ Monitor closely for S/S of tumor lysis syndrome (e.g., flank pain, hematuria, hyperkalemia, hyperphosphatemia, hyperuricemia, hypocalcemia, metabolic acidosis, urate crystalluria, and renal failure) and treat as appropriate. Allopurinol and alkalinization of urine may be indicated for prevention and/or treatment of hyperuricemia. ▪ Monitor for thrombocytopenia (platelet count less than 50,000/mm^3). Initiate precautions to prevent excessive bleeding (e.g., inspect IV sites, skin, and mucous membranes; use extreme care during invasive procedures; test urine, emesis, stool, and secretions for occult blood). ▪ Use prophylactic antiemetics to reduce nausea and/or vomiting and increase patient comfort. ▪ Observe closely for signs of infection. Prophylactic antibiotics may be indicated pending results of C/S in a febrile neutropenic patient.

Patient Education: A patient information guide is available from the manufacturer. ▪ Avoid pregnancy; nonhormonal birth control is recommended. ▪ Blood counts will be required at regular intervals. ▪ Take folic acid and vitamin B$_{12}$ as prescribed to help reduce side effects. ▪ Report soreness in the mouth, redness of mucous membranes, difficulty swallowing, or ulcerations in the mouth. Discuss ways to avoid and/or manage mucositis with a health care professional. ▪ Promptly report S/S of infection (e.g., fever) and S/S of bleeding. ▪ Promptly report S/S of skin reactions (e.g., blisters, peeling and loss of skin, rash, sores). ▪ Discuss medications (prescription and non-prescription) with a health care professional; see Drug/Lab Interactions. ▪ Avoid vaccination with live virus vaccines. ▪ See Appendix D, p. 1434.

Maternal/Child: Category D: avoid pregnancy. Can cause fetal harm. ▪ Discontinue breast-feeding. ▪ Safety and effectiveness for use in pediatric patients not established.

Elderly: No overall differences in effectiveness or safety based on age. ▪ No dose adjustment required in elderly patients with normal renal function.

DRUG/LAB INTERACTIONS

Coadministration with **probenecid** resulted in delayed renal clearance and an increase in pralatrexate exposure. ▪ Concomitant administration of drugs that are substantially cleared by the renal system (e.g., **NSAIDs** [e.g., ibuprofen (Advil, Motrin), naproxen (Aleve, Naprosyn)] **and sulfamethoxazole/trimethoprim**) may result in delayed clearance of pralatrexate. ▪ Do not administer **live virus vaccines** to patients receiving antineoplastic drugs. ▪ Not a substrate, inhibitor, or inducer of CYP$_{450}$ isoenzymes and has a low potential for drug-drug interactions with drugs metabolized by these isoenzymes.

SIDE EFFECTS

Most common side effects are fatigue, mucositis, nausea, and thrombocytopenia. Most common serious side effects are dehydration, dyspnea, febrile neutropenia, fever, mucositis (stomatitis or mucosal inflammation of the GI and GU tracts), sepsis, and thrombocytopenia. Mucositis and thrombocytopenia were the most common reasons for discontinuing treatment. Other reported side effects include abdominal pain, abnormal liver function tests (e.g., AST, ALT, transaminases), anemia, anorexia, asthenia, back pain, constipation, cough, diarrhea, edema, epistaxis, hypokalemia, leukopenia, neutropenia, night sweats, pain in extremities, pharyngolaryngeal pain, pruritus, rash, tachycardia, tumor lysis syndrome, upper respiratory infection, vomiting.

Post-Marketing: Dermatologic reactions (e.g., skin exfoliation, toxic epidermal necrolysis, and ulceration).

ANTIDOTE

Treatment of most side effects will be supportive and may require dose adjustment or discontinuation. Discontinue pralatrexate if toxicity from side effects occurs (e.g., dermatologic reactions, Grade 4 treatment-related toxicities [e.g., mucositis], hematologic toxicities [persisting for 3 weeks], uncontrolled tumor lysis syndrome) and notify the physician; see Dose Adjustments. Administration of blood products and/or blood modifiers (e.g., darbepoetin [Aranesp], epoetin alfa [Epogen], filgrastim [Neupogen], oprlevekin [Neumega], pegfilgrastim [Neulasta], sargramostim [Leukine]) may be indicated to treat bone marrow toxicity. Treat hypersensitivity reactions with epinephrine, antihistamines, and corticosteroids as needed. In addition to initiating supportive measures, leucovorin calcium (citrovorum factor, folinic acid) may be given PO, IM, or IV promptly to counteract inadvertent overdose. Resuscitate as indicated.

PRALIDOXIME CHLORIDE
(prah-lih-**DOX**-eem **KLOR**-eyed)

Protopam Chloride

Antidote
(anticholinesterase antagonist)

pH 3.5 to 4.5

USUAL DOSE

In poisonings, correct any existing hypoxemia, then administer atropine as directed in the following paragraphs. After the effects of atropine have become apparent, pralidoxime may be administered. See Contraindications. If IV administration is not possible, may be given IM or SC.

ORGANOPHOSPHATE PESTICIDE POISONING

Atropine: Must be given before pralidoxime and as soon as possible after adequate ventilation has been established (hypoxemia corrected). Ventricular fibrillation can occur if oxygenation is inadequate. Give atropine, 2 to 4 mg IV, after cyanosis disappears, then give initial dose of pralidoxime. Repeat atropine every 10 minutes until atropine toxicity (delirium, dilated pupils, dry mouth, muscle twitching, pulse 140 beats/min). Maintain atropinization for at least 48 hours.

Pralidoxime: 1 to 2 Gm initially after hypoxemia has been corrected, initial dose of atropine has been given, and effects of atropine are apparent (secretions are inhibited). Repeat in 1 hour if indicated. If muscle weakness continues, additional doses can be given with extreme caution, usually every 10 to 12 hours (has been given more frequently). Evidence suggests that a loading dose followed by a continuous infusion may maintain therapeutic levels longer than the traditional short intermittent infusion therapy; see prescribing information for studied regimens.

ORGANOPHOSPHATE CHEMICAL POISONING

Usually administered IM by an autoinjector system (survival technology). Atropine must be given first. After the effects of atropine are apparent (e.g., dry mouth), give pralidoxime 600 mg. Repeat both drugs at 15-minute intervals times 2 if indicated. If muscle weakness persists, seek medical help; IV doses may be required.

ANTICHOLINESTERASE OVERDOSE (E.G., NEOSTIGMINE, PYRIDOSTIGMINE)

1 to 2 Gm followed by 250 mg every 5 minutes.

PEDIATRIC DOSE

See Maternal/Child.

Organophosphate pesticide/chemical poisoning: Give **atropine** 0.05 to 0.1 mg/kg. See Usual Dose for order of administration and specific criteria.

Pralidoxime—Loading dose followed by a continuous infusion: Administer a loading dose of 20 to 50 mg/kg (not to exceed 2,000 mg) over 15 to 30 minutes. Follow with a continuous infusion of 10 to 20 mg/kg/hr.

Pralidoxime—Intermittent Infusion: Administer 20 to 50 mg/kg (not to exceed 2,000 mg) over 15 to 30 minutes. May repeat dose in 1 hour if muscle weakness has not been relieved. Repeat every 10 to 12 hours as needed.

DOSE ADJUSTMENTS

Reduce dose in renal impairment. ▪ Lower-end initial doses may be indicated in the elderly. Dose selection should be cautious in the elderly. Consider age-related organ impairment and concomitant disease or drug therapy.

DILUTION

Each 1 Gm of sterile powder is diluted with 20 mL of SW for injection. Should be further diluted in 100 mL of NS and given as an IV infusion. If reduced fluids are indicated (e.g., pulmonary edema is present) or rapid administration is required, a 5% solution (1 Gm in 20 mL SW) given over no less than 5 minutes may be used.

Storage: Store at CRT. Use promptly after reconstitution; discard remaining solution.

COMPATIBILITY

Specific information not available. Consider specific use; consult pharmacist.

RATE OF ADMINISTRATION

Too-rapid injection may cause laryngospasm, muscle rigidity, or tachycardia. Do not exceed a rate of 200 mg/min.

IV injection diluted in 20 mL SW: Each 1 Gm or fraction thereof over no less than 5 minutes. Used only if pulmonary edema present or infusion not practical.

Infusion (diluted in 100 mL NS, preferred): A single dose over 15 to 30 minutes.

ACTIONS

An anticholinesterase antagonist that reactivates cholinesterase inhibited by phosphate esters. Slows the conversion of phosphorylated cholinesterase to a nonreactivatable form and detoxifies certain organophosphates by direct chemical reaction. Its most critical effect is in relieving paralysis of the respiratory muscles. Because pralidoxime is less effective in relieving depression of the respiratory center, atropine is always required concomitantly to block the effect of accumulated acetylcholine at this site. Rapidly dispersed throughout body fluids. Onset of action is within 10 to 40 minutes; half-life is short (about 1.2 hours), requiring repeated doses as more poison is absorbed. Partially metabolized by the liver. Most of a single dose is excreted within 6 hours in the urine.

INDICATIONS AND USES

Principal indications for the use of pralidoxime are muscle weakness and respiratory depression. In severe poisoning, respiratory depression may be due to muscle weakness. ▪ An antidote (treatment adjunct) in organophosphate pesticide or chemical poisoning. Primarily useful for many phosphate ester insecticide poisons with anticholinesterase activity (e.g., diazinon, malathion) or chemicals with anticholinesterase activity (e.g., nerve gas). ▪ Control of overdose of anticholinesterase drugs used to treat myasthenia gravis. Confirm diagnosis with edrophonium (Tensilon).

CONTRAINDICATIONS
No known absolute contraindications to use of pralidoxime. Relative contraindications include known hypersensitivity to pralidoxime or any component of the product. ▪ See Precautions.

PRECAUTIONS
In poisoning: Most effective if administered immediately after poisoning. May be ineffective if more than 36 hours has passed since exposure; some response may be obtained in severe poisoning; see Contraindications. ▪ Not recommended in carbamate poisoning (increases toxicity of Sevin [carbamate insecticide]). ▪ Not effective for treatment of poisoning with phosphorus, inorganic phosphates, or organophosphates not having anticholinesterase activity. ▪ Rapid IV administration may lead to temporary worsening of cholinergic manifestations. Continuous or intermittent infusion is preferred; see Rate of Administration. ▪ Caregivers must protect themselves from contamination. Wear gowns and gloves. ▪ Remove contaminated clothing and cleanse contaminated skin surfaces, hair, and fingernails with water, sodium bicarbonate solution, or alcohol. ▪ Gently flush eyes with water for at least 15 minutes. ▪ Diazepam (Valium) may be required to stop convulsions. ▪ Use caution in myasthenia gravis; may cause a myasthenic crisis.
Monitor: Before any medication is given, establish and maintain an adequate airway and controlled respiration as indicated. Suctioning of secretions and oxygen usually required. Cardiovascular support, correction of metabolic abnormalities, and seizure control may be necessary. ▪ Draw blood samples for baseline RBC acetylcholinesterase and pseudocholinesterase concentrations. ▪ In suspected poisoning, initiate treatment without waiting for lab confirmation of diagnosis. Combined with a history of possible poisoning, a RBC cholinesterase concentration less than 50% of normal is indicative of organophosphate ester poisoning. ▪ Gastric lavage and activated charcoal are indicated if organophosphates are ingested; most effective if started within 30 minutes of ingestion. Avoid emesis as patient may lose consciousness and aspirate. ▪ Monitor vital signs and ECG continuously. ▪ Maintain adequate urine output. ▪ In cases of ingested poison, toxicity may recur as poison is absorbed from bowel; monitor for 48 to 72 hours. ▪ In all cases of organophosphate poisoning, patient should be observed for at least 48 to 72 hours. ▪ See Drug/Lab Interactions.
Maternal/Child: Category C: effects not known; use only if clearly needed. ▪ Safety for breast-feeding not established. ▪ Efficacy in pediatric patients is extrapolated from the adult population and is supported by nonclinical studies, pharmacokinetic studies in adults, and experience in pediatric patients. Muscle fasciculations, apnea, and convulsions have been reported; see Rate of Administration.
Elderly: Response similar to younger adults. ▪ Dose selection should be cautious; see Dose Adjustments.

DRUG/LAB INTERACTIONS
Used in combination with **atropine.** Signs of atropinization (e.g., dryness of mouth and nose, flushing, mydriasis, tachycardia) may occur earlier than

when atropine is used alone. ■ **CNS depressants** (e.g., anticonvulsants, antihistamines, muscle relaxants, narcotics, reserpine compounds, phenothiazines) and xanthines (e.g., aminophylline, caffeine) will intensify the effects of organophosphate poisoning and defeat effectiveness of treatment. ■ **Barbiturates** are potentiated by anticholinesterases; use with caution in treatment of seizures. ■ **Succinylcholine** may cause prolonged respiratory paralysis. ■ **Thiamine** delays excretion of pralidoxime.

SIDE EFFECTS

Blurred vision, diplopia, dizziness, drowsiness, headache, hyperventilation, impaired accommodation, increased diastolic and systolic BP, laryngospasm, muscle rigidity, muscular weakness, nausea, pharyngeal pain, tachycardia, transient elevated AST, ALT, and CPK. Excitement and manic behavior may occur (atropinization) if pralidoxime is delayed after atropine has been given.

ANTIDOTE

Has not been needed. Patient should be observed for atropine intoxication. Artificial ventilation and other supportive therapy should be administered as needed.

PROCAINAMIDE HYDROCHLORIDE   Antiarrhythmic
(proh-**KAYN**-ah-myd hy-droh-**KLOR**-eyed)
Pronestyl   pH 4 to 6

USUAL DOSE

Loading dose: 0.2 to 1 Gm (100 mg/mL). 100 mg every 5 minutes or 20 mg every 1 minute may be given as an infusion until arrhythmia is suppressed or 500 mg is administered. Wait 10 minutes to allow adequate distribution, then resume dosing until arrhythmia is suppressed, maximum initial dose of 1 Gm is reached, or side effects appear (e.g., hypotension, QRS complex widening by 50%). Dose cautiously to avoid a hypotensive response. AHA recommends 20 mg/min as an infusion to a maximum total dose of 17 mg/kg. **Maintenance dose:** After arrhythmia is suppressed or maximum dose is reached, follow initial dose with an infusion of 1 to 4 mg/min (may require up to 6 mg/min). Titrate to control arrhythmias. Maintain with oral procainamide as soon as possible but at least 4 hours after last IV dose. **Recurrent VT/VF:** AHA recommends 20 mg/min as an infusion. Up to 50 mg/min may be used in urgent situations. Maximum total dose is 17 mg/kg.

PEDIATRIC DOSE

See Maternal/Child; pediatric doses are unlabeled.

2 to 5 mg/kg of body weight. Do not exceed 100 mg/dose. Repeat as indicated every 10 to 30 minutes. Maximum dose in 24 hours is 30 mg/kg or 2 Gm. An alternate dose regimen is 2 to 6 mg/kg as a *loading dose* given over 5 minutes; follow with a *maintenance infusion* of 20 to 80 mcg/kg/min to control arrhythmias.

Supraventricular tachycardia (SVT), atrial flutter, VT with pulse: AHA recommends 15 mg/kg over 30 to 60 minutes.

DOSE ADJUSTMENTS

Maintenance dose may be reduced in impaired or reduced renal function and in individuals over 50 years of age. ■ See Drug/Lab Interactions.

DILUTION
IV injection: Dilute each 100 mg with 5 to 10 mL of D5W.
Infusion: Add 1 Gm of procainamide to 50, 250, or 500 mL of D5W. Yields 20 mg/mL, 4 mg/mL, or 2 mg/mL respectively. 20 mg/mL should only be used as a loading dose. 2 and 4 mg/mL dilutions may be used for loading or maintenance based on fluid restrictions. Solution should be clear; may be light yellow. Discard if darker than light amber.
Pediatric infusion: *Loading dose:* Add a calculated loading dose (2 to 5 mg/kg) to a minimum of 10 mL D5W for each 100 mg or fraction thereof. More diluent may be used based on size of child and fluid restriction. *Maintenance infusion:* See chart under Rate of Administration (Pediatric).
Storage: Photosensitive; protect from light. Store at CRT.

COMPATIBILITY   (Underline Indicates Conflicting Compatibility Information)
Consider any drug NOT listed as compatible to be INCOMPATIBLE until consulting a pharmacist; specific conditions may apply.
One source suggests the following **compatibilities:**
Additive: *Consider individualized rate adjustments necessary to achieve desired effects.* Amiodarone (Nexterone), atracurium (Tracrium), dobutamine, flumazenil (Romazicon), lidocaine, verapamil.
Y-site: Amiodarone (Nexterone), bivalirudin (Angiomax), cisatracurium (Nimbex), dexmedetomidine (Precedex), diltiazem (Cardizem), famotidine (Pepcid IV), fenoldopam (Corlopam), heparin, hetastarch in electrolytes (Hextend), hydrocortisone sodium succinate (Solu-Cortef), inamrinone (Amrinone), nitroprusside sodium, potassium chloride (KCl), ranitidine (Zantac), remifentanil (Ultiva), vasopressin.

RATE OF ADMINISTRATION
20 mg or fraction thereof over 1 minute. Use an infusion pump or a microdrip (60 gtt/mL) for infusion to deliver a constant rate. Up to 50 mg may be given by IV injection over 1 minute with extreme caution. After stabilized with loading dose, follow with a maintenance infusion at 1 to 6 mg/min.

Procainamide Infusion Rate (Adult)						
Desired Dose	1 Gm in 500 mL D5W 2 mg/mL			1 Gm in 250 mL D5W 4 mg/mL		
mg/min	mg/hr	mL/min	mL/hr	mg/hr	mL/min	mL/hr
1 mg/min	60	0.5	30	60	0.25	15
2 mg/min	120	1	60	120	0.5	30
3 mg/min	180	1.5	90	180	0.75	45
4 mg/min	240	2	120	240	1	60
5 mg/min	300	2.5	150	300	1.25	75
6 mg/min	360	3	180	360	1.5	90

Procainamide Infusion Rate (Pediatric)		
Desired Dose	200 mg in 500 mL D5W 400 mcg/mL	200 mg in 125 mL D5W 1,600 mcg/mL
mcg/kg/min	mL/kg/min × kg = mL/min	mL/kg/min × kg = mL/min
20 mcg/kg/min	0.05 × wt in kg	0.0125 × wt in kg
30 mcg/kg/min	0.075 × wt in kg	0.01875 × wt in kg
40 mcg/kg/min	0.1 × wt in kg	0.025 × wt in kg
50 mcg/kg/min	0.125 × wt in kg	0.03125 × wt in kg
60 mcg/kg/min	0.15 × wt in kg	0.0375 × wt in kg
70 mcg/kg/min	0.175 × wt in kg	0.04375 × wt in kg
80 mcg/kg/min	0.2 × wt in kg	0.05 × wt in kg

Example: To deliver 30 mcg/kg/min of a 400 mg/mL solution to a child weighing 20 kg, multiply 0.075 (mL/kg/min) × 20 (wt in kg) = an infusion rate of 1.5 mL/min.

ACTIONS

A procaine derivative. Exerts a depressing antiarrhythmic action on the heart, slowing the rate, slowing conduction, reducing myocardial irritability, and prolonging the refractory period. Decreases membrane permeability of the cell and prevents loss of sodium and potassium ions. Onset of action should occur in 2 to 3 minutes. Half-life is 3 to 4 hours. Crosses the placental barrier. Plasma levels decrease slowly; partially metabolized to the active metabolite NAPA; remaining drug excreted in the urine.

INDICATIONS AND USES

Suppress PVCs and recurrent ventricular tachycardia when lidocaine is contraindicated or has not suppressed ventricular arrhythmias. ▪ Treat wide-complex tachycardias difficult to distinguish from VT (lidocaine preferred). ▪ Rarely used in atrial fibrillation, paroxysmal atrial tachycardia, or arrhythmias caused by anesthesia. Safer drugs (e.g., verapamil, diltiazem) are readily available.

CONTRAINDICATIONS

Complete atrioventricular heart block, second- and third-degree AV block unless an electrical pacemaker is operative, pre-existing QT prolongation, torsades de pointes, known sensitivity to procainamide or any other local anesthetic of the ester type, myasthenia gravis, systemic lupus erythematosus.

PRECAUTIONS

Oral or IM administration is the route of choice; IV route for emergencies only. ▪ Use extreme caution in first- or second-degree blocks, ventricular tachycardia after a myocardial infarction, digoxin intoxication, CHF, any structural heart disease, and impaired liver or reduced kidney function. ▪ Predigitalize or cardiovert patients with atrial flutter or fibrillation to reduce incidence of sudden increase in ventricular rate as atrial rate is slowed. Use caution if used concurrently with other drugs that prolong QT interval (e.g., amiodarone [Nexterone]). ▪ Some clinicians recommend giving a dose the night before surgery and then discontinuing until after surgery. If an arrhythmia occurs, use lidocaine for ventricular arrhythmias and calcium channel blockers (e.g., diltiazem, verapamil) or beta-blockers (e.g., atenolol, propranolol) for supraventricular arrhythmias. Resume dosing after surgery and utilize oral dosing as soon as possible.

Monitor: Monitor the patient's ECG and BP continuously. Keep patient in a supine position. Avoid a hypotensive response. ▪ Discontinue IV use when the cardiac arrhythmia is interrupted or when the ventricular rate slows without regular atrioventricular conduction. ▪ Small emboli may be dislodged when atrial fibrillation is corrected. ▪ Monitor blood levels of procainamide and NAPA (active metabolite) in patients with renal impairment and in any patient receiving a constant infusion over 3 mg/min for more than 24 hours. ▪ Monitor CBC, including WBC, differential, and platelets with continued use; fatal blood dyscrasis have occurred with usual doses. ▪ See Drug/Lab Interactions.

Maternal/Child: Category C: safety for use in pregnancy and breast-feeding and in pediatric patients not established. Consider quinidine as an alternate for use during pregnancy.

Elderly: Half-life of parent drug and active metabolite is prolonged; renal excretion reduced about 25% at age 50 and 50% at age 75. ▪ Increased risk of hypotension.

DRUG/LAB INTERACTIONS

Potentiates or is potentiated by **neuromuscular blocking antibiotics** (e.g., kanamycin [Kantrex]), **anticholinergics** (e.g., atropine), **thiazide diuretics, antihypertensive agents, muscle relaxants, succinylcholine, cimetidine** (Tagamet), **and others.** ▪ May cause serious arrhythmias (e.g., prolongation of QT interval or other additive effects) with **other antiarrhythmic agents** (e.g., amiodarone (Nexterone), digoxin, disopyramide [Norpace], lidocaine, quinidine). Lower doses of both drugs may be required. ▪ Antagonizes **anticholinesterases** (e.g., neostigmine). ▪ **Alcohol** may increase hepatic metabolism. ▪ May **elevate AST levels.**

SIDE EFFECTS

Anorexia, bleeding, bruising, chills, dizziness, fever, flushing, giddiness, hallucinations, joint swelling or pain, mental confusion, nausea, skin rash, tremor, vomiting, weakness. May indicate onset of more serious side effects.

Major: Blood dyscrasias (e.g., agranulocytosis, bone marrow suppression, hypoplastic anemia, neutropenia, thrombocytopenia); hypotension with a BP drop over 15 mm Hg, lupus erythematosus-like symptoms, PR interval prolongation, QRS complex widening, QT interval prolongation, ventricular asystole, ventricular fibrillation, ventricular tachycardia.

ANTIDOTE

Notify the physician of any side effect. If minor symptoms progress or any major side effect appears, discontinue the drug immediately and notify the physician. Use dopamine or phenylephrine hydrochloride (Neo-Synephrine) to correct hypotension. Treatment of toxicity is symptomatic and supportive. Infusion of ⅙ M sodium lactate injection may reduce cardiotoxic effects. Hemodialysis may be indicated or urinary acidifiers may increase renal clearance. Resuscitate as necessary. Depending on arrhythmia, quinidine or lidocaine is an effective alternate. Consider insertion of a ventricular pacing electrode as a precautionary measure in case serious AV block develops.

PROCHLORPERAZINE EDISYLATE
(proh-klor-**PAIR**-ah-zeen eh-**DIS**-ah-layt)

Compazine

Phenothiazine
Antiemetic
Antipsychotic

pH 4.2 to 6.2

USUAL DOSE

A single IV dose should not exceed 10 mg. The maximum daily IV dose should not exceed 40 mg.

Control of severe nausea and vomiting: 2.5 to 10 mg; may be repeated one time in 1 to 2 hours if indicated.

Control of severe nausea and vomiting in adult surgical patients: 5 to 10 mg 15 to 30 minutes before induction of anesthesia or to control symptoms during or after surgery. Repeat once if necessary. Another source suggests 20 mg diluted in 1 L solution (see Dilution) during and/or after surgery.

Management of nausea and vomiting in emetic-inducing chemotherapy (unlabeled): One source suggests 10 to 20 mg 30 minutes before and 3 hours after treatment. Another source suggests 30 to 40 mg 30 minutes before and 3 hours after treatment. A third source suggests 0.8 mg/kg 30 minutes before and 3 hours after treatment and cites precipitous hypotension with larger doses; but another source suggests 2 mg/kg for highly emetogenic agents (e.g., cisplatin, dacarbazine) and 1 mg/kg for less emetogenic agents. Begin 30 minutes before chemotherapy, repeat every 2 hours for 2 doses, then every 3 hours for 3 doses. Treat extrapyramidal symptoms with diphenhydramine (Benadryl) IM. These doses have not been recommended by the manufacturer and exceed the recommended maximum daily IV dose of 40 mg/24 hr. In addition, recommended doses of newer agents (e.g., ondansetron [Zofran]) may be more effective.

Control of severe vascular and tension headaches (unlabeled): 10 mg given as an injection over 2 minutes. Sometimes given concurrently with dihydroergotamine 1 mg as an infusion over 30 minutes. Another regimen administers 3.5 mg of prochlorperazine over 5 minutes followed by dexamethasone 20 mg over 10 minutes.

PEDIATRIC DOSE

IV route not recommended for pediatric patients; safety has not been established; see Contraindications, Precautions, and Maternal/Child.

DOSE ADJUSTMENTS

Lower-end initial doses and more gradual adjustments may be indicated in the elderly and in debilitated or emaciated patients. ■ See Drug/Lab Interactions.

DILUTION

May be given undiluted or each 5 mg (1 mL) may be diluted with 9 mL of NS to facilitate titration. 1 mL will equal 0.5 mg. Larger amounts of NS may be used. May add doses over 10 mg to 50 mL to 1 liter of commonly used IV solution (e.g., D5W, NS, D5/½NS, Ringer's or LR), and give as an intermittent or prolonged infusion. Handle carefully; may cause contact dermatitis. Slightly yellow color does not affect potency. Discard if markedly discolored.

Storage: Store below 40° C and protect from light and freezing.

COMPATIBILITY   (Underline Indicates Conflicting Compatibility Information)
Consider any drug NOT listed as compatible to be INCOMPATIBLE until consulting a pharmacist; specific conditions may apply.
Manufacturer recommends not mixing with other agents in a syringe.

One source suggests the following **compatibilities:**

Additive: Amikacin (Amikin), ascorbic acid, calcium gluconate, dexamethasone (Decadron), dimenhydrinate, erthyromycin (Erythrocin), ethacrynic acid (Edecrin), lidocaine, nafcillin (Nallpen), penicillin G potassium, sodium bicarbonate.

Y-site: Calcium gluconate, cisatracurium (Nimbex), cisplatin (Platinol), cladribine (Leustatin), cyclophosphamide (Cytoxan), cytarabine (ARA-C), dexmedetomidine (Precedex), docetaxel (Taxotere), doxorubicin (Adriamycin), doxorubicin liposomal (Doxil), fluconazole (Diflucan), granisetron (Kytril), heparin, hetastarch in electrolytes (Hextend), hydrocortisone sodium succinate (Solu-Cortef), linezolid (Zyvox), melphalan (Alkeran), methotrexate, ondansetron (Zofran), oxaliplatin (Eloxatin), paclitaxel (Taxol), potassium chloride (KCl), propofol (Diprivan), remifentanil (Ultiva), sargramostim (Leukine), sufentanil (Sufenta), teniposide (Vumon), thiotepa, topotecan (Hycamtin), vinorelbine (Navelbine).

RATE OF ADMINISTRATION
IV injection: Each 5 mg or fraction thereof over 1 minute.
Infusion: May be given at ordered rate, or rate may be increased or decreased as symptoms indicate. Use an infusion pump for infusion.
Management of nausea and vomiting associated with emetic-inducing chemotherapy: A single dose over 15 to 20 minutes as an *intermittent IV.*

ACTIONS
A phenothiazine derivative approximately six times more potent than chlorpromazine (Thorazine), with effects on the central, autonomic, and peripheral nervous systems. Has weak anticholinergic effects, moderate sedative effects, and strong extrapyramidal effects. A potent antiemetic, acting both centrally at the chemoreceptor trigger zone and peripherally by blocking the vagus nerve in the GI tract. Onset of action is prompt and lasting. Metabolized in the liver and excreted in urine and feces. Crosses placental barrier. Secreted in breast milk.

INDICATIONS AND USES
Control of severe nausea and vomiting. ■ Used IM or PO in the treatment of schizophrenia and nonpsychotic anxiety.
Unlabeled uses: Use of higher doses to control nausea and vomiting associated with emetic-inducing chemotherapy. ■ Treatment of severe vascular and tension headaches.

CONTRAINDICATIONS
Pediatric patients under 2 years or 10 kg (22 lb); pediatric patients with conditions that do not have an established dose; comatose or severely depressed states or in the presence of large amounts of CNS depressants (e.g., alcohol, barbiturates, narcotics); hypersensitivity to phenothiazines; breast-feeding and pregnancy, except labor and delivery; do not use in pediatric surgery.

PRECAUTIONS
Use IV only when absolutely necessary. IV not recommended for pediatric patients. ■ Extrapyramidal symptoms caused by prochlorperazine may be confused with undiagnosed disease (e.g., Reye's syndrome, encephalopathy). ■ May mask diagnosis of other conditions including Reye's syn-

drome, brain tumor, drug intoxication, and intestinal obstruction. ■ May produce ECG changes (e.g., prolonged QT interval, changes in T waves). ■ Use caution in coronary disease, glaucoma, severe hypertension or hypotension, and in patients with bone marrow suppression. ■ Use caution in patients with epilepsy. May lower the seizure threshold. ■ Neuroleptic malignant syndrome, characterized by hyperpyrexia, muscle rigidity, autonomic instability, and altered mental status has been reported with phenothiazine use. ■ Tardive dyskinesia (potentially irreversible involuntary dyskinetic movements) may develop. Use the smallest doses and shortest duration of therapy to minimize risk. ■ Anticholinergic and cardiac effects may be troublesome during anesthesia. For patients receiving phenothiazines, taper and discontinue preoperatively if they will not be continued after surgery. ■ May discolor urine pink to reddish brown. ■ Photosensitivity of skin is possible. ■ May cause paradoxical excitation in pediatric patients and the elderly. ■ Do not re-expose patients who have experienced jaundice, skin reactions, or blood dyscrasias in reaction to a phenothiazine. Cross-sensitivity may occur. ■ May contain sulfites; use caution in patients with allergies.

Monitor: Keep patient in supine position and monitor BP and pulse before administration and between doses. ■ Cough reflex may be suppressed. Monitor closely if nauseated or vomiting to prevent aspiration. ■ See Drug/Lab Interactions.

Patient Education: Avoid use of alcohol or other CNS depressants (e.g., antihistamines, barbiturates). ■ Request assistance for ambulation; may cause dizziness or fainting. ■ Use caution performing tasks that require alertness. ■ May cause skin and eye photosensitivity. Avoid unprotected exposure to sun.

Maternal/Child: Safety for use in pregnancy, breast-feeding, and pediatric patients not established; see Contraindications. ■ Has been used during pregnancy, for intractable nausea and vomiting; physician must decide if benefit outweighs risk. ■ Use near term may cause maternal hypotension and adverse neonatal effects (e.g., extrapyramidal syndrome, hyperreflexia, hyporeflexia, jaundice). ■ Fetuses and infants have a reduced capacity to metabolize and eliminate. ■ Pediatric patients may metabolize antipsychotic agents more rapidly than adults. ■ Incidence of extrapyramidal reactions is relatively high in pediatric patients, especially in the presence of acute illness (e.g., measles, chickenpox, gastroenteritis).

Elderly: See Dose Adjustments and Precautions. ■ Have a reduced capacity to metabolize and eliminate and may have increased sensitivity to postural hypotension, anticholinergic and sedative effects. ■ Increased risk of extrapyramidal side effects (e.g., tardive dyskinesia, parkinsonism).

DRUG/LAB INTERACTIONS

Use with **epinephrine** not recommended; may cause precipitous hypotension. ■ Increased CNS respiratory depression and hypotensive effects with **narcotics, alcohol, anesthetics, barbiturates;** reduced doses of these agents usually indicated. ■ Additive effects with **MAO inhibitors** (e.g., selegiline [Eldepryl]), **anticholinergics, antihistamines, antihypertensives, hypnotics, muscle relaxants, phenytoin** (Dilantin), **propranolol, rauwolfia alkaloids, and thiazide diuretics;** dose adjustment may be necessary. ■ Risk of cardiotoxicity increased with **pimozide** (Orap) and **sparfloxacin** (Zagam); concurrent use not recommended. ■ Risk of additive QT interval prolongation, cardiac depressant effects, and cardiac arrhythmias increased with **amiodarone**

(Nexterone), **disopyramide** (Norpace), **erythromycin, probucol** (Lorelco), **procainamide** (Pronestyl), **and quinidine.** ▪ Concurrent use with **antidepressants** (e.g., fluoxetine [Prozac], paroxetine [Paxil]), **tricyclic antidepressants** (e.g., amitriptyline [Elavil], imipramine [Tofranil]), or **MAO inhibitors** may increase effects of both drugs; risk of neuroleptic malignant syndrome may be increased. ▪ Encephalopathic syndrome has been reported with concurrent use of **lithium;** monitor for S/S of neurologic toxicity. ▪ May diminish effects of **oral anticoagulants.** ▪ May lower seizure threshold. Dose adjustment of **anticonvulsants** may be necessary. ▪ Use with **metrizamide** (Amipaque) may lower seizure threshold; discontinue prochlorperazine 48 hours before **myelography,** and do not resume for 24 hours after test is completed. ▪ Use caution during anesthesia with **barbiturates** (e.g., methohexital, thiopental); may increase frequency and severity of hypotension and neuromuscular excitation. ▪ Capable of innumerable other interactions.

SIDE EFFECTS
Usually transient if drug discontinued but may require treatment if severe: anaphylaxis, blurring of vision, cardiac arrest, dermatitis, dizziness, drowsiness, dryness of mouth, dysphagia, elevated BP, extrapyramidal symptoms (e.g., abnormal positioning, extreme restlessness, pseudoparkinsonism, weakness of extremities), excitement, fever without etiology, hematologic toxicities (e.g., agranulocytosis, aplastic anemia, leukopenia, thrombocytopenia), hypersensitivity reactions, hypotension, photosensitivity, slurred speech, spastic movements (especially about the face), tachycardia, tardive dyskinesia, tightness of the throat, tongue discoloration, tongue protrusion, and many others. Overdose can cause convulsions, hallucinations, and death.

ANTIDOTE
Discontinue the drug at onset of any side effect and notify the physician. Discontinue prochlorperazine and all drugs not essential to concurrent therapy immediately if NMS occurs. Will require intensive symptomatic treatment, medical monitoring, and management of concomitant medical problems. Counteract hypotension with IV fluids and norepinephrine (Levophed) or phenylephrine (Neo-Synephrine) and extrapyramidal symptoms with benztropine mesylate (Cogentin), or diphenhydramine (Benadryl). Maintain a clear airway and adequate hydration. *Epinephrine is contraindicated for hypotension.* Further hypotension will occur. Use diazepam (Valium) for convulsions or hyperactivity. Follow with phenytoin. Phenytoin may be helpful in ventricular arrhythmias. In treating respiratory depression and unconsciousness, avoid analeptics such as doxapram (Dopram); they may cause convulsions. Not removed by dialysis. Resuscitate as necessary.

PROMETHAZINE HYDROCHLORIDE BBW
(proh-**METH**-ah-zeen hy-droh-**KLOR**-eyed)

Phenergan

Phenothiazine
Antiemetic
Sedative-hypnotic

pH 4 to 5.5

USUAL DOSE
A vesicant; see Dilution, Rate of Administration, Contraindications, Precautions, Monitor, and Antidote. Deep IM injection is the preferred route of administration.
All uses: The Institute for Safe Medication Practices (ISMP) recommends 6.25 to 12.5 mg as a starting IV dose and suggests considering the use of alternate drugs (e.g., 5-HT$_3$ receptor antagonists [e.g., dolasetron (Anzemet), granisetron (Kytril), ondansetron (Zofran)]).
Nausea and vomiting: 12.5 to 25 mg every 4 to 6 hours as needed.
Allergic conditions: 25 mg. May repeat in 2 hours if necessary. Change to oral therapy as soon as possible.
Sedation, nighttime: 25 to 50 mg.
Sedation, perioperative: 25 to 50 mg. May combine with a reduced dose of narcotic analgesic and an anticholinergic drug (e.g., atropine).
Sedation, labor and delivery: 50 mg during early stage of labor. When labor fully established, may administer 25 to 75 mg with a reduced dose of a narcotic analgesic. May repeat every 4 hours to a maximum dose of 100 mg in a 24-hour period.

PEDIATRIC DOSE
IV use is rare and is limited to pediatric patients 2 years of age or older; see Contraindications and Maternal/Child. Adjust dose to the age, weight, and severity of condition. Use the minimum effective dose and avoid concomitant administration with other drugs with respiratory depressant effects. Do not exceed one half of adult dose. One source suggests a maximum dose of 25 mg. If given IV, administer separately from other medications (e.g., appropriately reduced doses of barbiturates or narcotics, and an appropriate dose of an anticholinergic agent).
Adjunct to premedication: 1.1 mg/kg/dose.
Nausea and vomiting (unlabeled): 0.25 to 1 mg/kg/dose every 6 hours as needed.

DOSE ADJUSTMENTS
Reduced dose may be indicated in the elderly. See Drug/Lab Interactions.

DILUTION
May be given undiluted or may dilute with NS. Concentration should never exceed 25 mg/mL. 1 mL (25 to 50 mg) diluted with 9 mL of NS equals 2.5 to 5 mg/mL. The ISMP recommends further dilution with an additional 10 to 20 mL of NS or in a 50-mL minibag of NS. Slightly yellow color does not alter potency. Discard if greatly discolored. Administer through Y-tube or three-way stopcock of a free-flowing IV.
Storage: Store at CRT. Protect from light.

COMPATIBILITY   (Underline Indicates Conflicting Compatibility Information)
Consider any drug NOT listed as compatible to be INCOMPATIBLE until consulting a pharmacist; specific conditions may apply.
May form a precipitate with heparin; flush heparinized infusion sets with SW or NS before and after administration.

One source suggests the following **compatibilities:**
Additive: Amikacin (Amikin), ascorbic acid, hydromorphone (Dilaudid), penicillin G potassium.
Y-site: Amifostine (Ethyol), aztreonam (Azactam), bivalirudin (Angiomax), ciprofloxacin (Cipro IV), cisatracurium (Nimbex), cisplatin (Platinol), cladribine (Leustatin), cyclophosphamide (Cytoxan), cytarabine (ARA-C), dexmedetomidine (Precedex), docetaxel (Taxotere), doxorubicin (Adriamycin), etoposide phosphate (Etopophos), fenoldopam (Corlopam), filgrastim (Neupogen), fluconazole (Diflucan), fludarabine (Fludara), gemcitabine (Gemzar), granisetron (Kytril), heparin, hetastarch in electrolytes (Hextend), hydrocortisone sodium succinate (Solu-Cortef), linezolid (Zyvox), melphalan (Alkeran), ondansetron (Zofran), oxaliplatin (Eloxatin), palonosetron (Aloxi), pemetrexed (Alimta), potassium chloride (KCl), remifentanil (Ultiva), sargramostim (Leukine), teniposide (Vumon), thiotepa, vinorelbine (Navelbine).

RATE OF ADMINISTRATION
The ISMP recommends administration of a single dose over 10 to 15 minutes administered at a port furthest from the patient vein; observe continuously if given in a peripheral vein.

A maximum rate of 25 mg or fraction thereof over 1 minute is suggested by the manufacturer.

ACTIONS
A phenothiazine derivative with effects on the central, autonomic, and peripheral nervous systems. It has antihistaminic, antiemetic, anticholinergic, and sedative effects. As an antihistamine, it competitively blocks the H_1 histamine receptor, antagonizing most of the effects of histamine to at least some degree. Potentiates respiratory depression, sedative, and hypotensive effects of narcotics and other CNS depressants. Has no analgesic effects and does not potentiate analgesic effects of narcotics. Onset of action is prompt. Duration of action is 4 to 6 hours. Half-life ranges from 9 to 16 hours. Primarily metabolized in the liver and excreted in the urine.

INDICATIONS AND USES
Prophylaxis or treatment of minor transfusion reactions. ■ Treatment of or an adjunct to the treatment of hypersensitivity reactions (including anaphylaxis and other immediate-type reactions) after acute symptoms have been controlled with epinephrine and other standard measures. Consider for use if oral administration is impossible or contraindicated. ■ Treatment of acute nausea, vomiting, and motion sickness. ■ Sedation to meet surgical and obstetric needs. ■ Adjunct to analgesics for control of postoperative pain. ■ Sedation and relief of apprehension; production of a light sleep from which a patient can be easily aroused. ■ An adjunct to anesthesia and analgesia in selected surgical situations (e.g., repeated bronchoscopy, ophthalmologic surgery, and poor-risk patients). Given in conjunction with reduced amounts of narcotic analgesics.

CONTRAINDICATIONS

Comatose or severely depressed states, hypersensitivity or an idiosyncratic reaction to phenothiazines, and pediatric patients under 2 years of age. Never inject into an artery; may cause arteriospasm resulting in gangrene. *Do not* administer SC; chemical irritation may result in necrotic lesions.

PRECAUTIONS

Ampule must state "for IV use." Deep IM injection preferred. ▪ Use with extreme caution in pediatric patients and the elderly; see Maternal/Child and Elderly. ▪ Can cause severe chemical irritation and tissue damage regardless of route of administration. Irritation and damage can result from perivascular extravasation, unintentional intra-arterial injection, and intraneuronal or perineuronal infiltration. Adverse event reports include abscesses, burning, erythema, gangrene, pain, palsies, paralysis, sensory loss, severe spasm of the distal vessels, swelling, thrombophlebitis, tissue necrosis, and venous thrombosis. ▪ Use should be avoided in patients with compromised respiratory function or in patients at risk for respiratory failure (e.g., COPD, sleep apnea); risk of potentially fatal respiratory depression is increased. ▪ May cause paradoxical excitation in pediatric patients and the elderly. ▪ Use phenothiazines with extreme caution in pediatric patients with a history of sleep apnea, a family history of sudden infant death syndrome, or in the presence of Reye's syndrome. ▪ Use with caution in patients with asthma, bladder neck obstruction, bone marrow suppression, cardiovascular disease, glaucoma, liver dysfunction, prostatic hypertrophy, pyloroduodenal obstruction, or stenosing peptic ulcer disease. ▪ May produce ECG changes (e.g., prolonged QT interval, changes in T waves). ▪ May mask diagnosis of other conditions, including Reye's syndrome, brain tumor, drug intoxication, and intestinal obstruction. ▪ May lower seizure threshold; use extreme caution in patients with known seizure disorders and with narcotics or local anesthetics that also lower seizure threshold. ▪ May contain sulfites; use caution in patients with allergies. ▪ Neuroleptic malignant syndrome (NMS), a rare syndrome manifested by hyperpyrexia, muscle rigidity, irregular BP and HR, and altered mental status, has been reported in association with promethazine alone or in combination with antipsychotic drugs.

Monitor: A vesicant; determine absolute patency of vein; extravasation will cause necrosis; see Contraindications and Precautions. ISMP suggests administering through large-bore veins but prefers use of a central venous catheter. Administration through hand or wrist veins is strongly discouraged. ▪ Monitor frequently for S/S of extravasation (e.g., burning, erythema, pain, palsies, sensory loss, and swelling along IV site), especially along peripheral sites. ▪ Keep patient in supine position. Monitor BP and pulse before administration and between doses. ▪ Sedative effect may require ambulation to be monitored. ▪ See Drug/Lab Interactions.

Patient Education: Avoid use of alcohol or other CNS depressants (e.g., antihistamines, barbiturates). ▪ Request assistance for ambulation; may cause dizziness or fainting. ▪ Use caution performing tasks that require alertness. ▪ May cause skin and eye photosensitivity. Avoid unprotected exposure to sun. ▪ Report stinging or burning at IV site promptly. ▪ Report any involuntary muscle movements.

Maternal/Child: Category C: safety for use in pregnancy and pediatric patients not established. Use only when clearly needed. ▪ Discontinue breast-feeding. ▪ Contraindicated in pediatric patients under 2 years of age. Post-marketing cases of respiratory depression and death (not directly related to individualized weight-based dosing) have been reported. Concomitant administration with other respiratory depressants increases this risk. ▪ Use caution in pediatric patients 2 years of age or older. Use the minimum effective dose. ▪ Do not use for vomiting of unknown etiology in pediatric patients. Antiemetics are not recommended for treatment of uncomplicated vomiting in pediatric patients. Use should be limited to prolonged vomiting of known etiology. Extrapyramidal symptoms that can occur secondary to promethazine administration may be confused with CNS signs of an undiagnosed primary disease (e.g., encephalopathy or Reye's syndrome). ▪ Avoid use in pediatric patients with S/S suggestive of Reye's syndrome or other hepatic diseases. ▪ Excessively large doses of antihistamines in pediatric patients have caused hallucinations, convulsions, and death. ▪ Pediatric patients metabolize antipsychotic agents more rapidly than adults. ▪ Incidence of extrapyramidal reactions is relatively high in pediatric patients, especially in the presence of acute illness (e.g., measles, chickenpox, gastroenteritis). ▪ See Precautions and Contraindications.
Elderly: See Dose Adjustments and Precautions. ▪ Have a reduced capacity to metabolize and eliminate. ▪ May cause confusion, dizziness, hyperexcitability, hypotension, and/or sedation. ▪ Increased sensitivity to anticholinergic effects (e.g., dry mouth, urinary retention). ▪ Increased risk of extrapyramidal side effects (e.g., tardive dyskinesia, parkinsonism).

DRUG/LAB INTERACTIONS

Increased CNS depression and hypotensive effects with **narcotics, alcohol, anesthetics, and barbiturates;** reduced doses of these agents usually indicated. ▪ Additive effects with **MAO inhibitors** (e.g., selegiline [Eldepryl]), **anticholinergics, antihistamines, antihypertensives, hypnotics, muscle relaxants, and propranolol;** dose adjustments may be necessary. ▪ Use with **epinephrine** not recommended; may cause precipitous hypotension. ▪ Risk of cardiotoxicity increased with **pimozide** (Orap), **quinidine, and sparfloxacin** (Zagam); concurrent use not recommended. ▪ Risk of additive QT interval prolongation, cardiac depressant effects, and cardiac arrhythmias increased with **amiodarone** (Nexterone), **disopyramide** (Norpace), **erythromycin,**

procainamide (Pronestyl), **and quinidine.** ▪ Concurrent use with **antidepressants** (e.g., fluoxetine [Prozac], paroxetine [Paxil]), **tricyclic antidepressants** (e.g., amitriptyline [Elavil]), **or MAO inhibitors** may increase effects of both drugs. ▪ Concurrent use with **other neuroleptic agents** (e.g., haloperidol [Haldol]) may increase the risk of NMS. ▪ May lower seizure threshold. Dose adjustment of **anticonvulsants** may be necessary. ▪ Capable of innumerable other interactions. ▪ Selected **pregnancy tests** may show a false-negative or false-positive result. ▪ May cause an increase in blood glucose; consider when a **glucose tolerance test** is indicated.

SIDE EFFECTS

Average dose: Blurring of vision, bradycardia, confusion, dizziness, drowsiness, dryness of mouth, extrapyramidal symptoms, faintness, hallucinations, hematologic side effects (e.g., agranulocytosis, leukopenia, thrombocytopenia, thrombocytopenic purpura), hyperexcitability, hypersensitivity reactions, hypertension (rare), hypotension (mild), lassitude, nightmares, photosensitivity, sedation, somnolence, tachycardia, tinnitus, tremors.

Overdose: Anaphylaxis, cardiac arrest, coma, convulsions, deep sedation, respiratory depression. All side effects of phenothiazines are possible, but rarely occur. See prochlorperazine (Compazine).

ANTIDOTE

Discontinue the drug immediately at onset of any side effect and notify the physician. Sympathetic block and heparinization have been used during acute management of promethazine extravasation (unintentional intra-arterial injection or perivascular extravasation). In some cases surgical intervention, including fasciotomy, skin graft, and/or amputation, has been required. Counteract hypotension with IV fluids, Trendelenburg position, norepinephrine (Levophed), or phenylephrine (Neo-Synephrine); extrapyramidal symptoms with benztropine mesylate (Cogentin) or diphenhydramine (Benadryl). Epinephrine is contraindicated for hypotension; further hypotension will occur. Use diazepam (Valium) or phenobarbital for convulsions or hyperactivity. In treating respiratory depression and unconsciousness, avoid analeptics such as doxapram (Dopram); they may cause convulsions. Treatment of NMS includes discontinuation of all unnecessary drugs and intensive symptomatic treatment and monitoring. Dialysis does not appear to be helpful in overdose situations. Resuscitate as necessary.

PROPOFOL INJECTION
(**PROH**-poh-fohl in-**JEK**-shun)

General anesthetic
Anesthesia adjunct
Sedative-hypnotic

Diprivan

pH 7 to 8.5

USUAL DOSE

Lidocaine may be administered to minimize pain on injection of propofol. Administer before propofol injection or add to propofol immediately before administration. Do not exceed more than 20 mg lidocaine to 200 mg propofol.

INDUCTION OF ANESTHESIA

Must be individualized and titrated to desired response. Allow 3 to 5 minutes between dose adjustments to allow for and assess clinical effects.

Healthy adults less than 55 years of age: 40 mg every 10 seconds until induction onset (approximately 2 to 2.5 mg/kg).

Adults over 55 years of age, debilitated, or ASA III or IV risk patients: 20 mg every 10 seconds until induction onset (approximately 1 to 1.5 mg/kg).

Cardiac anesthesia: 20 mg every 10 seconds until induction onset (0.5 to 1.5 mg/kg).

Neurosurgical patients: 20 mg every 10 seconds until induction onset (approximately 1 to 2 mg/kg). Infusion or slow injection (20 mg over 10 seconds) is used to avoid significant hypotension and decrease in cerebral perfusion pressure. If increased intracranial pressure is suspected, hyperventilation and hypocarbia should accompany administration.

MAINTENANCE OF ANESTHESIA

Must be individualized and titrated to desired response. Allow 3 to 5 minutes between dose adjustments to allow for and assess clinical effects.

Adults less than 55 years of age: Immediately follow induction with an infusion of 100 to 200 mcg/kg/min (6 to 12 mg/kg/hr) or an intermittent bolus in increments of 25 to 50 mg as needed.

Adults over 55 years of age, debilitated, or ASA III or IV risk patients: Immediately follow induction with an infusion of 50 to 100 mcg/kg/min (3 to 6 mg/kg/hr). Do NOT use a rapid intermittent bolus in these patients.

Cardiac anesthesia: Most patients require 100 to 150 mcg/kg/min in combination with an opioid (primary propofol with an opioid secondary). An alternate regimen is an opioid primary with low-dose propofol 50 to 100 mcg/kg/min (3 to 6 mg/kg/hr).

Neurosurgical patients: Immediately follow induction with an infusion of 100 to 200 mcg/kg/min (6 to 12 mg/kg/hr). Do NOT use a rapid intermittent bolus in these patients.

INITIATION OF MAC SEDATION

Must be individualized and titrated to desired response. Allow 3 to 5 minutes between dose adjustments to allow for and assess clinical effects. MAC sedation rates are approximately 25% of those used for anesthesia.

Healthy adults less than 55 years of age: An infusion of 100 to 150 mcg/kg/min (6 to 9 mg/kg/hr) over 3 to 5 minutes or a slow injection of 0.5 mg/kg over 3 to 5 minutes. Slow infusion or slow injection techniques are preferable to rapid bolus administration.

Adults over 55 years of age, debilitated, or ASA III or IV risk patients: Most patients require doses similar to healthy adults. Must be given over 3 to 5 minutes as a slow infusion (preferred) or as a slow injection over 3 to 5 minutes. Do NOT give as a rapid bolus.

MAINTENANCE OF MAC SEDATION

Healthy adults less than 55 years of age: Maintain with an infusion (preferred) of 25 to 75 mcg/kg/min (1.5 to 4.5 mg/kg/hr) or incremental bolus doses of 10 to 20 mg.

Adults over 55 years of age, debilitated, or ASA III or IV risk patients: Reduce dose to 80% of usual dose; an infusion of 20 to 60 mcg/kg/min (1.2 to 3.6 mg/kg/hr). Do NOT use bolus doses.

SEDATION OF INTUBATED, MECHANICALLY VENTILATED ICU PATIENTS

Must be individualized and titrated to desired response. Given as a continuous infusion. Begin with an initial dose of 5 mcg/kg/min (0.3 mg/kg/hr) for 5 minutes. Allow at least 5 minutes between adjustments to reach peak drug effect and to avoid hypotension. Increase slowly over 5 to 10 minutes by 5 to 10 mcg/kg/min (0.3 to 0.6 mg/kg/hr) to desired level of sedation. Individualize to patient condition, response, blood lipid profile, and vital signs. Some clinicians recommend reducing dose by approximately one half for elderly (over 55 years) and debilitated. Check urinalysis and urine sediment before administration of propofol in patients at risk for renal failure; see Precautions and Monitor.

MAINTENANCE OF SEDATION IN MECHANICALLY VENTILATED OR RESPIRATORY-CONTROLLED ICU PATIENTS

5 to 50 mcg/kg/min (0.3 to 3 mg/kg/hr) or higher as a continuous infusion slowly titrated to desired level of sedation. Use caution with doses higher than 50 mcg/kg/min; may increase risk of hypotension. Bolus doses of 10 to 20 mg may be used to rapidly increase the depth of sedation in patients in whom hypotension is not likely to occur. Temporarily reduce dose once each day to assess neurologic and respiratory function and to determine minimum dose required for desired level of sedation. Average maintenance dose *under 55 years* is 38 mcg/kg/min; *over 55 years,* 20 mcg/kg/min. Average maintenance dose for *post–coronary artery bypass graft (CABG) patients* is usually low (median of 11 mcg/kg/min) because of high intraoperative opiates.

RELIEF OF PRURITUS ASSOCIATED WITH USE OF SPINAL OPIATES OR CHOLESTASIS (UNLABELED)

Subhypnotic doses of 10 to 15 mg as an IV injection or 0.5 to 1.5 mg/kg/hr as an infusion.

MANAGEMENT OF REFRACTORY STATUS EPILEPTICUS (UNLABELED)

Administer doses of 1 to 2 mg/kg as an IV injection over 5 minutes; may be repeated if seizure activity recurs. If indicated, follow with a maintenance infusion of 2 to 10 mg/hr. Adjust to achieve the lowest rate needed to suppress seizure activity. Decrease gradually to prevent withdrawal seizures.

PEDIATRIC DOSE

To minimize pain on injection of propofol in pediatric patients, administer through larger veins or pretreat smaller veins with lidocaine. See Maternal/Child.

INDUCTION OF ANESTHESIA IN HEALTHY PEDIATRIC PATIENTS 3 TO 16 YEARS OF AGE

Must be individualized and titrated to desired response. 2.5 to 3.5 mg/kg

Continued

administered over 20 to 30 seconds. *Induction with propofol is indicated only in pediatric patients 3 years of age or older. In pediatric patients from 2 months to 3 years of age, induction must be achieved by supplementing with another agent (literature suggests nitrous oxide 60% to 70%).* See Dose Adjustments.

MAINTENANCE OF ANESTHESIA IN HEALTHY PEDIATRIC PATIENTS FROM 2 MONTHS TO 16 YEARS OF AGE

Must be titrated to desired clinical effect. (See statement under induction in healthy pediatric patients in the previous paragraph, and see Indications and Uses.) Administered as a variable-rate infusion supplemented with nitrous oxide 60% to 70% for most pediatric patients.

Pediatric patients 2 months of age and older: Immediately follow induction dose with an infusion of 125 to 300 mcg/kg/min (7.5 to 18 mg/kg/hr). Initially, a rate of 200 to 300 mcg/kg/min may be indicated and can usually be reduced to 125 to 150 mcg/kg/min after the first half-hour. Decrease infusion rate if clinical signs of light anesthesia are not present after 30 minutes of maintenance; see Rate of Administration. Younger pediatric patients may require higher maintenance infusion rates than older pediatric patients. See Dose Adjustments.

DOSE ADJUSTMENTS

All situations: Reduce induction and maintenance doses for pediatric patients classified as ASA III or IV. ▪ See Usual Dose for specific reduced doses required for adults over 55 years of age; debilitated, ASA III, or IV risk patients; or patients with circulatory disorders. ▪ Reduced dose required in presence of other CNS depressants. See Drug/Lab Interactions. ▪ No dose adjustment required for gender, chronic hepatic cirrhosis, or chronic renal failure.

ICU sedation: Adjust infusion to maintain a light level of sedation through the wake-up assessment or weaning process.

DILUTION

Supplied in ready-to-use vials containing 10 mg/mL. Shake well before use. May be further diluted only with D5W. Do not dilute to a concentration less than 2 mg/mL (4 mL diluent to 1 mL propofol yields 2 mg/mL). More stable in glass than in plastic. Strict aseptic technique imperative; emulsion supports rapid growth of microorganisms. Failure to use strict aseptic technique has been associated with microbial contamination of the product with resultant fever, infection, sepsis, other life-threatening illnesses, and/or death. Do not use with evidence of emulsion separation. Prepare immediately before each use. Flush IV line at end of every 6 hours in extended procedures to remove residual propofol.

Filters: Use filters with caution. The pore size should be equal to or greater than 5 microns. Filters with a pore size less than 5 microns may impede the flow of propofol and/or cause a breakdown of the emulsion.

Storage: Protect from light and store below 22° C (72° F) but do not refrigerate. Discard infusion and tubing every 12 hours or every 6 hours if propofol has been transferred from the original container.

COMPATIBILITY (Underline Indicates Conflicting Compatibility Information)

Consider any drug NOT listed as compatible to be INCOMPATIBLE until consulting a pharmacist; specific conditions may apply.

Manufacturer states, "Should not be mixed with other therapeutic agents prior to administration. **Compatibility** with blood/serum/plasma has not been established."

Y-site: Manufacturer lists as **compatible** at the **Y-site** with the following solutions: D5W, LR, D5LR, D5½NS, D5¼NS. Other sources list acyclovir (Zovirax), alfentanil (Alfenta), aminophylline, ampicillin, atracurium (Tracrium), atropine, aztreonam (Azactam), bumetanide, buprenorphine (Buprenex), butorphanol (Stadol), calcium gluconate, carboplatin (Paraplatin), cefazolin (Ancef), cefepime (Maxipime), cefotaxime (Claforan), cefotetan, cefoxitin (Mefoxin), ceftazidime (Fortaz), ceftriaxone (Rocephin), cefuroxime (Zinacef), chlorpromazine (Thorazine), cisatracurium (Nimbex), cisplatin (Platinol), clindamycin (Cleocin), cyclophosphamide (Cytoxan), cyclosporine (Sandimmune), cytarabine (ARA-C), dexamethasone (Decadron), dexmedetomidine (Precedex), diphenhydramine (Benadryl), dobutamine, dopamine, doxycycline, droperidol (Inapsine), enalaprilat (Vasotec IV), ephedrine, epinephrine (Adrenalin), esmolol (Brevibloc), famotidine (Pepcid IV), fenoldopam (Corlopam), fentanyl (Sublimaze), fluconazole (Diflucan), fluorouracil (5-FU), furosemide (Lasix), ganciclovir (Cytovene), glycopyrrolate, granisetron (Kytril), haloperidol (Haldol), heparin, hydrocortisone sodium succinate (Solu-Cortef), hydromorphone (Dilaudid), ifosfamide (Ifex), imipenem-cilastatin (Primaxin), inamrinone (Amrinone), insulin (regular), isoproterenol (Isuprel), ketamine (Ketalar), labetalol (Trandate), lidocaine, lorazepam (Ativan), magnesium sulfate, mannitol, meperidine (Demerol), midazolam (Versed), milrinone (Primacor), morphine, nafcillin (Nallpen), nalbuphine, naloxone (Narcan), nitroglycerin IV, nitroprusside sodium, norepinephrine (Levophed), paclitaxel (Taxol), pancuronium, pentobarbital (Nembutal), phenobarbital (Luminal), phenylephrine (Neo-Synephrine), piperacillin, potassium chloride (KCl), prochlorperazine (Compazine), propranolol, ranitidine (Zantac), sodium bicarbonate, succinylcholine, sufentanil (Sufenta), thiopental (Pentothal), ticarcillin/clavulanate (Timentin), vancomycin, vecuronium.

RATE OF ADMINISTRATION

Use of a syringe pump or volumetric pump recommended to provide controlled infusion rates. See Usual Dose for specific rates for specific age and/or indication. Decrease rate based on age, debilitation, or calculated risk. Must be individualized and titrated to desired level of sedation and changes in vital signs. Monitor respiratory function continuously. Continuous administration preferable to intermittent to avoid periods of undersedation or oversedation. Too-rapid administration (bolus dosing, too-rapid increase in infusion rate, overdose) can cause severe cardiorespiratory complications, especially in pediatric patients, adults over 55 years, debilitated or ASA III or IV risk patients. In all anesthesia, higher rates are generally required for the first 15 minutes, then appropriate responses can usually be maintained with a decrease of 30% to 50%. Always titrate rates downward until there is a mild response to surgical stimulation. This avoids administration at rates higher than clinically necessary. Control increased response to surgical stimulation or lightening of anesthesia (increased pulse rate, BP, sweating and/or tearing) with bolus injections of 25 to 50 mg *(adults under 55 years of age only);* slow injection of reduced doses, or by increasing the infusion rate *(adults under or over 55 years of age)* or by increasing the infusion rate *(pediatric patients).* If control not effective within 5 minutes, consider use of an opioid, barbiturate, or inhalation agent.

ACTIONS

A potent emulsified IV sedative hypnotic agent. Action is dose and rate dependent. Can provide conscious (verbal contact maintained) or unconscious sedation, depending on dose. Produces hypnosis rapidly and smoothly with minimal excitation, usually within 40 seconds. Depth of sedation easily and rapidly controlled by adjusting rate of infusion. Rapid onset of action facilitates accurate titration and minimizes oversedation. Due to extensive redistribution from the central nervous system to other tissues and high metabolic clearance, recovery from anesthesia or sedation is rapid. Time to awakening is dependent on duration of infusion. Discontinuation of an infusion after maintenance of anesthesia for 1 hour or sedation in the ICU for 1 day will result in rapid awakening. Prolonged infusions (e.g., 10 days in ICU) will result in drug accumulation and an increased time to awakening. Terminal half-life after a 10-day infusion is 1 to 3 days. Other effects include decreased systemic vascular resistance, myocardial blood flow, and oxygen consumption; a decrease in cerebral blood flow and intracranial pressure; and a decrease in intraocular pressure. Also has antiemetic properties. Has minimal impact on cardiac output, but changes may occur because of assisted or controlled ventilation. Hypotension, oxyhemoglobin desaturation, apnea, and airway obstruction can occur. Addition of an opioid may further decrease cardiac output or respiratory drive. Metabolized in the liver and excreted as metabolites in urine. Crosses placental barrier. Secreted in breast milk.

INDICATIONS AND USES

Adults: Induce and/or maintain anesthesia as part of a balanced anesthetic technique for inpatient and outpatient surgery. ▪ Initiate and maintain monitored anesthesia care (MAC) during diagnostic procedures (e.g., colonoscopy, dental procedures) and in conjunction with local/regional anesthesia during surgical procedures. ▪ Continuous sedation and control of stress responses in intubated, mechanically ventilated ICU patients (e.g., post-CABG, post-surgical, neuro/head trauma, ARDS, COPD, asthma, status epilepticus, tetanus). Continuous infusions of low doses allows controlled recovery of consciousness when required and for assessment. **Pediatric patients:** Induction of anesthesia as a part of a balanced anesthetic technique for inpatient and outpatient surgery in pediatric patients over 3 years of age. ▪ Maintenance of anesthesia as part of a balanced anesthetic technique for inpatient and outpatient surgery in pediatric patients over 2 months of age. ▪ Not recommended for induction of anesthesia below the age of 3 years or for maintenance of anesthesia below the age of 2 months. ▪ Not indicated for use in pediatric patients for ICU sedation or for MAC sedation for surgical, nonsurgical, or diagnostic procedures. **Unlabeled uses:** Subhypnotic doses used for relief of pruritus associated with use of spinal opiates or cholestasis; treatment of status epilepticus refractory to standard anticonvulsant therapy.

CONTRAINDICATIONS

Known hypersensitivity to propofol or its components (e.g., soybean oil, glycerol, egg lecithin, sodium hydroxide) or any time general anesthesia or sedation is contraindicated.

PRECAUTIONS

All situations: For IV use only. ▪ Administered by or under the direct observation of the anesthesiologist. Must have responsibility only for anesthesia during surgery and/or procedures. In the ICU setting, may be administered to intubated, mechanically ventilated patients by persons skilled in medical management of critically ill patients and trained in cardiovascular resuscitation and airway management. Both life-threatening and fatal anaphylactoid and anaphylactic reactions have been reported. ▪ Strict aseptic technique required; see Dilution. ▪ Use caution in patients with compromised myocardial function, intravascular volume depletion, or abnormally low vascular tone (e.g., sepsis); may be more susceptible to hypotension. ▪ Avoid rapid bolus administration in the elderly, debilitated, or ASA-PS III or IV patients. May cause undesirable cardiopulmonary depression, including apnea, airway obstruction, hypotension, and oxygen desaturation. ▪ An emulsion; use caution in patients with lipid metabolism disorders (e.g., diabetic hyperlipidemia, pancreatitis, and primary hyperlipoproteinemia). ▪ May cause convulsions during recovery phase in patients with epilepsy. ▪ Use caution in patients with increased intracranial pressure or impaired cerebral circulation. Decrease in mean arterial pressure may cause decreases in cerebral perfusion. ▪ Propofol infusion syndrome has been reported and is characterized by severe metabolic acidosis, hyperkalemia, lipemia, rhabdomyolysis, hepatomegaly, and cardiac and renal failure. Deaths have occurred. Most often associated with prolonged, high-dose infusions in ICU but has been observed following large-dose, short-term infusions during surgical anesthesia. Consider alternative means of sedation when there is a prolonged need for sedation, when large doses of propofol are required to maintain a desired level of sedation, or if a patient develops metabolic acidosis. ▪ Has no analgesic properties; provide pain relief or local anesthetic as indicated. Has been used successfully with midazolam (Versed), 1 to 3 mg, for initial induction. Midazolam provides better amnesia and causes less pain on injection, whereas propofol sustains sedation and allows more rapid recovery. ▪ May contain sulfites; use caution in patients with allergies.

Monitor: All situations: Correct fluid volume deficiencies before administration. ▪ Will cause transient local pain during IV injection; minimize by using larger veins and lidocaine previous to injection. Use with midazolam reduces awareness of this pain. ▪ Apnea may occur during induction and last for more than 60 seconds. Intubation equipment, controlled ventilation equipment, oxygen, and facilities for resuscitation and life support must be available. Maintain a patent airway and ascertain adequate ventilation at all times. ▪ All vital signs must be monitored continuously. Use of a respiratory monitor required. ▪ Hypotension common during first 60 minutes; monitor closely. Significant hypotension or cardiovascular depression can be profound. ▪ To prevent profound bradycardia, anticholinergic agents (e.g., atropine, glycopyrrolate) may be required to modify increases in vagal tone due to concomitant agents (e.g., succinylcholine) or surgical stimulation. ▪ Bed rest required for a minimum of 3 hours after IV injection, or satisfy specific hospital rules for discharge. ▪ See Precautions and Drug/Lab Interactions.

ICU sedation: Observe for signs and symptoms of pain; may indicate need for opioids or analgesia, not an increase in propofol dose. ▪ Benzodiazepines (e.g., diazepam [Valium]) and/or neuromuscular blocking agents (e.g., atracurium [Tracrium], succinylcholine) may also be used. ▪ Monitor triglycerides with long-term use (ICU sedation). Adjust if fat is inadequately cleared from body and reduce other lipid administration.

1 mL of propofol contains approximately 0.1 Gm of fat (1.1 kcal). ▪ Dose may be reduced carefully to allow patient to awaken to a lighter level of sedation allowing neurologic and respiratory assessment daily. Avoid rapid awakening; will cause anxiety, agitation, and resistance to mechanical ventilation. ▪ Monitor urinalysis and urine sediment on alternate days in patients at risk for renal impairment. ▪ Some formulations contain EDTA, a trace metal chelator. Formulations containing EDTA should not be infused for longer than 5 days without providing a drug holiday to safely replace estimated or measured zinc losses. Consider zinc supplementation in patients who may be predisposed (e.g., patients with burns, diarrhea, or major sepsis). ▪ Discontinue opioids and paralytic agents and optimize respiratory function before weaning from mechanical ventilation. ▪ Maintain light sedation until 15 minutes before extubation.

Patient Education: Avoid alcohol or other CNS depressants (e.g., antihistamines, benzodiazepines) for 24 hours following anesthesia. ▪ Do not perform tasks requiring mental alertness (e.g., driving, operating hazardous machinery, or signing legal documents) until the day after surgery or longer. All effects must have subsided.

Maternal/Child: Category B: use during pregnancy only if clearly needed. ▪ Not recommended for use in obstetric procedures, including cesarean section; no assurance of safety for fetus. ▪ Not recommended for use during breast-feeding. ▪ Has been approved for induction of anesthesia in pediatric patients 3 years to 16 years of age. Has been approved for maintenance of anesthesia in pediatric patients 2 months to 16 years of age. ▪ Distribution and clearance in pediatric patients 3 years to 12 years of age is similar to that seen in adults. ▪ Serious bradycardia may result with concomitant administration of fentanyl. ▪ Serious adverse effects (e.g., metabolic acidosis) occurred during ICU sedation in pediatric patients with respiratory infections and/or with doses in excess of recommendations for adults. Fatalities have occurred. ▪ A recent study identified an increase in deaths with propofol versus standard sedative agents. Manufacturer has issued a warning letter stating that propofol should not be used for sedation of pediatric patients in ICU. ▪ See Side Effects.

Elderly: Dose requirements decrease after age 55 due to reduced clearance and volume distribution and higher blood levels. Minimize undesirable cardiorespiratory depression (hypotension, apnea, airway obstruction, and/or oxygen desaturation) by using reduced doses and rates of administration. Avoid rapid single or repeated bolus doses; see Precautions. See Usual Dose and Dose Adjustments.

DRUG/LAB INTERACTIONS

Potentiated by **inhalational anesthetics** (e.g., enflurane, halothane, isoflurane, nitrous oxide), **narcotics** (e.g., morphine, meperidine [Demerol], fentanyl [Sublimaze]), **sedatives** (e.g., barbiturates, benzodiazepines [e.g., diazepam (Valium), midazolam (Versed)], chloral hydrate, droperidol [Inapsine]). Anesthetic and sedative effects increased; systolic, diastolic, mean arterial pressure, and cardiac output are decreased. Dose adjustment may be indicated with concomitant use. ▪ No significant adverse interactions noted to date with neuromuscular blocking agents (e.g., atracurium [Tracrium], succinylcholine). ▪ Competition for chemoreceptor binding sites may occur if used in combination with **droperidol;** use of propofol as a single agent is suggested to control nausea and vomiting. ▪ In pediatric patients, serious bradycardia may result with concomitant administration of **fentanyl**.

SIDE EFFECTS

Adults and pediatric patients: More likely to occur during loading boluses, with supplemental boluses or higher rate of administration. Apnea; bradycardia (profound); cough; dyspnea; headache; hypotension; hypoventilation; injection site burning, pain, stinging; nausea, and upper airway obstruction are most common. Urine may be green. Abdominal cramping, anaphylaxis (including bronchospasm, erythema, and hypotension), bucking/jerking/thrashing, clonic/myclonic movement (rarely including convulsions and opisthotonus), dizziness, fever, flushing, hiccough, hypertension, tingling/numbness/coldness at injection site, twitching, and vomiting may occur.

Pediatric patients: Increased incidences of agitation, bradycardia, and jitteriness have occurred; apnea has been observed frequently. Abrupt discontinuation following prolonged infusion may result in agitation, flushing of the hands and feet, hyperirritability, and tremulousness.

Overdose: Cardiorespiratory depression (hypotension, apnea, airway obstruction, and/or oxygen desaturation).

ANTIDOTE

Keep physician informed of all side effects. Reduction of dose may be required or will be treated symptomatically. Discontinue the drug for major side effects, paradoxical reactions, or accidental overdose. A short-acting drug, a patent airway, and continuous controlled ventilation with oxygen until normal function assured should be adequate. Treat bradycardia and/or hypotension with increased rate of IV fluids, Trendelenburg position, vasopressors (e.g., dopamine). Anticholinergic agents (e.g., atropine or glycopyrrolate) may be required. Treat hypersensitivity reactions and resuscitate as necessary.

PROPRANOLOL HYDROCHLORIDE
(proh-**PRAN**-oh-lohl hy-droh-**KLOR**-eyed)

Beta-adrenergic blocking agent
Antiarrhythmic

pH 2.8 to 3.5

USUAL DOSE

1 to 3 mg given 1 mg at a time under careful monitoring (e.g., CVP, ECG); see Monitor and Rate of Administration. Do not give additional propranolol if the desired change in rate or rhythm is achieved. If there is no change in rhythm for at least 2 minutes after the initial dose, cycle may be repeated one time. (AHA recommends 0.5 to 1 mg over 1 minute, repeated as needed up to a total dose of 0.1 mg/kg). *No further propranolol may be given by any route for at least 4 hours.* Best results achieved if administered within 2 to 4 hours of symptom onset or thrombolytic therapy. Transfer to oral therapy as soon as possible.

PEDIATRIC DOSE (UNLABELED)

0.01 to 0.1 mg/kg/dose over 10 minutes. Maximum dose is 1 mg for infants and 3 mg for other pediatric patients. Repeat at 6- to 8-hour intervals if needed.

Tetralogy spells: 0.15 to 0.25 mg/kg/dose may be given slowly. May repeat once in 15 minutes.

DOSE ADJUSTMENTS

Lower-end initial doses may be indicated in the elderly based on potential for decreased organ function and concomitant disease or drug therapy. ■ Consider dose reduction in patients with impaired hepatic function. ■ See Drug/Lab Interactions. ■ Reduce dose gradually to avoid rebound angina, myocardial infarction, or ventricular arrhythmias.

DILUTION

May be given undiluted; however, further dilution of each 1 mg in 10 mL D5W or NS is preferred to facilitate titration of an exact dose while monitoring effect. May be diluted in 50 mL of D5W, D5/½NS, D5NS, or NS for infusion.

Storage: Store at CRT. Protect from freezing or excessive heat.

COMPATIBILITY

Consider any drug NOT listed as compatible to be INCOMPATIBLE until consulting a pharmacist; specific conditions may apply.

One source suggests the following **compatibilities:**

Additive: Dobutamine, verapamil.

Y-site: Alteplase (tPA, Activase), fenoldopam (Corlopam), heparin, hydrocortisone sodium succinate (Solu-Cortef), inamrinone (Amrinone), linezolid (Zyvox), meperidine (Demerol), milrinone (Primacor), morphine, nesiritide (Natrecor), potassium chloride (KCl), propofol (Diprivan), tacrolimus (Prograf), tirofiban (Aggrastat).

RATE OF ADMINISTRATION

Each 1 mg or fraction thereof must be given over 1 minute to avoid excessive hypotension and/or cardiac standstill. A single dose may be given as an infusion over 10 to 15 minutes. Allow adequate time for distribution; consider slow circulation time. Observe monitor and discontinue propranolol as soon as rhythm change occurs.

Pediatric rate: Extend rate of administration of a single dose by injection to a minimum of 5 minutes in pediatric patients.

ACTIONS

Propranolol is a nonselective beta-adrenergic blocker with antiarrhythmic effects. Cardiac response to sympathetic nerve stimulation is inhibited, slowing the HR (especially ventricular rate) by inhibiting atrioventricular conduction. Decreases the force of cardiac contractility, and decreases arterial pressure and cardiac output. Blockade of beta$_2$-adrenergic receptors found predominantly in smooth muscle (e.g., vascular, bronchial, gastrointestinal, and genitourinary); leads to constriction in these tissues. Well distributed throughout the body, the onset of action occurs within 1 to 2 minutes and lasts about 4 hours. Half-life is 2 to 5.5 hours. Metabolized in the liver. Excreted primarily in the urine. Secreted in breast milk.

INDICATIONS AND USES

Reserve IV use for life-threatening situations or for those occurring under anesthesia. ■ Short-term treatment to decrease the ventricular rate in supraventricular tachycardia, including Wolff-Parkinson-White syndrome and thyrotoxicosis. ■ Treatment of persistent and symptomatic PVCs that do not respond to conventional measures. ■ Use in patients with atrial flutter or atrial fibrillation should be reserved for arrhythmias unresponsive to standard therapy or when more prolonged control is required. ■ Control of ventricular rate in life-threatening, digoxin-induced arrhythmias (severe bradycardia may occur). ■ Treatment of tachyarrhythmias due to excessive catecholamine action during anesthesia when other measures fail. ■ Not the drug of first choice for treatment of ventricular arrhythmias unless the arrhythmia is induced by catecholamines or digoxin. In critical situations, when cardioversion or other drugs are not indicated or effective, propranolol may be used with caution. (Use a low dose and administer very slowly so the failing heart maintains some sympathetic drive to maintain myocardial tone. May respond with NSR, but a reduction in ventricular rate is more likely.) ■ Numerous other uses PO.

Unlabeled uses: Other beta-blockers (e.g., atenolol, esmolol) have been used in the perioperative period to reduce cardiac morbidity and mortality in patients at risk; propranolol was not used in these studies. ■ Has been used for adjunctive treatment of pheochromocytoma following primary treatment with an alpha-adrenergic blocking agent (e.g., phenoxybenzamine [Dibenzyline], phentolamine [Regitine]) and for treatment of other refractory arrhythmias when benefit outweighs risk.

CONTRAINDICATIONS

Cardiogenic shock, sinus bradycardia, greater than first-degree heart block, bronchial asthma, known hypersensitivity to propranolol.

PRECAUTIONS

Oral administration is preferred. Use IV administration only when necessary. ■ Not considered the drug of choice for arrhythmias in myocardial infarction. ■ Used concurrently with digoxin or alpha-adrenergic blockers as indicated. ■ Use with caution in overt CHF. May precipitate more severe failure. ■ Use with extreme caution in asthmatics, patients with lung disease or bronchospasm; can block bronchodilation produced by endogenous and exogenous catecholamine stimulation of beta receptors. ■ Use with caution in patients with diabetes or in patients with a history of hypoglycemia. May cause hypoglycemia and mask the symptoms. ▪ Beta blockade can mask symptoms of hyperthyroidism. Abrupt withdrawal of propranolol may be followed by exacerbation of symptoms, including thyroid storm. ▪ Use caution in patients with hepatic or renal impairment. ▪ May cause arrhythmia, angina, MI, or death if stopped abruptly. ▪ Beta-adrenergic receptor blockade can cause a reduction in intraocular pressure. Withdrawal of propranolol may lead to a return of elevated intraocular pressure. May also interfere with the screening test for glaucoma. ▪ IV dose used during surgery to replace an oral dose should be ¹⁄₁₀ of the oral dose. ▪ May cause severe bradycardia in patients with Wolff-Parkinson-White syndrome. See Drug/Lab Interactions.

Monitor: Continuous ECG and BP monitoring is mandatory during administration of IV propranolol. Monitoring of pulmonary wedge pressure or central venous pressure is recommended. Discontinue the drug when a rhythm change is noted and wait to note full effect before giving additional medication if indicated. ▪ See Precautions and Drug/Lab Interactions.

Patient Education: Report any breathing difficulty promptly.

Maternal/Child: Category C: safety for use in pregnancy and breast-feeding and in pediatric patients not established. Use only when clearly indicated. ▪ Bradycardia, hypoglycemia, and respiratory depression have been seen in neonates whose mothers received propranolol during labor or delivery. **Elderly:** Lower-end initial doses may be indicated; see Dose Adjustments. ▪ Response of elderly versus younger patients not documented. ▪ Use with caution in age-related peripheral vascular disease; risk of hypothermia increased. ▪ May exacerbate mental impairment.

DRUG/LAB INTERACTIONS

Metabolism involves multiple pathways in the **cytochrome P₄₅₀ system.** Interactions with inhibitors, inducers, or substrates of this system are documented. ▪ Blood levels of propranolol **increased** when administered concurrently **with substrates or inhibitors** such as amiodarone (Nexterone), cimetidine (Tagamet), ciprofloxacin (Cipro IV), delavirdine (Rescriptor), fluconazole (Diflucan), fluoxetine (Prozac), fluvoxamine (Luvox), imipramine (Tofranil), isoniazid (Nydrazid), paroxetine (Paxil), quinidine, ritonavir (Norvir), rizatriptan (Maxalt), teniposide (Vumon), theophylline, tolbutamide, zileuton (Zyflo), zolmitriptan (Zomig). ▪ Blood levels of propranolol **decreased** when administered concurrently with **inducers** such as cigarette smoke, ethanol, and rifampin (Rifadin). ▪ Concurrent use with **propafenone** may produce additive negative inotropic and beta-blocking effects. ▪ Concurrent administration with **quinidine** results in additive negative inotropic effects and beta-blockade and postural hypotension. ▪ Concurrent use with **disopyramide** (Norpace) has been associated with additive hypotension, severe bradycardia, asystole, and heart failure. ▪ Concurrent use with **amiodarone** (Nexterone) results in additive negative chronotropic properties. ▪ Decreases **lidocaine** clearance; lidocaine toxicity has been reported with concurrent use. ▪ Effects additive when given with **other agents that slow A-V nodal conduction** (e.g., digoxin [Lanoxin], lidocaine). ▪ Concurrent use with **calcium channel blockers** that have negative inotropic and/or chronotropic activity (e.g., diltiazem [Cardizem], verapamil) may further depress myocardial contractility and A-V nodal conduction. Bradycardia, heart failure, and cardiovascular collapse have been reported with verapamil and beta-blockers. Bradycardia, hypotension, heart block, and heart failure have been reported with coadministration of diltiazem and beta-blockers. ▪ Antihypertensive effects of **clonidine** may be antagonized by propranolol. Use with clonidine may precipitate acute hypertension or aggravate rebound hypertension if clonidine stopped abruptly; discontinue propranolol several days before gradual withdrawal of clonidine. Monitor BP with concurrent use. ▪ First-dose hypotension may be prolonged with **prazosin** (Minipress). Postural hypotension has been reported when used concurrently with **doxazosin** (Cardura) **and terazosin** (Hytrin). ▪ Coadministration with **reserpine** (a catecholamine-depleting drug) may result in hypotension, bradycardia, vertigo, syncope, or orthostatic hypotension. ▪ Avoid concurrent use with **epinephrine.** Beta-blockade may lead to unopposed alpha-receptor stimulation, resulting in uncontrolled hypertension. ▪ **Dobutamine or isoproterenol** (Isuprel) may be administered to reverse the effects of propranolol. However, patients may experience protracted, severe hypotension. ▪ **Anesthetic agents** (e.g., methoxyflurane [Penthrane] and trichloroethylene) may depress myocardial contractility when administered with propranolol. ▪ **ACE inhibitors** (enalapril [Vasotec, enalaprilat], lisinopril [Zestril]) may increase bronchial hyperactivity when given concurrently with propranolol. ▪ Hypotension and cardiac arrest have been reported with concurrent use of **haloperidol** and propranolol. ▪ Propranolol may increase serum levels of **theophylline and diazepam** (Valium). ▪ Potentiates **ergot alkaloids** (e.g., dihydroergotamine [D.H.E. 45]); monitor for peripheral ischemia; reduce ergot dose or discontinue beta-blocker. ▪ Added hypotensive effect with **diuretics** (e.g., furosemide), **other antihypertensive agents** (e.g., enalaprilat, nitroglycerin), some **phenothiazines** (e.g., chlorpromazine [Thorazine]), **and reserpine.** Reduced dose of one or both drugs may be indicated. ▪ May prolong effects of **nondepolarizing muscle relaxants** (e.g., pancuronium). ▪ May increase anticoagulant effects of **warfarin.** ▪ May mask symptoms of hypoglycemia with **insulin and sulfonylureas** and result in prolonged hypoglycemia. ▪ Can interfere with **numerous diagnostic and physiologic tests.** Consult literature. ▪ May alter **thyroid function tests** and cause **elevations in BUN, serum potassium, triglycerides, serum transaminases, and alkaline phosphatase.** ▪ Metabolism and release of catecholamines increased in **smokers;** increased doses may be required. May also interfere with therapeutic effects in **treatment of angina.** ▪ Patients taking beta-blockers who are exposed to a potential allergen may be unresponsive to the usual dose of **epinephrine** used to treat a hypersensitivity reaction.

SIDE EFFECTS

AV conduction delays, bradyarrhythmias, bronchospasm, cardiac failure, cardiac standstill, erythematous rash, hallucination, hypotension, laryngospasm, nausea, paresthesia of the hands, respiratory distress, syncopal attacks, vertigo, visual disturbances. Many other side effects have been reported with oral propranolol and could be seen with the IV route; see manufacturer's literature.

ANTIDOTE

For any side effect or excessive dosage, discontinue the drug and notify the physician immediately. Treat bradycardia with atropine 0.25 to 1 mg. Isoproterenol (Isuprel) may be used with caution if no response to vagal blockade. Serious bradycardia may require pacing. Treat cardiac failure with digitalization and diuretics. Treat hypotension or depressed myocardial function with glucagon. Administer 50 to 150 mcg/kg IV followed by an infusion of 1 to 5 mg/hr (see glucagon monograph for correct dilution). Isoproterenol (Isuprel) and dopamine may also be useful; see Drug/Lab Interactions. Treat bronchospasm with isoproterenol and aminophylline. Treat other side effects symptomatically. Monitor ECG, HR, neurobehavioral status, and intake and output until stable. Not significantly removed by hemodialysis or peritoneal dialysis. Resuscitate as necessary.

PROTAMINE SULFATE BBW

(**PROH**-tah-meen **SUL**-fayt)

Antidote
(heparin antagonist)

pH 6 to 7

USUAL DOSE

Following a serious heparin overdose, discontinue heparin and administer protamine immediately.

Pretreatment: Corticosteroids and antihistamines can be used for patients at risk for protamine hypersensitivity.

IV heparin overdose: 1 mg of IV protamine neutralizes approximately 100 USP units of heparin. May be repeated if needed in 10 to 15 minutes. Never exceed 50 mg in any 10-minute period. Dose adjusted as indicated by coagulation studies. Any dose over 100 mg in 2 hours should be justified by coagulation studies (has its own anticoagulant effect). Because heparin disappears rapidly from the circulation, the dose of protamine required decreases rapidly with the time elapsed after heparin injection (e.g., 30 minutes after IV heparin, 0.5 mg [or one half of the dose] of protamine may be sufficient to neutralize 100 USP units of heparin).

Subcutaneous heparin overdose: 1 to 1.5 mg IV protamine per 100 units of heparin. Some clinicians recommend a loading dose of 25 to 50 mg given slowly over 10 minutes followed by administration of the remainder of the calculated dose as a continuous infusion over 8 to 16 hours (the continuous infusion covers the absorption time seen with administration of SC heparin). See comments under IV heparin overdose.

Low-molecular-weight heparin overdose (unlabeled): 1 mg IV protamine for every 100 antifactor Xa units of LMWH. If PTT remains prolonged 2 to 4 hours after the first dose, or if bleeding continues, consider administration of a second dose of 0.5 mg protamine for every 100 antifactor Xa units. Only 60% to 75% of antifactor Xa activity is neutralized. Excessive protamine doses can worsen bleeding potential. See comments under IV heparin overdose.

DOSE ADJUSTMENTS

Because heparin disappears rapidly from the system, reduce dose of protamine based on length of time elapsed since heparin dose (up to one half if 30 minutes has elapsed). ▪ Prompt administration of protamine sulfate may also decrease dose requirements.

DILUTION

May be given undiluted or may be further diluted with NS or D5W.

Storage: Store at CRT. Do not freeze. Discard remaining medication or diluted solution.

COMPATIBILITY

Consider any drug NOT listed as compatible to be INCOMPATIBLE until consulting a pharmacist; specific conditions may apply.

Manufacturer recommends not mixing with other drugs unless **compatibility** is known, and lists as **incompatible** with some antibiotics, including several cephalosporins and penicillins. Consider individualized rate adjustment necessary to produce desired effects.

One source suggests the following **compatibilities:**

Additive: Ranitidine (Zantac), verapamil.

RATE OF ADMINISTRATION

50 mg (5 mL) or fraction thereof over 10 minutes. Do not exceed 50 mg in 10 minutes. As an infusion, may be given over 2 to 3 hours with dosage titrated according to coagulation studies. Increase duration of infusion to 8 to 16 hours for treatment of SC heparin overdose. Use infusion pump or microdrip (60 gtt/mL) to administer. Too-rapid administration, high doses, or repeated doses can cause anaphylaxis, bradycardia, cardiovascular collapse, catastrophic pulmonary vasoconstriction, pulmonary hypertension, dyspnea, flushing, noncardiogenic pulmonary edema, sensation of warmth, or severe hypotension. Hypertension has also occurred.

ACTIONS

An anticoagulant if administered alone. In the presence of heparin, protamine forms a stable salt, neutralizing the anticoagulant effect of both drugs. Does not bind to low-molecular-weight fragments of LMWH preparations, leading to incomplete neutralization of antifactor Xa. Each 1 mg of protamine can neutralize approximately 100 USP units of heparin. Onset of action is within 0.5 to 1 minute. Neutralization of heparin occurs within 5 minutes. Duration of action is about 2 hours.

INDICATIONS AND USES

To neutralize the anticoagulant activity of heparin in severe heparin overdosage.

Unlabeled uses: Neutralization of heparin administered during extracorporeal circulation in arterial and cardiac surgery or dialysis procedures. ■ Heparin neutralization in pregnant women near delivery. ■ Treatment of low-molecular-weight heparin (e.g., dalteparin, enoxaparin, tinzaparin) overdose. Neutralization of LMWH is not complete.

CONTRAINDICATIONS

Known hypersensitivity to protamine. ■ Do not use for bleeding that occurs without prior exposure to heparin.

PRECAUTIONS

For IV use only. Serious, life-threatening reactions have been reported. Risk increased in patients with allergies to fish, abnormal pulmonary hemodynamics, previous exposure to protamine or protamine-containing drugs (e.g., protamine insulin), infertile or vasectomized men (may have antiprotamine antibodies), and severe left ventricular dysfunction. Assess risk versus benefit in at-risk patients; see Rate of Administration and Usual Dose. ■ Must be administered in a facility equipped to monitor the patient and respond to any medical emergency. ■ Pulmonary edema and/or circulatory collapse may occur in patients undergoing cardiac bypass surgery; etiology unknown.

Monitor: Coagulation studies (e.g., aPTT, ACT, heparin titration test with protamine, plasma thrombin time) may be indicated to monitor therapeutic response. ■ Facilities to treat shock must be available; see Precautions. ■ After cardiac surgery or dialysis procedures, even with adequate neutralization, further bleeding may occur any time within 24 hours (heparin "rebound"). Observe the patient continuously. Additional protamine sulfate may be indicated.

Maternal/Child: Category C: safety for use in pregnancy, breast-feeding, or pediatric patients not established.

DRUG/LAB INTERACTIONS

Specific information not available.

SIDE EFFECTS

Occur more frequently with too-rapid injection; anaphylaxis, back pain, bradycardia, dyspnea, feeling of warmth, flushing, lethargy, nausea, vomiting, severe hypertension or hypotension. Acute pulmonary hypertension, noncardiogenic pulmonary edema, catastrophic pulmonary vasoconstriction, circulatory collapse, capillary leak, or pulmonary edema may occur.

ANTIDOTE

Discontinue the drug and notify the physician, who may recommend a decrease in rate of administration or, if side effects are severe, symptomatic treatment such as administration of whole blood, vasopressors (e.g., dopamine) for hypotension, atropine for bradycardia, and oxygen for dyspnea. Resuscitate as necessary.

PROTEIN (AMINO ACID) PRODUCTS
Nutritional therapy
(**PROH**-teen [ah-**MEE**-noh **AS**-id] **PROD**-ucks)

Aminess 5.2% with histadine ▪
Aminosyn 3.5%, 3.5% M, 5%, 7%, 8.5%, 10% ▪
Aminosyn 7%, 8.5%, and 10% with electrolytes ▪
Aminosyn (pH 6) 8.5% and 10% ▪ Aminosyn HBC 7% ▪
Aminosyn HF 8% ▪ Aminosyn II 7%, 8.5%, 10%, and 15% ▪
Aminosyn II 7%, 8.5%, and 10% with electrolytes ▪
Aminosyn II 3.5% in D5 or D25 ▪ Aminosyn II 5% in D25 ▪
Aminosyn II 4.25% in D10, D20, and D25 ▪
Aminosyn II 3.5% M and 4.5% M in D10 ▪
Aminosyn II 3.5% in D25 with electrolytes and calcium ▪
Aminosyn II 4.25% in D20, D25 with electrolytes and calcium ▪
Aminosyn PF 7% and 10% ▪
Aminosyn RF 5.2% ▪ 4% Branch Amin ▪
Clinimix 2.75% (sulfite free [SF]) in D5, D10, and D25 ▪
Clinimix 4.25% (SF) in D5, D10, D20, and D25 ▪
Clinimix 5% (SF) in D10, D15, D20, D25, and D35 ▪
Clinimix E 2.75% (SF) in D5, D10, D25 with electrolytes and
calcium ▪ Clinimix E 4.25% (SF) in D5, D10, D20, and D25 with
electrolytes and calcium ▪ Clinimix E 5% (SF) in D10, D15, D20,
D25, and D35 with electrolytes and calcium ▪
Clinisol 15% (SF) ▪ Crystalline amino acid infusions ▪
FreAmine HBC 6.9% ▪
FreAmine III 8.5%, 10%, and 3% and 8.5% with electrolytes ▪
HepatAmine 8% ▪ Hepatosol 8% ▪ Hyperalimentation ▪
NephrAmine 5.4% ▪ Novamine 11.4% and 15% ▪
Premasol 6% and 10% ▪
ProcalAmine ▪ ProSol 20% (sulfite free) ▪
Protein hydrolysates ▪ RenAmin without electrolytes ▪
Total parenteral nutrition ▪
Travasol 2.75% and 4.25% in D5, D10, and D25 ▪
Travasol 4.25% (SF) in D25 with electrolytes ▪
Travasol 5.5%, 8.5%, and 10% without electrolytes ▪
Travasol 3.5%, 5.5%, and 8.5% with electrolytes ▪
Travasol (SF) 3.5%, 5.5%, and 8.5% with electrolytes ▪
TrophaAmine 6% and 10%
pH 5 to 7

USUAL DOSE
0.5 to 2 Gm/kg of body weight/24 hr. Actual dose will depend on several factors, including daily protein and calorie requirements, disease state, physical condition, weight, and patient's metabolic and clinical response. Protein amino acid products are available in general, renal failure, hepatic failure/encephalopathy, and metabolic stress formulations. See Precautions/Monitor.

PEDIATRIC DOSE
Consult pharmacist; not all products are approved for use in pediatric patients. Amino acid formulations developed specifically for nutritional

support of infants and other pediatric patients are available (e.g., Aminosyn P/F sulfite free). Amino acid concentrations greater than 2.5% are too concentrated for infants; older pediatric patients may tolerate concentrations up to 5%. See Maternal/Child.

Actual dose and total volume will depend on several factors including age, protein requirements, disease state, physical condition, renal function, and weight. Infants and children require different percentages of all components. The primary source of calories is dextrose. IV fat emulsion may be used to supplement energy intake. Kcal requirements may be increased in malnutrition or stress.

One source indicates that normal energy requirements vary according to age and suggests the following:

1 to 7 years: 75 to 90 kcal/kg/day
7 to 12 years: 60 to 75 kcal/kg/day
12 to 18 years: 30 to 60 kcal/kg/day

Another source suggests a Gm/kg/day dose based on age:

1 to 3 years: 2 to 2.5 Gm/kg/day
4 to 12 years: 2 Gm/kg/day
13 to 15 years: 1.7 Gm/kg/day
16 years and older: 1.5 Gm/kg/day

A third source suggests a Gm/kg/day dose based on age and condition:
Pediatric patients from neonates to 10 years of age:
Unstressed and over 1 year of age: 1 to 1.2 Gm/kg/day
Unstressed and 1 year of age or under: 1.6 to 2.2 Gm/kg/day
Low stress or maintenance: 2 to 2.5 Gm/kg/day
Low-stress anabolism: 2.5 to 3 Gm/kg/day
Critically ill or severe burn injury: 2.5 to 3.5 Gm/kg/day

DILUTION

Dilute under strict aseptic techniques according to manufacturer's specific instructions. Some solutions are very concentrated; are for compounding only, not for direct infusion. Check label for aluminum content; see Precautions. Most commonly mixed with dextrose (nonprotein calorie source), electrolytes, vitamins, and trace elements to provide total parenteral nutrition (TPN) or peripheral parenteral nutrition (PPN). Intravenous lipids, providing a second nonprotein calorie source and a source of essential fatty acids, may be mixed with the dextrose/amino acid solution or run simultaneously. Use promptly after mixing; laminar flow hood preferred; refrigerate briefly if necessary, and discard any unused portion. Use only clear solutions; observe against adequate light for particulate matter or evidence of container damage.

Filters: Use of in-line filters is recommended. Use of 0.22-micron in-line microfilter for dextrose and amino acids. Use a 1.2-micron in-line microfilter for solutions with lipids (3 in 1). A precipitate is very difficult to detect in solutions that contain lipids.

Storage: Store unopened protein amino acid solutions at 20° to 25° C (68° to 77° F). Protect from freezing or excessive heat. Protect from light until use. Manufacturer recommends refrigeration after any additives (e.g., IV lipids, electrolytes, minerals) are added. Some preparations can be refrigerated for only short periods, preferably no more than 24 hours. When prepared for home use, some preparations have been refrigerated for up to 14 days (dextrose and amino acids) or up to 7 days with lipids added.

Leave vitamins (e.g., M.V.I.) out until time of administration. Consult pharmacist. Discard any single bottle after 24 hours at CRT.

COMPATIBILITY   (Underline Indicates Conflicting Compatibility Information)
Consider any drug NOT listed as compatible to be INCOMPATIBLE until consulting a pharmacist; specific conditions may apply.
Most **incompatibilities** relate to the preparation (chloride as opposed to phosphate), amount of medication added, other additives present, and thoroughness of mixing. Consult with the pharmacist before mixing any drugs in protein (amino acid) products. Many TPN solutions contain some phosphate. The addition of calcium salts may cause a precipitate. These additives must be mixed by the pharmacist. Specific amounts, calculations, temperature (precipitate forms more readily at room temperature), and order of dilution are required. Do not administer solutions containing calcium through the same administration set as blood; coagulation may occur.

Manufacturers suggest that only required nutritional products should be added, but H$_2$ receptors (e.g., ranitidine [Zantac]), insulin, and heparin are frequently added to selected products. Other drugs may be **compatible** for specific lengths of time. Mix thoroughly. Do not store.

One source suggests the following **compatibilities:**
Solution: Fat emulsion 10% IV.
Additive: *See general comments under Compatibility.* Amikacin (Amikin), aminophylline, ampicillin, aztreonam (Azactam), calcium gluconate, cefazolin (Ancef), cefepime (Maxipime), cefotaxime (Claforan), cefoxitin (Mefoxin), ceftazidime (Fortaz), cefuroxime (Zinacef), clindamycin (Cleocin), cyclophosphamide (Cytoxan), cyclosporine (Sandimmune), cytarabine (ARA-C), dopamine, epoetin alfa (Epogen), famotidine (Pepcid IV), fluorouracil (5-FU), folic acid, furosemide (Lasix), gentamicin, heparin, hydrochloric acid, insulin (regular), iron dextran, isoproterenol (Isuprel), kanamycin (Kantrex), lidocaine, meperidine (Demerol), methotrexate, methyldopate, methylprednisolone (Solu-Medrol), metoclopramide (Reglan), midazolam (Versed), morphine, multivitamins (M.V.I.), nafcillin (Nallpen), norepinephrine (Levophed), octreotide (Sandostatin), ondansetron (Zofran), oxacillin (Bactocill), penicillin G potassium and sodium, phytonadione (vitamin K$_1$), ranitidine (Zantac), sodium bicarbonate, tacrolimus (Prograf), tobramycin, vancomycin.
Y-site: Alprostadil, amikacin (Amikin), aminophylline, ampicillin, ampicillin/sulbactam (Unasyn), argatroban, ascorbic acid, atracurium (Tracrium), aztreonam (Azactam), bumetanide, buprenorphine (Buprenex), butorphanol (Stadol), calcium gluconate, carboplatin (Paraplatin), cefazolin (Ancef), cefotaxime (Claforan), cefotetan, cefoxitin (Mefoxin), ceftazidime (Fortaz), cefuroxime (Zinacef), chloramphenicol (Chloromycetin), chlorpromazine (Thorazine), ciprofloxacin (Cipro IV), cisplatin (Platinol), clindamycin (Cleocin), cyclophosphamide (Cytoxan), cyclosporine (Sandimmune), cytarabine (ARA-C), dexamethasone (Decadron), digoxin (Lanoxin), diphenhydramine (Benadryl), dobutamine, dopamine, doxycycline, droperidol (Inapsine), enalaprilat (Vasotec IV), epinephrine (Adrenalin), erythromycin (Erythrocin), famotidine (Pepcid IV), fentanyl (Sublimaze), fluconazole (Diflucan), fluorouracil (5-FU), folic acid, foscarnet (Foscavir), furosemide (Lasix), ganciclovir (Cytovene), gentamicin, granisetron (Kytril), haloperidol (Haldol), heparin, hydrocortisone sodium

succinate (Solu-Cortef), <u>hydromorphone (Dilaudid)</u>, idarubicin (Idamycin), ifosfamide (Ifex), imipenem/cilastatin (Primaxin), insulin (regular), isoproterenol (Isuprel), kanamycin (Kantrex), leucovorin calcium, lidocaine, linezolid (Zyvox), <u>lorazepam (Ativan)</u>, magnesium sulfate, mannitol, meperidine (Demerol), meropenem (Merrem IV), mesna (Mesnex), <u>methotrexate</u>, <u>methyldopate</u>, methylprednisolone (Solu-Medrol), <u>metoclopramide (Reglan)</u>, metronidazole (Flagyl IV), <u>micafungin (Mycamine)</u>, milrinone (Primacor), <u>mitoxantrone (Novantrone)</u>, <u>morphine</u>, <u>multivitamins (M.V.I.)</u>, nafcillin (Nallpen), <u>nalbuphine</u>, nitroglycerin IV, nitroprusside sodium, norepinephrine (Levophed), octreotide (Sandostatin), <u>ondansetron (Zofran)</u>, oxacillin (Bactocill), paclitaxel (Taxol), penicillin G, penicillin G potassium, <u>pentobarbital (Nembutal)</u>, <u>phenobarbital (Luminal)</u>, piperacillin, piperacillin/tazobactam (Zosyn), potassium chloride (KCl), prochlorperazine (Compazine), <u>promethazine (Phenergan)</u>, <u>propofol (Diprivan)</u>, ranitidine (Zantac), sargramostim (Leukine), <u>sodium bicarbonate</u>, sulfamethoxazole/trimethoprim, tacrolimus (Prograf), thiotepa, ticarcillin/clavulanate (Timentin), tobramycin, vancomycin, vecuronium, zidovudine (AZT, Retrovir).

RATE OF ADMINISTRATION

Begin parenteral nutrition at 0.5 to 2 mL/min and increase gradually as tolerated until the target rate is reached. The rate of a nutrient infusion is governed by the protein requirement and by the patient's glucose tolerance. With the correct parenteral nutrition formulation, fluid, protein, and calorie requirements should be met at the target rate. ***Total daily dose should be evenly distributed over the 24-hour period. Maintain a constant drip rate.*** Use of infusion pump and microfilter (0.22 micron for dextrose and amino acids, 1.2 micron for solutions with lipids [3 in 1]) recommended. Precipitate very difficult to detect in solutions that contain lipids. There are specific situations (e.g., cyclic TPN primarily used in home care patients) where a daily dose is given over less than 24 hours. Range is from 10 to 14 hours. Usually administered overnight, allowing individuals requiring prolonged TPN to maintain their daytime activities.

Pediatric rate: Usually begin with a one-half strength nutritional solution at 60 to 70 mL/kg/day. May be gradually increased over 48 hours until full strength and increased to 125 to 150 mL/kg/day. See all comments under Pediatric Dose, Rate of Administration/Adult, and Maternal/Child.

ACTIONS

Supplies essential and nonessential amino acids and calories with the intent of promoting protein production (anabolism) and preventing protein breakdown (catabolism). Promotes wound healing, and acts as a buffer in intracellular and extracellular body fluids. Various brands supply additional calories with alcohol, fructose, or glucose. These additional calories permit available protein to be used for repair of tissue in addition to meeting basic caloric needs.

INDICATIONS AND USES

To prevent nitrogen loss or to reverse negative nitrogen balance in severe illness when oral alimentation is not practical for prolonged periods; when normal GI absorption is impaired; when metabolic requirements for protein and calories are substantially increased, as with extensive burns; or when morbidity and mortality may be reduced by replacing amino acids lost from tissue breakdown, thereby preserving tissue reserves, as in acute renal failure.

CONTRAINDICATIONS

Hypersensitivity to any component, hepatic coma, or metabolic disorders involving impaired nitrogen utilization. Some manufacturers also list acidosis, anuria, azotemia, decreased circulating blood volume, severe liver disease, and metabolic disorders with impaired amino acid metabolization. ▪ Solutions containing dextrose may be contraindicated in patients with known allergies to corn or corn products.

PRECAUTIONS

Catheter insertion for administration of central parenteral nutrition is a sterile surgical procedure (must be a large vein [subclavian or superior vena cava preferred]; 50% glucose is a sclerosing solution). ▪ Peripheral veins are suitable for specific products (peripheral parenteral nutrition) when amino acid products are diluted with 2.5%, 5%, or 10% dextrose. ▪ Safe and effective use of central venous nutrition requires knowledge of nutrition as well as clinical expertise in recognition and treatment of the complications that can occur. Frequent clinical evaluation and laboratory determinations are necessary for proper monitoring of central venous nutrition; see Monitor. ▪ Amino acids given without carbohydrates may cause ketone accumulation. ▪ Use caution in impaired hepatic function; may cause serum amino acid imbalances, metabolic alkalosis, prerenal azotemia, hyperammonemia, stupor, and coma. ▪ Use caution in impaired renal function; may further increase BUN. ▪ Concentrated dextrose solutions, if administered too rapidly, may result in significant hyperglycemia and possible hyperosmolar syndrome characterized by mental confusion and loss of consciousness. ▪ Fatty infiltration of the liver, acute respiratory failure, and difficulty in weaning hypermetabolic patients from the respirator may be caused by excessive carbohydrate calories. ▪ Avoid circulatory overload, particularly in patients with cardiac insufficiency. ▪ Solutions containing electrolytes should be used with caution in selected patients (e.g., sodium ions, use caution in patients with CHF, renal insufficiency, and clinical states with edema with sodium retention; potassium ions, use caution in patients with hyperkalemia, renal insufficiency, and conditions with potassium retention; acetate ions from inorganic salts, use caution in patients with metabolic or respiratory alkalosis). ▪ Some solutions may contain aluminum. In impaired kidney function, aluminum may reach toxic levels. Premature neonates are particularly at risk because of their immature kidneys and requirement for calcium and phosphate, which also contain aluminum. Research indicates that patients with impaired renal function who receive greater than 4 to 5 mcg/kg/day of parenteral aluminum are at risk for developing CNS or bone toxicity associated with aluminum accumulation. ▪ Some solutions may contain sulfites; use caution in patients allergic to sulfites. ▪ Essential fatty acid deficiency has been observed in patients on long-term TPN (more than 5 days). The use of fat emulsion to provide 4% to 10% of total caloric intake as linoleic acid may help to prevent this deficiency.

Monitor: Specific baseline studies required before administration: CBC, platelet count, PT, BUN, SCr, electrolytes, glucose, triglycerides, cholesterol, albumin, bilirubin, liver function tests (e.g., AST, ALT, LDH), acid-base balance, fluid balance, weight, body length and head circumference (in infants), and immunocompetence. Frequent clinical evaluation and lab tests are indicated during therapy. ▪ Monitor intake and output and weight. More frequent monitoring of serum glucose and additional insulin may be indicated in patients with diabetes. After stabilization, measurement of urine glucose and ketones every 8 hours is suggested. ▪ Follow a strict, regular aseptic routine to care for insertion site. ▪ Single-port central venous catheters to be used only for the nutritional regimen. Do not draw blood samples, transfuse blood, or administer other medications. Pseudoagglutination and thrombosis can occur, risk of contamination is great, and validity of results is compromised. Multiple-port central venous catheters may be used for these additional procedures. Observe specific protocols. ▪ Monitor BUN frequently. Discontinue infusion if BUN exceeds normal postprandial limits and continues to rise. ▪ Blood ammonia levels important, especially in infants. ▪ Check frequently for any signs of extravasation. ▪ Observe for any signs of infection. ▪ Additional insulin coverage may be required, especially when dosage is increased too rapidly or with maximum doses. ▪ To prevent rebound hypoglycemia, may need to decrease rate gradually over 2 to 6 hours. ▪ Discard any single bottle after 24 hours. Replace administration set every 24 to 72 hours depending on formulation and facility-specific policies. ▪ See Precautions.

Maternal/Child: Category C: use during pregnancy only if clearly needed. ▪ Safety for use during breast-feeding not established; effects unknown. Use caution; has potential for adverse effects in nursing infants (e.g., hyperammonemia). ▪ Use with caution in pediatric patients with renal failure. ▪ Monitor neonates and very small infants carefully to maintain fluid and electrolyte balance, including monitoring of blood glucose. ▪ Use hypertonic dextrose (component of parenteral nutrition) with extreme caution in low-birth-weight or septic infants. May cause hyperglycemia, hypoglycemia, or increased serum osmolality with possible intracerebral hemorrhage. Monitor serum glucose frequently. Solutions should not exceed 718 mOsm/L. ▪ Amino acid concentrations greater than 2.5% are too concentrated for infants. ▪ Hyperammonemia is of particular significance in infants. Can cause mental retardation; measure blood ammonia frequently. **Elderly:** Differences in responses between elderly and younger patients have not been identified; however, incidence of fluid overload and electrolyte imbalance may be increased. Monitor closely. ▪ Lower end initial doses may be appropriate in the elderly based on the potential for decreased organ function and concomitant disease or drug therapy. Monitoring of renal function suggested.

DRUG/LAB INTERACTIONS

Tetracycline may reduce protein-sparing effects. ▪ **Magnesium-containing solutions** may have an additive CNS depressive effect with barbiturates, hypnotics, narcotics, or systemic anesthetics; dose adjustment of these agents may be indicated.

SIDE EFFECTS

Abdominal pains, anaphylaxis, bone demineralization, changes in levels of consciousness, convulsions, dehydration, edema at the site of injection, electrolyte imbalances, glycosuria, hyperammonemia, hyperglycemia, hyperpyrexia, hypertension, metabolic acidosis and/or alkalosis, osmotic dehydration, phlebitis and thrombosis, pulmonary edema, rebound hypoglycemia, septicemia, vasodilation, vomiting, weakness.

ANTIDOTE

Notify the physician of all side effects. An alternate brand may cause fewer problems, or amounts of glucose or additives may be adjusted to correct the problem. Many of the side effects listed will respond to a reduced rate. Some will require catheter insertion at a new site. Treat symptomatically and resuscitate as necessary. Stop infusion immediately for any signs of acute respiratory distress. May represent pulmonary embolus or interstitial pneumonitis, which may be caused by a precipitate of electrolytes (e.g., calcium and phosphates) in the solution.

PROTEIN C CONCENTRATE (HUMAN)
(**PROH**-teen C **KON**-sen-trayt)

Ceprotin

**Anticoagulant
Antithrombotic**

pH 6.7 to 7.3

USUAL DOSE

(International units [IU])

Dose, administration frequency, and duration of treatment depend on the severity of the protein C deficiency, the patient's age, the clinical condition of the patient, and the patient's plasma level of protein C. Initiate therapy as directed in the chart below and adjust the dosage regimen according to the pharmacokinetic profile for each patient. See Dose Adjustments and Monitor.

Protein C Concentrate Dosing Schedule for Acute Episodes, Short-Term Prophylaxis, and Long-Term Prophylaxis			
	Initial Dose*	Subsequent 3 Doses*	Maintenance Dose*
Acute episodes/ short-term prophylaxis†	100 to 120 IU/kg	60 to 80 IU/kg every 6 hours	45 to 60 IU/kg every 6 or 12 hours
Long-term prophylaxis	N/A	N/A	45 to 60 IU/kg every 12 hours

*Dose regimen should be adjusted according to the pharmacokinetic profile for each individual patient.
†Continue therapy until the desired anticoagulation is achieved.

PEDIATRIC AND NEONATAL DOSE

See Usual Dose and Maternal/Child.

DOSE ADJUSTMENTS

For treatment of acute episodes or with short-term prophylaxis, adjust dose according to the pharmacokinetic profile of the patient. Adjust to maintain a target peak protein C activity of 100%. After resolution of the acute episode, continue patient on the same dose to maintain a trough protein C activity above 25% for the duration of treatment. ■ Higher peak protein C activity levels may be required for situations in which there is an increased risk of thrombosis (e.g., infection, surgical intervention, trauma). Maintaining trough protein C activity levels above 25% is recommended. ■ Use in renal and hepatic impairment has not been studied. See Precautions.

DILUTION (International units [IU])

Available in single-dose vials that contain 500 or 1,000 International Units (IU) of protein C. Reconstitute the 500-IU vial with 5 mL of SWI and the 1,000-IU vial with 10 mL of SWI to provide a single dose of human protein C at a concentration of 100 IU/mL. Vials also contain human albumin, trisodium citrate dihydrate, and sodium chloride as excipients. Bring the vials of protein C and SWI (supplied diluent) to room temperature. Remove tops of vials and cleanse stoppers. Insert one end of the manufacturer-supplied double-ended transfer needle through the center of the diluent vial stopper. Invert the diluent vial and insert the free end of the double-ended transfer needle into the protein C vial. The vacuum in the vial should pull in the diluent. If a vacuum is not present, do not use the vial. Remove the double-ended transfer needle from the diluent vial, then from the protein C vial. Gently swirl the protein C vial until the powder is completely dissolved. The powder must be completely dissolved to prevent active materials from being removed by the filter needle during infusion. Solution should be colorless to slightly yellowish and clear to slightly opalescent. Attach manufacturer-supplied filter needle to a disposable syringe. Withdraw plunger to admit air into the syringe and inject air into the protein C vial. Withdraw reconstituted solution from the vial into the syringe. Remove the filter needle and attach a suitable needle or infusion set for administration. The filter needle is intended to filter the contents of a single vial of protein C.

Filters: Filtering required; see Dilution.

Storage: Refrigerate unopened vials in original carton at 2° to 8° C (36° to 46° F); protect from light. Shelf life is 3 years. Do not use beyond expiration date. Do not freeze. Administer reconstituted product within 3 hours of reconstitution. Single-dose vial; discard any unused product after entry into vial.

COMPATIBILITY

Specific information not available. Consider specialized use.

RATE OF ADMINISTRATION

Administer as an infusion.

Adults and pediatric patients over 10 kg: Maximum rate 2 mL/min.

Pediatric patients less than 10 kg: Maximum rate 0.2 mL/kg/min.

ACTIONS

A precursor of the vitamin K–dependent anticoagulant glycoprotein (serine protease) that is synthesized in the liver. Manufactured from human plasma. Numerous processes are used during manufacturing to minimize the risk for viral transmission; see Precautions. Protein C is converted to activated protein C (APC), a serine protease with potent anticoagulant effects. APC exerts its effect by inactivation of the activated forms of factors V and VIII, which leads to a decrease in thrombin formation. APC also has been shown to have profibrinolytic effects. A complete absence of protein C is not compatible with life. A severe deficiency of this protein leads to unchecked coagulation activation, resulting in thrombin generation and intravascular clot formation and thrombosis. An increase in plasma levels of protein C can be seen within ½ hour after administration of protein C concentrate. Replacement of protein C in protein C–deficient patients is expected to control or, if given prophylactically, prevent thrombotic complications. In clinical studies, patients with severe congenital protein C deficiency were treated more effectively with protein C concentrate than those treated with modalities such as fresh frozen plasma or conventional anticoagulants. Half-life ranges from 4.9 to 14.7 hours, with a median of 9.8 hours. In patients with acute thrombosis, purpura fulminans, and skin necrosis, both the half-life and the increase in protein C plasma level may be reduced.

INDICATIONS AND USES
Prevention and treatment of venous thrombosis and purpura fulminans in patients with severe congenital protein C deficiency. A replacement therapy for pediatric and adult patients.

CONTRAINDICATIONS
None known.

PRECAUTIONS
Initiate treatment under the supervision of a physician experienced in replacement therapy with coagulation factors/inhibitors and in a facility where monitoring of protein C activity is available. ■ Half-life of protein C concentrate may be shortened in certain clinical conditions such as acute thrombosis, purpura fulminans, and skin necrosis. Patients treated during the acute phase of their disease may display much lower increases in protein C activity. ■ May contain trace amounts of mouse protein and heparin due to the manufacturing process. Hypersensitivity reactions are possible; see Monitor and Antidote. ■ Manufactured from pooled human plasma. Special screening and purification techniques are used to minimize the risk of transmitting infectious agents (e.g., hepatitis A, human parvovirus B19, Creutzfeldt-Jakob disease [CJD]), but transmission cannot be completely ruled out. Appropriate vaccination (hepatitis A and B) should be considered for patients receiving human-derived protein C. ■ Contains heparin. Discontinue if heparin-induced thrombocytopenia (HIT) is suspected; see Monitor. ■ Use with caution in patients who may be sensitive to a sodium load (e.g., patients with HTN or CHF); see Monitor. ■ Patients being started on anticoagulant therapy with a vitamin K–antagonist anticoagulant (e.g., warfarin) may experience a transient hypercoagulable state before desired anticoagulation is reached. Patients may be at increased risk for warfarin-induced skin necrosis. Initiate warfarin therapy at a low dose and adjust incrementally as indicated by INR monitoring. Continue protein C replacement until stable anticoagulation with warfarin is reached. ■ Bleeding episodes have been reported. Simultaneous administration with alteplase (Activase, tPA) and/or anticoagulants (e.g., warfarin, heparin) may increase the risk of bleeding; see Drug Interactions. ■ Use with caution in patients with renal and/or hepatic impairment. Has not been studied.

Monitor: Measure protein C activity using a chromogenic assay before and during treatment. ■ In the case of an acute thrombotic event, it is recommended that protein C activity measurements be obtained immediately before the next injection until the patient is stabilized. Once stabilized, continue monitoring to maintain the trough protein C level above 25%. ■ Coagulation parameters (e.g., INR/PT) should be monitored. However, a correlation between coagulation parameters and protein C activity levels has not been determined. ■ Discontinue therapy and check platelet count if heparin-induced thrombocytopenia is suspected. ■ Contains more than 200 mg of sodium. Monitor fluid and electrolyte status, especially in patients on a low-sodium diet and/or in patients with renal impairment. ■

Monitor for S/S of hypersensitivity reactions (e.g., anaphylaxis, hives, hypotension, generalized itching, tightness of the chest, and/or wheezing). **Patient Education:** Manufactured from pooled human plasma. Risk of transmission of infectious agents cannot be ruled out. Discuss risk versus benefit of therapy with physician. ▪ Review vaccination status with physician. Vaccination against hepatitis A and B should be considered. ▪ Contains sodium. ▪ Report S/S of hypersensitivity reaction immediately (e.g., hives, generalized itching, tightness of the chest, wheezing). ▪ Consultation with a physician is required if abdominal pain, chills, drowsiness, fever, jaundice, nausea and vomiting, prolonged poor appetite, runny nose, tiredness, or dark urine occur.

Maternal/Child: Category C: safety for use in pregnancy and lactation has not been established. ▪ Has been used in patients as young as 2 days of age. ▪ Pharmacokinetics in the very young may differ from that of older pediatric patients and adults. Systemic exposure (Cmax and AUC) may be reduced due to a faster clearance, larger volume of distribution, and/or shorter half-life. Doses must be individualized based on protein C activity levels; see Dose Adjustments.

Elderly: Specific differences in safety and efficacy have not been identified.

DRUG/LAB INTERACTIONS

Formal drug interaction studies have not been conducted. ▪ Simultaneous use with **alteplase** (Activase, tPA) and **anticoagulants** (e.g., warfarin, heparin) may increase the risk of bleeding. ▪ Patients being started on anticoagulant therapy with a **vitamin K–antagonist anticoagulant** (e.g., warfarin) may experience a transient hypercoagulable state before desired anticoagulation is reached; see Precautions.

SIDE EFFECTS

The most commonly reported side effects are rash, itching, and light-headedness.

Post-Marketing: Fever, hemothorax, hyperhidrosis, hypotension, and restlessness.

ANTIDOTE

Notify physician of any side effects; most will be treated symptomatically. Discontinue protein C concentrate for any serious reaction (e.g., HIT, hypersensitivity). Treat hypersensitivity reactions as indicated (e.g., oxygen, diphenhydramine, epinephrine, corticosteroids, vasopressors, and/or fluids). Resuscitate as necessary.

PYRIDOXINE HYDROCHLORIDE
(peer-ih-**DOX**-een hy-droh-**KLOR**-eyed)

Nutritional supplement
(vitamin)
Antidote

Vitamin B$_6$

pH 2 to 3.8

USUAL DOSE

Pyridoxine dependency syndrome: 30 to 600 mg/day.

Drug-induced pyridoxine deficiency: 50 to 200 mg/day for 3 weeks. Follow with 25 to 100 mg/day as needed.

Prophylaxis or treatment of pyridoxine deficiency in patients receiving parenteral nutrition: May be added to parenteral nutrition; dose will depend on patient condition.

INH poisoning (greater than 10 Gm) (unlabeled): 4 Gm IV followed by 1 Gm IM every 30 minutes. Total pyridoxine dose should equal ingested INH dose.

Cycloserine poisoning (unlabeled): 300 mg/day. Higher doses may be required.

Hydrazine poisoning (unlabeled): 25 mg/kg. Give one third of dose IM and remainder as a 3-hour infusion.

Gyrometra mushroom poisoning (unlabeled): 25 mg/kg over 15 to 30 minutes. Repeat as needed.

PEDIATRIC DOSE

See Maternal/Child.

Pyridoxine-dependent seizures: 10 to 100 mg.

DOSE ADJUSTMENTS

Removed by hemodialysis. Dialysis patients may require higher doses.

DILUTION

May be given by IV injection undiluted or added to most IV solutions and given as an infusion. See chart on inside back cover.

Storage: Store below 40° C unless otherwise stated by manufacturer. Deteriorates in excessive heat; protect from heat and light.

COMPATIBILITY

Consider any drug NOT listed as compatible to be INCOMPATIBLE until consulting a pharmacist; specific conditions may apply.

Manufacturer lists as **incompatible** with alkaline solutions, iron salts, oxidizing solutions.

One source suggests the following **compatibilities:**

Solution: Fat emulsion 10% IV.

RATE OF ADMINISTRATION

50 mg or fraction thereof over 1 minute if given undiluted.

ACTIONS

Vitamin B$_6$ is water soluble. It is a coenzyme necessary for the metabolism of proteins, carbohydrates, and lipids. Involved in many reactions including the conversion of tryptophan to nicotinamide and serotonin, breakdown to glucose-1-phosphate, synthesis of gamma aminobutyric acid (GABA) in the CNS (energy transformation in brain and nerve cells), and synthesis of heme. Metabolized by the liver, and excreted in the urine.

INDICATIONS AND USES
Prophylaxis and treatment of pyridoxine deficiency. Deficiency may be due to inadequate diet, inborn error of metabolism or concomitant drug use. **Unlabeled uses:** Treatment of INH, hydrazine, and cycloserine poisoning. Treatment of neurologic effects of Gyrometra mushroom poisoning. Nausea and vomiting associated with pregnancy.

CONTRAINDICATIONS
Known sensitivity to pyridoxine.

PRECAUTIONS
Used IV only when oral dosage not acceptable. ▪ Deficiency can cause abnormal EEG. ▪ Need for pyridoxine increases with amount of protein in diet. Chronic administration of large doses may cause adverse neurologic effects. **Maternal/Child:** Category A: requirements are increased in pregnancy and breast-feeding. Do not exceed RDA. ▪ Large doses in utero can cause pyridoxine-dependency syndrome in newborn. ▪ May inhibit breast-feeding. ▪ Safety for use in pediatric patients not established.

DRUG/LAB INTERACTIONS
An antagonist to **levodopa**. Does not antagonize carbidopa/levodopa combination (Sinemet). ▪ **Isoniazid** is a vitamin B_6 antagonist and will cause deficiency disease. ▪ **Cycloserine, penicillamine, hydralazine, oral contraceptives** may increase pyridoxine requirements. ▪ May decrease **phenobarbital and phenytoin** (Dilantin) levels. ▪ Excessive doses **may elevate AST.**

SIDE EFFECTS
Almost nonexistent; some slight flushing or feeling of warmth may occur. With larger doses, ataxia, low folic acid levels, paresthesias, somnolence, and withdrawal seizures in infants with high maternal doses may occur.

ANTIDOTE
No antidote is known or has been needed. Symptomatic treatment of side effects may be indicated.

QUINIDINE GLUCONATE INJECTION BBW
(**KWIN**-ih-deen **GLOO**-ko-nayt in-**JEK**-shun)

Antiarrhythmic

pH 5.5 to 7

USUAL DOSE

Cardiac monitoring required with IV administration; see Monitor. *All doses are for quinidine gluconate only. See prescribing information for doses by other routes (e.g., quinidine sulfate PO).*

Test dose: 200 mg PO or IM is recommended by some sources to determine the possibility of idiosyncratic reactions.

Symptomatic atrial fibrillation/flutter: Given as an infusion not to exceed a rate of 0.25 mg/kg/min. Most arrhythmias that will respond to IV quinidine will respond to a total dose of less than 5 mg/kg, but some patients may require a total dose of up to 10 mg/kg. If conversion has not occurred after a dose of 10 mg/kg, discontinue infusion and consider other means of conversion (e.g., direct current cardioversion). Maintain with an oral quinidine preparation.

Life-threatening ventricular arrhythmias: Dosing regimens for use in controlling life-threatening ventricular arrhythmias have not been adequately studied. Regimens are usually similar to the regimen for treatment of symptomatic atrial fibrillation/flutter.

***Plasmodium falciparum* malaria:** A loading dose should not be used if the patient has received more than 40 mg/kg of quinine in the previous 48 hours or mefloquine in the previous 12 hours. If appropriate, administer a loading dose of 24 mg/kg of quinidine gluconate in 250 mL NS as an infusion over 4 hours. Follow with a maintenance dose of 12 mg/kg quinidine gluconate in 125 to 250 mL NS over 4 hours. Begin maintenance dose 8 hours after initiation of loading dose. Repeat every 8 hours for 7 days or transfer to oral therapy. An alternate regimen is a loading dose of 10 mg/kg of quinidine gluconate in approximately 5 mL/kg NS over 1 to 2 hours. Follow with a maintenance infusion of 20 mcg/kg/min quinidine gluconate. Transfer to oral therapy if possible. Continue quinidine therapy (IV or oral) for up to 72 hours or until parasitemia is less than 1%, whichever comes first. After completion of quinidine course, therapy is continued with other antimalarial medications.

PEDIATRIC DOSE

***Plasmodium falciparum* malaria:** See Usual Dose.

Antiarrhythmic (unlabeled): One source recommends a test dose of 2 mg/kg (60 mg/M^2) of quinidine gluconate (up to 200 mg) IM or PO. If no reaction, follow with 2 to 10 mg/kg/dose of quinidine gluconate every 3 to 6 hours. Use IV only when oral routes not possible; see Maternal/Child.

DOSE ADJUSTMENTS

Reduce dose in patients with renal or hepatic impairment or in patients with CHF. ▪ Another source suggests administering 75% of the normal dose to patients with a CrCl less than 10 mL/min and suggests that a larger initial dose may be indicated in hepatic impairment, but maintenance doses should be reduced by 50% with close monitoring of serum levels. ▪ Reduced dose may be indicated in the elderly based on potential for decreased organ function and concomitant disease or drug therapy. ▪ See Drug/Lab Interactions.

DILUTION

Symptomatic atrial fibrillation/flutter: 800 mg (10 mL) must be diluted with 40 mL of D5W to provide a final concentration of 16 mg/mL.

***Plasmodium falciparum* malaria:** Add loading dose to 250 mL of NS and maintenance dose to 125 to 250 mL of NS. In the alternative regimen, the loading dose is added to 5 mL/kg of NS. The maintenance infusion is prepared by mixing 800 mg (10 mL) with 40 mL of D5W to provide a final concentration of 16 mg/mL. Use only clear, colorless solutions. May be adsorbed to PVC tubing; minimize tubing length.

Storage: Store at CRT. Protect from light. Infusion solution containing 16 mg/mL in D5W is stable for 24 hours at RT or up to 48 hours at 4° C (40° F).

COMPATIBILITY (Underline Indicates Conflicting Compatibility Information)

Consider any drug NOT listed as compatible to be INCOMPATIBLE until consulting a pharmacist; specific conditions may apply.

One source suggests the following **compatibilities:**

Additive: Milrinone (Primacor), ranitidine (Zantac), verapamil.

Y-site: <u>Diazepam (Valium)</u>, <u>heparin</u>, milrinone (Primacor), nesiritide (Natrecor).

RATE OF ADMINISTRATION

Symptomatic atrial fibrillation/flutter: Do not exceed a rate of 0.25 mg/kg/min (1 mL/kg/hr) of properly diluted solution. Another source suggests not exceeding a rate equal to or less than 10 mg/min.

***Plasmodium falciparum* malaria:** See rates outlined in Usual Dose. Use of an infusion pump recommended. Too-rapid administration may cause peripheral vascular collapse and severe hypotension.

For all indications: Decrease rate or interrupt infusion if corrected QT interval exceeds 0.6 seconds, corrected QT interval exceeds baseline by more than 25%, QRS widening exceeds 50% of baseline, or symptomatic hypotension that does not respond to fluid expansion develops.

ACTIONS

An antimalarial schizonticide and an antiarrhythmic with Class 1a activity. A dextro-isomer of quinine. Decreases myocardial excitability and conduction velocity. May suppress atrial fibrillation or flutter by increasing the effective refractory period and increasing the action potential duration in atrial and ventricular muscle and in the His-Purkinje system. Has anticholinergic, vasodilating, and negative inotropic actions. As an antimalarial agent, it acts primarily as an intra-erythrocytic schizonticide, with little effect on sporozoites or pre-erythrocytic parasites. Rapidly distributed into all tissues except the brain. 80% to 88% bound to plasma proteins. Metabolized in the liver by CYP3A4 to several metabolites, some of which have antiarrhythmic activity. Half-life is 6 to 8 hours. Eliminated mainly in urine. Less than 5% of dose excreted in feces. Crosses placental barrier. Secreted in breast milk.

INDICATIONS AND USES

Treatment of life-threatening *Plasmodium falciparum* malaria. ▪ Conversion of atrial fibrillation/flutter. Indicated when rapid therapeutic effect is required or when oral therapy is not feasible as a means of restoring normal sinus rhythm in patients with symptomatic atrial fibrillation/flutter. ▪

Treatment of ventricular arrhythmias (e.g., sustained ventricular tachycardia) that in the judgment of the physician are life threatening. Because of the proarrhythmic effects of quinidine, its use for treatment of less severe arrhythmias is not recommended. *(The use of quinidine for treatment of arrhythmias has largely been replaced by more effective, safer antiarrhythmics [e.g., amiodarone (Nexterone)] and/or nonpharmacologic therapies [e.g., ablation]).*

CONTRAINDICATIONS

Known hypersensitivity to quinidine or cinchona (e.g., febrile reactions, skin eruption, thrombocytopenia), myasthenia gravis, history of thrombocytopenic purpura with quinidine administration. ▪ In the absence of a functioning artificial pacemaker, quinidine is also contraindicated in any patient whose cardiac rhythm is dependent on a junctional or idioventricular pacemaker, including patients in complete atrioventricular block. ▪ *Contraindicated with ritonavir (Norvir).*

PRECAUTIONS

A meta-analysis of data from several randomized, controlled studies in patients with atrial flutter and fibrillation indicates that quinidine therapy may be associated with a mortality rate greater than 3 times higher than that associated with placebo. ▪ A meta-analysis of patients with various non–life-threatening ventricular arrhythmias showed that mortality associated with quinidine was consistently greater than that associated with various other antiarrhythmic agents (e.g., flecainide, mexiletine, propafenone, tocainide). ▪ Risk associated with antiarrhythmic drug therapy probably is greatest in patients with structural heart disease. ▪ IM injection of quinidine is not recommended; the kinetics of absorption may vary with the patient's peripheral perfusion. ▪ Causes prolongation of the QTc interval, which can lead to torsades de pointes. Risk increased in patients with bradycardia, hypokalemia, hypomagnesemia, and high serum quinidine levels. Best predictor of this arrhythmia appears to be the length of the QTc interval. Use quinidine with extreme caution in patients who have pre-existing long QT syndromes, who have a history of torsades de pointes, or who have previously responded to quinidine (or other antiarrhythmics) with marked lengthening of the QTc. ▪ Other ventricular arrhythmias (e.g., frequent extrasystoles, ventricular tachycardia, ventricular flutter, and ventricular fibrillation) have been reported. ▪ Has been associated with marked sinus node depression and bradycardia in patients with sick sinus syndrome. ▪ Use extreme caution with first- or second-degree blocks, extensive myocardial damage, digoxin intoxication, impaired liver or kidney function, and CHF. ▪ Use caution in atrial flutter or fibrillation; may require pretreatment with conduction-reducing drugs such as digoxin, verapamil, diltiazem, or beta-blockers to prevent progressive reduction of AV block and an extremely rapid ventricular rate. ▪ Even in patients without pre-existing cardiac disease, antimalarial use of quinidine has caused hypotension, increased QRS and QT intervals, and cinchonism (e.g., dizziness, ringing in ears). ▪ Because quinidine opposes the atrial and AV nodal effects of vagal stimulation, physical or pharmacologic vagal maneuvers used to terminate paroxysmal supraventricular tachycardia may be ineffective in patients taking quinidine. ▪ See Drug/Lab Interactions.

Monitor: Monitor patient's ECG and BP continuously (plus parasitemia in malaria). Too-rapid administration may cause marked hypotension or peripheral vascular collapse. ■ Keep patient in supine position. ■ Discontinue IV use when the normal sinus rhythm returns, HR falls to 120 beats/min, or any signs of cardiac toxicity occur (QRS complex widens to 130% of its pretreatment duration, QTc interval widens to 130% of its pretreatment duration and is then longer that 500 msec, P waves disappear, or patient develops significant tachycardia, symptomatic bradycardia, or hypotension). ■ Monitor serum levels if quinidine is used over 48 hours. ■ See Drug/Lab Interactions.

Patient Education: Promptly report breathing difficulty, dizziness, headache, nausea, ringing in the ears, skin rash, or visual disturbances.

Maternal/Child: Category C: safety for use in pregnancy not established. ■ Safety for use in breast-feeding not established. Present in breast milk. Avoid breast-feeding if possible. ■ Safety and effectiveness for antiarrhythmic use in pediatric patients not established. ■ In antimalarial trials, was as safe and effective in pediatric patients as in adults. ■ Half-life in pediatric patients is 3 to 4 hours.

Elderly: Reduced dose may be indicated; see Dose Adjustments. ■ Half-life prolonged; frequency and severity of side effects may be increased. ■ Response of elderly versus younger patients not documented.

DRUG/LAB INTERACTIONS

Interacts with many medications. Consult pharmacist. ■ Drugs that alkalinize urine (e.g., **sodium bicarbonate, carbonic-anhydrase inhibitors, thiazide diuretics**) reduce renal elimination of quinidine. ■ Quinidine levels increased with coadministration of **cimetidine** (Tagamet) **or amiodarone** (Nexterone). ■ Quinidine levels decreased with coadministration of **nifedipine** (Procardia). ■ Hepatic elimination increased with coadministration of **phenobarbital** (Luminal), **phenytoin** (Dilantin), **and rifampin** (Rifadin). ■ Hepatic clearance reduced when coadministered with **diltiazem** (Cardizem) **or verapamil.** ■ Metabolism may be decreased and serum levels increased with concurrent use of **ketoconazole** (Nizoral) **and itraconazole** (Sporanox); monitoring of quinidine levels suggested. Causes marked increase in **digoxin** (Lanoxin) levels. Digoxin dose reduction and monitoring required. ■ Potentiates **warfarin** (Coumadin). Warfarin dose reduction and monitoring required. ■ Increases serum levels of **haloperidol** (Haldol) **and procainamide** (Pronestyl). ■ Causes variable slowing of the metabolism of **nifedipine** (Procardia) and most likely of **felodipine** (Plendil), **nicardipine** (Cardene), **and nimodipine.** ■ Potentiates the action of **depolarizing and nondepolarizing neuromuscular blockers** (e.g., succinylcholine [Anectine], pancuronium). ■ Therapeutic levels of quinidine inhibit cytochrome P2D6. Use with caution with drugs that are metabolized by this enzyme (e.g., mexiletine, some phenothiazines, most polycyclic antidepressants). ■ **Contraindicated** with **ritonavir** (Norvir); may cause life-threatening arrhythmias. ■ Quinidine does not affect the pharmacokinetics of diltiazem (Cardizem), flecainide (Tambocor), mephenytoin, metoprolol (Lopressor), propafenone (Rhythmol), propranolol, quinine, timolol (Betimol), or tocainide (Tonocard). ■ Pharmacokinetics of quinidine are not affected by caffeine, ciprofloxacin (Cipro), digoxin (Lanoxin), felodipine (Plendil), omeprazole (Prilosec), or quinine. ■ **Grapefruit juice** may affect certain enzymes of the P450 enzyme system and should be avoided.

SIDE EFFECTS

Most common side effects include diarrhea, nausea, upper GI distress, and vomiting. Less commonly reported side effects include angina-like pain, apprehension, ataxia, autoimmune syndromes, change in sleep habits, cinchonism (a syndrome that may include blurred vision, confusion, deafness, delirium, diplopia, headache, photophobia, reversible high-frequency hearing loss, tinnitus, and vertigo), diaphoresis, discoordination, fatigue, fever, headache, inflammatory syndromes, nervousness, rash, tremor, urge to defecate, urge to void, vertigo, visual disturbances, weakness.

Major: Potentially fatal arrhythmias (including atrioventricular heart block, cardiac standstill, prolonged PR or QT intervals, or 50% widening of QRS complex; tachycardia; ventricular fibrillation), acidosis, arthralgia, coma, confusion, hypokalemia, hypotension (acute), lethargy, myalgia, paresthesia, respiratory depression or arrest, thrombocytopenia purpura, seizures, urticaria.

Overdose: Blurred vision, confusion, delirium, diarrhea, diplopia, headache, high-frequency hearing loss, hypotension, photophobia, tinnitus, ventricular arrhythmias, vertigo, and vomiting.

ANTIDOTE

Notify the physician of any side effects. If minor symptoms progress or if any major side effect appears, discontinue the drug immediately and notify the physician. Discontinue IV use when the normal sinus rhythm returns, HR falls to 120 beats/min, or any signs of cardiac toxicity occur (QRS complex widens to 130% of its pretreatment duration, QTc interval widens to 130% of its pretreatment duration and is then longer than 500 msec, P waves disappear, or patient develops significant tachycardia, symptomatic bradycardia, or hypotension). Another source suggests decreasing the rate or interrupting the infusion if corrected QT interval exceeds 0.6 seconds, corrected QT interval exceeds baseline by more than 25%, QRS widening exceeds 50% of baseline, or hypotension that does not respond to fluid expansion develops. Treatment of hemodynamically unstable polymorphic ventricular tachycardia (including torsades de pointes) is either immediate cardioversion or, if a cardiac pacemaker is in place or is immediately available, immediate overdrive pacing. After cardioversion or pacing, further management must be guided by the length of the QTc interval. Continuous electrocardiographic monitoring required. Use fluid replacement and Trendelenburg positioning and dopamine or norepinephrine (Levophed) to correct hypotension. In overdose, monitoring of blood gases and electrolytes are indicated. Treatment of toxicity is symptomatic and supportive. Resuscitate as necessary.

QUINUPRISTIN/DALFOPRISTIN
(kwin-oo-**PRIS**-tin/**DAL**-foh-**pris**-tin)

Synercid

Antibacterial
(Streptogramin)

pH 4.5 to 4.75

USUAL DOSE
Complicated skin and skin structure infection: 7.5 mg/kg every 12 hours. Minimum recommended duration of therapy is 7 days.

PEDIATRIC DOSE
Safety and effectiveness for use in pediatric patients under 16 years of age not established. Doses of 7.5 mg/kg every 8 or 12 hours have been used under emergency-use conditions in a limited number of pediatric patients; dose adjustment does not seem to be required.

DOSE ADJUSTMENTS
No dose adjustments required in the elderly, pediatric patients, patients with renal insufficiency, or patients undergoing hemodialysis or peritoneal dialysis. See Maternal/Child. ■ Dose reduction may be required in patients with hepatic cirrhosis (Child Pugh A or B). Exact recommendations are not currently available, but one source recommends decreasing dose to 5 mg/kg in patients who cannot tolerate the usual dose. ■ Patients experiencing arthralgias and myalgias may respond to a reduction in dose frequency to every 12 hours; see Precautions. ■ See Drug/Lab Interactions.

DILUTION
Reconstitute the 500-mg single-dose vial by slowly adding 5 mL of D5W or SW. Swirl gently to limit foam formation. Do not shake. Allow solution to sit until foam has disappeared. Final concentration of reconstituted solution is 100 mg/mL. Must be further diluted, withdraw calculated dose and add to 250 mL of D5W. Desired concentration is approximately 2 mg/mL. If moderate to severe venous irritation occurs following peripheral administration, consideration should be given to increasing infusion volume to 500 to 750 mL of D5W; see Precautions. An infusion volume of 100 mL may be used for central line infusions.

Storage: Store unopened vials in refrigerator at 2° to 8° C (36° to 46° F). Reconstituted solution should be used within 30 minutes. Diluted solution is stable for 5 hours at RT and for 54 hours if refrigerated.

COMPATIBILITY   (Underline Indicates Conflicting Compatibility Information)
Consider any drug NOT listed as compatible to be INCOMPATIBLE until consulting a pharmacist; specific conditions may apply.

Manufacturer lists saline solutions and heparin as **incompatible** and recommends administering quinupristin/dalfopristin separately. Always flush line with D5W before and after administration of any other drug through the same IV line.

Manufacturer lists **Y-site compatibility** with specific concentrations of aztreonam (Azactam [20 mg/mL]), ciprofloxacin (Cipro IV [1 mg/mL]), fluconazole (Diflucan [2 mg/mL]), haloperidol (Haldol [0.2 mg/mL]), metoclopramide (Reglan [5 mg/mL]), and potassium chloride (KCl [40 mEq/L]). Another source adds anidulafungin (Eraxis), caspofungin (Cancidas), and fenoldopam (Corlopam).

RATE OF ADMINISTRATION

Flush IV line with D5W before and after administration. A single dose properly diluted over 60 minutes. Use of an infusion pump or device to control rate of infusion is recommended. In animal studies toxicity was higher when administered as a bolus. Studies in humans have not been performed.

ACTIONS

A streptogramin antimicrobial agent composed of two semisynthetic pristinamycin derivatives, quinupristin and dalfopristin, in a ratio of 30:70 (w:w). Quinupristin and dalfopristin bind to the bacterial ribosome, thereby inhibiting protein synthesis. When combined, the two components act synergistically. The compound is bactericidal against strains of methicillin-susceptible and methicillin-resistant staphylococci. Cross-resistance between quinupristin/dalfopristin and other antibacterial agents such as beta-lactams, aminoglycosides, glycopeptides, quinolones, macrolides, lincosamides and tetracyclines has not been reported. Metabolized in the liver via non-enzymatic processes to several active metabolites. Elimination half-life of quinupristin and dalfopristin is approximately 0.85 and 0.7 hours, respectively. Although the elimination half-life for each component is short, the combination exhibits a prolonged post-antibiotic effect of 10 hours with *Staphylococcus aureus* and 9.1 hours with *Streptococcus pneumoniae*. Fecal excretion is the primary elimination route for both components and their metabolites. Urinary excretion accounts for about 15% of the quinupristin and 19% of the dalfopristin dose.

INDICATIONS AND USES

Treatment of complicated skin and skin structure infections caused by *Staphylococcus aureus* (methicillin susceptible) or *Streptococcus pyogenes*.

CONTRAINDICATIONS

Known hypersensitivity to quinupristin/dalfopristin or to other streptogramins (e.g., pristinamycin or virginiamycin).

PRECAUTIONS

C/S indicated to determine susceptibility of causative organism to quinupristin/dalfopristin. ▪ Flush line with D5W after completion of peripheral infusion to minimize vein irritation. If moderate to severe venous irritation occurs with 250-mL infusion, consider increasing volume to 500 or 750 mL of D5W, changing the infusion site, or infusing by a peripherally inserted central catheter (PICC) or a central venous catheter; see Dilution. Concomitant administration of hydrocortisone or diphenhydramine does *not* appear to alleviate venous irritation. ▪ Episodes of arthralgia and myalgia have been reported. In some patients, improvement was noted with a reduction in dose frequency to every 12 hours; see Dose Adjustments. ▪ Superinfection caused by the overgrowth of nonsusceptible organisms may occur with antibiotic use. Treat as indicated. ▪ *Clostridium difficile*–associated diarrhea (CDAD) has been reported. May range from mild diarrhea to fatal colitis. Consider in patients who present with diarrhea during or after treatment with quinupristin/dalfopristin.

Monitor: Monitor total bilirubin. Levels greater than 5 times the upper limit of normal were reported in approximately 25% of patients. ▪ Monitor infusion site for any sign of irritation or inflammation; see Precautions.

Patient Education: Report pain at injection site or any other side effect promptly. ▪ Promptly report diarrhea or bloody stools that occur during treatment or up to several months after an antibiotic has been discontinued; may indicate CDAD and require treatment.
Maternal/Child: Category B: safety for use in pregnancy and breast-feeding not established. Use caution. ▪ Safety and effectiveness in pediatric patients under 16 years of age not established. Has been used in a limited number of pediatric patients under emergency-use conditions. Dose adjustment does not appear to be required; see Pediatric Dose.
Elderly: No apparent differences in frequency, type, or severity of side effects. Dose adjustment not required.

DRUG/LAB INTERACTIONS
Quinupristin/dalfopristin significantly inhibits cytochrome P_{450} 3A4 metabolism of **cyclosporin A** (Sandimmune), **midazolam** (Versed), **nifedipine** (Procardia), **and tacrolimus** (Prograf) and increases their plasma concentrations, dose adjustments may be indicated. Monitoring of cyclosporine and/or tacrolimus serum levels to determine therapeutic dose should be performed when cyclosporine or tacrolimus must be used concomitantly with quinupristin/dalfopristin. ▪ It is reasonable to expect that quinupristin/dalfopristin would **inhibit other drugs that are metabolized by the P_{450} 3A4 enzyme system.** Use caution if being coadministered with **drugs that have a narrow therapeutic index** (e.g., cyclosporine) and are metabolized via this pathway. Effects may be prolonged, side effects may be increased, dose adjustments may be indicated. Some drugs that are predicted to have elevated plasma concentrations when coadministered with quinupristin/ dalfopristin are **carbamazepine** (Tegretol), **cisapride** (Propulsid), **delavirdine** (Rescriptor), **diazepam** (Valium), **dihydropyridines** (e.g., nifedipine [Procardia]), **diltiazem** (Cardizem), **disopyramide** (Norpace), **docetaxel** (Taxotere), **HMA-CoA reductase inhibitors** (e.g., lovastatin [Mevacor], simvastatin [Zocor]), **lidocaine, quinidine, indinavir** (Crixivan), **methylprednisolone** (Solu-Medrol), **nevirapine** (Viramune), **paclitaxel** (Taxol), **ritonavir** (Norvir), **verapamil, vinca alkaloids** (e.g., vinblastine). ▪ Concomitant medications metabolized by the P_{450} 3A4 enzyme system that **may prolong the QTc interval** should be avoided. ▪ May increase **digoxin** levels. If S/S of digoxin toxicity occur, monitor digoxin levels. ▪ In vitro combination testing of quinupristin/dalfopristin with aztreonam, cefotaxime (Claforan), ciprofloxacin, and gentamicin against *Enterobacteriaceae* and *Pseudomonas aeruginosa* did not show antagonism. ▪ In vitro combination testing of quinupristin/dalfopristin prototype drugs of the following classes: aminoglycosides (gentamicin), beta-lactams (cefepime, ampicillin, and amoxicillin), glycopeptides (vancomycin), quinolones (ciprofloxacin), tetracyclines (doxycycline), and also chloramphenicol against enterococci and staphylococci did not show antagonism. See Actions.

SIDE EFFECTS
Allergic reaction; arthralgia; diarrhea; edema, inflammation, and/or pain at infusion site; edema, elevated total and conjugated bilirubin; headache; myalgia; nausea; pain; pruritus; rash; thrombophlebitis; thrombus; and vomiting are reported most frequently. Numerous other side effects have been reported in fewer than 1% of patients. CDAD has been reported. ▪ Numerous laboratory abnormalities were noted during studies but were not significantly different than those seen in the comparator group. See literature.

ANTIDOTE

Notify physician of any side effects. Discontinue drug if indicated. Treat hypersensitivity reactions as indicated. Observation and supportive therapy are indicated in an overdose situation. Is not removed by hemodialysis or peritoneal dialysis. Treat CDAD with fluids, electrolytes, protein supplements, and oral vancomycin (Vancocin) or metronidazole (Flagyl) as indicated. In severe cases, surgical evaluation may be indicated. Resuscitate as necessary.

RANITIDINE
(rah-**NIH**-tih-deen)

H₂ antagonist
Antiulcer agent
Gastric acid inhibitor

Zantac

pH 6.7 to 7.3

USUAL DOSE

IV injection or intermittent infusion: 50 mg (2 mL) every 6 to 8 hours. Increase frequency of dose, not amount, if necessary for pain relief. 50 mg every 8 to 12 hours may be used short term to replace an oral dose of 150 mg every 12 hours in patients unable to take oral meds. Do not exceed 400 mg/day.

Continuous infusion: 150 mg may be given as a continuous infusion equally distributed over 24 hours. To maintain intergastric acid secretion rates at 10 mEq/hr or less, dose range may be higher in patients with pathologic hypersecretory syndrome (Zollinger-Ellison). Literature suggests an initial dose of 1 mg/kg/hr. Measure gastric acid output in 4 hours. If above 10 mEq/hr or symptoms recur, adjust dose upward in 0.5 mg/kg/hr increments. Up to 2.5 mg/kg/hr has been used.

Additive for total parental nutrition (TPN [unlabeled]): 70% to 100% of an average 24-hour dose has been used equally distributed over 24 hours as a continuous infusion. May be supplemented with intermittent doses as needed.

Perioperatively to prevent pulmonary aspiration during anesthesia (unlabeled): 45 to 50 mg 60 minutes before anesthesia.

Prophylaxis and/or control of GI hemorrhage associated with stress ulcers (unlabeled): 150 mg over 24 hours.

PEDIATRIC DOSE

Safety for selective use in pediatric patients from 1 month to 16 years of age established; see Indications.

One source suggests:

Infants and other pediatric patients: 2 to 4 mg/kg/24 hr in equally divided doses every 6 to 8 hours (0.5 to 1 mg/kg every 6 hours or 0.67 to 1.3 mg/kg every 8 hours). Do not exceed 50 mg/dose.

NEONATAL DOSE

Safety for use of IV ranitidine in neonates less than 1 month of age not established; see Maternal/Child.

2 mg/kg every 12 to 24 hours or as a continuous infusion.

Another source suggests 2 mg/kg/24 hr in equally divided doses every 6 to 8 hours (0.5 mg/kg every 6 hours or 0.67 mg/kg every 8 hours).

DOSE ADJUSTMENTS
Dose selection should be cautious in the elderly. ■ If the CrCl is less than 50 mL/min, reduce dose to 50 mg every 18 to 24 hours. Gradually increase to 50 mg every 12 hours, or 6 hours with caution if indicated. Adjust schedule to be given after dialysis.

DILUTION
IV injection: Each vial containing 50 mg (2 mL) must be diluted with 18 mL of NS or other **compatible** infusion solution for injection (D5W, D10W, LR, 5% sodium bicarbonate). Concentration of solution must be no greater than 2.5 mg/mL. Additional diluent may be used.
Intermittent infusion: Available premixed as a 1 mg/mL solution in 50 mL. May be given without further dilution. Or each 50 mg may be diluted in 100 mL (0.5 mg/mL) of D5W or other **compatible** infusion solution and given piggyback. Concentration of solution should be no greater than 0.5 mg/mL. Manufacturer recommends discontinuing primary IV during intermittent infusion to avoid incompatibilities. Do not use premixed plastic containers in series connections; may cause air embolism.
Continuous infusion: Total daily dose may be diluted in 250 mL of D5W or other **compatible** infusion solution. For Zollinger-Ellison patients, concentration of solution must be no greater than 2.5 mg/mL. In all situations, avoid any contact with aluminum during administration (e.g., needles). Inspect for color and clarity. Slight darkening of solution does not affect potency. **Compatible** in selected TPN solutions for 24 hours (consult pharmacist).
Storage: Store at CRT protected from light. Stable at room temperature for 48 hours after dilution.

COMPATIBILITY   (Underline Indicates Conflicting Compatibility Information)
Consider any drug NOT listed as compatible to be INCOMPATIBLE until consulting a pharmacist; specific conditions may apply.
Manufacturer states, "Additives should not be introduced into the premixed solution, and the primary IV should be discontinued during ranitidine infusion."
Solution: D5½NS, <u>IV fat emulsion 10%</u>, selected TNA and TPN solutions; see Dilution.
One source suggests the following **compatibilities:**
Additive: *See previous comments under Compatibility.* Acetazolamide (Diamox), amikacin (Amikin), aminophylline, <u>ampicillin</u>, chloramphenicol (Chloromycetin), chlorothiazide (Diuril), ciprofloxacin (Cipro IV), <u>clindamycin (Cleocin)</u>, colistimethate (Coly-Mycin M), dexamethasone (Decadron), digoxin (Lanoxin), dobutamine, dopamine, doxycycline, epinephrine (Adrenalin), erythromycin (Erythrocin), flumazenil (Romazicon), furosemide (Lasix), gentamicin, heparin, <u>insulin (regular)</u>, isoproterenol (Isuprel), lidocaine, lincomycin (Lincocin), meropenem (Merrem IV), methylprednisolone (Solu-Medrol), midazolam (Versed), nitroprusside sodium, <u>norepinephrine (Levophed)</u>, penicillin G potassium and sodium, potassium chloride (KCl), protamine sulfate, quinidine gluconate, tobramycin, vancomycin, zidovudine (AZT, Retrovir).
Y-site: Acyclovir (Zovirax), aldesleukin (Proleukin), allopurinol (Aloprim), amifostine (Ethyol), aminophylline, <u>anidulafungin (Eraxis)</u>, atracurium (Tracrium), aztreonam (Azactam), bivalirudin (Angiomax), cefazolin

(Ancef), cefepime (Maxipime), cefoxitin (Mefoxin), ceftazidime (Fortaz), ciprofloxacin (Cipro IV), cisatracurium (Nimbex), cisplatin (Platinol), cladribine (Leustatin), cyclophosphamide (Cytoxan), cytarabine (ARA-C), dexmedetomidine (Precedex), diltiazem (Cardizem), dobutamine, docetaxel (Taxotere), dopamine, doripenem (Doribax), doxapram (Dopram), doxorubicin (Adriamycin), doxorubicin liposomal (Doxil), enalaprilat (Vasotec IV), epinephrine (Adrenalin), esmolol (Brevibloc), etoposide phosphate (Etopophos), fenoldopam (Corlopam), fentanyl (Sublimaze), filgrastim (Neupogen), fluconazole (Diflucan), fludarabine (Fludara), foscarnet (Foscavir), furosemide (Lasix), gallium nitrate (Ganite), gemcitabine (Gemzar), granisetron (Kytril), heparin, hetastarch in electrolytes (Hextend), hydromorphone (Dilaudid), idarubicin (Idamycin), labetalol (Trandate), linezolid (Zyvox), lorazepam (Ativan), melphalan (Alkeran), meperidine (Demerol), methotrexate, midazolam (Versed), milrinone (Primacor), morphine, nicardipine (Cardene IV), nitroglycerin IV, norepinephrine (Levophed), ondansetron (Zofran), oxaliplatin (Eloxatin), paclitaxel (Taxol), pancuronium, pemetrexed (Alimta), piperacillin, piperacillin/ tazobactam (Zosyn), procainamide (Pronestyl), propofol (Diprivan), remifentanil (Ultiva), sargramostim (Leukine), tacrolimus (Prograf), teniposide (Vumon), theophylline, thiopental (Pentothal), thiotepa, tigecycline (Tygacil), vecuronium, vinorelbine (Navelbine), warfarin (Coumadin), zidovudine (AZT, Retrovir).

RATE OF ADMINISTRATION

Too-rapid administration has precipitated rare instances of bradycardia, tachycardia, and PVCs.

IV injection: Each 50 mg or fraction thereof at a rate not to exceed 4 mL/min diluted solution (20 mL over 5 min).

Intermittent infusion: Each 50-mg dose over 15 to 20 minutes.

Continuous infusion: Total daily dose equally distributed over 24 hours. Should not exceed a rate of 6.25 mg/hr (10.7 mL/hr if 150 mg [6 mL ranitidine] is diluted in 250 mL). Use of infusion pump preferred to avoid complications of overdose or too-rapid administration.

ACTIONS

A histamine H_2 antagonist, it inhibits both daytime and nocturnal basal gastric acid secretion. It also inhibits gastric acid secretion stimulated by food, histamine, bentazole, and pentagastrin. Not an anticholinergic agent. Does not lower calcium levels in hypercalcemia. Onset of action is prompt and effective for 6 to 8 hours. 5 to 12 times more potent than cimetidine. Half-life is 2 to 2.5 hours. Metabolized in the liver. Excreted in the urine. 70% of a dose is recovered in urine as unchanged drug. Crosses placental barrier. Secreted in breast milk.

INDICATIONS AND USES

Short-term treatment of intractable duodenal ulcers and pathologic hypersecretory conditions in the hospitalized patient. ▪ Treatment of active benign gastric ulcers in those patients unable to take oral medication. ▪ Treatment of duodenal ulcers in pediatric patients from 1 month to 16 years of age. Safety for use in pathologic hypersecretory conditions not established. ▪ Oral dosing for treatment of duodenal and gastric ulcers, maintenance of healing of duodenal and gastric ulcers, and treatment of GERD and erosive esophagitis has been approved for pediatric patients from 1 month to 16 years of age; see package insert.

Unlabeled uses: Perioperatively to suppress gastric acid secretion, prevent stress ulcers, and prevent aspiration pneumonitis. ▪ Reduce the incidence of GI hemorrhage associated with stress ulcers. ▪ Additive to TPN to simplify fluid and electrolyte management (decreases the volume and chloride content of gastric secretions).

CONTRAINDICATIONS
Known hypersensitivity to ranitidine or its components.

PRECAUTIONS
Use antacids concomitantly to relieve pain. ▪ Gastric malignancy may be present even though patient's symptoms improve on ranitidine therapy. ▪ Use caution in patients with impaired hepatic or renal function. ▪ Avoid use in patients with acute porphyria; may precipitate acute porphyric attacks. ▪ Gastric pain and ulceration may recur after medication stopped. ▪ Effects maintained with oral dosage. Total treatment usually discontinued after 6 weeks.

Monitor: Observe frequently; monitor vital signs and pain levels. ▪ Obtain baseline SCr. Monitor periodically during extended course of treatment. ▪ Monitor ALT if therapy exceeds 400 mg for over 5 days. ▪ Change to oral dose when appropriate. ▪ See Drug/Lab Interactions.

Patient Education: Stop smoking or at least avoid smoking after the last dose of the day. ▪ May increase blood alcohol levels.

Maternal/Child: Category B: use during pregnancy or breast-feeding only when clearly needed. ▪ No significant difference in pharmacokinetic parameter values between pediatric patients over 1 month of age and healthy adults when correction is made for body weight. ▪ Safety for use of IV ranitidine in neonates less than 1 month of age not established; however, limited data suggest that ranitidine may be useful and safe in increasing gastric pH for infants at risk of GI hemorrhage. ▪ Half-life in neonates averages 6.6 hours.

Elderly: Use caution in dose selection; monitoring of renal function suggested; see Dose Adjustments. ▪ Half-life is prolonged (3.1 hours) and total clearance is decreased due to reduced renal function. ▪ Differences in response between elderly and younger patients not identified; greater sensitivity of some elderly cannot be ruled out. ▪ Agitation, confusion (reversible), depression, and hallucination have been reported.

DRUG/LAB INTERACTIONS
Concurrent use with **warfarin** may result in increased or decreased PT and/or INR. Close monitoring is recommended. ▪ High doses of ranitidine may reduce the renal excretion of **procainamide;** monitoring for procainamide toxicity is suggested if ranitidine doses exceed 300 mg/day. ▪ May increase serum concentrations of **sulfonylureas** (e.g., glipizide); monitor blood glucose and adjust dose as indicated. ▪ Increased pH may reduce the antibiotic effectiveness of selected **cephalosporins** (e.g., cefpodoxime [Vantin], cefuroxime [Zinacef]). ▪ Increased pH may impair the absorption of **atazanavir** (Reyataz) **and delavirdine** (Rescriptor). ▪ Effectiveness of **gefitinib** (Iressa) may be reduced if coadministered with ranitidine and sodium bicarbonate. ▪ Reduces the plasma concentrations and antibiotic effectiveness of **enoxacin** (Penetrex). ▪ Monitor for excessive sedation with concurrent administration of selected **benzodiazepines** (e.g., midazolam [Versed], triazolam [Halcion]). ▪ May potentiate the effects of **alcohol.** ▪ May inhibit gastric absorption of **ketoconazole** (Nizoral) and reduce antifungal effects. ▪ Clinical effect (inhibition of nocturnal gastric secre-

tions) may be reversed by **cigarette smoking.** ▪ **Elevated ALT, slight elevation in SCr,** and a **false-positive for urine protein** with Multistix may occur.

SIDE EFFECTS

Abdominal discomfort, burning and itching at IV site, constipation, diarrhea, headache (severe), and nausea and vomiting are the most common side effects. Hypersensitivity reactions (bronchospasm, fever, rash, eosinophilia) can occur. Acute interstitial nephritis, agitation, alopecia, arthralgias, bradycardia, confusion, depression, dizziness, elevated ALT, erythema multiforme, galactorrhea (rare), gynecomastia (rare), hallucinations, hepatitis (reversible), impotence, insomnia, malaise, muscular pain, pneumonia, PVCs, somnolence, tachycardia, vasculitis, and vertigo occur rarely. See Drug/Lab Interactions.

ANTIDOTE

Notify physician of all side effects. May be treated symptomatically or may respond to decrease in frequency of dosage. Discontinue ranitidine if S/S of hepatitis with or without jaundice occur. Resuscitate as necessary for overdose. Hemodialysis or peritoneal dialysis may be indicated in overdose.

RASBURICASE   BBW

(ras-**BYOUR**-ih-kase)

Elitek

Antihyperuricemic

USUAL DOSE

Prehydration required; see Monitor.

0.15 or 0.2 mg/kg as a single daily dose each day for 5 days. Chemotherapy should be initiated 4 to 24 hours after the first dose. Safety and effectiveness of other schedules have not been evaluated. Dosing beyond 5 days and/or administration of more than one course of rasburicase is not recommended.

PEDIATRIC DOSE

Same as adult dose; see Maternal/Child.

DOSE ADJUSTMENTS

No dose adjustments recommended.

DILUTION

Each vial contains 1.5 mg of rasburicase. Determine the number of vials needed to provide the calculated dose. Reconstitute each vial with 1 mL of the diluent provided (SW and Poloxamer 188). Mix by swirling gently. *Do not shake.* Withdraw the calculated dose of reconstituted solution and inject into an infusion bag containing the appropriate volume of NS to achieve a final total volume of 50 mL. (For example a 20-kg child would receive a dose of 4 mg [20 kg × 0.2 mg/kg = 4 mg]. Reconstitute 3 vials, each with 1 mL of the diluent provided. Withdraw 2.7 mL of reconstituted solution and add to an infusion bag containing 47.3 mL of NS.)

Filters: *No filters should be used for the infusion.*

Storage: Refrigerate unopened lyophilized drug product and diluent. Do not freeze; protect from light. Both the reconstituted and diluted product may be stored for 24 hours if refrigerated. Discard any unused product.

COMPATIBILITY

Manufacturer states, "Should be infused through a different line than that used for the infusion of other concomitant medications. If use of a separate line is not possible, the line should be flushed with at least 15 mL of NS prior to and after infusion with rasburicase."

RATE OF ADMINISTRATION

A single dose as an infusion equally distributed over 30 minutes. *Do not administer as a bolus infusion. Do not filter infusion.*

ACTIONS

A recombinant urate-oxidase enzyme produced by genetic engineering. Catalyzes enzymatic oxidation of uric acid into an inactive and soluble metabolite (allantoin). Half-life is 18 hours.

INDICATIONS AND USES

Initial management of plasma uric acid levels in pediatric patients with leukemia, lymphoma, and solid tumor malignancies who are receiving anti-cancer therapy expected to result in tumor lysis and subsequent elevation of plasma uric acid.

CONTRAINDICATIONS

Glucose-6-phosphatase dehydrogenase (G6PD) deficiency or a history of hypersensitivity, hemolytic reactions, or methemoglobinemia reactions to rasburicase or any of its components.

PRECAUTIONS

May cause severe hypersensitivity reactions, including anaphylaxis. Reactions may occur at any time during treatment, including with the first dose; see Monitor and Antidote. ▪ Is immunogenic in healthy volunteers. May elicit antibodies that inhibit the activity of rasburicase. ▪ Has caused severe hemolytic reactions in patients with G6PD deficiency. It is recommended that patients at higher risk for G6PD deficiency (e.g., patients of African or Mediterranean descent) be screened before starting rasburicase therapy. See Contraindications and Antidote. ▪ Methemoglobinemia has been reported. Patients developed serious hypoxemia, requiring intervention and medical support. See Antidote.

Monitor: Monitor serum uric acid levels, electrolytes, and renal function before and during therapy. ▪ Patients should be hydrated intravenously according to standard medical practice for the management of plasma uric acid in patients at risk for tumor lysis syndrome (TLS). ▪ Maintain urine at neutral or slightly alkaline pH. To increase solubility of uric acid, alkalinity of urine may be increased with sodium bicarbonate. ▪ Observe for symptoms of TLS (e.g., hyperuricemia, hyperkalemia, hyperphosphatemia, and hypocalcemia). If untreated, may develop acute uric acid nephropathy, leading to renal failure. ▪ Monitor for S/S of a hypersensitivity reaction (e.g., anaphylaxis, bronchospasm, chest pain, dyspnea, hypotension, hypoxia, shock, urticaria). ▪ Will cause enzymatic degradation of uric acid within blood samples left at room temperature, resulting in falsely low uric acid levels. To ensure accurate measurement, blood must be collected into prechilled tubes containing heparin anticoagulant and immediately *immersed and maintained* in an ice water bath. Plasma samples must be prepared by centrifugation in a precooled centrifuge (4° C). Plasma samples must be analyzed within 4 hours of sample collection.

Patient Education: Report blood in urine, painful urination, or signs of a hypersensitivity reaction promptly.

Maternal/Child: Category C: studies have not been performed. Potential benefits must justify potential risks to fetus. ▪ Discontinue breast-feeding. ▪ Studied in pediatric patients from 1 month to 17 years of age. Pediatric patients less than 2 years of age had a higher mean uric acid AUC and a lower rate of success at achieving maintenance uric acid concentrations by 48 hours than older pediatric patients. They also experienced more toxicity (e.g., diarrhea, fever, rash, and vomiting).

Elderly: There are insufficient data to determine whether geriatric subjects, or adults in general, respond differently than pediatric patients.

DRUG/LAB INTERACTIONS

Studies have not been conducted. ▪ Does not metabolize allopurinol (Aloprim), cytarabine (ARA-C), methylprednisolone (Solu-Medrol), methotrexate, 6-mercaptopurine (Purinethol), thioguanine, etoposide (VePesid), etoposide phosphate (Etopophos), daunorubicin (Cerubidine), cyclophosphamide, or vincristine *in vitro*. Metabolic-based drug interactions are not anticipated with these agents. ▪ Did not affect the activity of P_{450} isoenzymes in preclinical *in vivo* studies. Clinically relevant P_{450}-mediated drug-drug interactions are not anticipated. ▪ Will cause enzymatic degradation of uric acid within blood samples left at room temperature, resulting in **falsely low uric acid levels;** see Monitor.

SIDE EFFECTS

The most serious adverse reactions observed are hemolysis, hypersensitivity reactions (e.g., anaphylaxis, chest pain, dyspnea, hypotension, urticaria), methemoglobinemia, and severe rash. Other, more commonly observed reactions include abdominal pain, acute renal failure, constipation, diarrhea, fever, headache, mucositis, nausea, neutropenia with or without fever, rash, respiratory distress, sepsis, and vomiting. Several other reactions have been observed in a small number of patients. Causality is uncertain. See product literature.

ANTIDOTE

Notify physician of all side effects. Should be immediately and permanently discontinued in patients who experience severe hypersensitivity reactions, hemolysis, or methemoglobinemia. Do not rechallenge. Treat anaphylaxis with epinephrine, corticosteroids (e.g., dexamethasone [Decadron]), oxygen, and antihistamines (diphenhydramine [Benadryl]). Hemolysis or methemoglobinemia may require transfusion support. Methylene blue may be required for treatment of methemoglobinemia. There is no specific antidote. Resuscitate as indicated.

REGADENOSON
(re-ga-**DEN**-oh-son)
Lexiscan

Diagnostic agent

pH 6.3 to 7.7

USUAL DOSE
0.4 mg (5 mL) as a rapid IV bolus. Given undiluted into a peripheral vein using a 22-gauge or larger catheter or needle. Immediately following dose, flush line with 5 mL of NS. Administer the radionuclide myocardial perfusion imaging agent 10 to 20 seconds after the NS flush. The radionuclide may be injected directly into the same catheter as the regadenoson.

DOSE ADJUSTMENTS
No dose adjustment is indicated based on age, gender, and race or for patients with hepatic or renal insufficiency. Has not been assessed in patients with end-stage renal disease.

DILUTION
Solution must be clear. Do not use if discolored or if particulate matter is present. Available in a single-use 0.4 mg/5 mL vial or syringe. Given undiluted into a peripheral vein using a 22-gauge or larger catheter or needle.
Filter: Information not available.
Storage: Store at CRT.

COMPATIBILITY
Specific information not available; see Dilution.

RATE OF ADMINISTRATION
Administer as a bolus injection over approximately 10 seconds.

ACTIONS
An adenosine receptor agonist that is a coronary vasodilator. It is a low-affinity agonist for the A_{2A} adenosine receptor. Activation of this receptor produces coronary vasodilation and a rapid increase in coronary blood flow that is sustained for a short duration. Mean average peak velocity of coronary blood flow increases to greater than twice the baseline level by 30 seconds and decreases to less than twice the baseline level within 10 minutes. Myocardial uptake of the radiopharmaceutical is proportional to coronary blood flow. Because regadenoson increases blood flow in normal coronary arteries with little or no increase in stenotic arteries, there is relatively less uptake of the radiopharmaceutical in areas of the heart supplied by stenotic arteries. Myocardial perfusion imaging intensity after administration is therefore greater in areas perfused by normal arteries than in areas perfused by stenosed arteries. Additional hemodynamic effects, which may be seen within 45 minutes of administration, include an increase in heart rate and a decrease in blood pressure. Peak plasma concentrations are achieved within 1 to 4 minutes. Half-life is approximately 2 hours. Metabolism is unknown. Excreted primarily as unchanged drug in the urine.

INDICATIONS AND USES
A pharmacologic stress agent indicated for radionuclide myocardial perfusion imaging (MPI) in patients unable to undergo adequate exercise stress.

CONTRAINDICATIONS

Second- or third-degree AV block or sinus node dysfunction unless a functioning artificial pacemaker is in place.

PRECAUTIONS

Pharmaceutical stress agents may induce myocardial ischemia, resulting in myocardial infarction, life-threatening ventricular arrhythmias, or fatal cardiac arrest. Patients with unstable angina may be at increased risk. Emergency resuscitation medications and equipment must be readily available. ■ May produce clinically significant increases in BP. These increases usually occur within minutes of administration and resolve within 10 to 15 minutes. These BP increases have lasted as long as 45 minutes in some patients; more often seen in patients with a history of hypertension and/or when myocardial perfusion imaging includes low-level exercise. ■ Can depress the SA and AV nodes and may cause sinus bradycardia or first-, second-, or third-degree AV block. Most episodes of AV block are asymptomatic and do not require intervention. ■ Induces arterial vasodilation and hypotension. Risk of serious hypotension may be higher in patients with autonomic dysfunction, hypovolemia, left main coronary artery stenosis, stenotic valvular heart disease, pericarditis or pericardial effusions, or stenotic carotid artery disease with cerebrovascular insufficiency. ■ May cause dyspnea, bronchoconstriction, and respiratory compromise. Use with caution in patients with known or suspected bronchoconstrictive disease, COPD, or asthma. Appropriate bronchodilator therapy and resuscitative measures should be readily available.

Monitor: ECG monitoring during administration and imaging is recommended. ■ Monitor BP and HR. ■ Monitor respiratory status.

Patient Education: Avoid consumption of any products containing methylxanthines for at least 12 hours before the study, including caffeinated coffee, tea, or other caffeinated beverages; caffeine-containing drug products; and theophylline. ■ Promptly report side effects such as shortness of breath, headache, and flushing. ■ Patients with COPD or asthma should discuss respiratory history and the administration of pre-study and post-study bronchodilator therapy before scheduling a study.

Maternal/Child: Category C: use in pregnancy only if the potential benefit justifies the risk to the fetus. ■ Consider interrupting breast-feeding for 10 hours after administration of regadenoson. ■ Safety and effectiveness for use in pediatric patients not established.

Elderly: Older patients have a similar side effect profile compared with younger patients but may have a higher incidence of hypotension.

DRUG/LAB INTERACTIONS

Formal pharmacokinetic drug interaction studies have not been conducted. ■ **Methylxanthines** (e.g., caffeine and theophylline) are nonspecific adenosine receptor antagonists and may interfere with the vasodilation activity of regadenoson. Separate the administration of theophylline preparations or the consumption of any products containing methylxanthines from the administration of regadenoson by at least 12 hours. ■ **Aminophylline** (a methylxanthine) may be used to attenuate severe or persistent adverse reactions to regadenoson. ■ **Dipyridamole** (Persantine) or **aspirin and dipyridamole** (Aggrenox) may change the effects of regadenoson. When possible, hold dipyridamole or aspirin and dipyridamole for at least 2 days before regadenoson administration. ■ Has been administered to patients taking other cardioactive drugs, including beta-blockers (e.g., metoprolol

[Lopressor]), calcium channel blockers (e.g., diltiazem [Cardizem]), ACE inhibitors (lisinopril [Zestril]), nitrates (nitroglycerin), cardiac glycosides (e.g., digoxin [Lanoxin]), and angiotensin receptor blockers (e.g., losartan [Cozaar]). ■ Does not appear to alter the pharmacokinetics of drugs metabolized by the cytochrome P_{450} system.

SIDE EFFECTS

Most side effects begin soon after dosing and generally resolve within approximately 15 minutes, except for headache, which resolves in most patients within 30 minutes. Side effects include abdominal discomfort, angina or ST segment depression, chest discomfort, chest pain, dizziness, dysgeusia, dyspnea, ECG abnormalities (e.g., first- or second-degree AV block, conduction abnormalities, PACs, PVCs), feeling hot, flushing, headache, nausea.

Overdose: Dizziness, flushing, increased heart rate.

Post-Marketing: Abdominal pain (may be severe) with myalgias, nausea, and vomiting; diarrhea and fecal incontinence; dyspnea and wheezing; heart block (including third-degree block) and asystole; marked hypertension; musculoskeletal pain in the arms, lower back, buttocks, and lower legs; seizures; and symptomatic hypotension, transient ischemic attack, and syncope requiring intervention with fluids and/or aminophylline.

ANTIDOTE

Notify physician of any side effects; most will be treated symptomatically. Aminophylline (50 to 250 mg IV) may be administered to attenuate severe and/or persistent side effects. Treat conduction abnormalities as indicated. Resuscitate as necessary.

RETEPLASE RECOMBINANT
(**REE**-teh-place re-**KOM**-buh-nant)

Retavase, r-PA

Thrombolytic agent
(recombinant)

pH 7 to 7.4

USUAL DOSE
Administered concomitantly with heparin. Give a 5,000-unit IV bolus of heparin before the initial injection of reteplase, then give 10 units (10 mL) of reteplase as an IV injection. Follow with a 1,000 unit/hr continuous IV infusion of heparin for at least 24 hours. Give a second 10-unit bolus of reteplase 30 minutes after the first. See Dilution, Compatibility, and Rate of Administration. Aspirin is also used either during or following heparin treatment; an initial dose of 160 to 350 mg is followed by doses of 75 to 350 mg.

DOSE ADJUSTMENTS
The second bolus should not be given if serious bleeding in a critical location (e.g., intracranial, gastrointestinal, retroperitoneal, pericardial) occurs before it is due to be given.

DILUTION
Supplied in a kit with all components for reconstitution. Each kit contains a package insert and two of each of the following: single-use reteplase vials (10.8 units each), single-use diluent vials of SW (10 mL each), sterile 10-mL syringes with 20-gauge needles attached, sterile dispensing pins, sterile 20-gauge needles for administration, and alcohol swabs. Withdraw diluent with 20-gauge needle. Discard needle and put dispensing pin on syringe of diluent. Transfer diluent to vial of reteplase. Pin and syringe should remain in place while vial is swirled to dissolve reteplase. *Do not shake.* When completely dissolved, withdraw 10 mL reconstituted solution into the syringe (vials are 0.7 mL overfilled). Remove dispensing pin and replace with a 20-gauge needle for administration.

Storage: Kit should remain sealed to protect contents from light. Store at 2° to 25° C (36° to 77° F). Do not use beyond expiration date. Contains no preservatives; should be reconstituted immediately before use, but may be stored at room temperature if used within 4 hours. Discard all unused solution and supplies.

COMPATIBILITY
Manufacturer states, "Should be given via an IV line in which no other medication is being simultaneously injected or infused. No other medication should be added to the injection solution containing reteplase. **Incompatible** with heparin; do not administer heparin in the same IV line unless the line is flushed through with NS or D5W before and after reteplase."

RATE OF ADMINISTRATION
Heparin: First 1,000 units over 1 minute. After this test dose, the balance of 4,000 units may be given over 1 minute. Follow with an infusion of 1,000 units/hr.

Reteplase: A single dose evenly distributed over 2 minutes. To avoid **incompatibilities** and ensure delivery of both doses, be sure to flush line with a minimum of 30 to 50 mL NS or D5W before and after each injection.

ACTIONS

A recombinant plasminogen activator. Exerts its thrombolytic action by generating plasmin from plasminogen through a specific process. Plasmin then degrades the fibrin matrix of the thrombus. Potency is expressed in units that are specific to reteplase. With therapeutic doses, a decrease in circulating fibrinogen makes the patient susceptible to bleeding. Onset of action is prompt, effecting patency of the vessel within 90 minutes in most patients. The FDA has allowed the manufacturer to claim superiority over alteplase at achieving patency within 90 minutes. Prompt opening of arteries increases probability of improved cardiac function. Half-life is 13 to 16 minutes. Cleared from the plasma by the liver and kidneys. Mean fibrinogen level should return to baseline value within 48 hours.

INDICATIONS AND USES

Management of acute myocardial infarction (AMI) in adults for the improvement of ventricular function following AMI, the reduction of the incidence of congestive failure, and the reduction of mortality associated with AMI. Treatment should begin as soon as possible after the onset of symptoms of AMI. ■ Current AHA and JAMA recommendations identify thrombolytic agents as Class 1 therapy in patients younger than 70 years with recent onset of chest pain (within 6 hours) consistent with AMI and at least 0.1 mV of ST segment elevation in at least two ECG leads. Use in all other patients based on age, accurate diagnosis, and time from onset of chest pain.

CONTRAINDICATIONS

Active internal bleeding, arteriovenous malformation or aneurysm, bleeding diathesis, history of cerebral vascular accident, intracranial or intraspinal surgery or trauma within 2 months, intracranial neoplasm, severe uncontrolled hypertension.

PRECAUTIONS

Administered under the direction of a physician knowledgeable in its use and with appropriate emergency drugs, diagnostic and laboratory facilities available. ■ Reperfusion arrhythmias occur frequently (e.g., sinus bradycardia, accelerated idioventricular rhythm, PVCs, ventricular tachycardia); have antiarrhythmic meds available at bedside. ■ A greater alteration of hemostatic status than with heparin. Strict bed rest indicated to reduce risk of bleeding. Use extreme care with the patient; avoid any excessive or rough handling or pressure (including too-frequent BPs); avoid invasive procedures (e.g., arterial puncture, venipuncture, IM injection). If these procedures are absolutely necessary, use extreme precautionary methods (use radial artery instead of femoral; small-gauge catheters and needles, and sites that are easily observed and compressible where bleeding can be controlled; avoid handling of catheter sites, and use extended pressure application of up to 30 minutes). Minor bleeding occurs often at catheter insertion sites. Avoid use of razors and toothbrushes. ■ Use extreme caution and weigh risks against anticipated benefits in the following situation: recent major surgery (e.g., coronary artery bypass graft, obstetric delivery, organ biopsy), previous puncture of noncompressible vessels (e.g., jugular, subclavian), cerebrovascular disease, recent GI or GU bleeding, recent trauma, hypertension (e.g., systolic BP equal to or greater than 180 mm Hg and/or diastolic BP equal to or greater than 110 mm Hg), high likelihood of left heart thrombus (e.g., mitral stenosis with atrial fibrillation), acute pericarditis, subacute bacterial endocarditis, hemostatic defects including those secondary to severe hepatic or renal disease, severe hepatic or renal dysfunction, pregnancy, diabetic hemorrhagic retinopathy or other hemorrhagic ophthalmic conditions, septic thrombophlebitis or occluded AV cannula at a seriously infected site, advanced age, patients currently receiving oral anticoagulants (e.g., warfarin [Coumadin]), any other condition in which bleeding constitutes a significant hazard or would be particularly difficult to manage because of its location. ▪ Simultaneous therapy with continuous infusion of heparin is used to reduce the risk of rethrombosis. Markedly increases risk of bleeding. ▪ Standard treatment for myocardial infarction continues simultaneously with reteplase therapy except if temporarily contraindicated (e.g., arterial blood gases) unless absolutely necessary. ▪ No experience with patients receiving repeat courses of reteplase. ▪ Cholesterol embolization has been reported and may be fatal.

Monitor: Best to establish separate IV lines for reteplase and heparin. If not appropriate, be sure to flush the IV line before and after each injection of reteplase. ▪ Baseline ECG, CPK, and clotting studies (TT, PTT, CBC, fibrinogen level, platelets) and baseline assessment (patient condition, pain, hematomas, petechiae, or recent wounds) should be completed before administration. Type and cross-match may also be ordered. ▪ Monitor ECG continuously, and record strips with greatest ST segment elevation initially and every 15 minutes for at least 4 hours. A 12-lead ECG is indicated when therapy is complete. ▪ Maintain strict bed rest; monitor the patient carefully and frequently for anginal pain and signs of bleeding; observe catheter sites at least every 15 minutes and apply pressure dressings to any recently invaded site; watch for hematuria, hematemesis, bloody stool, petechiae, hematoma, flank pain, muscle weakness; do neuro checks every hour. Continue until normal clotting function returns. ▪ Watch for extravasation. ▪ See Precautions and Drug/Lab Interactions.

Patient Education: Compliance with all measures to minimize bleeding (e.g., strict bed rest) is very important. ▪ Avoid use of razors, toothbrushes, and other sharp items. ▪ Use caution while moving to avoid excessive bumping. ▪ Report all episodes of bleeding and apply local pressure if indicated. Expect oozing from IV sites.

Maternal/Child: Category C: has resulted in hemorrhage leading to spontaneous abortions in rabbits. Safety for use in pregnancy, breast-feeding, and pediatric patients not established.

Elderly: See Indications and Precautions. ▪ May have poorer prognosis following AMI and pre-existing conditions that may increase risk of intracranial bleeding. Select patients carefully to maximize benefits.

DRUG/LAB INTERACTIONS

Interaction of reteplase with other cardioactive drugs has not been studied. Risk of bleeding may be increased by **any medicine that affects blood clotting** including anticoagulants (e.g., heparin, lepirudin [Refludan], warfarin [Coumadin]); **any medication that may cause hypoprothrombinemia, thrombocytopenia, or GI ulceration or bleeding** (e.g., selected antibiotics [e.g., cefotetan], aspirin, NSAIDs [e.g., ibuprofen (Advil, Motrin), naproxen (Aleve, Naprosyn)]); **and/or any other medication that inhibits platelet aggregation** (e.g., clopidogrel [Plavix], dipyridamole [Persantine], glycoprotein GPIIb/IIIa receptor antagonists [e.g., abciximab (ReoPro), eptifibatide (Integrilin), tirofiban (Aggrastat)], plicamycin [Mithracin], sulfinpyrazone [Anturane], ticlopidine [Ticlid], valproic acid [Depacon]). Concurrent use not recommended with the exception of heparin and aspirin (in AMI) to reduce the risk of rethrombosis. If concurrent or subsequent use indicated (e.g., management of acute coronary syndrome, percutaneous coronary intervention) monitor PT and aPTT closely. ▪ **Coagulation tests will be unreliable;** specific procedures can be used; notify the lab of reteplase use.

SIDE EFFECTS

Bleeding is most common: internal (GI tract, GU tract, intracranial, respiratory, or retroperitoneal sites), epistaxis, gingival, and superficial or surface bleeding (venous cutdowns, arterial punctures, sites of recent surgical intervention). Reperfusion arrhythmias are common; other serious arrhythmias may occur. A few hypersensitivity reactions, as well as fever, hypotension, nausea, and vomiting, have occurred. Cholesterol embolism has been reported and may be fatal. Clinical S/S may include acute renal failure, gangrenous digits, hypertension, infarctions (e.g., bowel, cerebral, myocardial, or spinal cord), pancreatitis, "purple toe" syndrome, renal artery occlusion.

ANTIDOTE

Notify physician of all side effects. Note even the most minute bleeding tendency. Oozing at IV sites is expected. Control minor bleeding by local pressure. For severe bleeding in a critical location, discontinue second dose of reteplase if it has not been given and any heparin therapy immediately. Whole blood, packed RBCs, cryoprecipitate, fresh-frozen plasma, platelets, desmopressin, tranexamic acid, and aminocaproic acid may all be indicated. Topical preparations of aminocaproic acid may stop minor bleeding. Consider protamine if heparin has been used. Treat bradycardia with atropine, reperfusion arrhythmias with lidocaine or procainamide; VT or VF may require cardioversion. Treat minor hypersensitivity reactions symptomatically. Discontinue drug and treat anaphylaxis as indicated; resuscitate as necessary. Discontinue therapy if any symptoms of cholesterol embolism occur.

Rh$_o$(D) IMMUNE GLOBULIN INTRAVENOUS (HUMAN) BBW
(ih-**MUNE GLAW**-byoo-lin **IN**-trah-ve-nes)

Rh$_o$(D)-IGIV, Rhophylac, WinRho SDF

Immunizing agent (passive)
Platelet count stimulator

pH 6.5 to 7.6

USUAL DOSE   (International units [IU])

Pregnancy, predelivery: *Rhophylac* and *WinRho SDF:* Confirm Rh$_o$(D) negative status of patient. May be given IV or IM. 1,500 IU (300 mcg) at 28 weeks' gestation. If *WinRho SDF* is administered early in the pregnancy, it should be repeated at 12-week intervals to maintain an adequate level of passively acquired anti-Rh.

Pregnancy, postdelivery: Confirm Rh$_o$(D) negative status of patient. May be given IV or IM. Administer as soon as possible after delivery of a confirmed Rh$_o$(D)-positive baby. Usually given no later than 72 hours postdelivery. If the Rh status of the infant is unknown at 72 hours, administer to the mother at that time. Should be given as soon as possible up to 28 days after delivery. This second dose postdelivery (first dose given predelivery; see above) can reduce treatment failure.

Rhophylac: 1,500 IU (300 mcg).

WinRho SDF: 600 IU (120 mcg).

Postabortion, amniocentesis (after 34 weeks' gestation), or any other manipulation late in pregnancy (after 34 weeks' gestation): Confirm Rh$_o$(D) negative status of patient. May be given IV or IM. Administer immediately after abortion or procedure associated with increased risk of Rh isoimmunization. Must be given within 72 hours. One half of a dose (a mini-dose [IM product]) may be given if a pregnancy terminates before 13 weeks' gestation, administration within 3 hours is preferred. According to the literature, this mini-dose can provide 100% effectiveness in preventing Rh immunization.

Rhophylac: 1,500 IU (300 mcg).

WinRho SDF: 600 IU (120 mcg).

Postamniocentesis before 34 weeks' gestation or after chorionic villus sampling: Confirm Rh$_o$(D) negative status of patient. May be given IV or IM. ***Rhophylac* and *WinRho SDF:*** 1,500 IU (300 mcg) immediately after the procedure. Repeat *WinRho SDF* every 12 weeks during the pregnancy.

Threatened abortion: Confirm Rh$_o$(D) negative status of patient. May be given IV or IM. ***Rhophylac* and *WinRho SDF:*** 1,500 IU (300 mcg) as soon as possible.

Transfusion or fetal hemorrhage: Confirm Rh$_o$(D) negative status of patient. May be given IV or IM. Administer within 72 hours of an incompatible event involving Rh$_o$(D) positive blood such as exposure to incompatible blood transfusions (Rh+ whole blood or Rh+ red blood cells) or massive fetal hemorrhage.

Rhophylac: Give 100 IU (20 mcg) per each 2 mL transfused blood or per 1 mL erythrocyte concentrate. In cases of known or suspected excessive feto-maternal hemorrhage, the number of fetal red blood cells in the maternal circulation should be determined. If testing is not feasible and excessive feto-maternal hemorrhage cannot be excluded, administer a dose of 1,500 IU (300 mcg).

WinRho SDF: Give up to 3,000 IU (600 mcg) every 8 hours IV or 6,000 IU (1,200 mcg) every 12 hours IM until the total dose is administered. Total IV dose is 45 IU (9 mcg) for every milliliter of Rh+ whole blood exposure or 90 IU (18 mcg) for every milliliter of Rh+ red blood cell exposure. Total IM dose is 60 IU (12 mcg) for every milliliter of Rh+ whole blood exposure or 120 IU (24 mcg) for every milliliter of Rh+ red blood cell exposure.

Treatment of immune thrombocytopenic purpura (ITP); Adults and pediatric patients: *WinRho SDF:* Confirm Rh$_o$(D)-positive status of patient. Must be given IV. Hemoglobin should be greater than 10 Gm/dL. Give 250 IU (50 mcg)/kg of body weight as the initial dose. May be given as a single dose or divided in half and given on two consecutive days. If response to the initial dose is adequate, maintenance doses of 125 to 300 IU (25 to 60 mcg)/kg may be given. If response to the initial dose is inadequate, see Dose Adjustments. Dose and frequency based on patient's clinical response (e.g., RBC, hemoglobin, reticulocyte levels, and platelet counts); see Dose Adjustments.

PEDIATRIC DOSE
Treatment of ITP: *WinRho SDF:* See Usual Dose and Dose Adjustments.

DOSE ADJUSTMENTS   (International units [IU])
Pregnancy and obstetrical conditions: *WinRho SDF* suggests protection must be maintained throughout pregnancy once Rh$_o$(D) immune globulin is administered. Level of passively acquired anti-Rh$_o$(D) should not fall below levels required to prevent an immune response to Rh$_o$(D)+ blood. Additional doses should be given every 12 weeks during pregnancy and at delivery unless the previous dose was administered within 3 weeks and there is less than 15 mL of fetomaternal red blood cell hemorrhage during delivery.

Suppression of Rh isoimmunization: *Rhophylac and WinRho SDF:* A large fetomaternal hemorrhage may cause an incorrect evaluation by standard tests of the amount of Rh$_o$(D) IGIV required. Assess the amount of hemorrhage and adjust dose accordingly.

Treatment of ITP: Adults and pediatric patients: *WinRho SDF:* If the hemoglobin level is less than 10 Gm/dL before or after the initial dose, reduce the initial dose and/or maintenance doses to 125 to 200 IU (25 to 40 mcg)/kg to minimize the risk of increasing the severity of anemia in the patient. ■ In patients with adequate platelet response to the initial dose, adjust maintenance doses based on platelet and hemoglobin levels. ■ If response to the initial dose is inadequate, adjust subsequent doses as follows:

Hemoglobin above 10 Gm/dL: redose with 250 to 300 IU (50 to 60 mcg)/kg.

Hemoglobin is 8 to 10 Gm/dL: redose with 125 to 200 IU (25 to 40 mcg)/kg.

Hemoglobin below 8 Gm/dL: use with caution, may increase severity of anemia.

DILUTION   (International units [IU])
Rhophylac: Available in a pre-filled 2-mL syringe containing 1,500 IU (300 mcg) for single-dose use. Bring to room or body temperature before use.

WinRho SDF: Available as a ready-to-use liquid. 5 IU equals 1 mcg. Withdraw the entire contents of the vial to obtain the labeled dose. If indicated, calculate a partial dose, then discard the excess from the syringe. The target fill volume of each vial is included in the following chart.

WinRho SDF Target Fill Volumes/Vial	
Vial Size	**Target Fill Volume**
600 IU (120 mcg)	0.5 mL
1,500 IU (300 mcg)	1.3 mL
2,500 IU (500 mcg)	2.2 mL
5,000 IU (1,000 mcg)	4.4 mL
15,000 IU (3,000 mcg)	13 mL

Storage: Rhophylac: Refrigerate syringes before use. Protect from light. Should not be used after expiration date. Discard unused product in syringe. **WinRho SDF:** Store unopened vials in refrigerator. Note expiration date. Do not freeze. Discard unused portion.

COMPATIBILITY
Rhophylac: Specific information not available.
WinRho SDF: Manufacturer states, "Should be administered separately from other drugs." Dilute only with NS.

RATE OF ADMINISTRATION
Rhophylac: A single dose as a slow IV injection.
WinRho SDF: A single dose as an IV injection over 3 to 5 minutes.

ACTIONS (International units [IU])
Rhophylac and WinRho SDF: Specialty immunoglobulins. A gamma globulin (IgG) fraction containing antibodies to the Rh$_o$(D) antigen (D Antigen). Reduces the incidence of Rh immunization of an Rh$_o$(D)-negative mother by an Rh$_o$(D)-positive infant before, during, and after delivery; reduces the likelihood of hemolytic disease in an Rh$_o$(D)-positive infant in present and future pregnancies. Has also been shown to increase platelet counts in nonsplenectomized Rh$_o$(D)-positive patients with immune thrombocytopenic purpura (ITP). A 1,500-IU vial or syringe contains 300 mcg of anti-Rh$_o$(D), which can effectively suppress the immunizing potential of approximately 15 to 17 mL of Rh$_o$(D)-positive blood cells, and, in addition, contains 25 to 40 mg of nonspecific gammaglobulin. Pooled from source plasma selected for high titers of Rh$_o$(D) antibody. Purified and standardized by several methods (e.g., solvent-detergent viral inactivation process to decrease the possibility of transmission of blood-borne pathogens [e.g., HIV, hepatitis]). Similar to native IgG that normally circulates in human plasma.
Rhophylac: Is thiomersol free, mercury free, and latex free. Contains albumin as a stabilizer. Half-life is 12 to 20 days. Anti-D IgG titers were measurable up to 9 weeks after injection.
WinRho SDF: Has also been shown to increase platelet counts in nonsplenectomized Rh$_o$(D)-positive patients with immune thrombocytopenic purpura (ITP). Platelet counts usually begin to rise in 1 to 2 days with peak effect in 7 to 14 days. Some effects last about 30 days. Contains 25 to 40 mg of nonspecific gammaglobulin. The liquid form contains maltose as a stabilizer; the lyophilized powder is stabilized with glycine, NaCl, and polysorbate 80. Half-life is 24 days. Crosses the blood-brain barrier.

INDICATIONS AND USES

Rhophylac and WinRho SDF: Suppression of Rh isoimmunization in non-sensitized $Rh_o(D)$-negative women during the normal course of pregnancy, within 72 hours after spontaneous or induced abortions, amniocentesis, chorionic villus sampling, ruptured tubal pregnancy, abdominal trauma or transplacental hemorrhage, unless the blood type of the fetus or father is known to be $Rh_o(D)$-negative (prophylaxis and Rh hemolytic disease of the newborn). ■ Suppression of Rh isoimmunization in $Rh_o(D)$-negative female pediatric patients and female adults in their childbearing years transfused with $Rh_o(D)$-positive red blood cells or blood components containing $Rh_o(D)$-positive RBCs.

WinRho SDF: Treatment of nonsplenectomized $Rh_o(D)$-positive pediatric patients with acute or chronic immune thrombocytopenic purpura (ITP), adults with chronic ITP, or pediatric patients and adults with ITP secondary to HIV infection in clinical situations requiring an increase in platelet counts to prevent excessive hemorrhage.

CONTRAINDICATIONS

Rhophylac and WinRho SDF: *All uses:* History of a prior severe hypersensitivity reaction to human immune globulin preparations or their components (*Rhophylac* contains albumin, *WinRho SDF* may contain thiomerosol); patients with isolated IgA deficiency or pre-existing IgA antibodies (benefits must outweigh risks; risk of anaphylaxis is greater).

Suppression of Rh isoimmunization in pregnancy: For suppression of Rh isoimmunization in the mother. *Do not administer to the infant.* Not recommended for use in $Rh_o(D)$-negative individuals shown to be Rh immunized by standard screening tests.

WinRho SDF: *Treatment of ITP:* Not recommended for use in $Rh_o(D)$-negative or splenectomized individuals.

PRECAUTIONS

All uses: Confirm vial or syringe label—must state for IV or IV/IM use; several similar products are for IM use only (e.g., RhoGam). ■ May risk transmission of infectious agents (e.g., hepatitis, HIV, possibly the Creutzfeldt-Jakob disease [CJD] agent); see Actions. ■ May contain trace amounts of anti-A, anti-B, anti-C, and anti-E blood group antibodies. ■ Use caution and weigh benefit versus risk in patients with known hypogammaglobulinemia or selective IgA deficiency; risk of severe allergic reactions or anaphylaxis is increased. ■ Not intended for use in Rh+ individuals (with the exception of *WinRho SDF* in the treatment of ITP). ■ Use with caution and monitor renal function in patients at risk for renal insufficiency. IGIV products have been reported to produce renal dysfunction in patients who are predisposed to acute renal failure or in those who have renal insufficiency. Most reports involve products that contain sucrose as a stabilizer. WinRho SDF does not contain sucrose.

Suppression of Rh isoimmunization in pregnancy: More than 1 dose of $Rh_o(D)$ immune globulin may be required. A fetal RBC count can be done on maternal blood to determine the required dose. ■ If a large fetomaternal hemorrhage occurs late in pregnancy or after delivery $Rh_o(D)$ IGIV should be administered in sufficient doses if there is any doubt about the mother's blood type (e.g., presence of passively administered anti-$Rh_o(D)$ in maternal or fetal blood [positive Coombs test]). ■ See Monitor. ■ Manufacturer recommends IM or IV use. Another source recommends IM injection when Rh$_o$(D) is used as an immunizing agent. ▪ Not effective in Rh$_o$(D)-negative females who have already been sensitized to the Rh$_o$(D) erythrocyte factor; however, if administered, the risk of side effects is not increased.

Treatment of ITP: IV route required for ITP. ▪ Rare cases of intravascular hemolysis have been reported. Usually occurs within 4 hours of administration. Complications may include clinically compromising anemia and multisystem organ failure, including ARDS. Fatalities have occurred. Serious complications, including severe anemia, acute renal insufficiency, renal failure, and DIC, have also been reported. Even if previous infusions have been uneventful, intravascular hemolysis and its complications may occur with subsequent infusions. ▪ If the hemoglobin level is less than 8 Gm/dL, use with extreme caution; may increase severity of anemia.

Monitor: *All uses:* See Precautions. ▪ Observe patient for at least 20 to 30 minutes after injection.

Suppression of Rh isoimmunization in pregnancy: Maintain accurate records of Rh factor and Rh$_o$(D)-IGIV. ▪ Obtain CBC and other appropriate lab work based on procedure or situation. ▪ Monitor vital signs if indicated.

Treatment of ITP: Obtain baseline RBC, hemoglobin, reticulocyte levels, and platelet counts. Monitor during therapy to determine clinical response. ▪ Given to Rh$_o$(D)-positive patients in this situation, interaction with RBC usually causes some degree of RBC hemolysis; observe carefully. Monitor for S/S of intravascular hemolysis (back pain, chills, fever, hemoglobinuria) for at least 8 hours after infusion. Perform a dipstick urinalysis at baseline, at 2 and 4 hours, and before the end of the monitoring period. ▪ Monitor for complications of intravascular hemolysis (IVH), including clinically compromising anemia (decreased hemoglobin, hypotension, pallor, and tachycardia), acute renal insufficiency (anuria, dyspnea, edema, or oliguria), or DIC (increased bruising and prolongation of bleeding or clotting time). ▪ If S/S of IVH or its complications occur, lab tests should be performed to confirm the diagnosis. Tests include but are not limited to CBC with platelets, haptoglobin, plasma hemoglobin, urine dipstick, BUN, SCr, LDH, direct and indirect bilirubin, and DIC-specific tests (e.g., D-dimer, fibrin degradation products [FDP], fibrin split products [FSP]). ▪ If transfusion is required, use Rh$_o$(D)-negative RBCs to avoid exacerbating ongoing IVH. Platelet products may contain RBCs; use caution if platelets from an Rh$_o$(D)+ donor are used.

Patient Education: Report S/S of a hypersensitivity reaction (e.g., feeling of fainting, hives, itching, tightness in the chest, wheezing). ▪ Report feelings of dizziness, tiredness, weakness. *ITP:* May cause a considerable drop in hemoglobin; follow-up testing important. ▪ Immediately report symptoms of back pain, chills, decreased urine output, discolored urine or hematuria, fever, sudden weight gain, fluid retention/edema, and/or shortness of breath. May indicate onset of intravascular hemolysis (IVH).

Maternal/Child: Category C: use only if clearly needed. ▪ Rhophylac is not secreted in breast milk. Specific information is not available for WinRho SDF on safety during breast-feeding. ▪ For the suppression of Rh isoimmunization in the mother; do not administer to the infant.

Elderly: When used for treatment of ITP, fatal outcomes associated with IVH and its complications occurred most frequently in patients over 65 years of age with co-morbid conditions.

DRUG/LAB INTERACTIONS

Interaction with other drugs has not been evaluated. ▪ Antibodies contained in $Rh_o(D)$ immune globulin may interfere with the body's immune response to certain **live virus vaccines.** Do not administer live virus vaccines (e.g., measles, mumps, polio, or rubella) for at least 3 months after $Rh_o(D)$ administration. ▪ Trace amounts of anti-A, anti-B, anti-C, and anti-E blood group antibodies may be detectable in **direct and indirect antiglobulin (Coombs') tests** following treatment with $Rh_o(D)$. ▪ May affect outcomes of **blood typing and antibody testing** in neonates. ▪ The liquid formulation of WinRho SDF contains maltose, which may give **falsely high blood glucose levels** with certain types of blood glucose testing systems. Only testing systems that are glucose specific should be used to monitor blood glucose levels in patients receiving maltose-containing parenteral products such as WinRho SDF.

SIDE EFFECTS

All uses: Abdominal or back pain, arthralgias, asthenia, chills, diarrhea, dizziness, fever, headache, hyperkinesia, hypertension, hypotension, increased LDH, pruritus, rash, somnolence, and sweating. Hypersensitivity reactions, including anaphylaxis, have been reported rarely. Made from human plasma donors, transmission of selected diseases possible but not probable; see Precautions.

Suppression of Rh isoimmunization in pregnancy: Side effects are infrequent in $Rh_o(D)$-negative individuals. Only a few women have had treatment failures resulting in development of $Rh_o(D)$ antibodies.

ITP: Destruction of $Rh_o(D)$ red cells resulting in decreased hemoglobin (range was 0.4 to 6.1 Gm/dL). IVH (back pain, shaking chills, hemoglobinuria), acute onset and exacerbation of anemia, and renal insufficiency have been reported in $Rh_o(D)$-positive patients. Has rarely resulted in death.

ANTIDOTE

Keep physician informed of side effects; may require symptomatic treatment. Discontinue immediately if an allergic reaction occurs; treat as indicated (e.g., maintain airway, administer fluids, oxygen, epinephrine [Adrenalin], diphenhydramine [Benadryl], corticosteroids [e.g., dexamethasone (Decadron)]). *ITP:* Treatment may have to be discontinued if drop in hemoglobin too severe. Transfusion may be required.

1212

RIFAMPIN
(rih-**FAM**-pin)

Rifadin

Antibacterial
(antituberculosis)

pH 7.8 to 8.8

USUAL DOSE
Dose and schedule may vary depending on treatment regimen selected. IV doses are the same as oral. Use oral dose form as soon as practical.

Tuberculosis: 10 mg/kg once a day. Do not exceed 600 mg/day. Another source suggests 600 mg once a day or 10 mg/kg not to exceed 600 mg/dose two or three times a week. Prescribed concurrently with other antituberculin drugs (e.g., ethambutol [Myambutol], isoniazid, pyrazinamide, or streptomycin). Consult current CDC guidelines for suggested treatment regimens.

Meningococcal carriers: 600 mg every 12 hours for 2 days.

Leprosy (unlabeled): 600 mg once a month for a minimum of 2 years or until smear is negative, whichever is longer. Given in combination with other antileprosy agents.

PEDIATRIC DOSE
Pediatric patients 1 month of age and older.

Tuberculosis: 10 to 20 mg/kg of body weight either once a day or two or three times a week depending on regimen. Do not exceed 600 mg. Prescribed concurrently with other antituberculin drugs (e.g., ethambutol [Myambutol], isoniazid, pyrazinamide, or streptomycin).

Meningococcal carriers: 10 mg/kg every 12 hours for 2 days.

NEONATAL DOSE
Tuberculosis: 10 to 20 mg/kg either once a day or two or three times a week depending on regimen. Prescribed concurrently with other antituberculin drugs (e.g., ethambutol [Myambutol], isoniazid, pyrazinamide, or streptomycin).

Meningococcal carriers; *under 1 month of age:* 5 mg/kg every 12 hours for 2 days. ***Over 1 month of age:*** 10 mg/kg every 12 hours for 2 days.

DOSE ADJUSTMENTS
To reduce hepatotoxicity, a reduced dose may be required in impaired hepatic function. ■ No dose adjustment is necessary in impaired renal function; serum concentrations do not change. ■ See Drug/Lab Interactions.

DILUTION
Each 600-mg vial must be initially diluted in 10 mL of SW for injection (60 mg/mL). Swirl gently to dissolve. Withdraw desired dose and further dilute in 500 mL or 100 mL of D5W or NS; see Storage. 100-mL dilution used only in selected situations.

Storage: Avoid excessive heat (temperatures above 40° C [104° F]). Protect from light. Reconstituted solution stable at CRT for 24 hours. Use solution diluted in D5W within 4 hours; solution diluted in NS stable for 24 hours.

COMPATIBILITY
Manufacturer states, "May form a precipitate with diltiazem (Cardizem) at the **Y-site.**"

RATE OF ADMINISTRATION

A single dose equally distributed as an infusion over 3 hours. In selected situations a single dose diluted in 100 mL may be administered over 30 minutes.

ACTIONS

A semisynthetic, antituberculosis antibiotic. Has a bactericidal action. Inhibits bacterial DNA-dependent RNA polymerase activity in susceptible *Mycobacterium tuberculosis* organisms but does not inhibit the mammalian enzyme. Rapidly distributed throughout the body and present in many organs and body fluids, including CSF. 80% protein bound. Metabolized in the liver. Undergoes enterohepatic circulation. Excreted in bile and urine. Half-life following repeated dosing is 2 to 3 hours. Crosses the placental barrier. Secreted in breast milk.

INDICATIONS AND USES

Treatment or retreatment of tuberculosis when the drug cannot be taken by mouth. ▪ Treatment of asymptomatic carriers of *Neisseria* meningitis. Not indicated for treatment of meningococcal infection because of rapid emergence of resistant meningococci. ▪ Used in combination with other agents in the treatment of certain atypical mycobacterial infections (e.g., *Mycobacterium avium*). Used in combination with other antistaphylococcal agents to treat serious staphylococcal infections.

Unlabeled uses: Used in combination with other agents in the treatment of certain atypical mycobacterial infections (e.g., *Mycobacterium avium*). ▪ Used in combination with other antistaphylococcal agents to treat serious staphylococcal infections. ▪ Leprosy.

CONTRAINDICATIONS

Hypersensitivity to rifampin or any of its components or to any rifamycins. Individuals with liver disease are at higher risk for complications. ▪ Contraindicated in patients receiving ritonavir-boosted saquinavir; risk for severe hepatocellular toxicity is increased. ▪ Concomitant use with atazanavir (Reyataz), darunavir (Prezista), fosamprenavir (Lexiva), saquinavir (Invirase), and tipranavir (Aptivus); see Drug/Lab Interactions.

PRECAUTIONS

For IV use only. Do not administer IM or SC. ▪ Obtain cultures before starting therapy to confirm susceptibility of the organism to rifampin. Repeat cultures periodically during therapy to monitor for the emergence of resistance. ▪ Resistance can emerge rapidly; appropriate susceptibility tests should be performed in the event of persistent positive cultures. ▪ Susceptibility tests also required before use as treatment for asymptomatic carriers of *Neisseria* meningitis. ▪ To reduce the development of drug-resistant bacteria and maintain its effectiveness, rifampin should be used to treat or prevent only those infections proven or strongly suspected to be caused by bacteria. ▪ Organisms resistant to rifampin are likely to be resistant to other rifamycins. ▪ Has been shown to produce liver dysfunction. Risk of liver damage is markedly increased if impaired liver function is present. Hepatotoxicity, hepatic encephalopathy, and death associated with jaundice have occurred in patients with liver disease and when rifampin is given with other hepatotoxic agents (e.g., isoniazid, halothane). Discontinue one or both drugs if signs of hepatocellular damage occur. ▪ May exacerbate porphyria. ▪ Use with caution in patients with diabetes; diabetes management may be more difficult. ▪ Not recommended for intermittent therapy; interruption of daily dosage regimen has resulted in rare renal hypersensitivity reactions when therapy was resumed. ▪ Urine, feces, saliva, sputum, sweat, and tears may be colored red-orange. Soft contact lenses may be permanently stained. CSF may be light yellow. ▪ Pseudomembranous colitis has been reported. May range from mild to life threatening. Consider in patients that present with diarrhea during or after treatment with rifampin.

Monitor: Obtain baseline measurements of hepatic enzymes (e.g., ALT and AST), bilirubin, SCr, CBC, and platelet count. Routine lab monitoring in patients with normal baseline labs is generally not necessary. However, patients should be seen monthly and questioned about symptoms that may indicate adverse reactions. ▪ Monitor liver function every 2 to 4 weeks in patients with pre-existing liver impairment. ▪ Monitor blood glucose closely in patients with diabetes. ▪ Notify physician immediately if flu-like symptoms develop; may be due to hepatotoxicity. ▪ Thrombocytopenia has occurred. Reversible if rifampin is discontinued as soon as purpura occurs. Cerebral hemorrhage has occurred when rifampin has been continued or resumed after the appearance of purpura. Contact physician immediately if purpura occurs. ▪ Confirm patency of IV; avoid extravasation. Restart IV at a new site for any signs of inflammation or irritation. ▪ Do all lab tests and affected radiology studies before daily dose of medication. ▪ See Drug/Lab Interactions.

Patient Education: Reliability of hormonal contraceptives may be affected; use of nonhormonal contraceptives recommended. ▪ Avoid use of alcohol or other hepatotoxic agents (e.g., acetaminophen [Anacin-3, Tylenol], NSAIDs [ibuprofen (Advil, Motrin) naproxen (Aleve, Naprosyn)], phenothiazines [e.g., promethazine (Phenergan)], some antineoplastic agents, sulfonamides). ▪ Review side effects with health care professional and promptly report any that occur. ▪ May cause reddish-orange discoloration of feces, saliva, sputum, sweat, urine, and tears. ▪ May discolor soft contact lenses. ▪ Do not interrupt daily dosage regimen.

Maternal/Child: Category C: has teratogenic potential. Safety for use during pregnancy not established. Benefit must outweigh risk. See literature for best combinations with least known risk. ▪ Administration during the last few weeks of pregnancy may cause postnatal hemorrhages in mother and infant; treatment with vitamin K may be required. ▪ Closely monitor neonates of rifampin-treated mothers for adverse effects. ▪ Discontinue breast-feeding if mother requires treatment.

Elderly: Differences in response between elderly and younger patients have not been identified. ▪ Risk of hepatitis increased after 50 years of age. ▪ See Dose Adjustments.

DRUG/LAB INTERACTIONS

Interactions are numerous and potentially life threatening. Review of drug profile by pharmacist imperative. ▪ Hepatotoxicity, hepatic encephalopathy, and death associated with jaundice have occurred when rifampin is given with **other hepatotoxic agents** (e.g., alcohol, isoniazid, halothane). Discontinue one or both drugs for signs of hepatocellular damage. ▪ Concurrent use of rifampin with **saquinavir/ritonavir** (ritonavir-boosted saquinavir) is *contraindicated;* significant hepatocellular toxicity with markedly increased transaminase elevations have been reported. ▪ Concurrent administration with **atazanavir** (Reyataz), **darunavir** (Prezista), **fosamprenavir** (Lexiva), **saquinavir** (Invirase), and **tipranavir** (Aptivus) is *contraindicated;* rifampin may substantially decrease plasma concentrations of these antiviral agents.

Loss of antiviral effectiveness and/or development of viral resistance may result. ▪ Rifampin increases metabolism and clearance and decreases serum levels and effectiveness of numerous drugs. Manufacturer lists **antiarrhythmics** (e.g., disopyramide [Norpace], mexiletine, quinidine, tocainide [Tonocard]), **anticonvulsants** (e.g., phenytoin [Dilantin]), **antifungals** (e.g., fluconazole [Diflucan], itraconazole [Sporanox], ketoconazole [Nizoral]), **barbiturates** (e.g., phenobarbital), **beta-blockers** (e.g., propranolol), **calcium channel blockers** (e.g., diltiazem [Cardizem], nifedipine [Procardia], verapamil), **cardiac glycoside preparations** (e.g., digoxin [Lanoxin], digitoxin), **chloramphenicol** (Chloromycetin), **clarithromycin** (Biaxin), **clofibrate** (Atromid-S), **corticosteroids** (e.g., prednisone), **cyclosporine** (Sandimmune), **dapsone, diazepam** (Valium), **doxycycline, fluoroquinolones** (e.g., ciprofloxacin [Cipro IV]), **haloperidol** (Haldol), **levothyroxine** (Synthroid), **methadone, narcotic analgesics, oral anticoagulants** (e.g., warfarin [Coumadin]), **oral hypoglycemic agents** (e.g., sulfonylureas [e.g., glyburide (DiaBeta), tolbutamide]), **oral or other systemic hormonal contraceptives, progestins** (e.g., megestrol [Megace], progesterone), **quinine, tacrolimus** (Prograf), **theophylline** (aminophylline), **tricyclic antidepressants** (e.g., amitriptyline [Elavil], nortriptyline [Aventyl]), **zidovudine.** Other sources add **acetaminophen** (Tylenol), **amiodarone** (Nexterone), **amprenavir** (Agenerase), **benzodiazepines** (e.g., midazolam [Versed], in addition to diazepam), **buspirone** (BuSpar), **clozapine** (Clozaril), **estrogens, lamotrigine** (Lamictal), **losartan** (Cozaar), **ondansetron** (Zofran), **propafenone** (Rythmol), **sildenafil** (Viagra), **and zolipidem** (Ambien). Increased doses of these drugs may be required. Monitor carefully; obtain prothrombin daily when used with **anticoagulants** (e.g., warfarin); use of **nonhormonal contraceptives** recommended during rifampin therapy; and **diabetes** may be more difficult to control. ▪ May reduce analgesic effects of **morphine and methadone.** Monitor carefully; an alternate analgesic may be required (see earlier statement). ▪ Treatment failure of **ketoconazole** (Nizoral) **or rifampin** may occur when given concomitantly. ▪ Concomitant use of rifampin and **macrolide antibiotics** (e.g., clarithromycin) may decrease the metabolism of rifampin and increase the metabolism of the macrolide antibiotic. ▪ Potentiated by **probenecid and cotrimoxazole.** ▪ May decrease concentrations of enalaprilat, the active metabolite of **enalapril** (Vasotec), resulting in hypertension. Adjust dose as required. ▪ When taken concomitantly, decreased concentrations of **atovaquone** (Mepron) and increased concentration of rifampin have been observed. ▪ May induce metabolism of endogenous substrates including **adrenal hormones, thyroid hormones, and vitamin D.** Reduced levels of vitamin D may be accompanied by decreased serum calcium and phosphate and increased parathyroid hormone. ▪ Cross-reactivity and false-positive urine screening **tests for opiates** have been reported when using certain assays. Gas chromatography or mass spectrometry will distinguish rifampin from opiates. ▪ May cause an early rise in bilirubin during initial days of treatment; should subside. Throughout treatment transient abnormalities in **liver function tests** will occur. ▪ Therapeutic levels inhibit assays of **serum folate and vitamin B$_{12}$.** ▪ Reduced biliary excretion of contrast media for **gallbladder studies** may occur. Perform test prior to dose of rifampin.

SIDE EFFECTS

Average dose: Anaphylaxis may occur even with repeat doses. Abnormal liver function tests, anorexia, ataxia, behavioral changes, conjunctivitis (exudative), cramps, diarrhea, dizziness, edema of face and extremities, epigastric distress, eosinophilia, fatigue, flushing, flu-like symptoms (e.g., chills, fever, headache, malaise, muscle and bone pain), gas, heartburn, hematuria, hemolytic anemia, hepatic reactions, hepatitis or a shocklike syndrome and abnormal liver function tests (rare), hypotension, leukopenia, menstrual disturbances, mental confusion, myopathy (rare), muscle weakness, nausea, numbness (generalized), pain in extremities, pseudomembranous colitis, psychosis purpura, pruritus, rash, renal failure (acute), shortness of breath, sore mouth and tongue, thrombocytopenia, urticaria, visual disturbances, vomiting, wheezing.

Overdose: Abdominal pain, bilirubin levels and/or liver enzymes may increase rapidly; brown-red discoloration of feces, skin, sweat, tears, and urine is proportional to amount of overdose; headache, lethargy, nausea, and vomiting are immediate; pruritus, unconsciousness. Liver enlargement, possibly with tenderness, can develop within a few hours after severe overdose; bilirubin levels may increase and jaundice may develop rapidly. Arrhythmias, cardiac arrest, hypotension, and seizures have been reported in fatal overdoses.

ANTIDOTE
With increasing severity of any side effect, alterations in liver function tests, flu-like symptoms, purpura, thrombocytopenia, or symptoms of overdose, discontinue the drug and notify the physician immediately. Antiemetics (e.g., ondansetron [Zofran], prochlorperazine [Compazine]) may be required to control nausea and vomiting. Forced diuresis will promote excretion. Bile drainage may be indicated in the presence of seriously impaired hepatic function lasting more than 24 to 48 hours. Hemodialysis may be indicated. If hemodialysis is not available, peritoneal dialysis can be used along with forced diuresis. In severe overdose or acute toxicity, maintain an adequate airway and confirm adequate respiratory exchange. Treat anaphylaxis and resuscitate as necessary.

RITUXIMAB [BBW]
(rih-**TUK**-sih-mab)
Rituxan

Recombinant monoclonal antibody
Antineoplastic

pH 6.5

USUAL DOSE
Premedication: *Use recommended for all indications.* Acetaminophen (Tylenol) and diphenhydramine (Benadryl) are recommended before each dose to prevent or attenuate severe hypersensitivity and/or infusion reactions. Additional premedication (e.g., methylprednisolone 100 mg IV (or equivalent) is required for patients with rheumatoid arthritis (RA). Patients with Wegener's granulomatosis (WG) and microscopic polyangiitis (MPA) require additional premedication with methylprednisolone IV 1,000 mg. Transient hypotension may occur during rituximab infusion; consider withholding antihypertensive medications 12 hours before rituximab infusion. See Precautions for PCP prophylaxis and/or antiherpetic viral prophylaxis required in specific indications.

Relapsed or refractory, low-grade or follicular, CD20-positive, B-cell non-Hodgkin's lymphoma (NHL): Single agent: *Initial therapy:* 375 mg/M^2 as an infusion once a week for 4 or 8 doses. See Drug/Lab Interactions. Risk of Grade 3 or 4 adverse events increased with treatment with 8 doses as compared to treatment with 4 doses. *Retreatment therapy:* Patients who subsequently develop progressive disease may be retreated with 375 mg/M^2 as an IV infusion once each week for 4 doses. Incidence of adverse events similar to initial therapy. Data on more than 2 courses are limited.

Previously untreated follicular, CD20-positive, B-cell NHL: 375 mg/M^2 as an infusion, given on Day 1 of each cycle of CVP chemotherapy for up to 8 doses. In patients with complete or partial response, initiate rituximab maintenance 8 weeks after completion of rituximab in combination with chemotherapy. Administer rituximab as a single agent every 8 weeks for 12 doses.

Non-progressing, low-grade, CD20-positive, B-cell NHL (after first-line CVP chemotherapy): In patients who have not progressed following 6 to 8 cycles of CVP chemotherapy (stable disease), 375 mg/M^2 may be administered as an infusion once a week for 4 doses every 6 months for up to 16 doses.

Diffuse large B-cell, CD20-positive NHL: 375 mg/M^2 as an infusion on Day 1 of each cycle of chemotherapy for up to 8 doses.

Chronic lymphocytic leukemia (CLL): 375 mg/M^2 the day before the initiation of FC chemotherapy (fludarabine [Fludara] and cyclophosphamide [Cytoxan]) in the first cycle, then 500 mg/M^2 on Day 1 of Cycles 2 through 6 (every 28 days); see Precautions.

Rheumatoid arthritis: Administer *glucocorticoids* (e.g., methylprednisolone [Solu-Medrol] 100 mg IV) 30 minutes before each infusion of rituximab to reduce the incidence and severity of infusion reactions. Follow with a *rituximab* infusion of 1,000 mg. Repeat entire sequence one time in 2 weeks. Given in combination with methotrexate. Subsequent courses should be administered every 24 weeks or based on clinical evaluation, but not sooner than every 16 weeks.

Wegener's granulomatosis (WG) and microscopic polyangiitis (MPA):
Methylprednisolone: 1,000 mg/day IV for 1 to 3 days followed by oral prednisone 1 mg/kg/day (not to exceed 80 mg/day and tapered per clinical need) is recommended to treat severe vasculitis symptoms. This regimen should begin within 14 days before or with the initiation of rituximab and may continue during and after the 4-week course of treatment.
Rituximab: 375 mg/M^2 as an infusion once weekly for 4 weeks. Safety and effectiveness of subsequent courses not established.

Therapeutic regimen with ibritumomab tiuxetan: 250 mg/M^2 as an IV infusion. Given in a specific protocol in combination with ibritumomab tiuxetan (Zevalin [In-111 ibritumomab and Y-90 ibritumomab]); see ibritumomab monograph.

DOSE ADJUSTMENTS

No dose adjustments recommended. See Rate of Administration.

DILUTION

Each single dose must be further diluted to a final concentration of 1 to 4 mg/mL with NS or D5W. 500 mg (50 mL) in 450 mL will yield 1 mg/mL; 500 mg (50 mL) in 75 mL will yield 4 mg/mL. Gently invert to mix solution. Contains no preservatives; discard any unused portion left in vial.

Storage: Refrigerate vials at 2° to 8° C (36° to 46° F); protect from light and freezing. Do not shake. Do not use beyond expiration date. Diluted solutions may be refrigerated for 24 hours and are stable at room temperature for an additional 24 hours.

COMPATIBILITY

Manufacturer states, "Rituximab should not be mixed or diluted with other drugs." No **incompatibilities** with polyvinylchloride or polyethylene bags have been observed.

RATE OF ADMINISTRATION

Must be given as an infusion. *Do not administer as an IV push or bolus.* Hypersensitivity (non–IgE-mediated) and/or infusion reactions are a common occurrence and may be prevented or lessened with premedication and a reduced rate of infusion.

First infusion: Begin with an initial rate of 50 mg/hr (at this rate a 500-mg dose would be infused over 10 hours). If no discomfort or adverse effects occur, may be gradually increased by 50-mg/hr increments at 30-minute intervals to a maximum rate of 400 mg/hr. At any time that discomfort or adverse effects occur, reduce the rate of infusion. Discontinue the infusion for severe reactions and treat as indicated; see Antidote. When symptoms have completely resolved, the infusion can be restarted at half the previous rate.

Subsequent infusions: If the patient did not tolerate the first infusion well, follow instructions under first infusion. If no discomfort or adverse effects occurred with the first infusion, subsequent infusions may begin with an initial rate of 100 mg/hr and increased by 100-mg/hr increments at 30-minute intervals to a maximum rate of 400 mg/hr. See all precautionary measures under First Infusion (see above). 90-minute infusions have been used in NHL patients who are receiving a corticosteroid as part of their combination chemotherapy regimen and tolerated the initial infusion at the recommended rate. Administer the corticosteroid, acetaminophen, and diphenhydramine; follow with rituximab. Administer 20% of rituximab dose equally distributed over the first 30 minutes and the remaining 80% of the dose equally distributed over 60 minutes.

ACTIONS

An antineoplastic agent. A humanized (Ig)G_1 monoclonal antibody produced by recombinant DNA technology. Designed to bind to the CD20 antigen found on the surface of normal and malignant B lymphocytes. CD20 is also expressed on more than 90% of B-cell non-Hodgkin's lymphomas but is not expressed on hematopoietic stem cells. CD20 regulates an early step(s) in the activation process for cell cycle initiation and differentiation. Rituximab binds to lymphoid cells in the thymus, the white pulp of the spleen, and a majority of B lymphocytes in peripheral blood and lymph nodes. There is little or no binding to nonlymphoid tissue. Results in a rapid and sustained depletion (cytotoxity) of circulating and tissue-based B cells. Cell lysis may be the result of complement-dependent cytotoxicity and antibody-dependent cellular cytotoxicity. May sensitize drug-resistant human B-cell lymphoma cell lines to cytotoxic chemotherapy. Detected in serum for 3 to 6 months after completion of therapy. B-cell depletion was sustained for 6 to 9 months posttreatment in 83% of patients. B-cell recovery begins at approximately 6 months, and most levels return to normal by 12 months following completion of treatment. Median half-life is 22 days (range 6.1 to 52 days). Clearance is increased in patients with higher CD19-positive cell counts or larger measurable tumor lesions. B-cells are believed to play a role in the pathogenesis of RA and associated chronic synovitis. In this setting, B-cells may act at multiple sites in the autoimmune/inflammatory process, including through production of rheumatoid factor and other auto-antibodies, antigen presentation, T-cell activation, and/or pro-inflammatory cytokine production. In RA it induces depletion of peripheral B-lymphocytes, with near-complete depletion occurring in most patients within 2 weeks of the first dose. This B-lymphocyte depletion lasted for at least 6 months, followed by a gradual recovery. A few patients had prolonged peripheral B-cell depletion lasting more than 3 years after a single course of treatment. Crosses the placental barrier. May be secreted in breast milk.

INDICATIONS AND USES

As a single agent in the treatment of patients with relapsed or refractory low-grade or follicular CD20-positive, B-cell NHL. ▪ In combination with CHOP (cyclophosphamide, doxorubicin [hydroxydaunorubicin], vincristine, and prednisone) or other anthracycline-based chemotherapy regimens for treatment in previously untreated diffuse large B-cell, CD20-positive NHL. ▪ Treatment of previously untreated follicular, CD20-positive, B-cell NHL in combination with first-line chemotherapy and as a single-agent maintenance therapy in patients achieving a complete or partial response to rituximab in combination with chemotherapy. ▪ Treatment of non-progressing (including stable disease), low-grade, CD20-positive, B-cell NHL as a single agent after first-line CVP chemotherapy. ▪ Treatment of patients with previously untreated and previously treated CD20-positive CLL. Used in combination with FC chemotherapy (fludarabine and cyclophosphamide). ▪ In combination with glucocorticoids for the treatment of adult patients with Wegener's granulomatosis (WG) and microscopic polyangiitis (MPA). ▪ In combination with ibritumomab tiuxetan as part of a therapeutic regimen for the treatment of patients with relapsed or refractory low-grade, follicular, or transformed B-cell NHL, including patients with rituximab-refractory follicular NHL. ▪ In combination with methotrexate to reduce S/S and to slow the progression of structural damage in adult patients with moderate to severe RA who have had an inadequate response to one or more TNF (tumor necrosis factor) antagonist therapies. ▪ Not indicated for use in patients with RA who have responded to treatment with TNF antagonists (e.g., adalimumab [Humira], etanercept [Enbrel]).

Unlabeled uses: To postpone relapses in patients with NHL.

CONTRAINDICATIONS

Known IgE-mediated hypersensitivity or anaphylactic reactions to murine proteins, rituximab, or any of its components.

PRECAUTIONS

Has been given on an outpatient basis; however, rituximab should be administered by or under the direction of the physician specialist in facilities equipped to monitor the patient and respond to any medical emergency. ▪ Severe infusion reactions and hypersensitivity reactions have occurred for up to 24 hours after initiating rituximab infusions, and some have been fatal. Most severe reactions occur within 30 minutes to 2 hours of beginning the first infusion. S/S of severe reactions may include hypotension, angioedema, hypoxia, urticaria, or bronchospasm. More severe manifestations may include anaphylactic and anaphylactoid events, pulmonary infiltrates, acute respiratory distress syndrome, myocardial infarction, ventricular fibrillation, and cardiogenic shock. ▪ Use caution in patients who either have or develop HAMA/HACA titers. RA patients may be at increased risk of developing HACA titers. Some tested positive as early as 16 weeks after the first course. Clinical relevance of HACA formation in rituximab-treated patients is unclear. ▪ Tumor lysis syndrome (TLS) has been reported within 12 to 24 hours after the first rituximab infusion in patients with NHL. S/S are rapid reduction in tumor volume, renal insufficiency, hyperkalemia, hypocalcemia, hyperuricemia, or hyperphosphatemia. May cause acute renal failure requiring dialysis and has been fatal. ▪ TLS occurs more often in patients with high numbers of circulating malignant cells or high tumor burden. Consider prophylactic measures; see Monitor. ▪ Renal toxicity occurs more frequently in patients with high numbers of circulating malignant cells, high tumor burden, and/or TLS. Severe, including fatal, renal toxicity has occurred in patients with NHL. ▪ Safety of immunization with vaccines, particularly live virus vaccines, and the ability of the patient to respond to vaccines following rituximab therapy has not been studied. Review vaccination status. Administration of live virus vaccines is not recommended. Weigh benefit versus risk in NHL patients if a delay in treatment may occur for vaccination. ▪ Administer any CDC-recommended, non–live virus vaccinations to RA patients at least 4 weeks before initiating treatment with rituximab. ▪ In CLL patients, *Pneumocystis jiroveci* pneumonia (PCP) and antiherpetic viral prophylaxis is recommended during treatment and for up to 12 months following treatment. ▪ In WG and MPA patients, *Pneumocystis jiroveci* pneumonia (PCP) prophylaxis is recommended during treatment and for at least 6 months following the last rituximab infusion. ▪ Mucocutaneous reactions (including lichenoid dermatitis, paraneoplastic pemphigus, Stevens-Johnson syndrome, toxic epidermal necrolysis, and vesiculobullous dermatitis), some with fatal outcomes, have been reported. Onset of reaction has occurred from 1 to 13 weeks following rituximab exposure. ▪ Hepatitis B virus reactivation with fulminant hepatitis, hepatic failure, and death has been reported. Persons at high risk for hepatitis B virus infections should be screened before initiation of rituximab. ▪ Carriers of hepatitis B should be closely monitored for clinical and laboratory S/S of hepatitis and/or active hepatitis B virus infection during and for several months following therapy. ▪ Not recommended for use in patients with severe active infections. ▪ Serious (including fatal) bacterial, fungal, and new or reactivated viral infections can occur during and up to 1 year after completion of therapy. New or reactivated viral infections have included JC virus (progressive multifocal leukoencephalopathy [PML], cytomegalovirus, herpes simplex virus, parvovirus B19, varicella zoster virus, West Nile virus, and hepatitis B and C). Deaths have occurred. ▪ PML is a rare, progressive, demyelinating disease of the CNS caused by infection of the JC virus. Usually leads to death or severe disability, and there is no effective treatment. Has been reported in patients receiving rituximab for both approved and unlabeled indications. Most of these patients received rituximab in combination with chemotherapy, prior to or concurrent with immunosuppressive therapy, or as part of a hematopoietic stem cell transplant. However, PML has also been reported in patients with autoimmune diseases (e.g., rheumatoid arthritis) who have been treated previously or concurrently with immunosuppressive therapy. ▪ RA patients may have an increased risk of cardiovascular events. ▪ Abdominal pain, bowel obstruction, and perforation have been reported in patients receiving rituximab in combination with chemotherapy. Death has occurred. ▪ Use of concomitant immunosuppressants other than corticosteroids has not been studied in WG or MPA patients exhibiting peripheral B-cell depletion following treatment with rituximab. ▪ See Rate of Administration, Drug/ Lab Interactions, and Antidote.

Monitor: In patients with lymphoid malignancies who are receiving rituximab monotherapy, obtain a baseline CBC and platelet count and repeat before each course of therapy. In patients treated with rituximab and chemotherapy, obtain baseline CBC and platelet count at weekly to monthly intervals. Repeat more frequently in patients who develop cytopenias (e.g., leukopenia, neutropenia, thrombocytopenia). Duration of cytopenias may extend months beyond the treatment period. In RA, WG, or MPA patients, obtain a baseline CBC and platelet count and repeat at 2- to 4-month intervals during therapy. ▪ Observe patient continuously for symptoms of hypersensitivity and/or infusion reactions, which are more common during the first infusion, but can occur at any time; see Antidote. ▪ Monitor HR and BP frequently. ▪ ECG and pulmonary monitoring required during and in the immediate posttreatment period in patients with pre-existing cardiac or pulmonary conditions, in any patient who develops or has previously developed a clinically significant cardiopulmonary adverse event during treatment, and in patients with RA. ▪ Monitor patients with high numbers of circulating malignant cells (greater than or equal to 25,000/mm^3) with or without other evidence of high tumor burden for infusion reaction and tumor lysis syndrome. Monitoring of serum electrolytes and renal function indicated. ▪ Prevention and treatment of hyperuricemia due to TLS may be accomplished with adequate hydration and, if necessary, allopurinol (Aloprim) and alkalinization of urine; see Drug/ Lab Interactions. ▪ Prevention and/or treatment of hyperphosphatemia, hyperkalemia, and hypocalcemia due to TLS is also indicated. ▪ Monitor closely for signs of renal failure, and discontinue rituximab in patients with a rising SCr or oliguria. ▪ Assess neurologic status frequently. Consider PML in patients with new-onset neurologic manifestations; consultation with a neurologist, brain MRI, and lumbar puncture may be required for diagnosis. ▪ Observe closely for signs of infection. Prophylactic antibiotics may be indicated pending results of C/S in a febrile neutropenic patient. ▪ Use prophylactic antiemetics to reduce nausea and vomiting and increase patient comfort. ▪ Monitor for thrombocytopenia (platelet count less than 50,000/mm^3). Initiate precautions to prevent excessive bleeding (e.g., inspect IV sites, skin, and mucous membranes; use extreme care during invasive procedures; test urine, emesis, stool, and secretions for occult blood). ▪ Monitor patients with diffuse large B-cell, CD20-positive NHL treated with R-CHOP closely for abdominal pain, especially early in the course of treatment. A thorough diagnostic evaluation is indicated; treat appropriately to prevent bowel obstruction and perforation. ▪ See Premedication in Usual Dose, Rate of Administration, Precautions, Drug/Lab Interactions, and Antidote.

Patient Education: Avoid pregnancy; nonhormonal birth control recommended; report a suspected pregnancy immediately. See Maternal/Child. ▪ Read manufacturer's patient information sheet before each infusion. ▪ Discuss health history (e.g., presence of an infection, carrier of or had a previous hepatitis B virus infection, heart or lung problems, recent or scheduled vaccinations, scheduled surgeries) and prescription and non-prescription medications with the health care provider administering the rituximab. ▪ Review monitoring requirements and potential side effects before therapy. ▪ Promptly report S/S of infection (e.g., fever), blisters, cough, difficulty breathing, dizziness, drowsiness, headache, hives, peeling skin, painful sores, ulcers, swelling, or wheezing; immediate medical treatment may be indicated. ▪ New neurologic S/S (e.g., changes in vision, loss of balance or coordination, disorientation, or confusion); could be warning signs of PML. Report them promptly. ▪ See Appendix D, p. 1434.

Maternal/Child: Category C: avoid pregnancy; women of childbearing age should use birth control during treatment and for up to 12 months after completion of treatment. B-cell lymphocytopenia generally lasting less than 6 months has occurred in infants exposed to rituximab in utero. Use only if clearly needed. ▪ Discontinue breast-feeding until circulating drug levels are no longer detectable. ▪ Safety and effectiveness for use in pediatric patients not established.

Elderly: No overall differences in effectiveness were observed between different age-groups of patients treated for diffuse large B-cell NHL. The numbers of elderly treated for low-grade or follicular NHL were insufficient to determine differences. ▪ Patients on the R-CHOP regimen 60 years of age and over reported increased incidences of cardiac events (e.g., supraventricular arrhythmias, tachycardia), chills, fever, and respiratory symptoms. ▪ The incidence of Grade 3 and 4 adverse reactions was higher in patients over 70 years of age treated for CLL with R-FC. No observed benefit was seen with the addition of rituximab to FC in patients over 65 years of age. ▪ In older patients being treated for RA, WG, or MPA, the incidence of side effects was similar to younger adults; however, the rates of serious side effects, including serious infection, malignancies, and cardiovascular events, was higher.

DRUG/LAB INTERACTIONS

Transient hypotension may occur during rituximab infusion; **consider withholding antihypertensive medications** 12 hours before rituximab infusion. ▪ May inhibit the generation of an anamnestic (immunologic memory) or humoral (development of antibodies in the blood) response to any **vaccine.** ▪ Pharmacokinetics of rituximab remained similar to rituximab alone when given in combination with CHOP chemotherapy (cyclophosphamide, doxorubicin, vincristine, prednisone). ▪ Risk of renal toxicity increased in patients receiving concomitant therapy with **cisplatin** (the combination of cisplatin and rituximab is not an approved treatment regimen). ▪ Concurrent use with **CHOP chemotherapy** has resulted in an increase in fatal infections in HIV-related lymphoma patients. ▪ Data on the safety of the use of biologic agents or **disease-modifying antirheumatic drugs** (DMARDs) other than methotrexate are limited. Monitor patients closely for signs of infection with concurrent use of biologic agents or DMARDs other than methotrexate.

SIDE EFFECTS

CD20-positive, B-cell NHL: The most common side effects are asthenia, chills, fever, infection, infusion reactions, and lymphopenia.

Diffuse large B-cell, CD20-positive NHL: In addition to the previously listed side effects, anemia, neutropenia, viral infection, and Grade 3 or 4 respiratory symptoms and thrombocytopenia occurred more frequently among patients on the R-CHOP regimen. Patients on this regimen 60 years of age and over reported increased incidences of cardiac events (e.g., supraventricular arrhythmias, tachycardia), chills, fever, and respiratory symptoms. **CLL:** The most common side effects during clinical trials were infusion reactions and neutropenia.

Major side effects for the previously listed indications include angina, bowel obstruction and perforation, cardiac arrhythmias (e.g., supraventricular and ventricular tachycardia, ventricular fibrillation), hepatitis B reactivation with fulminant hepatitis and other viral infections (including JC virus infection resulting in PML), hypersensitivity reactions (e.g., hypotension, bronchospasm, and angioedema), infusion reactions, mucocutaneous reactions (e.g., lichenoid dermatitis, paraneoplastic pemphigus, Stevens-Johnson syndrome, toxic epidermal necrolysis, and vesiculobullous dermatitis), renal failure, and tumor lysis syndrome (may occur within 12 to 24 hours). Hypersensitivity or infusion-related side effects generally occur within 30 minutes to 2 hours of beginning of first infusion. Other side effects include abdominal pain, angioedema, anorexia, anxiety, arthralgia, back pain, bone marrow suppression (e.g., anemia, leukopenia, neutropenia, thrombocytopenia, prolonged pancytopenia, and marrow hypoplasia), cough, diarrhea, dizziness, dyspnea, elevated LDH, flushing, headache, hyperglycemia, hypertension, hypotension, infections (with or without neutropenia), myalgia, nausea, night sweats, pain at disease sites, peripheral edema, pruritus, rash, respiratory symptoms (e.g., acute infusion-related bronchospasm, acute pneumonitis 1 to 4 weeks post-rituximab infusion, bronchiolitis obliterans [one case ended in death]), rhinitis, sinusitis, tachycardia, throat irritation, urticaria, and vomiting. Incidence of abdominal pain, anemia, dyspnea, hypotension, and neutropenia is higher in patients with bulky disease lesions equal to or greater than 10 cm.

Rheumatoid arthritis: Similar to those seen in patients with NHL. Major side effects include infusion reactions, cardiac events, immunogenicity, and infections (e.g., bronchitis, nasopharyngitis, sinusitis, URI, UTI). Other more frequently reported side effects include abdominal pain (upper), anxiety, arthralgia, asthenia, chills, dyspepsia, fever, hypercholesterolemia, hypertension, migraine headache, nausea, paresthesia, pruritus, rhinitis, throat irritation, urticaria.

WG and MPA: Most common side effects reported include anemia, arthralgia, cough, diarrhea, dyspnea, epistaxis, fatigue, headache, hypertension, increased ALT, insomnia, leukopenia, muscle spasm, nausea, peripheral edema, and rash. All major side effects associated with rituximab (e.g., infusion reactions, infections) may occur.

Post-Marketing: Bowel obstruction and perforation, bronchiolitis obliterans (fatal), cardiac failure (fatal), disease progression of Kaposi's sarcoma, hyperviscosity syndrome in Waldenström's macroglobulinemia, increase in fatal infections in HIV-associated lymphoma and a reported increased incidence of Grade 3 and 4 infections in patients with previously treated lymphoma without known HIV infection, lupus-like syndrome, marrow hyperplasia, mucocutaneous reactions (severe), neutropenia (late onset), optic neuritis, pancytopenia (prolonged), pleuritis, pneumonitis (including interstitial pneumonitis), polyarticular arthritis, serum sickness, systemic vasculitis, uveitis, vasculitis with rash, and viral infections, including PML.

ANTIDOTE

Keep physician informed of all side effects. May constitute a medical emergency or will be treated symptomatically as indicated. Hypersensitivity or infusion-related side effects generally resolve with slowing or interruption of the rituximab infusion and with supportive care (IV saline; diphenhydramine; bronchodilators such as albuterol [Ventolin] or aminophylline; and acetaminophen). Most patients who have had non–life-threatening reactions have been able to complete the full course of therapy. Restart the infusion at half the previous rate after symptoms have resolved completely. Discontinue the infusion immediately for any life-threatening side effect (e.g., clinically significant bronchospasm, cardiac arrhythmias, Grade 3 or 4 infusion reactions, hypersensitivity reactions, hypotension, tumor lysis syndrome). Discontinue rituximab in any patient who develops a serious infection. Initiate appropriate antiviral/anti-infective therapy as indicated. Discontinue treatment in patients who develop severe mucocutaneous reactions. Skin biopsy may be required to diagnose mucocutaneous reaction and guide treatment. Discontinue treatment in patients who develop PML; consider reduction or discontinuation of concomitant chemotherapy or immunosuppressive therapy. Discontinue treatment in patients with a rising SCr or oliguria. Treat anaphylaxis with oxygen, antihistamines (diphenhydramine), epinephrine, and corticosteroids. Maintain a patent airway. Treat arrhythmias if indicated and monitor ECG until recovery and with subsequent doses. Treat hypotension with IV fluids, Trendelenburg position, and, if necessary, vasopressors (e.g., norepinephrine [Levophed], dopamine). Blood modifiers (e.g., darbepoetin alfa [Aranesp], epoetin alfa [Epogen], filgrastim [Neupogen], oprelvekin [Neumega], pegfilgrastim [Neulasta], sargramostim [Leukine]) may be indicated to treat bone marrow toxicity. Tumor lysis syndrome requires correction of electrolyte abnormalities, monitoring of renal function and fluid balance, and supportive care including dialysis. Resuscitate if indicated.

ROMIDEPSIN
(ROE-mi-DEP-sin)

Istodax

Antineoplastic
(HDAC Inhibitor)

USUAL DOSE

14 mg/M^2 as an infusion over 4 hours. Administer on Days 1, 8, and 15 of a 28-day cycle; see Monitor. Cycles may be repeated every 28 days provided the patient continues to benefit from and tolerates the drug. Discontinuation or interruption with or without dose reduction to 10 mg/M^2 may be needed to manage adverse drug reactions; see Dose Adjustments.

DOSE ADJUSTMENTS

Romidepsin Dose Modification for Nonhematologic Toxicities Except Alopecia		
CTCAE* Grade on Day of Treatment	Action	Dose on Recovery
Grade 2 or 3 toxicity	Delay dose until toxicity returns to ≤ Grade 1 or baseline	14 mg/M^2
Grade 3 toxicity recurrence	Delay dose until toxicity returns to ≤ Grade 1 or baseline	Permanently reduce dose to 10 mg/M^2
Grade 4 toxicity	Delay dose until toxicity returns to ≤ Grade 1 or baseline	Permanently reduce dose to 10 mg/M^2
Grade 3 or 4 toxicities recur after dose reduction	Discontinue therapy	

*Per Common Terminology Criteria for Adverse Events (CTCAE), Version 3.

Romidepsin Dose Modification for Hematologic Toxicities		
CTCAE* Grade on Day of Treatment	Action	Dose on Recovery
Grade 3 or 4 neutropenia or thrombocytopenia	Delay dose until ANC ≥1,500/mm^3 and/or platelet count ≥75,000/mm^3	14 mg/M^2
Grade 4 febrile (≥38.5° C) neutropenia or thrombocytopenia that requires platelet transfusion	Delay dose until the specific cytopenia returns to ≤ Grade 1 or baseline	Permanently reduce dose to 10 mg/M^2

*Per Common Terminology Criteria for Adverse Events (CTCAE), Version 3.

No dose adjustments required based on age, gender, race, mild or moderate renal impairment, or mild hepatic impairment.

DILUTION

Special techniques required; see Precautions: Reconstitute each 10-mg vial with 2 mL of the supplied diluent. Inject diluent slowly into the vial of romidepsin and swirl contents until there are no visible particles. Concentration equals 5 mg/mL. Withdraw the calculated dose and further dilute in 500 mL NS.

Filters: Specific information not available.

Storage: Store vials in carton at CRT. Reconstituted solution is stable for 8 hours at RT. Diluted solutions are stable at RT for 24 hours, but use soon after dilution is recommended.

COMPATIBILITY

Manufacturer states, "The diluted solution is **compatible** with polyvinyl chloride (PVC), ethylene vinyl acetate (EVA), polyethylene (PE) infusion bags as well as glass bottles." No additional information available; consider specific use and consult pharmacist.

RATE OF ADMINISTRATION

A single dose as an infusion equally distributed over 4 hours.

ACTIONS

A histone deacetylase (HDAC) inhibitor. HDACs catalyze the removal of acetyl groups from acetylated lysine residues in histones, resulting in the modulation of gene expression. Induces cell cycle arrest and apoptosis of some cancer cell lines. Mechanism of antineoplastic effect not fully characterized. Highly protein bound. It undergoes extensive metabolism *in vitro* by CYP3A4 with minor contributions from other cytochrome P_{450} isoenzymes. Half-life is approximately 3 hours. No accumulation of plasma concentrations observed after repeated dosing.

INDICATIONS AND USES

Treatment of cutaneous T-cell lymphoma (CTCL) in patients who have received at least one prior systemic therapy.

CONTRAINDICATIONS

Manufacturer states, "None."

PRECAUTIONS

Follow guidelines for handling cytotoxic agents. See Appendix A, p. 1429. ■ Administered under the direction of a physician knowledgeable in its use in a facility with adequate diagnostic and treatment facilities to monitor the patients and respond to any medical emergency. ■ Bone marrow suppression can occur (e.g., anemia, lymphopenia, neutropenia, and thrombocytopenia). Dose modification based on ANC, and platelet count is required; see Dose Adjustments. ■ ECG changes have been reported (e.g., T-wave and ST-segment changes, QT prolongation). Use caution in patients with congenital long QT syndrome or a history of significant CV disease or in patients taking antiarrhythmic medicines that lead to significant QT prolongation; see Drug/Lab Interactions. ■ Use with caution in patients with moderate or severe hepatic impairment. ■ Renal impairment is not expected to influence romidepsin exposure. Effect on end-stage renal disease (ESRD) has not been studied; use with caution in patients with ESRD. **Monitor:** Due to the risk of QT prolongation, potassium and magnesium should be within the normal range before administration of romidepsin. ■ Obtain baseline CBC, platelets, and electrolytes. Baseline CrCl or SCr and liver function tests may be indicated. ■ Monitor CBC, platelets, and electrolytes during treatment and modify dose as indicated; see Dose Adjustments. ■ Consider ECG monitoring and more frequent monitoring of electrolytes in at-risk cardiac patients; see Precautions. ■ Monitor for thrombocytopenia (platelet count less than 50,000/mm^3). Initiate precautions to prevent excessive bleeding (e.g., inspect IV sites, skin, and mucous membranes; use extreme care during invasive procedures; test urine, emesis, stool, and secretions for occult blood). ■ Use prophylactic antiemetics to reduce nausea and/or vomiting and increase patient comfort. ■ Observe closely for signs of infection. Prophylactic antibiotics may be indicated pending results of C/S in a febrile neutropenic patient. **Patient Education:** Read patient insert carefully. ■ Avoid pregnancy; nonhormonal birth control recommended; see Drug/Lab Interactions. ■ Blood counts will be required at regular intervals. ■ Promptly report unusual bleeding, excessive nausea or vomiting, abnormal heartbeat, chest pain, or shortness of breath. ■ Report burning on urination, cough, fever, flulike symptoms, muscle aches, or worsening of skin problems. ■ Discuss medications (prescription, non-prescription, and herbal) with a health care professional; see Drug/Lab Interactions. ■ See Appendix D, p. 1434.

Maternal/Child: Category D: avoid pregnancy; may cause fetal harm. If the drug is used during pregnancy or the patient becomes pregnant during therapy, inform the patient of the potential hazard to the fetus. ▪ Discontinue breast-feeding. ▪ Safety and effectiveness for use in pediatric patients not established.

Elderly: No differences in safety and effectiveness compared with younger patients were noted; however; greater sensitivity of some older patients cannot be ruled out.

DRUG/LAB INTERACTIONS

Concurrent use with **warfarin** (Coumadin) may prolong PT and elevate INR. Monitoring of PT and INR recommended. ▪ **Strong CYP3A4 inhibitors** (e.g., atazanavir [Reyataz], clarithromycin [Biaxin], indinavir (Crixivan), itraconazole [Sporanox], ketoconazole [Nizoral], nefazodone, nelfinavir [Viracept]. ritonavir [Norvir], saquinavir [Invirase], telithromycin [Ketek], and voriconazole [VFEND]), may increase concentrations of romidepsin; avoid concurrent use if possible. Use caution with concomitant use of **moderate CYP3A4** inhibitors (aprepitant [Emend], verapamil). ▪ **Potent CYP3A4 inducers** (e.g., carbamazepine [Tegretol], dexamethasone [Decadron], phenobarbital [Luminal], phenytoin [Dilantin], rifabutin [Mycobutin], rifapentine [Priftin], rifampin (Rifadin), and St. John's wort may decrease concentrations of romidepsin and should be avoided. ▪ Use caution with other **drugs that inhibit the efflux transporter P-glycoprotein (P-gp, ABCB1)** (e.g., protease inhibitors [e.g., nelfinavir (Viracept)]) may increase concentrations of romidepsin; use caution. ▪ Do not administer **live virus vaccines** to patients receiving antineoplastic drugs. ▪ Concurrent use with other **drugs that prolong the QT interval** (e.g., antiarrhythmics [e.g., amiodarone (Nexterone), disopyramide (Norpace), ibutilide (Corvert), mexiletine, procainamide (Pronestyl), quinidine], antihistamines, azole antifungals [e.g., itraconazole (Sporanox)], fluoroquinolones [e.g., levofloxacin (Levaquin)], phenothiazines [e.g., thioridazine (Mellaril)], and tricyclic antidepressants [e.g., amitriptyline (Elavil), imipramine (Tofranil)]) may cause torsades de pointes and could be fatal. ▪ May reduce the effectiveness of **estrogen-containing contraceptives.**

SIDE EFFECTS

Most common side effects are anorexia, bone marrow suppression (e.g., anemia, lymphopenia, neutropenia, thrombocytopenia), ECG T-wave changes, fatigue, infections, nausea, and vomiting. Serious adverse reactions reported included central line infection, edema, fatigue, fever, infection, leukopenia, nausea, neutropenia, sepsis, supraventricular arrhythmia, thrombocytopenia, and ventricular arrhythmia. Dyspnea, fatigue, infection, and QT prolongation were the most common reasons for discontinuing therapy. Other side effects reported include asthenia, constipation, dermatitis, diarrhea, dysgeusia, exfoliative dermatitis, elevated AST and ALT, hyperglycemia, hypermagnesemia, hyperuricemia, hypoalbuminemia, hypocalcemia, hypokalemia, hypomagnesemia, hypophosphatemia, hyponatremia, hypotension, and pruritus.

ANTIDOTE

Treatment of most side effects will be supportive and may require dose adjustment or discontinuation. Discontinue if Grade 3 or 4 toxicities recur after dose reduction. Keep physician informed. Administration of blood products and/or blood modifiers (e.g., darbepoetin [Aranesp], epoetin alfa [Epogen], filgrastim [Neupogen], oprelvekin [Neumega], pegfilgrastim [Neulasta], sargramostim [Leukine]) may be indicated to treat bone marrow toxicity. Treat hypersensitivity reactions with epinephrine, antihistamines, and corticosteroids as needed. No known antidote. Discontinue romidepsin and provide supportive therapy in overdose. Not known if romidepsin is dialyzable. Resuscitate if indicated.

SARGRAMOSTIM
(sar-**GRAM**-oh-stim)

GM-CSF, Human Granulocyte-Macrophage Colony-Stimulating Factor, Leukine

Colony-stimulating factor
Antineutropenic

pH 7.1 to 7.7

USUAL DOSE

Myeloid reconstitution after allogeneic or autologous bone marrow transplantation: 250 mcg/M^2/day as a 2-hour infusion daily for 21 days. Initial infusion must begin 2 to 4 hours after bone marrow infusion and not less than 24 hours after the last dose of chemotherapy and 12 hours after the last dose of radiation. Post–marrow infusion absolute neutrophil count (ANC) should be less than 500 cells/mm^3.

Engraftment delay or failure of bone marrow transplantation: 250 mcg/M^2/day as a 2-hour infusion daily for 14 days. Wait for 7 days; if engraftment has not occurred, repeat 14-day course of 250 mcg/M^2/day. Wait an additional 7 days; if engraftment has still not occurred, give a 14-day course of 500 mcg/M^2/day. If engraftment does not occur, further courses or dose increases are not indicated. Note time restrictions on chemotherapy and radiation above and in Drug/Lab Interactions.

Neutrophil recovery following chemotherapy in acute myelogenous leukemia (AML) in adults 55 years of age or older: 250 mcg/M^2/day as an infusion over 4 hours. Begin on day 11 or 4 days after induction chemotherapy is complete. Day 10 bone marrow should be hypoplastic with fewer than 5% blasts. Repeat sargramostim daily until absolute neutrophil count (ANC) is greater than 1,500/mm^3 for three consecutive days or a maximum of 42 days. Use same criteria if a second cycle of induction chemotherapy is indicated.

Mobilization of peripheral blood progenitor cells: 250 mcg/M^2/day as a 24-hour continuous infusion (or give SC once daily). Continue at the same dose until adequate numbers of progenitor stem cells are collected. Collection of progenitor cells (apheresis) usually begins about Day 5 and is repeated daily. All cells are stored until predetermined targets are achieved. After immunosuppression with selected antineoplastic bone marrow suppressant agents to neutralize remaining tumor cells or ineffective leukocytes, the collected progenitor stem cells are reinfused into the patient by IV infusion. This process has been used primarily in patients who were not candidates for bone marrow transplant; however, it is increasingly being used instead of bone marrow transplant.

Post–peripheral blood progenitor cell transplantation: 250 mcg/M^2/day as a 24-hour continuous infusion (or give SC once daily). Begin immediately following infusion of harvested progenitor cells and continue until an ANC is greater than 1,500/mm^3 for three consecutive days. Neutrophil recovery occurs somewhat sooner in patients receiving sargramostim stimulation. Results in a shorter time to platelet and RBC transfusion independence.

DOSE ADJUSTMENTS

May require reduced dose in impaired renal or hepatic function. Based on individual patient response. ■ For an ANC above 20,000 cells/mm^3, WBC above 50,000 cells/mm^3, or a platelet count above 500,000/mm^3, reduce dose by one half or temporarily discontinue. ■ See Antidote.

DILUTION

Now available in liquid form (reconstituted) or each 250- or 500-mcg vial of the dry product must be reconstituted with 1 mL SW for injection with or without preservative. Confirm expiration date to ensure valid product. Direct diluent to the side of the vial and swirl gently. Avoid foaming or vigorous agitation. Do not shake. Either product must be further diluted in NS for infusion. If the final concentration of sargramostim will be below 10 mcg/mL, albumin (human) must be added to the NS before addition of the sargramostim (1 mL of 5% albumin to each 50 mL NS). This will prevent adsorption of the drug into the components of the IV delivery system. Liquefied product contains benzyl alcohol. Use sterile technique; enter vial only to dilute and/or to withdraw a single dose. Discard any unused portion. Should be clear and colorless.

Filters: Manufacturer states, *"An in-line membrane filter should not be used for IV infusion of sargramostim."*

Storage: Must be refrigerated in all forms; do not freeze or shake. Reconstituted with SW without preservatives or any diluted solution should be used within 6 hours. Reconstituted with bacteriostatic SW (benzyl alcohol preservative) or the new liquid preparation can be refrigerated for up to 20 days.

COMPATIBILITY   (Underline Indicates Conflicting Compatibility Information)

Consider any drug NOT listed as compatible to be INCOMPATIBLE until consulting a pharmacist; specific conditions may apply.

Manufacturer recommends that no medication other than albumin be added to the infusion solution and that only NS be used to prepare IV solutions until specific **compatibility** data are available.

One source suggests the following **compatibilities:**

Y-site: Amikacin (Amikin), aminophylline, amphotericin B (generic), aztreonam (Azactam), bleomycin (Blenoxane), butorphanol (Stadol), calcium gluconate, carboplatin (Paraplatin), carmustine (BiCNU), cefazolin (Ancef), cefepime (Maxipime), cefotaxime (Claforan), cefotetan, ceftazidime (Fortaz), ceftriaxone (Rocephin), cefuroxime (Zinacef), cisplatin (Platinol), clindamycin (Cleocin), cyclophosphamide (Cytoxan), cyclosporine (Sandimmune), cytarabine (ARA-C), dacarbazine (DTIC), dactinomycin (Cosmegen), dexamethasone (Decadron), diphenhydramine (Benadryl), dopamine, doxorubicin (Adriamycin), doxycycline, droperidol (Inapsine), etoposide (VePesid), famotidine (Pepcid IV), fentanyl (Sublimaze), fluconazole (Diflucan), fluorouracil (5-FU), furosemide (Lasix), gentamicin, granisetron (Kytril), heparin, idarubicin (Idamycin), ifosfamide (Ifex), immune globulin IV (e.g., Gamunex-C), magnesium sulfate, mannitol, mechlorethamine (nitrogen mustard), meperidine (Demerol), mesna (Mesnex), methotrexate, metoclopramide (Reglan), metronidazole (Flagyl IV), mitoxantrone (Novantrone), pentostatin (Nipent), piperacillin/tazobactam (Zosyn), potassium chloride (KCl), prochlorperazine (Compazine), promethazine (Phenergan), ranitidine (Zantac), sulfamethoxazole/trimethoprim, teniposide (Vumon), ticarcillin/clavulanate (Timentin), <u>vancomycin</u>, vinblastine, vincristine, zidovudine (AZT, Retrovir).

RATE OF ADMINISTRATION

See Usual Dose. Each single dose must be evenly distributed over 2, 4, or 24 hours. Do not use an in-line membrane filter. Reduce rate or temporarily discontinue for onset of any side effects that cause concern (e.g., hypersensitivity reactions).

ACTIONS

Colony-stimulating factors are glycoproteins that bind to specific hematopoietic cell surface receptors and stimulate proliferation, differentiation commitment, and some end-cell functional activation. Utilizing recombinant DNA technology, sargramostim is produced in a yeast *(Saccharomyces cerevisiae)*. It differs slightly from endogenous G-CSF. It induces partially committed progenitor cells to divide and differentiate in the granulocyte-macrophage pathways. Can also activate mature granulocytes and macrophages. It is a multilineage factor and has dose-dependent effects. It increases the cytotoxicity of monocytes toward certain neoplastic cell lines and activates polymorphonuclear neutrophils to inhibit the growth of tumor cells. It significantly improves the time to neutrophil recovery (engraftment), decreases length of hospitalization, shortens the duration of infectious episodes, and decreases antibiotic usage. Patients with fewer impaired organs have the best opportunity for improvement in survival. Detected in the serum in 5 minutes; peak levels are reached 2 hours after injection and last at least 6 hours.

INDICATIONS AND USES

Acceleration of hematopoietic recovery (myeloid engraftment) in patients undergoing allogeneic or autologous bone marrow transplantation. ▪ Bone marrow transplantation failure or engraftment delay. ▪ Neutrophil recovery following chemotherapy in acute myelogenous leukemia (AML); safety for use in adults under 55 years not established. ▪ Mobilization of peripheral blood progenitor cells. ▪ Stimulate neutrophil recovery post–peripheral blood progenitor cell transplantation.
Unlabeled uses: Increase WBC in myelodysplastic syndromes and in AIDS patients receiving zidovudine. ▪ Correct neutropenia in aplastic anemia. ▪ Decrease transplantation-associated organ system damage, especially in kidney and liver transplants.

CONTRAINDICATIONS

Hypersensitivity to any components of sargramostim or yeast products; patients with leukemic myeloid blasts in the bone marrow or peripheral blood equal to 10% or more.

PRECAUTIONS

Should be administered under the direction of a physician knowledgeable about appropriate use. ▪ Use caution if considered for use in any malignancy with myeloid characteristics. Can act as a growth factor for any tumor type, particularly myeloid malignancies. ▪ Can be effective in patients receiving purged bone marrow if the purging process preserves a sufficient number of progenitors. ▪ Effects may be limited in patients previously exposed to intensive chemotherapy or radiation therapy. ▪ Neutralizing antibodies may form after receiving sargramostim and may inhibit therapeutic effect.

Monitor: Obtain a CBC with differential before administration and twice weekly thereafter to monitor for excessive leukocytosis (WBC above 50,000 cells/mm^3; or an absolute neutrophil count [ANC] above 20,000 cells/mm^3). ▪ If blast cells appear or disease progression occurs, treatment should be discontinued. ▪ Anemia, leukocytopenia, and thrombocytopenia occur as side effects of various procedures; monitor carefully. ▪ Observe for fluid retention; may cause peripheral edema, pleural effusion, and/or pericardial effusion. May occur more frequently in individuals with pre-existing lung disease or cardiac disease, including a history of arrhythmias. Use with caution. ▪ Use with caution in patients with preexisting renal or hepatic dysfunction; an increased SCr or increased bilirubin and hepatic enzymes may occur. Reversible if drug discontinued. Monitor renal and hepatic function biweekly. ▪ Flushing, hypotension, and syncope may occur, especially with the initial dose. Reduce rate or stop temporarily.

Patient Education: Promptly report any symptoms of infection (e.g., fever) or hypersensitivity reactions (e.g., itching, swelling, redness at the injection site).

Maternal/Child: Category C: safety for use in pregnancy and breast-feeding not established; use only if clearly needed. ▪ Has been used in more than 100 pediatric patients from 4 months to 18 years of age with similar experience to the adult population, even though literature says safety not established. ▪ Liquefied product contains benzyl alcohol; do not use in neonates.

DRUG/LAB INTERACTIONS

Do not administer within 24 hours preceding or following **chemotherapy** or within 12 hours preceding or following **radiotherapy.** Rapidly dividing cells and the success of the treatment would be adversely affected by chemotherapy and radiation. ▪ Myeloproliferative effects may be potentiated by **lithium or corticosteroids;** use with caution.

SIDE EFFECTS

Asthenia, diarrhea, malaise, peripheral edema, rash, and urinary tract disorders are most common. Hypersensitivity reactions, including anaphylaxis, are possible; arthralgia, capillary leak syndrome, dyspnea, fever, headache, hypoxia, local injection site reactions, myalgia, pericardial effusion, peripheral edema, pleural effusion, and supraventricular arrhythmias have been reported.

ANTIDOTE

Discontinue sargramostim for anaphylaxis, if blast cells appear, or there is progression of underlying disease. A maximum dose limit has not been determined; for accidental overdose, discontinue and monitor for WBC increase and respiratory symptoms. For an ANC above 20,000 cells/mm^3, WBC above 50,000 cells/mm^3, or a platelet count above 500,000/mm^3, reduce dose by one half or temporarily discontinue. Blood cell count should return to baseline level in 3 to 7 days. For any side effect that causes concern, reduce dose or temporarily discontinue. Keep physician informed. Treat anaphylaxis and resuscitate as necessary.

SILDENAFIL BBW *
(sil-**DEN**-a-fil)

Revatio

Vasodilating agent
Antihypertensive (pulmonary)

*This drug is on the Black Box Warning list; however, a BBW is not provided in the parenteral prescribing information.

USUAL DOSE
10 mg (12.5 mL) as an IV bolus 3 times daily (approximately 4 to 6 hours between doses). A 10-mg IV dose of sildenafil is equivalent to a 20-mg oral dose. Resume oral therapy as soon as tolerated.

DOSE ADJUSTMENTS
No dose adjustments required for age, gender, race, weight, renal impairment (mild, moderate, or severe), or hepatic impairment (mild or moderate). Has not been studied in patients with severe hepatic impairment.

DILUTION
May be given undiluted. Aseptically withdraw the calculated dose directly into a syringe for immediate use.

Filters: Specific information not available.

Storage: Store vials at CRT.

COMPATIBILITY
Specific information not available. Manufacturer made no recommendations.

RATE OF ADMINISTRATION
A single dose as an IV bolus.

ACTIONS
An inhibitor of cGMP-specific phosphodiesterase type 5 (PDE5) in the smooth muscle of the pulmonary vasculature where PDE5 is responsible for degradation of cGMP. Sildenafil increases cGMP within pulmonary vascular smooth muscle cells, resulting in relaxation. In patients with pulmonary hypertension, this can lead to vasodilation of the pulmonary vascular bed and, to a lesser degree, vasodilation in the systemic circulation. PDE5 is also found in other tissues, including vascular and visceral smooth muscle, and in platelets. Sildenafil and its major metabolite are approximately 96% protein bound. Metabolized in the liver predominantly by CYP3A4 and other hepatic microsomal isoenzymes. Terminal half-life is about 4 hours. Findings suggest a lower clearance and/or a higher bioavailability of sildenafil in patients with pulmonary hypertension compared with healthy volunteers. Primarily excreted in feces and approximately 13% in urine.

INDICATIONS AND USES
Treatment of pulmonary arterial hypertension (PAH) (WHO Group 1) in patients who are currently prescribed oral sildenafil and are temporarily unable to take oral medications. Intended to improve exercise ability and delay clinical worsening. Delay in clinical worsening demonstrated with concurrent use with epoprostenol (Flolan). Studies establishing effectiveness included predominantly patients with NYHA Functional Class II-III symptoms and etiologies of primary pulmonary hypertension or pulmonary hypertension associated with connective tissue disease.

CONTRAINDICATIONS

Known hypersensitivity to sildenafil or any component of the product. ■ Potentiates the hypotensive effects of nitrates. Do not use with organic nitrates in any form (medicines that treat chest pain [angina], nitroglycerin in any form, isosorbide mononitrate [Monoket, Imdur], or isosorbide dinitrate [Isordil, Dilatrate-SR], street drugs called "poppers" [amyl nitrate or nitrite]). ■ See Drug/Lab Interactions.

PRECAUTIONS

Has vasodilatory properties, resulting in mild and transient decreases in BP. Use with caution in patients with resting hypotension (BP less than 90/50 mm Hg), fluid depletion, severe left ventricular outflow obstruction, or autonomic dysfunction. ■ Not recommended for use in patients with pulmonary veno-occlusive disease (PVOD); it may significantly worsen their cardiac status. Consider the possibility of associated PVOD if signs of pulmonary edema occur. ■ Use with caution in patients who have had an MI, stroke, or life-threatening arrhythmia within the last 6 months; in patients with coronary artery disease (CAD) and unstable angina; in patients with hypertension (BP greater than 170/110 mm Hg); and in patients currently undergoing bosentan (Tracleer) therapy; safety and effectiveness not studied. ■ Epistaxis has been reported in patients with PAH secondary to connective tissue disease (CTD) and in patients treated with a concomitant oral vitamin K antagonist (warfarin [Coumadin]). ■ Safety for use in patients with bleeding disorders or active peptic ulceration is unknown. ■ Sudden loss of vision in one or both eyes has been reported and may lead to permanent loss of vision. Use with caution in patients with retinitis pigmentosa. ■ Retinal hemorrhage has occurred in patients with risk factors for hemorrhage, including concurrent **anticoagulant** therapy. ■ Sudden decrease or loss of hearing has been reported; may be accompanied by dizziness and tinnitus. ■ Use with caution in patients with an anatomic deformation of the penis (e.g., angulation, cavernosal fibrosis, or Peyronie's disease) or in patients with conditions that may predispose them to priapism (e.g., sickle cell anemia, multiple myeloma, or leukemia). Penile tissue damage and permanent loss of potency can result from priapism lasting more than 6 hours. ■ Effectiveness of sildenafil in pulmonary hypertension secondary to sickle cell anemia has not been established. Increased incidence of vaso-occlusive crisis requiring hospitalization has been reported in this patient population. ■ See Drug/Lab Interactions.

Monitor: Obtain baseline studies as indicated by specific patient history. ■ Monitor VS closely to note unsafe drops in BP. ■ Monitor for cardiovascular events, especially in patients with risk factors. ■ Monitor for vision and/or hearing loss. ■ See Precautions, Patient Education, and Drug/Lab Interactions.

Patient Education: Read manufacturers patient education booklet carefully. ■ Never take sildenafil with nitrate medicines; may cause a sudden and unsafe drop in BP. ■ Do not take Viagra or other similar medications for erectile dysfunction with sildenafil. ■ Seek immediate medical attention with a sudden loss of vision in one or both eyes. ■ Seek prompt medical attention in the event of a sudden decrease or loss of hearing. ■ Seek emergency help if an erection lasts for more than 4 hours. ■ Discuss medications (prescription, non-prescription, and herbal) with a health care professional; see Drug/Lab Interactions.

Maternal/Child: Category B: use during Pregnancy only if clearly needed. ▪ Use during labor and delivery has not been studied. ▪ Not known if sildenafil is secreted in human milk; use caution if required during breast-feeding. ▪ Safety and effectiveness for use in pediatric pulmonary hypertension patients not established.

Elderly: Major differences in response compared with younger adults have not been identified; however, healthy elderly volunteers had a reduced clearance resulting in higher plasma concentrations. Dosing should be cautious. Consider age-related organ impairment and concomitant disease or drug therapy.

DRUG/LAB INTERACTIONS

Sildenafil is also marketed as Viagra. Do not take **Viagra or other PDE5 inhibitors** (e.g., tadalafil [Cialis], vardenafil [Levitra]) concurrently with sildenafil (Revatio). ▪ Concurrent use with **nitrates** (e.g., amyl nitrate, nitroglycerin, nitroprusside) in any form (regularly or intermittently) is *contraindicated.* May result in an unsafe drop in BP. ▪ Concurrent use with **alpha-adrenergic blocking agents** (e.g., alfuzosin [Uroxatral], doxazosin [Cardura], phentolamine, prazosin [Minipress], tamsulosin [Flomax], terazosin [Hytrin]) can lower BP significantly and lead to symptomatic hypotension. BP may be lowered further with this combined use of vasodilators by other variables, including intravascular volume depletion and concomitant use of **antihypertensive drugs** (e.g., calcium channel blockers [amlodipine (Norvasc), diltiazem (Cardizem)]). ▪ Concomitant use of sildenafil with **ritonavir** (Norvir) **and other potent CYP3A4 inhibitors** (e.g., atazanavir [Reyataz], clarithromycin [Biaxin], indinavir [Crixivan], itraconazole [Sporanox], ketoconazole [Nizoral], nefazodone, nelfinavir [Viracept], saquinavir [Invirase], telithromycin [Ketek], and voriconazole [VFEND]) *is not recommended.* ▪ **Cimetidine** (Tagamet) and **erythromycin** may cause an increase in sildenafil plasma concentrations. ▪ **Potent CYP3A4 inducers** (e.g., carbamazepine [Tegretol], dexamethasone [Decadron], phenytoin [Dilantin], phenobarbital [Luminal], rifabutin [Mycobutin], rifapentine [Priftin], rifampin [Rifadin], and St. John's wort) may increase sildenafil clearance and reduce its effectiveness. ▪ **Bosentan** (Tracleer) may also increase sildenafil clearance. ▪ Concurrent use with epoprostenol (Flolan) did not have a significant effect on sildenafil pharmacokinetics, effect on epoprostenol not known. ▪ Does not potentiate the increase in bleeding time caused by aspirin. ▪ Did not potentiate hypotensive effects with alcohol in healthy volunteers. ▪ Has been given with atorvastatin [Lipitor], oral contraceptives, and tolbutamide without effect.

SIDE EFFECTS

Manufacturer does not distinguish between side effects caused by oral dosing versus injectable dosing. Most common side effects are dyspepsia, dyspnea, epistaxis, erythema, flushing, headache, insomnia, and rhinitis. Serious side effects include hearing loss, hypotension, indigestion, priapism, vaso-occlusive crisis, and vision loss. Other side effects reported include diarrhea, fever, gastritis, myalgia, paresthesia, and sinusitis. Sildenafil combined with epoprostenol (Flolan) added edema (including peripheral edema), nasal congestion, nausea, and pain in extremities. Retinal hemorrhage occurred in patients with risk factors for hemorrhage, including concurrent anticoagulant therapy. Most hypersensitivity reactions have been nonserious. Serious hypersensitivity reactions (e.g., anaphylaxis, shock) have been rare.

Post-Marketing: Serious cardiovascular, cerebrovascular, and vascular events, including MI, cerebrovascular hemorrhage, hypertension, pulmonary hemorrhage, subarachnoid and intracerebral hemorrhages, TIA, ventricular arrhythmia, and sudden cardiac death; sudden decrease or loss of hearing; seizure; and seizure recurrence.

ANTIDOTE

Treatment of most side effects will be supportive. Notify physician immediately if a serious side effect occurs (e.g., hearing loss, hypotension, hypersensitivity, priapism, vision loss). Treat hypersensitivity reactions with epinephrine, antihistamines, and corticosteroids as needed. Hemodialysis is not expected to be effective in overdose.

SIPULEUCEL-T
Provenge

Autologous cellular immunotherapy
Antineoplastic

USUAL DOSE

An autologous (derived from the same individual) cellular immunotherapy. Each infusion of sipuleucel-T is preceded by a leukapheresis procedure and a specific preparation procedure by the manufacturer; see Dilution and Actions. Three complete doses are administered at approximately 2-week intervals (range of 1 to 15 weeks in clinical trials).

Approximately 3 days before the desired infusion date: *Leukapheresis:* Peripheral blood mononuclear cells are obtained via a standard leukapheresis procedure. These cells are then sent to the manufacturer (Dendreon) to be prepared for reinfusion into the patient.

Day of infusion: *Premedication:* Administer oral acetaminophen and an antihistamine (e.g., diphenhydramine [Benadryl]) 30 minutes before administration to minimize potential acute infusion reactions (e.g., chills, fever).

Sipuleucel-T: For autologous IV use only. Do **not** use a cell filter. Confirm that the patient's identity matches the patient identifiers on the infusion bag and the Cell Product Disposition Form (CPDF). Each dose contains a minimum of 50,000,000 autologous CD54+ cells activated with PAP-GM-CSF and suspended in 250 mL of LR in a sealed, patient-specific infusion bag. Do **not** infuse until confirmation of product release has been received from Dendreon; see Dilution. Infusion must begin before the expiration date and time on the Cell Product Disposition Form (CPDF).

DILUTION

Will be shipped directly to the infusing provider in packaging intended to protect the infusion bag and maintain storage temperatures until infusion. Verify the product and patient-specific labels located on top of the insulated container. Do **not** remove from the shipping box or open the lid of the insulated container until the patient is ready for infusion. The manufacturer will send to the infusion site a CPDF that contains the patient identifiers, expiration date and time, and disposition status (approved for infusion or rejected). When all preparations have been made for infusion and the

CPDF has been received and verified, remove the sipuleucel-T infusion bag from the insulated container and inspect for signs of leakage. Contents will be slightly cloudy and a cream-to-pink color. Gently mix and resuspend contents, inspecting for clumps and clots. Small clumps of cellular material should disperse with gentle manual mixing. Do **not** administer if the bag leaks during handling or if clumps remain in the bag.

Filters: Do not use a cell filter.

Storage: After removal from the insulated container, the infusion must be complete within 3 hours at RT. Do not return to the shipping container. Do not initiate infusion of expired sipuleucel-T.

COMPATIBILITY

Specific information not available; however, specific use indicates it should be administered separately; consult pharmacist.

RATE OF ADMINISTRATION

A single dose of 250 mL as an infusion equally distributed over 1 hour. Do **not** use a cell filter. If an infusion reaction occurs, decrease rate or interrupt infusion depending on the severity of the reaction; see Antidote.

ACTIONS

An autologous cellular immunotherapy. The patient's own immune cells are obtained through leukapheresis. Active components of sipuleucel-T are autologous peripheral blood mononuclear cells, including antigen-presenting cells (APCs) and PAP-GM-CSF (prostatic acid phosphatase [PAP], an antigen expressed in prostate cancer tissue, linked to granulocyte-macrophage colony-stimulating factor [GM-CSF], an immune cell activator). The recombinant antigen can bind to and be processed by APCs into smaller protein fragments. The recombinant antigen is designed to target APCs and may help direct the immune response to PAP. The final product contains T-cells, B cells, natural killer (NK) cells and other cells.

INDICATIONS AND USES

Treatment of asymptomatic or minimally symptomatic metastatic hormone refractory prostate cancer.

CONTRAINDICATIONS

Manufacturer states, "None."

PRECAUTIONS

Intended solely for autologous use. For IV use only. ▪ Administered under the direction of a physician knowledgeable in its use in a facility with adequate diagnostic and treatment facilities to monitor the patient and respond to any medical emergency. ▪ Concurrent use of immunosuppressive agents may alter the effectiveness and/or safety of sipuleucel-T; see Drug/Lab Interactions. ▪ Health care professionals must use universal precautions when handling leukapheresis material and sipuleucel-T. Neither is routinely tested for transmissible infectious diseases and thus may carry the risk of infectious disease transmission to health professionals during handling of the products. ▪ Acute infusion reactions (reported within 1 day of infusion) occur frequently and range from mild to serious; see Monitor. Incidence increased with the second infusion and decreased after the third infusion.

Monitor: Obtain baseline vital signs and repeat as indicated. ▪ Observe the patient for S/S of an acute infusion reaction (e.g., bronchospasm, chills, fatigue, fever, hypertension, joint aches, nausea, tachycardia) during the infusion and for at least 30 minutes after the infusion. If an acute infusion reaction occurs, the infusion may be interrupted or slowed depending on the severity of the reaction. Do not resume the infusion if the bag will be held at RT for more than 3 hours. ■ Closely monitor patients with cardiac or pulmonary conditions. ■ If the patient is unable to receive a scheduled infusion, the patient will need to undergo an additional leukapheresis procedure. ■ Monitor for extravasation.

Patient Education: Maintain all scheduled appointments. ■ An additional leukapheresis procedure will be required if a scheduled infusion cannot be completed. ■ A central venous line may be required if peripheral venous access is not adequate to accommodate the leukapheresis procedure and/or the infusion. ■ Promptly report S/S of an infusion reaction (e.g., breathing problems, chills, dizziness, fatigue, fever, headache, hypertension, muscle aches, nausea, or vomiting). ■ Report S/S that may indicate a cardiac arrhythmia (e.g., very slow or rapid pulse). ■ Review prescription and non-prescription drug profile with a physician; see Drug/Lab Interactions.

Maternal/Child: Not indicated for use in these populations.

Elderly: Safety similar to that seen in younger adults.

DRUG/LAB INTERACTIONS

Drug interaction studies have not been performed. ■ Use of either **chemotherapy or immunosuppressive agents** (such as systemic corticosteroids) given concurrently with the leukapheresis procedure or sipuleucel-T has not been studied. ■ Sipuleucel-T is designed to stimulate the immune system, and concurrent use of **immunosuppressive agents** may alter the effectiveness and/or safety of sipuleucel-T. Evaluate patients carefully for the medical appropriateness of reducing or discontinuing immunosuppressive agents before treatment.

SIDE EFFECTS

The most common events of backache, chills, fatigue, fever, headache, joint aches, and nausea are usually mild or moderate and generally resolve within 2 days. Other side effects included anemia, anorexia, citrate toxicity, constipation, cough, diarrhea, hematuria, hot flush, influenza-like illness, insomnia, muscle aches and spasms, pain (bone, extremity, musculoskeletal, musculoskeletal chest, and neck), paresthesia (oral, extremity), peripheral edema, rash, sweating, tremor, URIs, UTIs, weight loss. Acute infusion reactions (mild to moderate) occur frequently. Severe acute infusion reactions (Grade 3) add asthenia, bronchospasm, dizziness, dyspnea, hypertension, hypoxia, and vomiting. Cerebrovascular events (e.g., hemorrhagic and ischemic strokes) and single reports of eosinophilia, myasthenia gravis, myositis, rhabdomyolysis, and tumor flare have been reported.

ANTIDOTE

Keep the physician informed of significant side effects and treat as appropriate. For acute infusion reactions, the infusion may be interrupted or slowed depending on the severity of the reaction. Do not resume the infusion if the bag will be held at RT for more than 3 hours. In controlled clinical trials, acute infusion reactions were treated with acetaminophen, IV antihistamines (e.g., diphenhydramine [Benadryl]) and/or H_2 blockers (e.g., ranitidine [Zantac]) and low-dose IV meperidine. Resuscitate as indicated.

SODIUM ACETATE
(**SO**-dee-um **AS**-ah-tayt)

Electrolyte replenisher
Antihyponatremic
Alkalizing agent

pH 6 to 7

USUAL DOSE

Determined by nutritional needs, evaluation of electrolytes, and degree of hyponatremia. Some solutions may contain aluminum; see Precautions. Available in 2 mEq and 4 mEq/mL concentrations. Each mL provides 2 or 4 mEq each of sodium and acetate.

DOSE ADJUSTMENTS

Lower-end initial doses may be appropriate in the elderly based on the potential for decreased organ function and concomitant disease or drug therapy.

DILUTION

Must be added to larger volumes of IV infusion solutions including total parenteral nutrition. Use only clear solutions. Check labels for aluminum content; see Precautions.

Storage: Store at room temperature. Discard unused portion.

COMPATIBILITY

Consider any drug NOT listed as compatible to be INCOMPATIBLE until consulting a pharmacist; specific conditions may apply.

One source suggests the following **compatibilities:**

Y-site: Enalaprilat (Vasotec IV), esmolol (Brevibloc), labetalol (Trandate), nicardipine (Cardene IV), ondansetron (Zofran).

RATE OF ADMINISTRATION

Administer at prescribed rate for infusion solutions. Rapid or excessive administration may produce sodium overload, water retention, alkalosis, or hypokalemia.

ACTIONS

An alkalizing agent and sodium salt. Sodium is the predominant cation of extracellular fluid. It controls water distribution throughout the body. Hypothalamus osmoreceptors, sensitive to osmolarity changes in the blood, control serum sodium concentration (142 mEq/L). Body fluid is lost when sodium content decreases and retained when sodium content increases. Sodium is excreted by the kidney. The acetate ion is metabolized to bicarbonate, thus providing a source of bicarbonate. It also acts as a hydrogen ion receptor.

INDICATIONS AND USES

To prevent or correct hyponatremia in patients with restricted intake, especially in individualized IV formulations when basic needs are not met by standard solutions. ■ Treatment of mild to moderate acidotic states. ■ Source of sodium ions in hemodialysis and peritoneal dialysis.

CONTRAINDICATIONS

Patients with hypernatremia or water retention.

PRECAUTIONS

Use with caution in impaired renal function, congestive heart failure, hypertension, peripheral or pulmonary edema, any condition resulting in salt retention, and in patients receiving corticosteroids. ■ Use acetate-containing solutions with extreme caution in patients with metabolic or respiratory alkalosis and/or impaired hepatic function. ▪ Temporary therapy in acidosis. Treatment of primary condition must be instituted. ▪ Sodium bicarbonate is the drug of choice for use in severe acidosis that requires immediate correction. ▪ Some solutions of sodium acetate contain aluminum. In impaired kidney function, aluminum may reach toxic levels. Premature neonates are particularly at risk because of their immature kidneys and requirement for calcium and phosphate, which also contain aluminum. Research indicates that patients with impaired renal function who receive more than 4 to 5 mcg/kg/day of parenteral aluminum are at risk for developing CNS or bone toxicity associated with aluminum accumulation.

Monitor: Evaluate electrolytes frequently during treatment. ▪ Evaluate fluid balance. ▪ Rapid or excessive administration may produce alkalosis or hypokalemia. Cardiac arrhythmias may result from an intracellular shift of potassium. Many other complications may arise from electrolyte imbalance.

Maternal/Child: Category C: safety not established; use only if clearly needed.

Elderly: Differences in response between elderly and younger patients have not been identified. Lower-end initial doses may be appropriate in the elderly; see Dose Adjustments.

DRUG/LAB INTERACTIONS

Alkalinization of urine may increase the renal elimination and decrease the effects of many drugs, including **tetracyclines, chlorpropamide, lithium carbonate, methotrexate, salicylates,** and may decrease the renal elimination and prolong the effects of others, including **anorexiants** (e.g., amphetamines), **flecainide, mecamylamine, quinidine, sympathomimetics** (e.g., ephedrine, dopamine).

SIDE EFFECTS

Hypernatremia, sodium level over 147 mEq/L, is most common (congestive heart failure, delirium, dizziness, edema, fever, flushing, headache, hypotension, oliguria, pulmonary edema, reduced salivation and lacrimation, respiratory arrest, restlessness, swollen tongue, tachycardia, thirst, weakness). Alkalosis and fluid or solute overload can occur.

ANTIDOTE

Notify the physician of any side effect. Reduce rate and notify physician at first sign of congestion or fluid overload. May be treated by sodium restriction and/or use of diuretics (e.g., furosemide [Lasix]) or dialysis. Resuscitate as necessary.

SODIUM BICARBONATE
(**SO**-dee-um bye-**KAR**-bon-ayt)

Electrolyte replenisher
Alkalizing agent

pH 7 to 8.5

USUAL DOSE

Adjusted according to pH, $Paco_2$, calculated base deficit, clinical response, and fluid limitations of the patient. In the presence of a low CO_2 content, adjust gradually to avoid unrecognized alkalosis. Correction to a CO_2 of 20 mEq/L within 24 hours will most likely result in a normal pH if the cause of acidosis is controlled and normal kidney function is present. Average dose for most indications is 2 to 5 mEq/kg/24 hr in adults and pediatric patients.

Cardiac arrest: 1 mEq/kg of body weight, only when appropriate (see Precautions; evidence supports little benefit and use may be detrimental). Repeat half dose in 10 minutes if indicated by blood pH and $Paco_2$.

PEDIATRIC DOSE

0.5 to 1 mEq/kg. For neonates and children up to 2 years of age, dose must never exceed 8 mEq/kg/24 hr of a 4.2% or more dilute solution; see Usual Dose, Monitor, and Maternal/Child.

DILUTION

4.2% sodium bicarbonate solution: 5 mEq/10 mL (0.5 mEq/mL).

5% sodium bicarbonate solution: 297.5 mEq/500 mL (0.595 mEq/mL).

7.5% sodium bicarbonate solution: 44.6 mEq/50 mL (0.892 mEq/mL).

8.4% sodium bicarbonate solution: 50 mEq/50 mL (1 mEq/mL).

neut (4% sodium bicarbonate solution): 2.4 mEq/5 mL (0.48 mEq/mL). Use limited to a buffering solution. Will raise pH of IV fluids and medications. Never used as a systemic alkalizer.

May be given in prepared solutions. 7.5% and 8.4% solutions should be diluted with equal amount of water for injection, or diluted with **compatible** IV solutions, depending on desired dosage and desired rate of administration. 4.2% or a more dilute solution is preferred for infants and children. Use only clear solutions.

COMPATIBILITY   (Underline Indicates Conflicting Compatibility Information)

Consider any drug NOT listed as compatible to be INCOMPATIBLE until consulting a pharmacist; specific conditions may apply.

Will form a precipitate with many drugs, including epinephrine. *If coadministration with epinephrine is indicated, give at separate sites.*

One source suggests the following **compatibilities:**

Additive: Amikacin (Amikin), aminophylline, amphotericin B (generic), atropine, calcium chloride, cefoxitin (Mefoxin), ceftazidime (Fortaz), chloramphenicol (Chloromycetin), clindamycin (Cleocin), cytarabine (ARA-C), erythromycin (Erythrocin), esmolol (Brevibloc), furosemide (Lasix), heparin, kanamycin (Kantrex), lidocaine, mannitol, meperidine (Demerol), methotrexate, methyldopa, multivitamins (M.V.I.), nafcillin (Nallpen), oxytocin (Pitocin), penicillin G potassium, phenylephrine (Neo-Synephrine), phytonadione (vitamin K_1), potassium chloride (KCl), prochlorperazine (Compazine), thiopental (Pentothal), verapamil.

Y-site: Acyclovir (Zovirax), amifostine (Ethyol), asparaginase (Elspar), aztreonam (Azactam), bivalirudin (Angiomax), cefepime (Maxipime), ceftriaxone (Rocephin), ciprofloxacin (Cipro IV), cisatracurium (Nimbex), cladribine (Leustatin), cyclophosphamide (Cytoxan), cytarabine (ARA-C), daunorubicin (Cerubidine), dexamethasone (Decadron), dexmedetomidine (Precedex), diltiazem (Cardizem), docetaxel (Taxotere), doripenem (Doribax), doxorubicin (Adriamycin), etoposide (VePesid), etoposide phosphate (Etopophos), famotidine (Pepcid IV), filgrastim (Neupogen), fludarabine (Fludara), gallium nitrate (Ganite), gemcitabine (Gemzar), granisetron (Kytril), heparin, ifosfamide (Ifex), indomethacin (Indocin IV), insulin (regular), levofloxacin (Levaquin), linezolid (Zyvox), melphalan (Alkeran), mesna (Mesnex), methylprednisolone (Solu-Medrol), milrinone (Primacor), morphine, paclitaxel (Taxol), pemetrexed (Alimta), piperacillin/tazobactam (Zosyn), potassium chloride (KCl), propofol (Diprivan), remifentanil (Ultiva), tacrolimus (Prograf), teniposide (Vumon), thiotepa, vancomycin, vasopressin.

RATE OF ADMINISTRATION

Flush IV line thoroughly before and after administration. Usual rate of administration of any solution is 2 to 5 mEq/kg over 4 to 8 hours. Do not exceed 50 mEq/hr. Decrease rate for pediatric patients. See Pediatric Dose. Rapid or excessive administration may produce alkalosis, hypernatremia, hypokalemia, and hypocalcemia. Cardiac arrhythmias may result from an intracellular shift of potassium. Will also produce pain and irritation along injection site.

Cardiac arrest: Up to 1 mEq/kg properly diluted over 1 to 3 minutes.

ACTIONS

An alkalizing agent and sodium salt. Helps to maintain osmotic pressure and ion balance. It is the buffering agent in blood. Bicarbonate ion elevates blood pH promptly. 99% reabsorbed with normal kidney function. Only 1% is excreted in the urine.

INDICATIONS AND USES

Metabolic acidosis (blood pH below 7.2 or plasma bicarbonate of 8 mEq/L or less) caused by circulatory insufficiency resulting from shock or severe dehydration, extracorporeal circulation of blood, severe renal disease, cardiac arrest (see Precautions), uncontrolled diabetes with ketoacidosis (low-dose insulin preferred), and primary lactic acidosis. ▪ Hyperkalemia. ▪ Hemolytic reactions requiring alkalinization of urine to reduce nephrotoxicity. ▪ Severe diarrhea. ▪ Barbiturate, methyl alcohol, or salicylate intoxication. ▪ Buffering solution to raise pH of IV fluids and medications.

CONTRAINDICATIONS

Diuretics known to produce hypochloremic alkalosis (e.g., thiazides), edema, hypertension, hypocalcemia (alkalosis may produce CHF, convulsions, hypertension, and tetany), hypochloremia (from vomiting, GI suction, or diuretics), hypernatremia, impaired renal function, metabolic alkalosis, respiratory alkalosis or acidosis, and any situation in which the administration of sodium could be clinically detrimental.

PRECAUTIONS

Temporary therapy in metabolic acidosis. Treatment of primary condition must be instituted. Best to partially correct acidosis and allow compensatory mechanisms to complete the correction. ▪ Use with caution in cardiac, liver, or renal disease; CHF, fluid/solute overload, elderly and postoperative patients with renal or cardiovascular insufficiency, and in patients receiving corticosteroids. ▪ Use in cardiac arrest indicated only if prolonged resuscitation with effective ventilation or after return of spontaneous circulation after a long arrest interval. ▪ Adequate alveolar ventilation should control acid-base balance in most arrest situations except prolonged cardiac arrest, arrested patients with pre-existing metabolic acidosis, hyperkalemia, or tricyclic or barbiturate overdose.

Monitor: Confirm absolute patency of vein. Extravasation may cause chemical cellulitis, necrosis, ulceration, or sloughing. ▪ Flush IV line thoroughly before and after administration; many incompatibilities. ▪ Determine blood pH, PO_2, PCO_2, and electrolytes several times daily during intensive treatment and daily in most other situations. Determine base excess or deficit in infants and children (dose = $0.3 \times$ kg $\times$ base deficit). Notify physician of all results. ▪ Rapid or excessive administration may produce alkalosis, hypokalemia, and hypocalcemia. Cardiac arrhythmias may result from an intracellular shift of potassium. Many other complications may arise from electrolyte imbalance. ▪ Use only 50-mL ampules in cardiac arrest to prevent accidental overdose. Recent practice indicates smaller doses may be appropriate when indicated in cardiac arrest and may prevent secondary alkalosis. Adequate alveolar ventilation is imperative. Evaluate patient response and blood gases.

Maternal/Child: Category C: safety for use in pregnancy not established; use only if clearly needed. ▪ Use caution in breast-feeding. ▪ Doses in excess of 8 mEq/kg/24 hr and/or given too rapidly (10 mL/min) may cause intracranial hemorrhage, hypernatremia, and decrease in cerebrospinal fluid pressure in neonates and children under 2 years.

Elderly: Contains sodium; use caution in the elderly with renal or cardiovascular insufficiency with or without CHF; see Precautions.

DRUG/LAB INTERACTIONS

Alkalinization of urine may increase the renal elimination and decrease the effects of many drugs, including **tetracyclines, chlorpropamide, lithium carbonate, methotrexate, salicylates,** and may decrease the renal elimination and prolong the effects of others, including **anorexiants** (e.g., amphetamines), **flecainide, mecamylamine, quinidine, sympathomimetics** (e.g., ephedrine, dopamine).

SIDE EFFECTS

Rare when used with caution: alkalosis (hyperirritability and tetany), hypernatremia (edema, CHF), hypokalemia, local site venous irritation.

ANTIDOTE

Discontinue the drug and notify the physician of any side effect. Hypokalemia usually occurs with alkalosis. Sodium and potassium chloride must be supplemented as indicated for correction. Treatment of alkalosis often results in more alkalosis. Rebreathing expired air from a paper bag may help to control beginning symptoms of alkalosis. Calcium gluconate may help in severe alkalosis. Administration of a balanced hypotonic electrolyte solution (Isolyte H, Normosol-M, Plasma-lyte 56) with sodium and potassium chloride added may help to excrete the bicarbonate ion in the urine. Ammonium chloride may be indicated. Treat tetany as indicated (calcium gluconate). For extravasation, discontinue infusion; aspirate fluid, drug, and/or 3 to 5 mL of blood through the in-place needle, then remove the needle. Elevate the extremity and apply warm moist compresses. Resuscitate as necessary.

SODIUM CHLORIDE
(**SO**-dee-um **KLOR**-eyed)

Electrolyte replenisher
Antihyponatremic

pH 4.5 to 7

USUAL DOSE

Highly individualized and dependent on age, weight, clinical condition of patient, concentration of salts in the plasma, and/or loss of body fluids.

Hypotonic: (0.45% [½NS], 4.5 Gm of sodium chloride/L or 77 mEq of sodium and 77 mEq of chloride [approximately 155 mOsm/L]) 2 to 4 L/24 hr.

Isotonic: (0.9% [NS], 9 Gm of sodium chloride/L or 154 mEq of sodium and 154 mEq of chloride [approximately 310 mOsm/L]), 1.5 to 3 L/24 hr. *Bacteriostatic isotonic NS* contains benzyl alcohol as a preservative. It is used in small amounts (usually 1 to 2 mL) as a diluent for injectable drugs (IV, IM, SC) or to flush IV lines. One study suggests that up to 30 mL/dose may be used in adults. However, the amount of benzyl alcohol that is tolerated within 24 hours in adults without toxic effects has not been determined. *Use only preservative-free sodium chloride in newborns for all indications.*

Hypertonic: Calculate sodium deficit. Total body water (TBW) is 45% to 50% in females and 50% to 60% in males.

Na deficit in mEq = TBW [desired − observed plasma Na]

Hypertonic (3%, 30 Gm of sodium chloride/L or 513 mEq of sodium and 513 mEq of chloride [approximately 1,030 mOsm/L] or 5%, 50 Gm of sodium chloride/L or 855 mEq of sodium and 855 mEq of chloride [approximately 1,710 mOsm/L]), 200 to 400 mL/24 hr. To correct *acute serious hyponatremia,* hypertonic sodium chloride is used to correct the serum sodium in 5 mEq/L/dose increments at a rate of no more than 0.5 mEq/hr until serum sodium is 125 mEq/L or neurologic symptoms improve. In the first 3 to 4 hours, an increase of plasma sodium at rates up to 1 mEq/L/hr may be tolerated in patients with distressing symptoms. To prevent an overly rapid correction, an increase in plasma sodium of less than 10 mEq/L in the first 24 hours and an increase of less than 18 mEq/L in the first 48 hours is desired. See Precautions.

Concentrated: To be used only as an additive in parenteral fluid therapy (14.6% contains 2.5 mEq of sodium and chloride/mL; 23.4% contains 4 mEq of sodium and chloride/mL).

DOSE ADJUSTMENTS

Dose selection should be cautious in the elderly, especially with hypertonic or concentrated solutions. Start at the lower end of the desired dosing range; consider the greater frequency of decreased organ function and of concomitant disease or drug therapy.

DILUTION

Available as *hypotonic* 25 mL, 50 mL, 150 mL, 250 mL, 500 mL, 1 L; *isotonic* (2 mL, 3 mL, 5 mL, 10 mL, 20 mL, 25 mL, 30 mL, 50 mL, 100 mL, 150 mL, 250 mL, 500 mL, 1 L); or *hypertonic* (500 mL) solution in vials and/or bottles for injection or infusion and ready for use. Isotonic and hypotonic sodium chloride are frequently combined with 5% or 10%

dextrose. **Concentrated** must be diluted before use. Used only as an additive in parenteral fluids. Permits specific mEq for mEq replacement of sodium and chloride without contributing to fluid overload. Available in 14.6% strength in 20 mL, 40 mL, and 200 mL; 23.4% strength in 30 mL, 50 mL, 100 mL, and 200 mL.

Bacteriostatic isotonic available in 2-mL, 10-mL, and 30-mL vials ready for use as a diluent. Never use in neonates.

Storage: Store at CRT. Do not freeze.

COMPATIBILITY

Consider any drug NOT listed as compatible to be INCOMPATIBLE until consulting a pharmacist; specific conditions may apply.

One source suggests the following **compatibilities:**

Additive: Potassium chloride (KCl).

Y-site: Ciprofloxacin (Cipro IV).

RATE OF ADMINISTRATION

Isotonic and hypotonic: A single daily dose equally distributed over 24 hours. Rate is dependent on age, weight, and clinical condition of the patient.

Hypertonic: One-half the calculated dose over at least 8 hours. Do not exceed 100 mL over 1 hour. Too-rapid infusion may cause local pain and venous irritation; reduce rate for tolerance.

Concentrated: Properly diluted in parenteral fluids and equally distributed over 24 hours. Never exceed hypertonic rate (see above) based on actual mEq of sodium chloride.

ACTIONS

Sodium: The predominant cation of extracellular fluid. It controls water distribution throughout the body. Hypothalamus osmoreceptors, sensitive to osmolarity changes in the blood, control serum sodium concentration (142 mEq/L). Body fluid is lost when sodium content decreases and retained when sodium content increases.

Chloride: The major extracellular anion. Closely follows the metabolism of sodium. Changes in the acid-base balance of the body are reflected by the changes in chloride concentration.

Distribution and excretion of sodium and chloride are largely under control of the kidney, which maintains a balance between intake and output.

INDICATIONS AND USES

Replace lost fluid or sodium and chloride ions in the body (e.g., hyponatremia, low salt syndrome, dehydration). ▪ Maintain fluid and electrolyte balance.

Hypotonic: Water replacement without increase of osmotic pressure or serum sodium levels; treatment of hyperosmolar diabetes requiring considerable fluid without excess sodium.

Isotonic: To replace sodium and chloride lost from vomiting because of obstructions and/or aspiration of GI fluids; treatment of metabolic alkalosis with fluid loss and sodium depletion. ▪ Diluent in parenteral preparations. ▪ To initiate and terminate blood transfusions without hemolyzing RBCs. ▪ Maintain patency and perform routine irrigations of many types of intravascular devices (e.g., catheters, implanted ports). ▪ Antidote for drug-induced hypercalcemia. Given concurrently with furosemide (Lasix). ▪ Priming solution in hemodialysis procedures.

Hypertonic: Used only when high sodium and/or chloride content without large amounts of fluid is required (e.g., electrolyte and fluid loss replaced with sodium-free fluids, excessive water intake resulting in drastic dilution of body water, emergency treatment of severe salt depletion, addisonian crisis, diabetic coma).

Concentrated: Used to meet the specific requirements of patients with unusual fluid and electrolyte needs (e.g., special problems of sodium electrolyte intake or excretion).

CONTRAINDICATIONS

Hypernatremia; fluid retention; situations where sodium or chloride could be detrimental. 3% and 5% sodium chloride solutions are contraindicated with elevated, normal, or slightly decreased serum sodium and chloride levels. Bacteriostatic sodium chloride is contraindicated in newborns.

PRECAUTIONS

Use caution in circulatory insufficiency, congestive heart failure, edema with sodium retention, kidney dysfunction, hepatic disease, hypoproteinemia, in the elderly or debilitated individuals, and in patients receiving corticosteroids. ■ Use with caution in surgical patients; see Monitor. ■ More than 1 liter of NS may cause hypernatremia, which can result in loss of bicarbonate ions and acidosis. ■ All uses require preservative-free solutions except the limited use of bacteriostatic NS as a diluent or flushing agent. ■ Inadvertent direct injection or absorption of concentrated sodium chloride may cause sudden hypernatremia, cardiovascular shock, CNS disorders, extensive hemolysis, cortical necrosis of the kidneys, and severe local tissue necrosis with extravasation. Use extreme caution; see Dilution. ■ Administration of IV solutions can cause fluid and/or solute overload, resulting in dilution of serum electrolyte concentrations, overhydration, congested states, or pulmonary edema. The risk of dilutional states is inversely proportional to the electrolyte concentration (increased fluids may dilute electrolyte concentration). The risk of solute overload causing congested states with peripheral and pulmonary edema is directly proportional to the electrolyte concentration (higher electrolytes pull in fluid, leading to fluid overload). ■ Overly rapid correction of severe hyponatremia (plasma sodium less than 110 to 115 mEq/L) may lead to a neurologic disorder (osmotic demyelination syndrome [central pontine myelinolysis]), which may be irreversible.

Monitor: Maintain accurate intake and output; monitor electrolytes and acid-base balance, especially in prolonged therapy. ■ Monitor vital signs as indicated. ■ Monitor for signs of hyponatremia (sodium less than 135 mEq/L [e.g., disorientation, headache, lethargy, nausea, weakness]). May progress to coma and seizures. ■ Excessive administration of potassium-free solutions may cause hypokalemia. ■ Before and during use of hypertonic or concentrated sodium chloride, determine osmolar concentrations and chloride and bicarbonate content of the serum. Observe patient continuously to prevent pulmonary edema. ■ Hypertonic solutions can cause vein damage; use a small needle and a large vein to reduce venous irritation and avoid extravasation; see Precautions.

Maternal/Child: Category C: safety for use during pregnancy not established; use only if clearly needed. ■ Use caution in breast-feeding. ■ Benzyl alcohol preservative in bacteriostatic sodium chloride has caused toxicity in newborns. Do not use. ■ Is used in pediatric patients. Safety and effectiveness based on similarity of clinical conditions of pediatric and adult populations. Use caution in neonates or very small infants; the volume of fluid may affect fluid and electrolyte balance.

Elderly: Lower-end initial doses may be indicated in the elderly; see Dose Adjustments. ■ Incidence of adverse reactions may be increased; monitor carefully, especially with renal or cardiac insufficiency with or without CHF. ■ See Precautions.

DRUG/LAB INTERACTIONS

High sodium intake may reduce serum **lithium** concentrations.

SIDE EFFECTS

Fever, hypovolemia, and injection site reactions may occur.

Osmotic demyelination syndrome (central pontine myelinolysis) secondary to too-rapid correction with hypertonic solutions.

Due to sodium excess: Aggravation of existing acidosis, anorexia, cellular dehydration, deep respiration, disorientation, distention, edema, hydrogen loss, hyperchloremic acidosis, hypertension, increased BUN, nausea, oliguria, potassium loss, pulmonary edema, water retention, weakness. Excessive excretion of crystalloids to maintain normal osmotic pressure will increase excretion of potassium and bicarbonate and further increase acidosis. Other salts (e.g., iodide and bromide) used for therapy will also be excreted rapidly.

ANTIDOTE

Discontinue or decrease rate of infusion; notify the physician of side effects. Sodium excess can be treated by sodium restriction and/or use of diuretics or hemodialysis to remove excessive amounts. Observe patient carefully and treat symptomatically. Save balance of fluid for examination.

SODIUM FERRIC GLUCONATE COMPLEX
(**SO**-dee-um **FAIR**-ick **GLUE**-koh-nayt **KOM**-pleks)

Ferrlecit

Antianemic
Iron supplement

pH 7.7 to 9.7

USUAL DOSE

Dose is represented in terms of mg of elemental iron. Given as an infusion and may be administered during the dialysis session.

Treatment of iron deficiency in hemodialysis patients: 125 mg (10 mL)/dose. Doses above 125 mg may be associated with a higher incidence and/or severity of adverse events; see Side Effects. A minimum cumulative dose of 1 Gm of elemental iron is required by most patients. May be administered over eight sessions at sequential dialysis treatments to achieve a favorable hemoglobin or hematocrit response. Additional doses as necessary are indicated to maintain target levels of hemoglobin, hematocrit, and laboratory parameters of iron storage within acceptable limits. Use the lowest dose that achieves this goal.

PEDIATRIC DOSE

1.5 mg/kg (0.12 mL/kg) of elemental iron as a 1-hour infusion. Do not exceed 125-mg dose. Administer at 8 sequential dialysis sessions. See Maternal/Child.

DOSE ADJUSTMENTS

Begin at the low end of the dosing range in elderly patients. Consider decreased cardiac, hepatic, or renal function, and concomitant disease or other drug therapy.

DILUTION

Available in ampules containing 62.5 mg/5 mL (12.5 mg/1 mL) of elemental iron.

Therapeutic dose: 125-mg (10-mL) dose may be diluted in 100 mL NS or may be given undiluted; see Rate of Administration.

Pediatric therapeutic dose: Dilute calculated dose in 25 mL of NS.

Filters: Specific studies not available from manufacturer. Filter needle not required by FDA for drug approval; however, use of a filter needle to withdraw it from an ampule should not have an adverse effect.

Storage: Store ampules at CRT. Use immediately after dilution in NS.

COMPATIBILITY

Manufacturer states, "Do not mix with other medications or add to parenteral nutrition solutions." Known to be **compatible** only with NS.

RATE OF ADMINISTRATION

Too-rapid administration may cause hypotension associated with fatigue; light-headedness; malaise; severe pain in the chest, back, flanks, or groin; and weakness.

Therapeutic dose: *Injection (adults only):* A single dose (undiluted) as a slow IV injection. May be given at a rate up to 12.5 mg/min (1 mL/min).

Infusion (adults and pediatric patients): A single dose as an infusion properly diluted and equally distributed over 60 minutes.

ACTIONS

A stable macromolecular complex in sucrose injection. Contains elemental iron as the sodium salt of a ferric ion carbohydrate complex. Free of ferrous ion and dextran polysaccharides. Used to replete the total body content of iron. Iron is critical for normal hemoglobin synthesis to maintain oxygen transport and necessary for metabolism and synthesis of DNA and various other processes. Total body iron content of an adult ranges from 2 to 4 Gm. Approximately two thirds is in hemoglobin and one third is in reticuloendothelial storage (bone marrow, spleen, liver) bound to intracellular ferritin. Half-life is approximately 1 hour. Doses of 1 mg/day are adequate to replenish losses in healthy non-menstruating adults. Iron complex is not dialyzable.

INDICATIONS AND USES
Treatment of iron deficiency anemia in adult patients and pediatric patients 6 years of age or older who are undergoing chronic hemodialysis and receiving supplemental erythropoietin therapy (e.g., EPO, Epogen, Procrit); see Maternal/Child.

CONTRAINDICATIONS
All anemias not associated with iron deficiency. Hypersensitivity to sodium ferric gluconate complex or any of its components. Evidence of iron overload.

PRECAUTIONS
Use only when truly indicated to avoid excess storage of iron. Not recommended for use in patients with iron overload. ▪ Too-rapid administration may cause hypotension; see Rate of Administration and Side Effects. ▪ Studies have included patients who have had prior iron dextran exposure with hypersensitivity reactions to at least one form of iron dextran (Infed or Dexferrum). The majority of these patients tolerated Ferrlecit therapy without a subsequent hypersensitivity reaction. ▪ There have been rare occurrences of severe hypersensitivity reactions to sodium ferric gluconate complex. ▪ Serum iron levels greater than 300 mcg/dL combined with transferrin oversaturation may indicate iron poisoning; see Side Effects.

Monitor: Recumbent position during and after injection may help to prevent postural hypotension. Hypotensive effects may be additive to transient hypotension during dialysis and/or from too-rapid rate of infusion; monitor closely. Hypotensive reactions associated with fatigue; light-headedness; malaise; severe pain in the back, chest, flanks, or groin; and weakness may occur with IV iron. These symptoms are not indicative of a hypersensitivity reaction and usually resolve within 1 or 2 hours. ▪ Observe continuously for a hypersensitivity reaction during an infusion. Monitor vital signs. ▪ Periodic monitoring of hemoglobin and hematocrit and iron storage levels recommended. Doses in excess of iron needs may lead to accumulation of iron in iron storage sites and iatrogenic hemosiderosis.

Patient Education: Report S/S of a hypersensitivity reaction (e.g., difficulty breathing, rash, shortness of breath) promptly. Report pain at injection site.

Maternal/Child: Category B: use during pregnancy only if potential benefit justifies potential risk to fetus. ▪ Safety for use during breast-feeding and in pediatric patients under 6 years of age not established. ▪ Contains benzyl alcohol; should not be used in neonates.

Elderly: No age differences identified. Caution in the elderly suggested; see Dose Adjustments.

DRUG/LAB INTERACTIONS

May reduce absorption of concomitantly administered **oral iron preparations.** ■ Concurrent administration of iron therapy with **dimercaprol** (BAL in Oil) will result in the formation of a toxic complex. Either postpone iron therapy to at least 24 hours after dimercaprol or consider transfusions.

SIDE EFFECTS

Hypotension associated with fatigue; light-headedness; malaise; severe pain in the chest, back, flanks, or groin; and weakness may be caused by too-rapid infusion. Severe hypersensitivity reactions (e.g., angioedema, bronchospasm, cardiac arrest, cardiovascular collapse, dyspnea, edema [oral or pharyngeal], muscle spasm, pain [back or chest], pruritus, urticaria) have been reported rarely. Most commonly reported side effects include abdominal pain, back pain, chest pain, diarrhea, fever, headache, hypersensitivity reactions, hypertension, hypotension, infection, nausea and vomiting, pain, pharyngitis, pruritus, rhinitis, tachycardia, and thrombosis. Many other side effects occurred in less than 1% of patients and may or may not be attributable to sodium ferric gluconate complex.

Post-Marketing: Convulsions, dysgeusia, hypoesthesia, loss of consciousness, pallor, phlebitis, skin discoloration, and shock have been identified. In addition, post-marketing reports have identified that individual doses exceeding 125 mg may result in a higher incidence and/or severity of side effects, including abdominal pain, chest pain, diarrhea, dizziness, dyspnea, hypotension, nausea, paresthesia, peripheral swelling, and urticaria.

Overdose: Serum iron levels greater than 300 mcg/dL may indicate iron poisoning. May result in hemosiderosis, and excess iron may increase susceptibility to infection. If acute toxicity is seen, it may present as abdominal pain, diarrhea, or vomiting progressing to pallor or cyanosis, lassitude, drowsiness, hyperventilation due to acidosis, iatrogenic hemosiderosis, and cardiovascular collapse.

ANTIDOTE

Reduce rate or temporarily discontinue infusion for hypotension; volume expanders (e.g., albumin, hetastarch [Hespan]) may be indicated. Restart when resolved. Discontinue drug and treat hypersensitivity reactions or resuscitate as necessary; notify physician. Epinephrine (Adrenalin) and diphenhydramine (Benadryl) should always be available. In overdose, monitor CBC, iron studies, vital signs, blood gases, and glucose and electrolytes. Maintain fluid and electrolyte balance. Correct acidosis with sodium bicarbonate. Iron complex is not dialyzable.

SODIUM PHENYLACETATE AND SODIUM BENZOATE

Ammonia detoxicant

(**SO**-dee-um fen-ill-**AH**-seh-tate and **SO**-dee-um **BEN**-zoh-ate)

Ammonul

pH 6 to 8

USUAL DOSE

Must be diluted and administered through a central line. Administration through a peripheral line may cause burns. Adjunctive to hemodialysis and given in combination with arginine (dose is dependent on the specific urea cycle disorder [UCD] and is contraindicated in patients with arginase deficiency); see Dilution, Rate of Administration, Precautions, and Monitor. Urea cycle disorders can result from decreased activity of any of the following enzymes: *N*-acetylglutamate synthetase (NAGS), carbamyl phosphate synthetase (CPS), argininosuccinate synthetase (ASS), ornithine transcarbamylase (OTC), argininosuccinate lyase (ASL), or arginase (ARG); dose and treatment may vary for each. Sodium phenylacetate and sodium benzoate (AMMONUL) infusion should be started as soon as the diagnosis of hyperammonemia is made.

Discontinue analogous oral drugs (e.g., sodium phenylbutyrate [Buphenyl]) before sodium phenylacetate and sodium benzoate (AMMONUL) infusion.

A **loading dose** as an infusion is administered over 90 to 120 minutes, followed by an **equivalent maintenance dose** as an infusion administered over 24 hours. Treatment also requires caloric supplementation and restriction of dietary protein. Non-protein calories should be supplied principally as glucose (8 to 10 mg/kg/min), with intravenous fat (e.g., Intralipid) added to maintain a caloric intake of greater than 80 cal/kg/day.

The dose of sodium phenylacetate and sodium benzoate (AMMONUL) is based on mg/kg in neonates, infants, and younger pediatric patients weighing up to 20 kg and on body surface area for older pediatric patients, adolescents, and adults weighing more than 20 kg as described in the following chart.

Dose and Administration Guidelines for Sodium Phenylacetate and Sodium Benzoate (AMMONUL)					
Patient Population	Components of Infusion Solution AMMONUL must be diluted with D10W at equal to or greater than 25 mL/kg before administration		Dosage Provided		
	Ammonul	Arginine HCl Injection, 10%	Sodium Phenylacetate	Sodium Benzoate	Arginine HCl
Weight equal to or less than 20 kg:					
CPS and OTC Deficiency					
Dose Loading: Over 90 to 120 minutes **Maintenance:** Over 24 hours	2.5 mL/kg	2 mL/kg	250 mg/kg	250 mg/kg	200 mg/kg
ASS and ASL Deficiency					
Dose Loading: Over 90 to 120 minutes **Maintenance:** Over 24 hours	2.5 mL/kg	6 mL/kg	250 mg/kg	250 mg/kg	600 mg/kg
Weight more than 20 kg:					
CPS and OTC Deficiency					
Dose Loading: Over 90 to 120 minutes **Maintenance:** Over 24 hours	55 mL/M^2	2 mL/kg	5.5 Gm/M^2	5.5 Gm/M^2	200 mg/kg
ASS and ASL Deficiency					
Dose Loading: Over 90 to 120 minutes **Maintenance:** Over 24 hours	55 mL/M^2	6 mL/kg	5.5 Gm/M^2	5.5 Gm/M^2	600 mg/kg

Repeat loading doses should not be administered because plasma levels achieved by phenylacetate are prolonged. Continue maintenance infusions until elevated plasma ammonia levels have been normalized or oral nutrition and medications can be tolerated. Mean duration of treatment was 4.6 days per episode and ranged from 1 to 72 days.

DOSE ADJUSTMENTS

No specific recommendations; see Precautions.

DILUTION
Must be diluted with D10W. Do not administer undiluted product.
A 0.22-micron filter must be used when injecting Ammonul into D10W. Particulate matter is present but may not be visible. The manufacturer is supplying the filter with Ammonul until further notice.
Loading dose: Dilute with an amount of D10W equal to or more than 25 mL/kg of body weight per dose.
Equivalent maintenance dose: Also requires dilution with an amount of D10W equal to or more than 25 mL/kg of body weight per dose.

A 4-kg neonate would require a minimum of 100 mL of D10W for dilution of the loading dose given over 90 to 120 minutes and a minimum of 100 mL of D10W for dilution of the maintenance dose given over 24 hours. An 80-kg adult would require a minimum of 2,000 mL of D10W for dilution of the loading dose over 90 to 120 minutes and a minimum of 2,000 mL D10W for dilution of the maintenance dose given over 24 hours.
Filters: Use of a 0.22-micron filter is required to inject Ammonul into D10W; see Dilution.
Storage: Store unopened vials at CRT. Diluted solutions are stable at CRT and room lighting conditions for up to 24 hours.

COMPATIBILITY
May be mixed in the same container with 10% arginine HCl injection. Manufacturer states, "Other infusion solutions and drug products should not be administered together with sodium phenylacetate and sodium benzoate." May be prepared in glass or PVC containers.

RATE OF ADMINISTRATION
Loading dose infusion rates are relatively high, especially for infants; monitor closely.
Loading dose: A single dose properly diluted as an infusion and equally distributed over 90 to 120 minutes.
Maintenance dose: Each single dose properly diluted as an infusion and equally distributed over 24 hours.

ACTIONS
Sodium phenylacetate and sodium benzoate are metabolically active compounds that can provide an alternative pathway for nitrogen disposal in patients without a fully functioning urea cycle. Two moles of nitrogen are removed per mole of phenylacetate when it is conjugated with glutamine, and one mole of nitrogen is removed per mole of benzoate when it is conjugated with glycine. Has been shown to decrease elevated plasma ammonia levels and improve encephalopathy and survival outcome. Considered to be the result of the reduction in nitrogen overload through glutamine and glycine scavenging by sodium phenylacetate and sodium benzoate (AMMONUL) in combination with appropriate dietary and other supportive measures.
Phenylacetate: Conjugates with glutamine in the liver and kidneys to form phenylacetylglutamine. It is then excreted by the kidneys via glomerular filtration and tubular secretion. Each mole of phenylacetylglutamine contains two moles of waste nitrogen. The nitrogen content of phenylacetylglutamine per mole is identical to that of urea (2 moles of nitrogen). Plasma levels remain higher and are present for a longer period of time than plasma levels of benzoate.

Benzoate: Conjugates with glycine to form hippuric acid, which is rapidly excreted by the kidneys by glomerular filtration and tubular secretion. One mole of hippuric acid contains one mole of waste nitrogen. The formation of hippurate from benzoate occurs more rapidly than that of phenylacetylglutamine from phenylacetate, and the rate of elimination of hippurate appears to be more rapid than that of phenylacetylglutamine.

INDICATIONS AND USES

Adjunctive therapy for the treatment of acute hyperammonemia and associated encephalopathy in patients with deficiencies in enzymes of the urea cycle. UCDs can result from decreased activity of any of the following enzymes: N-acetylglutamate synthetase (NAGS), carbamyl phosphate synthetase (CPS), argininosuccinate synthetase (ASS), ornithine transcarbamylase (OTC), argininosuccinate lyase (ASL), or arginase (ARG). Used in combination with dialysis (standard hemodialysis, peritoneal dialysis, arteriovenous hemofiltration, or other dialysis). Hemodialysis is most commonly used and is the most rapid and effective technique for removing ammonia in acute hyperammonemic coma, in moderate to severe episodes of hyperammonemic encephalopathy, and in episodes of hyperammonemia that fail to respond to an initial course of sodium phenylacetate and sodium benzoate (AMMONUL). Concomitant administration of sodium phenylacetate and sodium benzoate (AMMONUL) with hemodialysis can help prevent the re-accumulation of ammonia by increasing waste nitrogen excretion.

CONTRAINDICATIONS

Known hypersensitivity to sodium phenylacetate and sodium benzoate. ■ Concurrent use with 10% arginine HCl is contraindicated in patients with arginase deficiency.

PRECAUTIONS

For IV infusion only. Must be infused through a central line. Administration through a peripheral line may cause burns. ■ Acute symptomatic hyperammonemia should be treated as a life-threatening emergency. Treatment may require dialysis, preferably hemodialysis, to remove a large burden of ammonia. Uncontrolled hyperammonemia can rapidly result in brain damage or death, and prompt use of all therapies necessary to reduce ammonia levels is essential. ■ Administered under the direction of a physician knowledgeable in its use and in the treatment of diseases resulting from inborn errors in metabolism. Should be administered in a facility with adequate diagnostic and treatment facilities to monitor the patient and respond to any medical emergency. In addition, facilities for hemodialysis, nutritional support, and medical support are required. ■ Patients suspected of having a UCD based on family history should have documented hyperammonemia before administration of sodium phenylacetate and sodium benzoate (AMMONUL). ■ Patients with a large ammonia burden or patients who are not responsive to sodium phenylacetate and sodium benzoate (AMMONUL) require aggressive therapy, including hemodialysis. ■ The most commonly presented symptoms of UCDs in neonates include edema, lethargy, neurologic changes, poor feeding, respiratory distress, and seizures. Milder forms of UCDs may not present until late childhood, adolescence, or adulthood. Symptoms, including hyperammonemic crisis with coma, delirium, and/or lethargy, are often precipitated by viral illness, high-protein diet, stress, or trauma. ■

Metabolized in the liver and kidneys and excreted by the kidneys. Use caution in patients with impaired renal or hepatic function. ■ Use with extreme caution, if at all, in patients with CHF or severe renal insufficiency and in clinical states where there is sodium retention with edema; contains 30.5 mg of sodium/mL of undiluted product; see Antidote. ■ Bioavailability of both benzoate and phenylacetate may be slightly higher in females than in males. ■ See Monitor, Maternal/Child, and Drug/Lab Interactions.

Monitor: Plasma and urine amino acid analyses are used to diagnose ASS and ASL and to provide a preliminary diagnosis of CPS, OTC, or ARG. Blood citrulline levels are very low or absent in OTC and CPS, very high in ASS, and normal to moderately high in ASL and ARG. High urine levels of an unusual amino acid (argininosuccinic acid [ASA]) may distinguish ASL; however, ASA may be difficult to detect on initial examination. Specific studies are required to separate it from other amino acids. ARG is characterized by high urine levels of arginine. A liver biopsy is indicated for definitive diagnosis of CPS and OTC. RBC enzyme analysis is needed to confirm a diagnosis of ARG. ■ Monitor catheter infusion site closely. Extravasation may lead to skin necrosis. If extravasation is suspected, discontinue the infusion and, if necessary, resume at a different site. ■ Obtain baseline plasma ammonia levels, neurologic status, and laboratory tests, and observe clinical symptoms. Monitor all at frequent intervals along with clinical response. In patients responding to therapy, mean ammonia levels decreased significantly within 4 hours of initiation of therapy. ■ May be used in combination with dialysis. Hemodialysis is the most commonly used and can either be instituted immediately while waiting for a more definitive diagnosis or used as a recommended addition to treatment for those patients who fail to have a significant reduction in plasma ammonia levels within 4 to 8 hours after receiving sodium phenylacetate and sodium benzoate (AMMONUL). High levels of ammonia can be reduced quickly when sodium phenylacetate and sodium benzoate (AMMONUL) is used with dialysis. The ammonia scavenging of sodium phenylacetate and sodium benzoate (AMMONUL) suppresses the production of ammonia from catabolism of endogenous protein, and dialysis eliminates the ammonia and ammonia conjugates. ■ Monitor serum electrolytes and maintain with normal range. Monitor plasma potassium levels carefully and treat as indicated; urine potassium loss is enhanced by excretion of the non-resorbable anions phenylacetylglutamine and hippurate. ■ May cause side effects associated with salicylate overdose (e.g., hyperventilation, metabolic acidosis). Obtain baseline and monitor blood chemistry profiles, blood pH, and PCO_2. ■ Use with high-dose arginine may cause hyperchloremic acidosis. Obtain baseline and monitor chloride and bicarbonate levels; administer bicarbonate as indicated. ■ Use prophylactic antiemetics to reduce nausea and vomiting. ■ Neurotoxicity has been reported (e.g., disorientation, exacerbation of a pre-existing neuropathy, fatigue, headaches, hypoacusis [partial loss of hearing], impaired memory, light-headedness, somnolence). Onset may be acute, and symptoms should improve when therapy is discontinued. ■ Closely monitor patients with impaired renal function; drug therapy may be less effective due to poor clearance of drug metabolites and, subsequently, ammonia. ■ See Precautions, Maternal/Child, and Drug/Lab Interactions.

Patient Education: Compliance with dietary restrictions and supplemental medications is imperative. ▪ Obtain identification (e.g., a bracelet) with UCD diagnosis.

Maternal/Child: Category C: use during pregnancy and/or labor and delivery only if clearly needed. Effects on fetus unknown. ▪ Not known if it is secreted in human milk; use caution if required during breast-feeding. Has the potential for serious harm to infant. ▪ Is used as a treatment for acute hyperammonemia in pediatric patients, including patients in the early neonatal period. ▪ The most frequently presented symptoms of UCD in neonates include edema, lethargy, neurologic changes, poor feeding, respiratory distress, and seizures. ▪ Exchange transfusion is ineffective in the management of hyperammonemia. Hemodialysis may be repeated until the plasma ammonia level is stable at or near normal levels.

Elderly: Relevant information not available. Oldest patient in studies was 53 years of age. Average age in studies was 8.54 years. ▪ Monitoring of renal and hepatic function is suggested.

DRUG/LAB INTERACTIONS

Formal drug interaction studies have not been performed. ▪ Concurrent use with **corticosteroids** (e.g., dexamethasone [Decadron]) may cause the breakdown of body protein and increase plasma ammonia levels in patients with an impaired ability to form urea. ▪ Some **antibiotics** (e.g., penicillin) may compete with phenylacetylglutamine and hippurate for active secretion by renal tubules. This competition may affect the overall disposition of either of the infused drugs. ▪ **Probenecid** is known to inhibit the renal transport of many drugs and may inhibit the renal excretion of phenylacetylglutamine and hippurate, reducing its effectiveness. ▪ **Valproic acid** has been reported to induce hyperammonemia. Administration to patients with UCD may exacerbate their condition and antagonize the effectiveness of sodium phenylacetate and sodium benzoate (AMMONUL).

SIDE EFFECTS

Acidosis, agitation, anemia, coma, convulsions, diarrhea, DIC, edema of the brain, fever, hyperammonemia, hyperglycemia, hypocalcemia, hypokalemia, hypotension, injection site reactions, mental impairment, metabolic acidosis, nausea, respiratory distress, urinary tract infections, and vomiting were reported most frequently. Injection site reactions and metabolic acidosis were dose-limiting reactions in several patients. Incidence and severity of side effects tends to be increased in patients with enzyme deficiencies occurring earlier in the urea cycle (i.e., OTC and CPS). Incidence of side effects were also specific to age and diagnosis as follows.

Pediatric patients 30 days of age or less: Blood and lymphatic system disorders (e.g., anemia, DIC) and hypotension.

Patients more than 30 days of age: GI disorders (e.g., diarrhea, nausea, and vomiting).

Patients with OTC, ASS, CPS, and diagnoses characterized as other: Side effects were primarily the ones most frequently reported.

Patients with OTC and CPS: Nervous system disorders (e.g., coma, convulsions, edema of the brain, mental impairment) were most common.

Overdose: Cardiovascular collapse, encephalopathy (progressive), hypernatremia, hyperosmolarity, hyperventilation, large anion gap, metabolic acidosis (severe and compensated) with a respiratory component, obtundation (in the absence of hyperammonemia), and death. Causes of death from overdose were cardiorespiratory failure/arrest, error in dialysis procedure, hyperammonemia, hypotension (intractable) with probable sepsis, increased intracranial pressure, pneumonitis with septic shock and coagulopathy.

ANTIDOTE
Keep physician informed of all side effects. Many may be life threatening and immediate, and appropriate treatment is required. If an adverse reaction occurs due to sodium content, discontinue infusion, evaluate the patient, and treat as indicated. If extravasation is suspected, discontinue the infusion and, if necessary, resume at a different site. Treat extravasation by aspirating the residual drug from the catheter, elevating the limb (if a limb is involved), and applying intermittent cold packs. If overdose occurs, discontinue the drug, and monitor and treat as indicated by symptoms. In severe cases, hemodialysis (procedure of choice) and/or peritoneal dialysis (when hemodialysis is not available) may be indicated. Resuscitate as indicated.

SOTALOL HYDROCHLORIDE BBW
(**SO**-tuh-lol hy-droh-**KLOR**-eyed)

Beta-adrenergic
blocking agent
Antiarrhythmic

pH 6 to 7

USUAL DOSE
To minimize the risk of induced arrhythmia, patients initiated or reinitiated on sotalol and patients who are converted from IV to oral administration should be hospitalized in a facility that can provide cardiac resuscitation and continuous ECG monitoring. CrCl must be greater than 60 mL/min. Baseline studies and correction of electrolyte abnormalities required before initiating therapy; see Precautions, Monitor, and Dose Adjustments.
Initial dose: 75 mg twice daily. If symptomatic arrhythmia is not controlled and dose is tolerated without excessive QTc prolongation (i.e., greater than 500 msec), may increase dose to 112.5 mg twice daily after 3 days. Continuous ECG monitoring required during dose escalation.
Dose for ventricular arrhythmias: 75 mg twice daily. Dose may be increased in increments of 75 mg/day every 3 days. Usual therapeutic effect is seen with doses of 75 to 150 mg twice daily. However, doses as high as 225 to 300 mg have been required in patients with refractory life-threatening arrhythmias.
Dose for symptomatic atrial fibrillation/atrial flutter (AFIB/AFL): 112.5 mg twice daily was found to be the most effective dose in studies. If symptomatic arrhythmia is not controlled and this dose is tolerated without excessive QTc prolongation (i.e., greater than 520 msec), increase dose to 150 mg twice daily.
Conversion from oral to intravenous sotalol: Patients who have been stabilized on oral sotalol and are unable to take oral medications may be converted to IV sotalol using the following conversion table.

Conversion from Oral Sotalol to IV Sotalol	
Oral Dose	Intravenous Dose
80 mg	75 mg (5 mL sotalol injection)
120 mg	112.5 mg (7.5 mL sotalol injection)
160 mg	150 mg (10 mL sotalol injection)

DOSE ADJUSTMENTS

Increase dosing interval to every 24 hours in patients with a CrCl between 40 and 60 mL/min. Sotalol is not recommended in patients with a CrCl less than 40 mL/min. ■ Titrate dose upward or downward as needed based on clinical effect, QT interval, or adverse reactions as described in Usual Dose.

DILUTION

Available in vials containing 150 mg/10 mL. Dilute required dose with NS, D5W, or LR as described in the following table.

Sotalol Infusion Preparation to Compensate for Dead Space in the Infusion Set				
Target Dose	Sotalol Injection	Diluent	Volume Prepared	Volume to Infuse
75 mg	6 mL	114 mL	120 mL	100 mL
112.5 mg	9 mL	111 mL		
150 mg	12 mL	108 mL		
75 mg	6 mL	294 mL	300 mL	250 mL
112.5 mg	9 mL	291 mL		
150 mg	12 mL	288 mL		

Storage: Store at CRT. Protect from light and freezing.

COMPATIBILITY

Specific information not available. Consult pharmacist; specific conditions may apply.

RATE OF ADMINISTRATION

A single dose equally distributed over 5 hours. Use of an infusion pump recommended.

ACTIONS

An antiarrhythmic with Class II (beta-adrenoreceptor blocking) and Class III (cardiac action potential duration prolongation) properties. The beta-blocking effect is noncardioselective. Slows heart rate, decreases AV nodal conduction, and increases AV nodal refractoriness. ECG shows dose-related increase in QT and QTc. Produces a reduction in systolic and diastolic blood pressures and cardiac index and an increase in pulmonary capillary wedge pressure. Does not bind to plasma proteins and is not metabolized. Half-life is 12 hours. Excreted predominantly via the kidney in unchanged form. Crosses the placenta. Secreted in breast milk.

INDICATIONS AND USES

A substitute for oral sotalol in patients who are unable to take oral medications. ■ Maintenance of normal sinus rhythm in patients with a history of highly symptomatic AFIB/AFL. ▪ Treatment of documented life-threatening ventricular arrhythmias.

CONTRAINDICATIONS

Bradycardia (HR below 50 beats/min), sick sinus syndrome, or second- or third-degree AV block unless a functioning pacemaker is present. ▪ Congenital or acquired long QT syndromes, QT interval greater than 450 msec. ▪ Cardiogenic shock, uncontrolled heart failure. ▪ CrCl less than 40 mL/min. ▪ Serum potassium less than 4 mEq/L. ▪ Bronchial asthma or related bronchospastic conditions. ▪ Known hypersensitivity to sotalol.

PRECAUTIONS

To minimize the risk of induced arrhythmia, patients initiated or reinitiated on sotalol and patients who are converted from IV to oral administration should be hospitalized for at least 3 days (or until steady-state drug levels are reached) in a facility that can provide cardiac resuscitation and continuous ECG monitoring. Personnel trained in the management of serious ventricular arrhythmias must be present. ▪ Can cause serious ventricular arrhythmias, primarily torsades de pointes (TdP), a polymorphic ventricular tachycardia associated with QTc prolongation. QTc prolongation is directly related to the concentration of sotalol. Factors that may increase the risk of TdP include a reduced CrCl, larger doses, female gender, sustained VT, and a history of cardiomegaly or CHF. ▪ The use of sotalol in conjunction with other drugs that prolong the QT interval has not been studied and is not recommended; see Drug/Lab Interactions. ▪ May cause bradycardia, which increases risk of TdP. ▪ Increased risk of TdP in patients with AFIB and sinus node dysfunction, especially after cardioversion. Sotalol increases bradycardia and QTc following cardioversion. ▪ Produces significant reductions in both systolic and diastolic BP. May cause deterioration in cardiac performance in patients with marginal cardiac compensation. ▪ Use caution in CHF. Beta blockade may depress myocardial contractility and precipitate or exacerbate heart failure. ▪ Use caution in the presence of heart failure controlled by digoxin. Both drugs slow AV conduction. ▪ Experience with use following acute MI is limited. Use caution, titrate dose carefully, and monitor patient closely. ▪ May cause angina, arrhythmia, or MI if discontinued abruptly; gradually reduce over 1 to 2 weeks if possible. ▪ May mask tachycardia occurring with hypoglycemia in diabetes and tachycardia of hyperthyroidism. ▪ In general, patients with bronchospastic disease should not receive beta-blockers. If sotalol is to be administered, use the smallest effective dose; see Contraindications. ▪ Use caution in patients with renal impairment; see Dose Adjustments. ▪ Patients with atrial fibrillation should be anticoagulated according to usual medical practice.

Monitor: Obtain baseline ECG to determine the QT interval. If baseline QT interval is greater than 450 msec, sotalol is not recommended. Monitor QT interval after the completion of each infusion. If the QT interval increases to 500 msec or greater, reduce the dose, decrease the infusion rate, or discontinue therapy. ▪ Measure and normalize serum potassium and magnesium levels before initiating therapy and as required during therapy. Pay special attention to electrolytes and acid-base status in patients with prolonged diarrhea or in patients receiving concomitant diuretics. ▪ Obtain baseline SCr and calculate CrCl to establish dosing interval. ▪ Monitor HR and BP. Monitor hemodynamics in patients with marginal cardiac compensation. ▪ In patients with life-threatening ventricular arrhythmias, the response to treatment should be evaluated by a suitable method (e.g., programmed electrical stimulation [PES] or Holter monitoring) at steady-state blood levels of the drug before continuing the patient on chronic therapy. **Patient Education:** Do not discontinue therapy abruptly. ▪ Promptly report any breathing difficulty, syncope, or pain at injection site. **Maternal/Child:** Category B: use during pregnancy only if clearly needed. ▪ Discontinue breast-feeding. ▪ Safety for use in pediatric patients not established. See prescribing information for unlabeled suggested oral doses for use in pediatric patients.

Elderly: Age-related differences in safety and effectiveness not identified; however, greater sensitivity of some elderly cannot be ruled out. Dose with caution, taking into account decreased renal function: See Dose Adjustment.

DRUG/LAB INTERACTIONS

Proarrhythmic events were more common in sotalol-treated patients also receiving **digoxin.** Unclear as to whether this is a drug interaction or is related to the presence of heart failure, which is a known risk factor for arrhythmias. ▪ Concurrent use with **calcium channel blockers** (e.g., diltiazem [Cardizem], verapamil) is expected to have additive effects on AV conduction, ventricular function, and BP. ▪ Beta-adrenergic blocking agents may be continued during the perioperative period in most patients; however, use caution with **selected anesthetic agents** that may depress the myocardium. Protracted severe hypotension and difficulty in restoring and maintaining normal cardiac rhythm after anesthesia has been reported. ▪ Concurrent use with **clonidine** may precipitate acute hypertension if one or both agents is stopped abruptly. ▪ Coadministration with **catecholamine-depleting drugs** (e.g., reserpine and guanethidine) may result in hypotension, bradycardia, vertigo, syncope, or orthostatic hypotension. ▪ Hyperglycemia may occur. Dosage of **insulin and other antidiabetic drugs** may require adjustment. ▪ Symptoms of **hypoglycemia may be masked.** ▪ Increased doses of **beta-agonists** such as albuterol, terbutaline, and isoproterenol may be required when administered concomitantly with sotalol. ▪ Patients taking **beta-blockers** who are exposed to a potential allergen may be unresponsive to the usual dose of epinephrine used to treat a hypersensitivity reaction. ▪ The use of sotalol in conjunction with other **drugs that prolong the QT interval** has not been studied and is not recommended. Such drugs include some phenothiazines (e.g., prochlorperazine [Compazine], promethazine [Phenergan]), tricyclic antidepressants (e.g., amitriptyline [Elavil], imipramine [Tofranil]), certain oral macrolides (e.g., erythromycin [E-Mycin], clarithromycin [Biaxin]), Class I antiarrhythmic (e.g., disopyramide [Norpace], procainamide [Pronestyl], quinidine), and Class III antiarrhythmics (e.g., amiodarone [Nexterone]). **Class I and III antiarrhythmic agents** should be withheld for at least three half-lives before dosing with sotalol. In studies, sotalol was not administered to patients who had been previously treated with **oral amiodarone** (Nexterone) for a more than 1 month in the previous 3 months. ▪ Interactions with hydrochlorothiazide and warfarin were not observed. ▪ The presence of sotalol in the urine may result in **falsely elevated levels of urinary metanephrine** by certain methods.

SIDE EFFECTS

There is no clinical experience with IV sotalol. Side effects should be similar to those seen with oral sotalol therapy. The most common side effects (dose related) are asthenia, bradycardia, chest pain, dizziness, dyspnea, fatigue, headache, light-headedness, nausea, QT prolongation, and palpitations. Ventricular arrhythmia, primarily TdP, is the most common serious side effect. Other reported side effects include abdominal distension and pain, abnormal ECG, angina, bradycardia, cough, decreased appetite, diarrhea, dyspepsia, edema, fever, heart failure, hyperhidrosis, hypotension, infection, insomnia, musculoskeletal pain, tracheobronchitis, upper respiratory infection, visual disturbance, vomiting, and weakness. Other reactions have been reported.

Overdose: Bradycardia, bronchospasm, cardiac asystole, CHF, hypoglycemia, hypotension, premature ventricular complexes, prolongation of the QT interval, TdP, and ventricular arrhythmia.

ANTIDOTE

Notify physician of any side effects. If the QT interval increases to 500 msec or greater, reduce the dose, decrease the infusion rate, or discontinue therapy. Atropine, another anticholinergic drug, a beta-adrenergic agonist, or transvenous cardiac pacing may be used to treat bradycardia or cardiac asystole. A transvenous cardiac pacemaker may be required for second- or third-degree heart block. Epinephrine may be useful for treatment of hypotension. Aminophylline or aerosol beta-2–receptor stimulants (e.g., albuterol [Ventolin]) may be useful for treatment of bronchospasm. DC cardioversion, magnesium sulfate, and potassium replacement may be required for treatment of TdP. Once TdP is terminated, transvenous cardiac pacing or an isoproterenol infusion may be used to increase heart rate.

STREPTOMYCIN SULFATE BBW
(strep-toe-**MY**-sin **SUL**-fayt)

Antibacterial
(aminoglycoside)
Antituberculosis

pH 5 to 8

USUAL DOSE

ALL IV DOSES AND USES ARE UNLABELED.

Mycobacterium tuberculosis (unlabeled): 12 to 15 mg/kg daily. Calculation based on ideal body weight, not actual weight. 12 to 27 mg/kg has been used safely. Doses over 20 mg/kg are usually given every other day. Used in combination with isoniazid (INH), rifampin (Rifadin), and pyrazinamide. Maximum suggested total cumulative dose over course of therapy is 120 Gm.

Mycobacterium avium complex (unlabeled): 11 to 13 mg/kg daily. Part of a multiple drug regimen of three to five agents.

DOSE ADJUSTMENTS

Reduced dose required in renal impairment and/or nitrogen retention. ▪ Reduce dose in patients over 60 years based on age, renal function, and eighth nerve impairment. ▪ Elevated peak drug concentrations require a reduced dose. ▪ See Drug/Lab Interactions.

DILUTION

Prepared solution equals 400 mg/mL. Further dilute total daily dose to a volume of 100 mL with D5W or D5NS.

Storage: Refrigerate undiluted ampules. Diluted solution is stable for 24 hours at room temperature. According to the National Jewish Center guidelines, the current formulation from Pfizer is stable for up to 30 days after dilution if refrigerated.

COMPATIBILITY

Consider any drug NOT listed as compatible to be INCOMPATIBLE until consulting a pharmacist; specific conditions may apply.

Inactivated in solution with beta-lactam antibiotics (e.g., cephalosporins, penicillins) and vancomycin. Do not mix in the same solution. Appropriate spacing required because of physical **incompatibilities.** See Drug/Lab Interactions.

One source suggests the following **compatibilities:**

Additive: Bleomycin (Blenoxane).

Y-site: Esmolol (Brevibloc).

RATE OF ADMINISTRATION

Total daily dose, properly diluted, as an infusion over 30 minutes. Slow rate to 60 minutes if any tingling or dizziness occurs during administration or if elevated peak drug concentrations occur.

ACTIONS

An aminoglycoside antibiotic with potential neuromuscular blocking action. Inhibits protein synthesis in bacterial cells. Bactericidal against specific gram-negative organisms and bacilli. Well distributed through all organ tissues except the brain (unless meninges inflamed). Peak serum levels of 25 to 50 mcg/mL occur promptly and gradually decrease to 12.5 to 25 mcg/mL over 5 to 6 hours. Usual half-life is 2.5 hours. Half-life is prolonged in infants, postpartum females, liver disease and ascites, spinal cord injury, cystic fibrosis, and the elderly. May be prolonged up to 100 hours in end-stage renal disease. Half-life is shorter in anemia, severe burns, and fever. Crosses the placental barrier. 30% to 90% excreted in urine within 24 hours.

INDICATIONS AND USES

All IV uses are unlabeled. Treatment of *Mycobacterium* tuberculosis when one or more of the following drugs (ethambutol [Myambutol], isoniazid [INH], rifampin [Rifadin], or pyrazinamide) is contraindicated because of toxicity, intolerance, or drug resistance. Increased rates of drug resistance and/or concomitant HIV infection are more common than in previous times. Usual four-drug regimen is either ethambutol or streptomycin with isoniazid, rifampin, and pyrazinamide. IV administration is especially useful in cachectic patients or those needing prolonged streptomycin therapy. ■ *Mycobacterium avium* complex, a common infection in AIDS patients.

CONTRAINDICATIONS

Known streptomycin sensitivity. Known aminoglycoside sensitivity may be a contraindication due to cross-sensitivity.

PRECAUTIONS

Labeled for IM use only; probably due to impurities in early preparations. New formulations are being given IV safely; check your hospital's policy in case an informed consent or release is required. ■ Handle with care; may cause skin sensitivity reactions. ■ Used only when other, less hazardous agents are ineffective or contraindicated. ■ Adequate laboratory and audiometric testing facilities must be available. ■ Sensitivity studies necessary to determine susceptibility of causative organism to streptomycin. ■ Risk for neurotoxicity is sharply increased in patients with pre-existing renal damage or pre-renal azotemia. Manifestations include disturbances of vestibular and cochlear function. Arachnoiditis, encephalopathy, optic nerve dysfunction, and peripheral neuritis may also occur. Partial or total irreversible deafness may continue to develop after streptomycin is discontinued. ▪ Superinfection may occur from overgrowth of nonsusceptible organisms. ▪ *Clostridium difficile*–associated diarrhea (CDAD) has been reported. May range from mild diarrhea to fatal colitis. Consider in patients who present with diarrhea during or after treatment with streptomycin. ▪ May contain sulfites; use caution in patients with asthma. ▪ For additional questions, consultations may be obtained from the Division of Infectious Disease at National Jewish Center.

Monitor: Monitor serum BUN, creatinine, calcium, magnesium, potassium, and sodium before therapy and weekly. ▪ Calcium, magnesium, potassium, and sodium levels may decline and require replacement. ▪ Observe for any adverse effects including at the infusion site. ▪ High serum levels increase risk of ototoxicity and neurotoxicity. Assess adequacy of dose and clearance of drug with serum streptomycin concentrations (2 to 6 hours after a timed dose) initially and every 2 to 4 weeks. Peak therapeutic levels are between 20 and 30 mcg/mL. Serum levels over 50 mcg/mL may be toxic. ▪ Watch for decrease in urine output, rising BUN and SCr, and declining CrCl levels. A decrease in dose may be indicated; serum levels should not exceed 25 mcg/mL if any kidney damage is present. ▪ Assess vestibular function toxicity weekly (Romberg test, past point, heel-to-toe, and lateral nystagmus). ▪ Assess ototoxicity with audiograms every 2 to 4 weeks. ▪ All of the above monitoring may be done more frequently if indicated. Permanently implanted central venous catheters allow treatment on an outpatient basis. Blood work may be done every 2 weeks and all other tests every 4 weeks when stable enough to be treated as an outpatient. ▪ Maintain good hydration. Dehydration may increase risk of nephrotoxicity; monitor closely if vomiting, diarrhea, or other events that may cause dehydration occur. ▪ Closely monitor patients with impaired renal function for nephrotoxicity and neurotoxicity (e.g., auditory and vestibular ototoxicity); nephrotoxicity may be reversible. ▪ National Jewish Center uses chromatographic assay to determine streptomycin serum levels; concomitantly administered antibiotics do not have to be withheld when collecting samples for analysis. ▪ Usual length of treatment for tuberculosis is 1 year. Discontinue streptomycin therapy whenever toxic symptoms appear, impending toxicity is feared, organisms become resistant, or full therapeutic effect is achieved. ▪ In long-term therapy, alkalinization of urine may minimize renal irritation. ▪ See Drug/Lab Interactions.

Patient Education: Report promptly any changes in balance, dizziness, hearing loss or weakness. ▪ Consider birth control options. ▪ Promptly report diarrhea or bloody stools that occur during treatment or up to several months after an antibiotic has been discontinued; may indicate CDAD and require treatment.

Maternal/Child: Category D: avoid pregnancy; has caused total, irreversible, bilateral deafness in infants whose mothers received streptomycin during pregnancy. ▪ Discontinue breast-feeding. ▪ Has caused CNS depression, including stupor, flaccidity, coma, and deep respiratory depression in very young infants.

Elderly: Risk of toxicity increased; see Dose Adjustments.

DRUG/LAB INTERACTIONS

Synergistic when used in combination with **beta-lactam antibiotics** (e.g., cephalosporins, penicillins) **and vancomycin.** Synergism may be inconsistent; see Compatibility. ▪ Concurrent or sequential use with any other neurotoxic, ototoxic, or nephrotoxic agents should be avoided. May have dangerous additive effects with **other aminoglycosides** (e.g., gentamicin, tobramycin), **diuretics** (e.g., furosemide [Lasix], mannitol), **beta-lactam antibiotics** (e.g., cephalosporins), **colistin** (Coly-Mycin S), **polymyxin B, vancomycin, cyclosporine, and many others.** ▪ May be antagonized by **bacteriostatic antibiotics** (e.g., chloramphenicol, erythromycin, and tetracycline); bactericidal action may be affected. ▪ **Magnesium sulfate** may reduce antibiotic activity of streptomycin. ▪ Anesthetics (e.g., enflurane) and neuromuscular blocking muscle relaxants (e.g., atracurium [Tracrium], succinylcholine) are potentiated by aminoglycosides. Respiratory paralysis and apnea can occur. ▪ Aminoglycosides are potentiated by **anticholinesterases** (e.g., edrophonium), **antineoplastics** (e.g., nitrogen mustard, cisplatin). ▪ See Side Effects.

SIDE EFFECTS

Occur more frequently with impaired renal function, higher doses, prolonged administration, dehydration, in the elderly, and in patients receiving other ototoxic or nephrotoxic drugs. Apnea, azotemia, CDAD, cochlear ototoxicity (hearing loss and deafness), eosinophilia, exfoliative dermatitis, facial paresthesias, fever, hemolytic anemia, hypersensitivity reactions (e.g., angioneurotic edema, anaphylaxis, itching, rash, urticaria), leukopenia, muscular weakness, neuromuscular blockade, pancytopenia, roaring in the ears, seizures, thrombocytopenia, tinnitus, vestibular ototoxicity (nausea and vomiting, vertigo). Least nephrotic of the aminoglycosides but nephrotoxicity does occur. Has caused severe chilling (rigors) with penicillins if spacing is not adequate.

ANTIDOTE

Notify the physician of all side effects. Discontinue streptomycin with any evidence of renal impairment, ototoxicity, or vestibular toxicity. Tinnitus, roaring noises, or a sense of fullness in the ears indicate a need for audiometric examination. Auditory changes are usually irreversible and bilateral and may be partial or total. Vestibular symptoms are reversible if detected early. A reduction in dose may be required or an alternate drug used. In overdose hemodialysis may be indicated. Monitor fluid balance, CrCl, and plasma levels carefully. Complexation with ticarcillin may be as effective as hemodialysis. Calcium salts or neostigmine may reverse neuromuscular blockade. Treat CDAD with fluids, electrolytes, protein supplements, and oral vancomycin (Vancocin) or metronidazole (Flagyl) as indicated. In severe cases, surgical evaluation may be indicated. Resuscitate as necessary.

STREPTOZOCIN BBW

(strep-toe-**ZOH**-sin)

Zanosar

Antineoplastic
(alkylating agent/nitrosurea)

pH 3.5 to 4.5

USUAL DOSE

500 mg/M^2 for 5 consecutive days; see Monitor. Repeat every 6 weeks until maximum benefit or treatment-limiting toxicity observed. May also give 1,000 mg/M^2 weekly for 2 doses. May then increase up to 1,500 mg/M^2 to achieve therapeutic response if significant toxicity not observed. Overall cumulative dose to onset of response is 2,000 mg/M^2. Maximum response is usually achieved with 4,000 mg/M^2 total cumulative dose.

DOSE ADJUSTMENTS

Reduce dose in impaired renal function; see Precautions/Monitor. ▪ Reduce dose or discontinue drug if mild proteinuria occurs. Lower-end initial doses may be appropriate in the elderly; consider the potential for decreased organ function and concomitant disease or drug therapy. ▪ Can be used with other antineoplastic drugs in reduced doses to achieve tumor remission.

DILUTION

Specific techniques required; see Precautions. Each 1-Gm vial must be diluted with 9.5 mL NS or D5W (100 mg/mL). Usually further diluted in larger amounts (50 to 250 mL) of the same solutions.

Storage: Store in refrigerator before and after dilution. Discard within 12 hours of dilution. Contains no preservatives. Protect from light.

COMPATIBILITY

Consider any drug NOT listed as compatible to be INCOMPATIBLE until consulting a pharmacist; specific conditions may apply.

One source suggests the following **compatibilities:**

Y-site: Amifostine (Ethyol), etoposide phosphate (Etopophos), filgrastim (Neupogen), gemcitabine (Gemzar), granisetron (Kytril), melphalan (Alkeran), ondansetron (Zofran), teniposide (Vumon), thiotepa, vinorelbine (Navelbine).

RATE OF ADMINISTRATION

A single dose in minimum diluent given over 5 to 15 minutes is recommended. Increase injection time somewhat if additional diluent used or if indicated for patient comfort. Has been given as a continuous infusion over 5 days. Some side effects may be reduced, but CNS side effects (e.g., confusion, depression, lethargy) may be increased.

ACTIONS

An alkylating agent of the nitrosurea group with antitumor activity, cell cycle phase nonspecific. Has a diabetogenic (hyperglycemic) effect resulting from selective uptake into and toxicity to pancreatic islet beta cells. Disappears from the blood rapidly. Concentrates in the liver and kidneys. Excreted primarily in urine.

INDICATIONS AND USES

Suppress or retard neoplastic growth in metastatic pancreatic islet cell carcinoma. Use limited by renal toxicity to those with symptomatic or progressive metastatic disease.

Unlabeled uses: Treatment of adrenocortical and colon cancers and Hodgkin's lymphoma.

CONTRAINDICATIONS

Hypersensitivity to streptozocin. Severely impaired liver or renal function may be a contraindication.

PRECAUTIONS

Follow guidelines for handling cytotoxic agents. See Appendix A, p. 1429. ■ Administered by or under the direction of the physician specialist. ■ Adequate diagnostic and treatment facilities must be readily available. ■ Consider risk of known toxic effects versus benefit before initiating therapy. ■ Marked decrease in leukocyte and platelet counts has occurred and may be fatal. ■ Risk of nephrotoxicity may be reduced by decreasing renal and urinary concentration of streptozocin and its metabolites with adequate hydration. ■ Avoid concomitant use with other potential nephrotoxins (e.g., aminoglycosides [e.g., gentamicin], amphotericin B). ■ Liver dysfunction and diarrhea have been observed in some patients.

Monitor: Renal toxicity is dose related, cumulative, and can be fatal. Monitor renal function before, weekly, and for 4 weeks after each course of therapy (serial urinalysis, BUN, plasma creatinine, serum electrolytes, CrCl). Reduce dose or discontinue drug if mild proteinuria occurs. Further deterioration of renal function may occur; see Precautions. ■ Determine absolute patency and quality of vein and adequate circulation of extremity. Local inflammation (e.g., burning, edema, erythema, tenderness), severe cellulitis, and/or necrosis may result from extravasation. If extravasation occurs, discontinue injection; use another vein. ■ Have IV dextrose available especially with the first dose. Sudden release of insulin may precipitate hypoglycemia. Monitor serum glucose at periodic intervals. ■ Monitor CBC and liver function tests weekly. ■ Nausea and vomiting have occurred in all patients and can be severe. Prophylactic administration of antiemetics recommended. ■ Observe for any signs of infection. Use of prophylactic antibiotics may be indicated pending results of C/S in a febrile neutropenic patient. ■ Maintain hydration; see Precautions. ■ Monitor for thrombocytopenia (platelet count less than 50,000/mm^3). Initiate precautions to prevent excessive bleeding (e.g., inspect IV sites, skin, and mucous membranes; use extreme care during invasive procedures; test urine, emesis, stool, and secretions for occult blood). ■ See Drug/Lab Interactions.

Patient Education: Avoid pregnancy; nonhormonal birth control recommended. ■ Report IV site burning or stinging promptly. ■ Use caution in tasks that require alertness, such as driving or using complex machinery. ■ See Appendix D, p. 1434.

Maternal/Child: Category D: avoid pregnancy. Produces teratogenic effects in rats. Has mutagenic potential. ■ Discontinue breast-feeding.

Elderly: Differences in response compared to younger adults not observed. Lower-end initial doses may be appropriate; see Dose Adjustments.

DRUG/LAB INTERACTIONS

Do not administer **live virus vaccines** to patients receiving antineoplastic drugs. ■ Concurrent use with **hepatotoxic or nephrotoxic medications and radiation therapy** may increase toxicity and could be fatal. ■ Toxicity may be additive when used in combination with **other cytotoxic drugs** (e.g., cyclophosphamide [Cytoxan], doxorubicin [Adriamycin, Doxil]). ■ May prolong the elimination half-life of **doxorubicin** and lead to severe bone marrow suppression. A reduced dose of doxorubicin may be indicated. ▪ Concurrent use with **phenytoin** (Dilantin) may decrease therapeutic effects of streptozocin.

SIDE EFFECTS
Anemia, decreased platelet count (precipitous), diarrhea, elevated AST and LDH, hepatic toxicity (usually reversible), hypoalbuminemia, hypoglycemia, insulin shock, leukopenia (precipitous), nausea and vomiting (severe), proteinuria, thrombocytopenia. Two cases of diabetes insipidus have been reported.

ANTIDOTE
Notify physician of all side effects. Nausea and vomiting, hematologic changes, and renal toxicity (proteinuria) may require dose reduction or discontinuation of the drug. There is no specific antidote. Supportive therapy as indicated will help sustain the patient in toxicity. Administration of whole blood products (e.g., packed RBCs, platelets, leukocytes) and/or blood modifiers (e.g., darbepoetin alfa [Aranesp], epoetin alfa [Epogen], filgrastim [Neupogen], oprelvekin [Neumega], pegfilgrastim [Neulasta], sargramostim [Leukine]) may be indicated to treat bone marrow toxicity. For extravasation, elevate extremity, consider injection of long-acting dexamethasone (Decadron LA) throughout extravasated tissue. Use a 27- or 25-gauge needle. Apply warm, moist compresses.

SULFAMETHOXAZOLE AND TRIMETHOPRIM
(sul-fah-meh-**THOX**-ah-zohl and try-**METH**-oh-prim)

SMZ-TMP, TMP-SMZ

Antibacterial
Antiprotozoal

pH 10

USUAL DOSE
Doses listed are based on the trimethoprim component of the drug.
Severe urinary tract infections and shigellosis in adults and pediatric patients over 2 months of age: 8 to 10 mg/kg/24 hr in equally divided doses every 6, 8, or 12 hours (2 to 2.5 mg/kg every 6 hours, 2.67 to 3.33 mg/kg every 8 hours, or 4 to 5 mg/kg every 12 hours). Administer for 14 days (urinary tract infections) or 5 days (shigellosis). Maximum recommended dose is 960 mg trimethoprim and 4,800 mg sulfamethoxazole/24 hr (60 mL/24 hr).
***Pneumocystis jiroveci* pneumonitis in adults and pediatric patients over 2 months of age:** 15 to 20 mg/kg/24 hr in equally divided doses every 6 or 8 hours (3.75 to 5 mg/kg every 6 hours or 5 to 6.67 mg/kg every 8 hours) for up to 14 days.

DOSE ADJUSTMENTS
Reduce dose by one half for CrCl between 15 and 30 mL/min; see Contraindications. ▪ Reduced dose may be indicated in the elderly. ▪ See Monitor and Drug/Lab Interactions.

DILUTION

Each 5-mL ampule (16 mg trimethoprim/mL [80 mg/5 mL], 80 mg sulfamethoxazole/mL [400 mg/5 mL]) must be diluted in 125 mL D5W and given as an infusion. Reduce diluent to 75 mL for each ampule only if fluid restriction required. Standard dilution must be used within 6 hours; fluid restriction dilution must be used within 2 hours. Available in 5-, 10-, 20-, and 30-mL vials. Concentration per mL same as 5-mL ampule. Discard if cloudiness or crystallization is present.

Storage: Store at room temperature; do not refrigerate.

COMPATIBILITY   (Underline Indicates Conflicting Compatibility Information)

Consider any drug NOT listed as compatible to be INCOMPATIBLE until consulting a pharmacist; specific conditions may apply.

Manufacturer states, "Do not mix with other drugs or solutions."

One source suggests the following **compatibilities:**

Y-site: Acyclovir (Zovirax), aldesleukin (Proleukin), allopurinol (Aloprim), amifostine (Ethyol), amphotericin B cholesteryl (Amphotec), anidulafungin (Eraxis), atracurium (Tracrium), aztreonam (Azactam), bivalirudin (Angiomax), cefepime (Maxipime), cisatracurium (Nimbex), cyclophosphamide (Cytoxan), dexmedetomidine (Precedex), diltiazem (Cardizem), docetaxel (Taxotere), doxorubicin liposomal (Doxil), enalaprilat (Vasotec IV), esmolol (Brevibloc), etoposide phosphate (Etopophos), fenoldopam (Corlopam), filgrastim (Neupogen), fludarabine (Fludara), foscarnet (Foscavir), gallium nitrate (Ganite), gemcitabine (Gemzar), granisetron (Kytril), hetastarch in electrolytes (Hextend), hydromorphone (Dilaudid), labetalol (Trandate), lorazepam (Ativan), magnesium sulfate, melphalan (Alkeran), meperidine (Demerol), morphine, nicardipine (Cardene IV), pancuronium, pemetrexed (Alimta), piperacillin/tazobactam (Zosyn), remifentanil (Ultiva), sargramostim (Leukine), tacrolimus (Prograf), teniposide (Vumon), thiotepa, vecuronium, zidovudine (AZT, Retrovir).

RATE OF ADMINISTRATION

A single dose must be infused over 60 to 90 minutes. When administered by an infusion device, thoroughly flush all lines used to remove any residual sulfamethoxazole/trimethoprim. Avoid rapid infusion or bolus injection.

ACTIONS

A broad-spectrum antibacterial and antiprotozoal combination agent with bactericidal action effective against gram-positive and gram-negative organisms. Blocks sequential steps in the folic acid pathway, preventing the synthesis of nucleic acids and proteins essential to many bacteria. Combination contains 400 mg sulfamethoxazole and 80 mg trimethoprim per each 5 mL. Widely distributed in all body fluids and tissues, including cerebrospinal fluid, sputum, and bile. Onset of action is prompt and serum levels are maintained up to 10 hours. Metabolized in the liver and up to 60% is excreted in urine in 24 hours. Crosses placental barrier. Secreted in breast milk. Partially removed by hemodialysis.

INDICATIONS AND USES

Severe urinary tract infections. ▪ *Pneumocystis jiroveci* pneumonia. ▪ Shigellosis. ▪ Prophylaxis in neutropenic patients. ▪ Used orally in HIV and other immunocompromised patients to prevent pneumonia.

Unlabeled uses: Treatment of cholera and salmonella type infections. ▪ An alternative agent in the treatment of meningitis caused by susceptible organisms.

CONTRAINDICATIONS

CrCl less than 15 mL/min, hypersensitivity to trimethoprim or sulfonamides, megaloblastic anemia resulting from folate deficiency, nursing mothers, pregnancy at term and infants less than 2 months of age (may cause hemolytic anemia, jaundice, and kernicterus), streptococcal pharyngitis.

PRECAUTIONS

Sensitivity studies indicated to determine susceptibility of the causative organism to sulfamethoxazole/trimethoprim. ▪ Not for IM use. ▪ Use caution in impaired liver or renal function, possible folate deficiency, allergic individuals, bronchial asthma, porphyria, glucose 6-phosphate dehydrogenase (G-6PD) deficiency, and in the elderly. ▪ A sulfonamide drug; hypersensitivity reactions can occur. Use caution in patients with a history of hypersensitivity to furosemide (Lasix), thiazide diuretics (e.g., chlorothiazide), sulfonylureas (e.g., tolbutamide), or carbonic anhydrase inhibitors (e.g., acetazolamide). ▪ Some products contain bisulfites; use caution in patients with allergies. ▪ Incidence of side effects markedly increased in AIDS patients. May not tolerate or respond to this drug. ▪ *Clostridium difficile*–associated diarrhea (CDAD) has been reported. May range from mild diarrhea to fatal colitis. Consider in patients who present with diarrhea during or after treatment with sulfamethoxazole/trimethoprim.

Monitor: Maintain adequate hydration to prevent crystalluria and stone formation. ▪ CBC required before and during therapy. Discontinue for any significant reduction in a blood-forming element. Urinalysis and renal function tests also indicated. ▪ If extravasation occurs, discontinue and restart at a new site. May cause phlebitis. ▪ Monitor closely if any signs of rash appear or have appeared in previous infusions. Several cases of life-threatening reactions have occurred. ▪ See Precautions and Drug/Lab Interactions.

Patient Education: Maintain adequate hydration. ▪ Report bruising or bleeding, fever, rash, or sore throat promptly. ▪ Possible skin photosensitivity. Avoid unprotected exposure to sunlight. ▪ Promptly report diarrhea or bloody stools that occur during treatment or up to several months after an antibiotic has been discontinued; may indicate CDAD and require treatment.

Maternal/Child: Category C: no adequate studies. May interfere with folic acid metabolism in mother and fetus. Benefits must outweigh risks. ▪ May contain benzyl alcohol. ▪ See Contraindications. ▪ Discontinue breast-feeding. ▪ Two infants who developed a rash had life-threatening reactions when sulfamethoxazole/trimethoprim was restarted.

Elderly: See Dose Adjustments. ▪ Increased risk of severe side effects (e.g., bone marrow suppression, decrease in platelets with or without purpura, skin reactions), especially in impaired renal or liver function or with other drugs (e.g., diuretics).

DRUG/LAB INTERACTIONS

May be potentiated by **probenecid.** ▪ May inhibit **cyclosporine** (Sandimmune) and increase nephrotoxicity. ▪ May potentiate **warfarin** (Coumadin), **phenytoin** (Dilantin), **oral hypoglycemics, dapsone, and zidovudine** (AZT, Retrovir). ▪ The sulfa component may displace **methotrexate** from its binding sites, increasing free fraction of methotrexate and its potential for toxicity. The trimethoprim component inhibits methotrexate metabolism and increases toxicity. ▪ May decrease effectiveness of **tricyclic antidepres-**

sants (e.g., amitriptyline [Elavil]). ▪ Concurrent use with **folate antagonists** (e.g., hydantoins [e.g., phenytoin], methotrexate), is not recommended. May increase possibility of megaloblastic anemia. ▪ Concurrent use with **leucovorin calcium** may cause treatment failure and increased morbidity in HIV-infected patients being treated for *Pneumocystis jiroveci* pneumonia. ▪ Concurrent use with **bone marrow suppressants** (e.g., antineoplastics [e.g., busulfan, cisplatin], amphotericin B [all formulations], ganciclovir [Cytovene]) may increase leukopenic or thrombocytopenic effects. Monitor differential blood count. ▪ Serum levels of **digoxin** may be increased with concurrent use; monitor digoxin levels. ▪ Concurrent use with **hemolytics** (e.g., doxapram [Dopram], methyldopa, procainamide [Pronestyl], quinidine) may increase potential for toxic side effects. ▪ Concurrent use with **hepatotoxic agents** (e.g., amiodarone [Nexterone], erythromycins, fluconazole [Diflucan]) may increase incidence of hepatotoxicity. Risk increased with prolonged use or in patients with a history of liver disease. ▪ May form an insoluble precipitate in acid urine or cause crystalluria with **methenamine** (Mandelamine); concurrent use not recommended. ▪ May decrease clearance and increase serum concentrations of *N*-acetylprocainamide (NAPA) **and procainamide** (Pronestyl). ▪ Concurrent use with **rifampin** (Rifadin) will increase elimination, reduce serum concentrations, and shorten half-life of trimethoprim. ▪ Concurrent use with **thiazide diuretics** (e.g., chlorothiazide) in the elderly may result in an increased incidence of thrombocytopenia with purpura. ▪ May interfere with **serum methotrexate assay and Jaffe assay for creatinine.** ▪ See Precautions.

SIDE EFFECTS

All side effects of sulfonamides, including hypersensitivity reactions are possible. Nausea, vomiting, and rash occur most frequently. Ataxia, convulsions, tremors, and respiratory depression are symptoms of major toxicity. With high doses or administration over an extended period of time, bone marrow suppression (leukopenia, megaloblastic anemia, thrombocytopenia) may occur. CDAD has been reported.

ANTIDOTE

Notify the physician of any side effect. Discontinue the drug at any sign of major toxicity or bone marrow suppression. Some sources recommend leucovorin calcium 5 to 15 mg daily for treatment of bone marrow suppression. Peritoneal dialysis is not effective in toxicity; hemodialysis may be moderately effective in reducing serum levels. Acidification of urine may increase excretion. Treat anaphylaxis with epinephrine, corticosteroids, antihistamines, and vasopressors. Treat CDAD with fluids, electrolytes, protein supplements, and oral vancomycin (Vancocin) or metronidazole (Flagyl) as indicated. In severe cases, surgical evaluation may be indicated.

TACROLIMUS BBW
(tah-**KROH**-lih-mus)

Immunosuppressant

Prograf

USUAL DOSE

See Precautions. IV route used for patients unable to take oral medications; risk of anaphylaxis increased with IV administration.

For all indications: Dose regimens vary among transplant centers and approved or investigational use (range 0.01 to 0.05 mg/kg/day). Begin no sooner than 6 hours after transplantation. Adults usually receive doses at the lower end of the range. Pediatric patients may require doses at the upper end of the range. Individualized adjustment based on clinical assessment of rejection (e.g., trough blood concentrations) or patients' tolerance is imperative and may be required on a daily basis. Adjunctive adrenal corticosteroid therapy early post-transplant is recommended. Initiate oral tacrolimus therapy as soon as feasible. Oral doses vary with specific organ transplant and in adults and pediatric patients (see literature). Total dose in mg/kg/day is given in equally divided doses every 12 hours. Begin 8 to 12 hours after IV tacrolimus is discontinued. Lower doses may be sufficient for maintenance therapy.

Prophylaxis of organ rejection in heart transplant: The recommended starting dose is 0.01 mg/kg/day as a continuous infusion. Used in combination with azathioprine (Imuran) or mycophenolate (CellCept) in addition to adrenal corticosteroids. See all comments and protocol under For All Indications above.

Prophylaxis of organ rejection in kidney transplant: The recommended starting dose is 0.03 to 0.05 mg/kg/day as a continuous infusion. Used in combination with azathioprine (Imuran) or mycophenolate (CellCept) in addition to adrenal corticosteroids. See all comments and protocol under For All Indications above.

Prophylaxis of organ rejection in liver transplant: The recommended starting dose is 0.03 to 0.05 mg/kg/day as a continuous infusion. Used in combination with adrenal corticosteroids. See all comments and protocol under For All Indications above.

PEDIATRIC DOSE

Has been used successfully in pediatric patients up to 16 years of age in liver transplants. See Usual Dose for mg/kg/day dose recommendations. Studies indicate that higher doses may be required to maintain blood trough concentrations similar to adults. Experience in pediatric heart and kidney transplant patients is limited. See Dilution and Maternal/Child.

DOSE ADJUSTMENTS

Use lowest dosing range initially for patients with impaired renal or hepatic function (pre-transplant or post-transplant). Nephrotoxicity may be increased and further reductions may be required; should be based on tacrolimus trough levels in blood. Half-life and clearance decrease in patients with severe hepatic impairment (Child-Pugh greater than or equal to 10). Dose reduction may be required. Monitor blood concentrations. ■ Delay tacrolimus therapy up to 48 hours in patients with postoperative oliguria. ■ Lower doses may be appropriate for maintenance. ■ Black patients who have undergone a kidney transplant may require a higher dose to obtain trough concentrations comparable to those seen in white patients. ▪ See Monitor and Drug/Lab Interactions.

DILUTION
A 24-hour dose must be diluted with an appropriate amount of NS or D5W. Desired concentration is between 4 and 20 mcg/mL. May leach phthalate from polyvinylchloride containers; use diluents in glass or polyethylene infusion bottles. Use PVC-free IV tubing in pediatric patients. The following chart provides some dose and dilution examples.

Tacrolimus Dose and Dilution Examples				
Desired Dose	Weight	Total Dose	Amount of Diluent	mcg/mL
0.08 mg/kg	20 kg	1.6 mg/24 hr	250 mL	6.4 mcg/mL
			100 mL	16 mcg/mL
0.05 mg/kg	60 kg	3 mg/24 hr	500 mL	6 mcg/mL
			250 mL	12 mcg/mL
0.04 mg/kg	100 kg	4 mg/24 hr	1,000 mL	4 mcg/mL

Storage: Store between 5° and 25° C (41° and 77° F) before dilution. Discard diluted solution in 24 hours.

COMPATIBILITY   (Underline Indicates Conflicting Compatibility Information)
Consider any drug NOT listed as compatible to be INCOMPATIBLE until consulting a pharmacist; specific conditions may apply.
Manufacturer states, "Should not be mixed with solutions of pH 9 or greater (e.g., acyclovir [Zovirax], ganciclovir [Cytovene])." See Dilution.
   One source suggests the following **compatibilities:**
Y-site: Aminophylline, amphotericin B (generic), ampicillin, ampicillin/sulbactam (Unasyn), anidulafungin (Eraxis), benztropine (Cogentin), calcium gluconate, caspofungin (Cancidas), cefazolin (Ancef), cefotetan, ceftazidime (Fortaz), ceftriaxone (Rocephin), cefuroxime (Zinacef), chloramphenicol (Chloromycetin), ciprofloxacin (Cipro IV), clindamycin (Cleocin), dexamethasone (Decadron), digoxin (Lanoxin), diphenhydramine (Benadryl), dobutamine, dopamine, doripenem (Doribax), doxycycline, erythromycin (Erythrocin), esmolol (Brevibloc), fluconazole (Diflucan), furosemide (Lasix), gentamicin, haloperidol (Haldol), heparin, hydrocortisone sodium succinate (Solu-Cortef), hydromorphone (Dilaudid), imipenem-cilastatin (Primaxin), insulin (regular), isoproterenol (Isuprel), leucovorin calcium, lorazepam (Ativan), methylprednisolone (Solu-Medrol), metoclopramide (Reglan), metronidazole (Flagyl IV), micafungin (Mycamine), morphine, multivitamins (M.V.I.), mycophenolate (CellCept IV), nitroglycerin IV, nitroprusside sodium, oxacillin (Bactocill), penicillin G potassium, phenytoin (Dilantin), piperacillin, potassium chloride (KCl), propranolol, ranitidine (Zantac), sodium bicarbonate, sulfamethoxazole/trimethoprim, tobramycin, vancomycin.

RATE OF ADMINISTRATION
A single dose properly diluted and equally distributed over 24 hours as a continuous infusion. Use of a metriset (60 gtt/min) or infusion pump suggested.

ACTIONS

A potent immunosuppressive agent. Prolongs survival of allogeneic kidney and liver transplants. Suppresses some humoral immunity (within the body fluids) but suppresses cell-mediated reactions to a greater extent (e.g., allograft rejection, delayed type hypersensitivity, collagen-induced arthritis, experimental allergic encephalomyelitis, graft-versus-host disease). Inhibition of T-lymphocyte activation results in immunosuppression. Highly protein bound. Metabolized primarily by the P_{450} enzyme system. Half-life ranges from 32 to 54 hours. Primarily excreted in feces. Minimal excretion in urine. Crosses the placental barrier. Secreted in breast milk.

INDICATIONS AND USES

Prophylaxis of organ rejection in allogeneic heart, kidney, and liver transplants in conjunction with adrenal corticosteroids. In heart and kidney transplant patients, concomitant use with azathioprine or mycophenolate is recommended in addition to the adrenal corticosteroids.
Unlabeled uses: Treatment of autoimmune diseases (i.e., rheumatoid arthritis). ▪ Prevention and treatment of acute graft-versus-host disease.

CONTRAINDICATIONS

Hypersensitivity to tacrolimus or polyoxyl 60 hydrogenated castor oil.

PRECAUTIONS

For IV use only. Oral dosing preferred; begin as soon as feasible. Risk of anaphylaxis is increased by IV route versus oral route; use caution. *Reserve for patients unable to take oral medication.* ▪ Usually administered in the hospital by or under the direction of a physician experienced in immunosuppressive therapy and management of organ transplant patients. ▪ Adequate laboratory and supportive medical resources must be available. ▪ Use caution in impaired renal function; increases in SCr may require dose reduction or use of an alternate immunosuppressant. ▪ Use caution in severe hepatic dysfunction (mean Pugh score: greater than 10), clearance decreased. ▪ Can cause nephrotoxicity and neurotoxicity, particularly at higher doses; see Monitor. ▪ Posterior reversible encephalopathy syndrome (PRES) has been reported; see Monitor. ▪ Use combination immunosuppressant therapy with caution; may oversuppress the immune system and increase susceptibility to infection. ▪ Immunosuppressed patients are at increased risk for opportunistic infections, including latent viral infections such as BK virus–associated nephropathy and JC virus–associated progressive multifocal leukoencephalopathy (PML). PML is a serious progressive neurologic disorder caused by infection of the CNS by JC virus, a member of the papovavirus family. It typically occurs in immunocompromised patients. PML is rare but may result in irreversible neurologic deterioration and death, and there is no known effective treatment. Hemiparesis, apathy, confusion, cognitive deficiencies, and ataxia are the most commonly observed clinical signs. ▪ Concurrent use with sirolimus (Rapamune) is not recommended. Regimen is associated with an increased risk of wound healing complications, renal function impairment, and insulin-dependent, post-transplant diabetes mellitus in heart transplant patients. ▪ Post–liver transplant patients experiencing hepatic impairment may be at increased risk of developing renal insufficiency related to elevated tacrolimus concentrations. ▪ May cause lymphomas and other malignancies (especially of skin), and has been associated with a lymphoproliferative disorder (LPD) related to Epstein-Barr virus. ▪ Antiviral prophylaxis (e.g., acyclovir, ganciclovir, immune globulin) may be advisable in some patients. ▪ Insulin-dependent post-transplant diabetes mellitus has been reported in tacrolimus-treated heart, kidney, and liver transplant patients. May be reversible over 1 to 2 years in some patients. Black and Hispanic kidney transplant patients may be at an increased risk; see Monitor. ▪ Myocardial hypertrophy has been reported. Reversible in most cases with dose reduction or discontinuation of tacrolimus. ▪ See Drug/Lab Interactions.

Monitor: Obtain baseline CBC, differential, platelets, electrolytes, fasting glucose, BUN, SCr, and liver function tests. Monitor regularly during therapy. ▪ Contains a castor oil derivative and alcohol; observe continuously for signs of a hypersensitivity reaction for the first 30 minutes of the infusion and frequently thereafter. A source of oxygen and epinephrine must always be available. ▪ Monitor urine output and SCr carefully. Overt nephrotoxicity occurs more frequently early after transplant, resulting in increased SCr and decreased urine output. Consider changing to another immunosuppressive therapy in patients with persistent elevations of SCr who are unresponsive to dose adjustments. ▪ Monitor for S/S of neurotoxicity (e.g., changes in motor or sensory function, changes in mental status, coma, delirium, headache, tremor, seizures). ▪ Monitor for S/S of PRES (e.g., altered mental status, headache, hypertension, seizures, and visual disturbances). Diagnosis may be confirmed by MRI. Maintain BP control, and an immediate decrease of immunosuppression is advised. Symptoms have reversed when immunosuppression is reduced or discontinued. ▪ Monitor for S/S of PML; apathy, ataxia, cognitive deficiencies, confusion, and hemiparesis are the most commonly observed clinical signs. ▪ Monitor tacrolimus blood levels to evaluate rejection, toxicity, need for dose reduction, and patient compliance. Risk of toxicity (e.g., nephrotoxicity, neurotoxicity, post-transplant diabetes mellitus) is increased with higher trough concentrations. Whole blood median trough concentrations (measured by IMx or ELISA) may vary considerably during the first week but then stabilize. Most patients are stable when trough whole blood concentrations are between 5 and 20 ng/mL depending on indication and length of time since the transplant. ▪ Monitor all parameters to evaluate possibility of organ rejection. ▪ Monitor BP; antihypertensives may be indicated; see Drug/Lab Interactions. ▪ Monitor serum potassium and magnesium levels. May cause hyperkalemia or hypomagnesemia. ▪ May cause hyperglycemia. Monitor carefully; treatment may be required. ▪ Observe for signs of infection (e.g., fever, sore throat, tiredness) or unusual bleeding or bruising. ▪ Use of prophylactic antibiotics may be indicated pending results of C/S in a febrile neutropenic patient. ▪ Consider echocardiographic evaluation in patients who develop renal failure or clinical manifestations of ventricular dysfunction. ▪ See Precautions and Drug/Lab Interactions.

Patient Education: Nonhormonal birth control preferred to oral contraceptives to reduce complications of drug interactions. ▪ Emphasize need for frequent routine lab work; compliance imperative. ▪ Interacts with many medications. Discuss any changes in drug regimen (prescription or nonprescription) with doctor or pharmacist. ▪ Promptly report any side effects. ▪ Review S/S of diabetes mellitus. ▪ Inform patient of increased risk of neoplasia, including malignant skin changes. Limit exposure to sunlight and ultraviolet light. ▪ See Appendix D, p. 1434.

Maternal/Child: Category C: use only if necessary; benefits must outweigh risk to fetus. Has been associated with hyperkalemia and renal dysfunction in the fetus. ▪ Discontinue breast-feeding. ▪ Appears to be an increased risk for LPD and primary Epstein-Barr virus infection in immunosuppressed pediatric patients.

Elderly: Consider age-related organ impairment.

DRUG/LAB INTERACTIONS

May be used concurrently only with **adrenocorticosteroids.** *Do not use simultaneously with cyclosporine (Sandimmune).* If a change of immunosuppressants is indicated (tacrolimus to cyclosporine or cyclosporine to tacrolimus), avoid additive nephrotoxicity by waiting for at least 24 hours before starting the alternate drug. If elevated blood concentrations are present, further extend the interval between the two drugs. ▪ Concurrent use with **sirolimus** (Rapamune) is not recommended. Regimen is associated with an increased risk of wound healing complications, renal function impairment, and insulin-dependent post-transplant diabetes mellitus in heart transplant patients. ▪ Concurrent use with **muromonab-CD3** (Orthoclone) may increase the incidence of post-transplant lymphoproliferative disorder (PTLD). ▪ Use extreme caution with **other nephrotoxic agents** (e.g., aminoglycosides [gentamicin, tobramycin], amphotericin B [generic], cisplatin [Platinol]). ▪ Do not use **potassium-sparing diuretics** (e.g., spironolactone [Aldactone]); increases risk of hyperkalemia. ▪ **Calcium channel blockers** (e.g., diltiazem [Cardizem], nicardipine [Cardene], nifedipine [Procardia], verapamil), **antifungal agents** (e.g., clotrimazole [Mycelex], fluconazole [Diflucan], itraconazole [Sporanox], ketoconazole [Nizoral], voriconazole [VFEND]), **bromocriptine** (Parlodel), **chloramphenicol** (Chloromycetin), **cimetidine** (Tagamet), **clarithromycin** (Biaxin), **cyclosporine** (Sandimmune), **danazol** (Cyclomen), **erythromycin**, **estradiol** (Estrace), **methylprednisone** (Solu-Medrol), **metoclopramide** (Reglan), **metronidazole** (Flagyl), **omeprazole** (Prilosec), **protease inhibitors** (e.g., nelfinavir [Viracept], ritonavir [Norvir], saquinavir [Invirase]), **theophylline, and troleandomycin** (TAO) may inhibit the P_{450} enzyme system and increase tacrolimus blood levels, increasing toxicity potential. Tacrolimus toxicity may also be increased if given concurrently with **nefazodone.** ▪ **Anticonvulsants** (e.g., carbamazepine [Tegretol], phenobarbital, phenytoin [Dilantin]), **caspofungin** (Cancidas), **rifamycins** (e.g., rifabutin [Mycobutin], rifampin [Rifadin]), **sirolimus** (Rapamune), **and St. John's wort** may induce the P_{450} enzyme system, decreasing effectiveness and leading to decreased tacrolimus blood levels and organ rejection. ▪ Tacrolimus may increase serum concentrations of **mycophenolate** (CellCept). ▪ **Grapefruit juice** may affect certain enzymes of the P_{450} system and should be avoided. ▪ Avoid **vaccinations and do not use live virus vaccines** in patients receiving tacrolimus.

SIDE EFFECTS

Occur in a majority of patients and are more pronounced at higher doses. May improve somewhat over time. Nephrotoxicity (abnormal renal function with increased SCr and BUN, oliguria), and neurotoxicity (delirium, headache, insomnia, paresthesia, tremor, seizures) may be dose limiting. Abdominal pain, abnormal ECG, abnormal liver function tests, acute kidney failure, albuminuria, anemia, anorexia, arrhythmias, ascites, asthenia, atelectasis, back pain, blood dyscrasias, bronchitis, CHF, CMV infection, coma, constipation, cushingoid features, diabetes mellitus, diarrhea, dyspnea, fever, gastroenteritis, glycosuria, headache, hearing loss (including deafness), hemolytic-uremic syndrome, hyperglycemia, hyperkalemia or hypokalemia, hyperlipemia, hypertension, hypomagnesemia, impaired wound healing, infection, insomnia, leukopenia, leukocytosis, leukoencephalopathy, myocardial hypertrophy, nausea, neuralgia, pain, pancreatitis, peripheral edema, peritonitis, photosensitivity, plural effusion, pruritus, pulmonary edema, QT prolongation, rash, seizures, Stevens-Johnson syndrome, thrombocytopenia, thrombophlebitis, torsades de pointes, urinary tract infections, vertigo, vomiting. In heart transplant patients, abnormal renal function, CMV infection, diabetes mellitus, hyperglycemia, hyperlipemia, hypertension, infection, leukopenia, and tremor were reported most commonly. Many other side effects have occurred in fewer than 3% of patients.

Post-Marketing: Acute respiratory distress syndrome, BK nephropathy, cardiac arrhythmia, cerebral infarction, DIC, enterocolitis, gastroesophageal reflux disease, hepatotoxicity, interstitial lung disease, posterior reversible encephalopathy syndrome (PRES), primary graft dysfunction, and progressive multifocal leukoencephalopathy (PML) are some of the many additional side effects reported.

ANTIDOTE

Notify the physician of all side effects. Most will be treated symptomatically. Tacrolimus may be decreased or discontinued or alternate immunosuppressive agents substituted. Nephrotoxicity, neurotoxicity, or hematopoietic depression may require temporary reduction of dose or discontinuation of therapy. If S/S of PRES occur, maintain BP control, and an immediate decrease of immunosuppression is advised. Dialysis is not effective in overdose. Discontinue immediately if anaphylaxis occurs and treat with oxygen, epinephrine, corticosteroids, and/or antihistamines (e.g., diphenhydramine [Benadryl]). Resuscitate as necessary.

TELAVANCIN BBW
(tel-a-**VAN**-sin)

Vibativ

**Antibacterial
(lipoglycopeptide)**

pH 4 to 5

USUAL DOSE
10 mg/kg as an infusion once every 24 hours for 7 to 14 days. Duration of therapy is dependent on severity and site of infection and on the patient's clinical and bacteriologic progress.

DOSE ADJUSTMENTS
Dose adjustment required in renal impairment as outlined in the following chart.

Telavancin Dosage Adjustment in Adult Patients with Renal Impairment	
Creatinine Clearance (mL/min)	Telavancin Dosage Regimen
>50 mL/min	10 mg/kg every 24 hours
30 to 50 mL/min	7.5 mg/kg every 24 hours
10 to ≤30 mL/min	10 mg/kg every 48 hours

There is insufficient information to make specific dose recommendations for patients with end-stage renal disease (CrCl less than 10 mL/min), including patients undergoing hemodialysis. ■ Reduced doses may be indicated in the elderly based on age-related renal impairment. ■ No dose adjustment is recommended based on gender or in patients with mild or moderate hepatic impairment. Has not been studied in patients with severe hepatic impairment.

DILUTION
Reconstitute each 250-mg vial with 15 mL of D5W, SW, or NS (45 mL for a 750-mg vial). Resultant solution has a final concentration of 15 mg/mL. Reconstitution time is generally under 2 minutes but can occasionally take as long as 20 minutes. Mix thoroughly to dissolve contents completely. Discard vial if vacuum does not pull diluent into vial. Doses of 150 to 800 mg must be further diluted in 100 to 250 mL of D5W, NS, or LR. Doses less than 150 mg or greater than 800 mg must be diluted in a sufficient volume to provide a final concentration of 0.6 to 8 mg/mL.

Storage: Store unopened vials in refrigerator at 2° to 8° C (36° to 46° F). Excursions up to 25° C (77° F) are acceptable. Reconstituted and diluted solutions are stable for 4 hours at RT and for 72 hours refrigerated. Total time in the vial plus the time in the infusion bag should not exceed 4 hours at RT and 72 hours under refrigeration.

COMPATIBILITY
Manufacturer states, "Additives or other medications should not be added to telavancin single-use vials or infused simultaneously through the same IV line. If the same IV line is used for sequential infusion of additional medications, the line should be flushed before and after infusions of telavancin with D5W, NS, or LR."

RATE OF ADMINISTRATION

A singe dose equally distributed as an infusion over 60 minutes. Rapid IV infusions can cause "red man syndrome"–like infusion-related reactions, including flushing of the upper body, urticaria, pruritus, or rash.

ACTIONS

A lipoglycopeptide antibacterial that is a synthetic derivative of vancomycin. Bactericidal against gram-positive organisms, including susceptible strains of staphylococci, streptococci, and vancomycin-susceptible enterococci. Exerts bactericidal action through inhibition of cell wall synthesis. Highly protein bound, primarily to albumin. The metabolic pathway for telavancin has not been identified. Half-life is 6.6 to 9.6 hours. Primarily excreted by the kidney.

INDICATIONS AND USES

Treatment of adult patients with complicated skin and skin structure infections caused by susceptible isolates of Gram-positive microorganisms, including *Staphylococcus aureus* (including methicillin-susceptible and methicillin-resistant isolates), *Streptococcus pyogenes, Streptococcus agalactiae, Streptococcus anginosus* group, or *Enterococcus faecalis* (vancomycin-susceptible isolates only). Combination therapy may be clinically indicated if the documented or presumed pathogens include Gram-negative organisms.

CONTRAINDICATIONS

Manufacturer states, "None."

PRECAUTIONS

To reduce the development of drug-resistant bacteria and maintain its effectiveness, telavancin should be used to treat or prevent only those infections proven or strongly suspected to be caused by bacteria. ■ Sensitivity studies are necessary to determine susceptibility of the causative organism to telavancin. ■ Prolonged use of drug may result in superinfection caused by overgrowth of nonsusceptible organisms. ■ New-onset or worsening renal impairment has been reported. Patients with underlying renal dysfunction or risk factors for renal dysfunction (diabetes mellitus, CHF, or hypertension) may be at increased risk. Patients who received concomitant medications known to affect kidney function (e.g., NSAIDs, ACE inhibitors, and loop diuretics) may also be at higher risk; see Drug Interactions. ■ Data from clinical studies suggest that clinical cure rates were lower in patients with baseline CrCl less than or equal to 50 mL/min. These data should be considered when selecting antibacterial therapy for use in patients with baseline moderate/severe renal impairment. ■ *Clostridium difficile*–associated diarrhea (CDAD) has been reported. May range from mild diarrhea to fatal colitis. Consider in patients who present with diarrhea during or after treatment with telavancin. ■ Infusion-related reactions have been reported; see Rate of Administration and Monitor. ■ Has caused prolongation of the QTc interval. Use with caution in patients who are taking drugs known to prolong the QTc interval. Avoid use in patients with congenital long QT syndrome, known prolongation of the QTc interval, uncompensated heart failure, or severe left ventricular hypertrophy. ■ Does not interfere with coagulation. Increased risk of bleeding and effects on platelet aggregation have not been observed. However, has been shown to affect certain anticoagulation tests; see

Drug/Lab interactions. ■ There is no known cross-resistance between telavancin and other classes of antibiotics. Some vancomycin-resistant enterococci have a reduced susceptibility to telavancin. ■ See Maternal/Child.

Monitor: Obtain baseline CBC with differential and SCr. Monitor SCr every 48 to 72 hours, or more frequently if indicated, and at the end of therapy. If renal function deteriorates, the risk versus benefit of continuing therapy should be assessed. ■ Monitor for possible infusion-related reactions.

Patient Education: Women of childbearing potential should have a pregnancy test before initiating therapy. Effective birth control should be used throughout therapy. A pregnancy registry has been established to monitor the outcomes of women who become pregnant while receiving telavancin. ■ Report all side effects promptly. ■ Promptly report diarrhea or bloody stools that occur during treatment or up to several months after telavancin has been discontinued; may indicate CDAD and require treatment.

Maternal/Child: Category C: adverse developmental outcomes in three animal species at clinically relevant doses raise concerns about potential adverse developmental outcomes in humans. Avoid use during pregnancy unless potential benefit justifies potential risk. ■ Women with childbearing potential should have a serum pregnancy test before receiving telavancin. A pregnancy registry has been established to monitor pregnancy outcomes in women exposed to telavancin during pregnancy. ■ Safety for use in breast-feeding not established and effects unknown; use caution. ■ Safety and effectiveness for use in pediatric patients not been studied.

Elderly: Lower clinical cure rates were seen in patients over 65 years of age. Overall, treatment-emergent adverse events occurred with similar frequencies in patients of all age-groups studied. However, adverse events indicative of renal impairment occurred more frequently in the elderly. Consider age-related renal impairment; see Dose Adjustments.

DRUG/LAB INTERACTIONS

Use with caution in patients taking **medications known to prolong the QTc interval** (e.g., amiodarone [Nexterone], diphenhydramine [Benadryl], fosphenytoin [Cerebyx], furosemide [Lasix], itraconazole [Sporanox]). Effects may be additive. ■ Concomitant use with **other agents that can affect renal function** (e.g., NSAIDs [e.g., ibuprofen (Advil, Motrin), naproxen (Naprosyn, Aleve)], diuretics [e.g., furosemide (Lasix)], and ACE inhibitors [e.g., lisinopril (Zestril), enalaprilat (Vasotec)]) may increase risk of renal toxicity. ■ Telavancin clearance should not be affected by drugs that inhibit or induce the P_{450} system and should not affect the pharmacokinetics of drugs metabolized by the P_{450} system. ■ Has been administered with aztreonam (Azactam) and piperacillin/tazobactam (Zosyn). There was no effect on the pharmacokinetics of either drug. ■ Antagonism between telavancin and amikacin (Amikin), aztreonam (Azactam), cefepime (Maxipime), ceftriaxone (Rocephin), ciprofloxacin (Cipro), gentamicin, imipenem-cilastatin (Primaxin), meropenem (Merrem), oxacillin (Bactocil), rifampin (Rifadin), and sulfamethoxazole/trimethoprim has not been seen in *in vitro* studies. ■ May affect **certain anticoagulation tests.** Increases in PT, INR, aPTT, ACT and coagulation-based factor Xa tests have been observed. Effects dissipate over time. Interference seen when using samples drawn between 0 and 18 hours after telavancin administration. Collect blood samples for these coagulation tests immediately before a patient's next telavancin dose to minimize interaction. ▪ Interferes with **urine qualitative dipstick protein assays** and **quantitative dye methods** (e.g., pyrogallol red-molybdate). However, microalbumin assays are not affected and can be used to monitor urinary protein excretion.

SIDE EFFECTS

The most common side effects include foamy urine, nausea, taste disturbances, and vomiting. Most serious side effects include CDAD, infusion-related reactions, and renal impairment (increased SCr, renal insufficiency, renal failure). The most common events leading to discontinuation of therapy were nausea and rash. Other reported side effects include abdominal pain, decreased appetite, diarrhea, dizziness, infusion site pain and erythema, pruritus, QT prolongation, and rigors.

ANTIDOTE

Notify the physician of all side effects. Initiate supportive care as indicated. Infusion-related reactions may respond to temporarily discontinuing or slowing the rate of infusion. Consider alternative antimicrobial therapy in patients who develop renal toxicity. Treat CDAD with fluids, electrolytes, protein supplements, and oral vancomycin (Vancocin) or metronidazole (Flagyl) as indicated. In severe cases, surgical evaluation may be indicated. There is no information on the use of hemodialysis or continuous venovenous hemofiltration in toxicity.

TEMOZOLOMIDE
(te-moe-**ZOE**-loe-mide)

Temodar

Antineoplastic
(Alkylating agent)

USUAL DOSE

IV and oral doses are therapeutically equivalent if the IV dose is administered equally distributed over 90 minutes. The oral form should be used as soon as tolerated by the patient.

Newly diagnosed glioblastoma multiforme (GBM): *Concomitant phase:* 75 mg/M^2 for 42 days. Given concomitantly with focal radiotherapy. No dose reductions are recommended during the concomitant phase; however, dose interruptions or discontinuation may occur based on toxicity. The temozolomide dose should be continued throughout the 42-day concomitant period up to 49 days if all of the following conditions are met:

- Absolute neutrophil count must be equal to or greater than 1.5 × 10^9/L (1,500/mm^3).
- Platelet count must be equal to or greater than 100 × 10^9/L (100,000/mm^3).
- Nonhematologic toxicity must be equal to or less than Grade 1 (except for alopecia, nausea, and vomiting).
- CBC and platelet count should be obtained weekly.
- Interrupt or discontinue temozolomide dosing based on the hematologic and nonhematologic criteria in the following chart.

Temozolomide (TMZ) Dosing or Discontinuation During Concomitant Radiotherapy		
Toxicity	TMZ Interruption*	TMZ Discontinuation
Absolute neutrophil count	≥0.5 and <1.5 × 10^9/L	<0.5 × 10^9/L
Platelet count	≥10 and <100 × 10^9/L	<10 × 10^9/L
CTCAE nonhematologic toxicity (except for alopecia, nausea, vomiting)	CTCAE Grade 2	CTCAE Grade 3 or 4

TMZ, Temozolomide; *CTCAE,* Common Terminology Criteria for Adverse Events.
*Treatment with concomitant TMZ could be continued when all of the following conditions are met: ANC ≥1.5 × 10^9/L, platelet count ≥100 × 10^9/L, CTCAE nonhematologic toxicity Grade ≤1 (except for alopecia, nausea, vomiting).

Prophylaxis against *Pneumocystis jiroveci* **pneumonia (PCP):** Required for all patients during this concomitant therapy. PCP prophylaxis should be continued in patients who develop lymphocytopenia until they recover from lymphocytopenia (CTCAE Grade ≤1).

Newly diagnosed glioblastoma multiforme (GBM): *Maintenance phase:* 4 weeks after completing the temozolomide plus focal radiotherapy phase, temozolomide is administered for an additional 6 cycles of maintenance.

Cycle 1: The initial dose is 150 mg/M^2 once daily for 5 days followed by 23 days without treatment (a 28-day cycle).

Cycles 2 through 6: The dose can be increased to 200 mg/M^2 if the following conditions are met:

- Absolute neutrophil count is equal to or greater than 1.5×10^9/L (1,500/mm^3)
- Platelet count is equal to or greater than 100×10^9/L (100,000/mm^3)
- Nonhematologic toxicity is equal to or less than Grade 2 (except for alopecia, nausea, and vomiting).

The dose remains at 200 mg/M^2 per day for the first 5 days of each subsequent cycle except if toxicity occurs. If the dose was not increased at Cycle 2, it should not be increased for subsequent cycles. See Dose Adjustments for dose reduction or discontinuation during maintenance.

Refractory anaplastic astrocytoma: 150 mg/M^2 once daily for 5 consecutive days for each 28-day treatment cycle. This dose may be increased to 200 mg/M^2/day if both the nadir and day of dosing (Day 29, Day 1 of next cycle) ANC is equal to or greater than 1.5×10^9/L (1,500/mm^3) and the nadir and day of dosing (Day 29, Day 1 of next cycle) platelet count is equal to or greater than 100×10^9/L (100,000/mm^3). During treatment, a CBC should be obtained on Day 22 (21 days after the Day 1 dose of temozolomide) or within 48 hours of that day for each cycle. Repeat weekly until the ANC is above 1.5×10^9/L (1,500/mm^3) and the platelet count exceeds 100×10^9/L (100,000/mm^3). The next cycle of temozolomide should not be started until the ANC and platelet count exceed these levels. If the ANC falls to $<1 \times 10^9$/L (1,000/mm^3) or the platelet count is $<50 \times 10^9$/L (50,000/mm^3) during any cycle, reduce the next cycle by 50 mg/M^2 but not below 100 mg/M^2 (the lowest recommended dose). Therapy can be continued until disease progression. See the flow chart in Dose Adjustments.

DOSE ADJUSTMENTS

Newly diagnosed glioblastoma multiforme (GBM): Temozolomide dose must be adjusted according to the nadir ANC and platelet counts in the previous cycle and the ANC and platelet counts at the time of initiating the next cycle. Obtain a CBC and platelet count weekly during the concomitant phase and as indicated during the 4-week interim before beginning the maintenance phase. Obtain a baseline CBC and platelet count before beginning a cycle and repeat on Day 22 (21 days after the first dose of temozolomide in the cycle or within 48 hours of that day). Repeat weekly until the ANC is above 1.5×10^9/L (1,500/mm^3) and the platelet count exceeds 100×10^9/L (100,000/mm^3). The next cycle of temozolomide should not be started until the ANC and platelet count exceed these levels. This sequence is repeated for Cycles 1 through 6 of maintenance dosing. Base dose reductions during the next cycle on the lowest blood counts and worst nonhematologic toxicity during the previous cycle. Dose reductions or discontinuations during maintenance should be applied according to the following two charts.

Continued

Temozolomide Dose Levels for Maintenance Treatment		
Dose Level	Dose (mg/M²/day)	Remarks
−1	100 mg/M²/day	Reduction for prior toxicity
0	150 mg/M²/day	Dose during Cycle 1
1	200 mg/M²/day	Dose during Cycles 2 through 6 in absence of toxicity

Temozolomide Dose Reduction or Discontinuation During Maintenance Treatment		
Toxicity	Reduce TMZ by 1 Dose Level*	Discontinue TMZ
ANC	$<1 \times 10^9$/L	See † in footnote
Platelet count	$<50 \times 10^9$/L	See † in footnote
CTCAE nonhematologic toxicity (except for alopecia, nausea, vomiting)	CTCAE Grade 3	CTCAE Grade 4

TMZ, Temozolomide; *CTCAE*, Common Terminology Criteria for Adverse Events.
*See preceding chart for temozolomide dose levels for maintenance treatment.
†TMZ is to be discontinued if a dose reduction to <100 mg/M² is required or if the same Grade 3 nonhematologic toxicity (except for alopecia, nausea, vomiting) recurs after dose reduction.

Temozolomide Dose Modification Table for Refractory Anaplastic Astrocytoma:

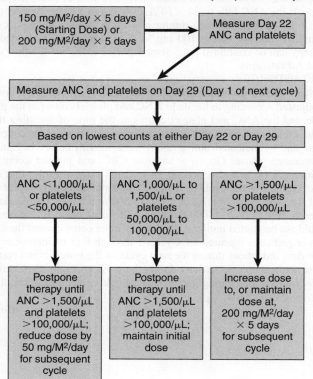

DILUTION

Specific techniques required; see Precautions. Bring vial(s) to room temperature before reconstitution. Reconstitute each 100-mg vial with 41 mL of SW. Swirl gently to dissolve; *do not shake;* will yield a concentration of 2.5 mg/mL of temozolomide. *Do not further dilute* the reconstituted solution. Withdraw up to 40 mL from each vial(s) and transfer into an empty 250-mL PVC infusion bag for delivery with an infusion pump. **Compatibility** with non-PVC bags has not been studied.

Filters: Specific information not available.

Storage: Refrigerate single-use vials at 2° to 8° C (36° to 46° F). Store reconstituted product at RT. Reconstituted solution must be used within 14 hours, including infusion time.

COMPATIBILITY

No **compatibility** data available. Manufacturer states, "Other medications should not be infused simultaneously through the same IV line." May be administered only in the same infusion line as NS.

RATE OF ADMINISTRATION

A single dose equally distributed over 90 minutes. Use of an infusion pump is recommended. Flush IV lines before and after temozolomide infusion. Infusion must be complete within 14 hours of reconstitution.

ACTIONS

An imidazotetrazine derivative and alkylating agent. It is not directly active but undergoes rapid nonenzymatic conversion, as dacarbazine does, to the reactive compound 5-(3-methyl triazen-1-yl)-imidazole-4-carboxamide (MTIC) and to temozolomide acid metabolite. Cytotoxicity is thought to be due primarily to alkylation of DNA. Weakly bound to plasma proteins. Rapidly eliminated with a mean elimination half-life of 1.8 hours. Some excretion in urine and a very small amount in feces.

INDICATIONS AND USES

Treatment of adults with newly diagnosed glioblastoma multiforme. Initially given concomitantly with radiotherapy and then continued as maintenance treatment. ■ Treatment of adults with refractory anaplastic astrocytoma (i.e., adults who have experienced disease progression on a drug regimen containing nitrosourea and procarbazine).

CONTRAINDICATIONS

Known history of hypersensitivity to dacarbazine. ■ Known history of hypersensitivity reaction to temozolomide or any of its components (e.g., urticaria, allergic reaction including anaphylaxis, toxic epidermal necrolysis, and Stevens-Johnson syndrome).

PRECAUTIONS

Follow guidelines for handling cytotoxic agents. See Appendix A, p. 1429.

■ Usually administered by or under the direction of the physician specialist in a facility with adequate diagnostic and treatment facilities to monitor the patient and respond to any medical emergency. ■ Myelosuppression may be severe and dose limiting. May include prolonged pancytopenia, which may result in aplastic anemia. Deaths have been reported. Risk may be increased with concomitant use of other medications associated with aplastic anemia (e.g., carbamazepine [Tegretol], phenytoin [Dilantin], sulfamethoxazole/trimethoprim [Bactrim]). ■ Risk of myelosuppression increased in women and the elderly. ■ Cases of myelodysplastic syndrome and secondary malignancies, including myeloid leukemia, have been observed. ■ Prophylaxis against *Pneumocystis jiroveci* pneumonia (PCP) is required for all patients being treated for newly diagnosed glioblastoma multiforme (a 42-day regimen). The longer dosing regimen may increase the risk of PCP; however, all patients, particularly those receiving steroids, should be monitored for symptoms of PCP regardless of the regimen. ▪ Use caution in patients with severe renal or hepatic impairment.

Monitor: Obtain a baseline CBC and platelet count. See Usual Dose for minimum levels required before administration of temozolomide.

Patients with newly diagnosed GBM: Obtain a CBC and platelet count weekly during the concomitant phase and as indicated during the 4-week interim before beginning the maintenance phase. Obtain a baseline CBC and platelet count before beginning a maintenance dose (28-day cycles) and repeat on Day 22 (21 days after the first maintenance dose of temozolomide or within 48 hours of that day). Repeat weekly until the ANC is above 1.5×10^9/L (1,500/mm^3) and the platelet count exceeds 100×10^9/L (100,000/mm^3). This sequence is repeated for Cycles 1 through 6 of maintenance dosing.

Patients with refractory anaplastic astrocytoma: Obtain a CBC and platelet count on Day 1 of each cycle. During treatment (28-day cycles), a CBC should be obtained on Day 22 (21 days after the Day 1 dose of temozolomide or within 48 hours of that day for each cycle). Repeat weekly until the ANC is above 1.5×10^9/L (1,500/mm^3) and the platelet count exceeds 100×10^9/L (100,000/mm^3).

All indications: Nausea and vomiting may be severe. Prophylactic antiemetics may reduce nausea and vomiting and increase patient comfort. ▪ Observe closely for signs of infection. Prophylactic antibiotics may be indicated pending results of C/S in a febrile neutropenic patient. ▪ Monitor for thrombocytopenia (platelet count less than 50,000/mm^3). Initiate precautions to prevent excessive bleeding (e.g., inspect IV sites, skin, and mucous membranes; use extreme care during invasive procedures; test urine, emesis, stool, and secretions for occult blood). ▪ Regardless of the regimen, monitor all patients, particularly those receiving steroids, for symptoms of PCP (dyspnea; fever; dry, nonproductive cough; characteristic x-ray).

Patient Education: Avoid pregnancy; use of nonhormonal birth control is recommended. ▪ Promptly report a rash; swelling of the face, throat, or tongue; severe skin reaction; or trouble breathing. ▪ Report IV site burning or stinging promptly. ▪ Secondary malignancies have been reported. ▪ See Appendix D, p. 1434. ▪ Additional precautions are required with the capsule form.

Maternal/Child: Category D: avoid pregnancy; can cause fetal harm. ▪ Discontinue breast-feeding. ▪ Safety and effectiveness for use in pediatric patients not established. An oral formulation of the 5-day regimen every 28 days has been used in selected pediatric patients from 3 to 18 years of age. Toxicity profile was similar to that seen in adults.

Elderly: Numbers in clinical studies are insufficient to determine if the elderly respond differently than younger subjects. Dose selection should be cautious based on the potential for decreased organ function and concomitant disease or drug therapy. *In newly diagnosed patients with glioblastoma multiforme,* side effects were similar to those seen in younger patients. *In the anaplastic astrocytoma study,* patients 70 years or older had a higher incidence of Grade 4 neutropenia and Grade 4 thrombocytopenia in the first cycle of therapy.

DRUG/LAB INTERACTIONS

Valproic acid decreases the oral clearance of temozolomide by about 5%; clinical significance is not known. Another source suggests the following interactions. ▪ Temozolomide may increase the effects of **leflunomide** (Arava), **natalizumab** (Tysabri), and **live vaccines** (may also decrease the effects of **live vaccines**); one source recommends that concomitant use be avoided. ▪ The effects of temozolomide may be increased by **divalproex** (Depakote), **trastuzumab** (Herceptin), and **valproic acid** (Depacon). ▪ May decrease the effects of **BCG and inactivated vaccines.** ▪ The effects of temozolomide may be decreased by **echinacea.**

SIDE EFFECTS

Newly diagnosed glioblastoma multiforme: Myelosuppression may be severe and dose limiting. May include prolonged pancytopenia, which may result in aplastic anemia; deaths have been reported. Alopecia, anorexia, constipation, headache, nausea and vomiting, and thrombocytopenia were the most frequently reported side effects. Abdominal pain, blurred vision, confusion, convulsions, coughing, diarrhea, dizziness, dry skin, dyspnea, erythema, fatigue, hypersensitivity reactions including anaphylaxis, insomnia, memory impairment, radiation injury, pruritus, rash, stomatitis, taste perversion, thrombocytopenia, and weakness have been reported.
Refractory anaplastic astrocytoma: Fatigue, headache, myelosuppression, and nausea and vomiting were the most frequently reported side effects. Abdominal pain, abnormal coordination, abnormal gait, abnormal vision (blurred vision, vision changes, visual deficit), adrenal hypercorticism, amnesia, anorexia, anxiety, asthenia, ataxia, back pain, breast pain (female), confusion, convulsions (local and general), coughing, depression, diarrhea, diplopia, dizziness, dysphasia, fever, hemiparesis, insomnia, myalgia, paresis, paresthesia, peripheral edema, pharyngitis, pruritus, rash, sinusitis, URI, urinary incontinence, UTI, viral infection, and weight increase have been reported.
Injection site reactions: Erythema, irritation, pain, pruritus, swelling, and warmth at the infusion site; hematoma; and petechiae.
Post-Marketing: The oral formulation has had reports of hypersensitivity reactions, including anaphylaxis; alveolitis; interstitial pneumonitis/pneumonitis; opportunistic infections, including *Pneumocystis jiroveci* pneumonia (PCP); prolonged pancytopenia, which may result in aplastic anemia with fatal outcomes; pulmonary fibrosis; and skin reactions (e.g., erythema multiforme, toxic epidermal necrolysis, and Stevens-Johnson syndrome).

ANTIDOTE

Keep physician informed of all side effects and CBC results. Temozolomide may need to be reduced or discontinued. Symptomatic and supportive treatment is indicated. Administration of whole blood products (e.g., packed RBCs, platelets, leukocytes) and/or blood modifiers (e.g., darbepoetin alfa [Aranesp], epoetin alfa [Epogen], filgrastim [Neupogen], oprelvekin [Neumega], pegfilgrastim [Neulasta], sargramostim [Leukine]) may be indicated to treat bone marrow toxicity. Precautions are indicated for cancer patients with erythropoietin-stimulating agents (ESAs); see darbepoetin alfa and epoetin alfa monographs. Treat hypersensitivity reactions and/or anaphylaxis as indicated (e.g., epinephrine, corticosteroids, oxygen, and antihistamines [diphenhydramine]). There is no specific antidote. Resuscitate as indicated.

TEMSIROLIMUS
(**TEM**-sir-**OH**-li-mus)
Torisel

Antineoplastic
(kinase inhibitor)

USUAL DOSE

Premedication: To minimize the incidence of hypersensitivity reactions, administer diphenhydramine (Benadryl) 25 to 50 mg IV (or similar antihistamine) 30 minutes before the start of each dose of temsirolimus; see Precautions and Monitor.

Temsirolimus: 25 mg as an infusion once a week until disease progression or unacceptable toxicity.

DOSE ADJUSTMENTS

Hold for absolute neutrophil count (ANC) less than 1,000/mm^3, platelet count less than 75,000/mm^3, or CTCAE Grade 3 or greater adverse reactions. Once toxicities have resolved to Grade 2 or less, restart therapy with the dose reduced by 5 mg/week to a dose no lower than 15 mg/week. ■ Consider dose reduction to 12.5 mg/week when coadministered with a strong CYP3A4 inhibitor; see Drug Interactions. If the strong inhibitor is discontinued, wait approximately 1 week before adjusting the temsirolimus dose upward to the indicated dose. ■ Consider a dose increase to 50 mg/week when coadministered with a strong CYP3A4 inducer; see Drug Interactions. If the strong inducer is discontinued, the temsirolimus dose should be returned to the dose used prior to initiation of the strong CYP3A4 inducer. ■ No dose adjustment indicated based on age, race, gender, or renal status. Not studied in hemodialysis patients. ■ No data available regarding the influence of hepatic impairment on temsirolimus pharmacokinetics.

DILUTION

Specific techniques required; see Precautions. Available as a kit containing a vial of temsirolimus and a vial of a manufacturer-supplied diluent. Temsirolimus vial contains overfill (30 mg/1.2 mL). A two-step dilution process is required. Reconstitute the temsirolimus vial with 1.8 mL of the provided diluent. Invert the vial several times to mix thoroughly. Allow time for foam to subside. Final concentration in temsirolimus vial is 10 mg/mL. Solution will be clear to slightly turbid and colorless to yellow. Withdraw the required amount of reconstituted temsirolimus and rapidly inject into a 250-mL container (glass, polyolefin, or polyethylene) of NS. Invert bag to mix. Avoid excessive shaking.

Filter: Use of an in-line polyethersulfone filter with a pore size not greater than 5 microns is recommended.

Storage: Store unopened vials at 2° to 8° C (36° to 46° F). Protect from light. During handling and preparation, protect from excessive room light or sunlight. The temsirolimus/diluent mixture is stable for 24 hours in the temsirolimus vial. Administration of the final product diluted in NS should be completed within 6 hours of adding the temsirolimus/diluent mixture to the NS.

COMPATIBILITY

Manufacturer states, "Final dilution for infusion should be stored in bottles (glass, polypropylene) or plastic bags (polypropylene, polyolefin) and administered through polyethylene-lined administration sets." Non–DEHP containing materials must be used for administration. Manufacturer also states that undiluted temsirolimus should not be added directly to aqueous infusion solutions. A precipitate will form. In addition, "The stability of temsirolimus in other infusion solutions has not been evaluated. Addition of other drugs or nutritional agents to admixtures of temsirolimus in NS has not been evaluated and should be avoided. Temsirolimus is degraded by both acids and bases, and thus combinations of temsirolimus with agents capable of modifying solution pH should be avoided."

RATE OF ADMINISTRATION

A single dose as an infusion equally distributed over 30 to 60 minutes. Use of an infusion pump is recommended. Increase duration of infusion to 60 minutes in patients who experience a hypersensitivity reaction.

ACTIONS

An inhibitor of mTOR (mammalian target of rapamycin). Binds to an intracellular protein (FKBP-12); this protein-drug complex inhibits the activity of mTOR that controls cell division. Results in a cell cycle–specific (G1) growth arrest in treated tumor cells. In *in vitro* studies, temsirolimus inhibited the activity of mTOR and resulted in reduced levels of hypoxia-inducible factors HIF-1 and HIF-2 α and the vascular endothelial growth factor. Both temsirolimus and sirolimus are extensively partitioned into formed blood elements. Extensively metabolized, primarily by cytochrome P_{450} 3A4. Sirolimus is the principal metabolite and is active. Elimination is primarily via the feces and to a small extent via urine. Mean half-lives of temsirolimus and sirolimus were 17.3 and 54.6 hours, respectively.

INDICATIONS AND USES

Treatment of advanced renal cell carcinoma.

CONTRAINDICATIONS

None; see Dose Adjustments and Precautions.

PRECAUTIONS

Follow guidelines for handling cytotoxic agents. See Appendix A, p. 1429.
■ Should be administered by or under the direction of the physician specialist in facilities equipped to monitor the patient and respond to any medical emergency. ■ Hypersensitivity reactions have been reported. Premedication required to minimize the chance of a reaction; see Usual Dose. Use with caution in patients with known hypersensitivity to temsirolimus or its metabolites (including sirolimus) or to any components of the product. Use caution in patients who cannot receive prophylactic treatment with an antihistamine for medical reasons; see Monitor. ■ Hyperglycemia/ glucose intolerance is common. Initiation of or an increase in the dose of insulin and/or oral hypoglycemic agent therapy may be required. ■ Elevated cholesterol and triglycerides are common. Initiation or adjustment of existing therapy may be required. ■ May cause immunosuppression, thus increasing the risk of infections, including opportunistic infections. ■ Cases of interstitial lung disease, some resulting in death, have been reported. ■ Cases of fatal bowel perforation have been reported. ■ Rapidly progressive and sometimes fatal acute renal failure has occurred. ■ Has been associated with abnormal wound healing. Exercise caution when temsirolimus is used in the perioperative period. ■ Patients who have CNS tumors and/or are receiving anticoagulation therapy may be at increased risk of intracerebral bleeding. ■ The use of live virus vaccines and close

contact with those who have received live virus vaccines should be avoided. See Drug Interactions.

Monitor: Obtain baseline and weekly CBC with differential and platelet count. Obtain a baseline chemistry panel and repeat every 2 weeks. ▪ Monitor for S/S of a hypersensitivity reaction (e.g., anaphylaxis, bronchospasm, chest pain, dyspnea, flushing, rash). If a reaction occurs, the infusion should be stopped and the patient should be observed for at least 30 to 60 minutes (depending on the severity of the reaction). At the discretion of the physician, treatment may be resumed with the administration of an H_1-receptor antagonist (such as diphenhydramine [Benadryl]) if not previously administered and/or an H_2-receptor antagonist (e.g., ranitidine [Zantac] 50 mg IV or famotidine [Pepcid] 20 mg IV) approximately 30 minutes before restarting the temsirolimus infusion. The infusion may be resumed at a slower rate; see Rate of Administration. ▪ Monitor serum glucose, cholesterol, and triglycerides before and during therapy. ▪ Monitor for S/S of infection. ▪ Monitor respiratory status. Patients may present with symptoms such as dyspnea, cough, hypoxia, and fever or may be asymptomatic. ▪ Monitor for S/S of bowel perforation (abdominal pain, acute abdomen, bloody stools, diarrhea, fever, metabolic acidosis). ▪ Monitor for thrombocytopenia (platelet count less than $50,000/mm^3$); see Dose Adjustments and Contraindications. Initiate precautions to prevent excessive bleeding (e.g., inspect IV sites, skin, and mucous membranes; use extreme care during invasive procedures; test urine, emesis, stool, and secretions for occult blood).

Patient Education: Review medical history with health care provider. Temsirolimus may affect existing medical conditions (e.g., diabetes, high cholesterol, hyperlipidemia). Therapy may need to be adjusted. ▪ Review medication list (prescription, over-the-counter, and herbal) with health care provider. Interactions are possible. ▪ Promptly report any S/S of a hypersensitivity reaction (chest tightness, dyspnea, flushing, pruritus, rash, urticaria). ▪ Avoid pregnancy during and for 3 months after completion of therapy. Men with partners of childbearing potential should use reliable contraception during treatment and for 3 months after completion of therapy. ▪ Report excessive thirst or any increase in volume or frequency of urination. ▪ Promptly report S/S of infection, new or worsening respiratory symptoms, new or worsening abdominal pain, or blood in stools. ▪ Wound healing complications may occur while on therapy. ▪ The use of live virus vaccines and close contact with those who have received live virus vaccines should be avoided. ▪ Increased risk of intracerebral bleed in patients who have CNS tumors and/or are receiving anticoagulants.

Maternal/Child: Category D: avoid pregnancy; may cause fetal harm. ▪ Potential for tumorigenicity. Discontinue breast-feeding. ▪ Safety and effectiveness for use in pediatric patients not established.

Elderly: Numbers of elderly insufficient to establish differences in response; see Dose Adjustments.

DRUG/LAB INTERACTIONS

Use of concomitant **strong CYP3A4 inhibitors** (e.g., amprenavir [Agenerase], atazanavir [Reyataz], clarithromycin [Biaxin], delavirdine [Rescriptor], indinavir [Crixivan], itraconazole [Sporanox], ketoconazole [Nizoral], nefazodone, nelfinavir [Viracept], ritonavir [Norvir], saquinavir [Invirase], telithromycin [Ketek], or voriconazole [VFEND]) may increase plasma concentrations of the active metabolite sirolimus. Avoid concomitant use if possible. If required, consider a dose reduction of temsirolimus to 12.5 mg/week and monitor closely for acute toxicity. If the strong inhibitor is discontinued, a washout period of approximately 1 week should be allowed before adjusting the temsirolimus dose upward to the indicated dose; see Dose Adjustments. ■ **Grapefruit juice** may increase plasma concentrations of temsirolimus and should be avoided. ■ **CYP3A4/5 inducers** (e.g., carbamazepine [Tegretol], dexamethasone [Decadron], phenobarbital [Luminal], phenytoin [Dilantin], rifabutin [Mycobutin], rifampin [Rifadin]) may decrease plasma concentrations of the active metabolite sirolimus, thus decreasing effectiveness. Avoid concomitant use if possible. If required, consider a dose increase to 50 mg/week. If the strong inducer is discontinued, the temsirolimus dose should be returned to the dose used before initiating the strong CYP3A4 inducer; see Dose Adjustments. ■ **St. John's wort** may decrease temsirolimus plasma concentrations, decreasing effectiveness. Avoid use. ■ No clinically significant effect is anticipated when temsirolimus is coadministered with agents that are metabolized by CYP2D6 or CYP3A4.

SIDE EFFECTS
The most common side effects include abdominal pain, anemia, anorexia, asthenia, constipation, edema, elevated alkaline phosphatase and AST, elevated SCr, hyperglycemia, hyperlipemia, hypertriglyceridemia, hypophosphatemia, leukopenia, lymphopenia, mucositis, nausea, rash, and thrombocytopenia. Less commonly reported side effects include acne, arthralgia, bowel perforation, chest pain, chills, cough, depression, diarrhea, dry skin, dysgeusia, dyspnea, edema, epistaxis, fever, headache, hypokalemia, increased bilirubin, increased total cholesterol, increased triglycerides, infection, insomnia, nail disorder, neutropenia, pain, pruritus, rash, vomiting, and weight loss. The most serious side effects include bowel perforation, hyperglycemia/glucose intolerance, hyperlipemia, hypersensitivity reactions, interstitial lung disease, and renal failure.

ANTIDOTE
Keep physician informed of all side effects. Most minor side effects will be treated symptomatically. Monitor patient closely. Discontinue temsirolimus at the first sign of a hypersensitivity reaction. Monitor patient for 30 to 60 minutes. Treatment may be resumed at the discretion of the physician; see Monitor. Treat severe hypersensitivity reactions as indicated; may require epinephrine, airway management, oxygen, IV fluids, antihistamines (e.g., diphenhydramine [Benadryl]), corticosteroids (e.g., hydrocortisone sodium succinate [Solu-Cortef]) and pressor amines (e.g., dopamine). Treat the development of interstitial lung disease as indicated. May require discontinuation of temsirolimus and/or treatment with corticosteroids and/or antibiotics. Some patients have been able to continue therapy without additional intervention.

TENECTEPLASE
(teh-**NECK**-teh-plays)

TNKase

**Thrombolytic agent
(recombinant)**

pH 7.3

USUAL DOSE

Initiate therapy as soon as possible after the onset of acute myocardial infarction (AMI) symptoms. Total dose is based on patient weight and should not exceed 50 mg. See the following chart.

Tenecteplase Dosing Guidelines		
Patient Weight (kg)	Tenecteplase (mg)	Volume of Tenecteplase* to Be Administered (mL)
<60 kg	30 mg	6 mL
≥60 to <70 kg	35 mg	7 mL
≥70 to <80 kg	40 mg	8 mL
≥80 to <90 kg	45 mg	9 mL
≥90 kg	50 mg	10 mL

*From one vial of tenecteplase reconstituted with 10 mL of SW.

Concurrent administration of heparin and aspirin has been used in MI patients receiving tenecteplase therapy. In the ASSENT-2 trial, the following doses were used.

Aspirin: 150 to 325 mg as soon as possible was followed by 150 to 325 mg daily.

Heparin IV: Was administered based on weight. *Patients weighing 67 kg or less* received a heparin loading dose of 4,000 units followed by an infusion at 800 units/hr. *Patients weighing more than 67 kg* received a heparin loading dose of 5,000 units followed by an infusion at 1,000 units/hr. Heparin was continued for 48 to 72 hours with the infusion rate adjusted to maintain the aPPT at 50 to 75 seconds.

DOSE ADJUSTMENTS

None noted.

DILUTION

Remove the shield assembly from the manufacturer-supplied B-D® 10 mL syringe with TwinPak™ dual Cannula Device. Aseptically withdraw 10 mL of SW from the supplied diluent vial using the red hub cannula syringe filling device. Do not use bacteriostatic water for injection. Do not discard the shield assembly. Inject the 10 mL of SW into the tenecteplase vial, directing the diluent stream into the powder. Slight foaming may occur. Allow product to stand for several minutes. Gently swirl until contents are completely dissolved. Do not shake. The reconstituted preparation is colorless to pale yellow and contains tenecteplase 50 mg/10 mL. Withdraw the desired dose from the vial using the syringe. Once the appropriate dose is drawn into the syringe, stand the shield vertically on a flat surface with the green side down and passively recap the red hub cannula. Remove the entire shield assembly, including the red hub cannula, by twisting counterclockwise. **Note:** The shield assembly also contains the clear-ended blunt plastic cannula; retain for split septum IV access. The supplied syringe is compatible with a conventional needle and with needleless IV systems. See package insert for complete instructions for administration.

Storage: Store unopened vial at CRT or under refrigeration (at 2° to 8° C [(36° to 46° F]). Reconstitution immediately before use preferred, or may be refrigerated for up to 8 hours.

COMPATIBILITY

Manufacturer states, "Precipitation may occur when tenecteplase is administered in an IV line containing dextrose. Dextrose-containing lines should be flushed with a saline-containing solution prior to and following single bolus administration of tenecteplase."

RATE OF ADMINISTRATION

A single bolus dose over 5 seconds. Flush line with saline-containing solution to ensure delivery of entire dose.

ACTIONS

A tissue plasminogen activator and enzyme produced by recombinant DNA technology. Binds to fibrin in a thrombus and converts plasminogen to plasmin. Plasmin digests fibrin and dissolves the clot. Onset of action is prompt. Cleared via hepatic metabolism. Terminal half-life is 90 to 130 minutes.

INDICATIONS AND USES

For use in the reduction of mortality associated with acute myocardial infarction (AMI). Treatment should be initiated as soon as possible after the onset of AMI symptoms.

CONTRAINDICATIONS

Active internal bleeding, history of cerebrovascular accident, intracranial or intraspinal surgery or trauma within the past 2 months, intracranial neoplasm, arteriovenous malformation, or aneurysm, known bleeding diathesis, and severe uncontrolled hypertension.

PRECAUTIONS

Administered under the direction of a physician knowledgeable in its use and with appropriate emergency drugs and diagnostic and laboratory facilities available. ■ Most common complication is bleeding. May be internal bleeding or superficial or surface bleeding. Strict bed rest indicated to reduce risk of bleeding. Use extreme care with the patient; avoid any excessive or rough handling or pressure; avoid invasive procedures (e.g., arterial puncture, venipuncture, IM injection). If these procedures are absolutely necessary, use extreme precautionary methods (use radial artery instead of femoral; use small-gauge catheters and needles, and sites that are easily observed and compressible where bleeding can be controlled; avoid handling catheter sites; and use extended pressure application of up to 30 minutes). Minor bleeding occurs often at catheter insertion sites. Avoid use of razors and toothbrushes. If serious bleeding (not controlled by local pressure) occurs, discontinue any concomitant heparin or antiplatelet agents immediately. ■ Use extreme caution in the following situations: recent major surgery (e.g., CABG), previous puncture of noncompressible vessels, organ biopsy, or trauma, cerebrovascular disease, recent GI or GU bleeding, hypertension (systolic BP above 180 and/or diastolic BP above 110), high likelihood of left heart thrombus (e.g., mitral stenosis with atrial fibrillation), acute pericarditis, subacute bacterial en-docarditis, hemostatic defects (including those secondary to severe hepatic or renal disease), severe hepatic dysfunction, pregnancy or recent child-birth, diabetic hemorrhagic retinopathy, septic thrombophlebitis or oc-cluded AV cannula at a seriously infected site, advanced age, patients currently receiving oral anticoagulants (e.g., warfarin), recent administra-tion of GPIIb/IIIa inhibitors (e.g., abciximab [ReoPro], eptifibatide [Inte-grilin]), any other condition in which bleeding constitutes a significant hazard or would be particularly difficult to manage because of its location. In the presence of any of these situations, the risk versus benefit of tenecteplase therapy must be evaluated. ■ Cholesterol embolism has been reported rarely in patients treated with all types of thrombolytic agents. See Side Effects. ■ Reperfusion arrhythmias (e.g., sinus bradycardia, acceler-ated idioventricular rhythm, ventricular premature depolarization, ventric-ular tachycardia) may occur following coronary thrombolysis. Manage with standard antiarrhythmic measures. Have antiarrhythmic meds readily available. ■ Standard management of MI should be implemented concom-itantly with tenecteplase therapy. Simultaneous therapy with heparin and aspirin is used to reduce the risk of rethrombosis. Increases risk of bleeding; see Usual Dose. ■ Readministration of tenecteplase to patients who have received prior plasminogen activator therapy has not been studied. Use caution if deemed necessary, and monitor for signs of hypersensitivity or anaphylactic reactions.

Monitor: Obtain appropriate clotting studies (e.g., PT, PTT, aPTT, fibrin-ogen levels), CBC, and platelet count. ■ Diagnosis-specific baseline stud-ies (e.g., ECG, CPK with isoenzymes, troponin) are indicated. Baseline assessment (patient condition, pain, hematomas, petechiae, or recent wounds) should be completed before administration. ■ Type and cross-match may also be ordered. ■ Maintain strict bed rest; monitor the patient carefully and frequently for pain and signs of bleeding; observe catheter sites at least every 15 minutes and apply pressure dressings to any recently invaded site; watch for hematuria, hematemesis, bloody stool, petechiae, hematoma, flank pain, muscle weakness; and do neuro checks every hour (or more frequently if indicated). Continue until normal clotting function returns. ■ Monitor ECG continuously. ■ See Precautions and Drug/Lab Interactions.

Patient Education: Compliance with all measures to minimize bleeding (e.g., strict bed rest) is very important. ■ Avoid use of razors, toothbrushes, and other sharp items. Use caution while moving to avoid excessive bumping. ■ Report all episodes of bleeding and apply local pressure if indicated. Expect oozing from IV sites.

Maternal/Child: Category C: safety for use in pregnancy, breast-feeding and pediatric patients not established.

Elderly: See Indications and Precautions. May have poorer prognosis following AMI and pre-existing conditions that may increase risk of adverse events, including bleeding. Select patients carefully to maximize benefits.

DRUG/LAB INTERACTIONS

Formal studies have not been performed. ■ Risk of bleeding may be increased by **any medicine that affects blood clotting** including anticoagu-lants (e.g., heparin, lepirudin [Refludan], warfarin [Coumadin]); **any med-ication that may cause hypoprothrombinemia, thrombocytopenia, or GI ulcera-**

tion or bleeding (e.g., selected antibiotics [e.g., cefotetan], aspirin, NSAIDs [e.g., ibuprofen (Advil, Motrin), naproxen (Aleve, Naprosyn)]); **and/or any other medication that inhibits platelet aggregation** (e.g., clopidogrel [Plavix], dipyridamole [Persantine], glycoprotein GPIIb/IIIa receptor antagonists [e.g., abciximab (ReoPro), eptifibatide (Integrilin), tirofiban (Aggrastat)], plicamycin [Mithracin], sulfinpyrazone [Anturane], ticlopidine [Ticlid], valproic acid [Depacon, Depakene]). Concurrent use not recommended with the exception of heparin and aspirin to reduce the risk of rethrombosis. If concurrent or subsequent use indicated (e.g., management of acute coronary syndrome, percutaneous coronary intervention) monitor PT and aPTT closely. ▪ **Coagulation test will be unreliable;** specific procedures can be used; notify the lab of tenecteplase use.

SIDE EFFECTS

Bleeding is most common: internal (GI tract, GU tract, retroperitoneal, or intracranial), epistaxis, gingival, and superficial or surface bleeding (venous cutdowns, arterial punctures, sites of recent surgical intervention). Hypersensitivity reactions (e.g., anaphylaxis, angioedema, laryngeal edema, rash, and urticaria) have been reported rarely. Fever, hypotension, nausea and vomiting, and reperfusion arrhythmias have occurred. Cholesterol embolization can occur with thrombolytic therapy, but has been reported rarely. Clinical features may include livedo reticularis, "purple toe" syndrome, acute renal failure, gangrenous digits, hypertension, pancreatitis, MI, cerebral, spinal cord or bowel infarction, retinal artery occlusion, and rhabdomyolysis. Several other adverse events have been reported. These reactions are frequently sequelae of the underlying disease, and the effect of tenecteplase on the incidence of these events is unknown.

ANTIDOTE

Notify physician of all side effects. Note even the most minute bleeding tendency. Oozing at IV sites is expected. Control minor bleeding by local pressure. For severe bleeding in a critical location or suspected intracranial bleeding, discontinue any heparin therapy immediately. Obtain PT, aPTT, platelet count, and fibrinogen. Draw blood for type and cross-match. Platelets and cryoprecipitate are most commonly used but whole blood, packed red blood cells, fresh-frozen plasma, desmopressin, tranexamic acid, or aminocaproic acid may be indicated. Topical preparations of aminocaproic acid may stop minor bleeding. Consider protamine if heparin has been used. Treat bradycardia with atropine, reperfusion arrhythmias with lidocaine, procainamide, or other standard antiarrhythmic therapy; VT or VF may require cardioversion. If hypotension occurs, vasopressors (e.g., dopamine), Trendelenburg position, and suitable plasma expanders (e.g., albumin, plasma protein fraction [Plasmanate], or hetastarch) may be indicated. Treat minor hypersensitivity reactions symptomatically. Discontinue drug and treat anaphylaxis as indicated; resuscitate as necessary.

TENIPOSIDE BBW

(teh-**NIP**-ah-side)

VM-26, Vumon

**Antineoplastic
(mitotic inhibitor)**

pH 4 to 6.5

USUAL DOSE

Adults: *All indications and doses are unlabeled;* however, teniposide has been used in several adult protocols. Doses range from 50 to 180 mg/M^2 given once or twice weekly for 4 to 6 weeks. 20 to 60 mg/M^2/day for 5 days has also been used.

PEDIATRIC DOSE

See Precautions and Maternal/Child.

Acute lymphocytic leukemia (ALL): 165 mg/M^2 in combination with cytarabine 300 mg/M^2. Both drugs are given twice weekly for 8 to 9 doses. An alternate regimen includes teniposide 250 mg/M^2 and vincristine 1.5 mg/M^2 once each week for 4 to 8 weeks plus predisone 40 mg/M^2 PO daily for 28 days.

DOSE ADJUSTMENTS

Reduce dose by one half in patients with Down syndrome and leukemia (increased sensitivity to myelosuppressive chemotherapy). Higher doses may be used in subsequent courses based on degree of myelosuppression and mucositis. Must be individualized. ▪ Reduced dose may be necessary in severe renal or hepatic impairment. ▪ Reduced dose may be indicated in combination therapy. Withhold dose if platelets less than 50,000/mm^3 or absolute neutrophil count less than 500/mm^3. Do not restart until adequate recovery.

DILUTION

Specific techniques required; see Precautions. Must be diluted and given as an infusion. May leach the toxic plasticizer DEHP from PVC infusion bags or sets; prepare and store in bottles (glass, polypropylene) or plastic bags (polypropylene, polyolefin) and administer through polyethylene-lined administration sets (e.g., lipid administration sets or low DEHP–containing nitroglycerin IV sets). Undiluted tenoposide has caused acrylic or ABS plastic devices to crack and leak; handle carefully during dilution process. **Compatible** with NS or D5W. Final concentration of 0.1, 0.2, 0.4, or 1 mg/mL desired. Contains 10 mg/mL. 100 mg (10 mL) in 990 mL yields 0.1 mg/mL, in 490 mL yields 0.2 mg/mL, in 240 mL yields 0.4 mg/mL, in 90 mL yields 1 mg/mL. Precipitation may occur at recommended concentrations, especially with excessive agitation. Avoid contact of diluted solution with any other drugs or fluids; flush IV line with D5W or NS before and after administration.

Storage: Refrigerate unopened ampules in original packaging. Do not refrigerate diluted solutions; 1 mg/mL should be administered within 4 hours; all other dilutions are stable at CRT for up to 24 hours.

COMPATIBILITY

Consider any drug NOT listed as compatible to be INCOMPATIBLE until consulting a pharmacist; specific conditions may apply.

Manufacturer states, "Heparin solution can cause precipitation of teniposide; flush IV line thoroughly with D5W or NS before and after administration of teniposide. Because of potential for precipitation, **compatibility** with other drugs, infusion materials, or IV pumps cannot be ensured." See Dilution, Rate of Administration, and Precautions/Monitor.

One source suggests the following **compatibilities:**

Y-site: *Not recommended by manufacturer.* Acyclovir (Zovirax), allopurinol (Aloprim), amifostine (Ethyol), amikacin (Amikin), aminophylline, amphotericin B (generic), ampicillin, ampicillin/sulbactam (Unasyn), aztreonam (Azactam), bleomycin (Blenoxane), bumetanide, buprenorphine (Buprenex), butorphanol (Stadol), calcium gluconate, carboplatin (Paraplatin), carmustine (BiCNU), cefazolin (Ancef), cefotaxime (Claforan), cefotetan, cefoxitin (Mefoxin), ceftazidime (Fortaz), ceftriaxone (Rocephin), cefuroxime (Zinacef), chlorpromazine (Thorazine), ciprofloxacin (Cipro IV), cisplatin (Platinol), cladribine (Leustatin), clindamycin (Cleocin), cyclophosphamide (Cytoxan), cytarabine (ARA-C), dacarbazine (DTIC), dactinomycin (Cosmegen), daunorubicin (Cerubidine), dexamethasone (Decadron), diphenhydramine (Benadryl), doxorubicin (Adriamycin), doxycycline, droperidol (Inapsine), enalaprilat (Vasotec IV), etoposide (VePesid), etoposide phosphate (Etopophos), famotidine (Pepcid IV), fluconazole (Diflucan), fludarabine (Fludara), fluorouracil (5-FU), furosemide (Lasix), gallium nitrate (Ganite), ganciclovir (Cytovene), gemcitabine (Gemzar), gentamicin, granisetron (Kytril), haloperidol (Haldol), hydrocortisone sodium succinate (Solu-Cortef), hydromorphone (Dilaudid), ifosfamide (Ifex), imipenem-cilastatin (Primaxin), leucovorin calcium, lorazepam (Ativan), mannitol, mechlorethamine (nitrogen mustard), melphalan (Alkeran), meperidine (Demerol), mesna (Mesnex), methotrexate, methylprednisolone (Solu-Medrol), metoclopramide (Reglan), metronidazole (Flagyl IV), mitomycin (Mutamycin), mitoxantrone (Novantrone), morphine, nalbuphine, ondansetron (Zofran), piperacillin, potassium chloride (KCl), prochlorperazine (Compazine), promethazine (Phenergan), ranitidine (Zantac), sargramostim (Leukine), sodium bicarbonate, streptozocin (Zanosar), sulfamethoxazole/trimethoprim, thiotepa, ticarcillin/clavulanate (Timentin), tobramycin, vancomycin, vinblastine, vincristine, vinorelbine (Navelbine), zidovudine (AZT, Retrovir).

RATE OF ADMINISTRATION

Total desired dose, properly diluted and evenly distributed over at least 30 to 60 minutes. Infusion time may be extended. Flush IV line with D5W or NS before and after administration to avoid precipitation of teniposide in IV catheter. Rapid infusion may cause marked hypotension or increased nausea and vomiting.

ACTIONS

An antineoplastic agent. A semisynthetic derivative of podophyllotoxin related to etoposide. Cell cycle–specific for the late S or early G_2 phase. Cytotoxic effects are related to the relative number of single- and double-strand DNA breaks produced in cells. Active against certain murine leukemias with acquired resistance to cisplatin, doxorubicin, amsacrine, daunorubicin, mitoxantrone, or vincristine. Highly protein bound; limits distribution within the body (a beneficial effect). Plasma levels increase with dose. Terminal half-life is 5 hours. Metabolized primarily in the liver. Only about 10% excreted as unchanged drug in urine.

INDICATIONS AND USES

Induction therapy in refractory childhood acute lymphoblastic leukemia. Used in combination with other antineoplastic agents.

Unlabeled uses: Has been used as an unlabeled agent in several adult protocols (e.g., non-Hodgkin's lymphoma in patients refractory to other regimens and small-cell lung cancer).

CONTRAINDICATIONS

Hypersensitivity to teniposide, etoposide (no cross-sensitivity to date), or a history of prior severe hypersensitivity reactions to other drugs formulated in Cremophor EL (e.g., cyclosporine, paclitaxel).

PRECAUTIONS

Follow guidelines for handling cytotoxic agents. See Appendix A, p. 1429. ▪ Usually administered by or under the direction of the physician specialist. ▪ Adequate diagnostic and treatment facilities must be readily available. ▪ May cause severe myelosuppression with resulting infection or bleeding. ▪ Use caution in patients with impaired hepatic or renal function; may reduce plasma clearance and increase toxicity. ▪ Hypersensitivity reactions, including anaphylaxis, may occur with initial dosing or with repeated exposure. ▪ Incidence of hypersensitivity may be increased in patients with brain tumors or neuroblastoma. ▪ Acute CNS depression and hypotension occurred in patients receiving high-dose teniposide pretreated with antiemetic drugs; use caution. ▪ Pediatric patients with ALL in remission on teniposide maintenance therapy have shown an increased risk of developing secondary acute nonlymphocytic leukemia (ANLL). ▪ Plasma drug levels decline following IV infusion in pediatric patients; in adults levels increase with dose. No cumulative toxicity has been reported. ▪ Reduce dose in patients with Down's syndrome.

Monitor: Use caution to prevent bone marrow suppression; occurs early with indicated doses and can be profound. Obtain baseline hemoglobin, WBC count with differential, and platelet count. Monitor frequently during therapy, before each dose, and after therapy. See Dose Adjustments. ▪ Severe hypersensitivity reactions can occur with the first dose of teniposide and may be life threatening. Epinephrine, oxygen, and other emergency supplies must be at the bedside. Monitor patient continuously and take vital signs very frequently during the first hour and at intervals thereafter. ▪ Monitor renal and hepatic function tests before and during therapy. ▪ Determine absolute patency and quality of vein and adequate circulation of extremity. Avoid extravasation; can cause local tissue necrosis and thrombophlebitis. ▪ Precipitation sufficient to occlude central venous access catheters has occurred; monitor infusion closely, and flush thoroughly before and after administration. ▪ Use prophylactic antiemetics to increase patient comfort. ▪ Steady-state volume of distribution increases with a decrease in plasma albumin levels; monitor pediatric patients with hypoalbuminemia carefully. ▪ If severe myelosuppression occurs, bone marrow examination should be repeated before a decision to continue therapy is made. ▪ Monitor for thrombocytopenia (platelet count less than 50,000/mm^3). Initiate precautions to prevent excessive bleeding (e.g., inspect IV sites, skin, and mucous membranes; use extreme care during invasive procedures; test urine, emesis, stool, and secretions for occult blood). ▪ Observe closely for signs of infection. Prophylactic antibiotics may be indicated pending results of C/S in a febrile neutropenic patient.

Patient Education: Report IV site burning or stinging promptly. ■ Avoid pregnancy; nonhormonal birth control recommended. ■ Report any signs of hypersensitivity promptly (e.g., chills, difficult breathing, fever, flushing, rapid heartbeat, rash). ■ Secondary acute nonlymphocytic leukemia (ANLL) has been reported (see Precautions). ■ Interacts with many medications. Discuss all drugs (prescription or nonprescription) with doctor or pharmacist. ■ See Appendix D, p. 1434.

Maternal/Child: Category D: avoid pregnancy. May cause fetal harm. ■ Potential for serious adverse reactions in nursing infants; discontinue breast-feeding. ■ Contains benzyl alcohol; not recommended for use in premature infants. ■ Intended for use in pediatric patients, but see Precautions/Monitor. ■ When used as a single agent, side effects in pediatric patients from 2 weeks to 20 years of age are similar to other age-groups.

Elderly: Monitor renal, hepatic, and hematologic function closely.

DRUG/LAB INTERACTIONS

Sodium salicylate, sulfamethizole, and tolbutamide displace teniposide from protein-binding sites. Can cause substantial increases in free drug levels and increase toxicity of teniposide. ■ May result in clinically significant drug interactions with **other drugs highly bound to protein** (e.g., buprenorphine, calcium channel blocking agents [e.g., diltiazem, verapamil], phenothiazines [e.g., prochlorperazine (Compazine)]). ■ May increase plasma clearance and increase intracellular levels of **methotrexate.** ■ **Phenobarbital, fosphenytoin** (Cerebyx), **and phenytoin** (Dilantin) increase clearance of teniposide; may reduce effectiveness. ■ Depressant and hypotensive effects of **antiemetics** may be additive with alcohol in teniposide. ■ May cause additive effects with **bone marrow–suppressing agents or agents that cause blood dyscrasias** (e.g., amphotericin B, antithyroid agents [Methimazole (Tapazole)], azathioprine [Imuran], chloramphenicol, ganciclovir [Cytovene], interferon, plicamycin [Mithracin], zidovudine [AZT, Retrovir]) **and radiation therapy.** ■ Do not administer **live virus vaccines.**

SIDE EFFECTS

Most are reversible if detected early. Hypersensitivity reactions (e.g., bronchospasm, chills, dyspnea, facial flushing, fever, hypertension, hypotension, tachycardia, urticaria) have occurred in 5% of patients and can be fatal if not treated promptly. Myelosuppression (anemia [88%], leukopenia [89%], neutropenia [95%], thrombocytopenia [85%]) occurs early, can be profound, and recovery can be delayed. Alopecia (9%), bleeding (5%), diarrhea (33%), fever (3%), hypotension/cardiovascular (2%), infection (12%), mucositis (76%), nausea and vomiting (29%), rash (3%), thrombophlebitis. Hepatic dysfunctions, metabolic abnormalities, neurotoxicity, and renal dysfunction have occurred in less than 1% of patients.

ANTIDOTE

Keep physician informed of all side effects. Symptomatic treatment is often indicated. Discontinue teniposide and treat hypersensitivity reactions immediately (epinephrine [Adrenalin], antihistamines [e.g., diphenhydramine (Benadryl)], cimetidine [Tagamet], corticosteroids [e.g., dexamethasone (Decadron)], bronchodilators [e.g., theophylline (Aminophylline)], IV fluids). Consider risk/benefit before rechallenging any patient who has had a severe hypersensitivity reaction. Pretreatment with corticosteroids and antihistamines and constant observation are imperative. For other severe side effects (e.g., myelosuppression), drug dose may be reduced or it may be discontinued. Administration of whole blood products (e.g., packed RBCs, platelets, leukocytes) and/or blood modifiers (e.g., darbepoetin alfa [Aranesp], epoetin alfa [Epogen], filgrastim [Neupogen], oprelvekin [Neumega], pegfilgrastim [Neulasta], sargramostim [Leukine]) may be indicated to treat bone marrow toxicity. Consider diazepam (Valium) or phenytoin (Dilantin) for seizures. Hypotension is usually due to a rapid infusion rate; discontinue temporarily. Trendelenburg position and IV fluids should reverse the hypotension; vasopressors (e.g., dopamine) may be required. In addition to antiemetics (e.g., ondansetron [Zofran]), rate reduction may reduce nausea and vomiting. For extravasation, discontinue the drug immediately and administer into another site. Consider injection of long-acting dexamethasone (Decadron LA) throughout extravasated tissue. Use a 27- or 25-gauge needle. Elevate extremity; moist heat may be helpful. Resuscitate as necessary.

THIAMINE HYDROCHLORIDE   Nutritional supplement (vitamin)
(**THIGH**-ah-min hy-droh-**KLOR**-eyed)

Vitamin B$_1$ pH 2.5 to 4.5

USUAL DOSE

Transfer to PO doses when practical; see Precautions. Administer before dextrose solutions in the poorly nourished to avoid the development of acute symptoms of thiamine deficiency.

Thiamine deficiency (prophylaxis): Administered as part of a TPN program and based on individual patient needs (average daily requirement in a normal healthy adult is 1 mg). Average supplementation in TPN is 6 mg/day; may be increased to 25 to 50 mg/day in patients with a history of alcohol abuse. In critically ill adults, an initial dose of up to 100 mg has been used. May be followed with 50 to 100 mg daily until a regular balanced diet can be eaten. IV dextrose solutions or high carbohydrate diets increase thiamine requirements and may worsen symptoms in patients who are thiamine deficient.

Beriberi: 5 to 30 mg IV or IM 3 times daily for up to 2 weeks. Continue PO for 1 month.

Alcohol withdrawal syndrome: 100 mg IV or IM daily for several days. Administer concurrently with IV glucose. Follow with 50 to 100 mg/day PO.

Wernicke's encephalopathy: An initial dose of 100 mg IV. Larger doses may be required in the first 24 hours with extreme caution. Follow with 50 to 100 mg daily until a normal diet is resumed.

PEDIATRIC DOSE

Thiamine deficiency (prophylaxis and/or treatment): Administered as part of a TPN program and based on individual patient needs (average daily requirement in a normal healthy infant or child ranges from 0.2 mg in infants to 0.9 mg in 9- to 13-year-olds). Up to 10 to 25 mg/24 hr may be used in critically ill pediatric patients. See comments under Usual Dose.

Beriberi: 10 to 25 mg/24 hr. Follow with 10 to 50 mg PO daily for 2 weeks, then 5 to 10 mg PO daily for 1 month.

DILUTION

May be given by IV injection or added to most IV solutions and given as an infusion. See chart on inside back cover.

Storage: Can be refrigerated; protect from freezing and from light.

COMPATIBILITY

Consider any drug NOT listed as compatible to be INCOMPATIBLE until consulting a pharmacist; specific conditions may apply.

Manufacturer states, "Unstable in neutral or alkaline solutions. Do not use in combination with alkaline solutions (e.g., acetates, barbiturates [e.g., phenobarbital (Luminal)], carbonates, citrates, copper ions). **Incompatible** with solutions containing sulfites and other oxidizing and reducing agents."

One source suggests the following **compatibilities:**

Y-site: Famotidine (Pepcid IV).

RATE OF ADMINISTRATION

100 mg or fraction thereof over 5 minutes. For 100 mg or larger doses, equal distribution over an extended time as an infusion is preferred.

ACTIONS

A water-soluble vitamin, thiamine is necessary to most metabolic processes in humans, especially carbohydrate metabolism. Widely distributed in all body tissues, metabolized in the liver, and excreted in urine.

INDICATIONS AND USES

Prophylaxis or treatment of thiamine deficiency syndromes including beriberi (wet or dry), Wernicke's encephalopathy, or peripheral neuritis.

CONTRAINDICATIONS

Known hypersensitivity to thiamine hydrochloride.

PRECAUTIONS

Not commonly administered IV; PO or IM is preferred. ■ Rarely used alone, it is more often administered as a multiple B vitamin. ■ In thiamine deficiency, administer thiamine before giving any glucose load to prevent the sudden onset of Wernicke's encephalopathy or add 100 mg to each of the first few liters of IV fluid to avoid precipitating heart failure. ■ Requirements may be increased in certain conditions (e.g., alcoholism, burns, GI disease, or malabsorption). ■ Supplementation is necessary in patients receiving total parenteral nutrition (usually administered as a multivitamin). ■ S/S of thiamine deficiency (e.g., ataxia, edema, heart failure, neuritis, ocular signs) may respond within hours of thiamine administration and disappear within days. Confusion and psychosis may be slower to respond and may not improve if nerve damage has occurred.

Patient Education: Dietary consultation indicated to prevent relapse.

Maternal/Child: Category A: use only if clearly needed. ■ Use caution in breast-feeding.

SIDE EFFECTS

Anaphylaxis and death caused by hypersensitivity reaction can occur with IV administration. Recent studies have shown that hypersensitivity reactions can occur with equal frequency by any route. Incidence after IV administration is less than 0.1%. May increase in frequency with repeat injections. Other reactions include feeling of warmth, nausea, pruritus, pain, sweating, urticaria, and weakness.

ANTIDOTE

Discontinue the drug, treat hypersensitivity reactions or resuscitate as necessary, and notify the physician.

THIOTEPA

(thigh-oh-**TEP**-ah)

TSPA

Antineoplastic
(alkylating agent/nitrosurea)

pH 7.6

USUAL DOSE

0.3 to 0.4 mg/kg every 1 to 4 weeks. Maintenance dose and frequency adjusted according to blood cell counts before and after treatment. Dose based on average weight in presence of ascites or edema.

DOSE ADJUSTMENTS

Reduce dose or discontinue if WBC or platelet count falls rapidly. ■ Usually contraindicated but can be used with extreme caution and in low doses in patients with existing hepatic, renal, or bone marrow damage if benefits outweigh risks.

DILUTION

Specific techniques required; see Precautions. Each 15 mg of drug is reconstituted with 1.5 mL of SW for injection (10 mg/mL). Shake solution gently and allow to stand until clear. A hypotonic solution; further dilute with NS before administration. Must be filtered through a 0.22-micron filter before administration. May then be given through Y-tube or three-way stopcock of a free-flowing IV infusion. Final solution should be clear; do not use if hazy, opaque, or a precipitate is present.

Filters: Filter through a 0.22-micron filter before administration. See Dilution.

Storage: Must be refrigerated before and after reconstitution. Protect from light at all times. Use reconstituted solution within 8 hours. Use diluted solution immediately.

COMPATIBILITY

Consider any drug NOT listed as compatible to be INCOMPATIBLE until consulting a pharmacist; specific conditions may apply.

One source suggests the following **compatibilities:**

Y-site: Acyclovir (Zovirax), allopurinol (Aloprim), amifostine (Ethyol), amikacin (Amikin), aminophylline, amphotericin B (generic), ampicillin, ampicillin/sulbactam (Unasyn), aztreonam (Azactam), bleomycin (Blenoxane), bumetanide, buprenorphine (Buprenex), butorphanol (Stadol), calcium gluconate, carboplatin (Paraplatin), carmustine (BiCNU), cefazolin (Ancef), cefepime (Maxipime), cefotaxime (Claforan), cefotetan, cefoxitin (Mefoxin), ceftazidime (Fortaz), ceftriaxone (Rocephin), cefuroxime (Zinacef), chlorpromazine (Thorazine), ciprofloxacin (Cipro IV), clindamycin (Cleocin), cyclophosphamide (Cytoxan), cytarabine (ARA-C), dacarbazine (DTIC), dactinomycin (Cosmegen), daunorubicin (Cerubidine), dexamethasone (Decadron), diphenhydramine (Benadryl), dobutamine, dopamine, doxorubicin (Adriamycin), doxycycline, droperidol (Inapsine), enalaprilat (Vasotec IV), etoposide (VePesid), etoposide phosphate (Etopophos), famotidine (Pepcid IV), fluconazole (Diflucan), fludarabine (Fludara), fluorouracil (5-FU), furosemide (Lasix), gallium nitrate (Ganite), ganciclovir (Cytovene), gemcitabine (Gemzar), gentamicin, granisetron (Kytril), haloperidol (Haldol), heparin, hydrocortisone sodium succinate (Solu-Cortef), hydromorphone (Dilaudid), idarubicin (Idamycin), ifosfamide (Ifex), imipenem-cilastatin (Primaxin), leucovorin calcium, lorazepam (Ativan), magnesium sulfate, mannitol, melphalan (Alkeran), meperidine (Demerol), mesna (Mesnex), methotrexate, methylprednisolone (Solu-Medrol), metoclopramide (Reglan), metronidazole (Flagyl IV), mitomycin (Mutamycin), mitoxantrone (Novantrone), morphine, nalbuphine, ondansetron (Zofran), paclitaxel (Taxol), piperacillin, piperacillin/tazobactam (Zosyn), potassium chloride (KCl), prochlorperazine (Compazine), promethazine (Phenergan), ranitidine (Zantac), sodium bicarbonate, streptozocin (Zanosar), sulfamethoxazole/trimethoprim, teniposide (Vumon), ticarcillin/clavulanate (Timentin), tobramycin, vancomycin, vinblastine, vincristine, zidovudine (AZT, Retrovir).

RATE OF ADMINISTRATION
A single dose as a rapid IV injection.

ACTIONS
An alkylating agent of the nitrosurea group with antitumor activity. Cell cycle phase–nonspecific. Thought to have a radiomimetic action, which releases ethylenimine radicals that disrupt DNA bonds and destroy actively dividing cells. Well distributed, it is metabolized in the liver and excreted as metabolites in the urine.

INDICATIONS AND USES
To suppress or retard neoplastic growth in adenocarcinomas of the breast and ovary. ■ Treatment of Hodgkin's lymphomas. ■ Also used intracavitary to treat some bladder cancers and to control intracavitary effusions (pericardial or pleural) secondary to neoplastic disease (toxicity still occurs from systemic absorption).

CONTRAINDICATIONS
Hepatic, renal, or bone marrow damage unless need is greater than the risk; known hypersensitivity to thiotepa.

PRECAUTIONS
Follow guidelines for handling cytotoxic agents. See Appendix A, p. 1429. ■ Administered by or under the direction of the physician specialist. ■ Use caution in leukopenia, thrombocytopenia, recent radiation therapy, and infection. ■ See Dose Adjustments and Side Effects.

Monitor: Daily blood cell and platelet counts are necessary during initial treatment and weekly thereafter until 3 weeks after therapy is discontinued. Very toxic to hematopoietic system. ■ Obtain baseline SCr, BUN, and/or liver function tests in patients with renal or hepatic impairment and monitor during treatment. ■ Be alert for signs of bone marrow suppression or infection. Use of prophylactic antibiotics may be indicated pending results of C/S in a febrile neutropenic patient. ■ May induce hyperuricemia, increased doses of antigout agents may be necessary (e.g., allopurinol, probenicid). Allopurinol preferred to reduce risk of uric acid nephropathy associated with uricosuric antigout agents. ■ Prophylactic antiemetics may increase patient comfort. ■ Monitor for thrombocytopenia (platelet count less than 50,000/mm^3). Initiate precautions to prevent excessive bleeding (e.g., inspect IV sites, skin, and mucous membranes; use extreme care during invasive procedures; test urine, emesis, stool, and secretions for occult blood). ■ See Drug/Lab Interactions.

Patient Education: Nonhormonal birth control recommended for patient and partner. ■ See Appendix D, p. 1434.

Maternal/Child: Category D: avoid pregnancy. Will produce teratogenic effects on the fetus. Has a mutagenic potential. ■ Discontinue breast-feeding. ▪ Safety for use in pediatric patients up to 12 years of age not established.

Elderly: Consider possibility of impaired organ function.

DRUG/LAB INTERACTIONS

May cause irreversible bone marrow damage with **other antineoplastic drugs, radiation therapy, or any drugs that cause bone marrow suppression** (e.g., amphotericin B [all formulations], ganciclovir [Cytovene]). Allow complete recovery verified by WBC count before using a second agent. ▪ Potentiates **succinylcholine.** May cause prolonged apnea. ▪ Do not administer **live virus vaccines** to patients receiving antineoplastic drugs.

SIDE EFFECTS

Alopecia, amenorrhea, anorexia, asthenia, dizziness, fatigue, fever, headache, hives, hyperuricemia, nausea, pain at injection site, skin rash, throat tightness, vomiting.

Major: Anaphylaxis, hemorrhage, intestinal perforation, septicemia. Bone marrow suppression (anemia, leukopenia, thrombocytopenia) may be life threatening, is dose related, and does occur with usual doses.

ANTIDOTE

Minor side effects will be treated symptomatically if necessary. Discontinue the drug and notify the physician of major side effects. If platelet count below 150,000/mm^3 or WBCs below 3,000/mm^3, discontinue use and notify physician. Administration of whole blood products (e.g., packed RBCs, platelets, or leukocytes) and/or blood modifiers (e.g., darbepoetin alfa [Aranesp], epoetin alfa [Epogen], filgrastim [Neupogen], oprelvekin [Neumega], pegfilgrastim [Neulasta], sargramostim [Leukine]) may be indicated to treat bone marrow toxicity. Treat hypersensitivity reactions as indicated.

TICARCILLIN DISODIUM AND CLAVULANATE POTASSIUM

(tie-kar-**SILL**-in dye-**SO**-dee-um and klav-you-**LAN**-ate poe-**TASS**-ee-um)

Timentin

Antibacterial (extended-spectrum penicillin and β-lactamase inhibitor)

pH 5.5 to 7.5

USUAL DOSE

3.1 Gm of preparation available contains 3 Gm ticarcillin to 0.1 Gm clavulanate. Doses vary depending on the severity of the infection, susceptibility of the organism, and condition of the patient. Treatment usually continued for 10 to 14 days; may be extended if required. Continue for at least 2 days after signs and symptoms of infection have disappeared.

Systemic and urinary tract infections: *60 kg (130 lb) or more:* 3.1 Gm every 4 to 6 hours. Some sources extend interval to 6 to 8 hours.

Under 60 kg: 200 to 300 mg/kg of body weight/24 hr in equally divided doses every 4 to 6 hours (33.3 to 50 mg/kg every 4 hours or 50 to 75 mg/kg every 6 hours). Base dose on the ticarcillin component.

Moderate gynecologic infections: 200 mg/kg/day in divided doses every 6 hours (50 mg/kg every 6 hours). Base dose on the ticarcillin component.

Severe gynecologic infections: 300 mg/kg/day in divided doses every 4 hours (50 mg/kg every 4 hours). Base dose on the ticarcillin component.
Surgical prophylaxis (unlabeled): 3.1 Gm 30 to 60 minutes before start of surgery or as soon as the umbilical cord is clamped in cesarean section. Repeat at 4-hour intervals for 3 doses.

PEDIATRIC DOSE

Infants and other pediatric patients 3 months to 12 years of age and less than 60 kg: 50 mg/kg every 6 hours. Base dose on the ticarcillin component. In serious infections, increase to 50 mg/kg every 4 hours. See Contraindications.
Pediatric patients greater than 60 kg: 3.1 Gm every every 6 hours for mild to moderate infections. Increase frequency to every 4 hours for severe infections.
Pediatric patients with cystic fibrosis: 300 to 600 mg/kg/24 hr. Give in equally divided doses every 4 to 6 hours (50 to 100 mg/kg every 4 hours or 75 to 150 mg/kg every 6 hours). Maximum dose is 24 Gm/24 hr.

NEONATAL DOSE

Safety for use in infants under 3 months of age not established but has been used. Base dose on ticarcillin component. See Contraindications.
75 mg/kg/dose, with interval adjusted based on age and weight as follows:
Up to 4 weeks of age and under 1,200 Gm: Every 12 hours.
0 to 7 days of age and under 2,000 Gm: Every 12 hours.
Over 7 days of age and 1,200 to 2,000 Gm: Every 8 hours.
0 to 7 days of age and over 2,000 Gm: Every 8 hours.
Over 7 days of age and over 2,000 Gm: Every 6 hours.

DOSE ADJUSTMENTS

After an initial loading dose of 3.1 Gm, reduce dose in impaired renal function according to the following chart.

Ticarcillin/Clavulanate Dose in Impaired Renal Function	
Creatinine Clearance (mL/min)	Dosage
>60 mL/min	3.1 Gm q 4 hr
30-60 mL/min	2 Gm q 4 hr
10-30 mL/min	2 Gm q 8 hr
<10 mL/min	2 Gm q 12 hr
<10 mL/min with hepatic dysfunction	2 Gm q 24 hr
Patients on peritoneal dialysis	3.1 Gm q 12 hr
Patients on hemodialysis	2 Gm q 12 hr supplemented with 3.1 Gm after each dialysis

■ Reduce dose in impaired hepatic function. ■ Reduced dose may be indicated in the elderly.

DILUTION

Each 3.1 Gm or fraction thereof is reconstituted with 13 mL of SW or NS (200 mg/mL of ticarcillin). Shake well. A single dose must be further diluted to a final concentration between 10 and 100 mg/mL. Dilute in 50 to 100 mL or more of D5W, NS, or LR and given as an intermittent infusion.

Also available prediluted and frozen and in ADD-Vantage vials for use with ADD-Vantage infusion containers.

Storage: Store unopened vials below 24° C (75° F). Reconstituted solutions (200 mg/mL) are stable at room temperature for 6 hours or up to 72 hours under refrigeration. Stability extended after further dilution (see literature).

COMPATIBILITY   (Underline Indicates Conflicting Compatibility Information)
Consider any drug NOT listed as compatible to be INCOMPATIBLE until consulting a pharmacist; specific conditions may apply.

May be inactivated in solution with aminoglycosides (e.g., amikacin [Amikin], gentamicin). Do not mix in the same solution. Appropriate spacing and/or separate sites required. See Drug/Lab Interactions. Manufacturer lists as **incompatible** with sodium bicarbonate.

One source suggests the following **compatibilities:**
Y-site: Allopurinol (Aloprim), amifostine (Ethyol), <u>anidulafungin (Eraxis)</u>, aztreonam (Azactam), bivalirudin (Angiomax), cefepime (Maxipime), <u>cisatracurium (Nimbex)</u>, cyclophosphamide (Cytoxan), dexmedetomidine (Precedex), diltiazem (Cardizem), docetaxel (Taxotere), doxorubicin liposomal (Doxil), etoposide phosphate (Etopophos), famotidine (Pepcid IV), fenoldopam (Corlopam), filgrastim (Neupogen), fluconazole (Diflucan), fludarabine (Fludara), foscarnet (Foscavir), gallium nitrate (Ganite), gemcitabine (Gemzar), granisetron (Kytril), heparin, hetastarch in electrolytes (Hextend), insulin (regular), melphalan (Alkeran), meperidine (Demerol), milrinone (Primacor), morphine, ondansetron (Zofran), pemetrexed (Alimta), propofol (Diprivan), remifentanil (Ultiva), sargramostim (Leukine), teniposide (Vumon), theophylline, thiotepa, <u>topotecan (Hycamtin)</u>, <u>vancomycin</u>, vinorelbine (Navelbine).

RATE OF ADMINISTRATION
Intermittent infusion: A single dose over 30 minutes. May be given through Y-tube or three-way stopcock of infusion set. Discontinue primary IV during administration. Too-rapid injection may cause seizures. Slow infusion rate for pain along venipuncture site.

ACTIONS
An extended-spectrum penicillin combined with a β-lactamase inhibitor. Bactericidal for many gram-negative, gram-positive, and anaerobic organisms. This specific formulation extends activity by protecting ticarcillin from degradation by β-lactamase enzymes. Large doses with high blood levels are well tolerated. Widely distributed in all body fluids and tissues. Distributes into cerebrospinal fluid only if inflammation is present. Peak serum levels achieved by end of infusion. Half-life is 1.1 hours. Crosses the placental barrier. Primarily excreted in the urine.

INDICATIONS AND USES
Treatment of infections caused by susceptible strains of specific microorganisms in the following conditions caused by β-lactamase–producing organisms: bacterial septicemia; acute and chronic infections of the lower respiratory tract, skin and skin structures, bone and joint, endometrium, urinary tract; and peritonitis. Useful in mixed infections as presumptive therapy before identifying the causative organism, in infections complicated by impaired renal functions, or in patients receiving immunosuppressive or oncolytic drugs.

Unlabeled use: Surgical prophylaxis.

CONTRAINDICATIONS

Known hypersensitivity to penicillins, cephalosporins, or β-lactamase inhibitors (not absolute); see Precautions. ▪ Not recommended in infants and children under 16 years of age for the treatment of septicemia or infections where the suspected or proven pathogen is *Haemophilus influenzae* type B.

PRECAUTIONS

Hypersensitivity reactions, including fatalities, have been reported in patients undergoing penicillin therapy; most likely to occur in patients with a history of penicillin allergy or sensitivity to multiple allergens. There have been reports of individuals with a history of penicillin hypersensitivity experiencing severe reactions when treated with cephalosporins. Check history of previous hypersensitivity reactions to penicillins, cephalosporins, or other allergens. Actual incidence of cross-allergenicity not established but may be more common with first-generation cephalosporins. ▪ Specific sensitivity studies indicated to determine susceptibility of the causative organism to ticarcillin and clavulanate. ▪ To reduce the development of drug-resistant bacteria and maintain its effectiveness, ticarcillin/clavulanate should be used to treat or prevent only those infections proven or strongly suspected to be caused by bacteria. ▪ Superinfection caused by overgrowth of nonsusceptible organisms can occur. ▪ Use caution in patients with CHF or a history of bleeding disorders or GI disease (e.g., colitis). ▪ *Clostridium difficile*–associated diarrhea (CDAD) has been reported. May range from mild diarrhea to fatal colitis. Consider in patients who present with diarrhea during or after treatment with ticarcillin/clavulanate. ▪ Seizures have been reported. More common with very high doses, especially in patients with impaired renal function.

Monitor: Periodic evaluation of renal, hepatic, and hematopoietic systems and serum potassium is recommended in prolonged therapy. Observe for electrolyte imbalance and cardiac irregularities. Observe for hypokalemia. Contains 4.51 mEq sodium/Gm. May aggravate CHF. ▪ Observe for increased bleeding tendencies in all patients but especially those with impaired renal function. Monitor coagulation tests as indicated (bleeding time, INR, PT). ▪ May cause thrombophlebitis; observe carefully and rotate infusion sites. ▪ Test patients with syphilis for HIV. ▪ See Drug/Lab Interactions.

Patient Education: Report promptly: fever, rash, sore throat, unusual bleeding or bruising, seizures. ▪ Promptly report diarrhea or bloody stools that occur during treatment or up to several months after an antibiotic has been discontinued; may indicate CDAD and require treatment. ▪ May require alternate birth control.

Maternal/Child: Category B: use only if clearly needed. Studies in rats have not shown adverse effects on the fetus. ▪ May cause diarrhea, candidiasis, or allergic response in nursing infants. ▪ Has been used in infants under 3 months of age but safety for use not established.

Elderly: Safety and effectiveness similar to that seen in younger adults; however, greater sensitivity of some elderly patients cannot be ruled out. ▪ Monitoring of renal function suggested. ▪ Use care in dose selection. Consider age-related organ function and concomitant disease or drug therapy; see Dose Adjustments.

DRUG/LAB INTERACTIONS
Probenecid decreases rate of ticarcillin elimination, resulting in higher and more prolonged blood levels of ticarcillin; will not affect clavulanate levels. May be desirable or may cause toxicity. ▪ Synergistic when used in combination with **aminoglycosides** (e.g., amikacin [Amikin], gentamicin). Synergism may be inconsistent; see Compatibility. ▪ May be antagonized by **bacteriostatic antibiotics** (e.g., chloramphenicol, erythromycin, tetracyclines); may interfere with bactericidal action. ▪ Concomitant use with **beta-adrenergic blockers** (e.g., propranolol) may increase risk of anaphylaxis and inhibit treatment. ▪ Use caution with **anticoagulants** (e.g., heparin), **thrombolytic agents** (e.g., alteplase [tPA]), **platelet aggregation inhibitors** (e.g., aspirin, NSAIDs, dextran, dipyridamole, **glycoprotein GPIIb/IIIa receptor antagonists** [e.g., abciximab (ReoPro), eptifibatide (Integrilin), tirofiban (Aggrastat)], plicamycin). Risk of bleeding may be increased. Monitoring of coagulation tests may be indicated. Concurrent use with thrombolytic agents is not recommended; may increase risk of severe hemorrhage. ▪ May inhibit effectiveness of **oral contraceptives;** breakthrough bleeding or pregnancy could result. ▪ Monitoring of serum **lithium** indicated with concurrent use; increased sodium may alter renal excretion. ▪ May decrease clearance and increase toxicity of **methotrexate.** ▪ Clavulanic acid may cause a **false-positive Coombs' test.** ▪ May cause **false urine protein reactions** with various tests; see Side Effects and/or literature.

SIDE EFFECTS
Anaphylaxis; anemia; arthralgia; CDAD; chest discomfort; chills; convulsions; diarrhea; disturbances of taste and smell; elevated alkaline phosphatase, BUN, LDH, serum bilirubin, AST, and ALT; eosinophilia; fever; flatulence; epigastric pain; headache; hemorrhagic cystitis; hypernatremia; hypokalemia; increased bleeding time; leukopenia; myalgia; nausea; neutropenia; phlebitis; prolonged clotting time or PT; pruritus; skin rash; stomatitis; thrombocytopenia; urticaria; vomiting. Hypersensitivity myocarditis can occur (fever, eosinophilia, rash, sinus tachycardia, ST-T changes, and cardiomegaly). Higher than normal doses may cause neurologic adverse reactions including convulsions; especially with impaired renal function.

ANTIDOTE
Notify the physician immediately of any adverse symptoms. For severe symptoms, discontinue the drug; treat hypersensitivity reactions (epinephrine, antihistamines, corticosteroids), and resuscitate as necessary. Mild cases of CDAD may respond to discontinuation of ticarcillin/clavulanate. Treat CDAD with fluids, electrolytes, protein supplements, and oral vancomycin (Vancocin) or metronidazole (Flagyl) as indicated. In severe cases, surgical evaluation may be indicated. Hemodialysis may be indicated in overdose.

TIGECYCLINE FOR INJECTION
(tye-ge-**SYE**-kleen)

Tygacil

Antibacterial
(glycylcycline)

pH 7.8

USUAL DOSE
100 mg as an initial dose. Follow with 50 mg every 12 hours. Recommended duration of treatment is 5 to 14 days for complicated skin and skin structure infections and complicated intra-abdominal infections and 7 to 14 days for community-acquired bacterial pneumonia. Duration of treatment is based on the severity and site of the infection and the patient's clinical and bacteriologic progress.

DOSE ADJUSTMENTS
In patients with severe impaired liver function (Child Pugh C [score 10 to 15]), the initial dose remains the same, but subsequent doses should be reduced to 25 mg every 12 hours. ■ No dose adjustment is indicated for impaired renal function, for mild to moderate impaired liver function (Child Pugh A and Child Pugh B [score 5 to 9]), or in patients undergoing hemodialysis. ■ No dose adjustment is indicated based on age, gender, or race.

DILUTION
Reconstitute each 50-mg vial with 5.3 mL of NS, D5W, or LR (yields 10 mg/mL). Use 2 vials for the 100-mg dose. Swirl gently until lyophilized powder is dissolved. Reconstituted solution should be yellow to orange in color. Immediately withdraw 5 mL from two vials for the 100-mg dose (vials are overfilled) or from one vial for the 50-mg dose and add to a 100-mL IV bag of D5W, NS, or LR for infusion. Maximum concentration should be 1 mg/mL. Reconstituted solution has a pH of 7.8. When fully diluted, tigecycline assumes the pH of its diluent.

Filters: No data available from manufacturer.

Storage: Store unopened vials at CRT. Reconstituted solution may be stored at RT for up to 6 hours. Fully diluted solution in the IV bag may be stored at RT for up to 24 hours or for 6 hours in the vial and the remaining time in the IV bag, or the fully diluted solution in either D5W or NS may be refrigerated at 2° to 8° C (36° to 46° F) for up to 48 hours following immediate transfer of the reconstituted solution into the IV bag.

COMPATIBILITY
Consider any drug NOT listed as compatible to be INCOMPATIBLE until consulting a pharmacist; specific conditions may apply.

Manufacturer states, "The following drugs should not be administered simultaneously through the same **Y-site** as tigecycline: amphotericin B (generic), amphotericin B lipid complex (Abelcet), diazepam (Valium), esomeprazole (Nexium IV), and omeprazole (Prilosec)."

Y-site: Manufacturer lists as **compatible** at the **Y-site** with amikacin (Amikin), dobutamine, dopamine, gentamicin, haloperidol (Haldol), LR solution, lidocaine, metoclopramide (Reglan), morphine, norepinephrine (Levophed), piperacillin/tazobactam (Zosyn), potassium chloride, propofol (Diprivan), ranitidine (Zantac), theophylline (Aminophylline), and tobramycin.

Another source adds **compatibility** at the **Y-site** with azithromycin (Zithromax), aztreonam (Azactam), cefepime (Maxipime), cefotaxime (Claforan), ceftazidime (Fortaz), ceftriaxone (Rocephin), ciprofloxacin (Cipro IV), doripenem (Doribax), epinephrine (Adrenalin), ertapenem (Invanz), fluconazole (Diflucan), heparin, imipenem-cilastatin (Primaxin), linezolid (Zyvox), metoclopramide (Reglan), tobramycin, vancomycin.

RATE OF ADMINISTRATION

Flush IV line with D5W, NS, or LR before and after infusion of tigecycline if other drugs are administered through the same line; see Compatibility. Consider **compatibility** of other drugs when flushing the line.

A single dose as an infusion over 30 to 60 minutes.

ACTIONS

A broad-spectrum glycylcycline antibiotic, bacteriostatic against specific aerobic gram-positive and gram-negative microorganisms and specific anaerobic microorganisms; see prescribing information. Inhibits protein translation in bacteria by binding to a specific ribosomal subunit and blocking entry of specific molecules into the A site of the ribosome. Chemical structure has similarities to tetracyclines; however, it is not affected by the two major tetracycline resistance mechanisms of ribosomal protection and efflux. Plasma protein binding is approximately 71% to 89%. Extensively distributed beyond the plasma volume and into tissues. For example, concentrations have been identified in the bone, colon, gallbladder, synovial fluid, and lung. Mean half-life is 42.4 hours. Not extensively metabolized. 59% of a dose is excreted in bile and feces, and 33% is excreted in urine. Crosses the placental barrier in animals.

INDICATIONS AND USES

Treatment of adults with infections caused by susceptible strains of designated microorganisms in complicated skin and skin structure infections, complicated intra-abdominal infections, and community-acquired bacterial pneumonia.

CONTRAINDICATIONS

Known hypersensitivity to tigecycline. Contains no excipients or preservatives.

PRECAUTIONS

Sensitivity studies are indicated to determine susceptibility of the causative organism to tigecycline. Treatment may begin after culture and sensitivity studies are drawn. Re-evaluate after results are known. ■ To reduce the development of drug-resistant bacteria and maintain its effectiveness, tigecycline should be used to treat or prevent only those infections proven or strongly suspected to be caused by bacteria. ■ Cross-resistance and/or antagonism between tigecycline and other antibiotics has not been observed. ■ Not affected by resistance mechanisms seen with other antibiotics (e.g., β-lactamases). ■ Structurally similar to the tetracycline class of antibiotics; may have similar side effects (e.g., anti-anabolic action [which has led to acidosis, azotemia, hypophosphatemia, and increased BUN], pancreatitis, photosensitivity, and pseudotumor cerebri). ■ An increase in all-cause mortality has been observed across Phase 3 and 4 clinical trials in tigecycline-treated patients versus comparator groups. The cause of this increase has not been established and should be considered when selecting among treatment options. ■ Anaphylaxis/anaphylactoid reactions have been reported. Use caution in patients with a history of hypersensitivity to tetracyclines; may have cross-sensitivity. ■

Lower cure rates and higher mortality rates were seen in patients with ventilator-associated pneumonia treated with tigecycline versus comparator groups. Particularly high mortality rates were seen in tigecycline-treated patients with ventilator-associated pneumonia and bacteremia at baseline. ▪ Acute pancreatitis, including fatalities, have been reported. ▪ Use caution when considering tigecycline monotherapy in patients with complicated intra-abdominal infections secondary to clinically apparent intestinal perforation; sepsis/septic shock has occurred. ▪ Abnormalities in total bilirubin, PT, and transaminases have been seen in patients treated with tigecycline. Has also caused isolated cases of significant hepatic dysfunction and hepatic failure; see Monitor. ▪ May cause permanent discoloration of the teeth during tooth development; see Maternal/Child. ▪ Avoid prolonged use of drug; superinfection caused by overgrowth of nonsusceptible organisms may result. ▪ Use caution in patients with severe liver impairment. Monitoring for treatment response is indicated. ▪ *Clostridium difficile*–associated diarrhea (CDAD) has been reported. May range from mild diarrhea to fatal colitis. Consider in patients who present with diarrhea during or after treatment with tigecycline.

Monitor: Monitor vital signs carefully. ▪ Obtain baseline CBC with differential, and monitor as indicated. ▪ Monitor patients with impaired liver function carefully. If abnormal liver function tests develop, monitor closely for worsening hepatic function and evaluate for risk/benefit of continuing therapy. May occur after tigecycline is discontinued. ▪ Observe for signs of hypersensitivity reactions (e.g., chills, fever, hives, rash, shortness of breath). ▪ See Precautions and Drug/Lab Interactions.

Patient Education: Avoid pregnancy; use effective contraceptive measures; see Drug/Lab Interactions. Should pregnancy occur, notify physician immediately and discuss potential hazards. ▪ Promptly report diarrhea or bloody stools that occur during treatment or up to several months after an antibiotic has been discontinued; may indicate CDAD and require treatment. ▪ Promptly report S/S of hypersensitivity (e.g., chills, fever, hives, rash, shortness of breath) and/or S/S of liver dysfunction (e.g., jaundice or yellow sclera).

Maternal/Child: Category D: avoid pregnancy. May cause fetal harm; use of effective contraception required; see Drug/Lab Interactions. Use during pregnancy only if benefits justify potential risk to the fetus. ▪ Use during tooth development (the last half of pregnancy, infancy, and childhood to the age of 8 years) may cause permanent discoloration of the teeth. ▪ Not known if tigecycline is secreted in breast milk; use caution. Is secreted in the milk of lactating rats. ▪ Safety and effectiveness in pediatric patients less than 18 years of age not established.

Elderly: Response similar to that seen in younger adults; however, the potential for greater sensitivity to side effects cannot be disregarded.

DRUG/LAB INTERACTIONS

Digoxin (Lanoxin) and tigecycline do not affect each other's pharmacokinetics; no dose adjustment of either drug is indicated. ▪ Concurrent use of tigecycline with **warfarin** (Coumadin) does not significantly affect INR; however, monitoring of PT or other anticoagulation tests is recommended. ▪ Inhibits **oral contraceptives;** may result in pregnancy or breakthrough bleeding. ▪ Tigecycline does not inhibit the metabolism of any of the following six cytochrome P_{450} (CYP) isoforms: 1A2, 2C8, 2C9, 2C19, 2D6, and 3A4; it is not expected to alter the metabolism of drugs metabolized by these enzymes. In addition, because tigecycline is not extensively metabolized, its clearance is not expected to be affected by drugs that induce or inhibit the activity of these P_{450} isoforms. ▪ No reported interactions with lab tests.

SIDE EFFECTS

Nausea and vomiting are the most common side effects and are the primary reason for discontinuing therapy. Other commonly reported side effects include abdominal pain, diarrhea, headache, and increased ALT. Less commonly reported side effects include abnormal healing; abscess; acute pancreatitis; anemia; asthenia; back pain; bilirubinemia; CDAD; constipation; cough; dizziness; dyspepsia; dyspnea; fever; hyperglycemia; hypertension; hypokalemia; hypoproteinemia; hypotension; increased alkaline phosphatase, amylase, AST, BUN, and lactic dehydrogenase; infection; insomnia; leukocytosis; local injection reaction; pain; peripheral edema; phlebitis; pruritus; pulmonary findings; rash; sweating; thrombocytopenia. Sepsis/septic shock and death occurred in a few patients with complicated infections.

Post-Marketing: Acute pancreatitis, anaphylaxis/anaphylactoid reactions, hepatic cholestasis, jaundice.

Overdose: Increased incidence of nausea and vomiting. Estimated lethal dose in rats was 106 mg/kg.

ANTIDOTE

Keep physician informed of all side effects. Most minor side effects will be treated symptomatically; monitor closely. If minor side effects are progressive or if any major side effect occurs, discontinue the drug, treat hypersensitivity reactions, or resuscitate as necessary. Mild cases of CDAD may respond to discontinuation of tigecycline. Treat CDAD with fluids, electrolytes, protein supplements, and oral vancomycin (Vancocin) or metronidazole (Flagyl) as indicated. In severe cases, surgical evaluation may be indicated. Not removed by hemodialysis.

TIROFIBAN HYDROCHLORIDE
(ty-roh-**FYE**-ban hy-droh-**KLOR**-eyed)

Platelet aggregation inhibitor

Aggrastat

pH 5.5 to 6.5

USUAL DOSE

Tirofiban: A *loading infusion* of 0.4 mcg/kg/min for 30 minutes, followed by a *maintenance infusion* of 0.1 mcg/kg/min. Unless contraindicated, give in conjunction with *aspirin* and *heparin.*

Aspirin: 325 mg/day.

Heparin: Administer a heparin bolus of 5,000 units, followed by an infusion titrated to maintain an aPTT of 2 times control. Heparin and tirofiban may be administered through the same intravenous catheter. Duration of therapy will vary depending on patient condition and procedures performed. In one major study, infusion was continued for 48 to 108 hours. The infusion should be continued through angiography and for 12 to 24 hours after angioplasty or arthrectomy.

DOSE ADJUSTMENTS

Patients with severe renal insufficiency (CrCl less than 30 mL/min) should receive half the usual rate of infusion. See Rate of Administration. ■ Differences in plasma clearance based on age, race, gender, or mild to moderate hepatic insufficiency do not require dose adjustment.

DILUTION

Available premixed in a plastic container in a 50 mcg/mL concentration (12.5 mg/250 mL). Remove overwrap. Plastic may be somewhat opaque due to sterilization process. Opacity should diminish. Squeeze inner container to check for leak. Discard if leakage noted; sterility is impaired. Also available in vials containing 6.25 mg/25 mL or 12.5 mg/50 mL (both equal a 250 mcg/mL concentration). Vials must be diluted to the same concentration as a premixed solution before administration (50 mcg/mL). Manufacturer suggests three methods for dilution. One is to withdraw 100 mL from a 500-mL bag of NS or D5W and replace this volume with 100 mL of tirofiban (four 25-mL vials or two 50-mL vials). A second choice is to withdraw 50 mL from a 250-mL bag of NS or D5W and replace this volume with 50 mL of tirofiban (two 25-mL vials or one 50-mL vial). A third choice is to add the contents of one 25-mL vial to 100 mL of NS or D5W. Mix well. Concentration of all three of these solutions is 50 mcg/mL. Do not use plastic containers in a series connection.

Filters: Studies found no loss of drug potency through most standard 5-micron or larger filters.

Storage: Store unopened or premixed containers at 25° C (77° F). Variations from 15° to 30° C (59° to 86° F) are acceptable for short periods. Protect from light during storage. Do not freeze. Discard unused solution.

COMPATIBILITY

Consider any drug NOT listed as compatible to be INCOMPATIBLE until consulting a pharmacist; specific conditions may apply.

Manufacturer states, "Do not add other drugs or remove solution directly from the bag with a syringe. Should not be administered in the same IV line as diazepam (Valium)."

Manufacturer indicates **compatibility** at the **Y-site** with atropine, dobutamine, dopamine, epinephrine (Adrenalin), famotidine (Pepcid IV), furosemide (Lasix), lidocaine, midazolam (Versed), morphine, nitroglycerin IV, potassium chloride, propranolol. Another source adds amiodarone (Nexterone), argatroban (Acova), bivalirudin (Angiomax), and heparin.

RATE OF ADMINISTRATION

Loading infusion: 0.4 mcg/kg/min for 30 minutes.
Maintenance infusion: 0.1 mcg/kg/min.

	Tirofiban Infusion Rates			
	Most Patients		Severe Renal Impairment	
Patient Weight (kg)	30-Min Loading Infusion Rate (mL/hr)	Maintenance Infusion Rate (mL/hr)	30-Min Loading Infusion Rate (mL/hr)	Maintenance Infusion Rate (mL/hr)
30-37	16 mL/hr	4 mL/hr	8 mL/hr	2 mL/hr
38-45	20 mL/hr	5 mL/hr	10 mL/hr	3 mL/hr
46-54	24 mL/hr	6 mL/hr	12 mL/hr	3 mL/hr
55-62	28 mL/hr	7 mL/hr	14 mL/hr	4 mL/hr
63-70	32 mL/hr	8 mL/hr	16 mL/hr	4 mL/hr
71-79	36 mL/hr	9 mL/hr	18 mL/hr	5 mL/hr
80-87	40 mL/hr	10 mL/hr	20 mL/hr	5 mL/hr
88-95	44 mL/hr	11 mL/hr	22 mL/hr	6 mL/hr
96-104	48 mL/hr	12 mL/hr	24 mL/hr	6 mL/hr
105-112	52 mL/hr	13 mL/hr	26 mL/hr	7 mL/hr
113-120	56 mL/hr	14 mL/hr	28 mL/hr	7 mL/hr
121-128	60 mL/hr	15 mL/hr	30 mL/hr	8 mL/hr
129-137	64 mL/hr	16 mL/hr	32 mL/hr	8 mL/hr
138-145	68 mL/hr	17 mL/hr	34 mL/hr	9 mL/hr
146-153	72 mL/hr	18 mL/hr	36 mL/hr	9 mL/hr

ACTIONS

A non-peptide antagonist of the platelet glycoprotein GPIIb/IIIa receptor. It inhibits platelet aggregation by preventing the binding of fibrinogen to the receptor site on activated platelets. Inhibits platelet aggregation in a dose- and concentration-dependent manner. When given according to the recommended regimen, greater than 90% inhibition is attained by the end of the 30-minute infusion. Bleeding time is prolonged. Inhibition is reversible, with aggregation returning to baseline in more than 90% of patients within 4 to 8 hours following cessation of the infusion. Has been shown to decrease the rate of a combined endpoint of death, new myocardial infarction, or refractory ischemia/repeat cardiac procedure (see literature). Half-life is approximately 2 hours. Cleared from the plasma primarily by renal excretion, with about 65% of the unchanged drug appearing in the urine and about 25% appearing in feces. Metabolism is limited.

INDICATIONS AND USES

Used in combination with heparin and aspirin for the prevention of acute cardiac ischemic complications in patients with acute coronary syndrome (characterized by prolonged [more than 10 minutes] or repetitive symptoms of cardiac ischemia occurring at rest or with minimal exertion, associated with either ischemic ST-T wave changes on electrocardiogram [ECG] or elevated cardiac enzymes. Includes "unstable angina" and "non–Q-wave myocardial infarction" but excludes myocardial infarction that is associated with Q-waves or nontransient ST-segment elevation). May be used in patients who are being medically managed and in those undergoing percutaneous coronary intervention (PCI) or arthrectomy.

CONTRAINDICATIONS

Known hypersensitivity to any component of the product; active internal bleeding or history of bleeding diathesis within the previous 30 days (a second source indicates within the previous year); a history of intracranial hemorrhage, intracranial neoplasm, arteriovenous malformation, or aneurysm; a history of thrombocytopenia following prior exposure to tirofiban; a history of stroke within 30 days or any history of hemorrhagic stroke, major surgical procedure or severe physical trauma within the previous month; history, symptoms, or findings suggestive of aortic dissection; severe hypertension (systolic BP above 180 mm Hg and/or diastolic BP above 110 mm Hg); concomitant use of another parenteral GPIIb/IIIa inhibitor (e.g., abciximab [ReoPro]); acute pericarditis; liver disease.

PRECAUTIONS

Use with caution in patients with platelet count less than 150,000/mm^3, in patients with hemorrhagic retinopathy, and in patients with a history of cerebrovascular disease. ■ Use caution when given with drugs that affect hemostasis (e.g., warfarin [Coumadin]). Safety when used in combination with thrombolytic agents (e.g., alteplase [tPA, Activase], reteplase [Retavase], streptokinase [Streptase]) has not been established. See Drug/Lab Interactions. ■ Use with caution in patients with renal insufficiency. See Dose Adjustments. ■ Bleeding is the most common complication encountered during therapy. Incidence may be slightly higher in females and the elderly. ■ Most major bleeding occurs at the arterial access site for cardiac catheterization. Care should be taken when attempting vascular access that only the anterior wall of the femoral artery is punctured.

Monitor: Obtain platelet count, hemoglobin, and hematocrit before therapy, within 6 hours following the loading infusion, and at least daily thereafter. More frequent monitoring may be indicated. ■ If platelet count drops to below 90,000/mm^3, additional platelet counts should be performed to exclude pseudothrombocytopenia. If thrombocytopenia is confirmed, heparin and tirofiban should be discontinued and appropriate therapy initiated. ■ Obtain an aPTT 6 hours after the start of the heparin infusion. Adjust heparin infusion rate to maintain an aPTT 2 times control. ■ Patients receiving percutaneous coronary intervention who have a sheath in place should be maintained on complete bed rest with the head of the bed elevated 30 degrees and the affected limb restrained in a straight position. Monitor sheath insertion site(s) and distal pulses of affected leg(s) frequently while sheath is in place and for 6 hours after removal. Measure any hematoma and monitor for enlargement. ■ Monitor the patient for signs of bleeding; take vital signs (avoiding automatic BP cuffs), observe any invaded sites at least every 15 minutes (e.g., sheaths, IV sites, cutdowns, punctures, Foleys, NGs); watch for hematuria, hematemesis, bloody stool, petechiae, hematoma, flank pain, muscle weakness. Perform neuro checks frequently. If during therapy bleeding cannot be controlled with pressure, tirofiban and heparin infusions should be discontinued. ▪ Use care in handling patient; minimize use of urinary catheters, nasotracheal intubation, and nasogastric tubes. Avoid arterial puncture, venipuncture, epidural procedures, and IM injection. Use extreme precautionary methods and only compressible sites if these procedures are absolutely necessary (i.e., avoid subclavian or jugular veins). Apply pressure for 30 minutes to any invaded site and then apply pressure dressings. Saline or heparin locks suggested to facilitate blood draws. ▪ In patients receiving percutaneous coronary intervention, heparin should be discontinued 3 to 4 hours before pulling the sheath and an activated clotting time (ACT) less than 180 seconds or an aPTT less than 45 seconds should be documented. ▪ Care should be taken to obtain proper hemostasis after removal of the sheath using standard compressive techniques followed by close observation. Sheath hemostasis should be achieved at least 4 hours before hospital discharge.

Patient Education: Compliance with all measures to minimize bleeding (e.g., strict bed rest, positioning) is imperative. ▪ Avoid use of razors, toothbrushes, and other sharp items. ▪ Use caution while moving to avoid excessive bumping. ▪ Report all episodes of bleeding and apply local pressure if indicated. ▪ Expect oozing from IV sites.

Maternal/Child: Category B: safety for use in pregnancy not established. Benefits must outweigh risks. ▪ Discontinue breast-feeding until 24 hours after completion of tirofiban therapy. ▪ Safety and efficacy for use in pediatric patients not established.

Elderly: Clearance is reduced in the elderly, possibly due to age-related renal impairment. Dose adjustment is not necessary unless renal impairment severe; see Dose Adjustments. Incidence of bleeding complications increase somewhat but are similar to use of heparin as a single agent. Incidence of non-bleeding side effects also increased.

DRUG/LAB INTERACTIONS

All studies with tirofiban included the use of **aspirin** and **heparin.** Concomitant use, although indicated, increases the risk of bleeding. ▪ Use caution when given with drugs that affect hemostasis (e.g., **thrombolytics** [e.g., alteplase (tPA, Activase), reteplase (Retavase), streptokinase (Streptase)], **anticoagulants** [e.g., warfarin (Coumadin)], **NSAIDs** [e.g., ibuprofen (Advil, Motrin), naproxen (Aleve, Naprosyn)], **platelet aggregation inhibitors** [e.g., dipyridamole (Persantine), ticlopidine (Ticlid)], **glycoprotein GPIIb/IIIa receptor antagonists** [e.g., abciximab (ReoPro), eptifibatide (Integrilin)], **or selected antibiotics** [e.g., cefotetan]). ▪ Patients receiving **omeprazole** (Prilosec) **or levothyroxine** (Synthroid) concurrently with tirofiban had a higher clearance of tirofiban. Clinical significance of this observation is not known. ▪ The following drugs were coadministered with tirofiban in clinical trials: acebutolol (Monitan), acetaminophen (Tylenol), alprazolam (Xanax), amlodipine, aspirin, atenolol (Tenormin), bromazepam, captopril (Capoten), diazepam (Valium), digoxin, diltiazem (Cardizem), docusate sodium, enalapril (Vasotec), furosemide (Lasix), glyburide, heparin, insulin, isosorbide, lorazepam (Ativan), lovastatin (Mevacor), metoclopramide

(Reglan), metoprolol (Lopressor), morphine, nifedipine (Procardia), nitrate preparations (e.g., nitroglycerin), oxazepam (Serax), potassium chloride, propranolol, ranitidine (Zantac), simvastatin (Zocor), sucralfate (Sulcrate), and temazepam (Restoril). Plasma clearance of tirofiban was not affected by coadministration.

SIDE EFFECTS

Bleeding is the most frequent adverse event and is usually reported as mild oozing. Laboratory findings related to bleeding include decrease in hemoglobin, hematocrit, and platelet count and occult blood in urine and feces. Decreased platelet count may be associated with chills and fever. Other side effects that occur at an incidence of greater than 1%, regardless of drug relationship, are bradycardia, dissection of the coronary artery, dizziness, edema, fever, headache, hypersensitivity reactions (e.g., hives, rash), leg pain, nausea, pelvic pain, sweating, thrombocytopenia, and vasovagal reflex.

Post-Marketing: Acute decreases in platelet counts, intracranial bleeding, pulmonary (alveolar) hemorrhage, retroperitoneal bleeding, spinal-epidural hematoma, hemopericardium, and fatal bleeding events have been reported.

ANTIDOTE

Keep physician informed of laboratory values and side effects. Discontinue the infusion of tirofiban and heparin if any serious bleeding not controllable with pressure occurs. If platelet count drops to below 90,000 mm^3, obtain additional platelet counts to exclude pseudo-thrombocytopenia. If thrombocytopenia is confirmed, discontinue tirofiban and heparin. Platelet transfusion may be required. If a hypersensitivity reaction should occur, discontinue the infusion and treat as indicated by severity (e.g., epinephrine, dopamine, theophylline, antihistamines [e.g., diphenhydramine (Benadryl)], and/or corticosteroids as necessary).

No specific antidote is available. Overdosage should be treated by assessment of the patient's clinical condition and cessation or adjustment of the drug infusion as appropriate. Hemodialysis may be useful in an overdose situation.

TOBRAMYCIN SULFATE BBW
(toe-brah-**MY**-sin **SUL**-fayt)

Antibacterial (aminoglycoside)

pH 3 to 6.5

USUAL DOSE

3 mg/kg of body weight/24 hr equally divided into 3 doses and given every 8 hours (1 mg/kg every 8 hours). Up to 5 mg/kg equally divided into 3 or 4 doses may be given in life-threatening infections (1.25 mg/kg every 6 hours or 1.67 mg/kg every 8 hours). Reduce to usual dose as soon as feasible. For obese patients, the dosing weight used to calculate the mg/kg dose is achieved by adding the ideal or lean body weight (IBW) to 40% of the excess over IBW.

Dosing weight = IBW + 0.4 (Total body weight − IBW)

Do not exceed 5 mg/kg/day unless serum levels are monitored.

Studies suggest that a single daily dose of 5 to 7 mg/kg (instead of divided into 2 to 3 doses) may provide higher peak levels and enhance drug effectiveness while actually reducing or having no adverse effects on risk of toxicity. Various procedures for monitoring blood levels are in use. Some health facilities are monitoring with trough levels; others may draw levels at predetermined times and plot the concentration on nomograms. Depending on the protocol in place, doses or intervals may be adjusted. See Precautions.

Patients with cystic fibrosis: One source suggests 7.5 to 10.5 mg/kg/24 hr equally divided into 3 doses and given every 8 hours for 7 to 21 days (2.5 to 3.5 mg/kg every 8 hours).

PEDIATRIC DOSE

In pediatric and neonatal patients, monitor serum levels. Wide interpatient variability; see Monitor and Maternal/Child.

Over 1 week of age: 6 to 7.5 mg/kg of body weight/24 hr in 3 or 4 equally divided doses (1.5 to 1.89 mg/kg every 6 hours or 2 to 2.5 mg/kg every 8 hours). Another source suggests the same as adult dose.

A single daily dose is also being used in pediatric patients. See comments under Usual Dose.

Severe cystic fibrosis: 10 mg/kg/day in equally divided doses every 6 hours (2.5 mg/kg every 6 hours).

NEONATAL DOSE

1 week of age or less: Up to 4 mg/kg of body weight/24 hr in two equal doses every 12 hours (up to 2 mg/kg every 12 hours). Lower doses may be safer because of immature kidney function. 2.5 mg/kg every 18 hours or 3 mg/kg every 24 hours may provide acceptable peak and trough levels in neonates weighing less than 2,000 Gm. See Maternal/Child.

DOSE ADJUSTMENTS

Reduce daily dose commensurate with amount of renal impairment and/or increase intervals between injections. Measurement of serum concentrations following a loading dose of 1 mg/kg is suggested. Adjust subsequent doses accordingly. ■ Reduced doses or extended intervals may be required in the elderly. ■ See Drug/Lab Interactions.

DILUTION

Prepared solutions equal 10 or 40 mg/mL. Further dilute each single dose in 50 to 100 mL of NS or D5W and administer through an additive tubing. Also available in ADD-Vantage vials for use with ADD-Vantage infusion containers. Reduce volume of diluent proportionately for pediatric patients.

Storage: Store at CRT.

COMPATIBILITY   (Underline Indicates Conflicting Compatibility Information)

Consider any drug NOT listed as compatible to be INCOMPATIBLE until consulting a pharmacist; specific conditions may apply.

Manufacturer states, "Do not physically premix with other drugs; administer separately." Inactivated in solution with beta-lactam antibiotics (e.g., cephalosporins, penicillins) and vancomycin; do not mix in the same solution. Appropriate spacing required because of physical **incompatibilities**. See Drug/Lab Interactions.

One source suggests the following **compatibilities:**

Additive: *Not recommended by manufacturer.* Aztreonam (Azactam), bleomycin (Blenoxane), calcium gluconate, cefoxitin (Mefoxin), ciprofloxacin (Cipro IV), clindamycin (Cleocin), furosemide (Lasix), linezolid (Zyvox), metronidazole (Flagyl IV), ranitidine (Zantac), verapamil.

Y-site: Acyclovir (Zovirax), alprostadil, amifostine (Ethyol), amiodarone (Nexterone), anidulafungin (Eraxis), aztreonam (Azactam), bivalirudin (Angiomax), caspofungin (Cancidas), cefepime (Maxipime), ceftazidime (Fortaz), ciprofloxacin (Cipro IV), cisatracurium (Nimbex), cyclophosphamide (Cytoxan), dexmedetomidine (Precedex), diltiazem (Cardizem), docetaxel (Taxotere), doripenem (Doribax), doxorubicin liposomal (Doxil), enalaprilat (Vasotec IV), esmolol (Brevibloc), etoposide phosphate (Etopophos), fenoldopam (Corlopam), filgrastim (Neupogen), fluconazole (Diflucan), fludarabine (Fludara), foscarnet (Foscavir), furosemide (Lasix), gemcitabine (Gemzar), granisetron (Kytril), hetastarch in electrolytes (Hextend), hydromorphone (Dilaudid), insulin (regular), labetalol (Trandate), linezolid (Zyvox), magnesium sulfate, melphalan (Alkeran), meperidine (Demerol), midazolam (Versed), milrinone (Primacor), morphine, nicardipine (Cardene IV), remifentanil (Ultiva), tacrolimus (Prograf), teniposide (Vumon), theophylline, thiotepa, tigecycline (Tygacil), vinorelbine (Navelbine), zidovudine (AZT, Retrovir).

RATE OF ADMINISTRATION

Each single dose, properly diluted, over a minimum of 20 and a maximum of 60 minutes.

ACTIONS

An aminoglycoside antibiotic with potential neuromuscular blocking action. Inhibits protein synthesis in bacterial cells. Bactericidal against specific gram-negative and bacilli, including *Escherichia coli, Klebsiella, Proteus,* and *Pseudomonas.* Well distributed through all body fluids. Usual half-life is 2 to 2.5 hours. Half-life is prolonged in infants, postpartum females, fever, liver disease and ascites, spinal cord injury, cystic fibrosis, and the elderly; shorter in severe burns. Crosses the placental barrier. Excreted in the kidneys.

INDICATIONS AND USES

Short-term treatment of serious infections caused by susceptible organisms. Indicated infections include septicemia, lower respiratory tract infections, CNS infections (meningitis), intra-abdominal infections (including peritonitis and skin, bone, and skin structure infections), and complicated and recurrent urinary tract infections. ▪ Primarily used when penicillin and other less toxic antibiotics are ineffective or contraindicated. ▪ Concurrent therapy with a penicillin or cephalosporin sometimes indicated.

CONTRAINDICATIONS
Known tobramycin or aminoglycoside sensitivity. Sulfite sensitivity may be a contraindication.

PRECAUTIONS
Use extreme caution if therapy is required over 7 to 10 days. ▪ Sensitivity studies necessary to determine susceptibility of causative organism to tobramycin. ▪ To reduce the development of drug-resistant bacteria and maintain its effectiveness, tobramycin should be used to treat or prevent only those infections proven or strongly suspected to be caused by bacteria. ▪ Superinfection may occur from overgrowth of nonsusceptible organisms. ▪ Use caution in infants, children, the elderly, and patients with congestive heart failure, extensive burns, or muscular disorders. ▪ May contain sulfites; use caution in patients with asthma. ▪ Risk for neurotoxicity (e.g., auditory and vestibular ototoxicity) increased in patients with pre-existing renal damage or in normal renal function with prolonged use. Partial or total irreversible deafness may continue to develop after tobramycin is discontinued. ▪ Aminoglycosides are nephrotoxic; risk for nephrotoxicity increased in patients with impaired renal function and in patients who receive high doses or prolonged therapy. ▪ Single daily dosing has been used effectively in abdominal, pelvic inflammatory, and GU infections in patients with normal renal function. Not recommended in bacteremia caused by *Pseudomonas aeruginosa,* endocarditis, meningitis, during pregnancy, or in patients less than 6 weeks postpartum. Limited data available for use in all other situations (e.g., burns, pediatric patients or the elderly, cystic fibrosis, renal impairment). ▪ *Clostridium difficile*–associated diarrhea (CDAD) has been reported. May range from mild diarrhea to fatal colitis. Consider in patients who present with diarrhea during or after treatment with tobramycin.

Monitor: Watch for decrease in urine output, rising BUN and SCr, and declining CrCl levels. Dose may require decreasing. ▪ Closely monitor renal and eighth cranial nerve function, especially in patients with known or suspected reduced renal function at onset of therapy and in patients who develop signs of renal dysfunction during therapy. Monitor urine for decreased specific gravity, increased protein, and the presence of cells or casts. Serial audiograms are recommended, particularly in high-risk patients. ▪ Closely monitor patients with impaired renal function for nephrotoxicity and neurotoxicity (e.g., auditory and vestibular ototoxicity, convulsions, muscle twitching, numbness, tingling); nephrotoxicity may be reversible. ▪ Routine evaluation of hearing is recommended. ▪ Narrow range between toxic and therapeutic levels. Periodically monitor peak and trough concentrations to avoid peak serum concentrations above 12 mcg/mL and trough concentrations above 2 mcg/mL (indicates accumulation). With traditional dosing, therapeutic levels are between 4 and 8 mcg/mL depending on site and severity of infection. Accumulation, excessive peak concentrations, advanced age, cumulative doses, and dehydration may contribute to ototoxicity and nephrotoxicity. ▪ Maintain good hydration. ▪ Monitor serum calcium, magnesium, potassium, and sodium; levels may decline. ▪ Closely monitor patients with impaired renal function for nephrotoxicity and neurotoxicity (e.g., auditory and vestibular ototoxicity); nephrotoxicity may be reversible. ▪ In extended treatment, monitoring of serum levels, electrolytes, renal, auditory, and vestibular functions daily is recommended. ▪ See Drug/Lab Interactions.

Patient Education: Report promptly dizziness, hearing loss, weakness, or any changes in balance. ▪ Consider birth control options. ▪ Promptly report diarrhea or bloody stools that occur during treatment or up to several months after an antibiotic has been discontinued; may indicate CDAD and require treatment.

Maternal/Child: Category D: avoid pregnancy; use during pregnancy and breast-feeding only when absolutely necessary. Potential hazard to fetus. ▪ Peak concentrations are generally lower in infants and young children. ▪ Use extreme caution in premature infants and neonates; immature kidney function will result in prolonged half-life. ▪ See Precautions.

Elderly: Consider less toxic alternatives. ▪ Monitor renal function and drug levels carefully. Measurement of CrCl more useful than BUN or SCr to assess renal function. ▪ Half-life prolonged; longer intervals between doses may be more important than reduced doses. ▪ See Precautions, Dose Adjustments, and Side Effects.

DRUG/LAB INTERACTIONS

Synergistic when used in combination with **beta-lactam antibiotics** (e.g., cephalosporins, penicillins) **and vancomycin.** Synergism may be inconsistent; see Compatibility. ▪ Concurrent and/or sequential use topically or systemically with any other neurotoxic, ototoxic, or nephrotoxic agents should be avoided. May have dangerous additive effects with **anesthetics** (e.g., enflurane), **other neuromuscular blocking antibiotics** (e.g., other aminoglycosides [e.g., kanamycin (Kantrex)]), **diuretics** (e.g., furosemide [Lasix]), **beta-lactam antibiotics** (e.g., cephalosporins), **vancomycin, and many others.** ▪ Neuromuscular blocking muscle relaxants (e.g., atracurium [Tracrium], succinylcholine) are potentiated by aminoglycosides. *Apnea can occur.* ▪ May be antagonized by **bacteriostatic antibiotics** (e.g., chloramphenicol, erythromicin, and tetracycline); bactericidal action may be affected. ▪ **Magnesium sulfate** may reduce the antibiotic activity of tobramycin. ▪ Aminoglycosides are potentiated by **anticholinesterases** (e.g., edrophonium), **antineoplastics** (e.g., nitrogen mustard, cisplatin). ▪ See Side Effects.

SIDE EFFECTS

Occur more frequently with impaired renal function, higher doses, prolonged administration, dehydration, in the elderly, and in patients receiving other ototoxic or nephrotoxic drugs.

Dizziness; fever; headache; increased AST, ALT, and serum bilirubin; itching; lethargy; rash; roaring in the ears; seizures; urticaria; vomiting.

Major: Apnea; blood dyscrasias; CDAD; cylindruria; elevated BUN, nonprotein nitrogen (NPN), and creatinine; hearing loss; leukocytosis; neuromuscular blockade; oliguria; proteinuria; seizures (large doses); tinnitus; vertigo.

ANTIDOTE

Notify the physician of all side effects. If minor side effects persist or any major symptom appears, discontinue the drug and notify the physician. Evidence of impaired renal, vestibular, or auditory function requires discontinuation of tobramycin or a dose adjustment. Treatment is symptomatic or a reduction in dose may be required. Mild cases of CDAD may respond to discontinuation of drug. Treat CDAD with fluids, electrolytes, protein supplements, and oral vancomycin (Vancocin) or metronidazole (Flagyl) as indicated. In severe cases, surgical evaluation may be indicated. In overdose hemodialysis may be indicated. Monitor fluid balance, CrCl, and plasma levels carefully. Complexation with ticarcillin may be as effective as hemodialysis. Consider exchange transfusion in the newborn. Calcium salts or neostigmine may reverse neuromuscular blockade. Resuscitate as necessary.

TOCILIZUMAB BBW

(**TOE**-si-**LIZ**-oo-mab)

Actemra

Antirheumatic
Monoclonal Antibody

pH 6.5

USUAL DOSE

Before initial use, the absolute neutrophil count (ANC) should be equal to or greater than 2,000/mm^3, platelet count should be equal to or greater than 100,000/mm^3, and ALT and AST should be no more than 1.5 times the ULN.

Initial adult dose in rheumatoid arthritis: 4 mg/kg as an IV infusion once every 4 weeks. Increase dose to 8 mg/kg based on clinical response. May be used in combination with disease-modifying anti-rheumatic drugs (DMARDs) such as methotrexate or as monotherapy. Doses above 800 mg per infusion are not recommended.

Systemic juvenile idiopathic arthritis (SJIA): Administer as an IV infusion once every 2 weeks. May be used alone or in combination with methotrexate. Do not adjust dose based on a single-visit body weight; weight may fluctuate.

Weight less than 30 kg: 12 mg/kg.

Weight equal to or more than 30 kg: 8 mg/kg.

DOSE ADJUSTMENTS

There is a trend toward a higher clearance with increasing body weight; see Usual Dose. No specific dose adjustments required based on age, gender, race, or mild renal impairment. ■ Withhold therapy in patients with severe infections, an opportunistic infection, or sepsis. ■ Dose reduction has not been studied in SJIA. Dose interruptions are recommended for liver enzyme abnormalities, low neutrophil counts, and low platelet counts in patients with SJIA at levels similar to those outlined in the following charts for patients with rheumatoid arthritis (RA). May require interrupting or discontinuing tocilizumab and/or other concomitant medications (e.g., methotrexate) until evaluation of the clinical situation. ■ The effects of moderate to severe renal impairment or hepatic impairment have not been studied. The following charts outline dose adjustments for adults with RA based on ANC, platelets, and liver function tests.

Tocilizumab Dose Recommendations for Low Absolute Neutrophil Count (ANC)	
Lab Value (cells/mm^3)	Recommendation
ANC >1,000/mm^3	Maintain dose.
ANC 500 to 1,000/mm^3	Interrupt tocilizumab dosing. When ANC >1,000/mm^3, resume tocilizumab at 4 mg/kg and increase to 8 mg/kg as clinically appropriate.
ANC <500/mm^3	Discontinue tocilizumab.

Tocilizumab Dose Recommendations for Low Platelet Count	
Lab Value (cells/mm^3)	Recommendation
Platelet count 50,000 to 100,000/mm^3	Interrupt tocilizumab dosing. When platelet count is >100,000/mm^3, resume tocilizumab at 4 mg/kg and increase to 8 mg/kg as clinically appropriate.
Platelet count <50,000/mm^3	Discontinue tocilizumab.

Tocilizumab Dose Recommendations for Liver Enzyme Abnormalities	
Lab Value	Recommendation
>1 to 3 × ULN	Dose modify concomitant DMARDs if appropriate. For persistent increases in this range, reduce tocilizumab dose to 4 mg/kg or interrupt dosing until ALT and/or AST have normalized.
>3 to 5 × ULN (confirmed by repeat testing)	Interrupt tocilizumab dosing until <3 × ULN, and follow recommendations above for >1 to 3 × ULN. For persistent increases >3 × ULN, discontinue tocilizumab.
>5 × ULN	Discontinue tocilizumab.

DILUTION

Available as a solution for single use (20 mg/mL). For adults and SJIA patients weighing 30 kg or more, the solution must be further diluted to 100 mL in NS. For SJIA patients weighing less than 30 kg, dilute to 50 mL in NS. From a 100-mL (or 50-mL) infusion bag or bottle, withdraw a volume of NS equal to the volume of solution required for the calculated dose. Slowly add tocilizumab and avoid foaming by gently inverting the bag or bottle. Bring fully diluted solution to RT before administration.
Filters: Specific information not available.
Storage: Refrigerate unopened vials in original carton at 2° to 8° C (36° to 46° F). Do not use beyond expiration date. Protect from light. Do not freeze. Fully diluted solution may be refrigerated or stored at RT for up to 24 hours. Protect from light. Discard unused solution.

COMPATIBILITY

Manufacturer states, "Fully diluted solutions are **compatible** with polypropylene, polyethylene, and polyvinyl chloride infusion bags and glass infusion bottles. Tocilizumab should not be infused concomitantly in the same intravenous line with other drugs."

RATE OF ADMINISTRATION
A single dose as an infusion equally distributed over 60 minutes.

ACTIONS
A recombinant humanized anti-human interleukin 6 (IL-6) receptor monoclonal antibody. Binds specifically to both soluble and membrane-bound IL-6 receptors. Inhibits IL-6–mediated signaling through these receptors. IL-6 is a pro-inflammatory cytokine produced by a variety of cell types. IL-6 is also produced by synovial and endothelial cells leading to local production of IL-6 in joints affected by inflammatory processes such as rheumatoid arthritis. IL-6 has been shown to be involved in diverse physiologic processes such as T-cell activation, induction of immunoglobulin secretion, initiation of hepatic acute phase protein synthesis, and stimulation of hematopoietic precursor cell proliferation and differentiation. Following administration, increases in hemoglobin and decreases in C-reactive protein, rheumatoid factor, erythrocyte sedimentation rate, and serum amyloid A were observed. ANC counts decreased to the nadir 3 to 5 days after administration, and neutrophils recovered toward baseline in a dose-dependent manner. Steady state is reached with the first administration. It undergoes biphasic elimination from the circulation. Half-life is concentration dependent and ranges from 11 to 13 days depending on the dose administered.

INDICATIONS AND USES
Treatment of adults with moderately to severely active rheumatoid arthritis who have had an inadequate response to one or more TNF antagonist therapies (e.g., adalimumab [Humira], etanercept [Enbrel], infliximab [Remicade]). ■ Treatment of patients 2 years of age and older with active systemic juvenile idiopathic arthritis.

CONTRAINDICATIONS
Known hypersensitivity to tocilizumab.

PRECAUTIONS
Administered under the direction of a physician knowledgeable in its use in a facility with adequate diagnostic and treatment facilities to monitor the patients and respond to any medical emergency. ■ Serious and sometimes fatal infections due to bacterial, mycobacterial, invasive fungal, viral, protozoal, or other opportunistic pathogens have been reported. Deaths have occurred. The most common serious infections included bacterial arthritis, cellulitis, diverticulitis, gastroenteritis, herpes zoster, pneumonia, sepsis, and UTIs. Opportunistic infections reported with tocilizumab include aspergillosis, candidiasis, cryptococcus, pneumocystosis, and tuberculosis (TB). Patients were often taking concomitant immunosuppressants such as methotrexate or corticosteroids, which may have predisposed them to infection. ■ Tocilizumab should not be administered in patients with an active infection, including localized infections. Assess the risks and benefits of tocilizumab before initiating in patients with chronic or recurrent infection, patients who have been exposed to tuberculosis, patients with a history of a serious or an opportunistic infection, patients who have resided or traveled in areas of endemic tuberculosis or endemic mycoses, or patients with underlying conditions that may predispose them to infection. ■ Evaluate patients for TB risk factors and latent TB before initiating therapy; see Monitor. ■ Antirheumatic therapies have been associated with hepatitis B reactivation.

Viral reactivation (e.g., herpes zoster) occurred during clinical studies; patients who screened positive for hepatitis were excluded. ▪ Has not been studied in patients with active hepatic disease or hepatic impairment, including patients with positive HBV (hepatitis B virus) or HCV (hepatitis C virus) serology. Use is not recommended. ▪ Has not been studied in patients with moderate to severe renal impairment. ▪ Use caution in patients who may be at risk for GI perforation (e.g., diverticulitis) and in patients with pre-existing or recent-onset demyelinating disorders (e.g., multiple sclerosis, chronic inflammatory demyelinating polyneuropathy). ▪ Hypersensitivity reactions, including anaphylaxis and death, have been reported. Emergency medical equipment and medications for treating these reactions must be readily available. ▪ Tocilizumab is associated with increases in lipids. ▪ Infusion-related reactions have occurred; see Side Effects. ▪ A small number of patients have developed binding antibodies to tocilizumab. Hypersensitivity reactions leading to withdrawal have been reported. ▪ Treatment may result in an increased risk of malignancy.

Monitor: Evaluate patients for TB risk factors and latent TB with a TB skin test before tocilizumab use and during therapy. Patients testing positive in TB screening should be treated with a standard TB regimen before initiating therapy with tocilizumab. Include patients with a history of latent or active TB when an adequate course of treatment cannot be confirmed and patients who have a negative test for latent TB but have risk factors for TB. Consultation with a specialist in TB diagnosis and treatment is encouraged. ▪ Screening for viral hepatitis may be indicated. ▪ In RA patients, obtain baseline CBC, platelets, and liver function tests (e.g., ALT, AST, bilirubin). Consider obtaining a baseline bilirubin. Monitor neutrophils, platelets, ALT, and AST every 4 to 8 weeks. In SJIA patients, obtain baseline CBC, platelets, and liver function tests. Monitor neutrophils, platelets, ALT, and AST before the second infusion and every 2 to 4 weeks. ▪ In both RA and SJIA patients, obtain baseline lipid studies (e.g., cholesterol [HDL, LDL, and total], triglycerides). Repeat in 4 to 8 weeks and then at 24-week intervals. Elevated lipids respond to lipid-lowering agents (e.g., simvastatin [Zocor]). ▪ Closely monitor for S/S of infection during and after treatment with tocilizumab; may present with disseminated, rather than localized, disease; S/S may be lessened due to suppression of the acute phase reactants. Therapy should be interrupted if a serious infection, an opportunistic infection, or sepsis develops, and appropriate evaluation and treatment should be initiated promptly. ▪ Monitor for S/S of hypersensitivity or infusion-related reactions (e.g., anaphylaxis, hypotension, pruritus, rash, urticaria, or wheezing); most hypersensitivity reactions have occurred between the second and fourth infusion; see Side Effects. ▪ Monitor for S/S of GI perforation (e.g., new-onset abdominal pain). ▪ Monitor for S/S potentially indicative of demyelinating disorders. ▪ Do not administer live virus vaccines. All patients, especially SJIA patients, should be brought up-to-date with all immunizations before beginning therapy. ▪ See Precautions and Drug/Lab Interactions.

Patient Education: Read manufacturer's medication guide before starting therapy. ▪ Promptly report S/S of an allergic reaction (e.g., rash, itching, wheezing), infusion reaction (e.g., dizziness, headache), or infection (e.g., chill, cough, fever). Report severe, persistent abdominal pain promptly. ▪ Discuss previous infections, current infections, or exposure to TB. ▪ Routine laboratory monitoring required.

Maternal/Child: Category C: use during pregnancy only if the potential benefit justifies the potential risk to the fetus. ▪ A pregnancy registry has been established; contact manufacturer. ▪ Discontinue breast-feeding. ▪ Safety and effectiveness for use in pediatric patients not established.
Elderly: Incidence of infection is higher in the elderly. Use caution; see Precautions.

DRUG/LAB INTERACTIONS

Formal drug interaction studies have not been conducted. Avoid concurrent use with a **TNF antagonist** (e.g., adalimumab [Humira], etanercept [Enbrel], infliximab [Remicade]); may increase immunosuppression and risk of infection. ▪ Methotrexate, NSAIDs (e.g., naproxen [Naprosyn, Aleve], ibuprofen [Advil, Motrin]), and corticosteroids (e.g., prednisone) do not appear to influence tocilizumab clearance. ▪ Has no clinically significant effect on methotrexate exposure. ▪ Inhibition of IL-6 signaling in patients treated with tocilizumab may restore CYP450 activities to higher levels, resulting in an increased metabolism of drugs that are CYP450 substrates. Concurrent use showed an increase in metabolism and lower serum concentrations of **omeprazole** (Prilosec) and **simvastatin** (Zocor). This effect may be clinically relevant with CYP450 substrates with a narrow therapeutic index, in which the dose is individually adjusted (e.g., **warfarin** [Coumadin], **cyclosporine** [Sandimmune], **theophylline**). Therapeutic monitoring of effect (INR) and/or serum concentrations is indicated to adjust the dose of these drugs with initiation or termination of tocilizumab. Use caution with CYP3A4 substrate drugs in which a decrease in effectiveness is undesirable (e.g., **atorvastatin** [Lipitor], **lovastatin** [Mevacor], **oral contraceptives**). The effect of tocilizumab on CYP450 enzyme activity may persist for several weeks after therapy is discontinued. ▪ Do not administer **live virus vaccines.**

SIDE EFFECTS

RA: Most common adverse reactions include headache, hypertension, increased transaminases (ALT, AST), nasopharyngitis, and upper respiratory tract infections. The most common serious infections include bacterial arthritis, cellulitis, diverticulitis, gastroenteritis, herpes zoster, pneumonia, sepsis, and UTIs. Most common side effects that required discontinuation of therapy were increased hepatic transaminase values and serious infections. Infusion-related reactions have been reported. Headache frequently occurred during infusion, and skin reactions (e.g., pruritus, rash, urticaria) were reported within the next 24 hours. Hypersensitivity reactions (e.g., anaphylactoid and anaphylactic) did occur in a few patients. Other side effects reported include bronchitis, dizziness, elevated lipids, gastritis, GI perforation, mouth ulceration, neutropenia, thrombocytopenia, and upper abdominal pain.
SJIA: Most common adverse reactions included diarrhea, headache, nasopharyngitis, and upper respiratory tract infections. Anaphylaxis, decreased platelet count, development of anti-tocilizumab antibodies, increased liver function tests and lipids, infections, infusion reactions, and neutropenia have been reported.
Post-Marketing: Fatal anaphylaxis.

ANTIDOTE

Notify physician of any side effects; most will be treated symptomatically. During clinical studies, most infusion-related reactions were mild to moderate. Interrupt therapy for decreases in ANC and platelets and increases in liver function studies as outlined in Dose Adjustments. Therapy may need to be interrupted in patients who develop infections. Discontinue tocilizumab for any serious reaction or infection. Treat infusion and hypersensitivity reactions as indicated (e.g., oxygen, diphenhydramine, epinephrine, corticosteroids, vasopressors, and/or fluids). Resuscitate as necessary.

TOPOTECAN HYDROCHLORIDE BBW   Antineoplastic
(toh-poh-**TEE**-kan hy-droh-**KLOR**-eyed)   **(topoisomerase I inhibitor)**

Hycamtin
pH 2.5 to 3.5

USUAL DOSE

Before giving the initial dose, the baseline neutrophil count must be at least 1,500/mm^3 and baseline platelet count must be at least 100,000/mm^3.

Ovarian cancer and small-cell lung cancer: 1.5 mg/M^2/day as an infusion each day for 5 consecutive days (Days 1 through 5 of a 21-day course). Begin the second course on Day 22. A minimum of four courses is recommended; median time to response has been 9 to 12 weeks for ovarian cancer and 5 to 7 weeks for small-cell lung cancer. See Dose Adjustments.

Cervical cancer: 0.75 mg/M^2 as an infusion on Days 1, 2, and 3. On Day 1 follow with cisplatin 50 mg/M^2. Repeat every 21 days. See cisplatin monograph for prehydration requirements.

Non–small-cell lung cancer (unlabeled): 1.5 mg/M^2/day as an infusion each day for 5 consecutive days. Repeat every 21 days.

Myelodysplastic syndrome/chronic myelomonocytic leukemia (unlabeled): 2 mg/M^2/day as a continuous 24-hour infusion. Repeat every day for 5 consecutive days. Repeat every 3 to 4 weeks until remission, then repeat once a month.

DOSE ADJUSTMENTS

Do not begin subsequent courses of topotecan until neutrophils recover to more than 1,000/mm^3, platelets recover to 100,000/mm^3, and hemoglobin recovers to 9 mg/dL (with transfusion if necessary). ■ No dose adjustment required in patients with impaired hepatic function (bilirubin between 1.5 and 10 mg/dL). ■ Reduce dose to 0.75 mg/M^2 in patients with moderate impaired renal function (CrCl 20 to 39 mL/min). There are inadequate data at this time to recommend a dose in severe renal impairment. ■ Dose adjustment may be required in the elderly because of age-related renal impairment.

Ovarian cancer and small-cell lung cancer: If severe neutropenia occurs (neutrophils less than or equal to 500/mm^3) during any course, either reduce dose for all subsequent courses by 0.25 mg/M^2 (to 1.25 mg/M^2) or, before resorting to dose reduction, give G-CSF (filgrastim) starting with Day 6 (must be at least 24 hours after the final dose of that course). ■ If platelet count falls below 25,000/mm^3, reduce dose for all subsequent courses by 0.25 mg/M^2 (to 1.25 mg/M^2). *Continued*

Cervical cancer: Dose adjustment in subsequent cycles is drug specific.
Topotecan: If severe febrile neutropenia occurs (neutrophils less than 1,000 cells/mm^3, temperature equal to or greater than 38° C [100.4° F]), either reduce the dose of topotecan by 20% to 0.6 mg/M^2 for subsequent courses or give G-CSF (filgrastim) starting on Day 4 (24 hours after completion of topotecan). If febrile neutropenia occurs despite the use of filgrastim, further reduce dose to 0.45 mg/M^2 for subsequent courses. ▪ If platelet count falls below 10,000 cells/mm^3, reduce dose to 0.6 mg/M^2.
Cisplatin: See cisplatin monograph for specific dose adjustments. ▪ Topotecan in combination with cisplatin for treatment of cervical cancer should be initiated only in patients with a SCr equal to or less than 1.5 mg/dL. Discontinue cisplatin for a SCr greater than 1.5 mg/dL. Insufficient data available regarding continuation of topotecan as monotherapy after discontinuation of cisplatin.

DILUTION
Specific techniques required; see Precautions. Reconstitute each 4-mg vial with 4 mL of SW (1 mg/mL). Withdraw the calculated dose and further dilute in 50 to 100 mL of NS or D5W.
Filters: No data available from manufacturer.
Storage: Store unopened vials in cartons protected from light at CRT. Reconstituted solutions contain no preservative; use immediately. Solutions diluted for infusion are stable at room temperature in soft light for 24 hours.

COMPATIBILITY   (Underline Indicates Conflicting Compatibility Information)
Consider any drug NOT listed as compatible to be INCOMPATIBLE until consulting a pharmacist; specific conditions may apply.
One source suggests the following **compatibilities:**
Y-site: Carboplatin (Paraplatin), cisplatin (Platinol), cyclophosphamide (Cytoxan), doxorubicin (Adriamycin), etoposide (VePesid), gemcitabine (Gemzar), granisetron (Kytril), ifosfamide (Ifex), methylprednisolone (Solu-Medrol), metoclopramide (Reglan), ondansetron (Zofran), oxaliplatin (Eloxatin), paclitaxel (Taxol), palonosetron (Aloxi), prochlorperazine (Compazine), ticarcillin/clavulanate (Timentin), vincristine.

RATE OF ADMINISTRATION
A single dose as an infusion evenly distributed over 30 minutes.
Myelodysplastic syndrome/chronic myelomonocytic leukemia (unlabeled): See Usual Dose.

ACTIONS
A new class of antineoplastic agent that inhibits the enzyme topoisomerase I required for DNA replication. A topoisomerase I inhibitor, it is a semisynthetic derivative of camptothecin. Hydrolyzed to its active lactone form. Causes cell death by damaging DNA produced during the S-phase of cell synthesis. Distributes evenly between plasma and blood cells and is found in significant quantities in CSF. Minor additional metabolism occurs in the liver. Terminal half-life is from 2 to 3 hours. Moderately bound to plasma protein (35%). Some excretion in urine and bile.

INDICATIONS AND USES
Treatment of metastatic carcinoma of the ovary after failure of initial or subsequent chemotherapy. ▪ Treatment of small-cell lung cancer sensitive disease after failure of first-line chemotherapy. ▪ In combination with cisplatin for treatment of stage IV-B, recurrent or persistent cervical cancer not amenable to curative treatment with surgery and/or radiation therapy.

Unlabeled uses: Treatment of non–small-cell lung cancer. ▪ Treatment of myelodysplastic syndrome and chronic myelomonocytic leukemia (CMML).

CONTRAINDICATIONS
Severe hypersensitivity reactions (e.g., anaphylactoid) to topotecan or any of its components. Not recommended for use during pregnancy, breast-feeding, or in patients with severe bone marrow suppression.

PRECAUTIONS
Follow guidelines for handling cytotoxic agents. See Appendix A, p. 1429. ▪ Administered by or under the direction of the physician specialist. ▪ Adequate diagnostic and treatment facilities must be available to meet any medical emergency. ▪ Must have adequate bone marrow reserves. Bone marrow suppression (primarily neutropenia) is the dose-limiting toxicity. Anemia, Grade 3 and 4 neutropenia, pancytopenia, and thrombocytopenia have been reported; see Monitor. ▪ Use with caution in patients who have received previous cytotoxic drug therapy or radiation therapy. ▪ Use with caution in impaired renal function; clearance decreased. ▪ Use caution in patients with a history of allergies. ▪ Fatalities have occurred from neutropenia that resulted in neutropenic colitis; see Monitor. ▪ Fatalities have occurred from interstitial lung disease (ILD); risk increased in patients with a history of ILD, lung cancer, pulmonary fibrosis, thoracic exposure to radiation, and the use of pneumotoxic drugs and/or colony-stimulating factors.

Monitor: Baseline neutrophil count must be at least 1,500 cells/mm^3 and platelets at least 100,000 cell/mm^3 before the initial dose. ▪ Obtain a baseline CBC with differential and platelets. ▪ Monitor before each course and frequently during treatment. Platelet count must be 100,000/mm^3, neutrophils 1,000/mm^3, and hemoglobin 9 mg/dL before a course of therapy can be repeated. Anemia is frequent and transfusion is often indicated. ▪ Baseline CrCl and BUN suggested. ▪ Monitor vital signs. ▪ Maintain adequate hydration. ▪ Nausea and vomiting are frequent and may be severe; use prophylactic administration of antiemetics to increase patient comfort. ▪ Observe closely for S/S of infection. Prophylactic antibiotics may be indicated pending results of C/S in a febrile or nonfebrile neutropenic patient. ▪ Not a vesicant, but monitor injection site for inflammation and/or extravasation. ▪ Median duration of neutropenia is 7 days. Expected nadir for neutrophils is 12 days, 15 days for platelets and hemoglobin. ▪ Monitor for S/S of ILD (e.g., cough, dyspnea, fever, and/or hypoxia). ▪ Monitor for signs of neutropenic colitis (e.g., fever, neutropenia, and abdominal pain). ▪ Monitor for thrombocytopenia (platelet count less than 50,000/mm^3). Platelet transfusions may be required. Initiate precautions to prevent excessive bleeding (e.g., inspect IV sites, skin, and mucous membranes; use extreme care during invasive procedures; test urine, emesis, stool, and secretions for occult blood).

Patient Education: Nonhormonal birth control recommended. ▪ Report any unusual or unexpected symptoms or side effects as soon as possible (e.g., signs of infection [e.g., chills, fever, night sweats] or signs of bleeding [e.g., bruising, black tarry stools]). ▪ May cause loss of strength or fatigue. Use caution when driving or operating machinery. ▪ See Appendix D, p. 1434.

Maternal/Child: Category D: avoid pregnancy; can cause fetal harm. ▪ Discontinue breast-feeding. ▪ Safety and effectiveness for use in pediatric patients not established. One study showed that severe myelotoxicity may occur at lower doses in pediatric patients than in adults.

Elderly: Safety and effectiveness similar to younger adults; however, greater sensitivity of some older adults cannot be ruled out. ■ Consider age-related renal impairment; see Dose Adjustments. Monitoring of renal function may be useful.

DRUG/LAB INTERACTIONS

May cause severe prolonged myelosuppression and Grade 3 or 4 nonhematologic effects (e.g., diarrhea, lethargy, nausea, vomiting) with **cisplatin**. Interaction on myelosuppression is sequence dependent. Coadministration of a platinum agent on day 1 of topotecan therapy required lower doses of each agent compared to coadministration on day 5 of topotecan therapy. ■ Concurrent administration of **G-CSF (filgrastim)** can prolong the duration of neutropenia. If used, do not administer before day 6, at least 24 hours after the final dose of topotecan. ■ Concurrent or consecutive administration of **other bone marrow suppressants** (e.g., cyclophosphamide [Cytoxan], paclitaxel [Taxol]), **radiation therapy or agents that cause blood dyscrasias** (e.g., amphotericin B, anticonvulsants [e.g., phenytoin, valproic acid], NSAIDs [e.g., ibuprofen (Advil, Motrin), naproxen (Aleve, Naprosen)]) may produce additive bone marrow suppression. Dose reduction may be required based on blood cell counts. ■ Concurrent use of **immunosuppressants** (e.g., tacrolimus [Prograf], **corticosteroids, muromonab CD-3** [Orthoclone]) may increase the risk of infection. ■ **Probenecid** may decrease renal clearance and increase the risk of toxicity. ■ Do not administer **live or killed virus vaccines.**

SIDE EFFECTS

Bone marrow suppression, primarily neutropenia, is the dose-limiting toxicity of topotecan. Abdominal pain; alopecia; anorexia; asthenia; bone marrow toxicity such as anemia (less than 10 mg/dL [96%], less than 8 mg/dL [40%]), leukopenia (less than 3,000/mm^3 [98%], less than 1,000/mm^3 [32%]), neutropenia (less than 1,500/mm^3 [98%], less than 500/mm^3 [81%]), thrombocytopenia (less than 75,000/mm^3 [63%], less than 25,000/mm^3 [26%]); coagulation; constipation; coughing; diarrhea; dyspnea; fatigue; fever; headache; hemorrhage; infection with neutropenia less than 500/mm^3 (26%); nausea (77%); neuropathy; pain; paresthesia; rash; stomatitis; transient increases in AST and ALT; vomiting (58%); weakness.

Post-Marketing: Abdominal pain associated with neutropenic colitis, hypersensitivity reactions (including anaphylaxis), interstitial lung disease, severe bleeding, skin and subcutaneous tissue disorders (e.g., angioedema, severe dermatitis, severe pruritus).

ANTIDOTE

Keep physician informed of all side effects. Withhold topotecan until myelosuppression has improved to minimum requirements. Neutropenia recovery may be aided by G-CSF (filgrastim, pegfilgrastim [Neulasta]) under specific conditions; see Dose Adjustments or Drug/Lab Interactions. Anemia required RBC or whole blood tranfusions in 50% of patients. Thrombocytopenia may require platelet transfusion. Death can result from the progression of many side effects. Discontinue topotecan if a new diagnosis of ILD is confirmed. No known antidote for overdose. Symptomatic and supportive treatment is indicated. Treat hypersensitivity reactions with oxygen, epinephrine, corticosteroids, and antihistamines.

TORSEMIDE INJECTION
(**TOR**-seh-myd in-**JEK**-shun)

Demadex

Diuretic (loop)
Antihypertensive

pH over 8.3

USUAL DOSE
IV and oral doses are therapeutically equivalent. Oral dose can replace an IV dose at any time. If diuretic response is not adequate, titrate the recommended dose upward by doubling the dose until desired response achieved or maximum suggested dose reached.

Edema of congestive heart failure: 10 to 20 mg once daily. See general instructions above; single doses over 200 mg have not been adequately studied.

Edema of chronic renal failure: 20 mg once daily. See general instructions above; single doses over 200 mg have not been adequately studied.

Hepatic cirrhosis with ascites: 5 to 10 mg once daily. To prevent hypokalemia and metabolic alkalosis give in combination with an aldosterone antagonist (e.g., spironolactone [Aldactone]) or a potassium-sparing diuretic (e.g., dyazide). See general instructions above; single doses over 40 mg have not been adequately studied.

Hypertension: 5 mg once daily. May be increased to 10 mg in 4 to 6 weeks if BP reduction is inadequate. If response is still inadequate, the addition of other antihypertensive agents is recommended instead of larger doses of torsemide. Usually given PO.

Continuous infusion: Studies used a 100-mg dose divided as follows. A *loading dose* of 25 mg (2.5 mL) as an IV injection over 2 minutes (25% of total daily dose). Follow with an infusion at 3.1 mg/hr (10 mL/hr) or 75% of total daily dose equally distributed over 24 hours.

DOSE ADJUSTMENTS
Higher doses may be required in renal failure. See Drug/Lab Interactions.

DILUTION
Available as 10 mg/mL. May be given undiluted. May be given through Y-tube or three-way stopcock of infusion set. May be further diluted in NS, ½NS, or D5W. For a 75-mg dose (75% of the 100-mg total daily dose), dilute 7.5 mL to a total volume of 240 mL. 200 mg in 250 mL diluent yields 0.8 mg/mL. 50 mg in 500 mL diluent yields 0.1 mg/mL.

Storage: Store at CRT. Do not freeze.

COMPATIBILITY
Consider any drug NOT listed as compatible to be INCOMPATIBLE until consulting a pharmacist; specific conditions may apply.

Manufacturer recommends flushing the IV line before and after torsemide injection to avoid **incompatibilities** caused by alkaline pH.

One source suggests the following **compatibilities:**

Y-site: Milrinone (Primacor), nesiritide (Natrecor).

RATE OF ADMINISTRATION
Ototoxicity (usually reversible) has occurred with too-rapid injection and doses over 200 mg. Flush IV line with NS before and after administration.

IV injection: Each 200 mg or fraction thereof over 2 minutes.

Continuous infusion: Balance of daily dose after loading dose equally distributed over 24 hours. For a 75-mg dose, the rate would be 3.1 mg (10 mL/hr) for 24 hours.

ACTIONS

A sulfonamide type loop diuretic. Acts from within the ascending portion of the loop of Henle to excrete water, sodium, chlorides, and some potassium. Diuretic action correlates better with the rate of drug excretion in urine than with plasma concentration. Will produce diuresis in alkalosis or acidosis. Effects begin within 10 minutes and peak within 1 hour. Diuresis lasts 6 to 8 hours. Highly protein bound. Metabolized by the liver (80%). 20% eliminated via urinary excretion. Other loop diuretics cross the placental barrier and are secreted in breast milk; specific information not available for torsemide.

INDICATIONS AND USES

Treatment of edema associated with congestive heart failure, cirrhosis of the liver with ascites, and chronic renal failure. Used when a rapid onset of diuresis is desired or when oral administration is impractical. ▪ Treatment of hypertension.

CONTRAINDICATIONS

Known hypersensitivity to torsemide or to sulfonylureas and in anuric patients.

PRECAUTIONS

Tests to determine serum levels of torsemide not widely available. ▪ In patients with congestive heart failure and/or renal failure, a smaller dose is actually delivered to the ascending loop of Henle, resulting in less response at any given dose. ▪ Use caution and improve basic condition first in hepatic coma, electrolyte depletion, and advanced cirrhosis of the liver. Initiation of therapy in the hospital is preferred. ▪ Use extreme caution in patients sensitive to bumetanide, furosemide (Lasix), or sulfonamides (including thiazide diuretics); may also be sensitive to torsemide. ▪ In patients with hepatic disease with cirrhosis and ascites use a potassium-sparing diuretic (e.g., dyazide) or an aldosterone antagonist (e.g., spironolactone) concurrently to prevent hypokalemia and metabolic alkalosis. ▪ Use caution in acute MI; excessive diuresis may precipitate shock. ▪ In nonanuric renal failure, may cause marked increases in water and sodium excretion without impacting steady-state fluid retention. High doses (500 to 1,200 mg) have caused seizures. ▪ May activate or exacerbate systemic lupus erythematosus. Chronic use in renal or hepatic disease has not been adequately studied. ▪ Antihypertensive effects greater in black patients. **Monitor:** Monitor BP frequently, especially during initial therapy. May precipitate excessive diuresis with water and electrolyte depletion. Dehydration, electrolyte imbalance, hypovolemia, prerenal axotemia, embolism, or thrombosis can occur. Routine checks on electrolyte panel, CO_2, and BUN are necessary during therapy. Potassium chloride and/or magnesium replacement may be required. ▪ Risk of hypokalemia greatest in patients with cirrhosis of the liver, during brisk diuresis, with inadequate oral electrolyte intake, or with concurrent administration of corticosteroids (e.g., prednisone). ▪ May increase blood glucose, serum cholesterol, and triglycerides. ▪ Slight increases in BUN, SCr, and uric acid may occur, usually reverse when therapy discontinued. Sudden changes in fluid and electrolyte balance may precipitate hepatic coma in patients with hepatic disease and ascites. ■ Rarely precipitates an attack of gout. ■ See Drug/ Lab Interactions.

Patient Education: Hypotension may cause dizziness; request assistance with ambulation. ■ May cause a decrease in potassium levels and require a supplement. ■ Possible skin photosensitivity. Avoid unprotected exposure to sunlight. ■ Report cramps, dizziness, muscle weakness, or nausea promptly.

Maternal/Child: Category B: use only if clearly needed during pregnancy; safety for use not established. ■ Safety for use during breast-feeding not established; other loop diuretics suggest discontinuing breast-feeding. ■ Safety and effectiveness for use in pediatric patients under 18 years of age not established. Administration of other loop diuretics to premature infants with edema due to patent ductus arteriosus and hyaline membrane disease may have caused renal calcifications; also other loop diuretics may have increased the risk of persistent patient ductus arteriosus in premature infants with hyaline membrane disease. Torsemide has not been studied in these situations.

Elderly: No specific age-related differences; dose adjustment not indicated. May be more susceptible to dehydration; observe carefully. ■ Avoid rapid contraction of plasma volume and hemoconcentration. May cause thromboembolic episodes (e.g., CVA, pulmonary emboli).

DRUG/LAB INTERACTIONS

Concurrent administration with **high-dose salicylates** may cause salicylate toxicity. ■ Probenicid decreases the diuretic activity of torsemide. ■ May reduce renal clearance of spironolactone, but dose adjustment not required. ■ Has been administered with beta-blockers (e.g., atenolol), ACE inhibitors (e.g., captopril), calcium-channel blockers (e.g., diltiazem), cimetidine (Tagamet), digoxin, and nitrates (e.g., nitroglycerin) without new or unexpected adverse events; however, torsemide has caused severe hypotension with **ACE inhibitors** in sodium- or volume-depleted patients. ■ Does not affect protein binding of glyburide (DiaBeta) or coumarin derivatives (e.g., warfarin). ■ May cause excessive potassium depletion with **amphotericin B** (generic, Abelcet), **corticosteroids, thiazide diuretics** (e.g., hydrochlorothiazide [HydroDiuril]). Monitor electrolytes closely. ■ May cause cardiac arrhythmias with **digoxin and other antiarrhythmic agents** secondary to potassium and magnesium depletion. ■ **NSAIDs** (e.g., indomethacin [Indocin], ibuprofen [Advil, Motrin], naproxen [Aleve, Naprosyn]) **or salicylates** (e.g., aspirin) may cause retention of sodium and water and may decrease diuretic and antihypertensive effects. ■ Antihypertensive effects may be increased by any **hypotension-producing agent** (e.g., lidocaine, nitroglycerin, nitroprusside sodium, paclitaxel); reduced dose of the antihypertensive agent or both drugs may be indicated. ■ May potentiate **propranolol, salicylates, muscle relaxants** (e.g., atracurium [Tracrium]), and hypotensive effect of **other diuretics.** ■ May increase ototoxicity in doses exceeding the usual or in conjunction with **ototoxic drugs** (e.g., cisplatin, aminoglycosides [e.g., amikacin, streptomycin, gentamicin], ethacrynic acid [Edecrin]). ■ May increase nephrotoxicity if given concurrently with **any other nephrotoxic agent** (e.g., amphotericin B, aminoglycosides [e.g., gentamicin], foscarnet [Foscavir], rifampin [Rifadin]). Concurrent use with **amphotericin B** is not recommended, especially in patients with some impaired renal function. ■ Effects of **warfarin** (Coumadin) are increased; may require dose adjustment. ■ May be inhibited by **phenytoin** (Dilantin). ■ May reduce excretion of **lithium** and cause lithium toxicity. ■ May increase or decrease effectiveness of **theophyllines.**

SIDE EFFECTS

Arthralgia, constipation, cough, diarrhea, dizziness, dyspepsia, ECG abnormalities, edema, electrolyte imbalance, esophageal hemorrhage, excessive thirst, excessive urination, headache, hyperglycemia, hyperuricemia, hypokalemia, impotence, insomnia, myalgia, nervousness, ototoxicity (usually reversible), rhinitis, sore throat, and tinnitus have all been reported. Hypersensitivity reactions can occur. Hypocalcemia and hypomagnesemia have been minimal with usual doses.

Major: Anorexia, dizziness, drowsiness, dryness of the mouth, hypotension, increased BUN, lethargy; mental confusion, muscle cramps, fatigue, or pain; nausea and vomiting, oliguria, restlessness, tachycardia, thirst, or weakness may indicate severe electrolyte imbalance, hypovolemia, or prerenal azotemia.

Overdose: Circulatory collapse, dehydration, excessive diuresis, hemoconcentration, hypochloremic alkalosis, hyperchloremia or hypochloremia, hyperkalemia or hypokalemia, hypomagnesemia, hypernatremia or hyponatremia, hypotension, hypovolemia, vascular thrombosis, and embolism.

ANTIDOTE

Notify the physician of any side effect. Depending on severity the physician may treat the side effects symptomatically and either continue or discontinue torsemide. Fluid and electrolyte replacement may be indicated. If side effects are progressive or any major side effects or signs of overdose appear, discontinue the drug immediately and notify the physician. Treatment of overdose is symptomatic and aggressive. Hemodialysis is not effective in overdose. Resuscitate as necessary. Torsemide may be restarted at a lower dose after the patient is stable.

TOSITUMOMAB AND IODINE-131 TOSITUMOMAB BBW

(toes-ih-**TOO**-moh-mab)

Radiopharmaceutical
Monoclonal antibody
Antineoplastic

Bexxar

pH 7.2 and 7

USUAL DOSE

A therapeutic regimen consisting of pretesting and premedication followed by four components administered in two specific steps: the dosimetric step, followed 7 to 14 days later by a therapeutic step. Each step consists of a sequential infusion of tositumomab followed by iodine-131 (I-131) tositumomab. Intended as a single course of treatment; safety of multiple courses of this regimen or combination with other forms of irradiation or chemotherapy have not been evaluated.

PRETESTING

Pretesting required; see Monitor. Do not administer to patients with a platelet count less than 100,000 cells/mm^3, neutrophils less than 1,500 cells/mm^3, or greater than 25% lymphoma marrow involvement and/or impaired bone marrow reserve.

PREMEDICATION

Prophylaxis to reduce the risk of hypothyroidism: Thyroid-protective agents *must be started at least 24 hours before the dosimetric step begins and continued daily until 2 weeks after the therapeutic dose is completed.* May be *one of three* agents: saturated solution of potassium iodide (SSKI) 4 drops PO three times daily, Lugol's solution 20 drops PO three times daily, or potassium iodide tablets 130 mg PO daily. Patients who cannot tolerate these thyroid-blocking agents may not begin the regimen. *Do not give dosimetric dose unless the patient has received at least 3 doses of SSKI, three doses of Lugol's solution, or one 130-mg potassium iodide tablet.*

Prophylaxis to prevent or reduce infusion reactions: Administer 30 minutes before both the dosimetric step and the therapeutic step.

Acetaminophen: 650 mg PO
and
Diphenhydramine: 50 mg PO

DAY BEFORE DOSIMETRIC STEP (DAY −1)

Begin **thyroid-protective regimen** with one of the three agents listed under Premedication. Continue daily through 14 days post-therapeutic dose.

DAY OF DOSIMETRIC STEP (DAY 0)

Premedicate with *acetaminophen* 650 mg and *diphenhydramine* 50 mg. Both are given PO 30 minutes before infusion begins.

Tositumomab: 450 mg as an infusion over 60 minutes. Follow with I-131 tositumomab (containing 5 mCi I-131 and 35 mg tositumomab) as an infusion over 20 minutes. *Specific process required;* see Dilution and Rate of Administration.

Biodistribution: Whole-body dosimetry and biodistribution. The therapeutic dose will be based on information from three scans taken during the dosimetric step:

1st image (scan): Within 1 hour of the end of the infusion of I-131 tositumomab. Do not allow patient to void; must have urine in the bladder when this image is taken.

2nd image (scan): 2 to 4 days after I-131 tositumomab infusion and immediately following patient voiding.

3rd image (scan): 6 to 7 days after I-131 tositumomab infusion and immediately following patient voiding.

DAY 6 OR 7

Assessment of biodistribution of I-131 tositumomab: *If biodistribution is not acceptable, stop therapy now.* If biodistribution is acceptable, therapy with the therapeutic dose can proceed. On this day the radiation oncologist must calculate the exact dose activity to be ordered based on patient parameters (e.g., CBC, differential, platelets). May be given on any day from Day 7 to Day 14. Specific date may be selected based on patient parameters, availability of the radioactive component, or patient or physician convenience.

THERAPEUTIC STEP: DAY 7 TO DAY 14 (SELECT ONE DAY)

Do not administer if biodistribution is altered.

Thyroid-protective agents: Have been administered every day and will continue for at least 2 more weeks.

Premedicate with *acetaminophen* 650 mg and *diphenhydramine* 50 mg. Both are given PO 30 minutes before infusion begins.

Tositumomab: 450 mg as an infusion over 60 minutes. Follow with calculated therapeutic dose of I-131 tositumomab (calculated dose of I-131 and 35 mg tositumomab) as an infusion over 20 minutes. *Specific process required;* see Dilution and Rate of Administration.

Dose of I-131 is administered based on platelet count as follows:

Platelets equal to or greater than 150,000/mm³: Activity of I-131 calculated to deliver 75 cGy total-body irradiation.

Platelets equal to or greater than 100,000/mm³ but less than 150,000/mm³: Activity of I-131 calculated to deliver 65 cGy total-body irradiation.

Do not treat patients with a platelet count less than 100,000/mm³.

DOSE ADJUSTMENTS

See Usual Dose under Therapeutic Step.

DILUTION

Tositumomab is supplied in a carton containing two single-use 225-mg vials and one single-use 35-mg vial for both the dosimetric and therapeutic steps (14 mg/mL). Available from McKesson Biosciences. *I-131 tositumomab* for the dosimetric step is supplied in a package containing one single-use vial (0.61 mCi/mL at calibration). For the therapeutic step, it is supplied in a package containing one or two single-use vials (5.6 mCi/mL at calibration). Both are supplied by NDS Nordion. Availability of supplies must be confirmed by the radiation specialist before scheduling therapy.

Tositumomab: To prepare for the dosimetric and therapeutic steps of the 450-mg tositumomab dose, additional supplies needed include 50-mL syringe(s), 18-gauge needle(s), and a 50-mL infusion bag of NS. Withdraw 32 mL of NS from the 50-mL infusion bag of NS and discard (approximately 18 mL will remain). Withdraw entire contents from each of the two

225-mg vials (450 mg tositumomab in 32 mL) and transfer to the infusion bag containing 18 mL of NS. Final volume is 50 mL. Gently mix by inverting and rotating the bag; *do not shake.* Solution may contain some white particles (expected). Additional supplies are needed for administration; see Rate of Administration.

I-131 tositumomab: All supplies, preparation, calibration, confirmation of radiochemical purity, and administration of these doses in both the dosimetric and therapeutic steps will be provided by personnel authorized to handle radiopharmaceuticals and certified to administer this therapeutic regimen. Each requires a specific order and specific timing of preparation. For additional information, see prescribing information.

Filters: Must be administered through a 0.22-micron in-line filter. The same primary IV tubing set and filter must be used throughout the entire dosimetric step. A change in filter during the procedure can result in loss of drug. Another IV tubing and filter must be used throughout the entire therapeutic step.

Storage: *Tositumomab:* Prior to dilution, refrigerate 35-mg and 225-mg vials at 2° to 8° C (36° to 46° F). Diluted solutions are stable for 24 hours refrigerated or 8 hours at CRT. In all concentrations, protect from strong light. *Do not shake.* Do not freeze. Discard any unused portions. *I-131 tositumomab:* Stored in radiation therapy freezer at −20° C or below in original lead pots until removed for thawing before administration. Thawed doses are stable for up to 8 hours refrigerated or at room temperature. Do not use beyond expiration date. Discard unused portions according to specific regulations.

COMPATIBILITY

A radiopharmaceutical. Use only as directed. Should not be mixed or diluted with other drugs.

RATE OF ADMINISTRATION

Reduce rate by 50% for mild infusion reactions. Discontinue for severe infusion reactions.

Tositumomab 450-mg dose (dosimetric and therapeutic): If unit staff will be administering these doses, correlate timing with the radiation oncologist directing the procedure. Supplies required include the following:

A. One IV filter set (0.22-micron filter) with injection site (port) and Luer-Lok.
B. One primary IV infusion set.
C. One 100-mL bag of NS for infusion.
D. Two secondary IV infusion sets.
E. One IV extension set, 30-inch Luer-Lok.
F. One 3-way stopcock.
G. One 50-mL bag of NS for infusion.
H. One infusion pump for tositumomab infusion.
I. One syringe pump for I-131 tositumomab infusion.
J. Lead shielding for use in administration of dosimetric dose of I-131.

The procedure is as follows:

Attach the primary IV infusion set (B) to the 0.22-micron in-line filter set (A) and the 100-mL bag of NS for infusion (C).

After priming the primary IV infusion set (B) and IV filter set (A), connect the infusion bag containing 450 mg tositumomab (50 mL) via a secondary IV infusion set (D) to the primary IV infusion set (B) to a port distal to the 0.22-micron in-line filter. Carefully prime this second infusion set from the 50-mL solution of tositumomab so as not to waste any drug. A single dose must be administered evenly distributed over 60 minutes via an infusion pump.

After completion of the infusion, disconnect the secondary IV infusion set (D) and flush the primary IV infusion set (B) and the in-line filter set (A) with NS. Leave the primary line and filter extension intact; the pre-wetted filter must be used for delivery of the radioactive component. Discard the tositumomab bag and secondary IV infusion set.

I-131 tositumomab 35-mg dose: Preparation, calibration, confirmation of radiochemical purity, administration, and disposal of these doses and the equipment used to deliver them in both the dosimetric and therapeutic steps will be provided by personnel authorized to handle radiopharmaceuticals and certified to administer this therapeutic regimen. Administration will be via a syringe pump using an appropriate shield, new secondary IV tubing, and the same primary line and pre-wetted filter used for the previously administered (450-mg) dose. A single dose must be administered evenly distributed over 20 minutes. Actual delivered dose will be calculated by the radiation oncologist. All materials must be discarded according to federal regulations.

ACTIONS

An antineoplastic, radioimmunotherapeutic, monoclonal antibody–based regimen composed of the monoclonal antibody, tositumomab, and the radiolabeled monoclonal antibody (I-131 tositumomab). Tositumomab is a murine IgG_{2a} monoclonal antibody directed against the CD20 antigen found on the surface of normal and malignant B lymphocytes. I-131 tositumomab is tositumomab that has been covalently linked to I-131. Tositumomab binds to the CD20 antigen. This antigen is expressed on pre-B lymphocytes and mature B lymphocytes. It is also expressed in more than 90% of non-Hodgkin's lymphomas (NHL). Thought to act by inducing cell self-destruction through fragmentation of DNA. Additional cell death may be caused by the radioisotope, complement-dependent cytotoxicity, and antibody-dependent cellular toxicity. Regimen results in sustained depletion of circulating CD20-positive cells. Lymphocyte recovery began at approximately 12 weeks following treatment. Eliminated in urine and through decay. Radioiodine is secreted in breast milk.

INDICATIONS AND USES

Treatment of patients with CD20-positive, follicular, non-Hodgkin's lymphoma, with and without transformation, whose disease is refractory to rituximab and has relapsed following chemotherapy. ▪ Not indicated for the initial treatment of patients with CD20-positive non-Hodgkin's lymphoma.

CONTRAINDICATIONS

Known hypersensitivity to murine proteins or any component of the regimen. ▪ Patients who cannot tolerate the thyroid-blocking agents may not begin the regimen. ▪ Should not be administered to patients with greater than 25% lymphoma marrow involvement and/or impaired bone marrow reserve. ▪ Do not administer a therapeutic dose to patients with altered biodistribution as determined by imaging with I-131 tositumomab.

PRECAUTIONS

Radiopharmaceuticals are administered by or under the direction of the physician specialist whose experience and training in the safe use and handling of radionuclides have been approved by the appropriate government agency. In addition, the specific physician administering I-131 tositumomab should either be participating in a certification program or have been certified in the preparation and administration of this therapeutic regimen. ▪ Administer in a facility with adequate personnel, equipment, and supplies to monitor the patient and respond to any medical emergency. ▪ Safety for use in patients with a platelet count less than 100,000 cells/mm³ or a neutrophil count less than 1,500 cells/mm³ has not been established. ▪ During and after radiolabeling, care should be taken to minimize radiation exposure to patients and to medical personnel consistent with institutional good radiation safety practices and patient management procedures. Contact the radiation safety officer. ▪ Use of rubber gloves is recommended if handling of radioactive materials or supplies is necessary. If a splash occurs, flush eyes for at least 15 minutes. For skin contact, wash affected areas thoroughly with soap and water and blot dry; do not abrade skin. In both situations, notify the radiation safety officer and continue the process until no more radiation can be detected. ▪ May cause severe hypersensitivity reactions, including anaphylaxis; see Monitor, Side Effects, and Antidote. ▪ Biodistribution of I-131 tositumomab on the first day occurs mainly in the blood pool (heart and major blood vessels), liver, and spleen. Second and third imaging time points reflect decreased accumulation in the blood pool, liver, and spleen and may show uptake by the thyroid, kidneys, and other organs. Tumors show areas of increased intensity. Altered biodistribution on the first day may be visualized as little or no activity in the blood pool, intense uptake in the liver or spleen, greater uptake in the lungs than in the blood pool, or uptake suggestive of urinary obstruction. Altered biodistribution on the second and third imaging time points may suggest urinary obstruction, diffuse lung uptake greater than the blood pool, or total-body residence times of less than 50 hours and more than 150 hours. ▪ Patients with a high tumor burden, splenomegaly, or bone marrow involvement were noted to have a faster clearance, shorter terminal half-life, and larger volume of distribution. ▪ May cause prolonged, severe, and life-threatening cytopenias (neutropenia, thrombocytopenia); see Contraindications, Monitor, Side Effects, and Antidote. ▪ Impaired renal function may decrease the rate of excretion of the radiolabeled iodine and increase patient exposure to this radioactive component. ▪ Has a potential for immunogenicity; patients who have received murine proteins should be screened for human anti-mouse antibodies (HAMA); may be at increased risk for hypersensitivity reactions. ▪ Many individuals are allergic to shellfish and may have a hypersensitivity reaction to iodine. ▪ Myelodysplastic syndrome and secondary malignancies have been reported. ▪ Safety of immunization with live virus vaccines not studied. Ability to generate a primary or anamnestic humoral response to any vaccine has not been studied. ▪ See Contraindications.

Monitor: Obtain baseline CBC with differential and platelets, thyroid-stimulating hormone (TSH) levels, and SCr. ▪ Monitor CBC with differential and platelets weekly for 10 to 12 weeks or more frequently if indicated (e.g., cytopenias, concurrent drugs). Continue until recovery. Cytopenias (e.g., neutropenia and thrombocytopenia) can be severe and may be fatal. Time to nadir was 4 to 7 weeks, and the duration of cytopenias was approximately 30 days. Anemia, neutropenia, and thrombocytopenia may persist for more than 90 days, and some patients died without recovering. ▪ Monitor for S/S of hypersensitivity reactions and/or infusion reactions (e.g., bronchospasm, chills, dyspnea, fever, hypotension, injection site hypersensitivity, itching, nausea, rash, serum sickness); see Precautions and Antidote. Have occurred during or within 48 hours of infusion or up to 2 weeks after infusion. ▪ To reduce unnecessary radiation exposure to vital organs (e.g., thyroid, kidneys, bladder), patients should be well hydrated before, during, and for at least 1 day after the final dose. Encourage fluid intake and frequent voiding. Impaired renal function may decrease the rate of excretion of the radiolabeled iodine and increase patient exposure to the radioactive component. ▪ Establish a free-flowing IV line before administration; avoid extravasation. Monitor closely; if any signs of extravasation occur, discontinue immediately and restart in another vein. ▪ Monitor for thrombocytopenia (platelet count less than 50,000/mm^3) for up to 3 months. Initiate precautions to prevent excessive bleeding (e.g., inspect IV sites, skin, and mucous membranes; use extreme care during invasive procedures; test urine, emesis, stool, and secretions for occult blood). ▪ Observe closely for signs of infection for up to 3 months. Prophylactic antibiotics may be indicated pending results of C/S in a febrile neutropenic patient. ▪ Monitor for S/S of hypothyroidism (e.g., cold intolerance, drooping eyelids, facial puffiness, thinning hair). Screen for biochemical evidence of hypothyroidism by monitoring TSH annually. ▪ See Precautions, Drug/Lab Interactions, and Antidote.

Patient Education: Avoid pregnancy; effective birth control is recommended for males and females during treatment and for up to 12 months following therapy. Women should report a suspected pregnancy immediately. ▪ Increased fluid intake and frequent voiding are important to aid in excretion of the drug. ▪ Promptly report S/S of a hypersensitivity reaction (e.g., chills, fever, difficulty breathing, faintness, itching, rash), S/S of infection (e.g., fever, sore throat), or S/S of bleeding (e.g., bruising, nosebleed, dark stools). ▪ Compliance with daily medications for thyroid protection imperative; monitoring for hypothyroidism will continue. ▪ Side effects, especially reduced blood counts, may persist for many weeks; close follow-up with physician is imperative. ▪ Radiation department should provide instructions for minimizing exposure of family members, friends, and the general public. ▪ Review all Precautions before treatment begins.

Maternal/Child: Category X: avoid pregnancy; may cause harm to the fetal thyroid gland, and radioiodide may cause severe, and possibly irreversible, hypothyroidism in neonates. ▪ Women of childbearing potential should avoid becoming pregnant. ▪ Could cause toxic effects on testes and ovaries. Effective contraceptive methods are recommended for men and women during treatment and for up to 12 months following therapy. ▪ Discontinue breast-feeding. ▪ Safety and effectiveness for use in pediatric patients not established.

Elderly: Preliminary data suggests that the overall response rate was lower in patients age 65 and over and the duration of response was shorter. ▪ Incidence of severe hematologic toxicity was lower, but the duration was longer. ▪ Greater sensitivity of some older individuals cannot be ruled out.

DRUG/LAB INTERACTIONS

Drug interaction studies have not been performed. ▪ Risk of bleeding may be increased by **any medicine that affects blood clotting,** including anticoagulants (e.g., heparin, lepirudin [Refludan], warfarin [Coumadin]); **any medication that may cause hypoprothrombinemia, thrombocytopenia, or GI ulceration or bleeding** (e.g., selected antibiotics [e.g., cefotetan], aspirin,

NSAIDs [e.g., ibuprofen (Advil, Motrin), naproxen (Aleve, Naprosyn)]); **and/or any other medication that inhibits platelet aggregation** (e.g., dipyridamole [Persantine], glycoprotein GPIIb/IIIa receptor antagonists [e.g., abciximab (ReoPro), eptifibatide (Integrilin), tirofiban (Aggrastat)], plicamycin [Mithracin], sulfinpyrazone [Anturane], ticlopidine [Ticlid], valproate [Depacon]). ■ Safety of immunization with live virus vaccines has not been studied. ■ Potential for additive effects with previously administered bone marrow–suppressing agents and/or radiation therapy has not been studied.

SIDE EFFECTS

Most common side effects included anemia, neutropenia, and thrombocytopenia (prolonged and severe). Dehydration, pleural effusion, and pneumonia were severe but less common. Other reported side effects that may or may not be related to tositumomab and may be reported within days or be delayed included abdominal pain, anorexia, arthralgia, asthenia, back pain, chest pain, chills, constipation, cough, diarrhea, dizziness, dyspepsia, dyspnea, fever, headache, hypotension, hypothyroidism, infection, myalgia, nausea and vomiting, neck pain, pain, peripheral edema, pharyngitis, pruritus, rash, rhinitis, somnolence, sweating, vasodilation, weight loss. Abdominal pain and nausea and vomiting often occur days after the infusion. Diarrhea may occur days to weeks after the infusion. Other delayed side effects may include HAMA, hypothyroidism, myelodysplastic syndrome (MDS), secondary leukemia, and secondary malignancies. **Major:** Severe and prolonged cytopenias and the sequelae of cytopenias, including infections (sepsis) and hemorrhage in thrombocytopenic patients, allergic reactions and infusion-related reactions (e.g., bronchospasm, chills, dyspnea, fever, hypotension, injection site hypersensitivity, itching, nausea, rash, serum sickness), secondary leukemia, and myelodysplasia.

ANTIDOTE

Keep physician informed of all side effects. May constitute a medical emergency or will be treated symptomatically as indicated. Hypersensitivity or infusion-related side effects to any component of the regimen may resolve by slowing the rate of infusion by 50% or interrupting the infusion and by providing supportive care (IV saline; diphenhydramine; bronchodilators such as albuterol [Ventolin], or aminophylline; and acetaminophen). Discontinue entire regimen in patients who develop severe hypersensitivity reactions. Treat anaphylaxis with oxygen, antihistamines (diphenhydramine), epinephrine, and corticosteroids. Maintain a patent airway. If overdose occurs, monitor closely for cytopenias and radiation-related toxicity. Autologous stem cell transplantation has not been studied; consider timing in relation to dosing to minimize the possibility of irradiation of infused hematopoietic stem cells. Administration of whole blood products (e.g., packed RBCs, platelets, leukocytes) and/or blood modifiers (e.g., darbepoetin alfa [Aranesp], epoetin alfa [Epogen], filgrastim [Neupogen], oprelvekin [Neumega], pegfilgrastim [Neulasta], sargramostim [Leukine]) may be indicated to treat bone marrow toxicity or to treat moderate to severe bleeding. Control minor bleeding by local pressure. For severe bleeding, delay or discontinue therapy and obtain PT, aPTT, platelet count, and fibrinogen. Draw blood for type and cross-match. Antibiotic therapy is indicated for infections and may be indicated prophylactically. Death may occur from the progression of some side effects. Resuscitate as indicated.

TRACE METALS
(tras **MET**-als)

Chromium	MulTE-PAK-5
Copper	Multiple Trace Element With
Iodine	Selenium
Manganese	Multiple Trace Element With
Molybdenum	Selenium Concentrated
M.T.E.-4, 5, 6, & 7	Multitrace-5 Concentrated
M.T.E.-4, 5, & 6 Concentrated	Selenium
MulTE-PAK-4	Zinc

Multiple Trace Element Neonatal, Neotrace-4, PedTE-PAK-4, P.T.E.-4, P.T.E.-5

USUAL DOSE

Available as single elements, selected combined elements in various strengths, and in combination with electrolytes. *Some preparations may contain aluminum; see Precautions.* Selection of correct product based on minimum daily requirement and individual needs.

Chromium: 10 to 15 mcg/day. Increase to 20 mcg/day with intestinal fluid loss.

Copper: 0.5 to 1.5 mg/day.

Iodine: 1 to 2 mcg/kg of body weight/day. Increase to 2 to 3 mcg/kg/day in growing children, pregnant and lactating women.

Manganese: 0.15 to 0.8 mg/day. May contain up to 100 mcg/L of aluminum; see Precautions.

Molybdenum: 20 to 120 mcg/day. Increase to 163 mcg/day for 21 days in deficiency states resulting from prolonged TPN.

Selenium: 20 to 40 mcg/day. Increase to 100 mcg/day for 31 days in deficiency states resulting from prolonged TPN.

Zinc: 2.5 to 4 mg/day; add 2 mg in acute catabolic states. Increase to 12.2 mg/L of total parenteral nutrition (TPN) if there is fluid loss from the small bowel. May contain aluminum.

PEDIATRIC DOSE

Chromium: 0.14 to 0.2 mcg/kg/day.

Copper: 20 mcg/kg/day.

Manganese: 2 to 10 mcg/kg/day. May contain up to 100 mcg/L of aluminum; see Precautions.

Molybdenum: Must calculate dosage by extrapolation; consult pharmacist.

Selenium: 3 mcg/kg/day.

Zinc: 100 mcg/kg/day for full-term infants and other pediatric patients up to 5 years of age. 300 mcg/kg/day for premature infants with birth weights from 1,500 Gm to 3 kg. May contain aluminum.

DOSE ADJUSTMENTS

Reduce or omit dose in impaired renal function. ■ Caution and lower-end dosing may be appropriate in the elderly; consider decreased organ function and concomitant disease or drug therapy.

DILUTION

Must be added to daily volume of IV infusion fluids including TPN. Check labels for aluminum content; see Precautions.

COMPATIBILITY

Specific trace metals may present **compatibility** problems. Check **incompatibilities** of each agent to be admixed or delivered to the **Y-site.**

RATE OF ADMINISTRATION

Administer properly diluted at rate prescribed for IV infusion fluids or TPN.

ACTIONS

All are basic elements present in the human body. Specific amounts required to initiate, facilitate, or maintain appropriate body systems.

INDICATIONS AND USES

Nutritional supplement to IV solutions given for total parenteral or central nutrition.

CONTRAINDICATIONS

Do not give direct IV; hypersensitivity to any component (especially iodides). Manganese contraindicated in presence of high manganese levels. Molybdenum without copper supplementation contraindicated in copper-deficient patients.

PRECAUTIONS

Selenium enhances vitamin E and decreases the toxicity of mercury, cadmium, and arsenic. ▪ Patients with biliary tract obstruction may retain copper and manganese. ▪ Avoid copper in patients with Wilson's disease (genetic disorder of copper metabolism). ▪ Assess possibility of diabetes mellitus when giving chromium supplements to maintain normal glucose metabolism. ▪ Some solutions may contain aluminum (e.g., manganese, zinc). In impaired kidney function, aluminum may reach toxic levels. Premature neonates are particularly at risk because of their immature kidneys and requirement for calcium and phosphate, which also contain aluminum. Research indicates that patients with impaired renal function who receive more than 4 to 5 mcg/kg/day of parenteral aluminum are at risk for developing CNS or bone toxicity associated with aluminum accumulation.

Monitor: Monitor serum trace metal concentration to avoid accumulation. Results will also determine use of a single element or a combined product.

Maternal/Child: Category C: use in pregnancy only if clearly indicated. Use manganese with caution in the nursing mother. ▪ May contain benzyl alcohol; may cause fatal "gasping" syndrome in premature infants.

Elderly: Differences in response compared to younger adults not identified. ▪ Dosing should be cautious; see Dose Adjustments.

DRUG/LAB INTERACTIONS

Therapeutic serum levels of **copper and zinc** will decrease if not given together.

SIDE EFFECTS

Toxicity is rare at recommended doses. Iodine may cause anaphylaxis.

ANTIDOTE

Dosage will be adjusted based on serum levels. Keep physician informed. Resuscitate as necessary.

TRASTUZUMAB BBW

(traz-**TOO**-zah-mab)

Herceptin

Monoclonal antibody
Antineoplastic

pH 6

USUAL DOSE

Premedication: Pretreatment with antihistamines (e.g., diphenhydramine [Benadryl]) and/or corticosteroids (e.g., dexamethasone [Decadron]) may be indicated and is suggested for patients being retreated after a hypersensitivity reaction or a severe infusion reaction; see Precautions. Pretreatment may not be successful; hypersensitivity reaction and/or infusion reaction may recur. Preassessment required; see Monitor. Combination therapies may require additional premedication; refer to product monographs.

Adjuvant treatment of breast cancer: Administer according to one of the following dose regimens and schedules for a total of 52 weeks of trastuzumab therapy:

1. *During and following paclitaxel, docetaxel, or docetaxel/carboplatin:* Administer an initial dose of **trastuzumab** 4 mg/kg as an infusion over 90 minutes. Follow with a dose of 2 mg/kg as an infusion over 30 minutes at weekly intervals for the first 12 weeks when given in combination with *paclitaxel or docetaxel* or for 18 weeks when given in combination with *docetaxel/carboplatin.* Beginning 1 week after the last 2-mg/kg weekly dose of **trastuzumab,** administer **trastuzumab** 6 mg/kg as an infusion over 30 to 90 minutes every 3 weeks.

2. *As a single agent within 3 weeks of completion of multimodality, anthracycline-based chemotherapy regimens,* administer an initial dose of **trastuzumab** 8 mg/kg as an infusion over 90 minutes. Follow with a dose of 6 mg/kg as an infusion over 30 to 90 minutes every 3 weeks.

3. See clinical studies in prescribing information for different treatment regimens used. In all studies, **trastuzumab** was initiated *after completion of the doxorubicin and cyclophosphamide treatment cycles.*

Metastatic breast cancer: *Initial dose:* 4 mg/kg as an infusion over 90 minutes. Follow with a *maintenance dose* of 2 mg/kg as an infusion over 30 minutes at weekly intervals. Trastuzumab is administered until tumor progression.

Metastatic breast cancer in combination therapy with paclitaxel: *Trastuzumab* dose as above. *Paclitaxel dose:* 175 mg/M^2 over 3 hours every 21 days for at least 6 cycles. See paclitaxel monograph.

Metastatic gastric cancer in combination with cisplatin and capecitabine or 5-fluorouracil: *Initial dose:* 8 mg/kg as an infusion over 90 minutes. Follow with a dose of 6 mg/kg as an infusion over 30 to 90 minutes every 3 weeks until disease progression. See individual monographs and specific protocol for doses of cisplatin and capecitabine (Xeloda) or 5-fluorouracil (5-FU).

DOSE ADJUSTMENTS

Withhold trastuzumab dose for at least 4 weeks for either of the following:
- Equal to or greater than a 16% absolute decrease in left ventricular ejection fraction (LVEF) from baseline assessment.
- LVEF below institutional limits of normal and equal to or greater than 10% absolute decrease in LVEF from baseline assessment.

May resume trastuzumab if within 4 to 8 weeks the LVEF returns to normal limits and the absolute decrease from baseline is equal to or less than 15%. Discontinue permanently for a persistent (more than 8 weeks) LVEF decline or for suspension of trastuzumab dosing on more than three occasions for cardiomyopathy.

DILUTION

Manufacturer supplies a vial of bacteriostatic water for injection (BWFI). Confirm content of vial; 20 mL is required to obtain the correct concentration. Inject diluent slowly directed at the lyophilized cake. Swirl gently; **do not shake** (is sensitive to agitation or rapid expulsion from a syringe). Allow vial to stand for 5 minutes, slight foaming is permissible. Will yield a multidose solution containing 21 mg/mL. Label vial immediately with a "do not use after" date 28 days from date of reconstitution. SW may be used to reconstitute trastuzumab for patients with a known hypersensitivity to benzyl alcohol, but the calculated dose must be withdrawn, used immediately, and the balance of the reconstituted solution discarded. Reconstituted solution must be further diluted and given as an infusion. Withdraw the calculated dose from the reconstituted vial (21 mg/mL) and add it to an infusion bag containing 250 mL of NS. Gently invert to mix the solution.

Filters: In-line filters are not necessary but may be used (0.2-micron filters were evaluated).

Storage: Refrigerate unopened and reconstituted vials at 2° to 8° C (36° to 46° F). Vials reconstituted in supplied diluent are stable for 28 days after reconstitution. Discard remaining diluent. Discard reconstituted trastuzumab after expiration date written or stamped on vial. Solutions diluted in NS may be refrigerated for 24 hours before use. Do not freeze reconstituted trastuzumab.

COMPATIBILITY

Manufacturer states, "Do not reconstitute with drugs other than BWFI or SW. Further dilute infusion with NS. Infusions should not be administered or mixed with dextrose solutions Do not mix with other drugs." Is **compatible** with polyethylene and polyvinylchloride infusion bags and tubing.

RATE OF ADMINISTRATION

Use of a microdrip (60 gtt/min) or other IV controller suggested. For infusion only, **do not administer** as an IV push or bolus. Decrease rate of infusion for mild or moderate infusion reactions.

Initial dose: A single dose as an infusion over a minimum of 90 minutes. Observe for chills, fever, or other infusion-associated symptoms; see Precautions/Monitor.

Maintenance dose: If the initial dose was well tolerated, administer a single dose as an infusion over 30 to 90 minutes (based on regimen; see Usual Dose).

ACTIONS

A recombinant DNA–derived humanized monoclonal antibody that selectively binds with high affinity to the extracellular domain of the human epidermal growth factor receptor 2 (HER2) protein. Inhibits proliferation and mediates an antibody-dependent cellular toxicity in cancer cells that overexpress the HER2 protein. Half-life increases and clearance decreases with increasing doses. May cross the placental barrier. May be secreted in breast milk.

INDICATIONS AND USES

Indicated for adjuvant treatment of breast cancer that is HER2-overexpressing, node-positive or node-negative (ER/PR-negative or with one high-risk feature). May be used as part of a treatment regimen that may consist of (1) doxorubicin (Adriamycin), cyclophosphamide (Cytoxan), and either paclitaxel (Taxol) or docetaxel (Taxotere); (2) a regimen with docetaxel and carboplatin (Paraplatin); or (3) a single agent following multimodal anthracycline-based therapy. ▪ As a single agent for treatment of patients with metastatic breast cancer whose tumors overexpress the HER2 protein and who have received one or more chemotherapy regimens for their metastatic disease. ▪ In combination with paclitaxel (Taxol) for the first-line treatment of patients with metastatic breast cancer whose tumors overexpress the HER2 protein and who have not received chemotherapy for their metastatic disease. ▪ In combination with cisplatin and capecitabine (Xeloda) or 5-fluorouracil (5-FU) for treatment of patients with HER2-overexpressing metastatic gastric or gastroesophageal junction adenocarcinoma who have not received prior treatment for metastatic disease. ▪ Trastuzumab is not indicated for any other patients, including those with newly diagnosed, operable breast cancer.

CONTRAINDICATIONS

None known when used as indicated; see Precautions.

PRECAUTIONS

Trastuzumab should be used only in patients whose tumors have HER2 overexpression. Beneficial treatment effects were largely limited to patients with the highest level of HER2 protein overexpression (3+). Tumor histology differs; use FDA-approved tests for specific tumor type (breast or gastric/gastroesophageal adenocarcinoma) to assess HER2 overexpression and HER2 gene amplification. HER2 protein overexpression can be determined or inferred using immunohistochemistry (IHC) or fluorescence in situ hybridization (FISH). Must be performed in laboratories with demonstrated proficiency in the specific technology. ▪ Administered by or under the direction of the physician specialist. May be given on an outpatient basis. ▪ Adequate laboratory and supportive medical resources must be available. ▪ Emergency equipment and drugs for treatment of left ventricular dysfunction and/or hypersensitivity reactions must be immediately available; see Antidote. ▪ Use with caution in patients with known hypersensitivity to trastuzumab, Chinese hamster ovary cell proteins, benzyl alcohol, or any component of this product. ▪ Hypersensitivity reactions and infusion reactions (including some with a fatal outcome) and pulmonary toxicity (including ARDS and death) have occurred. Retreatment after full recovery from a hypersensitivity or infusion reaction has been tried following pretreatment with antihistamines and/or corticosteroids. Some tolerated treatment; others had another severe reaction. ▪ Can cause subclinical and clinical cardiac failure. Incidence of cardiac dysfunction was highest in patients who received trastuzumab with an anthracycline-containing chemotherapy regimen (e.g., doxorubicin [Adriamycin]) and in the elderly. ▪ Can cause left ventricular cardiac dysfunction, arrhythmias, hypertension, disabling cardiac failure, cardiomyopathy, and cardiac death. May also cause asymptomatic decline in left ventricular ejection fraction (LVEF). Congestive heart failure may be severe; has been associated with disabling cardiac failure, mural thrombosis leading to stroke, and death. ▪ Use extreme caution in treating patients with pre-existing cardiac dysfunction or pulmonary compromise. Pre-existing cardiac disease or prior cardiotoxic therapy (e.g., anthracyclines), radiation therapy to the chest or pre-existing pulmonary compromise secondary to intrinsic lung disease and/or malignant pulmonary involvement may decrease ability to tolerate trastuzumab. ▪ May exacerbate chemotherapy-induced neutropenia. Septic deaths have been reported. ▪ Low titers of human anti-human antibodies (HAHA) were detected in one patient who had no symptoms of a hypersensitivity reaction. **Monitor:** Obtain baseline CBC with differential and platelet count and repeat as needed. ▪ Monitor all vital signs before and during therapy. ▪ Treatment with trastuzumab can result in the development of ventricular dysfunction and CHF. For all treatment regimens (monotherapy and/or combination therapies), patients should have a thorough baseline cardiac assessment to evaluate left ventricular function, including a history and physical exam, determination of LVEF, and an echocardiogram or a MUGA scan. Monitoring and assessment may not identify all patients at risk for developing cardiotoxicity. ▪ Monitor closely throughout treatment for S/S of deteriorating cardiac function (e.g., cough, dyspnea, paroxysmal nocturnal dyspnea, peripheral edema, S_3 gallop, or reduced ejection fraction [symptomatic or asymptomatic]). Suggested monitoring schedule includes a repeat evaluation of left ventricular function (echocardiogram or MUGA scan) every 3 months during treatment with trastuzumab and at least every 6 months for 2 years after completion of treatment if trastuzumab was used as a component of adjuvant therapy. More frequent monitoring should be used for patients with pre-existing cardiac dysfunction and/or if S/S of deteriorating cardiac function develop. ▪ Onset and clinical course of infusion reactions are variable. Most occur during or immediately following the infusion or within 24 hours; however, delayed infusion events (up to 1 week post-infusion) have also been reported. Chills and/or fever occur in 40% of patients during the first infusion. May be treated with acetaminophen (Tylenol), diphenhydramine (Benadryl), and meperidine (Demerol) with or without reduction in the rate of infusion. During infusion, monitor closely; asthenia, bronchospasm, dizziness, dyspnea, headache, hypotension (may be severe), hypoxia, nausea, pain (may be at tumor site), rash, rigors, and vomiting have also occurred. Recurrence of this syndrome is infrequent with subsequent infusions. Fatal serious infusion reactions have been reported (rare); death occurred within hours to days. ▪ Monitor closely; in addition to the symptoms of infusion reaction previously noted, severe and sometimes fatal hypersensitivity reactions (e.g., anaphylaxis, angioedema, bronchospasm, hypotension, urticaria) and pulmonary reactions (e.g., dyspnea, pulmonary infiltrates, pleural effusions, pneumonitis, non-cardiogenic pulmonary edema, pulmonary fibrosis, pulmonary insufficiency, hypoxia, and ARDS) have occurred during and after the infusion. Monitor until symptoms completely resolve. ▪ Monitor for thrombocytopenia (platelet count less than 50,000/mm^3). Initiate precautions to prevent excessive bleeding (e.g., inspect IV sites, skin, and mucous membranes; use extreme care during invasive procedures; test urine, emesis, stool, and secretions for occult blood). ▪ Not a vesicant; if extravasation occurs, discontinue infusion and restart using another vein.

Patient Education: During infusion, promptly report chills and/or fever and other S/S of infusion reaction. ▪ Promptly report cough, difficulty breath-

ing, weight gain, and swelling of extremities. ▪ Avoid pregnancy; nonhormonal birth control is preferred during and for 6 months following treatment. ▪ See Appendix D, p. 1434.
Maternal/Child: Category D: avoid pregnancy; can cause fetal harm. Increases the risk for oligohydramnios and oligohydramnios sequence manifesting as pulmonary hypoplasia, skeletal abnormalities, and neonatal death during the second and third trimesters. Pregnant women with breast cancer who receive trastuzumab are encouraged to enroll in the Cancer and Childbirth Registry. ▪ Discontinue breast-feeding during trastuzumab therapy. ▪ Safety and effectiveness for use in pediatric patients not established. **Elderly:** Advanced age may increase the risk of cardiac dysfunction.

DRUG/LAB INTERACTIONS
No formal drug interaction studies have been done. Use with **paclitaxel** may decrease trastuzumab clearance and increase serum levels. Paclitaxel concentration is not affected. ▪ Use in combination with capecitabine, cisplatin, docetaxel, doxorubicin, or cyclophosphamide did not suggest any interactions; however, risk of cardiotoxicity increased with concurrent use or previous use of **anthracyclines** (e.g., doxorubicin). ▪ Bone marrow toxicity may be additive with **other antineoplastic agents** (e.g., anthracyclines, cyclophosphamide).

SIDE EFFECTS
Cardiomyopathy, pulmonary toxicity, infusion reactions, and febrile neutropenia are the most serious side effects. Anemia, cough, diarrhea, dysgeusia, dyspnea, fatigue, fever, headache, infections, infusion reactions, myalgia, nausea, neutropenia, rash, stomatitis, thrombocytopenia, vomiting, and weight loss are most common. Side effects that cause interruption or discontinuation of therapy include severe infusion reactions, pulmonary toxicity, congestive heart failure, and a decline in left ventricular cardiac function. Abdominal pain, accidental injury, acne, anorexia, arthralgia, asthenia, back pain, bone pain, depression, dizziness, edema, flu syndrome, headache, herpes simplex, hypersensitivity reactions, hypotension, insomnia, neuropathy, pain (may be at tumor site), paresthesia, peripheral edema, peripheral neuritis, pharyngitis, rash, rhinitis, sinusitis, and tachycardia have been reported in more than 5% of patients. Many other serious side effects have been reported in some patients (e.g., cardiac arrest, coagulation disorder, death; hypersensitivity reactions [e.g., angioedema, bronchospasm, dyspnea, urticaria, wheezing]; hypertension, hypotension, non-cardiogenic pulmonary edema, pancytopenia, pericardial or pleural effusion, pulmonary infiltrates, pulmonary insufficiency and hypoxemia requiring O_2 and/or ventilatory support, shock arrhythmia, syncope, vascular thrombosis).
Post-Marketing: Serious adverse events including hypersensitivity reactions and infusion reactions, including some with a fatal outcome; and pulmonary events including ARDS and death. Symptoms occurred most commonly during the infusion, but some occurred 24 hours or more after the infusion. Renal toxicity (glomerulopathy) has also been reported. Cases of oligohydramnios, and oligohydramnios sequence manifesting as pulmonary hypoplasia, skeletal abnormalities, and neonatal death, have been reported when trastuzumab has been administered to pregnant women.

ANTIDOTE

Notify physician of all side effects. Most will be treated symptomatically. Decrease rate of infusion for mild or moderate infusion reactions. Temporarily discontinue infusion if dyspnea or clinically significant hypotension occurs. Discontinue infusion and strongly consider discontinuing trastuzumab therapy in patients who experience a severe infusion reaction. Discontinue infusion in patients who develop anaphylaxis, angioedema, ARDS, interstitial pneumonitis, and/or a clinically significant decrease in left ventricular function. Strongly consider discontinuation of trastuzumab therapy in patients who develop clinically significant congestive heart failure. Safety of continuation or resumption of therapy has not been studied. Treatment may include diuretics, ACE inhibitors (e.g., lisinopril [Prinivil, Zestril], enalaprilat [Vasotec]), inotropic agents (e.g., digoxin, inamrinone [Amrinone], isoproterenol [Isuprel]), beta-blockers (e.g., atenolol [Tenormin], propranolol), and/or supplemental oxygen. Infusion reaction is treated with acetaminophen, diphenhydramine, and meperidine. Administration of whole blood products (e.g., packed RBCs, platelets, leukocytes) and/or blood modifiers (e.g., darbepoetin alfa [Aranesp], epoetin alfa [Epogen], filgrastim [Neupogen], oprelvekin [Neumega], pegfilgrastim [Neulasta], sargramostim [Leukine]) may be indicated to treat bone marrow toxicity from concurrent antineoplastics. Treat hypersensitivity reactions (may be more frequent with coadministration of paclitaxel) with epinephrine, antihistamines, corticosteroids, bronchodilators, and oxygen. To treat extravasation, apply cold compresses and elevate extremity. Resuscitate as indicated.

TROMETHAMINE
(troh-**METH**-ah-meen)

Tham-E

Alkalizing agent

pH 8.6

USUAL DOSE

Limit dose to amount needed to increase blood pH to normal limits (7.35 to 7.45) and to correct acid-base derangements. Evaluate the need for repeat doses by serial determinations of existing base deficit, pH, and clinical observations. Tham-E contains electrolytes.

Acidosis: Required dose (mL of 0.3 molar solution) equal to body weight in kilograms × base deficit in mEq/L × 1.1.

Acidosis in cardiac bypass surgery: 9 mL/kg (324 mg/kg) of body weight. 500 mL (18 Gm) is an average adult dose. Up to 1,000 mL has been used. Never exceed 500 mg/kg in any individual dose over less than 1 hour.

Correct acidity of ACD priming blood: Stored blood has a pH of 6.22 to 6.8. An average of 60 mL (15 to 77 mL) tromethamine to each 500 mL of stored blood is required to correct pH to 7.4.

Acidosis in cardic arrest: Use only if indicated. Never inject into cardiac muscle. Initial dose in an open chest is 62 to 185 mL (2 to 6 Gm). Additional doses should be based on evaluation of base deficit. If the chest is not open, give 111 to 333 mL (3.6 to 10.8 Gm); use a large peripheral vein. After arrest is reversed, additional amounts may be needed to control persistent acidosis.

PEDIATRIC DOSE

Correction of metabolic acidosis associated with RDS in neonates and infants: 1 mL/kg of body weight for each pH unit below 7.4. Repeat doses may be given according to changes in PaO_2, pH, and PCO_2.

DOSE ADJUSTMENTS

Lower-end initial doses may be appropriate in the elderly based on the potential for decreased organ function and concomitant disease or drug therapy.

DILUTION

Supplied as a 0.3 molar solution. Each 100 mL contains tromethamine 3.6 Gm in water for injection. May be given undiluted as an infusion or added to pump oxygenator blood, other priming fluid, or ACD blood.

Storage: Store at CRT. Single use container, discard unused solution.

COMPATIBILITY

Specific information not available. Consider specific use; consult pharmacist.

RATE OF ADMINISTRATION

Slow IV infusion recommended. 5 mL or less/min would deliver up to 300 mL in 1 hour. Rate dictated by patient's condition and intended use; see Usual Dose and Precautions. Reduced rate may control venospasm.

ACTIONS

Acts as a proton acceptor. Prevents or corrects acidosis by actively binding hydrogen ions in metabolic acids and carbonic acid. Releases bicarbonate anions. Rapidly excreted in the urine, it has an osmotic diuretic effect, increases urine output, urine pH, and excretion of fixed acids, CO_2, and electrolytes. Also capable of neutralizing acidic ions of the intracellular fluid.

INDICATIONS AND USES

Prevention and correction of metabolic acidosis; particularly metabolic acidosis associated with cardiac bypass surgery, correction of acidity of ACD blood in cardiac bypass surgery, and cardiac arrest.

CONTRAINDICATIONS

Hypersensitivity to tromethamine, anuria, and uremia. In neonates it is also contraindicated in chronic respiratory acidosis and salicylate intoxication.

PRECAUTIONS

Intended for short-term use only (1 day). ■ Sodium bicarbonate or sodium lactate is effective in most acidotic situations and has fewer side effects. ■ Use extreme caution in impaired renal function or decreased urine output. **Monitor:** Determine blood pH, PCO_2, bicarbonate, glucose, and electrolytes before, during, and after administration. ■ Avoid overdose (total drug or too-rapid rate). Severe alkalosis and/or prolonged hypoglycemia may result. ■ May cause fluid and/or solute overload, resulting in dilution of serum electrolyte concentrations, overhydration, congested states, or pulmonary edema. ■ Use a large peripheral vein. Determine absolute patency of vein; necrosis may result from extravasation. ■ May severely depress respiration. Incidence may be increased in patients who have chronic hypoventilation or those who have been treated with drugs that depress respiration. Oxygen and controlled ventilation equipment must always be available. ■ ECG monitoring and frequent serum potassium measurements are required to rule out hyperkalemia in impaired renal function or decreased urine output. Decreased excretion of tromethamine may also occur, resulting in toxicity.

Maternal/Child: Category C: safety for use not established. Benefits must outweigh risks. ■ Use caution or discontinue breast-feeding. ■ Has been used to treat severe cases of metabolic acidosis with concurrent respiratory acidosis because it does not raise PCO_2 as bicarbonate does in neonates and infants with respiratory failure. It has also been used in neonates and infants with hypernatremia and metabolic acidosis to avoid the additional sodium given with the bicarbonate. However, because the osmotic effects of tromethamine are greater and large continuous doses are required, bicarbonate is preferred to tromethamine in the treatment of acidotic neonates and infants with RDS. ■ Severe hypoglycemia may occur in premature or full-term infants. ■ Infusion via low-lying umbilical venous catheters has been associated with hepatocellular necrosis.

Elderly: Lower-end initial doses may be appropriate in the elderly; see Dose Adjustments. Differences in response between elderly and younger patients have not been identified.

DRUG/LAB INTERACTIONS

Potentiates **amphetamines, ephedrine, and quinidine.** ■ Inhibits **lithium, methotrexate, and salicylates.** ■ Incidence of respiratory depression may be increased in patients receiving **drugs that depress respiration** (e.g., narcotic analgesics [morphine]). ■ May **increase coagulation time.**

SIDE EFFECTS

Hyperkalemia, hypoglycemia, phlebitis, respiratory depression, and thrombosis.

Overdose: Alkalosis, overhydration, severe prolonged hypoglycemia, solute overload. May be due to total drug or too-rapid rate of administration.

ANTIDOTE

Notify physician of all side effects. Reduced rate of infusion may prevent hypoglycemia. Use glucose if indicated. Discontinue drug immediately for hyperkalemia or extravasation. Local infiltration with 1% procaine with phentolamine may reduce tissue necrosis. Use a number 25 needle. Symptomatic treatment is indicated. Alternate drugs are indicated (sodium bicarbonate, sodium lactate).

VACCINIA IMMUNE GLOBULIN INTRAVENOUS (HUMAN) BBW   Immunizing agent (passive)

(vack-**SIN**-ee-ah ih-**MUNE GLAW**-byoo-lin IV)

VIGIV

USUAL DOSE

100 mg/kg (2 mL/kg) as a single-dose IV infusion; see Monitor. May be repeated based on the severity of symptoms and on individual patient response. Higher doses (200 mg/kg or 500 mg/kg) may be considered in patients who do not respond to the initial 100 mg/kg dose; see Precautions.

DOSE ADJUSTMENTS

Because of sucrose content, doses higher than 400 mg/kg are not recommended in patients with potential renal problems.

DILUTION

Contains sucrose; see Precautions. A ready-to-use liquid preparation supplied in a 50-mL vial containing 50 mg VIGIV/mL or 2,500 mg VIGIV/vial. Solution should be colorless, free of particulate matter, and not turbid. *Do not shake vial; avoid foaming.* Further dilution before or during administration is not recommended. Infusion should begin within 6 hours of entering the vial and be complete within 12 hours of entering the vial. Use of a dedicated IV line, a 0.22-micron in-line filter, and a constant infusion pump is recommended. If necessary, it may be piggybacked into a pre-existing IV line containing NS or D2½W, D5W, D10W, or D20W with or without NaCl added; see Compatibility. VIGIV should not be diluted more than 1:2 (v/v) with any of these solutions.

Filters: Use of a 0.22-micron in-line filter is recommended; see Dilution.

Storage: Store between 2° and 8° C (35.6° and 46.4° F). Do not use after expiration date. Infusion must begin within 6 hours and be complete within 12 hours of entering the vial. Discard partially used vials. Do not use if turbid or has been frozen.

COMPATIBILITY

Manufacturer states, "Administer separately from other drugs or medications." If necessary, it may be piggybacked into a pre-existing IV line containing NS or D2½W, D5W, D10W, or D20W with or without NaCl added. Flush line before and after administration. VIGIV should not be diluted more than 1:2 (v/v) with any of these solutions.

RATE OF ADMINISTRATION

Flush line before and after administration.

Administer 1 mL/kg/hr for the first 30 minutes. If no discomfort or adverse effects, it may be increased to 2 mL/kg/hr for the next 30 minutes and then to 3 mL/kg/hr for the remainder of the infusion, as tolerated. Infusion of 100 mg/kg (2 mL/kg) should take approximately 70 minutes in a 70-kg patient. Do not exceed these rates. Too-rapid infusion may cause infusion rate–related reactions (e.g., arthralgia, back pain, chills, fever, flushing, muscle cramps, nausea, vomiting, wheezing). *In patients at risk for developing renal dysfunction, administer at the minimum concentration available and the minimum rate of infusion practicable.* Use of a dedicated IV line, a 0.22-micron in-line filter, and a constant infusion pump (i.e., an IVAC pump or equivalent) is recommended.

ACTIONS

An immunoglobulin (Ig). Obtained from human plasma, purified, and standardized. Donors had received booster immunizations with the Dryvax smallpox vaccine. Specific methods (e.g., cold ethanol fractionation, detergents, nanofiltration, solvents) inactivate bloodborne viruses (e.g., hepatitis, HIV). Tested and found negative for antibodies against HIV, hepatitis, Creutzfeldt-Jakob disease, and others. Contains increased levels of protective antibodies against the vaccinia virus—the live virus used in the currently available smallpox vaccine. When use is necessary, can help to minimize possible risks associated with this highly effective smallpox vaccine. Half-life is approximately 22 days but may be decreased by fever or infection (increased catabolism or consumption).

INDICATIONS AND USES

Treatment and/or modification of the following conditions: aberrant infections induced by the vaccinia virus that include accidental implantation in the eyes (excluding isolated keratitis; see Contraindications), mouth, or other areas where vaccinia infection would be hazardous; eczema vaccinatum; progressive vaccinia; severe generalized vaccinia; and vaccinia infections in individuals who have skin conditions such as burns, impetigo, varicella-zoster, or poison ivy or in individuals who have eczematous skin lesions because of the activity or extensiveness of such lesions.

CONTRAINDICATIONS

Presence of isolated vaccinia keratitis. ▪ Individuals known to have an allergic response to this or other human immunoglobulin preparations. ▪ Contains trace amounts of IgA. Patients with isolated or selective IgA deficiency can develop antibodies to IgA and have an increased risk of anaphylactic reactions with subsequent exposure to blood products that contain IgA. ▪ Not considered effective for the treatment of postvaccinal encephalitis.

PRECAUTIONS

For IV infusion only. ▪ Hypersensitivity reactions are possible and have occurred with other IGIV preparations; administer in a facility with adequate equipment and supplies to monitor the patient and respond to any medical emergency. ▪ Use extreme caution in individuals with a history of prior systemic hypersensitivity reactions. Incidence of anaphylaxis may be increased, especially with repeated injections. ▪ Use caution when treating complications that include vaccinia keratitis; may cause increased corneal scarring. ▪ IGIV products have been associated with renal dysfunction, acute renal failure, osmotic nephrosis, and death. Use extreme caution in patients with any degree of renal insufficiency; in patients 65 years of age and older; in patients with diabetes mellitus, paraproteinemia, sepsis, or volume depletion; and/or in patients receiving known nephrotoxic drugs. If used, should be administered at the minimum concentration available and at the minimum rate of infusion practicable. *Products containing sucrose as a stabilizer have demonstrated an increased risk of renal dysfunction.* Consider benefit versus risk before use. ■ May cause aseptic meningitis syndrome (AMS), which may begin from 2 hours to 2 days after treatment. Symptoms are drowsiness, fever, headache (severe), nausea and vomiting, nuchal rigidity, painful eye movements, and photophobia. Symptoms resolve if VIGIV is discontinued. A neurologic exam to rule out other causes of meningitis is indicated. ■ IGIV products have been associated with thrombotic events; use caution in patients with a history of cardiovascular disease or thrombotic episodes and in patients with thrombotic risk factors (e.g., cerebrovascular disease, coronary artery disease, diabetes, hypertension). Baseline assessment of blood viscosity should be made in patients at risk for hyperviscosity, including chylomicronemia, markedly high triglycerides, or monoclonal gammopathies. ■ Hemolysis and hemolytic anemia may develop. ■ Noncarcinogenic pulmonary edema (transfusion-related acute lung injury ([TRALI]) has been reported with other IGIV preparations; see Monitor. ■ Interacts with some glucose-monitoring systems; see Monitor and Drug/Lab Interactions.

Monitor: Use of larger veins may reduce infusion site discomfort. ■ Correct volume depletion before administration. ■ Recording the lot number on vials is helpful. ■ Monitor vital signs and observe patient continuously during infusion. A precipitous drop in BP or anaphylaxis can occur at any time. Emergency equipment and supplies must be at bedside. ■ Monitor renal function (e.g., BUN, SCr) and urine output in patients at increased risk for renal failure. Obtain baseline studies, monitor at intervals, and discontinue future VIGIV therapy if renal function deteriorates. See Precautions. ■ Monitor for S/S of hemolysis (e.g., anemia, lysis of red blood cells, liberation of hemoglobin). ■ Monitor for S/S of TRALI (e.g., fever, hypoxemia, normal left ventricular function, pulmonary edema, severe respiratory distress). Usually occurs within 1 to 6 hours after completion of the transfusion. Manage with oxygen and adequate ventilatory support. If TRALI is suspected, test for the presence of anti-neutrophil antibodies in product and patient serum. ■ Some types of blood glucose testing systems (e.g., those based on the glucose dehydrogenase pyrroloquinolinequinone [GDH-PQQ] or glucose-dye-oxidoreductase methods) could falsely interpret the maltose contained in VIGIV as glucose. To avoid this interference by maltose contained in VIGIV, blood glucose measurements in patients receiving VIGIV must be done with a glucose-specific method (monitor and test strips); see Drug/Lab Interactions.

Patient Education: Report a burning sensation in the head, chills, cyanosis, diaphoresis, dyspnea, faintness or light-headedness, fatigue, fever, hives, itching or rash, neck pain or difficulty moving neck, tachycardia, wheezing. ■ Report chest pain or tightness, difficulty passing urine, decreased urine output, fluid retention, edema, shortness of breath, or sudden weight gain.

Maternal/Child: Category C: use during pregnancy only if clearly needed. ■ Safety for use in breast-feeding not established. ■ Safety and effectiveness for use in pediatric patients not established.

Elderly: Not tested for safety and effectiveness in the elderly. Use with caution. Incidence of renal insufficiency and other side effects may be increased due to age, potential for decreased organ function, and pre-existing medical conditions; see Precautions.

DRUG/LAB INTERACTIONS

Defer administration of **live virus vaccines** for approximately 6 months after administration of VIGIV. ▪ Concurrent use with **nephrotoxic drugs** (e.g., aminoglycosides [e.g., gentamicin], amphotericin B [Amphotec, generic], cidofovir [Vistide], rifampin [Rifadin]) may increase the risk of renal insufficiency. ▪ Maltose in IVIG products has been shown to give falsely high blood glucose levels. Use could result in inappropriate doses of insulin, resulting in life-threatening hypoglycemia or untreated hypoglycemia masked by falsely elevated glucose readings. Review product information of the blood glucose testing system, including test strips, to determine if the system is appropriate for use with maltose-containing parenteral products. ▪ Additional drug/lab interaction studies have not been completed.

SIDE EFFECTS

Headache and mild to moderate urticaria are most frequently observed. A full range of hypersensitivity symptoms, including anaphylaxis, is possible. Backache, dizziness, injection site reaction, nausea, and upper respiratory infections also occur. A precipitous hypotensive reaction can occur and is most commonly associated with a too-rapid rate of injection. Serious side effects reported with other IGIV products should be considered and include acute renal failure, acute tubular necrosis, osmotic nephrosis, and proximal tubular nephropathy (may result in death); aseptic meningitis syndrome; hemolytic anemia (reversible); increased BUN and SCr (may occur as soon as 1 to 2 days following infusion); noncarcinogenic pulmonary edema (transfusion-related acute lung injury ([TRALI]); severe reactions (e.g., circulatory collapse, fever, loss of consciousness, nausea and vomiting, sudden onset of dyspnea) are more common in patients with antibody deficiencies; thromboembolism. Made from human plasma; the manufacturing process attempts to eliminate the risk of bloodborne viruses (e.g., hepatitis, HIV infection, Creutzfeldt-Jakob disease), but the potential for infection cannot be ruled out.

ANTIDOTE

Reduce rate or temporarily interrupt infusion for patient discomfort or any sign of adverse reaction. Reduce rate in patients at risk for renal insufficiency. Loop diuretics (e.g., furosemide [Lasix]) may be helpful in the management of fluid overload. If patient continues to experience adverse reactions after rate has been reduced, other IGIV preparations suggest premedicating with hydrocortisone 1 to 2 mg/kg 30 minutes before the immune globulin infusion. Pretreatment with acetaminophen (Tylenol) and diphenhydramine (Benadryl) may also be useful. Discontinue the drug immediately for any signs of a hypersensitivity reaction. Notify the physician. May be treated symptomatically and infusion resumed at slower rate if symptoms subside. Treat anaphylaxis immediately. Epinephrine (Adrenalin), diphenhydramine (Benadryl), oxygen, vasopressors (e.g., dopamine), corticosteroids, and ventilation equipment must always be available. Manage TRALI with oxygen and ventilatory support. Resuscitate as necessary.

VALPROATE SODIUM BBW

(val-**PROH**-ayt **SO**-dee-um)

Depacon

Anticonvulsant

pH 7.6

USUAL DOSE

Adults and pediatric patients 10 years of age or older: For all indications optimal clinical response is usually achieved with doses less than 60 mg/kg/24 hr. Usual therapeutic range of plasma levels is 50 to 100 mcg/mL. A total daily dose exceeding 250 mg should be given in divided doses every 6 hours (studies used an every-6-hour regimen). See Precautions, Monitor, and Drug/Lab Interactions. Transfer to oral dosing as soon as practical. Oral and IV doses are considered to be equivalent and should be given at previously established intervals (e.g., every 6 or 8 hours). See Precautions.

Complex partial seizures (monotherapy [initial]): Begin with an initial dose of 10 to 15 mg/kg/24 hr. May be increased by 5 to 10 mg/kg/week until desired clinical response achieved or side effects are dose limiting.

Complex partial seizures (conversion to monotherapy): Begin with an initial dose of 10 to 15 mg/kg/24 hr. May be increased by 5 to 10 mg/kg/week until desired clinical response achieved or side effects are dose limiting. Concomitant antiepilepsy drug (AED) dosage can usually be reduced by 25% every 2 weeks. Dose of AEDs may be decreased at the beginning of valproate therapy or decrease may be delayed for 1 to 2 weeks to avoid unwanted seizures.

Complex partial seizures (adjunctive therapy): Begin with an initial dose of 10 to 15 mg/kg/24 hr. May be increased by 5 to 10 mg/kg/week until desired clinical response achieved. Has been used in combination with either carbamazepine (Tegretol) or phenytoin (Dilantin). Dose adjustment of these drugs is not usually needed; however, drug interactions may occur; monitor plasma concentrations, especially during early therapy.

Simple and complex absence seizures: Begin with an initial dose of 15 mg/kg/24 hr. May be increased by 5 to 10 mg/kg/week until seizures are controlled or side effects are dose limiting.

PEDIATRIC DOSE

No IV dose recommendations available for pediatric patients under 10 years of age. See Maternal/Child.

DOSE ADJUSTMENTS

Monitor plasma concentrations when transferring from oral to IV or IV to oral; dose increases or decreases may be indicated. ■ Reduce initial dose in the elderly; base subsequent doses on clinical response and/or development of side effects. ■ Reduced dose or discontinuation of therapy may be indicated if there is evidence of bruising, hemorrhage, or a disorder of hemostasis/coagulation. ■ Reduced doses and increased monitoring are indicated in hyperammonemia with or without lethargy or coma. Reduce dose further or discontinue if clinically significant symptoms occur (e.g., abnormal liver function tests, lethargy, coma). ■ No dose adjustments required for impaired renal function, gender, or race. ■ See Maternal/Child.

DILUTION

Each single dose should be diluted with at least 50 mL of D5W, NS, or LR. **Storage:** Store vials at CRT. Diluted solutions stable at CRT for 24 hours. No preservative added; discard unused contents of vial.

COMPATIBILITY

Consider any drug NOT listed as compatible to be INCOMPATIBLE until consulting a pharmacist; specific conditions may apply.

One source suggests the following **compatibilities**:

Y-site: Cefepime (Maxipime), ceftazidime (Fortaz).

RATE OF ADMINISTRATION

A single dose as an infusion over 60 minutes. Manufacturer has recommended that a rate of 20 mg/min not be exceeded; however, results of a single study suggest that selected patients tolerated rates from 1.5 to 3 mg/kg/min, allowing administration of up to 15 mg/kg/dose over 5 to 10 minutes. Incidence of side effects may be increased with too-rapid infusion.

ACTIONS

An anticonvulsant. A sodium salt of valproic acid. Therapeutic effect in epilepsy may result from increased brain concentrations of gamma-aminobutyric acid (GABA). Peak effect occurs at the end of a 60-minute infusion or 4 hours after an oral dose. Plasma protein binding is high and is concentration dependent. Concentration in CSF is similar to unbound concentrations in plasma (10%). Half-life range is 13 to 19 hours. The half-life will be in the lower part of the range in patients receiving other enzyme-inducing antiepileptic agents (e.g., carbamazepine [Tegretol], phenobarbital [Luminal], phenytoin [Dilantin]). Metabolized in the liver. 30% to 50% excreted in changed form in urine. Crosses placental barrier. Secreted in breast milk.

INDICATIONS AND USES

Use of IV product indicated in the following specific conditions when oral administration of valproate products (e.g., divalproex sodium [Depakote]) is temporarily not feasible. ■ Treatment of complex partial seizures occurring in isolation or with other seizures (monotherapy or adjunctive therapy). ■ Treatment of simple and complex absence seizures (monotherapy or adjunctive therapy). ■ Adjunctive treatment of multiple seizure types that include absence seizures.

Unlabeled uses: Used alone or in combination with other antiepileptic drugs for treatment of absence, myoclonic and grand mal seizures and for treatment of patients with intractable status epilepticus who have not responded to other therapies.

CONTRAINDICATIONS

Known hypersensitivity to valproate products, patients with hepatic disease or significant hepatic dysfunction, and patients with known urea cycle disorders. ■ Not recommended for use in patients with acute head trauma for the prophylaxis of posttraumatic seizures.

PRECAUTIONS

Use of IV valproate for more than 14 days has not been studied. Safety of doses above 60 mg/kg/day is not known. ■ Use caution in patients with a history of hepatic disease. Has caused fatal hepatic failure. Pediatric patients under 2 years of age are at the greatest risk, especially if they are on multiple anticonvulsants or have congenital metabolic disorders, severe seizure disorders with mental retardation, or organic brain disease. If valproate is used in pediatric patients under 2 years of age with or without these increased risk factors, benefits must outweigh risks; use only as a sole agent with extreme caution. Most cases of hepatic failure have occurred during the first 6 months of treatment. Incidence of fatal hepatotoxicity decreases in progressively older patient groups. ■ Cases of life-threatening pancreatitis have been reported in both pediatric patients and adults receiving valproate. Some of the cases have been described as hemorrhagic with rapid progression from initial symptoms to death. May occur at any time from shortly after initiation of therapy to years later. If pancreatitis is diagnosed, valproate should be discontinued. ■ Hyperammonemic encephalopathy has been reported in patients with urea cycle disorders (UCD); has been fatal. Before starting valproate, consider a possible diagnosis of UCD in patients with a history of unexplained encephalopathy or coma, encephalopathy associated with a protein load, pregnancy-related or postpartum encephalopathy, unexplained mental retardation, a history of elevated plasma ammonia or glutamine, cyclical vomiting or lethargy, episodic extreme irritability, ataxia, low BUN, protein avoidance, a family history of UCD or unexplained infant deaths, or any other S/S of UCD. ■ Hyperammonemia may be present even with normal liver function tests. Hyperammonemic encephalopathy should be considered in patients who present with lethargy and vomiting or altered mental status. Hyperammonemia should also be considered in patients who present with hypothermia (unintentional drop in body temperature to less than 35° C [95° F]). Elevation of ammonia may also be asymptomatic. ■ Hyperammonemia with or without encephalopathy has been reported with concomitant administration of valproic acid and topiramate (Topamax). Has occurred in patients who have tolerated either drug alone. S/S in most cases are abated with discontinuation of either drug. ■ Hypothermia has occurred with valproate therapy both in conjunction with and in the absence of hyperammonemia. Can also occur in patients using concomitant topiramate with valproate after starting topiramate therapy or after increasing the dose of topiramate. ■ Some adverse effects (e.g., elevated liver enzymes and thrombocytopenia) appear to be dose-related. Must weigh benefit of improved therapeutic effect with higher doses against the possibility of an increased incidence of adverse effects. ■ Psychotic symptoms and other behavioral changes have been reported and may include aggression, agitation, anger, anxiety, apathy, depersonalization, depression, emotional lability, hallucinations, hostility, irritability, and suicidal tendencies. Some resolved without intervention. Others required dose reduction or discontinuation of valproate. ■ Incidence of thrombocytopenia increases at total trough concentrations greater than 110 mcg/mL in females and greater than 135 mcg/mL in males. ■ Multiorgan hypersensitivity reactions have been reported rarely when beginning valproate therapy. Onset may range from 1 to 40 days (median 21 days), and initial S/S include fever and rash associated with other organ system involvement (e.g., arthralgia, hepatitis, lymphadenopathy, nephritis). Discontinue valproate and use alternative therapy. ■ Plasma protein binding is decreased and free fraction is increased in the elderly, in hyperlipidemic patients, in chronic hepatic disease, in impaired renal function, and in the presence of other drugs; see Drug/Lab Interactions. Total plasma concentrations may be normal, but free concentrations may be substantially elevated in these patients. ■ Reduce AED doses gradually to prevent status epilepticus in patients treated for major seizure activity. ■ Can produce teratogenic effects. Consider benefit versus risk to the fetus in women of childbearing age. Do not use to treat non–life-threatening conditions (e.g., migraine); see Maternal/Child. ■ In vitro studies suggest that valproate may stimulate the replication of the HIV and CMV viruses under certain experimental conditions. The clinical significance of this is unknown but should be kept in mind when evaluating patients with HIV or CMV.

Monitor: Thrombocytopenia, inhibition of the secondary phase of platelet aggregation, and abnormal coagulation parameters have been reported. Obtain baseline platelet counts and coagulation tests and monitor during therapy. Repeat before planned surgery. ■ Obtain baseline liver function tests and monitor frequently during therapy, especially during the first 6 months. ■ Observe closely for S/S of hepatotoxicity (e.g., anorexia, facial edema, lethargy, loss of seizure control, malaise, weakness, vomiting). ■ Abdominal pain, anorexia, nausea, and vomiting may be symptoms of pancreatitis and should be evaluated promptly. ■ Therapeutic serum levels for most patients will range from 50 to 100 mcg/mL; however, a good correlation has not been established between daily dose, serum levels, and therapeutic effect. ■ Monitor antiepileptic concentrations more frequently whenever concomitant AEDs are being introduced or withdrawn and observe closely for seizure activity. ■ Monitor serum concentrations more frequently if an asymptomatic elevation of ammonia occurs; may need to discontinue valproate sodium if hyperammonemia appears. ■ Monitor serum concentrations more frequently if any of the risk factors listed in Dose Adjustments or Precautions are present, and when any drugs that affect hepatic enzymes are introduced or discontinued; see Drug/Lab Interactions. ■ Evaluate for S/S of UCD; see Precautions and Antidote. ■ Consider hyperammonemia encephalopathy in patients who develop unexplained lethargy and vomiting or changes in mental status. Consider hyperammonemia in patients who present with hypothermia. Elevations of ammonia may be asymptomatic; monitor plasma ammonia levels closely; see Antidote. Treat hyperammonemia and assess for underlying UCD. ■ Observe patient closely for signs of CNS side effects; see Precautions. ■ Total serum valproic acid concentration is affected by variable free-fractions of drug; consider hepatic metabolism and protein binding when interpreting valproic acid concentrations. ■ See Dose Adjustments, Precautions, and Drug/Lab Interactions for additional monitoring requirements.

Patient Education: May cause drowsiness; determine effects before driving or operating any machinery. ■ Avoid pregnancy; consider birth control options. ■ Read the patient information leaflet provided by manufacturer, and discuss your medical history and concurrent prescription and nonprescription medications with your health care provider. ■ Report symptoms such as abdominal pain, anorexia, changes in mental state, fever, jaundice, lymphadenopathy, nausea, rash, unexplained lethargy, or vomiting promptly. ■ May cause alterations in mood (e.g., aggression, agitation, anger, anxiety, apathy, decreased ability to cope, depression, hostility, irritability, thoughts of suicide); report these changes promptly. ■ Women who are pregnant or who become pregnant should be encouraged to enroll in the North American Antiepileptic Drug (NAAED) Pregnancy Registry.

Maternal/Child: Category D: avoid pregnancy. There is an increased risk for neural tube defects (e.g., spina bifida) and other birth defects, such as craniofacial defects and cardiovascular malformation, in infants exposed to valproate sodium and related products in utero. The incidence of congenital malformations associated with the use of valproate by women with seizure disorders during pregnancy is higher than in women with seizure disorders who use other AEDs. The increased teratogenic risk from valproate in women with epilepsy is expected to be reflected in an increased risk in other indications (e.g., bipolar disorder, migraine). Use during pregnancy only if essential for management of a serious medical condition (e.g., seizures). Tests to detect neural tube and other defects should be considered as part of routine prenatal care in pregnant women receiving valproate. ▪ When used during pregnancy, valproate has caused clotting abnormalities, including afibrinogenemia in a newborn; monitor clotting parameters carefully. Has also caused hepatic failure in a newborn and an infant. ▪ Effects on testicular development and sperm production not known. ▪ Discontinue breast-feeding. ▪ Neonates under 2 months have a markedly decreased ability to eliminate valproate compared to older pediatric patients and adults. ▪ Pediatric patients 3 months to 10 years of age have 50% higher clearance rates based on weight. ▪ Younger pediatric patients, especially those receiving enzyme-inducing drugs (e.g., carbamazepine, phenobarbital, phenytoin) will require larger maintenance doses to achieve therapeutic valproic acid concentrations. ▪ IV product has not been studied in pediatric patients under 2 years of age. If used, use as a sole agent with extreme caution. ▪ Children under 2 years of age are at an increased risk for developing fatal hepatotoxicity. ▪ See Precautions and Monitor.

Elderly: May be more prone to adverse events. Initial dose should be lower, and dosage should be increased slowly. Rate of clearance decreased, free fraction increased; see Dose Adjustments. ▪ Monitor for fluid, nutritional intake, dehydration, somnolence, and other adverse events.

DRUG/LAB INTERACTIONS

Clearance increased and effectiveness reduced by **drugs that induce hepatic enzymes** (e.g., phenytoin [Dilantin], carbamazepine [Tegretol], phenobarbital [Luminal], primidone [Mysoline]); increased monitoring of valproate and concomitant drug concentrations indicated. ▪ **Aspirin** decreases protein binding, inhibits metabolism, and increases free concentration of valproate; use caution and monitor valproate concentrations if administered concomitantly. ▪ Peak concentrations increased if coadministered with **felbamate** (Felbatol); reduced dose of valproate indicated. ▪ Metabolism may be decreased and serum levels increased when given concurrently with **chlorpromazine** (Thorazine) **or erythromycin.** ▪ **Carbapenem antibiotics** (e.g., doripenem [Doribax], ertapenem [Invanz], meropenem [Merrem]) may reduce serum valproic acid concentrations to subtherapeutic levels, resulting in loss of seizure control. Monitor valproic acid levels. Consider alternative antibacterial therapy. If administration of a carbapenem is necessary, supplemental anticonvulsant therapy should be considered. ▪ **Rifampin** (Rifadin) may increase clearance of valproate and require dose adjustment. ▪ Inhibits metabolism of **barbiturates** (e.g., phenobarbital) **and primidone,** increasing their effects. Monitor for neurologic toxicity; obtain barbiturate serum levels and reduce barbiturate dose as indicated. ▪ May increase or decrease serum levels of carbamazepine. **Carbamazepine** decreases plasma concentrations of valproate, and a loss of seizure control may occur; monitor carefully and increase valproate dose if indicated. ▪ Concomitant use with **clonazepam** (Klonopin) may induce absence status in patients with a history of absence-type seizures. ▪ **Displaces some protein-bound drugs,** inhibits their metabolism, and increases their effects (e.g., carbamazepine, diazepam [Valium], phenytoin, tolbutamide, warfarin [Coumadin]). Dose adjustments and serum concentrations may be indicated. **Phenytoin** with valproate has caused breakthrough seizures in patients with epilepsy; adjust dose of phenytoin as indicated by serum concentrations. ▪ Hyperammonemia with or without encephalopathy has been reported with concomitant administration of valproic acid and **topiramate** (Topamax); see Precautions. ▪ Monitor coagulation tests if administered with **anticoagulants** (e.g., warfarin). ▪ CNS effects may be increased when given concurrently with **CNS depressants** (e.g., benzodiazepines [e.g., diazepam (Valium)] **and tricyclic antidepressants** [e.g., amitriptyline (Elavil)]). ▪ May decrease clearance and increase effects of **amitriptyline** (Elavil) **and nortriptyline** (Aventyl). Dose reduction of these drugs may be required. ▪ Inhibits metabolism of **ethosuximide** (Zarontin); monitor serum concentrations of both drugs with concomitant administration. ▪ Concurrent administration of **lamotrigine** (Lamictal) and valproate may decrease valproate levels and increase lamotrigine levels. Serious skin reactions have been reported. Dose adjustments may be required. ▪ Decreases clearance and may increase toxicity of **zidovudine** (AZT, Retrovir). ▪ See package insert for additional information about many drugs that do not present significant clinical interactions. ▪ May alter **thyroid function tests.** ▪ May cause **false-positive urine ketone test.**

SIDE EFFECTS

Abdominal cramps and/or pain; abnormal gait; acute pancreatitis; anaphylaxis; anorexia with weight loss or increased appetite with weight gain; asterixis (spots before the eyes); chest pain; confusion; constipation; diarrhea; diplopia; dizziness; elevated serum amylase; euphoria; headache; hyperesthesia; indigestion; injection site reaction; insomnia; nausea; nervousness; nystagmus; parkinsonism; psychotic symptoms including aggression, agitation, anger, anxiety, apathy, depersonalization, depression, emotional lability, hallucinations, hostility, irritability, and suicidal tendencies; pharyngitis; pneumonia; somnolence; taste perversion; thrombocytopenia; tremor; vasodilation; vertigo; vomiting. Frequency of elevated liver enzymes and thrombocytopenia may be dose related. Fatal hepatotoxicity (anorexia, facial edema, lethargy, loss of seizure control, malaise, sweating, weakness, vasodilation, vomiting) has occurred. Coma has occurred with or without concurrent phenobarbital. Encephalopathy with or without fever has caused fatalities in patients with hyperammonemic encephalopathy and/or underlying UCD disorder.

Overdose: Somnolence, deep coma, heart block. Some fatalities have been reported.

ANTIDOTE

Keep physician informed of all side effects. Some may respond to a decrease in the rate of administration. Discontinue immediately if signs of suspected or apparent significant hepatic dysfunction appear (e.g., hyperammonemia, elevated liver function tests) or S/S of underlying UCD. Hepatic dysfunction may progress after valproate is discontinued. Discontinue if S/S of multi-organ hypersensitivity reaction occur. Initiate alternate therapy. Reduce dose or discontinue if bruising, hemorrhage, or abnormal coagulation parameters occur (e.g., thrombocytopenia). Discontinue if S/S of pancreatitis occur. All of the above situations may be life threatening and will require immediate symptomatic treatment. Maintain a patent airway and resuscitate as indicated. Support patient as required in treatment of overdose; monitor and maintain adequate urine output. Hemodialysis is effective in overdose. Naloxone (Narcan) may reverse CNS depressant effects in overdose but may also reverse antiepilepsy effects of valproate. Psychotic symptoms may require dose reduction or discontinuation of valproate.

VANCOMYCIN HYDROCHLORIDE
(van-koh-**MY**-sin hy-droh-**KLOR**-eyed)

**Antibacterial
(tricylic-glycopeptide)**

pH 2.4 to 5

USUAL DOSE

7.5 mg/kg or 500 mg every 6 hours or 15 mg/kg or 1 Gm every 12 hours for 7 to 10 days. Maximum dosage of 3 to 4 Gm/24 hr used only in extreme situations. Normal renal function required.

Prevention of bacterial endocarditis in selected penicillin-allergic patients having GI, biliary, or GU surgery or instrumentation:

Adults and adolescents: 1 Gm IV before the procedure. Give gentamicin 1.5 mg/kg IV concurrently in high-risk patients (not to exceed 120 mg). Infusion must be administered over at least 60 minutes and should be completed within 30 minutes of starting the procedure. Gentamicin may not be necessary in moderate-risk patients. Both doses may be repeated in 8 to 12 hours for high-risk patients. Vancomycin alone may be indicated in selected patients having dental procedures or upper respiratory tract surgery or instrumentation. Consult recent recommendations of the American Heart Association or the American Dental Association.

Treatment of patients with methicillin-resistant or methicillin-susceptible staphylococcal endocarditis who have a native cardiac valve: 30 mg/kg/24 hr equally divided into 2 doses (15 mg/kg every 12 hours) for 6 weeks or longer. If more than 2 Gm/day are required, monitoring of serum concentrations of vancomycin is recommended.

Treatment of patients with methicillin-resistant or methicillin-susceptible staphylococcal endocarditis who have a prosthetic valve or other prosthetic material: 30 mg/kg/24 hr equally divided into 2 doses (15 mg/kg every 12 hours) or 4 doses (7.5 mg/kg every 6 hours) for 6 weeks or longer. If more than 2 Gm/day are required, monitoring of serum concentrations of vancomycin is recommended. Given in conjunction with oral rifampin 300 mg every 8 hours for 6 weeks or longer and IM or IV gentamicin 1 mg/kg every 8 hours during the first 2 weeks of vancomycin therapy.

Treatment of endocarditis caused by viridans streptococci or *Streptococcus bovis:* 30 mg/kg/24 hr equally divided into 2 doses (15 mg/kg every 12 hours) for 4 weeks. If more than 2 Gm/day are required, monitoring of serum concentrations of vancomycin is recommended.

Treatment of enterococcal endocarditis: 30 mg/kg/24 hr equally divided into 2 doses (15 mg/kg every 12 hours) for 4 to 6 weeks. If more than 2 Gm/day are required, monitoring of serum concentrations of vancomycin is recommended. Given in conjunction with IM or IV gentamicin 1 mg/kg every 8 hours for 4 to 6 weeks.

Perioperative prophylaxis in selected surgeries (e.g., cardiac, prosthetic valve, coronary artery bypass, joint replacement, craniotomy) when a cephalosporin cannot be used or there is a high incidence of methicillin-resistant staphylococci at the institution (unlabeled use): 1 Gm IV over 1 to 2 hours; should be completed within 30 minutes before the start of surgery. May be repeated one or more times if surgery is prolonged or major blood loss occurs. Postoperative doses are considered generally unnecessary and are not recommended.

Prevention of neonatal Group B streptococcal disease: Used for women with penicillin hypersensitivity who should not receive β-lactam anti-infectives or if resistance to clindamycin or erythromycin is known or suspected. 1 Gm every 12 hours until delivery. Initiate at the beginning of labor or rupture of membranes.

PEDIATRIC DOSE

Pediatric patients 1 month of age or older: *Mild to moderate infections:* 40 mg/kg of body weight/24 hr equally divided and given every 6, 8, or 12 hours (10 mg/kg every 6 hours, 13.33 mg/kg every 8 hours, or 20 mg/kg every 12 hours) for 7 to 10 days.

Severe infections: Up to 60 mg/kg/24 hr (15 mg/kg every 6 hours, 20 mg/kg every 8 hours, or 30 mg/kg every 12 hours) has been used if there is CNS involvement. Do not exceed 2 Gm in 24 hours.

Prevention of bacterial endocarditis in selected penicillin-allergic patients having GI, biliary, or GU surgery or instrumentation: 20 mg/kg before the procedure. Give gentamicin 1.5 mg/kg concurrently in high-risk patients (not to exceed 120 mg). Gentamicin may not be necessary in moderate-risk patients. Infusion must be administered over at least 60 minutes and should be complete within 30 minutes of starting the procedure. Both doses may be repeated in 8 to 12 hours for high-risk patients. Note comments about dental and upper respiratory surgery or instrumentation under Usual Dose.

NEONATAL DOSE

15 mg/kg as an initial dose. See Maternal/Child. Follow with 10 mg/kg. Adjust interval based on age and/or weight as follows:

Infants up to 1 week of age: Give every 12 hours.

Infants 1 week to 1 month of age: Give every 8 hours.

Continued

The American Academy of Pediatrics recommends 10 to 15 mg/kg. Adjust dose and interval based on weight and/or age as follows:

Postnatal Weight and Age	Dose and Interval
Less than 1.2 kg and less than 7 days of age	15 mg/kg/dose every 24 hours
Less than 1.2 kg and 7 days of age or older	15 mg/kg/dose every 24 hours
1.2 to 2 kg and less than 7 days of age	10 to 15 mg/kg/dose every 12 to 18 hours
1.2 to 2 kg and 7 days of age or older	10 to 15 mg/kg/dose every 8 to 12 hours
Over 2 kg and less than 7 days of age	10 to 15 mg/kg/dose every 8 to 12 hours
Over 2 kg and 7 days of age or older	15 to 20 mg/kg/dose every 6 to 8 hours

DOSE ADJUSTMENTS

Reduce total daily dose in premature infants and the elderly. Greater dose reductions than expected may be necessary in these patients because of impaired renal function. ■ Dose reduction required in impaired renal function. In all renal impaired patients (including functionally anephric and anuric patients), the initial dose should be no less than 15 mg/kg. *See prescribing information;* dose is reduced for every decrease of 10 mL/min in the CrCl. Subsequent doses of 250 to 1,000 mg every several days are suggested for functionally anephric patients. Subsequent doses of 1,000 mg every 7 to 10 days are suggested for anuric patients. Monitoring of serum levels is recommended.

DILUTION

Available premixed, premixed and frozen, or reconstitute each 500-mg vial with 10 mL of SW for injection. Each 500 mg must be further diluted with 100 mL of NS or D5W and given as an intermittent infusion. Also **compatible** in D5NS, LR, D5LR, D5 Normosol-M, Isolyte E, and acetated Ringer's injection. Concentrations greater than 5 mg/mL are not recommended. If absolutely necessary, 1 to 2 Gm may be further diluted in sufficient amounts of the same infusion fluids and given over 24 hours. Not recommended. Also available in ADD-Vantage vials for use with ADD-Vantage infusion containers.

Storage: Store in refrigerator after initial dilution. Maintains potency for 2 weeks in D5W or NS, 96 hours for other infusion solutions. Solutions prepared from ADD-Vantage vials stable at room temperature for 24 hours.

COMPATIBILITY   (Underline Indicates Conflicting Compatibility Information)

Consider any drug NOT listed as compatible to be INCOMPATIBLE until consulting a pharmacist; specific conditions may apply.

Several sources recommend not admixing with other drugs. They suggest it is **incompatible** with alkaline solutions (e.g., aminophylline, aztreonam [Azactam], barbiturates [e.g., pentobarbital (Nembutal)], chloramphenicol [Chloromycetin], dexamethasone [Decadron], sodium bicarbonate) and may form a precipitate with heavy metals. May inactivate aminoglycosides; should also not be combined in the same solution with albumin, selected cephalosporins, foscarnet (Foscavir), or selected penicillins; if administered concurrently, administer at separate sites or separate intervals (flush IV line with a **compatible** solution before and after administration). One source suggests the following **compatibilities:**

Additive: *See general comments under Compatibility.* Amikacin (Amikin), aminophylline, atracurium (Tracrium), aztreonam (Azactam), calcium gluconate, cefepime (Maxipime), dimenhydrinate, famotidine (Pepcid IV), heparin, hydrocortisone sodium succinate (Solu-Cortef), meropenem (Merrem IV), potassium chloride (KCl), ranitidine (Zantac), verapamil.

Y-site: *See general comments under Compatibility.* Acyclovir (Zovirax), aldesleukin (Proleukin), allopurinol (Aloprim), alprostadil, amifostine (Ethyol), amiodarone (Nexterone), ampicillin, ampicillin/sulbactam (Unasyn), anidulafungin (Eraxis), atracurium (Tracrium), aztreonam (Azactam), caspofungin (Cancidas), cefazolin (Ancef), cefepime (Maxipime), cefotaxime (Claforan), cefotetan, cefoxitin (Mefoxin), ceftazidime (Fortaz), ceftriaxone (Rocephin), cefuroxime (Zinacef), cisatracurium (Nimbex), cyclophosphamide (Cytoxan), dexmedetomidine (Precedex), diltiazem (Cardizem), docetaxel (Taxotere), doripenem (Doribax), doxapram (Dopram), doxorubicin liposomal (Doxil), enalaprilat (Vasotec IV), esmolol (Brevibloc), etoposide phosphate (Etopophos), fenoldopam (Corlopam), filgrastim (Neupogen), fluconazole (Diflucan), fludarabine (Fludara), foscarnet (Foscavir), gallium nitrate (Ganite), gemcitabine (Gemzar), granisetron (Kytril), heparin, hetastarch in electrolytes (Hextend), hydromorphone (Dilaudid), insulin (regular), labetalol (Trandate), levofloxacin (Levaquin), linezolid (Zyvox), lorazepam (Ativan), magnesium sulfate, melphalan (Alkeran), meperidine (Demerol), meropenem (Merrem IV), methotrexate, midazolam (Versed), milrinone (Primacor), morphine, mycophenolate (CellCept IV), nafcillin (Nallpen), nicardipine (Cardene IV), ondansetron (Zofran), paclitaxel (Taxol), palonosetron (Aloxi), pancuronium, pemetrexed (Alimta), piperacillin, piperacillin/ tazobactam (Zosyn), propofol (Diprivan), remifentanil (Ultiva), sargramostim (Leukine), sodium bicarbonate, tacrolimus (Prograf), teniposide (Vumon), theophylline, thiotepa, ticarcillin/clavulanate (Timentin), tigecycline (Tygacil), vecuronium, vinorelbine (Navelbine), warfarin (Coumadin), zidovudine (AZT, Retrovir).

RATE OF ADMINISTRATION
Severe hypotension, with or without red blotching of the face, neck, chest, and extremities, and cardiac arrest can occur with too-rapid injection.

A single dose properly diluted (concentration of no more than 5 mg/mL) at a rate not to exceed 10 mg/min or 60 minutes, whichever is longer. Another reference suggests infusion over 1 to 2 hours. This intermittent infusion is the preferred route of administration because of high incidence of thrombophlebitis.

Pediatric rate: A single dose over a minimum of 60 minutes.

ACTIONS
A very potent tricyclic glycopeptide antibiotic, it is bactericidal against gram-positive organisms. Bactericidal action results from the inhibition of cell wall synthesis. Also alters bacterial cell-membrane permeability and RNA synthesis. Well distributed in most body tissues and fluids, including pleural, pericardial, acitic, and synovial fluids; in urine; in peritoneal dialysis fluid; and in atrial appendage tissue. Penetration into the CSF occurs when the meninges are inflamed. Half-life is 4 to 6 hours in patients with normal renal function. Vancomycin is excreted in biologically active form in the urine. Crosses the placental barrier. Secreted in breast milk.

INDICATIONS AND USES

Serious gram-positive infections (e.g., staphylococcal) infections including endocarditis, septicemia, bone, lower respiratory tract, and skin and skin structure infections that do not respond or are resistant to other less toxic antibiotics, such as penicillins or cephalosporins (e.g., methicillin-resistant staphylococci). ▪ Penicillin-allergic patients. ▪ Treatment of endocarditis caused by *Streptococcus viridans* or *S. bovis* concurrently with an aminoglycoside antibiotic; endocarditis caused by diphtheroids or *S. epidermidis* concurrently with rifampin and/or an aminoglycoside. ▪ Parenteral form used orally for pseudomembranous colitis/staphylococcal enterocolitis caused by *C. difficile.*

Unlabeled uses: Prophylaxis against bacterial endocarditis in moderate or high-risk (prosthetic heart valves, congenital or rheumatic heart disease) penicillin-allergic patients undergoing GI, biliary or GU surgery or instrumentation. Given in combination with gentamicin in GI or GU procedures.

CONTRAINDICATIONS

Known hypersensitivity to vancomycin. Solutions containing dextrose may be contraindicated in patients with allergies to corn or corn products.

PRECAUTIONS

To reduce the development of drug-resistant bacteria and maintain its effectiveness, vancomycin should be used only to treat or prevent infections proven or strongly suspected to be caused by bacteria. ▪ Sensitivity studies necessary to determine susceptibility of the causative organism to vancomycin. ▪ Prolonged use of drug may result in superinfection caused by overgrowth of nonsusceptible organisms. ▪ May be ototoxic and nephrotoxic. Some clinicians feel the risk of ototoxicity and nephrotoxicity is minimal in patients with normal renal function who receive vancomycin as a single agent. ▪ Use caution in impaired hearing, impaired renal function, pregnancy, breast-feeding, neonates, and the elderly. ▪ *Clostridium difficile*–associated diarrhea (CDAD) has been reported. May range from mild diarrhea to fatal colitis. Consider in patients who present with diarrhea during or after treatment with vancomycin. ▪ Oral vancomycin has a local effect only (e.g., in the bowel); not for systemic use. ▪ A syndrome of chemical peritonitis has been reported in patients receiving intraperitoneal vancomycin during CAPD.

Monitor: Monitoring of serum levels and SCr may be indicated in patients at increased risk for developing nephrotoxicity and/or ototoxicity (e.g., underlying renal dysfunction, or receiving concomitant aminoglycosides [e.g., gentamicin]). ▪ Determine absolute patency of vein. Necrosis and sloughing will result from extravasation. Rotate injection sites every 2 to 3 days. ▪ Observe for furry tongue, diarrhea, and foul-smelling stools. ▪ Severe hypotension, with or without red blotching of the face, neck, chest, and extremities, and cardiac arrest can occur with too-rapid injection (red man or red neck syndrome). ▪ Monitor BP continuously during infusion to prevent a precipitous drop. ▪ Auditory testing indicated with prolonged use. ▪ Periodic monitoring of leukocyte count recommended in prolonged therapy. ▪ See Drug/Lab Interactions.

Patient Education: Report all side effects promptly. ▪ Promptly report diarrhea or bloody stools that occur during treatment or up to several months after an antibiotic has been discontinued; may indicate CDAD and require treatment.

Maternal/Child: Category C: studies not conclusive. Use only if clearly needed. ■ Safety for use in breast-feeding not established; discontinue breast-feeding. ■ Neonates have immature renal function; blood levels may be excessive. Confirmation of desired serum concentrations suggested in premature and full-term neonates.
Elderly: Systemic and renal clearance may be reduced; dosage reduction required.

DRUG/LAB INTERACTIONS

Synergistic with **aminoglycosides** (e.g., amikacin [Amikin], gentamicin, tobramycin) against many strains of *Staphylococcus aureus* and streptococci; see package insert. Combined use may increase risk of ototoxicity and nephrotoxicity. ■ Use caution with **dimenhydrinate**, which can mask ototoxicity. ■ Additive toxicities may occur with *systemic or topical* use of **other nephrotoxic, neurotoxic, or ototoxic drugs** (e.g., aminoglycosides, amphotericin B, bacitracin, cisplatin, colistin, ethacrynic acid [Edecrin], furosemide [Lasix], polymyxin B). Use with caution in combination with vancomycin; serial monitoring of renal and auditory systems indicated. ■ May enhance neuromuscular blockade with **nondepolarizing muscle relaxants** (e.g., pancuronium). ■ May cause erythema and histamine-like flushing in pediatric patients with **anesthetics.** Use with anesthetics may also increase the risk of hypersensitivity reactions, including anaphylaxis and infusion reactions. Administration of vancomycin as a 1-hour infusion before anesthetic induction may reduce this interaction. ■ May inhibit **methotrexate** excretion and increase methotrexate toxicity. May occur even if 10 days have elapsed since vancomycin administered. Adjust methotrexate dose as indicated.

SIDE EFFECTS

Chills, dizziness, fever, macular rashes, pain at injection site, pruritus, tinnitus, urticaria.
Major: Anaphylaxis, cardiac arrest, CDAD, dyspnea, eosinophilia, hearing loss, hypotension, infusion-related events (anaphylactoid reactions, dyspnea, flushing of the upper body, pruritus, urticaria, wheezing), interstitial nephritis, neutropenia, red neck or red man syndrome, renal failure, Stevens-Johnson syndrome (erythema multiforme [flu-like symptoms that can be fatal]), thrombophlebitis, wheezing.
Post-Marketing: Drug Rash with Eosinophilia and Systemic Symptoms (DRESS).

ANTIDOTE

Notify the physician of all side effects. Hearing loss may progress even if drug is discontinued. If minor side effects are progressive or any major side effect occurs, discontinue the drug, treat hypersensitivity reaction, or resuscitate as necessary. Prevent severe hypotension by slowing infusion rate to 2 hours. Fluids, antihistamines, corticosteroids, and vasopressors (e.g., dopamine) may be required. Mild cases of CDAD may respond to discontinuation of drug. Treat CDAD with fluids, electrolytes, protein supplements, and oral vancomycin (Vancocin) or metronidazole (Flagyl) as indicated. In severe cases, surgical evaluation may be indicated. Hemodialysis or CAPD will not decrease blood levels in toxicity.

VASOPRESSIN INJECTION
(vay-so-**PRESS**-in in-**JEK**-shun)

Hormone
Antidiuretic
Vasopressor (unlabeled)

Pitressin, ✚ Pressyn

pH 2.5 to 4.5

USUAL DOSE
ALL IV DOSES AND USES ARE UNLABELED.

Treatment of shock-resistant VF or pulseless VT during cardiac arrest in adult patients: AHA Emergency Cardiovascular Care recommends 40 units by IV push or through the endotracheal tube for 1 dose only (may replace the first or second dose of epinephrine).

Hemodynamic support during vasodilatory shock (e.g., septic shock): AHA guidelines recommend a continuous infusion of 0.02 to 0.04 units/min. Other sources in the literature recommend low-dose vasopressin infusions in vasodilatory shock refractory to catecholamines. 0.04 units/min as an infusion (range was 0.01 to 0.1 units/min). Doses greater than 0.08 units/min showed no added benefit. Continue infusion until the patient is stabilized. Mean duration in a study was 18 to 168 hours.

Hypotension unresponsive to norepinephrine following cardiopulmonary bypass: In 2002, Masetti and colleagues conducted an open-label study of vasopressin in 16 adults with hypotension following cardiopulmonary bypass. All had failed to respond to maximum norepinephrine doses (greater than 30 mcg/kg/min). Vasopressin was administered at rates of 0.1 to 1 unit/min for an average of 58.8 ± 37.3 hours. Systolic blood pressure increased from 89.6 ± 7.9 to 119 ± 10.5 mm Hg with treatment, and systemic vascular resistance increased from 688 ± 261.7 to $1,043.3 \pm 337.1$ dynes • sec/cm^5. Vasopressin use permitted discontinuation of other vasopressors in 13 of the patients within an average of 5.8 ± 7.8 hours. Seven of the 16 patients survived to discharge. (Source: Buck ML [PharmD, FCCP]: Low-dose vasopressin infusions for vasodilatory shock, *Journal of Cardiac Surgery,* 17:485-489, 2002.)

GI hemorrhage: 0.2 units/min as an infusion. Increase each hour by 0.2 units/min until hemorrhage is controlled. Doses up to 1 unit/min are suggested. Another source suggests 0.2 to 0.4 units/min as an infusion. Gradually increase dose as needed to a maximum dose of 0.9 units/min.

PEDIATRIC DOSE
All IV doses and uses are unlabeled; however, studies in pediatric patients have been conducted.

Hemodynamic support during vasodilatory shock: 0.0003 to 0.002 units/kg/min as an infusion (range is 0.018 to 0.12 units/kg/hr). Continue infusion until the patient and concurrently administered catecholamine infusions are stabilized. Mean duration in a study was 6 to 144 hours. AHA guidelines recommend a continuous infusion of 0.0002 to 0.002 units/kg/min (0.2 to 2 milliunits/kg/min).

Treatment of shock-resistant VF or pulseless VT during cardiac arrest: Recommended for use in adult patients only. AHA guidelines recommend 0.4 to 1 unit/kg IV push (maximum dose 40 units).

GI hemorrhage: 0.002 to 0.005 units/kg/min as an infusion. Gradually increase dose as needed to a maximum dose of 0.01 units/kg/min.

DILUTION

AHA Guidelines do not mention the use of a diluent, which suggests that vasopressin may be given undiluted. Another source recommends dilution for IV use to a 0.1 to 1 unit/mL dilution with NS or D5W. 38 mL diluent with 2 mL vasopressin (40 units) yields 1 unit/mL. 398 mL diluent with 2 mL vasopressin (40 units) yields 0.1 unit/mL.

Storage: Store unopened vials at CRT.

COMPATIBILITY   (Underline Indicates Conflicting Compatibility Information)

Consider any drug NOT listed as compatible to be INCOMPATIBLE until consulting a pharmacist; specific conditions may apply.

Consider specific use and unlabeled IV use.

Sources suggest the following **compatibilities:**

Additive: One source lists it as **compatible** as an additive with verapamil.

Y-site: Another source suggests **Y-site compatibility** with amiodarone (Nexterone), argatroban, caspofungin (Cancidas), ciprofloxacin (Cipro IV), diltiazem (Cardizem), dobutamine, dopamine, drotrecogin alfa (Xigris), epinephrine (Adrenalin), fluconazole (Diflucan), gentamicin, heparin, imipenem-cilastatin (Primaxin), insulin (regular), lidocaine, linezolid (Zyvox), meropenem (Merrem IV), metronidazole (Flagyl IV), micafungin (Mycamine), milrinone (Primacor), moxifloxacin (Avelox), nitroglycerin IV, norepinephrine (Levophed), pantoprazole (Protonix IV), phenylephrine (Neo-Synephrine), piperacillin/tazobactam (Zosyn), procainamide (Pronestyl), sodium bicarbonate, voriconazole (VFEND IV).

RATE OF ADMINISTRATION

Injection: A single dose IV push; see Precautions.

Infusion: See Usual Dose for recommended rates for each diagnosis. Use of a central venous catheter is recommended. Titrate rate so that perfusion remains adequate while BP is optimized. Do not discontinue abruptly; one source recommends tapering over 2 to 3 hours while monitoring effects.

ACTIONS

Synthetic vasopressin of the posterior pituitary gland standardized to 20 units/mL. An antidiuretic. Also a potent vasoconstrictor. Causes smooth muscle contraction of all parts of the vascular bed (e.g., capillaries, small arterioles, and venules). Has a lesser effect on the smooth muscles of larger arteries and veins. This direct contractile effect on the smooth muscle of the vascular system is not antagonized by adrenergic blocking agents (e.g., atenolol [Tenormin], metoprolol [Lopressor]) and is not prevented by vascular denervation (loss of nerve impulse to the vascular system). Its IV use is as an alternative pressor agent to epinephrine. Not effective in normotensive patients; however, promotes an effective increase in BP in hypotensive patients, even when other agents have failed. Rapidly degraded by enzymes in the liver and kidneys. Plasma half-life is 10 to 35 minutes. A small amount is excreted unchanged in the urine.

INDICATIONS AND USES

Used IM or SC as an antidiuretic in central diabetes insipidus or as a diagnostic aid in diabetes insipidus.

Unlabeled uses: The AHA Handbook of Emergency Cardiovascular Care recommends use in the treatment of adult shock-refractory ventricular fibrillation (class IIb) (an alternative pressor agent to epinephrine) and for hemodynamic support in vasodilatory shock (e.g., septic shock). Has also been used for treatment of GI hemorrhage.

CONTRAINDICATIONS

Hypersensitivity to vasopressin or any of its components; see Precautions. AHA Guidelines state "not recommended for responsive patients with coronary heart disease."

PRECAUTIONS

IV uses are unlabeled. ■ May cause ischemia of other organs (e.g., GI tract, kidneys) if fluid intake is not adequate. ■ Use with extreme caution in patients with vascular disease, especially coronary artery disease; may cause cardiac ischemia. Small doses may precipitate anginal pain, and larger doses may cause myocardial infarction. ■ May produce water intoxication; use with caution in patients with asthma, chronic nephritis and nitrogen retention, epilepsy, heart failure, migraine, or any conditions in which a rapid addition to extracellular water could be hazardous.

Monitor: In addition to management of airway, oxygenation, and blood gas determinations, the continuous monitoring of ECG, vital signs, and fluid and electrolyte status is mandatory. ■ Monitor IV site very closely, especially if it is a peripheral site; a central venous catheter is preferred. Produces intense vasoconstriction. Avoid extravasation; vasoconstriction that may result in severe tissue necrosis and gangrene can occur. ■ Maintain adequate fluid intake to avoid ischemia of other organs. ■ Use of vasopressin in vasodilatory shock may permit reduction or discontinuation of other vasopressors. ■ Use an indwelling urinary catheter to confirm urine output and monitor closely. ■ Fluid restriction may be indicated; initial signs of water intoxication include drowsiness, listlessness, and headache, which can rapidly progress to terminal coma and convulsions. ■ See Rate of Administration, Precautions, and Drug/Lab Interactions.

Maternal/Child: Category C: safety for use during pregnancy not established; use only if clearly needed. ■ Safety for use during breast-feeding not established. ■ Safety and effectiveness for use in pediatric patients not established; however, it has been used successfully in selected critically ill pediatric patients with catecholamine-resistant hypotension.

Elderly: See Precautions; elderly may be more sensitive to adverse effects.

DRUG/LAB INTERACTIONS

Vasodilators (e.g., nitroglycerin, nitroprusside sodium) counteract the vasoconstrictive effects of vasopressin. ■ Additive pressor response with **ganglionic blocking agents** (e.g., trimethaphan [Arfonad (rarely used antihypertensive)]). ■ Antidiuretic effect may be increased with concurrent use of **carbamazepine** (Tegretol), **chlorpropamide** (Diabinese), **clofibrate** (Atromid-S), **fludrocortisone** (Florinef), **tricyclic antidepressants** (e.g., amitriptyline [Elavil]), **urea.** ■ Antidiuretic effect may be decreased with concurrent use of **alcohol, demeclocycline** (Declomycin), **heparin, lithium** (Carbolith), **norepinephrine** (Levophed).

SIDE EFFECTS

Arrhythmias, bradycardia, hypertension, and MI have resulted from high doses. Abdominal cramps, angina, arrhythmias, bronchial constriction, cardiac arrest, circumoral pallor, cutaneous gangrene, decreased cardiac output, diaphoresis, flatus, gangrene, headache (pounding), hypersensitivity reactions (including anaphylaxis), hyponatremia, injection site ischemia resulting in severe tissue necrosis and gangrene, ischemic skin and mucous membrane lesions, myocardial ischemia, nausea, organ ischemia (e.g., GI, kidney), peripheral vasoconstriction, shock, sweating, tremor, urticaria, venous thrombosis, vertigo, and vomiting.

Overdose: Water intoxication.

ANTIDOTE

In an emergency cardiac care situation, all side effects can present life-threatening additional problems. Monitor the patient closely and observe all S/S that may indicate further deterioration. Treat symptomatically according to AHA Guidelines. Monitor fluid intake and urine output to ensure adequate hydration. Extravasation and/or ischemia at the injection site should be reported immediately to prevent tissue necrosis and gangrene. If water intoxication should occur, treat with water restriction and discontinue vasopressin. If possible, discontinue gradually as described in Rate of Administration to prevent a rapid fall in BP. If severe, may require osmotic diuresis with mannitol, hypertonic dextrose, or urea alone or with furosemide (Lasix).

VECURONIUM BROMIDE BBW
(veh-kyour-**OH**-nee-um **BRO**-myd)

Neuromuscular
blocking agent
(nondepolarizing)
Anesthesia adjunct

pH 4

USUAL DOSE
Adjunct to general anesthesia: Must be individualized, depending on previous drugs administered and degree and length of muscle relaxation required. 0.08 to 0.1 mg/kg (80 to 100 mcg/kg) of body weight initially as an IV bolus. Must be used with adequate anesthesia and/or sedation and after unconsciousness induced. One source suggests using IBW for obese patients (equal to or greater than 30% of IBW). Determine need for *maintenance dose* based on beginning symptoms of neuromuscular blockade reversal determined by a peripheral nerve stimulator. *IV bolus injection:* 0.01 to 0.015 mg/kg (10 to 15 mcg/kg) will be required in approximately 25 to 40 minutes and every 12 to 20 minutes thereafter to maintain muscle relaxation. Higher doses (0.15 to 0.28 mg/kg) at longer intervals have been given with proper ventilation without causing adverse cardiac effects. *Continuous infusion:* 1 mcg/kg/min. Begin in 20 to 40 minutes after initial bolus dose.

Support of intubated, mechanically ventilated, or respiratory-controlled adult ICU patients (unlabeled): *IV bolus injection:* 0.1 to 0.2 mg/kg (100 to 200 mcg/kg) every 1 hour. *Continuous infusion:* Begin with a loading dose of 0.1 mg/kg (100 mcg/kg) followed by a *maintenance dose* of 0.05 to 0.1 mg/kg/hr (50 to 100 mcg/kg/hr). A lower-end or reduced dose may be indicated if administered more than 5 minutes after the start of an inhalation agent, when steady-state has been achieved, or in patients with organ dysfunction (e.g., impaired liver function). Adjust dose according to clinical assessment of the patient's response. Use of a peripheral nerve stimulator is recommended. Vecuronium may be the preferred agent for patients with renal failure.

PEDIATRIC DOSE
Adjunct to general anesthesia: 1 to 10 years of age: May require high end of initial adult dose, and maintenance dose may be required on a more frequent basis.

DOSE ADJUSTMENTS
Reduce dose by 15% if administered more than 5 minutes after inhalation general anesthetics. ▪ Reduce dose to 0.04 to 0.06 mg/kg if following succinylcholine administration. Succinylcholine must show signs of wearing off before vecuronium is given. Use caution. ▪ Reduced dose required with numerous drugs; see Drug/Lab Interactions. ▪ Reduced dose may be required in renal or hepatic impairment. Preparation by dialysis before surgery is recommended for patients with renal failure. In an emergency surgery when dialysis cannot be accomplished, consider a lower initial dose. ▪ Infants between 7 weeks and 1 year may require a slightly lower dose, and recovery time will be extended.

DILUTION

Each 10 mg must be diluted with 5 mL SW for injection (supplied). May be given by IV injection or 10 (20) mg may be further diluted in up to 100 mL NS, D5W, D5NS, or LR and given as an infusion 0.1 (0.2) mg/mL concentration. Titrated to symptoms of neuromuscular blockade reversal. **Storage:** Stable at room temperature before reconstitution. Store under refrigeration. Discard after 24 hours except if reconstituted with bacteriostatic water; stable refrigerated up to 5 days.

COMPATIBLE WITH   (Underline Indicates Conflicting Compatibility Information)

Consider any drug NOT listed as compatible to be INCOMPATIBLE until consulting a pharmacist; specific conditions may apply.

Manufacturer states, "Has an acid pH. Reconstituted vecuronium should not be mixed with alkaline solutions (e.g., barbiturates [thiopental (Pentothal)]) in the same syringe or administered simultaneously during IV infusion through the same needle or the same IV line."

One source suggests the following **compatibilities:**

Additive: Ciprofloxacin (Cipro IV).

Y-site: Alprostadil, aminophylline, amiodarone (Nexterone), cefazolin (Ancef), cefuroxime (Zinacef), diltiazem (Cardizem), dobutamine, dopamine, epinephrine (Adrenalin), esmolol (Brevibloc), fenoldopam (Corlopam), fentanyl (Sublimaze), fluconazole (Diflucan), gentamicin, heparin, hetastarch in electrolytes (Hextend), hydrocortisone sodium succinate (Solu-Cortef), hydromorphone (Dilaudid), isoproterenol (Isuprel), labetalol (Trandate), linezolid (Zyvox), lorazepam (Ativan), midazolam (Versed), milrinone (Primacor), morphine, nicardipine (Cardene IV), nitroglycerin IV, nitroprusside sodium, norepinephrine (Levophed), palonosetron (Aloxi), propofol (Diprivan), ranitidine (Zantac), sulfamethoxazole/trimethoprim, vancomycin.

RATE OF ADMINISTRATION

Adjunct to general anesthesia: A single dose as an IV bolus over 30 to 60 seconds. If maintenance dose is given as an infusion, adjust rate to specific dose desired, usually 1 mcg/kg/min. See the following chart.

Vecuronium Guidelines for Infusion During General Anesthesia		
Desired Vecuronium Delivery Rate (mcg/kg/min)	Vecuronium Infusion Delivery Rate (mL/kg/min)	
	0.1 mg/mL*	0.2 mg/mL†
0.7 mcg/kg/min	0.007 mL/kg/min	0.0035 mL/kg/min
0.8 mcg/kg/min	0.008 mL/kg/min	0.0040 mL/kg/min
0.9 mcg/kg/min	0.009 mL/kg/min	0.0045 mL/kg/min
1.0 mcg/kg/min	0.010 mL/kg/min	0.0050 mL/kg/min
1.1 mcg/kg/min	0.011 mL/kg/min	0.0055 mL/kg/min
1.2 mcg/kg/min	0.012 mL/kg/min	0.0060 mL/kg/min
1.3 mcg/kg/min	0.013 mL/kg/min	0.0065 mL/kg/min

*10 mg of vecuronium in 100 mL solution.
†20 mg of vecuronium in 100 mL solution.

Mechanical ventilation support in ICU: Dose must be calculated; the preceding chart is for use during general anesthesia only. See Usual Dose for specific rates and criteria.

ACTIONS

A nondepolarizing skeletal muscle relaxant about one-third more potent than pancuronium with a shorter duration of neuromuscular blockade. Acts by competing for cholinergic receptors at the motor end-plate. Onset of action is within 30 seconds, is dose dependent, produces maximum neuromuscular blockade (paralysis) within 3 to 5 minutes, and lasts about 25 minutes. It may take up to 60 minutes or more before complete recovery occurs. Up to three times the therapeutic dose has been given without significant changes of hemodynamic parameters in good-risk surgical patients. Excreted as metabolites in bile and urine. Crosses the placental barrier.

INDICATIONS AND USES

Adjunctive to general anesthesia, to facilitate endotracheal intubation and to relax skeletal muscles during surgery or mechanical ventilation.

Unlabeled uses: Support of intubated, mechanically ventilated, or respiratory-controlled patients in ICU.

CONTRAINDICATIONS

Known hypersensitivity to vecuronium.

PRECAUTIONS

For IV use only. ■ Administered by or under the direct observation of the anesthesiologist. ■ Appropriate emergency drugs and equipment for monitoring the patient and responding to any medical emergency must be readily available. ■ Repeated doses have no cumulative effect if recovery is allowed to begin before administration. ■ Use extreme caution in patients with cirrhosis, cholestasis, obesity, or circulatory insufficiency. ■ Myasthenia gravis and other neuromuscular diseases increase sensitivity to drug. Can cause critical reactions. ■ Severe anaphylactic reactions have been reported with neuromuscular blocking agents; some have been fatal. Use caution in patients who have had an anaphylactic reaction to another neuromuscular blocking agent (depolarizing or nondepolarizing); cross-reactivity has occurred. ■ Acid base and/or electrolyte imbalance, debilitation, hypoxic episodes, and/or the use of other drugs (e.g., broad-spectrum antibiotics, narcotics, steroids) may prolong the effects of vecuronium.

Monitor: All uses: This drug produces apnea. Controlled artificial ventilation with oxygen must be continuous and under direct observation at all times. Maintain a patent airway. ■ Use a peripheral nerve stimulator to monitor response to vecuronium and avoid overdose. Have reversal agents available (e.g., edrophonium, neostigmine, pyridostigmine with atropine or glycopyrrolate); see Antidote. ■ Patient may be conscious and completely unable to communicate by any means. Has no analgesic or sedative properties. Respiratory depression with morphine may be preferred in some patients requiring mechanical ventilation. ■ Action is altered by dehydration, electrolyte imbalance, body temperatures, and acid-base imbalance. ■ Recovery time extended in infants 7 weeks to 1 year. ■ See Drug/Lab Interactions. **Mechanical ventilation support in ICU:** Physical therapy is recommended to prevent muscular weakness, atrophy, and joint contracture. Muscular weakness may be first noticed during attempts to wean patients from the ventilator.

Maternal/Child: Category C: use in pregnancy only if use justifies potential risk to fetus. Has been used during cesarean section; monitor infant carefully. Action may be enhanced by magnesium administered for the management of toxemia of pregnancy. ■ Use caution during breast-feeding. ■ Safety for use in infants under 7 weeks of age not established. ■ Some preparations contain benzyl alcohol; do not use in premature infants. ■ See Dose Adjustments.

Elderly: Differences in response compared to younger adults not observed. Lower-end initial doses may be appropriate based on the potential for decreased organ function and concomitant disease or drug therapy. ■ Duration of neuromuscular block may be prolonged.

DRUG/LAB INTERACTIONS

Potentiated by **acidosis, hypokalemia, some carcinomas, general anesthetics** (e.g., enflurane, isoflurane, halothane), **many antibiotics** (e.g., clindamycin [Cleocin]), **aminoglycosides** (e.g., kanamycin [Kantrex], gentamicin), **poly-peptide antibiotics** (e.g., bacitracin, colistimethate), **tetracyclines, diuretics, diazepam** (Valium) **and other muscle relaxants, magnesium sulfate, quinidine, morphine, meperidine, succinylcholine, verapamil, and others.** May need to reduce dose of vecuronium. Use with caution. ■ Effects may be decreased by **acetylcholine, alkalosis, anticholinesterases, azathioprine, carbamazepine, phenytoin, and theophylline.** ■ **Succinylcholine** must show signs of wearing off before vecuronium is given. Use caution.

SIDE EFFECTS

No side effects have occurred except with overdose: prolonged action resulting in respiratory insufficiency or apnea, airway closure caused by relaxation of epiglottis, pharynx, and tongue muscles. Hypersensitivity reactions including anaphylaxis are possible. Muscular weakness and atrophy may occur with long-term use (1 to 3 weeks).

ANTIDOTE

All side effects are medical emergencies. Treat symptomatically. Controlled artificial ventilation must be continuous until full muscle control returns. Edrophonium (Enlon), pyridostigmine (Regonol) or neostigmine given with atropine or glycopyrrolate will probably reverse the muscle relaxation but should not be required because of short time of effectiveness. Not effective in all situations; may aggravate severe overdose. Resuscitate as necessary.

VERAPAMIL HYDROCHLORIDE
(ver-**AP**-ah-mil hy-droh-**KLOR**-eyed)

Calcium channel blocker
Antiarrhythmic

pH 4.1 to 6

USUAL DOSE

5 to 10 mg initially (0.075 to 0.15 mg/kg of body weight). May cause transient bradycardia or hypotension. 10 mg (0.15 mg/kg) may be repeated in 30 minutes if needed to achieve appropriate response. Maximum total dose is 20 mg. AHA recommendation is 2.5 to 5 mg as an initial dose. Repeat 5 to 10 mg if needed every 15 to 30 min. Maximum dose 20 mg. Alternately, give 5 mg every 15 min to a total dose of 30 mg.

PEDIATRIC DOSE

ECG and BP monitoring mandatory. See Maternal/Child.

Infants up to 1 year of age: 0.1 to 0.2 mg/kg of body weight (usually 0.75 to 2 mg). Repeat in 30 minutes if indicated.

1 to 15 years of age: 0.1 to 0.3 mg/kg (usually 2 to 5 mg). Do not exceed 5 mg. Repeat in 30 minutes if response not adequate. Repeat dose should not exceed 10 mg as a single dose.

DOSE ADJUSTMENTS

Reduced dose may be required in hepatic or renal disease, especially with repeat dosing. ▪ Dose selection should be cautious in the elderly. Reduced doses may be indicated based on the potential for decreased organ function and concomitant disease or drug therapy. ▪ See Drug/Lab Interactions.

DILUTION

IV injection: May be given undiluted through Y-tube or three-way stopcock of tubing containing D5W, NS, or Ringer's solution for infusion or further diluted for infusion (1 mg/mL).

Filters: No data available from manufacturer.

Storage: Store between 15° and 30° C (59° and 86° F). Protect from light and freezing. Do not use if discolored or particulate matter present. Discard unused solution.

COMPATIBILITY   (Underline Indicates Conflicting Compatibility Information)

Consider any drug NOT listed as compatible to be INCOMPATIBLE until consulting a pharmacist; specific conditions may apply.

Manufacturer states, "Not recommended for dilution with sodium lactate in polyvinyl chloride bags. Will precipitate in any solution with a pH greater than 6." Lists as **incompatible** with albumin, amphotericin B (generic), hydralazine, sulfamethoxazole/trimethoprim.

One source suggests the following **compatibilities:**

Additive: Amikacin (Amikin), amiodarone (Nexterone), ampicillin, ascorbic acid, atropine, calcium chloride, calcium gluconate, cefazolin (Ancef), cefotaxime (Claforan), cefoxitin (Mefoxin), chloramphenicol (Chloromycetin), clindamycin (Cleocin), dexamethasone (Decadron), diazepam (Valium), digoxin (Lanoxin), dobutamine, dopamine, epinephrine (Adrenalin), erythromycin (Erythrocin), furosemide (Lasix), gentamicin, heparin, hydrocortisone sodium succinate (Solu-Cortef), hydromorphone (Dilaudid), insulin (regular), isoproterenol (Isuprel), lidocaine, magnesium sulfate, mannitol, meperidine (Demerol), methyldopa, methylprednisolone

(Solu-Medrol), metoclopramide (Reglan), morphine, multivitamins (M.V.I.), <u>nafcillin (Nallpen)</u>, naloxone (Narcan), nitroglycerin IV, nitroprusside sodium, norepinephrine (Levophed), <u>oxacillin (Bactocill)</u>, oxytocin (Pitocin), pancuronium, penicillin G potassium and sodium, <u>pentobarbital (Nembutal)</u>, <u>phenobarbital (Luminal)</u>, phentolamine (Regitine), <u>phenytoin (Dilantin)</u>, piperacillin, potassium chloride (KCl), potassium phosphate, procainamide (Pronestyl), propranolol, protamine sulfate, quinidine gluconate, <u>sodium bicarbonate</u>, theophylline, tobramycin, vancomycin, vasopressin.

Y-site: Argatroban, bivalirudin (Angiomax), ciprofloxacin (Cipro IV), dexmedetomidine (Precedex), dobutamine, dopamine, famotidine (Pepcid IV), fenoldopam (Corlopam), hetastarch in electrolytes (Hextend), hydralazine, inamrinone (Amrinone), linezolid (Zyvox), meperidine (Demerol), milrinone (Primacor), nesiritide (Natrecor), oxaliplatin (Eloxatin), penicillin G potassium, piperacillin.

RATE OF ADMINISTRATION

IV injection: A single dose over 2 minutes for adults and pediatric patients. Extend to 3 minutes in the elderly.

Infusion: Infusion pump required; separate IV line preferred to ensure accuracy and prevent accidental bolusing during addition of other fluids. Rate may be constant (e.g., 5 to 10 mg/hr) or titrated to HR.

ACTIONS

A calcium (and possibly sodium) ion inhibitor through slow channels into conductile and contractile myocardial cells and vascular smooth muscle cells. Slows conduction through SA and AV nodes, prolongs effective refractory period in the AV node, and reduces ventricular rates. Prevents reentry phenomena through the AV node. Reduces myocardial contractility, afterload, arterial pressure, vascular tone, and oxygen demand. Effective within 1 to 5 minutes. Hemodynamic effects last about 20 minutes, but antiarrhythmic effects may last up to 6 hours. Does not alter total serum calcium levels. Metabolized in the liver. Half-life range is 2 to 5 hours. Crosses the placental barrier. Excreted in urine and feces. Secreted in breast milk.

INDICATIONS AND USES

Treatment of supraventricular tachyarrhythmias including conversion to normal sinus rhythm of paroxysmal supraventricular tachycardia (includes Wolff-Parkinson-White and Lown-Ganong-Levine syndromes). ■ Temporary control of rapid ventricular rate in atrial flutter or atrial fibrillation.

Unlabeled uses: Alternative drug after adenosine to terminate re-entry SVT with narrow QRS complex and adequate BP and preserved LV function (AHA guidelines).

CONTRAINDICATIONS

SA nodal function impairment or atrial fibrillation or flutter when associated with an accessory bypass tract (e.g., Wolff-Parkinson-White or Lown-Ganong-Levine syndromes), cardiogenic shock, congestive heart failure (severe) unless secondary to supraventricular tachyarrhythmia treatable with verapamil, known hypersensitivity to verapamil, second- or third-degree AV block (unless functioning artificial pacemaker is in place), severe hypotension, sick sinus syndrome (unless functioning artificial pacemaker in place), patients receiving IV beta-adrenergic blocking drugs (e.g., propranolol) within 2 to 4 hours, and ventricular tachycardia.

PRECAUTIONS

Administer in a facility with adequate personnel, equipment, and supplies to monitor the patient and respond to any medical emergency. ■ Valsalva maneuver recommended before use of verapamil in all paroxysmal supraventricular tachycardias if clinically appropriate. ■ May produce hypotension. Usually transient and asymptomatic, but can cause dizziness. ■ Has rarely caused second- and third-degree AV block and, in extreme cases, asystole. ■ Caution required in hepatic and renal disease, especially if repeated dosing is required. ■ Use extreme caution in patients with hypertrophic cardiomyopathy. ■ May cause ventricular fibrillation in patients with wide-complex ventricular tachycardia. ■ May precipitate respiratory muscle failure in patients with muscular dystrophy or increase intracranial pressure during anesthesia induction in patients with supratentorial tumors. Use caution and monitor closely. ■ Use with caution in patients with severe aortic stenosis and acute MI with pulmonary congestion documented by x-ray. ■ Reduction of myocardial contractility may worsen CHF in patients with severe left ventricular dysfunction. ■ Continue regular dosing on day of surgery and thereafter unless otherwise specified by physician. May cause severe angina or MI if discontinued. ■ Recent studies indicate that verapamil inhibits thrombus formation and platelet aggregation.

Monitor: Continuous ECG and BP monitoring recommended. ■ Document cardiac rhythm before therapy, with any significant change in type or rate, and at least every 4 hours. See PR interval. ■ Monitor BP and HR very closely, every 5 minutes times 3 or until reasonably stabilized, every 15 minutes times 4 and hourly thereafter. May need more frequent checks with increased drip rate. ■ Emergency resuscitation drugs and equipment must always be available. ■ Treat heart failure with digoxin and diuretics before using verapamil. ■ Patients with pulmonary wedge pressure above 20 mm Hg and/or ejection fraction below 20% to 30% may experience acute worsening of heart failure. ■ Maintain bed rest until effects on HR, BP, and potential dizziness evaluated. ■ Monitor for side effects (AV block) and digoxin levels when used concurrently with digoxin. ■ Monitor for any unusual bleeding or bruising. ■ See Drug/Lab Interactions.

Maternal/Child: Category C: safety for use in pregnancy not yet established; use only when clearly indicated. ■ Discontinue breast-feeding. ■ Severe hemodynamic side effects (e.g., bradycardia, hypotension, or a rapid ventricular rate in atrial flutter/fibrillation) can occur in infants and neonates. Use caution and monitor closely.

Elderly: May have an increased hypotensive effect; see Rate of Administration. ■ Half-life may be prolonged; see Dose Adjustments. ■ May cause drug-induced tinnitus.

DRUG/LAB INTERACTIONS

Potentiates **digoxin;** lower dose may be appropriate. Both drugs slow AV conduction. Monitor for AV block and bradycardia. ■ Do not give comcomitantly (within a few hours) with **IV beta-adrenergic blocking drugs** (e.g., propranolol); see Contraindications. Use with extreme caution with **oral or ophthalmic beta blockers.** Both drugs depress myocardial contractility and AV node conduction; monitor patient closely. ■ Do not administer **disopyramide** (Norpace) within 48 hours before or 24 hours after verapamil. ■ Use caution with **inhalation anesthetics.** Both depress cardiovascular activity. Titrate each carefully to avoid excessive cardiovascular depression. ■ Coadministration with **amiodarone** (Nexterone) may result in bradycardia and decreased cardiac output. Monitor closely. ■ Potentiates **cyclosporine, carbamazepine, and theophyllines.** Monitor serum levels of these drugs and adjust dose as needed. ■ Potentiates **nondepolarizing muscle relaxants** (e.g., vecuronium); dose reduction of either drug may be required. ■ Metabolism may be decreased and serum concentrations may be increased by **cimeti-dine** (Tagamet) **and itraconazole** (Sporanox). ■ Verapamil may increase serum concentrations of **dofetilide** (Tikosyn). One source says avoid use; another says concurrent use contraindicated. ■ Verapamil may increase serum concentrations of **HMG-CoA reductase inhibitors** (e.g., atorvastatin [Lipitor], simvastatin [Zocor]), **imipramine** (Tofranil), **prazosin** (Minipress), **sirolimus** (Rapamune), **tacrolimus** (Prograf). Monitor serum levels and/or monitor for S/S of toxicity; adjust dose as needed. ■ May increase effects of certain **benzodiazepines** (e.g., midazolam [Versed], triazolam [Halcion]) and **buspirone** (BuSpar); monitor and adjust doses as indicated. ■ May cause excessive hypotension with **other antihypertensive drugs** (vasodilators and diuretics). ■ Serum concentrations and effectiveness of verapamil may be decreased by **barbiturates** (e.g., phenobarbital), **calcium salts, phenytoin** (Dilantin), **sulfinpyrazone** (Anturane). ■ Concomitant use with **IV dan-trolene** (Dantrium) may result in cardiovascular collapse. ■ Use with **quin-idine** may cause AV block, bradycardia, hypotension, ventricular tachy-cardia, and pulmonary edema. ■ Hypotension and bradycardia have been observed with concurrent telithromycin (Ketek). ■ Highly protein bound; use with caution with **other highly protein-bound drugs** (e.g., oral hypogly-cemics, warfarin). Use caution. ■ Variable effects when administered with **lithium.** Has caused decreased effectiveness of lithium and may cause neurotoxicity. ■ May have additive effects with **flecainide** (Tambocor). ■ Monitor heart rate with concurrent use of verapamil with **clonidine;** has resulted in sinus bradycardia requiring pacemaker insertion. ■ **Grapefruit juice** may affect certain enzymes of the P_{450} enzyme system and should be avoided.

SIDE EFFECTS

Abdominal discomfort, asystole, bradycardia, dizziness, headache, second- and third-degree heart block, heart failure, hypersensitivity reac-tions including anaphylaxis, hypotension (symptomatic), increased ven-tricular response in atrial flutter, fibrillation (Wolff-Parkinson-White and Lown-Ganong-Levine syndromes), nausea, PVCs, skin eruptions (includ-ing rare reports of erythema multiforme), tachycardia.

ANTIDOTE

Discontinue verapamil and notify physician promptly if hypotension, bradycardia, or second- or third-degree heart block occurs. Keep physician informed of all side effects. Treatment will depend on clinical situation. Calcium chloride may reverse effects of verapamil and can be used in toxicity. Glucagon may also be used in toxicity; see glucagon monograph. Rapid ventricular response in atrial flutter/fibrillation should respond to cardioversion, procainamide, and/or lidocaine. Treat bradycardia, AV block, and asystole with standard AHA protocol (atropine, pacing). Norepinephrine (Levarterenol) or dopamine will reverse hypotension. Treat hypersensitivity reactions or resuscitate as necessary. Not removed by hemodialysis.

VERTEPORFIN
(ver-teh-**POR**-fin)

Visudyne

Photosensitizing agent
Macular degeneration therapy adjunct

USUAL DOSE

A course is a ***two-stage process*** requiring administration of both drug and light. Each course may be repeated every 3 months as indicated. Body surface area, lesion size determination, and spot size determination of the choroidal neovascularization (CNV) are used by the retina specialist to calculate dosing of verteporfin. The greatest linear dimension of the lesion is estimated by fluorescein angiography and color fundus photography. The treatment spot size should be 1,000 microns larger than the greatest linear dimension of the lesion on the retina to allow a 500-micron border. The nasal edge of the treatment spot must be positioned at least 200 microns from the temporal edge of the optic disc.

First stage: 6 mg/M^2 of verteporfin as a single IV infusion.

Second stage: Activation of verteporfin using a recommended light dose of 50 J/cm^2 of neovascular lesion administered at an intensity of 600 mW/cm^2 over 83 seconds. Initiate 689 ± 3 nm wavelength laser light delivery 15 minutes after the start of the verteporfin infusion. Light is delivered to the retina as a single circular spot via a fiber optic and a slit lamp, using a suitable ophthalmic magnification lens. Light dose, light intensity, ophthalmic lens magnification factor, and zoom lens setting are important parameters for the appropriate delivery of light to the predetermined treatment spot. Follow the laser system manuals for procedure set up and operation.

Concurrent bilateral treatment: In patients who present with eligible lesions in both eyes without prior verteporfin therapy, treat only one eye (the most aggressive lesion) during the first course. One week after the first course, if no significant safety issues are identified, the second eye can be treated, using the same treatment regimen including a verteporfin infusion and light activation. Approximately 3 months later, both eyes can be evaluated and concurrent treatment following a new verteporfin infusion can be started if both lesions still show evidence of leakage. When treating both eyes concurrently, the more aggressive lesion should be treated first, at 15 minutes after the start of infusion. Immediately at the end of light application to the first eye, the laser settings should be adjusted to introduce the treatment parameters for the second eye, with the same light dose and intensity as for the first eye, starting no later than 20 minutes from the start of the infusion.

DOSE ADJUSTMENTS

No adjustments required. See Precautions.

DILUTION

Specific techniques required; see Precautions. Reconstitute each vial of verteporfin with 7 mL of SW to provide 7.5 mL of opaque, dark green solution containing 2 mg/mL. Withdraw the desired dose from the vial and further dilute with D5W to a total infusion volume of 30 mL.

Filters: Use of a 1.2-micron in-line filter is required for administration.

Storage: Store between 20° and 25° C (68° and 77° F). Reconstituted and diluted solution must be protected from light and used within 4 hours.

COMPATIBILITY

Manufacturer states, "May precipitate in saline solutions. Do not use NS or other parenteral solutions. Do not mix in same solution with other drugs." Use only SW and D5W as listed under Dilution.

RATE OF ADMINISTRATION

A 30-mL infusion equally distributed over 10 minutes (3 mL/min) using an appropriate syringe pump and a 1.2-micron in-line filter.

ACTIONS

A light activated drug (photosensitizing agent) for use in photodynamic therapy (PDT). Transported in the plasma by lipoproteins. Endothelial cells of the abnormal choroidal blood vessels which have high concentrations of lipoprotein receptors take up the lipoprotein-verteporfin complex. Light activation in the presence of O_2, induces a photochemical reaction, generating highly reactive singlet oxygen and reactive oxygen radicals that cause local damage to the neovascular endothelium. The damaged endothelium releases procoagulant and vasoactive factors through the lipooxygenase (leukotriene) and cyclo-oxygenase (eicosanoids such as thromboxane) pathways, resulting in platelet aggregation, fibrin clot formation, vasoconstriction, and ultimately, vessel occlusion. Verteporfin appears to preferentially accumulate in neovasculature, including chorioidal neovasculature. However, animal models indicate that the drug is also present in the retina. Therefore, there may be collateral damage to retinal structures following photoactivation. Terminal elimination half-life of verteporfin is 5 to 6 hours. It is metabolized to a small extent by liver and plasma esterases and is eliminated primarily by the fecal route as unchanged drug. May be secreted in breast milk.

INDICATIONS AND USES

Treatment of patients with predominantly classic subfoveal choroidal neovascularization due to age-related macular degeneration, pathologic myopia, or presumed ocular histoplasmosis. Slows retinal damage, does not reverse loss of vision in eyes damaged by AMD. ▪ Not recommended for use in treatment of predominantly occult subfoveal choroidal neovascularization; evidence insufficient.

Unlabeled uses: Treatment of psoriasis, psoriatic arthritis, rheumatoid arthritis, non-melanoma skin cancers, and circumscribed choroidal hemangioma.

CONTRAINDICATIONS

Patients with porphyria or a known hypersensitivity to any component of this preparation.

PRECAUTIONS

Use rubber gloves and eye protection during preparation and administration. Avoid any skin or eye contact since that area will become photosensitive. Wipe up spills with a damp cloth. Dispose of all contaminated materials in a polyethylene bag to avoid accidental contact by others. Protection from light will be necessary if accidental exposure or overexposure occurs. Note process in Patient Education. ▪ Administered by or under the direction of the physician specialist with appropriate knowledge of the selected laser system. Facilities for monitoring the patient and responding to any medical emergency must be available. ▪ Requires laser systems and a fiber-optic diffuser to activate. *Coherent Opal Photoactivator Laser Console and LaserLink Adapter, Zeiss VISULAS 690s laser and VISILINK PDT adapter, Ceralas I laser system and Ceralink Slit*

Lamp Adapter, and Quantel Activis laser console and the ZSL30 ACTTM, ZSL120 ACTTM, and HSBMBQ ACTTM slit lamp adapters are the laser systems that have been tested for **compatibility** with verteporfin and are approved for delivery of a stable power output at a wavelength of 689 ± 3 nm. Use of **incompatible** lasers that do not provide the required characteristics of light could result in incomplete treatment due to partial photoactivation, overtreatment due to overactivation, or damage to surrounding normal tissue. ▪ Following verteporfin administration, care should be taken to avoid exposure of skin or eyes to direct sunlight or bright indoor light for 5 days. If emergency surgery is necessary within 48 hours after treatment, as much of the internal tissue as possible should be protected from intense light. ▪ Patients who experience severe decrease of vision of 4 lines or more within 1 week after treatment should not be retreated, at least until their vision completely recovers to pretreatment levels. Potential risk versus benefit of any subsequent treatment should be considered. ▪ Use with caution in patients with moderate to severe hepatic impairment or biliary obstruction, and in anesthetized patients. There is no clinical experience with these patient populations. ▪ Older patients, patients with dark irides, patients with occult lesions or patients with less than 50% classic CNV may be less likely to benefit from verteporfin therapy. ▪ Safety and efficacy of verteporfin beyond 2 years has not been demonstrated; however, it has been used up to 5 years in extension studies.

Monitor: Standard precautions should be taken to avoid extravasation (e.g., establish a free-flowing IV line in a large arm vein, preferably the antecubital vein). If extravasation occurs, the infusion should be stopped immediately and cold compresses applied. The extravasation area must be thoroughly protected from direct light until the swelling and discoloration have faded in order to prevent the occurrence of a local burn, which could be severe. Oral analgesics may be indicated. ▪ Monitor patient during infusion. Verteporfin has caused a concentration-dependent increase in complement activation in human blood in vitro. S/S consistent with complement activation (chest pain, dyspnea, flushing, syncope) have been reported. ▪ Patient should be reevaluated every 3 months and if choroidal neovascular leakage is detected on fluorescein angiography, therapy should be repeated. ▪ See Usual Dose, Precautions, Patient Education, and Drug/Lab Interactions.

Patient Education: ▪ Must observe precautions to avoid exposure of skin and eyes to direct sunlight or bright indoor light for 5 days. Photosensitivity is due to residual drug, which is present in all parts of the skin. Ambient indoor light is beneficial as it gradually inactivates the remaining drug through a photobleaching reaction. Do not remain in a darkened room. Do expose skin to ambient indoor light. Avoid bright indoor light from examination lamps, dental lamps, operating room lamps, bright halogen lighting, and unshaded light bulbs. Limit time outdoors to necessary excursions and completely cover body with clothing and shade face before going out. Ultraviolet sunscreens are of no value because photoactivation is caused by visible light, not UV rays. Eyes will be sensitive to sun, bright lights, and car headlights; wear dark sunglasses with an average white light transmittance of less than 4%. ▪ Visual disturbances may develop and interfere with the ability to drive or operate machinery. Avoid these activities as long as visual symptoms persist.

Maternal/Child: Category C: use during pregnancy only if benefits justify potential risk to fetus. Effective contraception necessary for women of childbearing age. Has caused maternal and fetal toxicity in rats and rabbits. ■ Discontinue breast-feeding. ■ Safety and effectiveness for use in pediatric patients not established.

Elderly: Reduced treatment effect was seen with increasing age (75 years of age or older).

DRUG/LAB INTERACTIONS

Formal drug interaction studies have not been performed. Based on the mechanism of action of verteporfin, many drugs used concomitantly could influence the effect of verteporfin therapy. ■ **Calcium channel blockers** (e.g., diltiazem [Cardizem], verapamil, nicardipine [Cardene]), **polymyxin B, or radiation therapy** could enhance the rate of verteporfin uptake by the vascular endothelium. ■ Use with **other photosensitizing agents** (e.g., griseofulvin, phenothiazines [e.g., prochlorperazine (Compazine)], sulfonamides [sulfisoxazole (Gantrisin)], ophthalmic solutions (AK-Sulf)], sulfonylurea hypoglycemic agents [tolbutamide], tetracyclines [doxycycline], thiazide diuretics [chlorothiazide (Diuril)]) could increase the photosensitivity reaction. ■ Compounds that quench active oxygen species or scavenge radicals (e.g., **dimethyl sulfoxide** [DMSO], **beta-carotene, ethanol, formate, mannitol**) would be expected to decrease verteporfin activity. ■ Effectiveness may be reduced by **drugs that decrease clotting** (e.g., heparin, alteplase [tPA]), **vasoconstriction** (e.g., nicardipine [Cardene]) **or platelet aggregation** (e.g., clopidogrel [Plavix], dipyridamole [Persantine], ticlopidine [Ticlid]). ■ **Glucocorticoid hormones** (e.g., dexamethasone [Decadron]) given before or with PDT may reduce the effectiveness of verteporfin by inhibiting the production of thromboxane A_2.

SIDE EFFECTS

The most frequently reported side effects are headache, injection site reactions (e.g., edema, extravasation, hemorrhage with discoloration, pain, and rashes), visual disturbances (e.g., blurred vision, decreased visual acuity and visual field defects), and self-resolving photosensitivity. Less frequently reported side effects include abnormal white blood cell count (decreased or increased), albuminuria, anemia, arthralgia, arthrosis, asthenia, atrial fibrillation, back pain (primarily during infusion), blepharitis, cataracts, chest pain, conjunctivitis, constipation, decreased hearing, diplopia, dizziness, dry eyes, dyspnea, elevated liver function tests, eye hemorrhage (subconjunctival, subretinal, or vitreous), eczema, fever, flu-like syndrome, flushing, hypertension, hyperesthesia, hypersensitivity reactions, increased creatinine, lacrimation disorder, malaise, myasthenia, nausea, ocular itching, peripheral vascular disorder, pharyngitis, photosensitivity, pneumonia, prostatic disorder, pruritus, severe vision loss (may be equivalent of 4 lines or more within 7 days of treatment and occur with or without subretinal/retinal or vitreous hemorrhage), sleep disturbance, sweating, syncope, urticaria, varicose veins, vasovagal reactions, and vertigo.

Overdose: Overdose of drug and/or light may result in nonperfusion of normal retinal vessels with the possibility of severe decrease in vision that could be permanent. May also result in prolongation of the time during which the patient will be photosensitive.

ANTIDOTE

Keep the physician informed of all side effects; most will be treated symptomatically. In the event of an overdose of drug and/or light, extend the photosensitivity precautions for a time proportional to the overdose.

VINBLASTINE SULFATE `BBW`
(vin-**BLAS**-teen **SUL**-fayt)

VLB

Antineoplastic
(mitotic inhibitor-vinca alkaloid)

pH 3.5 to 5

USUAL DOSE

Auxiliary labeling required; see Precautions.

3.7 mg/M^2 initially. Administered once every 7 days, increasing the dose to specific amounts (5.5, 7.4, 9.25, 11.1 mg/M^2) a single step each week until the WBC count is decreased to 3,000 cells/mm^3, remission is achieved, or a maximum dose of 18.5 mg/M^2 is reached. Maintenance dose is one step below any dose that causes leukopenia (3,000 cells/mm^3 or less), once every 7 to 14 days. Usually 5.5 to 7.4 mg/M^2. Continue treatment for 4 to 6 weeks. Up to 12 weeks often necessary.

PEDIATRIC DOSE

See Maternal/Child.

One source suggests 2.5 mg/M^2 initially. Use same procedure as for adult dose using steps to 3.75, 5, 6.25, and 7.5 mg/M^2. Maximum dose is 12.5 mg/M^2. Maintenance dose is calculated by same parameters as Usual Dose (above). Usually differs with each individual. Other sources suggest that initial doses vary depending on the schedule used, use of vinblastine as a single agent, or in a combination regimen. Some suggested doses are:

Letterer-Siwe disease (unlabeled): As a single agent, an initial dose of 6.5 mg/M^2.

Hodgkin's disease: An initial dose of 6 mg/M^2 in combination with other chemotherapeutic agents.

Testicular cancer: An initial dose of 3 mg/M^2 in combination with other chemotherapeutic agents.

DOSE ADJUSTMENTS

Reduce dose by 50% if serum bilirubin above 3 mg/dL. ▪ Often used with other antineoplastic drugs and corticosteroids in reduced doses and/or extended intervals to achieve tumor remission.

DILUTION

Specific techniques required; see Precautions. Each 10 mg is diluted with 10 mL of NS for injection. 1 mg equals 1 mL. Also available in liquid form (1 mg/mL). May be given by IV injection or through Y-tube or three-way stopcock of a free-flowing IV infusion.

Storage: Store in refrigerator before and after dilution. Potency maintained for 28 days after dilution if reconstituted with bacteriostatic NS.

COMPATIBILITY

Consider any drug NOT listed as compatible to be INCOMPATIBLE until consulting a pharmacist; specific conditions may apply.

Manufacturer suggests that the pH not be altered from between 3.5 to 5 by an additive or a diluent, and it recommends NS as a diluent and not admixing with other drugs in the same container.

One source suggests the following **compatibilities:**

Additive: *Not recommended by manufacturer.* Bleomycin (Blenoxane).

Y-site: Allopurinol (Aloprim), amifostine (Ethyol), amphotericin B cholesteryl (Amphotec), aztreonam (Azactam), bleomycin (Blenoxane), cisplatin (Platinol), cyclophosphamide (Cytoxan), doxorubicin (Adriamycin), doxorubicin liposomal (Doxil), droperidol (Inapsine), etoposide phosphate (Etopophos), filgrastim (Neupogen), fludarabine (Fludara), fluorouracil (5-FU), gemcitabine (Gemzar), granisetron (Kytril), heparin, leucovorin calcium, melphalan (Alkeran), methotrexate, metoclopramide (Reglan), mitomycin (Mutamycin), ondansetron (Zofran), paclitaxel (Taxol), pemetrexed (Alimta), piperacillin/tazobactam (Zosyn), sargramostim (Leukine), teniposide (Vumon), thiotepa, vincristine, vinorelbine (Navelbine).

RATE OF ADMINISTRATION

IV injection: Total desired dose, properly diluted, over 1 minute.

ACTIONS

An alkaloid of the periwinkle plant with antitumor activity. Cell cycle–specific for M phase. Thought to interfere with the metabolic pathways of amino acids. Sometimes pharmacologically effective without any noticeable improvement in symptoms of malignancy. Cell energy production and synthesis of nucleic acid may also be inhibited. Half-life is 24.8 hours. Metabolism mediated by the hepatic cytochrome P_{450} isoenzymes in the CYP 3A subfamily. Some excretion through bile and urine.

INDICATIONS AND USES

To suppress or retard neoplastic growth. Remission and probable cure has been achieved with bleomycin and cisplatin in testicular malignancies. Response has been noted in Hodgkin's disease, non-Hodgkin's lymphomas, choriocarcinoma, Kaposi's sarcoma, mycosis fungoids, breast and renal cell malignancies. ▪ Used to treat many other malignancies.

CONTRAINDICATIONS

Bacterial infection or leukopenia below 3,000 cells/mm³.

PRECAUTIONS

Follow guidelines for handling cytotoxic agents. See Appendix A, p. 1429. ▪ Usually administered by or under the direction of the physician specialist. ▪ Manufacturer provides an auxillary sticker labeled "Fatal if given intrathecally, for IV use only" and an overwrap labeled "Do not remove covering until moment of injection. Fatal if given intrathecally. For intravenous use only." Each and every syringe(s) containing a specific dose and prepared in advance of actual administration must be labeled with the provided auxiliary sticker and packaged in this overwrap. If intrathecal injection should occur, immediate neurosurgical intervention is required, consult package insert for immediate steps to be taken. ▪ May cause corneal ulceration with accidental contact to the eye. ▪ Use caution in presence of ulcerated skin areas, cachexia, or impaired liver function. ▪ Leukocyte and platelet counts have fallen precipitously in patients with malignant-cell infiltration of the bone marrow following moderate doses of vinblastine. Further administration is not recommended. ▪ Acute pulmonary reactions including acute shortness of breath and severe broncho-spasm have been reported in patients receiving vinca alkaloids. Occurs most frequently when given in combination with mitomycin C. Onset of reaction may occur minutes to hours after vinca administration and up to 2 weeks following the mitomycin dose. **Monitor:** Determine absolute patency, quality of vein, and adequate circulation of extremity. Severe cellulitis may result from extravasation. Rinse syringe and needle with venous blood before withdrawal from the vein; see Antidote. ▪ Leukopenia is dose-limiting toxicity. Nadir occurs 5 to 10 days after therapy. Recovery occurs within another 7 to 14 days. ▪ WBC count must be checked before each dose. Must be above 4,000 cells/mm^3. ▪ Be alert for signs of bone marrow suppression or infection. ▪ Prophylactic antibiotics may be indicated pending results of C/S in a febrile neutropenic patient. ▪ Thrombocytopenia is rare, but may occur in patients whose bone marrow has been impaired by prior radiation therapy or other bone marrow suppressants. If platelet count is less than 50,000/mm^3, initiate precautions to prevent excessive bleeding (e.g., inspect IV sites, skin, and mucous membranes; use extreme care during invasive procedures; test urine, emesis, stool, and secretions for occult blood). ▪ Observe for increased uric acid levels; may require increased doses of antigout agents; allopurinol (Aloprim) preferred. ▪ Maintain adequate hydration. ▪ Prophylactic antiemetics may increase patient comfort. ▪ See Drug/Lab Interactions.

Patient Education: Avoid pregnancy; nonhormonal birth control recommended. ▪ Report IV site burning or stinging promptly. ▪ Report chills, fever, sore mouth, or throat promptly. ▪ Maintain adequate hydration; avoid constipation. ▪ See Appendix D, p. 1434.

Maternal/Child: Category D: avoid pregnancy. May produce teratogenic effects on the fetus. Has a mutagenic potential. ▪ Discontinue breast-feeding. ▪ Do not use diluents containing benzyl alcohol in premature infants.

Elderly: Leukopenic response may be increased in malnutrition or with skin ulcers.

DRUG/LAB INTERACTIONS

Inhibited by **some amino acids, glutamic acid, and tryptophan.** ▪ Potentiated by **other bone marrow suppressants** (e.g., antineoplastics, radiation therapy). ▪ Do not administer **live virus vaccines** to patients receiving antineoplastic drugs. ▪ Acute pulmonary reactions can occur with **Mitomycin-C;** see Precautions. ▪ May inhibit effects of **phenytoin** (Dilantin); increased doses of phenytoin may be needed. ▪ **Erythromycin** decreases metabolism and increases toxicity of vinblastine. ▪ Use caution with **any drug that inhibits P$_{450}$ enzymes** (e.g., calcium channel blockers [e.g., diltiazem (Cardizem), nicardipine (Cardene), verapamil], antifungal agents [e.g., fluconazole (Diflucan), itraconazole (Sporanox), ketoconazole (Nizoral)], bromocriptine [Parlodel], cimetidine [Tagamet], clarithromycin [Biaxin], cyclosporine [Sandimmune], danazol [Medrol], metoclopramide [Reglan]); may increase vinblastine blood levels and increase toxicity. ▪ Effect of **bleomycin** is significantly enhanced if vinblastine is administered 6 to 8 hours prior to bleomycin administration.

SIDE EFFECTS

Usually dose related and not always reversible: abdominal pain, alopecia, anorexia, cellulitis, constipation, convulsions, diarrhea, dizziness, extravasation, gonadal suppression, headache, hemorrhage, ileus, leukopenia (severe), malaise, mental depression, myelosuppression, nausea, numbness, oral lesions, paresthesias, peripheral neuritis, pharyngitis, Raynaud's syndrome, reflex depression (deep tendon), skin lesions, thrombophlebitis, tumor site pain, vomiting, weakness.

ANTIDOTE

For extravasation, discontinue the drug immediately and administer into another vein. Hyaluronidase should be injected locally into extravasated area. Use a fine hypodermic needle. Elevate extremity. Moist heat may be helpful. Notify the physician of all side effects; symptomatic treatment is often indicated. Administration of whole blood products (e.g., packed RBCs, platelets, leukocytes) and/or blood modifiers (e.g., darbepoetin alfa [Aranesp], epoetin alfa [Epogen], filgrastim [Neupogen], oprelvekin [Neumega], pegfilgrastim [Neulasta], sargramostim [Leukine]) may be indicated to treat bone marrow toxicity. Glutamic acid blocks toxicity of vinblastine but also blocks its antineoplastic activity.

VINCRISTINE SULFATE   `BBW`
(vin-**KRIS**-teen **SUL**-fayt)

VCR, Vincasar PFS

Antineoplastic
(mitotic inhibitor-vinca alkaloid)

pH 3.5 to 5.5

USUAL DOSE

Auxiliary labeling required; see Precautions.

Neurotoxicity appears to be dose related. Use extreme care in calculating and administering vincristine. Overdose may be fatal.

1.4 mg/M^2 administered once every 7 days. Various dosage schedules have been used with caution.

PEDIATRIC DOSE

Weight 10 kg or more with a body surface area of more than 1 M²: 1.5 to 2 mg/M^2 once each week.

Weight less than 10 kg (22 lb) or with a body surface area less than 1 M²: 0.05 mg/kg of body weight once a week. See comments under Usual Dose.

DOSE ADJUSTMENTS

In impaired hepatic function, reduce initial doses to 0.05 to 1 mg/M^2 or by 50% if direct bilirubin above 3 mg/dL. May be increased gradually based on individual response. ■ Usually given with other antineoplastic drugs and corticosteroids in reduced doses to achieve tumor remission. ■ See Drug/Lab Interactions.

DILUTION

Specific techniques required; see Precautions. Available in preservative-free solutions (1 mg/mL). May be given by IV injection or through Y-tube or three-way stopcock of a free-flowing IV infusion. Occasionally further diluted in 50 mL or more NS or D5W and given as an infusion.

Storage: Store in refrigerator before and after dilution. Potency maintained for 14 days after dilution. Label vial pertaining to mg/mL.

COMPATIBILITY   (Underline Indicates Conflicting Compatibility Information)
Consider any drug NOT listed as compatible to be INCOMPATIBLE until consulting a pharmacist; specific conditions may apply.
Manufacturer suggests that the pH not be altered from between 3.5 to 5.5 by an additive or a diluent, and it recommends NS or D5W as a diluent and not admixing with other drugs in the same container.

One source suggests the following **compatibilities:**
Additive: *Not recommended by manufacturer.* Bleomycin (Blenoxane), cytarabine (ARA-C), doxorubicin (Adriamycin), fluorouracil (5-FU), methotrexate.

Y-site: Allopurinol (Aloprim), amifostine (Ethyol), amphotericin B cholesteryl (Amphotec), anidulafungin (Eraxis), aztreonam (Azactam), bleomycin (Blenoxane), caspofungin (Cancidas), cisplatin (Platinol), cladribine (Leustatin), cyclophosphamide (Cytoxan), doxorubicin (Adriamycin), doxorubicin liposomal (Doxil), droperidol (Inapsine), etoposide phosphate (Etopophos), filgrastim (Neupogen), fludarabine (Fludara), fluorouracil (5-FU), gemcitabine (Gemzar), granisetron (Kytril), heparin, leucovorin calcium, linezolid (Zyvox), melphalan (Alkeran), methotrexate, metoclopramide (Reglan), mitomycin (Mutamycin), ondansetron (Zofran), oxaliplatin (Eloxatin), paclitaxel (Taxol), pemetrexed (Alimta), piperacillin/tazobactam (Zosyn), sargramostim (Leukine), teniposide (Vumon), thiotepa, topotecan (Hycamtin), vinblastine, vinorelbine (Navelbine).

RATE OF ADMINISTRATION
IV injection: Total desired dose, properly diluted, over 1 minute.
Infusion: A single dose over 20 to 30 minutes or as a continuous infusion prolonged over up to 96 hours.

ACTIONS
An alkaloid of the periwinkle plant with antitumor activity. Cell cycle–specific for the M phase. Well distributed except in spinal fluid, it is primarily excreted through bile and feces.

INDICATIONS AND USES
To suppress or retard neoplastic growth; good response experienced in leukemia, Hodgkin's disease, lymphosarcoma, oat cell, Wilms' tumor and others.
Unlabeled uses: Treatment of idiopathic thrombocytopenic purpura; treatment of Kaposi's sarcoma, breast and bladder cancer.

CONTRAINDICATIONS
Demyelinating form of Charcot-Marie-Tooth syndrome.

PRECAUTIONS
Follow guidelines for handling cytotoxic agents. See Appendix A, p. 1429.
■ Administered by or under the direction of the physician specialist. ■ Manufacturer provides an auxiliary sticker labeled "Fatal if given intrathecally, for IV use only" and an overwrap labeled "Do not remove covering until moment of injection. Fatal if given intrathecally. For intravenous use only." Each and every infusion bag(s) or syringe(s) containing a specific dose and prepared in advance of actual administration must be labeled with the provided auxiliary sticker and packaged in this overwrap. If intrathecal injection should occur, immediate neurosurgical intervention is required, consult package insert for immediate steps to be taken. ■ Use extreme

caution in combination with radiation therapy. ■ May cause corneal ulceration with accidental contact to the eye; flush eyes with water immediately. ■ Use caution in pre-existing neuromuscular disease or impaired liver function. ■ Not recommended for use in patients receiving radiation therapy that involves the liver.

Monitor: Determine absolute patency and quality of vein and adequate circulation of extremity. Severe cellulitis may result from extravasation; see Antidote. ■ Monitor CBC and platelets and evaluate neuro status before therapy and at frequent intervals. ■ Be alert for signs of bone marrow suppression or infection. ■ Prophylactic antibiotics may be indicated pending results of C/S in a febrile neutropenic patient. ■ Observe for increased uric acid levels; may require increased doses of antigout agents; allopurinol (Aloprim) preferred. ■ Maintain adequate hydration. ■ Prophylactic antiemetics may increase patient comfort. ■ Monitor for hyponatremia and inappropriate secretion of antidiuretic hormone (ADH); may require fluid limitation. ■ Use a laxative to prevent constipation. ■ Monitor for thrombocytopenia (platelet count less than 50,000/mm³). Initiate precautions to prevent excessive bleeding (e.g., inspect IV sites, skin, and mucous membranes; use extreme care during invasive procedures; test urine, emesis, stool, and secretions for occult blood). ■ See Drug/Lab Interactions.

Patient Education: Avoid pregnancy; nonhormonal birth control recommended. ■ Report IV site burning or stinging promptly. ■ See Appendix D, p. 1434. ■ Use laxatives to avoid constipation.

Maternal/Child: Category D: avoid pregnancy. May produce teratogenic effects on fetus. Has a mutagenic potential. ■ Discontinue breast-feeding.

Elderly: Neurotoxicity may be more severe (observe closely for constipation, ileus, and urinary retention).

DRUG/LAB INTERACTIONS

May cause severe bone marrow suppression with **other antineoplastic drugs or radiation therapy.** ■ Use with **asparaginase or doxorubicin** not recommended. Asparaginase inhibits the elimination of vincristine and increases its toxicity. The manufacturer suggests giving vincristine 12 to 24 hours before asparaginase; use caution. ■ Concurrent use with **itraconazole** (Sporanox) may increase vincristine toxicity. ■ Acute pulmonary reactions can occur with **mitomycin-C.** ■ Inhibited by **glutamic acid.** ■ Do not administer **live virus vaccines** to patients receiving antineoplastic drugs. ■ Inhibits **digoxin and phenytoin.** Monitor serum levels of digoxin and phenytoin; increased doses of these drugs may be required. ■ Use with **filgrastim** may induce a severe atypical neuropathy (foot pain, severe motor weakness). ■ Use caution with concurrent use of **drugs known to inhibit drug metabolism by hepatic cytochrome P$_{450}$ isoenzymes** such as azole antifungals (e.g., fluconazole [Diflucan], itraconazole [Sporanox]), cimetidine (Tagamet), diltiazem (Cardizem), verapamil, macrolide antibiotics (e.g., erythromycin), omeprazole (Prilosec), and ranitidine (Zantac).

SIDE EFFECTS

Frequently dose related and not always reversible: abdominal pain, alopecia, anaphylaxis, ataxia, bronchospasm, cellulitis, constipation, convulsions, cranial nerve damage, diarrhea, dysuria, extravasation, fever, foot-drop, gonadal suppression, headache, hypertension, hypotension, leukopenia (rare), muscle wasting, nausea, neuritic pain, oral lacerations, paralytic ileus, paresthesias, polyuria, reflex changes, sensory impairment, shortness of breath, SIADH, thrombocytopenia (rare), thrombophlebitis, tingling and numbness of extremities, upper colon impaction, uric acid nephropathy, vomiting, weakness, weight loss.

ANTIDOTE

For extravasation, discontinue the drug immediately and administer into another vein. Hyaluronidase may be injected locally into extravasated area. Use a fine hypodermic needle. Elevate extremity; moist heat may be helpful. Notify the physician of all side effects; symptomatic treatment is often indicated. Will probably reduce dose at earliest signs of neurologic toxicity (tingling and numbness of extremities). Discontinue for inappropriate ADH secretion or hyponatremia. Treat with fluid restriction and diuretics. Phenobarbital may be needed for convulsions. Use enemas or cathartics to treat constipation or prevent ileus. Glutamic acid blocks toxicity of vincristine, but also blocks its antineoplastic activity. Folinic acid, 100 mg IV every 3 hours for 24 hours and then every 6 hours for at least 48 hours, may be helpful in overdose. Supportive measures still required. Administration of whole blood products (e.g., packed RBCs, platelets, leukocytes) and/or blood modifiers (e.g., darbepoetin alfa [Aranesp], epoetin alfa [Epogen], filgrastim [Neupogen], oprelvekin [Neumega], pegfilgrastim [Neulasta], sargramostim [Leukine]) may be indicated to treat bone marrow toxicity.

VINORELBINE TARTRATE   BBW

(vin-**OR**-el-been   **TAHR**-trayt)

Navelbine, NVB

Antineoplastic
(mitotic inhibitor-vinca alkaloid)

pH 3.5

USUAL DOSE

Auxiliary labeling required; see Precautions.

30 mg/M^2 administered once each week until disease progression or dose-limiting toxicity. Calculate carefully in presence of edema or ascites. Vinorelbine 25 mg/M^2 weekly has been used in combination with cisplatin 100 mg/M^2 every 4 weeks. Vinorelbine 30 mg/M^2 weekly has also been used in combination with cisplatin 120 mg/M^2 on Days 1 and 29 and then once every 6 weeks. Premedication with dexamethasone (Decadron) may be beneficial in patients who experience acute or subacute pulmonary reactions. See cisplatin monograph.

DOSE ADJUSTMENTS

Reduce or withhold dose based on hematologic toxicity or hepatic insufficiency (e.g., hyperbilirubinemia) on the day of treatment. For patients with both hematologic toxicity and hepatic insufficiency, administer the lower of the doses determined appropriate from the following charts.

Vinorelbine Dose Adjustments for Hematologic Toxicity	
Granulocytes (cells/mm³) on Day of Treatment	Dose of Vinorelbine
≥1,500 cells/mm³	100%
1,000 to 1,499 cells/mm³	50%
<1,000 cells/mm³	Do not administer. Repeat count in 1 week. If 3 consecutive weekly doses are held because granulocyte count is <1,000 cells/mm³, discontinue vinorelbine.

For patients who during treatment with vinorelbine have experienced fever and/or sepsis while granulocytopenic or had 2 consecutive weekly doses held due to granulocytopenia, subsequent doses of vinorelbine should be:

≥1,500 cells/mm³	75%
1,000 to 1,499 cells/mm³	37.5%
<1,000 cells/mm³	Same as <1,000 above

Vinorelbine Dose Adjustments for Impaired Hepatic Function	
Total Bilirubin (mg/dL)	Dose of Vinorelbine
≤2 mg/dL	100%
2.1 to 3 mg/dL	50%
>3 mg/dL	25%

Appropriate dose reductions for cisplatin should be made when vinorelbine is used in combination. During studies, most patients required a 50% dose reduction of vinorelbine by Day 15 and a 50% dose reduction of cisplatin by Cycle 3. ▪ No dose adjustment is required for impaired renal function. ▪ If Grade 2 or greater neurotoxicity develops, discontinue vinorelbine.

DILUTION
Specific techniques required; see Precautions.
IV injection: Each 10 mg (1 mL) must be further diluted with a minimum of 2 to 5 mL NS or D5W. Desired concentration is 1.5 to 3 mg/mL (2 mL diluent yields 3 mg/mL concentration, 5 mL yields 1.5 mg/mL concentration). Must be given into the side-arm port of a free-flowing IV infusion. **Intermittent infusion:** Each 10 mg (1 mL) must be further diluted with 4 to 19 mL NS or D5W, ½NS, D5/½NS, R, or LR. Desired concentration is 0.5 to 2 mg/mL (4 mL diluent yields 2 mg/mL concentration, 19 mL yields 0.5 mg/mL concentration). Other references recommend diluting a single dose to a minimum total volume of 100 mL. Must be given into the side-arm port of a free-flowing IV infusion or may be given directly into a large central vein.
Storage: Refrigerate vials and protect from light; are stable at room temperature for up to 72 hours. Diluted solution stable for 24 hours at 5° to 30° C (41° to 86° F).

COMPATIBILITY   (Underline Indicates Conflicting Compatibility Information)
Consider any drug NOT listed as compatible to be INCOMPATIBLE until consulting a pharmacist; specific conditions may apply.
Manufacturer recommends mixing only with solutions listed under Dilution.

One source suggests the following **compatibilities:**
Y-site: Amikacin (Amikin), aztreonam (Azactam), bleomycin (Blenoxane), bumetanide, buprenorphine (Buprenex), butorphanol (Stadol), calcium gluconate, carboplatin (Paraplatin), carmustine (BiCNU), cefotaxime (Claforan), ceftazidime (Fortaz), chlorpromazine (Thorazine), cisplatin (Platinol), clindamycin (Cleocin), cyclophosphamide (Cytoxan), cytarabine (ARA-C), dacarbazine (DTIC), dactinomycin (Cosmegen), daunorubicin (Cerubidine), dexamethasone (Decadron), diphenhydramine (Benadryl), doxorubicin (Adriamycin), doxorubicin liposomal (Doxil), doxycycline, droperidol (Inapsine), enalaprilat (Vasotec IV), etoposide (VePesid), famotidine (Pepcid IV), filgrastim (Neupogen), fluconazole (Diflucan), fludarabine (Fludara), gallium nitrate (Ganite), gemcitabine (Gemzar), gentamicin, granisetron (Kytril), haloperidol (Haldol), heparin, hydrocortisone sodium succinate (Solu-Cortef), hydromorphone (Dilaudid), idarubicin (Idamycin), ifosfamide (Ifex), imipenem-cilastatin (Primaxin), lorazepam (Ativan), mannitol, mechlorethamine (nitrogen mustard), melphalan (Alkeran), meperidine (Demerol), mesna (Mesnex), methotrexate, metoclopramide (Reglan), metronidazole (Flagyl IV), mitoxantrone (Novantrone), morphine, nalbuphine, ondansetron (Zofran), oxaliplatin (Eloxatin), potassium chloride (KCl), prochlorperazine (Compazine), promethazine (Phenergan), ranitidine (Zantac), streptozocin (Zanosar), teniposide (Vumon), ticarcillin/clavulanate (Timentin), tobramycin, vancomycin, vinblastine, vincristine, zidovudine (AZT, Retrovir).

RATE OF ADMINISTRATION
Inadequate flushing of the vein after administration may increase the risk of phlebitis.
IV injection: Total desired dose, properly diluted over 6 to 10 minutes through the side-arm port of a free-flowing IV. After administration, flush with at least 75 to 125 mL of diluent solution over 10 minutes or more. Up to 300 mL has been used as a flush.
Intermittent infusion: Total desired dose, properly diluted over 6 to 10 minutes. Other references recommend over 20 minutes. Must be given into the side-arm port of a free-flowing IV infusion or may be given directly into a large central vein. Flush according to directions for IV injection.

ACTIONS
An antineoplastic agent. A semisynthetic vinca alkaloid with chemical differences from other vinca alkaloids that may provide unique clinical benefits with a lower incidence of clinical neurotoxicity. Causes depolymerization of microtubules and inhibits microtubule assembly. May be more specific to mitotic microtubules. Cell cycle–specific and produces a blockade in the cell-cycle progression in G_2 and M phase. Widely distributed in the body. Elimination half-life is 27 to 43 hours. Metabolized in the liver by hepatic cytochrome P_{450} isoenzymes in the CYP3A subfamily. Excreted in bile, feces, and urine.

INDICATIONS AND USES

Treatment of unresectable advanced non–small-cell lung cancer (ANSCLC), in ambulatory patients. Used as a single agent or in combination with cisplatin. ▪ Indicated as a single agent or in combination with cisplatin in patients with Stage IV NSCLC and in combination with cisplatin in patients with Stage III NSCLC.

Unlabeled uses: Treatment of breast, cervical, and epithelial ovarian cancers; treatment of desmoid tumors and fibromatosis, and advanced Kaposi's sarcoma.

CONTRAINDICATIONS

Patients with pretreatment granulocyte counts less than 1,000 cells/mm³.

PRECAUTIONS

Follow guidelines for handling cytotoxic agents. See Appendix A, p. 1429. ▪ Severe irritation of the eye has been reported with accidental exposure to another vinca alkaloid. If exposure occurs, thoroughly flush eye with water immediately. ▪ Administered by or under the direction of the physician specialist. ▪ Manufacturer provides an auxiliary sticker labeled "Fatal if given intrathecally, for IV use only" and an overwrap labeled "Do not remove covering until moment of injection. Fatal if given intrathecally. For Intravenous use only." Each and every syringe(s) containing a specific dose and prepared in advance of actual administration must be labeled with the provided auxiliary sticker and packaged in this overwrap. If intrathecal injection should occur, immediate neurosurgical intervention is required, consult package insert for immediate steps to be taken. ▪ Adequate diagnostic and treatment facilities must be readily available. ▪ May cause severe granulocytopenia resulting in increased susceptibility to infection. ▪ Use extreme caution in patients with hepatic impairment, pre-existing neuromuscular disease, pre-existing peripheral neuropathies, or those taking other neurotoxic drugs (e.g., antineoplastics [cisplatin], phenothiazines [prochlorperazine]). ▪ Acute SOB and severe bronchospasm have been reported, most commonly when vinorelbine was used with mitomycin. May require treatment with oxygen, bronchodilators (e.g., albuterol), and/or corticosteroids (e.g., hydrocortisone). Incidence may be increased when there is pre-existing pulmonary dysfunction. ▪ Prior radiation therapy or treatment with other antineoplastic agents may cause an increase in myelotoxicity; use with extreme caution. ▪ Administration to patients with prior radiation therapy may result in radiation recall reactions. ▪ See Monitor and Drug/Lab Interactions.

Monitor: Monitor CBC, differential, platelets, and bilirubin on each day of treatment to determine correct dose and 1 or 2 times weekly, granulocytopenia is dose-limiting. Temporary leukopenia is an expected effect. Maximum depression usually occurs in 7 to 10 days after the dose, and recovery should occur within the following 7 to 14 days. ▪ Cases of interstitial pulmonary changes and adult respiratory distress syndrome (ARDS), most of which were fatal, have been reported. Onset of symptoms has occurred in 3 to 8 days. Promptly evaluate patients with alterations in their baseline pulmonary symptoms or with new onset of cough, dyspnea, hypoxia, or other symptoms. ▪ Monitor AST frequently. ▪ Evaluate neurologic status frequently (e.g., constipation, decreased deep tendon reflexes, paresthesia). ▪ Closely monitor patients who have had symptoms of neuropathy with previous drug regimens (e.g., paclitaxel [Taxol]) for new or worsening neuropathy. ▪ Determine absolute patency and quality of vein and adequate circulation of extremity. Local tissue necrosis and/or thrombophlebitis can result from extravasation; see Antidote. ▪ Be alert for any sign of infection. Infections must be brought under control before beginning therapy with vinorelbine. ▪ Use of prophylactic antibiotics may be indicated pending results of C/S in a febrile neutropenic patient. ▪ Maintain adequate hydration. ▪ Prophylactic antiemetics may increase patient comfort; haloperidol and oral dexamethasone have benefited some patients. ▪ May cause severe (Grade 3-4) constipation, paralytic ileus, intestinal obstruction, necrosis, and/or perforation. Use a laxative to prevent constipation. Monitor bowel sounds. ▪ Monitor for hyponatremia and syndrome of inappropriate secretion of antidiuretic hormone (SIADH). ▪ Monitor for thrombocytopenia (platelet count less than 50,000/mm^3). Initiate precautions to prevent excessive bleeding (e.g., inspect IV sites, skin, and mucous membranes; use extreme care during invasive procedures; test urine, emesis, stool, and secretions for occult blood). ▪ See Precautions and Drug/Lab Interactions.

Patient Education: Report burning or stinging at IV site promptly. ▪ Report chills, fever, difficulty breathing, or shortness of breath promptly. ▪ Avoid pregnancy; nonhormonal birth control recommended. ▪ Take laxatives consistently to avoid constipation. ▪ See Appendix D, p. 1434.

Maternal/Child: Category D: avoid pregnancy; may cause fetal harm. ▪ Discontinue breast-feeding. ▪ Safety and effectiveness for use in pediatric patients has not been established but has been investigated. In one study, vinorelbine was considered to be ineffective when used in doses similar to those used in adults in a limited number of pediatric patients with recurrent solid malignant tumors (e.g., rhabdomyosarcoma/undifferentiated sarcoma, neuroblastoma, and CNS tumors). Toxicities were similar to those reported in adults.

Elderly: The pharmacokinetics of vinorelbine in elderly and younger adult patients are similar. No relationship between age, systemic exposure, and hematologic toxicity has been observed.

DRUG/LAB INTERACTIONS

Neurotoxicity may be increased by **other neurotoxic drugs** (e.g., antineoplastics [such as cisplatin, paclitaxel (Taxol)] and phenothiazines [prochlorperazine]); may require dose reduction or discontinuation of vinorelbine. Vestibular and auditory deficits have been observed, usually when vinorelbine is used in combination with cisplatin. ▪ Do not administer **live virus vaccines** to patients receiving antineoplastic drugs. ▪ **Mitomycin-C** may cause or aggravate acute pulmonary reactions (e.g., acute shortness of breath, bronchospasm). May require oxygen, bronchodilators, and/or corticosteroids. ▪ Granulocytopenia significantly higher when used in combination with **cisplatin.** ▪ Additive bone marrow suppression may occur with **radiation therapy and/or other bone marrow-suppressing agents** (e.g., azathioprine [Imuran], chloramphenicol, melphalan [Alkeran]); dose reductions may be required. ▪ Leukopenic effects may be increased by **agents that cause similar blood dyscrasias** (e.g., anticonvulsants, antidepressants, phenothiazines). ▪ **Drugs that inhibit the cytochrome P$_{450}$ isoenzymes in the CYP3A subfamily** (e.g., azole antifungals [e.g., itraconazole (Sporanox)], macrolides [e.g., erythromycin (Erythrocin), troleandomycin (TAO)]) may inhibit the metabolism of vinorelbine and increase its toxicity. *Other vinca alkaloids cause interactions with the following drugs; vinorelbine has not been studied.* ▪ Use with **asparaginase or doxorubicin** may not be recommended or may require specific scheduling. ▪ May be potentiated by **calcium channel blockers** (e.g., verapamil). ▪ May inhibit **digoxin and phenytoin;** increased doses of these drugs may be required. ▪ See Precautions.

SIDE EFFECTS

Granulocytopenia is the major dose-limiting toxicity and may be significantly greater in combination regimens. Alopecia (12%, mild); anemia (87%, mild to moderate); ARDS, auditory deficits, bronchospasm, chest pain (7%); constipation (35%); diarrhea; dyspnea [2%] (acute and reversible shortness of breath may occur within a few hours); elevated total bilirubin and AST; fatigue; hematologic toxicity [99%] (leukopenia and neutropenia are the most frequent and are dose-limiting); hemorrhagic cystitis (rare); hypertension; hypotension; intestinal obstruction, necrosis, and/or perforation; jaw pain; loss of deep tendon reflexes (5%); nausea and vomiting (50% [23%]); pain and redness at injection site (38%); pancreatitis, paralytic ileus (less than 2%); peripheral neuropathy (31%), mild to moderate paresthesia and hypesthesia, phlebitis (10%); pulmonary edema; radiosensitizing effects in patients with prior or concomitant radiation therapy; SIADH (few); subacute pulmonary reactions (4%, e.g., cough, dyspnea, hypoxemia, and interstitial infiltrates on chest x-ray); thrombocytopenia (rare), thrombocytosis (asymptomatic), tumor pain, vestibular deficits. Pattern of side effects similar when vinorelbine is used as a single agent or in combination.

ANTIDOTE

For severe reactions, discontinue vinorelbine or reduce subsequent doses. If Grade 2 or greater neurotoxicity develops, discontinue vinorelbine. For extravasation, discontinue the drug immediately and administer into another vein. Elevate the extremity. Moist heat may be helpful. Notify the physician of all side effects; symptomatic treatment is often indicated. Discontinue for hyponatremia or SIADH, may require fluid limitation and diuretics (e.g., furosemide [Lasix]). Bone marrow toxicity is reversible after discontinuing vinorelbine. Administration of whole blood products (e.g., packed RBCs, platelets, leukocytes) may be indicated. Darbepoetin alfa (Aranesp), epoetin alfa (Epogen), filgrastim (Neupogen), oprelvekin (Neumega), pegfilgrastim (Neulasta), or sargramostim (Leukine) may be used to promote bone marrow recovery but may not be given within 24 hours of a dose of cytotoxic therapy or until 24 hours after a dose of cytotoxic therapy. Acute or chronic pulmonary reactions may be an allergic phenomena, corticosteroids (e.g., hydrocortisone sodium succinate [Solu-Cortef]), oxygen and bronchodilators (e.g., albuterol [Ventolin, Proventil]) may be helpful. Neurologic toxicity may be reversible.

VON WILLEBRAND FACTOR/COAGULATION FACTOR VIII COMPLEX (HUMAN)

(von **WILL**-a-brand **FAK**-tor VIII/
an-tee-hee-moe-**FIL**-ik **KOM**-plex) (**HYOO**-man)

Antihemorrhagic

Wilate

USUAL DOSE

(International Units [IU])

Completely individualized. One IU of von Willebrand factor:Ristocetin Cofactor (VWF:RCo) or 1 IU of Factor VIII (FVIII) is approximately equal to the level of VWF:RCo or FVIII activity found in 1 mL of fresh pooled human plasma. The ratio between VWF:RCo and FVIII activities in Wilate is approximately 1:1. When using a FVIII-containing VWF product, continued treatment may cause an excessive rise in FVIII activity; see Monitor. The following chart provides estimated doses for minor and major hemorrhages.

Guide to Wilate Dosing for Treatment of Minor and Major Hemorrhages			
Type of Hemorrhage	Loading Dose (IU VWF:RCo/kg)	Maintenance Dose (IU VWF:RCo/kg)	Therapeutic Goal
Minor Hemorrhages	20 to 40 IU/kg	20 to 30 IU/kg every 12 to 24 hours*	VWF:RCo and FVIII activity trough levels of >30%
Major Hemorrhages	40 to 60 IU/kg	20 to 40 IU/kg every 12 to 24 hours*	VWF:RCo and FVIII activity trough levels of >50%

*Maintenance doses may need to be continued for up to 3 days for minor hemorrhages and 5 to 7 days for major hemorrhages. Repeat doses may be administered for as long as needed based on repeated monitoring of appropriate clinical and laboratory measures.

PEDIATRIC DOSE

Unlabeled: For immediate control of bleeding, follow the general recommendations for dosing and administration for adults. See Usual Dose and Maternal/Child.

DOSE ADJUSTMENTS

Adjust dose according to the extent and location of bleeding. Higher doses may be required in von Willebrand (vWD) Type 3 patients, especially those with GI bleeding. ■ If a dose is missed, consider administration of a dose based on the level of coagulation factors measured, extent of the bleeding, and patient's clinical condition.

DILUTION

Provided as a kit containing a single-dose vial of powder, a vial of diluent, a Mix2Vial transfer device, a 10-mL syringe, an infusion set, and 2 alcohol swabs. Consult instructions for reconstitution and injection in the package insert. Warm to room temperature (25° C) before dilution and maintain throughout reconstitution. If a water bath is used for warming (temperature should not exceed 37° C [98° F]), do not allow water to come into contact with the latex-free rubber stopper or vial caps. The total number of IUs available is clearly marked on each vial. Concentration is 90 IU/mL. Record the batch number of each vial. Should be used immediately after reconstitution. Solution should be slightly opalescent. Contents of multiple vials may be pooled in a single administration device. Use a new Mix2Vial transfer set for each vial of drug.

Filters: Incorporated into the Mix2Vial.

Storage: Store in original carton to protect from light. Stable for 36 months from date of manufacture when refrigerated at $2°$ to $8°$ C ($36°$ to $46°$ F). Avoid freezing. May be stored at RT (maximum of $25°$ C [$77°$ F]) for up to 6 months. Label vial with date removed from refrigeration. Once stored at RT, do not return to refrigeration. Shelf life expires with date of manufacture or 6 months from date of removal from refrigeration, whichever comes first. Confirm expiration date on vial. Administer immediately after reconstitution. Discard any unused solution.

COMPATIBILITY

Manufacturer states, "Must not be mixed with other medicinal products or administered simultaneously with other IV preparations in the same infusion set."

RATE OF ADMINISTRATION

A single dose as an infusion at 2 to 4 mL/min. Reduce rate of administration or interrupt the infusion if a marked increase in pulse occurs.

ACTIONS

A purified, sterile, lyophilized concentrate of von Willebrand Factor (VWF) and antihemophilic factor (Factor VIII) that is obtained from pooled human plasma. Multiple methods of purification are used to inactivate infectious agents, including viruses. VWF and FVIII are normal constituents of human plasma. Patients with vWD have a deficiency or abnormality of VWF; this results in low FVIII activity and an abnormal platelet function, which causes excessive bleeding. VWF re-establishes platelet adhesion at the site of vascular damage, providing primary hemostasis (shortening of bleeding time occurs immediately), and stabilizes FVIII by binding to it and preventing its rapid degradation. This latter action is slightly delayed. However, administration of a FVIII-containing VWF preparation rapidly restores FVIII activity to normal. VWF activity is measured with an assay that uses an agglutinating cofactor called Ristocetin (RCo). The VWF:RCo assay provides a quantitative measurement of VWF function by determining how well VWF helps platelets adhere to one another. Reduced VWF:RCo activity indicates a deficiency of VWF. Half-life varies based on type of VWF (1, 2, or 3). Half-life range is 10.9 to 34.7 hours. Clearance may be slightly higher in females; clinical significance unknown.

INDICATIONS AND USES

Treatment of spontaneous and trauma-induced bleeding episodes in patients with severe von Willebrand disease (vWD), as well as patients with mild or moderate vWD in which the use of desmopressin is known or suspected to be ineffective or contraindicated. ■ Not indicated for the prevention of excessive bleeding during and after surgery in vWD patients (see Alphanate [type 1 or 2], Humate-P [type 1, 2, or 3]). ■ Not indicated for hemophilia A (see Alphanate, Humate-P). ■ Studies to determine safety and effectiveness of prophylactic dosing to prevent spontaneous bleeding have not been conducted.

CONTRAINDICATIONS
History of anaphylactic or severe systemic response to plasma-derived products, any ingredient in the formulation, or components of the container.

PRECAUTIONS
For IV use only. ▪ Administered under the direction of a physician knowledgeable in the treatment of coagulation disorders in a facility with adequate diagnostic and treatment facilities to monitor the patient and respond to any medical emergency. ▪ Hypersensitivity reactions, including anaphylaxis, have occurred; see Monitor. ▪ Important to establish that coagulation disorder is caused by vWD. Not useful in treatment of other deficiencies. ▪ Manufactured from human plasma. Risk of transmitting infectious agents (e.g., HIV, hepatitis and, theoretically, Creutzfeldt-Jakob disease) has been greatly reduced by screening, testing, and manufacturing techniques. However, risk of transmission cannot be totally eliminated. Health care professionals should use caution during administration; may have risk of exposure to viral infection. ▪ Hepatitis A and B vaccines are recommended for patients receiving plasma derivatives. ▪ Thrombotic events have been reported. Use caution in patients with known risk factors for thrombosis. ▪ Inhibitors may develop with large or frequent doses; see Monitor.

Monitor: Monitor BP and pulse during infusion. If a marked increase in pulse occurs, either reduce rate of infusion or interrupt the infusion. ▪ Throughout the infusion, monitor for S/S of a hypersensitivity reaction (e.g., angioedema, burning and stinging at injection site, chills, flushing, headache, hives, hypotension, tachycardia, tightness of the chest, urticaria, wheezing). Evaluate for the presence of inhibitors if an anaphylactic reaction occurs. ▪ When using a FVIII-containing VWF product, continued treatment may cause an excessive rise in FVIII activity. Appropriate laboratory tests should be performed on the patient's plasma at suitable intervals to ensure that adequate VWF:RCo and FVIII activity levels have been reached and are maintained. Excessive activity levels may increase the risk of thrombotic events. ▪ Monitor for development of VWF and FVIII inhibitors (neutralizing antibodies). Consider formation of inhibitors and perform assays if bleeding is not controlled with usual doses.

Patient Education: Prophylactic hepatitis A and hepatitis B vaccines recommended. ▪ Promptly report S/S of a hypersensitivity reaction (e.g., dizziness, hives, itching, rash, tightness of the chest). ▪ Frequent blood tests (e.g., monitoring of VWF:RCo and FVIII activity) are required to reduce the risk of thrombotic events. ▪ Report symptoms of possibly transmitted viral infections immediately. Symptoms may include anorexia, arthralgias, fatigue, jaundice, low-grade fever, nausea, or vomiting.

Maternal/Child: Category C: use during pregnancy or labor and delivery only if clearly needed. ▪ Safety for use during breast-feeding has not been studied. ▪ Has been used in pediatric patients between 5 and 16 years of age. No dose adjustment is required.

Elderly: Numbers insufficient to determine differences in response compared with younger adults.

DRUG/LAB INTERACTIONS

Manufacturer states, "No interactions with other medicinal products are known."

SIDE EFFECTS

Most common side effects reported are dizziness, facial edema, headache, paresthesia, pruritus, and urticaria. The most serious effect is a hypersensitivity reaction.

Post-Marketing: Cough, dyspnea, hypersensitivity reactions, nausea, and vomiting.

ANTIDOTE

Keep the physician informed of side effects. Slow or interrupt infusion for a marked increase in pulse rate or mild hypersensitivity reaction. Discontinue the infusion immediately if a severe hypersensitivity reaction or thrombotic event (e.g., chest pain, dyspnea, leg pain, MI) occurs and evaluate for the presence of inhibitors. Treat hypersensitivity as necessary (e.g., antihistamines, epinephrine, corticosteroids), and treat thrombotic events with appropriate measures. Resuscitate as necessary.

VORICONAZOLE
(**vor**-ih-**KOH**-nah-zohl)
VFEND IV

Antifungal

USUAL DOSE

IV and oral doses are therapeutically equivalent. Oral dose can replace an IV dose as soon as practical; see Precautions and Patient Education. Duration of treatment is based on severity of the underlying disease, recovery from immunosuppression, and clinical response. Pretesting required; see Precautions and Monitor. Obtain baseline electrolytes and correct calcium, magnesium, and potassium deficiencies before initiating voriconazole.

	Voriconazole Dose Guidelines		
Infection	Loading Dose	IV Maintenance Dose	Oral Maintenance Dose
Invasive aspergillosis	6 mg/kg q 12 hr for the first 24 hours	4 mg/kg q 12 hr	200 mg q 12 hr[c]
Candidemia in non-neutropenic patients and in other deep tissue *Candida* infections	6 mg/kg q 12 hr for the first 24 hours	3 to 4 mg/kg q 12 hr[a, b]	200 mg q 12 hr[a, b, c]
Esophageal candidiasis			200 mg q 12 hr[c, d]
Scedosporiosis and fusariosis	6 mg/kg q 12 hr for the first 24 hours	4 mg/kg q 12 hr	200 mg q 12 hr[c]

[a]In clinical trials, patients with candidemia received 3 mg/kg q 12 hr as primary therapy, and patients with other deep tissue *Candida* infections received 4 mg/kg as salvage therapy. Appropriate dose should be based on the severity and nature of the infection.
[b]Treat for at least 14 days following resolution of symptoms or following last positive culture, whichever is longer.
[c]Patients who weigh 40 kg or more should receive an oral maintenance dose of 200 mg q 12 hr. Adult patients who weigh less than 40 kg should receive an oral maintenance dose of 100 mg q 12 hr.
[d]Treat for a minimum of 14 days and for at least 7 days following the resolution of symptoms.

DOSE ADJUSTMENTS

Reduce the maintenance dose to 3 mg/kg every 12 hours in patients unable to tolerate treatment. ▪ Increase the maintenance dose to 5 mg/kg every 12 hours if phenytoin (Dilantin) is being administered concurrently; see Drug/Lab Interactions. ▪ When voriconazole is coadministered with efavirenz (Sustiva), increase voriconazole maintenance dose to 400 mg every 12 hours and decrease efavirenz dose to 300 mg every 24 hours. ▪ No dose adjustment is indicated based on age or gender or in patients with baseline liver function tests (ALT, AST) up to 5 times the ULN (see Precautions and Monitor). ▪ In patients with mild to moderate hepatic cirrhosis (Child-Pugh Class A and B), use the standard loading dose but reduce the maintenance dose by one half and administer every 12 hours based on tolerance of treatment and/or concurrent medication. ▪ No dose adjustment is required in patients with a CrCl of 50 mL/min or greater; however, the intravenous vehicle, sulfobutyl ether beta-cyclodextrin sodium (SBECD), accumulates in patients with a CrCl of less than 50 mL/min. Use of oral voriconazole is recommended in these patients; see Precautions and Monitor. ■ A 4-hour hemodialysis session does not remove a sufficient amount of voriconazole to warrant dose adjustment.

DILUTION

Reconstitute each vial with exactly 19 mL SW. Use of a standard 20-mL (nonautomated) syringe is recommended to facilitate exact measurement. Volume will be 20 mL (10 mg/mL). Discard the vial if a vacuum is not present to pull the diluent into the vial. Shake until all powder is dissolved. Calculate the required dose based on patient weight (see the following chart). Must be further diluted for infusion in D5W, D5LR, LR, NS, D5/½NS, D5NS, ½NS, or D5W with 20 mEq KCl. Withdraw a volume equal to the calculated dose of voriconazole from an infusion bag or bottle (30 mL in the following example). The volume of diluent left in the infusion bag or bottle should be enough to allow a final concentration of not less than 0.5 mg/mL or greater than 5 mg/mL after voriconazole is added. Withdraw the required volume of reconstituted drug and add to the infusion bag or bottle. For example, a patient weighing 50 kg will require a loading dose of 300 mg (6 mg/kg × 50 kg), which equals 30 mL of reconstituted drug (1½ vials). Withdraw and discard 30 mL of solution from a 100-mL infusion bag and add the 30 mL of reconstituted drug. Final concentration equals 3 mg/mL.

Required Volumes of 10 mg/mL Voriconazole Concentrate			
	Volume of Voriconazole Concentrate (10 mg/mL) required for:		
Body Weight (kg)	3 mg/kg Dose (number of vials)	4 mg/kg Dose (number of vials)	6 mg/kg Dose (number of vials)
30 kg	9 mL (1 vial)	12 mL (1 vial)	18 mL (1 vial)
35 kg	10.5 mL (1 vial)	14 mL (1 vial)	21 mL (2 vials)
40 kg	12 mL (1 vial)	16 mL (1 vial)	24 mL (2 vials)
45 kg	13.5 mL (1 vial)	18 mL (1 vial)	27 mL (2 vials)
50 kg	15 mL (1 vial)	20 mL (1 vial)	30 mL (2 vials)
55 kg	16.5 mL (1 vial)	22 mL (2 vials)	33 mL (2 vials)
60 kg	18 mL (1 vial)	24 mL (2 vials)	36 mL (2 vials)
65 kg	19.5 mL (1 vial)	26 mL (2 vials)	39 mL (2 vials)
70 kg	21 mL (2 vials)	28 mL (2 vials)	42 mL (3 vials)
75 kg	22.5 mL (2 vials)	30 mL (2 vials)	45 mL (3 vials)
80 kg	24 mL (2 vials)	32 mL (2 vials)	48 mL (3 vials)
85 kg	25.5 mL (2 vials)	34 mL (2 vials)	51 mL (3 vials)
90 kg	27 mL (2 vials)	36 mL (2 vials)	54 mL (3 vials)
95 kg	28.5 mL (2 vials)	38 mL (2 vials)	57 mL (3 vials)
100 kg	30 mL (2 vials)	40 mL (2 vials)	60 mL (3 vials)

Filters: No data available from manufacturer.
Storage: Store unopened vials at CRT. Immediate use of reconstituted vials is preferred; however, they may be refrigerated up to 24 hours at 2° to 8° C (37° to 46° F). Discard partially used vials.

COMPATIBILITY   (Underline Indicates Conflicting Compatibility Information)
Consider any drug NOT listed as compatible to be INCOMPATIBLE until consulting a pharmacist; specific conditions may apply.
Manufacturer states, "Must not be infused concomitantly with any blood product or short-term infusion of concentrated electrolytes, even if the two infusions are running in separate IV lines or cannulas. Electrolyte disturbances such as hypokalemia, hypomagnesemia, and hypocalcemia should be corrected before initiation of voriconazole; see Precautions." Voriconazole can be infused at the same time as other IV solutions containing (non-concentrated) electrolytes but must be infused through a separate line. Voriconazole can be infused at the same time as total parenteral nutrition (TPN) but must be infused in a separate line. If infused through a multiple-lumen catheter, TPN needs to be administered using a different port from the one used for voriconazole. Manufacturer states that voriconazole should not be diluted with 4.2% sodium bicarbonate solution. **Compatibility** with other concentrations of sodium bicarbonate is unknown; do not use.

One source suggests the following **compatibilities:**
Y-site: Anidulafungin (Eraxis), caspofungin (Cancidas), doripenem (Doribax), vasopressin.

RATE OF ADMINISTRATION
A single dose as an infusion over 1 to 2 hours. Do not exceed a rate of 3 mg/kg/hr.

ACTIONS
A triazole antifungal agent. Inhibits a fungal cytochrome P_{450}-mediated essential step in fungal ergosterol biosynthesis. With a loading dose regimen, peak and trough plasma concentrations close to steady-state concentrations are achieved within the first 24 hours. Extensively distributed into tissues. Plasma protein binding (estimated at 58%) is not affected by varying degrees of hepatic and renal insufficiency. Metabolized by cytochrome P_{450} enzymes (CYP2C19 is significantly involved). Terminal half-life is dose dependent and is not useful in predicting accumulation or elimination. Eliminated via hepatic metabolism; less than 2% is excreted unchanged in urine.

INDICATIONS AND USES
Treatment of invasive aspergillosis caused by *Aspergillus fumigatus* and other species of *Aspergillus*. ■ Treatment of candidemia in nonneutropenic patients and the following *Candida* infections: disseminated infections in the skin and infections in the abdomen, kidney, bladder wall, and wounds.
■ Treatment of serious fungal infections caused by *Scedosporium apiospermum* and *Fusarium* species, including *Fusarium solani,* in patients intolerant of or refractory to other therapy. ■ Treatment of esophageal candidiasis.

CONTRAINDICATIONS
Hypersensitivity to voriconazole or any of its components. Use caution in patients exhibiting hypersensitivity to other azoles (e.g., fluconazole [Diflucan], itraconazole [Sporanox], ketoconazole [Nizoral]); see Precautions.
■ Coadministration is specifically **contraindicated** with CYP3A4 substrates

(e.g., cisapride [Propulsid], pimozide [Orap], and quinidine [astemizole and terfenadine would be included but are no longer commercially available]); increased plasma concentrations of these drugs may result in QT prolongation and torsades de pointes. ▪ Coadministration is **contraindicated** with the following drugs: barbiturates (long-acting [e.g., phenobarbital (Luminal)]), carbamazepine (Tegretol), a *standard dose* of efavirenz (Sustiva) with a *standard dose* of voriconazole, ergot alkaloids (ergotamine and dihydroergotamine [D.H.E. 45]), rifabutin (Mycobutin), rifampin (Rifadin), high-dose (400 mg every 12 hours) ritonavir (Norvir), sirolimus (Rapamune), and St. John's wort; see Drug Interactions.

PRECAUTIONS
Do not give as an IV bolus, for infusion only. ▪ Specimens for fungal culture, serologic testing, and histopathologic testing should be obtained before therapy to isolate and identify causative organisms. Therapy may begin as soon as all specimens are obtained and before results are known. Reassess after test results are known. ▪ Correct electrolyte disturbances such as hypokalemia, hypomagnesemia, and hypocalcemia before initiation of voriconazole. ▪ Infusion-related hypersensitivity reactions, including anaphylaxis, chest tightness, dyspnea, faintness, fever, flushing, nausea, pruritus, rash, sweating, and tachycardia have occurred. Usually appear at the beginning of the infusion. If a hypersensitivity reaction occurs, discontinue the infusion. ▪ Consider use in patients with severe hepatic insufficiency only if the benefit outweighs potential risk; monitor carefully for drug toxicity. ▪ Serious hepatic reactions (including clinical hepatitis, cholestasis, and fulminant hepatic failure, including fatalities) have occurred. Usually occur in patients with serious underlying medical conditions (e.g., hematologic malignancy); however, hepatic reactions, including hepatitis and jaundice, have occurred in patients with no other identifiable risk factors. Liver function usually improves with discontinuation of voriconazole. ▪ Pancreatitis has been reported; see Monitor. ▪ Consider use of IV formulation in patients with a CrCl less than 50 mL/min only if the benefit outweighs potential risk. Accumulation of SBECD may occur with the IV formulation; use of the oral formulation is recommended. ▪ Acute renal failure has been reported, usually in patients receiving concomitant nephrotoxic drugs or in patients who have concurrent medical conditions that may result in decreased renal function; see Drug/Lab Interactions. ▪ May cause prolongation of the QT interval on ECG and rarely torsades de pointes. Use with caution in patients with proarrhythmic conditions (e.g., cardiotoxic chemotherapy, cardiomyopathy, hypokalemia, and concomitant medications that may also prolong the QT interval). ▪ Because of the enzymes involved in metabolism, Asian populations may be poor metabolizers, and serum concentrations may be elevated from 2 to 4 times higher than normal metabolizers. Some Caucasians and Blacks are also poor metabolizers. ▪ Blurred vision, color vision changes, and/or photophobia are common but may be associated with higher serum concentrations and/or doses. Usually resolves within 2 weeks of the end of voriconazole therapy. If therapy continues beyond 28 days, the effects of voriconazole therapy on visual function is not known. Prolonged visual adverse effects, including optic neuritis and papilledema, have been reported. ▪ Fungi with reduced susceptibility to one azole antifungal agent may also be less susceptible to other azole derivatives. Cross-resistance may occur and may

require alternative antifungal therapy. ▪ Oral maintenance doses adjusted based on weight (above or below 40 kg); see product literature.
Monitor: Obtain baseline electrolytes and make rigorous attempts to correct calcium, magnesium, and potassium before initiating voriconazole. Monitor electrolytes during therapy; may cause hypocalcemia, hypokalemia, and hypomagnesemia. ▪ ▪ Obtain baseline liver function tests (e.g., alkaline phosphatase, ALT, AST, bilirubin), serum creatinine, and electrolytes in all patients. Monitor liver function tests during therapy, more frequently in patients with increasing or pre-existing elevated liver function tests and/or impaired hepatic function, and any time S/S suggestive of liver dysfunction develop (e.g., jaundice, lethargy). ▪ Monitor pancreatic function (e.g., serum amylase) in adults and children with risk factors for acute pancreatitis (e.g., recent chemotherapy, hematopoietic stem cell transplantation [HSCT]). ▪ Monitor serum creatinine during therapy, more frequently in patients with a CrCl less than 50 mL/min. If an increase in serum creatinine occurs, consider changing to the oral formulation. ▪ Monitor for S/S of hypersensitivity reactions; see Precautions and Antidote. ▪ Monitor visual acuity, visual field, and color perception if treatment continues beyond 28 days. ▪ If a rash develops, serious cutaneous reactions (e.g., Stevens-Johnson syndrome) may develop; monitor closely and consider discontinuing voriconazole. ▪ See Precautions, Drug/Lab Interactions, and Antidote.
Patient Education: Review of health history and medication profile is imperative. ▪ Avoid pregnancy; nonhormonal birth control recommended. Should pregnancy occur, notify physician immediately and discuss potential hazards. ▪ Do not drive at night; changes to vision, including blurring and/or photophobia, may occur. Ophthalmologic monitoring is required with prolonged use. ▪ If a change in vision occurs, avoid hazardous tasks, such as driving or operating machinery. ▪ Avoid strong, direct sunlight. ▪ Promptly report S/S of a hypersensitivity reaction (e.g., itching, hives, shortness of breath). ▪ Additional precautions required with transfer to oral voriconazole.
Maternal/Child: Category D: avoid pregnancy; may cause fetal harm. Teratogenic in rats and embryotoxic in rabbits. Use of effective contraception is required in women of childbearing age. ▪ Discontinue breast-feeding. ▪ Safety and effectiveness for use in pediatric patients less than 12 years of age not established; however, 22 pediatric patients between 12 and 18 years of age with invasive aspergillosis were included in studies.
Elderly: Safety profile similar to younger adults. ▪ Peak plasma concentrations slightly higher in elderly males; however, dose adjustment is not indicated. ▪ Use caution; consider decreased cardiac, hepatic, or renal function and effects of concomitant disease or other drug therapy. ▪ Monitor liver and renal function closely.

DRUG/LAB INTERACTIONS
Interactions are numerous and potentially life threatening. Review of drug profile by pharmacist is imperative.
Contraindicated with CYP3A4 substrates (e.g., **cisapride** [Propulsid], **pimozide** [Orap], and **quinidine** [astemizole and terfenadine would be included but are no longer commercially available]); increased plasma concentrations of these drugs may result in QT prolongation and torsades de pointes. ▪ **Contraindicated** with **long-acting barbiturates** (e.g., phenobarbital [Luminal]), **carbamazepine** (Tegretol), **rifampin** (Rifadin), **and St.**

John's wort; these drugs may significantly increase metabolism and decrease serum concentrations of voriconazole. ▪ **Contraindicated** with **high-dose (400 mg every 12 hours) ritonavir** (Norvir); decreases serum concentrations of voriconazole. **Low-dose ritonavir (100 mg every 12 hours)** reduces voriconazole concentration to a lesser extent. Coadministration should be avoided unless assessment of the benefit versus risk to the patient justifies voriconazole use. ▪ **Contraindicated** with **sirolimus** (Rapamune); metabolism of sirolimus is decreased, and serum concentrations are significantly increased by voriconazole. ▪ **Contraindicated** with **rifabutin** (Mycobutin); voriconazole significantly increases the serum concentrations of rifabutin, and rifabutin significantly decreases voriconazole serum concentrations. ▪ **Contraindicated** with ***standard doses* of efavirenz** (Sustiva); voriconazole increases serum concentrations of efavirenz, and efavirenz decreases serum concentrations of voriconazole. If coadministration is required, dose adjustment of both drugs is indicated. Increase voriconazole to 400 mg every 12 hours and decrease efavirenz to 300 mg every 24 hours. Restore the initial dose of efavirenz when treatment with voriconazole is discontinued. ▪ **Contraindicated** with **ergot alkaloids** (e.g., ergotamine and dihydroergotamine [D.H.E. 45]); serum concentrations of ergot alkaloids may be increased and may lead to ergotism. ▪ Avoid concomitant use with **fluconazole** (Diflucan). Potential for voriconazole toxicity remains if voriconazole is initiated within 24 hours of the last dose of fluconazole. ▪ May decrease the metabolism and increase serum levels of **cyclosporine** (Sandimmune). If concurrent administration with voriconazole is indicated, reduce the dose of cyclosporine by one half and monitor cyclosporine serum levels frequently. When voriconazole is discontinued, monitor cyclosporine levels frequently and increase the dose as necessary. ▪ May decrease the metabolism and increase serum levels of **methadone** (Dolophine) and increase risk of QT prolongation. If concurrent administration with voriconazole is indicated, monitor closely and decrease dose of methadone as necessary. ▪ Increases concentration and half-life of **alfentanil** (Alfenta), **fentanyl** (Sublimaze), **oxycodone** (ETH-Oxydose), **and sufentanil** (Sufenta). Dose reduction and extended monitoring recommended. ▪ May decrease the metabolism and increase serum levels of **tacrolimus** (Prograf). If concurrent administration with voriconazole is indicated, reduce the dose of tacrolimus by one third and monitor tacrolimus serum levels frequently. When voriconazole is discontinued, monitor tacrolimus levels frequently and increase the dose as necessary. ▪ Concurrent use with **warfarin** (Coumadin) or oral coumarin preparations may cause a significant increase in PT or INR. Monitor PT or INR closely and adjust warfarin dose as necessary. ▪ May decrease the metabolism and increase serum concentrations of CYP3A4 substrates, such as selected **HMG-CoA reductase inhibitors** (statins such as lovastatin [Mevacor]), **selected benzodiazepines** (e.g., alprazolam [Xanax], midazolam [Versed], triazolam [Halcion]), **selected calcium channel blockers** (e.g., felodipine [Plendil]), **vinca alkaloids** (e.g., vinblastine, vincristine), and CYP2C9 substrates such as **sulfonylureas** (e.g., glipizide [Glucotrol XL], glyburide [DiaBeta], tolbutamide) and **NSAIDs** (e.g., ibuprofen [Motrin], diclofenac [Voltaren]). To reduce the potential for toxic effects that may be caused by these drugs (e.g., rhabdomyolysis, prolonged sedative effect, cardiac toxicity, GI toxicity, neurotoxicity, hypoglycemia), close monitoring for toxic effects of all of these drugs is indicated, and in most cases dose reduction is indicated during concomitant administration of voriconazole. ▪ Concurrent use with **phenytoin** (Dilantin) may require dose adjustments of both drugs. Phenytoin increases metabolism and decreases serum concentrations of voriconazole. An increased dose of voriconazole is indicated; see Dose Adjustments. Voriconazole decreases the metabolism of phenytoin and increases serum concentrations. Monitor phenytoin serum concentrations and reduce dose as necessary to avoid toxicity. ▪ May decrease the metabolism and increase serum levels of **selected HIV protease inhibitors** (e.g., amprenavir [Agenerase], nelfinavir [Viracept], saquinavir [Invirase]). Selected HIV protease inhibitors (e.g., amprenavir, saquinavir) may decrease the metabolism of voriconazole and increase its serum levels. Monitor frequently for drug toxicity with coadministration of voriconazole and HIV protease inhibitors. No dose adjustment is required with indinavir (Crixivan). ▪ May decrease the metabolism and increase serum levels of **omeprazole** (Prilosec). If concurrent administration with voriconazole is indicated, reduce a dose of omeprazole of 40 mg or more by one half. The metabolism of other selected proton pump inhibitors may react similarly. ▪ **Non-nucleoside reverse transcriptase inhibitors** (NNRTIs) such as delavirdine (Rescriptor) may decrease the metabolism of voriconazole and increase its serum concentrations. Voriconazole may inhibit the metabolism of the same NNRTIs and increase their serum levels. Monitor frequently for drug toxicity with coadministration of voriconazole and NNRTIs. ▪ Concurrent use with **other nephrotoxic drugs** (e.g., aminoglycosides, cyclosporine) may result in decreased renal function or acute renal failure. ▪ Concurrent use with **oral contraceptives** may increase concentrations of both drugs. Monitor for adverse events related to each drug. Should not reduce the effectiveness of oral contraception. ▪ May have minor interactions with **cimetidine** (Tagamet), **macrolide antibiotics** (e.g., azithromycin, erythromycin), **and ranitidine** (Zantac); however, no dose adjustments are required. ▪ No significant interactions have been observed with indinavir (Crixivan), prednisolone, digoxin (Lanoxin), and mycophenolate (CellCept).

SIDE EFFECTS

Abdominal pain, diarrhea, dyspnea, fever, headache, hypokalemia, increases in liver function tests, nausea, peripheral edema, rash, respiratory disorders, sepsis, visual disturbances, and vomiting occur most frequently. Side effects that most often led to discontinuation of therapy include elevated liver function tests, rash, and visual disturbances. Blurred vision, color vision change, and/or photophobia are common but may be associated with higher serum concentrations and/or doses. Hypersensitivity reactions, including anaphylaxis, have been reported. Rarely, Stevens-Johnson syndrome and photosensitivity skin reactions have been reported. In patients with photosensitivity reactions, squamous cell cancer and melanoma have been reported. Numerous other side effects may occur, including QT prolongation and, rarely, torsades de pointes.

Post-Marketing: Pancreatitis in pediatric patients, prolonged visual adverse events, including optic neuritis and papilledema.

ANTIDOTE

Notify physician of all side effects; most will be treated symptomatically. If a hypersensitivity reaction (e.g., an infusion reaction) occurs, discontinue the infusion and treat with oxygen, epinephrine, antihistamines (e.g., diphenhydramine [Benadryl]), corticosteroids (e.g., dexamethasone [Decadron]), or bronchodilators (e.g., albuterol [Ventolin]) as indicated. Consider discontinuation of voriconazole if liver function tests are elevated and/or clinical S/S of liver disease attributable to voriconazole develop, if visual disturbances occur, if an increase in serum creatinine occurs, or if a rash develops (may be the first sign of an exfoliative skin disorder). No known specific antidote. Hemodialysis may assist in the removal of some voriconazole in accidental overdose and in the removal of SBECD. Resuscitate as indicated.

WARFARIN SODIUM **BBW**

(**WAR**-far-in **SO**-dee-um)

Coumadin

Anticoagulant

pH 8.1 to 8.3

USUAL DOSE

Used primarily for patients on Coumadin when oral dosing is not feasible. IV and oral doses are the same, and administration of the IV formulation should not provide any increased effect or an earlier onset of action. Dose must be individualized and adjusted based on PT/International Normalized Ratio (INR). An INR of greater than 4 appears to provide no additional benefit in most patients and is associated with a higher risk of bleeding. Loading doses may increase the incidence of complications and do not offer greater prompt anticoagulation protection. Heparin is preferred in situations requiring prompt anticoagulation because the anticoagulant actions for warfarin are not effective for at least 60 hours after initial dosing begins (60 hours is the half-life of the last clotting factor [II] to be affected by warfarin). Conversion to warfarin therapy may begin concomitantly with heparin therapy or may be delayed 3 to 6 days. To ensure continuous anticoagulation, overlap therapy until warfarin has produced a therapeutic response as determined by PT/INR. Discontinue heparin when therapeutic response is achieved. Duration of treatment is individualized. In general, it should continue until the danger of thrombosis and embolism has passed. See prescribing information for suggested durations of therapy for different indications and/or risk factors. Aspirin may or may not be a component of therapy depending on indication and risk factors. Not all factors causing warfarin dose variability are known. The maintenance dose needed to achieve a target PT/INR is influenced by clinical factors that include age, race, body weight, gender, concomitant medications, co-morbidities, and genetic factors (CYP2C9 and VKORC1 genotypes). See prescribing information and Dose Adjustments for dosing related to specific genotypes.

Initial dose: Select the starting dose based on the expected maintenance dose, taking into account the above factors. If the patient's CYP2C9 and VKORC1 genotypes are not known, the initial dose is usually 2 to 5 mg/day. Adjust dose based on patient-specific clinical factors and PT/INR determination. The American College of Chest Physicians (ACCP) suggests 5 to 10 mg/day for the first 1 to 2 days, then adjust dose based on PT/INR determination.

Maintenance dose: 2 to 10 mg/day. Adjust dose to maintain desired INR.

Atrial fibrillation, prophylaxis and treatment of venous thromboembolism, prophylaxis and treatment of pulmonary embolism: Adjust dose to maintain an INR of 2 to 3 (target INR 2.5).

Postmyocardial infarction: Current ACCP guidelines recommend that moderate-risk and low-risk patients be treated with aspirin alone instead of warfarin plus aspirin. High-risk patients with MI should be treated with low-dose aspirin (100 mg or less/day) and warfarin for 3 months after the MI. Adjust dose to maintain an INR of 2 to 3 (target INR 2.5).

Mechanical heart valves: Adjust dose to maintain an INR of 2.5 to 3.5 (target INR 3). Maintained long term. Use in combination with aspirin 75 to 100 mg/day may be indicated.

Bioprosthetic heart valves: Adjust dose to maintain an INR of 2 to 3.5 (target INR 3) for 12 weeks after valve insertion. Use in combination with aspirin 75 to 100 mg/day may be indicated. Longer-term therapy may be required in patients with additional risk factors (e.g., atrial fibrillation, prior thromboembolism).

PEDIATRIC DOSE

Safety for use in pediatric patients under 18 years of age not established, but is used. Usually given PO. See Maternal/Child.

DOSE ADJUSTMENTS

Use low initial doses in the elderly, debilitated, and those with expected increased PT/INR responses. ■ Patients with genetic factors (CYP2C9 and VKORC1 genotypes) may require a reduced dose because these alleles may be associated with reduced clearance of warfarin. ■ Use lower end of dose range in patients at increased risk of bleeding or those on aspirin therapy. ■ Reduced dose is required in impaired hepatic function. ■ No dose adjustment is required in impaired renal function. ■ Higher doses may be required in selected situations (e.g., patients with recurrent systemic embolism or mechanical prosthetic valves). The ACCP and National Heart, Lung, and Blood Institute (NHLBI) suggest that maintaining an INR of 3 to 4.5 may be indicated.

DILUTION

Reconstitute the 5-mg vial with 2.7 mL of SW (2 mg/mL).

Storage: Protect from light by storing in carton at CRT. Store reconstituted solution at room temperature and use within 4 hours. Do not refrigerate; discard any unused solution.

COMPATIBILITY   (Underline Indicates Conflicting Compatibility Information)

Consider any drug NOT listed as compatible to be INCOMPATIBLE until consulting a pharmacist; specific conditions may apply.

Some adsorption may occur in PVC containers and tubing when diluted in D5W or NS.

One source suggests the following **compatibilities:**

Y-site: Amikacin (Amikin), ammonium chloride, ascorbic acid, bivalirudin (Angiomax), cefazolin (Ancef), ceftriaxone (Rocephin), dopamine, epinephrine (Adrenalin), heparin, lidocaine, morphine, nitroglycerin IV, oxytocin (Pitocin), potassium chloride (KCl), ranitidine (Zantac), vancomycin.

RATE OF ADMINISTRATION

A single dose as an injection over 1 to 2 minutes.

ACTIONS

An anticoagulant that acts by inhibiting vitamin K–dependent coagulation factors (e.g., Factor II, VII, IX, and X) and the anticoagulant proteins C and S in the liver, resulting in a depression of their activities. An anticoagulant effect occurs within 24 hours; however, peak anticoagulant effect may be delayed for 72 to 96 hours. Approximately 99% bound to plasma proteins. Effective half-life ranges from 20 to 60 hours. Effects may be more pronounced as daily maintenance doses overlap. Well-established clots are not dissolved, but growth is prevented. Metabolized by hepatic microsomal enzymes (cytochrome P_{450} system) to inactive metabolites and reduced metabolites. Excreted primarily in urine with small amounts excreted in bile. Crosses the placental barrier.

INDICATIONS AND USES

Prophylaxis and/or treatment of venous thrombosis and pulmonary embolism. ▪ Prophylaxis and/or treatment of the thromboembolic complications of atrial fibrillation and/or cardiac valve replacement. ▪ Reduce the risk of death, recurrent myocardial infarction, and thromboembolic events such as stroke or systemic embolization after myocardial infarction. ▪ Treatment of patients receiving oral warfarin who are unable to take oral medication.

CONTRAINDICATIONS

Localized or general physical condition or circumstance in which the hazard of hemorrhage might be greater than the potential clinical benefits of anticoagulation (e.g., bleeding tendencies associated with active ulceration or overt bleeding of GI, GU, or respiratory tracts, CVA, aneurysms [cerebral or aortic], pericarditis, pericardial effusions, bacterial endocarditis; hemorrhagic tendencies or blood dyscrasias, inadequate laboratory facilities; major regional or lumbar block anesthesia; malignant hypertension; pregnancy; spinal puncture or other procedures with potential for uncontrollable bleeding; threatened abortion, eclampsia, preeclampsia; unsupervised patients who would find it difficult to cooperate [e.g., senility, alcoholism, or psychosis]; and recent or contemplated surgery of the CNS, eye, or traumatic surgery resulting in large open surfaces).

PRECAUTIONS

For IV use only; do not administer IM. ▪ Hemorrhage in any tissue or organ is one of the most serious risks associated with warfarin therapy. Fatalities have occurred. Bleeding is more likely to occur during initiation of therapy and with higher doses (resulting in a higher INR). Risk factors for hemorrhage include an INR greater than 4 or highly variable INRs, elderly patients age 65 or older, history of GI bleed, hypertension, cerebrovascular disease, serious heart disease, anemia, malignancy, trauma, renal insufficiency, concomitant drugs that affect hemostasis, and a long duration of therapy. Necrosis and/or gangrene is another serious risk associated with warfarin therapy. Necrosis appears to be associated with local thrombosis. In severe cases, débridement or amputation may be required. ▪ Limit IM injections of concomitant medications to upper extremities to permit easy access for manual compression, inspection for bleeding, and use of pressure bandages. ▪ Anticoagulation with warfarin may enhance the release of atheromatous plaque emboli, increasing the risk of complications from systemic cholesterol microembolization. May present with a variety of S/S, including abdominal, back, or flank pain; abrupt and intense pain in the leg, foot, or toes; cerebral ischemia; foot ulcers; gangrene; hematuria; hypertension; livedo reticularis (reddish blue mottling of skin on exposure to cold); myalgias; pancreatitis; purple toe syndrome; rash; and renal insufficiency. The kidney is the most commonly involved visceral organ, followed by the pancreas, spleen, and liver. Some cases have progressed to necrosis and death. ▪ Use with caution in patients with heparin-induced thrombocytopenia and deep vein thrombosis. Cases of venous limb ischemia, necrosis, and gangrene have occurred when heparin was discontinued and warfarin was started. ▪ Determinations of whole blood clotting and bleeding times are not an accurate measurement to adjust dose. ▪ Warfarin may increase the aPTT, even in the absence of heparin. A severe aPTT elevation (greater than 50 seconds) with a PT/INR in the normal range is an indicator of increased risk of postoperative hemorrhage. ▪ Use caution in the elderly or debilitated, severe to moderate impaired hepatic or renal function, severe to moderate hypertension, severe diabetes, with indwelling catheters, infectious diseases or disturbances of intestinal flora (e.g., sprue, antibiotic therapy), surgery or trauma involving large raw surfaces or that may result in internal bleeding, patients with a history of allergic problems, polycythemia vera, vasculitis, and known or suspected deficiency in protein C anticoagulant response. ▪ Increased PT/INR response may occur in patients with blood dyscrasias (see Contraindications), cancer, collagen vascular disease, congestive heart failure, diarrhea, elevated temperature, hyperthyroidism, infectious hepatitis, jaundice, poor nutritional state, steatorrhea, or vitamin K deficiency. ▪ Decreased PT/INR response may occur in patients with edema, hereditary coumarin resistance, hyperlipidemia, hypothyroidism, or nephrotic syndrome. Patients who are protein C or S deficient (inherited thrombotic conditions) must be covered with heparin and warfarin. ▪ If dental procedures or surgery or other minor surgical procedures are necessary, the PT/INR should be adjusted to the lower end of the therapeutic range. Monitor PT/INR just before treatment. Operative site should be limited so local procedures for hemostasis can be used. Warfarin therapy may have to be interrupted; consider risks versus benefits.

Monitor: PT/INR must be done before initial injection. Frequent monitoring of PT/INR required (very accurate bedside monitoring units are now available). Usually repeated daily during initiation of therapy, every 1 to 4 weeks after PT/INR has stabilized in the therapeutic range. Monitor with any change in patient regimen that may affect treatment (e.g., diet, illness, change in drug regimen). Draw blood for prothrombin just before a heparin dose being given concomitantly. If heparin is given as a continuous infusion, PT/INR may be drawn at any time; see Precautions. ▪ Because heparin may affect the PT/INR in patients receiving both heparin and warfarin, PT/INR determinations should be drawn 5 hours after the last IV bolus dose of heparin, 4 hours after a heparin infusion has been discontinued, or 24 hours after the last SC injection of heparin. ▪ Patients at high risk for bleeding may benefit from more frequent monitoring of INR, careful dose adjustments to desired INR, and a shorter duration of therapy. ▪ Monitor for S/S of hemorrhage, necrosis, cholesterol microembolization, and the possible sequelae; see Precautions. ▪ Has a narrow therapeutic range that can be affected by other drugs and dietary vitamin K. See Drug/Lab Interactions.

Patient Education: Nonhormonal birth control recommended. ▪ Adhere to dose schedule; do not take or discontinue any prescription or over-the-counter medication, including herbal products, without physician's approval. ▪ Confirm procedure for missed dose. ▪ Avoid alcohol. Eat a normal balanced diet, maintaining a consistent vitamin K intake. Avoid cranberry products. ▪ Avoid any activity or sport that may result in traumatic injury. ▪ Regular PT/INR testing and physician visits are imperative. ▪ Notify physician of unusual bleeding (e.g., increased menstrual flow, nosebleeds, tarry stools), any illness (e.g., diarrhea, infection, fever), headache, dizziness, or weakness. ▪ Carry an ID stating that warfarin is being taken.

Maternal/Child: Category X: avoid pregnancy. May cause fatal hemorrhage, has caused birth deformities, and may cause abortion and/or stillbirth. Low birth weight and growth retardation have also been reported. ▪ In mothers requiring warfarin, consider alternative methods of infant feeding, or use extreme caution if decision is made to breast-feed. Prolonged PTs have been reported in breast-fed infants. Careful monitoring of coagulation tests and vitamin K status in the breast-fed infant and the mother's PT/INR is required. ▪ Safety and effectiveness for use in pediatric patients not established; however, use is well documented for prevention and treatment of thromboembolic events. Difficulty in achieving and maintaining a therapeutic PT/INR in pediatric patients has been reported. More frequent PT/INR determinations are recommended.

Elderly: Less warfarin is required to produce a therapeutic level of anticoagulation in patients over 60 years of age; may have a greater-than-expected PT/INR response; see Dose Adjustments and Precautions. ▪ Not recommended for use in an unsupervised patient with senility.

DRUG/LAB INTERACTIONS

Monitor PT/INR carefully when drugs are added or discontinued. *Interactions are numerous and potentially life threatening. Review of drug profile by pharmacist is imperative.* ▪ Listed are some of the most significant. ▪ Not recommended for concurrent use with **streptokinase or urokinase**; may be hazardous. ▪ **Increased PT/INR response** (risk of bleeding increased) may occur with numerous drugs, including **amiodarone** (Nexterone), **anticoagulants** (e.g., argatroban, bivalirudin [Angiomax], lepirudin [Refludan]), **antifungal agents** (e.g., fluconazole [Diflucan], itraconazole [Sporanox], miconazole [Monistat (intravaginal or systemic)]), **aspirin, atenolol** (Tenormin), **capecitabine** (Xeloda), **cephalosporins** (e.g., cefazolin [Ancef], cefotetan, cefoxitin [Mefoxin], ceftriaxone [Rocephin]), **cimetidine** (Tagamet), **cisapride** (Propulsid), **clofibrate** (Atromid-S), **cyclophosphamide** (Cytoxan), **ezetimibe** (Zetia), **fenofibrate** (Tricor), **fluoroquinolones** (e.g., ciprofloxacin [Cipro IV], levofloxacin [Levaquin], moxifloxacin [Avelox], norfloxacin [Noroxin]), **fluvastatin** (Lescol), **gefitinib** (Iressa), **heparin, herbal medicines** (e.g., bromelains, cranberry products, danshen, dong quai, garlic, ginkgo biloba, and ginseng), **HMG-CoA reductase inhibitors** (e.g., atorvastatin [Lipitor], fluvastatin [Lescol], pravastatin [Pravachol], simvastatin [Zocor]), **isoniazid** (Nydrazid), **levothyroxine** (Synthroid), **macrolide antibiotics** (e.g., azithromycin [Zithromax], clarithromycin [Biaxin], erythromycin), **metronidazole** (Flagyl), **NSAIDs** (e.g., celecoxib [Celebrex], ibuprofen [Advil, Motrin], ketorolac [Toradol], naproxen [Aleve, Naprosyn], rofecoxib [Vioxx]), **oxandrolone** (Oxandrin), **propafenone** (Rhythmol), **propoxyphene** (Darvon-N), **propranolol, proton pump inhibitors** (e.g., esomeprazole [Nexium], omeprazole [Prilosec], pantoprazole [Protonix], rabeprazole [Aciphex]), **sertraline** (Zoloft), **sulfinpyrazone** (Anturane), **sulfonamides** (e.g., sulfamethoxazole/trimethoprim [Bactrim]), **tamoxifen** (Nolvadex), **ticlopidine** (Ticlid), **tolterodine** (Detrol), **tramadol** (Ultram), **zafirlukast** (Accolate). ▪ Concomitant treatment with **thrombolytics** (e.g., alteplase [Activase, tPA], reteplase [Retavase, rPA], streptokinase [Streptase]) may increase the risk of bleeding. ▪ Concomitant treatment with **drugs that affect platelet function,** such as dipyridamole (Persantine), glycoprotein GPIIb/IIIa receptor antagonists (e.g., abciximab [ReoPro], eptifibatide [Integrilin], tirofiban [Aggrastat]), and NSAIDs (e.g., ibuprofen [Advil, Motrin], naproxen [Aleve, Naprosyn]), may also increase the risk of bleeding. ▪ **Decreased PT/INR response** (anticoagulant effects decreased and risk of blood clots increased) may occur with numerous drugs, including **ascorbic acid** (high-dose vitamin C), **barbiturates** (e.g., phenobarbital), **carbamazepine** (Tegretol), **cholestyramine** (Questran), **griseofulvin** (Fulvicin), **nevirapine** (Viramune), **penicillins** (e.g., nafcillin [Nallpen]),

protease inhibitors (e.g., ritonavir [Norvir]), **rifampin** (Rifadin), **spironolactone** (Aldactone), **sucralfate** (Carafate), **trazodone** (Desyrel), and increased oral **vitamin K** intake (e.g., leafy greens, supplements). ■ **Atorvastatin** (Lipitor) **and pravastatin** (Pravachol) may increase or decrease PT/INR. ■ May inhibit metabolism and increase effects of **oral antidiabetic agents** (e.g., tolbutamide), **and phenytoin** (Dilantin); may cause toxicity. ■ **Herbal medicines** should be used with caution. May have anticoagulant, coagulant, or fibrinolytic properties; see literature for specific examples.

SIDE EFFECTS

Bleeding when the PT/INR is within the therapeutic range (may unmask an unsuspected lesion [e.g., tumor, ulcer]), hemorrhage in any tissue or organ, necrosis and/or gangrene of skin and other tissues. Complications from systemic cholesterol microembolization (e.g., "purple toes syndrome") from release of atheromatous plaque emboli. Less frequently reported side effects include anemia, angina, chest pain, coma, hypotension, loss of consciousness, pallor, and syncope. Hypersensitivity reactions, including anaphylaxis, do occur. Protein C deficiency may occur if not covered by heparin long enough.

ANTIDOTE

Keep physician informed of all side effects; some may be life threatening. Discontinue if warfarin is suspected to be the cause of developing necrosis (e.g., "purple toes syndrome"); consider heparin therapy if anticoagulation required. Phytonadione (vitamin K_1) is a specific antagonist and is indicated in overdose or desired warfarin reversal (e.g., severe bleeding). May be given via the parenteral or oral route; the usual dose is 5 to 25 mg (rarely up to 50 mg). In one small study, IV phytonadione (vitamin K_1) decreased the INR more rapidly in 24 hours than SC phytonadione; however, within 72 hours, results were similar. See phytonadione monograph for precautions surrounding IV administration. The use of phytonadione will impede subsequent anticoagulant therapy, and patients are at risk of returning to a pretreatment thrombotic status following rapid reversal of a prolonged PT/INR. Fresh whole blood, fresh frozen plasma, Factor IX complex (not purified Factor IX preparations, they increase PT levels) may be indicated.

ZIDOVUDINE BBW

(zye-**DOH**-vyou-deen)

Azidothymidine, AZT, Retrovir

Antiviral

pH 5.5

USUAL DOSE

Treatment of HIV infection (symptomatic or asymptomatic): 1 mg/kg every 4 hours (5 or 6 times daily) is the most frequent dose used in the United States. Dose recommendation in Canada is 1 to 2 mg/kg every 4 hours. Initiate oral therapy as soon as possible (100 mg PO approximately equal to 1 mg/kg IV). Impaired renal or hepatic function may increase toxicity. Usually part of a multi-drug regimen (e.g., zidovudine, zalcitabine [HIVID], saquinavir [Invirase]); see Drug/Lab Interactions.

Prevention of maternal-fetal HIV transmission: 2 mg/kg of total body weight over 1 hour when labor begins. Follow with an infusion of 1 mg/kg/hr (of total body weight) until umbilical cord is clamped.

PEDIATRIC DOSE

See Maternal/Child.

Treatment of HIV infections in infants up to 3 months of age (unlabeled): 1.5 mg/ kg every 6 hours.

Treatment of HIV infections in pediatric patients 3 months to 12 years of age (unlabeled): 120 mg/M^2 every 6 hours as an intermittent infusion or a continuous infusion of 20 mg/M^2/hr. See Dose Adjustments. Follow with oral therapy; see comments in Usual Dose.

NEONATAL DOSE

See Maternal/Child.

Prevention of maternal-fetal HIV transmission: 1.5 mg/kg infused over 30 minutes every 6 hours. Oral dosing preferred. Consider impaired hepatic or renal function. Begin within 12 hours of birth and continue until 6 weeks of age. Another source suggests 1.5 mg/kg/dose every 12 hours in premature infants from birth to 2 weeks of age, then increase to 2 mg/kg/dose every 8 hours.

DOSE ADJUSTMENTS

Dose selection should be cautious in the elderly based on the potential for decreased organ function and concomitant disease or drug therapy. ▪ Reduce dose to 1 mg/kg every 6 to 8 hours in patients with ESRD. ▪ Reduce the 120 mg/M^2 dose to 90 mg/M^2 in pediatric patients with granulocytopenia. ▪ May be required in anemia and/or with other drugs. See Monitor, Drug/Lab Interactions, and Antidote.

DILUTION

Each 1 mg of the calculated dose must be diluted in at least 0.25 mL of D5W (4 mg/mL). For a 70-kg patient at 1 mg/kg, a 70-mg dose would be diluted in 17.5 mL (equals 4 mg/mL [70 mg in 35 mL equals 2 mg/mL]). More dilute solutions are preferred (e.g., 1 mg/mL).

Infusion: Dilute 1 Gm in 1,000 mL D5W (1 mg/mL), 500 mg in 500 mL (1 mg/mL), 1 Gm in 500 mL (2 mg/mL), or 1 Gm in 250 mL (4 mg/mL).

Filters: Not required by manufacturer; no further data available from manufacturer.

Storage: Store undiluted vials at CRT. Protect from light. Chemically and physically stable after dilution for 24 hours at CRT or 48 hours refrigerated. However, as an added precaution against microbial contamination, manufacturer recommends use within 8 hours at CRT and 24 hours if refrigerated.

COMPATIBILITY   (Underline Indicates Conflicting Compatibility Information)
Consider any drug NOT listed as compatible to be INCOMPATIBLE until consulting a pharmacist; specific conditions may apply.
Manufacturer states, "Admixture in biologic or colloidal fluids (e.g., blood products, protein solutions) is not recommended."
 One source suggests the following **compatibilities:**
Additive: Dobutamine, meropenem (Merrem IV), ranitidine (Zantac).
Y-site: Acyclovir (Zovirax), allopurinol (Aloprim), amifostine (Ethyol), amikacin (Amikin), amphotericin B (generic), amphotericin B cholesteryl (Amphotec), anidulafungin (Eraxis), aztreonam (Azactam), cefepime (Maxipime), ceftazidime (Fortaz), ceftriaxone (Rocephin), cisatracurium (Nimbex), clindamycin (Cleocin), dexamethasone (Decadron), dobutamine, docetaxel (Taxotere), dopamine, doripenem (Doribax), doxorubicin liposomal (Doxil), erythromycin (Erythrocin), etoposide phosphate (Etopophos), filgrastim (Neupogen), fluconazole (Diflucan), fludarabine (Fludara), gemcitabine (Gemzar), gentamicin, granisetron (Kytril), heparin, imipenem-cilastatin (Primaxin), linezolid (Zyvox), lorazepam (Ativan), melphalan (Alkeran), meropenem (Merrem IV), metoclopramide (Reglan), morphine, nafcillin (Nallpen), ondansetron (Zofran), oxacillin (Bactocill), oxytocin (Pitocin), paclitaxel (Taxol), pemetrexed (Alimta), pentamidine, phenylephrine (Neo-Synephrine), piperacillin, piperacillin/ tazobactam (Zosyn), potassium chloride (KCl), ranitidine (Zantac), remifentanil (Ultiva), sargramostim (Leukine), sulfamethoxazole/ trimethoprim, teniposide (Vumon), thiotepa, tobramycin, vancomycin, vinorelbine (Navelbine).

RATE OF ADMINISTRATION
Intermittent infusion: Each single dose properly diluted must be delivered at a constant rate over 1 hour. Avoid rapid infusion or IV bolus.
Continuous infusion: Prevention of maternal-fetal HIV transmission: 2 mg/kg equally distributed over 1 hour, followed by 1 mg/kg/hr until umbilical cord clamped.
Pediatric continuous infusion: 0.5 to 1.8 mg/kg/hr.
Neonatal in prevention of maternal-fetal HIV transmission: A single dose infused over 30 min.

ACTIONS
An antiviral agent. Through a specific process this thymidine analog inhibits the in vitro replication and terminates the DNA chain of some retroviruses, including HIV (HTLV III, LAV, or ARV). May also have antiviral activity against the Epstein-Barr virus. Metabolized by glucuronidation in the liver and excreted through the kidneys. Half-life is approximately 1 hour. Crosses the placental barrier. Secreted in breast milk.

INDICATIONS AND USES
Treatment of HIV infection in combination with other anti-retroviral agents. ■ Prevention of maternal-fetal HIV transmission. Protocol includes oral zidovudine beginning with week 14 to week 34 of gestation, continuing until labor begins, IV dosing during labor, and zidovudine syrup or IV dosing to the newborn.

CONTRAINDICATIONS
Life-threatening hypersensitivity reactions to any of the components.
PRECAUTIONS
Do not give IM. ▪ Zidovudine has not been shown to reduce the risk of transmission to others. ▪ Incidence of adverse reactions appears to increase with disease progression. ▪ Has been associated with hematologic toxicity, including neutropenia and severe anemia, particularly in patients with advanced HIV. ▪ Use with extreme caution in patients with bone marrow compromise as indicated by a granulocyte count of less than 1,000/mm³ or hemoglobin below 9.5/dL. ▪ Zidovudine resistance seems to develop more quickly in patients with advanced disease. ▪ Decrease in CD4 count or clinical deterioration may be reversed with a switch to didanosine. ▪ Prolonged use of zidovudine has been associated with myopathy and myositis with pathologic changes similar to those produced by HIV disease. ▪ Rare cases of lactic acidosis (without hypoxemia) and severe hepatomegaly with steatosis have been reported with the use of some antiretroviral nucleoside analogs, including zidovudine when used alone or in combination. Deaths have occurred. Female gender, obesity, and prolonged exposure to antiretroviral nucleoside analogs may increase risk of lactic acidosis. Lactic acidosis should be considered, and therapy suspended, in patients who develop unexplained tachypnea, dyspnea, or a fall in serum sodium bicarbonate. ▪ Use with caution in any patient (especially obese women) with hepatomegaly, hepatitis, or other risk factors for liver disease. Suspend therapy with rapidly elevating aminotransferase levels (ALT), progressive hepatomegaly, or metabolic/lactic acidosis of unknown etiology. ▪ Use with caution in patients with severe hepatic impairment; may be at increased risk for hematologic toxicity. ▪ Hepatic decompensation has occurred in HIV/HCV co-infected patients receiving combination antiretroviral therapy for HIV and interferon alfa with or without ribavirin (Rebetol) for HVC. ▪ Use with caution in patients with severely impaired renal function (CrCl less than 15 mL/min); see Dose Adjustments. ▪ Immune reconstitution syndrome has been reported in patients treated with combination antiretroviral therapy, including zidovudine. Patients may develop an inflammatory response to indolent opportunistic infections (e.g., *Mycobacterium avium*, CMV, PCP, or tuberculosis). May require further evaluation and treatment. ▪ See Drug/Lab Interactions.
Monitor: Observe closely; not a cure for HIV infections. Patients may acquire illnesses associated with AIDS or ARC, including opportunistic infections. ▪ Frequent blood cell counts are required. Hematologic toxicity, including granulocytopenia, severe anemia, and occasionally reversible pancytopenia are common. Anemia may occur as early as 2 to 4 weeks. Neutropenia usually occurs after 6 to 8 weeks of therapy; dosage adjustments and/or transfusions may be required. ▪ Monitor liver function. ▪ Closely monitor patients receiving zidovudine and interferon alfa, with or without ribavirin (Rebetol), for treatment-associated toxicities, especially hepatic decompensation, neutropenia, and anemia. Dose reduction or discontinuation of interferon, ribavirin, or both may be required if worsening clinical toxicities are seen (e.g., hepatic decompensation [e.g., Child-Pugh score greater than 6]). ▪ Monitoring of zidovudine serum concentrations has been used to individualize therapy. May increase effectiveness while decreasing toxicity. ▪ Monitor CD4 lymphocyte count at diagnosis and every 3 to 6 months. ▪ Drug resistance testing and moni-

toring of (HIV) RNA, an indicator of viral load, are recommended to help guide treatment. ▪ See Drug/Lab Interactions.

Patient Education: Zidovudine is not a cure. ▪ Report abdominal pain, jaundice, muscle weakness, shortness of breath, or rapid breathing promptly. ▪ Major side effects are neutropenia and/or anemia. ▪ Requires frequent lab work and close follow-up with physician; keep all appointments. ▪ Check with physician before taking any other meds.

Maternal/Child: Category C: safety for use during pregnancy has been evaluated. Risk versus benefit appears justified only in HIV-infected mothers. Congenital deformities not increased in studies. ▪ Discontinue breastfeeding to reduce incidence of HIV transmission and potential for serious adverse reactions in nursing infants. ▪ Has been studied in HIV-infected pediatric patients over 3 months of age who have HIV-related symptoms or are asymptomatic with abnormal lab values, indicating significant HIV-related immunosuppression. Has also been studied in neonates perinatally exposed to HIV. To monitor maternal-fetal outcomes, an Antiretroviral Pregnancy Registry has been established. See prescribing information.

Elderly: Dose selection should be cautious; see Dose Adjustments. Consider impaired hepatic and renal function.

DRUG/LAB INTERACTIONS

Toxicity may be increased by **nephrotoxic and/or cytotoxic drugs and/or drugs that interfere with RBC or WBC number and function** (e.g., amphotericin B [generic], dapsone, doxorubicin [Adriamycin], flucytosine, interferons, pentamidine, vinblastine, vincristine). ▪ *Do not use in combination with other products that contain zidovudine (e.g., lamivudine/zidovudine [Combivir], abacavir/lamivudine/zidovudine [Trizivir]).* ▪ Use caution with any drug metabolized by **glucuronidation** (e.g., acetaminophen, diazepam [Valium], morphine); toxicity of both drugs may be increased. ▪ **Probenicid** may inhibit glucuronidation or reduce renal excretion of zidovudine, increasing zidovudine toxicity. ▪ Use with **atovaquone** (Mepron), **fluconazole** (Diflucan), or **sulfamethoxazole/trimethoprim** (Bactrim) may increase zidovudine serum levels. ▪ **Acetaminophen** (Anacin-3, Tylenol), **clarithromycin** (Biaxin), and **rifamycins** (e.g., rifampin [Rifadin], rifabutin [Mycobutin]) may increase clearance, reduce zidovudine serum levels, and reduce effectiveness. ▪ **Acetaminophen** has increased the incidence of granulocytopenia. ▪ Antagonized by **doxorubicin** (Adriamycin), **stavudine** (Zerit), **and ribavirin** (Rebetol). Avoid concurrent use. ▪ Hematologic toxicity may be increased by **nucleoside analogs** being evaluated in AIDS and ARC patients (e.g., didanosine [DDI]) because of their effect on RBC or WBC numbers or function. These analogs can affect DNA replication and may antagonize effects of zidovudine. Avoid concomitant administration. ▪ Hematologic toxicity increased with **ganciclovir** (Cytovene), **interferons, or other bone marrow suppressants or cytotoxic agents.** ▪ **Phenytoin** levels may increase or decrease; monitor carefully to ensure proper dosing. ▪ **Phenytoin** may also increase zidovudine levels by decreasing clearance. ▪ Use with **acyclovir** may cause neurotoxicity (drowsiness, lethargy). ▪ Combination therapy with zidovudine and **interferon alfa,** with or without **ribavirin** (Rebetol), may increase risk of hepatic decompensation.

SIDE EFFECTS

Frequency and severity of adverse events are greater in patients with more advanced infection at the time of initiation of treatment. Directly related to pretreatment bone marrow reserve, dose and duration and inversely related to T4 lymphocyte numbers. Abdominal pain, anaphylaxis, anemia (severe), anorexia, arthralgia, asthenia, chills, constipation, diaphoresis, diarrhea, dizziness, dyspepsia, dysphagia, dyspnea, fatigue, fever, flatulence, GI pain, granulocytopenia, gynecomastia, headache, hepatomegaly (severe), hyperbilirubinemia, increased liver function tests (e.g., ALT, AST, alkaline phosphatase), insomnia, malaise, mouth ulcers, myalgia, myopathy and myositis, nausea, neuropathy, neutropenia, pancytopenia (reversible), paresthesia, pure red cell aplasia, rash, somnolence, taste perversion, thrombocytopenia, vomiting. Suspect lactic acidosis if dyspnea, a fall in serum bicarbonate level, or tachypnea occurs.

ANTIDOTE

Notify physician of all side effects; most will be treated symptomatically. Moderate anemia or granulocytopenia may respond to a reduction in dose. Discontinue zidovudine for severe anemia (less than 7.5 Gm/dL or a 25% reduction from baseline) or severe granulocytopenia (less than 750/mm^3 or 50% reduction from baseline). Transfusions may be required. If marrow recovery occurs following dose interruption, resumption of therapy may be appropriate using adjunctive measures such as epoetin alfa (Epogen). Rash may be the first sign of anaphylaxis; notify physician and treat with diphenhydramine (Benadryl), epinephrine (Adrenalin), and corticosteroids as indicated. Sulfamethoxazole/trimethoprim (Bactrim), pyrimethamine (Daraprim), and acyclovir (Zovirax) may be indicated to treat opportunistic infections.

ZOLEDRONIC ACID
(**ZOH**-leh-dron-ick **AS**-id)

Reclast ▪ **Zometa**

Bone resorption inhibitor
Antihypercalcemic
(bisphosphonate)

pH 6 to 7 ▪ pH 2

USUAL DOSE
(International Units [IU])

RECLAST AND ZOMETA
Prehydration required. Always used with adequate hydration and appropriate monitoring. See Dose Adjustments, Precautions, and Monitor.

RECLAST
Premedication: Administration of acetaminophen after Reclast administration may reduce the incidence of acute phase reaction symptoms; see Side Effects. In clinical studies, a standard dose of acetaminophen was given with the infusion and for the next 72 hours as needed.

Treatment of Paget's disease: One dose of 5 mg as an infusion over no less than 15 minutes. A CrCl greater than 35 mL/min and supplemental calcium and vitamin D are required, particularly during the 2 weeks following administration.

Calcium: 1,500 mg daily in divided doses (750 mg two times a day or 500 mg three times a day).

Vitamin D: 800 IU/day.

An extended remission period has been observed after a single treatment. Specific retreatment data not available; however, retreatment may be considered for patients who have relapsed based on increases in serum alkaline phosphatase, for patients who did not achieve normalization of their serum alkaline phosphatase, and for patients with symptoms.

Treatment of osteoporosis in men and post-menopausal women and treatment and prevention of glucocorticoid-induced osteoporosis: A single dose of 5 mg given once a year as an infusion over at least 15 minutes. 1,200 mg of calcium and 800 to 1,000 IU of vitamin D daily are recommended. If the calcium and vitamin D are not obtained by dietary means, oral supplementation is indicated.

Prevention of osteoporosis in postmenopausal women: A single dose of 5 mg given every 2 years as an infusion over at least 15 minutes.

ZOMETA
Hypercalcemia of malignancy (corrected serum calcium equal to or greater than 12 mg/dL [3 mmol/L]): One dose of 4 mg as an infusion over no less than 15 minutes.

Experience is limited, but retreatment with the same dose may be considered if serum calcium does not return to normal or remain normal after initial treatment. Wait at least 7 days from completion of the first infusion to allow full response.

Multiple myeloma and metastatic bone lesions from solid tumors: 4 mg as an infusion over no less than 15 minutes every 3 to 4 weeks. A CrCl greater than 60 mL is required; see Dose Adjustments. Optimal duration of therapy is unknown. Concurrent daily administration of PO calcium 500 mg and a multivitamin with 400 units vitamin D is recommended.

Continued

DOSE ADJUSTMENTS
RECLAST AND ZOMETA
Dose adjustment is not indicated based on age or race. Studies have not been conducted in patients with hepatic or severe renal impairment; see Precautions and Elderly.

RECLAST
No dose adjustment required in patients with a CrCl greater than 30 mL/min. Not recommended for use in patients with a CrCl less than 35 mL/min; clinical experience insufficient.

ZOMETA
Hypercalcemia of malignancy: Dose adjustments are not necessary in patients with mild to moderate renal impairment before beginning treatment (SCr less than 4.5 mg/dL). If renal function deteriorates, consider if the potential benefit of continued treatment outweighs the possible risk.

Multiple myeloma and metastatic bone lesions from solid tumors: Reduce the initial and following doses in patients with mild to moderate renal impairment based on the following chart:

Zometa Dose Adjustments in Multiple Myeloma and Metastatic Bone Lesions	
Baseline Creatinine Clearance	Zoledronic Acid Recommended Dose
Greater than 60 mL/min	4 mg
50 to 60 mL/min	3.5 mg
40 to 49 mL/min	3.3 mg
30 to 39 mL/min	3 mg

Measure SCr before each Zometa dose and withhold if renal condition deteriorates; see Monitor. When the CrCl has returned to within 10% of the baseline value, resume dosing at the same dose administered before treatment interruption.

In patients who experience a decrease in renal function after receiving the initial dose of Zometa, delayed dosing is required before retreatment as follows:

Normal serum creatinine (SCr) before treatment: If SCr has increased 0.5 mg/dL within 2 weeks of planned retreatment, withhold retreatment dose until recovery to within 10% of baseline SCr value.

Abnormal SCr before treatment: If SCr has increased 1 mg/dL within 2 weeks of planned retreatment, withhold retreatment dose until the SCr is within 10% of baseline value.

DILUTION
RECLAST
A 5-mg dose is available prediluted in 100 mL of water for injection for administration as an infusion. If previously refrigerated, allow solution to reach room temperature before administration.

ZOMETA
Vials contain overfill; measure accurately. Withdraw desired volume from vial. Must be further diluted immediately in 100 mL of NS or D5W.

Zometa Dilution Recommendations	
Recommended Dose (mg)	Volume of Diluent (mL)
4 mg	5 mL
3.5 mg	4.4 mL
3.3 mg	4.1 mL
3 mg	3.8 mL

Filters: Not required by manufacturer; however, use of a filter should not have an adverse effect.

Storage: *Reclast:* Store at CRT. Stable for 24 hours refrigerated at 2° to 8° C (36° to 46° F) after opening. *Zometa:* Store vials in carton at CRT. Use immediately after dilution is preferred. Diluted solution may be refrigerated but must be used and the infusion completed within 24 hours of mixing. Do not store undiluted solution in a syringe (to avoid inadvertent injection).

COMPATIBILITY

RECLAST AND ZOMETA

Novartis manufactures both Reclast and Zometa and states, "Must not be mixed with calcium or other divalent cation–containing infusion solutions (e.g., LR). Should be administered as a single IV solution in a line separate from all other drugs."

RECLAST

A vented IV set is required.

RATE OF ADMINISTRATION

A single dose equally distributed over no less than 15 minutes. After infusion is finished, flush IV line with 10 mL NS. An increase in renal toxicity that can progress to renal failure can result from shorter infusion times.

ACTIONS

ZOLEDRONIC ACID

A bisphosphonate that inhibits osteoclast-mediated bone resorption. Used as a bone resorption inhibitor in Paget's disease (Reclast) and as a hypocalcemic agent to reduce hypercalcemia in oncology patients (Zometa). Inhibits osteoclastic (destructive to bone) activity and induces osteoclast apoptosis (fragmentation of a cell into particles for elimination). Blocks the osteoclastic resorption of mineralized bone and cartilage through its binding to bone and inhibits the increased osteoclastic activity and skeletal calcium release induced by various tumors. Decreases serum calcium and phosphorus and increases urinary calcium and phosphorus excretion. Not metabolized. Most bound to bone and slowly released back into the systemic circulation. Primarily excreted intact via the kidney. Half-life is triphasic with a terminal half-life of 146 hours.

RECLAST

In Paget's disease, it localizes preferentially at sites of high bone turnover and promotes bone of normal quality with no evidence of impaired bone remodeling or mineralization effect. Returns patients to normal levels of bone turnover; see Indications.

ZOMETA

In oncology patients with hypercalcemia, it reduces serum calcium concentrations by inhibiting bone resorption. Reduction in calcium levels is seen in 24 to 48 hours, but maximum response may take up to 7 days.

INDICATIONS AND USES

RECLAST

Treatment of Paget's disease of the bone in men and women. Treatment indicated to induce remission (normalization of serum alkaline phosphatase) in patients with elevations in serum alkaline phosphatase of two times or higher than the upper limit of the age-specific reference range and in patients who are symptomatic or are at risk for complications from their disease. Paget's disease of the bone is a chronic focal skeletal disorder characterized by greatly increased and disorderly bone remodeling. Excessive osteoclastic bone resorption is followed by irregular osteoblastic new bone formation, which leads to replacement of the normal bone architecture by disorganized, enlarged, and weakened bone structure. ■ Prevention and treatment of osteoporosis in post-menopausal women. In osteoporosis diagnosed by a bone mineral density test or prevalent vertebral fractures, Reclast reduces the incidence of hip, vertebral, and non-vertebral osteoporosis-related fractures. In patients at high risk for fracture (defined as a recent low-trauma hip fracture), Reclast reduces the incidence of new clinical fractures. ■ Treatment to increase bone mass in men with osteoporosis. ■ Treatment and prevention of glucocorticoid-induced osteoporosis in men and women who are initiating or continuing systemic glucocorticoids in a daily dose that is equivalent to 7.5 mg or more of prednisone and who are expected to remain on glucocorticoids for at least 12 months.

ZOMETA

Treatment of hypercalcemia of malignancy (HCM) (defined as an albumin-corrected calcium [cCa] of greater than 12 mg/dL [3 mmol/L] using the following formula: cCa = Ca in mg/dL + 0.8 [mid-range of measured albumin in mg/dL]). ■ Treatment of patients with multiple myeloma and patients with documented bone metastases from solid tumors in conjunction with chemotherapy. Prostate cancer should have progressed after treatment with at least one hormonal therapy. ■ Safety for use in the treatment of hypercalcemia associated with hyperparathyroidism or with other non–tumor related conditions has not been established.

CONTRAINDICATIONS

RECLAST AND ZOMETA

Hypersensitivity to zoledronic acid or any of its components.

RECLAST

Hypocalcemia, pregnancy, and lactation.

PRECAUTIONS

RECLAST AND ZOMETA

A patient being treated with Zometa should not be treated with Reclast. A patient being treated with Reclast should not be treated with Zometa. ■ Bisphosphonates have been associated with deterioration of renal function and potential renal failure. Multiple cycles of zoledronic acid, doses over 4 or 5 mg, and/or a rate of administration less than 15 minutes increase this risk. Patients who are dehydrated, are receiving diuretics or other nephrotoxic drugs, or have pre-existing renal impairment may also be at increased risk. ▪ Use in patients with severe renal impairment (CrCl less than 35 mL/min) has not been adequately studied. ▪ Use with caution in patients with aspirin-sensitive asthma; bronchoconstriction has been reported in these patients. ▪ Osteonecrosis of the jaw (ONJ) has been reported in patients receiving bisphosphonates. The majority of cases have been in cancer patients undergoing dental procedures. Risk factors include cancer, concomitant therapy (e.g., chemotherapy, radiotherapy, corticosteroids), and co-morbid conditions (e.g., anemia, coagulopathies, infection, pre-existing oral disease). Post-marketing experience suggests a greater frequency of reports based on tumor type (advanced breast cancer or multiple myeloma). ▪ Consider a dental exam and appropriate preventive dentistry before beginning therapy with bisphosphonates. Avoid invasive dental procedures during bisphosphonate therapy. Dental surgery may exacerbate ONJ in patients who develop ONJ while undergoing bisphosphonate therapy. ▪ Severe and occasionally incapacitating bone, joint, and/or muscle pain has been reported. Onset of symptoms may be days to months after initiation of therapy. Symptoms usually resolve when zoledronic acid is discontinued; however, in some patients symptoms resolved slowly or persisted. ▪ Atypical, low-energy, or low trauma fractures of the femoral shaft have been reported in bisphosphonate-treated patients. May be bilateral. Many patients report prodromal pain in the affected area (usually presenting as dull, aching thigh pain) weeks to months before a complete fracture occurs. Patients presenting with thigh or groin pain should be evaluated to rule out an incomplete femur fracture. Patients presenting with an atypical fracture should also be assessed for S/S of fracture in the contralateral limb. ▪ See Monitor.

RECLAST

Hypocalcemia may occur. Pre-existing hypocalcemia must be treated by adequate intake of calcium and vitamin D before initiating therapy. Concurrent dosing with calcium and vitamin D during therapy is required and is especially important in the 2 weeks following Reclast administration. ▪ Effectively treat disturbances of calcium and mineral metabolism (e.g., hypoparathyroidism, thyroid surgery, parathyroid surgery, malabsorption syndromes, excision of the small intestine) before initiating therapy with Reclast. ▪ Safety and effectiveness for treatment of osteoporosis based on 3 years of clinical data. Optimum duration of use has not been determined. Re-evaluate need for continued therapy on a periodic basis.

ZOMETA

Calcium is bound to serum protein; concentration fluctuates with changes in blood volume. Changes in serum calcium (especially during rehydration) may not reflect true plasma levels. Measurement with ionized calcium levels is preferred. If unavailable, all calcium measurement should be corrected for albumin to establish a basis for treatment and evaluation of treatment. ▪ Mild or asymptomatic hypercalcemia will be treated with conservative measures (e.g., saline hydration, with or without diuretics [after correcting hypovolemia]). Consider patient's cardiovascular status. Corticosteroids may be indicated if the underlying cancer is sensitive (e.g., hematologic cancers). ▪ Not recommended for patients with bone metastases with a SCr greater than 3 mg/dL (265 micromol/L) or for patients with hypercalcemia of malignancy with a SCr equal to or greater than 4.5 mg/dL (400 micromol/L). These patients were excluded from the studies. After considering other treatment options, use only if benefit outweighs risk of renal failure. ■ Retreatment may increase potential for renal failure; before retreatment, consider other available treatment options and risk versus benefit; evaluate serum creatinine before each dose. ■ May be used adjunctively with chemotherapy, radiation, or surgery.

Monitor: RECLAST AND ZOMETA: Serum phosphate levels will decrease (hypophosphatemia) and may require treatment. Short-term supplemental therapy may also be required for hypocalcemia or hypomagnesemia. ■ See Precautions and Drug/Lab Interactions.

RECLAST: S/S of Paget's disease range from no symptoms to severe morbidity due to bone pain, bone deformity, pathologic fractures, and neurologic and other complications. Serum alkaline phosphatase provides an objective measure of disease severity and response to therapy. Diagnosis can be confirmed by radiographic evidence. ■ Obtain baseline measurement of serum alkaline phosphatase, serum calcium, electrolytes, phosphate, magnesium, and SCr. Monitor as indicated. Obtain serum creatinine before each dose. ■ Supplemental calcium and vitamin D required; see Usual Dose. Very important in the 2 weeks following Reclast administration. ■ Adequate hydration required; a minimum of two glasses of liquid is recommended before dosing on day of administration. Additional hydration is required in patients undergoing diuretic therapy. ■ Monitor calcium and mineral levels closely in patients with disturbances of calcium and mineral metabolism (e.g., hypoparathyroidism, thyroid surgery, parathyroid surgery, malabsorption syndromes, excision of the small intestine).

ZOMETA: Obtain baseline measurements of serum calcium (corrected for serum albumin), electrolytes, phosphate, magnesium, SCr, and CBC with differential and hematocrit/hemoglobin. Monitor all closely as indicated by baseline results (may be daily). ■ Monitor SCr before each dose to identify renal deterioration. During clinical studies, deterioration was considered as an increase of 0.5 mg/dL if the patient had a normal baseline; if the patient had an abnormal baseline, deterioration was considered as an increase of 1 mg/dL. ■ Patients with cancer-related hypercalcemia are often dehydrated. Must be adequately hydrated orally and/or IV before treatment is initiated. Hydration with saline is preferred to facilitate the renal excretion of calcium and correct dehydration. A pretreatment urine output of 2 L/day is recommended. Maintain adequate hydration and urine output throughout treatment. ■ Correct hypovolemia before using diuretics. ■ Avoid overhydration in patients with compromised cardiovascular status. Observe frequently for signs of fluid overload. ■ Monitor patients with pre-existing anemia, leukopenia, or thrombocytopenia very carefully during treatment and the first 2 weeks following treatment.

Patient Education: RECLAST AND ZOMETA: Avoid pregnancy; use of nonhormonal birth control recommended. Report a suspected pregnancy; may cause fetal harm. ■ Regular visits and assessment of lab tests imperative. ■ Take only prescribed medications. ■ Adequate hydration required. Drink at least two glasses of fluid before infusion. ■ Report abdominal cramps, chills, confusion, fever, muscle spasms, sore throat, and/or any new medical problems promptly. ■ Flu-like symptoms may occur within the first 3 days of therapy. Usually resolve within 3 days of onset but may last for up to 7 to 14 days. ▪ Good dental hygiene and routine dental care required. Obtain a dental exam before initiating therapy, and avoid invasive dental procedures during therapy. ▪ Report development of bone, joint, or muscle pain promptly. Onset of pain is variable. ▪ Report thigh or groin pain promptly.

RECLAST: Calcium and vitamin D supplementation required to maintain calcium levels. ▪ Tell your physician if you have had surgery to remove some or all of the parathyroid glands in your neck, have had sections of your intestine removed, or are unable to take calcium supplements. ▪ Promptly report muscle spasms and/or numbness or tingling sensations (especially around the mouth); may indicate hypocalcemia.

ZOMETA: Dietary restriction of calcium and vitamin D may be required in hypercalcemia of malignancy. ▪ An oral calcium supplement of 500 mg and a multivitamin with 400 IU of vitamin D are recommended for patients with multiple myeloma and bone metastasis of solid tumors.

Maternal/Child: Category D: avoid pregnancy; may cause fetal harm. ▪ Discontinue breast-feeding. ▪ Not indicated for use in pediatric patients. Because of long-term retention in bone, zoledronic acid should be used in pediatric patients only when potential benefit outweighs potential risk. Has been used in pediatric patients with severe osteogenesis imperfecta; see manufacturer's prescribing information.

Elderly: Response similar to that seen in younger patients. ▪ Use with caution based on age-related impaired organ function and concomitant disease or other drug therapy; monitor renal function closely. ▪ Monitor fluid and electrolyte status carefully to avoid overhydration. ▪ Acute phase reactions occur less frequently in the elderly; see Side Effects.

DRUG/LAB INTERACTIONS

RECLAST AND ZOMETA

Concurrent use with **loop diuretics** (e.g., furosemide [Lasix]) may increase risk of hypocalcemia or nephrotoxicity. ▪ Concurrent use with **aminoglycosides** (e.g., gentamicin) may have an additive hypocalcemic effect that may persist for a prolonged period. ▪ Use caution when administered with other potentially **nephrotoxic drugs** (e.g., aminoglycosides [gentamicin, tobramycin], cisplatin [Platinol], NSAIDs [ibuprofen (Advil), naproxen (Aleve)]); the risk of renal deterioration is increased. Consider monitoring of SCr. ▪ Concurrent administration with **renally eliminated drugs** (e.g., digoxin) may lead to increased exposure of these drugs. Use caution and consider monitoring of SCr. ▪ Thought not to inhibit cytochrome P_{450} enzymes; however, no specific drug interaction studies have been completed.

ZOMETA

Does not interfere with any known primary cancer therapy. ▪ Concurrent use with **thalidomide** does not result in a significant change in the pharmacokinetics or creatinine clearance of zoledronic acid; no dose adjustment indicated. ▪ Effects may be antagonized by **calcium-containing preparations or vitamin D**; avoid use.

SIDE EFFECTS

RECLAST AND ZOMETA

Abdominal pain, anorexia, atypical femur fracture, conjunctivitis, constipation, dehydration, diarrhea, dyspnea, episcleritis, flu-like syndrome (e.g., arthralgias and/or bone pain, chills, fever, flushing, and myalgias), headache, hypersensitivity reactions (including rare case of anaphylaxis, angioedema, and urticaria), hypocalcemia (abdominal cramps, confusion, muscle spasms), hypomagnesemia, hypophosphatemia, hypotension, injection site reactions, nausea, ocular inflammation (e.g., iritis, uveitis, scleritis, orbital inflammation and edema), osteonecrosis (primarily of the jaw), rash, renal impairment, and vomiting.

RECLAST

Hypocalcemia is the most serious side effect. Dizziness, fatigue, and nausea were commonly reported. In addition to the previously noted side effects, an acute-phase reaction (e.g., chills; fever; headache; muscle, bone, or joint pain) and nausea and vomiting were reported. Symptoms may be significant and lead to dehydration. May occur within the first 3 days; is usually mild to moderate and lasts only a few days. Abdominal distention, anemia, asthenia, atrial fibrillation, back pain, dyspepsia, lethargy, musculoskeletal stiffness, pain, paresthesia, and peripheral edema have also been reported.

ZOMETA

The most commonly reported side effects are anemia, constipation, dyspnea, fever, and nausea. In addition to the previously noted side effects, agitation, anxiety, bronchoconstriction, chest pain, confusion, cough, dehydration, dysphagia, edema, granulocytopenia, hypokalemia, increased serum creatinine, musculoskeletal pain (e.g., bone pain and/or arthralgia and myalgias, which may be severe), pancytopenia, pleural effusion, pruritus, somnolence, thrombocytopenia, urinary tract infection, and weakness have occurred in 10% or more of patients. Fluid overload, hypokalemia, hypomagnesemia, and hypophosphatemia may occur more often with the use of concurrent fluid and diuretics.

Post-Marketing: Acute renal failure; angioneurotic edema; blurred vision; bradycardia; dehydration secondary to diuretic therapy, fever, or GI losses; dry mouth; hematuria; hyperesthesia; hyperkalemia; hypernatremia; hypersensitivity reactions; hypertension; increased SCr; increased sweating; influenza-like illness (asthenia, fatigue or malaise, fever persisting for more than 30 days); proteinuria; and weight increase.

Overdose: Clinically significant hypocalcemia (e.g., abdominal cramps; confusion; irregular heartbeats; muscle cramps in the hands, arms, feet, legs, or face; numbness and tingling around the mouth, fingertips, or feet), hypophosphatemia (e.g., unusual tiredness or weakness), and hypomagnesemia (e.g., muscle trembling or twitching) may occur. Elevated SCr levels and renal tubular necrosis may occur with excessive dose or rate of administration.

ANTIDOTE

RECLAST AND ZOMETA

Keep physician informed of side effects. According to the manufacturer, no specific treatment was required in most cases of flu-like syndrome, GI symptoms, and infusion site reactions, and the symptoms subsided in 24 to 48 hours. Some side effects may respond to symptomatic treatment. IV fluids may be required for dehydration. Magnesium and phosphorus may require replacement if depletion is too severe. If mild, all will probably return toward normal in 7 to 10 days. For asymptomatic or mild to moderate hypocalcemia (6.5 to 8 mg/100 mL [1 dL] corrected for serum albumin), short-term calcium therapy (e.g., calcium gluconate) may be indicated. Discontinue drug for any symptoms of hypersensitivity or overdose. Discontinue for severe bone, joint, or muscle pain. Treat anaphylaxis and resuscitate as indicated.

ZOMETA

Monitor serum calcium and use vigorous IV hydration, with or without diuretics, for 2 to 3 days. Monitor intake and output to ensure adequacy and balance. Use short-term IV calcium therapy if indicated. Potassium phosphate and/or magnesium sulfate may be required to treat hypophosphatemia and hypomagnesemia. High fever may respond to steroids. RBC transfusions may be required in anemia.

APPENDIX A

Recommendations for the Safe Use of Handling of Cytotoxic Drugs

INTRODUCTION

Cytotoxic drugs are toxic compounds and are known to have carcinogenic, mutagenic, and/or teratogenic potential. With direct contact they may cause irritation to the skin, eyes, and mucous membranes, and ulceration and necrosis of tissue. The toxicity of cytotoxic drugs dictates that the exposure of health care personnel to these drugs should be minimized. At the same time, the requirement for maintenance of aseptic conditions must be satisfied.*

POTENTIAL ROUTES OF EXPOSURE

This brochure reviews the routes through which exposure may occur and presents recommendations for the safe handling of parenteral cytotoxic drugs by pharmacists, nurses, physicians, and other personnel who participate in the preparation and administration of these drugs to patients. These guidelines apply in any setting where cytotoxic drugs are prepared—including pharmacies, nursing units, clinics, physicians' offices and the home health care environment. The primary routes of exposure during the preparation and administration phases are through the inhalation of aerosolized drug or by direct skin contact.

During drug preparation, a variety of manipulations are used which may result in aerosol generation, spraying, and splattering. Examples of these manipulations include: the withdrawal of needles from drug vials; the use of syringes and needles or filter straws for drug transfer; the opening of ampules; and the expulsion of air from the syringe when measuring the precise volume of a drug. Pharmaceutical practice calls for the use of aseptic techniques and a sterile environment. Many pharmacies provide this sterile environment by using a horizontal laminar flow work bench. However, while this type of unit provides product protection, it may expose the operator and other room occupants to aerosols generated during drug preparation procedures. Therefore, a Class II laminar flow (vertical) biological safety cabinet that provides both product and operator protection is needed for the preparation of cytotoxic drugs. This is accomplished by filtering incoming and exhaust air through a high-efficiency particulate air (HEPA) filter. It should be noted that these filters are not effective for volatile materials because they do not capture vapors and gases. Personnel should be familiar with the capabilities, limitations, and proper utilization of the biological safety cabinet selected.

During administration, clearing air from a syringe or infusion line and leakage at tubing, syringe, or stopcock connections should be avoided to prevent opportunities for accidental skin contact and aerosol generation. Dispose of syringes and unclipped needles into a leakproof and puncture-resistant container.

From U.S. Department of Health and Human Services, Public Health Service, National Institutes of Health: NIH Publication No. 92-2621. Prepared by the NIH Division of Safety and the NIH Clinical Center Pharmacy Department and Cancer Nursing Service.
*Although it is no longer included in these guidelines, some authorities recommend avoiding exposure to cytotoxic agents during pregnancy and using caution or avoiding exposure during breast-feeding or if trying to conceive.

The disposal of cytotoxic drugs and trace contaminated materials (e.g., gloves, gowns, needles, syringes, vials) presents a possible source of exposure to pharmacists, nurses, and physicians as well as to ancillary personnel, especially the housekeeping staff. Excreta from patients receiving cytotoxic drug therapy may contain high concentrations of the drug. All personnel should be aware of this source of potential exposure and should take appropriate precautions to avoid accidental contact.

The potential risks to pharmacists, nurses, and physicians from repeated contact with parenteral cytotoxic drugs can be effectively controlled by using a combination of specific containment equipment and certain work techniques which are described in the recommendations sections. For the most part, the techniques are merely an extension of good work practices by health care and ancillary personnel, and similar in principle and practice to *Universal Precautions*.[1] These may be supplemented as deemed appropriate for the work being performed. By using these precautions, personnel are better able to minimize possible exposure to cytotoxic drugs.

RECOMMENDED PRACTICES FOR PERSONNEL PREPARING CYTOTOXIC DRUGS

Professionally accepted standards concerning the aseptic preparation of parenteral products should be followed. Only properly trained personnel should handle cytotoxic drugs. Training sessions should be offered to new professionals as well as to technical and housekeeping personnel who may come in contact with these drugs. Safe handling should be the focus of such training. To speed loading time, the information regarding safe preparation has been divided into 3 sections:
- Steps A, B, C
- Steps D, E, F, G
- Steps H, I, J, K, L

SAFE PREPARATION OF CYTOTOXIC DRUGS

A. Part 1—All procedures involved in the preparation of cytotoxic drugs should be performed in a Class II, Type A or Type B laminar flow biological safety cabinet. The cabinet exhaust should be discharged to the outdoors in order to eliminate the exposure of personnel to drugs that may volatilize after retention on filters of the cabinet. The cabinet of choice is a Class II, Type B which discharges exhaust to the outdoors and can be obtained with a bag-in/bag-out filter to protect the personnel servicing the cabinet and to facilitate disposal.

Part 2—Alternatively, a Class II, Type A cabinet can be equipped with a canopy or thimble unit which exhausts to the outdoors. For detailed information about the design, capabilities, and limitations of various types of biological safety cabinets, refer to the National Sanitation Foundation Standard 49.[2]

1. Centers for Disease Control. 1988. Update: Universal precautions for prevention of transmission of human immunodeficiency virus, hepatitis B virus, and other blood-borne pathogens in health-care settings. *Morbidity and Mortality Weekly Report,* 37(24): 377-382, 387-388.
2. National Science Foundation. Standard 49 for Class II (Laminar Flow) Biohazard Cabinetry.

B. The work surface of the safety cabinet should be covered with plastic-backed absorbent paper. This will reduce the potential for dispersion of droplets and spills and facilitate cleanup. This paper should be changed after any overt spill and at the end of each work shift.

C. Personnel preparing the drugs should wear unpowdered latex surgical gloves and a disposal gown with elastic or knit cuffs. Gloves should be changed regularly and immediately if torn or punctured. Protective clothing should not be worn outside of the drug preparation area. Overtly contaminated gowns require immediate removal and replacement. In case of skin contact with any cytotoxic drug, thoroughly wash the affected area with soap and water. However, do not abrade the skin by using a scrub brush. Flush the affected eye(s), while holding back the eyelid(s), with copious amounts of water for at least 15 minutes. Then seek medical evaluation by a physician.

D. Vials containing drugs requiring reconstitution should be vented to reduce the internal pressure with a venting device using a 0.22-micron hydrophobic filter or other appropriate means such as a chemotherapy dispensing pin. This reduces the probability of spraying and spillage.

E. If a chemotherapy dispensing pin is not used, a sterile alcohol pad should be carefully placed around the needle and vial top during withdrawal from the septum.

F. The external surfaces contaminated with a drug should be wiped clean with an alcohol pad before transfer or transport.

G. When opening the glass ampule, wrap it and then snap it at the break point using an alcohol pad to reduce the possibility of injury and to contain the aerosol produced. Use a 5-micron filter needle or straw when removing the drug solution.

H. Syringes and IV bottles containing cytotoxic drugs should be labeled and dated. Before these items leave the preparation area, an additional label reading, *"Caution—Chemotherapy, Dispose of Properly"* is recommended.

I. After completing the drug preparation process, wipe down the interior of the safety cabinet with water (for injection or irrigation) followed by 70% alcohol using disposable towels. All wastes are considered contaminated and should be disposed of properly.

J. Contaminated needles and syringes, IV tubing, butterfly clips, etc., should be disposed of intact to prevent aerosol generation and injury. *Do not recap needles.* Place these items in a puncture-resistant container along with any contaminated bottles, vials, gloves, absorbent paper, disposable gowns, gauze, and other waste. The container should then be placed in a box labeled, *"Cytotoxic waste only,"* sealed and disposed of according to Federal, state, and local requirements. Linen contaminated with drugs, patient excreta, or body fluids should be handled separately.

K. Hands should be washed between glove changes and after glove removal.

L. Cytotoxic drugs are categorized as regulated wastes and therefore, should be disposed of according to Federal, state, and local requirements.

RECOMMENDED PRACTICES FOR PERSONNEL ADMINISTERING PARENTERAL CYTOTOXIC DRUGS

A. A protective outer garment such as a closed-front surgical-type gown with elastic or knit cuffs should be worn. Gowns may be of the disposable or washable variety.

B. Disposable latex surgical gloves should be worn during those procedures where exposure to the drugs may result and when handling patient body fluids or excreta. When bubbles are removed from syringes or IV tubing, an alcohol pad should be placed carefully over the tip of such items in order to collect any of the cytotoxic drugs which may be inadvertently discharged. Discard gloves after each use and wash hands.

C. Contaminated needles and syringes and IV apparatus should be disposed of intact into a labeled, puncture-resistant container in order to minimize aerosol generation and risk of injury. *Do not recap needles.* The container, as well as other contaminated materials should be placed in a box labeled, *"Cytotoxic waste only."* Linen overtly contaminated with any cytotoxic agent or excreta from a patient within 48 hours following drug administration, may be safely handled by using the procedures prescribed for isolation cases. For example, place the contaminated articles in a "yellow" cloth bag lined with a water-soluble plastic bag and then place into the washing machine. Linen without overt contamination can be handled by routine laundering procedures.

D. In case of skin contact with any cytotoxic drug, thoroughly wash the affected area with soap and water. However, do not abrade the skin by using a scrub brush. Flush affected eye(s), while holding back the eyelid(s), with copious amounts of water for at least 15 minutes. Then seek evaluation by a physician. Always wash hands after removing gloves.

   Pictures illustrating each of the prescribed actions and accompanied by this text may be found at the NIH website in one of three ways:

1. http://dohs.ors.od.nih.gov/pdf/Recommendations_for_the_Safe_
    Use_of_Handling_of_Cytotoxic_Drugs.pdf

2. http://www.nih.gov/
    In the search box, type in Recommendations for the Safe Use of Handling of Cytotoxic Drugs. Select the first choice that comes up with that wording.

3. http://www.nih.gov/
    In the search box, type in 92-2621 (this is the NIH publication number). Select the first choice that comes up with that wording.

FDA Pregnancy Categories

No drug should be used during pregnancy unless clearly needed and the risks to the fetus are outweighed by the benefits to the mother.

Category A   Adequate studies have not demonstrated a risk to the fetus in any trimester.

Category B   May have caused adverse effects in animals, but no adverse effects have been demonstrated in humans in any trimester or no demonstrated risk in animals but there are no adequate studies in pregnant women.

Category C   Animal studies have shown an adverse effect but there are no adequate studies in pregnant women or no animal studies and no studies in pregnant women.

Category D   Definite fetal risks. May be given in spite of risks if needed in life-threatening conditions.

Category X   Will cause fetal abnormalities. Risk of use outweighs benefits. Not recommended for use at any time during pregnancy. Consider alternatives before treating a pregnant woman.

Consider all men and women capable of conception when any drug in Category D or Category X is to be administered. Discuss birth control options to avoid pregnancy if a specific drug in these categories must be administered. Some drugs require birth control for months after all dosing is complete. Research complete information and keep patient informed.

U.S. Department of Health and Human Services, National Institutes of Health, National Cancer Institute Common Terminology Criteria for Adverse Events (CTCAE)

In Appendix D we have in the past incorporated the Common Toxicity Criteria (CTC) provided by the U.S. Department of Health and Human Services, the National Institutes of Health, and the National Cancer Institute. It was referred to throughout the text as the National Cancer Institute Common Toxicity Grading Criteria (NCI CTGC). This listing has been expanded and updated by these organizations and is too expansive to be included in an appendix. Web access to this material is available at www.cancer.gov. Search for CTCAE (Common Terminology Criteria for Adverse Events Version 3.0). Printed copies are available free of charge; call 1-800-4-CANCER (1-800-422-6237).

Information for Patients Receiving Immunosuppressive Agents

- Report allergic or sensitivity reactions you may have had to drugs or food.
- Report other medical problems you may have (e.g., exposure to chickenpox, herpes zoster, infections, bone marrow, heart, kidney, or liver problems).
- Provide a complete list of all medications you take, prescription and over the counter.
- In most situations birth control is essential and may be required for both patient and partner. Nonhormonal birth control reduces the possibility of drug interactions, but compliance is imperative. If there is any possibility you or your partner may be pregnant, inform your physician promptly.
- Discontinue breast-feeding.
- Take only prescribed medication(s) in the exact amounts prescribed and at the times prescribed. This will help to maintain correct blood levels and avoid drug interactions.
- Confirm procedure if you should miss a dose. If any questions, notify physician.
- Confirm procedure for correct storage of your medication(s).
- Close monitoring by your physician is very important; keep all appointments and have all required lab work done on schedule. Your medications may interfere with some test results. Discuss with your physician.
- Do not take any immunizations without your physician's approval. Polio vaccine is especially virulent in your condition; request family members to defer immunization and either avoid friends who have been immunized or wear a protective mask covering your nose and mouth while visiting.
- Dental procedures may need to be completed before starting therapy or deferred until therapy is completed. Use caution with your toothbrush, toothpicks, or dental floss. Alternate methods of dental hygiene may be necessary should your gums become tender, inflamed, or bleed.
- Review all side effects with your physician. Confirm those that may be a special problem for you and discuss solutions and expectations.
- Avoid anyone with an infection or fever. Report symptoms such as: chills, fever, cough, hoarseness, lower back or side pain, painful or difficult urination.
- Wash hands before touching your eyes or the inside of your nose.
- Report unusual bleeding, bruising, black tarry stools, blood in urine, or pinpoint red spots on your skin (petechiae).
- Report redness, swelling, or soreness in the mouth (symptoms of stomatitis).
- Report mild hair loss, nausea and vomiting, rash, tiredness, weakness.
- Avoid accidental cuts whenever possible (e.g., razors, fingernail and toenail clippers).
- Avoid contact sports where you might be bruised or injured.
- Drink adequate amounts of fluids to prevent increases in serum uric acid concentrations. Allopurinol (Zyloprim) and/or alkalinization of urine may be required.
- Anesthesia during dental, surgical, or emergency treatment may be a problem. Best to consult with your physician, but inform all health care professionals of the medications you are taking before they treat you in any way.

Recently Approved Drugs

BELIMUMAB
Monoclonal antibody
(be-**LIM**-ue-mab)

Benlysta
pH 6.5

USUAL DOSE

Premedication: Consider premedication (e.g., antihistamines [e.g., diphenhydramine (Benadryl)], H_2 antagonists [e.g., ranitidine (Zantac)], and/or corticosteroids [e.g., dexamethasone (Decadron)]) to help prevent or minimize hypersensitivity/infusion reactions.

Belimumab: 10 mg/kg as an infusion at 2-week intervals for the first 3 doses. Administer at 4-week intervals thereafter.

DILUTION

Available in two strengths (120 mg or 400 mg). Allow vial to reach RT before reconstitution (approximately 10 to 15 minutes). Reconstitute the 120-mg vial with 1.5 mL SWFI and the 400-mg vial with 4.8 mL SWFI. Concentration for both will equal 80 mg/mL. Direct the SW toward the side of the vial to minimize foaming. Gently swirl for 60 seconds. Allow to sit at RT and gently swirl for 60 seconds every 5 minutes until completely dissolved. **Do not shake.** Reconstitution may take up to 30 minutes. Protect from sunlight. Solution should be opalescent and colorless to pale yellow. Small air bubbles are expected and are acceptable. If reconstituted with a mechanical swirler, do not exceed 500 rpm and/or a duration of 30 minutes. Desired dose of the reconstituted solution must be further diluted to 250 mL with NS by withdrawing and discarding a volume equal to the desired dose from a 250-mL infusion bag or bottle of NS. Add the desired dose of belimumab to the infusion bag or bottle and invert to mix the solution; see Storage.

Filters: No data available from manufacturer.

Storage: Before use, refrigerate vials (2° to 8° C [36° to 46° F]) in original carton, protected from light. Do not freeze. Avoid exposure to heat. Do not use beyond expiration date. Reconstituted solution, if not used immediately, should be refrigerated protected from direct sunlight. Solution diluted in NS may be refrigerated or kept at RT. Total time from reconstitution to completion of the infusion should not exceed 8 hours. Discard any unused product.

COMPATIBILITY

Manufacturer states, "**Incompatible** with dextrose solutions," "No **incompatibilities** with polyvinylchloride or polyolefin bags observed," and "Should not be infused concomitantly in the same IV line with other agents."

RATE OF ADMINISTRATION

A single dose, properly diluted, as an infusion equally distributed over 1 hour. Slow or interrupt infusion rate if an infusion reaction develops.

ACTIONS

A recombinant, DNA-derived, humanized monoclonal antibody. It is a B-lymphocyte stimulator (BLyS)–specific inhibitor that blocks the binding of soluble BLyS (a B-cell survival factor) to its receptors on B-cells. Does not bind with B-cells directly. However, by binding BLyS, it inhibits the survival of B-cells (including auto-reactive B-cells) and reduces the differentiation of B-cells into immunoglobulin-producing plasma cells. Significantly reduces circulating CD19+, CD20+, naïve, and activated B-cells, plasmacytoid cells, and the SLE B-cell subset. Reductions in IgG and anti-dsDNA and increases in complement (C3 and C4) were observed as early as Week 8 and sustained through Week 52. Terminal half-life is 19.4 days.

INDICATIONS AND USES

Treatment of adult patients with active, autoantibody-positive, systemic lupus erythematosus (SLE) who are receiving standard therapy. ▪ Not recommended in patients with severe active lupus nephritis or severe active central nervous system lupus; has not been studied in these situations.

CONTRAINDICATIONS

Patients who have experienced an anaphylactic hypersensitivity reaction with belimumab.

PRECAUTIONS

For IV infusion only. ▪ Administered under the direction of a physician knowledgeable in its use in a facility with adequate diagnostic and treatment facilities to monitor the patient and respond to any medical emergency. ▪ Serious hypersensitivity/infusion reactions, including anaphylaxis, have occurred. ▪ Serious and sometimes fatal infections have been reported. Use with caution in patients with chronic infections. Therapy should not be started if a patient is receiving any therapy for a chronic infection. ▪ Depression and suicidality have been reported. Most patients had a history of depression or other serious psychiatric disorders and were receiving psychoactive medications. ▪ More deaths were reported with belimumab than with placebo during the controlled period of clinical trials. Etiologies included cardiovascular disease, infection, and suicide. No single cause of death predominated. ▪ The impact of treatment with belimumab on the development of malignancies is not known. ▪ Anti-belimumab antibodies developed in a small percentage of patients. Clinical relevance is unknown. ▪ Response rates were lower in Black/African-American patients; use with caution. ▪ Use in patients with impaired renal or hepatic function has not been studied.

Monitor: Obtain a baseline CBC, including a differential and platelet count. Monitor as indicated. ▪ Monitor for hypersensitivity reactions carefully during and for an appropriate period of time after administration. S/S reported include anaphylaxis, angioedema, dyspnea, hypotension, pruritus, rash, and urticaria. ▪ On the day of the infusion, monitor for S/S of an infusion reaction (e.g., bradycardia, headache, hypotension, myalgia, nausea, rash, urticaria). ▪ Consider interrupting therapy if a new infection develops during treatment with belimumab.

Patient Education: Women of childbearing potential should use effective contraceptive methods during treatment and for a minimum of 4 months after the final treatment. ▪ Manufacturer has established a pregnancy registry, and patients who are or who become pregnant are encouraged to register. ▪ Promptly report difficulty breathing, peri-oral or lingual edema, and rash; may indicate a hypersensitivity/infusion reaction. ▪ Promptly report bloody diarrhea, chest discomfort or pain, chills, cold sweats, coughing up mucus, dizziness, fever, nausea, new or worsening depression or suicidal thoughts, pain or burning with urination, unusual changes in behavior or mood.

Maternal/Child: Category C: use during pregnancy only if the potential benefit justifies the potential risk to the fetus. ▪ Discontinue breast-feeding. ▪ Safety and effectiveness for use in pediatric patients not established.

Elderly: Numbers in clinical studies are insufficient to determine if the elderly respond differently than younger subjects; use with caution.

DRUG/LAB INTERACTIONS

Formal drug interaction studies have not been performed. ▪ Has not been studied in combination with other **biologics, including B-cell-targeted therapies or IV cyclophosphamide;** concurrent use is not recommended. ▪ Do not administer **live virus vaccines** for 30 days before or concurrently with belimumab. ▪ Has been administered concomitantly with corticosteroids, antimalarials, immunomodulatory and immunosuppressive agents (including azathioprine, methotrexate, and mycophenolate), angiotensin-pathway antihypertensives, HMG-CoA reductase inhibitors (statins), and NSAIDs without meaningful clinical effect on belimumab pharmacokinetics.

SIDE EFFECTS

Bronchitis, depression, diarrhea, fever, insomnia, nasopharyngitis, migraine, nausea, pain in extremities, and pharyngitis were most commonly reported. The most common serious infections included bronchitis, cellulitis, pneumonia, and urinary tract infections. Anxiety, cystitis, depression, hypersensitivity/infusion reactions, influenza, leukopenia, sinusitis, and viral gastroenteritis also were reported.

ANTIDOTE

Notify physician of all side effects. Treatment of most side effects will be supportive. Consider interrupting therapy if a new infection develops during treatment with belimumab. Slow or interrupt infusion rate if an infusion reaction develops. Infusion reactions may be treated with acetaminophen, antiemetics (e.g., ondansetron [Zofran]), antihistamines (e.g., diphenhydramine [Benadryl]), H_2 antagonists (e.g., ranitidine [Zantac]), or corticosteroids (e.g., hydrocortisone sodium succinate [Solu-Cortef]) as indicated. Discontinue if a serious hypersensitivity reaction occurs. Treat hypersensitivity reactions as indicated; may require epinephrine, airway management, oxygen, IV fluids, antihistamines (e.g., diphenhydramine [Benadryl]), corticosteroids (e.g., hydrocortisone sodium succinate [Solu-Cortef]), and pressor amines (e.g., dopamine).

IPILIMUMAB BBW

(ip-i-**LIM**-ue-mab)

Yervoy

Monoclonal antibody
Antineoplastic

pH 7

USUAL DOSE

3 mg/kg administered as an IV infusion over 90 minutes every 3 weeks for a total of 4 doses.

DOSE ADJUSTMENTS

Withhold scheduled dose for any moderate (Grade 2), immune-mediated, adverse reaction or for symptomatic endocrinopathy. Patients with complete or partial resolution of adverse reactions (Grade 0 to 1) who are receiving less than 7.5 mg of prednisone or the equivalent per day may resume ipilimumab at a dose of 3 mg/kg every 3 weeks until administration of all 4 doses or until 16 weeks after the first dose, whichever occurs earlier. ■ Permanently discontinue ipilimumab for persistent moderate adverse reactions, an inability to reduce the corticosteroid dose to 7.5 mg prednisone or equivalent per day, or a failure to complete a full-treatment course within 16 weeks from administration of the first dose. ■ Permanently discontinue ipilimumab for severe or life-threatening adverse reactions; see Precautions and Antidote.

DILUTION

Available as a 5 mg/mL solution in 50-mg and 200-mg vials. Solution may have a clear to pale yellow color and may contain translucent-to-white amorphous particles. Discard vial if solution is cloudy. *Do not shake.* Allow vials to stand at RT for approximately 5 minutes. Withdraw required volume of ipilimumab and transfer into a infusion bag containing NS or D5W. Final concentration of diluted solution should range from 1 to 2 mg/mL. Mix diluted solution by gentle inversion. For example, a dose for a 70-kg patient would be 70 kg × 3 mg/kg dose = 210 mg. Withdraw 210 mg (42 mL of a 5 mg/mL solution) and transfer to a 100-mL bag of NS or D5W. Final concentration = 210 mg ÷ 142 mL = 1.5 mg/mL.

Filters: Administer through a separate line equipped with a sterile, non-pyrogenic, low–protein binding in-line filter.

Storage: Refrigerate vials at 2° to 8° C (36° to 46° F). Do not freeze. Protect from light. Store diluted solution for no more than 24 hours under refrigeration (2° to 8°C [36° to 46°F]) or at RT. Discard partially used vials.

COMPATIBILITY

Manufacturer states, "Do not mix with, or administer as an infusion with, other medicinal products." Flush IV line with NS or D5W after each dose.

RATE OF ADMINISTRATION

A single dose equally distributed as an infusion over 90 minutes. Administer through a separate line equipped with a low–protein binding terminal filter. Flush line with NS or D5W after each dose; see Filters.

ACTIONS

An IgG1 kappa immunoglobulin. A recombinant, human monoclonal antibody that binds to the cytotoxic, T-lymphocyte–associated antigen 4

(CTLA-4). CTLA-4 is a negative regulator of T-cell activation. Ipilimumab binds to CTLA-4 and blocks the interaction of CTLA-4 with its ligands, CD80/CD86. Blockade has been shown to augment T-cell activation and proliferation. The mechanism of action of ipilimumab's effect in patients with melanoma is indirect, possibly through T-cell–mediated anti-tumor immune responses. Terminal half-life is 14.7 days. Renal impairment (CrCl equal to or greater than 29 mL/min) and various degrees of hepatic impairment did not have a clinically important effect on the pharmacokinetics of ipilimumab.

INDICATIONS AND USES

Treatment of unresectable or metastatic melanoma.

CONTRAINDICATIONS

Manufacturer states, "None."

PRECAUTIONS

May result in severe and fatal immune-mediated adverse reactions due to T-cell activation and proliferation. Reactions may involve any organ system; however, the most common severe immune-mediated adverse reactions are enterocolitis, hepatitis, dermatitis (including toxic epidermal necrolysis), neuropathy, and endocrinopathy. Most reactions are manifested during treatment; however, a minority occurred weeks to months after discontinuation of ipilimumab. Consider the risk for severe and fatal immune-mediated adverse reactions versus benefit before initiating therapy with ipilimumab. ■ Severe, life-threatening, or fatal immune-mediated enterocolitis, hepatotoxicity, and dermatitis have been reported. ■ Severe, life-threatening, or fatal motor or sensory neuropathy, Guillain-Barré syndrome, or myasthenia gravis have been reported. ■ Severe to life-threatening immune-mediated endocrinopathies that require hospitalization or urgent medical intervention or that interfere with activities of daily living have been reported. Endocrinopathies have included hypopituitarism, adrenal insufficiency, hypogonadism, hypothyroidism, hyperthyroidism, and Cushing's syndrome. ■ Severe immune-mediated reactions involving other organ systems (e.g., nephritis, pneumonitis, pancreatitis, non-infectious myocarditis, uveitis, iritis) have been reported rarely. ■ A small number of patients have tested positive for binding antibodies against ipilimumab. Infusion-related or peri-infusional reactions consistent with hypersensitivity or anaphylaxis were not reported in these patients, and neutralizing antibodies against ipilimumab were not detected. ■ Immune-mediated ocular disease unresponsive to topical immunosuppressive therapy has been reported.

Monitor: Obtain baseline clinical chemistries, including liver function tests and thyroid function tests. Repeat before each dose and as indicated based on symptoms. ■ Assess patients for signs and symptoms of enterocolitis (diarrhea [greater than 6 to 7 stools/day above baseline], abdominal pain, mucus or blood in stool, with or without fever), GI hemorrhage or perforation (peritoneal signs and ileus), and/or the need for IV hydration for more than 24 hours. In symptomatic patients, rule out infectious etiologies or malignant causes and consider endoscopic evaluation for persistent or severe symptoms. ■ Monitor for severe immune-mediated hepatitis (AST or ALT elevations of more than 5 times the ULN or total bilirubin elevations more than 3 times the ULN). In patients with hepatotoxicity, rule out infectious or malignant causes and increase the frequency of liver function test monitoring until resolution of symptoms. ▪ Monitor for severe immune-mediated dermatitis (e.g., Stevens-Johnson syndrome, toxic epidermal necrolysis, rash complicated by full-thickness dermal ulceration, or necrotic, bullous, or hemorrhagic manifestations). Median time to immune-mediated dermatitis was 3.1 weeks. Unless an alternate etiology has been identified, S/S of dermatitis should be considered immune mediated. ▪ Monitor for symptoms of severe motor or sensory neuropathy (e.g., unilateral or bilateral weakness, sensory alterations, or paresthesia that interfere with daily activities). ▪ Monitor for clinical signs and symptoms of endocrinopathies, including hypophysitis (inflammation of the pituitary gland), adrenal insufficiency (including adrenal crisis), and hyperthyroidism or hypothyroidism. Patients may present with fatigue, headache, mental status changes, abdominal pain, unusual bowel habits, and hypotension. Median time to onset of immune-mediated endocrinopathy was 11 weeks. Unless an alternate etiology has been identified, S/S of endocrinopathies should be considered immune mediated. ▪ Monitor for clinical S/S of immune-mediated ocular disease. ▪ See Precautions.

Patient Education: Review Medication Guide before each dose. Severe immune-mediated reactions have been reported. ▪ Promptly report any side effects. ▪ May cause fetal harm. Birth control recommended.

Maternal/Child: Category C: based on animal data; may cause fetal harm. Use during pregnancy only if the potential benefit justifies the potential risk to the fetus. ▪ Discontinue breast-feeding. ▪ Safety and effectiveness for use in pediatric patients not established.

Elderly: No overall differences in safety or efficacy were reported between elderly patients and younger patients.

DRUG/LAB INTERACTIONS

Formal drug interaction studies have not been performed.

SIDE EFFECTS

The most common side effects are colitis, diarrhea, fatigue, pruritus, and rash. Severe to fatal immune-mediated reactions included dermatitis, endocrinopathy (adrenal insufficiency and hypopituitarism), enterocolitis (including intestinal perforation), eosinophilia, hepatotoxicity, meningitis, nephritis, pericarditis, and pneumonitis. Other reported side effects include acute respiratory distress syndrome, esophagitis, infusion reaction, intestinal ulcer, renal failure, and urticaria. Other immune-mediated adverse reactions were reported in fewer than 1% of patients; see manufacturer's prescribing information.

ANTIDOTE

Keep physician informed of all side effects. Permanently discontinue ipilimumab and initiate systemic high-dose corticosteroid therapy (e.g., 1 to 2 mg/kg/day of prednisone or equivalent) for severe immune-mediated reactions (e.g., Grades 3 to 5). With improvement to Grade 1 or less, initiate corticosteroid taper and continue to taper over at least 1 month. In one clinical study, infliximab (Remicade) was administered to patients with moderate or severe enterocolitis following an inadequate response to corticosteroids. Withhold ipilimumab dosing for moderate enterocolitis; administer antidiarrheal treatment (e.g., loperamide [Imodium]) and, if persistent for more than 1 week, initiate systemic corticosteroids at a dose of 0.5 mg/kg/day of prednisone or the equivalent. Mycophenolate (CellCept) may be considered in patients with persistent, severe hepatitis despite high-dose corticosteroids. Withhold ipilimumab dosing in patients with moderate hepatotoxicity, dermatitis, or neuropathy (neuropathy not interfering with daily activities). For mild to moderate dermatitis, such as localized rash and pruritus, treat symptomatically with topical or systemic steroids if no improvement of symptoms within 1 week. Initiate appropriate hormone replacement therapy in patients with symptomatic endocrinopathies. Administer corticosteroid eyedrops to patients who develop uveitis, iritis, or episcleritis. Resuscitate as necessary.

INDEX

Color type indicates generic drug name.
Italic type indicates drug categories and listings.
*See http://evolve.elsevier.com/IVMeds for detailed information.

Color type indicates generic drug name.
Italic type indicates drug categories and listings.
*See http://evolve.elsevier.com/IVMeds for detailed information.

Color type indicates generic drug name.
Italic type indicates drug categories and listings.
*See http://evolve.elsevier.com/IVMeds for detailed information.

Color type indicates generic drug name.
Italic type indicates drug categories and listings.
*See http://evolve.elsevier.com/IVMeds for detailed information.

Color type indicates generic drug name.
Italic type indicates drug categories and listings.
*See http://evolve.elsevier.com/IVMeds for detailed information.

Color type indicates generic drug name.
Italic type indicates drug categories and listings.
*See http://evolve.elsevier.com/IVMeds for detailed information.

Color type indicates generic drug name.
Italic type indicates drug categories and listings.
*See http://evolve.elsevier.com/IVMeds for detailed information.

Color type indicates generic drug name.
Italic type indicates drug categories and listings.
*See http://evolve.elsevier.com/IVMeds for detailed information.

Color type indicates generic drug name.
Italic type indicates drug categories and listings.
*See http://evolve.elsevier.com/IVMeds for detailed information.

Color type indicates generic drug name.
Italic type indicates drug categories and listings.
*See http://evolve.elsevier.com/IVMeds for detailed information.

Color type indicates generic drug name.
Italic type indicates drug categories and listings.
*See http://evolve.elsevier.com/IVMeds for detailed information.

Color type indicates generic drug name.
Italic type indicates drug categories and listings.
*See http://evolve.elsevier.com/IVMeds for detailed information.

Color type indicates generic drug name.
Italic type indicates drug categories and listings.
*See http://evolve.elsevier.com/IVMeds for detailed information.

Color type indicates generic drug name.
Italic type indicates drug categories and listings.
*See http://evolve.elsevier.com/IVMeds for detailed information.

Color type indicates generic drug name.
Italic type indicates drug categories and listings.
*See http://evolve.elsevier.com/IVMeds for detailed information.

Color type indicates generic drug name.
Italic type indicates drug categories and listings.
*See http://evolve.elsevier.com/IVMeds for detailed information.

Solution Compatibility Chart

Intravenous Medication	D2½W	D5W	D10W	D5/¼NS	D5/½NS	D5NS	NS	½NS	R	LR	D5R	D5LR	Dextran 6%/D5W/NS	Fruc 10%/W/NS	Invert sug 10%/W/NS	Na Lactate ⅙ M
Acetazolamide	C	C	C	C	C	C	C	C	C	C	C	C	C	C	C	C
Acyclovir		C		C	C	C	C			C						
Aminophylline	C	C	C	C	C	C	C	C	C	C	C	C	C			C
Antithymocyte Globulin	C	C	C	C	C	C	C	C								
Ascorbic Acid	C	C	C	C	C	C	C	C	C	C	C	C	C	C	C	C
Aztreonam		C	C	C	C	C	C		C	C		C				C
Calcium Chloride		C	C	C	C	C	C		C	C	C	C				
Calcium Gluconate		C	C			C	C			C		C		W		C
Cefazolin Na		C	C	C	C	C	C		C	C		C			W	
Cefoperazone Na		C	C	C		C	C			C		C				
Cefotaxime Na		C	C	C	C	C	C			C					W	C
Cefotetan		C					C									
Cefoxitin Na		C	C	C	C	C	C		C	C		C			C	C
Ceftazidime		C	C	C	C	C	C		C	C					W	
Ceftriaxone Na		C	C		C		C								W	
Cefuroxime Na		C	C	C	C	C	C		C	C					W	C
Clindamycin		C	C		C	C	C			C	C					
Dexamethasone		C					C									
Dobutamine HCl		C	C		C	C	C	C		C		C				C
Dopamine HCl		C	C		C	C	C			C		C				C
Doxycycline		C					C			C					W	
Epinephrine	C	C	C	C	C	C	C		C	C	C	C	C	C	C	C
Famotidine		C	C				C			C						
Fentanyl		C					C									
Folic Acid		C					C									
Furosemide		C	C			C	C			C		C				C
Gentamicin		C	C				C		C	C						
Heparin Na	C	C[*]		C	C	C	C[*]	C	C		C	C	C	C	C	
Hydrocortisone Phosphate		C	C				C	C								
Hydrocortisone Na Succinate	C	C	C	C	C	C	C	C	C	C	C	C	C	C	C	C
Hydromorphone HCl		C	C		C	C	C	C	C	C	C	C			W	C
Imipenem-Cilastatin		C[4]	C[4]	C[4]	C[4]	C[4]	C[10]									
Insulin (Regular)		C[P]	C		C		C[P]			C	C					
Isoproterenol	C	C[P]	C	C	C	C	C[P]	C	C	C	C	C	C	C	C	C
Kanamycin		C	C			C	C			C						
Labetalol		C		C		C	C		C	C	C	C				
Lidocaine		C[P]			C	C	C	C		C		C				
Magnesium Sulfate		C					C			C						
Meperidine HCl	C	C	C	C	C	C	C	C	C	C	C	C	C	C	C	C
Meropenem		C[1]	C[1]	C[1]		C[1]	C[4]		C[4]	C[4]		C[1]				C[2]